HEALTH SCIENCES LIBRARY
MAINEGENERAL MEDICAL CENTER
6 EAST CHESTNUT STREET
AUGUSTA, MAINE 04330

AIDS Therapy

SECOND EDITION

AIDS Therapy

Raphael Dolin, MD
Maxwell Finland Professor of Medicine
Dean for Clinical Programs
Harvard Medical School
Boston, Massachusetts

Henry Masur, MD
Chief, Critical Care Medicine
Clinical Center
National Institutes of Health
Bethesda, Maryland

Michael S. Saag, MD
Professor of Medicine
Director, AIDS Outpatient Clinic
University of Alabama at Birmingham
Birmingham, Alabama

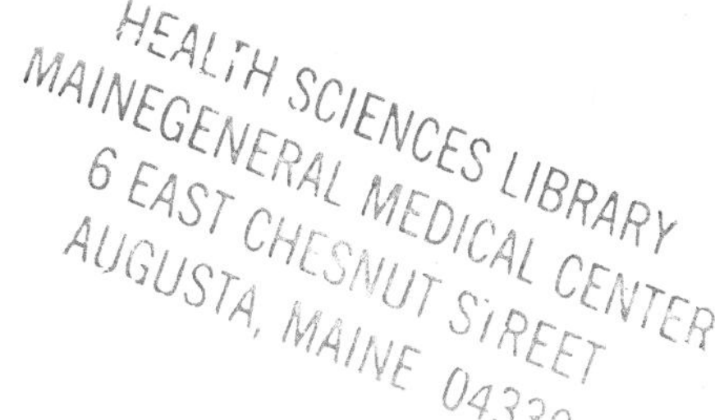

WC 503.2 A2885 2003
$148.50

CHURCHILL LIVINGSTONE
An Imprint of Elsevier Science
New York • Edinburgh • London • Philadelphia • San Francisco

CHURCHILL-LIVINGSTONE
An Imprint of Elsevier Science

The Curtis Center
Independence Square West
Philadelphia, PA 19106

AIDS THERAPY ISBN 0-443-06594-2
Copyright 2003, Elsevier Science (USA). All rights reserved.

No part of this publication may be reproduced, stored in a retrieval system, or transmitted in any form or by any means, electronic, mechanical, photocopying, recording, or otherwise, without prior permission of the publisher (Churchill, The Curtis Center, Independence Square West, Philadelphia, PA 19106-3399).

Notice

Infectious Disease is an ever-changing field. Standard safety precautions must be followed, but as new research and clinical experience broaden our knowledge, changes in treatment and drug therapy become necessary or appropriate. Readers are advised to check the product information currently provided by the manufacturer of each drug to be administered to verify the recommended dose, the method and duration of administration, and contraindications. It is the responsibility of the treating physician relying on experience and knowledge of the patient to determine dosages and the best treatment for the patient. Neither the Publisher nor the editors assume any responsibility for any injury and/or damage to persons or property.

The Publisher

First Edition 1999

Library of Congress Cataloging-in-Publication Data

AIDS therapy / [edited by] Raphael Dolin, Henry Masur, Michael S. Saag—2nd ed.
p. cm.
Includes bibliographical references and index.
ISBN 0–443–06594–2
1. AIDS (Disease)—Treatment. I. Dolin, Raphael. II. Masur, Henry. III. Saag, Michael S.
[DNLM: 1. Acquired Immunodeficiency Syndrome–therapy. WC 503.2 A2885 2002]
RC606.6.A37 2002
616.97'9206–dc21 2001055272

PIT / MVY

Printed in the United States of America

Last digit is the print number 9 8 7 6 5 4 3 2 1

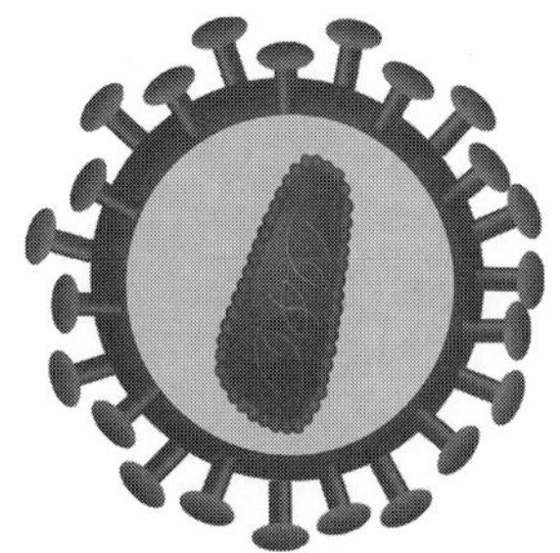

Contributors

Judith A. Aberg, MD
Assistant Professor of Medicine, Washington University School of Medicine, St. Louis, Missouri
Cryptococcosis

Donald I. Abrams, MD
Professor of Clinical Medicine, University of California San Francisco; Assistant Director, University of California San Francisco, Positive Health Program, San Francisco General Hospital, San Francisco, California
Complementary and Alternative Therapies

Neil M. Ampel, MD
Professor of Medicine, University of Arizona; Staff Physician, Southern Arizona Veterans Affairs Health Care System, Tucson, Arizona
Coccidioidomycosis

John A. Bartlett, MD
Professor of Medicine, Duke University Medical Center, Durham, North Carolina
Zalcitabine; Emtricitabine

Constance A. Benson, MD
Professor of Medicine, University of Colorado Health Sciences Center, Denver, Colorado
Mycobacterium avium
Complex and Other Atypcial Mycobacterial Infections

William Bonnez, MD
Associate Professor of Medicine, University of Rochester School of Medicine and Dentistry; Attending Physician, Strong Memorial Hospital, Rochester, New York
Sexually Transmitted Human Papillomavirus Infection

R. Pat Bucy, MD, PhD
Professor of Pathology, Microbiology and Medicine, University of Alabama at Birmingham, Birmingham, Alabama
Approach to HIV Antigen-Specific Immune Enhancement

Michael P. Busch, MD, PhD
Adjunct Professor of Laboratory Medicine, University of California San Francisco, San Francisco, California; Vice President of Research and Scientific Affairs, Blood Centers of the Pacific, San Francisco, California, and Blood Systems, Inc., Scottsdale, Arizona
Establishing the Diagnosis of HIV Infection

Raymond T. Chung, MD
Assistant Professor of Medicine, Harvard Medical School; Medical Director, Liver Transplant Program, Massachusetts General Hospital, Boston, Massachusetts
Hepatic and Hepatobiliary Diseases

Daniel E. Cohen, MD
Attending Physician, Beth-Israel-Deaconess Medical Center and Fenway Community Health, Boston, Massachusetts
Primary Care: Daily Management of HIV-Infected Patients

Ann C. Collier, MD
Professor of Medicine, University of Washington School of Medicine; Director, Adult AIDS Clinical Trials Unit, University of Washington, Seattle, Washington
Saquinavir

Richard A. Colvin, MD, PhD
Graduate Assistant in Medicine, Harvard University, Cambridge; Graduate Assistant in Medicine, Massachusetts General Hospital, Boston, Massachusetts
HIV/AIDS-Related Internet Resources

Sven A. Danner, MD, PhD
Professor of Medicine, Vrije Universiteit Medical Centre, Amsterdam, The Netherlands
Ritonavir

Richard T. D'Aquila, MD
Addison B. Scoville Professor of Medicine, Chief, Infectious Disease Division, Vanderbilt University School of Medicine, Nashville, Tennessee
HIV Resistance Testing in Clinical Practice

Lisa M. Demeter, MD
Associate Professor of Medicine and Microbiology and Immunology, University of Rochester School of Medicine and Dentistry, Rochester, New York
Delavirdine

Raphael Dolin, MD
Maxwell Finland Professor of Medicine and Dean for Clinical Programs, Harvard Medical School, Boston, Massachusetts
Didanosine

Joseph J. Eron, Jr., MD
Associate Professor of Medicine, Division of Infectious Diseases, University of North Carolina at Chapel Hill School of Medicine, Chapel Hill, North Carolina
Lamivudine

Carl J. Fichtenbaum, MD
Associate Professor of Clinical Medicine, University of Cincinnati College of Medicine; Infectious Diseases Consultant, University Hospital, Cincinnati, Ohio
Candidiasis

Margaret A. Fischl, MD
Professor of Medicine, and Director, AIDS Clinical Research Unit, University of Miami School of Medicine, Miami, Florida
Zidovudine

Stacy D. Fisher, MD
Adult Congenital Heart Disease Fellow, University of Rochester School of Medicine and Dentistry, Rochester, New York; Attending Physician in Medicine and Cardiology, The Sinai Hospital of Baltimore, Mid Atlantic Cardiovascular Associates, Baltimore, Maryland
Cardiac Disease

Timothy P. Flanigan, MD
Associate Professor of Medicine, Brown University School of Medicine; Director, Division of Infectious Diseases, The Miriam Hospital, Providence, Rhode Island
Cryptosporidium, Isospora, *and* Cyclospora *Infections*

Charles Flexner, MD
Associate Professor of Medicine, Pharmacology and Molecular Sciences, and International Health, Johns Hopkins University, Johns Hopkins School of Medicine and Bloomberg School of Public Health; Johns Hopkins Hospital, Baltimore, Maryland
Drug Administration and Interactions

Julie Louise Gerberding, MD, MPH
Director, Center for Disease Control and Prevention, Atlanta, Georgia
Occupational and Nonoccupational Exposure Management

John W. Gnann, Jr., MD
Professor of Medicine and Microbiology, Division of Infectious Diseases, Department of Medicine, University of Alabama at Birmingham and The Birmingham Veterans Administration Medical Center, Birmingham, Alabama
Varicella-Zoster Virus Infections; Human Herpesvirus-6 and Herpesvirus-7 Infections

Fred Gordin, MD
Professor of Medicine, George Washington University; Chief, Infectious Diseases, Veterans Affairs Medical Center, Washington, DC
Mycobacterium Tuberculosis *Infection*

John R. Graybill, MD
Professor of Medicine, Department of Medicine, University of Texas Health Science Center, San Antonio, Texas
Mycoses Caused by Moulds

Steven Grinspoon, MD
Associate Professor of Medicine, Harvard Medical School; Director, Program in Nutritional Metabolism, Massachusetts General Hospital, Boston, Massachusetts
Diabetes, Insulin Resistance, Lipid Disorders, and Fat Redistribution Syndromes

Roy Gulick, MD, MPH
Associate Professor of Medicine, Weill Medical College of Cornell University; Associate Attending Physician, New York Presbyterian Hospital, New York, New York
Indinavir

Colleen Hadigan, MD, MPH
Assistant Professor in Pediatrics, Harvard Medical School; Assistant in Pediatrics, Division of Nutritional Metabolism, Department of Pediatric Gastroenterology and Nutrition, Massachusetts General Hospital, Boston, Massachusetts
Diabetes, Insulin Resistance, Lipid Disorders, and Fat Redistribution Syndromes

Colin D. Hall, MB, ChB
Professor of Neurology and Medicine, and Vice Chair of Neurology, University of North Carolina School of Medicine, Chapel Hill, North Carolina
JC Virus Neurologic Infection

George J. Hanna, MD
Assistant Professor of Medicine, University of Pittsburgh, Pittsburgh, Pennsylvania
New Drugs in Development

Richard H. Haubrich, MD
Associate Adjunct Professor of Medicine, University of California San Diego, San Diego, California
Nelfinavir

Diane V. Havlir, MD
University of California San Francisco; Director, Positive Health Program, San Francisco General Hospital, San Francisco, California
Nelfinavir

David K. Henderson, MD
Deputy Director for Clinical Care and Hospital Epidemiologist, Warren G. Magnuson Clinical Center, National Institutes of Health, Bethesda, Maryland
Occupational and Nonoccupational Exposure Management

Jeffery D. Hill, DMD
Instructor of Dentistry, 1917 Dental Clinic, University of Alabama School of Dentistry, Birmingham, Alabama
Oropharyngeal Disease

Martin S. Hirsch, MD
Professor of Medicine, Harvard Medical School; Director of Clinical AIDS Research, Massachusetts General Hospital, Boston, Massachusetts
New Drugs in Development

Craig J. Hoesly, MD
Assistant Professor of Medicine, University of Alabama at Birmingham, Birmingham, Alabama
Tenofovir Disoproxil Fumarate

Mark Holodniy, MD
Associate Professor of Medicine, Stanford University, Stanford; Director, AIDS Research Center, VA Palo Alto Health Care System, Palo Alto, California
Establishing the Diagnosis of HIV Infection

Edward W. Hook, III, MD
Professor of Medicine, University of Alabama at Birmingham, Birmingham, Alabama
Sexually Transmitted Diseases

Laurence Huang, MD
Associate Professor of Medicine, University of California San Francisco; Medical Director, Inpatient AIDS Unit and Consultation Service, and Chief, AIDS Chest Clinic, San Francisco General Hospital, San Francisco, California
Respiratory Disease

Douglas A. Jabs, MD
Professor of Ophthalmology and Medicine, and Epidemiology, The Johns Hopkins University School of Medicine, The Johns Hopkins University Bloomberg School of Public Health; Director, Division of Ocular Immunology, Department of Ophthalmology, Johns Hopkins Hospital, Baltimore, Maryland
Ophthalmologic Disease

Eric C. Johannsen, MD
Instructor in Medicine, Harvard Medical School; Associate Physician, Division of Infectious Diseases, Brigham and Women's Hospital, Boston, Massachusetts
Epstein-Barr Virus and Kaposi's Sarcoma-Associated Herpesvirus

Richard A. Johnson, MD
Instructor in Dermatology, Harvard Medical School; Associate Dermatologist, Massachusetts General Hospital, Boston, Massachusetts
Dermatologic Disease

Steven C. Johnson, MD
Associate Professor of Medicine, Division of Infectious Diseases, University of Colorado Health Sciences Center; Director, Infectious Disease Group Practice, University of Colorado Hospital, Denver, Colorado
Lopinavir

Victoria A. Johnson, MD
Associate Professor of Medicine and Microbiology, and Associate Scientist, University of Alabama at Birmingham Center for AIDS Research, University of Alabama School of Medicine, Birmingham, Alabama
Abacavir

Christine Katlama, MD
Assistance Hopitaux Publique de Paris, Paris, France
Toxoplasmosis

Harold A. Kessler, MD
Professor of Medicine and Immunology/Microbiology, Rush Medical College; Associate Director, Section of Infectious Disease, Rush-Presbyterian-St. Luke's Medical Center, Chicago, Illinois
Herpes Simplex Virus Infections

J. Michael Kilby, MD
Associate Professor of Medicine, and Medical Director, University of Alabama at Birmingham HIV Out-Patient Clinic, University of Alabama at Birmingham, Birmingham, Alabama
Inhibitors of HIV Attachment and Fusion

David W. Kimberlin, MD
Assistant Professor of Pediatrics, The University of Alabama at Birmingham, Birmingham, Alabama
Human Herpesvirus-6 and Herpesvirus-7 Infections

Paul E. Klotman, MD
Murray M. Rosenberg Professor of Medicine, and Chairman, Department of Medicine, Mount Sinai School of Medicine, New York, New York
Renal Disease

Jane E. Koehler, MD
Associate Professor of Medicine, Division of Infectious Diseases, University of California San Francisco, San Francisco, California
Bartonellosis

Joseph A. Kovacs, MD
Associate Clinical Professor of Medicine, The George Washington University School of Medicine and Health Sciences, Washington, DC; Head, AIDS Section, Critical Care Medicine Department, Clinical Center, National Institutes of Health, Bethesda, Maryland
General Immune-Based Therapies in the Management of HIV-Infected Patients

Susan E. Krown, MD
Professor of Medicine, Weill Medical College of Cornell University; Attending Physician and Member, Memorial Sloan-Kettering Cancer Center, New York, New York
Kaposi's Sarcoma

Daniel R. Kuritzkes, MD
Associate Professor of Medicine, Harvard Medical School; Head, Section of Retroviral Therapeutics, Harvard Medical School Division of AIDS; Director of AIDS Research, Brigham and Women's Hospital, Boston, Massachusetts
Lopinavir

Joep M.A. Lange, MD, PhD
Professor of Internal Medicine, Academic Medical Centre, University of Amsterdam; Director, National AIDS Therapy Evaluation Centre (NATEC), Amsterdam, The Netherlands
Nevirapine

Steven E. Lipshultz, MD
Professor of Pediatrics and Oncology, University of Rochester School of Medicine and Dentistry; Chief of Pediatric Cardiology, University of Rochester Medical Center and Golisano Children's Hospital at Strong, Rochester, New York
Cardiac Disease

Joan C. Lo, MD
Assistant Professor of Medicine, University of California San Francisco; Staff Physician, San Francisco General Hospital, San Francisco, California
Adrenal, Gonadal, and Thyroid Disorders

Henry Masur, MD
Clinical Professor of Medicine, George Washington University School of Medicine, Washington, DC; Chief, Critical Care Medicine Department, Warren G. Magnuson Clinical Center, National Institutes of Health, Bethesda, Maryland
Pneumocystosis

Kenneth H. Mayer, MD
Professor of Medicine and Community Health, Brown University; Attending Physician, Division of Infectious Diseases, Department of Medicine, The Miriam Hospital, Providence, Rhode Island
Primary Care: Daily Management of HIV-Infected Patients

Douglas L. Mayers, MD
Head, Division of Infectious Diseases, Henry Ford Hospital, Detroit, Michigan
Efavirenz

Howard Minkoff, MD
Professor of Obstetrics and Gynecology, State University of New York, Downstate; Chairman, Department of Obstetrics and Gynecology, Maimonides Medical Center, Brooklyn, New York
Managing Pregnant Patients

Ronald Mitsuyasu, MD
Professor of Medicine, UCLA School of Medicine; Director, UCLA Center for Clinical AIDS Research and Education (CARE Center), University of California Los Angeles, Los Angeles, California
Hematologic Disease

Klaus E. Mönkemüller, MD
Assistant Professor of Medicine, University of Alabama at Birmingham; Chief of Endoscopy, Birmingham Veterans Affairs Medical Center, Birmingham, Alabama
Diseases of the Esophagus, Stomach, and Bowel

Julio S.G. Montaner, MD
Professor of Medicine and Chair of AIDS Research, University of British Columbia; Director of Clinical Activities, B.C. Centre for Excellence in HIV/AIDS, Vancouver, British Columbia, Canada
Nevirapine

Kathleen Mulligan, PhD
Assistant Professor of Medicine, Division of Endocrinology, University of California San Francisco; San Francisco General Hospital, San Francisco, California
Wasting Syndrome

Robert L. Murphy, MD
Professor, Feinberg School of Medicine, Northwestern University, Chicago, Illinois
Amprenavir

Henry W. Murray, MD
Professor and Associate Chairman, Department of Medicine, Weill Medical College of Cornell University; Attending Physician, New York Presbyterian Hospital, New York, New York
Toxoplasmosis

Thomas F. Patterson, MD
Professor of Medicine, University of Texas Health Science Center, San Antonio, Texas
Mycoses Caused by Moulds

Alice K. Pau, PharmD
Clinical Pharmacy Specialist, Clinical Center Pharmacy Department, National Institutes of Health, Bethesda, Maryland
AIDS-Related Medications; Antiretroviral Adult Dosage Guidelines

Andrew T. Pavia, MD
Professor of Pediatrics and Medicine, and Acting Chief, Division of Pediatric Infectious Disease, University of Utah, Salt Lake City, Utah
Stavudine

Stephen C. Piscitelli, PharmD
Formerly, Senior Pharmacokineticist, Pharmacy Department, Clinical Center, National Institutes of Health, Bethesda, Maryland; Presently, Director, Discovery Medicine-Viral Diseases, GlaxoSmithKline, Research Triangle Park, North Carolina
Drug Administration and Interactions; AIDS-Related Medications

Michael A. Polis, MD, MPH
Senior Investigator, Laboratory of Immunoregulation, National Institute of Allergy and Infectious Diseases, Bethesda, Maryland; Clinical Professor of Emergency Medicine, The George Washington University Medical Center, Washington, DC
Cytomegalovirus Disease

John C. Pottage, Jr., MD
Medical Director, Antivirals Vertex Pharmaceuticals Incorporated, Cambridge; Associate Attending Physician, New England Medical Center, Boston, Massachusetts
Herpes Simplex Virus Infections

William G. Powderly, MD
Professor of Medicine, and Chief, Division of Infectious Diseases, Washington University School of Medicine, St. Louis, Missouri
Cryptococcosis

Richard W. Price, MD
Professor and Vice Chair, Department of Neurology, University of California San Francisco; Chief, Neurology Service, San Francisco General Hospital, San Francisco, California
Neurologic Disease

Richard C. Reichman, MD
Professor of Medicine and Microbiology and Immunology, and Head, Infectious Diseases Unit, University of Rochester School of Medicine and Dentistry, Rochester, New York
Delavirdine

Gregory K. Robbins, MD, MPH
Instructor, Harvard Medical School; Assistant Physician, Massachusetts General Hospital, Boston, Massachusetts
Acute HIV Infection

Michael S. Saag, MD
Professor of Medicine, Director, AIDS Outpatient Clinic and Deputy Director, UAB Center for AIDS Research, University of Alabama at Birmingham, Birmingham, Alabama
Strategic Use of Antiretroviral Therapy

David T. Scadden, MD
Associate Professor of Medicine, Harvard Medical School; Director, Experimental Hematology, Massachusetts General Hospital, Dana Farber/Harvard Cancer Center, Partners AIDS Research Center, Boston, Massachusetts
Non-Hodgkin's Lymphoma

Morris Schambelan, MD
Professor of Medicine, University of California San Francisco; Chief Division of Endocrinology, San Francisco General Hospital, San Francisco, California
Adrenal, Gonadal, and Thyroid Disorders

Jane R. Schwebke, MD
Associate Professor of Medicine, University of Alabama at Birmingham, Birmingham, Alabama
Sexually Transmitted Diseases

Kenneth E. Sherman, MD, PhD
Associate Professor of Medicine, University of Cincinnati College of Medicine, Cincinnati Ohio
Hepatic and Hepatobiliary Diseases

Gail Skowron, MD
Associate Professor of Medicine, Boston University School of Medicine, Boston, Massachusetts; Chief, Division of Infectious Diseases, Roger Williams Medical Center, Providence, Rhode Island
Tenofovir Disoproxil Fumarate

Kathleen E. Squires, MD
Associate Professor of Medicine, University of Southern California Keck School of Medicine; Medical Director, Rand Schrader Clinic, Los Angeles County + University of Southern California Medical Center, Los Angeles, California
Saquinavir

Charles Steinberg, MD
Director, Beacon Clinic; Founder, AIDS Medicine and Miracles, Boulder, Colorado
Complementary and Alternative Therapies

Mark Sulkowski, MD
Assistant Professor of Medicine, Johns Hopkins School of Medicine, Baltimore, Maryland
Hepatitis Viruses

David L. Thomas, MD, MPH
Associate Professor of Medicine, Johns Hopkins School of Medicine, Baltimore, Maryland
Hepatitis Viruses

Jennifer E. Thorne, MD
Assistant, Division of Ocular Immunology, The Wilmer Eye Institute, The Johns Hopkins Medical Institutions, Baltimore, Maryland
Ophthalmologic Disease

Jamie H. Von Roenn, MD
Professor of Medicine, Division of Hematology/Oncology, Northwestern University Medical School; Member, Robert H. Lurie Comprehensive Cancer Center; Attending Physician, Northwestern Memorial Hospital, Chicago, Illinois
Wasting Syndrome

Bruce D. Walker, MD
Professor of Medicine, and Director, Division of AIDS, Harvard Medical School; Director, Partners AIDS Research Center, Massachusetts General Hospital, Boston, Massachusetts
Acute HIV Infection

Christine A. Wanke, MD
Associate Professor of Medicine, Tufts University School of Medicine; Infectious Disease Physician, New England Medical Center, Boston, Massachusetts
Cryptosporidium, Isospora, *and* Cyclospora *Infections*

D. Heather Watts, MD
Medical Officer, Pediatric, Adolescent, and Maternal AIDS Branch, Center for Research on Mothers and Children, National Institute of Child Health and Human Development, National Institutes of Health, Bethesda, Maryland
Managing Pregnant Patients

Louis M. Weiss, MD, MPH
Professor of Medicine and Pathology, Division of Infectious Diseases and Division of Parasitology and Topical Medicine, Albert Einstein College of Medicine; Attending Physician, Jack D. Weiler Hospital, Montefiore Medical Center, and Bronx Municipal Hospital (Jacobi Medical Center), Bronx, New York
Microsporidiosis

Melissa F. Wellons, MD
Medicine Resident, University of Alabama at Birmingham, Birmingham, Alabama
Emtricitabine

Joe Wheat, MD
Professor of Medicine, Indiana University School of Medicine; Director, Histoplasmosis Reference Laboratory, and Physician, Infectious Disease Division, Indiana University Medical Center, Veterans Affairs Hospital, Indianapolis, Indiana
Histoplasmosis

C. Mel Wilcox, MD
Professor of Medicine, and Director, Division of Gastroenterology and Hepatology, University of Alabama at Birmingham, Birmingham, Alabama
Diseases of the Esophagus, Stomach, and Bowel

Jonathan A. Winston, MD
Clinical Associate Professor of Medicine, Mount Sinai School of Medicine, New York, New York
Renal Disease

Andrew R. Zolopa, MD
Assistant Professor of Medicine, and Clinical Chief, Division of Infectious Diseases and Geographic Medicine, Stanford University, Palo Alto; Chief, AIDS Medicine, Santa Clara Valley Medical Center, San Jose, California
HIV Resistance Testing in Clinical Practice

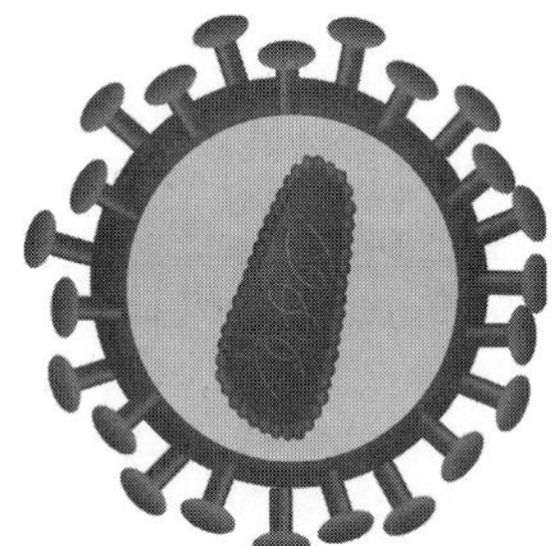

Preface

The field of HIV infection continues to undergo rapid evolution, and clinicians and their patients are faced with an ever greater complexity of issues. The second edition of *AIDS Therapy* is intended to provide current, comprehensive, and easily accessible information with which to address those issues. The editors are gratified that the first edition of *AIDS Therapy* was enthusiastically received and have attempted to build on that successful approach for this edition. The section on antiretroviral therapies contains chapters on individual drugs which have been newly approved since the last edition, as well as chapters on new classes of drugs under investigation. Sections on immune-based therapies and structured treatment interruptions have also been expanded. Chapters which deal with initiation of therapy, resistance testing, and management of failure of antiretroviral therapy have all been extensively revised. The sections on opportunistic infections have been updated to reflect new drugs, new diagnostic tests, and new approaches to management in the era of HAART. The chapters dealing with drug administration and interactions, which have been considered very useful by our readership, have been expanded as well.

We again wish to thank the many contributors to our book, each of whom are leaders in their particular field. Their commitment to the goals of the book and their willingness to devote time and effort to this task are very much appreciated. Finally, we would like to thank the organizational and editorial assistance in the preparation of this book that we have received from Stacy McGrath, as well as from Jennifer Candotti, and from our editor at Elsevier Science, Ann Ruzycka. We and our readers are the beneficiaries of their professionalism and excellence.

Raphael Dolin, M.D.
Henry Masur, M.D.
Michael S. Saag, M.D.

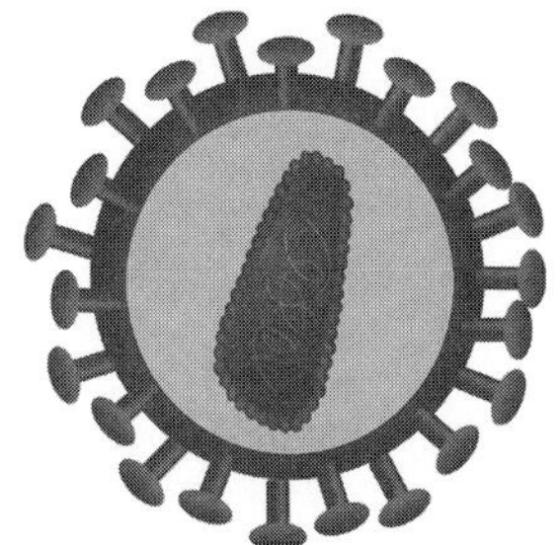

Preface to the First Edition

The treatment of patients with HIV infection and associated opportunistic infections and malignancies is an increasingly complex and fast-changing field. The editors believe that there is a need for a work which is comprehensive and up-to-date, yet presents material in a way which is practical and easy for clinicians to use. This book is intended to fulfill that need.

AIDS Therapy is organized into sections to facilitate use of the book. Sections address diagnosis of HIV infection (Section I), antiretroviral (Section II), immune-based (Section III), and alternative therapies (Section IV), and are followed by a section on strategies for managing antiretroviral therapies (Section V). Chapters 2 to 16 in Section II deal with individual drugs and include tables that summarize the major clinical trials carried out with these drugs, for easy reference by health care providers and students of the field. This format will facilitate rapid updating of chapters as new information becomes available.

The diagnosis, therapy, and prevention of opportunistic processes are presented in a separate section (VI), followed by a section on the approach to specific syndromes (VII). This latter section includes algorithms for the approach to the most common groups of illnesses and presenting complaints in patients with HIV infection, and we believe that this will be a particularly useful feature of this book.

The increasing number of drugs available for therapy and the complex interactions which can result present a particular challenge to clinicians. The last section (VIII) includes a chapter on drug interactions (Chapter 60), and a chapter which provides a profile of key prescribing information for commonly used medications (Chapter 61).

Finally, we have also included as appendices to the book two resources which we believe will be very useful to readers of our book: 1) a list of current HIV-related internet resources; and 2) a summary of dosage guidelines for antiretroviral drugs in adults.

The editors would like to express their appreciation to the many contributors to this book. The authors of each chapter are recognized authorities in their field who have devoted an extraordinary amount of time and effort to insure that their chapters not only meet the highest standards of scholarship, but also fulfill the purposes for which the book was intended. We would also like to thank the invaluable assistance in the preparation of this work that we have received from Bea Witmer, Candace Kurtz and Jane Garrison, as well as from our editors at Churchill Livingstone, Marc Strauss and Ann Ruzycka. Without these individuals, the existence of this book would not have been possible.

Raphael Dolin, M.D.
Henry Masur, M.D.
Michael S. Saag, M.D.

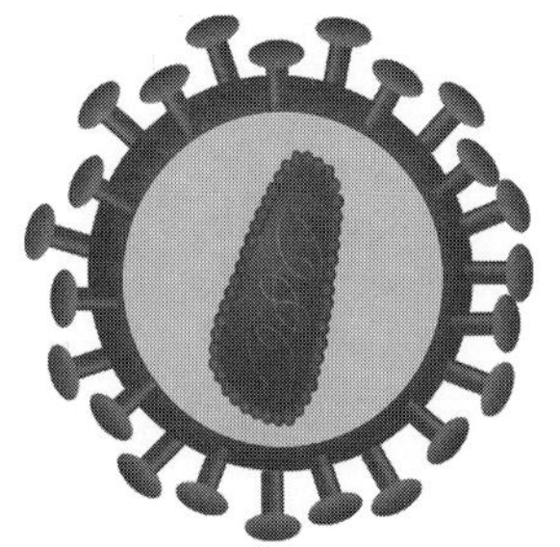

Contents

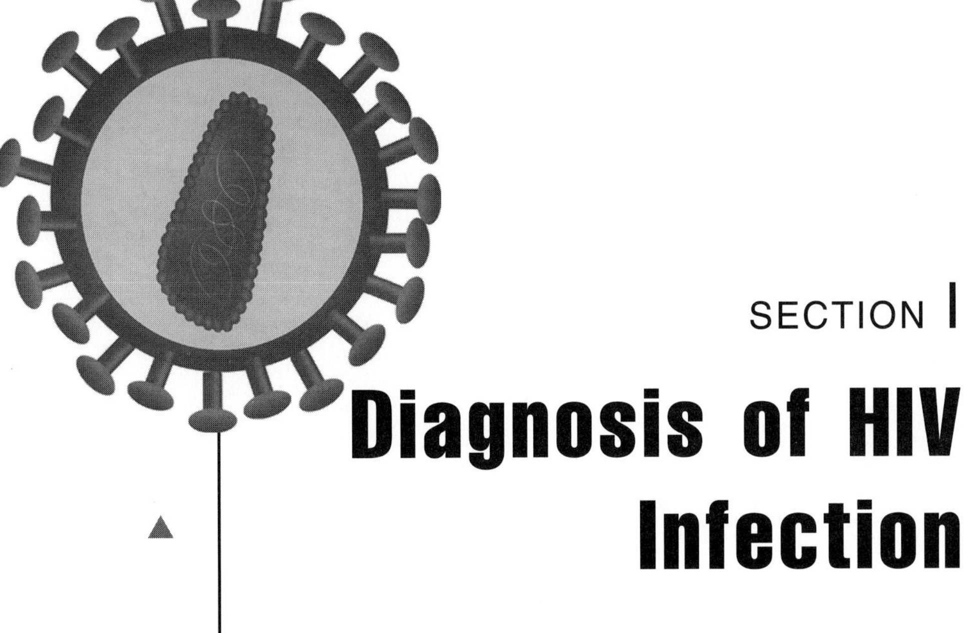

SECTION I

Diagnosis of HIV Infection

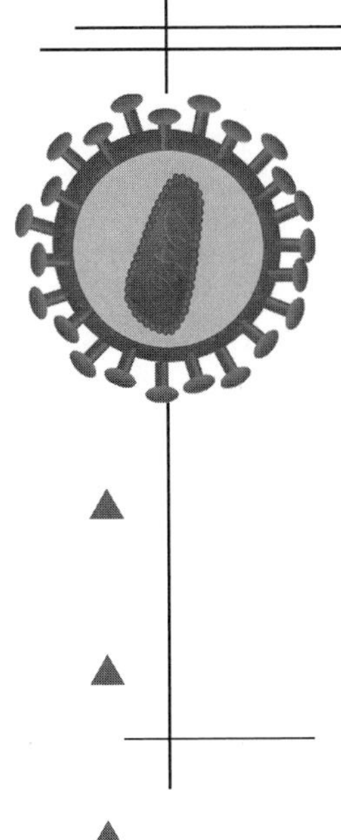

CHAPTER 1

Establishing the Diagnosis of HIV Infection

Mark Holodniy, MD
Michael P. Busch, MD, PhD

The diagnosis of human immunodeficiency virus (HIV) infection requires an understanding of the divergent characteristics of each patient including risk of infection, symptoms, and a thorough consideration of the performance characteristics of a wide array of HIV diagnostic tests. It is important for practitioners to be aware of what constitutes the clinical syndrome of acute HIV infection. An appropriate assessment of risk factors is critical to assess the probability that a syndrome represents acute HIV infection. Correct utilization of diagnostic tests is then necessary to substantiate the presence of an HIV infection.

Detection of HIV infection by standard serologic techniques may be difficult during the seroconversion period. Use of direct virus antigen assays such as p24 or RNA amplification tests may improve diagnostic capability. In contrast, the diagnosis of HIV infection during chronic asymptomatic or symptomatic disease is relatively straightforward. This chapter reviews various techniques currently used in the diagnosis of HIV infection (Tables 1–1, 1–2) and strategies for screening blood products for HIV infection.

▲ NATURAL HISTORY

After infection with HIV a flu-like syndrome may develop within days to weeks (see Chapter 24). Although some patients with acute infection are asymptomatic, most have a constellation of mild to moderate symptoms. A few patients require hospitalization. Primary HIV infection (PHI) often includes fever, fatigue, myalgias, lymphadenopathy, and a macular rash.[1,2] Clinical laboratory abnormalities during PHI include transient pancytopenia (including CD4+ lymphopenia) and elevated serum transaminases.[3] Symptoms may last for days to several weeks. Some adult and pediatric patients have experienced continued symptoms that in rare cases have proven fatal.[4,5]

Most patients are asymptomatic for several months to several years following PHI. Pathogenesis-based studies have determined that, despite clinical latency, viral replication is continuous and highly dynamic.[6,7] (For further discussion of pathogenesis, see Chapters 24, 26, and 27.) During clinical latency, progressive reductions in T-helper lymphocyte counts become evident. Non-life-threatening diseases related to immunodeficiency (e.g., oral candidiasis, oral hairy leukoplakia) and constitutional symptoms (e.g., fever, malaise, lymphadenopathy) can develop. Historically, this period of symptoms was referred to as the acquired immunodeficiency syndrome (AIDS)-related complex (ARC). With continued viral replication and destruction of CD4+ T lymphocytes there is further loss of immune function, which ultimately results in opportunistic infections such as *Pneumocystis* pneumonia, cytomegalovirus retinitis, and malignant neoplasms.

The duration of asymptomatic HIV infection has been observed to be several months to more than 15 years. Patients with high levels of HIV-1 replication and a high viral load set point experience much more rapid disease progression than those in whom viral replication is contained.[8] Certain patients have a predisposition for rapid progression based on specific mononuclear cell receptors (i.e., CCR5, CCR2, CXCR4).[9,10] Similarly, HLA class I and class II haplotypes have been associated with rapid (HLA B35) or delayed (HLA B57) HIV progression.[11–13] A switch in circulating viral strains, from non-syncytium-inducing to syncytia-inducing, has been shown to hasten the onset of

▲ **Table 1–1.** TESTS AVAILABLE FOR HIV-1 DIAGNOSIS

Antibody blood tests
HIV antibody enzyme immunoassay (EIA)
Immunofluorescent assay (IFA)
Western blot
Other blood tests
p24 Antigen
Culture of plasma or peripheral blood mononuclear cells (PBMCs)
PBMC DNA polymerase chain reaction (PCR)
Combination p24 antigen–HIV antibody assays
Plasma/serum viral load (RNA HIV-1)
Reverse transcriptase-polymerase chain reaction (RT-PCR) (Monitor)
Branched (b) DNA (Versant)
Nucleic acid sequence-based amplification (NASBA) (Nuclisens)
Other fluid tests
Oral HIV antibody EIA/Western blot
Urine antibody EIA/Western blot

clinical disease and to contribute to HIV disease progression.[14] Some patients, however, have rapidly progressing disease with non-syncytium-producing virus.[15,16]

▲ IMMUNE RESPONSE TO INFECTION

Both humoral and cellular responses develop against HIV within days of exposure to the virus (Fig. 1–1). The immunoglobulin M (IgM) class of antibodies against HIV appears first. These IgM antibodies are usually against HIV core (gag) or envelope (env) proteins.[17] The IgM response is usually transient and is followed by a long-lived IgG isotype response. Studies in acute seroconverters indicate that IgG antibodies to the gag (p24) and env (gp160, 120, 41) proteins appear first, followed within days to weeks by antibodies against HIV viral enzymes.[18] Antibodies to regulatory proteins, although not primarily screened for by commercial assays, also appear early in the seroconversion period.[19] The time when enough antibody bands become positive on a Western blot to meet diagnostic criteria varies from a few weeks to several months after acute infection.[20] Although the development of a full IgG immunologic response to all HIV proteins may take several weeks, enzyme immunoassays (EIAs) are usually positive within 3 months. Thus in cases in which either EIA or Western blot assays are found to be negative or indeterminate, repeat testing is recommended 8 to 12 weeks later. In rare cases patients do not manifest seroconversion or they have a prolonged process of seroconversion.[21,22] Usually, such immunosilent cases have extremely high-level viremia and rapid progression to clinical disease. It is unclear why this kind of humoral immunologic escape is possible. Perhaps it is due to B-lymphocyte loss or dysfunction, although most of these patients do appear to generate antibodies against other pathogens.[23] In such cases HIV infection can be documented by molecular techniques that demonstrate the presence of viremia (see below).

Viral proteins, such as p24 (gag) antigen, are readily detectable within the first few weeks of acute infection.[2,20] The presence of p24 antigen in serum is transient, and its disappearance coincides with the development of antibodies against p24.[24] More sensitive assays, which include acid dissociation of antigen from antibodies against p24, have only marginally improved p24 antigen detection during seroconversion. The p24 antigen typically disappears early (or is masked in immune complexes) after seroconversion and is not detectable for months to years. Its reappearance has been correlated with the loss of p24 antibody and progression of clinical HIV disease.[25]

Infectious HIV virus, from peripheral blood mononuclear cells (PBMCs) or in cell-free plasma, can be readily detected prior to seroconversion.[26] Infectious virus has also been recovered from other body compartments during primary infection (e.g., cerebrospinal fluid, lymph nodes, semen).[1,27,28] Plasma-associated and, to a lesser degree, PBMC-associated infectious virus levels drop precipitously within several days to weeks following seroconversion. Plasma virion-associated HIV RNA (viral load) or PBMC-associated HIV proviral DNA can be detected using sensitive molecular techniques in most untreated patients throughout the course of the infection.[29]

Cellular immune responses during PHI may include significant CD4+ lymphopenia and concomitant CD8+ lymphocytosis. Increased levels of activated CD8+ lymphocytes expressing CD45RA, CD38, or CD27 are seen.[30] In addition, cytokines such as interferons, tumor necrosis factor-α, neopterin, and β_2-microglobulin are elevated.[31,32] None of these immunologic responses occurs uniformly or predictably enough to use as a reliable diagnostic marker for HIV-1 infection.

▲ METHODOLOGIES

Enzyme Immunoassay

Tests for HIV diagnosis have historically used assays that detect antibodies against HIV-specific antigens/proteins (Table 1–1); the assays currently approved by the U.S. Food and Drug Administration (FDA) for diagnosis of HIV infection are listed in Table 1–2. Numerous non-FDA-approved tests are used for HIV diagnosis throughout the world. The characteristics of these assays vary, but in general the sensitivity and specificity are in the range of 96% to 99%. A complete list of these tests is maintained by the World Health Organization (WHO) at www.who.org (HIV Test Kit Evaluation).

Screening methods for HIV detection are based on techniques that capture circulating antibodies against HIV with solid surface-bound viral antigens. The antigen–antibody complex is then detected using an anti-human IgG antibody conjugated to an enzyme such as alkaline phosphatase or horseradish peroxidase. A substrate is then added from which the bound enzyme generates a colorimetric reaction. This method, formally known as an enzyme immunoassay, is the basis for most serologic assays (Fig. 1–2). EIAs for HIV-1 detection have been available since 1985. The assays have evolved from first-generation tests using crude HIV viral lysates as a source of viral antigens to third-generation tests using recombinant DNA proteins from immunodominant regions of HIV-1 and HIV-2 coated on paper strips, beads, and micro-plate wells. New “antigen

▲ **Table 1–2.** HIV DETECTION KITS AND ASSAYS

Trade name(s)	Format	Sample	Manufacturer	FDA Approval
HIV Antigen Assays for Serum and Plasma				
Abbott HIVAG-1 monoclonal	EIA	Serum/plasma	Abbott Laboratories	1996
Coulter HIV-1 p24 Ag assay	EIA	Serum/plasma	Coulter	1996
Abbott HIVAG-1	EIA	Serum/plasma	Abbott Laboratories	1989
Coulter HIV-1 p24 Ag Assay	EIA	Viral culture supernatant	Coulter	1996
Antibody Detection in Oral Specimen				
Epitope's OraSure	Oral specimen collection device	Oral fluid	Epitope	1991
Home Blood Collection for Laboratory Antibody Assay				
Home Access HIV-1 test system	Direct blood spot collection device	Dried blood specimen	Home Access Health	1996
HIV Viral Load Assay				
Roche Amplicor HIV-1 Monitor Assay	PCR	Plasma	Roche Molecular Systems	1999
NASBA NucliSens QT	NASBA RNA amplification	Plasma	Organon Teknika/BioMerieux	2001
Versant HIV-1 RNA 3.0 (bDNA)	bDNA signal amplification technology	Plasma	Bayer Nucleic Acid Diagnostics	Not approved
HIV Antibody Detection in Serum/Plasma				
HIVAB HIV-1 EIA	EIA	Serum/plasma	Abbott Laboratories	1985
Genetic Systems rLAV EIA	EIA	Serum/plasma	Bio-Rad Laboratories B	1998
Murex Single Use Diagnostic Test (SUDS)	EIA	Serum/plasma	Murex Diagnostics	1992
HIV-1 test Vironostika HIV-1	EIA	Serum/plasma	Organon Teknika/BioMerieux	1987
Microelisa Novapath HIV-1	WB	Serum/plasma	Bio-Rad Laboratories B	1990
Immunoblot Cambridge Biotech HIV-1 WB kit	WB	Serum/plasma	Calypte Biomedical	1991
Genetic systems HIV-1 Western blot	WB	Serum/plasma	Bio-Rad Laboratories B	1998
EPIblot HIV-1	WB	Serum/plasma	Epitope	1991
Fluorognost HIV-1 IFA	IFA	Serum/plasma	Waldheim Pharmazeutika G.m.b.H.	1992
HIVAB HIV-1 EIA	EIA	Dried blood spot	Abbott Laboratories	1992
HIV-1 urine EIA	EIA	Urine screen	Calypte Biomedical	1996
Genetic systems rLAV EIA	EIA	Dried blood spot	Bio-Rad Laboratories B	1998
Vironostika HIV-1 microelisa	EIA	Dried blood spot	Organon Teknika	1990
Oral fluid Vironostika HIV-1 microelisa system	EIA	Oral fluid	Organon Teknika	1994
Cambridge Biotech HIV-1 WB kit	WB	Urine screen	Calypte Biomedical	1998
Genetic Systems HIV-1 Western blot	WB	Dried blood spot	Bio-Rad Laboratories B	1998
OraSure HIV-1 Western blot kit	WB	Oral fluid	Epitope	1996
HIV antibody detection				
Fluorognost HIV-1 IFA	IFA	Dried blood spot	Waldheim Pharmazeutika G.m.b.H.	1996
Abbott HIVAB HIV-1/HIV-2 (rDNA) EIA	EIA	Serum/plasma	Abbott Laboratories	1992
Genetic Systems HIV-1/HIV-2 Peptide EIA	EIA	Serum/plasma/cadavaric serum	Bio-Rad Laboratories B	2000
Genetic Systems HIV-2 EIA	EIA	Serum/plasma	Bio-Rad Laboratories B	1990
Serostrip	Capillary EIA	Plasma/serum	Saliva Diagnostics Systems, The Medel, Singapore	Not approved
Multispot	Capillary EIA	Plasma/serum	Diagnostics Pasteur, Paris, France	Not approved
Combination Assays to Detect Antibody and/or P24 in Blood/Serum/Plasma				
Determine	EIA/p24	Dried blood	Abbott Laboratories	Not approved
AxSYM	EIA/p24	Serum/plasma	Abbott Laboratories	Not approved
Murex	EIA/p24		Murex Diagnostics	Not approved
Vidas Duo Ultra	Enzyme linked fluorescence/p24	Serum/plasma	Bio-Merieux	Not approved
Genescreen Plus	EIA/p24	Plasma	Sanofi Pasteur	Not approved
Enzygnost	EIA/p24	Plasma	Dade Behring	Not approved
Vironostika	EIA/p24	Plasma	Orgagnon Teknika	Not approved

EIA, enzyme immunoassay; WB, Western blot.

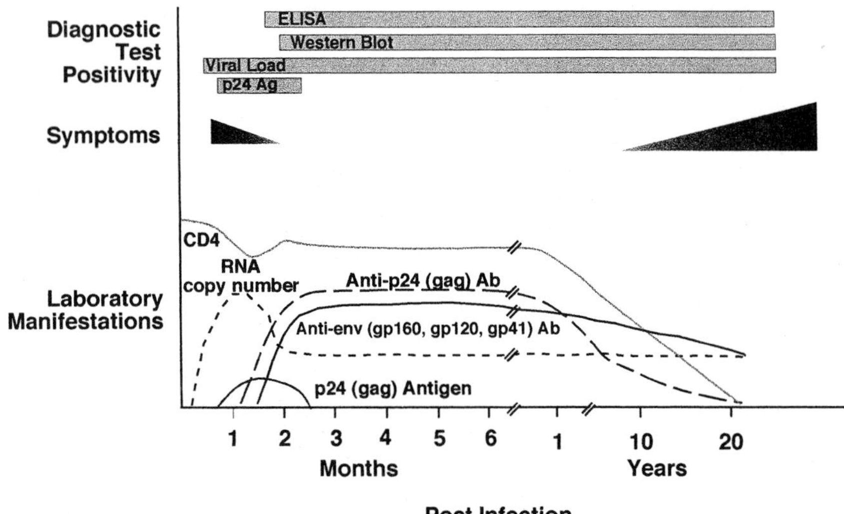

Figure 1–1. Viral and antiviral responses useful for establishing a diagnosis of HIV infection.

sandwich" EIA techniques also allow for the efficient capture of HIV-1 IgM and IgG antibodies and have sensitivities and specificities of more than 99.9% when assessing patients with chronic infection.[33] During PHI, when antibodies against HIV may not yet be present, these assays have much lower sensitivity.[34] Reported causes of false-positive and false-negative HIV-1 EIA results are listed in Table 1–3.[35] Newer assays may not have as significant a false- positive rate as older assays. The newer "fourth generation" assays have been developed that combine detection of p24 antigen and HIV-1 antibodies in the same assay, resulting in improved sensitivity and earlier detection of acute infection when compared to standard antibody assays.[36,37] These combination assays, however, may not be as sensitive for p24 antigen detection as p24 antigen testing alone, and there may not be uniform sensitivity of detection among all subtypes of HIV-1 (see below).[38]

Western Blot

A more specific assay for the presence of HIV antibodies in serum, which does not necessarily provide a test with high specificity, is the Western blot. An EIA does not delineate the specific antibodies that may be present in serum. Therefore, regardless of which antibodies are present, the assay is qualitatively scored as positive. To perform a Western blot, specific HIV proteins, derived from HIV viral lysates or from recombinant forms, are separated based on their molecular weight using electrophoresis. The proteins are then applied to nitrocellulose paper. Larger proteins are at the top of the strip and the smallest proteins at the bottom, in accordance with their electrophoretic migratory pattern. A Western blot for HIV-1 contains HIV-1 envelope proteins (gp160, gp120, gp41), gag core gene proteins (p55, p24, p17), and polymerase gene proteins (p66, p51, p31) (Table 1–4). HIV-2 Western blots are similar but differ slightly in terms of the molecular size of the three gene products (Table 1–4). If antibodies to any of these proteins are present in serum, they bind to the immobilized HIV protein on the strip. An enzyme and substrate are added to generate a colorimetric reaction and produce a colored band on the strip representing the antigen–antibody complex (Fig. 1–3).

If no colored bands are present, the Western blot is interpreted as negative. Depending on which organization's criteria for interpretation are used (Table 1–5),[39] a blot is scored as positive if one band is present against each of the gene products or when two bands (e.g., p24, gp41, gp120/160) are present.[40] If bands are present but do

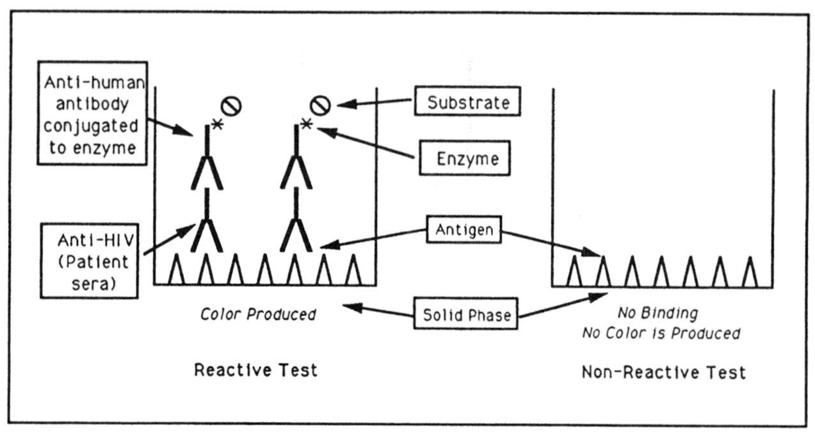

Figure 1–2. Principle of the indirect enzyme-linked immunosorbent assay (ELISA). (From Constantine NT, Callahan JD, Watts DM. Retroviral Testing: Essentials of Quality Control and Laboratory Diagnosis. Boca Raton, FL, CRC Press, 1992, p 40, with permission.)

▲ **Table 1–3.** CAUSES OF FALSE-POSITIVE OR FALSE-NEGATIVE HIV EIA RESULTS

Causes of False-Positive Results for HIV on EIA
Hematologic malignant disorders
DNA viral infections
Autoimmune disorders
Multiple myeloma
Primary biliary cirrhosis
Alcoholic hepatitis
Influenza vaccination
Hepatitis B vaccination
Rabies vaccination
Passively transferred antibodies
Antibodies to class II leukocytes
Renal transplantation
Chronic renal failure
Stevens-Johnson syndrome
Positive rapid plasma reagin test
Malaria
Dengue
Increased parity
Systemic lupus erythematosus
Causes of False-Negative Results for HIV on EIA
Incubation "window" period before antibody development
Immunosuppressive therapy
Replacement transfusion
Malignant disorders
B-lymphocyte dysfunction
Bone marrow transplantation
Kits that detect primarily antibody to p24
Starch powder from laboratory gloves

Adapted from Cordes RJ, Ryan ME. Pitfalls in HIV testing: application and limitations of current tests. Postgrad Med 98:177, 1995; Mylonakis E, Paliou M, Lally M, et al. Laboratory testing for infection with the human immunodeficiency virus: established and novel approaches. Am J Med 109:568, 2000. Related article: Daikh BE, Holyst MM. Lupus-specific autoantibodies in concomitant human immunodeficiency virus and systemic lupus erythematosus: case report and literature review. Semin Arthritis Rheum. 30:418, 2001.

not meet established criteria for a positive test, the blot is interpreted as being indeterminate.

Data from the Retrovirus Epidemiology Donor Study (REDS) indicate that the prevalence of false-positive Western blot results from blood donations was 4.8% of Western blot-positive donors and 0.0004% of all donors.[41] Patients with indeterminate Western blot tests (bands are present but they do not meet the criteria in Table 1–5) and without an evolution of bands indicative of HIV infection are usually not infected. A true positive is more likely in first-time donors, areas of high HIV-1 infection incidence, when a p31 band is present, or when three or more bands are present.[41] An indeterminate Western blot may be the result of nonspecific reactivity or the presence of primary HIV infection in an individual prior to seroconversion.[20,42] Other causes of false-positive or indeterminate Western blots are listed in Table 1–6.[35] In a long-term study of patients with nonreactive HIV EIAs and indeterminate Western blots, the most common indeterminate banding pattern usually had a p17 or p24 band. Independent risk factors for having an indeterminate Western blot test among male cases and controls were a tetanus booster during the last 2 years and sexual contact with a prostitute. Risk factors for women included parity and the presence of autoantibodies (e.g., rheumatoid factor or antinuclear antibodies).[43] In another study, increased detection of antibody to envelope or p24 on Western blot testing appeared related to enhanced sensitivity of enzyme immunoassays to gp41 and p24 antibodies.[44]

▲ **Table 1–4.** HIV PROTEINS REPRESENTED ON WESTERN BLOT TEST

HIV Gene and Products	Viral Protein/Glycoprotein Molecular Weight: HIV-1	HIV-2
env		
Precursor	gp160	gp140
External glycoprotein	gp120	gp105/125
Transmembrane glycoprotein	gp41	gp36/41
pol		
Reverse transcriptase	p66	p68
Reverse transcriptase	p51	p53
Endonuclease	p31	p31/34
gag		
Precursor	p55	p56
Core	p24	p26
Matrix	p17	p16

A few patients with indeterminate Western blot tests have demonstrated low CD4+/CD8+ cell ratios and cells that could be stained with p24 antibody. One group of investigators reported that HIV was detected in 3 of 20 subjects, but these viral isolates could not be transmitted to cell lines.[45] HIV RNA tests may be useful for resolving the true HIV status of persons with indeterminate or suspected false-positive Western blot patterns.

Immunofluorescence Assay

An alternative assay for HIV diagnosis is the immunofluorescence assay (IFA), although it is not often used. With this assay, HIV-infected lymphocytes are fixed on glass slides. Patient serum is then incubated with the cell preparations, washed, and further incubated with a fluorescein isothiocyanate-labeled anti-human IgG. If antibodies to HIV are present in serum, they bind to the viral antigens expressed by the infected lymphocytes. A positive test shows characteristic fluorescence of cells. IFA and Western blot results are usually concordant.[46] Although indeterminate results may occur with the IFA technique, the IFA may be useful to determine if a patient with an indeterminate Western blot test is truly infected.

Other Serologic Blood Tests

Other serologic assays include rapid screening tests (RSTs), such as agglutination assays. For these tests, gelatin or latex particles are coated with HIV antigen. In the presence of serum containing HIV antibodies, particles become crosslinked and agglutination occurs. Although somewhat quicker and easier to perform than enzyme-linked immunosorbent assays (ELISAs), these particle agglutination assays have been found to be slightly less sensitive or specific.[47] Other rapid screening blood HIV diagnostic tests have been developed that utilize dipsticks. Both the

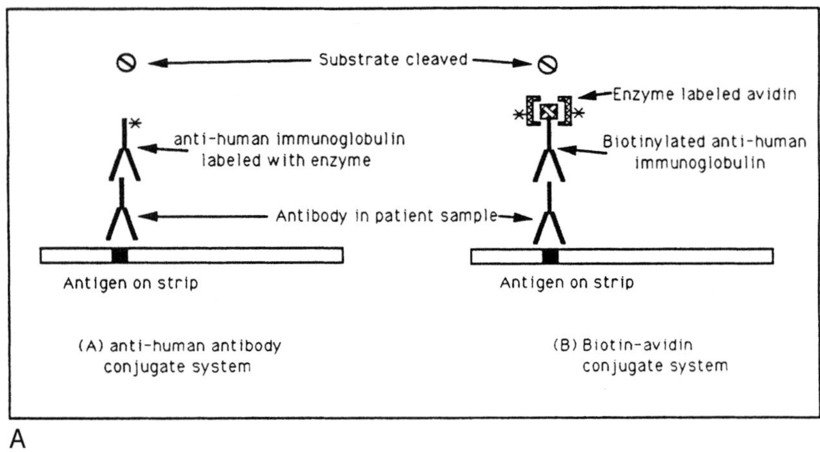

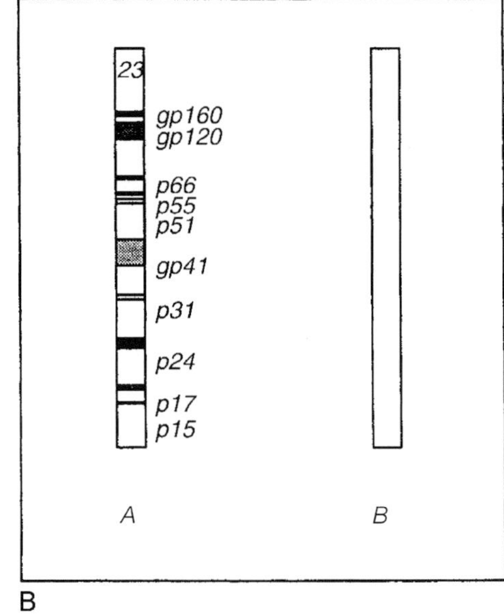

Figure 1–3. *A*, Anti-human and biotin–avidin conjugate systems. *B*, Western blot results: A, positive result (reactions to all antigens); B, negative result. (From Constantine NT, Callahan JD, Watts DM. Retroviral Testing: Essentials of Quality Control and Laboratory Diagnosis. Boca Raton, FL, CRC Press, 1992, p 63, with permission.)

sensitivity and specificity of a synthetic peptide dipstick EIA test exceeded 99% compared to the Abbott recombinant peptide HIV-1/HIV-2 EIA.[48] In another report, five standard EIA antibody tests and three rapid screening tests were evaluated using seroconversion and nonseroconversion low-titer panels. There was no significant difference in sensitivity between the five standard EIA antibody tests. However, the rapid screening tests were significantly less sensitive on the seroconversion panels and failed to detect some of the low-antibody-titer samples.[49]

At present, the Abbott (Murex) single-use diagnostic system (SUDS) is the only FDA-approved rapid screening test. Other rapid screening tests appear to give a performance superior to that of SUDS, but they may not produce uniform results for detecting all subtypes of HIV-1.[50]

Finally, recombinant immunoblot assays for HIV-1/HIV-2 have sensitivities comparable to that of the Western blot tests in chronically infected and seroconverting patients. Immunoblot testing has significantly reduced the number of indeterminate results found by Western blotting and can discriminate HIV-1 from HIV-2 infection with a single blot.[51,52]

Oral HIV Testing

It has been known for quite some time that oral fluids contain antibodies against HIV. Such oral antibodies are primarily of the IgG isotype and in some instances are present in higher concentration than concomitant serum levels.[53,54] Commercially available tests using saliva have been developed for HIV detection. An IgG antibody capture (GAC)

▲ **Table 1–5.** INTERPRETIVE CRITERIA FOR A POSITIVE HIV-1 WESTERN BLOT TEST

Organization	Criteria
ASTPHLD/CDC	Any two: p24, gp41, gp120/160
DuPont	p24 + p31 + gp41 or gp120/160
ARC	Three or more bands, one from each gene product group: *gag, pol, env*
CRSS	Two or more bands: p24 or p31 and gp41 or gp120/160
WHO	Two *env* bands with or without *gag* or *pol*

ARC, American Red Cross; ASTPHLD/CDC, Association of State and Territorial Public Health Laboratory Directors/Centers for Disease Control and Prevention; CRSS, Consortium for Retrovirus Serological Standardization; WHO, World Health Organization.

Data from Proffitt MR, Yen-Lieberman B. Laboratory diagnosis of human immunodeficiency virus infection. Infect Dis Clin North Am 7:203, 1993; George JR, Schochetman G. Serologic tests for the detection of human immunodeficiency virus infection. In: George JR, Schochetman G (eds) AIDS Testing: Methodology and Management Issues. New York, Springer-Verlag, 1992, p 48.

▲ **Table 1–6.** CAUSES OF FALSE-POSITIVE AND INDETERMINATE WESTERN BLOT RESULTS FOR HIV

Normal human ribonucleoproteins
Other human retroviruses
Antibodies to mitochondrial, nuclear, and T-lymphocyte antigens
Globulins produced during polyclonal gammopathy
Proteins on filter paper
Anti-carbohydrate antibodies
Heat-inactive serum
High concentration of bilirubin in serum
Passively acquired antibodies
Heterophil antibodies to bovine, ovine, caprine, and murine immunoglobulin G (IgG)
HIV vaccines

From Cordes RI, Ryan ME. Pitfalls in HIV testing: application and limitations of current tests. Postgrad Med 98:177, 1995; Willman JH, Hill HR, Martins TB, et al. Multiplex analysis of heterophil antibodies in patients with indeterminate HIV immunoassay results. Am J Clin Pathol. 115:764, 2001.

ELISA has been compared to a rapid test and showed comparable sensitivity and specificity.[55] Salivary testing has also been performed in HIV-infected children and was found to be 100% specific and sensitive relative to blood testing.[56]

The FDA has approved an oral salivary test called OraSure (Epitope, Beaverton, OR, USA). For this test a cotton swab is inserted into the mouth for 2 minutes to collect oral mucosal transudate. The swab is then placed in a transport container containing an antibacterial preservative and is sent to a referral laboratory for standard EIA and Western blot testing. The sensitivity and specificity of the OraSure test approach 100% when compared to standard Western blot confirmation.[57,58] Newer technologies have been developed in a kit format (Saliva-Strip HIV-1/2; Saliva Diagnostics Systems, Vancouver, WA, USA). This strip method was found to be highly concordant with blood testing methods.[59] Other studies indicate that antibodies in oral mucosal transudate are stable in preservative at ambient temperature for more than 1 month.[60] This advantage allows rapid, noninvasive HIV diagnosis in the field or clinic. Saliva-Strip has been employed extensively throughout the developing world but is not yet FDA-approved for use in the United States. Performance during seroconversion is not clear.

Urine HIV Testing

Urine contains antibodies against HIV, and so it has been studied for its diagnostic capability. Several studies have utilized IgG antibody capture particle adherence tests (GACPAT, GAC ELISA, SUDS, and standard commercially available EIA tests)[61–64] and have concluded that the performance of urine-based antibody screens is similar to that of serum tests, although there has been no rigorous analysis of early seroconversion samples. Currently, a Calypte HIV-1 urine EIA (Calypte Biomedical, Alameda, CA, USA) and a urine Western blot test have been approved by the FDA for HIV-1 diagnosis. Discordant responses demonstrating positive urine and negative serum results were found in 0.24% of patients; negative urine and positive serum results were found in 0.17% of 11,896 subjects. The false-positive rate for urine was 1.3%.[65]

Urine therefore provides an alternative testing medium for patients unwilling to provide serum. Compliance with HIV testing has been shown to be greater with urine testing than with serum testing.[66]

Home Sample Collection and Home Testing

Home HIV testing (i.e., obtaining the sample and the result at home) must be distinguished from home collection (i.e., sending the sample to a laboratory for processing). The FDA has approved one kit for home sample collection. Although home HIV testing kits are available through the Internet, none is FDA-approved. The Home Access System (Home Access Health Corporation, Hoffman Estates, IL, USA) utilizes standard EIA and confirmatory Western blot technology from blood collected by a person at home. Using a lancet, a person collects blood and places it on a test card, which is mailed to a testing center. If the EIA is positive, the sample is tested twice more by EIA, and the results are confirmed by Western blot. After 3 to 7 days the person calls the company for the results, referring to the number assigned to that specific kit. If the test is negative, the person hears a recording of the results. He or she can then access a counselor to discuss test results if desired. If the test is positive, the subject's call is referred to a counselor, who discusses the test results with the caller. The average cost for these "kits" is around $40 to $50. Two levels of service are available: express (results in 3 days) and regular (results in 7 days).

A recent study found that Home Access results had a 100% concordance with standard results from EIAs obtained from blood after venipuncture.[67] Subjects participated in pretest counseling by telephone. They called 3 days later for anonymous results and posttest counseling. Based on this preliminary study, it appears that home collection of HIV antibody screening along with pre- and posttest telephone counseling is a viable alternative to the conventional venous antibody testing available in clinics, although the anonymity of the test makes partner notification problematic. A study performed in San Francisco indicated that, compared to subjects using publicly funded testing centers, subjects utilizing home collection were more likely to be first-time testers, to be from low HIV risk groups, and be more likely to have had contact with an HIV-infected sexual partner.[68]

Other Diagnostic Blood Tests

As stated earlier, p24 antigen can be measured in the serum during primary HIV infection. Commercial assays for p24 quantification are available[69] that utilize a standard EIA micro-plate format where serum containing p24 antigen is incubated in the presence of anti-p24 antibodies. A subsequent enzymatic, colorimetric reaction is proportional to the amount of p24 antigen present in the sample. Natural history studies suggest that during primary HIV infection p24 antigen levels approach nanogram per milliliter concentrations. However, these levels are transient during seroconversion and rapidly become undetectable following the seroconversion period.

During seroconversion, antibodies against p24 result in the formation of immune complexes containing p24 antigen. Conventional p24 antigen assays do not detect p24 antigen complexed with antibodies. A modification has been developed that increases the sensitivity of p24 antigen detection by incorporating a preliminary acid hydrolysis step to dissociate complexes.[70] Free p24 antigen can then be measured. This step has resulted in improved sensitivity for p24 antigen detection and quantification in some patients.[71] However, even with this additional step, immune complex-dissociated p24 is not readily detectable in most patients after seroconversion.[20] Thus the p24 assay is only moderately useful as a diagnostic test before and during the seroconversion period. During the long period of clinical latency, p24 antigen is undetectable in virtually all patients. It reappears during late HIV infection when severe immune dysfunction results in increasing levels of HIV replication and overproduction of p24 antigen.[72] Even with late-stage disease the presence of p24 antigen is not uniform in all patients. Thus, this test has little utility for diagnostic purposes.

Infectious virus is present in both cell-free plasma and HIV-infected PBMCs. Standardized qualitative and quantitative micro-culture procedures for infectious HIV in the blood involve obtaining an aliquot of plasma or PBMCs and placing the sample in a co-culture with either established cell lines or activated HIV-seronegative donor PBMCs.[73,74] The presence of HIV is determined by sampling the cultured supernatant after a period of days for the presence of HIV p24 antigen or reverse transcriptase activity. In addition, specific phenotypic characteristics such as syncytia inducing versus non-syncytia-inducing or drug resistance patterns can be detected. Although not germane to the diagnosis of HIV infection, these phenotypic characteristics have important prognostic and management implications. The advantage of infectivity assays is that they provide definitive proof of infection. The disadvantages are several and include the requirement for special laboratories to handle highly infectious material; the duration of the assay, which requires 14 to 28 days of cell culture; lack of assay sensitivity; excessive cost; technical expertise for maintaining the cell culture; and differential infectability of HIV-seronegative donor cells. Because of these limitations, culture assays are not widely available for diagnostic purposes and are utilized in research settings.

Quantification of cell-free virion-associated HIV RNA in plasma is now a standard marker for assessing the risk of disease progression and monitoring the efficacy of antiretroviral therapy.[7,8] Three commercial assays are currently available to detect and quantitate plasma HIV RNA, although none is approved for diagnosing HIV infection in individuals.[75–77] One assay utilizes the reverse transcription-polymerase chain reaction (RT-PCR) (Amplicor HIV-1 Monitor; Roche Diagnostics, Branchburg, NJ, USA) to amplify plasma HIV RNA. After conversion of RNA to DNA, the amplified HIV *gag* gene PCR product is serially diluted in the presence of a known copy number standard, and an enzyme-linked DNA probe is hybridized to the amplified product. A subsequent colorimetric reaction is proportional to the input copy number. In contrast, nucleic acid sequence-based amplification (NASBA) (NucliSens; Organon-Teknika, Durham, NC, USA) utilizes repetitive rounds of RNA template transcription. After RNA extraction and amplification, the unknown patient RNA and three known internal standards generate an electroluminescent signal proportional to the input copy number. By comparison, the branched DNA (bDNA) assay (Versant; Bayer Diagnostics, Emeryville, CA, USA) utilizes a micro-plate to capture HIV RNA. Multiple DNA probes are hybridized to specific polymerase gene segments. Alkaline phosphatase is added in the presence of a substrate to generate a chemiluminescent reaction. The relative light units produced are compared to an external standard curve and are directly proportional to the amount of RNA in the sample. Thus in contrast to the RT-PCR and NASBA reactions, which are template (plasma RNA) amplification assays, the bDNA assay amplifies the signal from the RNA–DNA hybridization reaction. The (LCx) HIV RNA viral load assay (Abbott, Abbott Park, IL, USA) utilizes competitive RT-PCR and microparticle enzyme immunoassay technology for quantification.[78] Other viral load assays have been developed as well (Genprobe, San Diego, CA, USA; Digene, Gaithersburg, MD, USA).[79,80]

The FDA has approved the HIV-1 Monitor Standard version 1.0 and Monitor Ultra/Direct. These tests have a linear range of 400 to 750,000 and 50 to 75,000 copies per milliliter,[81] respectively. The COBAS Amplicor HIV-1 Monitor version 1.5 assays now automate amplification and detection. The FDA has also approved the Organon-Teknika NASBA Nuclisense QT assay, which produces linear results in the range of 176 to 3.47×10^6 copies RNA per milliliter of plasma. These assays are approved for the assessment of prognosis and antiretroviral response but are not approved for HIV-1 diagnosis. Although these assays all measure the same HIV RNA template, the copy numbers derived from each of these assays are not identical because of the differences in assay methodologies and inefficiency of sample preparation.[82]

The HIV viral load levels during primary HIV infection are extremely high, ranging from 10^5 to more than 2×10^7 copies per milliliter.[83] In addition, HIV RNA is detectable well before seroconversion (Fig. 1–1).[2,20] During seroconversion the HIV RNA levels drop precipitously within the first 4 to 8 weeks after infection.[3,20] Plasma RNA levels during seroconversion are not significantly different between patients who have symptoms and those who are asymptomatic.[84] Levels are significantly higher 6 to 12 months after seroconversion in patients who have symptoms during the time of seroconversion.[85]

During the period of clinical latency, HIV RNA levels remain relatively constant in clinically stable patients but increase gradually over the course of disease. Thus plasma RNA levels are detectable throughout the course of infection in the absence of effective antiretroviral therapy (Fig. 1–1).[86] In a study utilizing subjects from the multicenter AIDS cohort study, fewer than 2% of patients within 6 months of seroconversion had HIV RNA levels of less than 500 copies per milliliter.[8]

Although not FDA-approved for this indication, plasma HIV RNA testing is useful for diagnosing patients with primary HIV infection when the serum p24 antigen assay may be negative and HIV serology is not yet positive or is indeterminant.[2,20] During early chronic infection and thereafter, it can be expected that HIV serology will be positive, and so the need to utilize plasma viral load as a primary diagnostic test is unnecessary. Plasma RNA testing may be useful in cases with indeterminate or possibly false-positive Western blot results. It is important to note that some false positives have been described with viral load testing in patients manifesting acute viral symptoms.[87] These false-positive results generally demonstrate low HIV RNA levels (i.e., < 500 copies per microliter).

Polymerase chain reaction assays to detect the presence of proviral HIV DNA in PBMCs have also been used for diagnosing HIV infection. A commercial assay (Roche Molecular, Branchburg, NJ, USA) utilizes standard PCR techniques in a micro-plate format to amplify a segment of the HIV *gag* gene with subsequent probe hybridization and qualitative enzymatic, colorimetric readout. Because this methodology amplifies HIV genetic material in cells, it is an attractive alternative to serologic diagnosis. However, a recent meta-analysis comparing various PCR assay formats found that in documented

HIV infection the joint sensitivity and specificity of DNA PCR ranged from 97.0% to 98.1%. Corresponding false-positive and false-negative rates range between 1.9% and 3.0%.[88] Many assays exist, but they have not been standardized.

▲ PROBLEMS WITH INTERPRETATION OF SEROLOGIES AND VIRAL LOAD ASSAYS

The HIV-1 strains are categorized into major (M) and outlier (O) groups. Rare non-M, non-O ("N") group viruses have also been described.[89] Group M has been further divided (using sequence analysis) into subtypes (clades) A to J,[90] which have wide geographic diversity. Subtype (clade) B is currently most common in North America and western Europe, subtypes A and C are most common in Africa, and subtype E is common in Thailand. Other clades are also found in Africa and Asia. In areas where more than one subtype circulates, recombinants between HIV subtypes have been observed.

Many conventional assays for HIV detection were designed using a group M, subtype B strain and therefore detect subtype B strain extremely well, although they may not be as sensitive and specific for detecting other HIV-1 subtypes. In a study comparing FDA-approved EIA assays,[91] most assays, including the SUDS saliva test, detected 243 HIV isolates, including clades A to G and O, with 100% sensitivity.

Most plasma viral load assays do not have difficulty quantitating HIV across clades, although some clades may be more difficult to detect than others.[78–80,82,92,93] Nonclade B strains may not be readily detectable by molecular techniques that assay HIV DNA in cells. In a recent comparison of the standard Roche PBMC DNA PCR and the Amplicor HIV-1 Monitor v1.0 for quantitation of plasma HIV RNA, the standard Roche DNA assay did not detect non-clade B HIV DNA sequences in a significant number of HIV-infected Ugandan individuals.[94] Utilizing an HIV-1 *pol* gene primer pair in addition to the *gag* gene primer pair increased the sensitivity of the assay to 98%. The RNA assay qualitative positivity was significantly higher than that of the DNA-based assay. Detection of recombinant clades by current test kits remains under study.

Group O-infected individuals (seen primarily in western and central Africa) may not be reactive in the early-generation anti-HIV screening tests. With the introduction of an HIV-1 group O-specific peptide (gp41), a new version of an approved anti-HIV-1/HIV-2 diagnostic assay (Organon Teknika) successfully detected all group O-positive sera.[95] HIV antigen–antibody combination assays, such as the Abbott AXSYM assay, also detect group O infections. There have been further refinements to the Roche Molecular Systems PBMC DNA PCR assay; and using a new primer pair/probe system, this test detected 99% of genetically diverse group M and group O isolates.[96] The Amplicor HIV-1 Monitor v 1.5 plasma viral load assay can readily detect group M viral strains.

First identified in West Africa, HIV-2 subsequently spread to countries with traditional political and colonial ties to West Africa, including Portugal, Mozambique, and India.[97] HIV-2 infection has since been found in the United States, Europe, and Asia, including South Korea.[98] Some HIV-2 proteins are similar to those of HIV-1, which can produce potentially false-positive HIV-1 EIA results.[99] EIA tests for HIV-2 have been available since 1990, and combined EIA tests for HIV-1 and HIV-2 were introduced in 1992. EIA tests for HIV-2 detection or recombinant or Western blot tests for confirmation incorporate a specific recombinant envelope protein (gp36) that is unique to HIV-2. There are no commercially available HIV-2 viral load tests.

▲ NEONATAL/PEDIATRIC HIV DIAGNOSIS

Serologic diagnosis of HIV infection in newborns is difficult because maternal anti-HIV IgG antibodies cross the placenta into the fetal/neonatal circulation. Conventional EIA antibody and Western blot tests may be positive in uninfected newborns for more than 1 year as a result of maternal antibodies.[100] Some improvement in testing was found using EIA assays specific for IgA, IgM, or IgG3.[101] Other methods have been utilized to diagnose pediatric HIV infection. Several studies have evaluated HIV-specific IgA antibody as a possible HIV diagnostic test.[102–105] Despite excellent specificity (> 99%) and several performance-enhancing procedures (i.e., IgA-specific Western blotting, IgG depletion), its sensitivity ranged from only 40% to 80% during the first month and increased thereafter to 80% to 90%. Culture and the PCR appeared to be more sensitive than IgA in one study.[105] A sensitive assay to detect HIV-specific IgE has been reported. Because IgE does not cross the placenta, such an assay could provide an infant-specific diagnostic signal.[106,107]

Part of the controversy surrounding test performance of the various diagnostic assays and the difficulty establishing an HIV diagnosis in newborns relates to the timing of HIV infection. When HIV-infected pregnant women were assessed by ultrasound-guided fetal blood sampling, all 28 fetuses (mean 22 weeks' gestation) had negative cultures, PCR, and immune complex-dissociated (ICD) p24 antigen tests.[108] Most transmission appears to occur late in pregnancy, and early fetal testing is not recommended. Vertical transmission can be intrauterine (25% to 40%), peripartum (60% to 75%), or during breastfeeding (10% to 15%).[109,110] Vertical transmission is defined as intrauterine if the HIV viral culture or DNA PCR is positive within the first 48 hours of birth. Transmission is defined as being intrapartum if these studies are negative during the first week of life but positive within 1 month.[111]

The use of HIV cultures and p24 antigen EIAs for diagnosing HIV in newborns is largely determined by the timing of the infection. Several studies found that PBMC culture positivity ranged from 20% to 50% at birth and rose to 75% to 90% at 4 weeks.[112–114] This indicates that most infants are infected during the intrapartum period. PBMC DNA PCR has also been found to be significantly less sensitive in infants less than 4 weeks of age than after 1 month.[115–119] PBMC culture and DNA PCR have comparable sensitivities (50%) for infants infected at birth and after 1 to 2 months (> 95%).[114] Regular p24 antigen testing has been found to be highly specific but lacked sensitivity in HIV diagnosis.[112] ICD or heat-denatured p24 antigen assays have improved the sensitivity of this testing methodology but are clearly inferior for diagnosing HIV during the first month of life.[120–125]

Studies of vertical HIV transmission indicate that infected infants have a rapid rise of HIV plasma RNA over the first 1 to 2 months of life, followed by a slow decline over the next 22 months. The mean values throughout the first year of life are usually more than 10^5 copies per milliliter.[115] The median RNA levels at birth and at 1 month are much higher for infants infected in utero compared to peripartum (10,000 vs. 400 and 716,000 vs. 100,000 copies per milliliter at 1 month, respectively).[126,127] In contrast to most adults, whose levels decline 1 to 3 log copies per milliliter after seroconversion, perinatally infected children have levels that remain exceedingly high. The plasma RNA assay appears to be more sensitive than DNA PCR for diagnosis within 4 weeks of birth, although the two methods appear equally sensitive by 1 to 2 months.[128,129] In addition, HIV-1 diagnosis by DNA PCR does not appear to be affected by the mode of delivery or maternal or neonatal antiretroviral treatment.[130]

In summary, diagnosing HIV infection in neonates continues to be difficult. Routine ELISA and Western blot serologic assays are unreliable for providing a definitive diagnosis during the first year. Culture is not sufficiently sensitive and is logistically not feasible. Plasma RNA appears to be the diagnostic procedure of choice.

▲ PRE-HIV AND POST-HIV TESTING, COUNSELING, STRATEGIES

Counseling and testing guidelines for HIV patients have recently been issued by the Center for Disease Control and Prevention (CDC).[131] Risk groups to consider for HIV testing are listed in Table 1–7. Centers that offer testing services should provide the following elements: confidentiality; informed consent; optional anonymous testing; adherence to local, state, and federal regulations governing testing services; services responsive to community and client needs; services that are culturally, linguistically, and gender- and age-appropriate; and quality assurance of services.

Routine voluntary testing is recommended in areas where the prevalence of HIV infection is higher than 1%. Targeted voluntary testing is recommended in areas with lower prevalence if clients have behavioral risk.[132] After a decision to test for HIV is made, it is imperative that all clients undergo pretest and subsequent posttest counseling. According to the CDC guidelines, pretest counseling should include education about HIV disease, information about the specific test(s) available, personalized assessment of HIV risk factors, and education about risk reduction. Posttest counseling should include a discussion of the test results, an assessment of the patient's understanding of the results and psychological status, a discussion of behavioral modification, and the need for referral. Typical referral services include follow-up medical care (HIV, sexually transmitted diseases, viral hepatitis screening and treatment), psychological care, partner counseling and referral, reproductive health counseling, and substance abuse prevention and treatment.[132–134]

All pregnant women should be offered HIV testing regardless of their risk factors or the prevalence rates in their community. Counseling considerations for pregnant women include the interaction between pregnancy and HIV infection, the risk of perinatal HIV transmission, antiretroviral treatment options, and the prognosis for infants who are subsequently infected.[135] Women with indeterminate Western blot tests should undergo repeat testing 4 to 8 weeks after the first test. Use of additional testing procedures, including viral load testing, may facilitate early diagnosis during gestation. Testing incarcerated women, women in military service, those with mental illness, and victims of rape bring up complex issues of importance including spousal or partner notifications, insurance industry effects, and state and federal reporting requirements for HIV infection. For rape victims, consideration can be given to testing vaginal-cervical secretions for seminal fluid-containing HIV antibodies.[136]

Modern testing strategies are being employed to make the diagnosis of HIV-1/HIV-2 infection more efficient and accurate. Rapid screening tests can discriminate HIV-1, HIV-2, and HIV-1 subgroup M from subgroup O in 5 minutes. One assay (Abbott Laboratories) can be used for whole blood, urine, and saliva.[137,138] Rapid on-site HIV testing strategies result in decreased intervals between ordering tests and posttest counseling. This protocol has been successfully employed in emergency departments and field-testing centers, the latter of which demonstrated a significant cost savings for HIV screening and increased numbers of patients receiving posttest counseling.[139–143]

Identifying individuals with acute HIV infection is imperative from clinical and public health perspectives: (1) From a medical standpoint, evidence suggests that early therapy of HIV infection may result in substantial preservation of immunity; and (2) identifying acute HIV infection provides an opportunity to address high risk behavior and partner notification, potentially reducing overall HIV transmission.

Identification of acute HIV infection is often challenging because of the nonspecific clinical presentation and potentially confusing laboratory results. HIV-infected patients have been reported to have false-positive VDRL assays, *Borrelia* ELISA/Western blot tests, or Epstein-Barr virus (EBV) heterophile antibody tests.[144–148] Analyses, however, suggest that false positive EBV heterophile antibody tests for HIV are rare.[144–148] In addition, some diseases with a

▲ **Table 1–7.** RISK GROUPS IN WHOM HIV TESTING IS INDICATED

Persons with sexually transmitted diseases
High risk categories
Injection drug users
Homosexual and bisexual men
Hemophiliacs
Regular sexual partners of persons in these categories
Heterosexual persons with more than one sex partner during the past 12 months plus noncompliance with condom use in the past 6 months
Persons who consider themselves at risk
Pregnant women
Patients with active tuberculosis
Recipient and source of occupational exposures
Hospital admissions for patients ages 15 to 54 in areas of high prevalence
Health care workers who perform exposure-prone invasive procedures, depending on institutional policies
Donors of blood, semen, organs
Medical evaluations for clinical or laboratory findings suggesting HIV infection

clinical presentation similar to that of acute HIV (e.g., acute malaria, dengue, rheumatoid arthritis, systemic lupus erythematosus) may cause false-positive results in HIV ELISA assays.[149–152] Clearly, a high level of clinical suspicion, an appropriate use of screening and confirmatory tests, and a consideration for all alternative diagnoses are the essential elements for diagnosing acute HIV syndrome.

▲ ALGORITHM FOR HIV TESTING

A testing algorithm for HIV-1 and HIV-2 diagnostic testing is presented in Figure 1–4. A screening HIV-1/HIV-2 EIA should be performed first. If this test is negative, retest the patient in 3 to 6 months if clinically indicated. If the EIA is positive, a repeat EIA is performed on the same sample. If the repeat EIA is negative, retest the patient in 3 to 6 months. If the repeat EIA is positive, perform an HIV-1 Western blot test on the same sample. If the Western blot is positive, it confirms an HIV-1 infection. If the HIV-1 Western blot is negative, HIV-2-specific tests may be considered in the right clinical context (i.e., exposure to individuals in West or Central Africa). If the HIV-1 Western blot test is indeterminate, it is strongly recommended that repeat HIV-1 serotesting be performed 4 to 8 weeks later. It is possible that the patient is infected but is tested during the seroconversion period, in which case the Western blot assay may not yet be positive. If the patient is HIV-infected, 2 months is usually sufficient for further antibody production and hence a declaration of HIV positivity. Alternatively, one can use other tests (not FDA-approved for HIV diagnosis), such as plasma HIV-1 viral load tests, or fourth-generation combination HIV antibody–p24 antigen assays, as early definitive proof of infection.

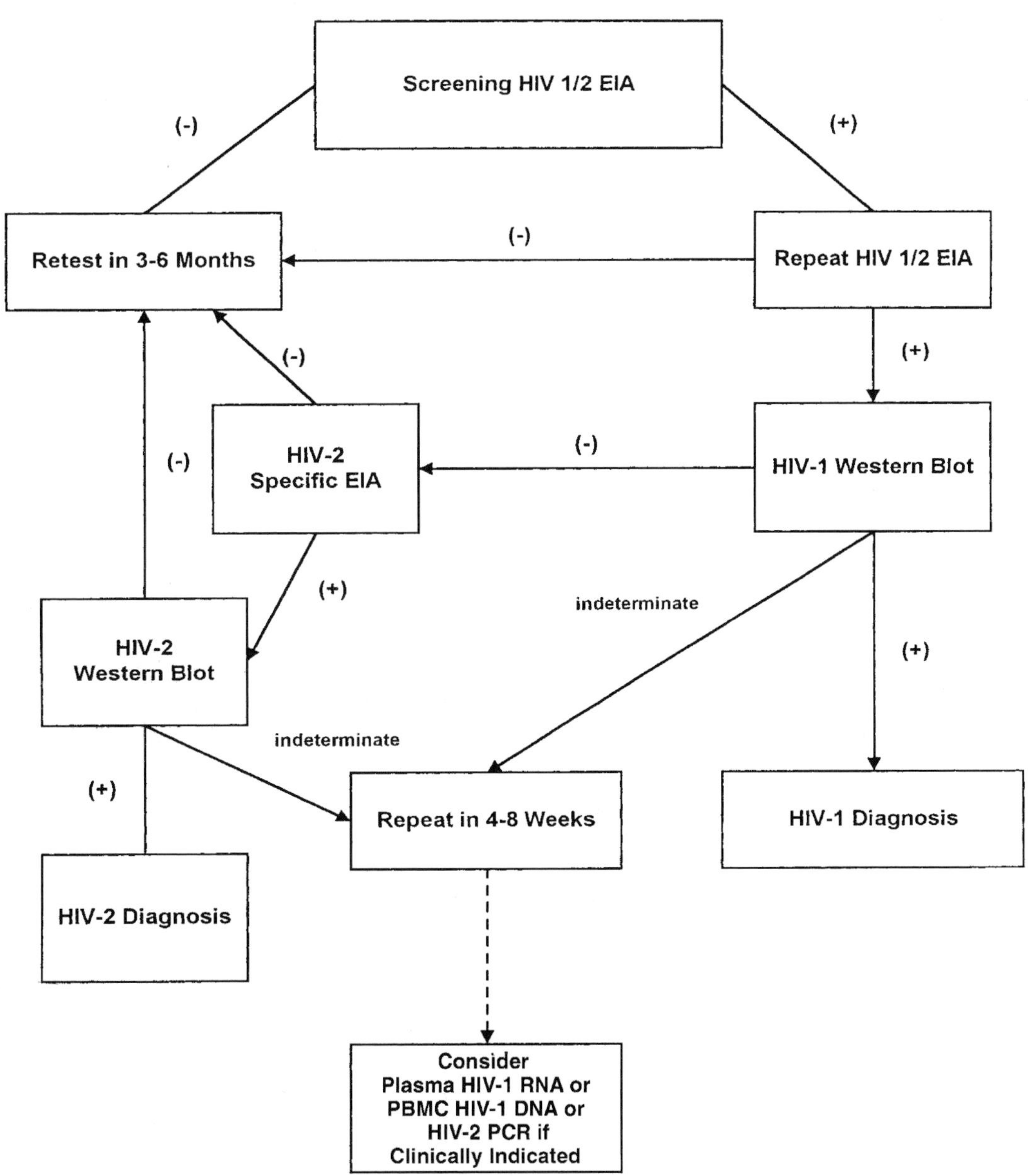

Figure 1–4. Algorithm for serologic diagnosis of HIV-1/HIV-2 infection.

The use of such tests permits consideration of early therapy if acute infection is documented. The duration of the seroconversion window continues to be reduced by increasingly sensitive and specific assays. A typical window period for detecting HIV infection by standard antibody testing is approximately 25 days. This period may be reduced to 14 to 21 days with p24 antigen testing, and nucleic acid-based testing may reduce the window by another 5 to 10 days.[153] Clearly, these boundaries for the HIV window period are based on limited data, and further investigation is required to assess the precise timing the HIV infection. An alternative algorithm utilizing these other testing strategies has been reported.[154]

▲ BLOOD DONOR TESTING FOR HIV-1/HIV-2

Screening donated blood (Fig. 1–5) relies on tests performed on samples from donated units. Initial testing is performed on serum or plasma from "pilot" tubes collected at the time of donation. If the initial test is reactive, repeat testing is performed on both the originally tested pilot tube serum/plasma and either a second pilot tube or an aliquot of plasma obtained from segmented tubing attached to the blood components. This element of the algorithm is designed as an additional safeguard to identify and resolve possible specimen labeling errors. If one or both repeat tests are reactive, the unit is designated "repeat reactive" and discarded. A process is also initiated to identify and quarantine all in-date components from any prior donation(s) by that donor and to notify recipients who received blood components from prior donations.[155]

Transmission of HIV has been reported from transfusion of seronegative blood later shown to contain p24 antigen. Because serum p24 antigen is found earlier than antibody during PHI, testing blood for p24 antigen became mandatory in the United States in March 1996.[156] Although models suggested that routine p24 antigen testing would detect one antigen-positive/antibody-negative donation in every 1.6 million units of blood tested,[157] only one in 9 million donations tested from volunteer donors were intercepted based on p24 antigen testing alone during the first 4 years of screening (a total of six such donors were detected).[158] A possible explanation for the underperformance of HIV-1 antigen testing to detect HIV-1 antibody-negative window period infections is that blood donors during the early phase of HIV-1 infection may be experiencing symptoms from PHI that deter them from donation or result in rejection during the predonation history and physical examination.

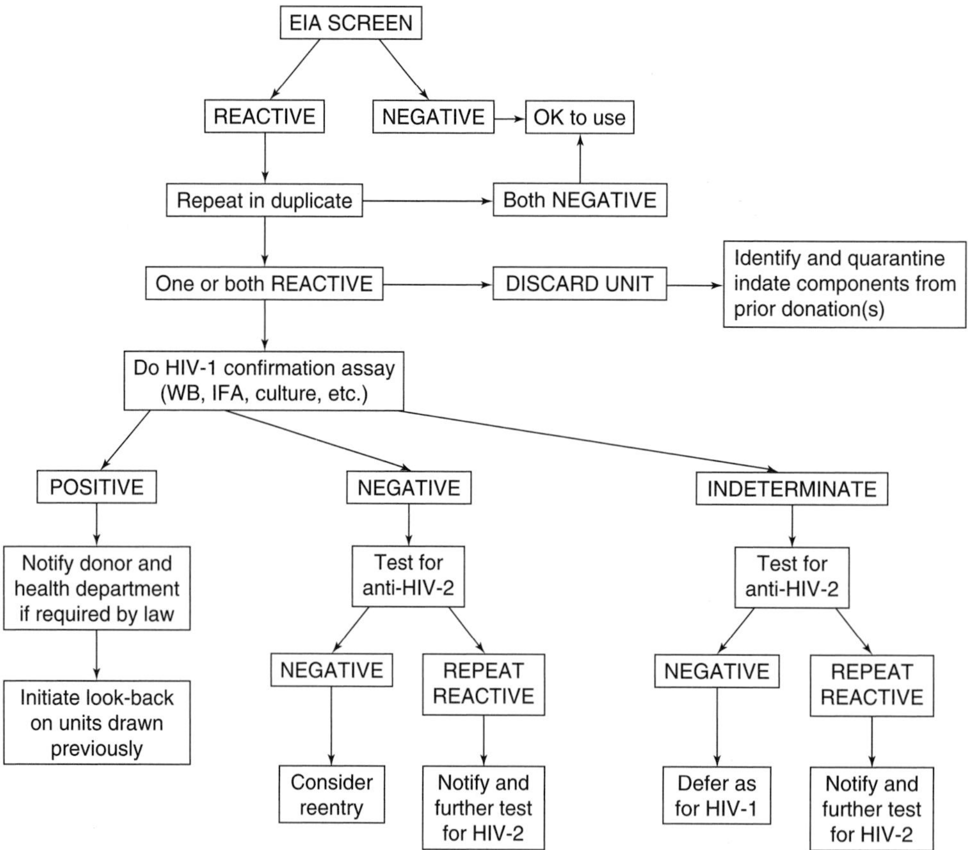

Figure 1–5. Decision tree for anti-HIV-1/HIV-2 testing of blood donors. In addition, nucleic acid testing is performed in parallel on all donations using pooled testing algorithms. IFA, immunofluorescence assay; WB, Western blot. (Figure redrawn from Fiebig W. Infectious complications of blood transfusion. In: Vengelen-Tyler, ed. Technical Manual, 13th ed. Bethesda, American Association of Blood Banks, 1999, p 613.)

Due to the exquisite sensitivity of HIV EIA assays used for blood donor screening and the low pretest probability of HIV infection among blood donors, most of the positive screening results are false positives despite the excellent specificity of the tests. Supplemental assays are therefore essential to confirm positive screening results and for donor counseling. Supplemental testing must use FDA-licensed reagents and rule out both HIV-1 and HIV-2 infection.[159] Although combination HIV-1/HIV-2 supplemental assays using recombinant DNA-derived or synthetic peptide antigens have been developed that appear to detect and discriminate anti-HIV-1 and anti-HIV-2 accurately,[155] they are not yet approved by the FDA. Therefore current confirmatory algorithms in U.S. blood banks employ HIV-1 viral lysate-based Western blots or IFA assays, in combination with a licensed anti-HIV-2 EIA and unlicensed HIV-2 supplemental assays.[159] Interpretive criteria for Western blots have evolved over time as tests have improved and our understanding of the meaning of various banding patterns has increased. Although these criteria are generally accurate, it is clear that some donors who show antibody reactivity limited to the gag and env glycoproteins are not infected with HIV-1.[41] Therefore, all initial positive Western blot results are confirmed using a separate follow-up sample to rule out specimen mix-up or testing errors and to discriminate nonspecific patterns from early seroconversion. Only a small proportion of donors who test "indeterminate" on the Western blot test are infected with HIV-1.[41,160] Our ability to clarify the infectious status has improved with the recent introduction of routine nucleic acid testing.

All repeat reactive donors are deferred from further blood donations and notified of their screening and supplemental test results. For confirmed positive donors, recipients of prior donations are traced by a process called "lookback."[161] Donors whose supplemental test results are completely negative are eligible for possible reentry into the donor pool according to an FDA-specified protocol,[159] although, in practice, logistical and legal considerations have generally prevented reinstatement of these donors.

Supplemental testing of HIV-1 antigen results relies on neutralization assays. When the EIA screening test for p24 antigen is repeatedly reactive, a confirmatory neutralization test should be performed to aid in counseling the donor and to determine the need for product quarantine, lookback, and deferral.[156] Although donors whose serum shows neutralization are classified as confirmed positive for HIV-1 antigen and must be permanently deferred, studies involving RT-PCR and follow-up of such donors have established that only a small proportion are actually infected with HIV; that is, most of their results are false-positive neutralizations.[158] Donors whose serum is not neutralizable are currently considered not confirmed but must be reported as HIV-1 antigen-indeterminate; they should be temporarily deferred from donation for a minimum of 8 weeks. Donors can be reentered in the donor pool if they are retested after this period and are found to be nonreactive by the HIV-1 antigen screening test and the HIV antibody test. Unfortunately, approximately 70% of donors with indeterminate results remain p24 antigen-indeterminate on follow-up and must be deferred indefinitely. As with antibody-reactive units, units from HIV-1 antigen repeatedly reactive donations cannot be used for transfusion or for preparing injectable products, and they must be quarantined and destroyed.

The risk of HIV-1 transmission from repeat donors and, with some adjustments, first-time donors can then be calculated. Window period estimates for HIV-1 infection in the United States dropped from a median of 45 days (95% confidence interval 34 to 55 days) for the overall period from 1985 to 1990 to approximately 22 to 25 days with routine introduction in 1992 of new-format anti-HIV-1/HIV-2 "combi-tests," which detect HIV-specific IgM antibody 10 to 15 days earlier than previously available assays.[155,162,163] By combining the 25-day window period estimate with data on the frequency of HIV seroconversions in large U.S. donor populations, two independent studies derived point estimates for the risk for HIV transmission during the 1992 to 1995 period of 1:450,000[164] and 1:495,000,[165] respectively. The introduction of HIV-1 antigen screening in 1995 further reduced the risk to an estimated 1:650,000. However, fewer than expected HIV-1 antigen-positive HIV1/HIV-2 antibody-negative units have been intercepted since the test was introduced. Therefore the contribution to risk reduction has been rather modest. Finally, the risk of HIV-2 transmission has been estimated at less than 1 in 15 million,[166] with other rare subtypes (e.g., HIV-1 subtype O)[167] being of even less concern. These combined risks are more than 5000-fold lower than that existing at the peak of the transfusion-AIDS epidemic between 1982 and 1984.[168]

Strategies to improve blood donor testing further focus on the introduction of new tests and enhancing the performance of existing assays. Nucleic acid testing, which was introduced in 1999 for HIV and hepatitis C virus (HCV) under FDA investigational new drug (IND) exemption, is the most recent advancement in blood donor screening. High-sensitivity, qualitative nucleic acid amplification testing assays have been developed based on RT-PCR and transcription mediated amplification (TMA) technologies.[169] To increase throughput and reduce cost, nucleic acid testing is performed in the donor screening setting on "minipools" of 16 to 24 donation samples. A pooled sample with a positive reaction is resolved by performing the assay on individual specimens. The current approach of testing pooled blood donor samples, although practical, is not optimal because sample dilution reduces assay sensitivity and because of the complexities involved in pooling algorithms and required identification of the source sample in case of a positive test on a pool. It is therefore expected that upgrading to single donation testing with nucleic acid testing will be phased in as soon as technically and financially feasible. Additionally, combination or "multiplex" nucleic acid amplification testing for simultaneous detection of HIV and HCV [and soon for HIV, HCV, and hepatitis B (HBV)] have been developed that are applied to either pooled or individual donor samples. Positive tests in multiplex assays are resolved when the positive specimen is further retested by single virus discriminatory tests for final resolution and confirmation.

Nucleic acid testing has already demonstrated in practice that it is capable of intercepting virus-containing blood units that are being missed by serologic assays.[170,171]

Studies conducted over the past several years have shown that these donor screening nucleic acid testing assays reduce the HIV window period by 10 to 15 days compared to HIV antibody and by 50 to 60 days compared to HCV antibody testing.[172,173] More than 16 million whole blood donations have been tested for HIV and HCV RNA since the implementation of nucleic acid testing into U.S. blood donor screening programs in April 1999. As of July 2000, nucleic acid testing screening had detected 5 HIV window-period donations (one in 3.1 million screened units) and 62 HCV window-period donations (one in 263,000 screened units); these numbers are close to the yield previously projected by mathematic modeling.[174] By multiplying the post-nucleic acid amplification testing per unit risk estimates × 18 million transfused components per year in the United States, it can be projected that up to 18 recipients per year may still be transfused with HIV-1-infected blood in the United States each year. This assumes that a person is infectious owing to exposure to RNA and hence is a worst-case estimate. Furthermore, fewer than five of these infected recipients would be expected to develop AIDS-related diseases prior to dying from other causes.[175]

The cost of universal nucleic acid testing screening is substantial (approximately $100 million per year in the United States) and the cost-effectiveness poor ($1.3 million per quality adjusted life-year).[176] Nonetheless, minipool nucleic acid testing screening has significantly decreased (although not eliminated) the infectious window period. Some delays in blood component availability are inevitable, which is a particular concern for platelets, which have only a 5-day shelf life. In addition, false-positive results, which can be expected with any new screening test, raise concern of unnecessary deferral of healthy blood donors at a time when blood shortages are becoming more frequent and severe.

Whereas the cost-effectiveness of routine donor screening using nucleic acid testing is controversial, the usefulness of nucleic acid testing to resolve discrepant or indeterminate antibody or p24 antigen test results is overwhelmingly clear. In the blood and plasma donor settings, where HIV prevalence is low, most HIV antibody EIA reactive donations are either negative or indeterminate upon supplemental Western blot testing. Such results are only rarely attributable to primary HIV infection. In a recent study, nucleic acid testing confirmed HIV-1 infection in all 20 Western blot-positive donors and ruled out infection in all 249 donors with indeterminate results.[41] This made it possible to reassure the individuals with indeterminate Western blot results at the time of initial notification and to reinstate donors who would otherwise have been permanently deferred.

Nucleic acid testing has also proven useful for identifying and resolving the infrequent but even more disturbing false-positive Western blot and p24 antigen neutralization results.[41] Nucleic acid testing systems are becoming the industry standard in the United States: In September 2001, the first nucleic acid testing systems for detecting HIV in pooled plasma samples were approved by the FDA; a draft FDA guidance document is currently being discussed that will require establishments to perform nucleic acid testing to reduce the risk of HIV transmission. Establishments that implement nucleic acid tests more sensitive than HIV p24 antigen assays may not be required to continue the p24 testing.[177]

Screening procedures are also required to evaluate the presence of HIV from cadaveric human tissue donors for transplantation.[178–184] At present, serum specimens obtained at the time of death may be utilized for this purpose: An HIV-1/HIV-2 synthetic peptide ELISA assay (Genetic Systems Corp.) has been FDA-approved and specifically labeled for testing cadaveric serum.[179] Testing for the p24 antigen is not required. The p24 antigen has been associated with false-positive results in cadaveric specimens and may delay tissue utilization.[180–184] Use of nucleic acid testing has been reported in skin transplant specimens.[181] Although nucleic acid testing may be useful in certain circumstances to evaluate "window-period" HIV infection in cadaveric donors, it has not been adequately evaluated to permit FDA approval.

Current blood donor screening and testing strategies have reduced the risk of HIV transmission in industrialized nations to near zero. Unfortunately, many developing nations, particularly those in sub-Saharan Africa and parts of Asia, do not employ these strategies. In some of the worst affected areas, a significant proportion of HIV infections are due to blood transfusion. These countries often lack the resources and supporting infrastructure to implement or maintain donor selection strategies that were developed in industrialized nations.[185,186]

REFERENCES

1. Shacker T, Collier AC, Hughes J, et al. Clinical and epidemiologic features of primary HIV infection. Ann Intern Med 125:257, 1996.
2. Daar ES, Little S, Pitt J, et al. Diagnosis of primary HIV-1 infection. Ann Intern Med 134:25, 2001.
3. Kinloch-De Loes S, Hirshel BJ, Hoen B, et al. A controlled trial of zidovudine in primary human immunodeficiency virus infection. N Engl J Med 333:408, 1995.
4. Montagnier L, Brenner C, Chamaret S, et al. Human immunodeficiency virus infection and AIDS in a person with negative serology. J Infect Dis 175:955, 1997.
5. Quinonez JM, Begue RE, Steele RW. HIV seronegativity in an infant with the acquired immunodeficiency syndrome. South Med J 91:879, 1998.
6. Pantaleo G, Graziosi C, Dmarest JF, et al. HIV infection is active and progressive in lymphoid tissue during the clinically latent stage of disease. Nature 362:355, 1993.
7. Perelson AS, Neumann AU, Markowitz M, et al. HIV-1 dynamics in vivo: virion clearance rate, infected cell life-span and viral generation time. Science 271:1582, 1996.
8. Mellors JW, Munoz A, Giorgi JV, et al. Plasma viral load and CD4+ lymphocytes as prognostic markers of HIV-1 infection. Ann Intern Med 126:946, 1997.
9. Dean M, Carrington M, Winkler C, et al. Genetic restriction of HIV-1 infection and progression to AIDS by a deletion allele of the CKR5 structural gene. Science 273:1856, 1996.
10. Fauci AS: Host factors and the pathogenesis of HIV-induced disease. Nature 384:529, 1996.
11. Carrington M, Nelson GW, Martin MP, et al. HLA and HIV-1: heterozygote advantage and B*35-Cw*04 disadvantage. Science 283:1748, 1999.
12. Hendel H, Caillat-Zucman S, Lebuanec H, et al. New class I and II HLA alleles strongly associated with opposite patterns of progression to AIDS. J Immunol 162:6942, 1999.
13. Migueles SA, Sabbaghian MS, Shupert WL, et al. HLA B*5701 is highly associated with restriction of virus replication in a subgroup of HIV-infected long term nonprogressors. Proc Natl Acad Sci USA 97:2709, 2000.
14. Roos MTL, Lange JMA, de Goede REY, et al. Viral phenotype and immune response in primary human immunodeficiency virus type 1 infection. J Infect Dis 8:1533, 1994.

15. De Roda Husman AM, van Rij RP, Blaak H, et al. Adaptation to promiscuous usage of chemokine receptors is not a prerequisite for human immunodeficiency virus type 1 disease progression. J Infect Dis 180:1106, 1999.
16. Koot M, Van Leeuwen R, De Goede REY, et al. Conversion rate towards a syncytium-inducing (SI) phenotype during different stages of human immunodeficiency virus type 1 infection and prognostic value of SI phenotype for survival after AIDS diagnosis. J Infect Dis 179:2548, 1998.
17. Lange JAM, Parry JV, De Wolf F, et al. Diagnostic value of specific IgM antibodies in primary HIV infection. AIDS 2:11, 1988.
18. Gaines H, von Sydow M, Sonnerberg A, et al. Antibody response in primary HIV infection. Lancet 1:1249, 1987.
19. Reiss P, de Ronde A, Dekker J, et al. Seroconversion to HIV-1 rev and tat gene-encoded proteins. AIDS 3:105, 1989.
20. Niu MT, Bethel J, Holodniy M, et al. Zidovudine treatment in patients with primary (acute) HIV-1 infection: a randomized, double-blind, placebo-controlled trial. J Infect Dis 178:80, 1998.
21. U.S. Department of Health and Human Services, Public Health Service. Persistent lack of detectable HIV-1 antibody in a person with HIV infection-Utah, 1995. MMWR Morb Mortal Wkly Rep 45:181, 1996.
22. Soriano V, Dronda F, Gonzalez-Lopez A, et al. HIV-1 causing AIDS and death in a seronegative individual. Vox Sang 67:410, 1994.
23. Ellenberger DL, Sullivan PS, Dorn J, et al. Viral and immunologic examination of human immunodeficiency virus type 1-infected, persistently seronegative persons. J Infect Dis 180:1033, 1999.
24. Von Sydow M, Gaiens H, Sonnerberg A, et al. Antigen detection in primary HIV infection. BMJ 296:238, 1988.
25. Pedersen C, Nielsen CM, Vestergaard BF, et al. Temporal relation of antigenaemia and loss of antibodies to core antigens to development of clinical disease in HIV infection. BMJ 295:567, 1987.
26. Daar ES, Moudgil T, Meyer RD, et al. Transient high levels of viremia in patients with primary human immunodeficiency virus type 1 infection. N Engl J Med 324:961, 1991.
27. Ferbas J, Daar ES, Grovit-Ferbas K, et al. Rapid evolution of human immunodeficiency virus strains with increased replicative capacity during the seronegative window of primary infection. J Virol 70:7285, 1996.
28. Tindall B, Evans LA, Cunningham P, et al. Identification of HIV-1 in semen following primary HIV-1 infection. AIDS 6:949, 1992.
29. Bagnarelli P, Valenza A, Menzo S, et al. Dynamics of molecular parameters of human immunodeficiency virus type 1 activity in vivo J Virol 68:2495, 1994.
30. Roos M, De Leeuw N, Claessen F, et al. Viro-immunological studies in acute HIV-1 infection. AIDS 8:1533, 1994.
31. Von Sydow M, Sonnerberg A, Gaines H, et al. Interferon-alpha and tumor necrosis factor in serum of patients in varying stages of HIV-1 infection. AIDS Res Hum Retroviruses 7:375, 1991.
32. Sonnerberg AB, von Stedingk L-V, Hansson L-O, et al. Elevated neopterin and beta2-microglobulin levels in blood and cerebrospinal fluid occur early in HIV-1 infection. AIDS 3:277, 1989.
33. Sloand E, Pitt E, Chiarello RJ, et al. HIV testing state of the art. JAMA 266:2861, 1991.
34. Kinloch-de Loes S, de Saussure P, Saurat J-H, et al. symptomatic primary infection due to human immunodeficiency virus type 1: review of 31 cases. Clin Infect Dis 17:59, 1993.
35. Cordes RJ, Ryan ME: Pitfalls in HIV testing: application and limitations of current tests. Postgrad Med 98:177, 1995.
36. Brust S, Duttmann H, Feldner J, et al. Shortening of the diagnostic window with a new combined HIV p24 antigen and anti-HIV-1/2/O screening test. J Virol Methods 90:153, 2000.
37. Saville RD, Constantine NT, Cleghorn FR, et al. Fourth-generation enzyme-linked immunosorbent assay for the simultaneous detection of human immunodeficiency virus antigen and antibody. J Clin Microbiol. 39:2518, 2001.
38. Labperche S, Maniez-Montreuil M, Courouce AM. Screening tests combined with p24 antigen and anti-HIV antibodies in early detection of HIV-1. Transfus Clin Biol 1 (suppl)1:18s, 2000.
39. George JR, Schochetman G. Serologic tests for the detection of human immunodeficiency virus infection. In: George JR, Schochetman G (eds) AIDS Testing: Methodology and Management Issues. New York, Springer-Verlag, 1992, p 48.
40. O'Gorman MRG, Weber D, Landis SE, et al. Interpretive criteria of the Western blot assay for serodiagnosis of human immunodeficiency virus type 1 infection. Arch Pathol Lab Med 115:26, 1991.
41. Kleinman S, Busch MP, Hall L, et al. False-positive HIV-1 test results in a low-risk screening setting of voluntary blood donation. JAMA 280:1080, 1998.
42. Sinicco A, Palestro G, Caramello P, et al. Acute HIV-1 infection: clinical and biological study of 12 patients. J Acquir Immune Defic Syndr 3:260, 1990.
43. Celum CL, Coombs RW, Jones M, et al. Risk factors for repeatedly reactive HIV-1 EIA and indeterminate Western blots: a population-based case-control study. Arch Intern Med 154:1129, 1994.
44. Sayre KR, Dodd RY, Tegtmeier G, et al. False-positive human immunodeficiency virus type 1 Western blot tests in noninfected blood donors. Transfusion 36:45, 1996.
45. Georgoulias VA, Malliaraki NE, Theodoropoulou M, et al. Indeterminate human immunodeficiency virus type 1 Western blot may indicate an abortive infection in some low-risk donors. Transfusion 37:65, 1997.
46. Carlson JR, Yee J, Hinrichs SH, et al. Comparison of indirect immunofluorescence and Western blot for detection of anti-human immunodeficiency virus antibodies. J Clin Microbiol 25:494, 1987.
47. Windsor IM, dos Santos MLG, Hunt LI, et al. An evaluation of the capillus HIV-1/HIV-2 latex agglutination test using serum and whole blood. Int J STD AIDS 8:192, 1997.
48. Ray CS, Mason PR, Smith H, et al. An evaluation of dipstick-dot immunoassay in the detection of antibodies to HIV-1 and 2 in Zimbabwe. Trop Med Int Health 2:83, 1997.
49. Kuun E, Brashaw M, Heyns AD. Sensitivity and specificity of standard and rapid HIV antibody tests evaluated by seroconversion and non-seroconversion low-titre panels. Vox Sang 72:11, 1997.
50. Phillips S, Granade TC, Pau CP, et al. Diagnosis of human immunodeficiency virus type infection with different subtypes using rapid tests. Clin Diagn Immunol 7:698, 2000
51. Zeeher HL, van Rixel T, van Exel-Oehler P, et al. New anti-human immunodeficiency virus immunoblot assays resolve nonspecific Western blot results. Transfusion 37:193, 1997.
52. Kline RL, McNairn D, Holodniy M, et al. Evaluation of Chiron HIV-1/HIV-2 recombinant immunoblot assay. J Clin Microbiol 34:2650, 1996.
53. Tamashiro H, Constantine NT: Serological diagnosis of HIV infection using oral fluid samples. Bull World Health Organ 72:135, 1994.
54. Lu XS, Delfraissy JF, Grangeot-Keros L, et al. Rapid and constant detection of HIV antibody response in saliva of HIV-infected patients: selective distribution of anti-HIV activity in the IgG isotype. Res Virol 145:369, 1994.
55. Martinez P, Ortiz deLejarazu R, Eiros JM, et al. Comparison of two assays for detection of HIV antibodies in saliva. J Clin Microbiol 14:330, 1995.
56. Tess BH, Granato C, Parry JV, et al. Salivary testing for human immunodeficiency virus type 1 infection in children born to infected mothers in Sao Paulo, Brazil: the Sao Paulo Collaborative Study for Vertical Transmission of HIV-1. Pediatr Infect Dis J 15:787, 1996.
57. Gallo D, George JR, Fitchen JH, et al. Evaluation of a system using oral mucosal transudate for HIV-1 antibody screening and confirmatory testing. JAMA 277:254, 1997.
58. King SD, Wynter SH, Bain BC, et al. Comparison of testing saliva and serum for detection of antibody to human immunodeficiency virus in Jamaica, West Indies. J Clin Virol 19:157, 2000.
59. Webber LM, Swanevelder C, Grabow WO, Fourie PB. Evaluation of a rapid test for HIV antibodies in saliva and blood. S Afr Med J 90:1004, 2000.
60. Thwe M, Frerichs RR, Oo KY, et al. Stability of saliva for measuring HIV in the tropics. J Trop Pediatr 45:296, 1999.
61. Sterne JA, Turner AC, Connell JA, et al. Human immunodeficiency virus: GACPAT and GACELISA as diagnostic tests for antibodies in urine. Trans R Soc Trop Med Hyg 87:181, 1993.
62. Hashida S, Hahinake K, Saitoh A, et al. Diagnosis of HIV-1 infection by detection of antibody IgG to HIV-1 in urine with ultrasensitive enzyme immunoassay (immune complex transfer enzyme immunoassay) using recombinant proteins as antigens. J Clin Lab Anal 8:237, 1994.
63. Constantine NT, Zhang X, Li L, et al. Application of a rapid assay for detection of antibodies to human immunodeficiency virus in urine. Am J Clin Pathol 101:157, 1994.
64. Berrios DC, Avins AL, Haynes-Sanstad K, et al. Screening for human immunodeficiency virus antibody in urine. Arch Pathol Lab Med 119:139, 1995.

65. Urnovitz HB, Sturge JC, Gottfried TD, Murphy WH. Urine antibody tests: new insights into the dynamics of HIV-1 infection. Clin Chem 45:1602, 1999.
66. Meehan MP, Sewankambo NK, Wawer MJ. Sensitivity and specificity of HIV-1 testing of urine compared with serum specimens: Rakai, Uganda; the Rakai Project Team. Sex Transm Dis 26:590, 1999.
67. Frank AP, Wandell MG, Headings MD, et al. Anonymous HIV testing using home collection and telemedicine counseling: a multicenter evaluation. Arch Intern Med 157:309, 1997.
68. McQuitty M, McFarland W, Kellogg TA, et al. Home collection versus publicly funded HIV testing in San Francisco: who tests where? J Acquir Immune Defic Syndr 21:417, 1999.
69. Constantine NT. Seriologic tests for the retroviruses: approaching a decade of evolution. AIDS 7:1, 1993.
70. Nishanian P, Huskins KR, Stehn S, et al. A simple method for improved assay demonstrates that HIV p24 antigen is present as immune complexes in most sera from HIV-infected individuals. J Infect Dis 162:21, 1990.
71. Bollinger RC, Kline RL, Francis HL, et al. Acid dissociation increases the sensitivity of p24 antigen detection for the evaluation of antiviral therapy and disease progression in asymptomatic human immunodeficiency virus-infected persons. J Infect Dis 165:913, 1992.
72. Porter M, Vitale F, La Licata R, et al. Free and antibody-complexed antigen and antibody profile in apparently healthy HIV-seropositive individuals and in AIDS patients. J Med Virol 30:30, 1990.
73. Lathey JL, Fiscus SA, Rasheed S, et al. Optimization of quantitative culture assay for human immunodeficiency virus from plasma: plasma viremia group laboratories of the AIDS Clinical Trials Group (National Institute of Allergy and Infectious Diseases). J Clin Microbiol 32:3064, 1994.
74. Fiscus SA, DeGruttola V, Gupta P, et al. Human immunodeficiency virus type: a quantitative cell microculture as a measure of antiviral efficacy in a multicenter clinical trial. J Infect Dis 171:305, 1995.
75. Mulder J, McKinney N, Christopherson C, et al. Rapid and simple PCR assay for quantitation of human immunodeficiency virus type 1 RNA in plasma: application to acute retroviral infection. J Clin Microbiol 32:292, 1994.
76. Pachl C, Todd JA, Kern DG, et al. Rapid and precise quantification of HIV-1 RNA in plasma using a branched DNA signal amplification assay. J Acquir Immune Defic Hum Retrovirol 8:446, 1995.
77. Van Gemen B, Wiel P, Van Beumingen R, et al. The one-tube quantitative HIV-1 RNA NASBA: precision, accuracy and application. PCR Methods Appl 4:5177, 1995.
78. Swanson P, Harris BJ, Holzmayer V, et al. Quantification of HIV-1 group M (subtypes A-G) and group O by the LCx HIV RNA quantitative assay. J Virol Methods 89:97, 2000.
79. Emery S, Bodrug S, Richardson BA, et al. Evaluation of performance of the Gen-Probe human immunodeficiency virus type 1 viral load assay using primary subtype A, C, and D isolates from Kenya. J Clin Microbiol 38:2688, 2000.
80. Schiltz H, Tang Y, Glock J, et al. Sensitive and accurate quantitation of diverse HIV-1 subtypes utilizing the Digene HIV RNA test. In: Abstracts of the 5th Conference on Retroviruses and Opportunistic Infections, Chicago. Alexandria, VA, Westover Management Group, 1998, abstract 118.
81. Sun R, Ku J, Jayakar H, et al. Ultrasensitive reverse transcription-PCR assay for quantitation of human immunodeficiency virus type 1 RNA in plasma. J Clin Microbiol 36:2964, 1998.
82. Murphy DG, Cote L, Fauvel M, et al. Multicenter Comparison of Roche COBAS AMPLICOR MONITOR version 1.5, Organon Teknika Nuclisens QT with Extractor, and Bayer Quantiplex Version 3.0 for Quantification of Human Immunodeficiency Virus Type 1 RNA in Plasma. J Clin Microbiol 38:4034, 2000.
83. Piatak M, Saag MS, Yang LC, et al. High levels of HIV-1 in plasma during all stages of infection determined by competitive PCR. Science 259:1749, 1993.
84. Katzenstein TL, Pederson C, Nielsen C, et al. Longitudinal serum HIV RNA quantification: correlation to viral phenotype at seroconversion and clinical outcome. AIDS 10:167, 1996.
85. Henrard DR, Daar E, Farzadegan H, et al. Virologic and immunologic characterizations of symptomatic and asymptomatic primary HIV-1 infection. J Acquir Immune Defic Syndr Hum Retrovirol 9:305, 1995.
86. Henrard DR, Phillips JF, Muenz LR, et al. Natural history of HIV-1 cell-free viremia. JAMA 274:554, 1995.
87. Rich J, Merriman MA, Mylonakis E, et al. Misdiagnosis of HIV infection by HIV-1 plasma viral load testing: a case series. Ann Intern Med 130:37,1999.
88. Owens DK, Holodniy M, Garber A, et al. Polymerase chain reaction for the diagnosis of HIV infection in adults: a meta-analysis with recommendations for clinical practice and study design. Ann Intern Med 124:803, 1996.
89. Simon F, Mauclere P, Roques P, et al. Identification of a new human immunodeficiency virus type 1 distinct from group M and group O. Nat Med 4:1032, 1998.
90. Hu DJ, Donder TJ, Rayfield MA, et al. The emerging genetic diversity of HIV. JAMA 275:210, 1996.
91. Koch WH, Sullivan PS, Roberts C, et al. Evaluation of United States-licensed human immunodeficiency virus immunoassays for detection of group M viral variants J Clin Microbiol 39:1017, 2001.
92. Todd J, Yeghiazarian T, Hoo B, et al. Quantitation of human immunodeficiency virus plasma RNA by branched DNA and reverse transcription coupled polymerase chain reaction assay methods: a critical evaluation of accuracy and reproducibility. Serodiagn Immunother Infect Dis 6:233, 1994.
93. Jacobs F, Brok M, de Ronde T, et al. Detection of a broad spectrum of HIV-1 group M and O viruses by NASBA. In: Abstracts of the 6th European Conference on Clinical Aspects and Treatment of HIV Infection, Hamburg, Germany, 1997, abstract 915.
94. Jackson JB, Piwowar EM, Parsons J, et al. Detection of human immunodeficiency virus type 1 (HIV-1) DNA and RNA sequences in HIV-1 antibody-positive blood donors in Uganda by the Roche AMPLICOR assay. J Clin Microbiol 35:873, 1997.
95. Van Binsbergen J, de Rijk D, Peels H, et al. Evaluation of a new third generation anti-HIV-1/anti-HIV-2 assay with increased sensitivity for HIV-1 group O. J Virol Methods 60:131, 1996.
96. Respess RA, Butcher A, Wang H, et al. Detection of genetically diverse human immunodeficiency virus type 1 group M and O isolates by PCR. J Clin Microbiol 35:1284, 1997.
97. George JR, Ou CY, Parekh B, et al. Prevalence of HIV-1 and HIV-2 mixed infections in Cote d'Ivoire. Lancet 340:337, 1992.
98. Kim SS, Kim EY, Park KY. Introduction of human immunodeficiency virus 2 infection into South Korea. Acta Virol 44:15, 2000.
99. Markovitz DM. Infection with the human immunodeficiency virus type 2. Ann Intern Med 118:211, 1993.
100. Chantry CJ, Cooper ER, Pelton SI, et al. Seroreversion in human immunodeficiency virus-exposed but uninfected infants. Pediatr Infect Dis J 14:382, 1995.
101. Madurai S, Moodley D, Coovadia HM, et al. Use of HIV-1 specific immunoglobulin G3 as a serological marker of vertical transmission. J Trop Pediatr 42:359, 1996.
102. McIntosh K, Comeau AM, Wara D, et al. The utility of IgA antibody to human immunodeficiency virus type 1 in early diagnosis of vertically transmitted infection: National Institute of Allergy and Infectious Disease and National Institute of Child Health and Human Development Women and Infants Transmission Study Group. Arch Pediatr Adolesc Med 150:598, 1996.
103. Moodley D, Coovadia HM, Bobat RA, et al. HIV-1 specific immunoglobulin A antibodies as an effective marker of perinatal infection in developing countries. J Trop Pediatr 43:80, 1997.
104. Parekh BS, Shaffer N, Coughlin R, et al. Human immunodeficiency virus 1-specific IgA capture enzyme immunoassay for early diagnosis of human immunodeficiency virus 1 infection in infants: NYC Perinatal HIV Transmission Study Group. Pediatr Infect Dis J 12:908, 1993.
105. Kline MW, Lewis DE, Hollinger FB, et al. A comparative study of human immunodeficiency virus immunoglobulin antibody detection in the diagnosis during early infancy of vertically acquired human immunodeficiency virus infection. Pediatr Infect Dis J 13:90, 1994.
106. Miguez-Burbano MJ, Hutto C, Shor-Posner G, et al. IgE-based assay for early detection of HIV-1 infection in infants. Lancet 350:782, 1997.
107. Fletcher M, Miguez-Burbano MJ, Shor-Posner G, et al. Diagnosis of human immunodeficiency virus infection using an immunoglobulin E-based assay. Clin Diagn Lab Immunol 7:55, 2000.
108. Mandelbrot L, Brossard Y, Aubin JT, et al. Testing for in utero human immunodeficiency virus infection with fetal blood sampling. Am J Obstet Gynecol 175:489, 1996.
109. Fowler MG, Simonds RJ, Roongpisuthipong A. Perinatal transmission of HIV-1. Pediatr Clin North Am 47:21, 2000.

110. Nduati R, John G, Mbori-Ngacha D, et al. Effect of breastfeeding and formula feeding on transmission of HIV-1: a randomized clinical trial. JAMA 283:1167, 2000.
111. Bryson YJ, Luzuriaga K, Sullivan JL, et al. Proposed definitions for in utero versus intrapartum transmission of HIV-1. N Engl J Med 327:1246, 1992.
112. Burgard M, Mayaux MJ, Blanche S, et al. The use of viral culture and p24 antigen testing to diagnose human immunodeficiency virus infection in neonates. N Engl J Med 327:192, 1992.
113. Kalish LA, Pitt J, Lew J, et al. Defining the time of fetal or perinatal acquisition of human immunodeficiency virus type 1 infection on the basis of age at first positive culture. J Infect Dis 175:712, 1997.
114. Borkowsky W, Krasinski K, Poolack H, et al. Early diagnosis of human immunodeficiency virus infection in children < 6 months of age: comparison of polymerase chain reaction, culture, and plasma antigen capture techniques. J Infect Dis 166:616, 1992.
115. Young NL, Shaffer N, Chaowanachan T, et al. Early diagnosis of HIV-1 infected infants in Thailand using RNA and DNA PCR assays sensitive to non-B subtypes. J Acquir Immune Defic Syndr 24:401, 2000.
116. Owens DK, Holodniy M, McDonald TW, et al. A meta-analytic evaluation of the polymerase chain reaction for the diagnosis of HIV infection in infants. JAMA 275:1342, 1996.
117. Bremer JW, Lew JF, Cooper E, et al. Diagnosis of infection with human immunodeficiency virus type 1 by a DNA polymerase chain reaction assay among infants enrolled in the Women and Infants Transmission Study. J Pediatr 129:198, 1996.
118. Nelson RP, Price LJ, Halsey AB, et al. Diagnosis of pediatric human immunodeficiency virus infection by means of a commercially available polymerase chain reaction gene amplification. Arch Pediatr Adoles' Med 150:40, 1996.
119. Dunn DT, Brandt CD, Krivine A, et al. The sensitivity of HIV-1 DNA polymerase chain reaction in the neonatal period and the relative contributions of intra-uterine and intrapartum transmission. AIDS 9:7, 1995.
120. Miles S, Balden E, Magpantay L, et al. Rapid serologic testing with immune complex dissociated HIV p24 antigen for early detection of HIV infection in neonates. N Engl J Med 328:297, 1993.
121. Schupbach J, Boni J, Tomasik Z, et al. Sensitive detection and early prognostic significance of p24 antigen in heat-denatured plasma of human immunodeficiency virus type-1 infected infants: Swiss Neonatal HIV Study Group. J Infect Dis 170:318, 1994.
122. Bulterys M, Farzadegan H, Chao A, et al. Diagnostic utility of immune-complex-dissociated p24 antigen detection in perinatally acquired HIV-1 infection in Rwanda. J Acquir Immune Defic Syndr Hum Retrovirol 10:186, 1995.
123. Lewis DE, Adu-Opong A, Hollinger FB, et al. Sensitivity of immune complex-dissociated p24 antigen testing for early detection of human immunodeficiency virus in infants. Clin Diagn Lab Immunol 2:87, 1995.
124. Lyamuya E, Bredberg-Raden U, Massawe A, et al. Performance of a modified HIV-1 p24 antigen assay for early diagnosis of HIV-1 infection in infants and prediction of mother-to-infant transmission of HIV-1 in Dar es Salaam, Tanzania. J Acquir Immune Defic Syndr Hum Retrovirol 12:421, 1996.
125. Paul MO, Toedter G, Hofheinz D, et al. Diagnosis of human immunodeficiency virus type 1 infection in infants by immune complex dissociation p24 antigen assay. Clin Diagn Lab Immunol 4:75, 1997.
126. Shearer WT, Quinn TC, LaRussa P, et al. Viral load and disease progression in infants infected with human immunodeficiency virus type 1. N Engl J Med 336:1337, 1997.
127. Palumbo PE, Kwok S, Waters S, et al. Viral measurement by polymerase chain reaction-based assays in human immunodeficiency virus-infected infants. J Pediatr 1267:592, 1995.
128. Steketee RW, Abrams EJ, Thea DM, et al. Early detection of perinatal human immunodeficiency virus (HIV) type 1 infection using HIV RNA amplification and detection: New York City Perinatal HIV Transmission Collaborative Study. J Infect Dis 175:707, 1997.
129. Cunningham CK, Charbonneau TT, Song K, et al. Comparison of human immunodeficiency virus 1 DNA polymerase chain reaction and qualitative and quantitative RNA polymerase chain reaction in human immunodeficiency virus 1-exposed infants. Pediatr Infect Dis J 18:30, 1999.
130. Dunn DT, Simonds RJ, Bulterys M, et al. Interventions to prevent vertical transmission of HIV-1: effect on viral detection rate in early infant samples. AIDS 14:1421, 2000.
131. Centers for Disease Control and Prevention revised guidelines for HIV counseling, testing, and referral and revised recommendations for HIV screening of pregnant women. MMWR Morb Mortal Wkly Rep 50(NORR 19): 1–53, 1–85, 2001.
132. Centers for Disease Control. Revised Guidelines for HIV counseling, testing, and referral. http://www.cdc.gov/pub, 2000, p 157.
133. Centers for Disease Control and Prevention, Recommendations for HIV testing services for inpatients and outpatients in acute-care hospital settings, and technical guidance on HIV counseling. MMWR Morb Mortal Wkly Rep 42(RR-12), 1993.
134. Centers for Disease Control and Prevention. U.S. Public Health Service guidelines for testing and counseling blood and plasma donors for human immunodeficiency virus type 1 P24 antigen. MMWR Morb Mortal Wkly Rep 45(RR-2), 5:1, 1996.
135. Centers for Disease Control and Prevention. Revised U.S. Public Health Service recommendations for human immunodeficiency virus screening of pregnant women. http://www.cdc.gov/pub, 2000.
136. Belec L, Matta M, Payan C, et al. Detection of seminal antibodies to human immunodeficiency virus in vaginal secretions after sexual intercourse: possible means of preventing the risk of human immunodeficiency virus transmission in a rape victim. J Med Virol 45:113, 1995.
137. Andersson S, da Silva Z, Norrgren H, et al. Field evaluation of alternative testing strategies for diagnosis and differentiation of HIV-1 and HIV-2 infections in an HIV-1 and HIV-2-prevalent area. AIDS 11:1815, 1997.
138. Vallari AS, Hickman RK, Hackett JR, et al. Rapid assay for simultaneous detection and differentiation of immunoglobulin G antibodies to human immunodeficiency virus type 1 (HIV-1) group M, HIV-1 group O, and HIV-2. J Clin Microbiol 36: 3657, 1998.
139. Wilkinson D, Wilkinson N, Lombard C, et al. On-site testing in resource-poor settings: is one rapid test enough? AIDS 11:377, 1997.
140. Kelen GD, Shahan JB, Quinn TC. Emergency department-based HIV screening and counseling: experience with rapid and standard serologic testing. Ann Emerg Med 33:147, 1999.
141. Kassler WJ, Dillon BA, Haley C, et al. On-site, rapid HIV testing with same-day results and counseling. AIDS 11:1045, 1997.
142. Bauserman RL, Ward MA, Eldred L, Swetz A. Increasing voluntary HIV testing by offering oral tests in incarcerated populations. Am J Public Health 1:1226, 2001.
143. Kallenborn JC, Price TG, Carrico R, Davidson AB. Emergency department management of occupational exposures: cost analysis of rapid HIV test. Infect Control Hosp Epidemiol 22:289, 2001.
144. Rompalo AM, Cannon RO, Quinn TC, Hook EW III. Association of biologic false-positive reactions for syphilis with human immunodeficiency virus infection. J Infect Dis 165:1124, 1992.
145. Oteo Revuelta JA, Elias Calvo C, Martinez de Artola V, Perez Surribas D. Infection by Borrelia burgdorferi in patients with the human immunodeficiency virus: diagnostic problem. Med Clin (Barc) 101:207, 1993.
146. Walensky RP, Rosenberg ES, Ferraro MJ, et al. Investigation of primary human immunodeficiency virus infection in patients who test positive for heterophile antibody. Clin Infect Dis 33:570, 2001.
147. Vidrih JA, Walensky RP, Sax PE, Freedberg KA. Positive Epstein-Barr virus heterophile antibody tests in patients with primary human immunodeficiency virus infection. Am J Med 111:192, 2001.
148. Rosenberg ES, Caliendo AM, Walker BD. Acute HIV infection among patients tested for mononucleosis. N Engl J Med 340:969, 1999.
149. Daikh BE, Holyst MM. Lupus-specific autoantibodies in concomitant human immunodeficiency virus and systemic lupus erythematosus: case report and literature review. Semin Arthritis Rheum 30:418, 2001.
150. Berman A, Cahn P, Perez H, et al. Human immunodeficiency virus infection associated arthritis: clinical characteristics. J Rheumatol 26:1158, 1999.
151. Gul A, Inanc M, Yilmaz G, et al. Antibodies reactive with HIV-1 antigens in systemic lupus erythematosus. Lupus 5:120, 1996.
152. Watt G, Chanbancherd P, Brown AE. Human immunodeficiency virus type 1 test results in patients with malaria and dengue infections. Clin Infect Dis 30:819, 2000.
153. Ling AE, Robbins KE, Brown TM, et al. Failure of routine HIV-1 tests in a case involving transmission with preseroconversion blood components during the infectious window period. JAMA 284:210, 2000.

154. Mylonakis E, Paliou M, Lally M, et al. Laboratory testing for infection with human immunodeficiency virus (HIV): established and novel approaches. Am J Med 109:568, 2000.
155. Food and Drug Administration. Current good manufacturing practices for blood and blood components: notification of consignees receiving blood and blood components at increased risk for transmitting HIV infection. Fed Reg 61: 47413, 1996.
156. Food and Drug Administration. Memorandum: Recommendation for Donor Screening with a Licensed test for HIV-1 Antigen. Rockville, MD, Congressional and Consumer Affairs, 1995.
157. Kleinman S, Busch MP, Korelitz JJ, Schreiber GB. The incidence/window period model and its use to assess the risk of transfusion-transmitted human immunodeficiency virus and hepatitis C virus infection. Transfus Med Rev 11:155, 1997.
158. Stramer S, Aberle-Grasse J, Brodsky J, et al. United States blood donor screening with p24 antigen; one-year experience. Transfusion 37:1S, 1997.
159. FDA Revised recommendations for the Prevention of Human Immunodeficiency Virus (HIV) Transmission by Blood and Blood Products. Rockville, MD, Center for Biologics Evaluation and Research, April 23, 1992.
160. Eble BE, Busch MP, Khayam-Bashi H, et al. Resolution of infection status of HIV-seroindeterminate and high-risk seronegative individuals using PCR and virus-culture: absence of persistent silent HIV-1 infection in a high-prevalence area. Transfusion 32:503, 1992.
161. Busch MP. Let's look at human immunodeficiency virus look back before leaping into hepatitis C virus lookback! Transfusion 31:655, 1991.
162. Busch MP, Lee LLL, Satten GA, et al. Time course of detection of viral and serological markers preceding HTV-1 seroconversion: implications for blood and tissue donor screening. Transfusion 38:189, 1998.
163. Busch MP. Retroviruses and blood transfusions: the lessons learned and the challenge yet ahead. In: Nance S (ed) Blood Safety: Current Challenges (Transcription of the Emily Cooley Award/AABB 1992 Annual Seminar). Bethesda, American Association of Blood Banks, 1992, p 1.
164. Lackritz EM, Satten GA, Aberle-Grasse J, et al. Estimated risk of transmission of the human immunodeficiency virus by screened blood in the United States. N Eng J Med 333: 1721, 1995.
165. Schreiber GB, Busch MP, Kleinman SH, Korelitz JJ. The risk of transfusion-transmitted viral infections. the Retrovirus Epidemiology Donor Study. N Engl J Med 334:1685, 1996.
166. Sullivan MT, Guido EA, Metler RP, et al. Identification and characterization of an HIV-2 antibody-positive blood donor in the United States. Transfusion 38:189, 1998.
167. Loussert-Ajaka I, Ly TD, Chaix ML, et al. HIV-1/HIV-2 seronegativity in HIV-1 subtype O infected patients. Lancet 343:1393, 1994.
168. Busch MP, Young MJ, Samson SM, et al. The Transfusion Safety Study Group: risk of human immunodeficiency virus transmission by blood transfusions prior to the implementation of HIV antibody screening in the San Francisco Bay area. Transfusion 31:4, 1991.
169. Busch MP, Stramer SL, Kleinman SH. Evolving applications of nucleic acid amplification assays for prevention of virus transmission by blood components and derivatives. In: Garratty G (ed) Applications of Molecular Biology to Blood Transfusion Medicine. Bethesda, American Association of Blood Banks, 1997.
170. Roth WK, Weber M, Seifried E, et al. Feasibility and efficacy of routine PCR screening of blood donations for hepatitis C virus, hepatitis B virus and HIV-1 in a blood bank setting. Lancet 353:359, 1999.
171. Stramer SL. Nucleic acid testing for transfusion-transmissible agents. Curr Opin Hematol 7:387, 2000.
172. Busch MP, Satten GA. Time course of viremia and antibody seroconversion following human immunodeficiency virus exposure. Am J Med 102:177, 1997.
173. Busch MP, Kleinman S, Jackson B. Nucleic acid amplification testing of blood donors for transfusion-transmitted infectious diseases: report of the Interorganizational Task Force on Nucleic Acid Amplification Testing of Blood Donors. Transfusion 40:143, 2000.
174. Stramer SL, Caglioti S, Strong DM. NAT of the United States and Canadian blood supply. Transfusion 40:1165, 2000.
175. Selik RM, Ward JW, Buehler JW. Trends in transfusion-associated acquired immune deficiency syndrome in the United States, 1982 through 1991. Transfusion 33:890, 1993.
176. Busch MP, Dodd RY. NAT and blood safety: what is the paradigm? Transfusion 40:1157, 2000.
177. Draft Guidance for Industry: Use of Nucleic Acid Tests on Pooled Samples from Source Plasma Donors to Adequately and Appropriately Reduce the Risk of Transmission of HIV-1 and HCV. Bethesda, US DHHS, CBER, December 2001.
178. 21CFR 1270.21(d).
179. Guidance for Industry Availability of Licensed Donor Screening tests labeled for use with Cadaveric Blood Specimens. Bethesda, U.S. DHHS, FDA, CBER June 2000.
180. Chung CW, Rapuano CJ, Laibson PR, et al. Human immunodeficiency virus p24 antigen testing in cornea donors. Cornea 20:277, 2001.
181. Gala JL, Vandenbroucke AT, Vandercam B, et al. HIV-1 detection by nested PCR and viral culture in fresh or cryopreserved postmortem skin: potential implications for skin handling and allografting. J Clin Pathol 50:481, 1997.
182. Guidance for industry: public health issues posed but the use of nonhuman primate xenografts in humans. 64 FR 16743–16744, April 1999.
183. PHS Guidelines on Infectious Disease Issues in Xenotransplantation. Bethesda, DHHS, FDA, CBER, January 2001.
184. Draft Guidance for Industry: Source Animal, Product, Preclinical, and Clinical Issues Concerning the Use of Xenotransplantation Products in Humans. Bethesda, DHHS, FDA, CBER, January 2001.
185. Lackritz EM. Prevention of HIV transmission by blood transfusion in the developing world: achievements and continuing challenges. AIDS 12(suppl A):s81, 1998.
186. Wake DJ, Cutting WA. Blood transfusion in developing countries: problems, priorities and practicalities. Trop Doct 28:4, 1998.

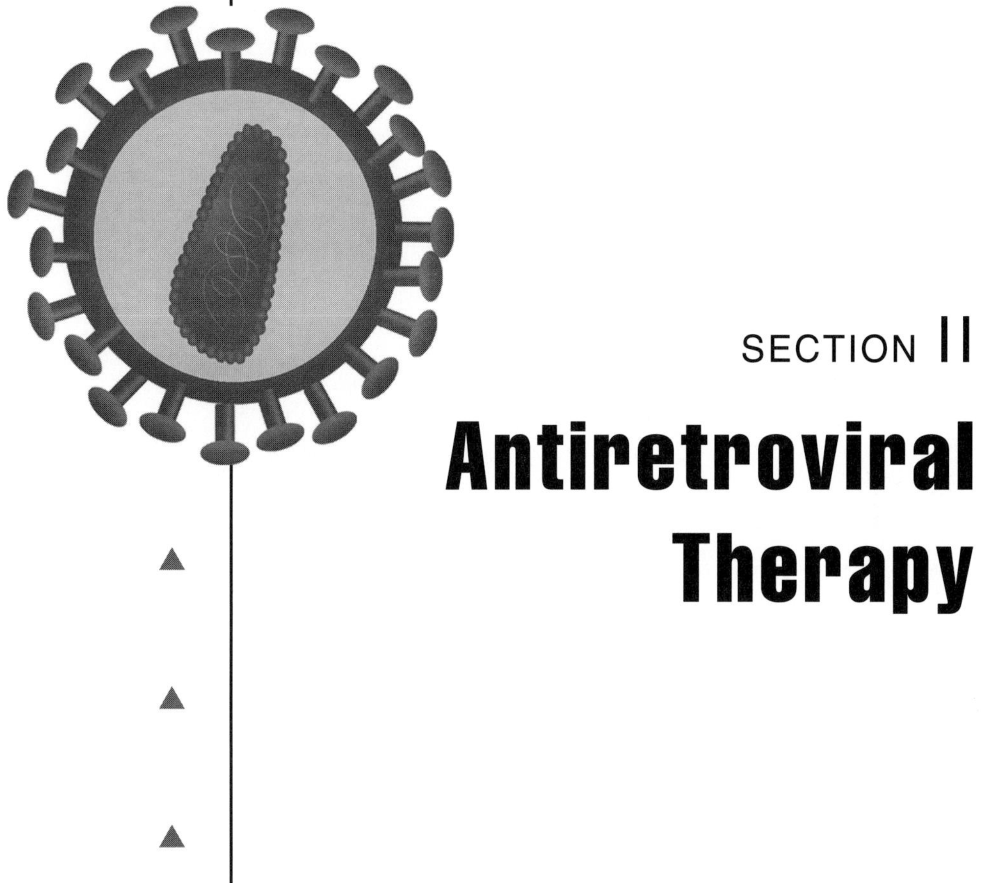

SECTION II

Antiretroviral Therapy

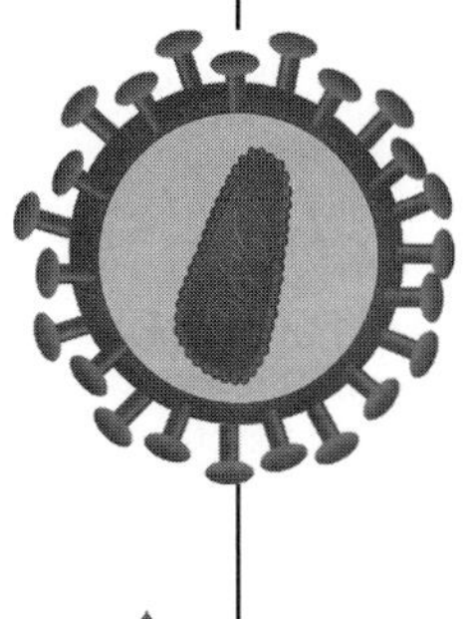

CHAPTER 2

Zidovudine

Margaret A. Fischl, MD

Zidovudine, a nucleoside reverse transcriptase inhibitor, was the first antiretroviral agent approved for the treatment of patients with human immunodeficiency virus (HIV) infection. Zidovudine was initially approved as monotherapy. Subsequently, zidovudine was approved in combination regimens with zalcitabine or lamivudine. Early studies demonstrated clinical and survival benefits in patients with acquired immunodeficiency syndrome (AIDS) and those with symptomatic or asymptomatic HIV disease who had a CD4+ T-lymphocyte count of 500 cells per cubic millimeter or less. Durable clinical benefits were limited in part because of the incomplete suppression of HIV replication and the emergence of resistant viral strains. Zidovudine is currently approved for the treatment of HIV infection in combination regimens with potent antiretroviral agents, including HIV-1 protease inhibitors (PIs), nonnucleoside reverse transcriptase inhibitors (NNRTIs), and potent nucleoside reverse transcriptase inhibitors (NRTIs) such as abacavir. Later studies demonstrated clinical and survival benefits when used in potent combination regimens with HIV-1 PIs. Such combination regimens can also achieve long-term viral suppression with partial reconstitution of the immunologic perturbations seen with HIV. Zidovudine remains an important component of multiple-drug regimens using other NRTIs, NNRTIs, and HIV-1 PIs (Table 2–1).

▲ MECHANISM OF ACTION

Zidovudine is a synthetic thymidine analogue that is phosphorylated to a monophosphate by thymidine kinase and converted to a diphosphate and then the active metabolite zidovudine 5′-triphosphate.[1,2] Zidovudine 5′-triphosphate inhibits the replication of HIV by interfering with viral transcriptase and elongation of the viral DNA chain (Fig. 2–1). Zidovudine 5′-triphosphate is also a weak inhibitor of cellular DNA polymerase-α and mitochondrial polymerase-γ and has been reported to be incorporated into the DNA of cells in culture. The 50% and 90% inhibitory concentrations (IC_{50} and IC_{90}) of HIV isolates from untreated patients range from 0.003 to 0.013 μg/ml and 0.03 to 0.30 μg/ml, respectively. Zidovudine is active in acutely infected cell lines and is less active in chronically infected lines.[3] In cell culture drug-combination studies, zidovudine demonstrated synergistic to additive inhibitor activity with other NRTIs (zalcitabine, didanosine, lamivudine, abacavir), NNRTIs (nevirapine, delavirdine, efavirenz), HIV-1 PIs (saquinavir, ritonavir, indinavir, nelfinavir, amprenavir, lopinavir), and interferon-α.[4–10] The combination of zidovudine and stavudine, however, shows antagonistic activity in vitro against several isolates of HIV.[7] In addition, ribavirin antagonizes the antiviral activity of zidovudine in vitro by inhibiting zidovudine phosphorylation.[11] The monophosphate form of zidovudine accumulates in cells as a result of slow conversion to the diphosphate, and high levels of the monophosphate have been shown to impair HIV-1 reverse transcriptase RNase H activity.[12]

▲ CLINICAL PHARMACOLOGY

Zidovudine is rapidly absorbed from the gastrointestinal tract after oral dosing and achieves peak serum concentrations within 0.5 to 1.5 hours.[13,14] Food decreases peak

▲ **Table 2–1.** INDICATIONS FOR USE OF ZIDOVUDINE

NRTI component of multiple-drug regimens for initial therapy in HIV infection
NRTI + NRTI + PI
NRTI + NRTI + NNRTI
NRTI + PI + PI
NRTI + NRTI + NRTI
Safe and effective NRTI combinations for initial multiple-drug therapy in HIV infection
ZDV/3TC
ZDV/ddI
ZDV/ddC
ZDV/abacavir
Dosage: 300 mg bid by mouth, with or without food

ddC, zalcitabine; ddI, didanosine; NNRTI, nonnucleoside reverse transcriptase inhibitor; NRTI, nucleoside reverse transcriptase inhibitor; PI, protease inhibitor; 3TC, lamivudine; ZDV, zidovudine.

plasma concentrations by more than 50%. However, total exposure as reflected by the area under the concentration curve (AUC) is unchanged. The mean half-life for zidovudine is approximately 1 hour (range 0.78 to 1.93 hours) following oral dosing. Zidovudine 5′-triphosphate, however, has an intracellular half-life of approximately 3 to 4 hours, and in treated patients it is stable for 6 hours after dosing. Zidovudine 5′-triphosphate levels do not appear to correlate well with plasma levels.[15]

Zidovudine is rapidly metabolized to 5′-glucuronylzidovudine (GZDV), which has an elimination half-life of about 1 hour (range 0.61 to 1.73 hours). Following oral administration, the urinary recovery of zidovudine and its major metabolite (GZDV) are 14% and 74%, respectively, with an average total urinary recovery of 90% (range 63% to 95%). As a result of first-pass metabolism, the bioavailability of zidovudine is about 0.63 ± 0.10 for an oral solution (5 mg/kg) and 0.64 ± 0.10 for an oral capsule. Zidovudine is not substantially metabolized by cytochrome P_{450} enzymes.

Following intravenous administration, zidovudine serum concentrations decay in a biexponential pattern. Total body clearance averages 1900 ml/min/70 kg. Renal clearance is approximately 400 ml/min/70 kg, indicating glomerular filtration and active tubular secretion. Zidovudine plasma protein binding is 34% to 38%.

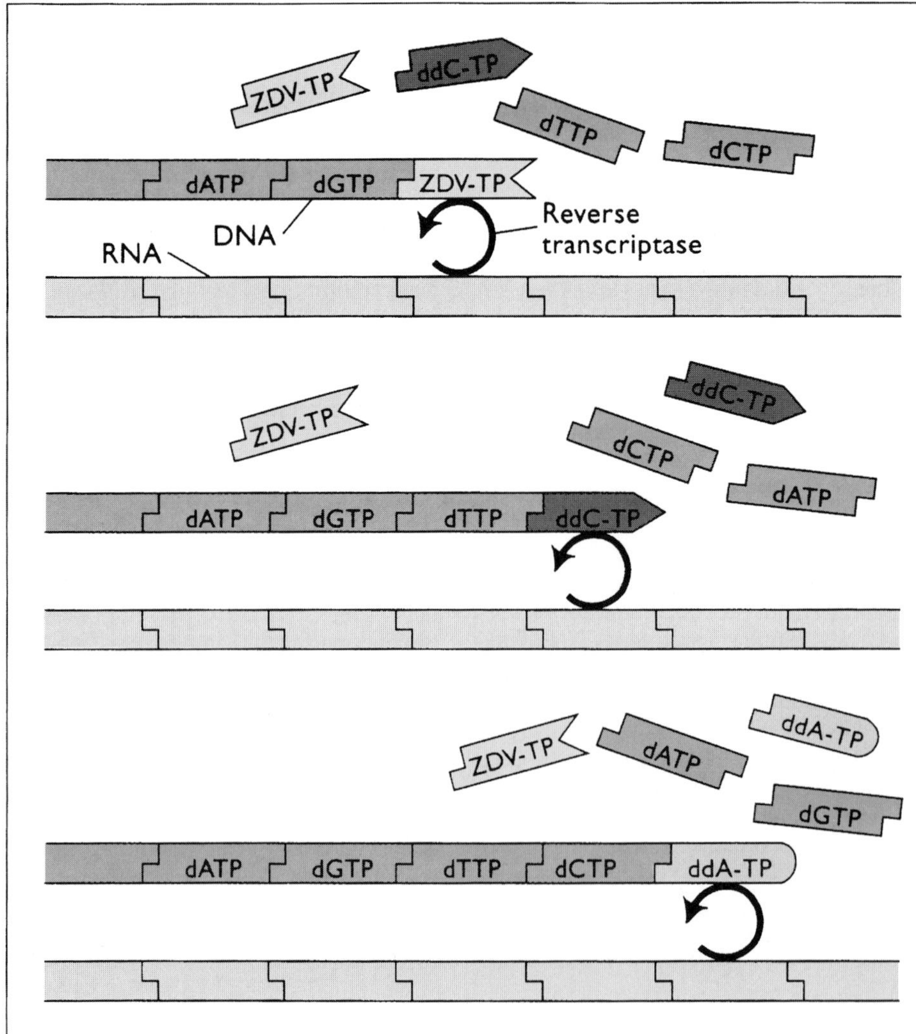

Figure 2–1. Zidovudine, like other dideoxynucleosides, exerts anti-HIV activity against reverse transcriptase. (From Fischl MA. Antiviral treatments. In: Mandell GL, Mildvan D [eds]. Atlas of Infectious Diseases. Philadelphia, Current Medicine, with permission.)

Zidovudine diffuses across the blood-brain barrier with a cerebrospinal fluid (CSF)/plasma ratio in adults of 0.6 (range 0.15 to 1.35).[16] The mean CSF zidovudine concentration in adults ranges from 0.14 to 2.30 mM over a dosage range of 2 to 15 mg/kg. Zidovudine is present in breast milk and crosses the placenta. Fetal glucuronidation of zidovudine appears impaired.[17] Zidovudine is also detected in semen, with a semen/serum ratio ranging from 1.3 to 20.0.[18]

Impaired Renal Function

Among patients with reduced creatinine clearance (18 ± 2 ml/min), the half-life of zidovudine is increased to 1.4 hours, and the AUC is increased approximately twofold. The half-life of the active metabolite (GZDV) is 8.0 hours compared to 9.0 hours in controls, and the AUC is increased approximately 17-fold.[19] Hemodialysis clearance does not contribute to zidovudine removal, although GZDV appears to be removed more efficiently.

Pregnancy

The pharmacokinetics of zidovudine appear unchanged during pregnancy.[20] Zidovudine crosses the placenta, and zidovudine concentrations in newborns are equivalent to maternal levels. Similarly, the mean concentration of zidovudine in breast milk and maternal serum is similar after a single dose.

▲ ADVERSE REACTIONS

Common toxicities seen with zidovudine include headache, fatigue, malaise, myalgia, anorexia, nausea, anemia, and neutropenia (Table 2–2).[21–23] Initial symptoms, particularly headache, insomnia, fatigue, and gastrointestinal problems, are mild and can be managed symptomatically. In a small percentage of patients, particularly those receiving three- and four-drug regimens, persistent symptoms may require modification of the dose of zidovudine or substitution by another nucleoside analogue. Rare cases of rash and fever have been described that necessitated discontinuing zidovudine.

Anemia is more prominent in advanced disease than in early disease (7% vs. 1%, respectively). Serum folate levels are normal or elevated, and vitamin B_{12} levels are normal or slightly decreased. The reticulocyte count is frequently depressed and may be the first sign of bone marrow toxicity. Bone marrow examinations in cases of severe anemia show a decrease or absence of red blood cell precursors. Erythropoietin levels are commonly elevated and in some cases are quite high (> 500 IU/L), suggesting that zidovudine-induced erythroid hypoplasia is not due to interference with erythropoietin production but is more likely due to inhibition of cell commitment to the erythroid line or direct toxic effects on committed erythroid stem cells.[24] Anemia can be seen as early as 4 to 6 weeks after initiation of zidovudine. Progressive declines in the hemoglobin concentration should signal the potential for severe anemia, particularly if the hemoglobin concentration declines to 7.5 to 8.0 g/dl. In cases of severe anemia, zidovudine (whenever possible) should be temporarily interrupted until the hemoglobin concentration increases, which typically takes 7 to 14 days. Recombinant human erythropoietin has been shown to be safe and to decrease blood transfusion requirements in patients without marked elevation in endogenous erythropoietin levels who develop severe anemia while receiving zidovudine.[25] Alternatively, the dose of zidovudine can be decreased or another antiretroviral agent substituted for zidovudine. Macrocytosis with an elevation in the mean corpuscular volume of 25 to 40 units is common and is typically not associated with anemia. Increases in mean corpuscular volume can occur within 6 to 8 weeks of starting zidovudine and are most prominent after 16 to 24 weeks.

Neutropenia also occurs more frequently during advanced HIV disease than in the early stages of the disease (37% vs. 8%, respectively) and is noted within 12 to 24 weeks of initiating zidovudine. Mild to moderate neutropenia, manifested by neutrophil counts of 750 to 1000 cells/mm^3, may be more frequent and do not require any adjustments in the zidovudine dose. Declines in the neutrophil count to less than 750 cells/mm^3 suggest a need to decrease the dose of zidovudine or temporarily interrupt the drug (when possible) until the neutrophil count increases. If persistent or recurrent neutropenia occurs, another antiretroviral agent can be substituted for zidovudine.

Long-term use of zidovudine may be associated with several toxicities, including nail hyperpigmentation,[26] hepatic toxicity, and muscle toxicity. The nail hyperpigmentation consists of multiple longitudinal streaks and diffuse pigment changes ranging from shades of blue to brown-black. Nails on both the hands and feet can be involved, and pigment changes appear to move distally from the base of the nail. Hyperpigmentation changes in the nail appear to occur more frequently among those of the black African population. Associated skin pigment changes have not been described.

Muscle toxicity manifested by myalgia, progressive muscle wasting, weakness, and elevation of the serum creatine kinase concentration has been described, as well as rare cases of cardiomyopathy. The lower extremities and gluteal muscles appear to be preferentially involved. Muscle biopsy histology is consistent with a destructive mitochondrial myopathy with ragged-red fibers and

▲ **Table 2–2.** SIDE EFFECTS ASSOCIATED WITH ZIDOVUDINE

Headache	Vomiting	Myopathy[a]
Fatigue	Anorexia	Fever[b]
Myalgia	Anemia	Rash[b]
Insomnia	Neutropenia	Hepatitis[b]
Nausea	Nail pigmentation[a]	Steatosis/lactic acidosis[b]

[a]Associated with long-term use.
[b]Rare events.

proliferation of abnormal mitochondria.[27] Reduction of mitochondrial DNA has been noted and is likely due to inhibition of mitochondrial DNA replication by DNA polymerase-γ.[28] Asymptomatic elevations in creatine kinase may also be seen.

Increased liver enzyme levels have been noted and in a subset of patients may be associated with severe steatosis, lactic acidosis, and death. This syndrome is typically characterized by progressive increases in liver aminotransferase levels and moderate to severe hepatomegaly. Scans and biopsy of the liver are consistent with steatosis. Associated symptoms of tachypnea, dsypnea, and severe acidosis with progressive liver and renal failure and death have been described and are mostly due to destruction of hepatic mitochondria. This syndrome has now been described with most NRTIs. Most of these cases have been in women. Obesity and prolonged administration may be risk factors. If this syndrome is suspected, antiretroviral therapy should be interrupted.

▲ CLINICAL EFFICACY

Zidovudine Monotherapy Trials

The zidovudine monotherapy trials are detailed in Table 2–3.

Zidovudine Placebo-Controlled Trials

Zidovudine was the first antiretroviral agent to indicate that treatment intervention can improve the outcome in HIV disease. For advanced HIV disease, the probability of surviving more than 24 weeks was significantly better for zidovudine recipients than for placebo recipients (0.98 vs. 0.78; $P < 0.001$).[29] Similarly, the risk of disease progression over 24 weeks was significantly lower for zidovudine recipients than for placebo recipients (0.23 vs. 0.43; $P < 0.001$). Subsequent placebo-controlled studies showed that the risk of disease progression was decreased more than threefold by 18 months for patients with symptomatic disease (3.23; $P = 0.0002$) and by 12 months for patients with asymptomatic disease (3.1; $P = 0.005$).[22,30] No differences in survival were demonstrable in either study. Early versus delayed use of zidovudine therapy has also been evaluated in patients with asymptomatic HIV infection.[31] The estimated 3-year survival probabilities were 92% for immediate therapy and 94% for delayed therapy. Similar findings were noted for progression to AIDS or death. These data confirmed the early benefit of zidovudine but pointed out the limited duration of the benefit.

Zidovudine Perinatal Transmission Trials

Zidovudine is approved for the prevention of perinatal transmission in pregnant women with HIV infection and newborns of women with HIV infection. In one study the estimated risk of HIV infection in the newborn was 8.3% for zidovudine recipients compared to 25.5% for placebo recipients, a 67.5% reduction in the relative risk of HIV transmission.[35] Chemoprophylaxis consisted of three components, including oral zidovudine administration to pregnant women during the second and third trimesters, intravenous administration to pregnant women during labor and delivery, and oral administration to infants during the first 6 weeks of life. Short antepartum and intrapartum regimens of zidovudine also reduced perinatal transmission by 50%.[36] (For a detailed discussion of the use of zidovudine and other antiretrovirals during pregnancy, see Chapter 28.)

Zidovudine Primary Infection Trials

Zidovudine has been evaluated for the treatment of primary HIV infection. In one study, disease progression among zidovudine recipients (one case) was significantly less than in placebo recipients (seven cases; $P = 0.009$).[32] The relative risk of disease progression for zidovudine recipients compared with placebo recipients was 0.008 ($P = 0.03$).

Zidovudine Comparative Trials

Comparing zidovudine and zalcitabine among patients with minimal prior therapy, zidovudine proved more effective. In patients with advanced HIV disease who had little or no prior zidovudine therapy, zidovudine provided a 1.5-fold decrease in disease progression compared with zalcitabine. Estimated 1-year survival rates were 85% for zalcitabine recipients and 92% for zidovudine recipients ($P = 0.007$).[37] Comparing zidovudine and didanosine among patients with extensive prior zidovudine therapy, didanosine provided a threefold decrease in disease progression compared with continuing zidovudine [relative risk (RR) 1.39; confidence interval (CI) 1.06–1.82; $P = 0.0015$).[34] However, for patients with advanced HIV disease and no or minimal prior zidovudine therapy, zidovudine provided a more than twofold decrease in disease progression compared with didanosine (RR 1.43, CI 1.02–2.00).[33]

Zidovudine-Nucleoside Combination Trials

The zidovudine-nucleoside combination trials are outlined in (Table 2–4). Several large studies have shown that nucleoside combination regimens with zidovudine provide improved and more durable clinical and survival benefits than monotherapy with zidovudine (Figs. 2–2, 2–3).[38,39] Zidovudine has been combined with several nucleoside analogues (zalcitabine, didanosine, lamivudine, abacavir) and was shown to be safe and effective. For treatment-naive patients, zidovudine in combination with zalcitabine provided a better clinical outcome than zidovudine combined with didanosine [hazard ratio (HR) 0.49 vs. 0.61] and a slightly better survival advantage (HR 0.59 vs. 0.61).[38] In treatment-experienced patients, zidovudine in combination with didanosine provided a better clinical outcome (HR 0.65 vs. 0.91) and a better survival advantage (HR 0.52 vs. 0.81). In another study, zidovudine in combination with didanosine decreased the mortality risk by 42% compared with 32% for zidovudine in combination with zalcitabine among treatment-naive patients (Delta 1 study) and by 23% compared with 9%, respectively, among treatment-experienced patients (Delta 2 study).[39] Among patients with extensive zidovudine therapy, one study showed no overall differences among patients receiving zidovudine, zalcitabine, or zidovudine in combination with zalcitabine; however, patients with CD4+ T-lymphocyte counts of 150 cells per cubic millimeter who received zidovudine and zalcitabine had better clinical outcomes.[40]

Zidovudine/lamivudine is a potent nucleoside combination (see Chapter 6). A 66% reduction in disease progression was noted with zidovudine/lamivudine compared with other treatments in a meta-analysis.[45] In several other studies, superior CD4+ T-lymphocyte and HIV RNA responses were noted among recipients of zidovudine in combination with lamivudine.[41,42] The addition of lamivudine to zidovudine-based regimens also showed a significant improvement in disease-free survival and overall survival in a large randomized trial.[45] Among 1840 patients, disease progression occurred in 20% of placebo recipients and 9% of lamivudine recipients ($P < 0.001$).

The combination of zidovudine/stavudine in treatment-experienced or treatment-naive patients proved to be antagonistic, with a detrimental effect on immunologic and virologic responses; these agents should not be used together. Among patients with prior zidovudine therapy experience, zidovudine/stavudine resulted in a decreased CD4+ T-lymphocyte count of 45 cells per cubic millimeter compared to an increase of 20 cells per cubic millimeter for stavudine alone, an increase of 70 cells per cubic millimeter for didanosine alone, and an increase of 5 cells per cubic millimeter for zidovudine/didanosine at 48 weeks. Plasma HIV RNA evaluations demonstrated a 0% decrease to less than 500 copies per millimeter for zidovudine/stavudine compared with 6% for stavudine alone, 45% for didanosine alone, and 36% for zidovudine/didanosine.[46] Among patients with no prior treatment experience, zidovudine/stavudine resulted in an increase of 14 cells per cubic millimeter in the CD4+ T-lymphocyte count compared to an increase of 65 cells per cubic millimeter for stavudine alone and an increase of 101 cells per cubic millimeter for zidovudine/lamivudine at 48 weeks. Plasma HIV RNA evaluations demonstrated an 8% decrease to less than 500 copies per milliliter for zidovudine/stavudine compared with 31% for stavudine alone and 38% for zidovudine/lamivudine.[46]

Fixed-Dose Combination of Lamivudine and Zidovudine (Combivir)

A fixed-dose combination (FDC) tablet of lamivudine 150 mg/zidovudine 300 mg is available. The bioequivalence of FDC lamivudine/zidovudine was evaluated in a Phase I open-label, randomized, three-way crossover study.[47] The FDC tablet was found to be bioequivalent to lamivudine/zidovudine tablets. The AUCs for lamivudine and zidovudine, respectively, were 6005 and 2299 ng/hr/ml when given as FDC tablets and 5932 and 2061 ng/hr/ml when given separately as lamivudine and zidovudine. Food did not affect the extent of absorption of lamivudine or zidovudine when given as FDC tablets but did slow absorption; the maximum plasma concentration geometric mean ratios for lamivudine and zidovudine were 0.85 and 0.90, respectively. No differences in side effects were noted for lamivudine or zidovudine whether given as FDC tablets or as separate tablets. The recommended dose is one FDC tablet twice per day, with or without food.

Fixed-Dose Combination of Lamivudine/Zidovudine/Abacavir (Trizivir)

An FDC tablet of abacavir 300 mg/lamivudine 150 mg/zidovudine 300 mg is available. In a single-dose, three-way crossover study of the FDC of abacavir/lamivudine/zidovudine versus each drug separately, there were no differences in the extent of absorption as measured by the AUC and the maximal peak concentration (C_{max}). The FDC tablet of abacavir/lamivudine/zidovudine was found to be bioequivalent to abacavir 300 mg, lamivudine 150 mg, and zidovudine 300 mg single tablets following single-dose administration to healthy volunteers in the fasted state. In a Phase III, open-label, randomized, parallel-group study, 195 subjects who had received prior therapy with FDC tablets of lamivudine/zidovudine/abacavir or FDC tablets of abacavir/lamivudine/zidovudine. At week 24, most of the subjects on either regimen (99% in the Trizivir group and 92% in the combivir/abacavir group) had HIV RNA levels of 400 copies per milliliter or less. Both regimens were well tolerated.[48] No differences in side effects have been noted for abacavir, lamivudine, or zidovudine whether given as FDC tablets or separately. The recommended dose is one FDC tablet twice a day, with or without food.

Zidovudine in Potent Combination Trials

Greater virologic and immunologic benefits are noted with increasingly potent combination regimens. In general, three-drug regimens appear more potent than two-drug regimens, and three-drug regimens containing HIV-1 PIs and NNRTIs appear to be the most potent. Regimens appear less effective in patients with advanced HIV disease and prior treatment experience. Patients with advanced HIV disease, particularly those with CD4+ T-lymphocyte counts of 50 cells per cubic millimeter or less and a plasma HIV RNA level of 100,000 copies per milliliter or more have a higher incidence of incomplete suppression of viral replication and are at greater risk for viral resistance and eventual drug failure.

Zidovudine/lamivudine/nelfinavir in antiretroviral-naive patients resulted in a decline in plasma HIV RNA to less than 400 copies per milliliter among 81% of patients after 6 months in one study and a decline to less than 500 copies per milliliter among 83% of patients after 28 weeks in another study.[49,50] Zidovudine in combination with lamivudine and indinavir resulted in a decline in plasma HIV RNA to less than 500 copies per millimeter in 90% of patients with CD4+ T-lymphocyte counts of more than 50 cells per cubic millimeter during prolonged therapy and among 51% of patients with CD4+ T-lymphocyte counts of less than 50 cells per cubic millimeter during prolonged therapy.[51,52] This combination regimen has also been associated with improved clinical and survival benefits.[44] Similar results have been described with combination

▲ **Table 2–3.** TRIALS OF ZIDOVUDINE MONOTHERAPY

Trial	Design	Dosage	No. of Subjects	Entry Criteria	CD4+/Lymphocytes on Entry (cells/mm³)
Fischl et al.[29] (BWO2)	Placebo controlled, randomized, double blind	ZDV 250 mg q4h	282	AIDS or ARC; CD4 <100, 101–499	49 and 54 (medians); 128 and 190 (medians)
Fischl et al.[30] (ACTG 016)	Placebo controlled, randomized, double blind	ZDV 200 mg q4h	711	Mildly sympto-matic; CD4 >200, <800	225 (median)
Volberding et al.[22] (ACTG 019)	Placebo controlled, randomized, double blind	300 mg 5×/day or 100 mg 5×/day	1338	Asymptomatic; CD4 <500	350
Concorde[31]	Placebo controlled, randomized, double blind	250 mg bid initially; or deferred until start of symptoms or low CD4 counts[a] (open label ZDV then)	1749	Asymptomatic	42% > 500 52% > 201, ≤ 500 6% ≤ 200
Kinloch-De Loes et al.[32]	Placebo controlled, randomized, double blind	ZDV 250 mg bid for 6 months	77	Acute retroviral syndrome, p24 antigenemia, and low or negative HIV ab tests	519–477 (mean)
Dolin et al.[33] (ACTG 116a)	ddI vs. ZDV; randomized, double blind	ddI: 500 or 750 mg/d ZDV: 600 mg/d	617	Symptomatic: CD4 <300 or Asymptomatic: CD4 <200; Previous ZDV experience of <16 wk	130 (median)
Kahn et al.[34] (ACTG 116b/117)	ddI vs ZDV; randomized, double blind	ddI: 500 or 750 mg/d ZDV: 600 mg/d	913	As for ACTG 116a above, but >16 wk of previous ZDV experi-ence	95 (median)

ab, antibody; ARC, AIDS-related complex; ddI, didanosine; OI, opportunistic infection; pt, patient; ZDV, zidovudine.
[a]CD4+ lymphocyte count.

regimens that include (1) zidovudine/zalcitabine or zidovudine/lamivudine with saquinavir soft gel capsules and (2) zidovudine/lamivudine/ritonavir.[53–55] Zidovudine/didanosine/nevirapine resulted in plasma HIV RNA declines to less than 20 copies per milliliter at week 52 among 51% of patients.[56] Similar results were noted with zidovudine/lamivudine/delavirdine. In a Phase II double-blind, placebo-controlled, dose-ranging study, zidovudine/lamivu-

<table>
<tr><th>CD4+ Lymphocyte Response</th><th>Antiviral Response</th><th>Clinical Outcome</th><th>Comments</th></tr>
<tr><td>Counts increased in ZDV recipients</td><td>p24 antigenemia decreased in ZDV recipients</td><td>ZDV increased survival and decreased OIs over 24 wk</td><td>Benefits demonstrated for CD4 count[a] <100; study was halted before effect on higher CD4 counts could be fully evaluated.</td></tr>
<tr><td>Counts increased by 44 in pts with entry counts of >200, but <500; no significant changes in counts for those with >500 on entry</td><td>Rate of p24 antigenemia decreased by 50% in 65% of ZDV recipients and in 15% of placebo recipients</td><td>ZDV decreased progression of disease in pts with CD4 >200, but <500; no effect on survival</td><td>Insufficient events occurred to assess effects on pts. With CD4 >500. Less toxicity than in pts with more advanced disease (BWO2).</td></tr>
<tr><td>Median increase of 26–39/mm^3</td><td>Decrease in rate of p24 antigenemia compared to placebo</td><td>ZDV decreased progression of disease; no effects on survival</td><td>ZDV dose of 1500 mg/d was more toxic than 500 mg/d dose.</td></tr>
<tr><td>Increase of 20/mm^3 in immediate ZDV and decrease of 9/mm^3 in deferred ZDV, at 3 mo</td><td>—</td><td>No difference in clinical outcomes between immediate and deferred ZDV at 3 yr; transient delay in disease progression at 1 yr with immediate ZDV therapy</td><td>Indicated that benefit of monotherapy with ZDV was temporally limited.</td></tr>
<tr><td>ZDV recipients gained 8.9 cells/mo; placebo lost 12.0 cells/mo</td><td>No difference in p24 or HIV RNA responses</td><td>Disease progression (primarily minor OI) was less frequent in ZDV group; no effect on acute retroviral syndrome</td><td>Long-term benefits not assessed. ZDV was relatively well tolerated.</td></tr>
<tr><td>ddI 500 mg group had slower decline in counts than ddI 750 mg or ZDV group</td><td>No difference in p24 declines among three treatment groups</td><td>
<table>
<tr><th>Group</th><th>Deaths (No.)</th><th>AIDS Events or Deaths (/100 pt-yr)</th></tr>
<tr><td>ZDV naive</td><td></td><td></td></tr>
<tr><td>500 ddI</td><td>10</td><td>32.3</td></tr>
<tr><td>750 ddI</td><td>10</td><td>36.6</td></tr>
<tr><td>ZDV</td><td>9</td><td>26.6</td></tr>
<tr><td>ZDV ≤8 wk</td><td></td><td></td></tr>
<tr><td>500 ddI</td><td>3</td><td>27.8</td></tr>
<tr><td>750 ddI</td><td>4</td><td>25.1</td></tr>
<tr><td>ZDV</td><td>3</td><td>24.1</td></tr>
<tr><td>ZDV >8, but ≤16 wk</td><td></td><td></td></tr>
<tr><td>500 ddI</td><td>4</td><td>24.8</td></tr>
<tr><td>750 ddI</td><td>3</td><td>31.5</td></tr>
<tr><td>ZDV</td><td>3</td><td>52.5</td></tr>
</table>
</td><td>ZDV more effective than 750 ddI in ZDV-naive patients; 500 ddI more effective than ZDV in patients with >8 but ≤16 wk ddI. No significant differences in efficacy between 500 and 750 ddI, but 750 ddI was more toxic.</td></tr>
<tr><td>CD4 change/mm^3 at 24 wk:
500 ddI: −10
750 ddI: −10
ZDV: −23</td><td>% of subjects with at least 50% p24 decrease at 24 wk:
500 ddI: 21
750 ddI: 32
ZDV: 21</td><td>
<table>
<tr><th>Group</th><th>Deaths (/100 pt-yr)</th><th>AIDS Events or Deaths (/100 pt-yr)</th></tr>
<tr><td>500 ddI</td><td>15.5</td><td>37.1</td></tr>
<tr><td>750 ddI</td><td>17.5</td><td>42.5</td></tr>
<tr><td>ZDV</td><td>16.9</td><td>52.8</td></tr>
</table>
</td><td>Dose of 500 ddI more effective than ZDV for reduction of risk of primary endpoints.</td></tr>
</table>

dine/efavirenz at 200, 400, and 600 mg/day resulted in declines in plasma HIV RNA levels to less than 50 copies per milliliter among 63% to 74% of patients.[57] Zidovudine/lamivudine/efavirenz resulted in a significantly greater proportion of subjects who achieved HIV RNA levels of less than 400 copies per milliliter compared with zidovudine/lamivudine/indinavir: 70% versus 48%, respectively, after 48 weeks of therapy ($P < 0.001$).[58]

▲ **Table 2–4.** TRIALS OF ZIDOVUDINE–NUCLEOSIDE COMBINATION THERAPY

Trial	Design	Dosage	No. of Subjects	Entry Criteria	CD4+/Lymphocytes on Entry (cells/mm³)
Hammer et al.[38] (ACTG 175)	ddI vs. ZDV vs. ddI + ZDV vs. ddC + ZDV; randomized, double blind	ddI: 400 mg/d ZDV: 600 mg/d Same in combination with ddC: 2.25 mg/d in combination	2467	CD4[a] 200–500; no AIDS-defining illness; antiretroviral naive or experienced	352 (mean)
Delta[39]	ZDV vs. ddI + ZDV vs. ddC + ZDV; randomized, double blind	As above for ACTG 175	3207	AIDS and CD4 >50; no or minimal symptoms and CD4 <350; may be ZDV experienced (Delta 2) or naive (Delta 1)	205 (mean)
Fischl et al.[40] (ACTG 155)	Randomized, double blind	ZDV: 600 mg/d *or* ddC 2.25 mg/d *or* both	1001	Symptomatic and <300 CD4, or asymptomatic and <200; on ZDV for ≥6 mo	112 and 127 (medians)
Eron et al.[41] (NUCA 3001)	Randomized, double blind	3TC: 300 mg q12h *or* ZDV: 200 mg q8h *or* 3TC: 150 mg q12h plus ZDV *or* 3TC: 300 mg q12h plus ZDV	366	CD4 200–500; 4 wk or less of ZDV	332 and 372 (medians)
Bartlett et al.[42] (NUCA 3002)	Randomized, double blind	3TC: 150 mg bid plus ZDV 200 mg tid *or* 3TC: 300 mg bid plus ZDV *or* ddC: 0.75 mg tid plus ZDV	254	CD4 100–300 and previous ZDV for >6 mo	203 and 229 (medians)
CAESAR[43]	Randomized, double blind	In addition to ZDV *or* ZDV + ddI *or* ZDV + ddC, add 3TC: 150 mg bid *or* 3TC + loviride: 100 mg tid *or* placebo	1840	CD4 25–250	126 (median)
Hammer et al.[44]	Randomized, double blind placebo controlled	ZDV: 600 mg/d + 3TC: 150 mg bid *or* ZDV: 600 mg/d + 3TC: 150 mg bid + (d4T could replace ZDV in either group)	1156	CD4 ≥200; ≥ of ZDV previously; naive to 3TC, IDV	87 (mean) (HIV-1 RNA: 5.0 $\log_{10}$ copies/ml)

ddC, zalcitabine; ddI, didanosine; pt, patient; 3TC, lamivudine; IDV, indinavir; d4T, stavudine.
[a]CD4, CD4+ lymphocyte count (cells per cubic millimeter).

In a multicenter, double-blind, placebo-controlled study in treatment-naive subjects, abacavir/lamivudine/zidovudine compared with lamivudine/zidovudine resulted in significantly more subjects with an HIV-1 RNA level of less than 400 copies per milliliter after 16 weeks of therapy.[59] In another study, 60% of patients who received zidovudine/lamivudine/abacavir had declines in plasma HIV RNA levels to less than 500 copies per milliliter and 48% to less than 50 copies per milliliter at 48 weeks.[60,61]

<table>
<tr><th>CD4 Response</th><th>Antiviral Response</th><th>Clinical Outcome</th><th>Comments</th></tr>
<tr><td>Significantly better for ddI or combination therapy than for ZDV ($P \le 0.006$)</td><td>Decrease in HIV RNA copies/ml $\log_{10}$ at 8 wk
ZDV—0.26
ddI—0.65
ddI + ZDV—0.93
ddI + ddC—0.89</td><td>Progression to AIDS-defining event or death or ≥ 50% decline in CD4 counts<table><tr><td>ZDV</td><td>32%</td></tr><tr><td>ddI</td><td>22%</td></tr><tr><td>ddI + ZDV</td><td>18%</td></tr><tr><td>ddC + ZDV</td><td>20%</td></tr></table>P <0.001 global</td><td>Survival benefit compared to ZDV noted for ddI, ddI + ZDV, and a trend for ddI + ddC ($P = 0.1$). Benefits for both antiretroviral naive and experienced, except for naive only for ddC + ZDV.</td></tr>
<tr><td>Better in combination therapy than in ZDV alone</td><td>—</td><td><table><tr><th>For Delta 1 and 2 vs. ZDV</th><th>Decrease in Mortality</th><th>Decrease in Disease Progression</th></tr><tr><td>ZDV</td><td>—</td><td>—</td></tr><tr><td>ddI + ZDV</td><td>33%</td><td>36%</td></tr><tr><td>ddC + ZDV</td><td>21%</td><td>17%</td></tr></table></td><td>Clinical benefit was seen largely in ZDV-naive subgroup (Delta 1).</td></tr>
<tr><td>Combination therapy had greater initial increase and slower decline than ZDV alone, but not ddC alone ($P = 0.06$)</td><td>Greater initial decrease in p24 levels in combination therapy</td><td>Combination therapy reduced disease progression in pts with CD4 >150; no differences among treatment groups if CD4 ≤150</td><td>Supports use of combination therapies earlier in disease.</td></tr>
<tr><td>Combination therapy increased median count by 41 or 66/mm^3, compared to 12 for ZDV, 24 for 3TC</td><td>Plasma RNA decreased in combination group by 1.12–1.15 logs, compared to 0.3 for ZDV and 0.6 for 3TC</td><td>Not designed to assess clinical endpoints</td><td>Adverse events no more frequent in combination therapy than with ZDV alone. 3TC well tolerated.</td></tr>
<tr><td>Median increases in count of 43 and 23/mm^3 with ZDV plus 3TC and decrease of 30/mm^3 with ZDV plus ddC at 52 wk</td><td>Changes in plasma RNA were similar in all 3 groups at 52 wk (decrease of 0.39–0.51 logs)</td><td>Trend toward less progression in combined 3TC groups compared to ddC groups ($P = 0.086$)</td><td>Low-dose 3TC was somewhat better tolerated than other two groups.</td></tr>
<tr><td>At wk 28
3TC: Increase of 23/mm^3
3TC + loviride: increase of 22
Placebo: decrease of 12
increase</td><td>$\log_{10}$ HIV RNA ml at wk 28
3TC: decrease of 0.1
3TC + loviride: decrease of 0.25
Placebo: slight</td><td>Progression in 9% of 3TC, 9% of 3TC + loviride, and 20% of placebo; survival benefit also seen</td><td>No differences in toxicities between groups.</td></tr>
<tr><td>At week 40, increase of 40/mm^3 for ZDV + 3TC, 121/mm^3 for ZDV + 3TC + IDV</td><td>At week 40, decrease by 1.0 $\log_{10}$ copies/ml for ZDV + 3TC; decrease by 2.1 $\log_{10}$ copies/ml for ZDV + 3TX + IDV</td><td><table><tr><th>Group</th><th>Progression to AIDS or Death</th><th>Death</th></tr><tr><td>ZDV + 3TC</td><td>11%</td><td>3.1%</td></tr><tr><td>ZDV + 3TC + IDV</td><td>06%</td><td>1.4%</td></tr><tr><td></td><td>$P = 0.001$</td><td>$P = 0.04$</td></tr></table></td><td>Three-drug regimen superior in clinical endpoints, CD4, and antiretroviral responses; rates of grade 3 or 4 adverse effects were similar for both regimens.</td></tr>
</table>

▲ ZIDOVUDINE RESISTANCE

Specific mutation sites on the HIV-1 *pol* gene, which codes for the reverse transcriptase, confer viral resistance to several nucleoside analogues, including zidovudine. Viral resistance to zidovudine is associated with a stepwise decrease in susceptibility with mutations (amino acid substitutions) at sites 41, 67, 70, 215, and 219; sites 41, 70, and 215 were the most important sites of mutation.[62,63] The rate of change in susceptibility of viral isolates to zidovudine is associated with the stage of HIV

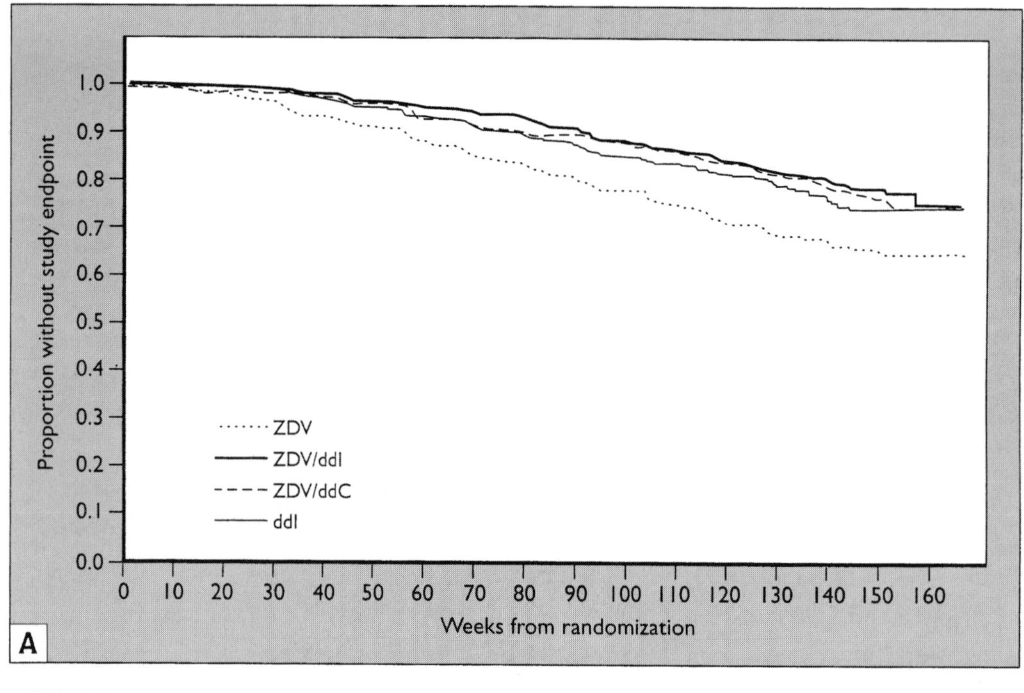

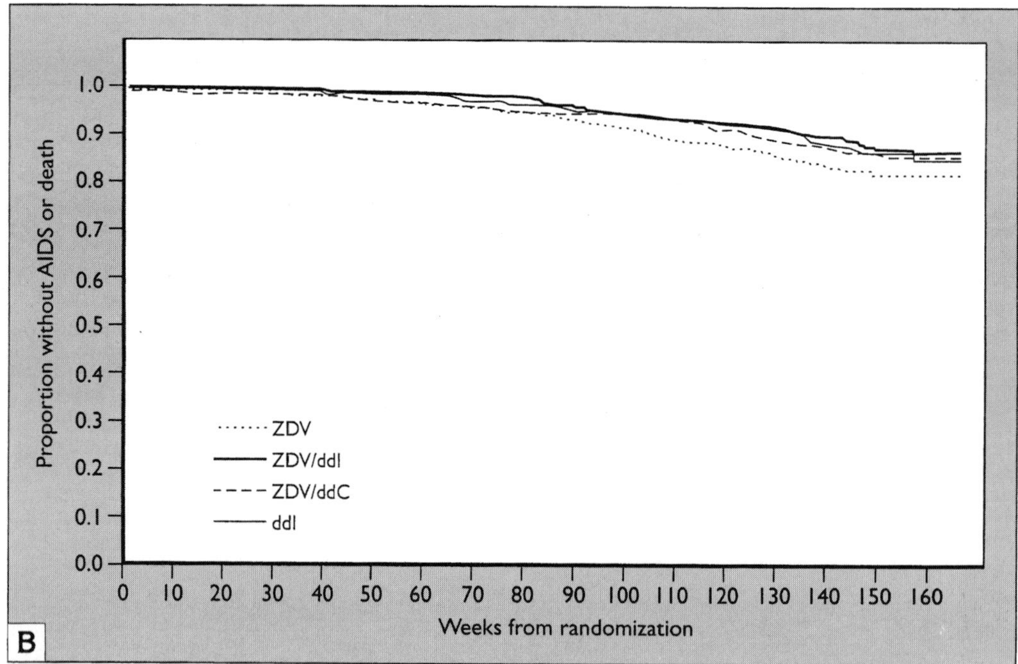

Figure 2–2. Proportion without disease progression, including deterioration in CD4+ T-lymphocyte count (**A**) and cumulative disease-free survival (**B**) among patients receiving combination therapy with zidovudine (ZDV) and either didanosine (ddI) or zalcitabine (ddC) or didanosine or zidovudine alone.[25] (From Fischl MA. Antiviral treatments. In: Mandell GL, Mildvan D [eds]. Atlas of Infectious Diseases. Philadelphia, Current Medicine, with permission.)

disease[64] (Fig. 2–4). After approximately 12 months of zidovudine monotherapy, 31% of viral isolates from patients with early HIV disease are resistant, and nearly all isolates from patients with advanced disease are resistant. Although most viral isolates from treatment-naive patients are susceptible to zidovudine, resistant strains have been transmitted between sexual partners and from mother to child during pregnancy.[65,66] High-level resistance is an independent risk factor for disease progression and compromises therapeutic regimens.[67] For the most part, isolates with decreased susceptibility to zidovudine remain sensitive to other nucleoside analogues, such as didanosine and zalcitabine.[68] Multiple resistance to nucleoside analogues has been described after long-term combination therapy. Mutations at amino acid residues 62, 75, 77, 116, and especially 151 have been

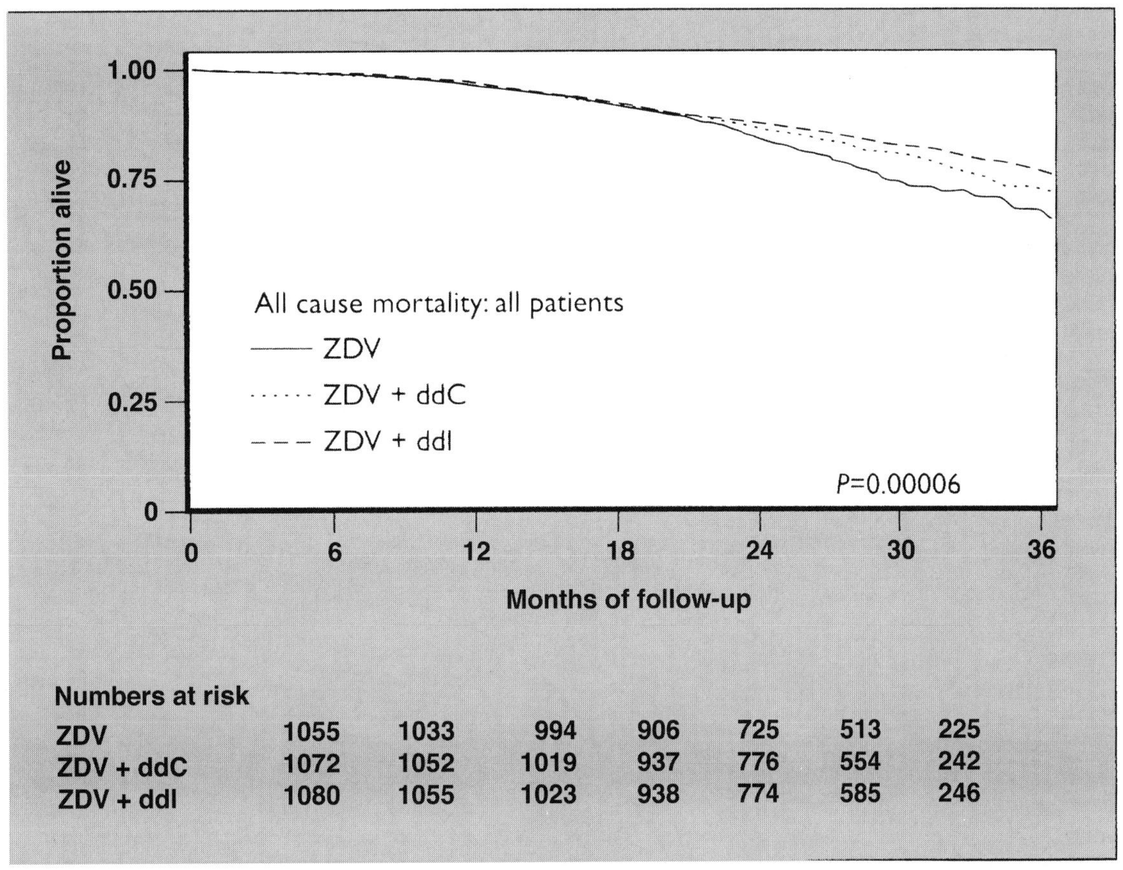

Figure 2–3. Proportion alive among patients receiving combination therapy with zidovudine (ZDV) and either didanosine (ddI) or zalcitabine (ddC) versus zidovudine alone.[38] (From Fischl MA. Antiviral treatments. In: Mandell GL, Mildvan D [eds]. Atlas of Infectious Diseases. Philadelphia, Current Medicine, with permission.)

noted and impart multiple resistance to zidovudine, didanosine, zalcitabine, and stavudine. The presence of the resistance mutation M184V, induced by lamivudine or abacavir therapy, results in increased zidovudine susceptibility for HIV-1 and a resensitization of zidovudine-resistant virus to zidovudine.[69,70]

▲ DRUG INTERACTIONS

Probenecid may increase zidovudine levels by inhibiting glucuronidation and reducing renal excretion.[19] Co-administration of zidovudine and phenytoin may result in decreased levels of phenytoin.[71] However, a pharmacokinetic study of a single 300 mg dose of phenytoin during steady-state zidovudine administration showed no change in phenytoin kinetics. Zidovudine appears to have no substantial effects on methadone kinetics.[72] Evaluation of the co-administration of fluconazole and zidovudine showed a 74% increase in the AUC of zidovudine and a 128% increase in its half-life. Atovaquone co-administration resulted in a 24% decrease in zidovudine oral clearance, leading to a 35% increase in AUC. In contrast, rifampin co-administration resulted in an increase in zidovudine clearance and a decrease in AUC; however, an increase in AUC and peak plasma concentrations were noted for the active metabolite (GZDV) (also see Chapter 66).

Zidovudine co-administration with other approved NRTIs does not appear to alter zidovudine or other NRTI kinetics. Plasma concentration is decreased by 25% when zidovudine is co-administered with nevirapine; co-administration with delavirdine does not appear to alter zidovudine kinetics. Zidovudine kinetics are minimally affected by concurrent use of saquinavir, indinavir, or nelfinavir. However, the zidovudine AUC is decreased by approximately 25% when zidovudine is co-administered with ritonavir, which induces glucuronidation. Zidovudine in combination with ganciclovir, interferon-α, and bone marrow suppressive agents or cytotoxic agents may result in increased hematologic toxicity.

▲ CLINICAL USE

Regimens

Zidovudine has been used alone and in various combination regimens for the treatment of patients with HIV infection. As a result of improved clinical outcomes with combination regimens and the decreased risk for viral

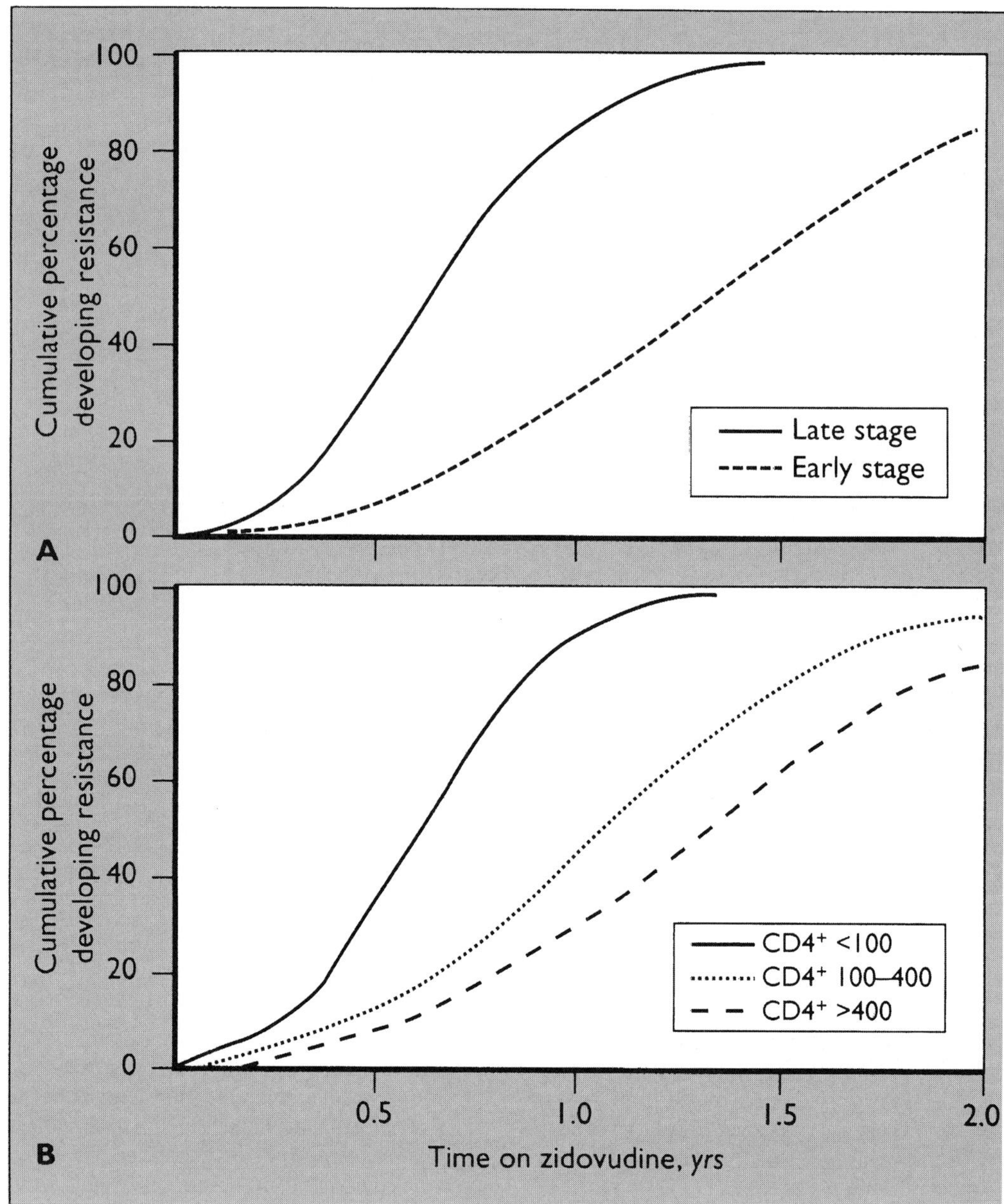

Figure 2–4. Proportion of patients developing viral resistance to zidovudine based on stage of disease (**A**) and CD4+ T-lymphocyte count (**B**). (From Fischl MA. Antiviral treatments. In: Mandell GL, Mildvan D [eds]. Atlas of Infectious Diseases. Philadelphia, Current Medicine, with permission.)

resistance, zidovudine monotherapy for the treatment of patients with HIV infection is no longer recommended.[38] Zidovudine is currently recommended for initial treatment regimens that include two NRTIs with an HIV-1 PI, two NRTIs with an NNRTI, or one or two NRTIs with two HIV-1 PIs (Table 2–1). Regimens under evaluation that may prove to be reasonable options for zidovudine inclusion include one or two NRTIs with an NNRTI and an HIV-1 PI or three NRTIs that include the drug abacavir.

Zidovudine has also been used to decrease the risk of HIV transmission when administered to HIV-infected pregnant women or uninfected individuals following an occupational exposure. It has also been used to improve platelet counts in patients with HIV-related thrombocytopenia and to improve cognitive function in patients with AIDS-related dementia.[35,73,74]

Dosage and Dose Frequency

Zidovudine was initially administered as 200 mg every 4 hours. This regimen was selected based on a rapid elimination half-life of 1 hour and target serum concentration of

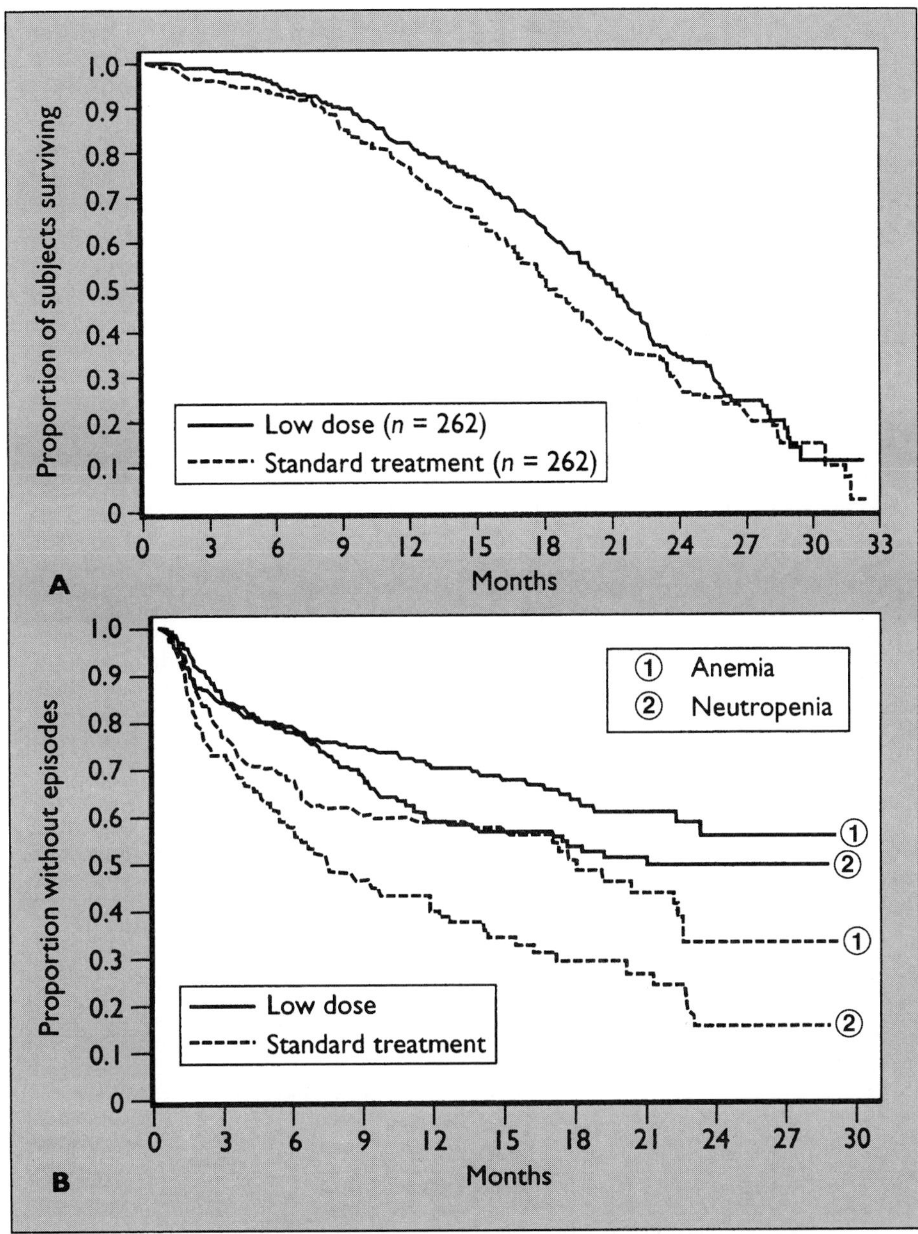

Figure 2–5. Proportion of patients surviving after two doses of zidovudine (standard dose 1500 mg/day versus low dose 600 mg/day) (**A**) and the proportion of patients with anemia or neutropenia receiving either the initial standard zidovudine dose (1500 mg/day) or the low dose (600 mg/day) (**B**). (From Fischl MA. Antiviral treatments. In: Mandell GL, Mildvan D [eds]. Atlas of Infectious Diseases. Philadelphia, Current Medicine, with permission.)

1 mM. Subsequent studies of early and advanced HIV disease utilizing lower daily doses (100 mg five or six times daily) demonstrated equivalent efficacy with less toxicity (Fig. 2–5).[21] Based on the estimated intracellular half-life for zidovudine 5′-triphosphate of 3 to 4 hours, zidovudine dosing was changed to 200 mg tid and most recently to 300 mg bid. Zidovudine, given as 100 mg every 4 hours or as 300 mg every 12 hours for 48 weeks in one study, resulted in no significant differences in adverse experiences.[75] Although the study was not designed as an efficacy study, no differences in clinical events were noted between the two regimens.

▲ CONCLUSIONS

Zidovudine was the first antiretroviral agent approved for use against HIV infection. It continues to be an important component of combination therapy and has been used extensively in regimens with lamivudine, for which a FDC tablet is available. A FDC tablet of zidovudine/lamivudine/abacavir is also available. Zidovudine monotherapy markedly reduces perinatal transmission of HIV[35] and has also provided benefit in the treatment of primary HIV infection,[32] although combination therapy with zidovudine-containing regimens will likely emerge as the preferred treatment in those settings as well. Zidovudine appears to be additive or synergistic with currently available nucleoside analogues, NNRTIs, and PIs. An important exception is stavudine, which is antagonistic in vitro and in vivo with zidovudine[46]; the two drugs should not be used in combination.

Toxicities associated with zidovudine, particularly anemia and neutropenia, occur more frequently in patients with advanced HIV disease and can generally be managed in those patients. Similarly, initial adverse effects such as constitutional symptoms, headache, and nausea are usually mild and respond to symptomatic therapy. Muscle and liver toxicities also occur; and on occasion they are severe, requiring discontinuation of the drug.

REFERENCES

1. Furman PA, Fyfe JS, St Clair MH, et al. Phosphorylation of 3′-azido-3′-deoxythymidine and selective interaction of the 5′-triphosphate with human immunodeficiency virus reverse transcriptase. Proc Natl Acad Sci USA 83:8333, 1986.
2. St Clair MH, Richards CA, Spector T, et al. 3′-Azido-3′-deoxythymidine triphosphate as an inhibitor and substrate of purified human immunodeficiency virus reverse transcriptase. Antimicrob Agents Chemother 31:1972, 1987.
3. Pincus SH, Wehrly K. AZT demonstrates anti-HIV activity in persistently infected cell lines: implications for combination chemotherapy and immunotherapy. J Infect Dis 162:1233, 1990.
4. Hayashi S, Fine RL, Chou T-C, et al. In vitro inhibition of the infectivity and replication of human immunodeficiency virus type 1 by combination of antiretroviral 2′,3′-dideoxynucleosides and virus-binding inhibitors. Antimicrob Agents Chemother 34:82, 1990.
5. Dornsife RE, St Clair MH, Huang AT, et al. Anti-human immunodeficiency virus synergism by zidovudine (3′-azidothymidine) and didanosine (dideoxyinosine) contrasts with their additive inhibition or normal human marrow progenitor cells. Antimicrob Agents Chemother 35:322, 1991.
6. Eron JJ Jr, Johnson VA, Merrill DP, et al. Synergistic inhibition of replication of human immunodeficiency virus type 1, including that of a zidovudine-resistant isolate, by zidovudine and 2′,3′-dideoxycytidine in vitro. Antimicrob Agents Chemother 36:1559, 1992.
7. Merrill DP, Moonis M, Chou T-C, et al. Lamivudine (3TC) or stavudine (d4T) in two- and three-drug combinations against HIV-1 replication in vitro. J Infect Dis 173:355, 1996.
8. Merluzzi VJ, Hargrave KD, Labadia M, et al. Inhibition of HIV-1 replication by a nonnucleoside reverse transcriptase inhibitor. Science 250:1411, 1990.
9. Richman D, Rosenthal AS, Skoog M, et al. BI-RG-587 is active against zidovudine-resistant human immunodeficiency virus type 1 and synergistic with zidovudine. Antimicrob Agents Chemother 35:305, 1991.
10. Johnson VA, Merrill DP, Chou T-C, et al. Human immunodeficiency virus type 1 (HIV-1) inhibitory interactions between protease inhibitor Ro 31-8959 and zidovudine, 2′,3′-dideoxycytidine, or recombinant interferon-α against zidovudine-sensitive or -resistant HIV-1 in vitro. J Infect Dis 166:1143, 1992.
11. Vogt MW, Hartshorn KL, Furman PA, et al. Ribavirin antagonizes the effect of azidothymidine on HIV replication. Science 235:1376, 1987.
12. Tan CK, Cival R, Mian AM, et al. Inhibition of RNase H activity of HIV reverse transcriptase by azidothymidine. Biochemistry 30:4831, 1991.
13. Blum MR, Liao SHT, Good SS, et al. Pharmacokinetics and bioavailability of zidovudine in humans. Am J Med 85(suppl 2A):189, 1988.
14. Klecker RW, Collins JM, Yarchoan R, et al. Plasma and cerebrospinal fluid pharmacokinetics of 3′-azido-3′-deoxythymidine: a novel pyrimidine analog with potential application for the treatment of patients with AIDS and related diseases. Clin Pharmacol Ther 41:407, 1987.
15. Rodman JH, Robbins B, Flynn PM, et al. A systemic and cellular model for zidovudine plasma concentrations and intracellular phosphorylation in patients. J Infect Dis 174:490, 1996.
16. Klecker RW Jr, Collins JM, Yarchoan R, et al. Plasma and cerebrospinal fluid pharmacokinetics of 3′-azido-3′-deoxythymidine: a novel pyrimidine analog with potential application for the treatment of patients with AIDS and related diseases. Clin Pharmacol Ther 41:407, 1987.
17. Gillet JY, Garraffo R, Abrar D, et al. Fetoplacental passage of zidovudine. Lancet 1:269, 1989.
18. Henry K, Chinnock BJ, Quinn RP, et al. Concurrent zidovudine levels in semen and serum determined by radioimmunoassay in patients with AIDS or AIDS-related complex. JAMA 259:3023, 1988.
19. DeMiranda P, Good SS, Yarchoan R, et al. Alteration of zidovudine pharmacokinetics by probenecid in patients with AIDS or AIDS-related complex. Clin Pharmacol Ther 46:494, 1989.
20. Watts DH, Brown ZA, Taraglione T, et al. Pharmacokinetic disposition of zidovudine during pregnancy. J Infect Dis 163:226, 1991.
21. Fischl MA, Parker CB, Pettinelli C, et al. A randomized controlled trial of a reduced daily dose of zidovudine in patients with the acquired immunodeficiency syndrome. N Engl J Med 323:1009, 1990.
22. Volberding PA, Lagakos SW, Koch MA, et al. Zidovudine in asymptomatic human immunodeficiency virus infection: a controlled trial in persons with fewer than 500 CD4-positive cells per cubic millimeter. N Engl J Med 322:941, 1990.
23. Richman DD, Fischl MA, Grieco MH, et al. The toxicity of azidothymidine (AZT) in the treatment of patients with AIDS and AIDS-related complex. N Engl J Med 317:192, 1987.
24. Walker RE, Parker RL, Kovacs JA, et al. Anemia and erythropoiesis in patients with acquired immunodeficiency syndrome (AIDS) and Kaposi's sarcoma treated with zidovudine. Ann Intern Med 108:372, 1988.
25. Fischl MA, Galpin JE, Levine JD, et al. Recombinant human erythropoietin for patients with AIDS treated with zidovudine. N Engl J Med 322:1488, 1990.
26. Don PC, Fusco F, Fried P, et al. Nail dyschromia associated with zidovudine. Ann Intern Med 112:145, 1990.
27. Dalakas MC, Illa I, Pezeshkpour GH, et al. Mitochondrial myopathy caused by long-term zidovudine therapy. N Engl J Med 322:1098, 1990.
28. Arnaudo E, Dalakas M, Shanske S, et al. Depletion of muscle mitochondrial DNA in AIDS patients with zidovudine-induced myopathy. Lancet 337:508, 1991.
29. Fischl MA, Richman DD, Grieco MH, et al. The efficacy of azidothymidine (AZT) in the treatment of patients with AIDS and AIDS-related complex: a double-blind, placebo-controlled trial. N Engl J Med 317:185, 1987.
30. Fischl MA, Richman DD, Hansen N, et al. The safety and efficacy of zidovudine (AZT) in the treatment of subjects with mildly symptomatic human immunodeficiency virus type I (HIV) infection: a double-blind placebo-controlled trial. Ann Intern Med 12:727, 1990.
31. Concorde. MRC/ANRS randomized double-blind controlled trial of immediate and deferred zidovudine in symptom-free HIV infection. Lancet 343:871, 1994.
32. Kinloch-De Loes S, Hirschel BL, Hoen B, et al. A controlled trial of zidovudine in primary human immunodeficiency virus infection. N Engl J Med 333:408, 1995.
33. Dolin R, Amato DA, Fischl MA, et al. Zidovudine compared with didanosine in patients with advanced HIV type 1 infection and little or no previous experience with zidovudine. Arch Intern Med 155:961, 1995.
34. Kahn JO, Legakos SW, Richman DD, et al. A controlled trial comparing continued zidovudine with didanosine in human immunodeficiency virus infection. N Engl J Med 327:581, 1992.
35. Connor EM, Sperling RS, Gelber R, et al. Reduction of maternal-infant transmission of human immunodeficiency virus type 1 with zidovudine treatment. N Engl J Med 331:1173, 1994.
36. Shaffer N, Chuachoowong R, Mock PA, et al. Short-course zidovudine for perinatal HIV-1 transmission in Bangkok, Thailand: a randomized controlled trial. Lancet 353:773, 1999.
37. Hofmann-La Roche. Letter to investigators. Nutley, NJ, Hofmann-La Roche, 1991.

38. Hammer SM, Katzenstein DA, Hughes MD, et al. A trial comparing nucleoside monotherapy with combination therapy in HIV-infected adults with CD4 cell counts from 200 to 500 per cubic millimeter. N Engl J Med 335:1081, 1996.
39. Delta Coordinating Committee. Delta. A randomized double-blind controlled trial comparing combinations with zidovudine plus didanosine or zalcitabine with zidovudine alone in HIV infected individuals. Lancet 348:283, 1996.
40. Fischl MA, Stanley K, Collier AC, et al. Combination and monotherapy with zidovudine and zalcitabine in patients with advanced HIV disease. Ann Intern Med 122:24, 1995.
41. Eron JJ, Benoit SL, Jemsek J, et al. Treatment with lamivudine, zidovudine, or both in HIV-positive patients with 200 to 500 CD4+ cells per cubic millimeter. N Engl J Med 333:1662, 1995.
42. Bartlett JA, Benoit SL, Johnson VA, et al. Lamivudine plus zidovudine compared with zalcitabine plus zidovudine in patients with HIV infection: a randomized, double-blind, placebo-controlled trial. Ann Intern Med 125:161, 1996.
43. CAESAR Coordinating Committee. Randomized trial of addition of lamivudine or lamivudine plus loviride to zidovudine-containing regimens for patients with HIV-1 infection: the CAESAR trial. Lancet 349:1413, 1997.
44. Hammer SM, Squires KE, Hughes MD, et al. A controlled trial of two nucleoside analogues plus indinavir in persons with human immunodeficiency virus infection and CD4 cell counts of 200 per cubic millimeter or less. N Engl J Med 337:725, 1997.
45. Staszewski K, Hill AM, Barlett J, et al. Reductions in HIV-1 disease progression for zidovudine/lamivudine relative to control treatments: a meta-analysis. AIDS 11:477, 1997.
46. Havlir DV, Friedland G, Pollard R, et al. Combination zidovudine and stavudine therapy versus other nucleosides: report of two randomized trials (ACTG 290 and 298). In: Abstracts of the 5th Conference on Retroviruses and Opportunistic Infections, Chicago. Alexandria, VA, Westover Management Group, 1998, abstract 2.
47. Moore KHP, Lloyd PP, Duncan B, et al. Bioequivalence of CombivirJ tablet and Epivir7 plus Retrovir7 tablets. In: Abstracts of the 5th Conference on Retroviruses and Opportunistic Infections, Chicago. Alexandria, VA, Westover Management Group, 1998, abstract 67.
48. Fischl M, Burnside A, Farthing C, et al. Efficacy of Combivir™ plus Ziagen™ bid compared with Trizivir™ bid for 24 weeks (ESS40005 study). In: Programs and Abstracts: 8th Conference on Retroviruses and Opportunistic Infections, Chicago, February 2001, p 315.
49. Clendeninn N, Quart B, Anderson R, et al. Analysis of long-term virologic data from the Viracept (nelfinavir, NFV) 511 using 3 HIV-RNA assays. In: Abstracts of the 5th Conference on Retroviruses and Opportunistic Infections, Chicago. Alexandria, VA, Westover Management Group, 1998, abstract 372.
50. Clumeck N, AVANTI Study Group. AVANTI 3: a randomized, double-blind, comparative trial to evaluate the efficacy, safety, and tolerance of AZT/3TC vs AZT/3TC/nelfinavir in anti-retroviral naive patients. In: Abstracts of the 5th Conference on Retroviruses and Opportunistic Infections, Chicago. Alexandria, VA, Westover Management Group, 1998, abstract 8.
51. Gulick RM, Mellors JW, Havlir D, et al. Treatment with indinavir, zidovudine and lamivudine in adults with human immunodeficiency virus infection and prior antiretroviral therapy. N Engl J Med 337:734, 1997.
52. Hirsch M, Meibohm A, Rawlins S, et al, for the Protocol 039 (Indinavir) Study Group. Indinavir (IDV) in combination with ZDV and 3TC in ZDV-experienced patients with CD4 cell count $\leq$ 50 cells: 3B60 week follow-up. In: Abstracts of the 5th Conference on Retroviruses and Opportunistic Infections, Chicago. Alexandria, VA, Westover Management Group, 1998, abstract 383.
53. Clumeck N, on behalf of the Saquinavir International Phase III Trial (SV14604) Group. Clinical benefit of saquinavir (SQV) plus zalcitabine (ddC) plus zidovudine (ZDV) in untreated/minimally treated HIV-infected patients. In: Abstracts of the 37th Interscience Conference on Antimicrobial Agents and Chemotherapy, Toronto. Washington, DC, American Society for Microbiology, 1997, abstract LB-4.
54. Borleffs JC, Boucher CA, Bravenboer B, et al. Saquinavir-soft gelatine capsules versus indinavir as part of AZT and 3TC containing triple therapy. In: Abstracts of the 37th Interscience Conference on Antimicrobial Agents and Chemotherapy, Toronto. Washington, DC, American Society for Microbiology, 1997, abstract I-92.
55. Cameron DW, Heath-Chiozzi M, Danner S, et al. Randomised placebo-controlled trial of ritonavir in advanced HIV-1 disease. Lancet 351:543, 1998.
56. Montaner JSG, Reiss P, Cooper D, et al. A randomized, double-blind trial comparing combinations of nevirapine, didanosine, and zidovudine for HIV-infected patients: the INCAS trial. JAMA 279:930, 1998.
57. Hicks C, Haas D, Seekins D, et al. A phase II, doubleblind, placebo-controlled, dose-ranging study to assess the antiretroviral activity and safety of efavirenz (DMP 266) in combination with open-label zidovudine (ZDV) with lamivudine (3TC). In: Abstracts of the 5th Conference on Retroviruses and Opportunistic Infections, Chicago. Alexandria, VA, Westover Management Group, 1998, abstract 920.
58. Staszewski S, Morales-Rameriz J, Tashima KT, et al. Efavirenz plus zidovudine and lamivudine, efavirenz plus indinavir, and indinavir plus zidovudine and lamivudine in the treatment of HIV-1 infection in adults. N Engl J Med 341:1865, 1999.
59. Fischl M, Watkins M, Fessel WJ, et al. Direct study: a multicenter, open-label, 24-week pilot study with a 24-week extension to evaluate the safety, tolerability and efficacy of indinavir (IDV)-ritonavir (RTV) (800/100) bid in combination with d4T plus 3TC in HIV-infected individuals (Merck protocol 094). In: Programs and Abstracts: Fifth International Congress on Drug Therapy in HIV Infection, Glasgow, October 2000, p 356.
60. Staszewski S, Keiser P, Montaner J, et al. Abacavir-lamivudine-zidovudine vs indinavir-lamivudine-zidovudine in antiretroviral-naive HIV-infected adults: a randomized equivalence trial. JAMA 285:1155, 2001.
61. Staszewski S, Katlama C, Harrer T, et al. Preliminary long-term open-label data from patients using abacavir (1592, ABC) containing, antiretroviral treatment regimens. In: Abstracts of the 5th Conference on Retroviruses and Opportunistic Infections, Chicago. Alexandria, VA, Westover Management Group, 1998, abstract 658.
62. Richman DD, Guatelli JC, Grimes J, et al. Detection of mutations associated with zidovudine resistance in human immunodeficiency virus by use of the polymerase chain reaction. J Infect Dis 164:1075, 1991.
63. Boucher C, O'Sullivan E, Mulder J, et al. Ordered appearance of zidovudine resistance mutations during treatment of 18 human immunodeficiency virus-positive subjects. J Infect Dis 165:105, 1992.
64. Richman DD, Grimes JM, Lagakos SW. Effect of stage of disease and drug dose on zidovudine susceptibilities of isolates of human immunodeficiency virus. J Acquir Immune Defic Syndr 3:743, 1990.
65. Erice A, Mayers D, Strike D, et al. Primary infection with zidovudine-resistant human immunodeficiency virus type 1. N Engl J Med 328:1163, 1993.
66. Frenkel L, Wagner LI, Demeter L, et al. Effects of zidovudine use during pregnancy on resistance and vertical transmission of human immunodeficiency virus type 1. Clin Infect Dis 20:1321, 1995.
67. D'Aquila R, Hughes M, Johnson V, et al. Nevirapine, zidovudine, and didanosine compared with zidovudine and didanosine in patients with HIV-1 infection: a randomized, double-blind, placebo-controlled trial. Ann Intern Med 124:10019, 1996.
68. Rooke R, Parniak M, Tremblay M, et al. Biological comparison of wild-type and zidovudine-resistant isolates of human immunodeficiency virus type 1 from the same subjects: susceptibility and resistance to other drugs. Antimicrob Agents Chemother 35:988, 1991.
69. Masquelier B, Descamps D, Carriere I, et al. Zidovudine resensitization and dual HIV-1 resistance to zidovudine and lamivudine in the delta lamivudine roll-over study. Antivir Ther 4:69, 1999.
70. Naeger LK, Margot NA, Miller RD. Increased drug susceptibility of HIV-1 reverse transcriptase mutants containing M184V and zidovudine-associated mutations: analysis of enzyme processivity, chain-terminator removal and viral replication. Antivir Ther 6:115, 2001.
71. Sharver P, Lampkin T, Dukes GE, et al. Effect of zidovudine on the pharmacokinetic disposition of phenytoin in HIVpositive asymptomatic patients. Pharmacotherapy 11:108, 1991.
72. Schwartz EL, Brechb ühl AB, Kahl P, et al. Pharmacokinetic interactions of zidovudine and methadone in intravenous drug-using patients with HIV infection. J Acquir Immune Defic Syndr 5:619, 1992.

73. Centers for Disease Control and Prevention. Case-control study of HIV seroconversion in health-care workers after percutaneous exposure to HIV-infected blood:France, United Kingdom, and United States, January 1988–August 1994. MMWR Morb Mortal Wkly Rep 44:929, 1995.
74. Gray F, Belec L, Keohane C, et al. Zidovudine therapy and HIV encephalitis: a 10-year neuropathological survey. AIDS 8:489, 1994.
75. Shepp DH, Ramirez-Ronda C, Dall L, et al. A comparative trial of zidovudine administered every 4 hours versus every twelve hours for the treatment of advanced HIV disease. J Acquir Immune Defic Syndr Hum Retrovirol 15:283, 1997.
76. Catucci M, Venturi G, Romano L, et al. Development and significance of the HIV-1 reverse transcriptase M184V mutation during combination therapy with lamivudine, zidovudine, and protease inhibitors. J Acquir Immune Defic Syndr 21:203, 1999.

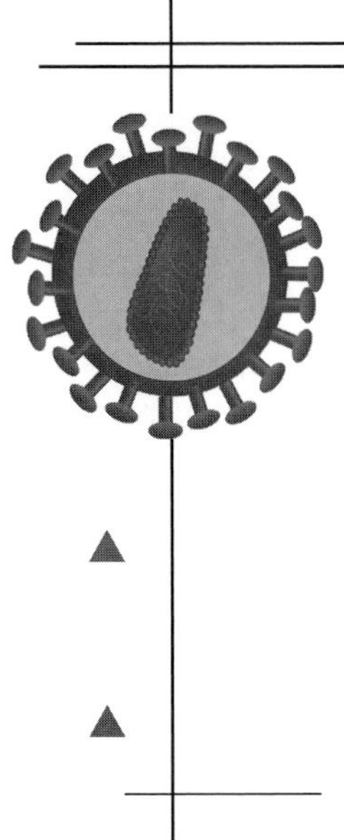

CHAPTER 3

Didanosine

Raphael Dolin, MD

▲ STRUCTURE

Didanosine (2′,3′-dideoxyinosine, ddI, Videx) is a nucleoside analogue active against human immunodeficiency virus type 1 (HIV-1), HIV-2, simian immunodeficiency virus, and human T cell leukemia virus-1 (HTLV-1)[1,2] (Fig. 3–1). It is acid-labile and under acidic conditions is hydrolyzed to 2′,3′-dideoxyribose and the base hypoxanthine.[3] Didanosine is also the deamination product in vivo of 2′,3′-dideoxyadenosine (ddA) through the action of the ubiquitous enzyme adenosine deaminase.[4] Didanosine was the second antiretroviral drug approved by the U.S. Food and Drug Administration (FDA) in 1991.

▲ MECHANISM OF ACTION

Didanosine exerts its antiviral action through its triphosphorylated metabolite 2′,3′-dideoxyadenosine 5′-triphosphate (ddATP), which competes with the naturally occurring nucleoside 2′-deoxyadenosine 5′-triphosphate (dATP) for binding to HIV-1 reverse transcriptase (RT).[5] In addition, ddATP serves as a chain terminator after incorporation into viral DNA because it lacks the requisite 3′-hydroxyl group for elongation of the DNA nascent chain.[6,7]

Didanosine enters the cell via nonfacilitated diffusion through a nucleobase carrier.[8] It is initially phosphorylated to the monophosphate form (ddIMP) by a 5′-nucleotidase and then converted to ddA monophosphate by an adenylosuccinate synthetase and adenylosuccinate lyase.[3] It is subsequently phosphorylated to the diphosphate (ddADP) and finally the triphosphate (ddATP), which is the active antiviral moiety. ddATP has a prolonged intracellular half-life, estimated to be 8 to 40 hours.[9,10] This provides the rationale for the prolonged dosing intervals of once or twice per day for didanosine used in clinical trials.

Didanosine is active against HIV-1 in both lymphocytes and macrophages, with a median inhibitory concentration (IC_{50}) of 0.24 to 0.6 mg/L in T cell cultures and 0.002 to 0.020 mg/L in monocyte/macrophage cultures.[6,11–13] Didanosine appears to have more activity in resting cells than in activated cells, in contrast to zidovudine or stavudine for which the reverse is true.[14,15] The antiviral activity of didanosine also appears to be relatively unaffected by the presence of endogenous nucleosides such as 2′-deoxyadenosine.[3] In vitro, didanosine almost completely inhibits HIV replication at concentrations of 4.8 mg/L.[16] Against HIV-1, didanosine demonstrates additive effects or synergy with nucleoside analogues such as zidovudine and stavudine,[17] nonnucleoside reverse transcriptase inhibitors (NNRTIs) such as delavirdine,[18] and protease inhibitors such as saquinavir[18] or indinavir.[19] Hydroxyurea demonstrates a synergistic effect against HIV-1 when combined with didanosine through inhibition of the ribonucleotide reductase enzyme. This results in the decrease of intracellular dATP with which the active metabolite of didanosine (ddATP) competes for binding to RT.[20] Didanosine is approximately 100-fold less toxic than zidovudine against bone marrow progenitor cells,[16] which likely accounts for the lack of hematopoietic toxicity of the drug observed in clinical trials.

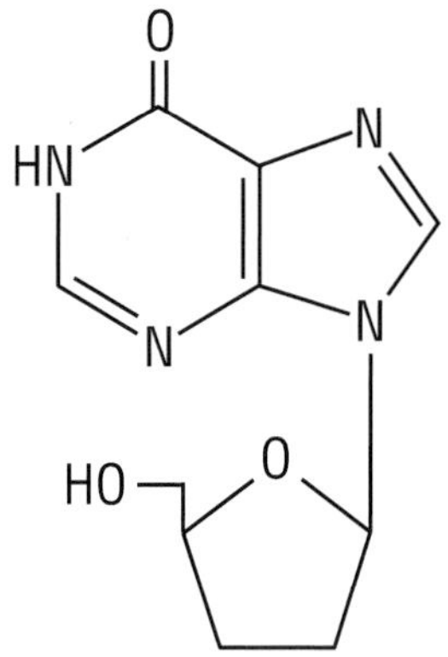

Figure 3–1. Structure of didanosine (2′,3′-dideoxyinosine, ddI, Videx).

▲ PHARMACOKINETICS

The *N*-glycocidic bond of didanosine is highly acid-labile, and significant degradation occurs at the low pH found in gastric fluid.[21] Thus oral preparations have been formulated with buffers to prevent degradation. The sachet (powder) form contains citrate phosphate buffer, and the chewable/dispersable tablet contains calcium carbonate and magnesium hydroxide as antacids. A pediatric powder formulation of didanosine is also available without buffer and must be reconstituted with water and administered with a concomitant antacid. A nonbuffered, enteric coated (EC), delayed-release formulation (Videx EC) has now been approved, consisting of a capsule with enteric coated beadlets that contain didanosine (see below).[22]

Oral bioavailability of didanosine has been reported to be somewhat variable and dose-dependent.[3,23] The buffered chewable/dispersable tablet is 20% to 25% more bioavailable than the sachet form, which accounts for the lower recommended daily dose of the tablet (usually 400 mg/day for patients weighing more than 60 kg) compared to the powder (500 mg/day).[4,10] Twice-a-day dosing of the buffered tablet is the regimen studied most extensively. However, once-daily administration of twice the dose given twice daily results in similar plasma concentration–time curves (area under the curve, or AUC),[24] as does administration of the enteric coated delayed-release formulation, which should be administrated only once a day (Table 3–1).[22] Once-a-day dosing has also been approved by the FDA, but twice-a-day dosing is recommended because of more extensive experience with the durability of effects (see below). The bioavailability of didanosine is decreased up to 50% when administered with food and so should be taken on an empty stomach.[22,25,26]

Oral absorption of buffered didanosine preparations is generally rapid, and time to peak plasma concentrations (T_{max}) occurs 0.50 to 1.13 hours after oral administration.[3,6,7,27] Peak concentrations range between 5 and 9 μmol/L when currently recommended doses are used.[3] The peak concentration for the EC delayed-release preparation is approximately 40% lower, and T_{max} is prolonged to 2.0 hours.[22] Approximately 5% of didanosine is bound to protein.[16] The plasma elimination half-life of didanosine after administration is relatively short, ranging from 0.50 to 2.74 hours after multiple oral doses.[6,7] Thirty to sixty percent of an oral dose is excreted unchanged by the kidneys via glomerular filtration and tubular secretion.[23,28] Reduction of dosage is recommended for patients with significant renal dysfunction (creatinine clearance is less than 60 mL/min), as shown in Table 3–2.[10,22] Didanosine is partially removed during hemodialysis, with an extraction ratio of 53%.[29] For buffered formulations, one-fourth of the total daily dose should be administered once a day to anuric patients requiring hemodialysis or continuous ambulatory peritoneal dialysis (CAPD). Patients taking the EC capsules should be given the dose appropriate for those with a creatinine clearance of less than 10 mL/min if hemodialysis or CAPD is used.[22]

As noted above, didanosine is converted to the active moiety ddATP and then further metabolized to hypoxanthine and eventually to uric acid. The volume of distribution of didanosine is 0.76 to 1.29 L/kg,[30] which is less than the distribution of zidovudine, likely reflecting the lower lipid solubility of didanosine. Mean cerebrospinal fluid concentrations have been reported to be 21% of serum concentrations (range 12% to 85%), although the concentrations were more variable in children.[28,30,31]

Pharmacokinetic measurements in pregnant patients were not significantly different from those obtained in nonpregnant patients.[32] Didanosine was found in placental and fetal circulations at concentrations that were 20% to 50% of those in the maternal circulation, presumably because of placental metabolism of the drug.[32–34] The pharmacokinetics of didanosine in pediatric patients are similar to those described in adults, although bioavailability was somewhat lower in some studies of children.[35–37] Once-daily dosing of didanosine (180 mg/m^2) in pediatric patients had similar bioavailability (90 mg/m^2) when given twice-daily.[38]

The currently available oral forms of didanosine are more palatable than earlier formulations. Hence, along with once-daily dosing, they have resulted in improved compliance with didanosine-containing regimens.

▲ **Table 3–1.** DIDANOSINE DOSAGE IN ADULTS

Patient weight	Buffered tablets[a]	Buffered powder	Enteric coated capsules
Recommended dosage			
≥60 kg	200 mg bid	250 mg bid	[c]
<60 kg	125 mg bid	167 mg bid	[c]
Dosage for patients whose management requires once-daily frequency			
≥60 kg	400 mg qd	[b]	400 mg qd
<60 kg	250 mg qd	[b]	250 mg qd

[a]The 200-mg strength tablet should only be used as a component of a once-daily regimen.

[b]Not suitable for once-daily dosing except for patients with renal impairment.

[c]The enteric coated capsule contains delayed release beadlets and should be administered no more frequently than once daily.

From Physicians' Desk Reference. Videx (Didanosine). Montvale, NJ, Medical Economics, 2001; and Prescribing Information, Videx EC. Bristol-Meyers Squibb, Princeton, NJ, November 2000.

▲ **Table 3–2.** DIDANOSINE DOSAGE DURING RENAL IMPAIRMENT

	≥60 kg			<60 kg		
Creatinine Clearance (ml/min)	**Buffered Tablet[a] (mg)**	**Buffered Powder[b] (mg)**	**Enteric Coated Capsule[d] (mg)**	**Buffered Tablet[a] (mg)**	**Buffered Powder[b] (mg)**	**Enteric Coated Capsule[d] (mg)**
>60	200 bid[c]	250 bid	400 qd	125 bid[c]	167 bid	250 qd
30–59	200 qd or 100 bid	100 bid	200 qd	150 qd or 75 bid	100 bid	125 qd
10–29	150 qd	167 qd	125 qd	100 qd	100 qd	125 qd
<10	100 qd	100 qd	125 qd	75 qd	100 qd	[e]

[a]Chewable/dispersible buffered tablet. Two tablets must be taken with each dose: different strengths of tablets may be combined to yield the recommended dose.
[b]Buffered powder for oral solution.
[c]400 mg qd (≥60 kg) or 250 mg qd (<60 kg) for patients whose management requires once-daily frequency of administration.
[d]Enteric coated capsule containing delayed release beadlets.
[e]Not suitable for use in patients <60 kg and creatinine clearance <10 ml/min.
From Physicians' Desk Reference. Videx (Didanosine). Montvale, NJ, Medical Economics, 2001; and Prescribing Information, Videx EC. Bristol-Meyers Squibb, Princeton, NJ, November 2000.

▲ TOXICITY

Didanosine has been a generally well tolerated drug as ascertained by large-scale clinical studies of HIV-infected patients at various stages of disease progression.[39–41] The most commonly encountered side effects associated with didanosine are listed in Table 3–3. The most well established side effects are peripheral neuropathy and pancreatitis, which have also been the dose-limiting toxicities encountered in Phase I dose-escalation studies.[41] Adverse effects occur most frequently in patients with advanced HIV disease and do not appear to differ significantly between once-a-day and twice-a-day regimens of ddI, except for rates of diarrhea, which may be decreased with the EC formulations.[10,22]

Peripheral neuropathy associated with didanosine is indistinguishable from that seen with other nucleoside analogues such as zalcitabine. It is primarily a sensory polyneuropathy that is usually symmetrical and distal; and it most commonly involves the lower extremities.[49–51] Initial symptoms are often dysesthesias, which are described as aching, burning, or tingling or numbness. They can progress to markedly disabling pain on ambulation or even at rest. Phase I studies indicated that the frequency of neuropathy was dose-related and decreased when doses below 12 mg/kg/day were used.[49] In the expanded access program in which patients with advanced HIV disease received didanosine, the reported frequency of peripheral neuropathy was 16%,[10] which undoubtedly includes a background of neuropathy caused by other drugs and by underlying HIV infection. In two large-scale clinical trials that compared didanosine and zidovudine monotherapy (ACTG 116a[39] and ACTG 116b/117[40]), the rates of peripheral neuropathy were not significantly different for the didanosine- and zidovudine-treated groups. Because zidovudine is not known to cause peripheral neuropathy, these studies indicate that peripheral neuropathy is uncommonly encountered when recommended doses of didanosine are employed. Nonetheless, clinicians must be aware of risk factors for the development of neuropathy with didanosine, which include the presence of underlying peripheral neuropathy from other causes, concurrent treatment with other potentially neurotoxic drugs,[52] and low CD4+ T-lymphocyte counts.[53] Rates of peripheral neuropathy appear to be increased when didanosine is combined with hydroxyurea or, to a lesser extent, stavudine (see below).[54,55] Peripheral neuropathy associated with didanosine generally resolves over several weeks after discontinuing the drug, although occasionally symptoms worsen for 1 to 2 weeks after the drug has been stopped. Some patients with didanosine-associated peripheral neuropathy have been able to tolerate reinstitution of the drug at lower doses,[56] but this is rarely necessary in an era when multiple alternative antiretroviral therapies are available. The pathogenesis of nucleoside-induced

▲ **Table 3–3.** TOXICITIES ASSOCIATED WITH DIDANOSINE

Toxicity	Frequency	Comment	Refs.
Peripheral neuropathy	9–15%	ZDV monotherapy in same studies had rates of 7–14%	39–42
Pancreatitis	4–7%	ZDV monotherapy in same studies had rates of 3–4%	39–42
Diarrhea	16% in expanded access program	Not significantly increased compared to ZDV monotherapy in some studies	39, 40, 43
Elevated serum amylase (>1.4 × normal)	13–20%	ZDV monotherapy in same studies had rates of 3–4%	39, 40, 42
Elevated AST, ALT (>5.1 × normal)	6–9%	Rare fulminant hepatitis has been noted	10, 39, 40, 44, 45
Lactic acidosis and hepatic steatosis[a]	Rare	As with other NRTIs	10, 22, 46–48

ALT, alanine transaminase; AST, aspartate transminase; NRTIs, nucleoside reverse transcriptase inhibitors; ZDV, zidovudine.
[a]Letter of warning has been issued regarding fatal cases of lactic acidosis that have occurred in pregnant women who were receiving didanosine and stavudine.[48]

peripheral neuropathy is not fully understood but appears to be related to inhibition of mitochondrial DNA polymerases in neurons by this class of drugs.[57]

Acute pancreatitis is a dose-related toxic effect of didanosine that is infrequently encountered at currently recommended doses.[58] As is the case with peripheral neuropathy, pancreatitis unrelated to didanosine can develop in HIV-infected patients because of opportunistic infections or neoplasms that involve the pancreas and the use of other pancreatotoxic drugs.[59] Among 7806 patients who participated in the expanded access program for didanosine, pancreatitis was noted in 5% who received the drug for at least 5 months.[10] Acute pancreatitis associated with didanosine can present with variable severity, ranging from mild abdominal pain to life-threatening illness on rare occasions.[58,60] Fatalities associated with pancreatitis occurred in 0.35% of patients in the expanded access program.[10] Asymptomatic elevations in serum amylase and, to a lesser extent, lipase and triglycerides have also been observed.[3,61] In the large-scale studies that compared zidovudine and didanosine monotherapy noted above (ACTG 116a[39] and ACTG 116b/117[40]), an excessive rate of pancreatitis (3% to 4%) was noted in the didanosine arm (500 mg/day) compared to the zidovudine monotherapy arm. In the ACTG 175 trial, which examined patients with somewhat less advanced HIV disease, the overall frequency of pancreatitis was 0.5% in the entire study population and was not increased in the didanosine-treated groups.[62] Risk factors for the development of pancreatitis include a history of pancreatitis, a history of alcohol or drug abuse, hypertriglyceridemia, and possibly renal dysfunction.[10,63] Clinicians who treat patients with didanosine should be alert to signs and symptoms of pancreatitis, and the drug should be stopped promptly if pancreatitis is suspected. Some patients with risk factors for the development of pancreatitis may benefit from periodic monitoring of amylase, lipase, and triglycerides. If amylase concentrations rise 1.5 to 2.0 times above the upper limit of normal or if triglycerides rise above 7 g/L, didanosine administration should be stopped.[52] Fractionation of serum amylase into total and salivary components may increase the specificity of such monitoring. Although some patients with didanosine-associated pancreatitis have been able to tolerate lower doses of the drug once the acute episode has resolved,[49,52] didanosine should be avoided in such patients unless there is no other alternative for antiretroviral therapy.

Diarrhea has also been associated with didanosine administration. It has been attributed, at least in part, to the citrate phosphate buffer in the powdered preparation and may be less frequent with the EC formulation.[22] Diarrhea was reported in 16% of patients in the didanosine expanded access program in which patients had far-advanced HIV disease and were receiving multiple other medications.[42] In studies of monotherapy with didanosine in which the chewable/dispersable tablet was employed, rates of diarrhea were not significantly different from those seen with zidovudine monotherapy arms in some studies. Elevations in aminotransferases (more than five times normal) were seen in 6% to 9% of subjects who received didanosine monotherapy,[10,39,40] and rare cases of fulminant hepatitis have been reported.[43,44]

As with other nucleoside analogues, life-threatening lactic acidosis and hepatic steatosis may occur with didanosine.[45,46] The FDA and the manufacturers of didanosine issued a letter of warning reporting three fatal cases of lactic acidosis in pregnant women who were receiving didanosine combined with stavudine and recommended that this combination be used in pregnant women only when the "potential benefit clearly outweighs the risk."[47] Asymptomatic elevations in uric acid have also been noted, primarily in patients with preexisting hyperuricemia.[42] Rarely, depigmented retinal lesions and optic neuritis have been reported in patients receiving didanosine.[64,65]

Of particular note has been the absence of hematopoietic toxicity associated with didanosine administration. In fact, in several studies, improvement in hemoglobin, white blood cell cells, and platelet counts occurred on didanosine therapy, presumably because of the beneficial effects of the drug in inhibiting replication of HIV.[4,66]

The recommended dosage schedule for didanosine was twice-a-day for the buffered formulation, but in 1999 the FDA approved once-a-day dosing,[10] as well as the EC delayed release formulation, which should be administered only once a day.[22] Comparative trials of twice- and once-a-day regimens of didanosine in combination with stavudine have demonstrated equivalent effects on virologic and CD4 cell count parameters,[67,68] and similar findings were noted when twice- and once-a-day regimens of didanosine were used in combination with zidovudine.[69] Once-a-day dosing of didanosine, in combination with stavudine and nelfinavir, had an antiretroviral effect equivalent to that of a combination of zidovudine, lamivudine, and nelfinavir.[10] Buffered didanosine preparations administered on a once-a-day regimen has also been employed in other comparative and noncomparative studies of didanosine in a wide variety of combination trials, including nucleoside reverse transcriptase inhibitors (NRTIs), nonnucleoside RT inhibitors (NNRTIs), and protease inhibitors.[7,70–73] The EC formulation of didanosine, administered once a day in combination with stavudine and nelfinavir, has given antiretroviral responses similar to those seen with the combination of zidovudine, lamivudine, and nelfinavir.[22]

At the time of the approval of once-a-day dosing for the buffered and EC formulations, the FDA pointed out that "there are limited data to support the long term durability of responses with a once-daily dosing regimen of didanosine," and therefore a twice-daily regimen was preferable. However, once-daily regimens were acceptable for "adults whose management requires once-daily administration of didanosine or an alternative didanosine formulation."[10,22]

▲ RESISTANCE

After didanosine monotherapy, 5- to 26-fold reductions in didanosine sensitivity have been reported; they are associated with a change in the *pol* gene at codon 74 (Leu → Val), which appears to be the predominant mutation associated with resistance.[13] Isolates from 60% to 65% of patients who have received didanosine therapy for at least 1 year demonstrate this mutation.[74–76] Viruses with the L74V mutation also manifested decreased virus replication ("fitness") in vitro.[77] A similar level of resistance with a change at codon 184 (Met → Val) has been reported.[78,79] A mutation at codon 65 (Lys → Arg) has resulted in a three- to fivefold decrease in sensitivity,[80]; and mutations at 135 (Ile → Val) and 200 (Thr → Ala), which confer resistance, have also been described.[81]

Mutations at codon 74 are also associated with partial restoration of susceptibility to zidovudine but with an approximately 10-fold reduction in sensitivity to zalcitabine.[12,82] The position 65 mutation is associated with a reduction in sensitivity to both zalcitabine and lamivudine.[83] The development of a mutation at codon 41, 67, 70, 215, or 219 conferred resistance to zidovudine in patients who received prolonged didanosine therapy but apparently had not received zidovudine therapy.[84] This suggests that viruses resistant to both zidovudine and didanosine occasionally emerge in patients on didanosine therapy alone. Resistance mutations at codon 74 have been associated with poorer CD4 responses and higher virus loads in patients receiving didanosine.[76]

Combination therapy with zidovudine and didanosine reduced the rate of emergence of genotypic didanosine resistance to less than 4% compared to patients who received didanosine monotherapy.[74,75,85–87] Combination therapy with didanosine and zidovudine did not decrease the emergence of viruses resistant to zidovudine in studies that examined the sensitivity of isolates to both drugs.[85,88]

Viruses resistant to both didanosine and zidovudine have been detected after prolonged combination therapy with both drugs, with amino acid substitutions at codons 62, 75, 77, 116, and 151.[85,89–91] These viruses are also resistant to zalcitabine and stavudine and are partially resistant to lamivudine. The inclusion of the mutation Glu to Met at codon 151 (Q151M) and three or four other mutations that result in broad NRTI resistance have been associated with loss of favorable effect on CD4+ T-lymphocyte counts.[92,93] A 6-basepair insert between codons 69 and 70 that confers broad resistance to NRTIs has also been identified in patients who received didanosine or zalcitabine alone or in combination with zidovudine.[94]

▲ DRUG INTERACTIONS

Drug interactions that occur with the buffered formulations of didanosine are most frequently related to the antacid activity in the tablet or powder or to the divalent calcium and magnesium cations present in the tablet form or in antacids added to the pediatric powder (Table 3–4). These interactions can be minimized by administering other drugs 2 hours before or 2 to 6 hours after administration of didanosine. An example of this type of interaction is the reduction in the absorption of drugs such as itraconazole[95,96] or ketoconazole,[97,98] which require gastric acidity for optimal absorption when these drugs are given concomitantly with didanosine. Dapsone also requires low gastric pH for optimal absorption, and there was concern that buffering by didanosine might account for the apparent failure of dapsone prophylaxis for *Pneumocystis carinii* infection when both drugs were administered to patients.[108] However, pharmacokinetic studies in humans receiving didanosine did not show a reduction of plasma dapsone levels.[10,22,109] Absorption of tetracycline[99] and ciprofloxacin[100] (and possibly other quinolone antibiotics) is decreased by chelation with divalent cations in didanosine tablets. Concurrent administration with ranitidine and presumably other H_2-blockers results in a small increase in bioavailability of buffered didanosine preparations by decreasing gastric acidity.[101] Concomitant ganciclovir administration increases plasma didanosine concentrations by 57.7% (C_{max}) and AUC values by 71.5%,[102–104] so clinicians should be alert for the possibility of increased didanosine toxicity when the two drugs are given together. Studies of interactions between didanosine and zidovudine have shown only minor changes in the pharmacokinetics of either drug.[110–112] When delavirdine and didanosine were administered simultaneously, reductions in the concentrations of both delavirdine (32% decrease in AUC) and didanosine (20% decrease in AUC) were noted[105,106]; hence the two drugs should be given at least 1 hour apart. Decreased absorption of indinavir has also been noted when the drug is administered simultaneously with didanosine[105,107] but not if didanosine is taken 1 hour before indinavir.[113] Minor interactions, without clinical significance, have been observed between didanosine and ritonavir.[114] Clinically significant interactions have not been observed between didanosine and the following drugs: trimethoprim-sulfamethoxazole,[115] rifabutin,[116] isoniazid,[117] foscarnet,[118] stavudine,[119] loperamide,[22] metoclopramide,[22]

▲ **Table 3–4.** DRUG INTERACTIONS WITH DIDANOSINE

Type of Interaction	Drug	Refs.
Decreased absorption of drugs requiring gastric acidity for optimal absorption[a]	Itraconazole Ketoconazole	95, 96 97, 98
Decreased absorption of drugs by chelation with cations[a]	Tetracycline Ciprofloxacin	99 100
Increased absorption of didanosine by block of gastric acid production	Ranitidine	101
Increased plasma concentration of didanosine	Ganciclovir	102–104
Decreased plasma concentration of drug when given at the same time as didanosine[a]	Delavirdine Indinavir	105, 106 105, 107
Decreased plasma concentration of didanosine when given with drug	Delavirdine Methadone	105, 106 107
Possibly increased rate of peripheral neuropathy when given with didanosine	Isoniazid Ethambutol Metronidazole Zalcitabine	52
	Hydroxyurea Stavudine	54, 55
Possibly increased pancreatic toxicity when given with didanosine	Pentamidine Azathioprine Zalcitabine	59
Increased plasma concentration of didanosine through inhibition of renal excretion	Allopurinol	10

[a]Interaction is avoided if didanosine is administered 1 to 2 hours before indinavir or if a nonbuffered preparation of didanosine (EC) is used.

clarithromycin,[120] nevirapine,[121] and nelfinavir.[122] Administration of allopurinol increases the AUC of didanosine approximately fourfold, so the two drugs should not be administered together.[10,22] Chronic methadone administration reduces the AUC of didanosine by 57% and the C_{max} by 66%.[123]

The EC formulation of didanosine, which does not contain buffer, should not be expected to result in drug interactions that depend on the antacid or cation contents of didanosine tablets. However, drug interactions with didanosine based on other mechanisms, such as those involving allopurinol, ganciclovir, or methadone, would be expected to occur with the EC formulation as well.[22]

As noted in the Toxicity section, clinicians should be alert to the development of didanosine toxicity when drugs that are known to cause or potentiate peripheral neuropathy[53] (e.g., isoniazid, ethambutol, metronidazole, vincristine, hydroxyurea, stavudine) or pancreatitis[58] (pentamidine, azathioprine) are co-administered, and alternative drugs should be considered. Because of the potential for additive toxicities involving peripheral neuropathy and pancreatitis, didanosine and zalcitabine should not be administered concurrently.

▲ EFFICACY

Didanosine Monotherapy or Dual Nucleoside Combination Therapy

Clinical studies of didanosine monotherapy or dual combination therapy were carried out at times when the use of one or two antiretrovirals was the standard of care. The major studies of this type are summarized in Table 3–5. Studies conducted by the AIDS Clinical Trial Group (ACTG) showed that changing to didanosine monotherapy was more effective than continuing zidovudine monotherapy in patients with advanced HIV infection who had previously received at least 8 weeks of zidovudine (ACTG 116a, ACTG 116b/117),[39,40] although zidovudine appeared to be somewhat more effective than didanosine in antiretroviral-naive patients.[39] Studies of patients who received at least 6 months of zidovudine and were either clinically stable[124] or deteriorating[42] also showed benefits after their therapy was changed to didanosine. A meta-analysis of the above studies and ACTG 175 (see below) supported the beneficial effect of switching from zidovudine to didanosine across a broad range of CD4 and HIV disease categories.[131] A comparison of didanosine with zidovudine as initial monotherapy in patients with "mildly symptomatic disease" and CD4 counts lower than 500/mm^3 showed that the clinical efficacies of the two drugs were similar.[132]

Three large-scale studies have examined the clinical benefit of didanosine as part of dual combination therapy with zidovudine in patients with a broad range of underlying CD4+ T-lymphocyte counts and previous experience with zidovudine (Table 3–5). Two of these studies, ACTG 175[62,126] and Delta,[127] found combination therapy to be superior to zidovudine monotherapy in the study population as a whole, and the third study, CPRA 007,[128] found the combination to be superior in a subgroup of patients with less than 12 months of previous zidovudine experience.

An additional study indicated that combinations of didanosine and zidovudine were superior to zidovudine alone in patients who were largely antiretroviral-naive and had CD4 counts of less than 300/mm^3.[88] A study of patients who had been receiving zidovudine for a median of 3 years showed a modest survival benefit if didanosine replaced or was added to zidovudine.[129]

The combination of didanosine and stavudine has been investigated in dose-range and comparative trials (Table 3–5). In antiretroviral-naive patients, didanosine (200 to 400 mg/day) plus stavudine (20 to 80 mg/day) resulted in a decrease in RNA levels of 0.9 to 1.3 $\log_{10}$ after 49 weeks. High-dose and low-dose combinations of didanosine and stavudine reduced the HIV RNA levels by 1.22 to 2.09 $\log_{10}$ copies/ml in a study in Thailand.[131] The ALBI trial found that 24 weeks of didanosine plus stavudine resulted in a greater drop in HIV RNA (2.26 $\log_{10}$ copies/ml) than either zidovudine plus lamivudine (1.26 $\log_{10}$ copies/ml) or alternating didanosine and stavudine followed by zidovudine plus lamivudine (1.58 $\log_{10}$ copies/ml).[130] Studies of didanosine and stavudine in highly antiretroviral-experienced patients have generally resulted in less profound decreases in HIV RNA levels than those seen in antiretroviral-naive patients.[69,125,134] An example is the Quintet study, in which didanosine and stavudine combination resulted in a mean reduction of 0.89 $\log_{10}$ copies/ml.[125] In antiretroviral-naive patients studied in ACTG 306, didanosine plus lamivudine did not increase antiretroviral effects compared to didanosine monotherapy, whose antiretroviral effects in turn were similar to those of lamivudine plus zidovudine.[135] Studies of combination therapy with didanosine and stavudine, and with didanosine and lamivudine are reviewed in Chapters 5 and 6, respectively.

Triple Combination Therapy with Didanosine

Dual nucleoside antiretroviral regimens have not been able to achieve the potency and durability of triple antiretroviral combinations, and the latter have generally become the standard of therapy in which didanosine is used most frequently. Didanosine has been studied as part of triple combination regimens with other nucleoside analogues, NNRTIs, and protease inhibitors in both noncomparative and comparative trials as reviewed below.

Didanosine in Regimens with NNRTIs

Triple regimens that include didanosine and NNRTIs have been compared with dual regimens in various stages of HIV infection. The ACTG 241 study evaluated the combination of didanosine/zidovudine/nevirapine versus didanosine/zidovudine in patients who had 350 or fewer CD4 cells/mm^3 and who had undergone more than 6 months of previous nucleoside therapy (Table 3–6).[136] The triple combination regimen resulted in higher mean CD4+ T-lymphocyte counts, lower mean infectious HIV-1 titers in peripheral blood mononuclear cells, and lower mean plasma HIV RNA levels than patients who received the

Table 3–5. TRIALS OF DIDANOSINE MONOTHERAPY AND DUAL NUCLEOSIDE COMBINATION THERAPY

Trial	Design	Dosage	No. of Subjects	Entry Criteria	CD4 cells/mm³ on Entry	CD4 Response	Antiviral Response	Clinical Outcome	Comments
ACTG 116a (Dolin et al.[39])	ddI vs. (ZDV; randomized, double-blind	ddI: 500 or 750 mg/d ZDV: 600 mg/d	617	Symptomatic: CD4 <300 *or* Asymptomatic: CD4 <200 Previous ZDV experience of <16 wk	130 (mean)	ddI 500 mg had slower decline in CD4 than ddI 750 mg or ZDV group	No difference in p24 declines among three treatment groups	Death (/100 pt-yr) / AIDS event or death (/100 pt-yr) 500 ddI: 17.7 / 30.0 750 ddI: 15.4 / 33.1 ZDV: 11.1 / 30.4	ZDV more effective than 750 ddI in ZDV-naive patients; 500 ddI more effective than ZDV in patients with >8 wks but ≤16 wks ddI
ACTG 116b/117 (Kahn et al.[40])	ddI vs. ZDV; randomized, double-blind	ddI: 500 or 750 mg/d ZDV: 600 mg/d	913	As for ACTG 116a but ≥16 wk of previous ZDV experience	95 (median)	CD4 change/mm³ at 24 wks 500 ddI: −10 750 ddI: −10 ZDV: −23	Percent of subjects with ≥50% p24 decrease at 24 wks: 500 ddI: 21 750 ddI: 32 ZDV: 21	Deaths (/100 pt-yr) / AIDS event or death (/100 pt-yr) 500 ddI: 15.5 / 37.1 750 ddI: 17.5 / 42.5 ZDV: 16.9 / 52.8	500 mg ddI more effective than ZDV in reducing risk of primary endpoints
BMS 010 (Spruance et al.[42])	Switch to ddI or continue ZDV; randomized, double-blind	ddI 600 mg/d (≥60 kg) 400 mg/d (<60 kg) ZDV: 600 mg/d	312	CD4 ≤300 ZDV for at least 6 months Clinical deterioration	70–75 (median)	Less decrease in CD4 in ddI group through week 24 ($P < 0.0001$)	No difference	New AIDS-defining event or death, or ≥50% CD4 decline ddI 53/100 pt-yr ZDV 75/100 pt-yr ($P = 0.02$)	Switching to ddI superior to continuation of ZDV in patients who are failing on ZDV
CTN 002 (Montaner et al.[124])	Switch to ddI or continue ZDV; double-blind, randomized	ddI 400 mg/d (≥60 kg) 200 mg/d (<60 kg) ZDV: 600 mg/d	246	CD4 200–500 ZDV for at least 6 months Clinically stable	324	Increase in CD4 in ddI, decrease in ZDV at 48 wks ($P < 0.01$)	—	New AIDS-defining event or death (no.) ddI 1 ZDV 8 ($P = 0.02$)	Switching to ddI superior to continuation of ZDV in patients clinically stable on ZDV
Quintet Trial (Raffi et al.[125])	ddI + d4T	ddI: 400 mg/d d4T: 80 mg/d	65	Heavily pretreated with ZDV or ddC	227	Increase of 70/mm³ at 24 wks	Decrease of HIV RNA of 0.89 $\log_{10}$ copies/ml at 24 wk	—	Response is less than in retroviral-naive patients

Table continued on following page

Table 3–5. TRIALS OF DIDANOSINE MONOTHERAPY AND DUAL NUCLEOSIDE COMBINATION THERAPY *Continued*

Trial	Design	Dosage	No. of Subjects	Entry Criteria	CD4 cells/mm^3 on Entry	CD4 Response	Antiviral Response	Clinical Outcome	Comments
ACTG 175 (Hammer et al.[62,126])	ddI vs. zidovudine (ZDV) vs. ddI + ZDV vs. ddC + ZDV; randomized, double-blind	ddI: 400 mg/d ZDV: 600 mg/d Same in combination ddC: 2.25 mg/d in combination	2467	CD4 200–500 No AIDS-defining illness Antiretroviral naive or experienced	352 (mean)	Significantly better for ddI or combination therapy than for ZDV ($P \leq 0.006$)	Decrease in HIV RNA copies/ml $\log_{10}$ at 8 wk: ZDV 0.26 ddI 0.65 ddI + ZDV 0.93 ddI + ddC 0.89	Progression to AIDS-defining event or death or ≥50% decline in CD4 counts ZDV 32% ddI 22% ddI + ZDV 18% ddC + ZDV 20% ($P < 0.001$ global)	Survival benefit for ddI, ddI + ZDV, and a trend for ddI + ddC ($P = 0.1$) Benefits for both antiretroviral naive and experienced, except for naive only for ddC + ZDV
Delta[127]	ZDV vs. ddI + ZDV vs. ddC + ZDV; randomized, double-blind	As for ACTG 175	3207	AIDS, and CD4 >50 No or minimal symptoms and CD4 <350 ZDV experienced (Delta 2) or naive (Delta 1)	205 (mean)	Better with combination therapy than with ZDV alone	—	For Delta 1 and 2 vs. ZDV / Decrease in mortality / Decrease in disease progression ZDV — — ddI + ZDV 33% 36% ddC + ZDV 21% 17%	Clinical benefit was seen largely in ZDV-naive subgroup (Delta 1)
CPCRA 007 (Saravolatz et al.[128])	ZDV vs. ZDV + ddI vs. ZDV + ddC; randomized, double-blind	As for ACTG 175	1102	CD4 <200 or <15% of total lymphocyte count	118 (mean)	At 2 months ZDV + ddI: +19.2/mm^3 ZDV + ddC: +12.9/mm^3 ZDV: −4.0/mm^3	—	Disease progression/100 pt-yr / Death/100 pt-yr ZDV + ddI 34.3 21.9 ZDV + ddC 36.2 22.7 ZDV 39.6 24.1	Combinations were superior to ZDV in patients with <12 mo or no previous ZDV experience
BMS 460 (Pollard et al.[129])	ddI + d4T five arms, dose ranging	ddI: 200–400 mg/d d4T: 20–80 mg/d	86	CD4 200–500 Antiretroviral-naive	343 (median)	Mean increase of 80–100/mm^3 sustained through wk 45 for all combination groups	Decrease in plasma RNA copies of 0.9–1.3 $\log_{10}$ after 49 wk	—	Well tolerated; 2pts. developed peripheral neuropathy (2.3%)
ALBI Trial (Molina et al.[130])	(1) ddI + d4T (2) ZDV + 3TC *or* (3) ddI + d4T followed by ZDV + 3TC	ddI: 400 mg/d d4T: 80 mg/d ZDV: 500 mg/d 3TC: 300 mg/d	151	CD4 ≥200 Antiretroviral-naive	382–384 (median)	Mean increase/mm^3 (1) 124 (2) 62 (3) 118	Decrease in HIV RNA copies/ml/ $\log_{10}$ at 24 wk (1) 2.26 (2) 1.26 (3) 1.58	—	Antiretroviral effect greater with ddI + d4T CD4 greater with both ddI and d4T regimens

ddC, dideoxycytidine; ddI, dideoxyinosine; d4T, stavudine; 3TC, lamivudine.

double-combination regimen. The risk for disease progression did not differ between the two groups, but the study may have been underpowered to detect clinical differences.[136] In the ISSIS 047[144] and INCAS[137] studies, the triple combination of didanosine, zidovudine, and nevirapine was superior for reducing HIV RNA levels compared to the combination of didanosine plus zidovudine. At weeks 48 to 52, HIV RNA was undetectable in 38% to 51% of patients, and CD4+ T-lymphocyte counts had increased by 117 and 139 cells/mm^3, respectively, which were also significantly better than in recipients of dual therapy (Table 3–6).[137,144] The VIRGO trial also showed marked reductions in HIV RNA levels (-2.5 log_{10} copies/ml) and increases in CD4+ T-lymphocyte counts (168 to 139 cells/mm^3) with a combination of didanosine/zidovudine/nevirapine (Table 3–6).[138] ACTG 261 compared a combination of didanosine/zidovudine/delavirdine with dual combinations of its components.[139] At 48 weeks recipients of triple therapy had a higher rate of undetectable HIV RNA in plasma (26%), although the mean reductions in plasma levels were relatively modest in all the treatment groups (Table 3–6).

A study of once-daily combination of didanosine/efavirenz/emtricitabine (an investigational NRTI) (see Chapter 7) in antiretroviral-naive patients also showed potent antiviral and CD4 responses (Table 3–6).[145] Didanosine and stavudine combined with the investigational NNRTI emivirine[145] or with the investigational protease inhibitor BMS-232632[146] have also been reported to have strong antiretroviral effects (see Chapter 19).

Didanosine in Regimens with Protease Inhibitors

Didanosine has been studied in combination with most of the available protease inhibitors (PIs). Combinations of didanosine/stavudine/indinavir were studied in the OZCOMBO 1,[141] START II,[142] and ATLANTIC[147,148] trials in patients who were largely antiretroviral-naive. In OZCOMBO 1 this combination resulted in a decrease in HIV RNA levels of 2.68 log_{10} copies/ml at week 52 and an increase in CD4 cells of 120/mm^3;[141] in the START II trial there was a decrease of 2.6 log_{10} copies/ml and an increase in CD4 cells of 214/mm^3 at 48 weeks (Table 3–7).[142] The ATLANTIC study found similar results for the combination of didanosine/stavudine/indinavir and for didanosine plus stavudine combined with either lamivudine or nevirapine.[147,148] Didanosine/lamivudine/indinavir therapy also demonstrated antiviral effects and improved CD4 counts at 24 weeks in another study of antiretroviral-naive patients among whom 41% were intravenous drug users.[149]

The combination of didanosine/stavudine/nelfinavir decreased the virus load (-1.36 log_{10} copies/ml) and increased CD4+ T-lymphocyte counts (111/mm^3) in patients without previous experience with any of the drugs in this regimen (Table 3–7).[122] A study carried out in 16 HIV-infected drug users with partly observed therapy with didanosine/stavudine/nelfinavir also showed either a more than 2 log_{10} drop in RNA levels or a more than 100/mm^3 in CD4 count in most of the subjects.[150] Didanosine and stavudine in combination with ritonavir resulted in a 3.1 log_{10} reduction of RNA copies/ml after 72 weeks, although nearly one-half of the subjects discontinued medication because of adverse side effects (Table 3–7).[143]

A triple combination of zidovudine/didanosine/lamivudine was employed to treat 10 patients with primary HIV-1 infection. This combination reduced plasma HIV RNA below detectable levels in all subjects after 108 ± 32 days of therapy. Infectious HIV could not be detected in lymph nodes from five patients on day 90, and HIV-1 RNA was at extremely low levels in lymph nodes after 1 year.[151]

Combinations of Didanosine and Hydroxyurea

As noted above, hydroxyurea does not inhibit HIV replication directly but, rather, potentiates the effects of didanosine.[20,152,153] Thus administration of hydroxyurea alone did not reduce HIV-1 RNA levels; but when given in combination with didanosine reductions of HIV RNA of 0.02 to 2.10 log_{10} copies/ml were achieved.[154–159] A greater effect on HIV RNA levels was seen when higher doses of hydroxyurea were used (1000 mg/day compared to 500 mg/day).[154] Because hydroxyurea also has antiproliferative cellular activity, CD4 responses generally have been absent or blunted, which is an important limitation on use of the drug. In a comparative study, combination therapy with didanosine and hydroxyurea was superior to monotherapy with either drug, with zidovudine alone, or with zidovudine plus hydroxyurea (Table 3–8).[160] Triple combination therapy with didanosine/stavudine/hydroxyurea was superior to that seen with didanosine/hydroxyurea[161,163] but appeared less effective than that observed with didanosine/stavudine/nelfinavir in another study.[162] Treatment of patients with primary infection with didanosine/indinavir/hydroxyurea resulted in undetectable (fewer than 50 copies/ml) levels of HIV RNA in 11 of 11 patients after 68 weeks.[164] Prolonged suppression of HIV RNA levels with didanosine/hydroxyurea also resulted in improvement of some immune parameters.[165] Triple combination therapy with didanosine/hydroxyurea/protease inhibitors has also been shown to suppress HIV RNA levels for up to 21 months.[166]

The combination of didanosine/hydroxyurea appeared to be generally well tolerated,[54,164,167–169] although in one long-term study most of the patients who had started with a hydroxyurea-containing regimen were no longer taking hydroxyurea at the end of the study.[163] Significant toxicities may be encountered. That most commonly encountered was reversible bone marrow suppression consistent with the drug's antiproliferative effect.[54,170] The addition of hydroxyurea also increased the rate of peripheral neuropathy when combined with either didanosine or stavudine[171] or when added to a combination of the two drugs.[55,163,172] Pancreatitis has also been reported in patients receiving hydroxyurea/didanosine.[173] A report from the FDA Adverse Event Reporting System suggested that the use of hydroxyurea in combination with an NRTI may enhance the risk of death caused by hepatoxicity, and that this risk may be further enhanced if hydroxyurea were used in combination with didanosine and stavudine. The report stated: "Interpretations of data from such voluntary reporting systems have limitations; however, clinicians should be particularly aware of this potential toxicity when combinations of these drugs are used."[174]

▲ **Table 3–6.** TRIPLE COMBINATION THERAPY WITH DIDANOSINE AND NONNUCLEOSIDE REVERSE TRANSCRIPTASE INHIBITORS

Trial	Design	Dosage	No. of Subjects	Entry Criteria
ACTG 241 (D'Aquila et al.[136])	ddI + ZDV vs. ddI + ZDV + NVP Double-blind, randomized	ddI: 400 mg/d ZDV: 600 mg/d NVP: 200 mg/d for 2 wk, then 400 mg/d	398	CD4: ≤350; >6 mo of prior nucleoside therapy
INCAS (Montaner et al.[137])	ddI + ZDV + NVP vs. ZDV + NVP vs. ZDV + ddI Double-blind, randomized	As for ACTG 241	153	CD4: 200–600 Antiretroviral-naive
Virgo I and II (Raffi et al.[138])	ddI + d4T + NVP Open label	ddI: 400 mg/d d4T: 80 mg/d NVP: 400 mg/d	100	Antiretroviral-naive
ACTG 261 (Friedland et al.[139])	ddI + ZDV + delavirdine (DLV) vs. ddI + ZDV vs. ddI + DLV vs. ZDV + DLV Double-blind, randomized	ddI: 400 mg/d ZDV: 600 mg/d DLV: 1.2 g/d	544	CD4: 100–500; <6 mo of monotherapy
Molina et al.[140]	ddI + efivarenz + emtricitabine	ddI: 400 mg/d Efivarenz: 600 mg/d Emitricitabine: 200 mg/d	40	Antiretroviral-naive

DLV, delavirdine; NVP, nevirapine.
[a]Log_{10} of copies of plasma HIV RNA/ml.

▲ STUDIES IN PEDIATRIC PATIENTS

Didanosine buffered formulations are approved for use in pediatric patients, and a powder for oral solutions is available for pediatric use. The recommended dose for pediatric administration is 120 mg/m^2 bid. Studies of the efficacy of once-daily dosing in children have not been reported, and the EC formulation is approved for adult use only.

Didanosine, alone or in combination with other antiretroviral agents, has been studied in children of various ages and HIV-related disease states; the major studies in this area are summarized in Table 3–9. Initial studies showed

▲ **Table 3–7.** TRIPLE COMBINATION THERAPY WITH DIDANOSINE AND PROTEASE INHIBITORS

Trial	Design	Dosage	No. of Subjects	Entry Criteria
OzCombo (Carr et al.[141])	ZDV + 3TC + IDV *or* d4T + 3TC + IDV *or* d4T + ddI +IDV Randomized	ddI: 400 mg/d d4T: 80 mg/d IDV: 2.4 g/d 3TC: 300 mg/d ZDV: 500 mg/d	109	CD4 <500/mm^3 or RNA >30,000 copies/ml Antiretroviral-naive
START II (Eron et al.[142])	ZDV + 3TC + IDV *or* d4T + ddI + IDV Randomized	As above, except ZDV given 600 mg/d	205	CD4 ≥200/mm^{3}and RNA ≥10,000 copies/ml, <4 wks of Rx; naive to 3TC and protease inhibitors
Elion et al.[122]	d4T + ddI + NFV Open label	ddI: 400 mg/d d4T: 80 mg/d NFV: 2250 mg/d	22	RNA >10,000 copies/ml; naive to d4T, ddI, or protease inhibitors
Saimot et al.[143]	ddI + d4T + ritonavir Open label	ddI: 200 mg bid d4T: 40 mg bid Ritonavir: NR	36	CD4: 5–350 Antiretroviral-naive

NR, not reported.
[a]Log_{10} of plasma HIV RNA copies/ml.

CD4 cells/mm³; HIV RNA[a] on Entry	CD4 Response	Antiviral Response[a]	Clinical Outcome	Comments
135–139 (median)	At 48 wks, triple combination had 18% higher mean CD4 counts	At 48 wks: triple combination had lower mean plasma RNA levels	No differences in disease progression	Severe rashes more common in NVP group
340 (median) 4.25–4.54 (median) RNA	At 52 wks Triple Rx: increase of 139/mm³ ZDV + ddI: increase of 87/mm³ ZDV + NVP: decrease of 6/mm³	At 52 wks: RNA levels $\log_{10}$ Triple Rx: −2.71 to −0.72 ZDV + ddI: −2.11 to −0.01 ZDV + NVP: −0.41 to −0.08	Disease progression or death Triple Rx: 12% ZDV + ddI: 25% ZDV + NVP: 23%	Trend toward improved clinical outcome in triple Rx (P = 0.08)
412–414 (mean) 4.59–4.87 (mean)	139–168 increase at wk 24	At wk 52: 67% of pts had <50 copies/ml	—	20% discontinued study because of an adverse event
2.95 (median) 4.45 (median)	At 40–48 wks, increase of 65 (mean) for triple Rx	At 40–48 wks: decrease of 0.73 for triple Rx	—	Generally better responses for triple Rx; 30% experienced rash (1 severe)
373 median 4.77 median	159 (median); increase at wk 24	At wk 24: 3.5 Decrease	—	Well tolerated; mild to moderate CNS symptoms in 73%

that didanosine monotherapy was well tolerated and associated with antiretroviral activity and improved CD4 counts.[175,182,183] Combination therapy with didanosine and zidovudine also demonstrated beneficial antiretroviral and CD4 count responses[176] and was superior to zidovudine monotherapy in terms of clinical endpoints in the ACTG 152 study.[177] In that study, didanosine/zidovudine combination therapy was not significantly better than didanosine monotherapy.

In the PACTG 300 study zidovudine/didanosine or zidovudine/lamivudine was associated with lower rates of disease progression than didanosine alone.[184] Didanosine/stavudine[185,186] or didanosine/lamivudine[179] also had a beneficial effect on HIV-1 virus markers. Marked decreases in HIV-1 RNA levels have been observed in pediatric studies of didanosine/stavudine as part of triple combinations with saquinavir,[187] indinavir,[180,188] or nelfinavir[181] and with zidovudine/nevirapine.[178]

CD4 cells/mm³; HIV RNA[a] at Entry	CD4 Response	Antiviral Response[a]	Comments
267–313 (mean) 5.00–5.21 (mean)	120–159/mm³ mean increase at wk 52	−2.68 to −3.28 mean decrease at wk 52	DTH responses improved but remained impaired; quality of life improved
422 (median) 4.5 (median)	214/mm³ median increase for ddI arm and 142 for ZDV arm at wk 48	−2.6 for both arms at wk 48	ddI + d4T + IDV comparable or superior to ZDV + 3TC + IDV
315 (median) 4.8 $\log_{10}$ (median)	+111 mean at wk 12	−1.36 mean at wk 12	Well tolerated; no pharmacokinetic interaction between ddI, d4T, and NFV
252 (mean)	At wk 12, mean CD4 increase of 138 cells/mm³	Decrease in plasma RNA levels by 3.1 $\log_{10}$ at wk 72	15/36 pts discontinued assigned dosage because of adverse effects

▲ **Table 3–8.** TRIALS OF DIDANOSINE AND HYDROXYUREA THERAPY

Trial	Design	Dosage	No. of Subjects	Entry Criteria
Foli et al.[160]	ddI *or* ZVD *or* HYD *or* HYD + ddI Randomized, nonblind	ddI: 200–600 mg/d ZVD: 500 mg/d HYD: 1000 mg/d	23	Asymptomatic infection; antiretroviral naive or experienced
Rutschmann et al.[161]	ddI + d4T vs. ddI + d4T + HYD Randomized, double-blind	ddI: 200 mg bid d4T: 40 mg bid HYD: 500 mg bid	144	CD4 >200 or <500/mm^3 RNA >1000 copies/ml Previous ddI Rx, 6 mos
Jaegel-Guedes et al.[162]	ddI + d4T + HYD; ddI + d4T + NFV	NR	26	Antiretroviral-naive

HYD, hydroxyurea; NR, not reported.
[a]Log_{10} of plasma HIV RNA copies/ml.

▲ **Table 3–9.** DIDANOSINE THERAPY IN CHILDREN

Trial	Design	Dosage	No. of Subjects	Entry Criteria
Mueller et al.[175]	ddI Dose ranging	20–180 mg/m^2 q8h	103	6 mo–18 yr: CD4 <500/mm^3
Husson et al.[176]	ddI + zidovudine (ZDV) Dose ranging	ddI: 90–180 mg/m^2 q12h ZDV: 60 mg/m^2 q6h	54	3 mo–18 yr: CD4 < 500/mm^3
ACTG 152 (Englund et al.[177])	ZDV vs. ddI vs. ZDV + ddI Double-blind, randomized	ZDV: 180 mg/m^2 q6h *or* ddI 120 mg/m^2 q12h *or* ZDV: 120 mg/m^2 q6h plus ddI 90 mg/m^2 q12h	831	3 mo– 18 yr: CD4 <1000/mm^3 if <15 mo; CD4 <500 if >15 mo but < 18 yr
Luzuriaga et al.[178]	ddI + ZDV + nevirapine Open label	ddI: 120 mg/m^2 q12h *plus* ZDV: 180 mg/m^2 q8h *plus* Nevirapine: 120 mg/m^2 qd × 28 days, then 200 mg/m^2 q12h	8	2–18 mo
PACTG 300[179]	ZDV + 3TC vs. ddI vs. ddI + ZDV; randomized, double-blind	ZDV: 160 mg/m^2 tid 3TC: 4 mg/kg q12h ddI monotherapy: 120 mg/m^2 q12h ddI combination: 90 mg/m^2 q12h	471	Immunosuppression or symptomatic infection; <56 days of prior Rx; ages 42 days to 15 yrs
Kline et al.[180]	ddI + d4T + IDV; open label	ddI: 90 mg/m^2 q12h d4T: 1 mg/kg q12h IDV: 500 mg/m^2 q12h	12	Symptomatic infection; ≥1 year of NRTI therapy; 4.2–13.5 yrs
Funk et al.[181]	ddI + d4T + NFV; open label	ddI: 180 mg/m^2 bid d4T: 2 mg/kg bid NFV: 60–90 mg/kg tid	8	CDC category A1, B1, or B3; no prior Rx; 14–132 mos

AUC, area under the curve; IDV, indinavir; URIs, upper respiratory infections.
[a]Log_{10} of plasma HIV RNA copies/ml.

CD4 cells/mm³; HIV RNA[a] at Entry	CD4 Response (cells/mm³)	Antiviral Response[a]	Comments
354–410 (mean); 30,827–71, 928 copies/ml (mean)	ddI: +60 ZDV: −15 HYD: −50 ddI + HYD: +50 At wk 24	ddI: no change ZDV: −0.3 HYD: −0.4 ddI + HYD: −1.1 At wk 24	—
364–375 (mean); 4.51–4.54 (mean)	d4T + ddI: +38 d4T + ddI + HYD: +28 Mean at wk 12	d4T + ddI: −1.5 d4T + ddI + HYD: −1.5 Mean at wk 12	Pts. were given option to add HYD at end of 12 wks; only 20–25% were still on HYD at 24 months 116 days
330–360 (mean) 25,000–33,000 mean copies/ml	HYD arm: +50 NFV arm: +100 Median values at 4.5 mos of Rx	HYD arm: −1.2 NFV arm: −1.7 Median at wk 4	Both regimens were comparable in tolerability

CD4 cells/mm³ on Entry	CD4 Response	Antiviral Response[a]	Clinical Outcome	Comments
10–37 (median)	>50 cell/ mm³ increases in 28/87 after 6 mo and in 11/27 after 3 yr	Decrease in p24 below 50 pg/ml in 17/40 at 6 mo and in 57–80% at >60 mo	Longer survival with entry CD4 >100	Interpatient variability in AUC
33 (median)	Median increase of 225/ mm³ at 24 wks	Median decrease of 64 pg/L	84% Gained weight; no overall increase in IQ	ZDV-intolerant patients tolerated lower doses of ZDV in combinations
809 (median)	At 96 wk, CD4 counts were 86% higher in ddI, and 76% were higher in ddI +ZDV than in ZDV monotherapy	At 48 wk, p24 levels were 40% lower for both ddI and ddI +ZDV than in ZDV group	Interim analysis for primary endpoint: ZDV: 27% ddI: 19% ddI +ZDV: 18% ($P = 0.007$) Final analysis: no difference between ddI and ddI +ZDV groups	More hematologic toxicity with ZDV + ddI than ddI alone
18–58% of peripheral lymphocytes	Stable or slightly increased CD4 counts	At 4 wks decrease of plasma RNA of ≥1.5 log_{10} in 7/8; during 6-mo treatment, RNA was undetectable in 2; 0.5–1.5 log_{10} decrease in 5/6	—	Well tolerated
699 (median); 5.1 (median)	ZDV +3TC: +73/mm³ ddI: +4/mm³ at 36–48 wks	ZDV +3TC: −0.80 ddI: −0.28 at wk 12	—	Randomization to ZDV + ddI stopped early because of ACTG152 results; both combination arms had lower rates of disease progression than HIV monotherapy
11–878 (range)	317/mm³ median increase at wk 48	−2.0 decrease at wk 48	—	9/12 completed 48-wk course; 6/12 had crystalluria
606 (median); 606,000 RNA copies/ml	183/mm³ median increase at wk 12	−2.4 decrease at wk 12	Some improvement in adenopathy, and possibly decreased URIs or otitis media	Generally well tolerated; mild diarrhea and elevated triglycerides were seen; no difference in results from a comparative group given ZDV 13TC 1 NFV

▲ CLINICAL INDICATIONS AND CONCLUSIONS

Didanosine is a potent antiretroviral agent whose efficacy has been demonstrated in large-scale clinical trials involving adults and children at various stages of HIV disease progression. In studies of monotherapy, didanosine was superior or equal to zidovudine in most studies when administered initially.[62,132,177] Beneficial effects have been noted when patients have been "switched" from zidovudine to didanosine therapy, irrespective of whether clinical deterioration was present.[40,42,119] Dual combinations of didanosine plus zidovudine or didanosine plus stavudine were generally superior to monotherapy with NRTIs.[62,127,128] Triple combination regimens that contain didanosine have demonstrated potent antiretroviral and CD4 responses. They have included various regimens of didanosine in combination with other NRTIs (zidovudine and lamivudine)[151] NNRTIs (nevirapine,[136] delavirdine), and protease inhibitors (indinavir,[141,142,147] nelfinavir,[122,150] ritonavir[143]). The addition of hydroxyurea potentiated the antiretroviral effect of didanosine, but the resultant CD4 responses were blunted because of the antiproliferative activity of hydroxyurea.[7,168] In vitro resistance to didanosine has been most frequently associated with a change in the *pol* gene at codon 74 (Leu → Val).[13]

Didanosine has an excellent safety profile overall. The major toxicities—pancreatitis and peripheral neuropathy—are infrequently encountered at currently recommended doses,[39,40,42] can be recognized early, and are generally reversible on discontinuation of the drug. As with any NRTI, lactic acidosis and hepatic injury can occur with didanosine and may be particularly severe in patients who receive the drug in combination with hydroxyurea or stavudine (or both),[174] and in pregnant patients.[48]

Drug interactions with didanosine are generally infrequent (Table 3–4), and those related to the antacid and cation content of buffered didanosine formulations can be minimized by appropriately spacing the administration of didanosine and other medications. Such interactions would not be present with the delayed-release EC formulation, which does not contain buffer.

Use of didanosine has been hampered by the poor palatability of the earlier tablet formulations. The currently available tablets and particularly the recently available EC capsules are significantly easier to tolerate. The once-daily dosage regimen of the EC capsules and the approval of once-daily dosing for the buffered formulations adds to the convenience of administration and should enhance adherence to didanosine-containing regimens.

REFERENCES

1. Hitchcock MJM. In vitro antiviral activity of didanosine compared with that of other dideoxynucleoside analogs against laboratory strains and clinical isolates of human immunodeficiency virus. Clin Infect Dis 16(suppl 1):S16, 1993.
2. McGowan JJ, Tomaszewski JE, Cradock J, et al. Overview of the preclinical development of an antiretroviral drug, 2′,3′-dideoxyinosine. Rev Infect Dis 12(suppl 5):S513, 1990.
3. Shelton MJ, O'Donnell AM, Morse GD. Didanosine. Ann Pharmacother 26:660, 1992.
4. Cooney DA, Ahluwalia G, Mitsuay H, et al. Initial studies on the cellular pharmacology of 2′,3′-dideoxyadenosine, an inhibitor of HTLV-III infectivity. Biochem Pharmacol 36:1765, 1987.
5. Reinke CM, Drach JC, Shipman C Jr. Differential inhibition of mammalian DNA polymerases α, β, and γ herpes simplex virus-induced DNA polymerase by the 5′-triphosphates of arabinosyladenine and arabinosylcytosine. In: de The G, Henle W, Rapp F (eds) Oncogenesis and Herpesviruses III. Lyon, IARC Scientific Publications, 1978, p 999.
6. Perry CM, Balfour JA. Didanosine: an update on its antiviral activity, pharmacokinetic properties and therapeutic efficacy in the management of HIV disease. Drugs 52:928, 1996.
7. Perry CM, Noble S. Didanosine: an updated review of its use in HIV infection. Drugs 58:1099, 1999.
8. Domin BA, Mahoney WB, Zimmerman TP. Membrane permeation mechanisms of 2′,3′-dideoxynucleosides. Biochem Pharmacol 46:725, 1993.
9. St Clair MH, Pennington KN, Rooney J. In vitro comparison of selected triple-drug combinations for suppression of HIV-1 replication: the inter-company collaboration protocol. J Acquir Immune Defic Syndr Hum Retrovirol 10(suppl 2):83, 1995.
10. Physicians' Desk Reference. Videx (Didanosine). Montvale, NJ, Medical Economics, 2001.
11. Reichman RC, Tejani N, Lambert LJ, et al. Didanosine (ddI) and zidovudine (ZDV) susceptibilities of human immunodeficiency virus (HIV) isolates from long-term recipients of ddI. Antiviral Res 20:267, 1993.
12. McLeod GX, McGrath JM, Ladd EA, et al. Didanosine and zidovudine resistance patterns in clinical isolates of human immunodeficiency virus type 1 as determined by a replication endpoint concentration assay. Antimicrob Agents Chemother 36:920, 1992.
13. St Clair MH, Martin JL, Tudor-Williams G, et al. Resistance to ddI and sensitivity to AZT induced by a mutation in HIV-1 reverse transcriptase. Science 253:1557, 1991.
14. Gao W-Y, Agbaria R, Driscoll JS, et al. Divergent anti-human immunodeficiency virus activity and anabolic phosphorylation of 2′3′-dideoxynucleoside analogs in resting and activated human cells. J Biol Chem 269:12633, 1994.
15. Aquaro S, Perno C-F, Balestra E, et al. Inhibition of replication of HIV in primary monocyte/macrophages by different antiviral drugs and comparative efficacy in lymphocytes. J Leukoc Biol 62:138, 1997.
16. Faulds D, Brodgen RN. Didanosine: a review of its antiviral activity, pharmacokinetic properties and therapeutic potential in human immunodeficiency virus infection. Drugs 44:94, 1992.
17. Merrill DP, Moonis M, Chou TC, et al. Lamivudine or stavudine in two- and three-drug combinations against human immunodeficiency virus type 1 replication in vitro. J Infect Dis 173:355, 1996.
18. Manion DJ, Hirsh MS. Mechanisms underlying combination anti-retroviral therapies In: Merigan TJ, Bartlett JG, Bolognes D (eds) Textbook of AIDS Medicine. Williams & Wilkins, Baltimore, 2000, p 886.
19. Hammer SM, Inouye RT. Antiviral agents. In: Richman DD, Whiteley RJ, Hayden FG (eds) Clinical Virology. New York, Churchill Livingstone, 1977, p 208.
20. Lori F, Malykh A, Cara A, et al. Hydroxyurea as an inhibitor of human immunodeficiency virus-type 1 replication. Science 266:801, 1994.
21. Burger DM, Meenhorst PL, Beijnen JH. Concise overview of the clinical pharmacokinetics of dideoxynucleoside antiretroviral agents. Pharm World Sci 17:25, 1995.
22. Prescribing Information, Videx EC. Bristol-Meyers Squibb, Princeton, NJ, November 2000.
23. Knupp CA, Shyu WC, Dolin R, et al. Pharmacokinetics of didanosine in patients with acquired immunodeficiency syndrome or acquired immunodeficiency syndrome complex. Clin Pharmacol Ther 49:523, 1991.
24. Hoetelmans RMW, van Heeswijk RPG, Profijt M, et al. Comparison of the plasma pharmacokinetics and renal clearance of didanosine during once and twice daily dosing in HIV-1 infected individuals. AIDS 12(suppl 1):F211, 1998.
25. Shyu WC, Knupp CA, Pittman KA, et al. Food-induced reduction in bioavailability of didanosine. Clin Pharmacol Ther 50:503, 1991.
26. Knupp CA, Milbrath R, Barbhaiya RH. Effect of time of food administration on the bioavailability of didanosine from a chewable tablet formulation. J Clin Pharmacol 33:568, 1993.
27. Dudley MN. Clinical pharmacokinetics of nucleoside antiretroviral agents. J Infect Dis 171(suppl 2):S99, 1995.

28. Hartman NR, Yarchoan R, Pluda JM, et al. Pharmacokinetics of 2′,3′-dideoxyadenosine and 2′,3′-dideoxyinosine in patients with severe human immunodeficiency virus infection. Clin Pharmacol Ther 47:647, 1990.
29. Singlas E, Taburet AM, Borsa Lebas LF, et al. Didanosine pharmacokinetics in patients with normal and impaired renal function: influence of hemodialysis. Antimicrob Agents Chemother 36:1519, 1992.
30. Klecker RW Jr, Collins JM, Yarchoan R, et al. Plasma and cerebrospinal fluid pharmacokinetics of 3′-azido-3′-deoxythimidine: a novel pyrimidine analog with potential application for the treatment of patients with AIDS and related diseases. Clin Pharmacol Ther 41:407, 1987.
31. Burger DM, Kraayeveld CL, Meenhorst PL, et al. Study on didanosine concentrations in cerebrospinal fluid: implications for the treatment and prevention of AIDS dementia complex. Pharm World Sci 17:218, 1995.
32. Wang Y, Livingston E, Patil S, et al. Pharmacokinetics of didanosine in antepartum and postpartum human immunodeficiency virus—infected pregnant women and their neonates: an AIDS clinical trials group study. J Infect Dis 180: 1536, 1999.
33. Dancis J, Lee JD, Mendoza S, et al. Transfer and metabolism of dideoxyinosine by the perfused human placenta. J Acquir Immune Defic Syndr 6:2, 1993.
34. Henderson GI, Perez AB, Yang Y, et al. Transfer of dideoxyinosine across the human isolated placenta. Br J Clin Pharmacol 38:237, 1994.
35. Balis FM, Pizzo PA, Butler KM, et al. Clinical pharmacology 2′,3′-dideoxyinosine in human immunodeficiency virus-infected children. J Infect Dis 165:99, 1992.
36. Stevens RC, Rodman JH, Yong FH, et al. Effect of food and pharmacokinetic variability on didanosine systemic exposure in HIV-infected children: pediatric AIDS Clinical Trials Group protocol 144 study team. AIDS Res Hum Retroviruses 16:415, 2000.
37. Marra CM, Booss J. Does brain penetration of anti-HIV drugs matter? Sex Transm Infect 76:1, 2000.
38. Abreu T, Plaisance K, Rexroad V, et al. Bioavailability of once- and twice-daily regimens of didanosine in human immunodeficiency virus-infected children. Antimicrob Agents Chemother 44:1375, 2000.
39. Dolin R, Amato DA, Fischl MA, et al. Zidovudine compared with didanosine in patients with advanced HIV type 1 infection and little or no previous experience with zidovudine. Arch Intern Med 155:961, 1995.
40. Kahn JO, Lagakos SW, Richman DD, et al. A controlled trial comparing continued zidovudine with didanosine in human immunodeficiency virus infection. N Engl J Med 327:581, 1992.
41. Dolin R. Didanosine (dideoxyinosine, ddI). In Mills J, Corey L (eds) Antiviral Chemotherapy: New Directions for Clinical Application and Research, vol 3. Englewood Cliffs, NJ, Prentice-Hall, 1993, p 363.
42. Spruance SL, Pavia AT, Peterson D, et al. Didanosine compared with continuation of zidovudine in HIV-infected patients with signs of clinical deterioration while receiving zidovudine: a randomized, double-blind clinical trial. Ann Intern Med 120:360, 1994.
43. Pike IM, Nicaise C. The didanosine expanded access program: safety analysis. Clin Infect Dis 16(suppl 1):S63, 1993.
44. Lai KK, Gang DL, Zawacki JK. Fulminant hepatic failure associated with 2′,3′-dideoxyinosine (ddI). Ann Intern Med 115:283, 1991.
45. Ware AJ, Berggren RA, Taylor WE. Didanosine-induced hepatitis. Am J Gastroenterol 95:2141, 2000.
46. Bissuel F, Bruneel F, Habersetzer F, et al. Fulminant hepatitis with severe lactate acidosis in HIV-infected patients on didanosine therapy. J Intern Med 235:367, 1994.
47. Ter Hofstede HJM, de Marie D, Foudraine NA, et al. Clinical features and risk factors of lactic acidosis following long-term antiretroviral therapy: 4 fatal cases. Int J STD AIDS 11:611, 2000.
48. Important Drug Warning [letter]. Princeton, NJ, Bristol-Meyers Squibb, January 5, 2001.
49. Lambert JS, Seidlin M, Reichman RC, et al. 2′,3′-Dideoxyinosine (ddI) in patients with the acquired immunodeficiency syndrome or AIDS-related complex: a phase I trial. N Engl J Med 322:1333, 1990.
50. Styrt BA, Piazza-Hepp TD, Chikami GK. Clinical toxicity of antiretroviral nucleoside analogs. Antivir Res 31:121, 1996.
51. Rozencweig M, McLaren C, Beltangady M, et al. Overview of phase I trials of 2′,3′-dideoxyinosine (ddI) conducted on adult patients. Rev Infect Dis 12(suppl 5):S570, 1990.
52. Yarchoan R, Mitsuya H, Pluda JM, et al. The National Cancer Institute phase I study of 2′,3′-dideoxyinosine administration in adults with AIDS or AIDS-related complex: analysis of activity and toxicity profiles. Rev Infect Dis 12(suppl 5):S522, 1990.
53. Kelleher T, Cross A, Dunkle L. Relation of peripheral neuropathy to HIV treatment in four randomized clinical trials including didanosine. Clin Ther 21:118, 1999.
54. Seminari E, Lisziewicz J, Tinelli C, et al. Hydroxyurea toxicity combined with didanosine (ddI) in HIV-1-seropositive asymptomatic individuals. Int J Clin Pharmacol Ther 37:514, 1999.
55. Moore RD, Wong WM, Keruly JC, McArthur JC. Incidence of neuropathy in HIV-infected patients on monotherapy versus those on combination therapy with didanosine, stavudine and hydroxyurea. AIDS 14:273, 2000.
56. Kieburtz KD, Seidlin M, Lambert JS, et al. Extended follow up of peripheral neuropathy in patients with AIDS and AIDS-related complex treated with dideoxyinosine. J Acquir Immune Defic Syndr 5:60, 1992.
57. Chen CH, Cheng YC. Delayed cytotoxicity and selective loss of mitochondrial DNA in cells treated with anti-human immunodeficiency virus compound 2′,3′-dideoxycytidine. J Biol Chem 264:11934, 1989.
58. Grasela TH, Walawander CA, Beltangady M, et al. Analysis of potential risk factors associated with the development of pancreatitis in phase I patients with AIDS or AIDS-related complex receiving didanosine. J Infect Dis 169:1250, 1994.
59. Schwartz MS, Brandt LJ. The spectrum of pancreatic disorders in patients with the acquired immunodeficiency syndrome. Am J Gastroenterol 84:459, 1989.
60. Jablonowski H, Arasteh K, Staszewski S, et al. A dose comparison study of didanosine in patients with very advanced HIV infection who are intolerant to or clinically deteriorate on zidovudine. AIDS 9:463, 1995.
61. Nguyen B-Y, Yarchoan R, Wyvill KM, et al. Five-year follow up of a phase I study of didanosine in patients with advanced human immunodeficiency virus infection. J Infect Dis 171:1180, 1994.
62. Hammer SM, Katzenstein DA, Hughes MD, et al. A trial comparing nucleoside monotherapy with combination therapy in HIV-infected adults with CD4 cell counts from 200 to 500 per cubic millimeter. N Engl J Med 335:1091, 1996.
63. Whitfield RM, Bechtel L, Schroeder G, et al. Pancreatitis in HIV/AIDS patients taking dideoxyinosine or dideoxycytosine who use ethanol, tobacco, or controlled substances [abstract]. Clin Res 42:46A, 1994.
64. Whitcup SM, Dastgheib K, Nussenblatt RB, et al. A clinicopathologic report of the retinal lesions associated with didanosine. Arch Ophthalmol 112:1594, 1994.
65. Whitcup SM, Butler KM, Pizzo PA. Retinal lesions in children treated with dideoxyinosine. N Engl J Med 326:1226, 1992.
66. Allan JD, Connolly KJ, Fitch H, et al. Long-term follow-up of didanosine administered orally twice daily to patients with advanced human immunodeficiency virus infection and hematologic intolerance of zidovudine. Clin Infect Dis 16(suppl 1):S46, 1993.
67. Monno L, Cargnel A, Soranzo ML, et al. Comparison of once- and twice-daily dosing of didanosine in combination with stavudine for the treatment of HIV-1 infection. Antivir Ther 4(4):195, 1999.
68. Mobley JE, Pollard RB, Schrader S, et al. Virological and immunological responses to once-daily dosing of didanosine in combination with stavudine. AIDS 13:F87, 1999.
69. Kazatchkine MD, Van PN, Costagliola D, et al. Didanosine dosed daily is equivalent to twice daily dosing for patients on double or triple combination antiretroviral therapy. J Acquir Immune Defic Syndr 24:418, 2000.
70. Youle M. Didanosine once daily: an overview. Antivir Ther 3(suppl 4):35, 1998.
71. Pollard RB. Didanosine once-daily: potential for expanded use [review]. AIDS 14:2421, 2000.
72. Van Heeswijk RPG, Veldkamp AI, Mulder JW, et al. Nevirapine plus didanosine: once or twice daily combination? J Acquir Immune Defic Syndr 25:93, 2000.
73. Garcia F, Knobel H, Sambeat MA, et al. Comparison of twice-daily stavudine plus once- or twice-daily didanosine and nevirapine in early stages of HIV infection: the scan study. AIDS 14:2485, 2000.
74. Mayers D, Bethel J, Wainberg MA, et al. Human immunodeficiency virus proviral DNA from peripheral blood and lymph nodes demonstrates concordance resistance mutations to zidovudine (codon 215) and didanosine (codon 74). J Infect Dis 177:1730, 1998.

75. Nielsen C, Bruun L, Mathiesen LR, et al. Development of resistance to zidovudine (ZDV) and didanosine (ddI) in HIV from patients in ZDV, ddI and alternating ZDV/ddI therapy. AIDS 10:625, 1996.
76. Kozal MJ, Kroodsma K, Winters MA, et al. Didanosine resistance in HIV-infected patients switched from zidovudine to didanosine monotherapy. Ann Intern Med 121:263, 1994.
77. Sharma PL, Crumpacker CS. Attenuated replication of human immunodeficiency virus type 1 with a didanosine-selected reverse transcriptase mutation. J Virol 71:8846, 1997.
78. Gu ZX, Gao Q, Li XG, et al. Novel mutation in the human immunodeficiency virus type-1 reverse transcriptase gene that encodes cross-resistance to 2′,3′-dideoxyinosine and 2′,3′-dideoxycytidine. J Virol 66:7128, 1992.
79. Gao Q, Gu Z, Parniak MA, et al. The same mutation that encodes low-level human immunodeficiency virus type 1 resistance to 2′,3′-dideoxyinosine and 2′,3′-dideoxycytidine confers high-level resistance to the (−) enantiomer of 2′,3′-dideoxy-3′-thiacytidine. Antimicrob Agents Chemother 37:1390, 1993.
80. Zhang D, Caliendo AM, Eron JJ, et al. Resistance to 2′,3′-dideoxycytidine conferred by a mutation in codon 65 of the human immunodeficiency virus type 1 reverse transcriptase. Antimicrob Agents Chemother 38:282, 1994.
81. Yerly S, Rakik A, Kaiser L, et al. Analyses of HIV-1 reverse transcriptase genotype in long-term ddI-treated patients. In: Abstracts of the HIV Drug Resistance 4th International Workshop, Sardinia, Italy, 1995, abstract 29.
82. Moyle G. Influence of emergence of viral resistance on HIV treatment choice [letter]. Int J STD AIDS 6:225, 1995.
83. Eron JJ, Chow Y-K, Caliendo AM, et al. Pol mutations conferring zidovudine and didanosine resistance with different effects in vitro yield multiply resistant human immunodeficiency virus type 1 isolates in vivo. Antimicrob Agents Chemother 37:1480, 1993.
84. Demeter LM, Nawaz T, Morse G, et al. Development of zidovudine resistance mutations in patients receiving prolonged didanosine monotherapy. J Infect Dis 172:1480, 1995.
85. Shafer RW, Kozal MJ, Winters MA, et al. Combination therapy with zidovudine and didanosine selects for drug-resistant human immunodeficiency virus type 1 strains with unique patterns of pol gene mutations. J Infect Dis 169:722, 1994.
86. Kojima E, Shirasaka T, Anderson BD, et al. Human immunodeficiency virus type 1 (HIV-1) viremia changes and development of drug-related mutations in patients with symptomatic HIV-1 infection receiving alternating or simultaneous zidovudine and didanosine therapy. J Infect Dis 102(suppl 5B):70, 1995.
87. Brun-Vezinet F, Boucher C, Loveday C, et al. HIV-1 viral load, phenotype, and resistance in a subset of drug-naive participants from the Delta trial: the National Virology Groups, Delta Virology Working Group and Coordinating Committee. Lancet 350:983, 1997.
88. Schooley RT, Ramirez-Ronda C, Lange JMA, et al. Virologic and immunologic benefits of initial combination therapy with zidovudine and zalcitabine or didanosine compared with zidovudine monotherapy. J Infect Dis 173:1354, 1996.
89. Shafer RW, Iversen AKN, Winters MA, et al. Drug resistance and heterogeneous long-term virologic responses of human immunodeficiency virus type 1-infected subjects to zidovudine and didanosine combination therapy. J Infect Dis 172:70, 1995.
90. Shirasaka T, Kavlick MR, Veno T, et al. Emergence of human immunodeficiency virus type 1 variants with resistance to multiple dideoxynucleosides in patients receiving therapy with dideoxynucleosides. Proc Natl Acad Sci USA 92:2398, 1995.
91. Garcia-Lerma JG, Gerrish PJ, Wright AC, et al. Evidence of a role for the Q151L mutation and the viral background in development of multiple dideoxynucleoside-resistant human immunodeficiency virus type 1. J Virol 74:9339, 2000.
92. Kavlick MF, Wyvill K, Yarchoan R, et al. Emergence of multi-dideoxynucleoside-resistant human immunodeficiency virus type 1 variants, viral sequence variation, and disease progression in patients receiving antiretroviral chemothapy. J Infect Dis 177:1506, 1998.
93. Shirasaka T, Kavlick MF, Ueno T, et al. Emergence of human immunodeficiency virus type 1 variants with resistance to multiple dideoxynucleosides in patients receiving therapy with dideoxynucleosides. Proc Natl Acad Sci USA 92:2398, 1995.
94. Winters MA, Coolley KL, Girard YA, et al. A 6-basepair insert in the reverse transcriptase gene of human immunodeficiency virus type 1 confers resistance to multiple nucleoside inhibitors. J Clin Invest 37:A61, 1998.
95. Moreno F, Hardin TC, Rinaldi MG, et al. Itraconazole-didanosine excipient interaction [letter]. JAMA 269:1508, 1993.
96. May DB, Drew RH, Yedinak KC, et al. Effect of simultaneous didanosine administration on itraconazole absorption in healthy volunteers. Pharmacotherapy 14:509, 1994.
97. Acosta EP, Fletcher CV. Antiretroviral drug interactions. Int J Antimicrob Agents 5:73, 1995.
98. Knupp CA, Brater DC, Relue J. Pharmacokinetics of didanosine and ketoconazole after coadministration to patients seropositive for the human immunodeficiency virus. J Clin Pharmacol 33:912, 1993.
99. American Hospital Formulary Service. Didanosine Prescribing Information, 1996.
100. Knupp CA, Barbhaiya RH. A multiple-dose pharmacokinetic interaction study between didanosine (Videx) and ciprofloxacin (Cipro) in male subjects seropositive for HIV but asymptomatic. Biopharm Drug Dispos 18:65, 1997.
101. Knupp CA, Graziano FM, Dixon RM, et al. Pharmacokinetic-interaction study of didanosine and ranitidine in patients seropositive for human immunodeficiency virus. Antimicrob Agents Chemother 36:2075, 1992.
102. Cimoch PJ, Lavelle J, Pollard R, et al. Pharmacokinetics of oral ganciclovir alone and in combination with zidovudine, didanosine, and probenecid in HIV-infected subjects. J Acquir Immune Defic Syndr Hum Retrovir 17:227, 1998.
103. Jung D, Griffy K, Dorr A, et al. Effect of high-dose oral ganciclovir on didanosine disposition in human immunodeficiency virus (HIV)-positive patients. J Clin Pharmacol 38:1057, 1998.
104. Trapnell CB, Cimoch P, Gaines K, et al. Altered didanosine pharmacokinetics with concomitant oral ganciclovir. In: Abstracts of the 95th Annual Meeting of the American Society of Clinical Pharmacology and Therapeutics, 1994, abstract 193.
105. Drugs for HIV infection. Med Lett 39:115, 1997.
106. Morse GD, Fischl MA, Shelton MJ, et al. Single-dose pharmacokinetics of delavirdine mesylate and didanosine in patients with human immunodeficiency virus infection. Antimicrob Agents Chemother 41:169, 1997.
107. Mummaneni V, Kaul S, Knupp CA. Single oral dose pharmacokinetic interaction study of didanosine and indinavir sulfate in healthy subjects [abstract]. J Clin Pharmacol 37:865, 1997.
108. Huengsberg M, Castelino S, Sherrard J, et al. Does drug interaction cause failure of PCP prophylaxis with dapsone? Lancet 341:48, 1993.
109. Sahai J, Garber G, Gallicano K, et al. Effects of the antacids in didanosine tablets on dapsone pharmacokinetics. Ann Intern Med 123:584, 1995.
110. Collier AC, Coombs RW, Fischl MA, et al. Combination therapy with zidovudine and didanosine compared with zidovudine alone in HIV-1 infection. Ann Intern Med 119:786, 1993.
111. Burger DM, Meenhorst PL, Kroon FP, et al. Pharmacokinetic interaction study of zidovudine and didanosine. J Drug Dev 6:187, 1994.
112. Barry M, Howe JL, Ormesher S, et al. Pharmacokinetics of zidovudine and dideoxyinosine alone and in combination in patients with the acquired immunodeficiency syndrome. Br J Clin Pharmacol 37:421, 1994.
113. Shelton MJ, Mei HJ, Hewitt RG. If taken 1 hour before indinavir (IDV), didanosine does not affect IDV exposure, despite persistent buffering effects. Antimicrob Agents Chemother. 45:298, 2001.
114. Pharmacokinetic interaction between ritonavir and didanosine when administered concurrently to HIV-infected patients. J Acquir Immune Defic Syndr Hum Retrovir 18:466, 1998.
115. Knupp C, Srinivas N, Batteiger B. A pK interaction study of didanosine coadministered with or without TMP and/or SMX in HIV seropositive patients [abstract]. Pharm Res 11(suppl):399, 1994.
116. Sahai J, Narang PK, Hawley-Foss N, et al. A phase I evaluation of concomitant rifabutin and didanosine in symptomatic HIV-infected patients. J Acquir Immune Defic Syndr Hum Retrovir 9:274, 1995.
117. Gallicano K, Sahai J, Zaror-Behrens G, et al. Effect of antacids in didanosine tablet on bioavailability of isoniazid. Antimicrob Agents Chemother 38:894, 1994.
118. Aweeka FT, Mathur V, Dorsey R, et al. Pharmacokinetics of concomitant foscarnet and didanosine in patients with HIV disease [abstract]. Clin Pharmacol Ther 57:143, 1995.
119. Seifert RD, Stewart MB, Sramek JJ, et al. Pharmacokinetics of co-administered didanosine and stavudine in HIV-seropositive male patients. Br J Clin Pharmacol 38:405, 1994.

120. Gillum JG, Bruzzese VL, Israel DS, et al. Effect of clarithromycin on the pharmacokinetics of 2′,3′-dideoxyinosine in patients who are seropositive for human immunodeficiency virus. Clin Infect Dis 22:716, 1996.
121. MacGregor TR, Lamson MJ, Cort S, et al. Steady state pharmacokinetics of nevirapine, didanosine, zalcitabine, and zidovudine combination therapy in HIV-1 positive patients [abstract]. Pharm Res 12(suppl):S101, 1995.
122. Elion R, Kaul S, Knupp C, et al. safety profile and antiviral activity of the combination of stavudine, didanosine and nelfinavir in patients with HIV infection. Clin Ther 21:1853, 1999.
123. Rainey PM, Friedland G, McCance-Katz EF, et al. Interaction of methadone with didanosine and stavudine. J Acquir Immune Defic Syndr 24:241, 2000.
124. Montaner JSC, Schechter MT, Rachlis A, et al. Didanosine compared with continuous zidovudine therapy for HIV infected patients, with 200–500 CD4 cells/mm^3. Ann Intern Med 123:561, 1995.
125. Raffi F, Reliquet V, Auger S, et al. Efficacy and safety of stavudine and didanosine combination therapy in antiretroviral-experienced patients. AIDS 12:1999, 1998.
126. Katzenstein DA, Hammer SM, Hughes MD, et al. The relation of virologic and immunologic markers to clinical outcomes after nucleoside therapy in HIV-infected adults with 200 to 500 CD4 cells per cubic millimeter. N Engl J Med 335:1091, 1996.
127. Delta Coordinating Committee. Delta: a randomised double-blind controlled trial comparing combinations of zidovudine plus didanosine or zalcitabine with zidovudine alone in HIV-infected individuals. Lancet 348:283, 1996.
128. Saravolatz LD, Winslow DL, Collins G, et al. Zidovudine alone or in combination with didanosine or zalcitabine in HIV-infected patients with the acquired immunodeficiency syndrome or fewer than 200 CD4 cells per cubic millimeter. N Engl J Med 335:1099, 1996.
129. Graham NMH, Hoover DR, Park LP, et al. Survival in HIV infected patients who have received zidovudine: comparison of combination therapy with sequential monotherapy and continued zidovudine monotherapy. Ann Intern Med 124:1031, 1996.
130. Molina J-M, Chene G, Ferchal F, et al. The ALBI trial: a randomized controlled trial comparing stavudine plus didanosine with zidovudine plus lamivudine and a regimen alternating both combinations in previously untreated patients infected with human immunodeficiency virus. J Infect Dis 180:351, 1999.
131. Raboud JM, Montaner JSG, Rae S, et al. Meta-analysis of five randomized controlled trials comparing continuation of zidovudine vs. switching to didanosine in HIV infected individuals. Antivir Ther 2:237, 1997.
132. Floridia M, Vella S, Seeber AC, et al. A randomized trial (ISS902) of didanosine versus zidovudine in previously untreated patients with mildly symptomatic human immunodeficiency virus infection. J Infect Dis 175:255, 1997.
133. Ruxruntham K, Kroon EDMB, Ungsedhapand C, et al. A randomized dose-finding study with didanosine plus stavudine versus didanosine (ddI) stavudine (d4T) in HIV-infected Thais. AIDS 14:1375, 2000.
134. Henry K, Erice A, Tierney C, et al. A randomized, controlled, double-blind study of d4T + ddI vs. ZDV+ddI as initial treatment HIV-infected subjects with CD4 counts < 500 cells/mm^3 [abstract]. Presented at the 37th Interscience Conference on Anti-microbial Agents and Chemotherapy, September 1997, p 266.
135. Kuritzkes DR, Marschner I, Johnson VA, et al. Lamivudine in combination with zidovudine, stavudine, or didanosine in patients with HIV-1 infection: a randomized double-blind, placebo-controlled trial. AIDS 13:685, 1999.
136. D'Aquila RT, Hughes MD, Johnson VA, et al. Nevirapine, zidovudine, and didanosine compared with zidovudine and didanosine in patients with HIV-1 infection. Ann Intern Med 124:1019, 1996.
137. Montaner JS, Reiss P, Cooper D, et al. A randomized, double-blind trial comparing combinations of nevirapine, didanosine, and zidovudine for HIV-infected patients: the INCAS trial: Italy, The Netherlands, Canada and Australian study. JAMA 279:930, 1998.
138. Raffi F, Reliquet V, Ferre V, et al. The VIRGO study: nevirapine, didanosine and stavudine combination therapy in anti-retroviral naive HIV-1 infected adults. Antivir Ther 5:267, 2000.
139. Friedland GH, Pollard R, Griffith B, et al. Efficacy and safety of delavirdine mesylate with zidovudine and didanosine compared with two-drug combinations of these agents in persons with HIV disease with CD4 counts of 100 to 500 cells/mm^3 (ACTG 261). J Acquir Immune Defic Syndr 21:281, 1999.
140. Molina JM, Ferchal F, Rancinan C, et al. Once-daily combination therapy with emtricitabine, didanosine, and efavirenz in human immunodeficiency virus-infected patients. J Infect Dis 182:599, 2000.
141. Carr A, Chauh J, Hudson J. A randomized, open-label comparison of three highly active antiretroviral therapy regimens including two nucleoside analogues and indinavir for previously untreated HIV-1 infection: the OzCombo 1 study. AIDS 14:1171, 2000.
142. Eron JJ, Murphy RL, Peterson D, et al. A comparison of stavudine, didanosine, and indinavir with zidovudine, lamivudine and indinavir for the initial treatment of HIV-1 infected individuals: selection of thymidine analog regimen therapy (START II). AIDS 14:1601, 2000.
143. Saimot AG, Landman R, Damond F, et al. Stavudine, didanosine and ritonavir as a triple therapy in antiretroviral-naive patients: results at 72 weeks [abstract]. Presented at the 12th World AIDS Conference, Geneva, 1998, p 344.
144. Floridia M, Bucciardini R, Ricciardulle D, et al. A randomized, double-blind trial on the use of a triple combination including nevirapine, a nonnucleoside reverse transcriptase HIV inhibitor, in antiretroviral-naive patients with advanced disease. J Acquir Immune Defic Syndr Hum Retrovir 20:11, 1999.
145. Raffi F, Arasteh K, Gathiram V, et al. 24-Week results of the antiviral activity, safety, and tolerability of emivirine (EMD, Coactinon) + stavudine (d4T, Zerit) + didanosine (ddI, Videx) in treatment-naive HIV-infected patients (MKC-302) [abstract 514]. In: Program and Abstracts of the 7th Conference on Retroviruses and Opportunistic Infections, San Francisco. Alexandria, VA, Foundation for Retrovirology and Human Health, 2000.
146. Squires K, Gatell J, Piliero P, et al. AI424-007: 48-week safety and efficacy results from a phase II study of a once-daily HIV-1 protease inhibitor (PI), BMS-232632 [abstract 15]. In: Program and Abstracts of the 8th Conference on Retroviruses and Opportunistic Infections, Chicago. Alexandria, VA, Foundation for Retrovirology and Human Health, 2001.
147. Gatell J, Murphy R, Katlama C, et al. The Atlantic study: a randomized open-label study comparing two protease inhibitors (PI)-sparing antiretroviral strategies versus a standard PI-containing regimen [abstract 18]. Presented at the 6th Conference on Retroviruses and Opportunistic Infections, Chicago, 1999.
148. Gatell J, Murphy R, Katlama C, et al. The Atlantic study: a randomized open-label study comparing two protease inhibitors (PI)-sparing antiretroviral strategies versus a standard PI-containing regimen, 48 week data. Presented at the 7th European Conference on Clinical Aspects and Treatment of HIV Infection, Lisbon, 1999, p 14.
149. De Mendoza C, Soriano V, Perez-Olmeda M, et al. Efficacy and safety didanosine and lamivudine both once daily plus indinavir in human immunodeficiency virus-infected patients. J Hum Virol 3:335, 2000.
150. Flepp XX, Wang J, Nigg C, et al. Nelfinavir, didanosine, and stavudine in HIV-infected drug users enrolled in opiate substitution programs at four outpatients clinics—the Zurich Prometheus Study [abstract]. AIDS 12(suppl 4):S41, 1998.
151. Lafeuillade A, Poggi C, Tamalet C, et al. Effects of a combination of zidovudine, didanosine, and lamivudine on primary human immunodeficiency virus type 1 infection. J Infect Dis 175:1051, 1997.
152. Luzzati R, Di Perri G, Fendt D, et al. Pharmacokinetics, safety and anti-human immunodeficiency virus (HIV) activity of hydroxyurea in combination with didanosine. J Antimicrob Chemother 42:565, 1998.
153. De BRJ, Boucher CAB, Perelson AS. Target cell availability and the successful suppression of HIV by hydroxyurea and didanosine. AIDS 12:1567, 1998.
154. Montaner JSG, Zala C, Raboud JM, et al. A pilot study of hydroxyurea (HO-urea) as adjuvant therapy among patients with advanced HIV disease receiving didanosine (ddI) therapy: Canadian HIV Trials Network protocol 080. J Infect Dis 175:801, 1997.
155. Hellinger JA, Iwane MK, Smith JJ, et al. A randomized study of the safety and antiretroviral activity of hydroxyurea combined with didanosine in persons infected with human immunodeficiency virus type 1. American Foundation for AIDS Research Community-Based Clinical Trials Network. J Infect Dis 181:540, 2000.
156. Clotet B, Ruiz L, Cabrerea C, et al. Short-term anti-HIV activity of the combination of didanosine and hydroxyurea. Antivir Ther 1:189, 1996.
157. Biron F, Lucht F, Peyramond D, et al. Pilot clinical trial of the combination of hydroxyurea and didanosine in HIV-1 infected individuals. Antivir Res 29:111, 1996.

158. Foli A, Lori F, Maserati R, et al. Hydroxyurea and didanosine is a more potent combination than hydroxyurea and zidovudine. Antivir Ther 2:31, 1997.
159. Lori F, Jessen H, Foli A, et al. Long-term suppression of HIV-1 by hydroxyurea and didanosine. JAMA 277:1437, 1997.
160. Foli A, Lori F, Maserati R, et al. Hydroxyurea and didanosine is a more potent combination than hydroxyurea and zidovudine. Antivir Ther 2:31, 1997.
161. Rutschmann OT, Opravil M, Iten A. A placebo-controlled trial of didanosine plus stavudine, with and without hydroxyurea, for HIV infection. AIDS 12:F71, 1998.
162. Jaegel-Guedes E, Wolf E, Goeppner S, et al. d4T/ddI plus hydroxyurea: an alternative to a PI containing triple regimen in ART-naive HIV^+ patients [abstract]. Presented at the 12th World AIDS Conference, Geneva, 1998, p 583.
163. Rutschmann OT, Vernazza PL, Bucher HC, et al. Long-term hydroxyurea in combination with didanosine and stavudine for the treatment of HIV-1 infection. AIDS 14:2145, 2000.
164. Lisziewicz J, Jessen H, Finzi D, et al. HIV-1 suppression by early treatment with hydroxyurea, didanosine, and a protease inhibitor. Lancet 352:199, 1998.
165. Lori F, Rosenberg E, Lieberman J, et al. Hydroxyurea and didanosine long-term treatment prevents HIV breakthrough and normalizes immune parameters. AIDS Res Hum Retroviruses 15:1333, 1999.
166. Lori F, Jessen H, Foli A. Long-term suppression of HIV replication and cell proliferation leads to minimal levels of proviral DNA and to immune recovery [abstract]. Presented at the 12th World AIDS Conference, Geneva, 1998, p 778.
167. Lori F, Lisziewicz J. Rationale for the use of hydroxyurea as an anti-human immunodeficiency virus drug. Clin Infect Dis 30(suppl 2):S193, 2000.
168. Zala C, Rouleau D, Montaner JS. Role of hydroxyurea in treatment of disease due to human immunodeficiency virus infection. Clin Infect Dis 30(suppl 2):S143, 2000.
169. Biron F, Ponceau B, Bouhour D. Long-term safety and antiretroviral activity of hydroxyurea and didanosine in HIV-infected patients. J Acquir Immune Defic Syndr 25:329, 2000.
170. Hydroxyurea in the treatment of HIV-1 infection: toxicity and side effects [review]. J Biol Regul Homeost Agents 13:181, 1999.
171. McCarthy WF, Gable J, Lawrence J, et al. A retrospective study to determine if hydroxyurea augmentation of antiretroviral drug regimens that contain ddI and/or d4T increases the risk of developing peripheral neuropathy in HIV-1 infected individuals. Pharmacoepidemiol Drug Safety 9:49, 2000.
172. Cepeda JA, Wilks D. Excess peripheral neuropathy in patients treated with hydroxyurea plus didanosine and stavudine for HIV infection [letter]. AIDS 14:332, 2000.
173. Longhurst HJ, Pinching AJ. Drug points: pancreatitis associated with hydroxyurea in combination with didanosine. BMJ 322:81, 2001.
174. Boxwell D, Toerner J. Fatal hepatoxicity associated with combination hydroxyurea and nucleoside reverse transcriptase inhibitors (NRTIs): cases from the FDA adverse event reporting system (AERS). Presented at the 8th conference on Retroviruses and Opportunistic Infections, Chicago, 2001, abstract 671.
175. Mueller BU, Butler KM, Stocker VL, et al. Clinical and pharmacokinetic evaluation of long-term therapy with didanosine in children with HIV infection. Pediatrics 94:724, 1994.
176. Husson RN, Mueller BU, Farley M, et al. Zidovudine and didanosine combination therapy in children with human immunodeficiency virus infection. Pediatrics 93:316, 1994.
177. Englund JA, Baker CJ, Raskino C, et al. Zidovudine, didanosine, or both as the initial treatment for symptomatic HIV-infected children. N Engl J Med 336:1704, 1997.
178. Luzuriaga K, Bryson Y, Krogstad P, et al. Combination treatment with zidovudine, didanosine, and nevirapine in infants with human immunodeficiency virus type 1 infection. N Engl J Med 336:1343, 1997.
179. Paediatric European Network for Treatment of AIDS. A randomized double-blind trial of the addition of lamivudine or matching placebo to current nucleoside analogue reverse transcriptase inhibitor therapy in HVI-infected children: the PENTA-4 trial. AIDS 12:F151, 1998.
180. Kline MW, Fletcher CV, Harris AT, et al. A pilot study of combination therapy with indinavir, stavudine (d4T), and didanosine (ddI) in children infected with the human immunodeficiency virus. J Pediatr 132:543, 1998.
181. Funk MB, Linde R, Wintergerst U, et al. Preliminary experiences with triple therapy including nelfinavir and two reverse transcriptase inhibitors in previously untreated HIV-infected children. AIDS 13:1653, 1999.
182. Butler KM, Husson RN, Balis FM, et al. Dideoxyinosine in children with symptomatic human immunodeficiency virus infection. N Engl J Med 324:137, 1991.
183. Blanche S, Calvez T, Rouzioux C, et al. Randomized study of two doses of didanosine in children infected with human immunodeficiency virus. J Pediatr 122:966, 1993.
184. McKinney RE Jr, Johnson GM, Stanley K, et al. A randomized study of combined zidovudine-naive HIV-1 infection: the pediatric AIDS Clinical Trials Group protocol 300 study team. J Pediatr 133:500, 1998.
185. Kline MW, Fletcher CV, Federici ME, et al. Combination therapy with stavudine and didanosine in children with advanced human immunodeficiency virus infection: pharmacokinetic properties, safety and immunologic and virologic effects. Pediatrics 97:886, 1996.
186. Kline MW, Van Dyke RB, Lindsey JC, et al. Combination therapy with stavudine (d4T) plus didanosine (ddI) in children with human immunodeficiency virus infection: the pediatric AIDS Clinical Trials Group 327 team. Pediatrics 103:e62, 1999.
187. Kline M, Fletcher CV, Brundage RC, et al. Combination therapy with saquinavir soft gelatin capsules plus nucleoside anti-retroviral agents in HIV-infected children [abstract]. Presented at the 12th World AIDS Conference, Geneva, 1998, p 64.
188. Fletcher CV, Brundage RC, Remmel RP, et al. Pharmacologic characteristics of indinavir, didanosine, and stavudine in human immunodeficiency virus-infected children receiving combination therapy. Antimicrob Agents Chemother 44:1029, 2000.

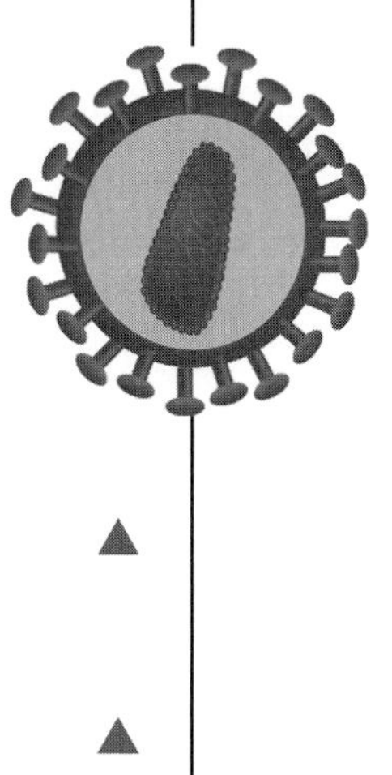

CHAPTER 4
Zalcitabine

John A. Bartlett, MD

Zalcitabine (2′, 3′-dideoxycytidine, ddC, HIVID) is a pyrimidine analogue whose synthesis was originally described by Horwitz et al. in 1966.[1] The antiretroviral activity of zalcitabine was first recognized in 1986,[2] and it was approved by the Food and Drug Administration (FDA) in 1992, initially only for use in combination with zidovudine. Of historical interest, zalcitabine was the third antiretroviral drug approved by the FDA and the first agent to receive licensure through the FDA's accelerated approval process.

▲ STRUCTURE

Zalcitabine is derived from cytidine (similar to lamivudine) and lacks the 3′-OH moiety on the ribose sugar (Fig. 4–1). Zalcitabine shares its nucleotide base with lamivudine, but they differ in their sugar moieties and stereochemistry. To become active as an antiretroviral agent, zalcitabine must undergo triphosphorylation to the 5′-triphosphate form.

▲ MECHANISMS OF ACTION AND IN VITRO ACTIVITY

Zalcitabine acts as an inhibitor of human immunodeficiency virus type 1 (HIV-1) reverse transcriptase and as a chain terminator.[2] It inhibits HIV-1 replication and protects against cytopathogenicity at concentrations of 0.5 μM.[2–4] Zalcitabine is active against HIV-1 in a variety of cell lines, including peripheral blood lymphocytes and those derived from lymphocytes or monocyte/macrophages, although its inhibitory activity and metabolism may be different across cell lines.[4] Zalcitabine is especially active against macrophage-tropic strains in monocyte/macrophage cell lines, with a median inhibitory concentration (IC_{50}) of 0.002 μM, compared to 0.01 μM for didanosine and 0.20 μM for zidovudine.[5] Zalcitabine is active against zidovudine-resistant HIV-1 isolates,[6–8] HIV-2,[9] and hepatitis B virus[10,11] but not against herpes simplex virus 1 or 2.[12] Zalcitabine has synergy with zidovudine, delavirdine, saquinavir, and interferon-α.[13–15] In contrast, zalcitabine has demonstrated antagonism with ribavirin, perhaps through ribavirin's inhibition of zalcitabine's phosphorylation.[16,17] In vitro cytotoxicity from zalcitabine has usually been demonstrated at concentrations of 10 μM or higher, although Molt-4 cells have demonstrated an increased doubling time, decreased cellular content of mitochondrial DNA, and decreased rate of glycolysis at 0.5 or 0.2 μM.[18]

The intracellular metabolism of zalcitabine begins with cellular entry through both nucleoside carrier-mediated and non-carrier-mediated mechanisms.[19–21] Zalcitabine then undergoes triphosphorylation by cellular kinases that are also used by 2′-deoxycytidine.[22] The process of triphosphorylation occurs in both HIV-infected and HIV-uninfected cell lines.[19,23,24] Anywhere from 2% to 40% of zalcitabine is converted to its triphosphate form, 2′,3′-dideoxycytidine 5′-triphosphate (ddCTP), depending on the cell line studied.[19,25,26] Zalcitabine is most efficiently triphosphorylated in resting peripheral blood mononuclear cells, in contrast to zidovudine, which is most efficiently triphosphorylated in activated cells.[27,28] The ddCTP binds to HIV-1 reverse transcriptase with a K_i of 0.2 to 0.9 μM.[29,30]; it does not bind efficiently to host α DNA polymerase, but it has been spec-

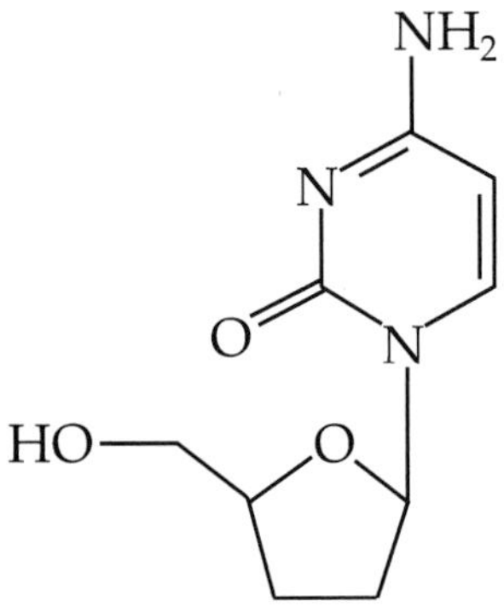

Figure 4–1. Biochemical structure of zalcitabine.

ulated that zalcitabine's neurotoxicity may be related to its inhibition of host β and γ DNA polymerases.[18] The efflux of ddCTP from Molt-4 cells follows a biphasic pattern with an initial retention half-life of 2.6 hours.[25]

▲ PHARMACOKINETICS

Zalcitabine has been administered over the dose range 0.007 to 0.50 mg/kg, although a clear dose–response relation with peripheral neuropathy at doses of more than 0.01 mg/kg has limited the use of higher doses.[31–34] Zalcitabine has linear pharmacokinetics over the dose range 0.03 to 0.5 mg/kg.[32,33] It is approximately 70% to 90% bioavailable following oral administration of zalcitabine oral solution or tablets.[32,33] The maximum plasma concentration of zalcitabine after an oral dose of 1.5 mg is 0.12 μM, which occurs 0.8 hour after dosing. Administration of zalcitabine with food decreases the maximum plasma concentration by 39%, prolongs the time to achieve maximum concentrations to 1.6 hours, and decreases the plasma concentration area under the curve (AUC) by 14%.[9]

Zalcitabine is rapidly eliminated, with a total body clearance of approximately 250 ml/min/m^2 after single and multiple doses. In patients with normal renal function, the plasma elimination half-life is 1 to 3 hours.[32,33] As a result, zalcitabine is recommended for every-8-hour oral dosing. The results of one study of zalcitabine dosed twice daily have been presented, but they are inconclusive given the small sample size, the lack of a comparator arm using zalcitabine dosed every 8 hours, and the preliminary nature of their results.[34] No significant drug accumulation was noted after 14 days of intravenous dosing.[32,33]

Zalcitabine reaches a steady-state volume of distribution of 0.5 to 0.6 L/kg in adults, and less than 4% is bound to plasma proteins.[9] Zalcitabine concentrations in cerebrospinal fluid approximate 20% of plasma levels.[31] Zalcitabine does not undergo hepatic metabolism, and approximately 75% and 62% of intravenous and oral doses, respectively, are recovered unchanged in the urine over 24 hours.[32] In seven patients with creatinine clearances of less than 55 ml/min, the plasma half-life of zalcitabine was prolonged to 8.5 hours.[9] Similar pharmacokinetics have been observed in HIV-infected children, although zalcitabine bioavailability is more variable in children (29% to 100%) than in adults.[35]

▲ TOXICITY

The reported toxicities of zalcitabine include peripheral neuropathy, stomatitis, rash, and pancreatitis. The major studies of zalcitabine that describe toxicities are summarized in Table 4–1.

Peripheral Neuropathy

The most common toxicity related to zalcitabine is a peripheral neuropathy.[36–39] The frequency of peripheral neuropathy is clearly dose-related and was reported in up to 100% of subjects receiving zalcitabine 0.03 mg/kg q4h.[36] Moderate peripheral neuropathy has been reported in 10% to 23% of patients taking zalcitabine, and severe peripheral neuropathy has been reported in 0% to 15%.[39,40,42–44] In randomized trials comparing zalcitabine-containing and didanosine-containing regimens, the frequency of zalcitabine-associated severe peripheral neuropathy was higher (5% vs. 1%[42] and 15.0% vs. 6.6%,[44] respectively). Baseline characteristics associated with a higher frequency of zalcitabine-associated peripheral neuropathy include a lower absolute CD4+ T-lymphocyte number,[38] diabetes mellitus,[45] lower baseline vitamin B_{12} levels, heavy alcohol consumption, and a history of symptomatic peripheral neuropathy.[46] Symptoms typically begin at a mean of 10 to 18 weeks after initiating zalcitabine[45–47] and most commonly involve the distal lower extremities.[45,46] The symptoms usually begin in a symmetrical stocking distribution, with numbness, aching, and burning dysesthesias. On examination, patients may have diminished sensation in response to light touch, pinprick, temperature, and vibration; and up to 60% may have absent ankle deep tendon reflexes.[45,48] Nerve conduction studies reveal a sensory axonal neuropathy with decreased to absent sensory nerve action potentials and normal distal latencies and velocities.[48] The symptoms of zalcitabine-associated peripheral neuropathy may worsen for up to 5 weeks following its discontinuation[31,48] but then slowly improve. More severe neuropathic symptoms may not return to baseline. If symptoms resolve, most patients are able to tolerate the careful reintroduction of half-dose zalcitabine.[45] Preexisting zalcitabine-associated peripheral neuropathy may predispose to neuropathic exacerbation on didanosine,[49] so didanosine should be substituted for zalcitabine with caution.

Stomatitis

Stomatitis was reported in 8 of 20 patients in the first dose-escalation Phase I trial of zalcitabine.[31] The ulcerations most commonly occur on the buccal mucosa, soft palate, tongue, or pharynx. They are usually self-limited and resolve with continued therapy. In large clinical trials utilizing zalcitabine at doses of 0.75 mg q8h, the reported frequency of moderate to severe oral ulcerations is 2% to

Table 4–1. TOXICITIES ASSOCIATED WITH ZALCITABINE

Trial	Dose	Entry Criteria	Peripheral Neuropathy	Stomatitis	Pancreatitis	Other Toxicities	Comments
Yarchoan et al.[31]	0.03–0.25 mg/kg IV and PO q8h	ARC or AIDS CD4 <350/mm^3	All 10 subjects treated for >6 wk	8/20	None reported	Rash 14/20	
Merigan et al.[36]	0.005–0.06 mg/kg PO q4h	Advanced ARC or AIDS p24 antigen ≥100 pg/ml	0.005 mg/kg q4h 17% 0.01 mg/kg q4h 80% 0.03 mg/kg q4h 100% 0.06 mg/kg q4h 100%	0.005 mg/kg q4h 7/15 0.01 mg/kg q4h 9/11 0.03 mg/kg q4h 11/15 0.06 mg/kg q4h 16/18	None reported	Rash 39/61	
ACTG 047 (Skowron et al.[37])	0.01–0.03 mg/kg PO q4h	ARC or AIDS p24 antigen >70 pg/ml	0.1 mg/kg 15% 0.03 mg/kg 34%* *$P = 0.04$	None reported	None reported	Anaphylactoid symptoms (1), fever (1) reversible hearing loss (1)	Dose-response relation with peripheral neuropathy; neuropathic symptoms occurred within first 24 weeks in 68%.
ACTG 119 (Fischl et al.[38])	0.75 mg PO q8h	Severe ARC or AIDS ≥ 48 wk prior ZDV	Severe peripheral neuropathy in 6/59 (10%) on ddC; 0/52 on ZDV	Mouth ulcers (1) and esophageal ulcers (1) leading to ddC discontinuation	1 Subject on ddC	Hepatotoxicity (1) leading to ddC discontinuation; (1) leading to ZDV discontinuation	
ACTG 155 (Fischl et al.[39])	0.75 mg PO q8h	ARC or AIDS with CD4 <300/mm^3 or asymptomatic with CD4 <200/mm^3 >6 mo prior ZDV	Moderate or worse neuropathy ZDV 13% ddC 23% ZDV + ddC 22% ($P < 0.005$) Severe neuropathy ZDV 4% ddC 6% ZDV + ddC 6% ($P = 0.51$)	ddC 4% ddC + ZDV 1% ZDV 1%	ddC 9 (3%) ddC + ZDV 8 (2%) ZDV 4 (1%) One fatal episode of pancreatitis in ZDV + ddC group	None reported	Increased frequency of peripheral neuropathy at lower baseline CD4; 1 fatal pancreatitis case.
					None reported	Arthralgias (1) Myalgias (1)	
ACTG 106 (Meng et al.[40])	0.005–0.01 mg/kg q8h	Advanced ARC or AIDS CD4 <200/mm^3 Treatment naive	1/29 severe neuropathy at 0.005 mg/kg; 1/18 severe neuropathy at 0.01 mg/kg	None reported	None reported	Transaminase elevations >5 × ULN in 4 subjects	
ACTG 175 (Hammer et al.[41])	0.75 mg q8h	Asymptomatic with CD4 200–500/mm^3	Not reported	Not reported	Not reported	Not reported	
Delta Coordinating Committee[42]	0.75 mg PO q8h	CD4 50–350/mm^3	Severe neuropathy ZDV + ddC 5% ZDV + ddC 1% ZDV 2%	Mouth ulcers ZDV + ddC 3%	ZDV + ddC 0.5% ZDV + ddI 1%	Transaminase elevations ZDV + ddC 7% ZDV + ddI 5% ZDV 5%	

ddI, didanosine; SQV, saquinavir; 3TC, lamivudine; ULN, upper limit of normal; ZDV, zidovudine.
CD4 indicates the CD4+ T-lymphocyte count.

4%.[39,40,42,43] One case of more severe esophageal ulceration that required discontinuation of zalcitabine has also been reported.[50]

Rash

Rash was reported in 14 of 20 patients in the first dose-escalation Phase I trial of zalcitabine.[31] The rash is most commonly an erythematous, maculopapular eruption over the trunk and extremities. It usually begins after 10 to 14 days of zalcitabine therapy and is self-limited. Larger trials have not reported the frequency of zalcitabine-associated rash, presumably because it is mild and self-limited. Skin biopsies of the rash reveal perivascular lymphocytic infiltrates.[51]

Pancreatitis

Pancreatitis has been reported infrequently in zalcitabine-treated patients. Large trials suggest a frequency of 0.5 to 3.0%.[37,38,40,42] Trials that have randomized subjects to either zalcitabine or didanosine suggest that zalcitabine-associated pancreatitis occurs less commonly (0.5% vs. 1%[40] and 0.5% vs. 2.2%, 42 respectively). One case of fatal zalcitabine-associated pancreatitis has been reported.[38]

Other Toxicities

Miscellaneous toxicities attributed to zalcitabine include cardiomyopathy,[9] anaphylactoid reactions,[37] fever,[37] reversible hearing loss,[37] arthralgias,[43] and myalgias.[43] Zalcitabine's potential to cause hepatotoxicity remains unclear; transaminase elevations led to drug discontinuation in one subject,[39] and a large randomized trial revealed transaminase elevations in 7.1% of subjects receiving zalcitabine/zidovudine, 5% of subjects receiving didanosine/zidovudine, and 5.1% of subjects receiving zidovudine alone.[42] There are no available data regarding the use of zalcitabine during pregnancy.

▲ EFFICACY

Zalcitabine has been evaluated extensively as monotherapy and two- and three-drug combinations in HIV-infected subjects. The results of major efficacy studies are summarized in Table 4–2.

Zalcitabine Monotherapy

Many early trials evaluated zalcitabine monotherapy in subjects with relatively late-stage HIV infection.[31,36–39,52,53] The designs of these trials included dose-escalation studies,[31,36] zalcitabine alternating with zidovudine,[37] and comparisons of zalcitabine monotherapy with zidovudine[38,39,52] or didanosine[53] monotherapies. Increases in absolute CD4+ T-lymphocyte number of zalcitabine-treated subjects were extremely small,[31] if they changed at all from baseline.[36] In patients with severe acquired immunodeficiency syndrome (AIDS)-related complex (ARC) or AIDS and 48 weeks or less of prior zidovudine, subjects randomized to zalcitabine had less decline in absolute CD4+ T-lymphocytes than zidovudine-treated subjects at 28 weeks.[38]

In contrast to the modest absolute CD4+ T-lymphocyte response in zalcitabine-treated subjects, serum p24 antigen levels responded more favorably.[31,36,37] In one dose-escalation study, most subjects experienced at least a 50% decline from baseline in serum p24 antigen levels.[36] Similar results were seen in subjects receiving alternating zalcitabine and zidovudine compared to those receiving zidovudine alone. Zidovudine-experienced subjects were less likely to have p24 antigen suppression, and in the ACTG 155 study no significant difference was noted between zalcitabine- and zidovudine-treated subjects.[39]

The clinical outcomes reported in zalcitabine-treated subjects are variable, and their inconsistency probably reflects the inadequacy of antiretroviral monotherapy. The ACTG 114 study, performed in subjects with ARC or AIDS and less than 3 months of prior zidovudine, reported more frequent progression to AIDS or death in zalcitabine-treated subjects compared to those receiving zidovudine.[51] Studies ACTG 119 and 155, both performed in subjects with ARC or AIDS and more zidovudine experience (ACTG 119: ≤48 weeks; ACTG 155: >6 months), revealed no differences in progression to AIDS or death, or survival, between zalcitabine- and zidovudine-treated subjects.[38,39] The CPCRA 002 study was performed in subjects with absolute CD4+ T-lymphocyte counts of less than 300 cells per cubic millimeter and either zidovudine intolerance or more than 6 months of prior zidovudine with disease progression. Subjects were randomized to zalcitabine or didanosine monotherapy, and the results suggested a possible survival advantage for zalcitabine over didanosine, with an adjusted relative risk of 0.65 (P = 0.003).[53]

Combination Therapy with Zalcitabine

Combination treatment with zalcitabine and zidovudine can clearly increase the absolute CD4+ T-lymphocyte number more than zidovudine monotherapy in treatment-naive subjects.[41–43] The magnitude of the absolute CD4+ T-lymphocyte increase in zalcitabine/zidovudine-treated subjects in these trials varied between 40 and 100 cells per cubic millimeter at 8 weeks. In one trial, the absolute CD4+ T-lymphocyte change from baseline was not significantly different at 72 weeks in subjects treated with zalcitabine/zidovudine or didanosine/zidovudine.[43]

Zidovudine-experienced subjects who add zalcitabine to their treatment may have higher absolute CD4+ T-lymphocyte increases than those who are randomized to continue on zidovudine monotherapy,[39,41] although one trial failed to show this difference.[42] The NUCA 3002 trial compared zalcitabine/zidovudine to lamivudine/zidovudine in experienced subjects. The results showed that adding zalcitabine to zidovudine provided an extremely small increase in absolute CD4+ T-lymphocyte number of short duration, and that the lamivudine/zidovudine group had greater absolute CD4+ T-lymphocyte increases.[56] Cumulatively, these results suggest that adding zalcitabine to zidovudine therapy can increase the absolute CD4+ T-lymphocyte number modestly, but the magnitude of this increase in experienced subjects is lower than in naive subjects and varies between 0 and 30 cells per cubic millimeter at 8 weeks.

Suppression of serum p24 antigen levels was greater in subjects receiving zalcitabine/zidovudine than in those receiving zalcitabine or zidovudine alone.[39] Serum p24 antigen suppression has shown a dose–response relation with zalcitabine and zidovudine doses, and the greatest suppression has been achieved at full doses of both drugs.[40] In more recent trials, plasma HIV RNA levels were monitored in subjects receiving zalcitabine/zidovudine. Treatment-naive subjects receiving both drugs achieved greater suppression of plasma HIV RNA levels than those receiving zidovudine alone.[40] In treatment-naive subjects, the magnitude of the change in plasma HIV RNA levels at 52 weeks was approximately 0.6 $\log_{10}$ copies per millimeter in the zalcitabine/zidovudine recipients and was not significantly different from those receiving didanosine/zidovudine.[43] In experienced subjects, no significant difference was seen in plasma HIV RNA suppression over 52 weeks between those receiving zalcitabine/zidovudine or lamivudine/zidovudine.[56] In treatment-experienced subjects receiving zalcitabine/zidovudine, the magnitude of suppression was approximately 0.4 $\log_{10}$ copies per milliliter over 52 weeks.

The clinical outcomes associated with zalcitabine/zidovudine have been studied in several large clinical trials. In treatment-naive subjects, progression to AIDS or death was less frequent for zalcitabine/zidovudine recipients compared with those receiving zidovudine alone[41,42] (relative risk 0.49[41] to 0.80[42]). Survival was improved in one trial[42] but did not achieve statistical significance in the other.[41] In one study, didanosine/zidovudine had a lower relative risk of progression to AIDS or death than zalcitabine/zidovudine, but survival was not significantly different.[42]

In treatment-experienced subjects it has been much more difficult to show improved clinical outcomes for any double nucleoside reverse transcriptase inhibitor (NRTI) combination. The ACTG 155, ACTG 175, CPCRA 007, and Delta 2 studies have all failed to show any improvement regarding progression to AIDS or death, or survival alone, in the recipients of zalcitabine/zidovudine compared to continued zidovudine monotherapy.[39,41,42,44] Only a stratified analysis in ACTG 155 identified improvements in disease progression or death in subjects with baseline absolute CD4+ T-lymphocyte counts higher than 150 cells per cubic millimeter. The CPCRA 007 and Delta 2 studies also showed no difference in clinical outcomes between zalcitabine/zidovudine recipients versus didanosine/zidovudine recipients.[42,44]

Three-drug combinations including zalcitabine have also undergone evaluation.[54,55,57] In the ACTG 229 study, the magnitude of absolute CD4+ T-lymphocyte increases was greater for the recipients of zalcitabine/zidovudine/saquinavir versus zalcitabine or zidovudine alone.[57] Plasma HIV RNA levels also achieved better suppression with three drugs than with two drugs in the same trial.[57] Clinical outcomes have been studied in two other trials, ACTG 193A and SV 14604. ACTG 193A studied two-drug combinations of didanosine alternating with zidovudine, didanosine/zidovudine, and zalcitabine/zidovudine versus a three-drug combination of didanosine/zidovudine/nevirapine in subjects with absolute CD4+ T-lymphocyte counts of more than 50 cells per cubic millimeter.[54] The three-drug combination offered improved clinical outcomes compared to didanosine alternating with zidovudine or zalcitabine/zidovudine. Finally, SV 14604 studied zidovudine alone, zalcitabine/zidovudine, saquinavir/zidovudine, and zalcitabine/zidovudine/saquinavir in 3485 subjects with zidovudine experience of 16 weeks or more.[55] The three-drug combination resulted in significantly less risk of the occurrence of a primary endpoint (disease progression or death) than zalcitabine/zidovudine but did not significantly affect survival when analyzed separately.

▲ RESISTANCE

Zalcitabine resistance is not easily identified from in vitro serial HIV passages or clinical isolates. High-level resistance (>100-fold changes in IC_{50}) has not been reported to date from in vitro studies or clinical trials.[58] Low-level to moderate-level resistance has been associated with five mutations in the *pol* gene: $Lys_{65} \rightarrow$ Arg, $Thr_{69} \rightarrow$ Arg, $Leu_{74} \rightarrow$ Val, $Gln_{151} \rightarrow$ Met, and $Met_{184} \rightarrow$ Val/Ile.[58] All five mutations are within or close to conserved motifs near the catalytic site of reverse transcriptase. All of these mutations may be associated with cross-resistance to didanosine, lamivudine, or zidovudine, except $Thr_{69} \rightarrow$ Asp.

The results of phenotypic and genotypic assays suggest the infrequent detection of zalcitabine resistance in subjects receiving zalcitabine/zidovudine. In the BW 34, 225–02 trial studying treatment-naive subjects, no change in phenotypic zalcitabine sensitivity was noted in 10 subjects receiving zalcitabine/zidovudine over 48 weeks.[43] However, two of these subjects did have codon 184 mutations when genotypic assays were performed. A subsequent study did not identify any M184V mutations in eight persons with treatment failure receiving zidovudine/zalcitabine.[59] Interestingly, zalcitabine/zidovudine therapy did not delay the onset of phenotypic zidovudine resistance in the BW 34, 225–02 study compared with zidovudine alone. Similar results in the ACTG 106 study documented a lack of zalcitabine resistance in phenotypic assays in 15 treatment-naive subjects receiving zalcitabine/zidovudine for 36 months.[60] In Delta 1 study subjects receiving zalcitabine/zidovudine, no zalcitabine resistance mutations were found in genotypic assays after 112 weeks.[61] Using the sensitive LiPA technique to detect point mutations, no L74V mutations were noted in eight patients who failed a zidovudine/zalcitabine regimen.[59]

In zidovudine-experienced patients, it is also difficult to detect zalcitabine resistance when zalcitabine is added, although these subjects can have zalcitabine-resistant strains prior to the initiation of zalcitabine therapy as a result of cross-resistance with zidovudine.[62,63] Zalcitabine resistance was not observed at baseline in the NUCA 3002 trial, and

▲ **Table 4–2.** MAJOR ACTIVITY AND EFFICACY TRIALS EVALUATING ZALCITABINE MONOTHERAPY AND COMBINATION THERAPY

Trial	Design	No. of Dose	Subjects	Entry Criteria	CD4 Response
ACTG 047 (Skowron et al.[37])	Alternating ddC + ZDV vs. continuous ZDV	0.01–0.03 mg/kg q4h ddC	131	ARC or AIDS p24 >70 pg/ml	Greatest in alternating limbs
ACTG 114[52]	ddC vs. ZDV	0.75 mg PO q8h ddC	635	ARC or AIDS CD4 ≤200/mm³ <3 mo prior ZDV	
ACTG 155 (Fischl et al.[39])	ddC vs. ZDV vs. ZDV + ddC	0.75 mg PO q8h	1001	ARC or AIDS with CD4 <300/mm³ or asymptomatic with CD4 <200/mm³ ZDV >6 mo	No significant difference vs. ZDV + ddC
CPCRA 002 (Abrams et al.[53])	ddC vs. ddI	0.75 mg PO q8h	467	CD4 <300/mm³ ZDV intolerant or ≥6 mo prior ZDV with disease progression	Not included
ACTG 175 (Hammer et al.[41]) Overall	ZDV vs. ddI vs. ddI + ZDV vs. ddC + ZDV	0.75 mg PO q8h	2467	Asymptomatic with CD4 200–500/mm³	Not reported
Naive subjects	ZDV vs. ddI vs. ddI + ZDV vs. ddC + ZDV	0.75 mg PO q8h	1067		Week 8 ZDV +14/mm³* ddI + ZDV +63/mm³* ddC + ZDV +41/mm³* *P <0.05 compared to ZDV
Experienced subjects	ZDV vs. ddI vs. ddI + ZDV vs. ddC + ZDV	0.75 mg PO q8h	1400		Week 8 ZDV −22/mm³ ddI +34/mm³* ddI + ZDV +40/mm³* ddC + ZDV +13/mm³* *P >0.05 compared to ZDV
Delta Coordinating Committee[42] Overall	ZDV vs. ddI + ZDV vs. ddC + ZDV	0.75 mg PO q8h	3207	CD4 50–350/mm³	Not provided
Naive subjects	ZDV vs. ddI + ZDV vs. ddC + ZDV	0.75 mg PO q8h	2124		Week 8 ZDV +30/mm³ ddI + ZDV +80/mm³* ddC + ZDV +67/mm³* *P <0.05 compared to ZDV
Experienced subjects	ZDV vs. ddI + ZDV vs. ddC + ZDV	0.7 mg PO q8h	1083		Week 8 ZDV −12/mm³ ddI + ZDV +20/mm³* ddC + ZDV +3/mm³ *P <0.05 compared to ZDV
CPCRA (Saravolatz et al.[44])	ZDV vs. ddI + ZDV vs. ddC + ZDV	0.75 mg PO q8h	1102	AIDS or CD4 <200/mm³	Month 2 ZDV −4/mm³ ddI + ZDV +19.2/mm³* ddC + ZDV +12.9/mm³ *P <0.001 compared to ZDV
ACTG 193A (Henry et al.[54])	ZDV alternating with ddI vs. ZDV + ddI vs. ZDV + ddI + NVP	0.75 mg PO q8h	1314	CD4 <50/mm³	Not available
SV 14604[55]	ZDV vs. ZDV + ddC vs. ZDV + SQV vs. ZDV + ddC + SQV	0.75 mg PO q8h	3485	≤ 16 wk prior ZDV	Not available

ddI, didanosine; LMV, lamivudine; NVP, nevirapine; RR, relative risk; SQV, saquinavir; ZDV, zidovudine.
CD4 indicates the CD4+ T-lymphocyte count.

<table>
<tr><th>Antiviral Response</th><th>Clinical Outcome</th><th>Comments</th></tr>
<tr><td>p24 Decline greatest in alternating limbs</td><td>Not studied</td><td>Alternating ddC and ZDV superior to intermittent ddC or ZDV</td></tr>
<tr><td></td><td><table><tr><th>Group</th><th>AIDS or Death</th><th>Death</th></tr><tr><td>ddC</td><td>41%</td><td>59</td></tr><tr><td>ZDV</td><td>30%</td><td>33</td></tr><tr><td>P</td><td>0.02</td><td>0.07</td></tr></table></td><td>ZDV monotherapy superior to ddC monotherapy</td></tr>
<tr><td>No significant difference in p24 decline vs. ZDV</td><td><table><tr><th>Group</th><th>AIDS or Death</th><th>Death</th></tr><tr><td>ddC</td><td>125</td><td>51</td></tr><tr><td>ZDV</td><td>11</td><td>43</td></tr><tr><td>ddC + ZDV</td><td>16</td><td>78</td></tr><tr><td>P</td><td>NS</td><td>NS</td></tr></table></td><td>No difference in clinical outcomes in ZDV-experienced subjects</td></tr>
<tr><td>Not included</td><td><table><tr><th>Group</th><th>AIDS or Death</th><th>Death</th></tr><tr><td>ddC</td><td>153</td><td>88</td></tr><tr><td>ddI</td><td>157</td><td>100</td></tr><tr><td>Adjusted RR</td><td>0.84</td><td>0.65</td></tr><tr><td>P</td><td>0.15</td><td>0.003</td></tr></table></td><td>Possible survival advantage for ddC over ddI</td></tr>
<tr><td>Not reported</td><td><table><tr><th>Treatment</th><th>AIDS or Death</th><th>Death</th></tr><tr><td>ddC + ZDV vs. ZDV</td><td>0.77</td><td>0.71</td></tr><tr><td>P</td><td>NS</td><td>NS</td></tr></table></td><td></td></tr>
<tr><td>Not reported</td><td><table><tr><th>Treatment</th><th>AIDS or Death</th><th>Death</th></tr><tr><td>ddC + ZDV vs. ZDV</td><td>0.49*</td><td>0.55</td></tr><tr><td>P</td><td><0.05</td><td>NS</td></tr></table></td><td>Combination therapy with ddC + ZDV offers improved clinical outcomes over ZDV alone in naive subjects.</td></tr>
<tr><td>Not reported</td><td><table><tr><th>Treatment</th><th>AIDS or Death</th><th>Death</th></tr><tr><td>ddC + ZDV vs. ZDV</td><td>0.91</td><td>0.81</td></tr><tr><td>P</td><td><0.05</td><td>NS</td></tr></table></td><td>No differences in clinical outcomes in ZDV-experienced subjects.</td></tr>
<tr><td>Not provided</td><td><table><tr><th>Treatment</th><th>AIDS or Death</th><th>Death</th></tr><tr><td>ddC + ZDV vs. ZDV</td><td>0.86*</td><td>0.79*</td></tr><tr><td>ddI + ZDV vs. ddC + ZDV</td><td>0.85*</td><td>0.85</td></tr></table>*$P < 0.05$</td><td></td></tr>
<tr><td>Not provided</td><td><table><tr><th>Treatment</th><th>AIDS or Death</th><th>Death</th></tr><tr><td>ddC + ZDV vs. ZDV</td><td>0.80*</td><td>0.68*</td></tr><tr><td>ddI + ZDV vs. ddC + ZDV</td><td>0.79*</td><td>0.85</td></tr></table>*$P < 0.05$</td><td>Combination therapy with ddC + ZDV offers improved clinical outcomes compared to ZDV but not ZDV + ddI in naive subjects.</td></tr>
<tr><td>Not provided</td><td><table><tr><th>Treatment</th><th>AIDS or Death</th><th>Death</th></tr><tr><td>ddC + ZDV vs. ZDV</td><td>0.95</td><td>0.91</td></tr><tr><td>ddI + ZDV vs. ddC + ZDV</td><td>0.92</td><td>0.84</td></tr></table></td><td>No differences in clinical outcomes in ZDV-experienced . subjects.</td></tr>
<tr><td>Not provided</td><td><table><tr><th>Treatment</th><th>AIDS or Death</th><th>Death</th></tr><tr><td>ddC + ZDV vs. ZDV</td><td>0.92</td><td>0.96</td></tr><tr><td>ddI + ZDV vs. ddC + ZDV</td><td>0.93</td><td>0.92</td></tr></table></td><td>No benefit to combination therapies; perhaps related to prior treatment in 77% of subjects.</td></tr>
<tr><td>Not available</td><td>AIDS or Death
ZDV + ddI + NVP vs. ZDV + ddC*
ZDV + ddI + NVP vs. ZDV alternating with ddI*
*$P < 0.05$</td><td>Three drugs improve clinical outcomes compared to ZDV + ddC in subjects with CD4 <50/mm³.</td></tr>
<tr><td>Not available</td><td><table><tr><th>Treatment</th><th>AIDS or Death</th><th>Death</th></tr><tr><td>ZDV + ddC</td><td>142</td><td>34</td></tr><tr><td>ZDV + ddC + SQV</td><td>116*</td><td>31</td></tr></table>*$P < 0.001$</td><td>Three drugs improve clinical outcomes compared to ZDV + ddC.</td></tr>
</table>

▲ **Table 4–3.** POTENTIAL DRUG INTERACTIONS: OVERLAPPING
▲ TOXICITIES WITH ZALCITABINE

Neuropathy
Didanosine
Stavudine
Dapsone
Disulfiram
Isoniazid
Lithium carbonate
Metronidazole
Pentamidine
Phenytoin
Ribavirin
Vincristine
Pancreatitis
Didanosine
Stavudine
Pentamidine
Azathioprine

more of 14 subjects treated with zalcitabine/zidovudine developed phenotypic zalcitabine resistance after 12 weeks of therapy.[64] In addition, none of these subjects had phenotypic evidence of cross-resistance to lamivudine. In contrast, among subjects treated with lamivudine/zidovudine who developed phenotypic lamivudine resistance at week 12, the median zalcitabine IC_{50} values increased 3.3- to 4.4-fold, suggesting the occurrence of cross-resistance to zalcitabine in lamivudine-treated subjects.[64]

▲ DRUG INTERACTIONS

Zalcitabine has few recognized drug interactions.[65] However, caution should be used when prescribing drugs that may have overlapping toxicities (Table 4–3). For example, other antiretroviral agents with neuropathic toxicities, such as didanosine and stavudine, should not be co-administered with zalcitabine. Other drugs that can cause neuropathy, such as dapsone, disulfiram, isoniazid, lithium carbonate, metronidazole, pentamidine, phenytoin, ribavirin, and vincristine, should be given with caution. Zalcitabine is predominantly eliminated through the kidneys; hence renal function should be monitored to avoid overdosage, especially in patients who may be receiving concurrent nephrotoxic medications.

▲ CONCLUSIONS

Zalcitabine is a nucleoside analogue that is used relatively infrequently in current antiretroviral regimens because other, less toxic and equally or more potent drugs are available. It has been demonstrated to have antiviral and clinical benefits, particularly in treatment-naive patients. Recipients of zalcitabine should be monitored carefully for peripheral neuropathy, which is the principal toxicity of the drug. Zalcitabine should not be used in combination regimens with didanosine or stavudine because of overlapping toxicities of the drugs. Cross-resistance between other nucleoside analogues and zalcitabine is common, particularly in patients treated with lamivudine.

REFERENCES

1. Horwitz JP, Chua J, DaRooge M, et al. Nucleosides. IX. The formation of 2′,3′-unsaturated pyrimidine nucleosides via a novel β-elimination reaction. J Org Chem 31:205, 1966.
2. Mitsuya H, Broder S. Inhibition of the in vitro infectivity and cytopathic effect of T-lymphotrophic virus type III/lymphadenopathy-associated virus (HTLV III/LAV) by 2′,3′-dideoxynucleosides. Proc Natl Acad Sci USA 82:7096, 1986.
3. Mitsuya H, Broder S. Strategies for antiviral therapy in AIDS. Nature 325:773, 1987.
4. Balzarini J, Pauwels R, Baba M, et al. The in vitro and in vivo antiretrovirus activity, and intracellular metabolism of 2′,3′-azido-2′,3′-dideoxythymidine and 2′,3′-dideoxcytidine are highly dependent on the cell species. Biochem Pharmacol 37:897, 1988.
5. Perno C-F, Yarchoan R, Cooney D. Replication of human immunodeficiency virus in monocytes: granulocyte/macrophage colony-stimulating factor (GMCSF) potentiates viral production yet enhances the antiviral effect mediated by 3′-azido-2′,3′-dideoxythymidine (AZT) and other dideoxynucleosides. J Exp Med 167:988, 1989.
6. Larder BA, Darby G, Richman D. HIV with reduced sensitivity to zidovudine (AZT) isolated during prolonged therapy. Science 243:1731, 1989.
7. Richman D. Susceptibility to nucleoside analogues of zidovudine-resistant isolates of human immunodeficiency virus. Am J Med 88 (suppl 5B):85, 1990.
8. Eron J, Johnson V, Merrill D, et al. Synergistic inhibition of replication of human immunodeficiency virus type 1, including that of a zidovudine-resistant isolate, by zidovudine and 2′,3′-dideoxycytidine in-vitro. Antimicrob Agents Chemother 35:394, 1991.
9. Zalcitabine package insert. Nutley, NJ, Roche Laboratories, 1996.
10. Kassianides C, Hoonagle J, Miller R, et al. Inhibition of duck hepatitis B virus replication by 2′,3′-dideoxycytidine. Gastroenterology 97:1276, 1989.
11. Yokota T, Mochizuki S, Kommo K, et al. Inhibitory effects of selected antiviral compounds on human hepatitis B virus DNA synthesis. Antimicrob Agents Chemother 35:394, 1991.
12. Balzarini J, Pauwels R, Herdewijn P, et al. Potent and selective anti-HTLV III/LAV activity of 2′,3′-dideoxycytidine, the 2N,3N-unsaturated derivative of 2′,3′-dideoxycytidine. Biochem Biophys Res Commun 140:735, 1986.
13. Vogt M, Durno A, Chou T-C. Synergistic interaction of 2′,3′-dideoxycytidine and recombinant interferon-alpha on replication of human immunodeficiency virus type 1. J Infect Dis 158:378, 1988.
14. Johnson V, Merrill D, Chou T-C. Human immunodeficiency virus type 1 (HIV-1) inhibitory interactions between protease inhibitor Ro 31-8959 and zidovudine, 2′,3′-dideoxycytidine, or recombinant interferon-alpha against zidovudine-sensitive or resistant HIV-1 in-vitro. J Infect Dis 166:1143, 1992.
15. Chong K-T, Pagano P, Hinshaw R. Bisheteroarylpiperazine reverse transcriptase inhibitor in combination with 3′-azido- 3′-deoxythymidine or 2′,3′-dideoxycytidine synergistically inhibits human immunodeficiency virus type 1 replication in vitro. Antimicrob Agents Chemother 38:288, 1994.
16. Vogt M, Hartshorn K, Furman P. Ribavirin antagonizes the effects of azidothymidine on HIV replication. Science 235:1376, 1987.
17. Baba M, Pauwels R, Balzarini J. Ribavirin antagonizes inhibitory effects of pyrimidine 2′,3′-dideoxynucleosides but enhances inhibitory effects of purine 2′,3′-dideoxynucleosides on replication of human immunodeficiency virus in-vitro. Antimicrob Agents Chemother 31:1613, 1987.
18. Chen C-H, Cheng Y-C. Delayed cytotoxicity and selective loss of mitochondrial DNA in cells treated with the anti-human immunodeficiency virus compound 2′,3′-dideoxycytidine. J Biol Chem 264:11934, 1989.
19. Cooney DA, Dala M, Mitsuga H, et al. Initial studies on the cellular pharmacology of 2′,3′-dideoxycytidine, an inhibitor of HTLV III infectivity. Biochem Pharmacol 35:2065, 1986.
20. Ullman B, Coons T, Rockwell S, et al. Genetic analysis of 2′,3′-dideoxycytidine incorporation into cultured human T lymphoblasts. J Biol Chem 263:12391, 1988.

21. Plagemann P, Woffendi C. Dideoxycytidine permeation and salvage by mouse leukemia cells and human erythrocytes. Biochem Pharmacol 38:3469, 1989.
22. Yarchoan R, Mitsuya H, Myers C, et al. Clinical pharmacology of 3′-azido-2′,3′-dideoxythymidine (zidovudine) and related dideoxynucleosides. N Engl J Med 321:726, 1989.
23. Broder S. Pharmacodynamics of 2′,3′-dideoxycytidine: an inhibitor of human immunodeficiency virus infection. Am J Med 88(suppl 5B):25, 1990.
24. Brandi G, Rossi L, Schiavano G, et al. In vitro toxicity and metabolism of 2′,3′-dideoxycytidine, an inhibitor of human immunodeficiency virus infectivity. Chem Biol Interactions 79:53, 1991.
25. Starnes M, Cheng Y. Cellular metabolism of 2N,3N-dideoxycytidine, a compound active against human immunodeficiency virus in vitro. J. Biol Chem 262:988, 1987.
26. Tornerik Y, Eriksson S. 2′,3′-Dideoxycytidine toxicity in cultured human CEM T lymphoblasts: effects of combination with 3′-azido-3N-deoxythymidine and thymidine. Mol Pharmacol 38:237, 1990.
27. Gao W-Y, Shirasaka T, Johns D. Differential phosphorylation of azidothymidine, dideoxycytidine and dideoxyinosine in resting and activated peripheral blood mononuclear cells. J Clin Invest 91:2326, 1993.
28. Gao W-Y, Agbaria R, Driscoll J. Divergent anti-human immunodeficiency virus activity and anabolic phosphorylation of 2′,3′-dideoxynucleoside analogs in resting and activated human cells. J Biol Chem 269:12633, 1994.
29. Chen M, Oshana S. Inhibition of HIV reverse transcriptase by 2′,3′-dideoxynucleoside triphosphates. Biochem Pharmacol 36:4361, 1987.
30. Hao Z, Cooney D, Hartman N, et al. Factors determining the activity of 2′,3′-dideoxynucleosides in suppressing human immunodeficiency virus in-vitro. Mol Pharmacol 34:431, 1988.
31. Yarchoan R, Devno C, Thomas R, et al. Phase I studies of 2′,3′-dideoxycytidine in severe human immunodeficiency virus infection as a single agent and alternating with zidovudine (AZT). Lancet 1:76, 1988.
32. Klecker R, Collins J, Yarchoan R, et al. Pharmacokinetics of 2′,3′-dideoxycytidine in patients with AIDS and related disorders. J Clin Pharmacol 28:835, 1988.
33. Gustavson L, Fukuda E, Rubio F, et al. A pilot study of the bioavailability and pharmacokinetics of 2′,3′-dideoxycytidine in patients with AIDS or AIDS-related complex. J Acquir Immune Defic Syndr 3:28, 1990.
34. Antunes F, Doroana M, on behalf of the HIVBID Study Group. Efficacy and tolerability of twice daily treatment with zalcitabine. Fifth International Congress on Drug Therapy in HIV Infection. Abstract P55. AIDS 14 (suppl 4): S32, 2000.
35. Pizzo P, Butler K, Balis F, et al. Dideoxycytidine alone and in an alternating schedule with zidovudine in children with symptomatic human immunodeficiency virus infection. J Pediatr 117:799, 1990.
36. Merigan T, Skowron G, Bozzette S, et al; ddC Study Group of the AIDS Clinical Trials Group. Circulating p24 antigen levels and responses to dideoxycytidine in human immunodeficiency virus (HIV) infections. Ann Intern Med 110:189, 1989.
37. Skowron G, Bozzette S, Lim L, et al. Alternating and intermittent regimens of zidovudine and dideoxycytidine in patients with AIDS or AIDS-related complex. Ann Intern Med 118:321, 1993.
38. Fischl M, Olson R, Follansbee S, et al. Zalcitabine compared with zidovudine in patients with advanced HIV-1 infection who received previous zidovudine therapy. Ann Intern Med 118:762, 1993.
39. Fischl M, Stanley K, Collier A, et al; NIAID AIDS Clinical Trials Group. Combination and monotherapy with zidovudine and zalcitabine in patients with advanced HIV disease. Ann Intern Med 122:24, 1995.
40. Meng T-C, Fischl M, Boota A, et al. Combination therapy with zidovudine and dideoxycytidine in patients with advanced human immunodeficiency virus infection. Ann Intern Med 116:13, 1992.
41. Hammer S, Katzenstein D, Hughes M, et al; AIDS Clinical Trials Group Study 175 Team. A trial comparing nucleoside monotherapy with combination therapy in HIV-infected adults with CD4 cell counts from 200 to 500 per cubic millimeter. N Engl J Med 335:1081, 1996.
42. Delta Coordinating Committee. Delta: a randomised double-blind controlled trial comparing combinations of zidovudine plus didanosine or zalcitabine with zidovudine alone in HIV-infected individuals. Lancet 348:283, 1996.
43. Schooley R, Ramirez-Ronda C, Lange J, et al; Wellcome Resistance Study Collaborative Group. Virologic and immunologic benefits of initial combination therapy with zidovudine and zalcitabine or didanosine compared with zidovudine monotherapy. J Infect Dis 173:1354, 1996.
44. Saravolatz L, Winslow D, Collins G, et al; Investigators for the Terry Beirn Community Programs for Clinical Research on AIDS. Zidovudine alone or in combination with didanosine or zalcitabine in HIV-infected patients with the acquired immunodeficiency syndrome or fewer than 200 CD4 cells per cubic millimeter. N Engl J Med 335:1099, 1996.
45. Blum A, Dal Pan G, Feinberg J, et al. Low dose zalcitabine (ddC)-related toxic neuropathy: frequency, natural history, and risk factors. Neurology 46:999, 1996.
46. Fichtenbaum C, Clifford D, Powderly W. Risk factors for dideoxynucleoside-induced toxic neuropathy in patients with human immunodeficiency virus infection. J Acquir Immune Defic Syndr 10:169, 1995.
47. Berger A, Arezzo J, Schaumberg H, et al. 2′,3′-Dideoxycytidine (ddC) toxic neuropathy: a study of 52 patients. Neurology 43:358, 1993.
48. Dubinsky R, Yarchoan R, Dalakas M, et al. Reversible axonal neuropathy from the treatment of AIDS and related disorders with 2′,3′-dideoxycytidine (ddC). Muscle Nerve 12:856, 1989.
49. LeLacheor S, Simon G. Exacerbation of dideoxycytidine-induced neuropathy with dideoxyinosine. J Acquir Immune Defic Syndr 4:538, 1991.
50. Indorf A, Pegram P. Esophageal ulceration due to zalcitabine (ddC). Ann Intern Med 117:133, 1992.
51. McNeely M, Yarchoan R, Broder S, et al. Dermatologic complications associated with administration of 2′,3′-dideoxycytidine in patients with human immunodeficiency virus infection. J Am Acad Dermatol 21:1213, 1989.
52. Letter to investigators. Nutley, NJ, Hoffman-LaRoche, 1991.
53. Abrams D, Goldman A, Launer C, et al; Terry Beirn Community Programs for Clinical Research on AIDS. A comparative trial of didanosine or zalcitabine after treatment with zidovudine in patients with human immunodeficiency virus infection. N Engl J Med 330:657, 1994.
54. Henry K, Tierney C, Kahn J, et al; ACTG 193A Study Team. A randomized double-blind, placebo-controlled study comparing combination nucleoside and triple therapy for the treatment of advanced HIV disease. In: Abstracts of the 4th Conference on Retroviruses and Opportunistic Infections, Washington, DC. Alexandria, VA, Westover Management Group, 1997, abstract LB6.
55. Letter to investigators. Nutley, NJ, Roche Laboratories, 1997.
56. Bartlett J, Benoit S, Johnson V, et al; North American HIV Working Party. Lamivudine plus zidovudine compared with zalcitabine plus zidovudine in patients with HIV infection. Ann Intern Med 125:161, 1996.
57. Collier A, Coombs R, Schoenfeld D, et al; AIDS Clinical Trials Group. Treatment of human immunodeficiency virus infection with saquinavir, zidovudine and zalcitabine. N Engl J Med 334:1011, 1996.
58. Craig C, Moyle G. The development of resistance of HIV-1 to zalcitabine. AIDS 11:271, 1997.
59. Rusconi S, La Seta Catamancio S, Sheridan F, Parker D. A genotypic analysis of patients receiving zidovudine, didanosine or zalcitabine dual therapy using the LiPA point mutations assay to detect genotypic variation at codons 41,69,70,74,184 and 215. J Clin Virol 3:135, 2000.
60. Richman D, Meng T-C, Spector S, et al. Resistance to AZT and ddC during long-term combination therapy in patients with advanced infection with human immunodeficiency virus. J Acquir Immune Defic Syndr 7:135, 1994.
61. Loveday C; Delta Virology Group. HIV-1 genotypic and phenotypic resistance in Delta patients. In: Abstracts of the XIth International Conference on AIDS, Vancouver, 1996, abstract Th.B 4354.
62. Cox S, Aperia K, Sandstrom E, et al. Cross-resistance between AZT, ddI and other antiretroviral drugs in primary isolates of HIV-1. Antivir Chem Chemother 5:7, 1994.
63. Mayers D, Japour A, Arduino J-M, et al; RV43 Study Group. Dideoxynucleoside resistance emerges with prolonged zidovudine monotherapy. Antimicrob Agents Chemother 38:307, 1994.
64. Johnson V, Quinn J, Benoit S, et al. Drug resistance and viral load in NUCA 3002: a randomized trial of lamivudine plus zidovudine versus zalcitabine plus zidovudine in zidovudine-experienced HIV-infected subjects. In: Abstracts of the 4th Conference on Retroviruses and Opportunistic Infections, Washington, DC. Alexandria, VA, Westover Management Group, 1997, abstract 580.
65. Shelton M, O'Donnell A, Morse G. Zalcitabine. Ann Pharmacother 27:480, 1993.

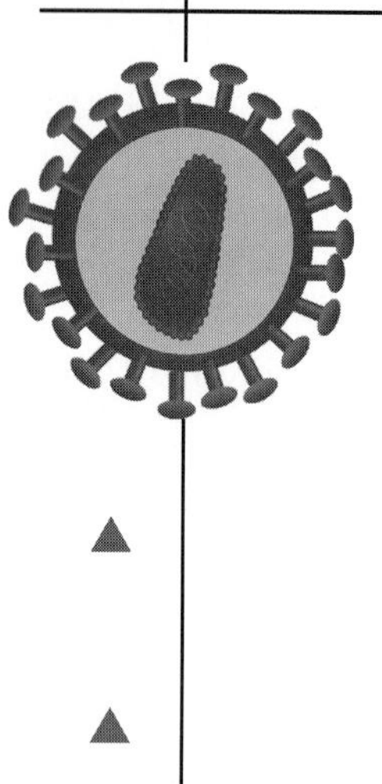

CHAPTER 5
Stavudine

Andrew T. Pavia, MD

▲ STRUCTURE

Stavudine (2′,3′-didehydro-2′,3′-didoxythymidine; d4T), like zidovudine, is an analogue of thymidine (Fig. 5–1). It differs from thymidine in that the hydroxyl group at the 3′ position is replaced by a hydrogen. It is relatively water-soluble, with a solubility of 83 mg/ml in water at 23°C.[1–3]

▲ MECHANISM OF ACTION AND IN VITRO ACTIVITY

Like other nucleoside analogues, stavudine is not active as the parent compound but must be phosphorylated to the active intracellular form, stavudine triphosphate.[1,4] The parent compound enters the cell by passive diffusion.[5] It is phosporylated by thymidine kinase, thymidylate kinase, and pyrimidine diphosphate kinase.[6] The initial phosphorylation by thymidine kinase appears to be the rate-limiting step in the activation of stavudine.[7] Unlike zidovudine, there is no accumulation of the monophosphate. The mono-, di-, and triphosphate forms of d4T are present in an approximately 1:1:1 ratio; and increasing the extracellular concentration of stavudine results in proportional increases in intracellular concentration of the active form.[6–8] The accumulation of zidovudine monophosphate and the difficulty achieving high levels of the active triphosphate may limit the antiviral activity of zidovudine and contribute to toxicity.[9,10] In contrast to zidovudine, stavudine does not result in depletion of the intracellular pools of thymidine-5′-triphosphate in bone marrow progenitor cells. This was hypothesized to explain the lack of hematologic toxicity,[11] but other studies have suggested that depletion of thymidine-5′-triphosphate does not explain zidovudine's bone marrow toxicity.[12,13]

The triphosphate form of stavudine acts as a competitive inhibitor of reverse transcriptase by competing with the natural substrate 2′-deoxy-thymidine-5′-triphosphate.[1,6,14,15] The alterations in the ribose ring at the 3′ position prevent formation of a new 3′-5′ phosphodiester bond with the next nucleotide. Therefore stavudine also acts as an obligate chain terminator.

Stavudine shows antiviral activity in vitro against human immunodeficiency virus type 1 (HIV-1) and HIV-2 but not against hepatitis B, herpes simplex, or cytomegalovirus (CMV).[8,16,17] The 50% inhibitory concentration (IC_{50}) for stavudine against laboratory and clinical isolates ranges from 0.009 to 4.100 μM (0.002 to 0.900 μg/ml) depending on the cell type and the assay system (Table 5–1).[1,8,11,13] Like zidovudine, stavudine is primarily active in HIV-infected activated cells, such as phytohemagglutinin-stimulated peripheral blood mononuclear cells, probably because thymidine kinase is an S phase-specific enzyme.[13,18,19] Stavudine exhibits partial cross resistance with zidovudine; isolates with multiple zidovudine-resistance mutations (M41L, D67N, T215Y) have reduced susceptibility.[20–23] Stavudine shows additive or synergistic activity in vitro when combined with didanosine, lamivudine, nevirapine, saquinavir, indinavir, or nelfinavir.[24–27] Zidovudine and stavudine compete for activation by thymidine kinase.[28] When they are co-administered in vivo, the amount of stavudine triphosphate is reduced relative to zidovudine triphosphate.[6] As might be predicted, the combination of zidovudine and stavudine shows antagonism in vitro against zidovudine-resistant strains of HIV.[24]

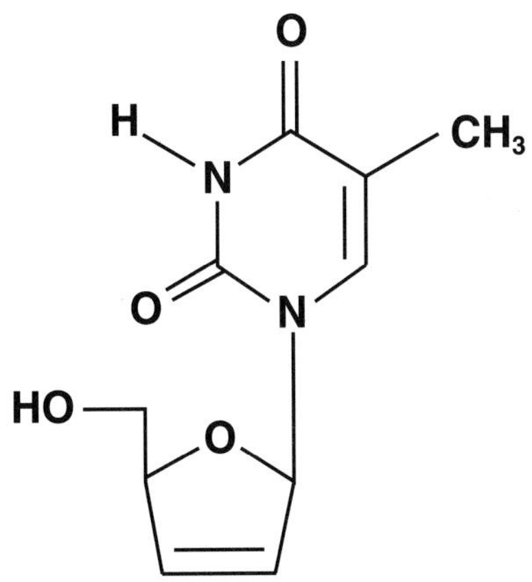

Figure 5–1. Structure of stavudine (2′,3′-didehydro-2′,3′-dideoxythymidine; d4T, Zerit).

▲ PHARMACOKINETICS

Stavudine is well absorbed. Initial studies suggested a bioavailability of 82% to 86%,[2,29,30] but population pharmacokinetic analysis on 33 patients calculated bioavailability of more than 99%,[31,32] consistent with the complete bioavailability observed in mice.[33] The area under the time-concentration curve (AUC) is identical when stavudine is taken while fasting or with a high-fat meal, but the maximum concentration (C_{max}) is reduced when given with a meal.[34] Peak plasma concentrations increase in a dose-related manner. After a 0.67 mg/kg dose, the peak serum concentration of 1.2 μg/ml is reached within 1 hour.[29] The estimated volume of distribution is 0.53 L/kg,[29,33] and there is negligible protein binding.

Plasma concentrations of stavudine decline in a biphasic manner, independent of dose. The mean plasma half-life following single oral doses in HIV-infected volunteers was 1.6 ± 0.8 hours. The intracellular half-life, however, is 3 to 4 hours.[19] Interpatient variation in the absorption and excretion of stavudine is relatively low.[35] About 40% of stavudine is excreted unchanged in the urine; therefore dose adjustment is necessary for patients with renal failure (creatinine clearance less than 50 ml/min). Patients with creatinine clearance of 26 to 50 ml/min should receive half of the usual dose (i.e., 20 mg for an adult) every 12 hours. For those with creatinine clearance of 10 to 25 ml/min, one-half of the usual dose is given every 24 hours. No formal guidelines exist for patients on dialysis; but based on the studies cited below, it is reasonable to dose patients on dialysis at the same dose as those with creatinine clearance less than 10 ml/min (i.e., 20 mg every 24 hours for patients weighing more than 60 kg).[36]

Two small studies have examined the clearance of stavudine in patients on hemodialysis (Bristol-Myers Squibb Investigational Drug Service, written communication, November 1996). The C_{max} was unchanged, but the terminal half-life was prolonged up to 12 hours. The mean hemodialysis clearance value of stavudine was 120 ± 18 ml/min. No dose adjustment is necessary in patients with hepatic impairment.[37]

Based on primate studies, the nonrenal metabolism is thought to involve cleavage of the sugar to yield thymine. Thymine, in turn, is degraded to β-aminoisobutyric acid or is used in the pyrimidine salvage pathway.[38]

Stavudine crosses the blood-brain barrier. Levels above the IC_{50} were measured in the brain tissue of rats, dogs, and monkeys after a single oral dose of 25 mg/kg.[33] Single-dose studies using a 40 mg PO dose in healthy volunteers demonstrated a mean concentration of 61 ng/ml at 4 to 5 hours, with a mean cerebrospinal fluid (CSF)/plasma ratio of 40% (Bristol-Myers Squibb Investigational Drug Service, written communication, April 1997). Foudraine et al. reported CSF concentrations of stavudine at week 12 in 17 HIV-infected patients treated with stavudine and lamivudine. The concentration of stavudine ranged from 0.20 to 0.27 μmol/L, and the mean CSF/plasma ratio was 38%.[39] The concentration exceeded the mean IC_{50} for clinical isolates. Foudraine et al. and others[40] also made the important observation that the CSF/plasma ratio can be misleading, as the ratio is highly dependent on the timing of the sampling. This is because the clearance rate from plasma is much faster than that from CSF. The absolute concentration of drug relative to antiviral activity may be a more reliable indicator. In HIV-infected children on stable dosing, CSF stavudine concentrations, obtained approximately 2 to 3 hours after oral doses, ranged from 16% to 97% of simultaneous plasma concentrations.[41] The clinical relevance of stavudine concentrations in the CSF was demonstrated in Prometheus, a trial that randomized patients to ritonavir and saquinavir with or without stavudine. Of 13 patients in the stavudine arm, 12 suppressed CSF HIV RNA to undetectable levels compared to only 4 of 14 of those not on stavudine.[42]

In pregnant macaques, stavudine reached the fetal circulation with a maternal/fetal ratio of 77% to 81%.[43] In ex vivo studies using human placenta, stavudine crossed the placenta via rapid, nonfacilitated, nonsaturable diffusion with pharmacokinetic properties similar to those of zidovudine.[44] Concentrations in placental tissue were approximately two-fold lower for stavudine than for zidovudine, probably reflecting stavudine's lower lipid solubility.[44]

Table 5–1. ANTIVIRAL ACTIVITY OF NUCLEOSIDE ANALOGUES AGAINST HIV IN VARIOUS CELL SYSTEMS

Cell System (Strain)	EC_{50} (μM)			
	Stavudine	Zidovudine	Zalcitabine	Didanosine
MT-4 (HTLV-III_B)	0.01	0.006	0.060	10.0
ATH-8 (HTLV-III_B)	4.10	2.400	0.200	7.0
PBMC (LAV-1)	0.04	0.0006	0.011	3.0–5.0
Monocytes/macrophages (HTLV-III_B)	0.30	0.200	0.002	0.01

Adapted from Sommadossi JP. Comparison of metabolism and in vitro antiviral activity of stavudine versus other 2′,3′-dideoxynucleoside analogues. J Infect Dis 171(suppl 2):S88, 1995, with permission.

▲ TOXICITY

Preclinical studies predicted the major clinical toxicities of stavudine. In vitro, stavudine is substantially less toxic to bone marrow precursors than zidovudine.[45,46] However, stavudine inhibits outgrowth of neurites in an *in vitro* model of neurotoxicity, with slightly less toxicity than didanosine or zalcitabine but substantially more than zidovudine.[47,48] The neurotoxicity of these nucleoside analogues is thought by some investigators to be due to inhibition of mitochondrial DNA polymerase-γ.[49] However, stavudine is significantly less potent at inhibiting mitochondrial DNA synthesis than zalcitabine in CEM cells (a T-cell-derived cell line).[50] In contrast to zalcitabine and didanosine, stavudine has no effect on mitochondria in PC-12 cells, a neuron-derived cell line.[48] This suggests that stavudine may cause peripheral neuropathy by a mechanism distinct from that of zalcitabine and didanosine.

Clinical toxicities of stavudine monotherapy from Phase III studies are shown in Table 5–2. Stavudine does not cause significant bone marrow suppression.[51–55] Initial Phase I and II dose-range trials demonstrated that peripheral neuropathy and, to a lesser extent, elevations of hepatic transaminases are the major dose-limiting toxicities of stavudine. The maximum tolerated dose of stavudine established in Phase 1 studies was 2 mg/kg/day.[51–54]

The risk of peripheral neuropathy is dose-related. In an analysis of data from three Phase 1 studies and one Phase II study, the incidence of neuropathy (of any severity) was 17 to 21 per 100 person-years in patients receiving doses of 0.5 mg/kg/day, 21 per 100 person-years at 1.0 mg/kg/day, and 41 to 66 per 100 person-years at 2.0 mg/kg/day. Patients receiving 4 mg/kg/day or more for extended periods had a 64% to 71% cumulative incidence of peripheral neuropathy.[55] In the BMS 019 study, a Phase III efficacy trial among zidovudine-experienced patients (using the currently recommended dose of 40 mg PO bid, roughly 1 mg/kg/day), the rate of neuropathy sufficient to require dose modification was 11.7 per 100 person-years among stavudine-treated patients compared to 3.9 per 100 person-years in the zidovudine group.[51] The occurrence of neuropathy was strongly associated with a baseline diagnosis of acquired immunodeficiency syndrome (AIDS), preexisting neuropathy, and low CD4 counts at study entry.

Neuropathy associated with stavudine is usually reversible when the drug is discontinued or the dose is modified. Among 56 stavudine-treated patients who developed neuropathy in the Phase III trial, 63% had complete resolution of neurologic symptoms within a median 17 days. These patients all tolerated rechallenge at half the original dose.[51] If neuropathic symptoms appear to be due to stavudine, the decision must be made whether to discontinue stavudine alone or to stop all antiretroviral drugs. In patients with fully suppressed plasma RNA on a robust regimen, it may be reasonable to stop stavudine alone. If symptoms resolve completely, stavudine may be restarted at one-half the original dose. However, if the cause of symptoms is unclear, or if HIV RNA remains detectable on therapy, stopping all drugs simultaneously may be less likely to select for drug-resistant HIV. Although early neuropathy due to stavudine usually resolves in 1 to 3 weeks, the neuropathy may be permanent, particularly if the drug is continued for prolonged periods in the face of worsening symptoms. In pediatric trials, peripheral neuropathy has been rare.[41,56–58] Higher rates of neuropathy have been observed in patients treated with stavudine in combination with didanosine and hydroxyurea.[59]

▲ **Table 5–2.** CLINICAL TOXICITIES OF STAVUDINE FROM A PHASE III RANDOMIZED CLINICAL TRIAL

	Rate per 100 person-years	
Adverse Event	Stavudine (40 mg bid) (n = 417)	Zidovudine (200 mg tid) (n = 405)
Headache	36	38
Chills/fever	34	40
Diarrhea	33	34
Rash	27	27
Nausea and vomiting	26	35
Abdominal pain	23	21
Myalgia	21	27
Insomnia	20	24
Pancreatitis	< 1	< 1
Neuropathy any grade	11.7	3.9
Neuropathy grade 3–4	2	1
Hyperamylasemia (>1.4 × ULN)	12.6	10.7
Elevated AST, any grade	65.6	44
Elevated AST, >5 × ULN	8.6	9.3
Elevated AST, any grade	69.1	41.3
Elevated ALT >5 × ULN	12.1	9.9
Anemia grade 3–4	0.6	14.2
Neutropenia grade 3–4	3.0	6.4

Events among patients on zidovudine are included for comparison. ALT, alanine transminase; AST, aspartate transminase; ULN, upper limits of normal.

From Spruance SL, Pavia AT, Mellors JW, et al. Clinical efficacy of monotheraphy with stavudine compared with zidovudine in HIV-infected, zidovudine-experienced patients: a randomized, double-blind, controlled trial; Bristol-Myers Squibb Stavudine/019 Study Group. Ann Intern Med 126:355, 1997 and Final Report of Protocol AI455-019.

Modest elevations of hepatic transaminases are common with stavudine therapy, but significant elevations and clinical hepatitis are uncommon. Grade III or IV elevations of hepatic transaminases (more than five times the upper limit of normal) occurred in 9% to 13% of patients receiving stavudine doses of 2.0 mg/kg/day or less in the Phase I and II studies.[54,60] Significant elevations were not apparently related to dose but were significantly associated with abnormal baseline levels. In the Phase III study, grade III or IV elevations of alaninine aminotransferase (ALT) or aspartate aminotransferase (AST) occurred at similar rates in the stavudine and zidovudine groups (12 vs. 10 per 100 person-years), but milder elevations were common and significantly more frequent in the stavudine group (69 vs. 44 per 100 person-years).[51]

Lactic acidemia, lactic acidosis, and hepatic steatosis were recognized early as rare but severe complications of nucleoside analogues, including zidovudine, zalcitabine, didanosine, and stavudine.[61–65] Severity ranges from asymptomatic lactic acidemia to fatal fulminant disease. Symptoms are nonspecific and include fatigue, nausea, vomiting, and abdominal pain. Mitochondrial dysfunction appears to be an underlying defect,[66–71] although other factors, including the rate of lactate clearance, may be critical.[72,73] A number of case reports and case series have implicated stavudine in lactic acidemia and lactic acidosis.[63,71,74–79] However, it has been difficult to determine if the risk is in fact higher with stavudine than with other nucleoside analogues. A cohort study of 233 patients from Amsterdam found that elevated lactate was significantly associated with nucleoside reverse transcriptose inhibitor (NRTI) therapy with odds ratio of 10.0 for stavudine use, 6.8 for zidovudine use, and 6.7 for abacavir use.[80] A study that involved 18 months of prospective monitoring of 349 patients found lactate levels to rise modestly after the initiation of stavudine- or zidovudine-based (HAART).[79] However, the increase was an average 0.23 mmol/L greater in those on stavudine. Severe hyperlactatemia and steatosis were rare. Another study looking at any level of elevated lactate found the highest incidence rate for stavudine-containing regimens, at 25.6 cases per 1000 person-years, of use.[81]

The U.S. Food and Drug Administration (FDA) and the manufacturers of stavudine issued a letter of warning reporting three fatal cases of lactic acidoses in pregnant women who were receiving stavudine combined with didanosine; they recommended that this combination be used in pregnant women only when the "potential benefit clearly outweighs the risk."[82]

It has been proposed that stavudine-induced mitochondrial dysfunction plays a role in lipodystrophy and fat atrophy,[83–85] but this remains controversial.[66,72] Many studies are plagued by the complexity of overlapping syndromes, cross-sectional design, and multiple confounders and interactions, both biologic and statistical. Nucleoside analogue use, duration of therapy, age, and gender have been consistent risk factors for lipoatrophy.[86,87] Many studies that have identified an association between stavudine and lipodystrophy have not been able to control adequately for common prescribing of stavudine or duration of therapy.[84,88] However, two prospective cohort studies do show an increased risk of lipodystrophy associated with stavudine use. Among 277 patients participating in the Western Australia cohort, stavudine-containing regimens were associated with an increased relative risk of fat wasting, as were protease inhibitor (PI) use, white race, age, and duration of nucleoside analogue therapy.[87] Among 1035 patients participating in the British Columbia drug treatment program, lipodystrophy was diagnosed based on prospectively collected self-reporting. Lipodystrophy syndrome was independently associated with age, use of PI therapy, being employed, use of alternative therapy, and duration of stavudine therapy.[89] It is likely that lipodystrophic syndromes result from a complex interaction between stavudine and other nucleosides, PI use, immunologic response, and host genetic factors.

In contrast to didanosine, stavudine alone is not clearly associated with an increased risk of pancreatitis or hyperamylasemia. The rates of these complications are similar among patients treated with stavudine or zidovudine,[51,90] confirmed in an analysis of 2613 patients followed at Johns Hopkins University.[91]

Stavudine is classified as FDA pregnancy category C. Long-term animal carcinogenicity studies are negative.[92] Animal toxicology studies of stavudine during pregnancy show no specific embryopathy. Exposure of early embryos to high levels of stavudine (10 μmol/L) inhibited blastocyst formation.[93] There was no reduction in fertility at doses 200 times higher than the human levels. Teratology studies showed that using 400 times the human serum concentrations in rats and 183 times the human serum concentration in rabbits produced no increase in birth defects. In rats exposed to the highest doses, there were decreases in sternal bone calcification and mild increases in neonatal mortality. These changes are consistent with nonspecific toxicity.[92,94,95]

▲ EFFICACY

Since 1996 there has been an explosion of clinical trials of combination regimens. Stavudine has been used as part of combination therapy in a large number. In many, however, it is not possible to discern the individual role of the nucleoside analogue component. Therefore it is useful to review data on monotherapy (Table 5–3) and dual therapy (Table 5–4) trials.

Monotherapy

In a Phase II dose-range study, beneficial effects on CD4+ T-lymphocyte count, p24 antigenemia, cellular viremia, and weight gain were observed at a dose of 0.5 or 2.0 mg/kg/day.[60] Little or no response was observed at 0.1 mg/kg/day. The median CD4+ T-lymphocyte count increase was 20 to 30 cells/mm^3; greater responses were observed in zidovudine-naive patients. The greatest antiviral response was seen at 2.0 mg/kg/day, with a 77% decrease in the median titer of infected peripherial blood mononuclear cells (PBMCs). Another small study of 15 patients demonstrated median drops in the infectious titer of 1 to 2 $\log_{10}$ and a median decrease in viral RNA of 0.5 $\log_{10}$ at 52 weeks.[104] Katlama and colleagues examined the short-term antiviral effect of stavudine among 66 treatment-naive subjects randomized to stavudine at 20 mg bid (roughly 0.5 mg/kg/day), stavudine 40 mg bid (1.0 mg/kg/day), or placebo.[105] Responses tended to favor the 40 mg bid dose compared to the 20 mg bid dose. The median CD4+ T-lymphocyte count increase at week 8 was 63 cells/mm^3 in the 40 mg bid group versus 33 cells in the low dose group and a 50-cell decline in the placebo group. The median decrease in cellular viremia was 1.0 $\log_{10}$ vs. 0.7 $\log_{10}$ copies/ml, and the median decrease in plasma HIV RNA at week 12 (measured by nucleic acid sequence-based amplification [NASBA]) was 0.8 $\log_{10}$ vs. 0.4 $\log_{10}$ copies/ml. In the ACTG 306 study, 34 treatment-naive patients were randomized to stavudine monotherapy at 40 mg bid. At 24 weeks the mean decrease in viral load was 0.55 $\log_{10}$ copies/ml, or 1.04 after adjustment for censoring.[98] In patients with prolonged zidovudine therapy, the response to stavudine is attenuated. Among patients with prolonged zidovudine monotherapy (mean 3.6 years) in the ACTG 175 trial who were switched to stavudine monotherapy, the virologic response at 48 weeks was modest (mean decrease 0.18 $\log_{10}$ copies/ml).[106]

The only clinical-endpoint study of stavudine monotherapy (BMS 019) compared stavudine (40 mg bid) with continued zidovudine in 822 patients with CD4+ T-lymphocyte counts of 50 to 500 at least 6 months of prior zidovudine treatment.[51] The median duration of follow-up was 115 weeks. Patients receiving stavudine reached clinical endpoints (AIDS-defining events or death) at a significantly lower rate than those randomized to continue

Table 5–3. SUMMARY OF MAJOR TRIALS INVOLVING STAVUDINE MONOTHERAPY

Study	Design	Arms	No. of Subjects	Patients	CD4 at Entry	Antiviral Response	Immunologic and Clinical Response
Phase II, dose range[60]	Three arms, dose escalation	d4T 0.1 mg/kg vs. d4T 0.5 mg/kg vs. d4T 2.0 mg/kg	152	Treatment-naive	250 (median)	Not done	CD4 and virologic response increased with increasing dose. Neuropathy more prominent at 2.0 mg/kg
Stavudine Parallel Track Program[90]	Simple trial; randomized, double-blind, dose comparison	d4T 20 mg bid vs. d4T 40 mg	15,000	ZDV-experienced, advanced disease, failing or intolerant to available drugs	41 (median)	Not done	Weight gain, hematologic improvement, and hospitalizations favored 40 mg dose. No difference in mortality. Neuropathy requiring dose modification 23% vs. 17%
BMS 019[51]	Double-blind RCT	d4T 40 mg bid vs. ZDV 200 mg tid	822	ZDV-experienced > 6 months	236 (median)	Not done	Decreased progression to AIDS or death in stavudine group. Improved CD4 count (30-50 cell difference). No difference in mortality
BMS 024[97]	Double-blind RCT	d4T 40 mg bid vs. d4T 20 mg bid vs. placebo	66	Treatment-naive; CD4 < 350	527 (median)	HIV RNA decrease 0.8 log_{10} copies/ml in 40 mg arm, decrease 0.4 log in 20 mg arm	CD4 increased 40 cells with 40 mg, 25 cells with 20 mg; decreased 50 cells with placebo
ACTG 240[57]	Initially double-blind RCT; unblinded early	d4T 1 mg/kg bid vs. ZDV 180 mg/m2 q 6h	266	Children 3 months to 6 yrs; treatment-naive	965 (median)	No difference in progression to endpoints (but underpowered due to early unblinding)	Clinical endpoints met in 19% on d4T vs. 24% on ZDV (NS). Better weight gain and maintenance of CD4 cell count in d4T group

NS, not significant; RCT, randomized controlled trial; ZDV, zidovudine.

zidovudine (26/100 vs. 32/100 person-years; relative risk 0.75; $P = 0.03$). This benefit was apparent in all strata of baseline CD4+ T-lymphocyte counts. Survival was not significantly different, but there was a trend favoring longer survival in the stavudine group (relative risk 0.74; $P = 0.66$). Patients assigned to stavudine remained on initial therapy significantly longer (79 weeks compared to 53 weeks). Quality of life as measured by the MOS SF-36 was significantly better among stavudine-treated patients at week 12, but by week 36 the difference was not significant.[107] Patients in the stavudine group had significantly less anemia and neutropenia and better weight gain. The CD4 count initially increased a median of 20 cells but then declined. The count remained 30 to 40 cells/mm^3 higher than that in the zidovudine group (Fig. 5–2). Viral RNA was not measured in this study.

Stavudine Combined with Lamivudine

Because of the convenient dosing and the favorable side effect profile, the combination of stavudine and lamivudine became popular before clinical trial data were available to demonstrate their efficacy.[108] In vitro, the combination shows additive to synergistic effects in vitro.[24] The combination appears at least as active as zidovudine and lamivudine.

In an open-label prospective study (ALTIS I) among 42 treatment-naive patients,[96] the combination of stavudine and lamivudine resulted in a median decrease in viral RNA of 1.96 $\log_{10}$ copies/ml at 4 weeks; it was sustained at −1.66 $\log_{10}$ at 24 weeks, with an increase in the CD4+ T-lymphocyte count of 108 cells/mm^3 at 24 weeks. RNA levels were below 500 copies/ml at week 24 in 30%. In a parallel study of 41 antiretroviral-experienced but stavudine- and lamivudine-naive patients (ALTIS II), more modest effects were observed. The median maximum change in HIV RNA was −1.3 $\log_{10}$ copies/ml at week 4 but only −0.55 $\log_{10}$ at week 24 accompanied by a CD4+ T-lymphocyte count increase of 46 cells/mm^3. Drug-related side effects were minimal. A pilot open-label study of 48 patients in Vancouver compared patients naive to both stavudine and lamivudine with others who were pretreated with one or the other drug. The study found that antiviral responses were substantial in naive patients (−1.47 $\log_{10}$ copies/ml at week 8) and more modest in stavudine- and lamivudine-experienced patients.[109]

Two studies have compared stavudine plus lamivudine with zidovudine plus lamivudine. ACTG 306 was a six-arm study among antiretroviral-naive patients.[97] The stavudine arm compared stavudine monotherapy, stavudine plus lamivudine, and zidovudine plus lamivudine. Adjusted for censoring, the change in plasma HIV RNA level at weeks 20 to 24 was −0.55 $\log_{10}$ copies/ml in the stavudine monotherapy arm, −1.59 $\log_{10}$ copies/ml in the stavudine/lamivudine arm, and −1.05 $\log_{10}$ copies/ml in the zidovudine/lamivudine arm. The difference favoring stavudine/lamivudine over zidovudine/lamivudine was of borderline statistical significance ($P = 0.052$) at week 24, but no difference was seen at week 48. A low baseline plasma HIV RNA level complicates the analysis. Using an ultrasensitive assay (lower limit 20 copies/ml), there was no difference between stavudine/lamivudine and zidovudine/lamivudine (−1.64 vs. −1.57 $\log_{10}$ copies/ml). In another randomized trial among 47 patients who received stavudine/lamivudine or zidovudine/lamivudine for 12 weeks, the plasma HIV RNA level decreased by −1.65 compared to −1.53 $\log_{10}$ copies/ml (Fig. 5–3). However, all patients had developed lamivudine resistance by 12 weeks.[98] In 28 patients who underwent lumbar puncture before and after therapy, both regimens resulted in CSF HIV RNA becoming undetectable by quantitative polymerase chain reaction (PCR) in all patients.[39]

A small randomized study compared adding lamivudine in zidovudine-experienced patients to changing to the combination of stavudine/lamivudine. After a mean follow-up of 24 weeks, decreases in plasma HIV RNA level were greater and more sustained in the group receiving stavudine/lamivudine.[110]

Other open label prospective studies[111] or retrospective studies[108,112] confirm the tolerability, antiviral efficacy and beneficial effects on CD4 count of stavudine plus lamivudine combination therapy.

Stavudine Combined with Didanosine

Additive synergistic antiviral effects are seen in vitro when stavudine is combined with didanosine.[24,26,27] There is no significant pharmacokinetic interaction.[113] Data from several trials suggests that this combination is clinically effective and well tolerated. A double-blind dose-range trial compared five regimens of stavudine plus didanosine among 76 treatment-naive patients with a median CD4+ T- lymphocyte count of 325 cells/mm^3 (stavudine/didanosine dose: 10/100 mg; 20/100 mg; 40/100 mg; 20/200 mg; or 40/200 mg, all dosed twice-daily).[99] The reduction in plasma viral RNA was −1.1 to −1.8 $\log_{10}$ copies/ml across groups. The reduction was sustained for 52 weeks, and patients receiving the two highest doses (close to full dose of each agent) had somewhat greater responses. CD4+ T-lymphocyte counts increased 42 to 112 cells/mm^3 across the groups. Increases of 80 to 100 cells/mm^3 were sustained at 52 weeks for the higher dose regimens. Only one episode of neuropathy occurred (grade 2), despite the concern over potential synergistic toxicity.

A double-blind randomized trial comparing stavudine/didanosine (at standard doses) with stavudine/didanosine/hydroxyurea (500 mg bid) confirmed the efficacy of stavudine/didanosine.[100] The trial enrolled 144 patients, 80% of whom were treatment-naive. In the stavudine/didanosine arm, the mean reduction in viral RNA was −1.6 $\log_{10}$ copies/ml at week 12 using the Roche PCR assay with a detection limit of 200 copies/ml. RNA levels were below the limit of detection in 28%. CD4+ T-lymphocyte counts increased by 91 cells/mm^3 at week 12. In an open-label extension, the viral load remained 1.5 $\log_{10}$ copies/ml below baseline at 24 months. In the group given hydroxyurea, the viral load reduction was slightly greater (−1.8 $\log_{10}$ copies/ml at week 12, $P = 0.06$), and 54% were below 200 copies/ml; the change in CD4+ T-lymphocyte count was less substantial (+10 cells at week 12, $P = 0.003$). This

▲ **Table 5–4.** SUMMARY OF MAJOR TRIALS INVOLVING STAVUDINE DUAL THERAPY

Study	Design	Arms	No. of Subjects
ALTIS 1[96]	Open label, 24 wks	d4T 40 mg+3TC 150 mg bid	42
ALTIS 2[96]	Open label, 24 wks	d4T 40 mg+3TC 150 mg bid	41
ACTG 306[97]	Double-blind RCT, 48 wks	d4T 40 mg bid vs. d4T+3TC 150 mg bid vs. ZDV 200 mg tid	146 (d4T limb)
Amsterdam Cohort[98]	Open label RCT	d4T/3TC vs. ZDV/3TC	47
BMS 460[99]	Randomized double-blind dose comparison, 48 wks	d4T 10 + ddI 100 d4T 20 + ddI 100 d4T 20 + ddI 200 d4T 40 + ddI 100 d4T 40 + ddI 400	94
Swiss HIV Cohort[100]	Double-blind RCT, 48 wks	d4T/ddI vs. d4T/ddI/hydroxyurea	142
ALBI[101]	Open label RCT, 24 wks	d4T/ddI vs.ZDV/3TC vs. d4T/ddI followed by ZDV/3TC	153
PACTG 327[102]	Partially randomized double-blind, 48 wks	d4T 1 mg/kg/ddI 90 mg/m^2 bid vs. d4T 1 mg/kg bid	108
ACTG 290[103]	Partially blinded, randomized 4-arm study	d4T vs. d4T/ZDV vs. ddI vs. ddI/ZDV	145

ddC, dideoxycytidine; ddI, didanosine; d4T, stavudine; 3TC, lamivudine.
[a]HIV RNA copies/ml.

was attributed to a decrease in the total lymphocyte count due to hydroxyurea rather than a change in the CD4+ T-lymphocyte percentage. In another trial among 151 naive patients, a stavudine/didanosine regimen was compared to zidovudine/lamivudine or alternating use of the two combinations. Stavudine/didanosine resulted in greater reductions of viral load than zidovudine/lamivudine (−2.26 vs. 1.26 $\log_{10}$ copies/ml; $P < 0.001$) (Fig. 5–4).[101]

Stavudine/didanosine dual therapy is active among patients with prior zidovudine treatment. In an open-label trial of 60 treatment-experienced patients, reductions in HIV RNA of −0.9 $\log_{10}$ copies/ml were sustained at 24 weeks.[114] In a study of treatment-experienced children, stavudine/didanosine in children also demonstrated sustained antiviral effect and minimal toxicity.[102]

Stavudine Combined with Protease Inhibitors or Nonnucleoside Reverse Transcriptase Inhibitors

A small number of studies used stavudine plus a protease inhibitor as a two-drug combination before it became clear that it was inadequate. Stavudine combined with nelfinavir was studied in a Phase II study dose-range study and a pivotal Phase III study. In Agouron Pharmaceuticals study 510, a series of 33 patients with moderately advanced disease (CD4+ T-lymphocyte count higher than 200 cells/mm^3, median HIV RNA about 80,000 copies/ml) who were naive to stavudine and protease inhibitors were randomized to receive stavudine alone or with nelfinavir (500, 750, or 1000 mg tid).[115] At 2 months the mean decrease in viral RNA was −0.9 $\log_{10}$ copies/ml in the stavudine monotherapy and

Patients	CD4 at Entry	Antiviral Response[a]	Immunologic and Clinical Response
Treatment-naive CD4 50–400; RNA > 15,000	258 (median)	HIV RNA decrease 1.66 log_{10} at wk 24; 21% < 200 copies;	CD4 increase 108 cells
ZDV-, ddI-, ddC-experienced; median 35 months; CD4, RNA as above	172 (median)	HIV RNA decrease 0.55 log_{10} at wk 24; 5% < 200 copies;	CD4 increase 46 cells
Nucleoside-naive; CD4 200–600; median HIV RNA 10,146 copies	407 (median)	HIV RNA decrease 1.59 log_{10} at wk 20-24 in d4T+3TC group vs. 1.05 log_{10} in ZDV+3TC group vs. 0.55 log_{10} in d4T monotherapy (analysis adjusted for censoring as 35–57% fell below 500 copies). At wks 40–48, RNA decrease 1.50 log_{10} in d4T+3TC group vs. 1.50 log_{10} in ZDV+3TC group vs.0.96 log_{10} in d4T monotherapy	Mean CD4 increase 80 cells with d4T monotherapy, 118 cells with d4T/3TC, 79 cells with ZDV/3TC at wk 40/48 (NS)
Treatment-naive	300 (median)	HIV RNA decrease 1.65 log_{10} at wk 12 in d4T+3TC group vs. 1.53 log_{10} in ZDV+ 3TC group (P<0.0001)	120 cell increase with d4T/3TC at 24 wks compared to 90 cell increase with in ZDV/3TC (P = 0.002)
Treatment-naive		HIV RNA decrease 1.2–1.4 log_{10} at wk 28 across group	CD4 increased 42 to 112 cells; better response with higher dose
d4T- and hydroxyurea-naive	370 (mean)	HIV RNA decrease 1.6 log_{10} in d4T/ddI arm vs. 1.9 log_{10} in d4T/ddI/HU arm at wk 12	CD4 increase 91 cells with d4T/ddI vs. 10 cells with d4T/ddI/HU
Treatment-naive	385 (median)	HIV RNA decrease 2.3 log_{10} in d4T+ddI arm vs. 1.26 log_{10} in ZDV/ 3TC arm vs. 1.58 log_{10} in sequential arm. Proportion less than 500 copies on treatment (bDNA) 91% vs. 42%.vs 60%	CD4 increase 124 cells in d4T+ddI arm vs. 62 ZDV/3TC arm vs. 118 in sequential
d4T or ZDV monotherapy-experienced children	730 (median)	HIV RNA decrease 0.51 log_{10} with d4T+ddI in ZDV-experienced group, 0.17 log_{10} with d4T monotherapy in ZDV-experienced (P = 0.026) and 0.3 log_{10} with d4T+ddI in d4T-experienced (NS)	No statistical difference in CD4 response
ZDV-experienced patients (median 135 weeks)	401 (median)	HIV RNA decrease 0.14 log_{10} in d4T and d4T/ZDV arms at wk 16 vs. 0.39 log_{10} in ddI arm and 0.56 log_{10} in ddI/ZDV arm	CD4 count decreased 22 cells in d4T/ZDV arm at wk 16 compared to 17 cell increase in d4T arm

[a]HIV RNA copies/ml.

-2.0 log_{10} copies/ml in the stavudine/nelfinavir groups. In study 506, a series of 308 patients were randomized to receive stavudine/placebo or stavudine/nelfinavir (500 or 750 mg tid).[116] Eighty percent had been extensively pretreated with nucleoside analogues. The mean CD4+ T-lymphocyte count was 279 cells/mm^3 and the mean HIV RNA 141,000 copies/ml. Among patients on combination therapy, viral RNA decreased -1.3 to -1.4 log_{10} copies/ml at week 8, associated with a 103- to 108-cell increase in CD4+ T-lymphocyte count. After 24 weeks of follow-up, 26% of patients had counts below the limit of detection. These results are less impressive and less sustained than those after using three-drug regimens. A trial of indinavir/stavdine compared to stavudine (sponsored by Merck) in heavily pretreated patients (Merck 037) compared stavudine/indinavir to either drug alone. At 52 weeks, 45.9% had counts below 400 copies/ml in the combination arm.[117]

Stavudine/lamivudine has been used as a backbone in a number of comparative trials.[118–120] Two trials have compared stavudine/lamivudine/indinavir versus zidovudine/lamivudine/indinavir. In START 1, a group of 204 antiretroviral-naive patients were enrolled in a randomized, open-label trial. At 48 weeks there was no significant difference between the arms in terms of the proportion below 500 copies/ml (62% vs. 54%; P = 0.2) or below 50 copies/ml (49% vs. 47%) or in the CD4 response (226 vs. 198 cells) (Fig. 5–5).[121] The OzCombo study randomized 109 therapy-naive patients to indinavir with either stavudine/ lamivudine, stavudine/didanosine, or zidovudine/lamivudine.[122]

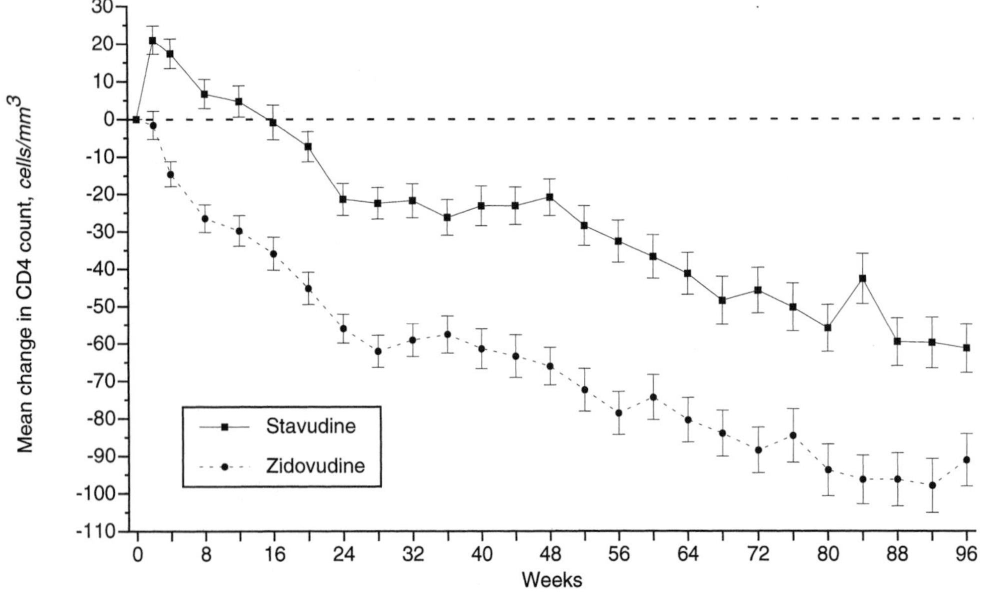

Figure 5–2. Mean change in CD4+ T-lymphocyte count from baseline by treatment group in BMS 019. *Bars* represent the standard error. (From Spruance SL, Pavia AT, Mellors JW, et al. Clinical efficacy of monotherapy with stavudine compared with zidovudine in HIV-infected, zidovudine-experienced patients: a randomized, double-blind, controlled trial; Bristol-Myers Squibb Stavudine/019 Study Group. Ann Intern Med 126:355, 1997, with permission.)

There were no significant differences in virologic outcome or CD4 response. Fewer patients in the stavudine/didanosine group discontinued therapy because of adverse events ($P = 0.06$).

Stavudine/didanosine has also been used as a backbone with PIs, nonnucleoside reverse transcriptase inhibitors (NNRTIs), and triple nucleoside regimens. Overall, it appears at least as potent as regimens using zidovudine and lamivudine.

Preliminary, noncomparative trials showed good efficacy and tolerability.[123–126] The START II trial compared indinavir with stavudine/didanosine or zidovudine/lamivudine in a randomized, open-label study of 205 therapy-naive patients.[127] At the 48-week primary endpoint, the plasma HIV RNA level reduction and the proportion of patients with less than 500 RNA copies/ml and less than 50 copies/ml were similar. Other analyses did show a benefit favoring the stavudine/didanosine arm. The patients in the stavudine/didanosine group had significantly larger increases in CD4 cell count (214 vs. 142; $P = 0.026$). The frequency of adverse events was similar. The Atlantic trial compared stavudine/didanosine with indinavir, nevirapine, or lamivudine. At 48 weeks, the plasma HIV RNA level reduction and the proportion with plasma HIV RNA levels less the 500 copies were similar in all three arms. Using the ultrasensitive RNA assay, the proportion of patients on the lamivudine arm below the limits of detection was lower in the lamivudine arm (Fig. 5–6).[128]

A trial comparing stavudine/didanosine/efavirenz with stavudine/didanosine/efavirenz/hydroxyurea showed excellent antiviral efficacy in both naive and zidovudine- and protease-experienced patients. About 90% of naive patients and 95% of experienced patients had plasma HIV RNA levels of less than 500 copies/ml at 24 weeks. However, the addition of hydroxyurea led to significantly more pancreatitis and neuropathy, causing premature closure of the trial.[129]

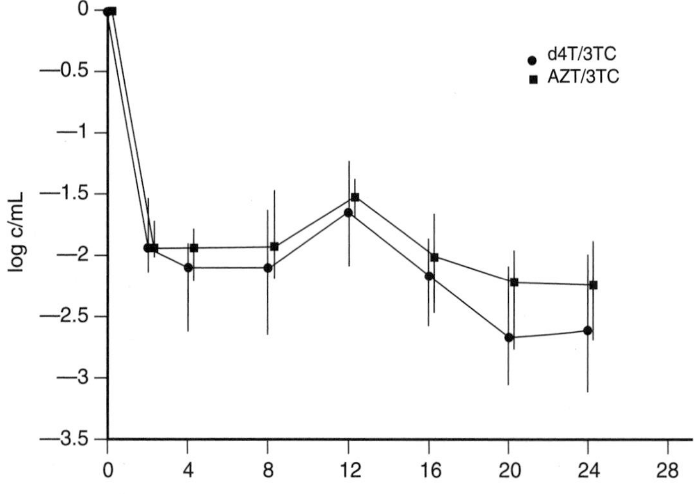

Figure 5–3. Mean change in HIV RNA from baseline in antiretroviral-naive patients on stavudine and lamivudine or zidovudine and lamivudine. (Redrawn from Foudraine NA, de Jong JJ, Jan Weverling G, et al. An open randomized controlled trial of zidovudine plus lamivudine versus stavudine plus lamivudine. AIDS 12:1513, 1998, with permission.)

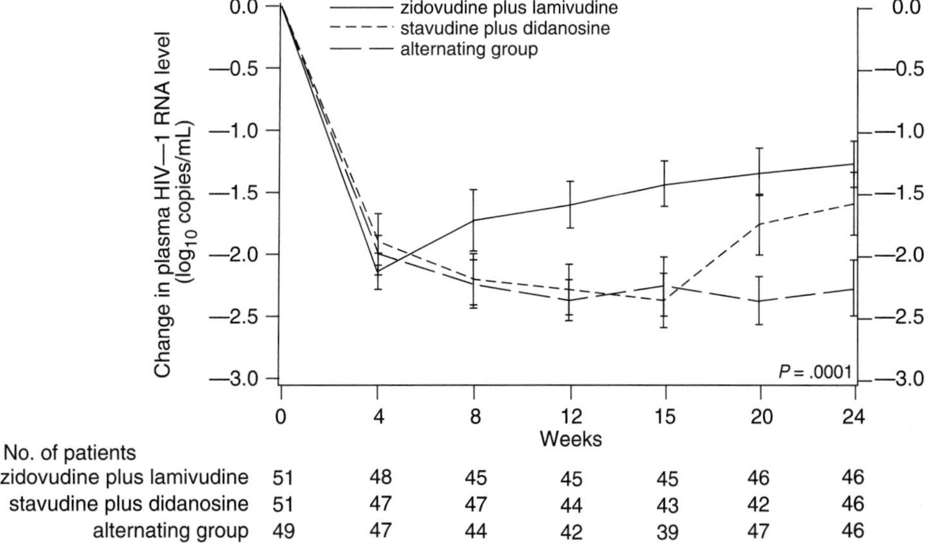

Figure 5–4. Mean change in HIV RNA from baseline in antiretroviral-naive patients on stavudine and didanosine, zidovudine and lamivudine, or stavudine and didanosine followed by zidovudine and lamivudine (alternating group). (Redrawn from Molina JM, Chene G, Ferchal F, et al. The ALBI trial: a randomized controlled trial comparing stavudine plus didanosine with zidovudine plus lamivudine and a regimen alternating both combinations in previously untreated patients infected with human immunodeficiency virus. J Infect Dis 180:351, 1999, with permission.)

A summary of the major trials of stavudine plus protease inhibitors or nonnucleoside reverse transcriptase inhibitors appears in Table 5–5.

Stavudine with Other Agents

No data are currently available on the in vitro activity or clinical efficacy of stavudine combined with the carbocyclic nucleoside analogue abacavir, although it has been widely prescribed.

▲ RESISTANCE

A number of HIV mutants resistant to all antiviral agents in current use have emerged with prolonged exposure in the presence of ongoing viral replication. It was noted early that stavudine-based regimens also lose effectiveness with time,[51] consistent with the evolution of resistance. Full understanding of resistance to stavudine was elusive, but great progress has finally been made. Initially, zidovudine-resistant isolates of HIV were noted to be susceptible to stavudine, within the limits of the

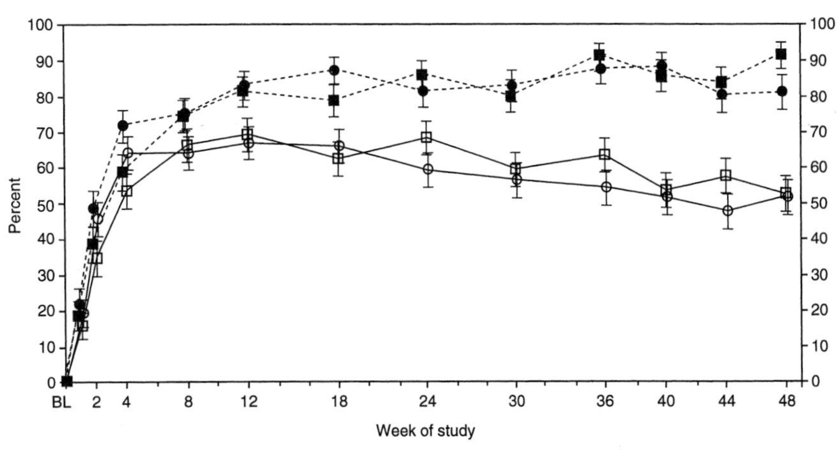

Figure 5–5. Proportion (with standard error bars) of patients with HIV RNA fewer than 500 copies/ml by both intent-to-treat and as-treated analyses among patients randomized to stavudine, lamivudine, and indinavir compared to zidovudine, lamivudine, and indinavir. (From Squires KE, Gulick R, Tebas P, et al. A comparison of stavudine plus lamivudine versus zidovudine plus lamivudine in combination with indinavir in antiretroviral naive individuals with HIV infection: selection of thymidine analog regimen therapy (START I). AIDS 14:1591, 2000, with permission.)

▲ **Table 5–5.** SUMMARY OF MAJOR TRIALS INVOLVING STAVUDINE WITH PROTEASE INHIBITORS OR NONNUCLEOSIDE REVERSE

Study	Design	Arms	No. of Subjects
De Truchis[130]	Open label	d4T/3TC bid/indinavir 800 mg tid	144
AG 506[116]	Double-blind RCT	d4T bid vs. d4T bid+nelfinavir 500 mg tid vs.d4T bid + nelfinavir 750 mg tid	308
PACTG 338[131]	Open label RCT	ZDV/3TC vs. ZDV/3TC/ritonavir vs. d4T/ritonavir	298
START 1[121]	Open label RCT	d4T/3TC/indinavi vs. ZDV/3TC/indinavir	204
START II[127]	Open label RCT	d4T/ddI/indinavir vs. ZDV/3TC/indinavir	205
Ozcombo[122]	Open label 3 arm RCT	d4T/3TC/indinavir vs. d4T/ddI/indinavir vs. ZDV/3TC/Indinavir	109
Atlantic[128]	Open label 2-arm RCT	D4T/ddI 400 mg qd/indinavir 800 mg tid vs. ddI/d4T/nevirapine 400 mg qd vs. ddI/d4T/3TC	298
Prometheus[42,132]	Open label RCT	Ritonavir 400 mg/saquinavir 400 mg/d4T vs. ritonavir/saquinavir (d4T added if not suppressed at wk 12)	208
DMP 043[43]	Open label, single arm	d4T/3TC/efavirenz	68

CSF, cerebrospinal fluid; IND, indinavir; ITT, intent to treat; PI, protease inhibitor; RTV, ritonavir; SQV, saquinavir.

assays.[133,134] Lacey and Larder reported that in vitro passage of HIV with increasing concentrations selected a strain mutant at codon 75 (substitution of threonine for valine) of the reverse transcriptase gene that conferred a sevenfold decrease in susceptibility.[135] Site-directed mutagenesis into an HXB2 background confirmed the change in stavudine susceptibility and demonstrated a moderate decrease in sensitivity to didanosine and zalcitabine. Another mutation was described during in vitro selection, substitution of threonine for isoleucine at codon 50 that conferred 30-fold resistance to stavudine, but no apparent cross resistance.[136]

TRANSCRIPTASE INHIBITORS

Patients	CD4/mm³ at Entry	Antiviral Response/ml	Immunologic and Clinical Response/mm³
Nucleoside-experienced protease-naive; AIDS in 51%	85 (mean)	HIV RNA decrease 1.4 $\log_{10}$ at week 24; 48% < 200 copies	CD4 increase 90 cells at wk 24
Nucleoside-experienced, d4T- and protease-naive (80%); naive (20%); CD4 50–500		HIV decrease 1.3–1.4 $\log_{10}$ in combination vs. 0.6 in d4T at wk 8; decreasing effect at wk 24	CD4 count increase 103–106 cells in combination vs. 51 on monotherapy
ZDV-experienced children, d4T- and PI-naive	680 (median)	8% < 500 copies on ZDV/3TC vs. 47% on ZDV/3TC/ritonavir vs. 34% on d4T/ritonavir at wk 24	No significiant difference in CD4 increase at wk 24
Antiretroviral-naive, viral load > 10,000 copies	400 (median)	62% < 500 copies on d4T/3TC/IND vs. 54% on AZT/3TC/IND (*P* = 0.21) at 40–48 wks; 49% < 50 copies on d4t/3TC arm vs.47%	CD4 increase 227 cells in d4T/3TC/IND vs. 198 in ZDV/3TC/IND (NS). CD4 response significantly better by area under the curve on d4t/3TC arm (*P* = 0.033)
Antiretroviral-naive, viral load > 10,000 copies	422 (median)	61% < 500 copies on d4T/ddI/IND vs. 45% on AZT/3TC/IND (*P* = 0.038) at 40–48 wks; 41% < 50 copies on d4t/ddI arm vs. 35%	CD4 increase 214 cells in d4T/ddI/IND vs. 142 in ZDV/3TC/IND (*P* = 0.026) CD4 response significantly better by area under the curve on d4t/ddI arm (*P* = 0.001)
Antiretroviral-naive, viral load > 30,000 copies or CD4 < 500 cells	285 (mean)	Proportion < 50 copies at wk 48 (ITT) 59% on d4T/3TC/IND vs. 48% on d4T/ddI/IND vs. 66% on ZDV/3TC/IND (NS)	CD4 increase 237 on d4T/3TC/IND vs. 176 on d4T/ddI/IND vs. 175 on ZDV/3TC/IND. No significant difference in time-weighted average CD4 count increase. Higher discontinuation on d4T/ddI arm
Antiretroviral-naive, viral load > 500 copies and CD4 >200 cells	406 (median)	Proportion < 500 copies at wk 48 (ITT) 57% on d4T/ddI/IND vs. 58% on d4T/ddI/NVP vs. 59% on d4T/ddI/I3TC Proportion < 50 (ITT) 55% vs. 54% vs. 46%	Mean CD4 increase 318 cells at wk 48 across all three groups (NS)
PI- and d4T-naive		By strict ITT analysis, 69% less than 400 copies in RTV/SQV/d4T group vs. 63% (*P* = 0.38); 31% in dual PI group 12) added nucleosides. In a CSF substudy, more patients in RTV/SQV/d4T had CSF HIV RNA < 400 or less than 50 copies than in RTV/SQV group 12/13 vs. 4/14 (*P* = 0.001)	No difference
Antiretroviral-naive	375 (mean)	By ITT analysis, 78% less than 400 copies, 73% less than 50 copies at 72 weeks. By as-treated analysis, 94% and 89% less than 400 and less than 50 copies	CD4 increase (mean) 283 cells 72 wks

In vivo, the situation is more complicated. Phenotypic resistance appears slowly without a consistent genotypic pattern.[137–139] The mutation at position 75 is rare in clinical isolates and often not associated with clinical resistance.[140] A mutation at position 50 has not been reported. In an important early study that was initially cited as evidence that stavudine did not select for resistance, Lin et al. studied 13 patients treated with stavudine for 18 to 22 months. Three patients had posttreatment isolates with decreased susceptibility to stavudine (4- to 12-fold).[138] The isolates demonstrated multiple mutations, including several associated with zidovudine resistance (T215Y, K219E, K70R). Five

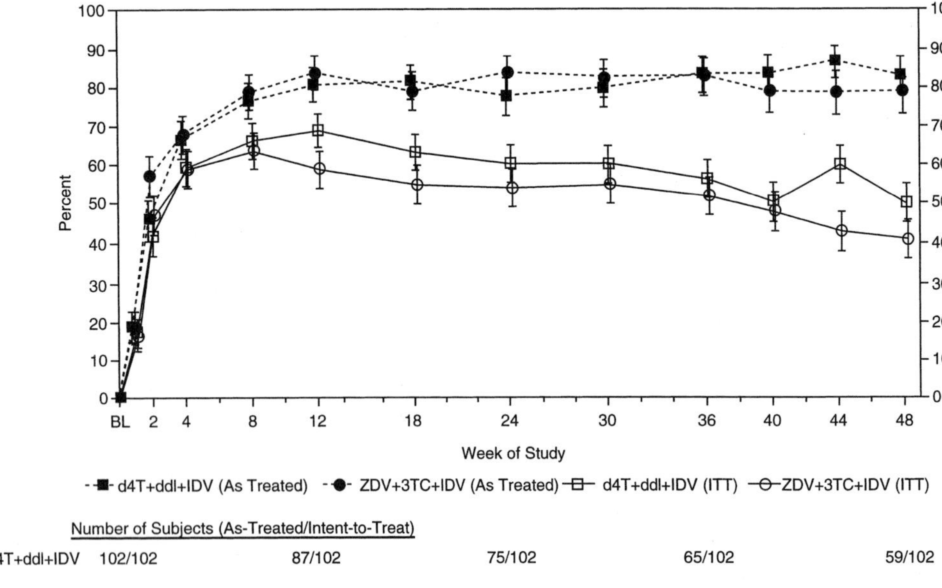

Figure 5-6. Proportion (with standard error bars) of patients with HIV RNA fewer than 500 copies/ml by both intent-to-treat and as-treated analysis among patients randomized to stavudine, lamivudine, and indinavir compared to zidovudine, lamivudine, and indinavir. (From Eron JJ Jr, Murphy RL, Peterson D, et al. A comparison of stavudine, didanosine and indinavir with zidovudine, lamivudine and indinavir for the initial treatment of HIV-1 infected individuals: selection of thymidine analog regimen therapy (START II). AIDS 14:1601, 2000, with permission.)

posttreatment isolates were resistant to zidovudine. Soriano et al. studied 24 patients who had received 2 years of stavudine monotherapy after prolonged zidovudine use.[139] None was mutant at position 50 or 75. However, 83% maintained zidovudine resistance mutations for more than 2 years on stavudine.

Although the clues were present in early studies, it has become clear that resistance to stavudine can develop along three pathways. The most common one involves the development of mutations classically associated with zidovudine resistance, including M41L, D77N, K70R, and T215Y/F. Because these mutations not only confer resistance to zidovudine but contribute to resistance to abacavir, didanosine, zalcitabine, lamivudine, and stavudine, they have been referred to as thymidine-associated mutations (TAM) or, more accurately, nucleoside-associated mutations (NAMs). Treatment with stavudine alone or in combination with lamivudine or didanosine may select for NAMs.[140–145] These mutations have been detected in 15% to 38% of stavudine failures. In contrast to zidovudine, they confer modest phenotypic resistance to stavudine, in the range of a 1.9-fold change in IC_{50} in one study,[140] but this change appears to have a measurable effect on the antiviral response. In another study NAMs were detected in 38% of patients on stavudine/lamivudine compared to 50% of those on zidovudine/lamivudine.[143] The presence of mutations at K70 and T215 were similar, but the zidovudine-based regimen was significantly more likely to select for M41L. This suggests that although stavudine and zidovudine select for similar mutations, the selection may be slower and less potent with stavudine.

The presence of NAMs in zidovudine-experienced patients is associated with a decreased virologic response to stavudine.[22,146,147] In the ALTIS 2 study, the magnitude of response to stavudine was associated with the presence of T215Y or F mutation, the number of previously used nucleosides, and a phenotypic sensitivity to stavudine. A modest change in IC_{50} of more than 1.8-fold over control isolates was associated with decreased response. Purified reverse transcriptase from zidovudine-resistant viruses shows decreased inhibition by stavudine triphosphate, providing in vitro correlation.[148] Interestingly, the V75T mutation may have a role in increasing pyrophosphorolysis, similar to the effect of NAMs.[149]

A second pathway is through a multidrug resistance pathway involving a signature mutation Q151M with multiple mutations. Additional mutations include A62V, V75I, F77L, F116Y, and M184V.[150–152] These strains exhibit high-level resistance to multiple nucleoside analogues including didanosine, lamivudine, stavudine, zalcitabine, and zidovudine. The third pathway, described in 1998, involves insertion of two amino acids between codons 67 and 70 of reverse transcriptase, most often a double insertion of six basepairs coding for two threonines at codon 69.[153–156] This multidrug resistance pathway (also referred to as MDR-2) confers high level resistance to stavudine, lamivudine, zalcitabine, and zidovudine and variable resistance to abacavir and didanosine. Both the Q151M and the T69SSS pattern are selected for at lower frequency than zidovudine mutations.

▲ DRUG INTERACTIONS

There are relatively few significant drug–drug interactions documented with stavudine.[157] Stavudine has no effect on the cytochrome P_{450} system. The most clinically relevant drug interaction is with zidovudine. Stavudine and zidovudine compete for phosphorylation by thymidine kinase.[6,28] At initial concentrations of 1 μM this leads to decreased intracellular levels of stavudine triphosphate, although if the initial concentration of both drugs is increased to 10 μM the concentration of stavudine triphosphate is increased relative to zidovudine triphosphate.[6,7] In vitro this can result in antagonism, at least with zidovudine-resistant strains of HIV, although additive effects have been reported for some strains.[24,25] In vivo antagonism was demonstrated in the ACTG 290 trial.[103] This study randomized patients with more than 12 weeks of prior zidovudine to didanosine alone, didanosine plus zidovudine, stavudine alone, or stavudine plus zidovudine. Patients in the stavudine/zidovudine arm had decreases in their CD4+ T-lymphocyte count, in contrast to modest increases in all other arms, leading to closure of the stavudine/zidovudine arm.

In vitro, ribavirin and doxorubicin also interfere with the phosphorylation of stavudine, although the clinical relevance is unknown.[28] Co-administration with methadone results in a 27% reduction in stavudine area under the concentration curve (AUC), which is an amount thought not to be clinically significant.[158] Because of the potential for additive neurotoxicity, most experts advise against the use of stavudine with zalcitabine. Other agents that cause neuropathy, including vincristine, isoniazid, ethambutol, and ethanol, might be expected to have additive neurotoxicity with stavudine, although there are no clear data to support this hypothesis.

▲ RECOMMENDATIONS FOR USE

Stavudine is a well tolerated drug with a simple dosing regimen. It is available as capsules or a pediatric oral solution. The drug may be taken fasting or with food. Stavudine should administered at a dose of 40 mg PO bid for persons weighing at least 60 kg and 30 mg PO bid for adults weighing less than 30 kg. Lower doses may result in a less potent antiviral effect.[105] The recommended dose for children who weigh less than 30 kg is 1 mg/kg bid. Children weighing more than 30 kg should receive the adult dose. Dose adjustment is necessary for significant renal impairment (see Pharmacokinetics section). Stavudine is now available as an enteric coated (EC) formulation that allows once daily dosing.

The major role of stavudine is in combination with lamivudine or didanosine as part of combination therapy.[159,160] Clinical trial data support the use of either a stavudine-based combination with PIs or NNRTIs. Much attention has been devoted to the issue of whether to use stavudine or zidovudine as part of an initial regimen and how to sequence nucleoside analogues. This debate may have more marketing implications than clinical ones. Arguments in favor of using stavudine in initial regimens include tolerability, the slower selection of resistance mutations relative to zidovudine, and the better response to stavudine/lamivudine in zidovudine-naive compared to zidovudine-experienced patients.[161] Arguments in favor of using stavudine after zidovudine include the demonstrated virologic benefit of stavudine in zidovudine-experienced patients,[51,96] the selection of similar mutations, the convenience of co-formulated preparations with zidovudine, and the possible increased risk of lipoatrophy with stavudine. There are no data from well designed strategy trials to address this point, although several are in progress.

Peripheral neuropathy is the major dose-limiting toxicity. A previous history of neuropathy, whether due to antiretrovirals or other causes, is a risk factor for neuropathy on stavudine. Careful monitoring is important if stavudine is prescribed for persons with a history of neuropathy. Care should be taken to discriminate distal symmetrical painful neuropathy due to nucleosides from other causes of neuropathy.[162,163] Neuropathy caused by stavudine usually resolves on discontinuing the drug (see Toxicity section).

Many experts suggest substituting stavudine for zidovudine in pregnant women who are unable to take zidovudine. The rationale is based on the fact that both are thymidine analogues; moreover, there is similar placental passage and similar activity in activated cells, and there is a lack of significant animal toxicity and a lack of reported toxicity to date in pregnant women. Preliminary results from a study comparing various nucleoside analogue regimens suggested that stavudine was well tolerated and at least as effective as zidovudine.[164] Lactic acidosis and hepatic steatosis has been reported with the use of stavudine and didanosine during pregnancy, and a warning letter has been issued regarding the use of this combination in pregnant women, as noted above.[82] Whether the risk during pregnancy is more severe than with other nucleoside combinations is unknown; but if this combination must be used during pregnancy, monitoring the serum lactate concentration is prudent.

REFERENCES

1. Mansuri MM, Starrett JE Jr, Ghazzouli I, et al. 1-(2,3-Dideoxy-beta-D-glycero-pent-2-enofuranosyl)thymine: a highly potent and selective anti-HIV agent. J Med Chem 32:461, 1989.
2. Bristol Myers Squibb. Package insert: Zerit (stavudine) (revised October 1996).
3. Moyle GJ. Stavudine: pharmacology, clinical use and future role. Exp Opin Invest Drugs 6:191, 1997.
4. August EM, Marongiu ME, Lin TS, et al. Initial studies on the cellular pharmacology of 3′-deoxythymidine-2′-ene (d4T): a potent and selective inhibitor of human immunodeficiency virus. Biochem Pharmacol 37:4419, 1988.
5. August EM, Birks EM, Prusoft W. 3′-Deoxythymidine-2′ene permeation of human lymphocyte H9 cells by nonfacilitated diffusion. Mol Pharmacol 39:441, 1991.
6. Ho HT, Hitchcock MJ. Cellular pharmacology of 2′,3′-dideoxy-2′,3′-didehydrothymidine, a nucleoside analog active against human immunodeficiency virus. Antimicrob Agents Chemother 33:844, 1989.
7. Balzarini J, Herdewijn P, De Clercq E. Differential patterns of intracellular metabolism of 2′,3′-didehydro-2′,3′-dideoxythymidine and 3′-azido-2′,3′-dideoxythymidine, two potent anti-human immunodeficiency virus compounds. J Biol Chem 264:6127, 1989.
8. Martin JC, Hitchcock MJ, Fridland A, et al. Comparative studies of 2′,3′-didehydro-2′,3′-dideoxythymidine (d4T) with other pyrimidine nucleoside analogues. Ann NY Acad Sci 616:22, 1990.
9. Lavie A, Schlichting I, Vetter IR, et al. The bottleneck in AZT activation. Nat Med 3:922, 1997.
10. Hazuda D, Kuo L. Failure of AZT: a molecular perspective. Nat Med 3:836, 1997.
11. Hitchcock M. 2′,3′-Didehydro-2′,3′-dideoxythymidine, an anti-HIV agent. Antivir Chem Chemother 2:125, 1991.
12. Fridland A, Connelly M, Ashmun R. Cellular pharmacology of anti-HIV agents azidothymidine (AZT) and 2′,3′-didehydrothymidine (d4T) in human T cells. Presented at the International Conference on AIDS, 1989, p 561 (abstract M.C.P.120).
13. Sommadossi JP. Comparison of metabolism and in vitro antiviral activity of stavudine versus other 2′,3′-dideoxynucleoside analogues. J Infect Dis 171(suppl 2):S88, 1995.
14. Huang P, Farquhar D, Plunkett W. Selective action of 2′,3′-didehydro-2′,3′-dideoxythymidine triphosphate on human immunodeficiency virus reverse transcriptase and human DNA polymerases. J Biol Chem 267:2817, 1992.
15. Chen MS, Suttmann RT, Wu JC, et al. Metabolism of 4′-azidothymidine: a compound with potent and selective activity against the human immunodeficiency virus. J Biol Chem 267:257, 1992.

16. Lin TS, Schinazi RF, Prusoff WH. Potent and selective in vitro activity of 3′-deoxythymidine-2′-ene (3′-deoxy-2′,3′-didehydrothymidine) against human immunodeficiency virus. Biochem Pharmacol 36:2713, 1987.
17. Hamamoto Y, Nakashima H, Matsui T, et al. Inhibitory effect of 2′,3′-didehydro-2′,3′-dideoxynucleosides on infectivity, cytopathic effects, and replication of human immunodeficiency virus. Antimicrob Agents Chemother 31:907, 1987.
18. Gao WY, Shirasaka T, Johns DG, et al. Differential phosphorylation of azidothymidine, dideoxycyidine, and dideoxyinosine in resting and activated peripheral blood mononuclear cells. J Clin Invest 91:2326, 1993.
19. Zhu Z, Ho HT, Hitchcock MJM, et al. Cellular pharmacology of 2′,3′-didehydro-2′,3′-dideoxythymidine (d4T) in human peripheral blood mononuclear cells. Biochem Pharmacol 39:R15, 1990.
20. Milazzo L, Rusconi S, Testa L, et al. Evidence of stavudine-related phenotypic resistance among zidovudine-pretreated HIV-1-infected subjects receiving a therapeutic regimen of stavudine plus lamivudine [letter]. J Acquir Immune Defic Syndr 22:101, 1999.
21. Izopet J, Bicart-See A, Pasquier C, et al. Mutations conferring resistance to zidovudine diminish the antiviral effect of stavudine plus didanosine. J Med Virol 59:507, 1999.
22. Shulman N, Shafer R, Winters M, et al. Genotypic predictors of virologic response to stavudine after zidovudine monotherapy (ACTG 302). In: Abstracts of the 8th Conference on Retroviruses and Opportunistic Infections, Chicago, 2001. abstract 437.
23. Calvez V, Descamps D, Valantin MA, et al. Genotypic analysis of experienced patients treated by d4T/3TC combination (ALTIS 2). In: Abstracts of the 5th Conference on Retroviruses and Opportunistic Infections, Chicago, 1998, p 206 (abstract 676).
24. Merrill DP, Moonis M, Chou TC, et al. Lamivudine or stavudine in two- and three-drug combinations against human immunodeficiency virus type 1 replication in vitro. J Infect Dis 173:355, 1996.
25. Sorensen AM, Nielsen C, Mathiesen LR, et al. Evaluation of the combination effect of different antiviral compounds against HIV in vitro. Scand J Infect Dis 25:365, 1993.
26. Brankovan V, Tarantini K, Datema R, et al. Strong synergistic anti-HIV activity of a purine and a pyrimidine nucleoside analog, ddI and d4T. In: Abstracts of the 5th International Conference on AIDS, 1989, abstract M.C.P.128.
27. Deminie C, Bechtold C, Stock D, et al. Evaluation of d4T, ddI and BMS-186,318, in two-drug combinations against HIV replication. In: Abstracts of the 3rd Conference on Retroviruses and Opportunistic Infections, Washington, DC, 1996, abstract 107.
28. Back D, Haworth S, Hoggard P, et al. Drug interactions with d4T phosphorylation in vitro. In: Abstracts of the 11th International Conference on AIDS, Vancouver, BC, 1996, p 88 (abstract mo.B.1194).
29. Dudley MN, Graham KK, Kaul S, et al. Pharmacokinetics of stavudine in patients with AIDS or AIDS-related complex. J Infect Dis 166:480, 1992.
30. Lea AP, Faulds D. Stavudine: a review of its pharmacodynamic and pharmacokinetic properties and clinical potential in HIV infection. Drugs 51:846, 1996.
31. Horton CM, Dudley MN, Kaul S, et al. Population pharmacokinetics of stavudine (d4T) in patients with AIDS or advanced AIDS-related complex. Antimicrob Agents Chemother 39:2309, 1995.
32. Grasela TH, Haworth SJ, Fiedler-Kelley J, et al. Population pharmacokinetic (PK) analysis of stavudine (d4T) in HIV-infected patients with CD4 counts between 50 and 500 cells/mm^3. In: Abstracts of the 11th International Conference on AIDS, Vancouver, 1996, abstract 287.
33. Russell JW, Whiterock VJ, Marrero D, et al. Disposition in animals of a new anti-HIV agent: 2′,3′-didehydro-3′-deoxythymidine. Drug Metab Dispos 18:153, 1990.
34. Kaul S, Christofalo B, Raymond RH, et al. Effect of food on the bioavailability of stavudine in subjects with human immunodeficiency virus infection. Antimicrob Agents Chemother 42:2295, 1998.
35. Dudley MN. Clinical pharmacokinetics of nucleoside antiretroviral agents. J Infect Dis 171(suppl 2):S99, 1995.
36. Grasela DM, Stoltz RR, Barry M, et al. Pharmacokinetics of single-dose oral stavudine in subjects with renal impairment and in subjects requiring hemodialysis. Antimicrob Agents Chemother 44:2149, 2000.
37. Schaad HJ, Petty BG, Grasela DM, et al. Pharmacokinetics and safety of a single dose of stavudine (d4T) in patients with severe hepatic impairment. Antimicrob Agents Chemother 41:2793, 1997.
38. Cretton EM, Zhou Z, Kidd LB, et al. In vitro and in vivo disposition and metabolism of 3′-deoxy-2′,3′-didehydrothymidine. Antimicrob Agents Chemother 37:1816, 1993.
39. Foudraine NA, Hoetelmans RM, Lange JM, et al. Cerebrospinal-fluid HIV-1 RNA and drug concentrations after treatment with lamivudine plus zidovudine or stavudine. Lancet 351:1547, 1998.
40. Haworth SJ, Christofalo B, Anderson RD, et al. A single-dose study to assess the penetration of stavudine into human cerebrospinal fluid in adults. J Acquir Immune Defici Syndr 17:235, 1998.
41. Kline MW, Dunkle LM, Church JA, et al. A phase I/II evaluation of stavudine (d4T) in children with human immunodeficiency virus infection. Pediatrics 96:247, 1995.
42. Gisolf EH, Enting RH, Jurriaans S, et al. Cerebrospinal fluid HIV-1 RNA during treatment with ritonavir/saquinavir or ritonavir/saquinavir/stavudine. AIDS 14:1583, 2000.
43. Odinecs A, Nosbisch C, Keller RD, et al. In vivo maternal-fetal pharmacokinetics of stavudine (2′,3′-didehydro-3′-deoxythymidine) in pig-tailed macaques (Macaca nemestrina). Antimicrob Agents Chemother 40:196, 1996.
44. Bawdon RE, Kaul S, Sobhi S. The ex vivo transfer of the anti-HIV nucleoside compound d4T in the human placenta. Gynecol Obstet Invest 38:1, 1994.
45. Inoue T, Tsushita K, Ito T, et al. In vitro bone marrow toxicity of nucleoside analog against human immunodeficiency virus. Antimicrob Agents Chemother 33:576, 1989.
46. Gogu SR, Beckman BS, Agrawal KC. Anti-HIV drugs: comparative toxicities in murine fetal liver and bone marrow erythroid progenitor cells. Life Sci 45:iii, 1989.
47. Sommadosi JP. Nucleoside analogs: similarities and differences. J Infect Dis 16(suppl 1):S7, 1993.
48. Cui L, Locatelli L, Xie MY, et al. Effect of nucleoside analogs on neurite regeneration and mitochondrial DNA synthesis in PC-12 cells. J Pharmacol Exp Ther 280:1228, 1997.
49. Chen CH, Vazquez Padua M, Cheng YC. Effect of anti-human immunodeficiency virus nucleoside analogs on mitochondrial DNA and its implication for delayed toxicity. Mol Pharmacol 39:625, 1991.
50. Medina DJ, Tsai CH, Hsiung GD, et al. Comparison of mitochondrial morphology, mitochondrial DNA content, and cell viability in cultured cells treated with three anti-human immunodeficiency virus dideoxynucleosides. Antimicrob Agents Chemother 38:1824, 1994.
51. Spruance SL, Pavia AT, Mellors JW, et al. Clinical efficacy of monotherapy with stavudine compared with zidovudine in HIV-infected, zidovudine-experienced patients: a randomized, double-blind, controlled trial; Bristol-Myers Squibb Stavudine/019 Study Group. Ann Intern Med 126:355, 1997.
52. Browne MJ. Phase I study of 2′3′-didehydro-2′,3′-dideoxythymidine (d4T) in patients (Pts.) with AIDS or ARC. In: Abstracts of the 6th International Conference on AIDS, 1990, p 200 (abstract S.B.456).
53. Squires K, Sacks H, Sledz S, et al. Findings from a phase I study of stavudine (d4T). In: Abstracts of the 8th International Conference on AIDS, 1992, p B92 (abstract PoB 3030).
54. Murray HW, Squires KE, Weiss W, et al. Stavudine in patients with AIDS and AIDS-related complex: AIDS clinical trials group 089. J Infect Dis 171(suppl 2):S123, 1995.
55. Skowron G. Biologic effects and safety of stavudine: overview of phase I and II clinical trials. J Infect Dis 171(suppl 2):S113, 1995.
56. Kline MW, Fletcher CV, Federici ME, et al. Combination therapy with stavudine and didanosine in children with advanced human immunodeficiency virus infection: pharmacokinetic properties, safety, and immunologic and virologic effects. Pediatrics 97:886, 1996.
57. Kline MW, Van Dyke RB, Lindsey JC, et al. A randomized comparative trial of stavudine (d4T) versus zidovudine (ZDV, AZT) in children with human immunodeficiency virus infection. AIDS Clinical Trials Group 240 team. Pediatrics 101:214, 1998.
58. Kline MW. Pediatric stavudine (d4T) studies. In: Abstracts of the 3rd Conference on Retroviruses and Opportunistic Infection, Washington, DC, 1996, p 173.
59. Moore RD, Wong WM, Keruly JC, et al. Incidence of neuropathy in HIV-infected patients on monotherapy versus those on combination therapy with didanosine, stavudine and hydroxyurea. AIDS 14:273, 2000.
60. Petersen EA, Ramirez-Ronda CH, Hardy WD, et al. Dose-related activity of stavudine in patients infected with human immunodeficiency virus. J Infect Dis 171(suppl 2):S131, 1995.

61. Freiman JP, Helfert KE, Hamrell MR, et al. Hepatomegaly with severe steatosis in HIV-seropositive patients. AIDS 7:379, 1993.
62. Bissuel F, Bruneel F, Habersetzer F, et al. Fulminant hepatitis with severe lactate acidosis in HIV-infected patients on didanosine therapy. J Intern Med 235:367, 1994.
63. Brinkman K, Ter Hofstede H, Veerkamp MJ, et al. Fatal lactic acidosis following HAART containing stavudine (d4T), lamivudine (3TC) and saquinavir. In: Abstracts of the 12th International Conference on AIDS, Vancouver, BC, 1998, p 1182 (abstract 60998).
64. Fortgang IS, Belitsos PC, Chaisson RE, et al. Hepatomegaly and steatosis in HIV-infected patients receiving nucleoside analog antiretroviral therapy. Am J Gastroenterol 90:1433, 1995.
65. Sundar K, Suarez M, Banogon PE, et al. Zidovudine-induced fatal lactic acidosis and hepatic failure in patients with acquired immunodeficiency syndrome: report of two patients and review of the literature. Crit Care Med 25:1425, 1997.
66. Moyle G. Toxicity of antiretroviral nucleoside and nucleotide analogues: is mitochondrial toxicity the only mechanism? Drug Saf 23:467, 2000.
67. Moyle G. Clinical manifestations and management of antiretroviral nucleoside analog-related mitochondrial toxicity. Clin Ther 22:911, 2000.
68. Pan-Zhou XR, Cui L, Zhou XJ, et al. Differential effects of antiretroviral nucleoside analogs on mitochondrial function in HepG2 cells. Antimicrob Agents Chemother 44:496, 2000.
69. Kakuda TN. Pharmacology of nucleoside and nucleotide reverse transcriptase inhibitor-induced mitochondrial toxicity. Clin Ther 22:685, 2000.
70. Chariot P, Drogou I, de Lacroix-Szmania I, et al. Zidovudine-induced mitochondrial disorder with massive liver steatosis, myopathy, lactic acidosis, and mitochondrial DNA depletion. J Hepatol 30:156, 1999.
71. Brivet FG, Nion I, Megarbane B, et al. Fatal lactic acidosis and liver steatosis associated with didanosine and stavudine treatment: a respiratory chain dysfunction [letter]? J Hepatol 32:364, 2000.
72. Moyle G. Mitochondrial toxicity hypothesis for lipoatrophy: a refutation. AIDS 15:413, 2001.
73. Brinkman K. Editorial response: hyperlactatemia and hepatic steatosis as features of mitochondrial toxicity of nucleoside analogue reverse transcriptase inhibitors. Clin Infect Dis 31:167, 2000.
74. Bleeker-Rovers CP, Kadir SW, van Leusen R, et al. Hepatic steatosis and lactic acidosis caused by stavudine in an HIV-infected patient. Neth J Med 57:190, 2000.
75. Gerard Y, Maulin L, Yazdanpanah Y, et al. Symptomatic hyperlactataemia: an emerging complication of antiretroviral therapy. AIDS 14:2723, 2000.
76. Lonergan JT, Behling C, Pfander H, et al. Hyperlactatemia and hepatic abnormalities in 10 human immunodeficiency virus-infected patients receiving nucleoside analogue combination regimens. Clin Infect Dis 31:162, 2000.
77. Miller KD, Cameron M, Wood LV, et al. Lactic acidosis and hepatic steatosis associated with use of stavudine: report of four cases. Ann Intern Med 133:192, 2000.
78. Mokrzycki MH, Harris C, May H, et al. Lactic acidosis associated with stavudine administration: a report of five cases. Clin Infect Dis 30:198, 2000.
79. John M, Moore CB, James IR, et al. Chronic hyperlactatemia in HIV-infected patients taking antiretroviral therapy. AIDS 15:717, 2001.
80. Vrouenraets SM, Treskes M, Regez RM, et al. Hyperlactatemia in HIV-infected patients: the role of NRTI treatment. In: Abstracts of the 8th Conference on Retroviruses and Opportunistic Infections, Chicago, 2001, abstract 625.
81. Lonergan JT, Havlir D, Barber E, et al. Incidence and outcome of hyperlactatemia associated with clinical manifestations in HIV-infected adults receiving NRTI-containing regimens. In: Abstracts of the 8th Conference on Retroviruses and Opportunistic Infections, Chicago, 2001, abstract 624.
82. Important drug warning [letter]. Bristol-Myers Squibb, Princeton, NJ, January 5, 2001.
83. Saint-Marc T, Partisani M, Poizot-Martin I, et al. Fat distribution evaluated by computed tomography and metabolic abnormalities in patients undergoing antiretroviral therapy: preliminary results of the LIPOCO study. AIDS 14:37, 2000.
84. Carr A, Miller J, Law M, et al. A syndrome of lipoatrophy, lactic acidaemia and liver dysfunction associated with HIV nucleoside analogue therapy: contribution to protease inhibitor-related lipodystrophy syndrome. AIDS 14:F25, 2000.
85. Brinkman K, Smeitink JA, Romijn JA, et al. Mitochondrial toxicity induced by nucleoside-analogue reverse-transcriptase inhibitors is a key factor in the pathogenesis of antiretroviral-therapy-related lipodystrophy. Lancet 354:1112, 1999.
86. Lichtenstein KA, Delaney KM, Ward DJ, et al. Clinical factors associated with incidence and prevalence of fat atrophy and accumulation. Antivir Ther 5(suppl 5):61, 2000.
87. Mallal SA, John M, Moore CB, et al. Contribution of nucleoside analogue reverse transcriptase inhibitors to subcutaneous fat wasting in patients with HIV infection. AIDS 14:1309, 2000.
88. Saint-Marc T, Partisani M, Poizot-Martin I, et al. A syndrome of peripheral fat wasting (lipodystrophy) in patients receiving long-term nucleoside analogue therapy. AIDS 13:1659, 1999.
89. Heath KV, Hogg RS, Chan KJ, et al. Lipodystrophy-associated morphological, cholesterol and triglyceride abnormalities in a population-based HIV/AIDS treatment database. AIDS 15:231, 2001.
90. Gottlieb M, Peterson D, Adler M, et al. Comparison of safety and efficacy of two doses of stavudine (Zerit, d4T) in a large simple trial in the US parallel track program. In: Abstracts of the 35th Interscience Conference on Antimicrobial Agents and Chemotherapy, San Francisco, 1995, abstract I171.
91. Moore RD, Keruly JC, Chaisson RE. Incidence of pancreatitis in HIV-infected patients receiving nucleoside reverse transcriptase inhibitor drugs. AIDS 15:617, 2001.
92. Kaul S, Dandekar KA, Schilling BE, et al. Toxicokinetics of 2′,3′-didehydro-3′-deoxythymidine, stavudine (d4T). Drug Metab Dispos 27:1, 1999.
93. Toltzis P, Mourton T, Magnuson T. Comparative embryonic cytotoxicity of antiretroviral nucleosides. J Infect Dis 169:1100, 1994.
94. Schilling B, Diamond S, Proctor J, et al. Nonclinical toxicity profile of BMY 27857 (d4T, stavudine). In: Abstracts of the 8th International Conference on AIDS, 1992, p B91 (abstract PoB 3027).
95. Minkoff H, Augenbraum M. Antiviral therapy for pregnant women. Am J Obstet Gynecol 176:478, 1997.
96. Katlama C, Valantin MA, Matheron S, et al. Efficacy and tolerability of stavudine plus lamivudine in treatment-naive and treatment-experienced patients with HIV-1 infection. Ann Intern Med 129:525, 1998.
97. Kuritzkes DR, Marschner I, Johnson VA, et al. Lamivudine in combination with zidovudine, stavudine, or didanosine in patients with HIV-1 infection: a randomized, double-blind, placebo-controlled trial; National Institute of Allergy and Infectious Disease AIDS Clinical Trials Group Protocol 306 Investigators. AIDS 13:685, 1999.
98. Foudraine NA, de Jong JJ, Jan Weverling G, et al. An open randomized controlled trial of zidovudine plus lamivudine versus stavudine plus lamivudine. AIDS 12:1513, 1998.
99. Pollard RB, Peterson D, Hardy D, et al. Safety and antiretroviral effects of combined didanosine and stavudine therapy in HIV-infected individuals with CD4 counts of 200 to 500 cells/mm^3. J Acquir Immune Defic Syndr 22:39, 1999.
100. Rutschmann OT, Opravil M, Iten A, et al. A placebo-controlled trial of didanosine plus stavudine, with and without hydroxyurea, for HIV infection: the Swiss HIV Cohort Study. AIDS 12:F71, 1998.
101. Molina JM, Chene G, Ferchal F, et al. The ALBI trial: a randomized controlled trial comparing stavudine plus didanosine with zidovudine plus lamivudine and a regimen alternating both combinations in previously untreated patients infected with human immunodeficiency virus. J Infect Dis 180:351, 1999.
102. Kline MW, Van Dyke RB, Lindsey JC, et al. Combination therapy with stavudine (d4T) plus didanosine (ddI) in children with human immunodeficiency virus infection: the pediatric AIDS Clinical Trials Group 327 team. Pediatrics 103:e62, 1999.
103. Havlir DV, Tierney C, Friedland GH, et al. In vivo antagonism with zidovudine plus stavudine combination therapy. J Infect Dis 182:321, 2000.
104. Griffith BP, Brett-Smith H, Kim G, et al. Effect of stavudine on human immunodeficiency virus type 1 virus load as measured by quantitative mononuclear cell culture, plasma RNA, and immune complex-dissociated antigenemia. J Infect Dis 173:1252, 1996.
105. Katlama C, Molina JM, Rozenbaum W, et al. Stavudine (d4T) in HIV infected patients with CD4 less than 350/mm^3: results of a double-blind randomized placebo controlled study. In: 3rd Conference on Retroviruses and Opportunistic Infections, Washington, DC, 1996, p 89.

106. Katzenstein DA, Hughes M, Albrecht M, et al. Virologic and CD4+ cell responses to new nucleoside regimens: switching to stavudine or adding lamivudine after prolonged zidovudine treatment of human immunodeficiency virus infection: ACTG 302 Study Team; AIDS Clinical Trials Group. AIDS Res Hum Retroviruses 16:1031, 2000.
107. Pavia AT, Gathe J, BMS-019 Study Group Investigators. Clinical efficacy of stavudine (d4T, Zerit) compared to zidovudine (ZDV, Retrovir) in ZDV-pretreated HIV positive patients. In: Abstracts of the 35th Interscience Conference on Antimicrobial Agents and Chemotherapy, San Francisco, 1995, abstract I169.
108. Cohen CJ, Shalit P, Conant M, et al. Lamivudine (3TC) and stavudine (d4T) combination therapy: HIV viral load and CD4 changes in a retrospective study of 330 patients. In: Abstracts of the 4th Conference on Retroviruses and Opportunistic Infections, Washington, DC, 1997, abstract 556.
109. Rouleau D, Conway B, Raboud J, et al. Stavudine plus lamivudine in advanced human immunodeficiency virus disease: a short-term pilot study. J Infect Dis 176:1156, 1997.
110. Novak RM, Colombo J, Linares-Diaz M, et al. Comparison of AZT/3TC vs. D4T/3TC for the treatment of HIV in persons with CD4 counts less than 300 and prior AZT experience. In: Abstracts of the 11th International Conference on AIDS, Vancouver, 1996, abstract Tu.B. 2132.
111. Cohen CJ, Skowron GF, Giordano M, et al. A prospective multicenter study of viral load changes in HIV$^+$ individuals, adding lamivudine to stable antiretroviral regiments other than AZT. In: Abstracts of the 4th Conference on Retrovirus and Opportunistic Infection, Washington, DC, 1997.
112. Steinhart CR, Jacobsen D, George S. Combination antiretroviral therapy with stavudine (d4T) and lamivudine (3TC): a retrospective analysis. In: Abstracts of the 11th International Conference on AIDS, Vancouver, 1996, abstract Tu.B. 2130.
113. Seifert RD, Stewart MB, Sramek JJ, et al. Pharmacokinetics of co-administered didanosine and stavudine in HIV-seropositive male patients. Br J Clin Pharmacol 38:405, 1994.
114. Raffi F, Reliquet V, Auger S, et al. Efficacy and safety of stavudine and didanosine combination therapy in antiretroviral-experienced patients. AIDS 12:1999, 1998.
115. Gathe J Jr, Burkhardt B, Hawley P, et al. A randomized phase II study of Viracept, a novel HIV protease inhibitor, used in combination with stavudine (d4T) vs. stavudine (d4T) alone. In: International Conference on AIDS. Vancouver, 1996, abstract Mo.B.413.
116. Powderly W, Sension M, Conant M, et al. The efficacy of Viracept (nelfinavir mesylate, NFV) in pivotal phase II/III double-blind randomized controlled trials as monotherapy and in combination with d4T or AZT/3TC. In: 4th Conferences on Retroviruses and Opportunistics Infections. Washington, DC, 1997, abstract 370.
117. Steigbigel RT, Cooper D, Clumeck N, et al. Indinavir with stavudine vs. IDV alone vs. stavudine alone in zidovudine experienced, HIV-infected patients. Merck Protocol 037 Study Group. In: Abstracts of the 12th International Conference on AIDS. Vancouver, 1998, p 80 (abstract 12335).
118. Murphy RL. Stavudine-based multiple agent combinations: initial studies and ongoing comparative trials. Antivir Ther 3:69, 1998.
119. Roca B, Gomez CJ, Arnedo A. A randomized, comparative study of lamivudine plus stavudine, with indinavir or nelfinavir, in treatment-experienced HIV-infected patients. AIDS 14:157, 2000.
120. Murphy RL, Brun S, Hicks C, et al. ABT-378/ritonavir plus stavudine and lamivudine for the treatment of antiretroviral-naive adults with HIV-1 infection: 48-week results. AIDS 15:F1, 2001.
121. Squires KE, Gulick R, Tebas P, et al. A comparison of stavudine plus lamivudine versus zidovudine plus lamivudine in combination with indinavir in antiretroviral naive individuals with HIV infection: selection of thymidine analog regimen therapy (START I). AIDS 14:1591, 2000.
122. Carr A, Chuah J, Hudson J, et al. A randomised, open-label comparison of three highly active antiretroviral therapy regimens including two nucleoside analogues and indinavir for previously untreated HIV-1 infection: the OzCombo1 study. AIDS 14:1171, 2000.
123. Saimot AG, Landman R, Damond F, et al. Stavudine (d4T), didanosine (ddI) and ritonavir as a triple therapy in antiretroviral-naive patients: results at 72 weeks. The IMEA 01 Study Group. In: Abstracts of the 12th International Conference on AIDS, Geneva, 1998, p 344 (abstract 22401).
124. Pednault L, Elion R, Adler M, et al. Stavudine (d4T), didanosine (ddI), and nelfinavir combination therapy in HIV-Infected subjects: antiviral effect and safety in an ongoing pilot study. In: Abstracts of the 4th Conference on Retroviruses and Opportunistic Infection, Washington, DC, 1997, abstract 241.
125. Elion R, Kaul S, Knupp C, et al. The safety profile and antiviral activity of the combination of stavudine, didanosine, and nelfinavir in patients with HIV infection. Clin Ther 21:1853, 1999.
126. Kline MW, Fletcher CV, Harris AT, et al. One-year follow-up of HIV-infected children receiving combination therapy with indinavir, stavudine (d4T), and didanosine (ddI). In: Abstracts of the 5th Conference on Retroviruses and Opportunistic Infection, Chicago, 1998, p 122 (abstract 232).
127. Eron JJ Jr, Murphy RL, Peterson D, et al. A comparison of stavudine, didanosine and indinavir with zidovudine, lamivudine and indinavir for the initial treatment of HIV-1 infected individuals: selection of thymidine analog regimen therapy (START II). AIDS 14:1601, 2000.
128. Squires K. The Atlantic study: a randomized, open-label trial comparing two protease inhibitor (PI)-sparing anti-retroviral strategies versusa standard PI-containing regimen, final 48 week data. In: Abstracts of the XIIIth International AIDS Conference, Durban, South Africa, 2000, abstract LbPeB7046.
129. Murphy R, Katlama C, Autran B, et al. The effects of hydroxyurea or placebo combined with efavirenz, didanosine, and stavudine in treatment naive and experienced patients: preliminary 24 week results from the 3d study. In: Abstracts of the XIIIth International AIDS Conference, Durban, South Africa, 2000, abstract WeOrB603.
130. De Truchis P, Zucman D, Dupont C, et al. Combination therapy with D4T + 3TC + indinavir (IDV) in nucleosides-experienced HIV-infected patients: an open-label study. In: Abstracts of the 4th Conference on Retroviruses and Opportunistic Infections, Washington, DC, 1997, p 109 (abstract 247).
131. Nachman SA, Stanley K, Yogev R, et al. Nucleoside analogs plus ritonavir in stable antiretroviral therapy-experienced HIV-infected children: a randomized controlled trial: pediatric AIDS Clinical Trials Group 338 study team. JAMA 283:492, 2000.
132. Gisolf EH, Jurriaans S, Pelgrom J, et al. The effect of treatment intensification in HIV infection: a study comparing treatment with ritonavir/saquinavir and ritonavir/saquinavir/stavudine: Prometheus study group. AIDS 14:405, 2000.
133. Larder BA, Darby G, Richman DD. HIV with reduced sensitivity to zidovudine (AZT) isolated during prologed therapy. Science 243:1731, 1989.
134. Richman DD. Susceptibilities of zidovudine-susceptible and -resistant human immunodeficiency virus isolates to antiviral agents determined by using a quantitative plaque reduction assay. Am J Med 88(suppl 5B):8S, 1990.
135. Lacey SF, Larder BA. Novel mutation (V75T) in human immunodeficiency virus type 1 reverse transcriptase confers resistance to 2′,3′-didehydro-2′,3′-dideoxythymidine in cell culture. Antimicrob Agents Chemother 38:1428, 1994.
136. Gu Z, Gao Q, Fang H, et al. Identification of novel mutations that confer drug resistance in the human immunodeficiency virus polymerase gene. Leukemia 8(suppl 1):S166, 1994.
137. Deminie C, Bechtold C, Riccardi K, et al. HIV-1 isolates from subjects on prolonged stavudine therapy remain sensitive to stavudine. In: Abstracts of the 11th International Conference on AIDS, Vancouver, 1996, p 74 (abstract Mo.A.1115).
138. Lin PF, Samanta H, Rose RE, et al. Genotypic and phenotypic analysis of human immunodeficiency virus type 1 isolates from patients on prolonged stavudine therapy. J Infect Dis 170:1157, 1994.
139. Soriano V, Dietrich U, Villalba N, et al. Lack of emergence of genotypic resistance to stavudine after 2 years of monotherapy. AIDS 11:696, 1997.
140. Coakley EP, Gillis JM, Hammer SM. Phenotypic and genotypic resistance patterns of HIV-1 isolates derived from individuals treated with didanosine and stavudine. AIDS 14:F9, 2000.
141. Pellegrin I, Izopet J, Reynes J, et al. Emergence of zidovudine and multidrug-resistance mutations in the HIV-1 reverse transcriptase gene in therapy-naive patients receiving stavudine plus didanosine combination therapy: STADI group. AIDS 13:1705, 1999.
142. Schuurman R, Nijhuis M, Keulen W, et al. Selection of zidovudine resistance mutations conferring low-level resistance to stavudine occurs

at low frequency in stavudine-treated patients and in vitro during prolonged selection experiments. Antivir Ther 5(suppl 3):39, 2000.

143. Johnson VA, Bassett RL, Koel JL, et al. Selection of zidovudine resistance mutations by zidovudine- or stavudine-based regimens and relationship to subsequent virologic response in ACTG 370. Antivir Ther 5(suppl 3):42, 2000.
144. De Mendoza C, Soriano V, Briones C, et al. Emergence of zidovudine resistance in HIV-infected patients receiving stavudine. J Acquir Immune Defic Syndr 23:279, 2000.
145. Moyle GJ, Gazzard BG. Differing reverse transcriptase mutation patterns in individuals experiencing viral rebound on first-line regimens with stavudine/didanosine and stavudine/lamivudine. AIDS 15:799, 2001.
146. Costagliola D, Descamps D, Calvez V, et al. Presence of thymidine-associated mutations and response to d4T, abacavir and ddI in the control arm of the Narval ANRS 088 trial. In: Abstracts of the 8th Conference on Retroviruses and Opportunistic Infections, Chicago, 2001, abstract 450.
147. Calvez V, Costagliola D, Descamps D, et al. Resistance and viral response to stavudine/lamivudine combination in zidovudine, didanosine and zalcitabine experienced patients in ALTIS 2 ANRS trial. Antivir Ther 5(suppl 3):83, 2000.
148. Duan C, Poticha D, Stoeckli T, et al. Biochemical evidence of cross-resistance to stavudine (d4T) triphosphate in purified HIV-1 reverse transcriptase (RT) derived from a zidovudine (AZT)- resistant isolate. In: Abstracts of the 8th Conference on Retroviruses and Opportunistic Infections, Chicago, 2001, abstract 442.
149. Selmi B, Boretto J, Navarro JM, et al. The valine-to-threonine 75 substitution in human immunodeficiency virus type 1 reverse transcriptase and its relation with stavudine resistance. J Biol Chem 276:13965, 2001.
150. Schmit JC, Cogniaux J, Hermans P, et al. Multiple drug resistance to nucleoside analogues and nonnucleoside reverse transcriptase inhibitors in an efficiently replicating human immunodeficiency virus type 1 patient strain. J Infect Dis 174:962, 1996.
151. Shafer RW, Winters MA, Iversen AK, et al. Genotypic and phenotypic changes during culture of a multinucleoside-resistant human immunodeficiency virus type 1 strain in the presence and absence of additional reverse transcriptase inhibitors. Antimicrob Agents Chemother 40:2887, 1996.
152. Iversen AK, Shafer RW, Wehrly K, et al. Multidrug-resistant human immunodeficiency virus type 1 strains resulting from combination antiretroviral therapy. J Virol 70:1086, 1996.
153. De Jong JJ, Goudsmit J, Lukashov VV, et al. Insertion of two amino acids combined with changes in reverse transcriptase containing tyrosine-215 of HIV-1 resistant to multiple nucleoside analogs. AIDS 13:75, 1999.
154. Larder BA, Bloor S, Kemp SD, et al. A family of insertion mutations between codons 67 and 70 of human immunodeficiency virus type 1 reverse transcriptase confer multinucleoside analog resistance. Antimicrob Agents Chemother 43:1961, 1999.
155. Sugiura W, Matsuda M, Matsuda Z, et al. Identification of insertion mutations in HIV-1 reverse transcriptase causing multiple drug resistance to nucleoside analogue reverse transcriptase inhibitors. J Hum Virol 2:146, 1999.
156. Winters MA, Coolley KL, Girard YA, et al. A 6-basepair insert in the reverse transcriptase gene of human immunodeficiency virus type 1 confers resistance to multiple nucleoside inhibitors. J Clin Invest 102:1769, 1998.
157. Piscitelli SC, Kelly G, Walker RE, et al. A multiple drug interaction study of stavudine with agents for opportunistic infections in human immunodeficiency virus-infected patients. Antimicrob Agents Chemother 43:647, 1999.
158. Rainey PM, McCance EF, Mitchell SM, et al. Interaction of methadone with didanosine (ddI) and stavudine (d4T). In: Abstracts of the 6th Conference on Retroviruses and Opportunistic Infection, Chicago, 1999, p 137 (abstract 371).
159. Carpenter CCJ, Cooper MDA, Fischl MA, et al. Antiretroviral therapy in adults: updated recommendations of the International AIDS Society—USA panel. JAMA 283:381, 2000.
160. DHHS Panel on Clinical Practices for the Treatment of HIV. Guidelines for the use of antiretroviral agents in HIV-infected adults and adolescents. http:\\www.hivatis.org. Updated April 23, 2001; accessed May 29, 2001.
161. Soriano V. Sequencing antiretroviral drugs. AIDS 15:547, 2001.
162. Simpson DM, Olney RK. Peripheral neuropathies associated with human immunodeficiency virus infection. Neurol Clin 10:685, 1992.
163. Simpson DM, Tagliati M. Nucleoside analogue-associated peripheral neuropathy in human immunodeficiency virus infection. J Acquir Immune Defic Syndr Hum Retrovirol 9:153, 1995.
164. Gray G, McIntyre J, Jivkov B, et al. Preliminary efficacy, safety, tolerability, and pharmacokinetics of short course regimens of nucleoside analogues for the prevention of mother-to-child transmission (MTCT) of HIV. In: Abstracts of the XIIIth International AIDS Conference, Durban, South Africa, 2000, abstract TuOrB355.

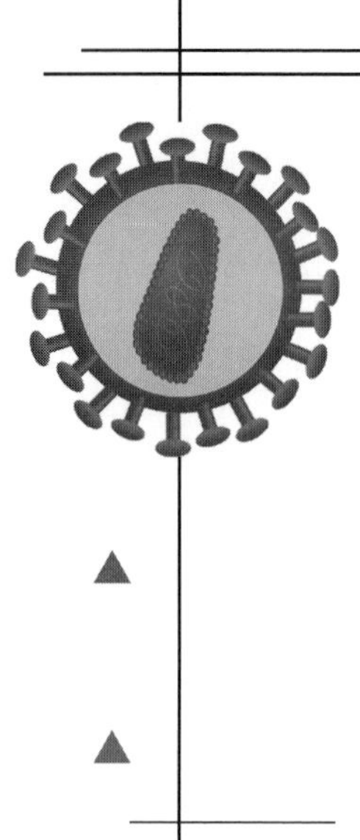

CHAPTER 6

Lamivudine

Joseph J. Eron, Jr., MD

STRUCTURE

Lamivudine (3TC, Epivir) is the negative or *cis* enantiomer of 2′-deoxy-3′-thiacytidine that has antiviral activity against human immunodeficiency virus types 1 and 2 (HIV-1, HIV-2) and hepatitis B virus. This compound is a pyrimidine nucleoside analogue that contains a sulfur atom in place of the 3′ carbon of the ribose ring (Fig. 6–1). 3TC was originally synthesized in a racemic mixture (BCH-189), and this racemic mixture was subsequently separated into positive and negative enantiomers. 3TC, the negative enantiomer, has its ribose ring in a position opposite to the ribose ring position in physiologic nucleosides and most nucleoside analogues.

MECHANISM OF ACTION AND IN VITRO ACTIVITY

Like all nucleoside analogues, 3TC must be metabolized to its triphosphorylated form, 3TC-triphosphate, to be an active antiviral compound. 3TC-triphosphate is a reverse transcriptase inhibitor that competes with deoxycytidine-triphosphate (dCTP), an endogenous nucleotide, for binding in the HIV reverse transcriptase binding site. Incorporation of 3TC-triphosphate into the elongating DNA molecule results in irreversible chain termination as 3TC lacks the 3′-hydroxyl group required for the 5′ to 3′ linkage required for DNA synthesis.[1] As mentioned above, 3TC was originally synthesized as a racemic mixture (BCH-189), and this mixture has potent activity in vitro against HIV-1 with a mean 50% inhibitory dose (IC_{50}) of 0.73 μM in an MT4 cell line assay.[2] The mixture was active against zidovudine (ZDV)-resistant isolates and had less cytotoxicity than ZDV.[2] When BCH-189 was separated into the positive and negative enantiomers, both compounds were discovered to have anti-HIV-1 activity.[3,4] The positive enantiomer, (+)-2′-deoxy-3-thiacytidine, has significantly more cytotoxicity than 3TC in vitro, and 3TC appeared to have more antiretroviral activity,[4, 5] with a median effect in the nanomolar range in some experiments.[3] 3TC has been tested against laboratory strains of HIV-1 and HIV-2 in a variety of lymphoid cell lines, and the IC_{50} ranged from 4 to 670 nM.[6] 3TC was also highly active against HIV-1 isolates in peripheral blood mononuclear cell assays (IC_{50} 2.5 to 90 nM).[6] In these experiments the IC_{50} for cytotoxicity was typically 1000-fold higher. That 3TC is more active than its positive enantiomer has been ascribed to the resistance of 3TC to cleavage from the 3′ terminals of RNA/DNA complexes by 3′-5′ cellular exonucleases.[5,7] In a series of experiments, Skalski and colleagues showed that the positive enantiomer has more inhibitory activity than 3TC-TP against the HIV reverse transcriptase, although a novel cellular exonuclease removed the positive enantiomer at a two- to six-fold higher rate.[5] This group also showed that 3TC was more readily phosphorylated in the cell than the positive enantiomer. In addition to in vitro activity against HIV-1 and HIV-2, 3TC inhibits the hepatitis B virus[8] and has antiviral activity in patients with chronic active hepatitis B.[9, 10]

Lamivudine has been shown to be synergistic in vitro with a variety of antiretroviral agents in inhibiting HIV-1. Against ZDV-sensitive isolates and in some studies against ZDV-resistant isolates[11] 3TC has been shown to be synergistic or additive with nucleoside analogues (zidovudine,[11–13] stavudine,[11,12] didanosine[12]), protease inhibitors,[11] and the nonnucleoside

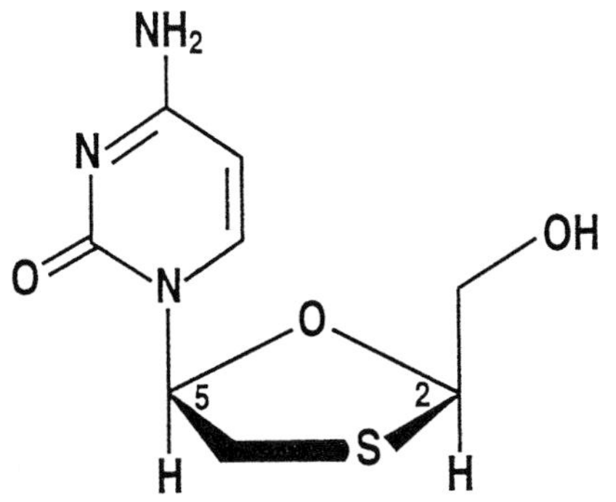

Figure 6–1. Structure of *cis* enantiomer of 2′-deoxy-3′-thiacytidine (3TC).

reverse transcriptase inhibitors.[11,14] Three-drug combinations of 3TC/ZDV/saquinavir,[11] 3TC/ZDV/d4T,[11] 3TC/ZDV/nevirapine,[11] and 3TC/ZDV/delavirdine[14] have also been shown to be synergistic or additive in vitro. The combination of 3TC/ZDV and indinavir demonstrates marked synergy in vitro,[15] which may help explain the clinical success of this regimen.[16,17] It is of note that 3TC interferes with phosphorylation of zalcitabine (ddC),[18] most likely because these agents are both cytosine analogues. These two agents may be antagonistic against HIV-1 replication, as has been shown in vitro for stavudine (d4T) and ZDV, which are both thymidine analogues.[11] Neither combination is recommended as a component of highly active antiretroviral therapy.[19]

▲ PHARMACOKINETICS

Favorable oral bioavailability was demonstrated during the initial in vivo studies of 3TC. When single doses of 3TC over a range of five doses (0.25 to 8.0 mg/kg) were given intravenously and orally to adult men who were HIV-infected, the bioavailability was 82%.[20] Food has no significant effect on the extent of 3TC absorption.[21] Other studies have shown similar oral bioavailability of tablet and oral solution formulations of 3TC,[22] although intrasubject variability in the bioavailability of the tablet was seen. The bioavailability of 3TC in infants, which was 66% in one study, is somewhat less than that seen in adults.[23]

In a phase I/II multiple-dose study, 97 subjects with acquired immunodeficiency syndrome (AIDS) or advanced HIV (median CD4+ T-lymphocyte count 128 cells per mm^3) were administered 3TC at 0.5, 1.0, 2.0, 4.0, 8.0, 12.0, and 20.0 mg/kg twice daily in sequential cohorts.[24] Pharmacokinetic parameters obtained at steady state after 2 weeks on therapy showed dose linearity with peak concentrations well above the in vitro IC_{90} of HIV-1, especially at the higher doses. The half-life of 3TC in serum was 3 to 4 hours. The pharmacokinetic parameters did not change after 24 weeks of continuous dosing. Other studies, which examined single doses of 3TC, have shown that the half-life in plasma was substantially longer than in the study of Pluda et al.,[24] ranging from 8 to 11 hours.[22,25] 3TC clearance is dependent on weight and renal function and is not influenced by gender, disease stage, CD4+ T-lymphocyte count or race.[26] 3TC has low protein binding in plasma and freely crosses the placenta and into breast milk[27]; it appears to be concentrated in the male genital tract.[28] 3TC clearance is prolonged in neonates compared to that in infants and older children.[27] 3TC is excreted predominantly by the kidney, with 70% excreted unchanged in the urine.[20] Dose adjustment is required with significant renal impairment (creatinine clearance < 50 ml/min).[25,29] 3TC is cleared by hemodialysis, though given the large volume of distribution of 3TC no increase in dose is required once an individual with chronic renal failure begins dialysis.[29] 3TC pharmacokinetics are unchanged in individuals with moderately to severely impaired hepatic function (cirrhosis).[30]

Lamivudine enters the cell by passive diffusion[8] and appears to be phosphorylated more efficiently in resting lymphocytes than in activated cells.[31] At steady state approximately 15% to 20% of 3TC in peripheral blood mononuclear cells is in the triphosphate form (3TC-TP) and 50% to 55% is in the diphosphate form, (3TC-DP), making the conversion of 3TC-DP to 3TC-TP the rate-limiting step during intracellular metabolism.[32] The intracellular half-life of 3TC-TP is approximately 12 to 16 hours[32,33] compared to 1.0 and 2.6 hours for ZDV-TP and ddC-TP, respectively. Once-daily dosing of 300 mg of 3TC is being evaluated in clinical studies and may become an acceptable dosing strategy.

In a dose-range Phase I/II study of 3TC, serum and cerebrospinal fluid (CSF) samples were obtained from some subjects and the CSF/serum drug concentration ratio was found to be low (0.06) similar to what was previously reported for ddI and ddC.[34] The concentration of 3TC in CSF relative to serum in nonhuman primates was significantly higher (41%), though levels in ventricular CSF in these animals was similar to those seen in humans.[35] In children the CSF/serum ratios were more than 0.1[34] and therefore higher than reported by van Leeuwen et al.[34] in adults.[36] It is of note that because 3TC has such favorable pharmacokinetics, reaching high levels in serum, the absolute concentrations of 3TC in CSF are as high or higher than the two thymidine nucleoside analogues d4T and ZDV.[37] In addition, CSF concentrations of nucleoside analogues are relatively stable over time, unlike plasma concentrations. Therefore CSF/serum drug ratios are highly time-dependent, with higher ratios when sampling is done later in the dosing interval.[37]

The penetration of 3TC into male genital secretions has also been examined. In 70 samples from nine men on 3TC and ZDV followed over time, the median seminal fluid/blood plasma 3TC concentration ratio was 9:1, demonstrating marked accumulation of 3TC in this compartment.[28] When the steady-state relation between the seminal fluid–blood plasma 3TC concentration was examined relative to the timing of drug ingestion, the 3TC concentrations in semen were remarkably constant over time, suggesting that 3TC is either actively taken up or trapped in this compartment.[38] The semen/blood concentration ratios for 3TC are higher than for other nucleosides,[28,38,39] nonnucleoside reverse transcriptase inhibitors (NNRTIs),[39,40] and single protease inhibitors[38,41,42] described to date. Whether these high concentrations of 3TC affect the likelihood of HIV-1 sexual transmission relative to other antiretroviral agents is not known.

▲ TOXICITY

Some of the toxicity seen with nucleoside analogues results from their affinity for human DNA polymerases, although for most nucleoside analogues the affinity for this enzyme is less than that for HIV-1 reverse transcriptase. The relative affinity of the nucleoside reverse transcriptase inhibitors (NRTIs) for specific human DNA polymerases varies by agent and may explain in part their differing toxicities. Significant attention has been given to the potential mitochondrial toxicity of nucleoside analogues, which may relate to their affinity for DNA polymerase -γ.[43–45]

Lamivudine has limited cytotoxicity in vitro,[4–6] possibly owing to the low affinity of 3TC-TP for human DNA polymerases.[8,46] For each of these human enzymes the positive enantiomer has greater affinity than 3TC,[8] and these enzyme affinities offer a likely explanation for the differences in cytotoxicity between these enantiomers. There was no evidence of a neuropathic effect of 3TC in an in vitro model of neuron toxicity,[47] and the potential for hematologic toxicity as measured in vitro is low.[48]

Significant toxicity that is clearly attributable to 3TC is uncommon (Table 6–1). Dose-limiting toxicity was not observed in early studies of 3TC monotherapy.[20,24,34] At doses higher than currently recommended, neutropenia was observed in a small number of subjects, and a general downward trend in absolute neutrophil counts was seen.[24,34] The subjects in these studies had relatively low CD4+ T-lymphocyte counts, and individuals with low counts may be at greater risk of hematologic toxicity, as has been shown for ZDV.[49] In comparative trials the addition of 3TC to ZDV in a double-blind placebo-controlled trial appeared to have no significant adverse effects other than those seen in subjects who were given ZDV alone.[50] In this study subjects given 3TC alone had significantly higher hemoglobin levels than the ZDV- and ZDV/3TC-treated subjects. In large clinical trials in subjects with more advanced disease and previous ZDV therapy for an average of 2 years, severe adverse effects of 3TC/ZDV were also uncommon.[51,52] In the study in which 3TC (at two doses)/ZDV was compared to ZDV alone, nausea was the most common adverse effect and was seen more commonly in the 3TC/ZDV arms (10% vs. 5% of subjects), though this difference was not significant.[52] Neutropenia occurred more commonly in subjects receiving 3TC (300 mg twice daily)/ZDV, but again the differences were not significant between arms. The number of subjects with severe neutropenia was the same in the 3TC (150 twice daily)/ZDV arm and the ZDV monotherapy arm. There were no episodes of pancreatitis and only one episode of peripheral neuropathy among the 223 subjects randomized. In a larger study of subjects with relatively advanced HIV disease (median CD4+ T-lymphocyte count approximately 210 cells per millimeter) in which two doses of 3TC/ZDV were compared with ddC/ZDV, the differences in cumulative moderate and severe toxicity between the treatment arms were not significant.[51]

▲ **Table 6–1.** TOXICITIES

Neutropenia
Headache
Nausea

The contribution of 3TC to antiretroviral adverse effects that may be due to mitochondrial toxicity (e.g., lipoatrophy and lactic acidosis) is not known. Among patients with hepatitis B treated with 3TC, there was no evidence of mitochondrial toxicity on liver biopsy after 6 months of therapy, albeit the 3TC dose was lower than is commonly used to treat HIV.[53] Some observational cohort studies have suggested that elevated lactate levels are more common in subjects treated with 3TC and d4T in contrast to other combinations,[54,55] but this finding has not been consistently observed.

Episodes of pancreatitis have been reported in pediatric patients receiving 3TC in clinical trials.[56] However, these HIV-infected children and infants had advanced HIV disease and had received or were currently receiving concomitant medications that are associated with pancreatitis. Increased frequency of pancreatitis has not been observed in subjects receiving 3TC in controlled trials in adults.

▲ ANTIRETROVIRAL ACTIVITY AND CLINICAL EFFICACY

Multiple trials of 3TC activity and efficacy have been completed. Initially, trials of 3TC monotherapy demonstrated the antiretroviral activity of this agent. Subsequent trials have evaluated 3TC in combination with other antiretroviral agents. Some trials have evaluated antiretroviral activity and the effect on the CD4+ T-lymphocyte count as the primary endpoint, and others have investigated the clinical efficacy of 3TC-containing regimens, as reviewed in the following sections.

3TC Monotherapy

Trials of 3TC as a single agent were predominantly small studies that were undertaken to evaluate the pharmacokinetic parameters of the drug.[24,34,57] An initial dose-range study of patients with advanced HIV disease showed only modest evidence of virologic or immunologic activity though HIV-1 RNA was not measured at that time.[24] Short-term increases in CD4+ T-lymphocyte counts were observed at higher doses (8 and 12 mg/kg/day) but subsequently decreased to baseline after 20 weeks. A similar study performed in Europe tested doses of 3TC ranging from 0.5 to 20.0 mg/kg and showed small, short-lived increases in CD4+ T-lymphocyte counts.[34] There were also changes in other surrogate markers of HIV infections, such as p24 antigen, β_2-microglobulin, and neopterin levels. These changes persisted for a longer duration than the changes in CD4+ T-lymphocyte counts, though there was no clear dose-response effect on these parameters.

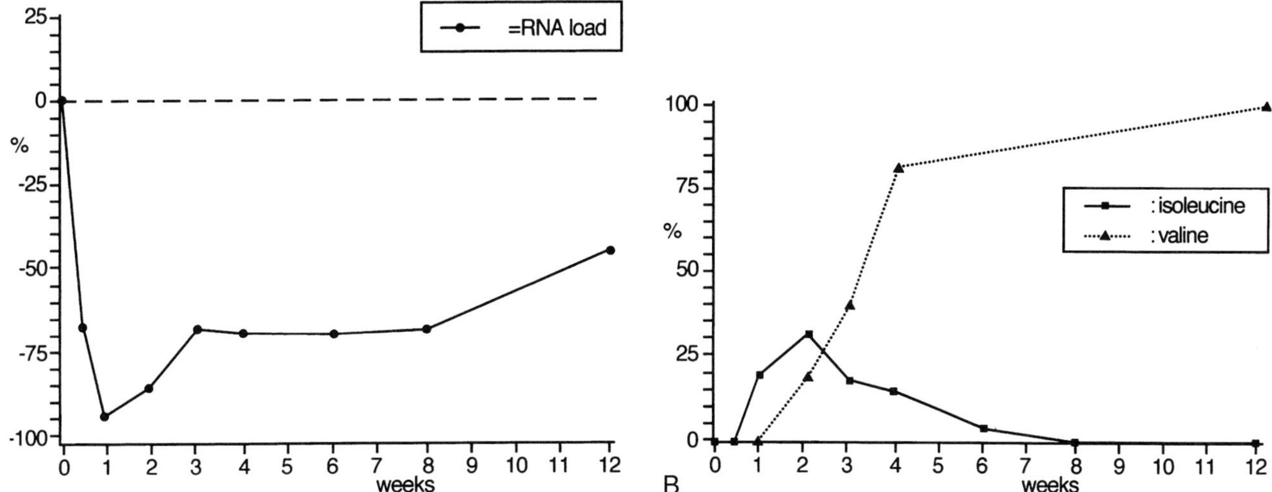

Figure 6-2. *A*, Percent change in HIV RNA from baseline over time achieved with 3TC monotherapy in HIV-infected subjects. *B*, Median percentage of HIV-1 variants (from 20 subjects) that contain a change in HIV-1 RT coding sequence at codon 184. Initially, mutants appear to have a substitution of isoleucine for the wild type, but these variants are rapidly replaced by variants with the methionine-to-valine change. (Adapted from Schuurman R, Nijhuis M, van Leeuwen R, et al. Rapid changes in human immunodeficiency virus type 1 RNA load and appearance of drug-resistant virus populations in persons treated with lamivudine (3TC). J Infect Dis 171:1411–1419, 1995.)

Schuurman and colleagues demonstrated that 3TC administered as a single agent resulted in a rapid decrease in serum HIV-1 RNA levels with an average decrease of more than 95% in 2 weeks[57] (Fig. 6–2*A*). This study was also one of the first to demonstrated in vivo emergence of resistance to 3TC (see below).

Monotherapy with 3TC was also studied in 90 subjects given 300 mg twice a day in a larger clinical trial done primarily to evaluate the combination of 3TC/ZDV.[50] Lamivudine monotherapy resulted in a peak mean increase in CD4+ T-lymphocyte count of 35 cells per microliter above baseline in subjects with CD4+ T-lymphocyte counts of 200 to 500 cells per mm^3. Mean CD4+ T-lymphocyte counts remained above baseline for approximately 8 months, an effect similar to that observed with ZDV monotherapy in the same study. HIV-1 RNA levels were decreased initially by a mean of 1.2 $\log_{10}$ copies/ml and remained below baseline through 52 weeks of observation (Fig. 6–3). HIV-1 RNA levels were reduced to a significantly greater extent with 3TC than with ZDV monotherapy.[50]

The limitations of 3TC monotherapy became apparent relatively early during laboratory and clinical studies of the drug. Resistance developed rapidly in vitro, with the initial effect of 3TC on CD4+ T-lymphocyte counts and p24 antigen levels being modest and transient.[24,58] In addition, the synergistic interactions of nucleoside analogues in vitro were being noted,[13,59,60] and the potential advantages of combination antiretroviral therapy were being recognized.[61,62]

Dual Nucleoside Therapy

The use of 3TC in combination with ZDV resulted from a convergence of observations and treatment concepts. As outlined, the modest effect of 3TC in vivo and the emergence of 3TC resistance in vitro were apparent. The clinical toxicity of 3TC was minimal, however. Importantly, it was noted that when the mutation associated with 3TC resistance (discussed in the next section) was added to HIV-1 variants resistant to ZDV, these variants regained sensitivity to ZDV.[63] In additional experiments, it was shown that resistance to a 3TC-like compound (FTC) developed more slowly in vitro in the presence of FTC and ZDV.[63]

Antiretroviral Activity and Effect on CD4+ T-Lymphocyte Count

The combination of lamivudine and ZDV was evaluated in two studies of patients who had received less than 4 weeks of ZDV and no other antiretroviral therapy. Both were randomized, double-blind, placebo-controlled multicenter trials comparing 3TC/ZDV with ZDV monotherapy. 3TC monotherapy was also evaluated in one of the studies.[50] Eron and colleagues evaluated subjects with CD4+ T-lymphocyte counts of 200 to 500 cells per mm^3 who remained on their original blinded therapy assignment through 52 weeks.[60] Primary study endpoints included the change (from baseline) of CD4+ T-lymphocyte counts and the plasma HIV-1 RNA levels. The primary metric for analysis of immunologic and HIV-1 RNA endpoints was the time-weighted area under the curve (AUC) of all postbaseline measurements minus the baseline value.[64] Sustained CD4+ T-lymphocyte increases were seen during 52 weeks of the 3TC/ZDV combination at two doses of 3TC (150 and 300 mg twice daily); there was a peak mean increase of 79 and 78 cells per microliter, respectively, with little trend toward baseline over time.[50] By week 52 the difference between the mean CD4+ T-lymphocyte count for either combination arm and ZDV monotherapy (200 mg three times a day) was more than 100 cells per mm^3. The combination arms showed a mean peak effect on HIV-1 RNA in plasma of almost 1.6 $\log_{10}$ copies/ml,

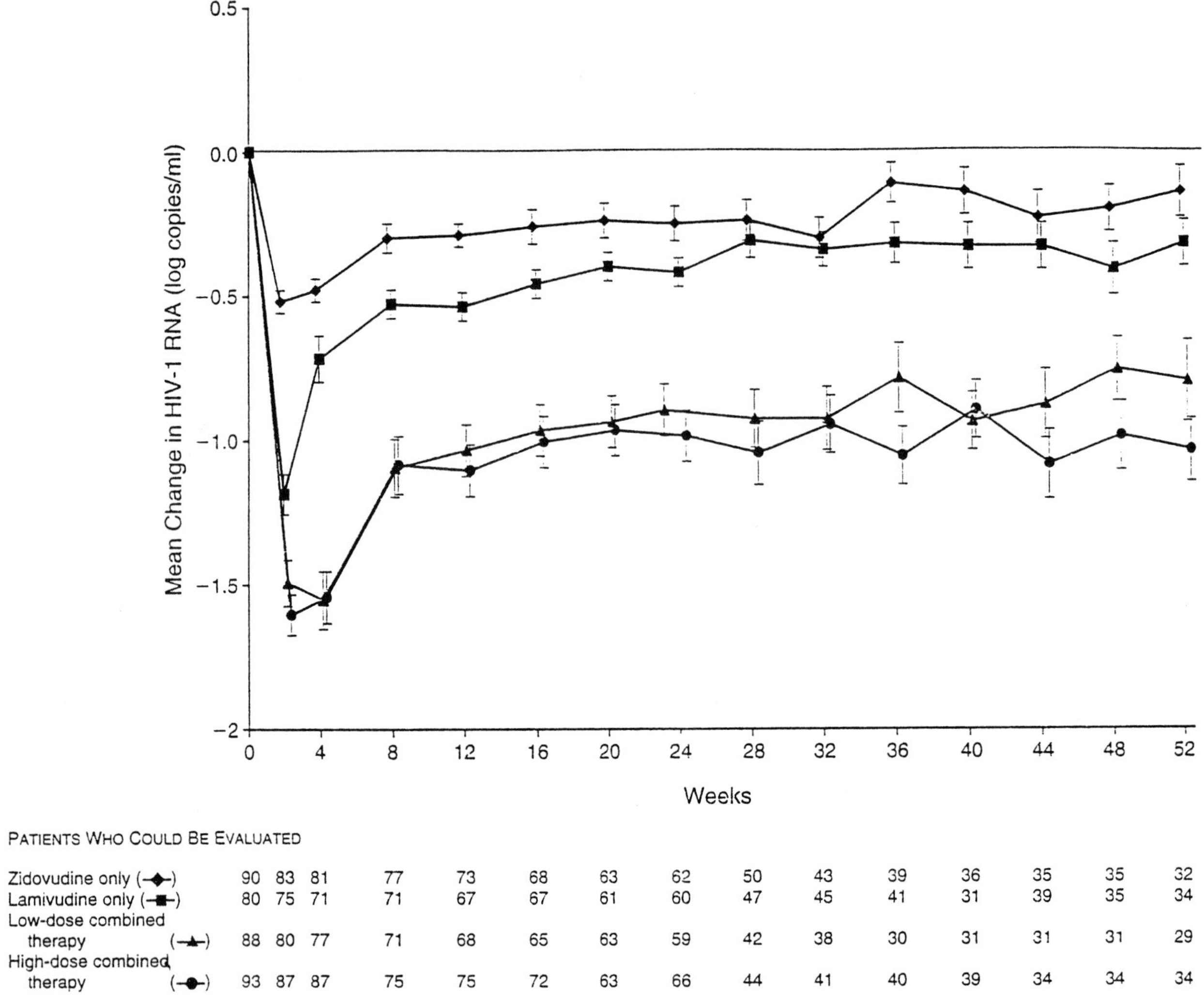

Figure 6–3. Change from baseline in HIV RNA levels over time in HIV-1-infected subjects naive to antiretroviral therapy who received zidovudine alone, lamivudine (3TC) alone, or one of two doses of lamivudine in combination with zidovudine. The numbers of subjects evaluated at each time point is listed below that time point. (Adapted from Eron J, Benoit S, Jemsek J, et al. Treatment with lamivudine, zidovudine or both in HIV-positive patients with 200–500 CD4+ cells per cubic millimeter. N Engl J Med 333:1662–1669, 1995.)

whereas the peak effect of ZDV was 0.5 $\log_{10}$ copies/ml. The median time-weighted change from baseline over 24 weeks were decreases of 1.1 and 1.2 $\log_{10}$ copies/ml for the low- and high-dose 3TC/ZDV combinations, respectively, compared to a decrease of 0.3 $\log_{10}$ copies/ml for ZDV monotherapy (Fig. 6–3). It is of note that in a subset of patients who began the study with a plasma HIV-1 RNA level of 20,000 copies per milliliter or more and therefore had the opportunity to experience a 2 $\log_{10}$ copies/ml decrease from baseline (the lower limit of detection of the HIV-1 RNA assay was 200 copies per milliliter) the combination of ZDV with either dose of 3TC showed a median peak decrease of more than 2.0 $\log_{10}$ copies/ml (100-fold reduction from baseline). Over the 52 weeks of the blinded therapy phase, the 3TC/ZDV combination had a persistent approximately 10-fold inhibitory effect on HIV-1 RNA levels. Clinical endpoints were also examined in this study, though the size of the study limits the interpretation of this information. Significantly fewer Centers for Disease Control and Prevention (CDC) class B and C endpoints occurred during 52 weeks in patients on combination therapy compared with patients on ZDV alone [J.J. Eron, unpublished observations].

Katlama et al. studied subjects with CD4+ T-lymphocyte counts of 100 to 400 randomized to one of two treatment arms: (1) ZDV 200 mg every 8 hours/placebo; (2) ZDV 200 mg every 8 hours/3TC 300 mg every 12 hours. The initial study period was 24 weeks, after which time patients were offered open-label 3TC and ZDV and were followed for an additional 24 weeks. In this study the peak mean change in CD4+ T-lymphocyte counts from baseline was 85 cells per mm^3 at 8 weeks for ZDV/3TC and 34 cells per mm^3 at week 4 for ZDV monotherapy.[65] At 24 weeks the mean CD4+ T-lymphocyte count was 78 cells above baseline for patients on 3TC/ZDV and had decreased to 9 cells below baseline in subjects on ZDV. Among the subjects who completed 24 weeks of study, 97% opted to continue on open-label 3TC and ZDV. Over the subsequent 24-week period the positive CD4+ T-lymphocyte effect of 3TC/ZDV persisted, though it declined somewhat to a mean of 48 cells above baseline at week 48. Using an immune-based capture technique,[66] HIV-1 RNA levels in plasma were evaluated in 29% of the patients. This assay measures only intact HIV-1 particles, and so a potentially smaller log reduction may be seen with this assay compared to other assays that measure HIV-1 RNA in plasma. The combination showed a 0.8 $\log_{10}$ copies/ml decrease at week 24. This antiretroviral effect persisted at 1.1 $\log_{10}$ copies/ml below baseline at week 48, though only a small number of samples were available at this time point. Despite 24 weeks of previous ZDV monotherapy the addition of 3TC to this group resulted in similar decreases in HIV-1 RNA at week 48.

These studies of 3TC and ZDV in antiretroviral treatment-naive patients yielded remarkably similar results. The 3TC/ZDV combination produced significant and prolonged effects on both CD4+ T-lymphocyte counts and HIV-1 RNA levels in plasma over the 48 to 52 weeks of the study. These effects were clearly superior to ZDV monotherapy and were obtained with no significant increase in adverse events when compared to ZDV alone.[50,65]

The 3TC/ZDV combination was also studied in patients who had undergone previous ZDV treatment. One study compared the addition of 3TC to ZDV versus continuing ZDV alone in 223 subjects with CD4+ T-lymphocyte counts of 100 to 400 cells per mm^3 who had been treated with ZVD for more than 6 months. Subjects either continued ZDV 200 mg three times daily or received 3TC at 150 or 300 mg bid/ZDV. Most (54%) of the subjects were asymptomatic, with a mean CD4+ T-lymphocyte count for the group of 251 cells per mm^3. The mean duration of previous ZDV therapy was 24 months. There were significant increases in CD4+ T-lymphocytes in the patients treated with ZDV/3TC, with a mean increase in CD4+ T-lymphocytes of approximately 40 cells per mm^3 above baseline at 24 weeks with either dose of 3TC and remained at approximately 30 cells per mm^3 above baseline through 48 weeks.[52] A mean decrease in plasma HIV RNA of approximately 1 $\log_{10}$ copies/ml was observed in either combination-therapy arm over 24 weeks.

In a study conducted in North America in ZDV-experienced patients with CD4+ T-lymphocyte counts of 100 to 300 cells per mm^3, the addition of two doses of 3TC (150 and 300 mg twice daily) were compared to adding ddC.[51] Altogether, 254 subjects with a median duration of previous ZDV treatment of 20 months, a median CD4+ T-lymphocyte count of 214 cells per mm^3, and a median plasma HIV RNA level of 4.7 $\log_{10}$ copies/ml were studied. Adding 3TC to ZDV resulted in significant increases in the CD4+ T-lymphocyte counts above baseline compared to adding ddC. The median change in CD4+ T-lymphocyte count after 52 weeks on 3TC (150 mg twice daily)/ZDV was an increase of 43 cells per mm^3, whereas subjects on ddC/ZDV experienced a decrease of 30 cells per mm^3. The effects on plasma HIV-1 RNA levels were similar in all three treatment arms, with median decreases of 0.4 to 0.5 $\log_{10}$ copies/ml at year. There were fewer new AIDS events in the 3TC/ZDV-treated arms than in the ZDV/ddC-treated group, but this trend did not reach statistical significance. These two studies of the addition of 3TC to the treatment of ZDV-experienced patients demonstrated significant immunologic and virologic effects. They also showed that the adding 3TC to the regimen of patients already receiving ZDV has a less potent effect than initiating the two agents simultaneously.

Evidence that 3TC and ZDV can have a prolonged, though incomplete, antiretroviral effect in selected patients, even in the presence of likely 3TC resistance, has also been demonstrated. In subjects treated with 3TC/ZDV for 2 years, the drugs were discontinued at the completion of the study period; the patients were then observed for 2 weeks before starting alternative antiretroviral therapy. Despite 2 years of treatment, these subjects experienced a rapid rise in HIV-1 RNA off therapy with the increases ranging from 2-fold to 50-fold[67] over the 2-week period; this increase suggests that a significant antiretroviral effect of 3TC/ZDV was present up to 2 years in some patients.

The combination of 3TC with other nucleosides has also been evaluated. Detailed comparisons of the effects of several nucleoside regimens on HIV-1 RNA levels and CD4+ T-lymphocyte counts have been carried out by the AIDS Clinical Trials Group (ACTG). ACTG 306 enrolled subjects naive to previous treatment and who had CD4+ T-lymphocyte counts of 200 to 600 cells per mm^3. The patients were randomized to one of two treatment limbs: one didanosine (ddI)-based and one stavudine (d4T)-based.[68] In the ddI limb subjects were randomized to ddI monotherapy, ddI/3TC, or ZDV/3TC. In the d4T limb subjects were randomized to d4T monotherapy, d4T/3TC, or ZDV/3TC. After 24 weeks subjects on either ddI or d4T monotherapy were also given 3TC. Altogether, 299 subjects were enrolled. The median baseline plasma HIV RNA levels were approximately 10,000 copies per milliliter, and the median CD4+ T-lymphocyte counts were approximately 400 cells per cubic millimeter. Using an HIV RNA assay with a lower limit of detection of 50 copies per milliliter, the mean $\log_{10}$ copies/ml decreases in RNA on the ddI limb at 24 weeks were 1.3, 1.2, and 1.4 for ddI, ddI/3TC, and ZDV/3TC, respectively.

None of the comparisons between treatment arms were significant. For the d4T limb the adjusted mean decreases in plasma HIV-1 RNA at 24 weeks were 0.5, 1.6, and 1.6 $\log_{10}$ copies per milliliter for d4T monotherapy, d4T/3TC, and ZDV/3TC, respectively. The difference between d4T and d4T/3TC was highly significant ($P = 0.001$), and the difference between d4T/3TC and 3TC/ZDV was not ($P = 0.77$). At 48 weeks the addition of 3TC to d4T and to ddI resulted in additional 0.44 and 0.79 $\log_{10}$ copies/ml adjusted decreases, respectively. After 48 weeks the decreases in HIV RNA ranged from 1.2 $\log_{10}$ copies/ml (d4T/3TC) to 1.8 $\log_{10}$ copies/ml (ddI/delayed 3TC) with both d4T/3TC and ZDV/3TC at 1.5 $\log_{10}$ copies/ml. None of the comparisons within arms were significant. During 48 weeks the CD4+ T-lymphocyte count increases were not significantly different between arms, with increases of 77 to 118 cells per mm^3. These results suggest that during 48 weeks in subjects with a relatively low viral load (mean HIV RNA at baseline approximately 10,000 copies per milliliter) 3TC/d4T is at least as effective at suppressing HIV RNA levels and increasing CD4+ T-lymphocyte counts as 3TC/ZDV. Data suggest that the genotypic resistance patterns for d4T and ZDV are similar, and therefore a mutational interaction between 3TC and d4T resistance similar to the 3TC–ZDV interaction may occur.[69] The antiviral activity of 3TC/ZDV compared to ddI/3TC and ddI monotherapy was more difficult to interpret, as activities over 24 and 48 weeks were quite similar. On one hand, the similarity of the 3TC/ddI and ddI arms suggests that adding 3TC to ddI affords little benefit. On the other hand, adding 3TC to ddI after 24 weeks resulted in a 0.8 $\log_{10}$ copies/ml decrease and supports the opposite conclusion. Resistance data from this study may shed further light on the utility of the ddI/3TC combination. The overall results from this study must be interpreted with some caution. The viral load of all the subjects at baseline was low, and the results may be less applicable to individuals with high viral loads. In addition, although the censoring of change in HIV RNA levels by the lower limits of the HIV RNA assays was taken into account, these methods may be imperfect and more censoring may have occurred in the dual nucleoside arms, which perhaps narrowed the differences.

The 3TC/d4T combination has also been investigated in an open-label study.[70] In treatment-naive subjects the antiretroviral effect of 3TC/d4T over a 6-month period was similar to effects seen with ZDV/3TC in previous studies and in the ACTG 306 trial (median decrease of 1.66 $\log_{10}$ copies/ml).[68] The effect of 3TC/d4T was much less potent in nucleoside treatment-experienced subjects who had not received 3TC or d4T, with a median decrease in HIV RNA of 0.55 $\log_{10}$ copies/ml at 24 weeks.

Effect on Disease Progression and Mortality

The effect of 3TC in combination with other nucleoside analogues on HIV disease progression and mortality has now been clearly demonstrated. After completion of four of the initial studies (reviewed in previous sections) that primarily examined antiretroviral efficacy, a meta-analysis of these studies was performed in an attempt to analyze effects on disease progression.[71] This analysis, which combined data from 972 subjects, showed a beneficial effect of 3TC/ZDV on disease progression compared to the control arms in various studies. There was a 49% reduction in all clinical events with ZDV/3TC therapy and a 66% reduction in progression to new AIDS events. This difference was seen when subjects were divided into subsets by treatment history, presence of symptoms, or CD4 cell counts. Few deaths occurred in these studies, and the number of AIDS-defining endpoints was limited. These factors, coupled with the retrospective design of the analysis, limited interpretation of the results.

To examine the effect of 3TC on disease progression, a large randomized, placebo-controlled trial of the addition of 3TC to zidovudine-containing nucleoside regimens was undertaken.[72] This study, referred to as the CAESAR trial to represent the locations. (Canada, Australia, Europe, South Africa) where the study took place, enrolled subjects receiving ZDV alone or in combination with ddI or ddC and with a CD4+ T-lymphocyte count of 25 to 250 cells per mm^3. More than 1800 subjects were randomized to receive placebo, 3TC (150 mg twice daily), or 3TC/loviride (100 mg three times daily), an NNRTI. Subjects were randomized in a 1:2:1 fashion so half the subjects added 3TC alone to their ZDV-containing regimen. The median duration of antiretroviral treatment prior to study entry was 28 months, and most subjects (62%) were on ZDV alone at baseline. The study was terminated prematurely at a second interim analysis because of the statistically significant benefit of 3TC in reducing the relative risk of disease progression compared to placebo. In the final intent-to-treat analysis, the relative reduction in risk of progression to AIDS or death was 57% (relative hazard [RH] = 0.43) for 3TC-containing arms compared to placebo. There was also a 60% reduction in mortality for the 3TC-containing arms compared to placebo. The addition of loviride to the 3TC regimen appeared to offer no benefit in the overall analysis of clinical progression. When the relative risk reduction of 3TC compared to placebo was examined for various subgroups (e.g., CD4+ T-lymphocyte count, AIDS versus non-AIDS, treatment at study entry, duration of antiretroviral experience), a consistent risk reduction of approximately 50% was seen (Fig. 6–4). The greatest risk reduction was seen in subjects who had received less than 6 months of previous antiretroviral therapy. The CAESAR study clearly demonstrated that the antiretroviral effects of 3TC that had been seen in earlier studies are translated into clinical benefit, as suggested by smaller studies[71,73] and seen with other antiretroviral therapies.[74]

3TC in HAART Combinations

3TC in Combination with Protease Inhibitors

Antiretroviral Effects and Effects on CD4+ T-Lymphocyte Counts

The demonstration of enhanced antiretroviral effect and clinical benefit of combination nucleoside therapy,[74,75] especially ZDV and 3TC,[50,-72] in conjunction with the clinical development of protease inhibitors[76-79] has dramatically altered the design of clinical research trials and ultimately of recommendations for clinical practice[80,81]. Highly active antiretroviral therapy (HAART) regimens, which most commonly consist of two nucleosides in combination with a protease inhibitor, an NNRTI, or the potent nucleoside abacavir, is the standard of care in developed countries.[19,82]

Multiple trials of 3TC in combination with ZDV or d4T and a protease inhibitor have demonstrated the potent activity of these combinations. One of the earliest of these studies was a trial that compared 3TC/ZDV/indinavir with ZDV/3TC and with indinavir alone.[83] In this double-blind study, 97 subjects who had previously received ZDV for at least 6 months (median previous treatment for 30 months) were randomized to have 3TC added to their ZDV, to have 3TC and indinavir added, or to switch to indinavir alone. Subjects had CD4+ T-lymphocyte counts of 50 to 400 cells per mm^3 and a plasma HIV-1 level of more than 20,000 copies per milliliter. The median CD4+ T-lymphocyte count at entry was 144 cells per mm^3, and the

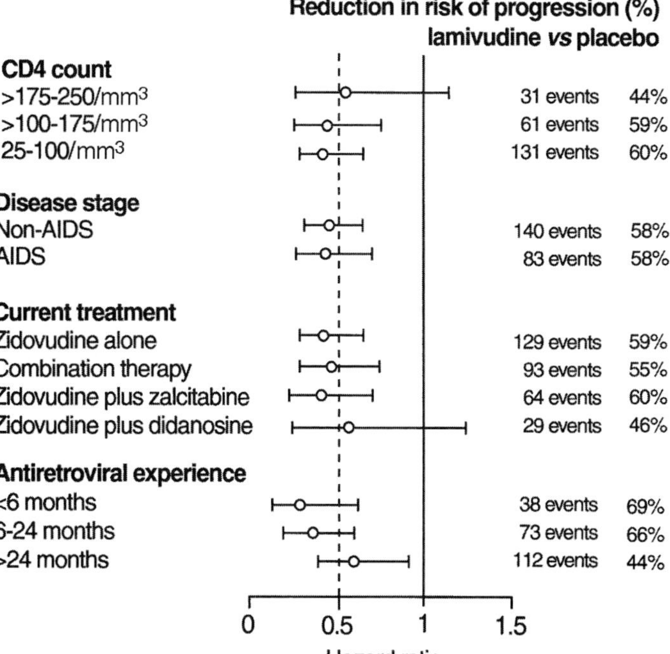

Figure 6–4. Reduction in relative risk of disease progression in subjects treated with 3TC-containing combinations compared to subjects treated with placebo. Subjects entered the study on ZDV, ZDV/ddI, or ZDV/ddC and had either placebo, 3TC, or 3TC plus loviride added to this regimen. Open circle represents the percent reduction in relative risk with 95% confidence intervals represented by the horizontal lines. Observations for which the confidence interval extends across unity (1) are not statistically significant. The number of subjects in some of the categories was small limiting the power of the observation. (Adapted from Anonymous. Randomised trial of addition of lamivudine or lamivudine plus loviride to zidovudine-containing regimens for patients with HIV-1 infection: the CAESAR trial. Lancet 349:1413–1421, 1997.)

median HIV-1 RNA level was 43,000 copies per milliliter. Subjects treated with the three-drug regimen had a more profound antiretroviral response than previously described. HIV RNA levels decreased to less than 500 copies per milliliter (the limit of quantification of the assay) in 90% of subjects after 24 weeks of therapy (Fig. 6–5). No subject who received only 3TC/ZDV had this level of response, whereas 43% of subjects on indinavir monotherapy were below quantification levels at 24 weeks. Approximately 70% of subjects on the three-drug therapy after 24 weeks were below detection limits when a more sensitive assay that could quantify HIV RNA in plasma to approximately 50 copies per milliliter was used (Fig. 6–5). CD4 cell changes were not significantly different between the indinavir arm and the three-drug therapy arm, although both were superior to ZDV/3TC. Follow-up of subjects on the three-drug therapy arm is ongoing, and two-thirds of subjects originally assigned to three-drug therapy have had their HIV RNA levels remain at less than 50 copies per milliliter through 3 years of therapy.[16,84] Similar results (although for a shorter time period) were seen with d4T/3TC and indinavir.[85]

In a population of HIV-infected individuals with more advanced disease, the combination of 3TC/ZDV/indinavir also had pronounced antiretroviral activity.[86] In a trial design similar to the one already described,[83] subjects were enrolled with CD4+ T-lymphocyte counts of less than 50 cells per mm^3 and more than 6 months of ZDV experience. In this trial more than half of the subjects (56%) on three-drug therapy had HIV RNA levels of less than 500 copies per milliliter and 45% were less than 50 copies per milliliter after 6 months of treatment.

The combinations 3TC/d4T and ZDV/3TC have been studied with each of the available protease inhibitors. Nelfinavir, a peptidomimetic protease inhibitor with good in vitro activity and a favorable toxicity profile in vivo, has been studied in several trials.[87–89] The largest of these trials enrolled subjects with no previous antiretroviral experience and compared 3TC/ZDV/nelfinavir to 3TC/ZDV alone with respect to the effect of treatment on HIV RNA levels and CD4+ T-lymphocyte counts.[88,89] Responses to 3TC/ZDV/nelfinavir were significantly better than those to 3TC/ZDV, as measured by changes in HIV RNA levels and the proportion of subjects with undetectable levels at 6 months.

The drugs 3TC and ZDV have also been studied with ritonavir (see Chapter 13), a potent protease inhibitor that has been shown to delay clinical progression in patients with advanced HIV disease.[90] These studies have been small and have focused on a specific patient subgroup or clinical question. Markowitz et al. investigated the effects of 3TC/ZDV/ritonavir in acutely infected HIV-positive patients using an open-label study design.[91] This three-drug combination was highly active in the 12 patients studied for up to 240 days on therapy. The effects of 3TC/ZDV/ritonavir on immune response, immune function, and viral dynamics were investigated in an intensive study of ZDV-experienced subjects.[92–94] At 48 weeks the HIV RNA levels were less than 100 copies per milliliter in 59% (20/34 subjects), and CD4+ T-lymphocytes increased by almost 200 cells per cubic millimeter.[93]

The antiretroviral effects of 3TC/ZDV or d4T have also been demonstrated with saquinavir soft gel capsules (SQV-SGC), amprenavir, and lopinavir/ritonavir. In a small study the combination of 3TC/ZDV/saquinavir had antiretroviral effects similar to those of a concurrent treatment group receiving 3TC/ZDV/indinavir. In that study 71% and 74% of subjects had HIV RNA levels of less than 50 copies per milliliter at 24 weeks.[95] When 3TC was combined with amprenavir and ZDV (50% of whom had had °previous nucleoside experience other than 3TC), 50% had HIV RNA levels of less than 500 copies per milliliter after 24 weeks of therapy.

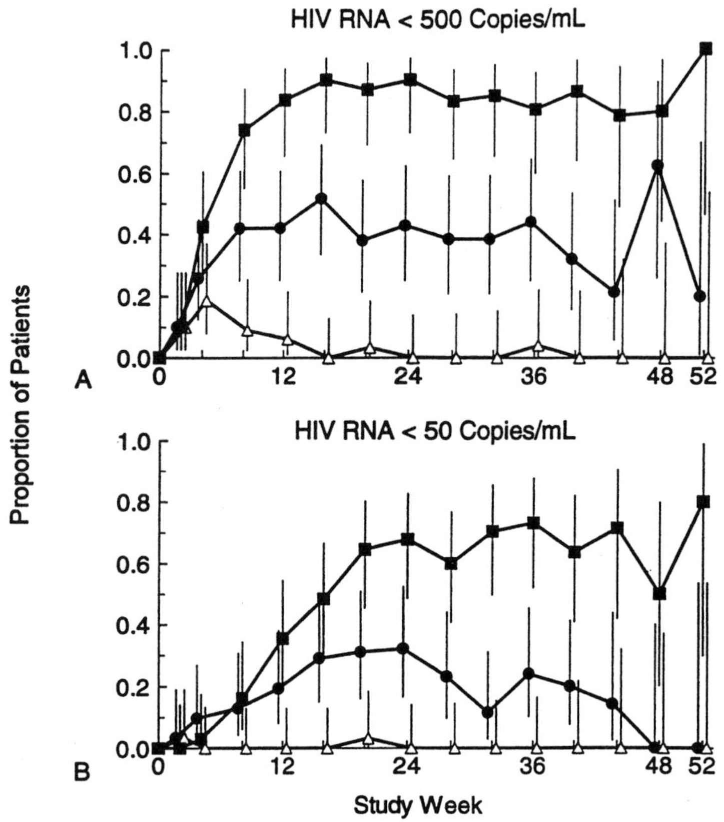

Number of Patients Evaluated					
Indinavir/Zidovudine/ Lamivudine	31	31	26	10	5
Indinavir	31	28	25	8	5
Zidovudine/Lamivudine	33	30	25	9	5

Figure 6–5. Proportion of subjects who achieved HIV-1 RNA levels of less than 500 copies per milliliter (top graph) or 50 copies per millimeter (lower graph) when treated with indinavir alone, ZDV/3TC, or ZDV/3TC/indinavir. Subjects in this study had received more than 6 months of ZDV prior to randomization. The number listed below the study week is the number of patients evaluated at that study week. The diminishing number reflects the number of subjects on study long enough to have reached that time point and does not represent dropout from the study. (Adapted from Gulick RM, Mellors JW, Havlir D, et al. Treatment with a combination of indinavir, zidovudine and lamivudine in HIV-1 infected adults with prior antiretroviral use. N Engl J Med 337:734–739, 1997.)

This was somewhat lower than other 3TC protease inhibitor (PI) studies, though the frequencies of treatment experience differ among studies, and cross-study comparisons should be interpreted cautiously.[96] Most recently the combination of lopinavir/ritonavir/3TC/d4T was shown to be superior to nelfinavir plus these two agents. Two-thirds of subjects on the lopinavir/ritonavir arm had HIV RNA levels of less than 50 copies per milliliter at 48 weeks compared to 52% with nelfinavir/3TC/d4T.[97] Overall, there appears to be no suggestion that the antiretroviral efficacy seen with 3TC containing PI-based regimens is better when 3TC is paired with a particular PI or with ZDV rather than d4T. Whether the antiretroviral potency of two NRTIs plus a PI is greater when one of the nucleosides is 3TC has also not been definitively demonstrated. 3TC/ZDV/indinavir was compared to ddI/d4T/indinavir, and the antiretroviral activities of the combinations were quite similar.[98] CD4 cell count increases were significantly greater in the ddI arm, although changes in CD4 percentage were similar. 3TC/d4T/indinavir was recently compared with the NNRTI nevirapine plus d4T and indinavir in treatment-naive or minimally nucleoside-experienced patients.[99] The 3TC-containing regimen was associated with a significantly higher rate of HIV RNA levels of less than 20 copies per milliliter at 72 weeks (81% vs. 62%) and fewer toxicities than the neviropine-containing arm.

Effect on Disease Progression and Mortality

The positive effect of 3TC/ZDV/indinavir on the clinical outcomes of disease progression and survival was established by ACTG 320.[17] In that study the subjects had CD4+ T-lymphocyte counts of 200 cells per mm^3 or less, had been treated with at least 3 months of zidovudine, were naive to 3TC and indinavir, and were randomized to receive ZDV/3TC or ZDV/3TC/indinavir. Of the 1156 subjects in the study, 38% had CD4+ T-lymphocyte counts of 50 cells per mm^3 or less and a mean HIV RNA level of 100,000 copies per milliliter. Stavudine could be substituted for ZDV if a subject was intolerant to ZDV. The study was halted prematurely when a predefined clinical benefit was noted at an interim analysis. In the final analysis, the proportion of subjects who progressed to a new AIDS endpoint or death was 6% (33 subjects) for 3TC/ZDV/indinavir compared to 11% (63 subjects) for 3TC (P = 0.001) indinavir (Table 6–2). Only 8 subjects (1.4%) died on the triple-therapy arm, whereas 18 subjects (3.1%) died on

▲ **Table 6–2.** RATES OF DISEASE PROGRESSION IN THE ACTG 320 TRIAL

Condition	ZDV/IDV/3TC (no.)	ZDV/3TC (no.)	Hazard Ratio[a]	P[b]
All subjects	577	579		
AIDS or death	33 (6%)	63 (11%)	0.50 (0.33–0.76)	0.001
Death	8 (1%)	18 (3%)	0.43 (0.19–0.99)	0.042
CD4+ count 50 cells/mm³	219	220		
AIDS or death	23 (11%)	44 (20%)	0.49 (0.30–0.82)	0.005
Death	5 (2%)	13 (6%)	0.37 (0.13–1.04)	0.51
CD4+ count 51–200 cells/mm³	358	359		
AIDS or death	10 (3%)	19 (5%)	0.51 (0.24–1.10)	0.08
Death	3 (1%)	5 (1%)	0.59 (0.14–2.46)	0.46

[a]Numbers in parentheses are 95% confidence intervals.
[b]Log-rank test.
[c]CD4+ T-lymphocyte count.
Adapted from Hammer SM, Squires K, Hughes M, et al. A randomized, placebo-controlled trial of indinavir in combination with two nucleoside analogs in human immunodeficiency virus infected persons with CD4 cell counts less than or equal to 200 per cubic millimeter. N Engl J Med 337:725–733, 1997.

3TC/ZDV ($P = 0.04$). The results were similar when the treatment arms were compared in subjects with less than 50 CD4+ T lymphocytes per cubic millimeter and in subjects with counts of 50 to 200 cells per cubic millimeter at baseline (Table 6–2). Effects on CD4+ T-lymphocyte counts and HIV-1 RNA levels in plasma paralleled the clinical results. These results confirmed the clinical benefit that was anticipated from the substantial antiretroviral effects of 3TC/ZDV/indinavir seen previously.

3TC in Combination with Other Reverse Transcriptase Inhibitors

Lamivudine has been studied with two other NRTIs or with one additional NRTI and an NNRTI. A significantly larger proportion of individuals treated with 3TC in combination with ZDV and efavirenz (EFV) had HIV RNA levels that fell below 400 copies per milliliter at 48 weeks than those treated with IDV/3TC/ZDV or with IDV/EFV (70% vs. 48% vs. 53%, respectively). The simplicity of this regimen with ZDV/3TC given twice daily without regard to meals and EFV given once daily compared with the more complex dosing of IDV-containing regimens may have contributed to the success of the 3TC/NNRTI-containing arm. 3TC has also been studied in combination with ZDV and delavirdine (DLV). In that study approximately two-thirds of subjects had HIV RNA levels below detectable limits at 52 weeks. This triple therapy was superior to either ZDV/3TC or DLV/ZDV.[100] Nevirapine with 3TC and ZDV has also been shown to be highly active therapy, even in individuals with HIV RNA levels of more than 100,000 copies per milliliter in a comparative study with NFV/3TC/ZDV.[101]

Lamivudine has been a key component of the relatively new HIV therapeutic approach using three nucleoside analogues. 3TC/ZDV/abacavir (ABV) has been compared to 3TC/ZDV/IDV in two randomized studies (one double-blind and one open label). In the double-blind study the two regimens were equivalent when the primary endpoint of HIV RNA levels of less than 400 copies per milliliter at 48 weeks was evaluated. However, in subjects with baseline HIV RNA levels higher than 100,000 copies per milliliter significantly fewer subjects on triple nucleoside had levels lower than 50 copies per milliliter at 48 weeks compared to those treated with 3TC/ZDV/IDV.[102] In contrast, when these two regimens were compared in an open-label fashion, the 3TC-containing triple-nucleoside therapy was at least as effective as 3TC/ZDV/IDV even in those with baseline HIV RNA levels of more than 100,000 copies per milliliter.[103] A clear suggestion from these two studies is that a convenient therapy such as 3TC/ZDV/ABV may make up with enhanced adherence what it may lose if antiretroviral potency is less. 3TC has also been tested with ddI and d4T as a triple nucleoside compared with ddI/d4T with either IDV or NVP.[104] Subjects in this study had low baseline HIV RNA levels (median 4.2 $\log_{10}$ copies/ml; interquartile range 3.8–4.8 $\log_{10}$ copies/ml). Nonetheless, there were no significant differences between treatment arms in the proportion of all subjects randomized who achieved HIV RNA levels of less than 50 copies per millimeter at 48 weeks. With higher viral loads [upper quartile with baseline values $> 4.8 \log_{10}$ (approximately 58,000) copies per milliliter] the proportions of subjects on both the 3TC- and NVP-containing arms with HIV RNA levels of less than 50 copies per milliliter at 48 weeks was less than with IDV (26% and 28% compared with 42%). When a less than 500 copies per milliliter cutoff was used, few differences were seen between arms.

The above studies do not answer the questions about whether the presence of 3TC in the NRTI regimens improves antiretroviral or clinical outcome. There are few direct comparative data between triple-NRTI regimens with and without 3TC for either of these endpoints, and comparisons across studies are hazardous.

3TC Co-formulations and Dosing Strategies

The results from the open-label trial of 3TC/ZDV/ABV compared to 3TC/ZDV/IDV support the hypothesis that among treatments of similar potency a simpler regimen would be more successful. To that end, simplification of 3TC-based therapy has been an important focus of HIV clinical research. 3TC has been combined with ZDV in a fixed-dose combination (FDC) tablet. Despite reducing the pill burden by only two pills per day, this FDC tablet is widely used. Switching from separate dosing of ZDV and 3TC to the FDC ZDV/3TC combine in the setting of ongoing HAART resulted in fewer virologic failures over 16 weeks than among those who remained on separate dosing, although the number of overall failures was small.[105] The FDC 3TC/ZDV/ABV (Trizivir) has now also been developed and is approved for use in the United States, providing an acceptable HAART regimen[82] as a single pill twice a day. In a trial design similar to the one used to test the FDC ZDV/3TC, switching to the FDC ZDV/3TC/ABV from the FDC ZDV/3TC and ABV did not compromise viral suppression.[106] Changing from successful combination therapy that predominantly contained a protease inhibitor to the FDC 3TC/ZDV/ABV also appeared not to compromise activity, and it improved blood lipids and adherence to the regimen.[107] Finally, using data suggesting that the intracellular half-life of 3TC-TP is well above 12 hours,[32] studies have been undertaken to examine 3TC given once daily. In a small study ($n = 81$) in which subjects on HAART with HIV RNA levels of less than 400 copies per milliliter were randomly assigned to switch to once-daily 3TC (300 mg qd) or remain on twice-daily 3TC (150 mg bid), 95% of subjects had less than 400 copies per milliliter on once-daily 3TC compared to 90% on the twice-daily regimen. No sustained rebounds in viral load to more than 1200 copies per milliliter were seen in either arm.[108] Larger studies are needed to evaluate once-daily 3TC as a component of initial therapy.

Pediatric Trials

The antiretroviral activity and the effect of 3TC on disease progression have also been evaluated in pediatric patients. The clinical activity of 3TC plus ZDV was assessed in ACTG 300[109] along with two other treatments: ddI monotherapy and ddI/ZDV. Didanosine and ddI/ZDV were included initially, but enrollment in the ddI/ZDV arm was stopped when the results of an earlier ACTG pediatric study (ACTG 152) suggested that treatment with ddI and ddI/ZDV I had comparable clinical efficacy. A total of 596 symptomatic children ages 6 weeks to 15 years and naive to antiretroviral treatment were enrolled. The primary endpoint was time to first progression of HIV disease or death. The 3TC/ZDV combination was significantly more effective that ddI alone in terms of both the overall combined endpoint (38 vs. 15 deaths; $P < 0.001$) and survival (15 vs. 3 deaths; $P = 0.004$). A mere profound effect of 3TC/ZDV on growth rates, CD4+ T-lymphocyte changes, and HIV-1 RNA levels were all consistent with the primary outcome.

As in the adult population, the combination of nucleoside analogues (including 3TC/ZDV) with a PI appears to have a more potent antiretroviral effect in HIV-infected children. In nucleoside-experienced children who had less than 4 weeks of ZDV/3TC, ZDV/3TC/ritonavir (RTV) had superior antiretroviral effects compared to either ZDV/3TC or d4T/RTV as measured by the proportion of subjects with HIV RNA levels less than 400 copies per milliliter at 48 weeks of therapy.[110] Overall, the experience with 3TC in HIV-1-infected children is similar to that in adults.

▲ RESISTANCE

High-level resistance to 3TC develops rapidly in vitro[63,111–113] and in vivo.[52,57,113–115] ZDV-sensitive and ZDV-resistant HIV-1 isolates passaged in vitro in the presence of 3TC (or a related compound 2′,3′-dideoxy-5-fluoro-3′-thiacytidine [FTC or emtricitabine]) (see Chapter 7) rapidly developed resistance to 3TC.[63,111–113] Some isolates in these experiments had more than 1000-fold decreases in sensitivity to 3TC and FTC. Sequence changes in the reverse transcriptase gene occurred only at codon 184, with a change from the wild-type methionine to either valine or isoleucine. Site-directed mutagenesis studies confirmed that these substitutions conveyed high-level resistance to 3TC.[63,111] The location of the 3TC resistance mutation in the reverse transcriptase enzyme lies within a highly conserved amino acid motif (YMDD), which is the polymerase active site of the enzyme.[116] Previous mutagenesis studies had shown that certain mutations in this location severely impaired function of the reverse transcriptase.[117,118] However, RNA transcriptases and RNA-dependent DNA transcriptases from many RNA viruses and retroviruses have conserved regions in their active site with a YXDD motif, where X can represent several amino acids.[119] These observations suggest that this position may "tolerate" the most variability in this highly conserved region. Subsequent studies suggest that the HIV that is wild type at codon 184 may have a small growth advantage over virus with the M184V mutation.[120,121] M184V variants do propagate in vitro in the absence of 3TC selective pressure, although growth may be attenuated.[122] HIV-1 with the M184V mutation, however, appears to have a significant growth advantage over virus with the methionine to isoleucine change.[120] Reverse transcriptase (RT) with the M184V mutation and the M184I mutation may have increased fidelity and decreased catalytic efficiency compared to wild-type RT.[121,123–125] The degree and importance of the increase in fidelity of HIV RT with the M184V mutation is uncertain, although some aspects of the treatment responses to 3TC might be explained by this phenomenon (see below).

In vivo, 3TC resistance was noted to occur rapidly when this drug was administered as monotherapy,[57] and it corresponds to an increase in HIV-1 RNA levels seen after 2 to 4 weeks (Figs. 6–2*A*, 6–3), although levels do not return immediately to baseline. The first mutation that appears is typically the M184I mutation. Variants with this mutation are in general rapidly replaced by resistant variants with the methionine-to-valine change.[57] (Fig. 6–2B). This observation may be explained by the fact that the isoleucine change requires only one nucleotide change from the wild type, and these variants may exist in extremely low numbers even in previously untreated patients, as has been postulated for resistance mutations to nevirapine.[126] The replacement of variants with the isoleucine change by variants with valine at codon 184 may occur because

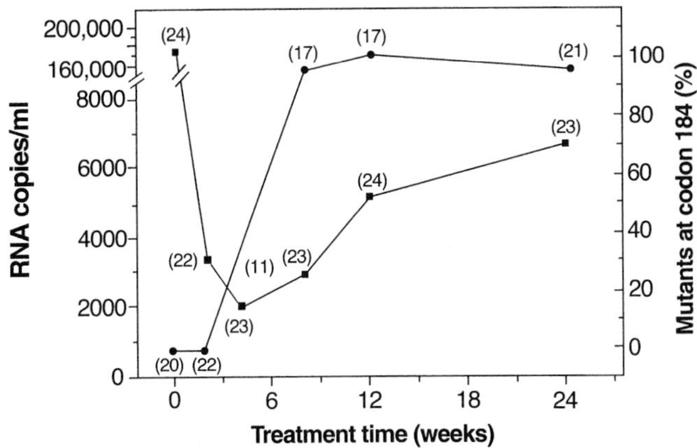

Figure 6–6. The change over time in HIV-1 RNA levels in subjects treated with 3TC plus ZDV (■). The proportion of subjects with mutant virus at codon 184 are also shown (●). The numbers in parentheses represent the number of subjects contributing data at each time point. (Adapted from Larder BA, Kemp SD, Harrigan PR. Potential mechanism for sustained antiretroviral efficacy of AZT-3TC combination therapy. Science 269:696–699, 1995.)

viruses with the M184V mutation have a growth advantage over virus with M184I.[120]

Emergence of viral variants with 3TC resistance also occurs rapidly in subjects treated with ZDV and 3TC[52,115,120] (Fig. 6–6). By 12 weeks of therapy most subjects treated with ZDV/3TC acquire variants with 3TC resistance if they were naive to previous therapy[115,120] (Fig. 6–6). Similar emergence of resistance to 3TC has been seen in subjects who had 3TC added to chronic ZDV therapy.[52]

In contrast to dual ZDV/3TC therapy, when 3TC is used in potent three-drug combinations, emergence of 3TC resistance is delayed in most subjects.[83] The likely explanation for this observation is that with marked suppression of viral replication the rate of mutation appearance, which is a result of the error rate of the RT multiplied by the replication rate, is substantially reduced. Resistance to 3TC occurs in a small number of individuals receiving three-drug combination therapy and appears to occur in the setting of incomplete suppression of replication.[83]

Despite the rapid emergence of 3TC resistance, combination therapy with 3TC/ZDV has potent, and prolonged antiretroviral effects.[50,127] Introduction of the 3TC resistance mutation at codon 184 into the genome of HIV-1 that contains ZDV resistance mutations results in virions that have regained susceptibility to ZDV.[63,120] The antiretroviral and clinical effects observed when 3TC is added to zidovudine therapy[51,52,72] and the fact that baseline ZDV resistance does not diminish the activity of ZDV/3TC and PI combinations[83,128] may be explained in part by this resensitization phenomenon. In addition, the prolonged effect of the ZDV/3TC combination may be due to persistent phenotypic sensitivity of HIV-1 to ZDV in treated individuals, despite the presence of ZDV resistance mutations.[127] Initiation of ZDV and 3TC simultaneously with the resultant selection of 3TC resistance would decrease the selective advantage of ZDV-resistance mutations, and indeed initial treatment with ZDV/3TC delays ZDV resistance[115] (Fig. 6–7). Subjects receiving this combination had a delay in the appearance of the codon 70 mutation, which is typically the first ZDV-resistance mutation to appear[129] and is associated with initial loss of antiretroviral activity of ZDV.[130] During a prolonged follow-up, the proportion of subjects with ZDV-resistance mutations was less when the ZDV/3TC-treated group was compared to those treated with ZDV alone.[127]

The mechanism by which 3TC resensitizes the ZDV-resistance virus is now becoming clearer. ZDV resistance has been incompletely understood. Multiple mutations in RT lead to HIV with high-level resistance to ZDV in cell culture,[131,132] although mutant RT enzymes remain sensitive to ZDV-TP, as measured by ZDV-MP incorporation.[133,134] However, the mutant RT has increased ability to remove ZDV-MP from blocked primers through a nucleotide-dependent or pyrophosphate-dependent reaction, which allows continued extension of the elongating HIV DNA and results in the phenotype of ZDV resistance.[135,136] The M184V mutation in the HIV RT impairs this rescue of chain termination[137] and therefore leads to increased susceptibility to ZDV in the presence of ZDV-resistance mutations. The resensitization of ZDV resistance by phosphonoformic acid- resistance mutations has been demonstrated to occur by this pathway.[138] The similar antiretroviral activity of 3TC/d4T when compared to 3TC/ZDV was difficult to explain if the mutational interaction

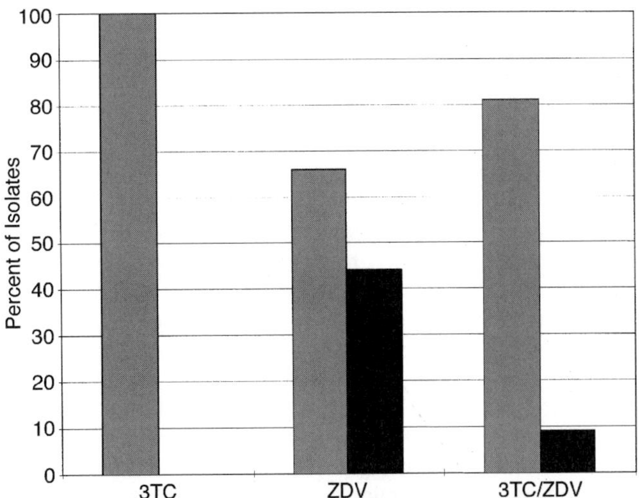

Figure 6–7. Isolates were obtained from subjects treated with 3TC or ZDV alone or 3TC/ZDV as part of a larger study.[32] The percentage of HIV-1 isolates obtained at week 12 of treatment that were found to be wild type (shaded bars) or mutants (solid bars) at codon 70 of the reverse transcriptase gene for each treatment regimen are shown. The proportion of subjects who acquired a mutation at codon 70 when treated with 3TC/ZDV was significantly lower than the proportion seen in subjects treated with ZDV alone (P = 0.009). (Adapted from Kuritzkes DR, Quinn JB, Benoit SL, et al. Drug resistance and virologic response in NUCA 3001, a randomized trial of lamivudine [3TC] versus zidovudine [ZDV] versus ZDV plus 3TC in previously untreated patients. AIDS 10:975–981, 1996.)

of 3TC with ZDV was responsible for the enhanced activity and prolonged effect of that combination.[68] Kuritzkes and his colleagues have demonstrated that "ZDV-resistance mutations" lead to a similar degree of resistance to d4T when inhibition of wild-type and mutant HIV RT is carefully studied.[69] Potentially, a similar mutational interaction between M184V and the thymidine resistance mutations that lead to d4T resistance might occur, explaining the potent and prolonged activity of this dual nucleoside combination.

There may be several other mechanisms for the activity of 3TC/ZDV and 3TC/d4T combinations, which have been shown to inhibit HIV-1 replication in a synergistic manner in vitro.[11,13] In addition, thymidine analogues and 3TC are converted to their respective active metabolites with different avidities depending on the state of activation of the cell the drugs are entering. Thymidine analogues enter and are phosphorylated preferentially in activated lymphocytes, whereas cytosine analogues are phosphorylated more efficiently in resting lymphocytes than in activated cells.[31,139]

Despite all of the above favorable interactions between 3TC and ZDV, dual resistance to ZDV and 3TC has been clearly documented.[127,140–143] This type of resistance has usually been demonstrated in the setting of adding 3TC to prolonged ZDV therapy,[140–143] but it can also be seen with prolonged combination therapy when the two agents are initiated simultaneously.[127] The pathway to dual resistance seems variable. Mutations at RT codons 333 and 210, among others, have been implicated.[140, 144]

Other pathways to 3TC resistance also exist. HIV-1 variants that are resistant to multiple nucleoside analogues, including 3TC, have been described. These variants typically have one of two mutation patterns: a family of insertions at or around codon 69[145] or a group of mutations anchored by a mutation at RT codon 151.[146] HIV-1 variants with these mutations may or may not also have the codon 184 mutation and have moderate to high 3TC resistance. Fortunately, these variants still have a low prevalence in the HIV-infected population in developed countries.[147] Novel mutations have been shown to be associated with low to moderate levels of 3TC resistance.[148] Mutations at codon 44 and 118 were associated with this level of 3TC resistance when a group of HIV-1 variants were examined. These mutations were typically associated with two well described thymidine-resistance mutations at codon 41 and 215. These observations were confirmed by site-directed mutagenesis,[148] and the occurrence of this pattern of mutations may be more common with a particular sequence of nucleoside administration.

The mutation that confers resistance to lamivudine at codon 184 has been shown in vitro to result in a low level of cross-resistance to ddI and ddC in some studies[112] but not in others.[63,113] A clinical impact of this possible low level of cross-resistance has been difficult to demonstrate. In a cross-sectional survey of HIV-1 variants from nucleoside-experienced patients in which both phenotype and genotype were determined, the presence of the M184V mutation was not associated with ddI or ddC cross-resistance.[149] However, the cutoff for phenotypic resistance was a fivefold increase in IC_{50} from the wild type, and smaller changes in IC_{50} may be clinically important for the dideoxynucleosides (ddI, d4T, ddC).

An aspect of 3TC antiretroviral activity and resistance that has yet to be fully explained is the apparent antiretroviral activity of 3TC despite emergence of the M184V mutation that results in extremely high-level resistance in vitro. In the initial study of 3TC monotherapy, persistent antiretroviral activity was noted after the appearance of the codon 184 mutation.[57] One treatment arm in the North American trial of 3TC/ZDV in treatment-naive individuals was 3TC monotherapy.[50] In a subset of these subjects from whom virology data were obtained, most subjects had acquired the 3TC resistance mutation at codon 184 of the RT by 12 weeks of therapy.[115] Despite this observation, the mean decrease in HIV-1 RNA in this group had not returned to baseline even after 6 months of treatment (Fig. 6–3), which suggested there was a persistent antiretroviral effect of 3TC despite the appearance of resistance. Also subjects from this study who received ZDV/3TC had more potent antiretroviral effects on average than those who received ZDV long after the appearance of 3TC resistance.[115] Explanations for these observations are speculative, though the M184V mutation may modestly decrease the replication capacity of viral variants with this mutation.[120] In addition, the M184V mutation appears to improve the fidelity of the RT enzyme in some experimental models.[121,123–125,150] Increased fidelity might be expected to decrease the appearance of mutations in progeny virus.[121] Mechanisms for how increased RT fidelity might lead to persistent antiretroviral effects have been proposed.[121] For example, additional resistance mutations to other agents in combination therapy may appear more slowly, thereby preserving the activity of the combination; or variants that escape immune pressure may occur less frequently, allowing more prolonged control of viremia, an explanation that would help explain persistent activity of 3TC monotherapy.[121] These hypotheses are still speculative, and evidence to the contrary has been reported.[151–153]

▲ DRUG INTERACTIONS

Drug interactions between 3TC and other antiretroviral agents or other medications are uncommon (Table 6–3). A 43% increase in area under the concentration–time curve (AUC infinity) and a 35% decrease in renal clearance were observed when lamivudine was co-administered with trimethoprim-sulfamethoxazole compared with lamivudine alone.[154] 3TC did not significantly alter the pharmacokinetics of trimethoprim or sulfamethoxazole.

▲ RECOMMENDATIONS FOR USE

Lamivudine is an important component of many recommended highly active antiretroviral combinations used to treat HIV infection.[19,82] 3TC has been best studied in drug combinations that include the nucleoside analogues d4T and ZDV. However, combinations of 3TC with other nucleo-

▲ **Table 6–3.** IMPORTANT DRUG INTERACTIONS AND DOSE
▲ ADJUSTMENT WITH RENAL IMPAIRMENT

Creatinine Clearance (ml/min)	3TC Dose
50	150 mg q12h
30–49	150 mg q24h
15–29	150 mg single dose, then 100 mg q24h
5–14	150 mg single dose, then 50 mg q24h
< 5	50 mg single dose, then 25 mg q24h

There was a 43% increase in the AUC and a 35% decrease in renal clearance when lamivudine and trimethoprim-sulfamethoxazole were co-administered, compared to lamivudine alone.

sides (e.g., ddI and abacavir) also appear highly active. Whether 3TC must always be combined with another nucleoside RT inhibitor or inhibitors to be part of a potent multiple drug regimen is not known, and regimens using 3TC only in combination with two protease inhibitors or with a protease inhibitor and an NNRTI have not been tested extensively.

The currently recommended dose of 3TC is 150 mg PO bid for adolescents and adults weighing more than 50 kg and 2 mg/kg every 12 hours for adults weighing less than 50 kg. 3TC administered 300 mg once daily is now an approved dose in Europe. In children, the typical 3TC dose is 4 mg/kg every 12 hours up to 300 mg daily. Dose adjustment is required for renal disease, with a 50% decrease in dose when the creatinine clearance is less then 50 ml/min (Table 6–3).[155] 3TC can be administered with or without food. Given the potency of 3TC, its ease of administration, lack of frequent toxicity, incorporation into convenient combination tablets, and infrequent drug interactions, this drug has become an important component of combination antiretroviral therapy.

REFERENCES

1. Yarchoan R, Mitsuya H, Myers C, et al. Clinical pharmacology of 3′-azido-2′,3′-dideoxythymidine (zidovudine) and related dideoxynucleosides. N Engl J Med 321:726–738, 1989.
2. Soudeyns H, Yao XI, Gao Q, et al. Anti-human immunodeficiency virus type 1 activity and in vitro toxicity of 2′-deoxy-3′-thiacytidine (BCH-189), a novel heterocyclic nucleoside analog. Antimicrob Agents Chemother 35:1386–1390, 1991.
3. Schinazi RF, Chu CK, Peck A, et al. Activities of the four optical isomers of 2′,3′-dideoxy-3′-thiacytidine (BCH-189) against human immunodeficiency virus type 1 in human lymphocytes. Antimicrob Agents Chemother 36:672–676, 1992.
4. Coates JA, Cammack N, Jenkinson HJ, et al. The separated enantiomers of 2′-deoxy-3′-thiacytidine (BCH 189) both inhibit human immunodeficiency virus replication in vitro. Antimicrob Agents Chemother 36:202–205, 1992.
5. Skalski V, Chang CN, Dutschman G, et al. The biochemical basis for the differential anti-human immunodeficiency virus activity of two cis enantiomers of 2′,3′-dideoxy-3′-thiacytidine. J Biol Chem 268:23234–23238, 1993.
6. Coates JA, Cammack N, Jenkinson HJ, et al. (−)-2′-Deoxy-3′-thiacytidine is a potent, highly selective inhibitor of human immunodeficiency virus type 1 and type 2 replication in vitro. Antimicrob Agents Chemother 36:733–739, 1992.
7. Skalski V, Liu SH, Cheng YC. Removal of anti-human immunodeficiency virus 2′,3′-dideoxynucleoside monophosphates from DNA by a novel human cytosolic 3′ → 5′ exonuclease. Biochem Pharmacol 50:815–821, 1995.
8. Chang CN, Skalski V, Zhou JH, et al. Biochemical pharmacology of (+)- and (−)-2′,3′-dideoxy-3′-thiacytidine as anti-hepatitis B virus agents. J Biol Chem 267:22414–22420, 1992.
9. Dienstag JL, Perrillo RP, Schiff ER, et al. A preliminary trial of lamivudine for chronic hepatitis B infection. N Engl J Med 333:1657–1661, 1995.
10. Dienstag JL, Schiff ER, Wright TL, et al. Lamivudine as initial treatment for chronic hepatitis B in the United States. N Engl J Med 341:1256–1263, 1999.
11. Merrill DP, Moonis M, Chou TC, et al. Lamivudine or stavudine in two- and three-drug combinations against human immunodeficiency virus type 1 replication in vitro. J Infect Dis 173:355–364, 1996.
12. Bridges EG, Dutschman GE, Gullen EA, et al. Favorable interaction of beta-L(−) nucleoside analogues with clinically approved anti-HIV nucleoside analogues for the treatment of human immunodeficiency virus. Biochem Pharmacol 51:731–736, 1996. Erratum. Biochem Pharmacol 51:1415, 1996.
13. Mathez D, Schinazi RF, Liotta DC, et al. Infectious amplification of wild-type human immunodeficiency virus from patients' lymphocytes and modulation by reverse transcriptase inhibitors in vitro. Antimicrob Agents Chemother 37:2206–2211, 1993.
14. Chong KT, Pagano PJ. Synergistic inhibition of human immunodeficiency type 1 replication in vitro by two- and three-drug combination of delavirdine, lamivudine and zidovudine. Int Conf AIDS 11:1103, 1996.
15. Snyder S, D'Argenio DZ, Weislow O, et al. The triple combination indinavir-zidovudine-lamivudine is highly synergistic. Antimicrob Agents Chemother 44:1051–1058, 2000.
16. Gulick RM, Mellors JW, Havlir D, et al. 3-Year suppression of HIV viremia with indinavir, zidovudine, and lamivudine. Ann Intern Med 133:35–39, 2000.
17. Hammer SM, Squires K, Hughes M, et al. A randomized, placebo-controlled trial of indinavir in combination with two nucleoside analogs in human immunodeficiency virus infected persons with CD4 cell counts less than or equal to 200 per cubic millimeter. N Engl J Med 337:725–733, 1997.
18. Veal GJ, Hoggard PG, Barry MG, et al. Interaction between lamivudine (3TC) and other nucleoside analogues for intracellular phosphorylation. AIDS 10:546–548, 1996.
19. Carpenter CC, Cooper DA, Fischl MA, et al. Antiretroviral therapy in adults: updated recommendations of the International AIDS Society—USA Panel. JAMA 283:381–390, 2000.
20. Van Leeuwen R, Lange JM, Hussey EK, et al. The safety and pharmacokinetics of a reverse transcriptase inhibitor, 3TC, in patients with HIV infection: a phase I study. AIDS 6:1471–1475, 1992.
21. Angel J, Hussey E, Hall S, et al. Pharmacokinetics of 3TC (GR109714X) administered with and without food to HIV-infected patients. Drug Invest 6:70–74, 1993.
22. Yuen GJ, Morris DM, Mydlow PK, et al. Pharmacokinetics, absolute bioavailability, and absorption characteristics of lamivudine. J Clin Pharmacol 35:1174–1180, 1995. Erratum. J Clin Pharmacol 36:373, 1996.
23. Lewis LL, Venzon D, Church J, et al. Lamivudine in children with human immunodeficiency virus infection: a phase I/II study: the National Cancer Institute Pediatric Branch—Human Immunodeficiency Virus Working Group. J Infect Dis 174:16–25, 1996.
24. Pluda JM, Cooley TP, Montaner JS, et al. A phase I/II study of 2′-deoxy-3′-thiacytidine (lamivudine) in patients with advanced human immunodeficiency virus infection. J Infect Dis 171:1438–1447, 1995.
25. Heald AE, Hsyu PH, Yuen GJ, et al. Pharmacokinetics of lamivudine in human immunodeficiency virus-infected patients with renal dysfunction. Antimicrob Agents Chemother 40:1514–1519, 1996.
26. Moore KH, Yuen GJ, Hussey EK, et al. Population pharmacokinetics of lamivudine in adult human immunodeficiency virus-infected patients enrolled in two phase III clinical trials. Antimicrob Agents Chemother 43:3025–3029, 1999.
27. Moodley J, Moodley D, Pillay K, et al. Pharmacokinetics and antiretroviral activity of lamivudine alone or when coadministered with zidovudine in human immunodeficiency virus type 1-infected pregnant women and their offspring. J Infect Dis 178:1327–1333, 1998.
28. Pereira A, Kashuba A, Fiscus S, et al. Nucleoside analogues achieve high concentrations in seminal plasma: relationship

between drug concentrations and viral burden. J Infect Dis 180:2039–2043, 1999.
29. Johnson MA, Verpooten GA, Daniel MJ, et al. Single dose pharmacokinetics of lamivudine in subjects with impaired renal function and the effect of haemodialysis. Br J Clin Pharmacol 46:21–27, 1998.
30. Johnson MA, Horak J, Breuel P. The pharmacokinetics of lamivudine in patients with impaired hepatic function. Eur J Clin Pharmacol 54:363–366, 1998.
31. Gao WY, Agbaria R, Driscoll JS, et al. Divergent anti-human immunodeficiency virus activity and anabolic phosphorylation of 2′,3′-dideoxynucleoside analogs in resting and activated human cells. J Biol Chem 269:12633–12638, 1994.
32. Moore KH, Barrett JE, Shaw S, et al. The pharmacokinetics of lamivudine phosphorylation in peripheral blood mononuclear cells from patients infected with HIV-1. AIDS 13:2239–2250, 1999.
33. Cammack N, Rouse P, Marr CL, et al. Cellular metabolism of (−) enantiomeric 2′-deoxy-3′-thiacytidine. Biochem Pharmacol 43:2059–2064, 1992.
34. Van Leeuwen R, Katlama C, Kitchen V, et al. Evaluation of safety and efficacy of 3TC (lamivudine) in patients with asymptomatic or mildly symptomatic human immunodeficiency virus infection: a phase I/II study. J Infect Dis 171:1166–1171, 1995.
35. Blaney SM, Daniel MJ, Harker AJ, et al. Pharmacokinetics of lamivudine and BCH-189 in plasma and cerebrospinal fluid of nonhuman primates. Antimicrob Agents Chemother 39:2779–2782, 1995.
36. Mueller BU, Lewis LL, Yuen GJ, et al. Serum and cerebrospinal fluid pharmacokinetics of intravenous and oral lamivudine in human immunodeficiency virus-infected children. Antimicrob Agents Chemother 42:3187–3192, 1998.
37. Foudraine NA, Hoetelmans RM, Lange JM, et al. Cerebrospinal-fluid HIV-1 RNA and drug concentrations after treatment with lamivudine plus zidovudine or stavudine. Lancet 351:1547–1551, 1998.
38. Pereira AS, Smeaton LM, Gerber JG, et al. The pharmacokinetics of amprenavir zidovudine and lamivudine in the male genital tract of HIV-1 infected men (AIDS Clinical Trial Group Study 850). J Infect Dis, in press, 2002.
39. Taylor S, van Heeswijk RPG, Hoetelmans RMW, et al. Concentrations of nevirapine, lamivudine and stavudine in semen of HIV-1-infected men. AIDS 14:1979–1984, 2000.
40. Reddy S, Kim J, Eron J, et al. Efavirenz (EFV)- containing antiretroviral (ARV) therapy (T) effectively reduces HIV RNA in the seminal plasma (SP) of HIV-1-infected Men (M). In: 8th Conference on Retroviruses and Opportunistic Infections. Chicago, February 2001, abstract 750.
41. Taylor S, Back DJ, Workman J, et al. Poor penetration of the male genital tract by HIV-1 protease inhibitors. AIDS 13:859–860, 1999.
42. Van Praag R, Weverling GJ, Portegies P, et al. Enhanced penetration of indinavir in cerebrospinal fluid and semen after the addition of low-dose ritonavir. AIDS 14:1187–1194, 2000.
43. Brinkman K, Smeitink JA, Romijn JA, et al. Mitochondrial toxicity induced by nucleoside-analogue reverse-transcriptase inhibitors is a key factor in the pathogenesis of antiretroviral-therapy-related lipodystrophy. Lancet 354:1112–1115, 1999.
44. Honkoop P, Scholte HR, de Man RA, et al. Mitochondrial injury: lessons from the fialuridine trial. Drug Saf 17:1–7, 1997.
45. Carr A, Miller J, Law M, et al. A syndrome of lipoatrophy, lactic acidaemia and liver dysfunction associated with HIV nucleoside analogue therapy: contribution to protease inhibitor-related lipodystrophy syndrome. AIDS 14:F25–32, 2000.
46. Hart GJ, Orr DC, Penn CR, et al. Effects of (−)-2′-deoxy-3′-thiacytidine (3TC) 5′-triphosphate on human immunodeficiency virus reverse transcriptase and mammalian DNA polymerases alpha, beta, and gamma. Antimicrob Agents Chemother 36:1688–1694, 1992.
47. Cui L, Locatelli L, Xie MY, et al. Effect of nucleoside analogs on neurite regeneration and mitochondrial DNA synthesis in PC-12 cells. J Pharmacol Exp Ther 280:1228–1234, 1997.
48. Dornsife RE, Averett DR. In vitro potency of inhibition by antiviral drugs of hematopoietic progenitor colony formation correlates with exposure at hemotoxic levels in human immunodeficiency virus-positive humans. Antimicrob Agents Chemother 40:514–519, 1996.
49. McLeod GX, Hammer SM. Zidovudine: five years later. Ann Intern Med 117:487–501, 1992.
50. Eron J, Benoit S, Jemsek J, et al. Treatment with lamivudine, zidovudine or both in HIV-positive patients with 200-500 CD4+ cells per cubic millimeter. N Engl J Med 333:1662–1669, 1995.
51. Bartlett J, Benoit S, Johnson V, et al. Lamivudine plus zidovudine compared with zalcitabine plus zidovudine in patients with HIV infection. Ann Intern Med 125:161–172, 1996.
52. Staszewski S, Loveday C, Picazo J, et al. Safety and efficacy of lamivudine-zidovudine combination therapy in zidovudine-experienced patients: a randomized controlled comparison with zidovudine monotherapy. JAMA 276:111–117, 1996.
53. Honkoop P, de Man RA, Scholte HR, et al. Effect of lamivudine on morphology and function of mitochondria in patients with chronic hepatitis B. Hepatology 26:211–215, 1997.
54. Moore R, Keruly J, Chaisson R. Differences in anion gap with different nucleoside RTI combinations. In: 7th Conference on Retroviruses and Opportunistic Infections, San Francisco, 2000, abstract 55.
55. Chaisson RE, Keruly JC, Moore RD. Adverse effects of antiretroviral agents. In: 40th Interscience Conference on Antimicrob Agents and Chemotherapy, Toronto, September 2000, 543, abstract 1882.
56. FDA Antiviral Drugs Advisory Committee Meeting. Lamivudine. November 1995.
57. Schuurman R, Nijhuis M, van Leeuwen R, et al. Rapid changes in human immunodeficiency virus type 1 RNA load and appearance of drug-resistant virus populations in persons treated with lamivudine (3TC). J Infect Dis 171:1411–1419, 1995.
58. Schurmann D, Bergmann F, Jautzke G, et al. Acute and long-term efficacy of antituberculous treatment in HIV-seropositive patients with tuberculosis: a study of 36 cases. J Infect 26:45–54, 1993.
59. Johnson VA, Merrill DP, Videler JA, et al. Two-drug combinations of zidovudine, didanosine, and recombinant interferon-alpha A inhibit replication of zidovudine-resistant human immunodeficiency virus type 1 synergistically in vitro. J Infect Dis 164:646–655, 1991.
60. Eron JJ, Johnson VA, Merrill DP, et al. Synergistic inhibition of replication of human immunodeficiency virus type 1, including that of a zidovudine-resistant isolate, by zidovudine and 2′,3′-dideoxycytidine in vitro. Antimicrob Agents Chemother 36:1559–1562, 1992.
61. Caliendo AM, Hirsch MS. Combination therapy for infection due to human immunodeficiency virus type 1. Clin Infect Dis 18:516–524, 1994.
62. Hirsch MS, D'Aquila RT. Therapy for human immunodeficiency virus infection. N Engl J Med 328:1686–1695, 1993.
63. Tisdale M, Kemp SD, Parry NR, et al. Rapid in vitro selection of human immunodeficiency virus type 1 resistant to 3′-thiacytidine inhibitors due to a mutation in the YMDD region of reverse transcriptase. Proc Natl Acad Sci USA 90:5653–5656, 1993.
64. Dawson J. Comparing treatment groups on the basis of slopes, areas under-the-curve, and other summary measures. Drug Info J 28:723–732, 1994.
65. Katlama C, Ingrand D, Loveday C, et al. Safety and efficacy of lamivudine-zidovudine combination therapy in antiretroviral-naive patients: a randomized controlled comparison with zidovudine monotherapy. JAMA 276:118–125, 1996.
66. Semple M, Loveday C, Weller I, et al HIV Plasma viraemia quantification: a non-culture measurement needed for therapeutic trials. J Virol Methods 41:167–180, 1993.
67. Eron J, St Clair M, Gilbert C, et al. Rebound of plasma HIV-1 RNA after discontinuation of long-term lamivudine/zidovudine. In: International Workshop on HIV Drug Resistance, Treatement Strategies and Eradication. St Petersburg, FL, June, 1997, p 65.
68. Kuritzkes D, Marschner I, Johnson V, et al. Lamivudine in combination with zidovudine, stavudine or didanosine in patients with HIV-1 infection: a randomized, double-blind, placebo-controlled trial. AIDS 13:685–694, 1999.
69. Duan C, Poticha D, Stoeckli TC, et al. Inhibition of purified recombinant reverse transcriptase from wild-type and zidovudine-resistant clinical isolates of human immunodeficiency virus type 1 by zidovudine, stavudine and lamivudine triphosphates. J Infect Dis 184:1336–1340, 2001.
70. Katlama C, Valantin M, Matheron S, et al. Efficacy and tolerability of stavudine plus lamivudine in treatment-naive and treatment-experienced patients with HIV-1 infection. Ann Intern Med 129:525–531, 1998.
71. Staszewski S, Hill AM, Bartlett J, et al. Reductions in HIV-1 disease progression for zidovudine/lamivudine relative to control treatments: a meta-analysis of controlled trials. AIDS 11:477–483, 1997.
72. Anonymous. Randomised trial of addition of lamivudine or lamivudine plus loviride to zidovudine-containing regimens for patients with HIV-1 infection: the CAESAR trial. Lancet 349:1413–1421, 1997.

73. Phillips AN, Eron J, Bartlett J, et al. Correspondence between the effect of zidovudine plus lamivudine on plasma HIV level/CD4 lymphocyte count and the incidence of clinical disease in infected individuals. North American lamivudine HIV working group. AIDS 11:169–175, 1997.
74. Katzenstein D, Hammer S, Hughes M, et al. The relation of virologic and immunologic markers to clinical outcomes after nucleoside therapy in HIV-infected adults with 200 to 500 CD4 cells per cubic millimeter. N Engl J Med 335:1091–1098, 1996.
75. Hammer S, Katzenstein D, Hughes M, et al. A trial comparing nucleoside monotherapy with combination therapy in HIV-infected adults with CD4 cell counts from 200 to 500 per cubic millimeter. N Engl J Med 335:1081–1090, 1996.
76. Erickson J, Neidhart DJ, VanDrie J, et al. Design, activity, and 2.8 Å crystal structure of a C2 symmetric inhibitor complexed to HIV-1 protease. Science 249:527–533, 1990.
77. Markowitz M, Saag M, Powderly WG, et al. A preliminary study of ritonavir, an inhibitor of HIV-1 protease, to treat HIV-1 infection. N Engl J Med 333:1534–1539, 1995.
78. Danner SA, Carr A, Leonard JM, et al. A short-term study of the safety, pharmacokinetics, and efficacy of ritonavir, an inhibitor of HIV-1 protease: European-Australian Collaborative Ritonavir Study Group. N Engl J Med 333:1528–1533, 1995.
79. McDonald CK, Kuritzkes DR. Human immunodeficiency virus type 1 protease inhibitors. Arch Intern Med 157:951–959, 1997.
80. Carpenter CC, Fischl MA, Hammer SM, et al. Antiretroviral therapy for HIV infection in 1997: updated recommendations of the International AIDS Society—USA panel. JAMA 277:1962–1969, 1997.
81. Federal Register. HIV Infection, Principles of Therapy, NIH Panel Report; and HIV-Infected Adults, Antiretroviral Agents Use Guidelines. June 1997, p 33417.
82. Panel on Clinical Practices for the Treatment of HIV Infection: DHHS Guidelines. Guidelines for the Use of Antiretroviral Agents in HIV-Infected Adults and Adolescents, vol 2001, 2001.
83. Gulick RM, Mellors JW, Havlir D, et al. Treatment with a combination of indinavir, zidovudine and lamivudine in HIV-1 infected adults with prior antiretroviral use. N Engl J Med 337:734–739, 1997.
84. Gulick R, Mellors J, Havlir D, et al. Simultaneous vs. sequential initiation of therapy with indinair, zidovudine, and lamivudine for HIV-1 infection: 100 week follow-up. JAMA 280:35–41, 1998.
85. AVANTI Study Group. AVANTI 2: randomized, double-blind trial to evaluate the efficacy and safety of zidovudine plus lamivudine versus zidovudine plus lamivudine plus indinavir in HIV-infected antiretroviral-naive patients. AIDS 14:367–374, 2000.
86. Hirsch M, Steigbigel R, Staszewski S, et al. A randomized, controlled trial of indinavir, zidovudine, and lamivudine in adults with advanced human immunodeficiency virus type 1 infection and prior antiretroviral therapy. J Infect Dis 180:659–665, 1999.
87. Markowitz M, Cao Y, Hurley A, et al. Triple therapy with AZT and 3TC in combination with nelfinavir mesylate in 12 antiretroviral-naive subjects chronically infected with HIV-1. Int Conf AIDS 11:6031, 1996.
88. Powderly W, Sension M, Conant M, et al. The efficacy of Viracept (nelfinavir mesylate, NFV) in pivotal phase II/III double-blind randomized controlled trials as monotherapy and in combination with d4T or AZT/3TC. 4th Conf Retrovir Opportun Infect 132:370, 1997.
89. Saag MS, Tebas P, Sension M, et al. Randomized double-blind comparison of two nelfinavir doses plus nucleosides in HIV-infected patients (Agouron Study 511). AIDS 15:1971–1978, 2001.
90. Cameron DW, Heath-Chiozzi M, Danner S, et al. Randomised placebo-controlled trial of ritonavir in advanced HIV-1 disease: the Advanced HIV Disease Ritonavir Study Group. Lancet 351:543–549, 1998.
91. Markowitz M, Vesanen M, Tenner-Racz K, et al. The effect of commencing combination antiretroviral therapy soon after human immunodeficiency virus type 1 infection on viral replication and antiviral immune responses. J Infect Dis 179:527–537, 1999.
92. Wu H, Kuritzkes DR, McClernon DR, et al. Characterization of viral dynamics in human immunodeficiency virus type 1-infected patients treated with combination antiretroviral therapy: relationships to host factors, cellular restoration, and virologic end points. J Infect Dis 179:799–807, 1999.
93. Connick E, Lederman MM, Kotzin BL, et al. Immune reconstitution in the first year of potent antiretroviral therapy and its relationship to virologic response. J Infect Dis 181:358–363, 2000.
94. Smith KY, Valdez H, Landay A, et al. Thymic size and lymphocyte restoration in patients with human immunodeficiency virus infection after 48 weeks of zidovudine, lamivudine, and ritonavir therapy. J Infect Dis 181:141–147, 2000.
95. Cohen Stuart JW, Schuurman R, Burger DM, et al. Randomized trial comparing saquinavir soft gelatin capsules versus indinavir as part of triple therapy (CHEESE study). AIDS 13:F53–58, 1999.
96. Murphy RL, Gulick RM, DeGruttola V, et al. Treatment with amprenavir alone or amprenavir with zidovudine and lamivudine in adults with human immunodeficiency virus infection: AIDS Clinical Trials Group 347 study team. J Infect Dis 179:808–816, 1999.
97. King M, Bernstein B, Kempf D, et al. Comparison of time to achieve HIV RNA < 400 copies/ml and < 50 copies/ml in a phase III, blinded, randomized clinical trial of ABT-378/r vs. NFV in ARV-naive patients. In: 8th Conference on Retroviruses and Opportunistic Infections, Chicago, February 2001, abstract 329.
98. Eron J Jr, Murphy RL, Peterson D, et al. A comparison of stavudine, didanosine and indinavir with zidovudine, lamivudine and indinavir for the initial treatment of HIV-1 infected individuals: selection of thymidine analog regimen therapy (START II). AIDS 14:1601–1610, 2000.
99. Launay O, Gerard L, Morand-Joubert L, et al. Comparative antiviral activity and toxicity of nevirapine (NVP) versus lamivudine (3TC), in combination with stavudine (d4T) and indinavir (IDV), for the treatment of HIV-1-infected patients. In: 8th Conference on Retroviruses and Opportunistic Infections, Chicago, February 2001, abstract 326.
100. Green S, Para MF, Daly PW, et al. Interim analysis of plasma viral burden reductions and CD4 increases in HIV-1 infected patients with Rescriptor (DLV) + Retrovir (ZDV) + Epivir (3TC). In: 12th World AIDS Conference, Geneva, June–July 1998, abstract 12219.
101. Podzamczer D, Ferrer E, Consiglio E, et al. A randomized, open, multicenter trial comparing Combivir plus nelfinavir or nevirapine in HIV-infected naive patients (the combine study). In: 8th Conference on Retroviruses and Opportunistic Infections, Chicago, February 2001, abstract 327.
102. Staszewski S, Keiser P, Montaner J, et al. Abacavir-lamivudine-zidovudine vs indinavir-lamivudine-zidovudine in antiretroviral-naive HIV-infected adults: a randomized equivalence trial. JAMA 285:1155–1163, 2001.
103. Cahn P. Potential advantages of a compact triple nucleoside regimen; efficacy and adherence with Combivir/abacavir versus Combivir/indinavir in an open-label randomised comparative study (CNAB3014). In: 40th Interscience Conference on Antimicrobial Agents and Chemotherapy, Toronto, September 2000, p 293, abstract 695.
104. Squires K. The Atlantic Study: a randomized, open-label trial comparing two protease inhibitor (PI) sparing anti-retroviral strategies versus a standard PI-containing regimen, final 48 week data. In: 13th International AIDS Conference, Durban, South Africa, June–July 2000, p 43, abstract LbPeB7044.
105. Eron JJ, Yetzer ES, Ruane PJ, et al. Efficacy, safety, and adherence with a twice-daily combination lamivudine/zidovudine tablet formulation, plus a protease inhibitor, in HIV infection. AIDS 14:671–681, 2000.
106. Fischl M, Burnside A, Farthing C, et al. Efficacy of Combivir (COM) (lamivudine 150 mg/ zidovudine 300 mg) plus Ziagen [abacavir (ABC) 300 mg] bid compared to Trizivir (TZV) (3TC 150 mg/ZDV 300 mg/ABC 300 mg) bid in patients receiving prior COM plus ABC. In: 8th Conference on Retroviruses and Opportunistic Infections, Chicago, February 2001, abstract 315.
107. Katlama C, Clumeck N, Fenske S, et al. Use of Trizivir to simplify therapy in HAART- experienced patients with long-term suppression of HIV-RNA: TRIZAL Study (AZL30002): 24-week results. In: 8th Conference on Retroviruses and Opportunistic Infections. Chicago, February 2001, abstract 316.
108. Sension M, Bellos N, Johnson J, et al. Efficacy and safety of switch to 3TC 300 mg QD vs. continued 3TC 150 mg bid in subjects with virologic suppression on stable 3TC/d4T/ PI therapy (COLA4005): final 24-week results. In: 8th Conference on Retroviruses and Opportunistic Infections, Chicago, February 2001, abstract 317.
109. McKinney RE Jr, Johnson GM, Stanley K, et al. A randomized study of combined zidovudine-lamivudine versus didanosine monotherapy in children with symptomatic therapy-naive HIV-1 infection: the Pediatric AIDS Clinical Trials Group Protocol 300 study team. J Pediatr 133:500–508, 1998.

110. Nachman SA, Stanley K, Yogev R, et al. Nucleoside analogs plus ritonavir in stable antiretroviral therapy-experienced HIV-infected children: a randomized controlled trial: Pediatric AIDS Clinical Trials Group 338 study team. JAMA 283:492–498, 2000.
111. Boucher CA, Cammack N, Schipper P, et al. High-level resistance to (−)enantiomeric 2′-deoxy-3′-thiacytidine in vitro is due to one amino acid substitution in the catalytic site of human immunodeficiency virus type 1 reverse transcriptase. Antimicrob Agents Chemother 37:2231–2234, 1993.
112. Gao Q, Gu Z, Parniak MA, et al. The same mutation that encodes low-level human immunodeficiency virus type 1 resistance to 2′,3′-dideoxyinosine and 2′,3′-dideoxycytidine confers high-level resistance to the (−) enantiomer of 2′,3′-dideoxy-3′-thiacytidine. Antimicrob Agents Chemother 37:1390–1392, 1993.
113. Schinazi RF, Lloyd RMJ, Nguyen MH, et al. Characterization of human immunodeficiency viruses resistant to oxathiolane-cytosine nucleosides. Antimicrob Agents Chemother 37:875–881, 1993.
114. Wainberg MA, Salomon H, Gu Z, et al. Development of HIV-1 resistance to (−)2′-deoxy-3′-thiacytidine in patients with AIDS or advanced AIDS-related complex. AIDS 9:351–357, 1995.
115. Kuritzkes DR, Quinn JB, Benoit SL, et al. Drug resistance and virologic response in NUCA 3001, a randomized trial of lamivudine (3TC) versus zidovudine (ZDV) versus ZDV plus 3TC in previously untreated patients. AIDS 10:975–981, 1996.
116. Kohlstaedt LA, Wang J, Friedman JM, et al. Crystal structure at 3.5 Å resolution of HIV-1 reverse transcriptase complexed with an inhibitor. Science 256:1783–1790, 1992.
117. Larder BA, Kemp SD, Purifoy DJM. Infectious potential of human immunodeficiency type 1 reverse transcriptase mutants with altered inhibitor sensitivity. Proc Natl Acad Sci USA 86:4803–4807, 1989.
118. Boyer PL, Ferris AL, Hughes SH. Cassette mutagenesis of the reverse transcriptase of human immunodeficiency virus type 1. J Virol 66:1031–1039, 1992.
119. Halvas EK, Svarovskaia ES, Freed EO, et al. Wild-type and YMDD mutant murine leukemia virus reverse transcriptases are resistant to 2′,3′-dideoxy-3′-thiacytidine. J Virol 74:6669–6674, 2000.
120. Larder BA, Kemp SD, Harrigan PR. Potential mechanism for sustained antiretroviral efficacy of AZT-3TC combination therapy. Science 269:696–699, 1995.
121. Wainberg M, Drosopoulos W, Salomon H, et al. Enhanced fidelity of 3TC-selected mutant HIV-1 reverse transcriptase. Science 271:1282–1285, 1996.
122. Miller MD, Anton KE, Mulato AS, et al. Human immunodeficiency virus type 1 expressing the lamivudine-associated M184V mutation in reverse transcriptase shows increased susceptibility to adefovir and decreased replication capability in vitro. J Infect Dis 179:92–100, 1999.
123. Feng JY, Anderson KS. Mechanistic studies examining the efficiency and fidelity of DNA synthesis by the 3TC-resistant mutant (184V) of HIV-1 reverse transcriptase. Biochemistry 38:9440–9448, 1999.
124. Rezende LF, Drosopoulos WC, Prasad VR. The influence of 3TC resistance mutation M184I on the fidelity and error specificity of human immunodeficiency virus type 1 reverse transcriptase. Nucleic Acids Res 26:3066–3072, 1998.
125. Hsu M, Inouye P, Rezende L, et al. Higher fidelity of RNA-dependent DNA mispair extension by M184V drug-resistant than wild-type reverse transcriptase of human immunodeficiency virus type 1. Nucleic Acids Res 25:4532–4536, 1997.
126. Havlir DV, Eastman S, Gamst A, et al. Nevirapine-resistant human immunodeficiency virus: kinetics of replication and estimated prevalence in untreated patients. J Virol 70:7894–7899, 1996.
127. Kuritzkes DR, Shugarts D, Bakhtiari M, et al. Emergence of dual resistance to zidovudine and lamivudine in HIV-1-infected patients treated with zidovudine plus lamivudine as initial therapy. J Acquir Immune Defic Syndr 23:26–34, 2000.
128. Kuritzkes DR, Sevin A, Young B, et al. Effect of zidovudine resistance mutations on virologic response to treatment with zidovudine-lamivudine-ritonavir: genotypic analysis of human immunodeficiency virus type 1 isolates from AIDS clinical trials group protocol 315: ACTG Protocol 315 team. J Infect Dis 181:491–497, 2000.
129. Boucher CA, OSullivan E, Mulder JW, et al. Ordered appearance of zidovudine resistance mutations during treatment of 18 human immunodeficiency virus-positive subjects. J Infect Dis 165:105–110, 1992.
130. De Jong MD, Veenstra J, Stilianakis NI, et al. Host-parasite dynamics and outgrowth of virus containing a single K70R amino acid change in reverse transcriptase are responsible for the loss of human immunodeficiency virus type 1 RNA load suppression by zidovudine. Proc Natl Acad Sci USA 93:5501–5506, 1996.
131. Larder BA, Kemp SD. Multiple mutations in the HIV-1 reverse transcriptase confer high-level resistance to zidovudine (AZT). Science 246:1155–1158, 1989.
132. Kellam P, Boucher CA, Larder BA. Fifth mutation in human immunodeficiency virus type 1 reverse transcriptase contributes to the development of high-level resistance to zidovudine. Proc Natl Acad Sci USA 89:1934–1938, 1992.
133. Lacey SF, Reardon JE, Furfine ES, et al. Biochemical studies of the reverse transcriptase and RNase H activities from human immunodeficiency virus strains resistant to 3′-azido-3′-deoxythymidine. J Biol Chem 267:15789–15794, 1992.
134. Carroll SS, Geib J, Olsen DB, et al. Sensitivity of HIV-1 reverse transcriptase and its mutants to inhibition by azidothymidine triphosphate. Biochemistry 33:2113–2120, 1994.
135. Meyer PR, Matsuura SE, Mian AM, et al. A mechanism of AZT resistance: an increase in nucleotide-dependent primer unblocking by mutant HIV-1 reverse transcriptase. Mol Cell 4:35–43, 1999.
136. Arion D, Kaushik N, McCormick S, et al. Phenotypic mechanism of HIV-1 resistance to 3′-azido-3′-deoxythymidine (AZT): increased polymerization processivity and enhanced sensitivity to pyrophosphate of the mutant viral reverse transcriptase. Biochemistry 37:15908–15917, 1998.
137. Gotte M, Arion D, Parniak MA, et al. The M184V mutation in the reverse transcriptase of human immunodeficiency virus type 1 impairs rescue of chain-terminated DNA synthesis. J Viro 74:3579–3585, 2000.
138. Arion D, Sluis-Cremer N, Parniak MA. Mechanism by which phosphonoformic acid resistance mutations restore 3′-azido-3′-deoxythymidine (AZT) sensitivity to AZT-resistant HIV-1 reverse transcriptase. J Biol Chem 275:9251–9255, 2000.
139. Gao WY, Shirasaka T, Johns DG, et al. Differential phosphorylation of azidothymidine, dideoxycytidine, and dideoxyinosine in resting and activated peripheral blood mononuclear cells. J Clin Invest 91:2326–2333, 1993.
140. Miller V, Phillips A, Rottmann C, et al. Dual resistance to zidovudine and lamivudine in patients treated with zidovudine-lamivudine combination therapy: association with therapy failure. J Infect Dis 177:1521–1532, 1998.
141. Gass R, Shugarts D, Young R, et al. Emergence of dual resistance to zidovudine (ZDV) and lamivudine (3TC) in clinical HIV-1 isolates from patients receiving ZDV/3TC combination therapy. Antivir Ther 3:97–102, 1998.
142. Rusconi S, DePasquale M, Milazzo L, et al. Loss of antiviral effect owing to zidovudine and lamivudine double resistance in HIV-1 infected patients in an ongoing open-label trial. Antivir Ther 2:39–46, 1997.
143. Nijhuis M, Schuurman R, de Jong D, et al. Lamivudine-resistant human immunodeficiency virus type 1 variants (184V) require multiple amino acid changes to become co-resistant to zidovudine in vivo. J Infect Dis 176:398–405, 1997.
144. Kemp SD, Shi C, Bloor S, et al. A novel polymorphism at codon 333 of human immunodeficiency virus type 1 reverse transcriptase can facilitate dual resistance to zidovudine and L-2′,3′-dideoxy-3′-thiacytidine. J Virol 72:5093–5098, 1998.
145. Larder BA, Bloor S, Kemp SD, et al. A family of insertion mutations between codons 67 and 70 of human immunodeficiency virus type 1 reverse transcriptase confer multinucleoside analog resistance. Antimicrob Agents Chemother 43:1961–1967, 1999.
146. Shafer RW, Kozal MJ, Winters MA, et al. Combination therapy with zidovudine and didanosine selects for drug-resistant human immunodeficiency virus type 1 strains with unique patterns of pol gene mutations. J Infect Dis 169:722–729, 1994.
147. Tamalet C, Yahi N, Tourres C, et al. Multidrug resistance genotypes (insertions in the beta3-beta4 finger subdomain and MDR mutations) of HIV-1 reverse transcriptase from extensively treated patients: incidence and association with other resistance mutations. Virology 270:310–316, 2000.
148. Hertogs K, Bloor S, De Vroey V, et al. A novel human immunodeficiency virus type 1 reverse transcriptase mutational pattern confers phenotypic lamivudine resistance in the absence of mutation 184V. Antimicrob Agents Chemother 44:568–573, 2000.

149. Miller V, Sturmer M, Staszewski S, et al. The M184V mutation in HIV-1 reverse transcriptase (RT) conferring lamivudine resistance does not result in broad cross-resistance to nucleoside analogue RT inhibitors. AIDS 12:705–712, 1998.
150. Oude Essink BB, Back NK, Berkhout B. Increased polymerase fidelity of the 3TC-resistant variants of HIV-1 reverse transcriptase. Nucleic Acids Res 25:3212–3217, 1997.
151. Jonckheere H, Witvrouw M, De Clercq E, et al. Lamivudine resistance of HIV type 1 does not delay development of resistance to nonnucleoside HIV type 1-specific reverse transcriptase inhibitors as compared with wild-type HIV type 1. AIDS Res Hum Retroviruses 14:249–253, 1998.
152. Keulen W, van Wijk A, Schuurman R, et al. Increased polymerase fidelity of lamivudine-resistant HIV-1 variants does not limit their evolutionary potential. AIDS 13:1343–1349, 1999.
153. Balzarini J, Pelemans H, De Clercq E, et al. Reverse transcriptase fidelity and HIV-1 variation [letter]. Science 275:229–231, 1997.
154. Moore KH, Yuen GJ, Raasch RH, et al. Pharmacokinetics of lamivudine administered alone and with trimethoprim-sulfamethoxazole. Clin Pharmacol Ther 59:550–558, 1996.
155. McEvoy GK (ed). Lamivudine: American Society of Health System Pharmacists. American Hospital Formulary Service Drug Information, 1997.

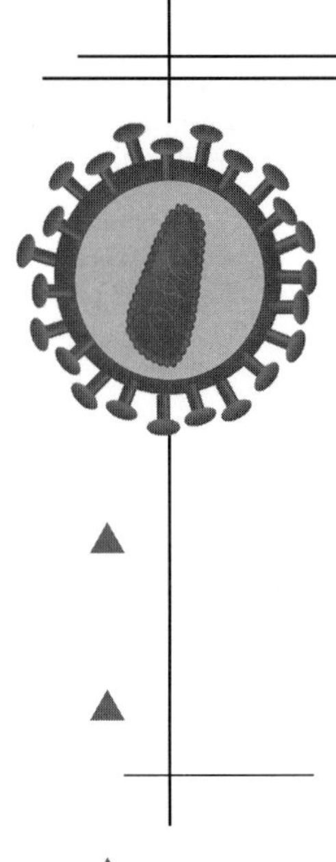

CHAPTER 7
Emtricitabine

Melissa F. Wellons, MD
John A. Bartlett, MD

Emtricitabine is a pyrimidine analogue whose antiviral activity was originally described by Schinazi et al. in 1992.[1] Emtricitabine is currently in development for use as a therapeutic agent for the treatment of human immunodeficiency virus (HIV) and hepatitis B virus (HBV) infections. It has not yet received approval from the U.S. Food and Drug Administration (FDA).

STRUCTURE

Emtricitabine (FTC), the negative or *cis* enatiomer of 2′,3′-dideoxy-5-fluoro-3′-thiacytidine, has antiviral activity against HIV-1, HIV-2, and HBV.[2] Similar to lamivudine, emtricitabine is a oxathiolane-cytosine analogue and has the unusual L configuration (1-β-L) rather than the D configuration found in natural nucleosides. Unlike lamivudine, emtricitabine has a fluorine in the 5-position of its cytosine ring (Fig. 7–1).

MECHANISM OF ACTION AND IN VITRO ACTIVITY

Like lamivudine and other nucleoside analogues, emtricitabine is a prodrug that must be metabolized intracellularly to exert its activity. After entering the cell through multiple transport mechanisms, emtricitabine is phosphorylated stepwise by cellular kinases to its active 5′-triphosphate form, emtricitabine 5′-triphosphate (E-TP) (Fig. 7–2).[3–5] E-TP competitively inhibits the binding of deoxycytidine triphosphate, an endogenous deoxynucleotide triphosphate, to the reverse transcriptase (RT) binding site.[6,7] E-TP is incorporated by RT into the nascent proviral DNA chain. This incorporation causes termination of DNA synthesis because E-TP lacks a hydroxyl group in the 3′ position of its sugar moiety and therefore does not allow the 5′ to 3′ linkage required for DNA synthesis. Thus incorporation of E-TP inhibits viral replication.[6–8]

Emtricitabine's antiviral activity has been evaluated in lymphocyte and monocyte/macrophage cell lines and peripheral blood mononuclear cell (PBMC) specimens. Emtricitabine is active against laboratory-adapted strains of HIV-1 and HIV-2 as well as clinical isolates of HIV-1, including zidovudine- and didanosine-resistant isolates. Depending on the cell type and viral isolate used, the concentration required to produce 50% inhibition (EC_{50}) of HIV ranged from 0.002 to 1.500 mM.[1,9,10] Emtricitabine's generally low EC_{50} values are attributed to its ability to bind efficiently to the RT–DNA complex. In a kinetic analysis of RT-catalyzed DNA synthesis, Feng and Anderson found that emtricitabine 5′-triphosphate bound 3.6-fold tighter to the enzyme–DNA complex and was incorporated into nascent chain DNA 2.5-fold faster than was lamivudine 5′-triphosphate.[11]

In addition to HIV-1 and HIV-2, emtricitabine also inhibits HBV in vitro. Its in vitro anti-HBV activity is comparable to that seen with lamivudine, inhibiting virus production with an EC_{50} of 0.01 to 0.04 μM. Intracellularly, emtricitabine inhibits HBV DNA synthesis with an EC_{50} of 0.16 μM.[3,12,13]

When inhibiting HIV-1, emtricitabine is synergistic in vitro with the nucleoside analogues zidovudine[14] and stavudine.[15] Using MT-2 cells infected with HIV-1 strain IIIB (a zidovudine-sensitive isolate), synergistic antiviral activity was found when emtricitabine was combined with

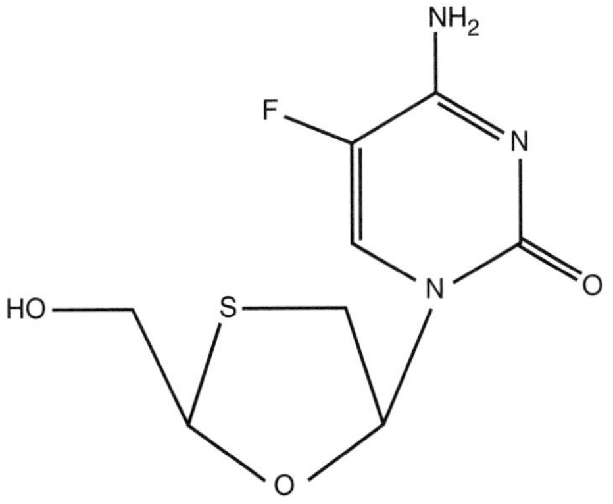

Figure 7–1. Structure of emtricitabine.

zidovudine or stavudine. Additive antiviral activity was found when emtricitabine was combined with zalcitabine or didanosine.[15]

▲ PHARMACOKINETICS

Emtricitabine is rapidly and well absorbed following oral doses. When single doses of emtricitabine were given orally to HIV-infected volunteers over the dose range of 100 to 1200 mg, emtricitabine disposition followed linear kinetics, and the steady-state emitricitabine concentrations were predictable based on single-dose data. Plasma emitricitabine concentrations reached levels above the in vitro IC_{50} and IC_{90} values even after single-dose administration. Emtricitabine's bioavailability was not significantly affected by food intake.[16]

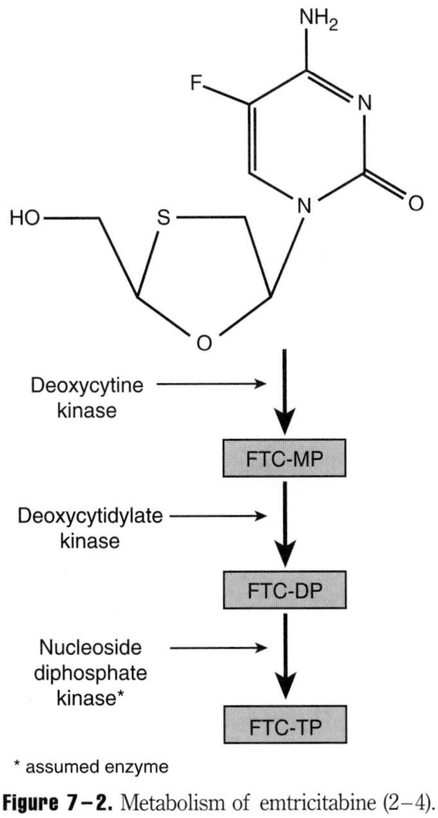

* assumed enzyme

Figure 7–2. Metabolism of emtricitabine (2–4).

Based on various studies in healthy or HIV-infected adults following administration of the therapeutic dose of 200 mg emtricitabine once daily, the mean steady-state peak plasma emtricitabine concentration of approximately 2 μg/ml occurs within 2 hours after the dose. The mean steady-state peak plasma area under the curve (AUC) over the 24-hour dosing interval is 9 to 10 hr/μg/ml and mean half-life ($t_{1/2}$) is 8 to 9 hours.[17] Comparable pharmacokinetic parameters are seen in children administered a dose of 6 mg/kg in preliminary analyses, but further analyses are needed (unpublished data on FTC 105 provided by Triangle Pharmaceuticals).

Emtricitabine is excreted predominantly in the urine. Following a single oral dose, 86% of the emtricitabine dose was recovered in the urine and 13% in the feces. More than 85% of the dose was excreted in the urine as unchanged emitricitabine. Hence there should be minimal potential for drug interactions with other hepatically metabolized drugs. The effect of renal impairment and hemodialysis on emtricitabine's pharmacokinetic parameters has been studied, and analyses of these data are pending.

Emtricitabine triphosphate has a prolonged intracellular half-life compared to its plasma half-life and the intracellular half-life of lamivudine triphosphate (L-TP). The estimated intracellular half-life of E-TP is estimated to be more than 20 hours,[18] compared with 10.5 to 15.5 hours for L-TP.[19]

Initially it was hypothesized that emtricitabine's fluorine would increase its lipophilicity and therefore increase its penetration into the central nervous system,[1] but emtricitabine's penetration into cerebrospinal fluid (CSF) is now estimated to be low. Animal studies have shown that emtricitabine does not effectively cross the blood-brain barrier; in monkeys, the concentration of emtricitabine in the CSF was found to be only 4.0% ± 0.7% of the corresponding plasma emtricitabine level.[20]

▲ TOXICITY

Emtricitabine, like other nucleoside analogues, has the potential for toxicity due to interaction with human DNA polymerases. Of particular concern is the potential for interactions with human mitochondrial DNA complexes, such as mitochondrial DNA polymerase-γ, as disruption of mitochondrial enzymes by nucleoside reverse transcriptase inhibitors (NRTIs) has been implicated as a cause of hepatomegaly-hepatic steatosis, primary lactic acidosis syndrome, myopathy, and neuropathy.[21–23] In light of this concern and because of the significant hepatotoxicity observed in subjects treated with another fluorinated nucleoside, fialuridine (FIAU),[24] particular emphasis has been placed on investigating emtricitabine's effects on cellular and mitochondrial DNA polymerases in vitro and emtricitabine's toxicities in clinical trials.

In in vitro investigations, E-TP does not appear to interfere significantly with cellular and mitochondrial DNA polymerase function. When the antiviral activity of E-TP against RT was compared with E-TP's activity against human (HeLa cell) DNA polymerases α, β, γ, and ε, E-TP was found to be a weak inhibitor of each of these enzymes when compared to its inhibition of HIV reverse transcriptase. Apparent K_i values were 6.0 μM for polymerase-α, 17 μM for polymerase-β, 6.0 μM for polymerase-γ, and 150 μM for polymerase-ε, compared to the K_i value of 0.17 μM for HIV-1 RT.[25] When the antiviral activity of E-TP against mitochondrial DNA polymerases (pol γ) was compared with lamivudine's effect, E-TP was found to incorporate into mitochondrial DNA at a rate that was 26 times lower than that of lamivudine.[26]

Short- and long-term animal toxicology studies in mice, rats, and cynomolgus monkeys have shown little toxicity with emtricitabine, with the only adverse finding being mild reversible anemia. In animals, emtricitabine had no adverse effects on reproduction, fertility, or teratogenesis; nor did it have adverse effects in a variety of in vitro mutagenesis assays.[25,27] In cynomolgus monkeys given emtricitabine for 3 months to 1 year in doses that exaggerated human doses by more than 25-fold, subcellular morphology including liver, heart, and skeletal muscle was unaffected (unpublished data provided by Triangle Pharmaceuticals, TPI DOC no. 3262).

In humans, emtricitabine has no significant effect on general behavior or on neurologic, autonomic, central nervous system, cardiovascular, renal, gastrointestinal, or smooth muscle function. Safety data have been obtained from 1586 HIV- and HBV-infected patients exposed to multiple doses (at least 14 consecutive days) of emtricitabine in controlled clinical trials. Of these 1586 patients, 885 had been treated with emtricitabine for at least 24 weeks. Selected adverse events occurring with at least a 10% frequency in controlled studies with a lamivudine comparator include abdominal pain (13% emtricitabine vs. 17% lamivudine), asthenia (15% vs. 13%), headache (22% vs. 25%), diarrhea (23% vs. 24%), nausea (20% vs. 18%), vomiting (12% vs. 13%), cough (14% vs. 13%), and pharyngitis (13% vs. 14%). Few serious adverse events with emtricitabine administration have been reported to date, and most of them have been non-life-threatening, such as anemia, diarrhea, vomiting, headache, and lactic acidosis. However, in the FTC-302 study there was an early onset of severe hepatotoxicity including two fatal cases.[28] Patients were randomized to emtricitabine (50%) or lamivudine (50%) in a blinded fashion, stavudine (100%), or either nevirapine (82%) or efavirenz (18%) depending on the baseline plasma HIV RNA level. Hepatotoxicity was observed in patients receiving nevirapine (64/385; 17%) but not among those receiving efavirenz (0/83). Among those with nevirapine-associated liver abnormalities, the incidence of grade 3 and 4 hepatic toxicities was not statistically different for the emtricitabine and lamivudine treatment groups (14% emtricitabine vs. 19% lamivudine; $P = 0.27$). Overall, the incidence of grade 3 or 4 liver toxicity was approximately twofold higher in females than in males (20% vs. 12%; $P < 0.03$).

▲ ANTIRETROVIRAL ACTIVITY AND CLINICAL EFFICACY

As of March 12, 2001, a total of 1856 subjects including healthy adult volunteers, adult HIV- and HBV-infected patients, and HIV-infected or exposed pediatric patients have received at least one dose of emtricitabine. Among them, 778 of these subjects have undergone at least 48 weeks of therapy (unpublished data provided by Triangle Pharmaceuticals).

Emtricitabine Monotherapy

As shown in Table 7–1, healthy, adult volunteers, adult HIV-infected patients, and HIV-infected or HIV-exposed pediatric patients have received emtricitabine in Phase I/II clinical trials. Most of these trials are pharmacokinetic (PK) and dose-finding trials (unpublished data provided by Triangle Pharmaceuticals[18]). However, studies FTC-101 and FTC-102[29,30] also evaluated the antiviral activity of emtricitabine alone and in comparison with lamivudine. FTC-101 was a Phase I/II, cross-sectional, dose-range study of 40 treatment-naive, HIV-infected subjects who were administered emtricitabine monotherapy at 25 mg bid, 100 mg qd, 100 mg bid, 200 mg qd, and 200 mg bid doses for 14 days. Antiretroviral suppression ($\geq$1.3 log) occurred in all dosage cohorts, with a strong trend toward greater activity at the high doses (200 mg bid and 200 mg qd).[29] Based on data from FTC-102, a 12-day monotherapy study, Delehanty et al.[30] reported that the in vivo activity of emtricitabine against HIV was greater than that of lamivudine. In this trial subjects receiving emtricitabine at a dose of 200 mg qd had a significantly steeper slope of HIV RNA decay over 7 days of treatment than subjects receiving lamivudine 150 mg bid ($P = 0.03$). These subjects also had a significantly greater change in plasma HIV RNA, as measured by the average AUC minus baseline plasma HIV RNA level (AAUCMB) ($P = 0.047$). These studies confirmed the potency of emtricitabine when used as a once-daily drug.

Emtricitabine in Three-Drug Combinations

As shown in Table 7–2, several studies of emtricitabine in combination with other antiretroviral medications are either complete or still underway. Most of these trials are evaluating the efficacy of once-daily regimens that include emtricitabine or are attempting to establish the equivalence of emtricitabine with lamivudine. In the ANRS 091/FTC-201 study, Molina et al.[31,32] assessed the activity of a once-daily antiretroviral regimen that combined emtricitabine, didanosine, and efavirenz in treatment-naive subjects. Among the 40 study subjects, the median baseline CD4+ T-lymphocyte count was 373 cells/mm^3, and the median baseline plasma HIV RNA was 4.8 $\log_{10}$ copies/ml. After 24 weeks of treatment, the median increase in CD4+ T-lymphocyte count was 159 cells/mm^3, and the median decrease in plasma HIV RNA was 3.4 $\log_{10}$. At 24 weeks, 98% of subjects had plasma HIV RNA levels of 400 copies/ml, and 93% had levels of 50 copies/ml. At 64 weeks the median increase in CD4+ T-lymphocyte count was 219 cells/mm^3, and 90% of subjects had plasma HIV RNA levels of 400 copies/ml. No significant toxicitites were reported during this trial.

Two randomized studies have compared the relative antiretroviral activity of emtricitabine and lamivudine.[33] In the

Table 7–1. MAJOR PHASE I/II SAFETY AND ACTIVITY TRIALS EVALUATING EMTRICITABINE THERAPY

Trial	Purpose	Design	Dose	No. of Subjects	Entry Criterion	Antiretroviral[a] Response	Comments
143-001	Safety and PK (with food and fasting) of emtricitabine	Randomized, single dose, placebo-controlled, dose-escalating	FTC 100–1200 mg	12	Adult, HIV-infected		Complete, emtricitabine had linear PK with small intersubject variabilities
FTC-101 (Delehanty et al.[29])	Safety, tolerance, PK, antiviral activity, dose finding	Open-label, dose-ranging, monotherapy, 14 days	25 mg bid, 100 mg qd, 100 mg bid, 200 mg qd, 200 mg bid	40 (N = 8 per dose group)	Adult, HIV-infected, treatment-naive	Decrease of 1.4 $\log_{10}$ (25 mg bid) $-2.0 \log_{10}$ (200 mg qd) at 14 days	Complete, greatest decrease in plasma HIV RNA was with 200 mg bid and qd dosing. Supported 200 mg once-daily dosing
FTC-102 (Delehanty et al.[30])	Safety, activity, dose-defining, comparison with LMV	Randomized, open-label, LMV-controlled, three doses of emtricitabine, 10-day monotherapy	FTC 25 mg qd, 100 mg qd, 200 mg qd *or* LMV 150 mg bid	81	Adult, HIV-infected, treatment-naive	Decrease $>1.4 \log_{10}$ for all groups; $1.7 \log_{10}$ for 200 mg qd. Slope of RNA decay over 7 days was significantly greater in emtricitabine group ($P = 0.03$), AAUCMB of emtricitabine significantly greater ($P = 0.047$)	Complete, suggested greater potency of emtricitabine vs. lamivudine
FTC-103	Assess interactions with NRTIs (ZDV, STV)	Randomized, single-dose, open label, three-way crossover	FTC, ZDV, STV	13	Healthy adult volunteers		Complete, PK of emtricitabine not affected to a clinically significant degree by ZDV or STV. C_{max} and AUC of ZDV mildly increased by emtricitabine (26% and 66%) PK of STV unaffected by emtricitabine
FTC-105 (Wiznia et al.[31])	Safety, tolerance, PK profile, dose-finding for pediatric patients	Open-label, two single escalating doses	FTC	25	Pediatric (1–17 yrs), HIV-infected or exposed		Complete; supported a 6 mg/kg pediatric dose for comparable exposure seen with 200 mg qd in adults
FTC-106	PK	Open-label, single dose and multiple doses	^{14}C-labeled FTC	6	Healthy adult volunteers		Complete, emtricitabine primarily excreted in the urine unchanged
FTC-107	PK in patients with renal insufficiency or on dialysis	Open label, single dose		29	Adult volunteers with renal insufficiency		Complete, analyses pending

AAUCMB, average area under the curve minus the baseline HIV RNA level; AUC, area under the curve; C_{max}, maximum concentration; FTC, emtricitabine; LMV, lamivudine; NRTIs, nucleoside reverse transcriptase inhibitors; PK, pharmacokinetics; STV, stavudine; ZDV, zidovudine.

[a]HIV RNA copies/ml.

Table 7–2. MAJOR PHASE II/III ACTIVITY AND EFFICACY TRIALS EVALUATING EMTRICITABINE THERAPY

Trial	Design	Dose	No. of Subjects	Entry Criterion	CD4+ T Lymphocyte Count Response	Antiretroviral[a] Response	Clinical Outcomes	Comments
ANRS 091/ FTC-201 (Molina et al.[31,32])	Open-label, single arm, qd regimen	FTC 200 mg qd, ddI 250 or 400 mg qd, EFV 600 mg qd	40	Adult, HIV-infected, treatment-naive, CD4 T lymphocyte count ≥ 100, HIV RNA ≥ 5000	+159 cells/mm^3 at 24 wks, +219 cells/mm^3 at 64 wks	Decrease of 3.5 $\log_{10}$ at 24 wks; 98% ≤ 400, 93% ≤ 50 at 24 wks; 90% ≤ 400 at 64 wks	No AIDS-defining events	Enrollment complete, follow-up ongoing. Supported the activity of a once-daily dosing regimen
FTC-301	Randomized, double-blind, STV-controlled	FTC vs. STV plus ddI, EFV	500 planned	Adult, HIV-infected, treatment-naive				Entirely once-daily regimen, ongoing
FTC-302 (van der Horst et al.[33]; Bartlett[28])	Randomized, double-blind, LMV-controlled	FTC 200 mg qd *or* LMV 150 mg bid; STV; nevirapine (*n* = 385), *or* efavirenz (*n* = 83)	468	Adult, HIV-infected, treatment-naive	+191 cells/mm^3 at 48 wks in FTC arm, +206 cells/mm^3 at 48 wks in LMV arm	65% ≤ 400, 60% ≤ 50 at wk 48 in FTC arm; 71% ≤ 400, 64% ≤ 50 in LMV arm		Complete, supported equivalence with LMV; observed hepatoxicity attributed to nevirapine
FTC-303/ FTC-350 (van der Horst et al.[33])	Randomized, double-blind, LMV-controlled, responders in emtricitabine-303 rollover to FTC-350	FTC 200 mg qd (*n* = 294) *or* continued 3TC 150 mg bid (*n* = 146)	440	Adult, HIV-infected, LMV-experienced, stable HIV-1 RNA (≤ 400)	+29 cells/mm^3 increase at 48 wks in FTC arm, 61 cells/mm^3 at 48 wks in LMV arm	73% ≤ 400, 68% ≤ 50 at wk 48 in FTC arm; 82% ≤ 400, 75% ≤ 50 at wk 48 in LMV arm		Supported equivalence with LMV
ALIZE	Randomized, open-label, switch	Switch to FTC, ddI, EFV	350	Adult, HIV-infected, treatment-experienced, stable HIV RNA				Ongoing
ACTG 5015	Open-label, single arm, two age cohorts	FTC, STV, lopinavir/rifonavir	90 planned	Adult, HIV-infected, treatment-naive				

ddI, didanosine; EFV, efavirenz.
[a]HIV RNA copies/ml.

FTC-302 trial, a total of 468 treatment-naive subjects were randomized to emtricitabine- or lamivudine-containing regimens in a double-blind, placebo-controlled study. The median plasma HIV RNA levels and CD4+ T-lymphocyte counts at baseline were 40,000 copies/ml and 373 cells/mm^3, respectively; 10% of subjects receiving emtricitabine and 10% of those given lamivudine withdrew owing to adverse events, and 12% of both groups withdrew for other reasons. After 48 weeks on study medications, the percentages of study subjects with plasma HIV RNA levels of less than 400 copies/ml and less than 50 copies/ml were not significantly different for the two groups, (emtricitabine: 65% <400 and 60% <50 copies/ml; lamivudine; 71% <400 and 65% <50 copies/ml). Virologic failure, defined as a lack of response (plasma HIV RNA >400 copies/ml at week 12) or loss of response (two consecutive plasma HIV RNA levels >400 copies/ml after having reached <400 copies/ml), occurred in 12.3% of the emtricitabine group and 7.3% of the lamivudine group ($P = 0.046$). Interestingly, when subjects with baseline plasma HIV RNA levels of more than 100,000 copies/ml were analyzed, 8% reached virologic failure in the emtricitabine group and 13% in the lamivudine group. In the FTC-303 study, 440 subjects on lamivudine-containing regimens with plasma HIV RNA levels of less than 400 copies/ml for at least 12 weeks were randomized in a 2:1 allocation to receive open-label emtricitabine or lamivudine. At baseline, subjects had received their lamivudine-containing regimen for a median of 35 months; 79% were on protease inhibitor (PI)-containing and 21% were on nonnucleoside reverse transcriptase inhibitor (NNRTI)-containing regimens. Baseline plasma HIV RNA levels were less than 50 copies/ml in 86% and 50 to 400 copies/ml in 14%. A significantly higher percentage of subjects receiving emtricitabine withdrew owing to adverse events compared to those receiving lamivudine (4% vs. 1%), and a significantly larger percentage of subjects receiving emtricitabine withdrew for other reasons compared to those receiving lamivudine (15% vs. 9%). After 48 weeks on study medications, the percentages of study subjects with plasma HIV RNA levels of less than 400 copies/ml and less than 50 copies/ml were not significantly different between the two groups (emtricitabine: 73% <400 and 68% <50; lamivudine: 82% <400 and 73% <50). Virologic failure, defined as plasma HIV RNA levels of more than 400 copies/ml on two consecutive measurements, occurred in 8% of subjects receiving emtricitabine and 8% of subjects receiving lamivudine.

▲ PEDIATRIC TRIALS

In the FTC-105 study, the single-dose pharmacokinetics of emtricitabine at 60 and 120 mg/m^2 were evaluated in HIV-infected children from birth to 18 years.[34] A total of 25 children completed the study; only 2 children were less than 2 years of age. The available pharmacokinetic data include only the 23 children over age 2. In this cohort plasma emtricitabine concentrations were dose-proportional for the two doses. The elimination $t_{1/2}$ was about 11 hours across all age groups. Based on the AUC data at a dose of 120 mg/m^2, it was projected that a emtricitabine dose of 6 mg/kg would produce plasma AUC concentrations in children comparable to that seen in adults given a 200 mg dose (i.e., 9 to 10 hr · μg/ml). Therefore, a therapeutic emtricitabine dose of 6 mg/kg was recommended for children and is currently being evaluated in a Phase II therapeutic trial (FTC-203).

▲ RESISTANCE

Emtricitabine-resistant HIV has been examined in vitro and in vivo in comparison with lamivudine-resistant virus. Drug resistance to emtricitabine develops rapidly and results from a single point mutation at position 184 of the highly conserved YMDD (Tyr-Met-Asp-Asp) motif of reverse transcriptase (RT), the RT polymerase domain.[35] The point mutation causes methionine to be replaced by valine or isoleucine (M184V and M184I mutations). Although this mutation confers cross resistance to lamivudine, viruses resistant to emtricitabine retain sensitivity to other nucleoside analogues and NNRTIs including zidovudine, zalcitabine, didanosine, and nevirapine.[9,10]

In an in vitro comparison of lamivudine and emtricitabine by Schinazi et al., HIV-infected PBMCs were exposed to equal concentrations of lamivudine or emtricitabine and were passaged weekly. With each weekly cell passage, HIV replication increased in both cell cultures. At the third week 50% of virus replication was inhibited by emtricitabine, whereas less than 5% was inhibited by an equal concentration of lamivudine. At week 7, however, viruses passaged with either drug were more than 1000-fold resistant to both drugs. DNA sequencing of the resistant virus generated by both drugs revealed the M184V or M184I mutations in the RT YMDD motif.[10]

Tisdale et al.[9] compared the antiviral activity of emtricitabine with that of zidovudine, zalcitabine, didanosine, lamivudine, and nevirapine in drug-resistant viral mutants. All viral mutants with the M184V substitution were markedly resistant to emtricitabine and lamivudine, showing a more than 1000-fold increase in EC_{50} values. The M184V substitution also led to a minor increase in the EC_{50} values for zalcitabine and didanosine but did not cause a change in susceptibility to zidovudine or nevirapine. In addition, in the presence of virus that was partially resistant to zidovudine (M41L and T215Y), the M184V substitution caused complete reversion to a zidovudine-sensitive phenotype.

The results of resistance testing in subjects experiencing virologic relapse on emitricitabine-containing regimens suggest that wild-type virus or M184V variants occur most commonly. In the FTC-302 study, 47 of 468 subjects experienced virologic failure, defined as a lack of response (plasma HIV RNA level >400 copies/ml at week 12) or loss of response (two consecutive plasma HIV RNA levels >400 copies/ml after having reached <400 copies/ml).[34,36] Virologic failure occurred in 12.3% of subjects receiving emtricitabine versus 7.3% of subjects receiving lamivudine ($P = 0.046$). Of 47 subjects experiencing virologic failure, 15 had viruses with M184V genotype, including 5 of 30 subjects receiving emtricitabine versus 10 of 17 subjects receiving lamivudine (17% emtricitabine vs. 59% lamivudine; $P = 0.003$). In a meta-analysis of 242 subjects with virologic relapse and available genotypes on emtricitabine and lamivudine-containing regimens, 124 failed with M184V genotypes.[37] There was a significantly lower incidence of M184V mutations in subjects relapsing on emtricitabine-containing regimens than on lamivudine-containing regimens. About 42% to 75% of subjects on emtricitabine-containing regimens failed with wild-type virus, and 12% to 40% of subjects on lamivudine-containing regimens failed with wild-type virus. A potential advantage of emtricitabine-containing regimens may be the frequency of wild-type relapse, although these results are preliminary and clinical trials to assess their virologic responses to changed regimens are not yet available.

A new variant of feline immunodeficiency virus (FIV) containing a proline to serine mutation at position 156 of FIV RT that confers resistance to lamivudine and zidovudine has been described.[38] A laboratory-adapted HIV RT containing the mutation in the analogous position, residue P157, has been developed. This P157S containing HIV RT has moderate resistance to emtricitabine and lamivudine and low-level resistance to zidovudine.[39]

P157 is one of several residues that comprise the template grip, a DNA polymerase structural motif that interacts with the template strand.[40–42] The mutation of P157 does not appear to affect overall polymerase activity; Klarmann et al.[39] found that P157S-containing RT grown in HeLa cells replicates at nearly wild-type levels. Although clinical isolates have not been identified to date, the P157S mutation has the potential to be clinically significant.

▲ DRUG INTERACTIONS

Because renal excretion of unchanged drug is the principal route of emtricitabine elimination from plasma, the potential for emtricitabine to cause metabolic drug interactions is thought to be low. In the few drug interaction studies conducted to date, emticitabine does not interact with other antiretroviral agents. In the FTC-103 study, the pharmacokinetics of emtricitabine in six subjects was unaffected by co-administration with either zidovudine or stavudine. In the same study, a single dose of emtricitabine caused a mild increase in the AUC and maximum concentration (C_{max}) of zidovudine (26% and 66%, respectively) but had no clinically significant effect on the pharmacokinetics of stavudine.

Because emtricitabine is eliminated unchanged in urine, a study was conducted that focused on potential interactions between emtricitabine and famciclovir at the site of urinary excretion. Famciclovir was chosen as a prototypical drug for this evaluation because its active form in plasma (penciclovir) is primarily eliminated in urine, and famciclovir may be commonly co-administered with emtricitabine. The results showed no clinically significant interactions between emtricitabine and famciclovir (unpublished data from FTC-108, provided by Triangle Pharmaceuticals).

▲ RECOMMENDATIONS FOR USE

- Emtricitabine has not yet received FDA approval.
- Emtricitabine demonstrates desirable pharmacokinetic properties, such as good oral bioavilability, linear kinetics over a wide dose range, potential lack of drug interaction, and high plasma and intracellular concentrations with a relatively long half-life.
- Emtricitabine has similar safety and tolerability to lamivudine. The safety of emtricitabine has been studied in more than 1500 HIV- or HBV-infected patients, and no life-threatening toxicities have been attributed to it. The most common side effects of emtricitabine are asthenia, headache, and nausea.
- In combination regimens, emtricitabine has activity similar to that of lamivudine, as documented by suppression of plasma HIV RNA levels and increases in absolute CD4+ T-lymphocyte counts.
- Emtricitabine offers once-daily dosing. The activity of emtricitabine in combination with that of didanosine and efavirenz in a once-daily dosing regimen appears outstanding in a pilot study.
- Viral isolates with M184V RT mutations display high-level emtricitabine resistance. Therefore emtricitabine's greatest use is in treatment-naive patients.

REFERENCES

1. Schinazi R, McMillan A, Cannon D, et al. Selective inhibition of human immunodeficiency viruses by racemates and enantiomers of cis-5-fluoro-1-[2-(hydroxymethyl)-1,3-oxathiolane-5-yl]cytosine. Antimicrob Agents Chemother 36:2423, 1992.
2. Van Roey P, Pangborn W, Schinazi R, et al. Absolute configuration of the antiviral agent (−)-cis-5-fluoro-1-[2-hydroxymethyl)-1,3-oxathiolan-5-yl]cytosine. Antivir Chem Chemother 4:369, 1993.
3. Furman P, Davis M, Liotta D, et al. The anti-hepatitis B virus activities, cytotoxicities, and anabolic profiles of the (−) and (+) enantiomers of cis-5-fluoro-1-[2-(hydroxymethyl)-1,3-oxathiolan-5-yl]cytosine. Antimicrob Agents Chemother 36:2686, 1992.
4. Furman P, Reardon J, Painter G. The role of absolute configuration in the anti-HIV and anti-HBV activity of nucleoside analogs. Antivir Chem Chemother 6:345, 1995.
5. Paff M, Averett D, Prus K, et al. Intracellular metabolism of (−) and (+)-cis-5-fluoro-1-[2-(hydroxymethyl)-1,3-oxathiolan-5-yl]cytosine in HepG2 derivative 2.2.15(subclone P5A)cells. Antimicrob Agents Chemother 38:1230, 1994.
6. Wilson J, Martin J, Borroto-Esoda K, et al. The 5′-triphosphates of the (−) and (+) enantiomers of cis-5-fluoro-1-[2-(hydroxymethyl)-1,3-oxathiolane-5-yl]cytosine equally inhibit human immunodeficiency virus type 1 reverse transcriptase. Antimicrob Agents Chemother 37:1720, 1993.
7. Wilson J, Aulabaugh A, Caligan B, et al. Human immunodeficiency virus type-1 reverse transcriptase contribution of Met-184 to binding of nucleoside 5′-triphosphate. J Biol Chem 271:13656, 1996.
8. Stein D, Moore K. Phosphorylation of nucleoside analog antiretrovirals: a review for clinicians. Pharmacotherapy 21:11, 2001.
9. Tisdale M, Kemp S, Parry N, Larder B. Rapid in vitro selection of human immunodeficiency virus type 1 resistant to 3′thiacytidine inhibitors due to a mutation in the YMDD region of reverse transcriptase. Proc Natl Acad Sci USA 90:5653, 1993.
10. Schinazi R, Lloyd R, Nguyen M, et al. Characterization of human immunodeficiency viruses resistant to oxathiolane-cytosine nucleosides. Antimicrob Agents Chemother 37:875, 1993.
11. Feng J, Anderson K. Mechanistic studies show that (−)-emtricitabine-TP is a better inhibitor of HIV-1 reverse transcriptase than lamivudine-TP. FASEB J 13:1511, 1999.
12. Jansen R, Johnson L, Averett D. High-capacity in vitro assessment of antihepatitis B virus compound selectivity by a virion-specific polymerase chain reaction assay. Antimicrob Agents Chemother 37:441, 1993.
13. Schinazi R, Gosselin G, Abdesslem F, et al. Pure nucleoside enantiomers of B-2′3′-dideoxycytidine analogs are selective inhibitors of hepatitis B virus in vitro. Antimicrob Agents Chemother 38:2172, 1994.

14. Mathez D, Schinazi R, Liotta D, Leibowitch J. Infectious amplification of wild-type human immunodeficiency virus from patients' lymphocytes and modulation by reverse transcriptase inhibitors in vitro. Antimicrob Agents Chemother 37:2206, 1993.
15. Bridges E, Dutschman G, Gullen E, Cheng Y. Favorable interaction of β-L(−) nucleoside analogues with clinically approved anti-HIV nucleoside analogues for the treatment of human immunodeficiency virus. Biochem Pharmacol 51:731, 1996.
16. Wang L, Gardner P, Frick L, et al. Pharmacokinetics (Pk) and safety of 524 W91 following single oral administration of escalating doses in HIV-infected volunteers. Presented at the 35th Interscience Conference on Antimicrobial Agents and Chemotherapy, San Francisco, 1995, abstract A129.
17. Wang L, Delehanty J, Blum M, et al. FTC: a potent and selective anti-HIV and anti-HBV agent demonstrating desirable pharmacokinetic characteristics. Presented at the 36th Annual Meeting of the Infectious Diseases Society of America, Denver, 1998, abstract 415.
18. Wang L, Delehanty J, Hulett L, et al. High levels of intracellular emtricitabine-triphosphate correlate with the potent antiviral activity of emtricitabine in vivo. Presented at the 38th Interscience Conference Antimicrobial Agents and Chemotherapy, San Diego, 1998, abstract LB-2.
19. Cammack N, Rouse P, Marr CL, et al. Cellular metabolism (−) enantiomeric 2′-deoxy-3′-thiacytidine. Biochem Pharmacol 43:2059, 1992.
20. Frick L, Lambe C, St John L, et al. Pharmacokinetics, oral bioavailability, and metabolism in mice and cynomolgus monkeys of (2′R,5′S)-cis-5-fluoro-1-[2-(hydroxymethyl)-1,3-oxathiolan-5-yl]cytosine and agent active against human immunodeficiency virus and human hepatitis B virus. Antimicrob Agents Chemother 38:2722, 1994.
21. Chen C, Cheng Y. Delayed cytotoxicity and selective loss of mitochondrial DNA in cells treated with anti-human immunodeficiency compound 2′,3′-dideoxycytidine. J Biol Chem 264:11934, 1989.
22. Dalakas M, Illa I, Pezeshkpour G, et al. Mitochondrial myopathy by long-term zidovudine therapy. N Engl J Med 332:1098, 1990.
23. Carr A, Cooper D. Adverse effects of antiretroviral therapy. Lancet 356:1423, 2000.
24. McKenzie R, Fried M, Sallie R, et al. Hepatic failure and lactic acidosis due to fialuridine (FIAU), an investigational nucleoside analogue for chronic hepatitis B. N Engl J Med 333:1099, 1995.
25. Schinazi R, Boudinot F, Ibrahim S, et al. Pharmacokinetics and metabolism of racemic 2′,3′-dideoxy-5-fluoro-3-thiacytidine in rhesus monkeys. Antimicrob Agents Chemother 36:2432, 1992.
26. Feng J, Johnson A, Johnson K, et al. Insights into the molecular mechanism of mitochondrial toxicity of antiviral drugs. Presented at the 2nd International Workshop on Adverse Drugs Reactions and Lipodystrophy in HIV, Toronto, 2000.
27. Frick L, St John L, Taylor L, et al. Pharmacokinetics, oral bioavailability, and metabolic disposition in rats of (—)-cis-5-fluoro-1-[2-(hydroxymethyl)-1,3-oxanthiolan-5-yl]cytosine, a nucleoside analog active against human immunodeficiency virus and hepatitis B virus. Antimicrob Agents Chemother 37:2285, 1993.
28. Bartlett J. Severe liver toxicity inpatients receiving two nucleoside analogues and a non-nucleoside reverse transcriptase inhibitor. Presented at the 8th Conference on Retroviruses and Opportunistic Infections, Chicago, 2001, abstract 19.
29. Delehanty J, Kahn J, Thompson M, et al. Selection of emtricitabine dose based on viral kinetics and pharmacokinetics in an accelerated clinical trial design. Presented at the 12th International Conference on AIDS, Geneva, 1998, abstract 12208.
30. Delehanty J, Wakeford C, Hulett L, et al. A phase I/II randomized controlled study of FTC versus 3TC in HIV infected patients. Presented at the 6th Conference on Retroviruses and Opportunistic Infections, Chicago, 1999, abstract 6.
31. Molina J, Ferchal F, Rancinan C, et al. Once-daily combination therapy with emtricitabine, didanosine, and efavirenz in human immunodeficiency virus-infected patients. J Infect Dis 182:599, 2000.
32. Molina J, Perusat S, Ferchal F, et al. Once-daily combination therapy with emtricitabine, didanosine and efavirenz in treatment-naive HIV-infected adults: 64 week follow-up of the ANRS091 trial. Presented at the 8th Conference on Retroviruses and Opportunistic Infections, Chicago, 2001, abstract 321.
33. Van der Horst C, Sanne I, Wakeford C, et al. Two randomized, controlled, equivalance trials of emtricitabine (emtricitabine) to lamivudine (3TC). Presented at the 8th Conference on Retroviruses and Opportunistic Infections, Chicago, 2001, abstract 18.
34. Wiznia A, Wang L, Rathore M, et al. An evaluation of the pharmacokinetics and safety of single oral doses of emtricitabine (FTC) in HIV-infected or exposed children. Presented at the 40th Interscience Conference on Antimicrobial Agents and Chemotherapy, Toronto, 2000, abstract 1665.
35. Kohlstaedt L, Wang J, Friedman J, et al. Crystal structure at 3.5Å resolution of HIV-1 reverse transcriptase complexed with an inhibitor. Science 256:1783, 1992.
36. Harris J, Shaw A, Borroto-Esoda K, et al. Genotypic analysis of HIV-1 infected ART naive patients receiving emitricitabine (FTC) or lamivudine (3TC) in a double-blinded equivalence trial. Presented at the 5th International Workshop on Drug Resistance and Treatment Strategies, Scottsdale, AR, 2001, abstract 104.
37. Borroto-Esoda K, Harris J, Shaw A, et al. Lower incidence of the M184V mutation in patients receiving combination therapy with emitricitabine (FTC) compared to lamivudine (3TC). Presented at the 5th International Workshop on Drug Resistance and Treatment Strategies, Scottsdale, AR, 2001, abstract 88.
38. Smith R, Remington K, Preston B, et al. A novel point mutation at position 156 of reverse transcriptase from feline immunodeficiency virus confers resistance to the combination of (−)-beta-2′,3′-dideoxy-3′-thiacytidine and 3′-azido-3′-deoxythymidine. J Virol 72:2335, 1998.
39. Klarmann G, Smith R, Schinazi R, et al. Site-specific incorporation of nucleoside analogs by HIV-1 reverse transcriptase and the template grip mutant P157S: template interactions influence substrate recognition at the polymerase active site. J Biol Chem 275:359, 2000.
40. Huang H, Chopra R, Verdine G, Harrison S. Structure of a covalently trapped catalytic complex of HIV-1 reverse transcriptase: implications for drug resistance. Science 282:1669, 1998.
41. Jacobo-Molina A, Ding J, Nanni R, et al. Crystal structure of human immunodeficiency virus type 1 reverse transcriptase complexed with double-stranded DNA at 3.0 A resolution shows bent DNA. Proc Natl Acad Sci USA 90:6320, 1993.
42. Ding J, Das K, Hsiou Y, et al. Structure and functional implications of the polumerase active site region in a complex of HIV-1 RT with a double-stranded DNA template-primer and an antibody Fab fragment at 2.7 A resolution. J Mol Biol 284:1095, 1998.

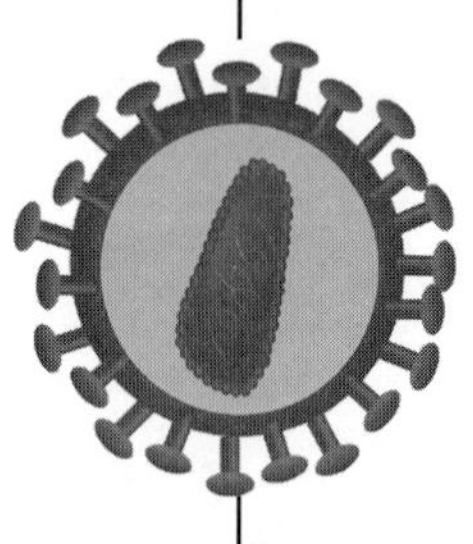

CHAPTER 8

Abacavir

Victoria A. Johnson, MD

▲ STRUCTURE

Abacavir sulfate, compound 1592U89 hemisulfate [(1*S*, *cis*)-4-(2-amino-6-(cyclopropylamino)-9H-purin-9-yl)-2-cyclopentene-1-methanol sulfate (salt)(2:1)]; (formerly also known as 1592), also known as Ziagen, is a carbocyclic nucleoside analogue with potent and selective activity against the human immunodeficiency virus (HIV).[1−8] This compound contains a novel 6-cyclopropylamino-substituted purine. The structure is shown in Figure 8−1*A*. The compound is activated by cellular enzymes to the triphosphate derivative of the guanine analogue [1144U88(1*R*,4*S*)-9-(4-(hydroxymethyl)-2-cyclopenten-1-yl)-guanine]; (-)-carbovir], shown in Figure 8−1*B*.

▲ IN VITRO ACTIVITY AND MECHANISMS OF ACTION

The active form of abacavir, 1144U88 triphosphate, is a potent inhibitor of HIV-1 reverse transcriptase in vitro, with a K_i of 0.02 μM.[1−7] In whole virus assays, abacavir has activity against HIV-1 (strain IIIB) cultured in MT-4 cells [a human leukemic cell line transformed with human T-lymphocyte leukemia virus type 1 (HTLV-1)], peripheral blood mononuclear cells (PBMCs), and macrophages. The 50% inhibitory concentration (IC_{50}) values in these cells were, respectively, 4.0, 3.7, and 0.65 μM.[5] The mean IC_{50} for abacavir against eight fresh clinical isolates of HIV-1 obtained from zidovudine-naive patients and amplified in PBMCs was 0.26 μM (i.e., potency equivalent to that of zidovudine).[1,3,5,7] Abacavir has also demonstrated synergistic activity in vitro against HIV-1 when used in combination with zidovudine, other nucleoside reverse transcriptase inhibitors (NRTIs) such as lamivudine and didanosine (but additive with stavudine), nonnucleoside reverse transcriptase inhibitors (NNRTIs) such as nevirapine, and protease inhibitors (PIs) such as amprenavir.[1,5,7−9]

▲ PHARMACOKINETICS

General Information

The cyclopropylamino moiety of abacavir is important for enhanced absorption and central nervous system penetration in vivo when compared to carbovir.[5,10] In contrast to the limited oral absorption of carbovir (e.g., 26% and 23% oral bioavailability in the rat and monkey, respectively), pharmacokinetic evaluation of abacavir showed good oral bioavailability (e.g., 92% and 77% in mice and monkeys, respectively).[5,11−13] In contrast to the poor brain penetration of carbovir (e.g., rat brain/plasma concentration ratios averaged 0.04), the penetration of abacavir into monkey cerebrospinal fluid (CSF) and rat brain were comparable to that of zidovudine.[5] Abacavir showed significant penetration into CSF in humans.[14]

Intracellular activation of abacavir to its active triphosphate form requires phosphorylation by cellular enzymes.[2,4,6,15] This involves a unique set of enzymes other than those involved in activation of other NRTIs that are currently approved for treatment of HIV infection. Abacavir sulfate is activated intracellularly to carbovir monophosphate by a novel phosphorylation pathway[2−6] involving adenosine phosphotransferase.[16] Carbovir monophosphate is then efficiently anabolized by cellular

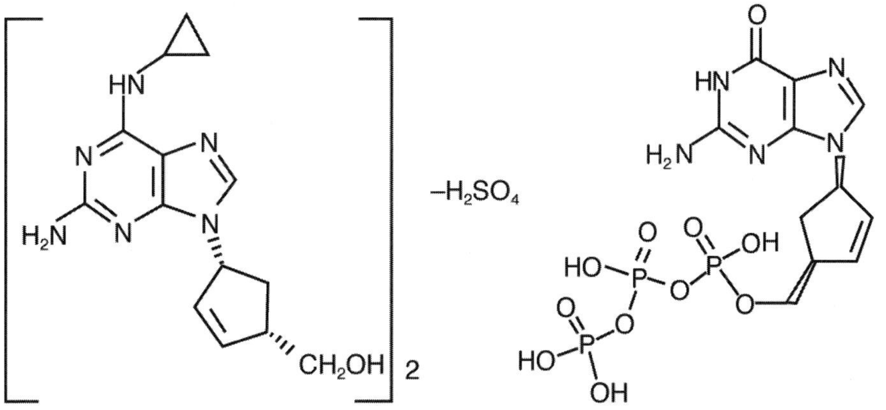

Figure 8–1. *A*, Structure of abacavir sulfate, compound 1592U89 hemisulfate [1*S*, *cis*)-4-[2-amino-6-(cyclopropylamino)-9H-purin-9-yl)-2-cyclopentene-1-methanol sulfate (salt)(2:1)], also known as Ziagen, a carbocyclic nucleoside analogue. The cyclopropylamino moiety of abacavir (1592U89) is important for absorption and central nervous system penetration in vivo. *B*, Structure of 1144U88 triphosphate. Compound 1592U89 (abacavir sulfate) is activated by cellular enzymes to the triphosphate derivative of the guanine analogue 1144U88 [(1*R*, 4*S*)-9-(4-(hydroxymethyl)-2-cyclopenten-1-yl)-guanine; (−)-carbovir].

enzymes to carbovir diphosphate, followed by anabolism to the active form carbovir triphosphate, which inhibits HIV reverse transcriptase. The existence of this unique activation pathway enables abacavir to overcome the deficiencies of carbovir (which include low oral bioavailability and minimal brain penetration) while maintaining potent, selective anti-HIV activity.[5,6] The intracellular half-life of carbovir triphosphate, produced from both abacavir and carbovir, is about 3.3 hours.[2,5,17]

The main route of elimination of abacavir is metabolism, with less than 2% of a dose recovered as unchanged drug in urine.[14] The catabolism of abacavir involves two pathways: (1) glucuronidation and (2) carboxylation through alcohol dehydrogenase.[12,13] The metabolism of abacavir is not dependent on cytochrome P_{450} liver enzymes. Physiologic concentrations of human albumin or α_1-acid glycoprotein do not markedly alter the anti-HIV activity of abacavir,[18] and food intake does not significantly affect abacavir's bioavailability. In an initial Phase I double-blind, parallel, dose-escalation trial evaluating safety and kinetics, the area under the concentration-time curve (AUC) for the 300 mg dose (tablets) was 99% of the oral solution AUC, and administration with food lowered the AUC by 5% and the maximum plasma concentration by 35%.[19] The main route of metabolite excretion is renal, with 83% of a dose recovered in urine.[14] There are no known significant drug interactions.[19,20] Abacavir demonstrated predictable pharmacokinetic characteristics when administered as single oral doses ranging from 100 to 1200 mg.[21] No significant pharmacokinetic interactions were detected after single-dose administration of abacavir in double or triple combinations with zidovudine, lamivudine, or both.[22] In multiple-dose studies abacavir showed predictable pharmacokinetic characteristics, and zidovudine co-administration had no effect on the abacavir AUC_{tau} (a parameter most closely associated with efficacy).[23]

In subjects with mild liver impairment (CNAB1006 study), there was a 1.9-fold increase in abacavir exposure and a 1.6-fold increase in abacavir half-life in the group with liver disease. Liver disease did not modify the extent of metabolite formation, although the rates of formation and elimination were decreased. The CNAB1006 study results suggested that patients with mild hepatic impairment should received 150 mg abacavir twice daily to achieve an AUC equivalent to that in patients without liver disease receiving the recommended 300 mg twice-daily dose.[24]

Pharmacokinetics in HIV-Infected Infants and Children

A Phase I single-dose pharmacokinetic study evaluated two oral abacavir doses (4 and 8 mg/kg body weight) in 22 HIV-infected children ages 3 months to 13 years.[25] Abacavir was rapidly absorbed, with time to peak concentration in plasma occurring within 1.5 hours after dosing. Abacavir was rapidly eliminated, with a mean elimination half-life of 0.98 to 1.13 hours. The extent of exposure to abacavir appears to be slightly lower in children than in adults, with the comparable unit doses being based on body weight.[25]

▲ TOXICITY

In Vitro Effects

Abacavir and carbovir are less myelotoxic than zidovudine, didanosine, or zalcitabine when tested in vitro using human and murine hematopoietic progenitor cells.[2,5] Carbovir triphosphate has relatively low inhibitory activity against cellular DNA polymerase γ when compared to the active triphosphates of other dideoxynucleoside analogues.[5] It is the inhibition of cellular DNA polymerase γ that has been associated with drug-induced peripheral neuropathy. Taken together, the preclinical development of abacavir sulfate was supported by both a relative lack of myelosuppressive effects and less inhibition of cellular enzymes involved in the development of peripheral neuropathy.

In Vivo Effects

In clinical trials to date, most adverse events were rated as mild or moderate. No specific hepatic, pancreatic, renal, or bone marrow toxicity patterns have been described.

Gastrointestinal and Neurologic Side Effects

The most common side effects seen during abacavir therapy are gastrointestinal and neurologic. Nausea, vomiting, and diarrhea have been ascribed to abacavir therapy. Nausea is common. All of these gastrointestinal complaints tend to abate over the first few weeks of abacavir therapy. Neurologic side effects are less common than gastrointestinal complaints. Headache, malaise, dizziness, insomnia, and rarely paresthesias have been noted during abacavir therapy. In placebo-controlled clinical trials, only nausea/vomiting and malaise/fatigue were statistically significantly more frequent in abacavir-containing regimens versus the control regimens.

Abacavir Hypersensitivity Syndrome

Hypersensitivity reactions occur in approximately 5% of patients receiving abacavir for the treatment of HIV-1 infection. The appearance of this syndrome demands immediate discontinuation and is an absolute contraindication to reinitiation of abacavir or an abacavir-containing medication (e.g., Trizivir). A total of 1015 cases have been described among 26,769 subjects enrolled in Phase II and III clinical trials and expanded access programs.[26] The median time to onset was 11 days, with 93% of cases appearing within 6 weeks of initiation of abacavir, although reactions may occur at any time during therapy. In a risk factor meta-analysis for hypersensitivity reactions to abacavir introduction, the incidence was 3.7%. The odds ratios (OR) for subjects with previous highly active antiretroviral therapy (HAART) and those of African descent were significantly lower [OR 0.41, 95% confidence intervals (CI) 0.23, 0.72; and OR 0.51, 95% CI 0.28, 0.92, respectively] than HAART-naive patients and those of other ethnic origins.[27] The mechanism is not fully understood but may involve an immunologic response. GlaxoSmithKline is conducting pharmacogenetic research to determine if genetic polymorphisms (variations) can be identified in HIV-infected patients who have developed hypersensitivity reactions following treatment with abacavir to help predict the risk of abacavir hypersensitivity in susceptible patients.[27a] An association between HLA-B*5701, HLA-DR7, and HLA-DQ3 and the hypersensitivity syndrome has been reported.[28]

The usual presentation includes symptoms indicating involvement of multiple organ systems.[29] The most common symptoms are fever, rash, gastrointestinal (GI) symptoms (nausea, vomiting, diarrhea, abdominal pain), and malaise or fatigue. *Fever is a key feature of the syndrome.* Less common symptoms include respiratory symptoms (cough, sore throat, dyspnea), musculoskeletal complaints (myalgia, myolysis, arthralgia, edema), headache, and paresthesias. Hypotension is present in 5% of reactions. In contrast to immunoglobulin E (IgE)-mediated anaphylactic reactions, wheezing is distinctly uncommon and edema less common. In contrast to the described reactions to NNRTIs, the rash is rarely severe, usually appearing later (e.g., 1 to 3 days) after the onset of the systemic symptoms; it is absent in up to 30% of cases.[30,31] The rash is usually maculopapular or urticarial. Morbidity is related more to the systemic symptoms than to the rash. Although the time course is variable, symptoms tend to occur in succession over the course of several days, with fever and GI symptoms appearing early and rash later. *The severity of symptoms tends to increase with each dose.* A delay in discontinuing abacavir in the face of an active hypersensitivity reaction may lead to a severe reaction and even death, although the risk of a fatal reaction is far more likely in the setting of a rechallenge (see below).

After discontinuing abacavir, symptoms diminish quickly and resolve over a few days, although the rash, if present, may persist longer. If abacavir is reinitiated (rechallenge), however, symptoms reappear within hours and are often more severe. Fever, rash, malaise, hypotension, facial or throat swelling (or both), and bronchospasm have been described. Symptoms not present with the initial reaction may also appear on rechallenge, and temperature elevations to 39° to 40°C may occur. One case report described severe anaphylactic shock after rechallenge with abacavir without preceding hypersensitivity.[32] Hypotension was present in approximately 25% of cases when abacavir was restarted after an initial reaction. Support with intravenous fluids with or without vasopressors (dopamine/dobutamine) may be necessary. Fatalities have been reported.[33] Among the reported cases where a rechallenge was attempted, 4% of patients have died. The rechallenge reaction has occurred even at reduced doses of 100 mg abacavir. Thus, *once hypersensitivity to abacavir has been diagnosed, do not rechallenge with abacavir or an abacavir-containing medication (e.g., Trizivir).*

Laboratory abnormalities observed during a hypersensitivity reaction to abacavir include elevated liver function test results and an acute, transient lymphopenia in some subjects. Occasionally, decreased platelet counts, elevated serum creatinine, and elevated creatine phosphokinase have been described. These laboratory abnormalities return to normal with prompt discontinuation of abacavir. No preexisting condition or screening laboratory abnormality has been identified that indicates an increased likelihood of developing this reaction.

Cutaneous reactions are common with other medications often prescribed to patients with HIV infection, such as NNRTIs or sulfamethoxazole. The appearance or characteristics of a rash without other symptoms are not sufficiently specific to differentiate the cause in most cases. However, the morbidity associated with hypersensitivity reactions to abacavir is not related to rash, and rash is not frequently an early sign of this reaction. Thus, for patients in whom rash is the only clinical symptom, abacavir may be continued with the warning to follow the patient carefully for the development of other symptoms. The patient should be counseled to report the appearance of any additional symptoms immediately. In cases where systemic symptoms and rash are present together, differentiation may not be possible and abacavir should be discontinued. The rash due to abacavir hypersensitivity is mild but may involve mucous membranes. However, Stevens-Johnson syndrome has been reported *only* when abacavir has been combined with NNRTIs.

In some cases the symptoms of a hypersensitivity reaction may resemble acute infections or reactions to other medications. Keiser et al. described the clinical features of diagnosed influenza infection with cases of hypersensitivity to abacavir.[34] Both rash and GI symptoms were strongly associated with the latter. Respiratory symptoms with hypersensitivity to abacavir appeared in conjunction with GI symptoms. Nevertheless, for some cases differentiating hypersensitivity to abacavir from an acute infection can be difficult. The symptoms increase in severity if dosing is continued. Moreover, the timing of the onset of symptoms with respect to drug exposure is critical for recognizing the syndrome. Abacavir hypersensitivity starts several days to 6 weeks after starting the drug in most cases. Furthermore, the symptoms diminish after stopping abacavir. Severe reactions and fatalities have occurred when symptoms of hypersensitivity to abacavir were ascribed to another cause and the discontinuation of abacavir was delayed or rechallenge was attempted. It is important not to ascribe the symptoms of abacavir hypersensitivity to nonspecific “flu” or “gastroenteritis.”[30,31]

There is no evidence to indicate that interruption of abacavir administration in the absence of any symptoms (i.e., for a reason other than a side effect) increases the frequency or severity of a subsequent hypersensitivity reaction.[35,36] However, there have been cases in which hypersensitivity reactions occurred within 1 day of restarting abacavir where no prior symptoms of an initial hypersensitivity reaction were recorded. This underscores the importance of advising a patient to contact the health care provider if abacavir is discontinued. The health care provider should then obtain a careful history to ensure that symptoms indicating a hypersensitivity reaction were not present at the time of interruption.

Common Adverse Events in Adult HIV-Infected Subjects Enrolled in CNAA2001

A summary of clinical toxicities associated with abacavir in the CNAA2001 trial is shown in Table 8–1.[37–40] In that study, abacavir was administered as monotherapy for 4 weeks followed by randomization to zidovudine or its matching placebo for an additional 8 weeks.[37–40] The most commonly reported adverse events were nausea, headache, asthenia, diarrhea, insomnia, fever, dizziness, vomiting, abdominal pain, and rash. Nausea was common, occurring in 9 of 20 subjects (45%) at 300 mg PO bid. Headache occurred in 8 of 20 subjects (40%) at 300 mg PO bid. A possible trend of an increase in the incidence of nausea and headache with increasing abacavir dose was observed. However, the small numbers of patients and the design of the study make it difficult to draw definitive conclusions about the significance of this preliminary observation. Only eight subjects (10%) withdrew from the study because of adverse events, all of which were considered possibly related to the study drug. The most common reasons for discontinuation were nausea (with or without vomiting) or a hypersensitivity reaction. The latter occurred within 4 weeks of dosing. Only four subjects experienced a serious adverse event, none of which were thought to be related to the study drug.

▲ **Table 8–1.** MOST COMMON ADVERSE EVENTS ASSOCIATED WITH ABACAVIR IN CNAA2001 TRIAL[a]

Toxicity	Frequency	Comment
Nausea	9/20 (45%)	A possible trend with increasing doses was noted
Headache	8/20 (40%)	A possible trend with increasing doses was noted
Asthenia	8/20 (40%)	—
Diarrhea	5/20 (25%)	—
Insomnia	5/20 (25%)	—
Fever	4/20 (20%)	—
Dizziness	2/20 (10%)	—
Vomiting	3/20 (15%)	—
Abdominal pain	3/20 (15%)	—
Rash	1/20 (5%)	—

[a]Adverse events experienced by the 300 mg bid cohort (n = 20 subjects) in the CNAA2001 trial, a Phase I/II trial to evaluates the effects of multiple dosing of abacavir alone and in combination with zidovudine capsules. Most adverse events were rated mild or moderate. The numbers of subjects listed experienced an event (regardless of association with abacavir) (see text).[37–40] This table does not specifically list the occurrence rate of the abacavir hypersensitivity reaction, which has been estimated at 5% in abacavir-treated subjects.

Abacavir did not demonstrate any evidence of bone marrow suppression, as evidenced by the lack of abnormalities in hematologic parameters during the study that were attributable to abacavir. Additionally, abacavir did not demonstrate any evidence of hepatic, renal, or pancreatic toxicity by biochemical analysis. Most treatment-emergent hematologic and clinical chemistry toxicities were rated as grade 1 or 2. No distinguishing pattern could be detected between the cohorts or treatment arms when clinical chemistry laboratory parameters were examined. The incidence of abnormal laboratory values was generally low, and no dose-related trends were observed. There was no evidence to indicate that abacavir used in combination with zidovudine was associated with an increase in the severity of clinical or laboratory toxicities compared with administration of the study drug alone.[37–40]

Safety in HIV-Infected Infants and Children

The side effects observed among children receiving abacavir are similar to those observed in adults. Hypersensitivity reactions to abacavir have been reported in children and appear at a frequency and with clinical characteristics similar to those observed among adults receiving abacavir.

▲ EFFICACY

Controlled clinical trials have been conducted in several patient populations, including antiretroviral-naive patients, NRTI-experienced or PI-experienced (or both) treatment failures, and people with acquired immunodeficiency syndrome (AIDS) dementia complex. In addition to controlled clinical trials, three broad patient populations have received compassionate use/open-label treatment: adults, children, and people with severe AIDS dementia complex. Findings of several pivotal clinical trials in antiretroviral-naive and antiretroviral-experienced HIV-infected patients are highlighted here.

Studies Conducted in Antiretroviral-Naive HIV-infected Adults

Several Phase I/II controlled clinical studies were conducted to determine the pharmacokinetics, safety, and antiviral activity of abacavir. A parallel, dose-range 12-week study (CNAA2001) has been completed in 79 antiretroviral-naive HIV-infected adults in the United States with limited prior antiretroviral experience (<12 weeks of zidovudine therapy).[37–40] This was the first multiple dosing study in humans. The doses of abacavir studied were 200, 400, and 600 mg tid or 300 mg bid. Patients received open-label abacavir monotherapy for 4 weeks, followed by 8 weeks of zidovudine (600 mg/day) or placebo in addition to abacavir. Abacavir given as monotherapy for 4 weeks resulted in median decreases in plasma HIV RNA of 1.11 to 1.77 $\log_{10}$ copies/ml and median CD4+ T-lymphocyte count increases of 63–111 cells/mm^3 in all groups. At week 12 the median decreases in plasma HIV RNA were 1.02 to 2.24 $\log_{10}$ copies/ml (abacavir monotherapy) and 1.81 to 2.01 $\log_{10}$ copies/ml (abacavir/zidovudine). At week 12 the median CD4+ T-lymphocyte counts increased by 79–195 cells/mm^3 (abacavir monotherapy) and by 93–142 cells/mm^3 (abacavir/zidovudine). The percentage of subjects who had plasma HIV RNA levels at week 12 of less than 400 and of 400 copies/ml were 28% and 11%, respectively (abacavir monotherapy) and 69% and 22%, respectively (abacavir/zidovudine). Eight subjects (10%) discontinued the regimen owing to adverse events; nausea (n = 4) and hypersensitivity (n = 3) were the most common reasons for withdrawal. There were no fatalities. After 12 weeks of abacavir/zidovudine or placebo, 72 of 79 patients were required to interrupt abacavir until essential preclinical studies were completed.

In a preliminary analysis, 43 of 72 subjects elected to restart therapy with abacavir following an interruption of up to 1 year. Six subjects received abacavir uninterrupted. During this extension phase, patients were offered open-label abacavir to use in appropriate combination antiretroviral regimens of abacavir plus either an NNRTI or a PI. The goal of this long-term open-label study was to monitor the long-term antiviral effects of abacavir therapy.[39] Altogether, 16 of 42 subjects had plasma HIV RNA levels of less than 400 copies/ml as extended therapy began. By the 12-week visit, 27 of 38 subjects had levels of less than 400 copies/ml. Of 22 subjects reaching 36 weeks, 16 had viral loads of less than 400 copies/ml. The proportions undetectable at week 24 for NRTI-only combination therapy and abacavir/PI/NRTI were 14 of 18 and 9 of 10, respectively.[39] Over 48 weeks of therapy, more than 50% of patients receiving either nucleoside-only therapy including abacavir (1592U89) or PI-containing therapy with abacavir were maintained below a plasma HIV RNA level of 400 copies per milliliter. Sustained increases in CD4+ T-lymphocyte counts were seen in both abacavir treatment groups while on therapy, with or without PI therapy.

A second randomized, double-blind, dose-ranging clinical trial (CNAB2002) of abacavir 100, 300, and 600 mg bid was conducted in Europe.[41] A total of 60 antiretroviral-naive patients with CD4+ T-lymphocyte counts of 100 cells/mm^3 or more and plasma HIV RNA levels of 30,000 copies/ml or more received up to 24 weeks of abacavir therapy alone; 55 then went into an open-label randomized study of abacavir 300 mg bid plus other antiretrovirals for 72 weeks. At week 24, all subjects who remained on abacavir alone were switched to abacavir 300 mg bid/lamivudine 150 mg bid/zidovudine 300 mg bid or other licensed antiretrovirals as determined by their treating physician. At week 4, greater reductions in plasma HIV RNA were seen in subjects receiving 300 or 600 mg abacavir twice daily (median changes −1.55 and −1.61 $\log_{10}$ copies/ml, respectively) than subjects receiving 100 mg abacavir twice daily (median change −0.63 $\log_{10}$ copies/ml). At 24 weeks, the 300 and 600 mg twice-daily groups had a median change of plasma HIV RNA of −0.70 and −1.30 $\log_{10}$ copies/ml, respectively. During the open-label phase in which zidovudine/ lamivudine was added to 300 mg abacavir twice daily, a further median reduction in plasma HIV RNA of 1.74 $\log_{10}$ copies/ml was seen. At week 48, a median 2.82 $\log_{10}$ copies/ml drop in the plasma HIV RNA level from randomized baseline was seen in pooled data from all abacavir-treated subjects. Sixty-five percent of patients had a plasma viral load of less than 400 copies/ml after 48 weeks of antiretroviral therapy containing abacavir, and 43% of patients had a plasma viral load of less than 50 copies/ml at the same time point. An additional decrease in HIV RNA of 2.16 $\log_{10}$ copies/ml was seen during the open-label phase from the reset open-label combination baseline. Most subjects (46/55, 87%) received abacavir combined with lamivudine 150 mg bid and zidovudine 300 mg bid since their switch to open-label. Overall, this study demonstrated that abacavir 100 mg bid was inferior to 300 mg bid or 600 mg bid, with the latter two doses showing similar viral load reductions. Most subjects (42/47, 90%) at week 72 remained on the triple combination of abacavir/lamivudine/zidovudine, four subjects were receiving PI(s) in addition to the triple combination, and one subject had substituted stavudine for zidovudine. By week 72 the median change in plasma HIV RNA was −2.8 $\log_{10}$ copies/ml. At week 72 about 72% of subjects had a plasma HIV RNA level of less than 400 copies/ml, and 50% of subjects had plasma HIV RNA levels less than 50 copies/ml.[42] The most frequently seen adverse experiences reported by 55 subjects during the long-term, open-label phase of the study were nausea/vomiting in 23 of the 55 (41%), malaise/fatigue in 10 (18%), headache in 9 (16%), muscle pain in 6 (11%), GI discomfort/pain in 7 (12%), sleep disorders in 4 (7%), and skin rashes in 4 (7%). These data included new adverse experiences that began once subjects switched to open-label abacavir, not those who may have been ongoing from the randomized phase.[42]

The CNAA3003 trial investigated the effect of zidovudine and lamivudine with or without abacavir in antiretroviral-naive adults located in the United States, Spain, Belgium, and the UK.[43] This double-blind, randomized phase III study was designed to assess the safety, tolerance, and antiviral activity of abacavir/lamivudine/zidovudine over 16 weeks, as well as the safety, tolerance, and durability of the abacavir/lamivudine/zidovudine response over 48 weeks. Subjects (n = 173 with CD4+ T-lymphocyte counts of 100 cells/mm^3 or more) were randomized 1:1 to receive abacavir 300 mg bid or placebo/lamivudine 150 mg bid/zidovudine 300 mg bid. Subjects were stratified based on plasma HIV RNA at screening: less than 10,000, 10,000 to 100,000, or more than 100,000 copies/ml. Both treatment groups had marked decreases in plasma HIV RNA by week 4, which was sustained in the abacavir/ lamivudine/zidovudine group. At week 16, the proportion of subjects with plasma HIV RNA levels below the limit of detection (less than 400 copies/ml) was significantly better in the abacavir/lamivudine/zidovudine group (75%) than in the lamivudine/zidovudine group (35%) ($P < 0.0001$ analyzed by the Cochran-Mantel-Haenzel test controlling for randomized plasma HIV RNA strata). In addition, the triple combination was effective irrespective of the baseline plasma HIV RNA strata. By contrast, the virologic response to lamivudine/zidovudine began to rebound toward baseline until week 16 when subjects were eligible to add abacavir plus other antiretroviral therapy. The virologic response to lamivudine/zidovudine at week 16 was also diminished at the higher plasma HIV RNA baseline strata. The mean increase in CD4+ T-lymphocyte counts was similar between the treatment groups at 16 weeks. The triple combination was generally well tolerated (3.0% of this group withdrew because of adverse experiences compared to 2.5% of subjects in the lamivudine/zidovudine group).[43]

To investigate the effect of treatment regimens in selected patient populations, a number of clinical trials have been undertaken. A Phase I/II study on the safety and antiviral efficacy of the combination of abacavir plus the PI amprenavir (141W94) was undertaken by the 141W94 International Study Group in HIV-infected patients with 150 to 400 CD4+ T lymphocytes/mm^3.[3,44] The combination was well tolerated and had potent antiviral activity. Five of six patients had decreases in the viral load to below the limits of detection (400 copies/ml). At 4 weeks the change in the viral load was $-1.97\ \log_{10}$ copies/ml from baseline, and the rise in the CD4+ T-lymphocyte count was +79 cells/mm^3 from baseline. In a separate study, 40 HIV-infected subjects were treated with abacavir 300 mg PO bid and amprenavir (1200 mg PO bid) for 72 weeks.[45,46] Subjects in the treatment cohort were antiretroviral-naive subjects with CD4+ T-lymphocyte counts of more than 400 cells/mm^3 and viral loads of more than 5000 copies/ml. Analysis of changes in HIV RNA plasma levels over time showed a rapid (2 to 4 weeks), dramatic decrease in viremia, reaching undetectable levels in 80% of subjects. After 8 weeks the viremia was undetectable. Among the 11 patients who reached 24 weeks of follow-up, plasma viremia was negative in all 11 patients: less than 5 copies/ml (in a boosted Amplicor Roche assay) in 6 of the 11 patients and less than 50 copies/ml in 9. This therapy was also able to restore CD4+ T-lymphocyte counts in blood and lymph nodes.[45]

The CNAA2004 open-label trial evaluated the role of abacavir plus PI therapy in 82 treatment-naive adults over 48 weeks.[47] This was a multicenter, randomized pilot study that evaluated abacavir combined with one of five PIs: indinavir (800 mg q8h), saquinavir soft-gel capsules (1200 mg qh), ritonavir (600 mg q12h), nelfinavir (750 mg q8h), or amprenavir (1200 mg q12h). All treatment arms demonstrated potent, durable antiviral activity. There did not appear to be differences between treatment arms, although the study was not powered to show differences statistically. In an intent-to-treat analysis at week 48, the proportions of subjects in the indinavir, saquinavir, ritonavir, nelfinavir, and amprenavir groups with plasma HIV RNA levels of 400 copies/ml or less were 53%, 50%, 50%, 41%, and 56%, respectively. The proportions with HIV RNA levels of 50 copies/ml or less were 47%, 56%, 50%, 47%, and 44%, respectively. The median CD4+ T-lymphocyte count increases from baseline were 195, 131, 116, 136, and 259 cells/μl, respectively. Increases in the total CD4+ T-lymphocyte number and "naive" CD4+ and CD8+ T lymphocytes were seen, as were increases in circulating B lymphocytes. The frequency of heightened expression of the immune activation markers CD38 and HLA-DR, which are associated with a poorer prognosis for HIV infection, was diminished toward normal levels during therapy.[48,49] More recently, 32-week data were presented for 82 HIV positive antiretroviral therapy-naive adults with CD4+ T-lymphocyte counts of more than 100 cells/mm^3 and plasma HIV RNA levels of 5000 copies/ml or more. Because most patients had achieved plasma HIV RNA levels of less than 400 copies/ml by week 16, samples during weeks 16 to 32 were analyzed using the Roche Ultrasensitive assay (limit of detection less than 50 copies/ml). All five combination treatment regimens reduced plasma HIV RNA levels below 50 copies/ml in approximately 50% to 70% of patients still on randomized treatment at 32 weeks. There were no differences in virologic response among the treatment arms. The combination of abacavir with the PIs examined in this study was safely administered.[50] Taken together, these results suggest that combined abacavir/PI therapy of treatment-naive individuals alleviated the abnormalities that characterize the immune dysfunction of HIV infection.

The CNAF3007/Ecureuil open label study evaluated the efficacy and safety of the triple nucleoside combination combivir/abacavir versus combivir/nelfinavir as first-line therapy in HIV-infected adults.[51] This randomized, open-label study in 195 HIV-infected adults with plasma HIV RNA levels of 1000 to 500,000 copies/ml compared combivir/abacavir to combivir/nelfinavir over 48 study weeks. At the intent-to-treat analysis at 48 weeks, 64% and 61% of subjects had plasma viral loads of less than 50 copies/ml in the combivir/abacavir and combivir/nelfinavir groups, respectively. The baseline viral load was comparable in the two groups with medians of $4.2\ \log_{10}$ copies/ml (combivir/abacavir) and $4.1\ \log_{10}$ copies/ml (combivir/nelfinavir). The median change in plasma viral load from baseline was $-2.3\ \log_{10}$ copies/ml in both groups. The median CD4+ T-lymphocyte count increases were 109 and 120 cells/mm^3 in the combivir/abacavir and combivir/nelfinavir arms, respectively. Possible hypersensitivity reactions to abacavir were reported in four subjects (4%). These results suggest that combivir/abacavir is a generally well tolerated first-line antiretroviral treatment for HIV-infected adults, with antiviral activity comparable to that of a PI-containing regimen over 48 weeks.

The CNA3014 study compared abacavir/combivir to yet another protease-containing regimen, abacavir/indinavir (800 mg q8h), in a 48-week open-label randomized study in 342 HIV-infected antiretroviral therapy-naive adults with CD4+ T-lymphocyte counts of 100 cells/mm^3 or more and plasma HIV RNA levels of more than 5000 copies/ml.[52] Subjects were stratified based on screening plasma HIV RNA: 5000 to 100,000 or more than 100,000 copies/ml. Results demonstrated that time to treatment failure over 48 weeks by intent-to-treat analysis was significantly longer in the abacavir/combivir group than in the indinavir/combivir group ($P < 0.001$). In the primary analysis (intent-to-treat, missing = failure, plasma HIV RNA less than 400 copies/ml), the abacavir/combivir regimen was superior. In the intent-to-treat analysis at week 48 by the baseline plasma HIV RNA stratum, abacavir/combivir was more effective than indinavir/combivir in patients with less than 100,000 copies/ml (70% vs. 49% with plasma HIV RNA less than 400 copies/ml). This difference was not observed in patients with plasma HIV RNA levels of more than 100,000 copies/ml (60% for abacavir/combivir vs. 51% for indinavir/combivir). Sustained increases in CD4+ T-lymphocytes were observed in both treatment groups over 48 weeks. Self-reported adherence to randomized treatment was significantly higher in the abacavir/combivir group: 72% of subjects reported that they took all of their doses or missed an average of less than one dose per week during the last month, compared with 45% of subjects in the indinavir/combivir group ($P < 0.001$). The percentages of drug-related adverse events during the study were 65% (108/165) in the abacavir/combivir group and 87% (142/164) in the indinavir/combivir group. Six percent (10/165) of subjects in the abacavir/combivir group had a possible abacavir hypersensitivity reaction, each of which occurred during the first 6 weeks of therapy.

Studies Conducted in Antiretroviral-Experienced HIV-Infected Adults

An abacavir open-label compassionate-use program evaluated patients with advanced HIV disease with CD4+ T-lymphocyte counts of less than 100 cells/mm^3 and plasma viral loads of 10,000 copies/ml or more. From July 1997 to March 1998, more than 2300 patients were enrolled worldwide. They had been heavily pretreated with antiretroviral drugs at screening: 99% were on NRTI therapy, 97% were on PIs, 46% were on NNRTIs, and 75% had been on treatment for at least 1 year (unpublished data). The program did not specify the regimens selected by investigators, but they included triple therapy with an NRTI and an NNRTI/PI/abacavir (25%). At least 38% of the patients received an abacavir/NNRTI regimen. The range of viral load responses to the therapy chosen was +1.30 to −3.68 $\log_{10}$ copies/ml in 151 patients. Overall, 25% of patients achieved a 0.5 $\log_{10}$ copies/ml or more decline in viral load. The mean change in plasma HIV RNA was −0.29 $\log_{10}$ copies/ml, with a median decline of −0.18 $\log_{10}$ copies/ml. The best response among these patients was seen in those who entered the program on no prior therapy or monotherapy, those who had high viral loads at baseline, and in those who added at least one (and preferably two) agents at enrollment. Interestingly, what did not obviously correlate with the response was the duration of prior therapy (more or less than 1 year), the CD4+ T-lymphocyte count at baseline, or the types of regimens used by category/class of agent. Abacavir is more effective in reducing viral load when the treatment history, disease process, or both are less advanced. Among the patients with advanced disease, 25% may respond to an abacavir-containing regimen, but combination with other new agents in the regimen is key. There were 191 deaths during 1422 person-years of follow-up, yielding a life expectancy of the subjects enrolled in the abacavir expanded access program (7.4 years, 95% CI 6.6, 8.6), which is similar to that of other patients with advanced HIV/AIDS and other observational cohorts.[53]

Several clinical trials have evaluated intensification of therapy by adding abacavir to existing therapy to achieve more virologic suppression. The best results were seen in subjects without extensive prior therapy or drug resistance. The CNA3002 study was a Phase II randomized, double-blind study designed to assess the potential effectiveness of abacavir in antiretroviral-experienced subjects by adding abacavir 300 mg bid to background therapy of subjects with detectable plasma HIV RNA.[54] Investigation of the usefulness of abacavir in patients previously exposed to lamivudine was another study goal. A total of 185 HIV-infected adults on stable background therapy for at least 12 weeks, with CD4+ T-lymphocyte counts of more than 100 cells/mm^3 and plasma HIV RNA of 400 to 50,000 copies/ml, were randomized to receive abacavir or placebo. At week 16, more subjects receiving abacavir plus stable background therapy had plasma HIV RNA levels of less than 400 copies/ml (36/92, 39%) than subjects receiving stable background therapy alone (7/93, 8%) ($P < 0.001$). A similar response was seen in lamivudine-naive versus lamivudine-experienced subjects. Most subjects (73%) with the M184V RT mutation in plasma had a virologic response, as demonstrated by a more than 1.0 $\log_{10}$ copies/ml reduction in plasma HIV RNA or ≤400 copies/ml by week 16. However, in heavily pretreated HIV-infected patients examined in the Swiss HIV Cohort Study, salvage therapy with abacavir/NNRTI/PI resulted in a low virologic success rate.[55] Of 23 HIV-infected patients with four (median) therapy changes before salvage, only 10 patients (43%) achieved a decrease in plasma HIV RNA of more than 0.5 $\log_{10}$ copies/ml after 6 months of therapy. After 6 months, only two subjects had undetectable plasma HIV RNA (less than 500 copies/ml). Only seven patients increased their CD4+ T-lymphocyte counts by more than 30% above baseline, whereas three patients with baseline CD4+ T-lymphocyte counts of less than 100 cells/mm^3 had a more than 30% decline. Almost all of the patients had extensive resistance-conferring mutations at study baseline.

Several studies have looked at the impact of switching treatment to abacavir-containing regimens. The TARGET study was an open-label, multicenter, single-arm clinical trial assessing the 48-week activity of a compact, twice-daily, triple-NRTI regimen containing abacavir/lamivudine in 87 treatment-experienced, PI-naive, HIV-infected adults.[56] These subjects had baseline plasma HIV RNA levels of less than 50,000 copies/ml and CD4+ T-lymphocyte counts of 50 cells/mm^3 or more and had been receiving single or double NRTIs immediately before screening. The median baseline plasma HIV RNA level was 3.10 $\log_{10}$ copies/ml, and the median CD4+ T-lymphocyte count was 506 cells/mm^3. In the intent-to-treat analysis at 48 weeks, the plasma HIV RNA level was less than 400 copies/ml in 45 (82%) of 55 patients and less than 50 copies/ml in 31 (56%) of 55 patients, respectively. Prior zidovudine or lamivudine use, as well as the presence of the M184V RT mutation, did not affect the virologic response. These investigators concluded that enhanced adherence by reducing the number of dosage forms to only four tablets daily translated to improved virologic response in these HIV-infected subjects with high CD4+ T-lymphocyte counts and relatively low plasma HIV RNA levels. Similar results were obtained in 209 patients randomized to receive Trizivir versus continued HAART in the TRIZAL study (AZL30002), with subjects reporting that taking one pill twice daily was easier than for subjects in the continued HAART group ($P < 0.0001$).[57] Other studies have looked at the impact of switching from protease-containing regimens to abacavir-based triple-nucleoside therapy in HIV-infected patients with undetectable plasma HIV RNA. The CNA30017 study concluded that replacement of a PI with abacavir in a triple-combination regimen following prolonged suppression of plasma HIV RNA could afford sustained virologic suppression, significant improvements in lipid abnormalities, and enhanced ease of dosing.[58]

Abacavir in the Treatment of HIV-1 Infected Infants and Children

Abacavir is indicated for the treatment of HIV-infected children, age 3 months to 13 years. The dose is 8 mg/kg up to a maximum of 300 mg bid and should be part of a multiple-drug antiretroviral treatment. Abacavir has been tested in patients in numerous studies including at least two well controlled randomized trials. In one study of children who had previously received nucleoside therapy for HIV infection, abacavir added to lamivudine and zidovudine was more efficacious in reducing plasma HIV RNA than the dual combination alone.[59] In the preliminary analysis of a second study of three double-nucleoside regimens, the abacavir-containing combinations, with or without nelfinavir, resulted in the greatest reduction of viral load for first-time treatment of HIV-infected children.[60]

▲ RESISTANCE

In vitro passage of virus in abacavir does not rapidly select for resistant virus.[61–67] The first RT mutation to arise upon in vitro passage of HIV in the presence of abacavir was M184V; and with further passage mutations K65R, L74V, and Y115F appeared. Although the M184V mutation alone produced only a two- to threefold shift in drug susceptibility, in combination with other mutations it caused increased resistance to abacavir. Alone or in combination, these mutations confer a maximum of about 10-fold reduction in abacavir susceptibility. In contrast, the M184 RT mutation is associated with a 100- to 1000-fold reduction in phenotypic susceptibility to lamivudine associated with the M184V. Abacavir is not cross-resistant with zidovudine in vitro. Some of the abacavir-resistant recombinant viruses were cross-resistant with zalcitabine, didanosine, and stavudine.[64]

The phenotypic abacavir susceptibility of 943 clinical isolates was determined in vitro.[68] These isolates were from subjects many of whom had received prior combined zidovudine/lamivudine. Abacavir susceptibility was categorized into three mutually exclusive groups: (1) susceptible (i.e., less than fourfold increase in IC_{50}); (2) intermediate resistant (i.e., four- to eightfold increase in IC_{50}); and (3) resistant (more than eightfold increase in IC_{50}). Interestingly, 95% of the isolates were susceptible to abacavir if they were resistant only to zidovudine or lamivudine (even if the M184V was present). Most isolates (71%) that are co-resistant to zidovudine and lamivudine remain susceptible to abacavir, although 25% show intermediate susceptibility, and 4% are resistant. If resistance to zidovudine, lamivudine, or zidovudine/lamivudine is associated with other NRTI resistance, the susceptibility to abacavir decreases. The decrease is more profound if resistance to one other NRTI is present. All multi-NRTI-resistant (e.g., lamivudine/zidovudine/all other NRTIs) isolates showed reduced susceptibility to abacavir. For example, if there was evidence of the nucleoside multidrug-resistance mutation at RT codon 151, fewer than 1% of isolates were susceptible to abacavir. It remains to be determined whether reduced abacavir susceptibility results mainly from exposure to lamivudine/zidovudine or it is a more general phenomenon resulting from NRTI regimens.[68] Abacavir resistance may be conferred by the following HIV RT mutations: (1) 41L, 210W, 215Y, and 184V; (2) the 151 multinucleoside drug resistance complex; and (3) codon 69 insertion mutations and ZDV resistance-conferring mutations.[66]

The resistance profile of HIV RT inhibitor abacavir (1592U89) after monotherapy and combination therapy with zidovudine was investigated in the dose-ranging CNA2001 clinical trial, the first trial to examine abacavir resistance in vivo.[61] The study evaluated HIV-infected, drug-naive subjects with 200 to 500 CD4+ T-lymphocytes/mm^3 who received four different dosing regimens of abacavir monotherapy (200 mg tid, 300 mg bid, 400 mg tid, and 600 mg tid for 4 weeks of monotherapy, after which they received 8 weeks of either continued abacavir/zidovudine/placebo or combined abacavir/zidovudine. Of the subjects with detectable HIV that could be polymerase chain reaction (PCR)-amplified for sequence analysis at week 12, mutations occurred at one or more of the codons K65R, L74V, or M184V in 66% of subjects receiving abacavir/placebo and in 17% of subjects receiving abacavir/zidovudine. Overall, mutations at codons K65R, L74V, or M184V were observed after 12 weeks in 51% of subjects assigned to the abacavir monotherapy arms (especially as double mutants) and in 11% of subjects assigned to the combined abacavir/zidovudine arm, mainly as single mutants. Small changes (two- to fourfold) in abacavir susceptibility were detected. With abacavir discontinuation, a wild-type sequence occurred within 4 weeks. In a separate trial in drug-naive subjects (CNA2002 study), 60 subjects were randomized to 100, 300, or 600 mg abacavir twice daily.[62] Mutant viruses were not detected prior to week 12 except in one patient. While on abacavir monotherapy at weeks 6 to 48, a total of 21 of 43 subjects had single, double, and triple combinations of K65R, L74V, Y115F, and M184V. The most common mutation pattern was L74V and M184V (11/24 cases). Altogether, 20 of 21 subjects with isolates containing abacavir-associated mutations reached week 48, yet achieved plasma HIV RNA levels of less than 400 copies/ml upon the addition of lamivudine/zidovudine.

The phenotypic sensitivity to abacavir in the presence of multiple genotypic mutations was correlated with viral load response in the CNAA2003 trial.[63] Abacavir was added to current NRTI therapy (defined as failing therapy with plasma HIV RNA levels of more than 10,000 copies/ml), CD4+ T-lymphocyte count of more than 100 cells/mm^3, and no active CDC class C problems. Patients had previously received stavudine for 6 months or more, didanosine/zidovudine for 6 months or more, zidovudine for 12 months or more, or zidovudine for 12 months or more combined with lamivudine for 6 months or more. A total of 32 patients were enrolled in the study, and 23 of 32 subjects' isolates were analyzed phenotypically and genotypically. Viruses were considered susceptible (i.e., less than fourfold increase in abacavir IC_{50}), intermediate (i.e., four- to eightfold increase in abacavir IC_{50}), or resistant (i.e., more than eightfold increase in abacavir IC_{50}). Based on mean changes in the viral load response from baseline over 12 weeks, patients with abacavir-sensitive and abacavir-intermediate viruses achieved higher peak reductions in viral load (e.g., -1.0 to -2.5 $\log_{10}$ copies/ml at week 2) when compared to patients with abacavir-resistant viruses (i.e., no reductions from baseline). The phenotypic resistance patterns also correlated with the week 4 viral load responses. However, there was a range of viral load responses within each category of abacavir phenotypic susceptibility, such that some individuals with baseline abacavir sensitivity did not achieve subsequent viral load reductions when started on abacavir in vivo. Interestingly, phenotypic resistance to lamivudine or the presence of the M184V RT mutation does not necessarily preclude the virologic activity of abacavir, and patients can still have virologic responses.[63,67,68,70] In general, the presence of high-level phenotypic abacavir resistance or multiple NRTI mutations prior to initiation of therapy in a patient's virus pool predicted a poorer subsequent virologic response than in patients harboring viruses with abacavir sensitivity.[63,67–70]

Lanier et al.[68] determined a "clinically" relevant phenotypic resistance "cutoff" for abacavir using the PhenoSense phenotypic assay with data combined from four GlaxoSmithKline studies: CNA3001, CNA2003, CNA3002, CNA3009.[71] In all of these studies, abacavir was added as a single agent to current therapy. The impact of the baseline abacavir phenotype on virologic response to abacavir addition after 24 weeks was investigated. This study determined that the plasma HIV RNA response was significantly reduced when four or more NRTI mutations were present at baseline. Reductions in susceptibility to abacavir of more than 4.5-fold significantly reduced the virologic response to abacavir. However, there appeared to be a continuum of virologic response with increasing resistance to abacavir, as some subjects whose baseline isolates showed 4.5- to 7.0-fold reductions also responded. If the baseline susceptibility to abacavir was reduced by more than sevenfold, the virologic response was severely affected.

▲ DRUG INTERACTIONS

There are no known significant drug interactions in studies that have been reported to date. The pharmacology of abacavir suggests that the potential for significant drug interactions with commonly prescribed antiretroviral and opportunistic infection medications is limited.

▲ RECOMMENDATIONS FOR USE

Abacavir

The U.S. Food and Drug Administration (FDA) approved the GlaxoSmithKline nucleoside analogue drug abacavir on December 18, 1998 for use in combination anti-HIV regimens for adults and children. The drug is taken twice daily, one 300 mg tablet per dose, with no food or water restrictions. Plasma HIV RNA levels have been documented to fall 1.5 to 2.0 $\log_{10}$ with CD4+ T-lymphocyte count rises of 90 to 145 cells/mm^3 in antiretroviral-naive patients treated with monotherapy for 12 weeks.

Abacavir is generally well tolerated, with the most common side effects being headache, nausea, vomiting, diarrhea, and malaise. The single most important treatment-limiting condition is severe hypersensitivity (allergy), in 3% to 5% of patients. The hypersensitivity syndrome usually occurs during the first month of therapy, with fever being the most common symptom of the syndrome. Nausea, rash, and malaise are also characteristic. When patients are taking multiple drugs, it is difficult to know whether fever, rash, or other manifestations are due to another drug, to abacavir, or to an unrelated process. People who experience increasing nausea, abdominal pain, fever, fatigue, or skin rash within 6 weeks after starting abacavir should contact their doctor immediately. The major decision is whether to stop the abacavir. Symptoms increase in severity if dosing is continued. Moreover, interrupting and restarting after a hypersensitivity reaction may result in a life-threatening return of symptoms within hours. Thus once abacavir is stopped because of manifestations compatible with the syndrome, it should not be restarted.

For clinicians, the proper place of abacavir in the antiretroviral armamentarium is increasingly clear. For initial therapy in antiretroviral-naive patients, a regimen containing abacavir is attractive from the perspective of potency and modest pill burden; whether abacavir-containing regimens are more advantageous than regimens containing other drugs in terms of long-term efficacy, safety, and tolerability remains to be established. When used as part of a triple-nucleoside regimen (e.g., Trizivir in antiretroviral-naive patients), the ability to achieve targeted viral loads of less than 50 copies/ml is reduced among patients with baseline (pretherapy) viral load levels of more 100,000 copies/ml. Therefore, triple-nucleoside regimens are best used in patients with lower (less than 80,000 to 100,000 copies/ml) baseline HIV RNA levels. Abacavir should be considered for salvage therapy, especially for patients who may not have isolates resistant to multiple nucleoside compounds and in subjects with low plasma HIV RNA levels. The hypersensitivity syndrome associated with abacavir requires that patients and physicians be educated in the recognition and management of this event.

Trizivir

On November 14, 2000, the FDA approved the use of Trizivir for treatment of HIV infection in adults and adolescents. Each dose of Trizivir is a fixed-dose combination of Ziagen (abacavir), Retrovir (zidovudine), and Epivir (lamivudine), three NRTIs already approved by the FDA. Trizivir is not recommended for treatment in adults or adolescents who weigh less than 40 kg because it is a fixed-dose tablet. It may be used alone or in combination with other antiretroviral agents for the treatment of HIV infection but should not be administered concomitantly with abacavir, lamivudine, or zidovudine, which are already contained in Trizivir. The recommended dose is one tablet twice daily. The same precautions about abacavir regarding the potential for a hypersensitivity reaction apply to Trizivir (see Recommendations for Use).

REFERENCES

1. Daluge SM, Good SS, Martin MT, et al. 1592U89 Succinate: a novel carbocyclic nucleoside with potent, selective anti-HIV activity. Presented at the 34th Interscience Conference on Antimicrobial Agents and Chemotherapy, 1994, abstract 16.
2. Faletto MB, Miller WH, Garvey EP, et al. Unique intracellular activation of a new anti-HIV agent (1S, 4R)-4-[2-amino-6-(cyclopropylamino)-9H-purin-9-yl]-2-cyclopentene-1-methanol (1592U89) in the human T-lymphoblastoid cell line CEM-T4. Presented at the 34th Interscience Conference on Antimicrobial Agents and Chemotherapy, 1994, abstract 184.
3. Daluge SM, Good SS, Faletto MB, et al. 1592U89 Succinate: a potent, selective anti-HIV carbocyclic nucleoside. Antiviral Res 26:A228, 1995.
4. Faletto MB, Miller WH, Garvey EP, et al. Unique purine crossover pathway for the potent anti-HIV agent 1592U89. Antiviral Res 26:A262, 1995.
5. Daluge SM, Good SS, Faletto MB, et al. 1592 Succinate: a novel carbocyclic nucleoside analog with potent, selective anti-HIV activity. Antimicrob Agents Chemother 41:1082, 1997.
6. Faletto MB, Miller WH, Garvey EP, et al. Unique intracellular activation of the potent antihuman immunodeficiency virus agent 1592U89. Antimicrob Agents Chemother 41:1099, 1997.
7. Tisdale M, Parry NR, Cousens D, et al. Anti-HIV activity of (1S,4R)-4-[2-amino-6-(cyclopropylamino)-9H-purin-9-yl]-2-cyclopentene-1-methanol (1592U89). In: Abstracts of the 34th Interscience Conference on Antimicrobial Agents and Chemotherapy. Washington, DC, American Society for Microbiology, 1994, abstract 182.
8. Bilello JA, Bilello PA, Symonds W, et al. 1592U89, A novel carbocyclic nucleoside analog with potent anti-HIV activity, is synergistic in combination with 141W94, an HIV protease inhibitor. In: Abstracts of the 4th Conference on Retroviruses and Opportunistic Infections, Washington, DC. Alexandria, VA, Westover Management Group, 1997, abstract 154.
9. St Clair MH, Millard J, Rooney J, et al. In vitro antiviral activity of 141W94 (VX-478) in combination with other antiretroviral agents. Antiviral Res 29:53, 1996.
10. Ravitch JR, Jarrett JL, White HR, et al. Central nervous system penetration of the antiretroviral abacavir (1592) in human and animal models. In: Abstracts of the 5th Conference on Retroviruses and Opportunistic Infections, Chicago. Alexandria, VA, Westover Management Group, 1998, abstract 636.
11. Ching SV, Ayers KM, Dornsife RE, et al. Nonclinical toxicology and in vitro toxicity studies with the novel anti-HIV agent (1592U89). In: Abstracts of the 34th Interscience Conference on Antimicrobial Agents and Chemotherapy. Washington, DC, American Society for Microbiology, 1994, abstract 188.
12. Good SS, Owens BS, Faletto MB, et al. Disposition in monkeys and mice of (1S, 4R)-4-[2-amino-6-(cyclopropylamino)-9H-purin-9-yl]-2-cyclopentene-1-methanol (1592U89) succinate, a potent inhibitor of HIV. Presented at the 34th Interscience Conference on Antimicrobial Agents and Chemotherapy, 1994, abstract 186.
13. Good SS, Daluge SM, Ching SV, et al. 1592U89 Succinate: preclinical toxicological and disposition studies and preliminary clinical pharmacokinetics. Antiviral Res 26:A229, 1995.
14. McDowell JA, Chittick GE, Ravitch JR, et al. Pharmacokinetics of [^{14}C]Abacavir, a human immunodeficiency virus type 1 (HIV-1) reverse transcriptase inhibitor, administered in a single oral dose to HIV-1-infected adults: a mass balance study. Antimicrob Agents Chemother 43:2855, 1999.
15. Miller WH, Daluge SM, Garvey EP, et al. Phosphorylation of carbovir enantiomers by cellular enzymes determines the stereoselectivity of antiviral activity. J Biol Chem 267:21220, 1992.
16. Garvey E, Krenitsky TA. A novel human phosphotransferase highly specific for adenosine. Arch Biochem Biophys 296:161, 1992.
17. Parker WB, Shaddix SC, Bowdon BJ, et al. Metabolism of carbovir, a potent inhibitor of human immunodeficiency virus type 1, and its effects on cellular metabolism. Antimicrob Agents Chemother 37:1004, 1993.
18. Bilello JA, Bilello PA, Symonds W, et al. Physiological concentrations of human albumin or α_1-acid glycoprotein do not markedly alter the anti-HIV activity of 1592U89, a novel inhibitor of the HIV-1 reverse transcriptase. In: Abstracts of the 36th Interscience Conference on Antimicrobial Agents and Chemotherapy. Washington, DC, American Society for Microbiology, 1996, abstract 18.
19. McDowell JA, Symonds WT, Kumar PN, et al. Initial phase I study of anti-HIV agent 1592U89: a single-dose escalation design including food effect and dosage form evaluation. In: Abstracts of the 35th Interscience Conference on Antimicrobial Agents and Chemotherapy. Washington, DC, American Society for Microbiology, 1995, abstract 1-109.
20. Ravitch JR, Walsh JS, Reese MJ, et al. In vivo and in vitro studies of the potential for drug interactions involving the antiretroviral abacavir (1592) in humans. In: Abstracts of the 5th Conference on Retroviruses and Opportunistic Infections, Chicago. Alexandria, VA, Westover Management Group, 1998, abstract 634.
21. Kumar PN, Sweet DF, McDowell JA, et al. Safety and pharmacokinetics of abacavir (1592U89) following oral administration of escalating single doses in human immunodeficiency virus type 1-infected adults. Antimicrob Agents Chemother 43:603, 1999.
22. Symonds A, McDowell J, Chittick G, et al. The safety and pharmacokinetics of GW1592U89, zidovudine, and lamivudine alone and in combination after single dose administration in HIV infected patients. AIDS 10(suppl 2):S23, 1996.
23. McDowell JA, Lou Y, Williams SS, et al. Multiple-dose pharmacokinetics and pharmacodynamics of abacavir alone and in combination with zidovudine in human immunodeficiency virus-infected adults. Antimicrob Agents Chemother 44:2061, 2000.
24. Raffi F, Benhantou Y, Sereni D, et al. Pharmacokinetics of, and tolerability to, a single, oral 600 mg dose of abacavir in HIV-positive subjects with or without liver disease (CNAB1006 Study). Presented at the 40th Interscience Conference on Antimicrobial Agents and Chemotherapy, 2000, abstract 1630.
25. Hughes W, McDowell JA, Shenep J, et al. Safety and single-dose pharmacokinetics of abacavir (1592U89) in human immunodeficiency virus type 1-infected children. Antimicrob Agents Chemother 43:609, 1999.
26. Hetherington S, Steel H, Naderer O. Hypersensitivity reactions during therapy with abacavir: clinical presentation and risk factors. In:

Abstracts of the 7th Conference on Retroviruses and Opportunistic Infections, San Francisco, 2000, abstract 60.

27. Cutrell A, Edwards A, Steel H, et al. Risk factor analysis for hypersensitivity reactions to abacavir introduction. In: Abstracts of the 1st IAS Conference on HIV Pathogenesis and Treatment, Buenos Aires, 2001, abstract 527.

27a. Hetherington S, Hughes A, Mosteller M, et al. HLA-B57 and TNF-alpha variants associated with hypersensitivity reactions to abacavir among HIV-1-positive subjects. Presented at the 9th Conference on Retroviruses and Opportunistic Infections, Seattle, 2002, abstract 92.

28. Mallal S, Nolan D, Witt C, et al. Association between presence of HLA-B*5701, HLA-DR7, and HLA-DQ3 and hypersensitivity to HIV-1 reverse-transcriptase inhibitor abacavir. Lancet 359: 727, 2002.

29. Hetherington S. Understanding drug hypersensitivity: what to look for when prescribing abacavir. AIDS Reader 11:620, 2001.

30. Letter to clinicians regarding abacavir hypersensitivity syndrome. Research Triangle Park, NC, Glaxo Wellcome, October 30, 1997.

31. Hetherington S, Steel H, Lafon S, et al. Safety and tolerance of abacavir (1592, ABC) alone and in combination therapy for HIV-1 infection. In: Abstracts of the 12th World AIDS Conference, Geneva, 1998, abstract 12353.

32. Frissen P, de Vries J, Weigel H, et al. Severe anaphylactic shock after rechallenge with abacavir without preceding hypersensitivity. AIDS 15:289, 2001.

33. Escaut L, Lioter JY, Albengres E, et al. Abacavir rechallenge has to be avoided in case of hypersensitivity reaction. AIDS 13:1419, 1999.

34. Keiser P, Andrews C, Yazdani B, et al. Comparison of symptoms of influenza A with abacavir-associated hypersensitivity reaction. In: Abstracts of the 8th Conference on Retroviruses and Opportunistic Infections, Chicago. Alexandria, VA, Westover Management Group, 2001, abstract 622.

35. Thompson M, Shaefer MS, Williams V, et al. Interruptions in abacavir dosing are not associated with increased risk of hypersensitivity in the HEART (NZT4006) study. In: Abstracts of the 40th Interscience Conference on Antimicrobial Agents and Chemotherapy, Toronto, 2000, abstract LB-14.

36. Loeliger AE, Steel H, McGuirk S, et al. The abacavir hypersensitivity reaction and interruptions in therapy. AIDS 15:1325, 2001.

37. Saag MS, Sonnerborg A, Torres RA, et al. Antiretroviral effect and safety of abacavir alone and in combination with zidovudine in HIV-infected adults. AIDS 12:F203, 1998.

38. McDowell JA, Symonds WT, LaFon SW, 1592U89 Clinical Trial Group. Single-dose and steady-state pharmacokinetics of escalating regimens of 1592U89 with and without zidovudine. In: Abstracts of the XIth International Conference on AIDS, Vancouver, 1996, abstract Mo.B.1140.

39. Torres R, Saag M, Lancaster D, et al. Antiviral effects of abacavir (1592) following 48 weeks of therapy. In: Abstracts of the 5th Conference on Retroviruses and Opportunistic Infections, Chicago. Alexandria, VA, Westover Management Group, 1998, abstract 659.

40. Harrigan R, Stone C, Griffin P, et al. Antiretroviral activity and resistance profile of the carbocyclic nucleoside HIV reverse transcriptase inhibitor 1592U89. In: Abstracts of the 4th Conference on Retroviruses and Opportunistic Infections, Washington, DC. Alexandria, VA, Westover Management Group, 1997, abstract 15.

41. Staszewski S, Katlama C, Harrer T, et al. A dose-ranging study to evaluate the safety and efficacy of abacavir alone or in combination with zidovudine and lamivudine in antiretroviral treatment-naive subjects. AIDS 12:F197, 1998.

42. Staszewski S, Katlama C, Harrer T, et al. Abacavir (ABC, 1592) in protocol CNAB 2002 provides effective, long-term, 72 week, art for patients on triple therapy regimens. In: Abstracts of the 12th World AIDS Conference, Geneva, 1988, abstract 12212.

43. Fischl M, Greenberg S, Clumeck N, et al. Safety and activity of abacavir (ABC, 1592) with 3TC/ZDV in antiretroviral naive subjects. In: Abstracts of the 12th World AIDS Conference, Geneva, 1998, abstract 12230.

44. Schooley RT, 141W94 International Study Group. Preliminary data from a phase I/II study on the safety and antiviral efficacy of the combination of 141W94 plus 1592U89 in HIV-infected patients with 150 to 400 CD4+ cells/mm^3. In: Abstracts of the 4th Conference on Retroviruses and Opportunistic Infections, Washington, DC. Alexandria, VA, Westover Management Group, 1997, abstract LB3.

45. Bart P-A, Rizzardi GP, Gallant S, et al. Combination abacavir (1592)/amprenavir (141W94) therapy in HIV-1-infected antiretroviral-naive subjects with CD4+ counts > 400 cells/μl and viral load > 5000 copies/ml. In: Abstracts of the 5th Conference on Retroviruses and Opportunistic Infections, Chicago. Alexandria, VA, Westover Management Group, 1998, abstract 365.

46. Bart P-A, Rizzardi GP, Gallant S, et al. Combination abacavir (1592, ABC)/amprenavir (141W947) therapy in HIV-1 infected antiretroviral naive subjects with CD4+ counts >400 cells/μl and viral load >5000 copies/ml. In: Abstracts of the 12th World AIDS Conference, Geneva, 1998, abstract 12204.

47. McMahon D, Lederman M, Haas DW, et al. Antiretroviral activity and safety of abacavir in combination with selected HIV-1 protease inhibitors in therapy-naive HIV-1-infected adults. Antivir Ther 6:105, 2001.

48. Lederman M, Mellors J, Haas D, et al. Early T-lymphocyte responses to antiretroviral therapy with abacavir (1592, ABC) and HIV protease inhibitors (PI). In: Abstracts of the 5th Conference on Retroviruses and Opportunistic Infections, Chicago. Alexandria, VA, Westover Management Group, 1998, abstract 364.

49. Kelleher D, Lederman M, Mellors J, et al. Early and sustained changes in lymphocyte sub-populations during abacavir (ABC) and PI therapy. In: Abstracts of the 12th World AIDS Conference, Geneva, 1998, abstract 12213.

50. Kelleher D, Mellors JW, Lederman M, et al. Activity of abacavir (1592, ABC) combined with protease inhibitors (PI) in therapy naive subjects. In: Abstracts of the 12th World AIDS Conference, Geneva, 1998, abstract 12210.

51. Matheron S, Brun-Vezinet F, Katlama C, et al. 48-Week results of the CNAF3007/Ecureuil open label study: efficacy and safety of the triple nucleoside combination abacavir/combivir versus nelfinavir/combivir as first line antiretroviral therapy in HIV-infected adult. In: 5th International Congress on Drug Therapy in HIV Infection, Glasgow, 2000, abstract 15.

52. Vibhagool A, Can 3015 International Study Team. Abacavir/combivir (ABC/COM) is comparable to indinavir/combivir (IDV/COM) in HIV-1-infected antiretroviral therapy naïve adults: results of a 48 week open-label study (CNA3014). In: 1st IAS Conference on HIV Pathogenesis and Treatment, Buenos Aires, 2001, abstract 063.

53. Funk ML, White AD, Cutrell A, et al. Life expectancy of patients with advanced HIV/AIDS enrolled in the abacavir expanded access program. In: 40th Interscience Conference on Antimicrobial Agents and Chemotheapy (ICAAC), Toronto, 2002, abstract 2042.

54. Katlama C, Clotet B, Plettenberg A, et al. The role of abacavir (ABC, 1592) in antiretroviral therapy-experienced patients: results from a randomized, double-blind trial. AIDS 14:781, 2000.

55. Khanna N, Klimkait T, Schiffer V, et al. Salvage therapy with abacavir plus a non-nucleoside reverse transcriptase inhibitor and a protease inhibitor in heavily pre-treated HIV-1 infected patients. AIDS 14:791, 2000.

56. Henry K, Wallace RJ, Bellman PC, et al. Twice-daily triple nucleoside intensification treatment with lamivudine-zidovudine plus abacavir sustains suppression of human immunodeficiency virus type 1: results of the TARGET study. J Infect Dis 183:571, 2001.

57. Katlama C, Clumeck N, Fenske S, et al. Use of Trizivir™ (abacavir, lamivudine, zidovudine) to simplify therapy in HAART-experienced subjects with long-term suppression of HIV-RNA: TRIZAL study (AZL30002) 24-week results. In: 8th Conference on Retroviruses and Opportunistic Infections, Chicago, 2001, abstract 316.

58. Clumeck N, Goebel F, Rozenbaum W, et al. Simplification with abacavir-based triple nucleoside therapy versus continued protease inhibitor-based highly active antiretroviral therapy in HIV-1-infected patients with undetectable plasma HIV-1 RNA. AIDS 15:1517, 2001.

59. Saez-Llorens X, Nelson RP, Emmanuel P, et al. A randomized, double-blind study of triple nucleoside therapy of abacavir, lamivudine, and zidovudine versus lamivudine and zidovudine in previously treated human immunodeficiency virus type 1-infected children: the CNAA3006 study team. Pediatrics 107:E4, 2001.

60. Gibb DM, PENTA 5 Executive Committee. A randomized trial evaluating three NRTI regimens with and without nelfinavir in HIV-1 infected children: 48-week follow-up from the PENTA 5 trial. In: 5th International Congress on Drug Therapy in HIV Infection, Glasgow, 2000, abstract PL6.8.

61. Harrigan PR, Stone C, Griffin P, et al. Resistance profile of the human immunodeficiency virus type 1 reverse transcriptase inhibitor

abacavir (1592U89) after monotherapy and combination therapy. J Infect Dis 181:912, 2000.
62. Miller V, Ait-Khaled M, Stone C, et al. HIV-1 reverse transcriptase (RT) genotype and susceptibility to RT inhibitors during abacavir monotherapy and combination therapy. AIDS 14:163, 2000.
63. Lanier ER, Stone C, Griffin P, et al. Phenotypic sensitivity to abacavir (1592, ABC) in the presence of multiple genotypic mutations: correlation with viral load response. In: Abstracts of the 5th Conference on Retroviruses and Opportunistic Infections, Chicago. Alexandria, VA, Westover Management Group, 1998, abstract 686.
64. Tisdale M, Najera I, Cousens D. Analysis of resistant variants isolated on passage with carbocyclic nucleoside analog 1592U89. J Acquir Immune Defic Hum Retrovirol 10(suppl 3):S5, 1995.
65. Harrigan PR, Tisdale M, Najera I, et al. Antiretroviral activity and resistance to 1592U89, a novel HIV RT inhibitor. In: Abstracts of the 5th International Workshop on HIV Drug Resistance, Treatment Strategies, and Eradication, 1997, abstract 16.
66. Tisdale M, Alnadaf T, Cousens D. Combinations of mutations in HIV-1 reverse transcriptase required for resistance to carbocyclic nucleoside 1592U89. Antimicrob Agents Chemother 41:1094, 1997.
67. Lanier R, Danehower S, Daluge S, et al. Genotypic and phenotypic correlates of response to abacavir (ABC, 1592) (abstract 52). Antivir Ther 3(suppl 1):36, 1998.
68. Lanier ER, Smiley ML, St Clair MH, et al. Phenotypic HIV resistance in vitro correlates with viral load response to abacavir (1592, ABC) in vivo. In: Abstracts of the 12th World AIDS Conference, Geneva, 1998, abstract 32289.
69. Mellors JW, Hertogs K, Peeters F, et al. Susceptibility profile (Antivirogram^{TM}) of 943 clinical HIV-1 isolates to abacavir (1592U89). In: Abstracts of the 5th Conference on Retroviruses and Opportunistic Infections, Chicago. Alexandria, VA, Westover Management Group, 1998, abstract 687.
70. Rozenbaum W, Katlama C, Bentata M, et al. Intensification with abacavir (1592, ABC) reduced viral load in lamivudine/zidovudine pretreated subjects with the 184V mutation (abstract 100). Antivir Ther 3(suppl 1):68, 1998.
71. Lanier ER, Hellman N, Scoot J, et al. Determination of a clinically relevant phenotypic resistance "cutoff" for abacavir using the PhenoSense^{TM} assay. In: Abstracts of the 8th Conference on Retroviruses and Opportunistic Infections, Chicago. Alexandria, VA, Westover Management Group, 2001, abstract 254.

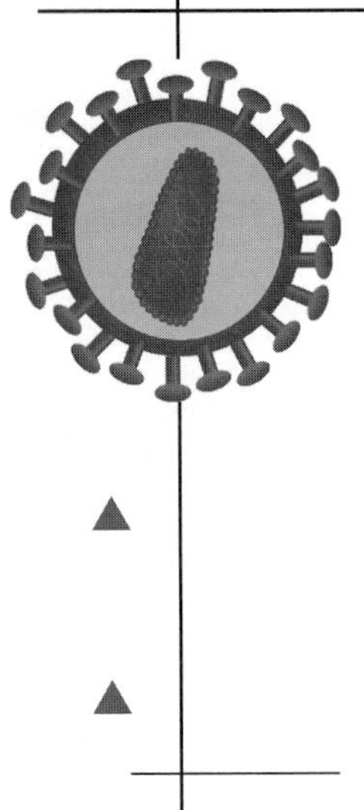

CHAPTER 9

Delavirdine

Lisa M. Demeter, MD
Richard C. Reichman, MD

▲ STRUCTURE

Delavirdine (Rescriptor, previously known as U-90152) (Fig. 9–1) is a member of the bisheteroarylpiperazine (BHAP) class of nonnucleoside reverse transcriptase inhibitors (NNRTIs).[1–3] Delavirdine was the second NNRTI approved by the U.S. Food and Drug Administration (FDA) for use in combination therapy for human immunodeficiency virus type 1 (HIV-1) infection.

▲ MECHANISMS OF ACTION AND IN VITRO ACTIVITY

Delavirdine and other NNRTIs selectively inhibit HIV-1 replication, displaying no significant activity against HIV-2, other retroviruses, or human DNA polymerases. Unlike nucleoside analogues, delavirdine and other NNRTIs do not require intracellular phosphorylation for activation.

Structural analyses of HIV-1 reverse transcriptase (RT) indicate that NNRTIs inhibit RT by binding to a hydrophobic pocket in the p66 subunit of HIV-1 RT near the catalytic site of the enzyme.[4–6] This process is thought to result in a switch to an inactive, stable form of the polymerase active site. In this inactive conformation, the catalytic aspartyl residues of RT are displaced relative to the nucleic acid binding groove of the enzyme. It is also thought that NNRTIs restrict the flexibility of some p66 subunit domains. Kinetic analyses have demonstrated that NNRTIs induce nonproductive binding of the nucleotide substrate to the enzyme but do not prevent nucleotide binding to RT or the subsequent nucleotide-induced conformational change in RT.[7]

The delavirdine molecule is larger than other NNRTIs, such as nevirapine and efavirenz. X-ray crystallographic analyses of delavirdine bound to HIV-1 RT indicate that delavirdine binds to the same hydrophobic pocket in the p66 subunit of RT as nevirapine, but that the enzyme–inhibitor complex is stabilized differently.[8] Because of its large size, delavirdine extends beyond the usual NNRTI binding pocket and projects into the solvent.[8] Delavirdine interacts with residues Tyr-188, Trp-229, Tyr-181, and Val-106, similar to other NNRTIs. In addition, delavirdine forms hydrogen bonds with Lys-103 and has strong hydrophobic interactions with Pro-236; these unique interactions stabilize the RT–delavirdine complex.[8] Binding by delavirdine appears to induce a distortion in the polymerase active site similar to that induced by other NNRTIs, suggesting that the specific binding characteristics of delavirdine do not substantially affect the mechanism of RT inhibition by this drug.

In vitro the concentrations of delavirdine required to inhibit cellular polymerases are at least 1000-fold higher than those required to inhibit HIV-1 RT.[2] The average median inhibitory concentration of delavirdine against a panel of laboratory and clinical HIV-1 isolates was 0.066μM (range <0.005 to 0.690 μM).[2] Delavirdine is also active against HIV-1 isolates resistant to zidovudine or didanosine. Delavirdine was more effective than zidovudine in preventing spread of HIV-1 from infected to uninfected lymphocytes, completely inhibiting viral spread in vitro at a concentration of 3 μM.[2]

In vitro delavirdine is synergistic in two-drug combinations with zidovudine, didanosine, dideoxycytidine, the protease inhibitor U-75875, and interferon-α.[9–11] Biochemical studies of the combination of delavirdine and nevirapine suggest that these drugs are antagonistic with respect to RT inhibition.[12]

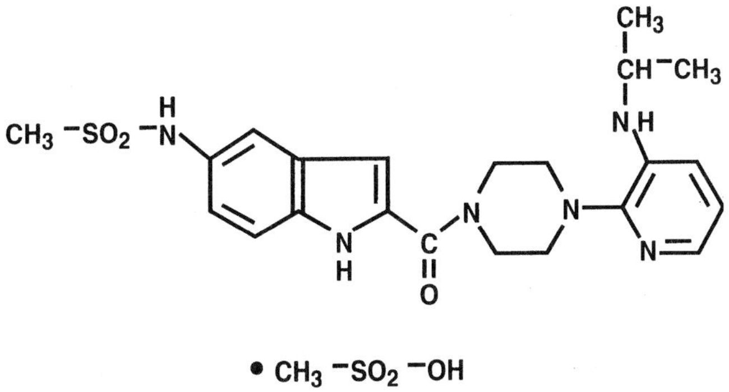

Figure 9–1. Structure of delavirdine.

▲ PHARMACOKINETICS

Delavirdine is rapidly absorbed after oral administration; most soluble at a pH of less than 2, its absorption is reduced by gastric hypoacidity.[13] Administration of orange juice in HIV-infected patients who have documented gastric hypoacidity reduces gastric pH and increases delavirdine absorption.[14] Nevertheless, delavirdine levels in these patients remain lower than in subjects without gastric hypoacidity.[14] Results of a single-dose study evaluating the bioavailability of delavirdine in healthy adults indicated that administration of a high-fat meal decreased the mean peak delavirdine plasma concentrations by 60% and the mean area under the concentration–time curve (AUC) by 26% compared to administration after fasting.[15] In the same study, administration of an antacid reduced the peak level by 48% and the AUC by 57%.[15] These results must be interpreted with caution, however, as the steady-state pharmacokinetics of delavirdine are nonlinear, leading to substantial prolongation of the apparent delavirdine half-life with increasing delavirdine doses.[16] Because of the nonlinearity of delavirdine pharmacokinetics, single-dose kinetic studies cannot always accurately predict steady-state concentrations of the drug. Thus when multiple doses of delavirdine were administered to HIV-infected subjects with meals, there was no difference in the AUC or the plasma trough levels of delavirdine compared to those achieved with drug regimens in which delavirdine was administered 1 hour before or 2 hours after meals.[17]

Delavirdine is bound extensively to plasma proteins, primarily albumin.[16,18] In most patients a delavirdine trough blood level of more than 10 μM can be easily achieved, which is approximately 100-fold higher than the delavirdine 90% inhibitory concentration (IC_{90}) of most clinical HIV isolates from NNRTI-naive patients.[15] There is a relatively large intersubject variability in steady-state delavirdine levels, presumably related to differences among patients in CYP3A activity. However, the intrasubject variability of steady-state delavirdine levels is low.

Delavirdine is metabolized by various pathways, producing several inactive metabolites. The major metabolic pathway of delavirdine is *N*-dealkylation, which is mediated by cytochrome P_{450} 3A (CYP3A). Studies in HIV-infected volunteers suggest that the metabolic pathway for *N*-dealkylation is saturable.[16] Delavirdine inhibits CYP3A activity, thereby inhibiting its own metabolism.[16] The maximum inhibitory effect of delavirdine on CYP3A activity has been seen at a plasma concentration of 5 μM or higher, which is exceeded by currently recommended dosing regimens.[16] Delavirdine is excreted primarily as dealkyl delavirdine and pyridine-cleaved delavirdine in both urine and feces.[13] In one study less than 5% of the drug was recovered unchanged in the urine.[13]

▲ DRUG INTERACTIONS

Interactions with Drugs Metabolized by Cytochrome P_{450}

Interactions with Drugs Other than Antiretrovirals

Because delavirdine is metabolized by the P_{450} system and inhibits CYP3A, its interactions with other drugs that are metabolized by similar mechanisms are complex and often difficult to predict. A list of observed and predicted interactions of delavirdine with other drugs is provided in Table 9–1. Rifampin increased the oral clearance of delavirdine approximately 27-fold, leading to negligible concentrations of delavirdine in all seven HIV-infected patients who received delavirdine 400 mg tid and rifampin, 600 mg qd.[19] Co-administration of delavirdine and rifampin is therefore not recommended.

Rifabutin increased oral clearance of delavirdine approximately fivefold, resulting in lower steady-state plasma delavirdine concentrations.[20] Delavirdine doses in excess of 600 mg tid were able to overcome this interaction and resulted in the same mean delavirdine exposure as a 400-mg tid dose of delavirdine given without rifabutin.[21] In addition, delavirdine was shown to inhibit rifabutin clearance and produced a more than 200% increase in rifabutin exposure.[21]

Clarithromycin is an inhibitor of CYP3A4 and was therefore predicted to have an effect on delavirdine metabolism. In a pharmacokinetic study of HIV-infected patients receiving clarithromycin, there were increases in delavirdine peak and trough concentrations, but these changes were not statistically different from concentrations seen when delavirdine was administered without clarithromycin.[22] Co-administration of delavirdine resulted in increased levels of clarithromycin and decreased levels of its 14-hydroxy metabolite, which has activity. However, the overall change in total levels of clarithromycin and its active metabolite were not significantly altered.[22]

Anticonvulsants such as phenobarbital, phenytoin, and carbamazepine induce CYP3A4 and therefore could potentially increase the metabolism of delavirdine. Limited unpublished data indicate that trough plasma delavirdine concentrations are reduced by concomitant administration of these agents.[13] Co-administration of delavirdine with these anticonvulsants is therefore not recommended.

▲ **Table 9–1.** IMPORTANT DRUG INTERACTIONS WITH
▲ DELAVIRDINE

Type of Interaction with Delavirdine
Inhibition of delavirdine absorption
Didanosine
Antacids
Acceleration of delavirdine metabolism
Carbamazepine
Phenobarbital
Phenytoin
Rifampin
Rifabutin
Inhibition of metabolism by delavirdine
Indinavir
Saquinavir
Nelfinavir
Lopinavir
Ritonavir
Amprenavir
Terfenadine
Astemizole
Clarithromycin
Dapsone
Rifabutin
Ergot derivatives
Alprazolam
Midazolam
Triazolam
Dihydropyridines (e.g., nifedipine)
Cisapride
Quinidine
Warfarin
Sildenafil

Interactions with Antiretroviral Drugs

Delavirdine has important interactions with currently available protease inhibitors, which are metabolized primarily by CYP3A4. The protease inhibitors also inhibit CYP3A4 to different extents, with ritonavir being the strongest inhibitor and saquinavir the weakest.[23,24] Both ritonavir and nelfinavir can induce some cytochrome P_{450} and glucuronosyl transferase enzymes and so reduce the levels of drugs metabolized by these pathways.[13] Thus the interactions of protease inhibitors with delavirdine are not always predictable. One potential advantage of delavirdine's interactions with protease inhibitors is that it may increase the levels of these drugs, allowing reduced dosing or increased regimen potency. This characteristic of delavirdine contrasts with those of efavirenz and nevirapine, both of which are inducers of cytochrome P_{450}.[13]

Neither saquinavir, ritonavir, nor indinavir appears to have a significant effect on delavirdine levels. In contrast, delavirdine, at a dose of 400 mg PO tid, significantly increased trough levels and AUC, but not the peak concentrations, of indinavir.[25–27] The recommended dose of indinavir when given in combination with delavirdine is 600 mg PO tid, instead of 800 mg PO tid. Theoretical modeling suggests that co-administration of delavirdine and indinavir may allow each to be given in twice-daily dosing regimens.[26] In HIV-infected patients receiving stable doses of ritonavir (600 mg bid) and two nucleoside inhibitors, addition of delavirdine 400 mg PO tid, increased the trough concentration and AUC of ritonavir by 84% and 60%, respectively.[28] Delavirdine increased the AUC of nelfinavir approximately twofold in healthy volunteers, whereas nelfinavir decreased the AUC of delavirdine approximately 40%.[29] Amprenavir inhibits CYP3A4 to a similar extent as indinavir and nelfinavir.[30] The optimal dose of amprenavir in combination with delavirdine has not yet been determined, but single-dose pharmacokinetic studies suggest that the dose of amprenavir should be reduced when given in combination with delavirdine.[13] Studies of delavirdine and saquinavir suggest that a twice-daily regimen, and a lower daily dose of saquinavir can be used.[13,32,33] The effects of delavirdine on the metabolism of the fixed dose of lopinavir/ritonavir have not been formally studied; although based on the fact that lopinavir is extensively metabolized by CYP3A4, one would expect that delavirdine would increase the levels of lopinavir and possibly ritonavir.

Other Drug Interactions

Significant pharmacokinetic interactions between delavirdine and zidovudine have not been observed. In a single-dose pharmacokinetic study of 12 HIV-infected patients, concurrent administration of delavirdine and didanosine resulted in reduced drug levels of each antiretroviral agent, although the extent of *N*-dealkylation of delavirdine was not affected. These effects were not seen when delavirdine was administered 1 hour before didanosine and presumably reflect inhibition of delavirdine absorption by the buffering agents in the didanosine formulation. The mechanism by which delavirdine lowers didanosine levels is not known.[34] A multiple-dose pharmacokinetic study of delavirdine and didanosine in nine HIV-infected individuals confirmed that, under steady-state conditions, the AUCs of both drugs were reduced approximately 20% when the drugs were administered simultaneously rather than 1 hour apart.[13]

▲ TOXICITY

Delavirdine was administered to more than 3500 patients before FDA approval was given in April 1997. The drug has been well tolerated, with the most frequent side effect of delavirdine being a maculopapular rash (Table 9–2). The National Institutes of Health (NIH)-sponsored AIDS Clinical Trials Group (ACTG) conducted a Phase I/II study of delavirdine monotherapy versus nucleoside monotherapy (ACTG 260).[35] Delavirdine doses in this study was adjusted to achieve one of three targeted trough concentration ranges (see discussion under Efficacy in Clinical Trials for a more detailed summary of the study design of ACTG 260). Approximately 36% of delavirdine recipients developed a rash, compared to none of the nucleoside-treated subjects.[35] The rash occurred a median of 10 days after initiating therapy. Altogether, 23 sub-

▲ **Table 9–2.** TOXICITIES ASSOCIATED WITH DELAVIRDINE

Toxicity	Frequency	Comments
Rash	18–36%	Rare after first month of therapy May be more common with higher delavirdine trough levels[35] Severe rash necessitating discontinuation of drug is uncommon (5–10%)
Hepatic enzyme elevations	Uncommon	4/30 Subjects receiving delavirdine + saquinavir had reversible increases in alanine transaminase and aspartate transaminase[25]
Neutropenia	Uncommon	Observed in 4/24 subjects receiving delavirdine + nelfinavir[29]

jects with less severe rashes (defined as the absence of fever, blistering, or mucosal lesions) were able to continue therapy uninterrupted or were successfully rechallenged. There was an association in ACTG 260 between the delavirdine trough level at week 1 and the subsequent risk of developing a rash. A rash attributable to delavirdine occurred in 18% of recipients receiving delavirdine 400 mg PO tid in Phase II and III controlled trials.[36] In studies M/0017 and M/0021, 42% to 50% of subjects developed a rash, compared with 24% to 32% of those receiving zidovudine or didanosine monotherapy.[36] In these studies 4.3% of patients discontinued delavirdine as a result of the rash.

The rash characteristically occurs within 1 to 3 weeks after initiation of therapy and often resolves despite continuating the drug.[35–37] The rash, which is uncommon after a month of therapy unless a prolonged interruption of treatment has intervened, is erythematous, maculopapular, and often pruritic, involving the upper body and proximal arms, with decreasing intensity on the neck, face, trunk, and limbs.[36] It can be managed successfully in more than 90% of patients. Serious delavirdine-related skin rashes, such as erythema multiforme and Stevens-Johnson syndrome, are rare (approximately 0.4%) and usually resolve after discontinuing the drug.

Occasionally, elevations of liver enzymes are seen in delavirdine recipients, most often in those who received other antiretroviral agents (Table 9–2). Significant but reversible elevations in alanine transaminase and aspartate transaminase occurred in 4 of 30 subjects during treatment with the combination of saquinavir and delavirdine.[25] Frank hepatitis has been rare.

In a study of 24 HIV-infected subjects receiving the combination of nelfinavir and delavirdine, 4 patients discontinued the study drugs because of neutropenia.[29] In these patients, neutropenia resolved within a few days of discontinuing both drugs (Table 9–2).

▲ EFFICACY IN CLINICAL TRIALS

The efficacy of delavirdine was evaluated initially in studies in which the drug was administered as monotherapy or in two- or three-drug combinations with zidovudine or didanosine (or both). Early studies of delavirdine in combination with zidovudine or didanosine (or both) did not demonstrate consistent, clinically significant virologic benefit from inclusion of delavirdine in these regimens. More recent data of the efficacy of delavirdine, when given in combination with zidovudine/lamivudine to subjects with limited nucleoside experience, or in combination with protease inhibitors as part of a salvage regimen for those with more extensive antiretroviral experience, have demonstrated that delavirdine can offer significant virologic and immunologic benefits. A summary of the major efficacy trials of delavirdine is provided in Table 9–3.

The ACTG 260 trial studied the efficacy and tolerability of delavirdine monotherapy.[35] Approximately one-half of the 113 subjects analyzed had no prior antiretroviral therapy; zidovudine-experienced subjects had a median duration of use of 21 months. Subjects were randomized to one of three delavirdine doses or nucleoside monotherapy; antiretroviral-naive patients randomized to the latter arm received zidovudine, and zidovudine-experienced patients received didanosine. Because of the intersubject variability of delavirdine pharmacokinetics that had been observed in earlier trials, ACTG 260 had a concentration-targeted design in which doses of delavirdine were chosen to achieve one of three delavirdine trough ranges: 3 to 10 μM, 11 to 30 μM, or 13 to 50 μM. No significant differences in the early plasma RNA responses of the three delavirdine arms were observed at week 2. The apparent lack of a dose response may have been due to the inability to achieve target trough delavirdine concentrations in approximately half of the subjects in the highest target trough concentration arm. The decline in mean plasma RNA in the three pooled delavirdine arms at week 2 was approximately 1.0 $\log_{10}$ copies/ml, which was significantly greater than the 0.67 $\log_{10}$ copies/ml decline in the nucleoside monotherapy arm. However, the effect of delavirdine monotherapy was short-lived, and a rapid rebound in plasma RNA levels was observed, with a return to near-baseline levels by week 8.[26] In the pooled delavirdine arms there was a transient median increase in CD4+ T-lymphocyte count of 25 cells/mm^3 at week 2, which declined to below baseline by week 8. The nucleoside arm demonstrated a median increase of 40 CD4+ T-lymphocyte cells/mm^3 at week 2 and remained above baseline at week 8. Although no differences in virologic response were seen among the three delavirdine arms, higher delavirdine levels at week 2 were associated with a significantly greater decline in plasma HIV RNA at week 2 independent of the treatment arm.[35]

An early Phase I/II study suggested that the three-drug combination of delavirdine/zidovudine/didanosine produced more sustained CD4+ T lymphocyte and plasma HIV RNA responses than the two-drug combination of didanosine/zidovudine.[37] This issue was further evaluated in ACTG 261,

Table 9–3. SUMMARY OF MAJOR EFFICACY TRIALS EVALUATING DELAVIRDINE

Clinical Trial	Phase	Entry Criteria[a]	Prior Antiretroviral Experience	Delavirdine Dose	Treatment Arms	Outcome
Para et al.[35] (ACTG 260)	I/II	CD4 200–500	<6 Months zidovudine experience; at least 50% naive	Dose chosen to achieve one of three DLV trough levels: 3–10 μM, 11–30 μM, or 31–50 μM	3–10 μM, 11–30 μM, or 31–50 μM DLV vs. ZDV or ddI	Mean decline in plasma RNA at week 2 in DLV arms was 1.0 $\log_{10}$ (no significant difference among DLV arms) vs. 0.67 $\log_{10}$ decline in nucleoside arm. Study stopped because RNA responses in DLV arms were not sustained beyond 8 weeks of therapy.
Friedland et al.[38] (ACTG 261)	II	CD4 100–500	<6 Months nucleoside experience	400 mg tid	DLV + ZDV vs. DLV + ddI vs. DLV + ZDV + ddI	There was a trend in CD4 and plasma RNA responses favoring the triple therapy arm over the ZDV/ddI arm that did not achieve statistical significance. Responses in the DLV/ZDV and DLV/ddI arms were inferior to triple therapy and ZDV/ddI arms.
Freimuth et al.[39] (M/0017)	II/III	CD4 < 300	ZDV experience (average 1 year; <4 months of ddI)	400 mg tid	DLV/ddI vs. ddI	Early RNA and CD4 response were greater in DLV/ddI arm, but these differences were not sustained. Study stopped by DSMB because of low likelihood that a significant difference in clinical outcome between the two arms would be detected.
Freimuth et al.[40] (M/0021 Part I)	II/III	CD4 200–500	<6 Months	200 mg tid 300 mg tid 400 mg tid	ZDV vs. ZDV/DLV (200 mg tid) vs. ZDV/DLV (300 mg tid) vs. ZDV/DLV (400 mg tid)	RNA and CD4 response superior in two higher DLV dose groups. Study stopped when data demonstrating inferiority of ZDV monotherapy became avaiable.
Sargent et al.[41] and Wathen et al.[42] (M/0021 Part II)	II/III	CD4 200–500	<6 Months	400 mg tid	ZDV/3TC vs. DLV/ZDV vs. DLV/3TC/ZDV	Interim analysis showed greatest RNA and CD4 responses in the triple-therapy arm; 71% of triple-therapy arm had <400 copies/ml RNA at 24 weeks vs.29% in ZDV/3TC arm. Study closed by DSMB; final analysis pending.

Kuritzkes et al.[43]	II	CD4 >200 HIV RNA >500	3TC/ZDV, d4T, or ddI for ≥6 months	400 mg tid	ZDV/3TC/IDV (800 mg tid) vs. ADV/DLV/IDV (600 mg tid)	73% of DLV and 58% of 3TC arms were suppressed to ≤200 copies/ml at 24 weeks ($P = 0.29$). 83% of DLV vs. 48% of 3TC arms were suppressed at 48 weeks ($P = 0.007$).
Eron et al.[44] (M/0074)	II	CD4 ≥ 50 HIV RNA >20,000	ZDV for <1 month; naive to 3TC, NNRTIs, PIs	400 mg tid	DLV/ZDV/IDV (600 mg tid) vs. DLV/3TC/IDV (600 mg tid) vs. DLV//ZDV/3TC/IDV (600 mg tid) vs. ZDV/3TC/IDV (800 mg tid)	ITT: 43% vs. 69% vs. 44% vs. 60%, respectively, were <400 copies/ml at 48 weeks. On-treatment analyses showed 43% vs. 97% vs. 87.5% vs. 82% were <400 copies/ml at 48 weeks.
Gulick et al.[45] (ACTG 359)	II	Any CD4 HIV RNA 2000–200,000	IDV for >6 months	600 mg bid	SQV/RTV/DLV vs. SQV/RTV/ADV vs. SQV/RTV/DLV/ADV vs. SQV/NFV/DLV vs. SQV/NFV/ADV vs. SQV/NFV/DLV/ADV	At 16 weeks, no significant differences between pooled RTV vs. NFV (28% vs. 33% with RNA < 500, $P = 0.50$) or DLV vs. DLV/ADV groups (40% vs. 33%, $P = 0.42$). Pooled DLV groups had a greater response rate than ADV groups (40% vs. 18%, $P = 0.002$).

ADV, adefovir; ddI, didanosine; DLV, delavirdine DSMB, Data and Safety Monitoring Board; IDV, indinavir; ITT, intent-to-treat analysis; NFV, nelfinavir; NNRTIs, nonnucleoside reverse transcriptase inhibitors; PIs, protease inhibitors; SQV, saquinavir; 3TC, lamivudine; ZDV, zidovudine.

[a]CD4+ T-lymphocytes/mm^3; HIV RNA copies/ml.

a Phase II randomized, double-blind, placebo-controlled trial that directly compared the safety and efficacy of four antiretroviral regimens: delavirdine/zidovudine, delavirdine/didanosine, delavirdine/zidovudine/didanosine, and zidovudine/didanosine.[38] A fixed delavirdine dose of 400 mg PO tid was used in this study. A total of 549 subjects with CD4+ T-lymphocyte counts of 100 to 500/mm^3 and less than 6 months of prior nucleoside monotherapy were randomized. Of the 544 evaluable subjects, 63% were treatment-naive, 36% were zidovudine-experienced (median duration 2 months), and 1% were didanosine-experienced (median duration 2 months). The plasma HIV RNA concentration was analyzed in a subset of 247 subjects.[38] In the delavirdine/zidovudine/didanosine arm, the change in plasma HIV-1 RNA was -1.13 $\log_{10}$ and -0.73 $\log_{10}$ copies/ml at weeks 4 to 12 and weeks 40 to 48, respectively. CD4+ T-lymphocyte counts responses in that arm were $+49$ and $+65$ cells/mm^3 at weeks 4 to 12 and 40 to 48, respectively. The differences in plasma RNA and CD4+ T-lymphocyte responses between the delavirdine/zidovudine/didanosine and didanosine/zidovudine arms were not statistically significant, although there was a trend favoring the three-drug arm.[38] A major limitation of this study was the high premature discontinuation rate of the study drugs (36% of all subjects), a factor that may have reduced the power to detect a difference between the three-drug and dual nucleoside regimens.

Protocols M/0017 and M/0021 were two Phase II/III clinical trials sponsored by Pharmacia Upjohn, the pharmaceutical company that initially developed delavirdine. Protocol M/0017 was a Phase II/III clinical trial comparing didanosine monotherapy with didanosine/delavirdine (400 mg PO tid) in subjects with 300 CD4+ T-lymphocyte cells/mm^3 or less and a history of nucleoside experience.[39] About one-fourth of study participants had a maximum of 4 months of prior didanosine therapy, and approximately 595 patients were randomized to each treatment group. The delavirdine/didanosine group showed a statistically significant improvement in plasma HIV RNA and CD4+ T-lymphocyte counts responses compared with the didanosine monotherapy arm. However, these differences were not sustained, and the trial was terminated by the Data and Safety Monitoring Board (DSMB) because of the unlikelihood that a significant difference in clinical outcome between the two groups would be detected.

Protocol M/0021 was a randomized, double-blind Phase II/III study of HIV-infected subjects with less than 6 months of prior zidovudine therapy and CD4+ T-lymphocyte counts of 200 to 500/mm^3. According to the original protocol (M/0021 Part I), 718 subjects with a median CD4+ T-lymphocyte count of 334/mm^3 and mean baseline RNA of 5.25 $\log_{10}$ copies/ml were randomized to receive zidovudine monotherapy or zidovudine/delavirdine (200, 300, or 400 mg PO tid).[40] Subjects who received zidovudine in combination with delavirdine at either of the two highest doses experienced reductions in plasma HIV RNA of 0.5 $\log_{10}$ copies/ml or more and increases in CD4+ T-lymphocyte count of 20 to 30/mm^3 for more than 1 year. These responses in the delavirdine/zidovudine arm were significantly greater than those in the zidovudine monotherapy arm.[40]

Because of this preliminary analysis as well as data from ACTG 175[46] and the Delta trial[47] that demonstrated the inferiority of zidovudine monotherapy when compared with dual nucleoside combination regimens, M/0021 was revised to eliminate the zidovudine monotherapy arm and to increase the delavirdine dose to 400 mg tid for all delavirdine recipients (M/0021 Part II)[41,42,48] Subjects with CD4+ T-lymphocyte counts of 200 to 500/mm^3 and less than 6 months of zidovudine experience who were not in Part I were initially randomized during Part II of the study to receive delavirdine/zidovudine, lamivudine/zidovudine, or delavirdine/lamivudine/zidovudine.

Interim analysis of M/0021 (Part II) in January 1998 showed that subjects receiving the three-drug combination of delavirdin/zidovudine/lamivudine had significantly greater declines in plasma HIV RNA concentrations than subjects in the zidovudine/lamivudine dual therapy arm beginning at 8 weeks of therapy. In the three-drug delavirdine/zidovudine/lamivudine arm, plasma HIV RNA levels were less than 400 copies/ml in 71% of patients at 24 weeks compared to 29% in the zidovudine/lamivudine arm.[41] Based on the interim analysis, the DSMB recommended closing the study to further enrollment. These results suggest that delavirdine, when given in combination with zidovudine/lamivudine can result in virologic suppression rates that approach those seen in combination antiretroviral regimens with protease inhibitors or other NNRTIs. The reasons for the differences in efficacy when delavirdine was given in combination with zidovudine/lamivudine in M/0021 versus zidovudine/didanosine in ACTG 261 are not fully understood but may relate in part to poor tolerance to the regimen in the latter study.

More recent studies have evaluated the efficacy of delavirdine using combination antiretroviral regimens designed to exploit the pharmacokinetic interactions between this drug and other antiretroviral agents metabolized by cytochrome P_{450}. ACTG 370 was a randomized, open-label, multicenter study in which subjects with plasma HIV-1 RNA level of more than 500 copies/ml who had previously received stavudine (d4T)/lamivudine (3TC) or didanosine (ddI)/3TC were randomized to receive zidovudine/3TC/indinavir (800 mg q8h) or zidovudine/delavirdine/indinavir (600 mg q8h).[43] There were no statistically significant differences between the delavirdine and 3TC arms in the proportion of subjects with 200 copies/ml or less at week 24 (73% vs. 58%, respectively, $P = 0.29$). However, there was more viral load suppression in the delavirdine arm at week 48 (83% vs. 48%, $P = 0.007$). Steady-state plasma indinavir levels were twofold higher in the delavirdine arm subjects than in those randomized to the 3TC-containing regimen, suggesting that pharmacokinetic interactions contributed to the greater benefit seen in the delavirdine arm. Although the control arm in this study does not reflect current clinical practice, this study does demonstrate that a relatively high frequency of virologic suppression can be achieved when using the zidovudine/delavirdine/indinavir combination in nucleoside-experienced patients.

Protocol M/0074 was an open-label study evaluating the efficacy of a regimen containing delavirdine in combination with a reduced indinavir dose (600 mg tid).[44] Altogether, 225 patients with less than 1 month of zidovudine experience, CD4+ T-lymphocyte counts of 50 cells/mm^3 or less, and a plasma HIV-1 RNA level higher than 20,000 copies/ml were randomized to receive: (1) delavirdine/lamivudine/indinavir, (2) delavirdine/zidovudine/indinavir, (3) delavirdine/zidovudine/ lamivudine/indinavir, or (4) zidovudine/lamivudine/indinavir (800 mg tid) (control arm). The mean baseline plasma HIV-1 RNA was 4.98 $\log_{10}$ copies/ml, and the CD4+ T-lymphocyte count was 276 cells/mm^3. On-treatment analyses at 24 weeks showed that approximately 97% of subjects in the delavirdine/lamivudine/indinavir arm maintained plasma HIV-1 RNA concentrations below 400 copies/ml compared to approximately 83% in the delavirdine/zidovudine/indinavir arm, 87% in the delavirdine/zidovudine/lamivudine/indinavir arm, and 82% in the zidovudine/lamivudine/indinavir control arm. Intent-to-treat analyses showed virologic suppression rates of 69%, 43%, 44%, and 60%, respectively, in these treatment arms. The delavirdine/lamivudine/indinavir and zidovudine/lamivudine/indinavir regimens were the best tolerated in this study.

ACTG 359 was a prospective, randomized, 2 × 3 factorial, partially placebo-controlled study in NNRTI-naive subjects who had had more than 6 months of prior treatment with indinavir and a plasma HIV-1 RNA level of 2000 to 200,000 copies/ml.[48] Subjects were randomized to receive: (1) saquinavir soft-gel formulation (saquinavir$_{sgc}$ 400 mg bid)/ritonavir (400 mg bid)/delavirdine (600 mg bid); (2) saquinavir$_{sgc}$ (400 mg bid)/ritonavir (400 mg bid)/adefovir; (3) saquinavir$_{sgc}$ (400 mg bid)/ritonavir (400 mg bid)/delavirdine (600 mg bid)/adefovir; (4) saquinavir$_{sgc}$ (800 tid)/nelfinavir (750 mg tid)/delavirdine (600 mg bid); (5) saquinavir$_{sgc}$ (800 mg tid)/nelfinavir (750 mg tid)/adefovir; or (6) saquinavir$_{sgc}$ (800 mg tid)/nelfinavir (750 mg tid)/delavirdine (600 mg bid)/adefovir. At week 16, virologic responses between the pooled nelfinavir and ritonavir groups were not significantly different (33% vs. 28%, $P = 0.50$). Pooled delavirdine groups had a higher frequency of virologic suppression than did the adefovir groups (40% vs. 18%, $P = 0.002$). There were no significant differences between the pooled delavirdine and delavirdine/adefovir groups. There are at least two potential reasons why the delavirdine/adefovir groups did no better than the delavirdine arms. First, all subjects were naive to NNRTIs and highly nucleoside-experienced before entering the study. The prior treatment experience of these subjects would be expected to maximize the impact of delavirdine and attenuate the effect of adefovir on virologic outcome. Second, an intensive pharmacokinetic substudy demonstrated that the delavirdine/adefovir combination arms had lower AUCs for both saquinavir and delavirdine than did the delavirdine-only arm(s).[45] The mechanism for this observed pharmacokinetic interaction is unknown.

▲ RESISTANCE OF HIV-1 TO DELAVIRDINE

Resistance to NNRTIs is largely mediated by mutations in the hydrophobic pocket of the p66 subunit of HIV-1 RT that binds this class of compounds. These mutations are thought to cause NNRTI resistance by altering the ability of HIV-1 RT to bind NNRTIs. The most common resistance mutations seen during in vitro passage in the presence of nevirapine and during monotherapy in patients are those at codons 103 (lysine to arginine mutation, K103N) and 181 (Y181C).[49–51]

In contrast to nevirapine, in vitro passage of HIV-1 in the presence of delavirdine selects for a P236L mutation in RT.[52,53] Unlike the Y181C and K103N mutations, which confer cross-resistance to most NNRTIs, P236L sensitizes HIV-1 to nevirapine and TIBO compounds.[52] The selective resistance of the P236L mutant to BHAPs is presumed to reflect the unique properties of binding of this class of compounds to HIV-1 RT.[8] Although HIV-1 mutants with the Y181C or K103N NNRTI resistance mutations each demonstrate decreased susceptibility to delavirdine, the P236L mutant is approximately twice as resistant to delavirdine than either Y181C or K103N.[52]

Similar to what was seen with monotherapy with other NNRTIs, monotherapy with delavirdine led to the rapid development of phenotypic resistance within 2 to 8 weeks of drug administration.[54] In contrast to in vitro studies in which P236L was the predominant delavirdine resistance mutation selected, most delavirdine-resistant clinical isolates in patients receiving delavirdine monotherapy had the K103N mutation, either alone or in combination with Y181C.[54] P236L occurred in fewer than 10% of patients studied. A trial of delavirdine in combination with zidovudine also found that K103N was the most common mutation.[55] In that study P236L occurred in 28% to 35% of subjects, and Y181C was seen only rarely. A potential explanation for the less frequent occurrence of P236L than K103N in clinical isolates is that P236L confers a replication defect when introduced into a laboratory strain relative to wild-type virus and virus with the K103N mutation.[56] This decrease in replication capacity is also a characteristic of most RT clinical sequences that contain the P236L mutation.[57]

Combination therapy with various nucleoside analogues appears to influence the development of phenotypic and genotypic delavirdine resistance. In vitro studies performed with isolates obtained from patients enrolled in a number of uncontrolled studies with other NNRTIs were unable to detect the Y181C mutation during combination therapy with NNRTIs and zidovudine, even though Y181C occurs quite commonly during NNRTI monotherapy.[50,51,55,58] The Y181C mutation was not observed during therapy with delavirdine/zidovudine in two studies,[53,55] yet Y181C occurred commonly in a pharmacokinetic study of delavirdine and didanosine,[59] suggesting that nucleoside analogues may differ in their effects on the development of NNRTI resistance. Analyses of ACTG 261, a randomized, double-blind, placebo-controlled trial comparing delavirdine/zidovudine and delavirdine/didanosine versus delavirdine/zidovudine/didanosine confirmed that combination therapy with delavirdine and zidovudine prevents development of the Y181C mutation, whereas combination therapy with delavirdine and didanosine does not.[60] Although the development of phenotypic delavirdine resistance in the dual-combination delavirdine arms was similar, the onset of phenotypic delavirdine resistance was delayed in the tripletherapy arm.[60] The effect of other nucleoside analogues, such as lamivudine and abacavir, on the development of delavirdine resistance is not known, but such information might be helpful for designing more effective delavirdine-containing combination regimens.

With the exception of the occasional isolate that develops the P236L mutation, it is expected that delavirdine-resistant isolates obtained from patients are also resistant to other NNRTIs such as nevirapine and efavirenz. Similarly, cross-resistance to delavirdine is frequent in isolates obtained from patients failing efavirenz- or nevirapine-containing regimens. There is no evidence of cross-resistance between delavirdine and either nucleoside analogues or protease inhibitors. However, some nucleoside and NNRTI resistance mutations may increase the susceptibility of HIV to NNRTIs and nucleoside analogues, respectively. For example, Y181C results in zidovudine hypersusceptibility.[61] Hypersusceptibility to delavirdine and other NNRTIs has been observed in patients who are NNRTI-naive and have extensive nucleoside experience. Phenotypic hypersusceptibility to NNRTIs correlates with phenotypic nucleoside resistance.[62] One study demonstrated that the presence of an NNRTI hypersusceptible HIV isolate at baseline is associated with improved virologic outcome to efavirenz[63]; analogous studies have not been performed to assess the response to delavirdine-containing regimens. The genetic basis for NNRTI hypersusceptibility has not been fully elucidated, but NNRTI hypersusceptibility is correlated with increasing numbers of nucleoside resistance mutations.[63] In one study, a reduction in the expected magnitude of phenotypic NNRTI resistance was observed in isolates that contained both NNRTI and nucleoside resistance mutations. However, patients who had such isolates before beginning an NNRTI-based regimen had minimal virologic response to an efavirenz-containing salvage regimen.[63]

▲ RECOMMENDATIONS FOR USE

Indications for Use Against HIV-1 Infection

Delavirdine is approved for use in combination with other appropriate antiretroviral agents for the management of HIV-1 infection in adults when antiretroviral therapy is warranted. The drug was approved by the FDA in April 1997 under the FDA's accelerated review policy that allows approval based on analysis of surrogate markers of response (e.g., changes in CD4+ T-lymphocyte counts and plasma HIV RNA concentrations) rather than clinical endpoints (e.g., disease progression or survival). To date, none of the Phase III studies has demonstrated a clinically significant impact of delavirdine on clinical outcome.

Dosing and Administration

Delavirdine mesylate is available in 100- or 200-mg tablets; the recommended dose in adults is 400 mg PO tid.[36] Pharmacokinetic modeling studies and preliminary clinical studies suggest that a dose of 600 mg PO bid provides steady-state drug exposure similar to that of the 400 mg tid regimen.[13] The pharmacokinetics of delavirdine in adults older than 65 years of age have not been studied, and it is not known if dosage adjustments are necessary for this age group. The safety and efficacy of delavirdine in neonates and children younger than 16 years of age have not been established, and data are insufficient to make a dosage recommendation in this age group. Delavirdine may be taken without regard to meals. The pharmacokinetics of delavirdine in patients with hepatic or renal insufficiency have not been studied, and it is not known if dosage adjustment of this drug is necessary under these circumstances. Because it undergoes extensive hepatic metabolism, the manufacturer recommends that delavirdine be used with caution in patients with impaired hepatic function.[36]

The manufacturer states that for patients unable to swallow delavirdine tablets the drug may be administered as a slurry or dispersion in water.[36] The bioavailability of the 100-mg delavirdine tablets is 20% greater when the tablets are allowed to disintegrate in water prior to administration, although this is not necessarily preferred in patients who are able to swallow the tablets. To prepare a suspension of delavirdine containing 400 mg, four 100-mg tablets should be placed in a glass containing at least 3 ounces of water, allowed to stand for a few minutes, then stirred until there is uniform dispersion of the drug. The dispersed drug should be swallowed promptly, followed by rinsing the glass and drinking the rinsing fluid to ensure that the entire dose is delivered.[36] The 200-mg tablets are not readily dispersed in water, and the bioavailability of the 200-mg tablet using this technique has not been determined.[36]

The manufacturer recommends that patients with achlorhydria take delavirdine with an acidic beverage such as cranberry or orange juice.[36] It is also recommended that delavirdine be taken at least 1 hour before or after an antacid because of studies demonstrating effects of antacids on delavirdine absorption.[36] Didanosine has been reported to decrease absorption of delavirdine, presumably as a result of the buffering agent in didanosine formulations.[34] Although the clinical significance of this reduction is unknown, it is recommended that the doses of delavirdine and didanosine be separated by at least 1 hour.[36]

Use of Delavirdine in Combination with Other Antiretroviral Agents

Because of the risk of developing resistance, delavirdine should be given in combination with at least two additional antiretroviral agents. Better responses appear to occur when lamivudine is also part of the antiretroviral regimen. Pharmacokinetic data suggest that delavirdine may increase the potency of regimens containing protease inhibitors, although more long-term data are needed on the efficacy and tolerability of such combination regimens. Patients treated with these combinations should be carefully monitored for signs of toxicity. There is no evidence to suggest that regimens containing two NNRTIs would be superior to regimens containing one NNRTI, and some in vitro data suggest that there may be antagonism between various NNRTIs.[12] Because of concerns about cross-resistance, patients who fail a regimen containing one NNRTI are unlikely to respond to a different NNRTI, and such a substitution is not generally recommended.

Concomitant Therapy with Delavirdine Plus Other Drugs

Use of rifampin or rifabutin concomitantly with delavirdine is not recommended because of the significant reduction in delavirdine levels induced by these drugs.[36] In addition, concomitant use of other drugs (e.g., the anticonvulsants carbamazepine, phenobarbital, and phenytoin) known to induce CYP3A and expected to accelerate delavirdine metabolism is not recommended.[13,36]

Delavirdine is predicted to result in clinically important increases in plasma concentrations of certain drugs metabolized by cytochrome P_{450} that may result in potentially serious or life-threatening adverse effects (Table 9–2). Examples are some nonsedating antihistamines (e.g., astemizole and terfenadine), antiinfective agents (e.g., rifabutin), sedative-hypnotics (e.g., alprazolam, midazolam, triazolam), and certain drugs used to treat gastrointestinal disorders (e.g., cisapride). Concomitant administration of delavirdine with these agents is not recommended.[13,36] In addition, delavirdine is predicted to increase plasma concentrations of antimicrobial agents (e.g., dapsone and clarithromycin), calcium channel blockers (e.g., dihydropyridine nifedipine), ergot derivatives, quinidine, warfarin, and sildenafil. Caution should be used when prescribing these drugs together with delavirdine, and dose adjustments or substitutions for these drugs may be necessary.

▲ CONCLUSIONS

Delavirdine is an NNRTI with potent activity against HIV-1 in vitro. When studied in clinical trials alone or in combination with zidovudine or didanosine, delavirdine's efficacy has been found to be limited. Use of delavirdine in combination with zidovudine and lamivudine may lead to greater plasma HIV RNA suppression than when delavirdine is given in combination with zidovudine and didanosine. Because of the disappointing results from early delavirdine clinical trials and the relative paucity of data directly comparing the potency of delavirdine-containing regimens to first-line antiretroviral regimens, delavirdine is used infrequently to treat patients with HIV infections compared to other NNRTIs, such as efavirenz or nevirapine. The need for three times a day dosing also is an obstacle to the more widespread use of this antiretroviral agent. Delavirdine has shown some promise when combined with protease inhibitors in regimens designed to take advantage of their pharmacokinetic interactions, although data are needed on how the efficacy and tolerability of delavirdine/protease inhibitor regimens compare with more widely used regimens in which ritonavir is used to augment protease inhibitor drug levels.

REFERENCES

1. Romero DL, Busso M, Tan C-K, et al. Nonnucleoside reverse transcriptase inhibitors that potently and specifically block human immunodeficiency virus type 1 replication. Proc Natl Acad Sci USA 88:8806, 1991.
2. Dueweke TJ, Poppe SM, Romero DL, et al. U-90152, a potent inhibitor of human immunodeficiency virus type 1 replication. Antimicrob Agents Chemother 37:1127, 1993.
3. Dueweke TJ, Kezdy FJ, Waszak GA, et al. The binding of a novel bisheteroarylipiperazine mediates inhibition of human immunodeficiency virus type 1 reverse transcriptase. J Biol Chem 267:27, 1992.
4. Kohlstaedt LA, Wang J, Friedman JM, et al. Crystal structure at 3.5 A resolution of HIV-1 reverse transcriptase coupled with an inhibitor. Science 256:1783, 1992.
5. Cohen KA, Hopkins J, Ingraham RH, et al. Characterization of the binding site for nevirapine (BI-RG-587), a nonnucleoside inhibitor of human immunodeficiency virus type-1 reverse transcriptase. J Biol Chem 266:14670, 1991.
6. Condra JH, Emini EA, Gotlib L, et al. Identification of the human immunodeficiency virus reverse transcriptase residues that contribute to the activity of diverse nonnucleoside inhibitors. Antimicrob Agents Chemother 36:1441, 1992.
7. Spence RA, Kati WM, Anderson KS, et al. Mechanism of inhibition of HIV-1 reverse transcriptase by nonnucleoside inhibitors. Science 267:988, 1995.
8. Esnouf RM, Ren J, Hopkins AJ. Unique features in the structure of the complex between HIV-1 reverse transcriptase and the bis(heteroaryl)piperazine (BHAP) U-90152 explain resistance mutations for this nonnucleoside inhibitor. Proc Natl Acad Sci USA 94:3984, 1997.
9. Chong K-T, Pagano PJ, Hinshaw RR. Bisheteroarylpiperazine reverse transcriptase inhibitor in combination with 3′-azido-3′-deoxythymidine or 2′,3′-dideoxycytidine synergistically inhibits human immunodeficiency virus type 1 replication in vitro. Antimicrob Agents Chemother 38:288, 1994.
10. Pagano PJ, Chong K-T. In vitro inhibition of human immunodeficiency virus type 1 by a combination of delavirdine (U-90152) with protease inhibitor U-75875 or interferon-alpha. J Infect Dis 171:61, 1995.
11. Chong K-T, Pagan PJ. Inhibition of human immunodeficiency virus type 1 infection in vitro by combination of delavirdine, zidovudine and didanosine. Antiviral Res 34:51, 1997.
12. Gu Z, Quan Y, Li A, et al. Effects of non-nucleoside inhibitors of human immunodeficiency virus type 1 in cell-free recombinant reverse transcriptase assays. J Biol Chem 270:31046, 1995.
13. Tran JQ, Gerber JG, Kerr BM. Delavirdine: clinical pharmacokinetics and drug interactions. Clin Pharmacokinet 40:207, 2001.
14. Shelton M, Adams J, Hewitt R, et al. Reduced delavirdine exposure in HIV+ subjects with gastric hypoacidity. In: Abstracts of the 35th Interscience Conference on Antimicrobial Agents and Chemotherapy, San Francisco. Washington, DC, American Society for Microbiology, 1995, abstract A30.
15. Cox SR, Della-Coletta AA, Turner SW, et al. Single-dose pharmacokinetic studies with delavirdine mesylate: dose proportionality and effects of food and antacid. Presented at the 34th Interscience Conference on Antimicrobial Agents and Chemotherapy, Orlando, FL, 1994, abstract A54.
16. Cheng C-L, Smith DE, Carver PL, et al. Steady-state pharmacokinetics of delavirdine in HIV-positive patients: effect on erythromycin breath test. Clin Pharmacol Ther 61:531, 1997.
17. Morse GD, Fishl MA, Cox SR, et al. Effect of food on the steady-state pharmacokinetics of delavirdine mesylate in HIV–positive patients. Presented at the 35th Interscience Conference on Antirmicrobial Agents and Chemotherapy, San Francisio, 1995, abstract I30.
18. Chaput AJ, D'Ambrosio R, Morse GD. In vitro protein-binding characteristics of delavirdine and its N-dealkylated metabolite. Antiviral Res 32:81, 1996.
19. Borin MT, Chambers JH, Carel BJ, et al. Pharmacokinetic study of the interaction between rifampin and delavirdine mesylate. Clin Pharmacol Ther 61:544, 1997.
20. Borin MT, Chambers JH, Carel BJ, et al. Pharmacokinetic study of the interaction between rifabutin and delavirdine mesylate in HIV-1 infected patients. Antiviral Res 35:53, 1997.
21. Cox SR, Herman BD, Batts DH, et al. Delavirdine and rifabutin: pharmacokinetic evaluation in HIV-1 patients with concentration-targeting of delavirdine. In: Abstracts of the 5th Conference on Retroviruses

and Opportunistic Infections, Chicago. Alexandria, VA, Westover Management Group, 1998, abstract 344.
22. Cox SR, Borin MT, Driver MR, et al. Effect of clarithromycin on the steady-state pharmacokinetics of delavirdine in HIV-1 patients. In: Abstracts of the 2nd National Conference of Human Retroviruses. Washington, DC, American Society for Microbiology, 1995, abstract 487.
23. Von Moltke LL, Greenblatt DJ, Grassi JM, et al. Protease inhibitors as inhibitors of hyman cytochromes P450: high risk associated with ritonavir. J Clin Pharmacol 38:106, 1998.
24. Eagling VA, Back DJ, Barry MG. Differential inhibition of cytochrome P450 isoforms by the protease inhibitors, ritonavir, saquinavir, and indinavir. Br J Clin Pharmacol 44:190, 1997.
25. Cox SR, Ferry JJ, Batts DH, et al. Delavirdine and marketed protease inhibitors: pharmacokinetic interaction studies in healthy volunteers. In: Abstracts of the 4th Conference on Retroviruses and Opportunistic Infections, Washington, DC. Alexandria, VA, Westover Management Group, 1997, abstract 372.
26. Ferry JJ, Herman BD, Carel BJ, et al. Pharmacokinetic drug–drug interaction study of delavirdine and indinavir in healthy volunteers. J Acquir Immune Defic Syndr Hum Retrovirol 18:252, 1998.
27. Para M, Beal J, Rathburn C, et al. Potent activity with lower doses of indinavir using delavirdine in combination with zidovudine: 48 week analysis. Presented at the 39th Interscience Conference on Antimicrobial Agents and Chemotherapy, San Francisco, 1999, abstract 1985.
28. Morse GD, Shelton MJ, Hewitt RG, et al. Ritonavir pharmacokinetics during combination therapy with delavirdine. In: Abstracts of the 5th Conference on Retroviruses and Opportunistic Infections, Chicago. Alexandria, VA, Westover Management Group, 1998, abstract 343.
29. Cox SR, Schneck DW, Herman BD, et al. Delavirdine and nelfinavir: a pharmacokinetic drug–drug interaction study in healthy adult volunteers. In: Abstracts of the 5th Conference on Retroviruses and Opportunistic Infections, Chicago. Alexandria, VA, Westover Management Group, 1998, abstract 345.
30. Woolley J, Studenberg S, Boehlert C, et al. Cytochrome P-450 isozyme induction, inhibition, and metabolism studies with the HIV protease inhibitor 141W94. Presented at the 37th Interscience Conference on Antimicrobial Agents and Chemotherapy, Toronto, 1997 abstract A60.
31. Tran JQ, Petersen C, Garrett M, et al. Delavirdine significantly increases plasma concentrations of amprenavir in healthy volunteers. AIDS 14(suppl 4):S92, 2000.
32. Cox SR, Batts DH, Stewart F, et al. Evaluation of the Pharmacokinetic interaction between saquinavir and delavirdine in healthy volunteers. Presented at the 4th Conference on Retroviruses and Opportunistic Infections, Washington, DC, 1997, abstract 381.
33. Cox S, Conway B, Freimuth W, et al. Pilot study of BID and TID combinations of saquinavir-SGC, delavirdine, zidvoudine, and lamivudine as initial therapy: pharmacokinetic interaction between saquinavir-SGC and delavirdine. Presented at the 7th Conference on Retroviruses and Opportunistic Infections, San Francisco, 2000, abstract 82.
34. Morse GD, Fischl MA, Shelton MJ, et al. Single dose pharmacokinetics of delavirdine mesylate and didanosine in patients with human immunodeficiency virus infection. Antimicrob Agents Chemother 41:169, 1997.
35. Para MF, Meehan P, Holden-Wiltse J, et al. ACTG 260: a randomized, phase I/II, dose-ranging, trial of the anti-HIV activity of delavirdine monotherapy. Antimicrob Agents Chemother 43:1373, 1999.
36. Rescriptor package insert. Agouron Pharmaceuticals, La Jolla, CA, 2001.
37. Davey RT, Chaitt DG, Reed GF, et al. Randomized, controlled phase I/II trial of combination therapy with delavirdine (U-90152S) and conventional nucleosides in human immunodeficiency virus type 1-infected patients. Antimicrob Agents Chemother 40:1657, 1996.
38. Friedland GH, Pollard RB, Griffith B, et al. Efficacy and safety of delavirdine mesylate with zidovudine and didanosine compared with two-drug combinations of these agents in persons with CD4+ T lymphocyte counts of 100 to 500 cells/mm^3 (ACTG 261). J Acquir Immune Defic Syndr 21:281, 1999.
39. Freimuth WW, Chuang-Stein CJ, Greenwald CA, et al. Delavirdine + didanosine combination therapy has sustained surrogate marker response in advanced HIV-1 population. In: Abstracts of the 3rd Conference on Retroviruses and Opportunistic Infections. Alexandria, VA, Westover Management Group, 1996, abstract LB8b.
40. Freimuth WW, Wathen LK, Cox SR, et al. Delavirdine in combination with zidovudine causes sustained antiviral and immunological effects in HIV-1 infected individuals. In: Abstracts of the 3rd Conference on Retroviruses and Opportunistic Infections. Alexandria, VA, Westover Management Group, 1996, abstract LB8c.
41. Sargent S, Green S, Para M, et al. Sustained plasma viral burden reductions and CD4+ T lymphocyte increase in HIV-1 infected patients with Rescriptor (DLV) + Retrovir (ZDV) + Epivir (3TC). In: Abstracts of the 5th Conference on Retroviruses and Opportunistic Infections, Chicago. Alexandria, VA, Westover Management Group, 1998, abstract 699.
42. Wathen L, Freimuth W, Getchel L, et al. Use of HIV-1 RNA PCR in patients on Rescriptor (DLV) + Retrovir (ZDV) + Epivir (3TC), ZDV + 3TC, or DLV + ZDV allowed early differentiation between treatment arms. In: Abstracts of the 5th Conference on Retroviruses and Opportunistic Infections, Chicago. Alexandria, VA, Westover Management Group, 1998, abstract 694.
43. Kuritzkes DR, Bassett RL, Johnson VA, et al. Continued lamivudine versus delavirdine in combination with indinavir and zidovudine or stavudine in lamivudine-experienced patients: results of Adult AIDS Clinical Trials Group Protocol 370. AIDs 14:1553, 2000.
44. Eron J, McKinley G, LeCrerq P, et al. Potent antiviral activity using delavirdine and reduced-dose indinavir combination therapies: a 48 week analysis. Presented at the 7th Conference on Retroviruses and Opportunistic Infections, San Francisco, 2000, abstract 535.
45. Gulick RM, Hu J, Fiscus SA, et al. Randomized study of saquinavir with ritonavir or nelfinavir together with delavirdine, adefovir, or both in HIV-infected adults with virologic failure on indinavir: ACTG study 359. J Infect Dis 182:1375, 2000.
46. Hammer SM, Katzenstein DA, Hughes MD, et al. A trial comparing nucleoside monotherapy with combination therapy in HIV-infected adults with CD4+ T lymphocyte cell counts from 200 to 500 per cubic millimeter. N Engl J Med 335:1081, 1996.
47. Delta Coordinating Committee. Delta: a randomized double-blind controlled trial comparing combinations of zidovudine plus didanosine or zalcitabine with zidovudine alone with HIV-infected individulas. Lancet 348:283, 1996.
48. Conway B. Initial therapy with protease inhibitor-sparing regimens: evaluation of nevirapine and delavirdine. Clin Infect Dis 30(suppl 2):S130, 2000.
49. Richman DD, Shih CK, Lowy I, et al. HIV-1 mutants resistant to nonnucleoside inhibitors of reverse transcriptase arise in tissue culture. Proc Natl Acad Sci USA 88:11241, 1991.
50. Saag MS, Emini EA, Lasin OL, et al. A short-term clinical evaluation of L-697,661, a nonnucleoside inhibitor of HIV-1 reverse transcriptase. N Engl J Med 329: 1065, 1993.
51. Richman DD, Havlir D, Corbeil J, et al. Nevirapine resistance mutations of human immunodeficiency virus type 1 selected during therapy. J Virol 68:1660, 1994.
52. Dueweke TJ, Pushkarskaya T, Poppe SM, et al. A mutation in reverse transcriptase of bis(heteroaryl)piperazine-resistant human immunodeficiency virus type 1 that confers increased sensitivity to other nonnucleoside inhibitors. Proc Natl Acad Sci USA 90:4713, 1993.
53. Beentiktak AMM, Joly V, Stibon G, et al. Combination therapy with delavirdine mesylate and AZT: virology data from a European phase II trial. J Acquir immune Defic Syndr Hum Retrovirol 10:S23, 1995.
54. Demeter L, Shafer R, Meehan P, et al. Delavirdine susceptibilities and associated reverse transcriptase mutations in human immunodeficiency virus type 1 isolates from patients in a phase I/II trial of delavirdine monotherapy (ACTG 260). Antimicrob Agents Chemother 44:794, 2000.
55. Joly V, Moroni M, Concia E, et al. Delavirdine in combination with zidovudine in treatment of HIV-1 infected patients: evaluation of efficacy and emergence of viral resistance in a randomized, comparative, phase III trial. Antimicrob Agents Chemother 44:3155, 2000.
56. Gerondelis P, Archer RH, Palaniappan C, et al. The P236L delavirdine-resistant HIV-1 mutant is replication defective and demonstrates alterations in both RNA 5′ end- and DNA 3′ end-directed RNase H activities. J Virol 73:5803, 1999.
57. Dykes C, Rox K, Lloyd A, et al. Impact of clinical reverse transcriptase sequences on the replication capacity of HIV-1 drug-resistant mutants. Virology 285:193, 2001.
58. Staszewski S, Massari FE, Kober A, et al. combination therapy with zidovudine prevents selection of human immunodeficiency virus type 1 variants expressing high-level resistance to L-697,661, a nonnucleoside reverse transcriptase inhibitor. J Infect Dis 171:1159, 1995.
59. Demeter LM, Meehan PM, Morse G, et al. HIV-1 drug susceptibilities and reverse transcriptase mutations in patients receiving combination

therapy with didanosine and delavirdine. J Acquir Immune Defic Syndr Hum Retrovirol 14:136, 1997.
60. Demeter L, Griffith B, Bosch R, et al. HIV-1 drug susceptibilities during therapy with delavirdine (DLV) + ZDV, DLV + ddI, or DLV + ZDV + ddI. In: Abstracts of the 5th Conference on Retroviruses and Opportunistic Infections, Chicago. Alexandria, VA, Westover Management Group, 1998, abstract 706.
61. Larder BA. 3′-Azido-3′-deoxythymidine resistance suppressed by a mutation conferring human immunodeficiency virus type 1 resistance to nonnucleoside reverse transcriptase inhibitors. Antimicrob Agents Chemother 36:2664, 1992.
62. Whitcomb J, Deeks S, Huang W, et al. Reduced susceptibility to NRTI is associated with NNRTI hypersensitivity in virus from HIV-1 infected patients. Presented at the 7th Conference on Retroviruses and Opportunistic Infections, San Francisco, 2000, abstract 234.
63. Shulman N, Zolopa AR, Passaro D, et al. Phenotypic hypersusceptibility to nonnucleoside reverse transcriptase inhibitors in treatment-experienced HIV-infected patients: impact on virological response to efavirenz-based therapy. AIDS 15:1125, 2001.

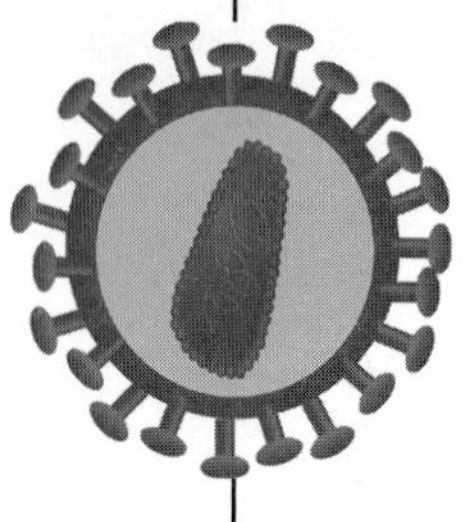

CHAPTER 10
Nevirapine

Julio S.G. Montaner, MD
Joep M.A. Lange, MD, PhD

Nevirapine (NVP) is a nonnucleoside reverse transcriptase inhibitor (NNRTI) of human immunodeficiency virus type 1 (HIV-1). It inhibits HIV-1 replication by binding directly to reverse transcriptase (RT) in a pocket adjacent to the catalytic site of the enzyme.[1] Once NVP has bound to RT, it causes a conformational change that inactivates the enzyme, thereby preventing the polymerization of viral RNA to DNA. NVP is highly specific for HIV-1 RT and does not interfere with human DNA polymerases. NVP freely enters the cell and is active in many cell lines, including T lymphocytes and macrophages, well known targets of HIV; this is in contrast to the nucleoside analogues (NRTIs), which have variable activity in different cell lines.[2,3] Unlike the NRTIs, NVP does not need to be phosphorylated intracellularly to become active; as a result, drug exposure is extremely consistent within and between cell lines. NVP can also bind to extracellular virion RT in the plasma. This means that the amount of cell-free viral reverse transcripts is decreased, leading to a reduction in infectivity.[4] NVP is a potent inhibitor of HIV-1, with a 90% inhibitory concentration (IC_{90}) of 60 nM.[5] The 90% inhibitory quotient for NVP (the concentration of free unbound drug in plasma relative to the IC_{90}) at the trough level is 113. NVP-resistant HIV-1 is usually resistant to the other licensed NNRTIs (efavirenz and delavirdine). NVP has no cross resistance with any of the protease inhibitors (PIs) or NRTIs, including multi-nucleoside-resistant strains. Nevirapine is available both as a tablet (200 mg) and an oral suspension (10 mg/ml).

HUMAN PHARMACOKINETICS

Distribution

Nevirapine is lipophilic and is essentially nonionized at physiologic pH. Following intravenous administration to healthy adults, the apparent volume of distribution (V_{dss}) of NVP was 1.21 ± 0.09 L/kg, suggesting that NVP is widely distributed in humans. NVP readily crosses the placenta and is found in breast milk; it has also been shown to be present in semen.[6–9] NVP is approximately 60% bound to plasma proteins in the plasma concentration range of 1 to 10 μg/ml. Penetration of NVP into the central nervous system has been extensively documented in experimental models and animal models. NVP concentration in human cerebrospinal fluid (CSF) is 45% ± 5% of that in plasma. It is of note that this ratio is approximately equal to the fraction not bound to plasma protein.[10] However, it is unknown to what extent CSF drug levels correlate with brain tissue drug levels.[11] Reduced CSF viral load has been demonstrated in patients taking NVP-based regimens.[12]

Plasma Pharmacokinetics

Nevirapine is readily absorbed (> 90%) after oral administration in healthy volunteers and in HIV-1-infected adults. Absolute bioavailability in 12 healthy adults following single-dose administration was more than 90%, whether given as a tablet or an oral solution.[13] Pooled data from several studies indicate that peak plasma concentrations of 2.0 ± 0.4 mg/ml (7.5 mM) were reached by 4 hours following a single 200 mg oral dose of NVP.[14] Following multiple doses, NVP peak concentrations appear to increase linearly in the dose range 200 to 400 mg/day.[15–17] Steady-state trough NVP concentrations of 4.5 ± 1.9 mg/ml (17 ± 7 mM) were attained at 400 mg/day. These parameters were not altered substantially whether the drug was given with or without food or with alkaline buffers (e.g., antacids).[18]

It is currently recommended that NVP be administered twice a day; however, because of its long half-life at steady state (25 to 30 hours), once-daily dosing is frequently used in clinical practice. An open-label, randomized, crossover study by van Heeswijk et al.[17] indicated that overall exposure to NVP (area under the time-concentration curve, or AUC) was not different when dosed as 400 mg once daily versus 200 mg twice daily.[19] The trough level of NVP, if dosed once a day was about 25% lower than if dosed twice a day but still substantially above the IC_{50}. The SCAN study found that once-daily NVP was as effective and well tolerated as twice-daily NVP in patients in the early stages of HIV infection.[20] Similarly, the Atlantic study showed that a triple drug combination including two nucleosides (didanosine and stavudine) plus NVP using a once-daily regimen had an antiviral and CD4+ T-lymphocyte effect similar to that of a triple combination regimen that included the same two nucleosides and a PI (indinavir).[21]

Metabolism/Elimination

Nevirapine is extensively metabolized via cytochrome P_{450} (CYP450) to several hydroxylated metabolites in vivo and in vitro. In vitro studies with human liver microsomes suggested that oxidative metabolism of NVP is mediated primarily by CYP450 isozymes from the CYP3A family, although other isozymes may play a secondary role. CYP450 metabolism, glucuronide conjugation, and urinary excretion of glucuronidated metabolites represent the primary routes of NVP metabolism and elimination in humans.[14]

Nevirapine has also been shown to be an inducer of CYP450 metabolic enzymes. As a result, the apparent oral clearance of NVP increases by approximately 1.5- to 2.0-fold from 2 to 4 weeks of dosing.[22] Autoinduction also results in a corresponding change in the terminal-phase half-life of NVP in plasma from approximately 45 hours after a single dose to approximately 25 to 30 hours following multiple dosing.[14] The pharmacokinetics of NVP in patients with renal impairment is unchanged. Nevirapine is cleared from the body during renal dialysis, and repeated dosing of nevirapine after dialysis should be considered. Patients with moderate or severe hepatic impairment (Child-Pugh score $\geq$ 8 ascites) are at risk of accumulating NVP and, more importantly, NVP-induced liver toxicity. NVP use in this setting is therefore not recommended. If NVP must be used in this setting, a decrease in the NVP dose should be considered.[23]

Gender, Race, Age

No substantial gender or race differences have been reported in NVP pharmacokinetics across several clinical trials. In one Phase I study that involved healthy volunteers (15 women, 15 men), the weight-adjusted V_{dss} of NVP was higher in women (1.54 L/kg) than in men (1.38 L/kg), suggesting that NVP was distributed more extensively in women. However, this difference was offset by a slightly shorter terminal-phase half-life in women, resulting in no significant gender difference in NVP oral clearance or plasma concentrations following single- or multiple-dose administration.[13] In adults, NVP pharmacokinetics do not change substantially with age (range 18 to 68 years). The apparent clearance rate of NVP in children reaches a maximum by the age of 1 to 2 years and subsequently decreases over time. As a result, the recommended dose for children 2 months to 8 years of age is 4 mg/kg once daily for the first 14 days followed by 7 mg/kg twice daily thereafter, whereas that for children 8 years of age and older is 4 mg/kg once daily for the first 14 days followed by 4 mg/kg twice daily.

Human Dose-Range Studies

Daily doses of 12.5, 50, 200, and 400 mg were studied in adult patients with CD4+ T-lymphocyte counts of less than 400 cells per cubic millimeter. Dose-proportional effects were found, with the 400 mg/day dose being superior in terms of magnitude and duration of effect.[14] In another study, daily doses of 600 mg were associated with increased toxicity and no substantial gain in antiretroviral activity.[19] The main dose-limiting toxicity observed was rash, although some liver enzyme elevations and occasional somnolence were described. As a result, a dose of 400 mg daily was selected for clinical development.

▲ TOXICITY

The most frequent drug-related adverse events reported as possibly related to NVP treatment in clinical trials include rash, fever, fatigue, headache, somnolence, nausea, liver enzyme elevations, and chemical hepatitis. Rash is the most prevalent adverse event that has been attributed to NVP therapy. In four controlled, combination therapy trials with NVP, the overall incidence of rash, regardless of causal association assigned by the investigator, was 35% in the NVP group and 19% in the control group. The difference was statistically significant, for a 16% overall incidence of rash attributable to NVP.[21–26] Rashes with NVP are generally mild and self-limited, and the risk of rash is greatest during the first 6 weeks of therapy. Among NVP-treated patients in four controlled clinical trials, a total of 6.5% experienced grade 3 or 4 rash as their most severe rash event, compared to 1.3% in the controls.[23–26] Only 7% of patients in the NVP group discontinued the drug because of rash, compared to 1% in the control groups; and most of them experienced a grade 3 or 4 rash. Based on 2861 NVP-treated patients in various clinical trials, 9 patients were confirmed to have Stevens-Johnson syndrome (SJS), including 2 reported to have SJS/toxic epidermal necrolysis (TEN). This represents an overall SJS incidence of 0.3%. Although most cases have been managed with supportive therapy, including fluid replacement and pain control, fatal cases have been reported in postmarketing surveillance. The incidence of rash in pediatric patients is not different from that in adults.

To date, no factors have been identified that might predispose a patient to the development of rash. Also, the mechanism of NVP-induced rash remains to be determined. Plasma concentrations of the drug do not correlate with the occurrence of rash. No relation to gender, race, concomitant medications, rash history, or disease stage has been proven. The currently recommended NVP dosing regimen is 200 mg qd for 2 weeks, followed by 200 mg bid thereafter. This is based on retrospective analyses suggesting that this regimen is less frequently associated with rash. Nevertheless, patients must be carefully warned about this potentially serious drug-related effect. In an NVP compassionate use program in The Netherlands, no rashes occurred in patients who had been pretreated with other antiretroviral agents and had plasma HIV-1 levels below the limit of detection.[27].

Table 10–1 provides a set of empiric rash management guidelines developed with input from an expert panel to provide appropriate direction for the continued use or discontinuation of NVP when a patient experiences rash. A number of protocols for rash prevention, including the use of corticosteroids, antihistamines, and slower dose escalation, have been investigated. Corticosteroids do not prevent NVP-related rashes and may even cause an increase in its incidence.[27,28] The role of antihistamines or slower dose escalation for the prevention of NVP-related rash require further evaluation in prospective controlled trials. Whether corticosteroids or antihistamines play a role in the treatment of established NVP-related rash remains unknown.[28,29]

Elevations of liver enzymes, including hepatitis, have also been reported in NVP-treated patients. Isolated γ-glutamyl transpeptidase increases are relatively frequent, but, they are of no clinical consequence and have been attributed to liver enzyme autoinduction of NVP metabolism. Drug-induced hepatitis was reported in 9 of 906 (1%) patients chronically treated with NVP in controlled clinical trials.[30] A similar result was obtained in the BI 1090 trial,[31] which was a randomized, placebo-controlled study involving 1121 patients taking NVP plus two NRTIs and 1128 patients taking placebo plus two NRTIs over 2 years. Using an expanded hepatitis definition (including viral hepatitis), 2.8% of patients in the NVP group and 1.4% in the placebo group had hepatitis over the course of the study ($P = 0.026$). No significant difference in the incidence of serious hepatic events was observed between the two groups. The overall rate of withdrawal as a result of hepatitis in adult NVP trials has been 0.8%. A limited number of fatal hepatitis cases associated with nevirapine use has been reported, however.

Concerning data have been reported from the blinded FTC-302 study,[32] a phase III study comparing the NRTIs emtricitabine and lamivudine, in which all patients also received stavudine and were stratified to receive either nevirapine or efavirenz, according to their baseline viral load. A total of 87% of the study subjects were black, and 59% were women. There was a high incidence of grade 3 and 4 hepatotoxicity, affecting 58 (12%) of 468 subjects, all of whom were receiving nevirapine; two cases were fatal. Most cases occurred within the first 8 weeks of therapy, with a temporal association with the dose escalation of nevirapine from 200 mg to 400 mg at day 14 of treatment. A statistically significant twofold greater incidence of hepatotoxicity was noted in women. The gender-adjusted incidence of hepatotoxicity was approximately 11%, not dissimilar to that reported in the nevirapine package insert.[32]

Although further study is required to identify risk factors that predispose patients to develop hepatitis, it has been suggested that patients with hepatitis C co-infection may be at higher risk for developing clinical hepatitis when receiving NVP-based therapy.[30,31] In a recent analysis of a clinical cohort (Athena study) covering approximately 70% of Dutch patients receiving highly active antiretroviral therapy (HAART), independent risk factors associated with the development of grade IV transaminase elevations were as follows: higher baseline alanine aminotransferase (ALAT) levels [hazard ratio

▲ **Table 10–1.** GUIDELINES FOR THE MANAGEMENT OF RASH

Rash Description	Action with Nevirapine
Mild/moderate rash (may include pruritus) Erythema Diffuse erythematous macular or maculopapular cutaneous eruption	Can continue dosing without interruption If rash or other suspected nevirapine toxicity occurs during lead-in, the dose should not be escalated until the rash resolves If nevirapine is interrupted for > 7 days, reintroduce with 200 mg/day lead-in
Urticaria	As above; however, if nevirapine is interrupted, do not reintroduce
Any rash with associated constitutional findings such as fever > 39°C, myalgia/arthralgia, blistering, facial edema, oral lesions, general malaise, conjunctivitis, severely increased, liver function tests	Permanent discontinuation; no reintroduction
Severe rash Extensive erythematous or maculopapular rash or moist desquamation Angioedema Serum sickness-like reactions Stevens-Johnson syndrome Toxic epidermal necrolysis	Immediate discontinuation; no reintroduction

From Pollard RB, Robinson P, Dransfield K. Safety profile of nevirapine, a nonnucleoside reverse transcriptase inhibitor for the treatment of human immunodeficiency virus infection. Clin Ther 20:1071, 1998. Copyright Excerpta Medica, Inc., with permission.

(HR) 1.06 per 10 units increase], chronic hepatitis B virus infection (HR 9.3), chronic hepatitis C virus infection (HR 5.2), recent start of nevirapine (HR 8.5) or ritonavir (HR 3.7), and female gender (HR 2.6). Furthermore, in patients chronically co-infected with hepatitis B virus, discontinuing the use of lamivudine (3TC) was associated with the development of grade 4 liver enzyme elevations (HR 4.8).[33]

To date, no previously unrecognized adverse events have been identified when using NVP in combination with various antiretroviral agents, including NRTIs and PIs. Furthermore, the rate of known adverse events has not increased when NVP was used in combination with these agents. Importantly, untoward lipid abnormalities (including hyperlipidemia and lipodystrophy) have not been associated with NVP. Indeed, it has been shown that lipid abnormalities at least partially revert following the switch from a PI to NVP.[34] In the Atlantic study, nevirapine-containing HAART resulted in an antiatherogenic lipid profile, with a striking increase in highdensity lipoprotein (HDL) cholesterol (49%) and a significant reduction (14%) in the total cholesterol/HDL cholesterol ratio.[35] Several cases have seen reported where NVP was given as part of a postexposure prophylaxis regimen resulting in severe liver toxicity. Although a number of potential confounders were noted in each case, it is at least likely that NVP may have contributed to the development of this serious toxicity. Until this issue is further clarified, therefore, NVP use in this setting is not recommended.[32,34,36]

▲ CLINICAL TRIALS

Treatment-Naive Patients

The INCAS trial was among the first to demonstrate that triple combination therapy was required to achieve a durable treatment response.[25] This study examined the activity, safety, and tolerance of three regimens—NVP/zidovudine (ZVD)/didanosine (ddI), NVP/ZDV, ZDV/ddI—in 151 antiretroviral-naive HIV-1-infected patients with 200 to 600 CD4+ T-lymphocytes per cubic millimeter. At baseline the mean plasma HIV RNA was 4.41 $\log_{10}$ copies per milliliter and the mean CD4+ T-lymphocyte count was 374 cells per cubic millimeter. The mean maximum viral load decrease from baseline for patients in the triple arm of the study was 2.94 $\log_{10}$ copies per milliliter. As shown in Figure 10–1, NVP/ZDV was associated with substantial but transient effects on virologic markers. However, NVP/ZDV/ddI was consistently superior to ZDV/ddI, providing a durable response in both virologic and immunologic markers, with 51% maintaining viral loads of less than 20 copies per milliliter at 52 weeks. Raboud et al. demonstrated that patients who achieve HIV-1 RNA levels of less

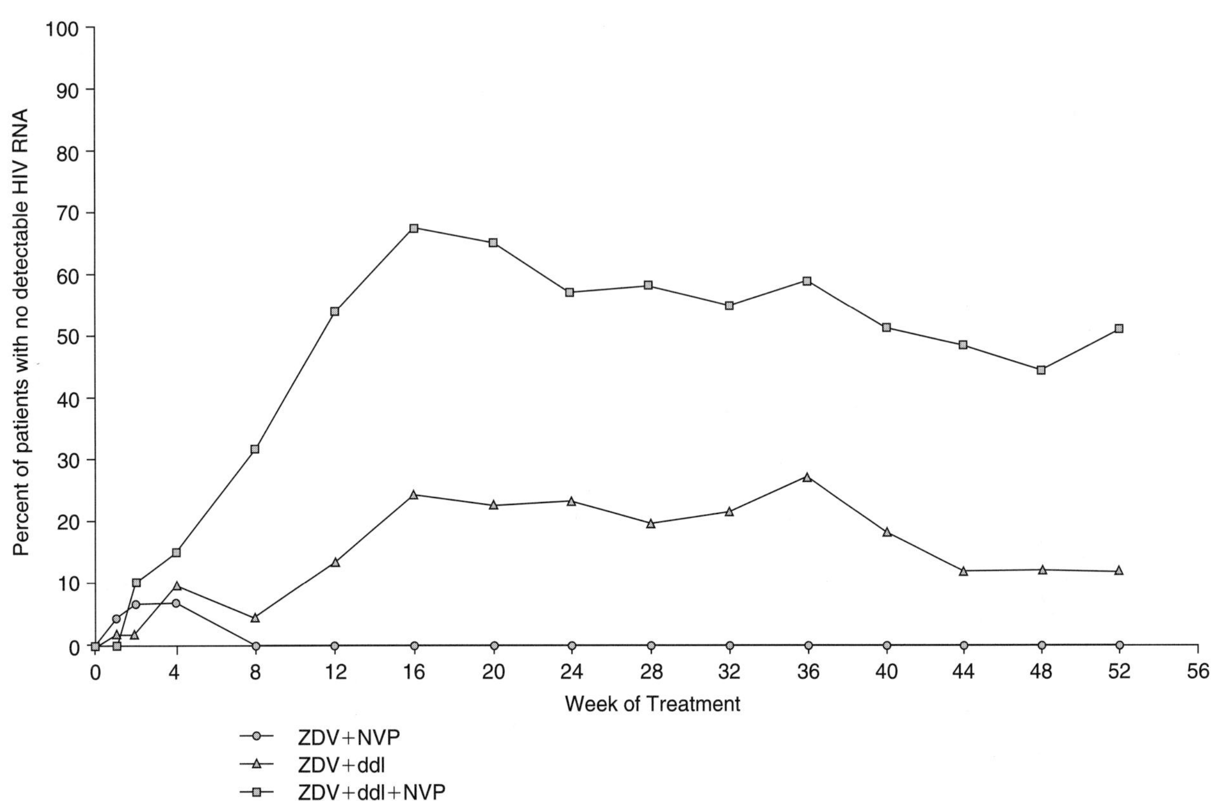

Figure 10–1. INCAS trial: percent of patients below the limit of detection through 52 weeks of treatment (limit of detection was 20 copies per milliliter). (Redrawn from Montaner JSG, Reiss P, Cooper D, et al. A randomized, double-blind trial comparing combinations of nevirapine, didanosine, and zidovudine for HIV-infected patients: the INCAS trial. JAMA 279:930, 1998. Copyright 1998, American Medical Association, with permission.)

than 20 copies per milliliter were able to maintain their antiretroviral response.[37] Indeed, long-term follow-up of patients from the INCAS study demonstrated that viral suppression could be sustained with NVP-based triple combination therapy for up to 4 years.[35] The INCAS study also demonstrated the need for high levels of adherence to the therapeutic regimen to achieve a sustained response. Adherence to the triple therapy regimen was associated with decreased recoverable virus and lessened the likelihood of developing resistance, whereas nonadherence was associated with virologic failure.[38] Although the study was not designed to evaluate clinical events, fewer NVP/ZDV/ddI-treated patients (12%) had HIV progression events, compared with patients who took ZDV/ddI (25%) or NVP/ZDV (23%).[25]

The INCAS trial was the first to demonstrate the powerful potential of NVP. A cross-study evaluation, using an intent-to-treat analysis, showed that the results of the INCAS trial were consistent with those of similar triple-combination regimens that included PIs or the NNRTI efavirenz.[38] Two other studies have further revealed the efficacy of NVP relative to PIs in comparative trials.[21,39] The Atlantic study, an international, multicenter, open-label, randomized trial, compared NVP/stavudine (d4T)/ddI with indinavir (IDV)/d4T/ddI and 3TC/d4T/ddI in antiretroviral-naive patients. This trial enrolled 298 patients with median baseline viral loads of 4.25 $\log_{10}$ copies per milliliter and baseline CD4+ T-lymphocyte counts of 406 cells per cubic millimeter. After 48 weeks, 58.4%, 57.0%, and 58.7% of patients in the NVP, IDV, and 3TC arms had less than 500 plasma HIV-1 RNA copies per milliliter in an intent-to-treat analysis (P = NS). After 96 weeks these figures were 59.6%, 50.0%, and 45.0%, respectively (P = NS). Looking at plasma HIV-1 RNA levels of less than 50 copies per milliliter, figures (percent undetectable) at 96 weeks in the intent-to-treat analysis were 81.8% for NVP, 79.0% for IDV, and 50.9% for 3TC, the 3TC arm being inferior to the other arms ($P = 0.001$). The Atlantic trial showed comparable efficacy for a triple combination including nevirapine or a PI (IDV) (Fig. 10–2).

More recently, preliminary results of the COMBINE study have been presented. This open label randomized study directly compared a simple twice-daily regimen of NVP/Combivir to twice-daily nelfinavir/Combivir.[39] The trial enrolled 142 HIV-infected, antiretroviral-naive patients. The median baseline viral load was 59,698 copies per milliliter in the NVP/Combivir arm and 65,806 copies per milliliter in the nelfinavir/Combivir arm. The median baseline CD4+ T-lymphocyte count was also similar in the two arms: 361 versus 351 cells per cubic millimeter in the NVP- and nelfinavir-containing arms, respectively. After 9 months there was no significant difference in outcome between the two arms, with 84% in the NVP/Combivir arm and 78% in the nelfinavir/Combivir arm having viral loads of less than 200 copies per milliliter. The results remain consistent whether an on-treatment or intent-to-treat approach was used. However, using the more sensitive viral load assay with a limit of quantitation of 20 copies per milliliter, 80% of patients in the NVP arm had undetectable viral loads, which is significantly more than the 56% who achieved this level in the nelfinavir arm ($P = 0.02$). The difference between the NVP and nelfinavir arms may be explained in part by greater adherence in the NVP arm. In summary, these two studies demonstrate that NVP-based triple-drug therapy is at least as effective as PI-based therapy in treatment-naive patients.

A substudy of the 1090 trial was reported that focused on the treatment response among treatment-naive patients with extremely high plasma viral loads and very low baseline CD4+ T-lymphocyte counts.[40] Patients were randomized to take NVP/ZDV/3TC or placebo/ZDV/3TC. Altogether, 77 patients in the NVP/ZDV/3TC arm had a mean baseline viral load of 138,986 copies per milliliter and a mean baseline CD4+ T-lymphocyte count of 101 cells per cubic millimeter. There were 94 patients in the placebo arm, with a mean baseline viral load of 146,332

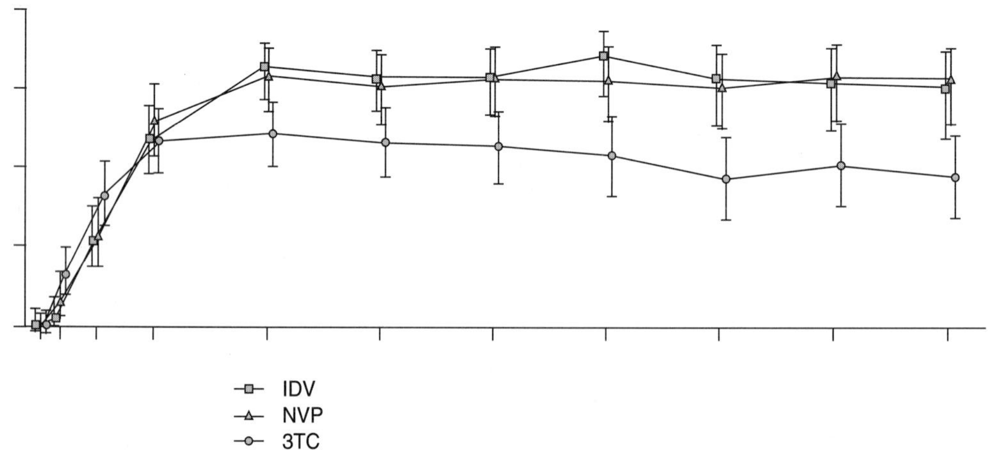

Figure 10–2. Atlantic trial: percent of patients below the limit of detection through 48 weeks of treatment (limit of detection was 50 copies per milliliter). (Redrawn from Squires K, Johnson V, Katlama C, et al. The Atlantic study: a randomized, open-label study to evaluate the efficacy and safety of three triple-combination therapies aimed at different HIV targets in antiretroviral naive HIV-1 infected patients (final 48 weeks analysis). In: Abstracts of the 13th International AIDS Conference, Durban, 2000, abstract LbPeB7046.)

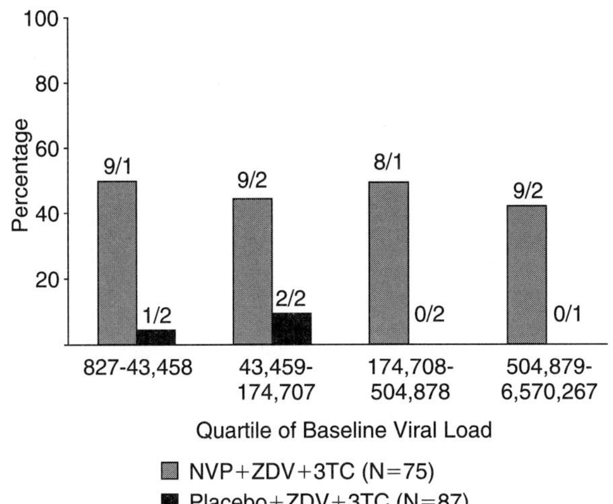

Figure 10–3. BI 1090 trial: percent of patients with sustained viral response through 48 weeks stratified by baseline viral load and CD4+ T-lymphocyte count (intent-to-treat analysis). (Redrawn from Pollard R, 1090 Team. Factors predictive of durable HIV suppression in a randomized double blind trial with nevirapine (NVP), zidovudine (ZDV) and lamivudine (3TC) in treatment-naive (ARV-n) patients with advanced AIDS. In: Abstracts of the 7th Conference on Retroviruses and Opportunistic Infections, San Francisco, 2000, abstract 517.)

copies per milliliter and a mean baseline CD4+ T-lymphocyte count of 93 cells per cubic millimeter. Figure 10–3 demonstrates that although the response in the placebo arm of this study was limited at 48 weeks in all viral load strata, NVP/ZDV/3TC was as effective in patients with viral loads higher than 500,000 copies per milliliter as in those with lower plasma viral load levels. Overall, 45% of patients in the NVP group had viral loads of less than 50 copies per milliliter at 48 weeks using an intent-to-treat analysis—comparable to that observed in the INCAS and Atlantic trials—confirming similar efficacy of NVP even in patients with advanced disease.[41] It is of note that patients with extremely low CD4+ T-lymphocyte counts at baseline ($<$ 38 cells per cubic millimeter) had a poor response to therapy compared with those with higher CD4+ T-lymphocyte counts. Overall, these results suggest that in this particular group of patients (with extremely high baseline plasma viral loads and extremely low baseline CD4+ T-lymphocyte counts) the antiviral effect of the regimen was dependent on the baseline CD4+ T-lymphocyte count but independent of the plasma viral load.

Additional analyses of a subset of patients in the INCAS trial indicate a statistically significant correlation between the cumulative antiviral response achieved over 1 year and the HIV-1 RNA load in lymphoid tissue at 1 year.[42] These data combined with similar results from a substudy of COMBINE[43], and Atlantic[44] support the concept that a high level of suppression of viral replication with NVP-based therapy can lead to a sustained antiviral response in plasma and a decrease in HIV-1 RNA load in tissue reservoirs, similar to the findings reported for PI-containing regimens.

Switch Studies

There are a number of reasons a patient succesfully treated with a PI-based regimen might consider a switch to a PI-sparing regimen. Possible rationales for such a switch include an attempt to improve or arrest morphologic or metabolic changes associated with the lipodystrophy syndrome, to improve adherence by avoiding food restrictions, to reduce the pill burden, or to change to a more convenient dosing schedule. Possible PI-sparing switch strategies currently tested include a switch to an NNRTI-containing regimen using efavirenz[45] or nevirapine[46–48] or to a triple-NRTI regimen using abacavir.[49,50] (See table Chapter 29).

Negredo et al. reported a randomized study of switching to nevirapine or efavirenz, or continuing with a PI-containing regimen, in 77 individuals whose HIV RNA has been suppressed below 50 copies per milliliter for at least 12 months (mean 29 to 31 months).[46] A total of 59% had clinically defined lipodystrophy as assessed by baseline dual energy x-ray absorptiometry (DEXA) scans and anthropometry. At baseline, 60% were receiving a stavudine-containing regimen (usually in combination with lamivudine), and 30% were receiving zidovudine/lamivudine. After 24 weeks there were two cases of virologic rebound in the efavirenz group (n = 25) and one each in the nevirapine group (n = 26) and the PI group (n = 26). Three patients in the efavirenz group stopped treatment owing to neurologic toxicity. Five cases of acute hepatitis and two grade 3/4 rashes were reported in the nevirapine arm, one of which necessitated a change of treatment. The NVP arm experienced the greater decline in low density lepoprotein (LDL) cholesterol and triglycerides, but none of the arms had experienced significant improvements in body fat distribution after 6 months.

Ruiz et al. conducted a randomized study in which patients with HIV RNA levels less than 400 copies per milliliter for longer than 9 months either maintained their PI-containing regimen or switched to didanosine/stavudine/ nevirapine, receiving antihistamine prophylaxis against rash during the first 15 days of therapy.[47] A statistically significant reduction in cholesterol and triglycerides occurred in the nevirapine group, but there was no significant improvement in body fat distribution in the nevirapine group. However, patient-reported quality of life was significantly better in the nevirapine group at week 48. In 60% of cases this was due to a simplified regimen, whereas 40% reported that it was primarily a consequence of either reduced side effects or improved physical status.

In summary, virologic responses in patients who switch to an NVP-based regimen are generally maintained, often associated with better adherence and better quality of life. However, significant improvement in lipodystrophy has not been reported, with the exception of reductions in fasting triglicerides and cholesterol with nevirapine (but not with efavirenz). Switching to a PI-sparing regimen (whether an NNRTI or abacavir-containing regimen) poses a significant risk of virologic rebound for patients with prior experience of mono-NRTI or dual-NRTI therapy and patients who have a history of virologic failure to any antiretroviral regimen.

Protease Inhibitor-Experienced Patients

Introduction of a new class of agents, such as an NNRTI, is recommended when changing treatment because of virologic failure.[51] A change to lopinavir plus an NNRTI-based therapy in NNRTI-naive patients who had failed PIs was explored in two studies, M97-965[52] and M98-957,[53] using concomitant nevirapine and efavirenz, respectively. In the M97-765 trial 32% of participants had a more than fourfold loss of susceptibility to at least three PIs; and in the M98-957 trial 68% had reduced susceptibility of a similar magnitude. Figure 10–4 shows the response to therapy at 96 weeks in the M97-965 study, with 49% of all patients enrolled having viral loads of less than 50 copies per milliliter using an intent-to-treat analysis and 63% having viral loads of less than 50 copies per milliliter using an on-treatment analysis. In the M98-957 study, 71% of individuals randomized to the higher lopinavir dose (533/133 mg) had an HIV RNA level of less than 400 copies per milliliter at week 48 using an intent-to-treat analysis. The virologic response at week 24 was strongly associated with the number of baseline genotypic PI mutations; the presence of more than seven mutations was associated with a decreased chance of suppression below 400 copies per milliliter (less than 40% versus approximately 70% of those with six or seven baseline mutations). In these two phase II studies, 40% of patients had cholesterol levels higher than 300 mg/dl at week 48, and 40% had triglycerides levels higher than 750 mg/dl at week 48. This figure includes individuals who had elevations to this level at baseline. Among single PI-experienced patients, the rates of cholesterol and triglyceride elevations above these levels were 29% and 26%, respectively, at 96 weeks. Discontinuations due to adverse events were rare, however.

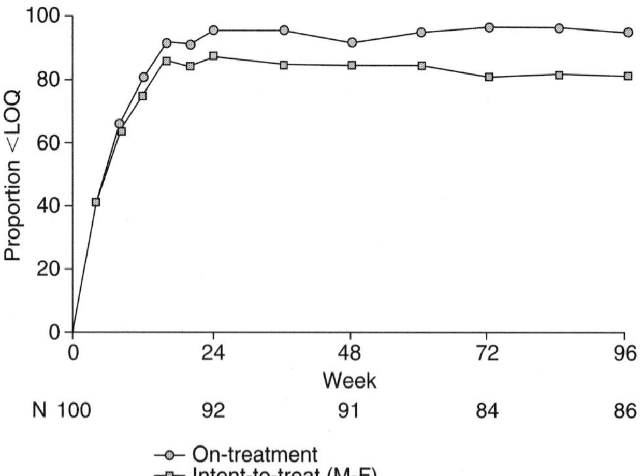

Figure 10–4. M97-765 trial: percent of patients below limit of quantification through 96 weeks of treatment (limit of detection was 400 copies per milliliter). This is an intent-to-treat analysis, with missing values counted as failures (M = F). (Redrawn from Feinberg J, Brun S, Xu Y, et al. Durable suppression of HIV+ RNA after 2 years of therapy with ABT-378/ritonavir (ABT-378/r) treatment in single protease inhibitor experienced patients. In: Abstracts of the 5th International Congress on Drug Therapy in HIV Infection, Glasgow, 2000, abstract P101.)

Rockstroh et al. reported 24-week data on 40 patients receiving expanded-access lopinavir in Germany.[54] A full 78% had received prior PIs, 78% were NNRTI-experienced, and they had taken a median of five prior NRTIs. After 24 weeks only 36% of patients had HIV RNA levels of less than 50 copies per milliliter. These results highlight the contribution of the new NRTIs or NNRTI to support lopinavir in PI-failing patients.

Pediatrics

Nevirapine has been demonstrated to be effective in pediatric populations with both advanced disease and prior PI experience.[55,56] In addition, in two studies of limited numbers of vertically infected children, treatment with NVP plus NRTIs from an early age led to seroconversion in a number of individuals and to the absence of an HIV-specific cytotoxic T-lymphocyte response.[57,58]

Mother-to-Child Transmission

The pharmacologic profile of NVP makes it suitable for preventing of perinatal transmission of HIV-1. NVP plasma levels remain well above the IC_{90} for NVP for up to 1 week after birth, after a single dose to the mother during labor followed by one dose to the infant 48 to 72 hours after birth.[7] Musoke et al. also showed that NVP was present in breast milk during that period and that maternal plasma viral load was decreased by a median 1.3 $\log_{10}$ copies per milliliter 7 days after a single dose.[7] These data suggested that short-course NVP could provide a simple regimen for the prevention of mother-to-child transmission. Two major clinical trials, HIVNET 012[59] and SAINT,[60] have investigated the use of NVP for preventing mother-to-child transmission in the developing world.

The HIVNET 012 trial was conducted in a breast-feeding population in Uganda. The study randomized 645 mothers to receive either NVP (200 mg to the mother at the onset of labor and 2 mg/kg to the infant after 72 hours), ZDV (600 mg at the onset of labor and 300 mg every 3 hours until delivery, with 4 mg/kg given to the infant twice daily for 7 days), or placebo. The placebo arm was discontinued after enrolling only 19 patients because a clear benefit for short-course ZDV had been demonstrated in the Thai study.[61] Figure 10–5 shows that significantly fewer infants in the NVP arm of HIVNET 012 became HIV-infected or died than in the ZDV arm. After 6 to 8 weeks only 11.9% in the NVP arm were HIV-infected compared with 21.3% in the ZDV arm ($P = 0.0027$). Long-term follow-up of patients in this study found that this benefit was maintained for more than 1 year, although 95% were still breastfeeding at 4 months.[62] Similar results were obtained from the SAINT trial, which revealed a 13.3% rate of transmission at 6 to 8 weeks with NVP compared with a 10.2% rate of transmission with ZDV/3TC. In this South African trial the mothers received an additional dose of NVP after delivery, and infants were given a fixed dose of 6 mg NVP. Mothers in the combination therapy arm underwent the same ZDV dosing schedule during labor as in the HIVNET 012 study but also

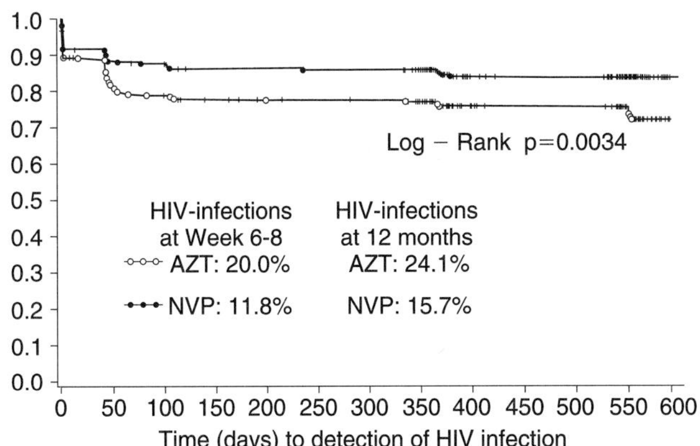

Figure 10–5. HIVNET 012 trial. Kaplan-Meier estimates of proportion of babies with HIV-free survival to 16 weeks. (Redrawn from Guay LA, Musoke P, Fleming T, et al. Intrapartum and neonatal single-dose nevirapine compared with zidovudine for prevention of mother-to-child transmission of HIV-1 in Kampala, Uganda: HIVNET 012 randomised trial. Lancet 354:795, 1999.)

received 150 mg 3TC every 12 hours during labor. Following delivery mothers and infants received 300 mg ZDV/150 mg 3TC twice daily, and 12 mg ZDV/6 mg 3TC twice daily, respectively. Based on the results of these studies, NVP is now indicated for prevention of mother-to-child transmission in a setting where more intensive regimens are not feasible, such as in the developing world.

▲ RESISTANCE

As with the other approved NNRTI agents, selection of drug-resistant virus in cell culture occurs readily with nevirapine, often after only three or four passages. Single-point mutations in the RT gene leads to high-level reduction in susceptibility, often on the order of more than 80-fold. The most common mutations are at the Y181C, Y188L and G190A positions of the RT gene product. Clinical studies have confirmed the rapid development of resistance when nevirapine is used as monotherapy.[63] In one study the appearance of resistant virus was detected as early as day 3 of treatment, with 50% of the wild-type population being replaced with resistant virus by day 14 and near-complete conversion to resistant virus by day 28 of monotherapy. Once a resistant virus has been established, it remains as a dominant viral variant while the patient remains on nevirapine therapy. When therapy is discontinued, there can be reversion to wild-type virus in the plasma compartment; however, archived resistant virus remains in chronically infected cells and can reemerge quickly after therapy with nevirapine or other approved NNRTI agents (delavirdine or efavirenz) is instituted. Therefore careful consideration should be given to the components of every NNRTI-containing regimen in order to have a highlevel of certainty that the regimen will be potent enough to lead to reduction of HIV RNA levels to less than 50 copies per milliliter. Failure to consider this possibility in patients being initiated on available NNRTI-containing antiretroviral regimens leads to the rapid loss of effectiveness of the new regimen and loss of effectiveness of the entire NNRTI class. Although early data indicate that novel NNRTI agents (e.g., capravirine or TMC-125) are potentially effective in the setting of preexistent NNRTI resistance-conferring mutations, the dictum to use all NNRTIs as part of a regimen that leads to high-level suppression remains a fundamental principle of antiretroviral therapy.

▲ DRUG INTERACTIONS

CYP450 Isoenzyme Inhibitors

Ketoconazole, a general inhibitor of CYP isoenzymes, should not be given in combination with NVP. In clinical studies the AUC and maximum concentration (C_{max}) of ketoconazole decreased by 63% and 40%, respectively. An increase in NVP plasma levels is also possible. In a retrospective subpopulation analysis of patients in NVP clinical trials, steady-state NVP trough plasma concentrations were evaluated in patients also on cimetidine or macrolide antibiotics. Steady-state NVP trough plasma concentrations increased by 21% in patients concomitantly receiving cimetidine and by 12% in those concomitantly receiving macrolide antibiotics. Currently, no NVP dosage adjustments are recommended when NVP is used in combination with cimetidine or macrolide antibiotics (e.g., erythromycin, clarithromycin).[51]

CYP450 Isoenzyme Inducers

CYP450 isoenzyme inducers may be expected to bring about a decrease in the plasma levels of NVP. A subgroup analysis detected a 16% average reduction in NVP steady-state trough plasma concentration in 19 patients receiving concomitant rifabutin. This interaction is thought not to be of clinical significance. A 37% reduction in NVP steady-state trough plasma concentration was also documented in three patients on rifampin and NVP. At this time, there are insufficient data to assess whether dosage adjustment is necessary when NVP and rifampin are co-administered. Therefore in tuberculosis co-infected patients rifampin should not be used in combination with NVP. Concomitant use of St. John's wort and NVP is to be avoided, as this herbal supplement is expected to produce a substantial decrease in the plasma levels of NVP.[51]

Antiretrovirals

When NVP was administered in various combinations with ZDV, ddI, and ddC, no substantial effect was detected on the steady-state concentrations of the NRTIs or NVP. Also, no significant drug interaction was detected between NVP and d4T. No substantial interaction between NVP and the other NRTIs, 3TC and abavacir is anticipated because these agents use metabolic pathways that are different from those of NVP.[64,65]

Currently approved PIs are metabolized by similar CYP450 pathways. Sahai et al. reported that co-administration of NVP and saquinavir hard gel capsule (SQV) led to a 27% decrease ($P = 0.03$) in the AUC of SQV and a 3% decrease in the NVP AUC.[66] Co-administration of NVP and ritonavir (RTV) led to an 11% decrease in the AUC for RTV that was not statistically significant. Likewise, there was a nonsignificant decrease in NVP levels compared to historical controls. A nonsignificant 4% increase in plasma nelfinavir levels was observed when it was dosed at 750 mg tid in combination with NVP.

Combinations containing NVP/RTV/SQV have proven to be effective in PI-experienced patients. The interaction between NVP and indinavir (IDV) has also been extensively characterized.[67–69] In these studies, the NVP AUC was not statistically significantly different than the AUC for historical controls, whereas the mean IDV AUC decreased by approximately one-fourth to one-third. Most of the decrease in IDV AUC was attributable to patients with the highest IDV serum levels before NVP dosing. It has been speculated, therefore, that the impact of NVP co-administration on the AUC for IDV may vary depending on the extent of prior CYP450 induction in a given patient. In general, the interaction of NVP with lopinavir, indinavir, and saquinavir is similar in nature and extent, but it is overcome by giving a low dose of ritonavir (as a pharmacokinetic booster of PI exposure).[70] However, as the IC_{90} of the virus increases (with an increasing number of PI-resistant mutations or an increasing number of PI failures) the therapeutic effect of the regimen increases when a higher dose of the PI is used, as illustrated by the M98-957 study. In that study a 30% dose increase of the PI was associated with a better response in patients with multiple PI failure.[71]

The interaction between NVP and efavirenz (EFV) has been characterized as a preliminary step for evaluating the efficacy and safety of this combination. A 22% decrease in the EFV AUC and a 36% decrease in the EFV C_{min} were observed in when the two NNRTIs were given in combination.[72] No change in NVP levels was noted relative to that of historical controls. The clinical significance of this interaction is not yet known, as the efficacy and safety of dual NNRTI combinations have not yet been characterized.

Other Agents

Oral contraceptives have the potential to interact with NVP. The effect of NVP on a single dose of ethinyl estradiol/norethindrone was measured and was found to decrease the AUC significantly, (by 29% and 18%, respectively), with no effect on NVP levels.[73] It is recommended, therefore, that supplemental barrier forms of contraception be used when oral contraceptives are given in conjunction with NVP.

As a CYP450 inducer NVP has the potential to reduce plasma levels of, and thus the requirement for, methadone.[69] The NNRTIs NVP and EFV similarly reduce plasma levels of methadone by 51% and 57%, respectively.[74–76] However, because methadone is dosed to achieve a certain clinical effect, it may be more informative to look at the change in methadone requirement in the presence of a CYP450 inducer. In this context, Altice et al. found that the methadone requirement was increased from 15 to 90 mg/day after initiation of NVP.[76]

▲ CONCLUSIONS

Nevirapine is a potent NNRTI. NVP has excellent bioavailability (90%) and a long half-life (25 to 30 hours). NVP is metabolized by the cytochrome P_{450} system and induces CYP450 enzymes. NVP induces its own metabolism (autoinduction) as well as the metabolism of other drugs metabolized by this system, including all currently marketed anti-HIV PIs. Thus the dose of NVP should be increased from 200 mg PO qd to 200 mg PO bid after 14 days to attain desired serum levels and avoid dose-related toxicity during the period of autoinduction.

The most important toxicities of NVP are skin rash and hepatic toxicity. The risk of rash is greatest during the initial 6 weeks of therapy. Reports of serious hepatotoxicity in several health care workers taking postexposure prophylaxis have led many experts to be reluctant to use NVP for postexposure prophylaxis regimens or in patients with underlying liver disease. Hyperlipidemia and lipodystrophies have not been associated with NVP, suggesting that NVP-based regimens could be a useful alternative for patients who need to switch regimens because of cholesterol or lipid-associated abnormalities.

The U.S. Public Health Service–Infectious Disease Society of America Antiretroviral Guidelines recommend that NVP can be the backbone for an initial antiretroviral regimen, or it can be used as part of a combination regimen for salvage regimens. Either NVP or efavirenz can be used in these settings. Many clinicians prefer efavirenz based on its once-daily dosing schedule and its toxicity profile, but there are no compelling data comparing NNRTI regimens, and other experts prefer NVP. For initial therapy, NVP can be combined with combivir for a convenient twice-daily regimen, as was done in the combine trial. For salvage regimens, NVP has been used successfully for patients who have failed PI-based regimens. There is considerable cross resistance with efavirenz and delavirdine: Patients who have experienced virologic failure on regimens containing the latter drugs are unlikely to benefit from NVP. A major use for NVP is to prevent mother-to-child transmission in the developed and the developing world. A regimen of 200 mg to the mother during labor and 2 mg/kg to the infant after 72 hours has been highly effective when the mother was antiretroviral-naive.

REFERENCES

1. Kohlstaedt LA, Wang J, Friedman JM, et al. Crystal structure at 3.5 Å resolution of HIV-1 reverse transcriptase complexed with an inhibitor. Science 256:1783, 1992.
2. Shirasaka T, Chokekijchai S, Yamada A, et al. Comparative analysis of anti-human immunodeficiency virus type 1 activities of dideoxynucleoside analogs in resting and activated peripheral blood mononuclear cells. Antimicrob Agents Chemother 39:2555, 1995.
3. Peterson P, Gekker F, Hu S, et al. Anti-human immunodeficiency virus type 1 activities of U-90152 and U-75875 in human brain cell cultures. Antimicrob Agents Chemother 38:2465, 1994.

4. Zhang H, Geethanjali D, Wu J, et al. Kinetic analysis of intravirion reverse transcription in the blood plasma of HIV-1 infected individuals. J Virol 70:628, 1996.
5. Shafer RW, Winters MA, Inversen AKN, et al. Genotypic and phenotypic changes during culture of a multinucleoside-resistant human immunodeficiency virus type 1 strain in the presence and absence of additional reverse transcriptase inhibitors. Antimicrob Agents Chemother 40:2887, 1996.
6. Mirochnick M, Fenton T, Gagnier P, et al. Pharmacokinetics of nevirapine in human immunodeficiency virus type 1-infected pregnant women and their neonates. J Infect Dis 178:368, 1998.
7. Musoke P, Guay LA, Bagenda D, et al. A phase I/II study of the safety and pharmacokinetics of nevirapine in HIV-1-infected pregnant Ugandan women and their neonates (HIVNET 006). AIDS 13:479, 1999.
8. Taylor S, van Heeswijk RPG, Hoetelmans RMW, et al. Concentrations of nevirapine, lamivudine and stavudine in semen of HIV-1-infected men. AIDS 14:1979, 2000.
9. Glynn SL, Yazdanian M. In vitro blood-brain barrier permeability of nevirapine compared to other HIV antiretroviral agents. J Pharm Sci 87:306, 1998.
10. Price RW, Brew B, Sidtis J, et al. The brain in AIDS: central nervous system HIV-1 infection and AIDS dementia complex. Science 239:586, 1988.
11. Kearney B, Price R, Sheiner L, et al. Estimation of nevirapine exposure within the cerebrospinal fluid using CSF:plasma area under the curve ratios. In: Abstracts of the 6th Conference on Retroviruses and Opportunistic Infections, Chicago, 1999, abstract 406.
12. Lamson MJ, Cort S, Sabo JP, et al. Absolute bioavailability of nevirapine in healthy volunteers following oral and intravenous administration. In: Abstracts of the American Association of Pharmaceutical Sciences Meeting, Miami, 1995, abstract PPDM 8356.
13. Lamson MJ, Cort S, Sabo JP, et al. Effects of gender on the single and multiple dose pharmacokinetics of nevirapine 200 mg/d. In: Abstracts of the American Association of Pharmaceutical Sciences Meeting, Miami, 1995, abstract CS 3004.
14. Cheeseman SH, Hattox SE, McLaughlin MM, et al. Pharmacokinetics of nevirapine: initial single-rising-dose study in humans. Antimicrob Agents Chemother 37:178, 1993.
15. Cheeseman SH, Havlir D, McLaughlin M, et al. Phase I/II evaluation of nevirapine alone and in combination with zidovudine for infection with human immunodeficiency virus. J Acquir Immune Defic Syndr Hum Retrovirol 8:141, 1995.
16. Lamson MJ, Cort S, Sabo JP, et al. Effects of food or antacid on the bioavailability of nevirapine 200 mg in 24 healthy volunteers. In: Abstracts of the American Association of Pharmaceutical Sciences Meeting, Miami, 1995, abstract CS 3003.
17. Van Heeswijk RPG, Veldkamp AI, Mulder JW, et al. The steady-state pharmacokinetics of nevirapine during once daily and twice daily dosing in HIV-1-infected individuals. AIDS 14:F77, 2000.
18. García F, Knobel H, Sambeat MA, et al. Comparison of twice-daily stavudine plus once- or twice-daily didanosine and nevirapine in early stages of HIV infection: the SCAN study. AIDS 14:2485, 2000.
19. Havlir D, Cheeseman SH, McLaughlin M, et al. High-dose nevirapine: safety, pharmacokinetics, and antiviral effect in patients with human immunodeficiency virus infection. J Infect Dis 171:537, 1995.
20. Lamson M, Maldonado S, Hutman H, et al. The effects of underlying renal or hepatic dysfunction on the pharmacokinetics of nevirapine (Viramune). In: Abstracts of the 13th International AIDS Conference, Durban, 2000, abstract TuPeB3301.
21. Squires K, Johnson V, Katlama C, et al. The Atlantic study: a randomized, open-label study to evaluate the efficacy and safety of three triple-combination therapies aimed at different HIV targets in antiretroviral naive HIV-1 infected patients (final 48 weeks analysis). In: Abstracts of the 13th International AIDS Conference, Durban, 2000, abstract LbPeB7046.
22. Carr A, Vella S, de Jong MD, et al. A controlled trial of nevirapine plus zidovudine versus zidovudine alone in p24 antigenaemic HIV-infected patients. AIDS 10:635, 1996.
23. D'Aquila RT, Hughes MD, Johnson VA, et al. Nevirapine, zidovudine, and didanosine compared with zidovudine and didanosine in patients with HIV-1 infection. Ann Intern Med 124:1019, 1996.
24. Henry K, Erice A, Tierney C, et al. A randomized, controlled, double-blind study comparing the survival benefit of four different reverse transcriptase inhibitor therapies (three-drug, two-drug, and alternating drug) for the treatment of advanced AIDS. J Acquir Immune Defic Syndr Hum Retrovirol 19:339, 1998.
25. Montaner JSG, Reiss P, Cooper D, et al. A randomized, double-blind trial comparing combinations of nevirapine, didanosine, and zidovudine for HIV-infected patients: the INCAS trial. JAMA 279:930, 1998.
26. Pollard RB, Robinson P, Dransfield K. Safety profile of nevirapine, a nonnucleoside reverse transcriptase inhibitor for the treatment of human immunodeficiency virus infection. Clin Ther 20:1071, 1998.
27. Wit FWN, for the Dutch HIV-Treating Physicians. Experience with nevirapine in previously treated HIV-1 infected individuals. Antivir Ther 5:257, 2000.
28. Wit FWNM, Wood R, Horban A, et al. Prednisolone does not prevent hypersensitivity reactions in antiretroviral drug regimens containing abacavir with or without nevirapine. AIDS 15:2423, 2001.
29. Barreiro P, Soriano V, Casas E, et al. Prevention of nevirapine-associated exanthema using slow dose escalation and/or corticosteroids. AIDS 14:2153, 2000.
30. Martinez E, Arnaiz JA, Cruceta A, et al. Nevirapine-induced liver toxicity: a prospective cohort study. In: Abstracts of the 5th International Congress on Drug Therapy in HIV Infection, Glasgow, 2000, abstract PL8.5.
31. Cahn P, Johnson M, Nusrat R, et al. Hepatic safety with nevirapine (NVP) and two nucleosides in patients with advanced HIV infection, from a placebo (PBO) controlled clinical endpoint trial (1090). In: Abstracts of the 5th International Congress on Drug Therapy in HIV Infection, Glasgow, 2000, abstract PL8.6.
32. Sanne I, FTC-302 Study Investigators, FTC-302 Independent Clinical Steering Committee. Severe liver toxicity in patients receiving two nucleoside analogues and a non-nucleoside reverse transcriptase inhibitor [abstract PL9.3]. AIDS 14(suppl 4):S12, 2000.
33. Wit FWNM, Weverling GJ, Weel J, et al. Incidence of and risk factors for severe hepatotoxicity associated with antiretroviral combination therapy. J Infect Dis 2002:186 (in press).
34. Martínez E, Conget I, Lozano L, et al. Reversion of metabolic abnormalities after switching from HIV-1 protease inhibitors to nevirapine. AIDS 13:805, 1999.
35. Van der Valk M, Kastelein JJP, Murphy RL, et al. Nevirapine-containing antiretroviral therapy in HIV-1 infected patients results in an anti-atherogenic lipid profile. AIDS 15:2407, 2001.
36. MMWR Weekly Report: serious adverse events attributed to nevirapine regimens for postexposure prophylaxis after HIV exposures—worldwide, 1997–2000. JAMA 285:402, 2001.
37. Raboud JM, Montaner JSG, Conway B, et al. Suppression of plasma viral load below 20 copies/ml is required to achieve a long-term response to therapy. AIDS 12:1619, 1998.
38. Montaner JSG, Hogg R, Raboud J, et al. Antiretroviral treatment in 1998. Lancet 352:1919, 1998.
39. Podzamczer D, Ferrer E, Consiglio E, et al. A randomized, open, multicenter trial comparing Combivir plus nelfinavir or nevirapine in HIV-infected naive patients (COMBINE study). In: Abstracts of the 40th Interscience Conference on Antimicrobial Agents and Chemotherapy, Toronto, 2000, abstract 694.
40. Pollard R, 1090 Team. Factors predictive of durable HIV suppression in a randomized double blind trial with nevirapine (NVP), zidovudine (ZDV) and lamivudine (3TC) in treatment-naive (ARV-n) patients with advanced AIDS. In: Abstracts of the 7th Conference on Retroviruses and Opportunistic Infections, San Francisco, 2000, abstract 517.
41. Floridia M, Bucciardini R, Ricciardulli D, et al. A randomized, double-blind trial on the use of a triple combination including nevirapine, a nonnucleoside reverse transcriptase HIV inhibitor, in antiretroviral-naive patients with advanced disease. J Acquir Immune Defic Syndr Hum Retrovirol 20:11, 1999.
42. Harris M, Patenaude P, Cooperberg P, et al. Correlation of virus load in plasma and lymph node tissue in human immunodeficiency virus infection. J Infect Dis 176:1388, 1997.
43. Podzamczer D, Ferrer E, Perez P, et al. Decrease of HIV-1 RNA levels in tonsillar lymphoid tissue of patients receiving Combivir/nevirapine (CNr) or Combivir/nelfinavir (CNf). In: Abstracts of the 13th International AIDS Conference, Durban, 2000, abstract TuPeB3213.
44. Murphy R. Lopinavir/ritonavir. Presented at the HIV DART 2000, Frontiers in Drug Development for Antiretroviral Therapies, Isla Verde, Puerto Rico, USA, 2000, abstract 042.
45. Rachlis A, Becker S, Gill J, et al. Successful substitution of protease inhibitors with Sustiva (efavirenz) in patients with undetectable

plasma HIV-1 RNA levels: results of a prospective, randomized, multicenter, open-label study (DMP 266-049). In: Program and Abstracts of the 40th Interscience Conference on Antimicrobial Agents and Chemotherapy, Toronto, 2000, abstract 475.
46. Negredo E, Cruz L, Ruiz L, et al. Impact of switching from protease inhibitors to nevirapine or efavirenz in patients with viral suppression. In: Program and Abstracts of the 40th Interscience Conference on Antimicrobial Agents and Chemotherapy, Toronto, 2000, abstract 473.
47. Ruiz L, Bonjoch A, Paredes R, et al. A multi-centre randomised open label comparative trial of the clinical benefits of switching the protease inhibitor by nevirapine in HAART-experienced patients suffering lipodystrophy. In: Program and Abstracts of the 6th Conference on Retroviruses and Opportunistic Infections, Chicago, 1999, abstract LB-14.
48. Raffi F, Esnault JL, Reliquet V, et al. The Maintavir study, substitution of a nonnucleoside reverse transcriptase inhibitor (NNRTI) for a protease inhibitor (PI) in patients with undetectable plasma HIV-1 RNA: 18 months follow-up. In: Program and Abstracts of the 40th Interscience Conference on Antimicrobial Agents and Chemotherapy, Toronto, 2000, abstract 474.
49. Opravil M, Hirschel B, Lazzarin A, et al. Simplified maintenance therapy with abacavir + lamivudine + zidovudine in patients with HAART-induced long-term suppression of HIV-1 RNA: final results. In: Program and Abstracts of the 40th Interscience Conference on Antimicrobial Agents and Chemotherapy, Toronto, 2000, abstract 476.
50. Youle M, CNA30017 Study Team. A novel use of abacavir to simplify therapy and reduce long-term toxicity in PI-experienced patients successfully treated with HAART: 48-week results (CNA30017). [abstract PL6.4]. AIDS 14(suppl 4):S7, 2000.
51. Carpenter C, Cooper DA, Fischl MA, et al. Antiretroviral therapy in adults: updated recommendations of the International AIDS Society—USA panel. JAMA 283:381, 2000.
52. Feinberg J, Brun S, Xu Y, et al. Durable suppression of HIV+ RNA after 2 years of therapy with ABT-378/ritonavir (ABT-378/r) treatment in single protease inhibitor experienced patients. In: Abstracts of the 5th International Congress on Drug Therapy in HIV Infection, Glasgow, 2000, abstract P101.
53. Becker S, Brun S, Bertz R, et al. ABT-378/ritonavir (ABT-378/r) and efavirenz: 24 week safety/efficacy evaluation in multiple PI experienced patients. In: Program and Abstracts of the 40th Interscience Conference on Antimicrobial Agents and Chemotherapy, Toronto, 2000, abstract 697.
54. Rockstroh J, Brun S, Sylte J, et al. ABT-378/ritonavir (ABT-378/r) and efavirenz: one year safety/efficacy evaluation in multiple PI experienced patients [abstract P43]. AIDS 14(suppl 4):S29, 2000.
55. Burchett SK, Khoury M, McIntosh K, et al. Viral load reduction (VLR) in children with advanced HIV disease treated with 4-drug antiretroviral treatment (ART) regimens including NRTIs, nevirapine (NVP), nelfinavir (NFV), and/or ritonavir (RTV) (PACTG 366). In: Abstracts of the 7th Conference on Retroviruses and Opportunistic Infections, San Francisco, 2000, abstract 698.
56. Wiznia A, Stanley K, Krogstad P, et al. Combination nucleoside analogs plus nelfinavir, nevirapine, or ritonavir in stable antiretroviral therapy-experienced HIV-infected children. In: Abstracts of the 7th Conference on Retroviruses and Opportunistic Infections, San Francisco, 2000, abstract 697.
57. Luzuriaga K, Bryson Y, Krogstad P, et al. Combination treatment with zidovudine, didanosine, and nevirapine in infants with human immunodeficiency virus type 1 infection. N Engl J Med 336:1343, 1997.
58. Luzuriaga K, McManus M, Catalina M, et al. Early therapy of vertical HIV-1 infection: evidence for cessation of viral replication and absence of virus-specific immunity. In: Abstracts of the 7th Conference on Retroviruses and Opportunistic Infections, San Francisco, 2000, abstract 211.
59. Guay LA, Musoke P, Fleming T, et al. Intrapartum and neonatal single-dose nevirapine compared with zidovudine for prevention of mother-to-child transmission of HIV-1 in Kampala, Uganda: HIVNET 012 randomised trial. Lancet 354:795, 1999.
60. Moodley D, SAINT Trial Team. The SAINT trial: nevirapine (NVP) versus zidovudine (ZDV) + lamivudine (3TC) in prevention of peripartum HIV transmission. In: Abstracts of the 13th International AIDS Conference, Durban, 2000, abstract LbOr2.
61. Shaffer N, Chuachoowong R, Mock PA, et al. Short-course zidovudine for perinatal HIV-1 transmission in Bangkok, Thailand: a randomised controlled trial. Lancet 353:773, 1999.
62. Owor M, Deseyve M, Duefield C, et al. The one year safety and efficacy data of the HIVNET 012 trial. In: Abstracts of the 13th International AIDS Conference, Durban, 2000, abstract LbOr1.
63. Wei X, Ghosh SK, Taylor ME, et al. Viral dynamics in human immunodeficiency virus type 1 infection. Nature 373:117, 1995.
64. MacGregor TR, Lamson MJ, Cort S, et al. Steady state pharmacokinetics of nevirapine, didanosine, zalcitabine and zidovudine combination therapy in HIV-1 positive patients. In: Abstracts of the American Association of Pharmaceutical Sciences Meeting, Miami, 1995, abstract CS 3002.
65. Skowron G, Leoung G, Dusek A, et al. Stavudine (d4T), nelfinavir (NFV) and nevirapine (NVP): preliminary safety, activity and pharmacokinetic (PK) interactions. In: Abstracts of the 5th Conference on Retroviruses and Opportunistic Infections, Chicago, 1998, abstract 350.
66. Sahai J, Cameron W, Salgo M, et al. Drug interaction study between saquinavir (SQV) and nevirapine (NVP). In: Abstracts of the 4th Conference on Retroviruses and Opportunistic Infections. Alexandria, VA, Westover Management Group, 1997, abstract no. 614.
67. Murphy RL, Sommadossi J-P, Lamson M, et al. Antiviral effect and pharmacokinetic interaction between nevirapine and indinavir in persons infected with human immunodeficiency virus type 1. J Infect Dis 179:1116, 1999.
68. Farthing C, Mess T, Ried C, et al. Ritonavir, saquinavir, and nevirapine as a salvage regimen for indinavir or ritonavir resistance. In: Abstracts of the 12th World AIDS Conference, Geneva, 1998, abstract 22356.
69. Harris M, Durakovic C, Rae S, et al. A pilot study of nevirapine, indinavir, and lamivudine among patients with advanced human immunodeficiency virus disease who had failure of combination nucleoside therapy. J Infect Dis 177:1514, 1998.
70. Ruane PJ, Tam JT, Libraty DH, et al. Salvage therapy using ritonavir/saquinavir with a non-nucleoside reverse transcriptase inhibitor after prolonged failure with indinavir or ritonavir. In: Abstracts of the 12th World AIDS Conference, Geneva, 1998, abstract 32308.
71. Kaletra: Prescribing Information. Abbott Park, IL, Abbott Laboratories
72. Veldkamp AI, Hoetelmans RMW, Beijnen JH, et al. DONUT: the pharmacokinetics (PK) of once daily nevirapine (NVP) and efavirenz (EFV) when used in combination. In: Abstracts of the 7th Conference on Retroviruses and Opportunistic Infections, San Francisco, 2000, abstract 80.
73. Leitz G, Mildvan D, McDonough M, et al. Nevirapine (Viramune, NVP) and ethinyl estradiol/norethindrone [Ortho-Novum 1/35 (21 pack) EE/NET] interaction study in HIV-1 infected women. In: Abstracts of the 7th Conference on Retroviruses and Opportunistic Infections, San Francisco, 2000, abstract 89.
74. Gourevitch MN, Friedland GH. Interactions between methadone and medications used to treat HIV infection: a review. Mt Sinai J Med 67:429, 2000.
75. Clarke S, Mulcahy F, Beck D, et al. Managing methadone and non-nucleoside reverse transcriptase inhibitors: guidelines for clinical practice. In: Abstracts of the 7th Conference on Retroviruses and Opportunistic Infections, San Francisco, 2000, abstract 88.
76. Altice FL, Friedland GH, Cooney EL. Nevirapine induced opiate withdrawal among injection drug users with HIV infection receiving methadone. AIDS 13:957, 1999.

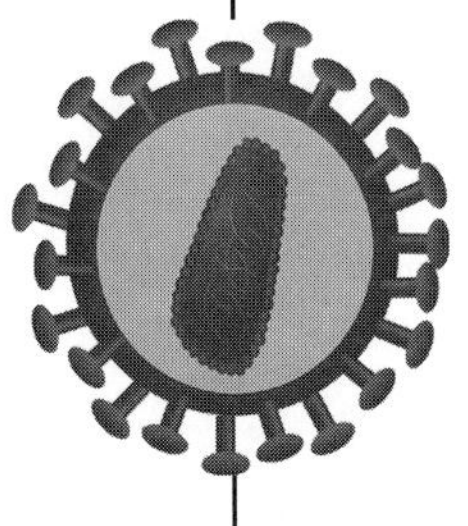

CHAPTER 11

Efavirenz

Douglas L. Mayers, MD

Among the drugs approved for use as antiretroviral agents, most target the reverse transcription step in the life cycle of the human immunodeficiency virus type 1 (HIV-1). Nucleoside agents such as zidovudine, didanosine, zalcitabine, stavudine, and lamivudine act by becoming incorporated in the growing DNA chain and interfering with continued transcription of the genomic RNA of the virus. Nonnucleoside agents, such as nevirapine and delavirdine, target the reverse transcriptase enzyme itself by binding to a unique site within the enzyme that alters its ability to function. Efavirenz (Sustiva) is a nonnucleoside reverse transcriptase inhibitor (NNRTI) that acts in a fashion similar to that of nevirapine and delavirdine. However, efavirenz has several unique properties that make it a highly attractive antiretroviral compound.

▲ STRUCTURE

Efavirenz (Sustiva, previously known as L-743,726 or DMP 266) is the first of a new class of NNRTIs, the 1,4-dihydro-2H-3,1-benzoxazin-2-ones. The drug has the chemical formula (*S*)-6-chloro-4-(cyclopropylethynyl)-1,4-dihydro-4-(trifluoromethyl)-2H-3, 1-benzoxazin-2-one (Fig. 11–1). The compound has a molecular weight of 315.68 and is packaged as an off-white to pink crystalline powder.

▲ IN VITRO ACTIVITY AND MECHANISM OF ACTION

Efavirenz is a potent NNRTI that acts by noncompetitive inhibition of HIV-1 reverse transcriptase with respect to template-primer and nucleotide substrates. Efavirenz is specific for HIV-1 reverse transcriptase, with an in vitro K_i value of 3 nM.[1,2] It does not inhibit the human cellular polymerases α, β, γ, or δ. Efavirenz inhibits laboratory strains of HIV-1 and clinical HIV-1 isolates with 90% to 95% inhibitory concentration (IC_{90-95}) values that range from 1.7 to 25 nM, including isolates resistant to zidovudine and indinavir.[1,3] Efavirenz demonstrated synergy against HIV-1 when combined with zidovudine, didanosine, or indinavir in vitro. The compound has also been shown to be active against recombinant viruses with many of the single-base mutations associated with NNRTI resistance, including Y181C, K101E, L100I, and K103N, with IC_{90} values of 1.5 μM or less. At least two mutations in the HIV-1 reverse transcriptase gene are necessary to produce high-level resistance to efavirenz (see Drug Resistance).[1,3,4]

▲ PHARMACOKINETICS

Efavirenz is well absorbed in humans, with a T_{max} at 3.0 to 5.0 hours using doses of 200 to 600 mg PO daily. The drug has a linear, but not proportional, increase in maximum plasma concentration (C_{max}) and plasma area under the time-concentration curve (AUC) with increasing oral doses, from a C_{max} of 4.6 μM at 200 mg qd to 8.9 to 10.2 μM at 400 mg qd to 12.5 to 14.3 μM at 600 mg qd at steady state (Fig. 11–2).[5] There appears to be diminished absorption of the drug as the dose is increased. The trough drug concentrations at 24 hours are 1.9 μM for the 200 mg dose, 4.2 to 4.3 μM for the 400 mg dose, and 4.5 to 5.5 μM for the 600 mg daily dose. Steady-state concentrations are reached after 6 to 10 days of receiving efavirenz, with a 22% to 42% decrease in AUC observed on day 10 compared with day 1.

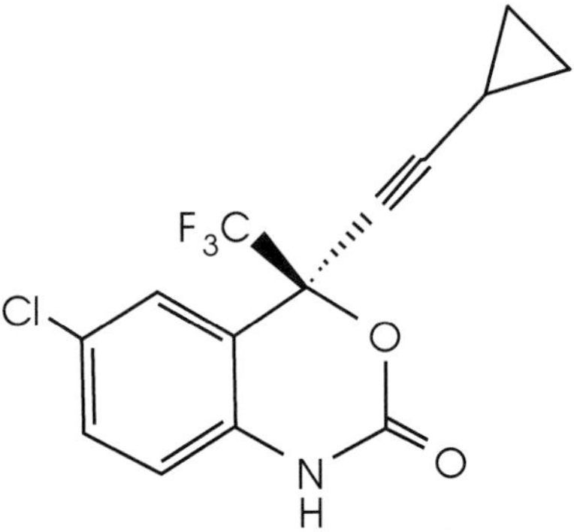

Figure 11–1. Structure of efavirenz.

The terminal half-life for efavirenz is 52 to 76 hours after single doses and 40 to 55 hours after multiple doses.[6]

The AUC and C_{max} of efavirenz given in a capsule were increased 22% and 39%, respectively, by a high-fat meal compared with an overnight fast. Regular meals increased the efavirenz AUC by 17% and C_{max} by 51% compared to fasted conditions. The AUC and C_{max} for the 600 mg efavirenz tablet were increased 28% and 79%, respectively, relative to fasted conditions.[6]

Efavirenz is 99.5% to 99.75% protein-bound such that only 0.5% of the measured drug level is available as free drug to inhibit HIV-1 in vivo.[6] Efavirenz is predominantly bound to albumin. Measurements of efavirenz in cerebrospinal fluid (CSF) are 0.69% (range 0.26% to 1.19%) of plasma levels, consistent with the estimated fraction of free drug.[7–9] Drug levels are not available for other tissue compartments. It is not known if efavirenz is excreted in human breast milk.

Efavirenz is metabolized in the liver via the P_{450} enzyme system. Efavirenz is slowly metabolized by CYP 3A4 and rapidly metabolized by CYP 2B6. Efavirenz appears to inhibit P_{450} isoenzymes 2C9, 2C19, and 3A4 in vitro. Human liver microsomes metabolize efavirenz to a phenolic metabolite (8-OH-efavirenz). The glucuronide conjugate of 8-OH-efavirenz is observed in both plasma and urine. In humans, 66% of a 400 mg dose of efavirenz is excreted in the urine as the glucuronide conjugate of 8-OH-efavirenz. The metabolites are not active against HIV-1. Pharmacokinetic studies suggest that the decreasing AUC observed during the initial weeks of therapy is due to hepatic enzyme induction.[5] In a 1-month mass balance study 14% to 34% of a radiolabeled dose of efavirenz was excreted as efavirenz metabolites in the urine, and 16% to 61% was excreted predominantly unchanged in the feces.[6]

No pharmacokinetic data are available for dose adjustments of efavirenz in patients with hepatic dysfunction. Because less than 1% of efavirenz is excreted unchanged in urine, the impact of renal insufficiency should be minimal.[6]

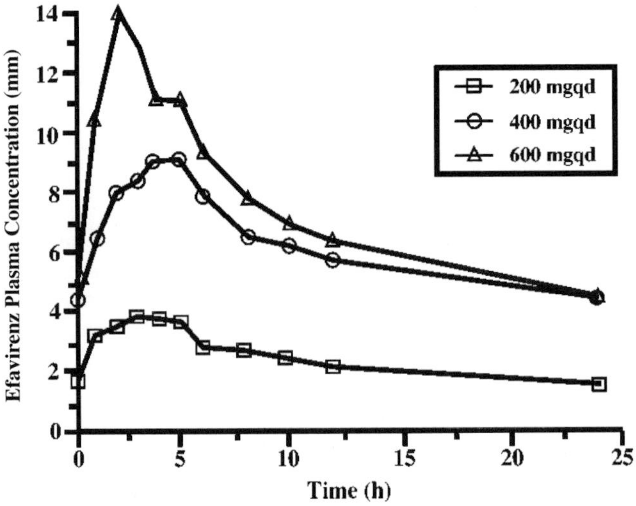

Figure 11–2. Pharmacokinetics of efavirenz in humans. Efavirenz plasma drug concentrations are shown for patients in the efavirenz-003 study who are at steady state after 2 weeks of dosing with efavirenz in combination with indinavir.

▲ TOXICITY

Animal Data

Efavirenz induces hepatic enzymes CYP 2B and CYP 3A in rats and rhesus monkeys and induces CYP 3A and UDP-glucuronyl transferase in cynomolgus monkeys.[5,10] Nephrotoxicity has been observed in rats given high doses of efavirenz but not in nonhuman primates; it is thought to be a species-specific effect.[11]

In cynomolgus monkeys treated with efavirenz for 1 year, mild biliary hyperplasia was observed in four of eight monkeys given 75 mg/kg bid (a dose that gives an AUC in monkeys sixfold greater than the proposed human dose of 600 mg qd). There was no evidence of associated cholestasis or fibrosis and no histologic evidence of hepatocellular injury in these monkeys. Minimal thyroid follicular cell hyperplasia was also seen and was thought to be related to the effect of hepatic enzyme induction on thyroid hormone metabolism in cynomolgus monkeys.[5]

Reproductive Toxicity

Efavirenz shows no evidence of genotoxicity in animal studies. Rat and rabbit studies of developmental and reproductive toxicity have demonstrated no evidence of effects on fertility other than a slight increase in fetal resorptions at 100 mg/kg bid and postnatal mortality at 50 mg/kg bid or more in efavirenz-treated rats. There are marked species differences in the disposition of efavirenz in rats versus humans that make these data difficult to interpret.[5]

Fetal malformations were detected in 3 of 20 fetuses of pregnant cynomolgus monkeys treated with efavirenz in developmental toxicology studies (versus 0 of 20 concomitant controls).[6] Plasma efavirenz concentrations in the monkeys were similar to those in humans receiving 600 mg/day. Efavirenz crossed the placenta and produced fetal blood concentrations similar to maternal blood levels.[6]

Barrier contraception should always be used in combination with other methods of contraception in women of childbearing potential. Women of childbearing potential should undergo pregnancy testing prior to initiating treatment with efavirenz. There are no adequate, well controlled studies of efavirenz use in HIV-infected pregnant women. Clinicians must consider the potential risk/benefit ratio of efavirenz in pregnant HIV-infected women, especially during the first trimester of pregnancy.[6]

Human Data

The most common new-onset adverse events in normal volunteers who received efavirenz were headache and dizziness. For HIV-infected patients who received efavirenz plus indinavir, the most common new-onset adverse events were diarrhea, dizziness, rash, headache, and impaired concentration. For patients who received efavirenz plus zidovudine (ZDV) and lamivudine (3TC), the most frequent new-onset adverse events were abnormal vision, anxiety, diarrhea, dizziness, headache, upper respiratory tract symptoms, nausea, and sinusitis.[12] It is of note that many of the moderate or severe adverse events were equally distributed across the efavirenz and placebo groups in these studies (Table 11–1).[6]

The two types of adverse events most clearly associated with efavirenz were rash and central nervous system symptoms. Rashes in patients receiving efavirenz therapy usually occur during the second week of therapy (median 11 days). In clinical trials, rashes occurred in 26.3% of adults and in 45.6% of children receiving efavirenz versus 17.5% of adult controls. Moderate to severe maculopapular rashes occurred in 15.6% of adults and in 37.0% of children receiving efavirenz compared to 7.7% of adult controls. Treatment with efavirenz can usually be continued with supportive therapy, and the rash usually resolves within 4 weeks (median duration 16 days). Efavirenz should be discontinued in patients who develop severe rash with blistering, desquamation, mucosal involvement, or fever.[6]

Central nervous system symptoms occur in 53% of patients receiving efavirenz. Symptoms include dizziness, insomnia, impaired concentration, somnolence, abnormal dreams, euphoria, confusion, agitation, amnesia, hallucinations, stupor, abnormal thinking, and depersonalization.[6,13] Symptoms are usually mild to moderate in intensity. The symptoms usually occur during the first 2 days of

Table 11–1. PERCENT OF PATIENTS WITH TREATMENT-EMERGENT[1] ADVERSE EVENTS OF MODERATE OR SEVERE INTENSITY REPORTED IN ≥2% OF PATIENTS IN STUDIES 006 AND ACTG 364

	Study 006 LAM, NNRTI and PI-Naive Patients			Study ACTG 364 NNRTI-Experienced/NNRTI-Naive/PI-Naive Patients		
Adverse Events	Sustiva[a] + ZDV/LAM (n = 412)	Sustiva[b] + Indinavir (n = 415)	Indinavir + ZDV/LAM (n = 401)	Sustiva[a] + Nelfinavir + NRTIs (n = 64)	Sustiva[b] + NRTIs (n = 65)	Nelfinavir + NRTIs (n = 66)
Body as a whole						
Fatigue	7	5	8	0	2	3
Pain	1	1	5	13	6	17
Central and peripheral nervous systems						
Dizziness	8	8	3	2	6	6
Headache	7	4	4	5	2	3
Concentration impaired	5	2	0	0	0	0
Inscemnia	6	7	3	0	0	2
Abnormal dreams	3	1	0	—	—	—
Somnolence	3	2	2	0	0	0
Anorexia	1	0	1	0	2	2
Gastrointestinal						
Nausea	12	7	25	3	2	2
Vomiting	7	6	14	—	—	—
Diarrhea	6	8	6	14	3	9
Dyspepsia	3	3	5	0	0	2
Abdominal pain	1	2	4	3	3	3
Psychiatric						
Anxiety	1	3	0	—	—	—
Depression	2	1	0	3	0	5
Nervousness	2	2	0	2	0	2
Skin and appendages						
Rash	13	20	7	9	5	9
Preritus	0	1	1	9	5	9
Increased sweating	2	1	0	0	0	0

[a]Includes adverse events at least possibly related to study drug or of unknown relationship for Study 006. Includes all adverse events regardless of relationship to study drug the Study ACTG 364.
[b]SUSTIVA provided as 600 mg once daily.
Reprinted with permission from Bristol-Myers Squibb Company. Full prescribing information for SUSTIVA® may be found at *www.sustiva.com.*,
—not specified; PI, protease inhibitor.

efavirenz therapy and last several hours. They usually resolve after the first 2 to 4 weeks of continued efavirenz therapy but can persist as mild symptoms for longer periods of time. Rarely, more serious psychiatric symptoms have been reported in patients on efavirenz including severe depression, suicidal ideation, suicide attempts, aggressive behavior, paranoid reactions, and manic reactions. These severe psychiatric reactions are more common in patients with a history of psychiatric illness.[6]

Liver enzymes should be monitored in patients with a history of hepatitis B or C infection or who are receiving medications associated with hepatotoxicity. Elevations of liver enzymes more than five times the upper limit of normal require clinical evaluation to determine the risk of significant liver toxicity versus the benefit of continued efavirenz. Asymptomatic elevations of serum amylase occurred in 10% of patients on efavirenz and 6% on control regimens.[6]

Elevation of nonfasting cholesterol and high density lipoprotein (HDL) occurred in, respectively, 20% and 25% of patients receiving efavirenz/ZDV/3TC and 40% and 35% of patients on efavirenz/indinavir. The effects of efavirenz on triglycerides and low density lipoprotein (LDL) are not well characterized.[6]

▲ EFFICACY: CLINICAL TRIALS RESULTS

Efavirenz has shown significant antiretroviral activity in combination drug regimens for both drug-naive and nucleoside-experienced patients. A summary of clinical studies involving efavirenz is presented in Table 11–2. In the Phase II study efavirenz-003, patients received 2 weeks of efavirenz monotherapy at 200 mg/day followed by combination therapy with efavirenz and indinavir at 800 or 1000 mg PO q8h.[13–19] In this study, efavirenz monotherapy at a dose of 200 mg PO daily produced a 1.68 log copies per milliliter reduction in plasma HIV RNA at 2 weeks. Long-term studies of efavirenz monotherapy were not conducted because of concerns about the emergence of drug-resistant virus with single-drug therapy.

The combination of efavirenz with indinavir has shown significant sustained antiviral activity. At 12 weeks of therapy, patients showed a mean reduction of plasma HIV

▲ **Table 11–2.** SUMMARY OF MAJOR TRIALS OF EFAVIRENZ

Trial	Drug Regimen	Patients	Status	Ref.
Phase I Studies				
Efavirenz-001	Efavirenz single dose 100–1600 mg	94 Healthy adult male volunteers: 70 efavirenz, 24 placebo	Completed	5
Efavirenz-002	Efavirenz multiple doses 200–400 mg qd × 10 days	23 Healthy adult male volunteers: 17 efavirenz, 6 placebo	Completed	5
Efavirenz-019	Efavirenz 400 mg qd + NFV 750 mg tid; 14-day study	20 Healthy volunteers	Completed	38
Phase II Studies				
Efavirenz-003	Efavirenz 200, 400, 600 mg qd + IDV 800, 1000, 1200 mg q8h; 8 cohorts	101 HIV-infected pts: all PI- and NNRTI-naive	Completed	13–19
Efavirenz-004	ZDV 300 mg PO bid + 3TC 150 mg PO bid + efavirenz 400 or 600 mg qd or placebo	97 HIV-infected pts; minimum 8 weeks of ZDV + 3TC	Completed	23
Efavirenz-005	ZDV 300 mg PO bid + 3TC 150 mg PO bid + efavirenz 200, 400, 600 mg qd or placebo	137 HIV-infected pts; antiretroviral drug-naive	Completed	12,22
Efavirenz-020	Blinded, 2 arms: two nucleoside agents + IDV 800 mg tid + efavirenz placebo qd *or* IDV 1000 mg tid + efavirenz 600 mg qd	184 HIV-infected pts	Completed	25
Efavirenz-024	Open label, two strata: NFV 750 mg tid + efavirenz 600 mg qd	62 HIV-infected pts: 32 antiretroviral drug-naive, 30 nucleoside-experienced	Completed	26
Phase III Studies				
Efavirenz-006	Open label, three arms: ZDV + 3TC + efavirenz 600 mg qd, IDV 1000 mg tid + efavirenz 600 mg qd, ZDV + 3TC + IDV 800 mg tid	1236 HIV-infected pts	Ongoing (Phase 3)	6,24
ACTG 364	Blinded, three arms: two NRTI + efavirenz 600 mg qd + NFV 750 mg tid *or* two NRTIs + efavirenz 600 mg qd *or* two NRTIs + NFV 750 mg tid	196 HIV-infected pts	Completed	27
Pediatric Studies				
PACTG 382	Open label: one or more NRTIs + efavirenz (dose adjusted) + NFV (dose adjusted)	57 HIV-infected children	Completed	30

IDV, indinavir; NFV, nelfinavir; NRTI, nucleoside agent; PI, protease inhibitor; 3TC, lamivudine; ZDV, zidovudine.

RNA of 2.3 $\log_{10}$ copies per milliliter with a CD4+ T-lymphocyte count increase of more than 100 cells per cubic millimeter. At this time, 6 of 11 patients (55%) had plasma HIV RNA levels of less than 400 copies per milliliter. During these initial studies, efavirenz was shown to reduce indinavir levels by 35%, whereas indinavir had no impact on the kinetics of efavirenz.[15,20] Indinavir doses were subsequently increased to 1000 mg PO q8h when indinavir was combined with efavirenz.

At 24 weeks the combination of efavirenz and indinavir produced an average reduction of plasma HIV RNA of 2.4 $\log_{10}$ copies per milliliter, with 82% of patients with plasma HIV RNA having less than 400 copies per milliliter compared to 43% of patients on indinavir alone. The average rise in CD4+ T-lymphocyte count remained higher than 100 cells per cubic millimeter. At 60 weeks of therapy, the mean reduction in plasma HIV RNA was 2.43 $\log_{10}$ copies per milliliter for efavirenz/indinavir, with 89% of patients having HIV RNA values of less than 400 copies per milliliter. The CD4+ T-lymphocyte count had increased to 267 cells per cubic millimeter above baseline values.[18] Patients on the indinavir-only arm had stavudine and efavirenz added at week 27. At week 60, the group on stavudine/efavirenz/indinavir had a mean reduction in plasma HIV RNA of 1.90 $\log_{10}$ copies per milliliter, with 68% of patients having plasma HIV RNA values less than 400 copies per milliliter, and a mean CD4+ T-lymphocyte count rise of 210 cells per cubic millimeter above baseline values.[18] These results have been maintained up to 72 weeks of follow-up with 85% of the patients on efavirenz/indinavir having HIV RNA values less than 400 copies per milliliter and a mean CD4+ T-lymphocyte count increase of 243 cells per cubic millimeter above baseline. The rate of decrease in plasma HIV RNA below 400 copies per milliliter was similar for patients with baseline plasma HIV RNA values above or below 100,000 copies per milliliter: 86% and 83%, respectively.[19]

Preliminary data suggest that a twice-a-day regimen of indinavir 1200 mg PO q12h/efavirenz 300 mg PO q12h may be as active as the standard regimen of indinavir 1000 mg PO q8h/efavirenz 600 mg PO qhs at 16 weeks.[21] Longer follow-up of this cohort is needed before these two regimens can be considered equivalent.

Efavirenz-005 is a study of three doses of efavirenz (200, 400, and 600 mg PO qd) versus placebo combined with ZDV 300 mg PO bid and 3TC 150 mg PO bid.[12,22] Patients were antiretroviral-naive with mean entry plasma HIV RNA levels of 52,500 copies per cubic millimeter and CD4+ T-lymphocyte counts of 367 cells per milliliter. Patients in the placebo arm of ZDV/3TC were allowed to add efavirenz and indinavir to their regimen at week 16 of the study. All three doses of efavirenz were well tolerated. There was a 12% rate of maculopapular rashes during the study. At week 24 there were 91% to 100% of patients in the efavirenz-containing arms who had plasma HIV RNA levels of less than 400 copies per milliliter versus 65% of patients in the placebo arm. CD4+ T-lymphocyte count rises ranged from 105 to 170 cells per cubic millimeter in the efavirenz-containing arms at week 24 versus 87 cells per cubic millimeter in the placebo arm.

Efavirenz was much less active when added to ZDV and 3TC in patients with detectable plasma HIV RNA values of more than 2500 copies per milliliter who had received at least 8 weeks of prior ZDV and 3TC (efavirenz-004).[23] In this trial, only 72% of patients on the 600 mg efavirenz arm achieved a plasma HIV RNA level of less than 400 copies per milliliter compared to 47% of patients on the 400 mg efavirenz arm. The median time to failure was 10 weeks in the 600 mg efavirenz arm. Based on this trial, efavirenz should not be added as monotherapy to a drug regimen with detectable viral replication. These data also support the decision to use the 600 mg dose as the standard dose of efavirenz in combination drug regimens.

Efavirenz-006 was a randomized open-label trial of ZDV/3TC/efavirenz 600 mg PO qhs versus ZDV/3TC/indinavir 800 mg PO q8h versus efavirenz 600 mg PO qhs/indinavir 1000 mg PO q8h. The study initially involved 450 patients who were naive to 3TC, NNRTI agents, and protease inhibitors with mean entry plasma HIV RNA levels of 58,900 copies per milliliter and mean CD4+ T-lymphocyte counts of 345 cells per cubic millimeter.[24] At 48 weeks of follow-up, using an intent-to-treat analysis for HIV RNA levels less than either 400 copies per milliliter or 50 copies per milliliter, the ZDV/3TC/efavirenz arm was clearly superior to the ZDV/3TC/indinavir arm. The efavirenz/indinavir arm had results similar to those of the ZDV/3TC/indinavir arm. By intent-to-treat analysis, 70% of patients on efavirenz versus 48% of patients on indinavir had plasma HIV RNA levels of less than 400 copies per milliliter ($P < 0.05$). These results were also seen for patients who entered the trial with plasma HIV RNA levels of more than 100,000 copies per milliliter and for a less than 50 copies of HIV RNA per milliliter endpoint at 48 weeks. The results of the intent-to-treat analysis were heavily influenced by a higher withdrawal rate from the ZDV/3TC/indinavir arm (with higher rates of nausea and vomiting) compared to the ZDV/3TC/efavirenz arm: 26 versus 10 patients, respectively.

Enrollment in this trial was expanded to 1266 patients with a mean CD4+ T-lymphocyte count of 341 cells cubic millimeter and a mean HIV RNA level of 60,250 copies per cubic milliliter.[6] The mean CD4+ T-lymphocyte count increase was approximately 200 cells per milliliter for all three arms of the trial. At 48 weeks those who met the HIV RNA criterion of less than 400 copies per cubic millimeter (or less than 50 copies per milliliter) amounted to 68% (62%) for the ZDV/3TC/efavirenz arm, 55% (49%) for the efavirenz/indinavir arm, and 49% (43%) for the ZDV/3TC/indinavir arm (Fig. 11–3).[6] A time to treatment failure Kaplan-Meier analysis was performed for patients followed up to 112 weeks in Study 006 (Fig. 11–4).[6]

Efficacy in Treatment-Experienced Adults

Efavirenz has been evaluated as a component of combination drug regimens used to treat highly treatment-experienced patient populations.[25–29]

Efavirenz-020 was a double-blind, placebo-controlled trial that compared the activity of efavirenz plus indinavir plus two nucleoside agents versus indinavir plus two nucleoside agents in nucleoside-experienced patients.[25] The study involved 327 patients who had a mean 2.8 years of prior nucleoside therapy but were naive to NNRTI agents and protease

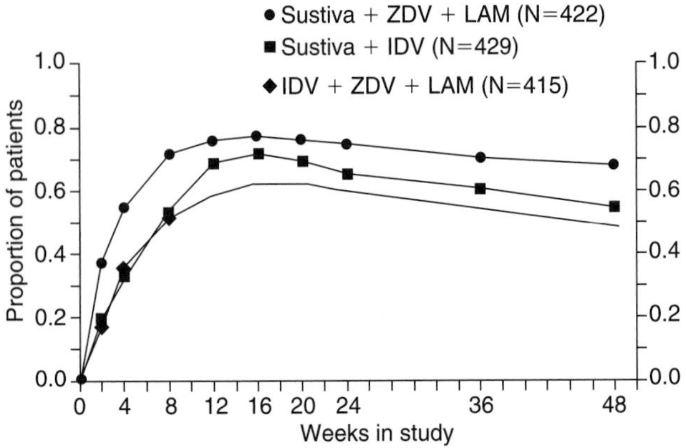

Figure 11–3. Results of the efavirenz-006 study: proportion of patients with an HIV RNA level of less than 400 copies per milliliter who are on their original study medication and who have not experienced an AIDS-defining event. Reprinted with permission from Bristol-Myers Squibb Company. Full prescribing information for SUSTIVA® may be found at *www.sustiva.com.*

inhibitors. The mean entry plasma HIV RNA levels were 25,557 copies per milliliter, and the mean CD4+ T-lymphocyte counts were 329 cells per cubic millimeter. At 24 weeks of follow-up, 68.2% of the patients on the four-drug regimen had plasma HIV RNA levels of less than 400 copies per milliliter compared to 52.4% on the three-drug regimen (P = 0.004).

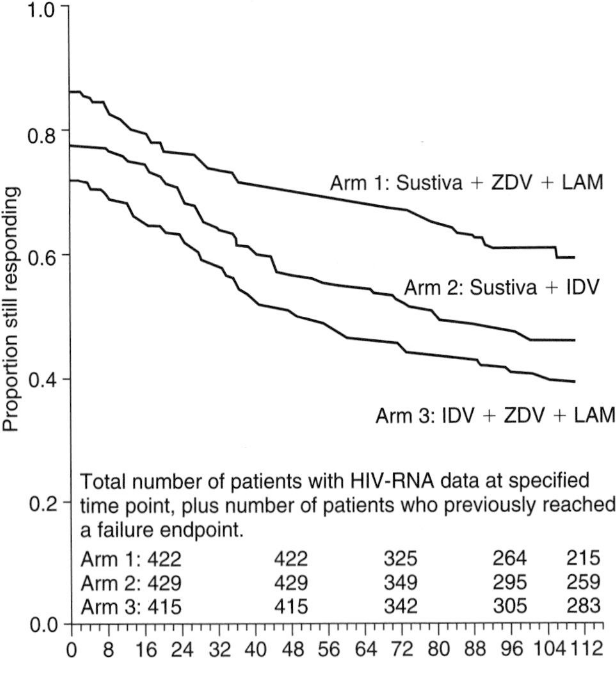

Figure 11–4. Results of the efavirenz-006 study: time to treatment failure. Patients were considered to have reached a study endpoint when they had a confirmed HIV RNA level of 400 copies per milliliter or more, an AIDS-defining event or discontinued study medication. Patients who never achieved an HIV RNA level of less than 400 copies per milliliter were assigned a study endpoint at time zero. Reprinted with permission from Bristol-Myers Squibb Company. Full prescribing information for SUSTIVA® may be found at *www.sustiva.com.*

CD4+ T-lymphocyte counts increased by 104 ± 9 cells per cubic millimeter on the four-drug regimen and 77 ± 10 cells per cubic millimeter on the three-drug regimen. Viral load responses were sustained at 48 weeks on the four-drug regimen.

Efavirenz-024 is an open-label evaluation of efavirenz 600 mg PO qhs/nelfinavir 750 mg PO q8h in both nucleoside-naive and nucleoside-experienced patients.[26] The study involved 62 patients (32 drug-naive, 30 nucleoside-experienced) with mean plasma HIV RNA levels of 38,900 copies per milliliter and mean CD4+ T-lymphocyte counts of 370 cells per milliliter at baseline. At 16 weeks of follow-up, 73% of patients had plasma HIV RNA levels of less than 400 copies per cubic millimeter, and 55% had less than 50 copies per milliliter. There were no significant differences in HIV RNA levels between the nucleoside naive and experienced groups. The mean increase in CD4+ lymphocyte count was 48 cells per cubic millimeter at 16 weeks. The combination was generally well tolerated, with diarrhea the most frequently reported side effect.

ACTG 364 was a randomized, double-blind, placebo-controlled comparison of nelfinavir versus efavirenz versus efavirenz plus nelfinavir combined with two nucleoside analogues (one of which was new) in nucleoside-experienced HIV-infected patients.[27] The study included 196 patients with a median 5.6 years of nucleoside therapy, a baseline mean CD4+ T-lymphocyte count of 389 cells per cubic millimeter, and a mean baseline HIV RNA level of 8130 copies per milliliter. The primary endpoint of the study was an HIV RNA level of less than 500 copies per milliliter at week 16 with a secondary endpoint of the composite HIV RNA levels measured at weeks 40 and 48. At weeks 16 and 48, respectively, 81% and 71% of patients on efavirenz/nelfinavir, 69% and 63% of patients on efavirenz, and 64% and 41% of patients on nelfinavir had HIV RNA levels of less than 500 copies per milliliter (Fig. 11–5).[6] There was no sig-

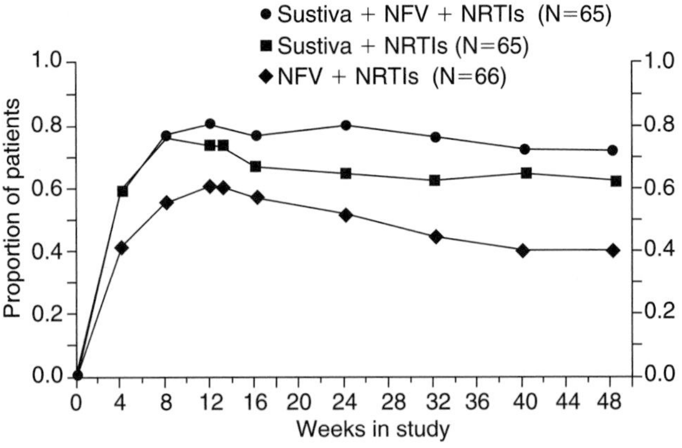

* Proportions of patients at each time pint who have HIV-RNA, 500 copies confirmed by two consecutive observations and are on their original study medication and who have not experienced an AIDS-defining event.

Figure 11–5. Results of the ACTG 364 study: proportion of patients with an HIV RNA level of less than 500 copies per milliliter confirmed by two consecutive observations, who are on their original study medication, and who have not experienced an AIDS-defining event. Reprinted with permission from Bristol-Myers Squibb Company. Full prescribing information for SUSTIVA® may be found at *www.sustiva.com.*

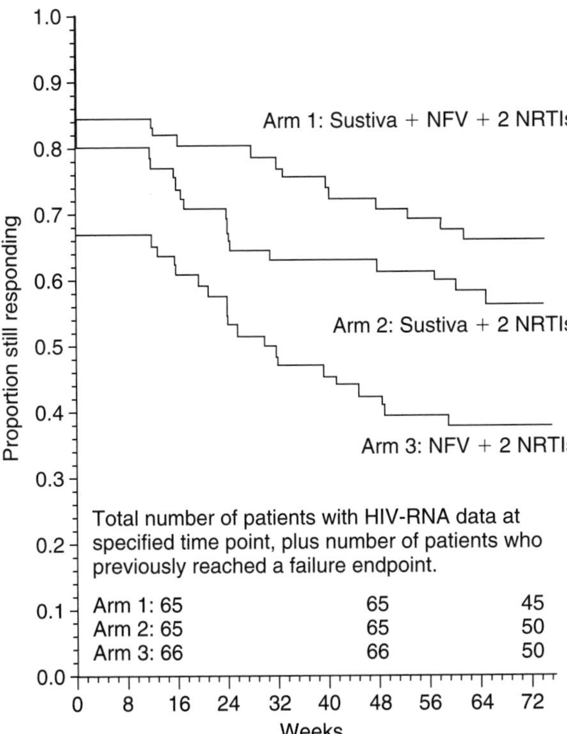

Figure 11–6. Results of the ACTG 364 study: time to treatment failure. Patients were considered to have reached a study endpoint when they had a confirmed HIV RNA level of 500 copies per milliliter or more, had an AIDS-defining event, or had discontinued the study medication. Patients who never achieved an HIV RNA level of less than 500 copies per milliliter were assigned a study endpoint at time zero. The plateaus observed through week 12 are due to the HIV RNA testing schedule and lack of dropouts during this period. Reprinted with permission from Bristol-Myers Squibb Company. Full prescribing information for SUSTIVA® may be found at *www.sustiva.com.*

nificant difference in the CD4+ T-lymphocyte counts among the treatment groups, with a mean overall increase of 100 cells at 48 weeks for patients who remained on their assigned treatment. The four-drug regimen was more effective than either three-drug regimen in this heavily nucleoside-experienced population during follow-up out to 72 weeks (Fig. 11–6).[6]

Pediatric Efficacy

The open-label combination of efavirenz, nelfinavir, and one or more nucleoside reverse transcriptase inhibitors (NRTIs) was evaluated in 57 nucleoside-experienced children (PACTG 382).[30] At baseline the HIV-infected children (age range 3.8 to 16.8 years) had median CD4+ T-lymphocyte counts of 699 cells per cubic millimeter and median plasma HIV RNA levels of 10,000 copies per milliliter. At 48 weeks of follow-up, 76% of patients had plasma HIV RNA levels of less than 400 copies per milliliter, and 63% had less than 50 copies per milliliter. The combination was generally well tolerated, with the most common side effects of at least moderate severity being rash (30%), diarrhea (18%), neutropenia (12%), and biochemical abnormalities (12%).

▲ DRUG RESISTANCE

In Vitro Data

Selection of drug-resistant virus in cell culture was significantly more difficult with efavirenz than with previous NNRTIs.[1,3] Initial studies with recombinant viruses demonstrated that most single-point mutations in the reverse transcriptase gene previously associated with NNRTI resistance had only a modest impact on susceptibility to efavirenz (Table 11–3).[4] The exception was Y188L, which caused a 500-fold decrease in susceptibility to efavirenz. In most instances, combinations of two or more mutations were necessary to produce high-level resistance to efavirenz. In MT-2 cells, 23 passages of HIV-1 in the presence of drug were necessary to produce high-level resistance to efavirenz. The virus selected had three mutations (L100I, V179D, Y181C) and an IC_{90} that was higher than 0.95 μM (> 300-fold decreased susceptibility to efavirenz). After 10 weeks of exposure to efavirenz, HIV-1 infected peripheral blood mononuclear cells produced a virus highly resistant to efavirenz with two mutations (L100I, V108I).[3] Similarly, investigators developed a highly efavirenz-resistant virus with serial passage of HIV-IIIb in the presence of drug that had two mutations (L100I, K103N).[1] The K103N and L100I mutated viruses show the highest resistance to efavirenz of all the single nucleotide substitutions (18-fold loss of potency). The viruses with K103N conferred cross-resistance to nevirapine and delavirdine.[31]

▲ **Table 11–3.** EFAVIRENZ IN VITRO DRUG RESISTANCE
▲ MUTATIONS

Source Mutation(s)	IC_{90-95} (μM)	Refs.
Recombinant viruses		
None (WT)	0.002–0.003	1, 3
A98G	0.012	
L100I	0.100	
K101E	0.025	
K103N	0.100	
V106A	0.012	
V108I	0.003	
V179D	0.003	
Y181C	0.006	
Y188L	1.500	
K101E + K103N	1.500	
K101E + L100I	1.500	
K103N + Y181C	0.400	
Viruses selected in vitro		
V179D	0.027	1, 3
L100I	0.089	
L100I + K103N	25.00	
L100I + V108I	>3.00	
L100I + V179D + Y181C	>0.95	
Viruses detected in vivo		
K103N	0.069–0.180	32, 33
K103N + V108I	0.390	

In Vivo Data

Genotypic data from patients with a rebound in viral load on efavirenz show that the most common mutation detected is K103N, with changes also detected at amino acid positions 98, 100, 101, 106, 108, 188, 190, and 225.[32,33] K103N is the predominant mutation associated with treatment failure with efavirenz. K103N is detected as the sole NNRTI-associated mutation in more than 90% of HIV isolates at the time of virologic rebound.[32,33] The subsequent addition of either a V108I or P225H mutation leads to higher level resistance to efavirenz. Viruses obtained at the time of virologic rebound on efavirenz demonstrate a mean 47-fold decrease in efavirenz susceptibility and high level cross-resistance to nevirapine and delavirdine.[6]

Some patients with extensive prior nucleoside exposure appear to have HIV-1 with nucleoside resistance-associated mutations that are hypersusceptible to NNRTI agents, by one phenotypic HIV-1 drug susceptibility assay. Short-term virologic responses to efavirenz-containing regimens appear to be enhanced in patients with these viruses.[34,35]

Responses to efavirenz were either transient or were significantly reduced for patients with prior NNRTI exposure and a virus containing either a K103N, Y181C, or G190A mutation or any two other NNRTI-associated mutations.[36,37]

▲ DRUG INTERACTIONS

Efavirenz is a modest inducer of CYP 3A4 and inhibits P_{450} isozymes 2C9, 2C19, and 3A4 at concentrations observed in vivo. Plasma concentrations of drugs primarily metabolized by CYP 2C9, 2C19, and 3A4 may be altered if co-administered with efavirenz. Drugs that induce CYP 3A4 can lower plasma efavirenz levels. Efavirenz is unlikely to affect the disposition of drugs excreted primarily by the kidney unchanged.[6]

HIV Protease Inhibitors

Efavirenz has been shown to decrease the area under the time-concentration curve (AUC) for indinavir by 31% (Table 11–4) such that the indinavir dose should be increased to 1000 mg PO tid when indinavir is co-administered with efavirenz.[20] Efavirenz increases the AUC for nelfinavir by 20%; no dose adjustment is recommended when efavirenz and nelfinavir are co-administered.[38–40] Efavirenz increases the AUC of ritonavir by 18%, and ritonavir increases the AUC of efavirenz by 21%.[41] No dosage adjustment is recommended unless there is intolerance attributed to ritonavir, but liver enzymes should be monitored. Efavirenz decreases the AUC of amprenavir by 36%.[42] Preliminary results indicate that efavirenz decreases the AUC of saquinavir by 62%, whereas saquinavir decreases the AUC of efavirenz by 12%. It is not recommended that saquinavir be given as the only protease inhibitor in combination with efavirenz.[6] Validated data are not yet available for the use of efavirenz in combination with ritonavir-boosted protease inhibitor combinations.[6]

Opportunistic Infection Drugs

Efavirenz has no significant impact on the pharmacokinetics of fluconazole[43] (Table 11–4). Rifampin induces efavirenz metabolism with a 26% decrease in the AUC of efavirenz. Because no doses of efavirenz higher than 600 mg have been evaluated, no dose adjustment is recommended at this time. Efavirenz does not appear to affect rifampin metabolism compared to that of historical controls.[44] Efavirenz decreases the AUC of rifabutin by 38%, but rifabutin does not affect efavirenz levels. Daily rifabutin doses should be increased by 50%, and two- to three-times-a-week doses should be doubled in the presence of efavirenz.[6] Efavirenz does not significantly affect the AUC of azithromycin.[45] Efavirenz decreases the AUC for clarithromycin by 39% and increases the AUC of the 14-OH metabolite of clarithromycin by 34%. The clinical impact of the changes in clarithromycin metabolism is not known, and clarithromycin is not currently recommended to be given with efavirenz.[45] No data are available for other drugs used to treat opportunistic infections at this time.

Commonly Used Medications

Aluminum/magnesium hydroxide antacids and famotidine do not appear to affect the levels of efavirenz[6] (Table 11–4). The AUC for ethinyl estradiol was increased by 37%. Women of childbearing potential are encouraged to add a barrier contraceptive when receiving efavirenz.[6,46] Cetirizine levels are not affected by efavirenz. Patients receiving methadone should be monitored carefully for withdrawal symptoms when efavirenz is co-administered. Methadone doses were increased 22% on average in patients receiving efavirenz.[6,47] Patients receiving warfarin, anticonvulsants, imidazole and triazole antifungals, quinidine, or clonazepam may need to have their dosage readjusted. St. John's wort is expected to substantially decrease plasma levels of efavirenz and should be avoided.[6]

Contraindicated Medications

Certain drugs that have narrow therapeutic indices and are metabolized by CYP3A should not be co-administered to patients receiving efavirenz. Examples of medications that should be avoided include astemizole, cisapride, midazolam, triazolam, and ergot derivatives (Table 11–4).

▲ RECOMMENDATIONS FOR USE

Efavirenz is a versatile drug that may be used as initial therapy or as part of a combination regimen for more heavily pretreated patients. The drug should *always* be used as part of a combination regimen, usually with at least two other agents, and never used alone as monotherapy. Owing to its convenient once-daily dosing and its relative potency, many experts recommend efavirenz as part of an initial regimen for newly diagnosed patients. The major drawbacks to the use of efavirenz as first-line treatment are the risks

▲ **Table 11–4.** IMPORTANT DRUG INTERACTIONS SEEN WITH EFAVIRENZ

Co-administered Drug	Drug Interaction		Dose Adjustment
	Co-administered Drug	Efavirenz	
Nucleoside Agents			
Zidovudine	None	None	None
Lamivudine	None	None	None
HIV-1 Protease Inhibitors			
Saquinavir SGC	Decreases AUC 62%	Decreases AUC 12%	Not recommended as sole PI
Indinavir	Decreases AUC 31%	None	Increase IDV to 1000 mg tid
Ritonavir	Increases AUC 18%	Increases AUC 21%	None; monitor liver enzymes
Nelfinavir	Increases AUC 20%	None	None
Metabolite AG-1402	Decreases AUC 37%		
Amprenavir	Decreases AUC 36%	Unknown	Unknown
Ritonavir/saquinavir	Unknown	Unknown	Unknown
Opportunistic Infection Agents			
Fluconazole	None	Increases AUC 16%	None
Rifampin	None	Decreases AUC 26%	Unknown
Rifabutin	Decreases AUC by 38%	None	Increase daily rifabutin dose by 50%, consider doubling dose if given two or three times a week
Azithromycin	None	None	None
Clarithromycin	Decreases AUC 39% Increases 14-OH CLR AUC 34%	None	Not recommended in combination
Commonly Used Medications			
Cetirizine	None	Decreased AUC 8%	None
Ethinyl estradiol	Increased AUC 37%	None	Use barrier contraception along with oral contraceptive
Lorazepam	Increased AUC 7%	Unknown	None
Methadone	Decreased AUC 52%	Unknown	Observe for withdrawl and increase methadone dose (mean dose increase 22%)
Antacids	Unknown	None	None
Famotidine	Unknown	None	None
Warfarin	Unknown	Unknown	Potential for drug interaction
Anticonvusants	Unknown	Unknown	Periodic drug level monitoring
Contraindicated Medications			
Astemizole (antihistamine)			
Midazolam, triazolam (benzodiazepines)			
Cisapride (gastrointestinal motility agent)			
Ergot derivatives (antimigraine)			

AUC, area under the time–concentration curve; 14-OH CLR, 14-OH metabolite of clarithromycin; PI, protease inhibitor; SGC, soft-gel capsules.

associated with a single point mutation (e.g., K103N) resulting in NNRTI-clan resistance and central nervous system (CNS) side effects, which lead to early discontinuation of therapy in a number of patients (approximately 8% to 10%). Other clinicians prefer to hold NNRTI therapy, including efavirenz, for later in the treatment course after the first or second regimen failure. When this approach is taken, efavirenz should be a component of a more potent regimen (e.g., a regimen containing all three classes of drugs).

Dose

The current recommended dose of efavirenz for adults is 600 mg PO once daily. Efavirenz is available as 50, 100, or 200 mg capsules or as a 600 mg film-coated tablet. The 600 mg single tablet allows much more convenient dosing of the drug (one tablet, once daily). The dose should be taken at bedtime on an empty stomach. Pediatric dose recommendations for efavirenz have been developed for children 3 years of age or older who weigh at least 10 kg (10 to <15 kg, 200 mg PO; 15 to <20 kg, 250 mg PO; 20 to <25 kg, 300 mg PO; 25 to <32.5 kg, 350 mg PO qd; 32.5 to <40 kg, 400 mg PO; and ≥40 kg, 600 mg PO.[6]

Food

Efavirenz levels are increased by both regular and high-fat meals. The manufacturer recommends that efavirenz be taken on an empty stomach prior to bedtime to decrease adverse events and improve the tolerability of CNS effects.[6]

Pregnancy

Efavirenz is a pregnancy category C drug that has produced fetal malformations in fetuses/infants of efavirenz-treated cynomolgus monkeys. Efavirenz should be used during pregnancy only if the potential benefit justifies the potential fetal risk such as a pregnant mother without other therapeutic options. Physicians are encouraged to register HIV-infected pregnant women exposed to efavirenz with the Antiviral Pregnancy Registry (phone: 800-258-4263) to monitor fetal outcomes. Mothers should be instructed not to breast-feed if they are receiving efavirenz.[6]

Overdose

Accidental ingestion of efavirenz of more than 600 mg/day has resulted in increased CNS symptoms. Involuntary muscle contractions were noted in one patient. Treatment of an overdose consists of supportive measures with close monitoring of vital signs and clinical status. Oral administration of activated charcoal can be considered. Dialysis is unlikely to be effective, and no specific antidote is available.[6]

▲ MANAGEMENT OF TOXICITIES

Rash

Rashes with efavirenz therapy usually occur during the second week of therapy. Approximately 8% to 18% of patients develop a maculopapular rash of mild to moderate severity. For most rashes, efavirenz can be continued at full dose or reduced to half-dose, along with symptomatic care with antihistamines. Rashes usually resolve over several days but can occur for up to a month. For severe rashes (<17% of patients), efavirenz should be discontinued until the rash resolves. Full-dose efavirenz can then usually be restarted several days later. Stevens-Johnson syndrome has been rare, occurring in 0.14% of patients receiving efavirenz. Efavirenz should be permanently discontinued in any patient who develops severe rash associated with blistering, desquamation, mucosal involvement, or fever. Prophylaxis with appropriate antihistamines should be considered in pediatric patients starting efavirenz.[6]

Central Nervous System Symptoms

Central nervous system symptoms of dizziness (28.1%), insomnia (16.3%), impaired concentration (8.3%), somnolence (7.0%), abnormal dreams (6.2%), and hallucinations (1.2%) have been reported at all doses of efavirenz. They appear in 53% of patients receiving efavirenz (compared to 25% of control patients) and are usually mild to moderate in intensity. The symptoms usually occur during the first 2 days of efavirenz therapy and last for several hours after each dose. They usually resolve after the first 2 to 4 weeks of continued efavirenz therapy but can persist as mild symptoms for a longer time. Symptoms were reported to be severe in 2.0% of patients, and 2.1% of patients discontinued efavirenz because of CNS symptoms. Taking efavirenz prior to bedtime can reduce symptoms. There have been no laboratory abnormalities associated with these subjective findings in clinical trial participants. Patients should be encouraged to continue efavirenz at the full dose at bedtime for 2 weeks. Patients should be informed of the potential for additive CNS effects when efavirenz is taken with alcohol or psychoactive drugs. Patients with impaired concentration or drowsiness should avoid potentially hazardous activities such as driving or operating heavy machinery.[6]

Psychiatric Symptoms

Serious psychiatric adverse experiences have been reported in patients treated with efavirenz. Rates for events (compared to control regimens) have included severe depression 1.6% (0.6%), suicidal ideation 0.6% (0.3%), nonfatal suicide attempts 0.4% (0%), aggressive behavior 0.4% (0.3%), paranoid reactions 0.4% (0.3%) and manic reactions 0.1% (0%). Patients with a history of psychiatric disorders appear to be at a greater risk of serious psychiatric adverse events. Patients with serious psychiatric adverse experiences should seek immediate medical evaluation to determine if the symptoms are related to efavirenz and if the risk of continued therapy outweighs the benefit.[6]

Cannabinoid Test Interaction

False-positive urine cannabinoid test results have been reported with the CEDIA DAU Multi-Level THC assay used for screening. This result has not been observed for cannabinoid assays used to confirm positive results.[6]

REFERENCES

1. Young SD, Britcher SF, Tran LO, et al. L-743,726 (DMP-266): a novel, highly potent nonnucleoside inhibitor of the human immunodeficiency virus type 1 reverse transcriptase. Antimicrob Agents Chemother 39:2602, 1995.
2. Young SD. DMP-266: a novel, highly potent nonnucleoside inhibitor of the human immunodeficiency virus type 1 reverse transcriptase. In: Abstracts of the XIth International Conference on AIDS, Vancouver, BC, 1996, abstract Mo.A.1077.
3. Winslow DL, Garber S, Reid C, et al. Selection conditions affect the evolution of specific mutations in the reverse transcriptase gene associated with resistance to DMP 266. AIDS 10:1205, 1996.
4. Winslow D, Anton R, Horlick R, et al. Construction of infectious molecular clones of HIV-1 containing defined mutations in the protease gene. Biochem Biophys Res Commun 205:1651, 1994.
5. Investigational Drug Brochure: DMP 266. Wilmington, DE, DuPont Merck Pharmaceutical Company, 1997.
6. Package Insert: Sustiva™ (Efavirenz) Capsules and Tablets. Princeton, NJ, Bristol-Myers Squibb, January 2002.
7. Fiske WD, Nibbelink DW, Brennan JM, et al. DMP 266 cerebrospinal fluid concentrations (CSF) after oral administration. In: Abstracts of the 37th Interscience Conference on Antimicrobial Agents and Chemotherapy, Toronto, 1997, abstract A-12.
8. Fiske WD, Brennan JM, Haines PJ, et al. Efavirenz (DMP 266) cerebrospinal fluid (CSF) concentrations after chronic oral administration to cynomolgus monkeys. In: Abstracts of the 5th Conference on Retroviruses and Opportunistic Infections, Chicago. Alexandria, VA, Westover Management Group, 1998, Abstract 640.
9. Tashima KT, Caliendo AMC, Ahmad MA, et al. Cerebrospinal fluid human immunodeficiency virus type 1 (HIV-1) suppression and efavirenz drug concentrations in HIV-1 infected patients receiving combination therapy. J Infect Dis 180:862, 1999.
10. Balani SK, Kauffman LR, deLuna FA, Lin JH. Nonlinear pharmacokinetics of efavirenz (DMP-266), a potent HIV-1 reverse transcriptase inhibitor, in rats and monkeys. Drug Metab Dispos 27:41, 1999.

11. Mutlib AE, Gerson RJ, Meunier PC, et al. The species-dependent metabolism of efavirenz produces a nephrotoxic glutathione conjugate in rats. Toxicol Appl Pharmacol 169:102, 2000.
12. Haas D, Hicks C, Seekins D, et al. A phase II, double-blind, placebo-controlled, dose-ranging study to assess the antiretroviral activity and safety of efavirenz (DMP 266) in combination with open-label zidovudine (ZDV) with lamivudine (3TC) at 24 weeks (DMP 266-005). In: Abstracts of the 5th Conference on Retroviruses and Opportunistic Infections, Chicago. Alexandria, VA, Westover Management Group, 1998, abstract 698.
13. Blanch J, Martinez E, Rousaud A, et al. Preliminary data of a prospective study of neuropsychiatric side effects after initiation of efavirenz. J Acquir Immuno Defic Syndr 27:336, 2001.
14. Wagner K, Kahn J, Mayers D, et al. Long-term anti-HIV-1 activity and tolerability of DMP 266 in combination with indinavir. In: Abstracts of the European Congress of Microbiology and Infectious Diseases, Lausanne, 1997.
15. Mayers D, Riddler S, Stein D, et al. A double-blind pilot study to evaluate the antiviral activity, tolerability, and pharmacokinetics of DMP 266 alone and in combination with indinavir. In: Abstracts of the 36th Interscience Conference on Antimicrobial Agents and Chemotherapy, New Orleans, 1996, abstract LB08A.
16. Mayers DL, Riddler S, Bach M, et al. Durable clinical anti-HIV-1 activity and tolerability for DMP 266 in combination with indinavir (IDV) at 24 weeks. In: Abstracts of the 37th Interscience Conference on Antimicrobial Agents and Chemotherapy, Toronto, 1997, abstract I-175.
17. Ruiz N, Dupont Merck Study Group. A double-blind pilot study to evaluate the antiretroviral activity, tolerability of DMP 266 in combination with indinavir (cohort III). In: Abstracts of the 4th Conference on Retroviruses and Opportunistic Infections, Washington, DC. Alexandria, VA, Westover Management Group, 1997, abstract LB2.
18. Kahn J, Mayers D, Riddler S, et al. Durable clinical anti-HIV-1 activity (60 weeks) and tolerability for efavirenz (DMP 266) in combination with indinavir (IDV): suppression to "< 1copy/ml" (OD = background) by Amplicor as a predictor of virologic treatment response (DMP 266-003, cohort IV). In: Abstracts of the 5th Conference on Retroviruses and Opportunistic Infections, Chicago. Alexandria, VA, Westover Management Group, 1998, abstract 692.
19. Riddler S, Kahn J, Hicks C, et al. Durable clinical anti-HIV-1 activity (72 weeks) and tolerability for efavirenz (DMP 266) in combination with indinavir (IDV) [DMP266-003, cohort IV]. In: Abstracts of the 12th World AIDS Conference, Geneva, 1998, abstract 12359.
20. Fiske WD, Mayers D, Wagner K, et al. Pharmacokinetics of DMP 266 and indinavir multiple oral doses in HIV-1 infected individuals. In: Abstracts of the 4th Conference on Retroviruses and Opportunistic Infections, Washington, DC. Alexandria, VA, Westover Management Group, 1997, abstract 568.
21. Isaacs R, Havlir D, Pottage J, et al. Sixteen week follow-up of indinavir sulfate (IDV) administered q8 hours (h) versus q12h in combination with efavirenz (EFV) (MSD protocol 067). In: Abstracts of the 12th World AIDS Conference, Geneva, 1998, abstract 12290.
22. Haas D, Seekens D, Cooper R, et al. A phase II, double-blind, placebo-controlled, dose-ranging study to assess the antiretroviral activity and safety of efavirenz (EFV, Sustiva, DMP 266) in combination with open-label zidovudine (ZDV) with lamivudine (3TC) at 36 weeks [DMP 266-005]. In: Abstracts of the 12th World AIDS Conference, Geneva, 1998, abstract 22334.
23. Mayers D, Jemesk J, Eyster E, et al. A double-blind, placebo controlled study to assess the safety, tolerability and antiretroviral activity of efavirenz (EFV, Sustiva, DMP 266) in combination with open-label zidovudine (ZDV) and lamivudine (3TC) in HIV-1 infected patients [DMP 266-004]. In: Abstracts of the 12th World AIDS Conference, Geneva, 1998, abstract 22340.
24. Staszewski S, Morales-Ramirez J, Tashima K, et al. Efavirenz plus zidovudine and lamivudine, efavirenz plus indinavir, and indinavir plus zidovudine and lamivudine in the treatment of HIV-1 infection in adults. N Engl J Med 341:1865, 1999.
25. Haas DW, Fessel WF, Delapenha RA, et al. Therapy with efavirenz plus indinavir in patients with extensive prior nucleoside reverse-transcriptase inhibitor experience: a randomized, double-blind, placebo-controlled trial. J Infect Dis 183:392, 2001.
26. Mildevan D, Martin G, Eyster M, et al. Initial effectiveness and tolerability of nelfinavir (NFV) in combination with efavirenz (EFV, Sustiva, DMP 266) in antiretroviral therapy naive or nucleoside experienced HIV-1 infected patients: characterization in a phase II, open label, multicenter study at 16 weeks [DMP 266-024]. In: Abstracts of the 12th World AIDS Conference, Geneva, 1998, abstract 22386.
27. Albrercht MA, Bosch RJ, Hammer SM, et al. Nelfinavir, efavirenz, or both after the failure of nucleoside treatment of HIV infedction. N Engl J Med 345:398, 2001.
28. Piketty C, Race E, Castiel P, et al. Efficacy of a five-drug combination including ritonavir, saquinavir and efavirenz in patients who failed on a conventional triple-drug regimen: phenotypic resistance to protease inhibitors predicts outcome of therapy. AIDS 13:F71, 1999.
29. Falloon J, Piscitelli S, Vogel S, et al. Combination therapy with amprenavir, abacavir, and efavirenz in human immunodeficiency virus (HIV)-infected patients failing a protease inhibitor regimen. Clin Infect Dis 30:313, 2000.
30. Starr S, Fletcher CV, Spector SA, et al. Combination therapy with efavirenz, nelfinavir, and nucleoside reverse-transcriptase inhibitors in children infected with human immunodeficiency virus type 1. N Engl J Med 341:1874, 1999.
31. Bacheler LT. Resistance to nonucleoside of HIV-1 reverse transcriptase. In: Drug Resistance Updates, vol. 2. Harcourt Brace, St Louis, 1999, pp 56–57.
32. Bachelor LT, Anton ED, Kudish P, et al. Human immunodeficiency virus type 1 mutations selected in patients failing efavirenz combination therapy. Antimicrob Agents Chemother 44:2475, 2000.
33. Bacheler L, Jeffrey S, Hanna G, et al. Genotypic correlates of phenotypic resistance to efavirenz in virus isolates from patients failing NNRTI combination therapy. J Virol 75:4999, 2001.
34. Haubrich R, Whitcomb J, Keiser P, et al. Non-nucleoside reverse transcriptase inhibitor hypersensitivity is common and improved short-term virological response. Antivir Ther 5(suppl 3):69, 2000.
35. Shulman N, Zolopa AR, Passaro D, et al. Phenotypic hypersusceptibility to non-nucleoside reverse transcriptase inhibitors in treatment-experienced HIV-infected patients: impact on virological response to efavirenz-based therapy. AIDS 15:1125, 2001.
36. Shulman N, Zolopa A, Passaro D, et al. Efavirenz and adefovir dipivoxil-based salvage therapy in highly treatment-experienced patient: clinical and genotypic predictors of virologic response. J Acquir Immuno Defic Syndr 23:221, 2000.
37. Walmsley SL, Kelly DV, Tseng AL, et al. Non-nucleoside reverse transcriptase inhibitor failure impairs HIV-RNA responses to efavirenz-containing salvage antiretroviral therapy. AIDS 15:1581, 2001.
38. Fiske WD, Benedek IH, White SJ, et al. Pharmacokinetic interaction between DMP 266 and nelfinavir mestylate (NFV) in healthy volunteers. In: Abstracts of the 37th Interscience Conference on Antimicrobial Agents and Chemotherapy, Toronto, 1997, abstract I-172.
39. Fiske WD, Benedek IH, White SJ, et al. Pharmacokinetic interaction between efavirenz (EFV) and nelfinavir mesylate (NFV) in healthy volunteers. In: Abstracts of the 5th Conference on Retroviruses and Opportunistic Infections, Chicago. Alexandria, VA, Westover Management Group, 1998, abstract 349.
40. Regazzi MB, Villani P, Maserati R, et al. Clinical pharmacokinetics of nelfinavir combined with efavirenz and stavudine during rescue treatment of heavily pretreated HIV-infected patients. J Antimicrob Chemother 45:343, 2000.
41. Fiske WD, Benedek IH, Joseph JL, et al. Pharmacokinetics of efavirenz (EFV) and ritonavir (RIT) after multiple oral doses in healthy volunteers. In: Abstracts of the 12th World AIDS Conference, Geneva, 1998, abstract 42269.
42. Piscitelli S, Vogel S, Sadler B, et al. Effect of efavirenz (DMP266) on the pharmacokinetics of 141W94 in HIV-infected patients. In: Abstracts of the 5th Conference on Retrovirus and Opportunistic Infections, Chicago. Alexandria, VA, Westover Management Group, 1998, abstract 346.
43. Benedek IH, Fiske WD, White SJ, et al. Plasma levels of fluconazole (FL) are not altered by co-administration of DMP 266 in healthy volunteers. In: Abstracts of the 37th Interscience Conference on Antimicrobial Agents and Chemotherapy, Toronto, 1997, abstract A-4.
44. Benedek IH, Joshi A, Fiske WD, et al. Pharmacokinetic interaction between efavirenz (EFV) and rifampin (RIF) in healthy volunteers. In: Abstracts of the 12th World AIDS Conference, Geneva, 1998, abstract 42880.
45. Benedek IH, Joshi A, Fiske WD, et al. Pharmacokinetic (PK) interaction studies in healthy volunteers with efavirenz (EFV) and the macrolide antibiotics, azithromycin (AZM) and clarithromycin (CLR).

In: Abstracts of the 5th Conference on Retroviruses and Opportunistic Infections, Chicago. Alexandria, VA, Westover Management Group, 1998, abstract 347.

46. Joshi AS, Fiske WD, Benedek IH, et al. Lack of pharmacokinetic interaction between efavirenz (DMP 266) and ethinyl estradiol in healthy female volunteers. In: Abstracts of the 5th Conference on Retroviruses and Opportunistic Infections, Chicago. Alexandria, VA, Westover Management Group, 1998, abstract 348.
47. Clarke SM, Mulcahy FM, Tjia J, et al. The pharmacokinetics of methadone in HIV-positive patients receiving the non-nucleoside reverse transcriptase inhibitor efavirenz. Br J Clin Pharmacol 51:213, 2001.

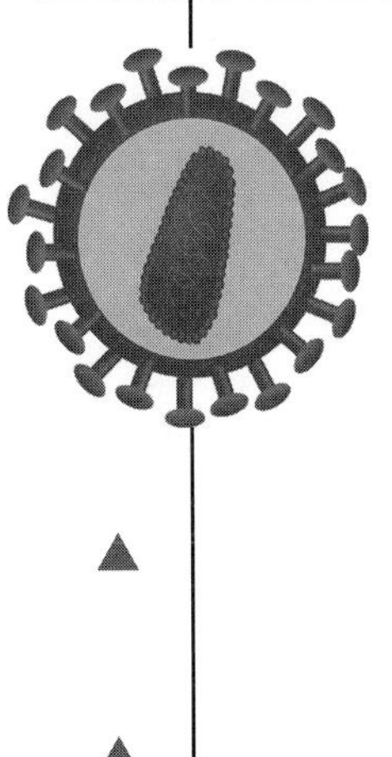

CHAPTER 12

Saquinavir

Ann C. Collier, MD
Kathleen E. Squires, MD

STRUCTURE

Saquinavir is a peptide-like, hydroxyethylamine transition-state analogue of the human immunodeficiency virus type 1 (HIV-1) protease. Its chemical name is *N*-tert-butyl-decahydro-2-[2(*R*)hydroxy-4-phenyl-3(*S*)-[[*N*-(2-quinolylcarbonyl)-L-asparaginyl]amino]butyl]-(4a*S*,8a*S*)-isoquinoline-3(*S*)-carboxamide (Fig. 12–1). Saquinavir has a molecular weight of 670.86. The formulation of saquinavir originally approved for treatment of HIV-1 infection was saquinavir mesylate formulated in hard gelatin capsules (Invirase), hereafter referred to as saquinavir-HGC. During its early development, saquinavir was known as Ro 31-8959 and compound XVII. A newer soft gelatin capsule (SGC) formulation of the free base of saquinavir (Fortovase) was made available for clinical use in late 1997; hereafter this is referred to as saquinavir-SGC.

IN VITRO ACTIVITY AND MECHANISMS OF ACTION

The HIV-1 protease is an aspartic protease.[1] It contains 99 amino acids and exists as a homodimer. HIV-1 protease functions to cleave small proteins from HIV-1's Gag-Pol polyprotein precursor (summarized by Deeks and Volberding[2] and Flexner[3]). This step is essential in the life cycle of HIV-1 and creates the individual structural and enzymatic proteins necessary for formation of mature virions.[4,5] Each component protein is cleaved in its core proteins, such as p24, p17, p9, and p7 for Gag. The functional core proteins contribute to the formation of infectious viral particles, which are released from infected cells. With inhibition of HIV-1 protease, noninfectious virions with abnormal structure are produced.[6]

Saquinavir was developed by rational drug design.[7] After the structure of HIV-1 protease became known, it was recognized that some of the cleavage sites (phenylalanine-proline and tyrosine-proline) were unique in comparison to eukaryotic proteases, which rarely have cleavage sites at a proline residue. This information and the results of mutagenesis experiments suggested that HIV-1 protease would be a useful target for inhibiting of HIV-1. A series of synthetic, peptide-like compounds were designed to mimic the transition state of the HIV-1 protease phenylalanine-proline dipeptide cleavage site.[7] The structures were modified to maximize the biochemical and biologic inhibitory activity against HIV-1.

Saquinavir is a potent in vitro inhibitor of the proteases of both HIV-1 and HIV-2, with a $K_i \leq 0.1$ nM.[6,8] It has virtually no activity against various mammalian proteases, such as pepsin and cathepsin, with K_i values higher than 10,000 nM.[7] In vitro, saquinavir has potent (nanomolar) anti-HIV activity—against a wide variety of laboratory and clinical isolates, including zidovudine-sensitive and zidovudine-resistant isolates; in acute and chronic infection systems; in infected T-lymphocyte lines, monocytic cell lines, and peripheral blood mononuclear cells (PBMCs)—using the outcome measures of inhibition of HIV-1 p 24 antigen production, inhibition of syncytium formation, or cell viability assays.[6,7,9–11] For example, in T-lymphocyte lines the range of 50% inhibitory concentration (IC_{50}) values was 0.5 to 7.0 nM, and the range of 90% inhibitory concentration (IC_{90}) values was 6 to 34 nM. In PBMCs the IC_{50} values range from 3.5 to 10.0 nM. In one monocyte/macrophage system, the IC_{50} was 20 nM and the IC_{90} was 200 nM.[12] However, specific IC_{50} and IC_{90} values from in vitro experiments may not directly reflect

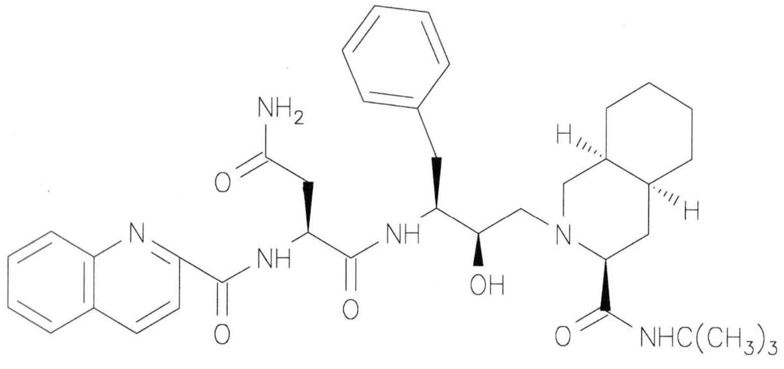

Figure 12–1. Chemical structure of saquinavir.

the in vivo activity of saquinavir because of issues such as plasma protein binding. Saquinavir is 97% bound to serum proteins, which is slightly less than that for lopinavir (98% to 99%) or nelfinavir (98%) but greater than that for amprenavir (90%) or indinavir (90%).[13] In vitro experiments suggested that acid glycoprotein binding resulted in a 10-fold decrease in saquinavir's anti-HIV activity.[9]

The in vitro effects of various concentrations of saquinavir on the development of mature virions has been assessed and has demonstrated decreasing amounts of mature particles with increasing concentrations of saquinavir.[7] For example, using the CEM T-lymphocyte line and HIV-1_{IIIB}, 10.0% and 0.4% of virions were mature at 10 nM and 100 nM concentrations of saquinavir, respectively.[6] In another study using a U1 promonocytic cell culture system, with 100 or 1000 nM of saquinavir, 0.3% or none, of the virions, respectively had a mature appearance.[14] In one model of chronic infection in MT-4 cells with the laboratory strain HIV-1_{IIIB}, 100 nM of saquinavir completely suppressed evidence of HIV-1 infection for 87 days when assayed using a variety of techniques, including HIV-1 p24 antigen, titers of infectious virus, and a DNA polymerase chain reaction (PCR) assay.[15] HIV-1 reemerged in this culture system when saquinavir was removed from the culture medium after 11 or 42 days postinfection.

A variety of in vitro studies have evaluated the anti-HIV-1 effects of saquinavir in double, triple, and quadruple antiviral combinations.[14,16–22] The clinical relevance of these data are not known, although in vivo data support the efficacy of some of these combinations. In general, use of increasing numbers of drugs in vitro resulted in increased antiviral efficacy.[18] Double combinations that have demonstrated additive to synergistic anti-HIV effects in vitro include saquinavir with the following agents: zidovudine, didanosine, zalcitabine, lamivudine, stavudine, interferon-α, nelfinavir, and ritonavir.[16,18,19,22] Triple combinations that have demonstrated additive to synergistic activity in vitro include saquinavir with zidovudine and lamivudine, zidovudine and stavudine, zidovudine and zalcitabine (additive effects were seen in some experiments), zidovudine and interferon-α, lamivudine and stavudine, and lamivudine and nevirapine.[12,17,22,23,33] Quadruple regimens with demonstrated in vitro synergy include saquinavir with zidovudine, didanosine, and interferon-α; zidovudine, lamivudine, and nevirapine; and saquinavir, zidovudine, interferon-α, and foscarnet.[12,17,18] At least one study suggested that the combination of indinavir with saquinavir had an antagonistic effect on HIV-1 in vitro.[20]

The concentrations of saquinavir that produce cytotoxicity are markedly higher than the concentrations that are inhibitory to HIV-1, with selectivity indices of more than 1000. For example, the concentration of saquinavir that produced toxicity in 50% of cells using the T-lymphocyte lines JM and C8166 ranged from 5 to 100 μM.[7]

▲ PHARMACOKINETICS

Saquinavir-HGC

Saquinavir-HGC is no longer used as monotherapy. For more information on the pharmacokinetics, toxicity, and efficacy of saquinavir-HGC, the reader is referred to the Invirase product package insert or the previous edition of this book.

Saquinavir-SGC

The administration of saquinavir-SGC gives rise to increased plasma levels of saquinavir compared to saquinavir-HGC. The pharmacokinetic properties of saquinavir-SGC have been studied in normal volunteers and HIV-infected individuals[25–31] (Table 12–1). Compared to saquinavir-HGC, the relative oral bioavailability of saquinavir-SGC is about threefold greater.

Food increases the absorption of saquinavir-SGC; the mean 12-hour area under the concentration-time curve (AUC) is at least sixfold greater when the drug is administered with a meal than when it is taken on an empty stomach.[32]

No significant differences were seen in a small single-dose study of saquinavir-SGC that compared the pharmacokinetics in women and men.[27] There is a dearth of information about the pharmacokinetics of saquinavir-SGC in persons with hepatic or renal dysfunction, and there is limited information available about the use of saquinavir-SGC in children. Additional data are needed before dosing recommendations can be made for these special populations.

In a randomized, nonblind, multicenter, close-ranging, 8-week study, 84 evaluable patients were given monotherapy with saquinavir-SGC (400, 800, or 1200 mg tid) or monotherapy with saquinavir-HGC (600 mg tid), and the exposure-response relationships for the administered therapies were determined using an empirical modeling approach.[33] When plasma HIV RNA levels were fitted to two measures of systemic drug exposure [AUC and minimum concentration

▲ **Table 12–1.** KEY SAQUINAVIR PHARMACOKINETIC PARAMETERS FOR REGIMENS CONTAINING SAQUINAVIR-HGC AND SAQUINAVIR-SGC

	Pharmacokinetics					
Regimen	AUC_{γ}[a] (ng.hr/ml)	AUC_{0-24} (ng.hr/ml)	C_{min} (ng/ml)	C_{max} (ng/ml)	**Subjects**	**Reference**
SQV-SGC 1200 mg tid	7,249	21,747	216	2181	P	27
SQV-HGC 400 mg bid + ritonavir 400 mg bid	699[b]	1,398[b]	230[b]	1280[b]	V	28
SQV-HGC 1000 mg bid + ritonavir 100 mg bid	14,607	29,214	317	2623	P	27
	23,440[b]	46,880	450[b]	3880[b]	V	27
	7,979	15,798	217	1318	V	29
SQV-SGC 400 mg bid + ritonavir 400 mg bid	–	30,920	840	2920	V	30
SQV-SGC 1000 mg bid + ritonavir 100 mg bid	19,085[b]	38,170[b]	433[b]	3344[b]	P	27
	5,745	11,655	153	1001	V	29
SQV-SGC 1600 mg qd + ritonavir 100 mg qd	48,100[b]	48,100[b]	170[b]	7000[b]	P	31

AUC, area under the time-concentration curve; C, concentration; min, minimum; max, maximum; P, HIV-infected patients; SQV-HGC, saquinavir—hard gel capsule; SQV-SGC, saquinavir—soft gel capsule; V, healthy volunteers.
Mean values are given unless otherwise indicated.
[a]The subscript γ indicates the dosing interval (i.e., 8 hours for bid, 12 hours for tid, and 24 hours for qd dosing).
[b]Median values.

(C_{min})], the pharmacokinetic-pharmacodynamic relationships were found to be best described by the two-parameter maximum effect (E_{max}) model, which predicted a typical maximum reduction in viral load of 1.94 $\log_{10}$ copies per milliliter with a half-maximal antiviral response occurring at a C_{min} of 50 mg/L.

Boosted Saquinavir with High-Dose Ritonavir

The use of highly active antiretroviral therapy (HAART), in which three or more antiretroviral agents are combined in a single regimen, has become routine in the management of HIV infection. HAART regimens often contain both reverse transcriptase inhibitors and protease inhibitors, with the objective of targeting the HIV at multiple sites. In some instances, however, the use of drug combinations can give rise to drug interactions, which may be desirable or undesirable.

As saquinavir is mainly metabolized by the cytochrome (CYP) 3A4 isoenzyme of the CYP P_{450} system, it has the potential to interact with any of the many other agents that are metabolized by (or induce or inhibit) this isoenzyme.[34,35] The most notable clinically relevant drug interaction with saquinavir is with ritonavir. This interaction can have desirable consequences when handled correctly.[36]

Saquinavir has minimal inhibitory effects on CYP3A4, even at high concentrations; but ritonavir is a potent inhibitor of this isoenzyme, even at low concentrations.[37] These phenomena have been exploited by using dual saquinavir/ritonavir therapy to increase plasma saquinavir concentrations and thereby improve the virologic response.[38,39]

When they are administered concurrently, ritonavir inhibits the metabolism of saquinavir; and plasma saquinavir concentrations are increased compared with those achieved with higher and more frequent doses of saquinavir alone.[38] Concurrent administration of ritonavir and saquinavir, as either saquinavir-HGC or saquinavir-SGC, allows a twice-daily or once-daily dosing regimen and lower than standard doses of saquinavir. Similar saquinavir exposure was seen when the same dose of either saquinavir-HGC or saquinavir-SGC was administered with ritonavir.[32] Saquinavir does not alter the pharmacokinetic parameters of ritonavir.

The "boosted" protease inhibitor (PI) combination of saquinavir-SGC/ritonavir is now frequently used. The dose regimen initially used was 400/400 mg bid. Several studies have therefore been performed to compare the pharmacokinetics of saquinavir following the administration of various saquinavir/ritonavir dose combinations (Table 12–1).

An open-label, randomized, parallel, multiple-dose study involving 64 healthy HIV-negative volunteers who were given saquinavir-SGC (800 mg bid) alone, ritonavir (400 mg bid) alone, or a combination of saquinavir (400 to 800 mg bid) with ritonavir (200 to 400 mg bid) for 14 days, has shown that concurrent administration of ritonavir substantially increases saquinavir exposure.[30] Among those given saquinavir at a dose of 800 mg bid, there were overall 17-, 22-, and 23-fold increases in saquinavir (AUC_{0-24}) when ritonavir was administered at doses of 200, 300, and 400 mg bid, respectively.

Boosted Saquinavir with Low-Dose Ritonavir

Although a variety of saquinavir/ritonavir dose regimens are currently used in clinical practice, to reduce the incidence of ritonavir-associated side effects it might be desirable to minimize the dose of ritonavir. Strategies in which 100 mg "minidoses" of ritonavir have been combined with saquinavir-SGC have therefore been investigated.

A retrospective analysis of pharmacokinetic data from two studies[30,40] involving 97 healthy HIV-negative volunteers has indicated that ritonavir 100 mg bid is adequate to increase saquinavir exposure.[40] In this analysis saquinavir exposure was shown to be related to the dose of saquinavir (either SGC or HGC), and the effect of ritonavir was similar for doses of 100 to 400 mg bid.

Another study has evaluated the pharmacokinetics of a saquinavir-SGC/ritonavir minidose regimen in healthy volunteers.[29] This study compared saquinavir-SGC/ritonavir (1000/100 mg bid) with saquinavir-HGC/ritonavir (1000/100 mg) in 24 healthy volunteers who were given each combination separately for 10 days. Saquinavir-HGC/ritonavir led to significantly higher plasma saquinavir levels than saquinavir-SGC/ritonavir (1000/100 mg bid) for all the pharmacokinetic variables evaluated, including mean differences of: AUC_{0-12} 38.9%, AUC_{12-24} 35.6%, AUC_{0-24} 36.0%, $C_{min_{12}}$ 41.9%, $C_{min_{24}}$ 40.0%, $C_{max_{0-12}}$ 35.0%, $C_{max_{12-24}}$ 28.8% (Table 12–1).

Although twice-daily dosing is currently used in clinical practice for combination saquinavir/ritonavir regimens, once-daily dosing might be a viable option. An open-label, randomized, parallel, multiple-dose study involving 44 healthy HIV-negative volunteers has indicated the feasibility of utilizing an all once-daily HAART regimen that incorporates saquinavir-SGC (1600 mg)/low-dose ritonavir (100 mg).[41] In this study, the addition of minidose ritonavir (100 mg qd) to saquinavir-SGC (1200 to 1800 mg qd) resulted in trough plasma saquinavir concentrations that were approximately fivefold higher than those achieved with saquinavir-SGC (1200 mg tid) alone. The AUC for saquinavir increased three- to sevenfold compared with that achieved with saquinavir-SGC (1200 mg tid) alone, and this difference was most apparent for the saquinavir-SGC/ritonavir (1600/100 mg qd) combination. Neither increasing the saquinavir-SGC dose to 1800 mg qd nor increasing ritonavir to 200 mg qd elevated the AUC beyond that achieved with saquinavir-SGC ritonavir (1600/100 mg qd).

Despite these promising observations, it remains to be verified beyond doubt that once-daily saquinavir/ritonavir dosing regimens are a reliable dosing strategy in HIV-infected individuals. It should be recognized that administration of a pharmacologically enhancing dose of ritonavir is critical to maintain adequate blood levels of saquinavir.

▲ TOXICITY

Information about the toxicities of saquinavir-HGC and saquinavir-SGC are available from clinical studies and from the experience in clinical settings. In controlled studies more than 5000 patients have received saquinavir-HGC, and more than 850 patients have received saquinavir-SGC. Data are available from early studies in which saquinavir-HGC was administered as monotherapy, but most available data are from the use of saquinavir-HGC or saquinavir-SGC in combination with other antiretroviral agents. The most frequent side effects with both formulations are gastrointestinal and include diarrhea, nausea, and abdominal discomfort or pain[42–44] Those for saquinavir-SCG are summarized in Table 12–2. Dyspepsia has also been linked to therapy with saquinavir-SGC. Most treatment-related side effects have been mild. As might be expected, because drug exposure is greater, the frequency of toxicities is higher with saquinavir-SGC than with saquinavir-HGC.[43] Overall, moderate or severe gastrointestinal side effects at least possibly related to treatment have occurred in 5% to 10% of patients receiving saquinavir-HGC and 10% to 20% of patients on saquinavir-SGC therapy; additional patients may have milder symptoms. Other toxicities that occurred in more than a few percent of patients treated with either formulation included headaches, fatigue, and hepatic toxicity manifested by elevations in serum transaminases. Elevations in creatine phosphokinase have also been observed but are believed to be related to HIV-1 or other therapies, rather than saquinavir.

Of 442 patients treated with saquinavir-SGC and other antiretroviral agents of their choice in the study NV15182, 8% discontinued treatment over a 1-year period, primarily because of gastrointestinal complaints.[44] The occurrence of moderate, severe, or life-threatening laboratory abnormalities has been low with saquinavir-SGC. Fewer than 1% of patients discontinued therapy because of laboratory abnormalities over a 1-year period in the NV15182 study.

▲ **Table 12–2.** MOST COMMON MODERATE AND SEVERE TOXICITIES IN SAQUINAVIR STUDIES

Adverse Event	Antiretroviral-Naive[a] SQV-SGC + 2 NRTIs (n = 90)	Antiretroviral-Naive[a] SQV-HGC + 2 NRTIs (n = 81)	Antiretroviral-Experienced[b] SQV-SGC + NRTIs (n = 442)
Symptoms			
Diarrhea	16	12	20
Nausea	18	14	11
Abdominal discomfort	13	5	9
Dyspepsia	9	0	8
Flatulence	12	7	6
Headache	9	5	5
Fatigue	7	6	5
Laboratory data			
Creatine phosphokinase > 4 × ULN	5	0	8
Alanine aminotransferase > 5 × ULN	2	1	6
Hypoglycemia (< 40 mg/dl)	4	3	6
Hyperglycemia (> 250 mg/dl)[c]	1	1	1

NRTI, nucleoside reverse transcriptase inhibitor; SQV-HGC, saquinavir-hard gel capsule, SQV-SGC, saquinavir-soft gel capsule; ULN, upper limit of normal range.

[a]Study NV15355, 16-week data.[43]

[b]Study NV15182, 48-week data.[44]

[c]Not one of the most common; presented for interest.

Metabolic complications have been increasingly described in patients receiving PI therapy. On the basis of postmarketing surveillance reports, the U.S. Food and Drug Administration (FDA) issued an alert in 1997 about a possible relation between PI use and the development or worsening of diabetes mellitus, hyperglycemia, and diabetic ketoacidosis; some of the reported cases occurred in persons receiving saquinavir.[45] The relative frequency of such events, their pathogenesis, and their relation to specific PIs are under active investigation (see Chapter 62). There have also been other metabolic complications recently described in persons receiving PIs, including body habitus changes, intraabdominal fat deposition, peripheral lipodystrophy, hypertriglyceridemia, hypercholesterolemia, and accelerated atherosclerosis; the frequency and relation of these events to treatment with either saquinavir formulation is unknown.[46–51] In this regard, it is of interest that the findings of the Prometheus study suggested a contributory role for nucleoside analogues in the development of antiretroviral therapy-associated lipodystrophy. During 96 weeks of follow-up, lipodystrophy was reported in 25% of patients randomized to saquinavir/ritonavir/stavudine but in only 8% of those allocated to saquinavir alone ($P = 0.003$).[52]

Insufficient data are available about the use of either saquinavir formulation during pregnancy to judge its safety, but voluntary reports of women using saquinavir during pregnancy are being collected in the Antiretroviral Pregnancy Registry.[24] Both formulations of saquinavir are classified in Pregnancy Category B of the FDA with respect to teratogenicity based on the available preclinical data. Saquinavir was not mutagenic in vitro in the Ames test in bacteria or in mammalian cells, and it did not induce chromosomal damage in vitro in PBMCs or in vivo in the mouse.[27,53] Carcinogenicity studies in rats and mice are underway.

Two cases of overdosage with saquinavir-HGC have been reported, but neither resulted in serious sequelae; no case of overdosage with saquinavir-SGC has been reported.[53] Preliminary data about quality-of-life assessments from the Phase III studies of saquinavir-HGC suggested better quality of life in saquinavir-HGC-treated patients than with the other regimens studied.[54,55]

The tolerability of the dual-PI regimen of saquinavir/ritonavir has been studied in 141 patients with HIV-1 infection treated for up to 60 weeks.[56] Subjects in this study received one of four dose combinations of saquinavir-HGC and ritonavir. The treatment groups were 400 mg bid of both drugs, 400 mg bid of saquinavir and 600 mg bid of ritonavir, 400 mg tid of both drugs, and 600 mg bid of both drugs. The regimen in which saquinavir-HGC and ritonavir were both administered at 400 mg bid was tolerated best. A total of 22 subjects (16%) discontinued study therapy because of adverse events. In addition, doses of the study drugs were decreased in 33 subjects (23%) to improve tolerability. The most common moderately severe or worse adverse events that were possibly, probably, or of unknown relation to study therapy were diarrhea, nausea, and asthenia. The most common laboratory abnormalities were elevations in transaminases; acquired immunodeficiency syndrome (AIDS) Clinical Trial Group (ACTG) grade III or IV transaminase elevations occurred in 14 subjects (2 in the 400 mg bid group), but most of these subjects had concurrent hepatitis B or C virus infections or entered the study with elevated transaminase levels.

An open-label, randomized, parallel group study has been performed to investigate the influence of saquinavir-SGC/ritonavir on saquinavir exposure and its relationship to tolerability.[30] In this study, healthy subjects were given either saquinavir-SGC 800 mg bid alone, ritonavir 400 mg bid alone, or six twice-daily combination regimens containing various doses of saquinavir-SGC/ritonavir, for 14 days. The most frequently reported adverse events were oral hypoesthesia, headache, nausea, taste disturbance and dizziness; none of the events was reported to be serious or severe. Among the various dosage groups, the most adverse events (83 in 8 subjects) occurred with saquinavir-SGC/ritonavir (400/400 mg bid) and the fewest (17 in 9 subjects) with saquinavir-SGC/ritonavir (800/200 mg bid). Intermediate frequencies of adverse events occurred in the other groups. This suggests that the incidence of adverse events with saquinavir-SGC/ritonavir combination therapy is more closely related to the dose of ritonavir than to the dose of saquinavir.

Another study has evaluated the safety of saquinavir-SGC/ritonavir in healthy volunteers using a higher dose of saquinavir-SGC and a lower, "minidose" of ritonavir.[29] This study specifically compared the safety of saquinavir-SGC/ritonavir (1000/100 mg) with that of saquinavir-HGC/ritonavir (1000/100 mg) in 24 healthy volunteers who received each combination separately for 10 days. A significantly larger number of subjects receiving the saquinavir-SGC combination reported gastrointestinal disorders compared with the saquinavir-HGC combination (23 vs. 8; $P < 0.05$). The incidence of diarrhea was significantly higher with saquinavir-SGC/ritonavir (1000/100 mg) than with saquinavir-HGC/ritonavir (1000/100 mg) (15 vs. 4; $P < 0.01$), but there was no significant correlation between this symptom and the saquinavir AUC. This suggests that in patients taking saquinavir-SGC who have a gastrointestinal side effect, a switch to saquinavir-HGC may be a desirable option, allowing continuation of saquinavir treatment with the opportunity for better tolerability.

The findings of another study have suggested that some gastrointestinal side effects associated with twice-daily saquinavir-SGC-containing therapy may be mainly associated with the large number of capsules rather than the drug itself.[57] In this study, 69 HIV-infected patients who had previously been treated with various doses of zidovudine/zalcitabine for 66 weeks followed by saquinavir-SGC 1400 mg bid plus either zidovudine/lamivudine or didanosine/stavudine for 112 weeks were switched to saquinavir-SGC/ritonavir 1600/100 mg qd plus continued nucleoside therapy. A comparison of the number of patients reporting gastrointestinal toxicity during the last 24 weeks before the switch with those during the first 24 weeks after the switch showed no significant difference between saquinavir-SGC 1400 mg bid and saquinavir-SGC/ ritonavir 1600/100 mg qd (50 vs. 41; $P = 0.124$). Separate comparisons of individual gastrointestinal events showed significant reductions after the switch—nausea (16 vs. 5; $P = 0.001$) and vomiting (10 vs. 1; $P = 0.004$)—but not diarrhea (22 vs. 15; $P = 0.210$), anorexia (10 vs. 11; $P = 1.000$), abdominal pain (5 vs. 8; $P = 0.453$), or indigestion (5 vs. 1; $P = 0.125$). Switching to saquinavir-SGC/ritonavir once-daily may therefore be a way to decrease the risk of gastrointestinal toxicity in patients taking twice-daily regimens of saquinavir-SGC.

▲ EFFICACY

Saquinavir-SGC

Saquinavir-SGC was approved by the FDA in November 1997 on the basis of data from two studies: NV15355, which compared saquinavir-SGC with saquinavir-HGC in HIV-1-infected, treatment-naive patients,[43] and NV15182, an open-label safety study of saquinavir-SGC in combination with other antiretroviral agents.[44] Since receiving approval, several more studies of saquinavir-SGC have been completed, including the NR15503/M61005 SUN, M61003 CHEESE, NV15436 SPICE, and NR15520/M61018 TIDBID studies and the first pediatric study of saquinavir[58–62] (Table 12–3). These studies suggest that saquinavir-SGC, in combination with other antiretroviral agents, provides increased activity compared to that seen with saquinavir-HGC. Both antiretroviral-naive and antiretroviral-experienced patients had substantial HIV RNA declines and CD4+ T-lymphocyte count increase in these studies.

NR15503/M61005 SUN Study

In this open-label, single-arm study (NR15503/M61005 SUN), 42 antiretroviral-naive HIV-1-infected patients with mean baseline CD4+ T-lymphocyte counts of 419 cells per cubic millimeter and mean baseline HIV-1 RNA values of 4.8 $\log_{10}$ copies per milliliter received saquinavir-SGC (1200 mg tid) in combination with zidovudine (300 mg bid) and lamivudine (150 mg bid).[58] At 48 weeks, 50% and 43% of patients in an intent-to-treat analysis achieved HIV-1 RNA titers of less than 400 and less than 20 copies per milliliter, respectively.

M61003 CHEESE Study

The M61003 CHEESE trial was a randomized, open-label, parallel-arm study that compared saquinavir-SGC (plus zidovudine and lamivudine) with indinavir (plus zidovudine and lamivudine) in antiretroviral-naive HIV-1-infected patients.[59] A total of 67 patients with less than 12 months of prior zidovudine experience and without prior PI or lamivudine therapy received either 1200 mg saquinavir tid or 800 mg indinavir q8h, both in combination with 300 mg zidovudine bid and 150 mg lamivudine bid. At 24 weeks there was no significant difference between the two groups in terms of virologic activity, but the saquinavir-SGC group had a better immunologic response (Table 12–3).

NV15436 SPICE Study

The NV15436 SPICE trial was a randomized, open-label, parallel-arm study that explored the utility of the double-PI combination of saquinavir-SGC and nelfinavir with or without two concurrent nucleoside reverse transcriptase inhibitors (NRTIs).[60] A total of 157 PI-naive patients were randomized to one of four treatment arms: (A) saquinavir-SGC 1200 mg tid + two NRTIs; (B) nelfinavir 750 mg tid + two NRTIs; (C) saquinavir-SGC 800 mg tid + nelfinavir 750 mg tid + two NRTIs; or (D) saquinavir-SGC 800 mg tid + nelfinavir 750 mg tid without NRTIs. At 48 weeks 61%, 63%, 65%, and 47% of patients in arms A, B, C, and D, respectively, achieved HIV-1 RNA titers of less than 50 copies per milliliter in an on-treatment analysis of those remaining in their original arm. Differences between the groups were not statistically significant.

NR15520/M61018 TIDBID Study

The NR15520/M61018 TIDBID study compared the antiviral activity and safety of saquinavir-SGC twice-daily regimens, either as the sole PI plus two nucleoside analogues or as a dual-PI regimen with nelfinavir plus one nucleoside analogue, with a saquinavir-SGC thrice-daily regimen containing two new nucleoside analogues.[61] A total of 840 antiretroviral-naive or nucleoside analogue-experienced patients were randomized to one of three treatment arms: (A) saquinavir-SGC 1200 mg tid plus two new nucleoside analogues; (B) saquinavir-SGC 1600 mg bid plus two nucleoside analogues; or (C) saquinavir-SGC 1200 mg bid plus nelfinavir 1250 mg bid plus one new nucleoside analogue. The mean baseline CD4+ T-lymphocyte counts were 307, 328, and 311 cells per cubic millimeter, and the mean baseline HIV-1 RNA titers were 4.8, 4.7, and 4.8 $\log_{10}$ copies per milliliter in arms A, B, and C, respectively. In an intent-to-treat analysis of week 48 data, 37%, 36%, and 35% of patients achieved HIV-1 RNA titers of less than 50 copies per milliliter in arms A, B, and C, respectively. The virologic responses in the saquinavir-SGC-containing twice-daily regimens were equivalent to the saquinavir-SGC-containing thrice-daily regimen.

Pediatric Study

The safety and effectiveness of saquinavir-SGC have not been established in HIV-infected patients younger than 16 years of age. However, the first study to evaluate the long-term efficacy of combination therapy including saquinavir-SGC in children has now been completed. It was an open-label study that evaluated the utility of saquinavir-SGC given in combination with nucleoside analogues with or without nelfinavir to HIV-infected, PI-naive children aged 3 to 16 years.[62] It was conducted in two parts, with part 1 lasting 72 weeks and part 2 lasting 48 weeks. In part 1 there were 14 children who were given saquinavir-SGC (initially 33 mg/kg tid, subsequently adjusted to 50 mg/kg tid based on initial pharmacokinetics) and two nucleoside antiretroviral agents (plus nelfinavir for the five children who did not achieve a predetermined steady-state target plasma saquinavir exposure). In part 2 another 13 children received saquinavir-SGC (33 mg/kg tid) in combination with nelfinavir (30 mg/kg tid) and one or two nucleoside analogues. In part 1, about 36% of patients achieved HIV-1 RNA titers of less than 50 copies per milliliter at 72 weeks, whereas in part 2 a total of 62% of patients achieved the HIV-1 RNA titer (Table 12–3).

Boosted Saquinavir

Since the impact of ritonavir on saquinavir concentrations was first recognized using saquinavir-HGC, several studies have been designed to evaluate the antiviral activity of ritonavir-boosted saquinavir-SGC therapy.[63–69] (Table 12–4).

Table 12–3. MAJOR CLINICAL STUDIES OF UNBOOSTED SAQUINAVIR-SGC

Study Name and Type	Regimens	Baseline Characteristics: Rx History	Mean HIV RNA	Mean CD4	Results: Mean HIV RNA	Change in Mean CD4	% Below LoQ	Comments
NV15355[43]: open label, randomized	SQV-SGC + 2 NRTIs (n = 90)	Naive[a]	4.8[a]	448	− 2.0	+97	80 (LoQ 400 copies/ml)	16-Week data
	SQV-HGC + 2 NRTIs (n = 80)							
NV15182[44]: open label, safety	SQV-SGC + 2 NRTIs (n = 444)	95% Prior NRTIs, < 12 months ZDV	4.1[a]	227[a]	–		43 (LoQ 400 copies/ml)	24-Week data
	Rx-naive					+200	75	
	Rx-experienced					+80	40	
NR 15503/ M61005 (SUN Study)[58]: open label	SQV-SGC + ZDV/3TC (n = 42)	Naive	4.8	419	− 3.3	+265	91 (LoQ 400 copies/ ml) 78 (LoQ 20 copies/ml)	48-Week data
M61003 (CHEESE Study)[59]: open label, randomized	SQV-SGC + ZDV/3TC (n = 33)	ZDV < 12 mo	5.0[a]	301	− 2.4	+162	74.3 (LoQ 50 copies/ ml)	24-Week data
	IDV + ZDV/3TC (n = 34)			301	− 2.4	+89	71.4 (LoQ 50 copies/ ml)	
NV15436 (SPICE Study)[60]: open label, randomized	SQV-SGC + 2 NRTIs (n = 26)	50% Naive, 50% prior NRTIs	4.8[a]	301[a]	− 2.4	+121	61 (LoQ 50 copies/ ml)	48-Week data
	NFV + 2 NRTIs (n = 26)				− 2.6	+127	63 (LoQ 50 copies/ ml)	
	SQV-SGC + NFV + 2 NRTIs[b] (n = 51)				− 2.5	+154	65 (LoQ 50 copies/ml)	
	SQV-SGC + NFV[b] (n = 54)				− 2.4	+207	47 (LoQ 50 copies/ ml)	
NR15520/ M61018 TIDBID Study[61]: open label, randomized	SQV-SGC 1200 mg tid + 2 NRTIs (n = 281)	Naive or prior NRTIs	4.8	307	− 2.63	+213	37 (LoQ 50 copies/ ml)	48-Week data
	SQV-SGC 1600 mg bid + 2 NRTIs (n = 279)		4.7	323	− 2.63	+184	36 (LoQ 50 copies/ ml)	

Table continued on following page

▲ **Table 12–3.** MAJOR CLINICAL STUDIES OF UNBOOSTED SAQUINAVIR-SGC *Continued*

Study Name and Type	Regimens	Baseline Characteristics: Rx History	Baseline Characteristics: Mean HIV RNA	Baseline Characteristics: Mean CD4	Results: Mean HIV RNA	Results: Change in Mean CD4	Results: % Below LoQ	Comments
	SQV-SGC + nelfinavir 1250 mg bid + 1 NRTI ($n = 280$)		4.8	311	− 2.55	+223	35 (LoQ 50 copies/ ml)	
Pediatric Study[62]: open label	SQV-SGC (initially 33 mg/ kg tid; subsequently adjusted to 50 mg/kg tid, based + 2 NRTIs[c] ($n = 14$)	100% Prior NRTIs but PI-naive	–	–	− 2.12	+292	36 (LoQ 50 copies/ ml)	72-Week data
	SQV-SGC (initially 33 mg/kg tid; subsequently adjusted to 50 mg/kg tid, based + 2 NRTIs + nelfinavir (30 mg/kg tid, maximum 750 mg) ($n = 13$)		–	–	− 2.58	+154	62 (LoQ 50 copies/ ml)	48-Week data

Doses of agents are as follows unless noted: SQV-SGC, 1200 mg tid; SQV-HGC, 600 mg tid; ZDV, 300 mg bid; 3TC, 150 mg bid; IDV, 800 mg q8h; NFV, 750 mg tid.

CD4, CD4+ T-lymphocyte count (cells/mm^3); HIV RNA, viral load (log_{10} copies/ml); IDV, indinavir; LoQ, limit of quantitation; NFV, nelfinavir; NRTIs, nucleoside reverse transcriptase inhibitors; PI, protease inhibitor; SQV-HGC saquinavir-HGC; SQV-SGC, saquinavir-soft gel capsules; 3TC, lamivudine; ZDV, zidovudine.

[a]For all enrollees.

[b]SQV-SGC dose was 800 mg tid.

[c]Five also had nelfinavir (30 mg/kg tid, maximum 750 mg).

▲ **Table 12–4.** MAJOR CLINICAL STUDIES OF BOOSTED SQV-SGC

Study Name and Type	Regimens	Baseline Characteristics: Rx History	Baseline Characteristics: Mean HIV RNA	Baseline Characteristics: Mean CD4	Results: Mean HIV RNA	Results: Change in Mean CD4	Results: % Below LoQ	Comments
MaxCmin1[63]: open label, randomized	SQV-SCG/RTV(1000/100 mg bid) (n = 148)	25% ART-naive, 39% PI-naive	4.0	275	–	+58	71 (LoQ 100 copies/ml)	24-Week data
	IDV/RTV (800/100 mg bid) (n = 158)		4.0	280	–	+40	66 (LoQ 100 copies/ml)	
French Five-Drug Combination Study[64]:open label	SQV-HGC/ritonavir (1000/100 mg bid) + EFV (600 mg/day) + 2 recycled NRTIs (n = 32)	Triple-drug regimen containing IDV or RTV	4.4	295	−1.21	+100	58 (LoQ 50 copies/ml)	48-Week data
Spanish Fortogene Trial[65]: open label, multicenter	SQV-SGC/ritonavir (1000/100 mg bid) (n = 144)	Multiple PI-containing regimens without SQV	5.0	367	75% (>1.0 log_{10} drop and/or < 50 copies/ml)	+97	60 (LoQ 50 copies/ml)	6-Month data
Focus[66]: open label, randomized, multicenter	SQV-SGC/RTV (1600/100 mg qd) + 2 NRTIs (n = 81)	All ART-naive	4.8	372	–	+166	60 (LoQ 50 copies/ml)	24-Week data
	EFV (600 mg qd) + 2 NRTIs (n = 80)		4.7	341	–	+144	78 (LoQ 50 copies/ml)	
HIV-NAT 001.3[67]: open label	SQV-SGC/ritonavir (1600/100 mg qd) (100 mg) plus continued dual NRTIs (n = 69)	ZDV/ddI + SQV-SGC + ZDV/3TC or ddI/d4T	4.7	534	–	+130	91 (LoQ 50 copies/ml)	48-Week data
Saquinavir-Lopinavir/Ritonavir Pilot Study[68]: open label, dose escalation	Individualized regimens, SQV-SGC, LPV/RTV + 2 NRTIs or tenofovir. All initiated SQV-SGC at 1000 mg bid 200 and LPV/RTV at 400/100 mg bid (n = 28)	All PI-experienced (71% SQV) and LPV-naive	4.4	216	–	+74	42 (LoQ 50 copies/ml)	24-Week data
Canadian Salvage Study[69]: open label	SQV-SGC (100 mg bid) + LPV/RTV (400/100 mg bid) + NRTIs (n = 36)	2 Prior HAARTs	5.1	91	−1.24	+16	–	24-Week data Intensification with efavirenz (600 mg qd) if < 0.8 log_{10} drop in the plasma HIV RNA level at week 4

ART, antiretroviral therapy; CD4, CD4+ T-lymphocyte count (cells/mm^3); d4T, stavudine; ddI, didanosine; EFV, efavirenz; HAART, highly active retroviral therapy; HIV RNA; Viral load (log_{10} copies/ml); LPV, lopinavir, LoQ, limit of quantitation; NRTIs, nucleoside reverse transcriptase inhibitors; PI, protease inhibitor; RTV, ritonavir; SQV-HGC saquinavir-hard gel capsules; SQV-SGC, saquinavir-soft gel capsules; ZDV, zidovudine.

Combining either formulation of saquinavir with ritonavir provided increased activity compared to that achieved with unboosted saquinavir-containing regimens. Regimens containing saquinavir-SGC/ritonavir 1000/100 mg bid have been shown to be superior, at least in terms of tolerability, to those containing higher doses of ritonavir. Recently completed and ongoing studies are evaluating potential alternative saquinavir-SGC/ritonavir regimens (e.g., 1600/100 qd) or exploring strategies such as "double boosting" in which plasma concentrations of more than one antiretroviral agent are boosted by concurrent ritonavir.

Saquinavir-HGC/Ritonavir 400/400 mg bid Combination Protocol

An open-label, multicenter study evaluated the safety and efficacy of four dosage regimens that combined saquinavir-HGC with ritonavir.[70] A total of 141 PI-naive patients were enrolled. The four regimens were 400 mg bid of each drug, saquinavir-HGC 400 mg bid with ritonavir 600 mg bid, 400 mg tid of each drug, and 600 mg bid of each drug. If subjects failed to achieve a plasma HIV RNA titer of less than 200 copies per milliliter by week 12 or subsequently had detectable plasma HIV RNA, concurrent reverse transcriptase therapy was added to the dual-PI therapy. Therapy was intensified in this manner in 27 subjects (19%), and 23 of the 27 subsequently had plasma HIV RNA titers below 200 copies per milliliter.

All four groups had prompt decreases in median HIV RNA titers of 2.7 to 3.1 $\log_{10}$ copies per milliliter (Roche Amplicor assay) and increased CD4+ T-lymphocyte counts; these trends were similar in all four groups at week 48.[70] After 48 weeks of the therapy, the subjects were offered the option to change to the best tolerated regimen: saquinavir-HGC/ritonavir 400/400 mg bid.

This study has now been ongoing for 5 years and is the longest trial of dual-PI therapy to be performed to date. The 5-year follow-up data indicate that dual-PI therapy containing saquinavir-HGC/ritonavir can have sustained virologic effects. Of the 66 subjects still participating at 5 years, 54 (82%) had plasma HIV RNA titers of less than 200 copies per milliliter.[71] Furthermore, between years 4 and 5, there was a median increase in CD4+ T-lymphocyte count of 54 cells per cubic millimeter even though only one subject (2%) required treatment intensification during this period.

Prometheus

Prometheus, an open-label, randomized, controlled trial, compared saquinavir-HGC/ritonavir (400/400 mg bid) with that of saquinavir-HGC/ritonavir (400/400 mg bid) plus stavudine (40 mg bid) in 208 PI- and stavudine-naive HIV-1-infected individuals. Intensification of reverse transcriptase inhibitor therapy was permitted if plasma HIV-RNA levels remained higher than 400 copies per milliliter after 12 weeks of treatment.[72] At 48 weeks, an intent-to-treat analysis revealed no significant difference between the two treatment groups in terms of the proportion of patients who achieved plasma HIV RNA levels of less than 400 copies per milliliter (63% in the saquinavir/ritonavir group vs. 69% in the saquinavir/ritonavir/stavudine group, $P = 0.379$).

Saquinavir/Ritonavir 1000/100 mg bid (MaxCmin1)

A Phase IV randomized, open-label, parallel group multicenter trial evaluated the safety and efficacy of saquinavir-SGC/ritonavir (1000/100 mg bid) versus indinavir/ritonavir (800/100 mg bid) in adult HIV-1-infected patients.[63] In an interim intent-to-treat analysis performed on 24-week data from 306 patients, no between-group differences were observed in terms of virologic or immunologic responses or in the proportion of patients with grade 3/4 adverse events. At baseline and at 4, 12, and 24 weeks, 36%, 48%, 66%, and 71% of patients in the saquinavir-SGC/ritonavir group, respectively, had HIV-1 RNA titers of less than 100 copies per milliliter compared with 35%, 47%, 61%, and 66% in the indinavir/ritonavir group. Virologic failure had occurred by week 24 in 16% of saquinavir-SGC/ritonavir recipients and 13% of those given indinavir/ritonavir. At weeks 4, 12, and 24 weeks, the CD4+ T-lymphocyte count increases from baseline were 33, 42, and 58 cells per cubic millimeter, respectively, in the saquinavir-SGC/ritonavir group and 30, 43, and 40 cells per cubic millimeter in the indinavir/ritonavir group. Among those who initiated study therapy, more on indinavir/ritonavir than on saquinavir-SGC/ritonavir had discontinued by week 24 (27% vs. 17%) (Table 12–4).

French Five-Drug Combination Study

The French five-drug combination trial was an open-label, single-arm study that assessed the safety and efficacy of a five-drug combination regimen that contained saquinavir-HGC/ritonavir (1000/100 mg bid), efavirenz (600 mg/day), and two recycled nucleosides in patients who had previously failed a conventional triple-drug regimen containing indinavir or ritonavir.[64] A total of 32 saquinavir- and efavirenz-naive, PI-experienced patients were enrolled. All but one remained in the study at 48 weeks. There was a decrease in the mean HIV RNA titer that remained at 1.21 $\log_{10}$ copies per milliliter below baseline at week 48. At this time point, 58% had an HIV RNA titer of less than 50 copies per milliliter. The median CD4+ T-lymphocyte count increased progressively throughout the study, reaching a peak of 100 cells per cubic millimeter above baseline at week 48. The lack of saquinavir phenotypic resistance at baseline was associated with a higher likelihood of achieving HIV RNA titers of less than 50 copies per milliliter at week 48. However, the lack of saquinavir genotypic resistance (L90M and G48V mutations) at baseline was not predictive of the virologic response.

Spanish Fortogene Trial

The Spanish Fortogene study, an ongoing, prospective, multicenter trial, is assessing the efficacy and safety of saquinavir-SGC/ritonavir (1000/100 mg bid) as salvage therapy in 144 HIV-infected, PI-experienced adults experiencing virologic failure.[65] Their mean plasma HIV RNA titer on entry was 100,047 copies per milliliter and their mean CD4+ T-lymphocyte count was 367 cells per cubic millimeter. Overall, a significant virologic response (defined as > 1 $\log_{10}$ drop, an HIV RNA titer < 50 copies per milliliter, or both) was seen in 76.6% of subjects, with 60.0% achieving HIV RNA titers of less than 50 copies per milliliter. By 6 months, the mean CD4+ T-lymphocyte count had increased by 97 cells per cubic millimeter. In a subanalysis involving 51 subjects, of whom 9 had virus with at least four saquinavir resistance-conferring mutations, a better virologic response was observed in subjects with saquinavir-sensitive viral genotypes than in subjects with saquinavir-resistant viral genotypes (four or more saquinavir resistance mutations) (89% vs. 57%; $P < 0.05$) (Table 12–4).

Switching From Saquinavir/Ritonavir 400/400 mg bid to 1000/100 mg bid

In a trial that switched doses of saquinavir/ritonavir, eligible patients with viral levels of less than 200 copies per milliliter, had been receiving saquinavir/ritonavir 400/400 mg bid for at least 6 months, without prior use of more than one other PI for more than 3 months.[73] Patients were randomized to continue their current therapy or to switch to saquinavir-SGC/ritonavir 1000/100 mg bid. None of the 23 patients in the study had HIV-1 RNA levels of more than 400 copies per milliliter through month 6. At 1 month after randomization the mean peak saquinavir levels were 1482 ± 1118 ng/ml in those continuing the 400/400 regimen compared with 1822 ± 2263 ng/ml in those switched to the 1000/100 mg regimen. Mean trough saquinavir levels with the 400/400 mg regimen were 545 ± 413 ng/ml compared with 1077 ± 2002 with the 1000/100 mg regimen. In the 1000/100 mg arm, fasting triglyceride levels fell from 635 mg/dl at baseline to 375 mg/dl at month 6 ($P = 0.038$). Cholesterol levels fell from 323 mg/dl at baseline to 236 mg/dl at month 6 (P = NS). Improved tolerability was also documented.

Saquinavir/Ritonavir 1600/100 mg qd

Focus Trial

The Fortovase Once Daily Canada US (FOCUS) trial is an ongoing, open-label, randomized, multicenter trial is that comparing the antiviral activity and safety of saquinavir-SGC/ritonavir (1600/100 mg qd) with that of efavirenz (600 mg qd), each in combination with two nucleoside analogues, in 159 HIV-positive, antiretroviral-naive patients.[66] Altogether, 60% of the saquinavir-SGC/ritonavir group and 78% of the efavirenz group achieved plasma HIV RNA titers of less than 50 copies per milliliter ($P = 0.008$) at 24 weeks. The mean increase in the CD4+ T-lymphocyte count was greater in the saquinavir-SGC/ritonavir group than in the efavirenz group (166 vs. 144 cells per cubic millimeter). Further analyses were planned for 48 weeks.

HIV-NAT 001.3

The HIV-NAT 001.3 trial was a prospective, open-label, single-arm study that evaluated the efficacy and safety of saquinavir-SGC/ritonavir (1600/100 mg qd) plus continued dual NRTI therapy.[67] A series of 69 Thai patients, were studied with plasma HIV RNA levels of less than 50 copies per milliliter. They had previously been treated with zidovudine/didanosine (half dose or full dose) for 66 weeks followed by saquinavir-SGC (1400 mg bid) plus zidovudine/lamivudine or didanosine/stavudine for 2 years. At 48 weeks 91.0% had a plasma viral load maintained at less than 50 copies per milliliter. The median CD4+ T-lymphocyte count increased significantly from 534 cells per cubic millimeter at the start of saquinavir-SGC/ritonavir once-daily therapy to 664 cells per cubic millimeter after 48 weeks.

Saquinavir-Lopinavir/Ritonavir Pilot Study

A prospective, open-label, single-arm, dose escalation study evaluated the antiviral activity of "double-boosting" with saquinavir-SGC plus lopinavir/ritonavir (Kaletra) in lopinavir-naive, PI-experienced patients.[68] A total of 28 individuals with plasma HIV RNA titers of more than 1000 copies per milliliter were given individualized regimens containing saquinavir-SGC, lopinavir/ritonavir, and two or more nucleosides (or tenofovir), guided by their virtual phenotypes. All initiated saquinavir-SGC at a dose of 1000 mg bid and lopinavir/ritonavir at 400/100 mg bid. At 24 weeks in the on-treatment analysis, 87% and 53% of patients had viral load levels < 40 copies per milliliter and < 400 copies per milliliter, respectively. By 24 weeks the median CD4+ T-lymphocyte count in the intent-to-treat sample had increased by 74 cells per cubic millimeter. Although the virtual phenotypes predicted resistance to saquinavir in 31% of the patients and to lopinavir in 42%, neither drug titers alone nor the virtual phenotype alone correlated with the virologic response. However, the combined normalized inhibitory quotient of lopinavir and saquinavir was significantly predictive of achieving a viral load of less than 50 copies per milliliter at week 12. Further analyses were planned for 48 weeks (Table 12–4).

Canadian Salvage Study

The Canadian salvage study, a prospective, open-label, single-arm trial, evaluated the antiviral activity of saquinavir-SGC plus lopinavir/ritonavir plus nucleosides in patients failing at least two prior HAART regimens.[69] A total of 36 patients were given saquinavir-SGC (100 mg bid) plus lopinavir/ritonavir (400/100 mg bid). Patients with a less than 0.8 $\log_{10}$ copies per milliliter drop in the plasma HIV RNA titer at week 4 were eligible for treatment intensification with efavirenz (600 mg qd) and lopinavir/ritonavir dose adjustment. By week 24 a total of 22 patients remained in the study, and there was a 1.24 $\log_{10}$ copies per milliliter reduction in HIV RNA compared with baseline and an increase in the CD4+ T-lymphocyte count of 59 cells per cubic millimeter (Table 12–4).

▲ RESISTANCE

In vitro experiments with saquinavir originally suggested that changes in codons at positions 48 and 90 of the protease gene were closely associated with decreased susceptibility to this inhibitor.[74–81] The protease codon changes in L90M and G48V are associated individually with about threefold and eightfold decreases in susceptibility to saquinavir, respectively. HIV isolates with both mutations have about a 20-fold decrease.[80,82]

In vivo experience from subjects in saquinavir treatment studies has confirmed the importance of these mutations with respect to saquinavir resistance during therapy.[10,82–86] The most common PI-associated codon change has been L90M, found in 18% to 42% of patients on saquinavir monotherapy. Codon G48V was found in fewer than 2% in Phase I and II studies; and fewer than 2% of patients were found to have codon changes at both positions 48 and 90.[87] In the Phase III study NV14256, G48V was present in none of the saquinavir monotherapy arm at 40 to 72 weeks, and both mutations occurred in only one patient analyzed (8%).[86] The frequency of mutations was higher in patients on saquinavir monotherapy than in those on combination regimens, and with increasing duration of saquinavir therapy.[83,86,87] Mutations were found to be similar in lymph nodes and plasma in 10 patients receiving high-dose saquinavir monotherapy.[88,89]

Similarly, the development of mutations at protease positions 48 and 90 was examined in 144 subjects assigned to a triple drug (zidovudine/zalcitabine/saquinavir) or a dual-drug (zidovudine/saquinavir), saquinavir-HCG-containing regimen in ACTG protocol 229.[90] At baseline, all subjects were wild type at codons 48 and 90. One-third of the subjects treated with the triple-drug regimen, and 46% of subjects in the dual-drug arm developed L90M at 24 weeks or more after starting the study regimen; 4% and 8%, respectively, developed both L90M and G48V. Only one subject was found to have an isolated mutation at position 48. The emergence of protease mutations was found to correlate with higher plasma HIV-1 RNA levels at baseline.

Secondary substitutions at other codons in HIV-1 protease have subsequently been described in patients treated with long-term saquinavir, including at positions 10, 36, 54, 63, 71, 82, and 84.[82,87,91] At least some of these secondary mutations (e.g., codons 10, 63, and 71) appear to compensate for reductions in HIV replicative capacity associated with the emergence of L90M without further decreasing viral susceptibility to saquinavir.[92,93]

The presence of L90M or G48V at baseline is not universally predictive of a poor virologic response to a saquinavir-containing combination regimen.[64,94] Indeed, L90M-containing isolates have been shown to exhibit a surprisingly broad range of susceptibilities to saquinavir and other PIs, modified by the presence of secondary mutations in protease.[94] In terms of phenotypic drug susceptibility, a significant and continuous correlation between saquinavir susceptibility and virologic suppression on a saquinavir-containing regimen has been observed.[95]

Early data suggested that the pattern of mutations associated with the use of saquinavir differed from that seen with ritonavir and indinavir, raising the possibility that cross resistance among these compounds would not be significant.[83] However, subsequent data indicate that cross resistance between saquinavir and most other PIs does occur.[96,97] More than 6000 recombinant HIV-1 isolates with protease and reverse transcriptase genes derived from HIV sequences in plasma from patients on PIs were tested for phenotypic resistance in vitro (Antivirogram assay).[97] Among the 1120 isolates that demonstrated more than a 10-fold decrease in susceptibility to saquinavir, more than 60% of isolates also had a 10-fold decrease in susceptibility to other PIs. The percentages of less sensitive isolates were 62% to indinavir, 72% to ritonavir, and 78% to nelfinavir. In addition, for isolates selected because of more than a 10-fold decrease in susceptibility to one of these three PIs, more than 60% also had more than a 10-fold decrease in susceptibility to saquinavir. The extent of in vitro cross resistance to other PIs associated with the emergence of protease changes under saquinavir drug pressure appears to be related to the type and number of mutations present in addition to L90M or G48V.[78,94,98–100]

The in vitro data on cross resistance is corroborated by in vivo studies that show an association between response to a subsequent PI following virologic failure on saquinavir and the number of mutations in the protease gene. One protocol (ACTG 333) found that the response to indinavir at a median of 112 weeks of saquinavir in patients with at least 48 weeks of prior saquinavir treatment, was inversely correlated with the number of protease mutations. The number of mutations, in turn, was correlated with the baseline CD4+ T-lymphocyte count, HIV-1 RNA levels, saquinavir experience, and phenotypic drug susceptibility.[91] Variable virologic responses to subsequent indinavir-, nelfinavir-, or ritonavir-based regimens following saquinavir exposure have also been described in other studies.[101–103]

Although there is some evidence that the G48V mutation is more common at higher doses of saquinavir,[98,101] it is not known whether the enhanced bioavailability and resultant increased systemic exposure of the soft gelatin formulation of saquinavir affects the type or frequency of mutations seen with the original formulation. Craig and colleagues sequenced the protease gene in plasma isolates from 74 patients before and after therapy with saquinavir-SGC 1200 mg tid from the early saquinavir-SGC studies NV15107, NV15182, and NV15355.[104,105] Although the key mutations seen were the same as those reported for the hard gelatin formulation, the incidence of the G48V mutation was increased, suggesting that treatment with saquinavir-SGC may favor this mutation. There did not appear to be an increased incidence of mutations in other sites in the protease gene that have been associated with cross resistance to other PIs. Further analyses are needed with specimens from patients receiving saquinavir-SGC in triple-combination regimens to determine the frequency of mutations in this setting.

▲ DRUG INTERACTIONS

The potential for drug interactions between either formulation of saquinavir and other drugs is significant because the CYP3A4 isoenzyme is a common metabolic pathway for many agents.[35] Drugs that are metabolized by or induce or inhibit the cytochrome P_{450} system, especially isoenzyme 3A4, may affect the metabolism, plasma levels, and systemic exposure of saquinavir-HGC and saquinavir-SGC.[3,34] In addition, saquinavir is a mild inhibitor of cy-

▲ **Table 12–5.** DRUG INTERACTIONS WITH SAQUINAVIR-HGC AND SAQUINAVIR-SGC

Class	Agents
Drugs that should not be administered with SQV-HGC or SQV-SGC	
H_1-receptor blockers	Astemizole, terfenadine
Antimigraine therapies	Ergot derivatives
Gastrointestinal motility agents	Cisapride
Sedative-hypnotics	Midazolam, triazolam
Herbal preparations	St. John's wort (*Hypericum perforatum*)
Co-administration may increase SQV-HGC or SQV-SGC plasma concentrations	
Antimicrobials	Clarithromycin, ketoconazole
Nonnucleoside reverse transcriptase inhibitors	Delavirdine
Protease inhibitors	Ritonavir, indinavir, nelfinavir, amprenavir[a]
H_2-receptor blockers	Ranitidine[a]
Co-administration may decrease SQV or SQV-SGC plasma concentrations	
Antimycobacterial agents	Rifabutin, rifampin
Nonnucleoside reverse transcriptase inhibitors	Nevirapine
Anticonvulsants	Carbamazepine, phenobarbital, phenytoin
Corticosteroids	Dexamethasone

[a]Not considered clinically significant.
Adapted from Roche Laboratories prescribing information,[27,53] except amprenavir data.[108]

tochrome P_{450} enzymes and may affect the metabolism of some other drugs.[106] Furthermore, as saquinavir is a substrate for P-glycoprotein, drugs that modify P-glycoprotein activity may modify the pharmacokinetics of saquinavir. Similarly, saquinavir has the potential to modify the pharmacokinetics of other drugs that are substrates for P-glycoprotein.[27,53]

Clinically significant interactions may occur between saquinavir-HGC or saquinavir-SGC (or both) and several drugs that are commonly used in HIV-infected persons. They are listed in Tables 12–5 and 12–6.[27,53,107–110] It should be noted that results from studies conducted with saquinavir-HGC may not be applicable to saquinavir-SGC and vice versa.[27,53]

Drug interactions with other antiretroviral agents that may be clinically significant for saquinavir-HGC and saquinavir-SGC include those with nelfinavir, indinavir, and the nonnucleoside reverse transcriptase inhibitors (NNRTIs) delavirdine and nevirapine. An interaction between saquinavir-SGC and the experimental PI atazanavir (BMS 232632) has been observed.[109] It appears to be less pronounced than that between saquinavir and ritonavir, requiring a therapeutic dose of atazanavir.[110] An interaction between the components of grapefruit juice and saquinavir has also attracted interest. Co-administration of 600 mg saquinavir-SGC and quadruple-strength grapefruit juice as a single administration in healthy volunteers results in a 54% increase in exposure to saquinavir, but the increase is

▲ **Table 12–6.** EFFECT OF SQV-SGC ON THE PHARMACOKINETICS OF CO-ADMINISTERED DRUGS

Co-administered Drug	Saquinavir Dose	Study Subjects	% Change for Co-administered Drug	
			AUC	C_{max}
Clarithromycin 500 mg bid × 7 days	1200 mg tid × 7days	12 Healthy volunteers		
Clarithromycin			↑45	↑39
14-OH clarithromycin metabolite			↓24	↓34
Nelfinavir 750 mg single dose	1200 mg tid × 4 days	14 Patients	↑18	↔
Ritonavir 400 mg bid × 14 days	400 mg bid × 14 days	8 Healthy volunteers	↔	↔
Amprenavir	Unknown	Unknown	↓40[b]	↓36[b]
Efavirenz	Unknown	Unknown	↓13	↓12
Sildenafil 100 mg single dose	1200 mg tid × 8 days	27 Healthy volunteers	↑210	↑140
Terfenadine 60 mg bid × 11 days[a]	1200 mg tid × 4 days	12 Healthy volunteers		
Terfenadine			↑368	↑253
Terfenadine acid metabolite			↑120	↑93

↑ Denotes an average increase in exposure by the percentage indicated. ↓ Denotes an average decrease in exposure by the percentage indicated.
↔ Denotes no statistically significant change in exposure.
[a]Saquinavir-SGC should not be co-administered with terfenadine.
[b]Compared with historical controls.
Adapted from Roche Laboratories prescribing information, except amprenavir and efavirenz data.[27,53,108]

not thought to be clinically relevant, and no dose adjustment of saquinavir is recommended.[27]

Another study involving 12 HIV-negative volunteers maintained on stable methadone (35 to 100 mg) has shown that the administration of saquinavir-SGC/ritonavir (1600/100 mg qd) for 14 days resulted in a small reduction in the free fraction of R-methadone.[111] However, it was not considered clinically significant, and no methadone dose changes were required.

Although specific studies have not been performed, co-administration with drugs that are mainly metabolized by CYP3A4 [e.g., calcium channel blockers, dapsone, disopyramide, quinine, amiodarone, quinidine, warfarin, tacrolimus, cyclosporine, ergot derivatives, carbamazepine, fentanyl, alfentanil, alprazolam, triazolam, nefazodone, 3-hydroxy-methylglutaryl coenzyme A (HMG-CoA) reductase inhibitors] may have elevated plasma concentrations when co-administered with saquinavir-SGC.[111] No data are available about interactions between either formulation of saquinavir and oral contraceptives.

▲ RECOMMENDATIONS FOR USE

Both saquinavir-HGC and saquinavir-SGC formulations should be used in conjunction with other antiretroviral agents. Current recommendations for first-line therapy suggest concurrent use of a potent PI (or more than one) and two NRTIs.[112,113] Saquinavir-SGC is one of the recommended options for first-line therapy as the sole PI.[113] However, the pill burden of this formulation is substantial. Saquinavir-HGC is not recommended for first-line therapy as the sole PI in a regimen because of its limited bioavailability. Saquinavir-HGC and saquinavir-SGC capsules are not bioequivalent and cannot be used interchangeably. A switch to saquinavir-SGC is not recommended in patients taking saquinavir-HGC who have not had an adequate response or who are failing therapy.[113] Saquinavir-HGC may be considered for first-line therapy if it is to be combined with antiretroviral agents that significantly inhibit the metabolism of saquinavir.[112]

The concomitant use of saquinavir-HGC or saquinavir-SGC and ritonavir is also one of the recommended options for a potent PI regimen; this regimen is attractive because of its twice-daily schedule, lower pill burden than saquinavir-SGC, and reasonable tolerability. If used, liver function tests should be carefully monitored. Other combinations of PIs with saquinavir formulations should be considered experimental until more data are available from ongoing studies. Concurrent use of nevirapine, rifampin, or rifabutin with either saquinavir formulation should be avoided to prevent a decrease in saquinavir concentrations. There are insufficient data about regimens that include saquinavir in combination with ritonavir or nelfinavir, along with NNRTIs, to make explicit treatment recommendations. Limited data are also available about the use of saquinavir-containing dual-PI regimens following treatment failure with other PIs. Saquinavir/ritonavir in combination with two other agents is in widespread use in this setting; variable results have been reported.[114–116]

▲ DOSING

Saquinavir-HGC

Saquinavir-HGC is available in 200 mg capsules. The dose of saquinavir-HGC originally recommended for use in adults was 600 mg tid, taken with or within 2 hours after food ingestion. Absorption is maximized if the food is a full meal. However, this formulation should not be used as a sole PI in a regimen. When used concurrently with ritonavir, two dosing regimens have achieved widespread acceptance: 1000/100 mg bid (12 capsules per day, not including the background regimen pill count) and 400/400 mg bid (12 capsules per day, not including the background regimen pill count). Data suggest that saquinavir-HGC/ritonavir provides therapeutic levels of saquinavir and has a better tolerability profile than saquinavir-SGC/ritonavir.[29] It is recommended that saquinavir/ritonavir be taken with or within 2 hours after food ingestion.

Saquinavir-SGC

Saquinavir-SGC is available in 200 mg capsules. The recommended dose of saquinavir-SGC, when used as a sole PI in adults, is 1200 mg tid, taken with or within 2 hours after food ingestion. The saquinavir pill burden with this regimen is 18 capsules per day. Studies have shown that regimens containing saquinavir-SGC 1600 mg bid are equivalent to those containing saquinavir-SGC 1200 mg tid. Absorption is maximized if the food is a full meal. When used concurrently with ritonavir, the recommended dose of saquinavir is 1000 mg bid with a ritonavir dose of 100 mg bid. Higher doses of ritonavir have been shown to be associated with an increase incidence of adverse events. This regimen has a total pill burden of 12 capsules per day (not including reverse transcriptase therapy). A 1600/100 mg qd regimen has also achieved promising results: it has a pill burden of 9 capsules per day (not including reverse transcriptase therapy). A logistical issue that may be relevant for saquinavir dosing in some settings or climates is that saquinavir-SGC should be stored in a refrigerator before being dispensed and should be stored at room temperature for only 3 months.

Acknowledgment. We are grateful to Jim Scott and Hoffmann LaRoche for providing updated materials for this chapter.

REFERENCES

1. Navia MA, Fitzgerald PM, McKeever BM, et al. Three-dimensional structure of aspartyl protease from human immunodeficiency virus HIV-1. Nature 337:615, 1989.
2. Deeks SG, Volberding PA. HIV-1 protease inhibitors. JAMA 277:145, 1997.
3. Flexner C. HIV-protease inhibitors. N Engl J Med 338:1281, 1998.
4. Ashorn P, McQuade TJ, Thaisrivongs S, et al. An inhibitor of the protease blocks maturation of human and simian immunodeficiency viruses and spread of infection. Proc Natl Acad Sci USA 87:7472, 1990.
5. McQuade TJ, Tomasselli AG, Liu L, et al. A synthetic HIV-1 protease inhibitor with antiviral activity arrests HIV-like particle maturation. Science 247:454, 1990.

6. Craig JC, Duncan IB, Hockley D, et al. Antiviral properties of Ro 31-8959, an inhibitor of human immunodeficiency virus (HIV) proteinase. Antiviral Res 16:295, 1991.
7. Roberts NA, Martin JA, Kinchington D, et al. Rational design of peptide-based HIV proteinase inhibitors. Science 248:358, 1990.
8. Bragman K. Saquinavir: an HIV proteinase inhibitor. Adv Exp Med Biol 394:305, 1996.
9. Lazdins JK, Mestan J, Goutte G, et al. In vitro effect of alpha1-acid glycoprotein on the antihuman immunodeficiency virus (HIV) activity of the protease inhibitor CGP 61755: a comparative study with other relevant HIV protease inhibitors. J Infect Dis 175:1063, 1997.
10. Eberle J, Bechowsky B, Rose D, et al. Resistance of HIV type 1 to proteinase inhibitor Ro 31-8959. AIDS Res Hum Retroviruses 11:671, 1995.
11. Galpin S, Roberts NA, O'Connor T, et al. Antiviral properties of the HIV-1 protease inhibitor Ro-31-8959. Antivir Chem Chemother 5:43, 1994.
12. Rusconi S, Merrill DP, Hirsch MS. Inhibition of human immunodeficiency virus type 1 replication in cytokine-stimulated monocytes/macrophages by combination therapy. J Infect Dis 170:1361, 1994.
13. Prescribing information for Kaletra, Viracept, Fortovase, Agenerase and Crixivan. In: Physician's Desk Reference. Montvale, NJ, Medical Economics, 2001.
14. Craig JC, Grief C, Mills JS, et al. Effects of a specific inhibitor of HIV proteinase Ro 31-8959 on virus maturation in a chronically infected promonocytic cell line UI. Antivir Chem Chemother 2:181, 1999.
15. Nitschko H, Lindhofer H, Schtzl H, et al. Long-term treatment of HIV-infected MT-4 cells in culture with HIV proteinase inhibitor Ro 31-8959 leads to complete cure of infection. Antivir Chem Chemother 5:236, 1994.
16. Johnson VA, Merrill DP, Chou TC, Hirsch MS. Human immunodeficiency virus type 1 (HIV-1) inhibitory interactions between protease inhibitor Ro 31-8959 and zidovudine, 2′,3′-dideoxycytidine, or recombinant interferon-alpha A against zidovudine-sensitive or -resistant HIV-1 in vitro. J Infect Dis 166:1143, 1992.
17. Oh M, Merrill DP, Sutton L, Hirsch MS. Sequential versus simultaneous combination antiretroviral regimens for the treatment of human immunodeficiency virus type 1 infection in vitro. J Infect Dis 176:510, 1997.
18. Mazzulli T, Rusconi S, Merrill DP, et al. Alternating versus continuous drug regimens in combination chemotherapy of human immunodeficiency virus type 1 infection in vitro. Antimicrob Agents Chemother 38:656, 1994.
19. Deminie CA, Bechtold CM, Stock D, et al. Evaluation of reverse transcriptase and protease inhibitors in two-drug combinations against human immunodeficiency virus replication. Antimicrob Agents Chemother 40:1346, 1996.
20. Merrill DP, Manion DJ, Chou TC, Hirsch MS. Antagonism between human immunodeficiency virus type 1 protease inhibitors indinavir and saquinavir in vitro. J Infect Dis 176: 265, 1997.
21. Patick AK, Boritzki TJ, Bloom LA. Activities of the human immunodeficiency virus type 1 (HIV-1) protease inhibitor nelfinavir mesylate in combination with reverse transcriptase and protease inhibitors against acute HIV-1 infection in vitro. Antimicrob Agents Chemother 41:2159, 1997.
22. Merrill DP, Moonis M, Chou TC, Hirsch MS. Lamivudine or stavudine in two- and three-drug combinations against human immunodeficiency virus type 1 replication in vitro. J Infect Dis 173:355, 1996.
23. Craig JC, Whittaker L, Duncan IB, et al. In vitro anti-HIV and cytotoxicological evaluation of triple combination: AZT and ddC with proteinase inhibitor saquinavir (Ro 31-8959). Antivir Chem Chemother 5:380, 1994.
24. Antiretroviral Pregnancy Registry for Didanosine, Indinavir, Lamivudine, Saquinavir, Stavudine, Zalcitabine, Zidovudine: Interim Report, January 1, 1989 through December 31, 1997. Pharmaresearch, Wilmington, NC, 1998.
25. Noble S, Faulds D. Saquinavir: a review of its pharmacology and clinical potential in the management of HIV infection. Drugs 52:93, 1996.
26. Perry CM, Noble S. Saquinavir soft-gel capsule formulation. a review of its use in patients with HIV infection. Drugs 1998:461, 1998.
27. Fortovase (saquinavir) soft gelatin capsules prescribing information. Nutley, NJ, Roche Laboratories, 1997.
28. Veldkamp AI, van Heeswijk RP, Mulder JW, et al. Steady-state pharmacokinetics of twice-daily dosing of saquinavir plus ritonavir in HIV-1-infected individuals. J Acquir Immun Defic Syndr 27:344, 2001.
29. Kurowski M, Sternfeld T, Hill A, et al. Comparative pharmacokinetics and short-term safety of Fortovase/ritonavir and Invirase/ritonavir 1000mg/100mg BID. In: Abstracts of the 9th Conference on Retroviruses and Opportunistic Infections, Seattle, 2002, abstract 432-W.
30. Buss N, Snell P, Bock J, et al. Saquinavir and ritonavir pharmacokinetics following combined ritonavir and saquinavir (soft gelatin capsules) administration. Br J Clin Pharmacol 52:255, 2001.
31. Van Heeswijk RPG, Cardiello P, Monhaphol T, et al. Once-daily dosing of 1,600 mg saquinavir gelatin capsules (SQV-SGC) plus low dose ritonavir (RTV; 100 mg) in HIV-1-infected Thai patients: pharmacokinetics and clinical experience (HIV-NAT 001). In: Abstracts of the 2nd International Workshop on Clinical Pharmacology of HIV Therapy, Noordwijk, The Netherlands, 2001, abstract 3.9.
32. Lalezari J. Selecting the optimum dose for a new soft gelatin capsule formulation of saquinavir; NV15107 Study Group. J Acquir Immune Defic Syndr Hum Retrovirol 19:195, 1998.
33. Gieschke R, Fotteler B, Buss N, Steimer JL. Relationships between exposure to saquinavir monotherapy and antiviral response in HIV-positive patients. Clin Pharmacokinet 37:75, 1999.
34. Fitzsimmons ME, Collins JM. Selective biotransformation of the human immunodeficiency virus protease inhibitor saquinavir by human small-intestinal cytochrome P4503A4: potential contribution to high first-pass metabolism. Drug Metab Dispos 25:256, 1997.
35. Van Cleef GF, Fisher EJ, Polk RE. Drug interaction potential with inhibitors of HIV protease. Pharmacotherapy 17:774, 1997.
36. Van Heeswijk RPG, Velkamp A, Mulder JW, et al. Combination of protease inhibitors for the treatment of HIV-1-infected patients: a review of pharmacokinetics and clinical experience. Antivir Ther 6:201, 2002.
37. Kumar GN, Dykstra J, Roberts EM, et al. Potent inhibition of the cytochrome P-450 3A-mediated human liver microsomal metabolism of a novel HIV protease inhibitor by ritonavir: a positive drug–drug interaction. Drug Metab Dispos 27:902, 1999.
38. Merry C, Barry MG, Mulcahy F, et al. Saquinavir pharmacokinetics alone and in combination with ritonavir in HIV-infected patients. AIDS 11:F29, 1997.
39. Kempf DJ, Marsh KC, Kumar G, et al. Pharmacokinetic enhancement of inhibitors of the human immunodeficiency virus protease by coadministration with ritonavir. Antimicrob Agents Chemother 41:654, 1997.
40. Kilby JM, Hill A, Buss N. The effect of ritonavir on increases in saquinavir plasma concentration independent of ritonavir dosage: combined analysis of data from 97 subjects. HIV Med 3:97, 2002.
41. Kilby JM, Sfakianos G, Gizzi N, et al. Safety and pharmacokinetics of once-daily regimens of soft-gel capsule saquinavir plus minidose ritonavir in human immunodeficiency virus-negative adults. Antimicrob Agents Chemother 44:2672, 2000.
42. Haubrich R, Lalezari J, Follansbee SE, et al. Improved survival and reduced clinical progression in HIV-infected patients with advanced disease treatment with saquinavir plus zalcitabine. Antivir Ther 3:33, 1998.
43. Mitsuyasu RT, Skolnik PR, Cohen SR, et al. Activity of the soft gelatin formulation of saquinavir in combination therapy in antiretroviral-naive patients. NV15355 Study Team. AIDS 12:F103, 1998.
44. Gill MJ. Safety profile of soft gelatin formulation of saquinavir in combination with nucleosides in a broad patient population. NV15182 Study Team. AIDS 12:1400, 1998.
45. Nightingale SL. From the Food and Drug Administration. JAMA 278:379, 1997.
46. Lo JC, Mulligan K, Tai VW, et al. "Buffalo hump" in men with HIV-1 infection. Lancet 351:867, 1998.
47. Miller KD, Jones E, Yanovski JA, et al. Visceral abdominal-fat accumulation associated with use of indinavir. Lancet 351:871, 1998.
48. Henry K, Melroe H, Huebsch J, et al. Severe premature coronary artery disease with protease inhibitors. Lancet 351:1328, 1998.
49. Hengel RL, Watts NB, Lennox JL. Benign symmetric lipomatosis associated with protease inhibitors. Lancet 350:1596, 1997.
50. Carr A, Samaras K, Burton S, et al. A syndrome of peripheral lipodystrophy (LD) hyperlipidemia and insulin resistance in patients receiving HIV protease inhibitors. AIDS 12:F51, 1998.
51. Carr A, Samaras K, Chisholm DJ, Cooper DA. Pathogenesis of HIV-1-protease inhibitor-associated peripheral lipodystrophy, hyperlipidaemia, and insulin resistance. Lancet 351:1881, 1998.

52. Van der Valk M, Gisolf EH, Reiss P, et al. Prometheus study group: increased risk of lipodystrophy when nucleoside analogue reverse transcriptase inhibitors are included with protease inhibitors in the treatment of HIV-1 infection. AIDS 15:847, 2001.
53. Invirase (saquinavir mesylate) capsules prescribing information. Nutley, NJ, Roche Laboratories, 1995.
54. Revicki D, Swartz C, Wu AW, et al. Quality of life outcomes of saquinavir, zalcitabine and combination saquinavir-zalcitabine therapy for adults with advanced HIV infection with CD4 counts between 50 and 300 cells/mm^3. Antivir Ther 4:35, 1999.
55. Revicki DA, Moyle G, Stellbrink HJ, Barker C. Quality of life outcomes of combination zalcitabine-zidovudine, saquinavir-zidovudine, and saquinavir-zalcitabine-zidovudine therapy for HIV-infected adults with CD4+ cell counts between 50 and 350 per cubic millimeter. PISCES (SV14604) Study Group. AIDS 13:851, 1999.
56. Cameron DW, Japur A, Mellors J, et al. Antiretroviral safety and durability of ritonavir (RIT)-saquinavir (SQV) in protease inhibitor-naive patients in year of follow-up. In: Abstracts of the 5th Conference on Retroviruses and Opportunistic Infections, Chicago, 1998, abstract 388.
57. Srasuebkul P, Cardiello P, Hassink E, et al. Gastrointestinal toxicity and triglyceride levels when switching from a twice daily to a once daily saquinavir soft gel regimen. In: Poster at the 3rd International Workshop on Adverse Drug Reactions Lipodystrophy in HIV, Athens, 2001, poster 118.
58. Sension MG, Farthing C, Shaffer AG, et al. Challenges of antiretroviral treatment in transient and drug-using populations: the SUN study. AIDS Patient Care STDS 15:129, 2001.
59. Cohen Stuart JW, Schuurman R, Burger DM, et al. Randomized trial comparing saquinavir soft gelatin capsules versus indinavir as part of triple therapy (CHEESE study). AIDS 13:F53, 1999.
60. Moyle G, Pozniak A, Opravil M, et al. The SPICE study: 48-week activity of combinations of saquinavir soft gelatin and nelfinavir with and without nucleoside analogues: study of protease inhibitor combinations in Europe. J Acquir Immune Defic Syndr 23:128, 2000.
61. Lalezari J, Feinberg JM, Sension M, et al. TIDBID study 48 week analysis: FORTOVASE (FTV) TID regimen compared to FTV BID or FTV + NFV BID regimens in HIV-1 infected patients. In: Poster at the XIII World AIDS Conference, Durban, South Africa, 2000, poster 12314.
62. Kline MW, Brundage RC, Fletcher CV, et al. Combination therapy with saquinavir soft gelatin capsules in children with human immunodeficiency virus infection. Pediatr Infect Dis J 20:666, 2001.
63. Castagna A, Dragsted UB, Chave JP, et al. The interim analysis of a phase IV randomised, open label, multicentre trial to evaluate safety and efficacy of indinavir/ritonavir (800/100 mg bid) vs. saquinavir/ritonavir (1000/100mg bid) in adult HIV-1 infection: the MaxCmin1 trial. In: Poster at the 9th Conference on Retroviruses and Opportunistic Infections, Seattle, 2002, poster 450-W.
64. Piketty C, Race E, Castiel P, et al. Phenotypic resistance to protease inhibitors in patients who fail on highly active antiretroviral therapy predicts the outcome at 48 weeks of a five-drug combination including ritonavir, saquinavir and efavirenz. AIDS 14:626, 2000.
65. Valer L, Gonzalez de Requena D, Mendoza C, et al. HIV genotyping and drug levels predict the response to a RTV-SQV sgc salvage therapy (Spanish Fortogene Trial). In: Poster at the 8th European Conference on Clinical Aspects and Treatment of HIV Infection, 2001, poster 1-670.
66. Montaner J, Saag M, Barylski C, Siemon-Hryczyk P. FOCUS study week 24 results (Fortovase® Once-daily Canada US): an open label, randomized, multicenter study to evaluate saquinavir SGC once-daily, ritonavir once-daily plus two nRTIs vs. efavirenz once-daily plus two nRTIs in HIV infected patients. In: Poster at the 41st Interscience Conference on Antimicrobial Agents and Chemotherapy, Chicago, 2001, poster I-670.
67. Cardiello P, Srasuebkul P, Hassink E, et al. The efficacy, safety and immunological changes of once-daily saquinavir soft-gel capsules 1600mg/ritonavir 100mg plus dual nucleosides in patients who had undetectable viral load after three years of treatment. In: Poster at the 9th Conference on Retroviruses and Opportunistic Infections, Seattle, 2002, poster 549-T.
68. Hellinger J, Cohen CJ, Morris AB, et al. Pilot study of the safety and antiviral activity of saquinavir 1000mg twice daily and lopinavir/ritonavir (Kaletra) combination therapy in HIV positive individuals. In: Poster at the 9th Conference on Retroviruses and Opportunistic Infections, Seattle, 2002, poster 451W.
69. Smith GHR, Klein MB, LeBlanc RP, et al. Salvage therapy for HIV-1 infection with lopinavir/ritonavir (LOP/RIT), saquinavir-SGC (SQR), and nucleoside analogues in patients having failed all three antiretroviral classes. Can J Infect Dis 12(suppl B):29B, 2002.
70. Cameron DW, Japour AJ, Xu Y, et al. Ritonavir and saquinavir combination therapy for the treatment of HIV infection. AIDS 13:213, 1999.
71. Cameron DW, Angel JB, Ryan J, et al. Durability of ritonavir (RTV) plus saquinavir (SQV) dual protease inhibitor therapy in HIV infection: 5-year follow-up. In: Abstracts of the 9th Conference on Retroviruses and Opportunistic Infections, Seattle, 2002, abstract 550-T.
72. Gisolf EH, Jurriaans S, Pelgrom J, et al. The effect of treatment intensification in HIV-infection: a study comparing treatment with ritonavir/saquinavir and ritonavir/saquinavir/stavudine; Prometheus Study Group. AIDS 14:405, 2000.
73. O'Brien WA, Rojo D, Acosta E, et al. Switch of saquinavir 400mg/ritonavir 400mg to saquinavir 1000mg/ritonavir 100mg during BID four drug antiretroviral therapy in patients with viral load suppression [abstract]. Third International Workshop on Clinical Pharmacology of HIV Therapy, Washington, DC, 2002.
74. Condra JH, Schleif WA, Blahy OM, et al. In vivo emergence of HIV-1 variants resistant to multiple protease inhibitors. Nature 374:569, 1995.
75. Schanazi RF, Larder BA, Mellors JW. Mutations in retroviral genes associated with drug resistance: 2000–2001 update. Int Antivir News 8:65, 2000.
76. Maschera B, Darby G, Palu G, et al. Human immunodeficiency virus: mutations in the viral protease that confer resistance to saquinavir increase the dissociation rate constant of the protease-saquinavir complex. J Biol Chem 271:33231, 1996.
77. Ermolieff J, Lin X, Tang J. Kinetic properties of saquinavir-resistant mutants of human immunodeficiency virus type 1 protease and their implications in drug resistance in vivo. Biochemistry 36:12364, 1997.
78. Craig C, Race E, Sheldon J, et al. HIV protease genotype and viral sensitivity to HIV protease inhibitors following saquinavir therapy. AIDS 12:1611, 1998.
79. Dianzani F, Antonelli G, Turriziani O, et al. In vitro selection of human immunodeficiency virus type 1 resistant to Ro 31-8959 proteinase inhibitor. Antivir Chem Chemother 4:329, 1993.
80. Jacobsen H, Yasargil K, Winslow DL, et al. Characterization of human immunodeficiency virus type 1 mutants with decreased sensitivity to proteinase inhibitor Ro 31-8959. Virology 206:527, 1995.
81. Turriziani O, Antonelli G, Jacobsen H, et al. Identification of an amino acid substitution involved in the reduction of sensitivity of HIV-1 to an inhibitor of viral proteinase. Acta Virol 38:297, 1994.
82. Ives KJ, Jacobsen H, Galpin SA, et al. Emergence of resistant variants of HIV in vivo during monotherapy with the proteinase inhibitor saquinavir. J Antimicrob Chemother 39:771, 1997.
83. Boucher C. Rational approaches to resistance: using saquinavir. AIDS 10(suppl 1):S15, 1996.
84. Eastman PS, Moffatt A, O'Sullivan E, et al. Evolution and stability of HIV-1 protease inhibitor resistance mutations during saquinavir monotherapy. In: Abstracts of the 5th Conference on Retroviruses and Opportunistic Infections, Chicago, 1998, abstract 397.
85. Jacobsen H, Hänggi M, Ott M, et al. In vivo resistance to a human immunodeficiency virus type 1 proteinase inhibitor: mutations, kinetics, and frequencies. J Infect Dis 173:1379, 1996.
86. Race E, Gilbert SM, Sheldon JG, et al. Correlation of response to treatment and HIV genotypic changes during phase III trials with saquinavir and reverse transcriptase inhibitor combination therapy. AIDS 12:1465, 1998.
87. Jacobsen H, Hänggi M, Ott M, et al. Reduced sensitivity to saquinavir: an update on genotyping from phase I/II trials. Antivir Res 29:95, 1996.
88. Schapiro JM, Winters MA, Vierra M, et al. Lymph node human immunodeficiency virus RNA levels and resistance mutations in patients receiving high-dose saquinavir. J Infect Dis 177:477, 1998.
89. Schapiro JM, Lawrence J, Speck R, et al. HIV RNA and resistance mutations to saquinavir and zidovudine in patients receiving dual versus triple combination therapy. In: Abstracts of the 5th Conference on Retroviruses and Opportunistic Infections, Chicago, 1998, abstract 401.
90. Schapiro JM, Lawrence J, Speck R, et al. Resistance mutations to zidovudine and saquinavir in patients receiving zidovudine plus

saquinavir or zidovudine and zalcitabine plus saquinavir in AIDS Clinical Trials Group 229. J Infect Dis 179:249, 1999.

91. Para MF, Glidden DV, Coombs RW, et al. Baseline human immunodeficiency virus type 1 phenotype, genotype, and RNA response after switching from long-term hard-capsule saquinavir to indinavir or soft-gel-capsule saquinavir in AIDS Clinical Trials Group protocol 333. J Infect Dis 182:733, 2000.
92. Roberts NA, Craig JC, Sheldon J. Resistance and cross-resistance with saquinavir and other HIV protease inhibitors: theory and practice. AIDS 12:453, 1998.
93. Martinez-Picado J, Savara AV, Sutton L, D'Aquila RT. Replicative fitness of protease inhibitor-resistant mutants of human immunodeficiency virus type 1. J Virol 73:3744, 1999.
94. Parkin NT Chappey C. Discordance between genotype-based predictions of protease inhibitor susceptibility and actual phenotype in HIV-1 isolates containing mutations at positions 82 or 90: modulatory effects of mutations at positions 46 and 54. Antiviral Ther 5(suppl 3):50, 2000.
95. Obry V, Costagliola D, Race E, et al. The extent of association between resistance phenotype and treatment response is highly dependent upon the drug. Antiviral Ther 6(suppl 1):61, 2001.
96. Tisdale M, Myers RE, Maschera B, et al. Cross-resistance analysis of human immunodeficiency virus type 1 variants individually selected for resistance to five different protease inhibitors. Antimicrob Agents Chemother. 39:1704, 1995.
97. Hertogs K, Bloor S, Kemp S, et al. Phenotypic and genotypic analysis of clinical HIV-1 isolates reveal extensive protease inhibitor cross-resistance: a survey of over 600 samples. AIDS 14:1203, 2000.
98. Winters MA, Schapiro JM, Lawrence J, Merigan TC. Human immunodeficiency virus type 1 protease genotypes and in vitro protease inhibitor susceptibilities of isolates from individuals who were switched to other protease inhibitors after long-term saquinavir treatment. J Virol 72:5303, 1998.
99. Dronda F, Casado JL, Moreno S, et al. Phenotypic cross-resistance to nelfinavir: the role of prior antiretroviral therapy and the number of mutations in the protease gene. AIDS Res Hum Retroviruses 17:211, 2001.
100. Servais J, Plesséria J-M, Lambert C, et al. Genotypic correlates of resistance to HIV-1 protease inhibitors on longitudinal data: the role of secondary mutations. Antiviral Ther 6:239, 2002.
101. Schapiro JM, Winters MA, Lawrence J, Merigan TC. Clinical cross-resistance between the HIV-1 protease inhibitors saquinavir and indinavir and correlations with genotypic mutations. AIDS 13:359, 1999.
102. Mayers DL, Neaton JD, Perez G, et al. Prior saquinavir therapy leads to a modest decrease in subsequent responses to drug regimens containing indinavir or ritonavir. In: Abstracts of the 5th Conference on Retroviruses and Opportunistic Infections, Chicago, 1998, abstract 400.
103. Bodsworth N, Slade M, Ewan J, et al. RTV and IDV therapy at 28 weeks after 32 weeks, SQV therapy-influence of HIV-1 protease mutations. In: Abstracts of the 5th Conference on Retroviruses and Opportunistic Infections, Chicago, 1998, abstract 396.
104. Craig C, O'Sullivan E, Cammack N. Increased exposure to the HIV protease inhibitor saquinavir (SQV) does not alter the nature key resistance mutations. In: Abstracts of the 5th Conference on Retroviruses and Opportunistic Infections, Chicago, 1998, abstract 398.
105. O'Sullivan E, Cammack N, Craig C, et al. Responsiveness to saquinavir is not affected by baseline protease genotype in protease-inhibitor naive patients. In: Abstracts of the 5th Conference on Retroviruses and Opportunistic Infections, Chicago, 1998, abstract 399.
106. Eagling VA, Back DJ, Barry MG. Differential inhibition of cytochrome P_{450} isoforms by the protease inhibitors, ritonavir, saquinavir and indinavir. Br J Clin Pharmacol 44:190, 1997.
107. Merry C, Mulcahy F, Barry M, et al. Saquinavir interaction with midazolam: pharmacokinetic considerations when prescribing protease inhibitors for patients with HIV disease. AIDS 11:268, 1997.
108. Jorga K, Buss NE. Pharmacokinetic drug interactions with saquinavir soft gelatin capsule. In: Poster at the 39th Interscience Conference on Antimicrobial Agents and Chemotherapy, San Francisco, 1999, poster 0339.
109. O'Mara E, Mummaneni V, Randall D, et al. BMS-232632: a summary of multiple dose pharmacokinetic, food effect and drug interaction studies in healthy subjects. In: Poster at the 7th Conference on Retroviruses and Opportunistic Infections, San Francisco, 2002, poster 504.
110. Hass D, Zala C, Schrader S, et al. Once-daily atazanavir plus saquinavir favorably affects total cholesterol (TC) and fasting triglyceride (TG) profiles in patients failing prior PI therapy (trial AI424-009, Wk 24). In: Abstracts of the 41st Interscience Conference on Antimicrobial Agents and Chemotherapy, Chicago, 2001, abstract LBI-16.
111. Shelton M, Cloen D, Berenson C, et al. Pharmacokinetics (PK) of once daily (QD) saquinavir/RTV (SQV/RTV): effects on unbound methadone and alpha 1-acid glycoprotein (AAG). In: Poster at the 41st Interscience Conference on Antimicrobial Agents and Chemotherapy, Chicago, 2001, poster A-492.
112. Centers for Disease Control and Prevention. Guidelines for the use of antiretroviral agents in HIV-infected adults and adolescents. Department of Health and Human Services and Henry J. Kaiser Family Foundation. HIV/AIDS Treatment Information Service website (http://www.hivatis.org) Updated February 4, 2002.
113. Carpenter CC, Cooper DA, Fischl MA, et al. Antiretroviral therapy in adults: updated recommendations of the International AIDS Society—USA panel. JAMA 283:381, 2000.
114. Cassano P, Hermans P Sommereijns B, et al. Combined quadruple therapy with ritonavir-saquinavir (RTV-SQV) + nucleosides in patients (p) who failed in triple therapy with RTV, SQV or indinavir (IDV). In: Abstracts of the 5th Conference on Retroviruses and Opportunistic Infections, Chicago, 1998, abstract 423.
115. De Truchis P, Force G, Zucman D, et al. Effects of "salvage" combination therapy with ritonavir + saquinavir in HIV-infected patients previously treated with protease-inhibitors (PI). In: Abstracts of the 5th Conference on Retroviruses and Opportunistic Infections, Chicago, 1998, abstract 425.
116. Gallant JE, Hall C, Barnett C, et al. Ritonavir/saquinavir (RTV/SQV) as salvage therapy after failure of initial protease inhibitor (PI) regimen. Presented at the 5th Conference on Retroviruses and Opportunistic Infections, Chicago, 1998, abstract 427.

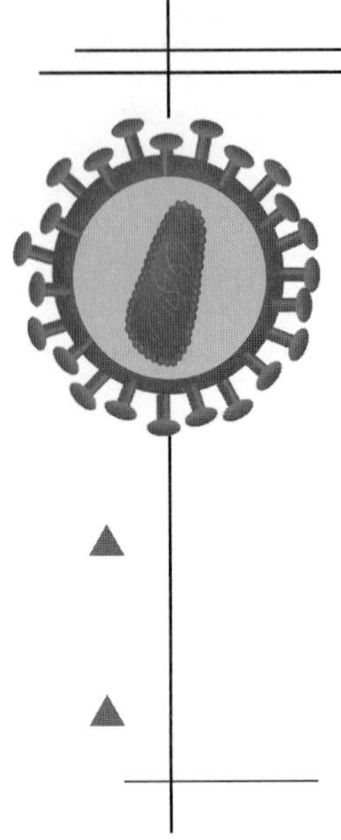

CHAPTER 13

Ritonavir

Sven A. Danner, MD, PhD

Ritonavir (RTV) is an inhibitor of the protease enzyme encoded by the human immunodeficiency virus (HIV) (Fig. 13–1). The chemical structure of the synthetic peptidomimetic antiviral agent RTV was designed based on the C_2 symmetry of this enzyme.[1,2] HIV protease cleaves the gag and gag-pol precursor molecules into smaller proteins. Without proper cleavage, the structural proteins of the virion core (p17, p24, p9, p7) and viral enzymes (reverse transcriptase, integrase, protease) cannot be formed adequately, which results in the formation of immature, noninfectious virions.[3,4] Early in vitro studies showed equal potency of RTV and zidovudine on a molar basis for several laboratory HIV-1 strains in MT-4 cells and eightfold less activity against an HIV-2 strain, with a median inhibitory concentration (IC_{50}) of 0.045 μmol/L against seven clinical HIV-1 isolates in peripheral blood lymphocytes.[1] The affinity of RTV for human aspartic proteases such as renin, pepsin, cathepsin D and E, and gastricin is low; and cytotoxic effects are seen only when RTV is administered in concentrations of more than 500 to 1000 times those required for antiretroviral activity.[1,2]

The spectrum of antiviral activity is limited. RTV is active against human retroviruses including HIV-1 and, to a lesser degree, HIV-2.[2,3,5]

▲ PHARMACOKINETICS

The pharmacokinetics of RTV have been studied in healthy volunteers and HIV-infected adults 18 to 63 years of age. Studies in children are currently underway. The pharmacokinetics in adults above the age of 63 and in persons with kidney or liver function disturbances have not been assessed.[6] So far the results do not reveal differences in pharmacokinetics between healthy individuals and HIV-infected persons or between individuals of different gender or race.

Following oral administration, RTV is well absorbed, with peak plasma concentrations appearing within 2 to 4 hours.[7] The maximal concentration (C_{max}) and area under the concentration-time curve (AUC) increased nonlinearly after single doses ranging from 100 to 1000 mg: The mean dose-normalized (per 100 mg) C_{max} and AUC increased from 0.416 μg/ml and 3.480 μg/hr/ml (100 mg) to 1.27 μg/ml and 12.31 μg/hr/ml (1000 mg), respectively. This points to a saturable metabolism.[7] In a Phase II clinical trial, after 3 weeks of treatment with RTV monotherapy, the C_{max} and AUC varied from 5.7 μg/ml and 29.7 μg/hr/ml, respectively, with a 300 mg bid dose to 11.2 μg/ml and 60.8 μg/hr/ml, respectively, with a 600 mg bid dose.[8] After oral dosing of 600 mg of ^{14}C-labeled RTV, 34% of the dose was recovered from the feces as unchanged drug, and virtually all of the RTV in the systemic circulation was unchanged, indicating an oral bioavailability of at least 60% and a small first-pass effect.[6]

Although the presence of food in the gastrointestinal tract affects the rate and extent of absorption of RTV, it does so only to a moderate degree and is dependent on the dosage form of the drug.[6] Administration of 600 mg of RTV as oral solution with food results in a delayed and decreased (by 23%) peak plasma concentration and 7% decreased overall absorption when compared to administration of the same dose in the fasting state. However, the overall absorption of RTV administered as capsules seems to be increased (by 15%) when taken simultaneously with a meal.[6]

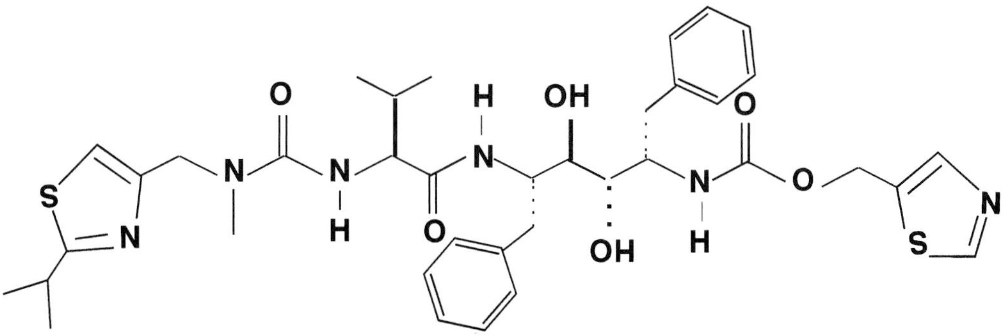

Figure 13–1. Chemical structure and chemical name of ritonavir. 10-Hydroxy-2-methyl-5-(1-methylethyl)-1-[2-(1-methylethyl)-4-thiazolyl]-3,6-dioxo-8,11-bis(phenylmethyl)-2,4,7,12-tetraazatridecan-13-oic-acid,5-thiazolylmethyl ester, [5S-(5R*,8R*,10R*11R*)]. (From Norvir [ritonavir] capsules and oral solution prescribing information. North Chicago, IL, Abbott Laboratories, 1996, with permission.)

Ritonavir is 98% to 99% bound to plasma proteins; most is bound to albumin and α_1-acid glycoprotein over a large concentration range (0.01 to 30 μg/ml). Currently it is not known if RTV crosses the placenta or is excreted in breast milk.[6]

The exact relation between plasma RTV concentrations and antiretroviral effects has not been determined. In patients receiving RTV 600 mg bid as an oral solution or as capsules, the plasma trough concentrations exceed the concentration of RTV (after adjustment for binding to human plasma proteins) required to inhibit 90% of detectable HIV-1 replication in vitro.[8]

Elimination of RTV is mainly by hepatic metabolism.[6,9] In patients receiving 600 mg bid, the systemic clearance was 8.8 L/hr, and the renal clearance has been reported to be less than 0.1 L/hr. Plasma half-life averages 3 to 5 hours.[6,8] In human liver microsomes, RTV metabolism is mediated by the cytochrome P_{450} (CYP) subsystems 3A4 and, to a lesser degree, 2D6. As stated above, after administration of 600 mg radiolabeled RTV as an oral solution, 34% of the drug was excreted in the unchanged form, and 86% of the dose was excreted in the feces. In total, 11% of the dose was excreted in the urine, of which only 3.5% was excreted as unchanged drug.[6] There are no data available on elimination by hemodialysis or peritoneal dialysis; but given the hepatic metabolism and the high degree of binding to proteins in the plasma, it seems unlikely that substantial amounts of the drug can be eliminated via these means.

▲ DRUG INTERACTIONS

Because RTV has a high affinity for several P_{450} isoenzymes, the compound exhibits clinically important drug interactions with a wide variety of other drugs. Isoenzymes CYP3A4, CYP2D6, CYP2C9, CYP2D19, and to a lesser degree CYP2A6, CYP1A2, and CYP2E1 are affected by RTV. Co-administration of RTV and drugs that are metabolized by these isoenzymes may result in competition for these enzymes, causing a decrease in metabolism and high plasma levels of the other agents. Conversely, RTV is metabolized by CYP3A4 and CYP2D6,[9] and therefore concomitant administration of RTV and drugs that induce these isoenzymes may result in decreased RTV plasma levels. Finally, RTV may increase the activity of glucuronyltransferase, and concomitant administration of RTV and drugs that are directly glucuronidated may result in loss of activity of these drugs.[6]

The manufacturer of RTV issues a regularly updated list of compounds that should not be used or be used with caution in conjunction with RTV. Pharmacokinetic interaction studies with RTV are available for some drugs (e.g., the antifungal fluconazole[10]), but for many others the recommendations are based on theoretical considerations. Table 13–1 lists recommendations for concomitant use of several drugs with RTV; this list is based on information from the manufacturer[6] and is by no means exhaustive.

The strong affinity of RTV for some P_{450} isoenzymes may also influence the pharmacokinetics of several other antiretroviral agents when given in combination with RTV. Concomitant administration of RTV (600 mg bid) and nucleoside analogue reverse transcriptase inhibitors (NRTIs) such as didanosine (200 mg bid) or zidovudine (ZDV) (200 mg tid) over 4 days decreased the C_{max} by 16% and 27%, and decreased the AUC by 13% and 25%, respectively.[11] The manufacturer does not advocate dose adjustments of either of these antiretroviral agents.

Co-administration of RTV and the nonnucleoside reverse transcriptase inhibitor (NNRTI) nevirapine resulted in a mean nonsignificant 11% decrease in RTV AUC in 12 HIV-infected individuals[12]; the change in nevirapine pharmacokinetics also was not significant. Co-administration with another NNRTI, delavirdine, likewise had no clinically relevant effects on the steady-state pharmacokinetics of either RTV or delavirdine in a study using RTV at a reduced dose.[13]

In contrast to the co-administration of RTV and reverse transcriptase (RT) inhibitors, the simultaneous use of RTV and other protease inhibitors leads to important pharmacokinetic interactions. RTV causes a highly significant increase in both the C_{max} and the AUC of saquinavir (SQV) when the two drugs are administered simultaneously. This information is useful because the oral bioavailability of SQV is poor as a result of, among other causes, an extensive first-pass effect.[14] Whereas the standard dose of SQV in combination with

▲ **Table 13–1.** DRUG INTERACTIONS WITH RITONAVIR

Drug Administered with RTV	Recommendation	Comments
Antifungals		
Fluconazole	No adjustment	Only small increase in C_{max} and AUC[10]
Itraconazole	Caution	
Ketoconazole	Caution	
Antimalarial and Antiprotozoals Agents		
Quinine	Caution	Threefold increase in AUC may be expected
Proguanil	No adjustment	
Chloroquine	Caution	
Primaquine	Caution	
Pyrimethamine	Caution	
Atovaquone	Caution	Possible decreased AUC as a result of enhanced glucuronidation
Antimycobacterials		
Rifabutin	Contraindicated	Large increase of AUC of rifabutin, and especially of its 25-*O*-desacetyl metabolite[6]
Rifampin	Caution	Threefold increase in AUC of rifampin, but large reduction in AUC of RTV[6]
Ethambutol	No adjustment	Anecdotal data only; no proper evalation done
Macrolide Antibiotics		
Clarithromycin	Depends on renal function	No adjustment in patients with normal renal function; 50% dose reduction when creatinine clearance is 30–60 ml/min, 75% dose reduction when <30 ml/min
Erythromycin	Caution	Threefold increase in AUC of erythromycin to be expected
Other Antiinfectives		
Cotrimoxazole	No adjustment	20% Decrease in AUC of sulfamethoxazole and 20% increase in AUC of trimethoprim expected
Metronidazole	Discouraged	Disulfiram-like reaction possible (RTV oral solution and capsules contain alcohol)
Anticoagulants		
Warfarin	Caution	Large increase in AUC of *R*-enantiomer and moderate decrease in AUC of *S*-enantiomer: monitor prothrombin time carefully
Antihistaminics		
Astemizole, terfenadine	Contraindicated	Very large increase in AUC expected
Antineoplastics		
Group I: etoposide, paclitaxel, tamoxifen, vincristine, vinblastine	Caution	These agents are metabolized by CYP3A4, so threefold or larger increase in AUC can be expected: monitor therapeutic and toxic effects carefully
Group II: cyclophosphamide, daunorubicin, doxorubicin	Caution	All these agents are metabolized by unidentified CYP isoenzymes, so changes in AUC are unpredictable: monitor therapeutic and toxic effects carefully
Cardiovascular Agents		
Group I: amiodarone, bepridil, encainide, flecainide, propafenone, quinidine	Contraindicated	
Group II: diltiazem, disopyramide, felodipine, isradipine, lidocaine, nicardipine, nefedipine, verapamil	Caution	All are metabolized by CYP3A4, so threefold or larger increase in AUC is expected
Group III: mexiletine, metoprolol, pindolol, propranolol, timolol	Caution	All are metabolized by CYP2C9/19 isoenzymes; moderate increase or decrease in AUC is to be expected
Group IV: acebutolol, digoxin, prazocin, tocainide	Caution	Metabolized by unidentified P_{450} isoenzymes; no data available
Antilipemic Agents		
Lovastatin, pravastatin fluvastatin, gemfibrozil	Caution	Metabolized by CYP3A4
Simvastatin	Contraindicated	Extensively metabolized by P_{450} isoenzymes
Clofibrate	Monitor effect	Metabolized by glucuronidation; might result in decrease of AUC
Central Nervous System Agents		
Pyroxicam	Contraindicated	
NSAIDs		
Diclofenac, ibuprofen, indomethacin	No adjustment	Only moderate increase in AUC expected
Ketoprofen, naproxen	Monitor effect	Metabolized by glucuronidation; might result in decrease of AUC
Opiate agonists		
Meperidine, propoxyphene	Contraindicated	
Alfentanyl, fentanyl	Caution	Threefold or larger increase in AUC expected
Methadone	Caution	Metabolized by unidentified P_{450} isoenzymes, so increase in AUC possible; also metabolized by glucuronidation, which might result in lowered AUC; net effect unknown

▲ **Table 13–1.** DRUG INTERACTIONS WITH RITONAVIR *Continued*

Drug Administered with RTV	Recommendation	Comments
Codeine, morphine	Monitor effect	Metabolized by glucuronidation; might result in decrease of AUC
Anticonvulsants		
Carbamazepine	Caution	Threefold or larger increase in AUC; decrease of RTV AUC
Phenobarbital	Caution	Metabolized by unidentified P_{450} isoenzymes, so increase in AUC possible; decrease in RTV AUC possible
Phenytoin	Caution	Moderate increase or decrease in AUC expected; decrease in RTV AUC possible
Sedatives and hypnotics		
Alprazolam, clorazepate, diazepam, estazolam, flurazepam, midazolam, triazolam, zolpidem	Contraindicated	
Lorazepam, oxazepam, propofol, temazepam	Caution	Metabolized by glucuronidation; might result in decrease of AUC
Gastrointestinal Agents		
Cisapride	Contraindicated	
Dronabinol, ondansetron	Caution	Metabolized by CYP3A4: threefold or larger increase in AUC
Lansoprazole, omeprazole	No adjustment	Moderate increase or decrease in AUC to be expected
Cimetidine, promethazine	Caution	Metabolized by unidentified P_{450} isoenzymes; increase in AUC possible
Corticosteroids		
Prednisone	Caution	Metabolized by CYP3A4: threefold or larger increase in AUC
Dexamethasone	Caution	Metabolized by CYP3A4: threefold or larger increase in AUC; also, induction of CYP3A4 possible, with resulting increase in RTV clearance and lowering of plasma RTV levels
Estrogens		
Ethinyl estradiol	Increase of dose or alternative contraceptive method	RTV 500 mg bid decreased C_{max} and AUC 32% and 40%, respectively[6]

AUC, area under the-time-concentration curve; NSAIDs, nonsteroidal antiinflammatory drugs.

NRTIs is 600 mg tid, when SQV is co-administered with RTV the AUC of SQV is so greatly increased that even 400 mg bid dosing results in a 20- to 40-fold increase without much effect on RTV pharmacokinetics.[15,16] The newly released soft gel capsule formulation of SQV (Fortovase) is administered at a dosage of 1200 mg tid. However, when used with RTV, the dose administered is the same as that recommended for the older formulation of SQV (Invirase): 400 to 600 mg bid. Several clinical trials with an RTV/SQV combination are now underway.

The pharmacokinetics of the protease inhibitor indinavir are heavily influenced by co-administration of RTV as well. In healthy volunteers, RTV increased the AUC and C_{max} of indinavir by 480% and 110%, respectively; even with a reduced, twice-daily dosing regimen of indinavir, without the usual administration of the drug in the fasting state, the combination of RTV and indinavir yielded a comparable AUC, with higher trough and slightly lower peak levels of indinavir compared to the standard three-times-a-day regimen. No effects on RTV pharmacokinetics were observed.[17] RTV also increased the AUC of the protease inhibitor nelfinavir by 150%, without affecting the AUC of RTV.[18] A thorough overview of drug interactions with antiretroviral drugs has been published.[19]

▲ CLINICAL TRIALS

Ritonavir monotherapy has been investigated in two Phase I/II trials[8,20] (Table 13–2). Danner et al., in a double-blind, randomized, placebo-controlled trial, studied 84 HIV-positive patients who had no prior exposure to a protease inhibitor and at least 50 CD4+ T-lymphocytes per cubic millimeter. They were assigned to one of four RTV dosing regimens (300, 400, 500, or 600 mg bid) or placebo for 4 weeks, then the placebo recipients were rerandomized to one of the RTV regimens.[8] During the first 4 weeks, increases in CD4+ T-lymphocytes and decreases in plasma HIV RNA were similar among the four RTV groups and significantly different from those in the placebo groups. Thereafter, however, a return to baseline values was noted after 16 weeks among the three lower dosage groups. In the highest dosage group, the HIV RNA load also partially increased after the nadir was reached at 4 to 8 weeks of treatment (1.2 $\log_{10}$ copies per milliliter decrease). After 32 weeks; among the patients in the 600 mg bid dosage group, the median increase from baseline in the CD4+ T-lymphocyte count was 230 cells per cubic millimeter, and the mean decrease in HIV RNA was 0.81 $\log_{10}$ copies per milliliter. However, this last parameter was assessed with the first-generation Chiron branched-chain DNA (bDNA) assay, which had a lower limit of detection of 10,000 RNA copies per milliliter.[21] When a more sensitive assay was utilized, decreases in the HIV RNA load turned out to be larger; applying the Roche polymerase chain reaction (PCR) assay[22] in the two highest dose groups, a mean maximal decrease of 1.91 $\log_{10}$ copies per milliliter was found, in contrast to 1.1 $\log_{10}$ copies per milliliter when measured with the bDNA assay. Adverse events included nausea, circumoral paresthesias, and elevated transaminase and triglyceride levels. Ten withdrawals from the study were judged to be RTV-related.[8]

Table 13–2. SUMMARY OF MAJOR CLINICAL TRIALS WITH RITONAVIR

Trial	Design	Dosage (mg)	No. of Subjects	Entry Criteria	CD+ T-Lymphocyte Count		Antiviral Response	Comments
					Cells/mm^3 on Entry	Response		
Danner[8]	Open label, nonrandomized	RTV: 300, 400, 500, 600 bid	84	PI-naive	>50	Initial inc with return toward BL in lower three dose groups	A 1.2 $\log_{10}$ dec with return toward BL in lower 3 dose groups	A 1.91 $\log_{10}$ dec when PCR (vs. bDNA) was used; 10 pts withdrew because of toxicity.
Markowitz[20]	Open label, nonrandomized	RTV: 200 tid, 200 qid, 300 tid, 300 qid	62	PI-naive, VL >25,000/ml	>50 and <500	Inc of 74 cells and 83 cells at 4 and 12 wk, respectively	A 0.86–1.18 $\log_{10}$ dec in VL at wk 2–4; 0.5 $\log_{10}$ dec at wk 12	10 Pts stopped therapy because of side effects, mostly N/V. Inc in triglycerides noted in some pts.
Mathez[23]	Open label, nonrandomized	RTV 600 bid + ZDV and ddC	32	Antiretroviral-naive	50–250	150-Cell inc at wk 60	A 2 $\log_{10}$ dec, sustained to 60 wk	15/32 Pts discontinued treatment by wk 36.
Notermans[25]	Open label, nonrandomized	RTV 600 bid + ZDV and 3TC	33	Antiretroviral-naive, VL >30,000/ml	>50	180-Cell inc at wk 24 in those receiving all drugs at once vs. 99-cell inc in those with RTV first	A 3.0 $\log_{10}$ dec by wk 16	8/33 Pts withdrew because of toxicity.
Cameron[30] (NA-Europe-Australia study)	Randomized, double blind	RTV 600 bid vs. placebo; add to existing Rx	1090	ART-experienced, failing existing regimen	<101	Initial inc in CD4+ cells in Rx group; no change in placebo group	A 1.5 $\log_{10}$ dec in RTV group (not sustained), no change in placebo group	Clinical events noted in 33% of placebo group vs. 16% of RTV group. Drug discontinued in 17% of RTV group vs. 6% of placebo group
Cameron[31] (RTV/SQV study)	Open label, nonrandomized	RTV/SQV: 400/400, 600/400, 600/600 bid; 400/400 tid	141	ART-experienced, PI-naive	273[a]	>100-Cell increase by 44 wk	A 80% achieved <200 copies by 44 wk	The tid regimen was poorly tolerated; lower dose bid regimen best tolerated.

ART, antiretroviral therapy; bDNA, branched-chain DNA assay; BL, baseline; ddC, zalcitabine; dec, decrease; inc, increase; NA, North America; N/V, nausea/vomiting; PCR, polymerase chain reaction; PI, protease inhibitor; pts, patients; Rx, therapy; SQV, saquinavir; 3TC, lamivudine; VL, viral load; ZDV, zidovudine.

[a]Median count at baseline.

In another Phase I/II trial, Markowitz et al. studied three- and four-times-a-day dosing regimens of RTV in 62 HIV-infected patients.[20] As in the prior study, a clear increase in CD4+ T-lymphocyte count and a decreased plasma HIV RNA load were found over 12 weeks, although the responses in these dosage groups were slightly inferior to those in the 600 mg bid regimen mentioned in the previous study. In this study pharmacokinetics were studied early (days 4 to 11) and later (days 22 to 29) during RTV administration. In all dosing groups the C_{max}, minimal concentration, and AUC decreased considerably during the period between the two time points, which is in agreement with preclinical studies suggesting that RTV induces its own metabolism.[1] The spectrum of adverse events was not different from that seen in the first Phase I/II study. Of the 62 patients, 3 withdrew because of adverse events thought to be related to RTV administration.[20]

On the basis of these two Phase I/II studies, the 600 mg bid dosage was chosen for use in subsequent studies.

Use in Antiretroviral-Naive HIV-Infected Patients

In an open-label study, Mathez et al. administered RTV (600 mg bid), ZDV (200 mg tid), and zalcitabine (0.75 mg tid) to 32 antiretroviral-naive HIV-infected patients who had CD4+ T-lymphocyte counts of 50 to 250 cells per cubic millimeter [23] (Table 13–2). During the first 2 weeks the patients received RTV monotherapy, after which the two NRTIs were added. The mean baseline peripheral CD4+ T-lymphocyte count was 173 cells per cubic millimeter, and the mean plasma HIV RNA load (Roche Amplicor assay) was 4.65 $\log_{10}$ copies per milliliter. After the first 2 weeks, RTV monotherapy resulted in a CD4+ T-lymphocyte rise of 113 cells per cubic millimeter and an HIV RNA decrease of 1 $\log_{10}$ copies per milliliter. After addition of the two NRTIs, the CD4+ T-lymphocytes continued to rise slowly to a mean increase of 150 cells per cubic millimeter after 60 weeks of triple treatment in the remaining 17 patients. A further decrease in HIV RNA load was observed, with a nadir of 2 $\log_{10}$ copies per milliliter after 8 weeks of treatment that was stable up to week 60. The percentage of patients with an undetectable plasma HIV RNA load (Roche Amplicor, lower limit of detection 200 copies per milliliter) was 50% after 60 weeks.[24] Many of the 32 patients discontinued the study prematurely. Two had stopped after 2 weeks, 11 after 24 weeks, and 15 after 36 weeks; the remaining 17 patients completed the 60 weeks. The same spectrum of adverse events was seen as in the Phase I/II studies described earlier. From week 36, the liquid formula, which was judged to be highly distasteful, was replaced by capsules, which clearly improved the compliance of the patients with the therapy regimen.

Notermans et al.[25] treated 33 antiretroviral-naive HIV-infected patients (31 men, 2 women) with a CD4+ T-lymphocyte count of more than 50 cells per cubic millimeter and a plasma HIV RNA load of more than 30,000 copies per milliliter (Roche Amplicor) with RTV, ZDV, and lamivudine (3TC) (Table 13–2). The patients were randomized into two groups: Group I started with all three antiretroviral agents simultaneously, and group II started with RTV monotherapy for 3 weeks; ZDV and 3TC were then added (this design was chosen to investigate whether quick development of resistance against the nucleoside analogues, especially against 3TC, could be prevented by prior lowering of the HIV replication rate by a protease inhibitor). A tonsillar biopsy was performed at baseline and after 2 days, 22 days, and 6 months of therapy to study changes in the HIV RNA load and lymphocyte subsets in lymphoid tissues.[26] Group I had a somewhat higher CD4+ T-lymphocyte count than group II (177 vs. 134 cells per cubic millimeter), but there were no differences in the baseline HIV RNA load (mean 5.3 $\log_{10}$ copies per milliliter) or in the Centers for Disease Control and Prevention (CDC) class of clinical HIV infection. Protease and RT gene sequencing at baseline showed only one case with a 41 and 215 RT codon change (known to confer resistance to ZDV) pretherapy, and in six cases two protease gene mutations (36, 71, or both) not known to be associated with resistance against RTV were observed. During treatment there was a quick initial rise in CD4+ T-lymphocytes, with a more gradual increase with a nonsignificant, slightly better result after 24 weeks in group I (an increase in CD4+ T lymphocytes of 180 vs. 99 cells per cubic millimeter in group II). A protease gene codon 82 mutation (known to confer resistance to RTV) developed in only one patient on therapy who did not comply with the regimen. No new RT gene mutations developed in any of the patients. The plasma HIV RNA load showed an initial rapid decline during the first 3 weeks, followed by a slower further decline, reaching its nadir of almost 3.0 $\log_{10}$ copies per milliliter at week 16 (Fig. 13–2).[25] The decreased plasma viral load was mirrored in the lymphoid tissue HIV RNA load. Both the amount of HIV trapped on the surface of follicular dendritic cells and the number of actively HIV-producing mononuclear cells decreased sharply, even after 2 days of therapy, and reached a decrease of more than 3.4 and more than 2.3 log units per gram of lymphoid tissue, respectively.[26] There were many adverse events, mainly gastrointestinal in nature, prompting 8 of 33 patients to withdraw from the study.

In contrast to the Phase I/II studies in which RTV was administered as monotherapy, in these last two studies the excellent HIV RNA response was maintained for at least 6 months. For example, in the RTV/ZDV/3TC study, 95% of the patients who were still on treatment after 52 weeks had no detectable plasma HIV RNA load in the Roche Amplicor assay (S.A. Danner, unpublished results). This clearly indicates that RTV should be used as part of a combination of antiretroviral agents, as now has been shown for all currently marketed antiretroviral drugs.

Saimot et al.[27] evaluated the efficacy and safety of RTV in combination with stavudine (d4T) and didanosine as first-line antiretroviral treatment in an open-label study in 33 patients with 50 to 350 CD4+ T-lymphocytes per cubic millimeter. After 2 weeks of RTV induction the nucleoside analogues were added. At 12 weeks of treatment, both infectious blood cells [cells per 10^7 peripheral blood mononuclear cells (PBMCs)] and plasma HIV RNA ($\log_{10}$ copies per milliliter) had decreased significantly, with reductions of 2.06 and 2.14, respectively. Six patients (18%) discontinued therapy during the first 5 weeks because of adverse events.[27]

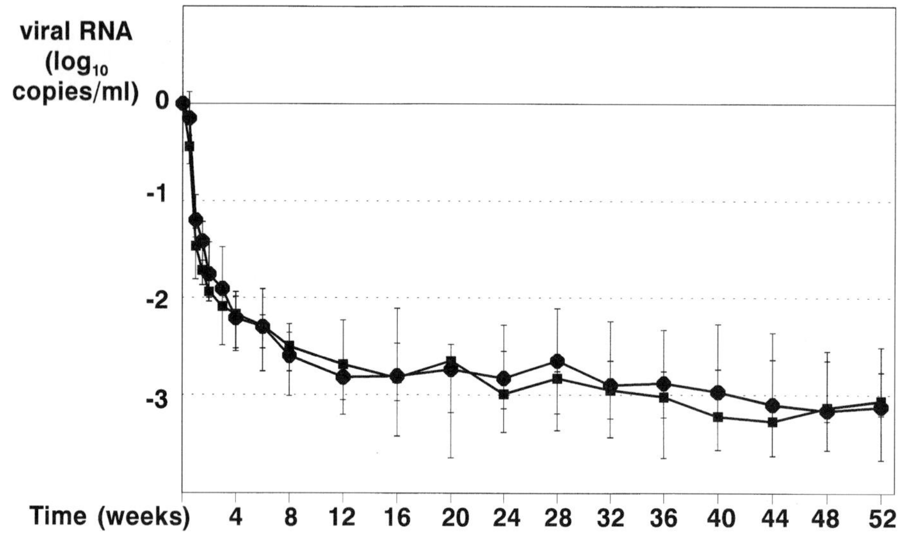

Figure 13–2. Plasma log HIV RNA response (mean ± SD) in 33 antiretroviral-naive HIV-infected patients who were treated for 52 weeks with ritonavir (RTV), zidovudine (ZDV), and lamivudine (3TC) administered simultaneously from the start of treatment (squares) or starting with RTV and adding ZDV and 3TC 3 weeks later (circles). (From Notermans D, Jurriaans S, de Wolf F, et al. Decreasing HIV-1 RNA levels in lymphoid tissue and peripheral blood during treatment with ritonavir, lamivudine and zidovudine. AIDS 12:167, 1998, with permission.)

Preliminary data from two studies with RTV in patients with primary HIV infection have been reported. Hoen et al.[28] studied the RTV/ZDV/3TC combination in 31 patients who were within 4 weeks of the onset of symptoms of the initial HIV infection (mean 25 days). Fifteen patients were enrolled for 12 weeks in the study; two of them were lost to follow-up. Of the remaining 13 patients, 9 had achieved an undetectable HIV RNA load (less than 200 copies per milliliter) from a median baseline viral load of 5.16 $\log_{10}$ copies per milliliter.

Markowitz et al. treated patients presenting with primary HIV infection with ZDV/3TC/RTV or indinavir.[29] The time from the onset of symptoms to the start of treatment was 55 days. In the RTV-treated group, 7 of 12 patients maintained their regimen for 10 to 16 months; in the indinavir group, 11 of 12 patients remained on therapy for 4 to 9 months. All subjects achieved undetectable levels of plasma HIV RNA (modified Chiron 2.0 assay, with a lower limit of detection of 100 copies per milliliter), and quantitative cultures went below the threshold of detection (0.1 $TCID_{50}/10^6$ PBMC) within months in all compliant subjects. Moreover, PBMCs isolated from semen collected from selected subjects did not express spliced or unspliced HIV-1 mRNA. No signs of viral replication could be found in lymphoid biopsy material from the sigmoid colon. The CD4+ T-lymphocyte count and the CD4/CD8 ratio increased, and reductions in env- and gag-specific antibody titers were noted. Clearly, early and aggressive treatment of primary HIV infection alters the virologic and immunologic course profoundly.[29]

Use in Antiretroviral-Experienced HIV-Infected Patients

In late 1994, the efficacy and safety of RTV were evaluated in a 68-center North American-European-Australian study in patients with clinically advanced disease for whom there were no other treatment options. The study enrolled 1090 HIV-infected persons with a CD4+ T-lymphocyte count of less than 101 cells per cubic millimeter and at least 9 months of prior antiretroviral treatment. Either RTV or placebo was added in a double-blind fashion to their existing antiretroviral medication[30] (Table 13–2). Crossover to open RTV for any acquired immunodeficiency syndrome (AIDS) outcome was permitted after 4 months. The patients had far-advanced HIV infection, with baseline median CD4+ T-lymphocyte counts of 18 and 22 cells per cubic millimeter for the RTV and placebo groups, respectively. The patients had been treated with antiretroviral drugs for a mean of 2.5 years, with an average of more than 2.5 drugs. Drug discontinuation because of adverse events occurred in 17% of the RTV group and 6% of the placebo group, mostly because of gastrointestinal symptoms during the first few weeks of the study. In the placebo group, no plasma HIV RNA-lowering effect was observed. In the RTV group, there was an initial decrease of ±1.5 $\log_{10}$ copies per milliliter that was not sustained after 6 months. The study was designed with clinical endpoints (death or occurrence of a new AIDS-defining event). Death or an AIDS-defining event occurred in 85 (15.7%) versus 181 (33.1%) patients in the RTV and placebo groups, respectively [$P <$ 0.001, hazard ratio 0.44%, 95% confidence interval (CI) 0.34 to 0.56]. Although the study was not powered to detect the presumed difference in deaths, it turned out that the number of deaths differed significantly between the two groups. After a median 6.1 months of follow-up, 26 (4.8%) patients died in the RTV group versus 46 (8.4%) patients in the placebo group, a highly significant difference [$P = 0.02$, hazard ratio 0.57, 95% CI 0.35 to 0.91).[30]

Given the long period of prior antiretroviral treatment, it can be assumed that many patients in this study must have been nucleoside analogue-resistant. As a result, these patients were treated with RTV monotherapy. This is in agreement with the transient nature of the plasma HIV RNA decrease, pointing to rapid development of viral resistance against the drug. Currently, with more antiretroviral agents available, monotherapy with RTV is no longer considered acceptable therapy even in patients with advanced disease. Because of expected rapid loss of viral susceptibility to the drug, a favorable clinical result of such a treatment must be judged remarkable. This study was instrumental in securing approval of the U.S. Food and Drug Administration's (FDA's) New Drug Application for RTV.

Use of Ritonavir in Pharmacologic "Boosting" of Other HIV-Protease Inhibitors

Ritonavir is not only an effective HIV-protease inhibitor, it is also one of the most powerful inhibitors of the P_{450} cytochrome system, especially of the isoenzyme CYP 3A4.[15,16] Because all other licensed HIV-protease inhibitors are largely metabolized by CYP3A4, ritonavir can be used to "boost" the efficacy of these compounds by enhancing their biologic availability. The combinations ritonavir/saquinavir and ritonavir/indinavir have been studied extensively, with different dosing schedules. Some data are also available on the combination of ritonavir with nelfinavir and amprenavir. Finally, there are substantial data on the combination ritonavir/lopinavir, which are co-formulated in one capsule (see Chapter 17).

When combining ritonavir and another protease inhibitor, two strategies can be chosen. In one the ritonavir dose is kept as low as possible (e.g., 100 or 200 mg bid) to avoid ritonavir-specific side effects, accepting the fact that the plasma ritonavir levels will be too low to exert antiretroviral activity, and so the antiretroviral activitity depends solely on the other protease inhibitor. Another strategy is to administer ritonavir in higher doses (e.g., 400 mg bid) so the drug itself inhibits HIV replication in addition to the inhibition by the other protease inhibitor.

The combination ritonavir/saquinavir has been studied in a dose-finding clinical trial.[31,32] A total of 141 patients with a median baseline CD4+ T-lymphocyte count of 273 cells per cubic millimeter and a median plasma HIV RNA load of 4.63 $\log_{10}$ copies per milliliter who discontinued their RT inhibitor therapy, took part in a multicenter, randomized, open-label study. The patients were randomized into four groups with various two- and three-times-a-day regimens: 400 mg RTV/400 mg SQV bid; 600 mg RTV/400 mg SQV bid; 400 mg RTV/400 mg SQV tid, and 600 mg RTV/600 mg SQV bid. All four dosage groups showed an excellent virologic and immunologic response: After 44 weeks, a median increase in CD4+ T-lymphocytes to more than 100 cells per cubic millimeter and a plasma RNA load decrease to less than 200 copies per milliliter were noted in more than 80% of the patients (intention-to-treat analysis). After 12 months, 90% of the patients on treatment still had low plasma RNA load values (Fig. 13–3). The most important difference between the four groups was tolerability: In the lowest-dose group (35 patients), few adverse events were noted, with only one discontinuation resulting from an adverse event. In seven patients who responded incompletely, d4T/3TC therapy was added at week 12, after which they also reached less than 200 copies per milliliter HIV RNA load.[31] Interestingly, the most important predictor of the duration of the viral response was the nadir in plasma viral load that was achieved. An HIV RNA load below 200 copies per milliliter at 6 months was predicted at 3 months by a level of less than 1000 copies per milliliter, [92% positive predictive value (PPV), 75% negative predictive value(NPV); $P = 0.005$] and a level of 200 copies per milliliter (93% PPV, 33% NPV; $P < 0.05$). This observation has been confirmed in studies with other antiretroviral drugs. For example, in the INCAS study with ZDV, didanosine (ddI), and nevirapine, the multivariate model revealed that neither the baseline plasma viral load, the viral response, the baseline CD4+ T-lymphocyte count, nor the CD4+ T-lymphocyte response was independently associated with the duration of the response; rather, the nadir of the plasma viral load was highly predictive and accounted for 78% of the treatment difference in duration of suppression.[33,34] The favorable antiviral effect in this study was even seen after 3 and 4 years of treatment, with a high virologic response in an intention-to-treat analysis.[35]. At the beginning of the fourth year, 48 of 84 patients were still being treated succesfully with only RTV/SQV.[36]

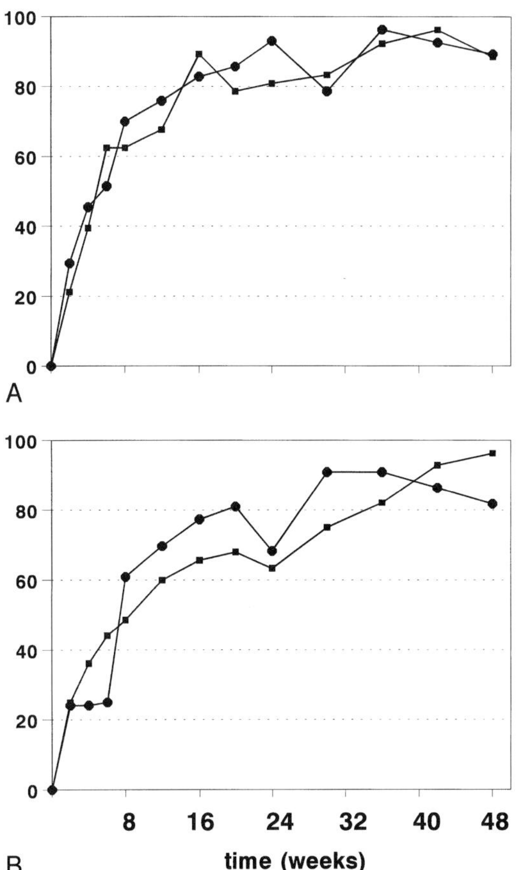

Figure 13–3. Percentage of patients reaching a plasma HIV RNA load below the limit of detection (200 copies per milliliter) during treatment with different ritonavir-saquinavir (RTV/SQV) combinations. *A*, Results during treatment with RTV 400 mg bid/SQV 400 mg bid (circles) and RTV 600 mg bid/SQV 400 mg bid (squares). *B*, Results during treatment with RTV 400 mg tid/SQV 400 mg tid (circles) and RTV 600 mg bid/SQV 600 mg (squares). (From Cameron W. Combining protease inhibitors for optimal HIV therapy. In: Proceedings of the Abbott Satellite Symposium During the 6th European Conference on Clinical Aspects and Treatment of HIV Infection, Hamburg, Germany, 1997, p 16, with permission.)

Another study investigating the efficacy of the RTV/SQV combination is the Dutch-Belgian Prometheus study. Combination therapy with RTV/SQV, each administered at 400 mg bid, is being compared with the same regimen plus d4T 40 mg bid.[37] Almost 200 patients who were protease inhibitor (PI)- and d4T-naive have been enrolled. Treatment intensification with NRTIs was allowed when at week 18 the virologic response still was unsatisfactory. In the RTV/SQV arm, more treatment intensification was seen. After 48 weeks, in patients who started treatment with a baseline serum HIV RNA concentration of more than 100,000 copies per milliliter treatment with RTV/SQV/d4T showed superior activity when compared with RTV/SQV alone. However, 52% of all patients on RTV/SQV never intensified their regimen and had an HIV RNA level of less than 400 copies per milliliter at week 48.

The tolerability for the regimens was good. The reported dropout rate of 22% that resulted from adverse events and virologic failure after 48 weeks is encouraging compared to most studies with RTV-containing triple regimens.[38]

In the Swiss Cohort Study, the RTV/SQV combination (600 mg RTV/600 mg SQV bid) was administered to patients with advanced disease who had failed RT inhibitor therapy or who were intolerant to it.[39] The results showed an unpredictable response. Among the 16 patients evaluable after 5 weeks, 11 were responders (decrease in plasma HIV RNA of 2 $\log_{10}$ copies per milliliter or more, or achieving a level below 200 copies per milliliter). Among these patients, 6 had a sustained response after 13 weeks, but only 2 patients achieved undetectable viral loads. There were several dropouts as a result of adverse events or according to patient choice. Plasma levels of both RTV and SQV were significantly higher in the responders than in nonresponders. Even in a few patients with good compliance and relatively high plasma drug levels, rapid accumulation of resistance-conferring mutations was observed, with resulting loss of viral response. No new life-threatening or irreversible side effects occurred in this group with far-advanced disease.[39] The higher dropout rate when compared to the previous study may be explained by the higher doses of RTV and SQV used (with a potential loss of patient compliance) or by the more advanced disease state.

Danish investigators compared three regimens in antiretroviral-naive patients: two NRTIs plus indinavir, ritonavir, or ritonavir/saquinavir (400/400 mg bid). The ritonavir/saquinavir arm was virologically superior to the other two; toxicity in that arm compared favorably with the arm containing ritonavir in the standard dose[40].

One concern about treatment with only protease inhibitors is whether HIV replication in the central nervous system is suppressed adequately because it is known that protease inhibitors penetrate the cerebrospinal fluid (CSF) poorly.[6] Experience in a few patients in one of the Phase I/II RTV studies showed that the CSF RTV level, sampled 2 hours after a 600 mg dose, is ±1% of the corresponding plasma level (S.A. Danner, unpublished results). The significance of this finding is not clear because the compound is 99% protein-bound in plasma. It is conceivable that the free, active RTV fraction may not differ much in the two compartments. Moreover, the CSF drug concentration might differ from the brain tissue concentration. In the above-mentioned dose-finding RTV/SQV study,[31] CSF analysis was carried out in 13 patients who maintained a plasma HIV RNA load of less than 200 copies per milliliter for at least 8 weeks. At a median of 60 weeks on RTV/SQV therapy, without addition of an RT inhibitor, 12 of 13 (92%) had a CSF HIV RNA level below 400 copies per milliliter. In the Prometheus study.[41] RTV and SQV levels in the CSF were extremely low; and in patients with detectable HIV RNA in the CSF, RTV/SQV therapy did not lower the load, in contrast to the CSF viral load in the RTV/SQV/d4T arm.

Several other studies with RTV/SQV were performed in patients with far-advanced disease. In the Desert AIDS Project (Palm Springs, CA), 32 patients with a CD4+ T-lymphocyte count of less than 250 cells per cubic millimeter and an HIV RNA level of more than 5000 copies per milliliter despite 4 months of triple-drug therapy (two nucleosides and one protease inhibitor) were treated with RTV/SQV plus two NRTIs. The mean $\log_{10}$ HIV RNA level decreased from 4.86 to 2.60 copies per milliliter after 12 weeks, with 97% of the patients reaching a level below 400 copies per milliliter. Two patients withdrew because of side effects.[42]

Less encouraging is a study in which Sampson et al. treated 54 HIV-1-infected patients with virologic or clinical failure despite at least 2 months of prior treatment with a protease inhibitor in a triple combination.[43] RTV was added to SQV-containing triple regimens; SQV was added to RTV-containing triple regimens; and RTV/SQV replaced indinavir in indinavir-containing regimens. Fifty-two percent of the patients had had previous opportunistic infections, and 63% had used more than five antiretroviral drugs prior to RTV/SQV. After 31 weeks (mean) of follow-up, 54% had either altered or discontinued their regimen, half of them because of virologic failure. The changes in plasma HIV RNA were at best moderate: 1.0 $\log_{10}$ copies per milliliter response (added RTV), 0.11 $\log_{10}$ copies per milliliter response (added SQV), and 0.34 $\log_{10}$ copies per milliliter response (switch to RTV/SQV). "Salvage" regimens containing RTV in heavily treated patients with advanced disease have only short- term virologic effects.[43] Mallolas et al. found a satisfactory response after using SQV(soft gel) 1600 mg/RTV 200 mg qd as salvage treatment after failure on a SQV(hard gel) 600 mg tid-containing highly active antiretroviral therapy (HAART) regimen. After 12 weeks the viral load had dropped to less than 200 copies per milliliter in 12 of 14 patients.[44]

There are ample data on the combination ritonavir/indinavir. Indinavir (IND), when given as the only protease inhibitor, must be administered three times daily with food restriction, and the resulting plasma levels are far from ideal. Trough levels are not far above the IC_{50} for wild-type HIV, whereas peak levels are extremely high, probably contributing to the nephrolithiasis frequently seen in indinavir-treated patients. Combining indinavir with ritonavir makes twice-daily dosing possible, lowers the peak levels, and considerably increases the trough levels (Fig. 13–4).

In a study applying population pharmacokinetics by Burger et al., IND/RTV 800/100 mg bid produced higher trough levels and more or less the same peak levels of indinavir as those in patients receiving a 800 mg tid indinavir dose. All levels measured were above the IC_{50} for wild-type HIV-1.[45]

Rockstroh et al. studied 92 treatment-naive patients with a high HIV RNA load (median 220,400 copies per milliliter)

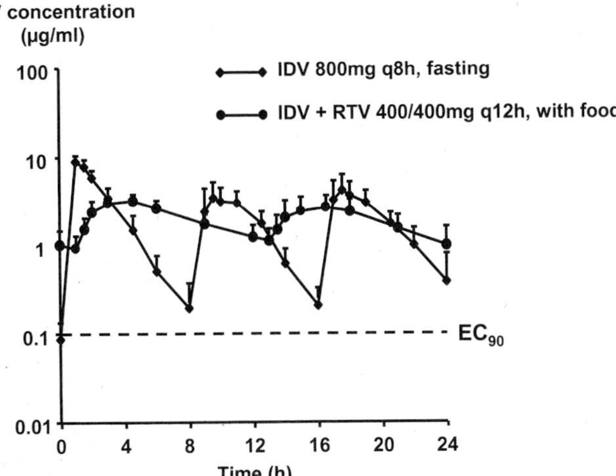

Figure 13–4. Effects on indinavir pharmacokinetics of addition of ritonavir. Indinavir 800 mg tid is compared with indinavir 400 mg bid/ritonavir 400 mg bid. (From Hsu et al., Geneva, 1998.)

who received two NRTIs plus RTV/IND 400/400 mg bid.[46] After 1 year 70% had an HIV RNA load of less than 80 copies per milliliter in an intention-to-treat analysis; there were 29 discontinuations, 8 of which were due to adverse events. No urolithiasis or flank pain had been noted. Boyd et al. studied IND/RTV 800/100 mg bid versus IND 800 mg tid in 104 patients in a randomized, open-label trial in Thailand. All patients received zidovudine/lamivudine in addition. Efficacy was equal in both study arms, but nausea and dry mouth were more often seen in the twice-daily regimen.[47]

In a "switch study," Shulman et al. showed that the viral load decreased in patients treated with IND 800 mg tid who had a detectable plasma HIV RNA load (50 to 50,000 copies per milliliter) after switching over to IND/RTV 400/400 mg bid (without a change in their NRTIs). After 3 weeks the percentage of patients with HIV RNA level of less than 50 copies per milliliter rose from 0% to 28%. After 3 weeks the NRTIs could be changed, which resulted in a 53% undetectable HIV RNA level (< 50 copies per milliliter) after 16 weeks.[48] Whether such an intensification of indinavir treatment is succesful depends largely on the degree of resistance against indinavir at the moment of intensification. Because indinavir and ritonavir have greatly overlapping resistance profiles, one can expect that this is true for both the low-dose ritonavir schedules (e.g., IND/RTV 800/100 mg bid) and the higher-dose ritonavir regimens (e.g., IND/RTV 400/400 mg bid).

Zolopa et al. looked at susceptibility for indinavir at the start of combination therapy. They studied RTV/IDV treatment when administered to patients who failed antiretroviral therapy in routine daily practice in a multicenter cohort. In a subgroup, phenotypic analysis was done at the start. In patients with less than 4-fold, 4- to 25-fold, and more than 25-fold loss of susceptibility to indinavir, the viral responses after 24 weeks were 80%, 75%, and 20%, respectively. Apparently, boosting the indinavir raises the inhibitory quotient to such high levels that even moderate loss of susceptibility is compensated.[49]

Kempf et al. correlated the response to such an intensification with the virtual inhibitory quotient (VIQ), which was defined as the ratio between the plasma trough level and the virtual phenotype times the serum-adjusted IC_{50} for wild-type HIV. The virtual phenotype was calculated from the genotype, and the interpretation was done by the HIV Resistance Collaborative Working Group. They found that a VIQ of more than 2 was the strongest predictor of succesful intensification with ritonavir.[50]

Finally, an IDV/RTV regimen can be expected to be associated with better patient compliance as a result of the more convenient medication schedule. Sension et al. studied 429 subjects on IDV 800 mg tid-containing regimens with a viral load of less than 400 copies per milliliter; they were randomized to either continue their regimen or switch to RTV/IDV 400/400 mg bid. Most of the subjects and their physicians preferred the RTV/IDV regimen because of improved adherence and convenience. Both arms provided durable HIV suppression in most subjects.[51]

Amprenavir (APV) has been combined with ritonavir as well to increase the trough concentration and lower the peak concentration (Fig. 13–5). Markowitz et al. studied 39 individuals with primary HIV infection (mean HIV RNA load of 5.3 $\log_{10}$ copies per milliliter, mean CD4+ T-lymphocyte count of 503 cells per cubic millimeter).[52] All patients started with an amprenavir-based HAART regimen; 33 of them switched after a median of 48 weeks to an APV/RTV 600/100 mg bid-based regimen. The adverse event profile improved, the number of "viral blips" (rises in viral loads) decreased slightly, and the plasma trough level of amprenavir rose fivefold compared to the preswitch APV 1200 mg bid dose.[52] Studies on the optimal doses of the AMP/RTV combination are somewhat conflicting. One of the reasons is that, especially in salvage therapy, NNRTIs frequently are added to the regimen, which by themselves might influence PI levels. Degen et al. found that AMP 450 mg bid/RTV 200 mg bid resulted in high, stable plasma levels, with or without concomitant NNRTIs.[53]

Katlama et al. administered APV/RTV 600/100 mg bid or 600/200 mg bid to 68 patients who had been heavily

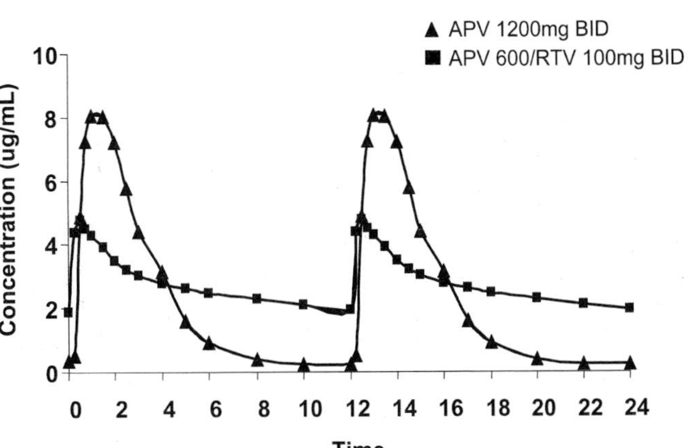

Figure 13–5. Effects of ritonavir on amprenavir pharmacokinetics. Amprenavir 1200 mg bid is compared with amprenavir 600 mg bid/ ritonavir 100 mg bid. (From Sadler, 7th Retroviral Conference, 2000, abstract 7.)

pretreated. Their mean period of treatment was 7.7 years, and 68% had used more than three PIs. At 48 weeks, an intention-to-treat analysis showed a viral load of less than 200 copies per milliliter in 36%.[54]

Pediatric Data

Data on the efficacy and safety of RTV in children are scarce. Mueller et al. treated 46 children who were intolerant or refractory to other antiretroviral regimens with ritonavir monotherapy in different dosages (liquid formula) in a Phase I/II study.[55] Among them, 37 completed 12 weeks of observation (median time on study 28 weeks). Six came off the study because of adverse events (three had liver enzyme elevations, and three had nausea and vomiting). Plasma HIV RNA decreased rapidly (0.5 to 2.0 $\log_{10}$ copies per milliliter) and remained below baseline up to 24 weeks. Tolerability thus seems reasonable, and these highly preliminary data point to a comparable virologic efficacy to that seen in adults.

Yogev et al. presented the final results of the Pediatric ACTG trial 338, a comparison between ZDV/3TC, d4T/RTV, and ZDV/3TC/RTV in stable, antiretroviral-experienced children 2 to 17 years of age. The results of an interim analysis, after which the ZDV/3TC group became unblinded, are presented in Table 13–3 for 162 of the 298 children who entered the study.[56] Of the 197 children on an RTV-containing treatment arm (treatment B or C), at 12 weeks 57% were on full dose and 10% had discontinued permanently. No clinical progression or unexpected toxicities were noted.

Chadwick et al. studied early therapy with ZDV/3TC/RTV [either 350 mg/m^2 (group 1) or 450 mg/m^2 (group 2) bid] in 39 children 1 to 24 months of age. After 48 weeks there were no grade 3 or 4 toxicities related to the study medication. Median RTV concentrations in group 1 were 16% to 57%, which were lower than predicted from adult data. Three children stopped therapy because of intolerance. Among those who could tolerate RTV, 10 of 11 in group 1 (or 91%) and 7 of 17 in group 2 (or 41%) had viral loads of less than 400 copies per milliliter at week 48. Most virologic failures were due to poor adherence.[57]

▲ ADVERSE EVENTS

Use of RTV is accompanied by adverse events in many patients. These effects, especially gastrointestinal symptoms, occur mainly during the first few weeks of RTV treatment and are associated with high plasma trough levels of the drug. RTV induces its own metabolism, and pharmacokinetic studies show that trough levels are initially high, not reaching a steady-state level before the end of the second week of administration.[6] Addition of some NRTIs sometimes increases toxicity, especially during the first weeks of treatment. This is reflected in a relatively high dropout rate after starting on RTV during routine patient care and in controlled clinical trials.[58,59] Several measures can help improve tolerability. One of the most important is gradual escalation to the full dose. Over the first 10 to 14 days, RTV metabolism is so slow that even a substantial dose reduction does not lead to drug levels below the IC_{90}; gradual escalation helps avoid high drug levels and resultant toxicity. Most physicians now start with 300 mg bid for a few days, increasing to 400 mg during the next 3 or 4 days, then 500 mg bid for 3 or 4 days, after which they administer the full dose of 600 mg bid (not before day 12 to 14). Careful dose escalation tailored to the symptoms in the individual, pharmacologic and nonpharmacologic interventions for side effects, and especially full disclosure to the patient of potential side effects and their transient nature can be helpful. Using these tools in a prospective study, 57 consecutive patients tolerated RTV during the first year in one study.[60]

The principal adverse effects are gastrointestinal, including nausea, diarrhea, vomiting, anorexia, abdominal pain, and taste perversion.[6] In addition, peripheral and perioral paresthesias occur frequently but are transient in nature. Asthenia and headache are noted more frequently in the RTV group in placebo-controlled monotherapy studies and even more so in studies with RTV/NRTI combinations.[6]

Substantial increases in the liver enzymes alanine transaminase and aspartate transaminase are seen in 5% to 6% of patients, mainly those who receive RTV plus nucleoside analogues. In one of the RTV/SQV studies, the incidence varied between 3% and 15%, depending on the dosage. In that study, a clear relation between liver toxicity and preexisting liver disease was found.[28] Elevations of creatine phosphokinase concentrations have been reported in 1% to 4% of patients on RTV monotherapy or combination therapies.

As reported to date, RTV has no negative effect on hemoglobin, leukocyte count, or platelet count. On the contrary, in the Phase III study in which either RTV or placebo was added to existing antiretroviral therapy, the RTV group showed improved hematologic parameters.[30,61]

Since protease inhibitors were introduced, physicians have become aware of more spontaneous bleeding episodes in patients with hemophilia than expected. Both

▲ **Table 13–3.** RESULTS OF CLINICAL TRIAL PEDIATRIC ACTG-338

	Plasma HIV RNA ($\log_{10}$ copies/ml)			% Patients with Viral Load <400 copies/ml		
Week	ZDV/3TC	Treatment B: d4T/RTV or ZDV/3TC/RTV	Treatment C: ZDV/3TC/RTV or d4T/RTV	ZDV/3TC	Treatment B: d4T/RTV or ZDV/3TC/RTV	Treatment C: ZDV/3TC/RTV or d4T/RTV
0	4.28	4.41	4.25	0	0	0
4	3.76	2.60	2.60	28	59	51
12	3.95	2.60	2.60	14	61	57

hematomas and hemarthroses have been reported. Most cases have been described in European patients with advanced HIV infection who are receiving multiple other drugs. It is not clear if this extra bleeding tendency in hemophiliacs is associated with one or more specific protease inhibitors or with the whole class of compounds. The FDA issued a warning to care providers to monitor closely any patients with hemophilia who are taking PIs.[62]

In a substantial number of patients on RTV, hypertriglyceridemia is seen, usually to a moderate degree. Fasting triglyceride concentrations exceeding 1500 mg/dl occurred in 2% to 8% of patients receiving RTV as monotherapy or in combination with dideoxynucleoside agents.[6] Although occasionally extreme hypertriglyceridemia is noted that resolves quickly after cessation of RTV, the incidence of pancreatitis is not higher than expected in these patients and does not seem to be associated with elevated plasma triglyceride levels. Hypercholesterolemia has been reported in fewer than 2% of the patients receiving RTV in clinical trials.[6] Extreme hypertriglycridemia and hypercholesterolemia seem to be dose-independent, as occasionally these elevations are also seen in the very low dose RTV schedules, where RTV is used only as a pharmacologic booster for other HIV-protease inhibitors.

During the last few years the poorly understood syndrome of redistribution of fat tissue (called lipodystrophy, consisting of both lipoatrophy and lipohypertrophy) has attracted a lot of attention (see Chapter 62). The exact prevalence is difficult to measure, mainly because there is no standardized definition. Treatment with both NRTIs and PIs seems to be involved in the pathogenesis. In the MACS study, Kingsley et al. found among HIV-positive men on no therapy or monotherapy/dual therapy a prevalence of less than 3% and 2%, respectively, but in patients on HAART it was 20%. The prevalence of lipodystrophy rose sharply during the first 2 years on HAART but remained stable thereafter.[63] The specific role of PIs in the development of this syndrome is far from clear at the moment. There are many studies on the prevalence of the syndrome, but there are few prospective data. Within the class of PIs, no differences in association with lipodystrophy between the individual PIs have been noted.

▲ RESISTANCE

Resistance to all PIs has been produced in vitro by serial passage of HIV-1 in the presence of increasing drug concentrations. When this class of compounds was first introduced, physicians and patients wondered if the problems with loss of efficacy as a result of resistance, as seen during treatment with NRTIs and NNRTIs, would be observed during treatment with these highly potent replication inhibitors. In monotherapy studies with all currently available PIs, efficacy was indeed lost after a few months, and mutations in the protease gene with decreased susceptibility of the patient's HIV isolate were found. Molla et al. studied clinical isolates from patients in Phase I/ II studies with RTV who showed virologic escape.[64] Mutations at several positions in HIV protease were found, always with a codon 82 change as the initial variation, regardless of time on therapy. Thereafter strains with more mutations were selected, with an ordered accumulation of mutations at positions 54, 71, and 36, after which other mutations were added at positions 10, 13, 20, 33, 63, 84, or 90, among others. Strains with the initial codon 82 mutation alone demonstrated only a small loss of susceptibility to RTV; but apparently the suppression of replication of these strains is incomplete enough to allow further selection of additional mutations. The occurrence of these strains with multiple mutations is unlikely to be the result of selection of preexisting strains. It is estimated that each amino acid substitution due to a single nucleotide change occurs in 1 of 10,000 basepairs.[65] Thus mutants with four or more codon changes occur by chance in fewer than 1 per 10^{16} basepairs, which is less than the estimated lifetime production.[66,67] Therefore it must be assumed that after selection of the first mutation (in the case of RTV, apparently at the protease gene codon 82) continuous selection of additional mutations takes place more easily than would be expected by chance. There is a clear relation between plasma trough levels of RTV and the selection rate, expressed as the number of mutations per week.[64]

The loss of RTV's efficacy as a result of the appearance of resistance-conferring mutations has been confirmed in other trials using combination therapy. Clavel et al. found multiple mutations in the protease gene and phenotypic resistance in patients treated with ZDV/ddC/RTV. Interestingly, they found that after more than 1 year of drug exposure in all patients with a resistant plasma HIV population there were no mutations in the HIV genomes from the patient's unstimulated PBMCs.[68] Pym et al. treated patients who failed virologically after prolonged SQV monotherapy by switching them to the RTV/SQV combination. Three patterns of response were seen: (1) patients who started the combination while lacking both the protease gene codon 48 and the codon 90 mutations (the two important mutations conferring resistance to SQV) showed a good, durable response; (2) patients starting with only the codon 90 mutation had a temporary response, which was lost after 16 weeks; and (3) patients starting with both SQV-induced mutations showed no response at all.[69]

Under selective drug pressure, the patient's HIV population may change not only in terms of susceptibility to the drug but also "fitness," and the two effects can work antagonistically or synergistically. Nijhuis et al. isolated protease genes from patients on prolonged RTV monotherapy during Phase I/II studies and introduced them into protease-deleted laboratory HIV-1 vectors via recombination. The first mutants were found to express increased drug resistance but reduced replication efficiency relative to the wild type. With prolonged treatment, variants dominated with other mutations that showed no further increase in resistance but increased replication efficiency relative to the wild type.[70]

One of the most important questions for physicians facing the initial selection of drugs for antiretroviral combination therapy in their patients is this: Suppose this combination fails as a result of resistance. Which options remain? Because most initial treatment regimens currently contain PIs, part of this question can be rephrased as: How extensive is the phenomenon of cross-resistance in this class of compounds? Unfortunately, the initial reports about cross-resistance, mainly published after completion of short-term Phase I/II studies, were more optimistic than recent results from long-term treatment periods and in routine patient care settings. Winters et al. studied patients who failed long-term (1 to 2 years) SQV antiretroviral therapy and found that more than one-third of the patients had acquired, in addition to the codon 48 and 90 mutations, several other mutations, conferring resistance to other PIs, such as indinavir and RTV.[71] In contrast, in another study of 27 patients treated with either SQV monotherapy or SQV plus nucleosides, the phenomenon of cross-resistance was also demonstrated, but it was confined to a much smaller percentage: 5% to 15%.[72] Calvez et al. found, in a heavily pretreated patient population (nucleoside analogues in monotherapy and dual therapy, as well as triple regimens), that switching to the RTV/SQV combination had only a short-term effect on CD4+ T-lymphocytes and the plasma HIV RNA load.[73] Also, Miller et al.[74] found extensive cross-resistance to RTV and SQV after triple therapy (with IND as the PI). Unanimous agreement exists that cross-resistance between indinavir and RTV approaches 100%.[75]

Amprenavir seems to harbor somewhat less cross-resistance. Lo Caputo et al. studied phenotypic resistance in 101 patients who were heavily PI-pretreated and who failed virologically when they were tested. The correlation coefficients between APV fold-resistance and that of individual PIs were as follows: IDV 0.23, RTV 0.42, nelfinavir (NFV) 0.43, SQV 0.31.[76]

Resistance to PIs can be caused by changes in the protease gene product, which affect binding of the inhibitor to the protease enzyme, or by changes in the substrate for the protease (i.e., the cleavage sites of the precursor polyproteins). It is conceivable that the latter changes can either facilitate or compromise the cleavage process, increasing or decreasing the degree of resistance, respectively. Considerable variation in cleavage sites has indeed been noted and has occurred in a setting of vertical transmission and during therapy with RTV or IND.[77,78]

Of particular concern are reports about simultaneous viral resistance to almost all available antiretroviral agents in patients who never had reached undetectable levels of plasma HIV RNA after nucleoside analogue therapy followed by PI-containing triple regimens. Shafer et al. found a specific set of 14 mutations in such patients: 6 in the protease gene (at condons 10, 48, 54, 63, 71, 82) and 8 in the RT gene (at codons 41, 43, 44, 67, 118, 184, 210, 215), regardless of which nucleosides and PIs had been used. The authors noted that "the striking concordance of mutations in these patients suggests that this set of RT and protease mutations provides a selective advantage in a variety of genetic contexts and in the presence of multiple different drug combinations."[79] In addition, in vitro studies have demonstrated that HIV-1 can readily develop resistance to several classes of antiretroviral drugs through genetic recombination of large viral genome segments, at least in the laboratory setting.[80]

▲ SUMMARY AND PLACE OF RTV IN ANTIRETROVIRAL TREATMENT

Evidence is mounting that the duration of the viral response depends heavily on whether maximal suppression (as reflected in an extremely low plasma HIV RNA load) can be reached.[81] Among the currently available antiretroviral agents, the PI RTV is highly potent. However, the specter of side effects when administered in its full dose (600 mg bid) precludes its widespread use. Instead, the compound is being used more and more as a pharmacologic booster for other PIs, as low or extremely low doses ("baby dose") such as 100 mg bid suffice to achieve the boosting effect. At those doses, side effects are minimal. A good example is found in the combination of RTV/lopinavir, which results in an extremely high inhibitory quotient, with remarkably good tolerability (see Chapter 17).

Regimens containing boosted PIs rank among the best first-line therapeutic options in antiretroviral therapy. Alternatives are found in the combination of NRTIs and an NNRTI, or a triple NRTI combination. The latter has not yet been studied thoroughly, and there is some concern that such a regimen may not be powerful enough in patients with high baseline viral loads. When comparing regimens of PI/NRTIs or NNRTI/NRTIs, both regimens are found to be powerful. However, an NNRTI/NRTIs regimen is more vulnerable to the development of resistance, and a PI/NRTIs regimen is associated with more adverse effects, especially metabolic disturbances and the ill-understood phenomenon of lipodystrophy (see Chapter 62). Currently it is not clear which of the components of this last combination are responsible for the different effects. It might be that lipoatrophy is associated with NRTIs and lipohypertrophy with PIs, as lipoatrophy is also seen in patients who have been treated only with NRTIs. NRTIs have formed the backbone of almost every antiretroviral regimen up to now, and so it is difficult to delineate their specific role. Maybe regimens consisting of (boosted) PIs and an NNRTI, without NRTIs, can be helpful for differentiating the contribution of the various classes of antiretroviral agents to the adverse effects. Studies on efficacy and adverse events of such regimens are currently lacking.

The Achilles heel of every antiretroviral therapy regimen is the development of viral resistance. There is little or no cross-resistance between different classes of antiretrovirals; but within the classes, especially the NNRTIs and PIs, cross-resistance occurs abundantly. Resistance against RTV usually begins with one specific mutation in the protease gene (codon 82); and if RTV therapy were to be halted at that moment, it is conceivable the patient's dominant HIV population would still be sensitive to another PI (e.g., SQV). However, during routine patient care, so much time has usually elapsed before the loss of viral response has been noted (or, even worse, has been confirmed at a next visit) that strains with more mutations have been selected, conferring resistance to most (or all) of the other PIs. One approach to this problem is to make the first treatment regimen as powerful as possible ("the first blow is half the battle"[82]) to stop replication as completely as possible, thereby postponing the selection of such resistant strains indefinitely. As stated above, a regimen containing drugs of which at least one can achieve a high inhibitory quotient, is important for reaching that goal. PIs boosted by ritonavir belong to that category.

The first experiences with RTV in pediatric treatment combinations suggest good efficacy. At this time, however, there are not enough data on safety and tolerance to make firm recommendations for pediatric treatment schedules. It is to be expected that RTV will be used more and more as a pharmacologic booster for other PIs in children as well as adults.

REFERENCES

1. Kempf DJ, Norbeck DW, Codacovi LM, et al. Structure-based, C_2 symmetric inhibitors of HIV protease. J Med Chem 33:2687, 1990.
2. Erickson J, Neidhart DJ, VanDrie J, et al. Design, activity, and 2.8 Å crystal structure of a C_2 symmetric inhibitor complexed to HIV-1 protease. Science 249:527, 1990.
3. Kempf DJ, Marsh KC, Denissen JF, et al. ABT-538 is a potent inhibitor of human immunodeficiency virus protease and has high oral bioavailability in humans. Proc Natl Acad Sci USA 92:2484, 1995.
4. Vella S. Rationale and experience with reverse transcriptase and protease inhibitors. J Acquir Immune Defic Syndr Hum Retrovirol 10(suppl 1):S58, 1995.
5. Markowitz M, Saag M, Powderly WG, et al. Selection and analysis of human immunodeficiency virus type 1 variants with increased resistance to ABT-538, a novel protease inhibitor. J Virol 69:701, 1995.
6. Norvir (ritonavir) capsules and oral solution prescribing information. North Chicago, IL, Abbott Laboratories, 1996.
7. Hsu A, Granneman R, Rienkiwicz K, et al. Kinetics of ABT-538, a protease inhibitor, after single oral rising doses (abstract). Pharmacol Res 11(suppl):400, 1994.
8. Danner SA, Carr A, Leonard JM, et al. A short-term study of the safety, pharmacokinetics, and efficacy of ritonavir, an inhibitor of HIV-1 protease. N Engl J Med 333:1528, 1995.
9. Kumar GN, Rodrigues AD, Buko AM, et al. Cytochrome P450-mediated metabolism of the HIV-1 protease inhibitor ritonavir (ABT-538) in human liver microsomes. J Pharmacol Exp Ther 277:423, 1996.
10. Cato A, Hsu A, Granneman R, et al. Assessment of pharmacokinetic interaction of the HIV-1 protease inhibitor ABT-538 and fluconazole. In: Proceedings of the 35th Interscience Conference on Antimicrobial Agents and Chemotherapy, San Francisco. Washington, DC, American Society for Microbiology, 1995, abstract 133.
11. Cato A, Hsu A, Granneman R, et al. Assessment of the pharmacokinetic interaction of the HIV-1 protease inhibitor ABT-538 and zidovudine. In: Proceedings of the 35th Interscience Conference on Antimicrobial Agents and Chemotherapy, San Francisco. Washington, DC, American Society for Microbiology, 1995, abstract 134.
12. Murphy R, Gagnier P, Lamson M, et al. Effect of nevirapine on pharmacokinetics of indinavir and ritonavir in HIV-1 infected patients. In: Proceedings of the 4th Conference on Retroviruses and Opportunistic Infections, Washington, DC. Alexandria, VA, Westover Management Group, 1997, abstract 374.
13. Cox SR, Ferry JJ, Batts DH, et al. Delavirdine and marketed protease inhibitors: pharmacokinetic interaction studies in healthy volunteers. In: Proceedings of the 4th Conference on Retroviruses and Opportunistic Infections, Washington, DC. Alexandria, VA, Westover Management Group, 1997, abstract 372.
14. Invirase (saquinavir mesylate) capsules prescribing information. Nutley, NJ, Roche Laboratories, 1995.
15. Hsu A, Granneman R, Sun E, et al. Assessment of single- and multiple-dose interactions between ritonavir and saquinavir. In: Proceedings of the XIth International Conference on AIDS, Vancouver, 1996, abstract LB.B 6041.
16. Merry C, Barry M, Mulcahy F, et al. Saquinavir pharmacokinetics alone and in combination with ritonavir in HIV-infected patients. AIDS 11:F29, 1997.
17. Hsu A, Granneman GR, Japour A, et al. Evaluation of potential ritonavir and indinavir combination bid regimens. In: Proceedings of the 37th Interscience Conference on Antimicrobial Agents and Chemotherapy, Toronto. Washington, DC, American Society for Microbiology, 1997, abstract A-57.
18. Kerr B, Lee C, Yuen G, et al. Overview of in-vitro and in-vivo drug interactions of nelfinavir mesylate, a new HIV-1 protease inhibitor. In: Proceedings of the 4th Conference on Retroviruses and Opportunistic Infections, Washington, DC. Alexandria, VA, Westover Management Group, 1997, abstract 373.
19. Burger DM, Hoetelmans RMW, Koopmans PP, et al. Clinically relevant drug interactions with antiretroviral agents. Antivir Ther 2:149, 1997.
20. Markowitz M, Saag M, Powderly WG, et al. A preliminary study of ritonavir, an inhibitor of HIV-1 protease, to treat HIV-1 infection. N Engl J Med 333:1534, 1995.
21. Pachl C, Todd JA, Kern DG, et al. Rapid and precise quantification of HIV-1 RNA in plasma using a branched DNA signal amplification assay. J Acquir Immune Defic Syndr Hum Retrovirol 8:446, 1995.
22. Mulder J, McKinney N, Christopherson C, et al. Rapid and simple PCR assay for quantification of human immunodeficiency virus type 1 RNA in plasma: application to acute retroviral infection. J Clin Microbiol 32:292, 1994.
23. Mathez D, Bagnarelli P, Gorin I, et al. Reductions in viral load and increases in T lymphocyte numbers in treatment-naive patients with advanced HIV-1 infection treated with ritonavir, zidovudine and zalcitabine triple therapy. Antivir Ther 2:175, 1997.
24. Mathez D, Schinazi RF, Liotta DC, et al. Infectious amplification of wild-type human immunodeficiency virus from patients' lymphocytes and modulation by reverse transcriptase inhibitors in vitro. Antimicrob Agents Chemother 37:2206, 1993.
25. Notermans D, Jurriaans S, de Wolf F, et al. Decreasing of HIV-1 RNA levels in lymphoid tissue and peripheral blood during treatment with ritonavir, lamivudine and zidovudine. AIDS 12:167, 1998.
26. Cavert W, Notermans D, Staskus C, et al. Kinetics of response in lymphoid tissue to antiretroviral therapy of HIV-1 infection. Science 276:960, 1997.
27. Saimot AG, Landman R, Damond F, et al. Ritonavir, stavudine (d4T), didanosine (ddI) as a triple combination treatment in antiretroviral-naive patients. In: Proceedings of the 4th Conference on Retroviruses and Opportunistic Infections, Washington, DC. Alexandria, VA, Westover Management Group, 1997, abstract 246.
28. Hoen B, Harzic M, Fleury HF, et al. ARNS053 trial of zidovudine, lamivudine and ritonavir combination in patients with symptomatic primary HIV-1 infection: preliminary results. In: Proceedings of the 4th Conference on Retroviruses and Opportunistic Infections, Washington, DC. Alexandria, VA, Westover Management Group, 1997, abstract 232.
29. Markowitz M, Cao Y, Vesamen M, et al. Recent HIV infection treated with AZT, 3TC and a potent protease inhibitor. In: Proceedings of the 4th Conference on Retroviruses and Opportunistic Infections, Washington, DC. Alexandria, VA, Westover Management Group, 1997, abstract LB8.
30. Cameron DW, Heath-Chiozzi M, Danner SA, et al. Prolongation of life and prevention of AIDS complications in a randomized controlled clinical trial of ritonavir in patients with advanced HIV disease. Lancet 352:543, 1998.
31. Cameron W. Combining protease inhibitors for optimal HIV therapy. In: Proceedings of the Abbott Satellite Symposium during the 6th European Conference on Clinical Aspects and Treatment of HIV Infection, Hamburg, Germany, 1997, p 16.
32. Cameron DW, Japour AJ, Xu Y, et al. Ritonavir and saquinavir combination therapy for the treatment of HIV infection. AIDS 13:213, 1998.
33. Kempf D, Molla A, Sun E, et al. The duration of viral suppression is predicted by viral load during protease inhibitor therapy. In: Proceedings of the 4th Conference on Retroviruses and Opportunistic Infections, Washington, DC. Alexandria, VA, Westover Management Group, 1997, abstract 603.
34. Raboud JM, Montaner JSG, Rae S, et al. Predictors of duration of plasma viral load suppression. In: Proceedings of the 37th Interscience Conference on Antimicrobial Agents and Chemotherapy, Toronto. Washington, DC, American Society for Microbiology, 1997, abstract A-57.
35. Cameron DW, Xu Y, Rode R, et al. Three years follow-up and conditional outcomes survival analysis of ritonavir plus saquinavir therapy in HIV infection. In: Proceedings of the 7th Conference of Retroviruses and Opportunistic Infections, San Francisco, 2000, abstract 533.

36. Farthing C, Ryan J, Rode R, et al. Durability of ritonavir (RTV) plus saquinavir (SQV) dual protease inhibitor therapy in HIV infection: four year follow-up. In: Proceedings of the 1st IAS Conference on HIV Pathogenesis and Treatment, Buenos Aires, 2001, abstract 223.
37. Gisolf EH, Colebunders R, van Wanzeele F, et al. Treatment with ritonavir/saquinavir versus ritonavir/saquinavir/stavudine. In: Proceedings of the 5th Conference on Retroviruses and Opportunistic Infections, Chicago. Alexandria, VA, Westover Management Group, 1998, abstract 576.
38. Gisolf EH, Jurriaans S, Pelgrom J, et al. The effect of treatment intensification in HIV infection: a study comparing treatment with ritonavir/saquinavir and ritonavir/saquinavir/stavudine. AIDS 14:405, 2000.
39. Lorenzi P, Yerli S, Abderrakim K, et al. Toxicity, efficacy, plasma drug concentrations and protease mutations in patients with advanced HIV infection treated with ritonavir plus saquinavir. AIDS 11:F95, 1997.
40. Kirk O, Katzenstein TL, Gerstoft J, et al. Combination therapy containing ritonavir plus saquinavir has superior short-term antiretroviral efficacy: a randomized trial. AIDS 13:F9, 1999.
41. Gisolf EH, Enting RH, Jurriaans S, et al. Cerebrospinal fluid HIV-1 RNA during treatment with ritonavir/saquinavir or ritonavir/saquinavir/stavudine. AIDS 14:1583, 2000.
42. Barbour CO II. Efficacy and safety of quadruple combination therapy in treatment experienced HIV/AIDS patients. In: Proceedings of the 4th Conference on Retroviruses and Opportunistic Infections, Washington, DC. Alexandria, VA, Westover Management Group, 1997, abstract 245.
43. Sampson M, Torres RA, Stein AJ, et al. Ritonavir-saquinavir combination treatment in protease inhibitor experienced patients with advanced HIV disease. In: Proceedings of the 37th Interscience Conference on Antimicrobial Agents and Chemotherapy, Toronto. Washington, DC, American Society for Microbiology, 1997, abstract I-104.
44. Mallolas J, Blanco J, Sarasa M, et al. Intensification therapy with saquinavir soft gel (SSG)/ritonavir (RIT) qd in patients failing on a saquinavir hard gel (SHG) containing HAART. In: Proceedings of the 1st IAS Conference on HIV Pathogenesis and Treatment, Buenos Aires, 2001, abstract 675.
45. Burger DM, Hugen PWH, Prins JM, et al. Pharmacokinetics of an indinavir/ritonavir 800/100 mg bid regimen. In: Proceedings of the 39th Interscience Conference on Antimicrobial Agents and Chemotherapy, San Francisco, 1999, abstract 363.
46. Rockstroh JK, Bergmann F, Wiesel W, et al. Efficacy and safety of twice daily first-line ritonavir/indinavir plus double nucleoside combination therapy in HIV-infected individuals. AIDS 14:1181, 2000.
47. Boyd M, Duncombe C, Newell M, et al. Indinavir/ritonavir vs indinavir in combination with AZT/3TC for treatment of HIV in nucleoside-experienced patients: a randomised, open-label trial. In: Proceedings of the 8th Conference on Retroviruses and Opportunistic Infections, Chicago, 2001, abstract 335.
48. Shulman N, Zolopa A, Havlir D, et al. Ritonavir intensification in indinavir recipients with detectable HIV RNA levels. In: Proceedings of the 7th Conference on Retroviruses and Opportunistic Infections, San Francisco, 2000, abstract 534.
49. Zolopa A, Rice H, Young B, et al. Ritonavir (RTV) boosting of indinavir (IDV) antiretroviral regimens in clinical practice: effectiveness, safety and exploration of phenotypic breakpoints. In: Proceedings of the 1st IAS Conference on HIV Pathogenesis and Treatment, Buenos Aires, 2001, abstract 678.
50. Kempf D, Hsu A, Jiang P, et al. Response to ritonavir (RTV) intensification in indinavir (IDV) recipients is highly correlated with virtual inhibitory quotient. In: Proceedings of the 8th Conference on Retroviruses and Opportunistic Infections, Chicago, 2001, abstract 523.
51. Sension M, Harley W, Dejesus E, et al. Final analysis of a 24-week randomized, controlled, open-label evaluation of adherence and convenience of continuing indinavir versus switching to ritonavir/indinavir 400 mg/400 mg bid (the NICE study). In: Proceedings of the 1st IAS Conference on HIV Pathogenesis and Treatment, Buenos Aires, 2001, abstract 417.
52. Markowitz M, Hurley A, Ramratnam B, et al. The safety and efficacy of a ritonavir-boosted amprenavir-based regimen after switch from amprenavir-based HAART. In: Proceedings of the 8th Conference on Retroviruses and Opportunistic Infections, Chicago, 2001, abstract 405.
53. Degen O, Kurowski M, van Lunzen J, et al. Amprenavir and ritonavir: intraindividual comparison of different doses and influence of concomitant NNRTI on steady-state pharmacokinetics in HIV-infected patients. In: Proceedings of the 8th Conference on Retroviruses and Opportunistic Infections, Chicago, 2001, abstract 739.
54. Katlama C, Schneider L, Agher R, et al. Ritonavir (RTV)/amprenavir (APV) combination therapy in HIV infected patients who failed several protease inhibitor containing regimens. In: Proceedings of the 1st IAS Conference on HIV Pathogenesis and Treatment, Buenos Aires, 2001, abstract 673.
55. Mueller BU, Zuckerman J, Nelson RT Jr, et al. Update on the pediatric phase I/II study of the protease inhibitor ritonavir (ABT-538). In: Proceedings of the 4th Conference on Retroviruses and Opportunistic Infections, Washington, DC. Alexandria, VA, Westover Management Group, 1997, abstract 722.
56. Yogev R, Stanley K, Nachman RA, et al. Virologic efficacy of ZDV + 3TC vs. D4T + ritonavir (RTV) vs. ZDV + 3TC + RTV in stable, antiretroviral experienced HIV-infected children (Pediatric ACTG Trial 338). In: Proceedings of the 37th Interscience Conference on Antimicrobial Agents and Chemotherapy, Toronto. Washington, DC, American Society for Microbiology, 1997, abstract LB-6.
57. Chadwick EG, Palumbo P, Rodman J, et al. Early therapy with ritonavir (RTV), ZDV and 3TC in HIV-1-infected children 1–24 months of age. In: Proceedings of the 8th Conference on Retroviruses and Opportunistic Infections, Chicago, 2001, abstract 677.
58. Clumeck N, Colebunders B, Vandercam K, et al. A comparative outcome trial of ritonavir and indinavir in HIV patients with CD4 cell count below 50. In: Proceedings of the 4th Conference on Retroviruses and Opportunistic Infections, Washington, DC. Alexandria, VA, Westover Management Group, 1997, abstract 196.
59. Gerard Y, Valette M, Ajana F, et al. Efficacy of proteinase inhibitors in combination with reverse transcriptase inhibitors: study in 177 HIV-1 infected patients in the North France AIDS Reference Center. In: Proceedings of the 4th Conference on Retroviruses and Opportunistic Infections, Washington, DC. Alexandria, VA, Westover Management Group, 1997, abstract 243.
60. Davis SM, Canniff JM, Andradas V, et al. Successful ritonavir induction: intensive patient management. In: Proceedings of the 4th Conference on Retroviruses and Opportunistic Infections, Washington, DC. Alexandria, VA, Westover Management Group, 1997, abstract 193.
61. De Wit S, Hermans P, Kabeya K, et al. Thrombocytopenia and leucopenia in HIV patients with CD4+ T lymphocyte counts below 50 treated with protease inhibitors. In: Proceedings of the 4th Conference on Retroviruses and Opportunistic Infections, Washington, DC. Alexandria, VA, Westover Management Group, 1997, abstract 200.
62. Feigal DW Jr. Dear healthcare provider letter: HIV protease inhibitors and patients with hemophilia. Rockville, MD, U.S. Food and Drug Administration, 1996.
63. Kingsley L, Smit E, Riddler S, et al. Prevalence of lipodystrophy and metabolic abnormalities in the Multicenter AIDS Cohort Study (MACS). In: Proceedings of the 8th Conference on Retroviruses and Opportunistic Infections, Chicago, 2001, abstract 536.
64. Molla A, Korneyeva M, Gao Q, et al. Ordered accumulation of mutations in HIV protease confers resistance to ritonavir. Nat Med 2:760, 1996.
65. Coffin JM. HIV population dynamics in vivo: implications for genetic variation, pathogenesis, and therapy. Science 267:483, 1995.
66. Ho DD, Neumann AU, Perelson AS, et al. Rapid turnover of plasma virions and CD4 lymphocytes in HIV-1 infection. Nature 373:123, 1995.
67. Perelson AS, Neumann AU, Markowitz M, et al. HIV-1 dynamics in vivo: virion clearance rate, infected cell lifespan, and viral generation time. Science 271:1582, 1996.
68. Clavel F, Paulos S, Mathez D, et al. HIV protease sequences selected during ZDV-DDC-ritonavir triple combination. In: Proceedings of the 4th Conference on Retroviruses and Opportunistic Infections, Washington, DC. Alexandria, VA, Westover Management Group, 1997, abstract 236.
69. Pym AS, Churchill DR, Galpin S, et al. Presence of mutation at codon 90 may predict response to ritonavir/saquinavir combination in HIV seropositive patients pretreated with saquinavir monotherapy. In: Proceedings of the International Workshop on HIV Drug Resistance, Treatment Strategies and Eradication, St. Petersburg, FL, 1997, abstract 84.
70. Nijhuis M, Schuurman R, De Jong D, et al. Selection of HIV- 1 variants with increased fitness during ritonavir therapy. In: Proceedings of the International Workshop on HIV Drug Resistance, Treatment Strategies and Eradication, St. Petersburg, FL, 1997, abstract 92.
71. Winters MA, Shapiro JM, Lawrence J, et al. Genotypic and phenotypic analysis of the protease gene in HIV-1-infected patients that failed long-term saquinavir therapy and switched to other protease inhibitors.

In: Proceedings of the International Workshop on HIV Drug Resistance, Treatment Strategies and Eradication, St. Petersburg, FL, 1997, abstract 17.

72. Craig C, Race E, Sheldon J, et al. A study of reduced sensitivity to inhibitors of HIV protease in virus isolates from selected patients after therapy with saquinavir. In: Proceedings of the International Workshop on HIV Drug Resistance, Treatment Strategies and Eradication, St. Petersburg, FL, 1997, abstract 27.
73. Calvez V, Coutellier A, Bossi P, et al. Failure of the association of ritonavir and saquinavir in multi-experienced HIV-1-infected patients. In: Proceedings of the International Workshop on HIV Drug Resistance, Treatment Strategies and Eradication, St. Petersburg, FL, 1997, abstract 76.
74. Miller V, Hertogs K, De Bèthune MP, et al. Incidence of HIV-1 resistance and cross-resistance to protease inhibitors after indinavir failure: impact on subsequent ritonavir/saquinavir combination therapy. In: Proceedings of the International Workshop on HIV Drug Resistance, Treatment Strategies and Eradication, St. Petersburg, FL, 1997, abstract 81.
75. Moyle GJ, Bartin SE. HIV-protease inhibitors in the management of HIV-infection. J Antimicrob Chemother 38:921, 1996.
76. Lo Caputo S, Gianotti N, Tomasoni L, et al. Phenotypic cross-resistance to amprenavir in HIV isolated from heavily pretreated patients (the Genpherex study). In: Proceedings of the 1st IAS Conference on HIV Pathogenesis and Treatment, Buenos Aires, 2001, abstract 575.
77. Bloom G, Perez E, Parikh S, et al. Comparison of gag-pol precursor cleavage in naturally arising HIV-1 variants. In: Proceedings of the International Workshop on HIV Drug Resistance, Treatment Strategies and Eradication, St. Petersburg, FL, 1997, abstract 29.
78. Perez E, Lamers S, Heath-Chiozzi M, et al. Emergence of resistant protease alleles and variant gag sequences in HIV-1-infected children enrolled in protease inhibitor phase I/II clinical trials. In: Proceedings of the International Workshop on HIV Drug Resistance, Treatment Strategies and Eradication, St. Petersburg, FL, 1997, abstract 75.
79. Shafer RW, Winters MA, Merigan TC. Multiple concurrent RT and protease mutations and multidrug resistance in heavily treated HIV-1-infected patients. In: Proceedings of the International Workshop on HIV Drug Resistance, Treatment Strategies and Eradication, St. Petersburg, FL, 1997, abstract 39.
80. Yusa K, Kavlick MF, Mitsuya H. HIV-1 acquires resistance to multiple classes of antiviral drugs through recombination. In: Proceedings of the 4th Conference on Retroviruses and Opportunistic Infections, Washington, DC. Alexandria, VA, Westover Management Group, 1997, abstract 585.
81. Carpenter CCJ, Fischl MA, Hammer SM, et al. Antiretroviral therapy for HIV infection in 1997: updated recommendations of the International AIDS Society—USA panel. JAMA 277:1962, 1997.
82. Lange JMA, Richman DD. The first blow is half the battle. Antivir Ther 2:132, 1997.

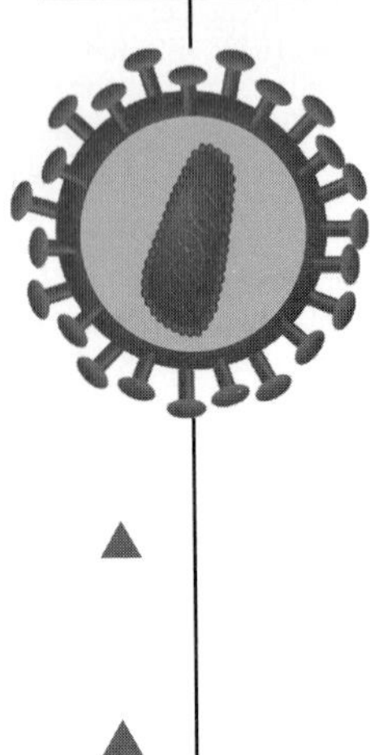

CHAPTER 14

Indinavir

Roy Gulick, MD, MPH

Indinavir sulfate (L-735,524; MK-639; Crixivan) is a member of the class of human immunodeficiency virus type 1 (HIV-1) protease inhibitors. The drug was approved by the U.S. Food and Drug Administration (FDA) in March 1996 and is labeled for the treatment of HIV infection in combination with antiretroviral agents.[1] Guidelines strongly recommend using an HIV protease inhibitor (e.g., indinavir, nelfinavir, or a combination of ritonavir with indinavir, lopinavir, or saquinavir) or the nonnucleoside reverse transcriptase inhibitor (NNRTI) efavirenz in combination with two nucleoside analogues as initial treatment for HIV disease.[2,3] HIV protease inhibitors have been associated with dramatic declines in HIV-related morbidity and mortality.[4,5]

▲ STRUCTURE

The chemical name for indinavir sulfate is [1(1*S*, 2*R*),5(*S*)]-2,3,4-trideoxy-*N*-(2,3-dihydro-2-hydroxy-1H-inden-1-yl)-5-[2-[{(1,1-dimethylethyl) amino}carbonyl]4-(3-pyridinylmethyl)-1-piperazinyl]-2-(phenylmethyl) *D*-erythro-pentonamide sulfate (1:1) salt (Fig. 14–1).[1,6] Indinavir is derived from the class of hydroxyethylene peptidomimetic protease inhibitors that display potent activity but have poor aqueous solubility in vitro and inadequate oral bioavailability in animal models.[6] By incorporating a basic amine group into the structural backbone of the hydroxyethylene protease inhibitors a new class of protease inhibitors, the hydroxyethylamine compounds, were developed. This class of compounds retains its peptide character but has improved aqueous solubility and enhanced oral bioavailability. Further improvements were achieved using a rational structure-based drug design to model and develop a series of structural analogues of these compounds in an attempt to retain potent antiretroviral activity while further improving oral bioavailability.[6–8] The modified hydroxyethylamine peptidomimetic compounds are exemplified by the HIV protease inhibitors saquinavir and indinavir.

▲ IN VITRO ACTIVITY

Indinavir potently and competitively inhibits both the HIV-1 and HIV-2 aspartyl protease enzymes with K_i (dissociation constant of the enzyme–inhibitor complex) values of 0.34 and 3.3 nM, respectively.[9] In concentrations higher than 10 μM, indinavir did not inhibit other clinically relevant proteolytic enzymes such as the aspartyl proteases human plasma renin, human cathepsin D, porcine pepsin, and bovine chymosin and the serine proteases factor Xa and elastase. Indinavir is a potent inhibitor of HIV replication in vitro.[9] In cell culture systems, indinavir showed potent activity against T lymphoid cell-adapted HIV variants (IIIb, MN, RFII) and a monocytotropic variant (SF162) with a 95% inhibitory concentration (IC_{95}) in the range of 12 to 100 nM. Indinavir also demonstrated potent activity against primary patient HIV isolates from peripheral blood mononuclear cells, including a zidovudine-resistant isolate and an NNRTI (L-697,661)-resistant isolate. Indinavir was also active in preventing acute infection in vitro by the simian immunodeficiency virus. Indinavir showed synergistic in vitro antiviral activity in combination with zidovudine, didanosine, or an NNRTI. The combination of indinavir and the protease inhibitor saquinavir showed mild antagonism in vitro,[10] and other

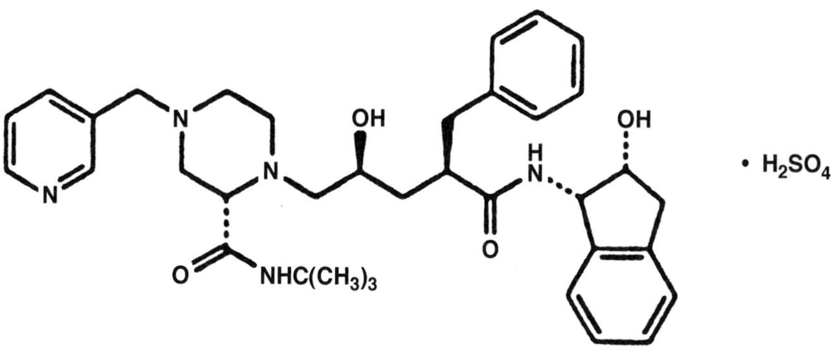

Figure 14–1. Structural formula of indinavir.

two- and three-protease inhibitor combinations have demonstrated synergy to mild antagonism.[11,12]

▲ MECHANISM OF ACTION

The HIV protease enzyme cleaves viral precursor polyproteins into structural proteins and enzymes, a step essential for the production of mature, infectious virions.[13] Retroviral proteases are unusual among proteolytic enzymes in terms of their ability to cleave protein substrates at the *N*-terminal side of proline residues. Phenylalanine-proline (Phe-Pro) residues constitute one of the important cleavage sites for the HIV-1 protease enzyme. The hydroxyethylamine peptidomimetic protease inhibitors, including saquinavir and indinavir, were designed to mimic the Phe-Pro dipeptide transition state of the substrate protein.[6–8] These inhibitors enter the cell without intracellular processing, bind at the active site of the protease enzyme, inhibit cleavage of the viral precursor proteins, and thereby prevent maturation of the virus. Immature, noninfectious viral particles are formed in the presence of the peptidomimetic protease inhibitors. The crystal structure of indinavir complexed to the HIV protease shows that binding causes closure of the flap domains of the enzyme. There are specific interactions between chemical groups of the inhibitor and the enzyme. The lipophilic groups of indinavir (with the exception of the pyridine ring) are confined inside the active site of the enzyme.[14]

Adding indinavir at concentrations of 500 to 12,000 nM to chronically HIV-infected cell culture systems decreased the amount of mature HIV proteins (p17 and p24) and increased the amount of the viral core protein precursor (p55) compared to untreated virions.[9] Indinavir also prevented incorporation of the HIV reverse transcriptase and integrase enzymes into viral particles. In parallel experiments, removing indinavir from the cell culture medium resulted in an increase in the amount of mature viral proteins and the subsequent production of infectious virions. Thus indinavir is a reversible inhibitor of the HIV protease enzyme.

▲ PHARMACOKINETICS

Preclinical Profiles

In initial animal studies, pharmacokinetic profiles were performed using intravenous and oral dosing of indinavir in rats, dogs, and monkeys.[6,9] In these animal models the plasma concentrations 6 hours after administration of oral indinavir solutions were twice the in vitro (IC_{95}). Oral bioavailability ranged from 14% in monkeys to 72% in dogs. Indinavir required an acidic pH environment for dissolution prior to absorption of the drug from the gastrointestinal tract and was less soluble at higher pH.[15] Other in vitro studies showed that indinavir was not highly bound to plasma proteins, with the unbound drug fraction ranging from 15% in dog plasma to 56% in human plasma at drug concentrations of 81 to 16,300 nM.[6,9] In vitro, in contrast to other protease inhibitors, the antiretroviral activity of indinavir was similar against wild-type and protease inhibitor-resistant isolates despite a fourfold increase in α_1-acid glycoprotein levels.[16]

Clinical Studies: Single-Dose Indinavir

The first clinical study of indinavir was an assessment of the safety, tolerability, and pharmacokinetics of single doses of the drug in 28 healthy volunteers.[17] Subjects were administered single doses ranging from 20 to 1000 mg of indinavir (free base formulation) in a double-blind, placebo-controlled manner. Alternate formulations also were given, including indinavir administered as the sulfate salt. A lower intersubject variation with comparable mean plasma concentrations seen with the sulfate formulation led to its further evaluation at doses of 400, 700, and 1000 mg. Results in 11 patients indicated rapid oral absorption of the drug in the fasting state, with peak plasma concentrations (C_{max}) achieved in approximately 0.8 hour. Plasma concentrations and urinary excretion were nonlinear, increasing more than proportionally to dose. The plasma half-life of the drug averaged 1.8 to 1.9 hours and was not dose-dependent. Calculated free drug concentrations exceeded the in vitro IC_{95} through 6 hours after the 700-mg dose and through 8 hours following the 1000-mg dose.

To investigate the nonlinear pharmacokinetics further, 12 healthy volunteers were administered single intravenous and oral doses of indinavir.[18] Although at low plasma concentrations indinavir clearance was extremely high, hepatic first-pass metabolism appeared to be saturable at higher doses of the drug (400- and 800-mg oral doses), resulting in reduced drug clearance and higher drug concentrations. In this study, oral bioavailability was estimated to be 60% to 65%. An intensive pharmacokinetic study in eight HIV-infected adults showed overall indinavir protein binding of 61% ± 6% (range 54% to 70%), with considerable variability among patients.[19] The fraction of bound drug was concentration-dependent in that indinavir binding was higher at the 8-hour postdose concentration than at the 1-hour time point.

Food Effects

Administration with food high in calories, fat, and protein reduced the absorption of indinavir.[17] Healthy volunteers fed a standard breakfast of eggs, toast with butter, bacon, potatoes, and whole milk (784 kcal, 49 g fat, 31 g protein, 57 g carbohydrate) together with a 400-mg dose of indinavir showed a 56% to 78% reduction in the area under the concentration–time curve (AUC) and a 73% to 86% reduction in maximum concentration (C_{max}) compared with levels obtained during fasted drug administration. Either of two lighter meals—toast with jelly, juice, and coffee with skim milk and sugar (292 kcal, 2 g fat, 5 g protein, 63 g carbohydrate) or corn flakes with skim milk and sugar (141 kcal, 1 g fat, 6 g protein, 29 g carbohydrate)—had no significant effect on the absorption of an 800-mg dose of indinavir. In eight HIV-infected subjects, 680-kcal meal treatments given with a 600-mg dose of indinavir significantly decreased absorption compared with fasted controls.[20] Reduction in indinavir AUC (0-infinity) by 68% (protein meal), 45% (carbohydrate meal), 34% (fat meal), and 30% (viscous cellulose meal) as well as similar reductions in C_{max} and a delayed time to C_{max} were noted. The greatest reductions in indinavir concentrations seen with the high-calorie protein meal suggest that an elevated gastric pH may promote drug precipitation, causing decreased absorption.

Clinical Studies: Multiple-Dose Indinavir

In a multidose study, indinavir was administered to 24 asymptomatic HIV-positive adults at doses of 100, 200, or 400 mg every 6 hours for up to 10 days.[21] There was a less than 30% increase in the AUC of indinavir in the plasma after multiple doses, suggesting little accumulation of the drug. Plasma drug concentrations again increased more than proportionally to the dose in the multiple-dose studies. The mean ± SD trough concentration (C_{min}) 6 hours postdose in six patients after 10 days of administration of indinavir at 400 mg q6h was 199 ± 139 nM, which exceeded the in vitro IC_{95}.

In further dose-escalation studies, indinavir was given at doses of 800 mg q8h, 1000 mg q8h, and 800 mg q6h in a study of 70 HIV-positive adults.[22] The geometric mean plasma AUCs over 24 hours for the three regimens were not statistically different. This led to selecting the 800-mg q8h dose for Phase III evaluation. In 16 patients at the 800-mg q8h dose, the steady-state AUC was 30,691 ± 11,407 nM/hn, the C_{max} was 12,617 ± 4037 nM, and the C_{min} 8 hours postdose was 251 ± 178 nM.[1] There was no significant accumulation with multiple doses at 800 mg q8h. Alternative dosing of indinavir at 1200 mg q12h was compared to 800 mg q8h in a combination regimen and found to have inferior virologic activity (64% vs. 91% of subjects with an HIV RNA level of less than 400 copies/ml at week 24).[23] Consequently, twice-daily dosing of indinavir is not recommended routinely.

Elimination

In one of the initial clinical studies, 1000-mg oral doses of indinavir were administered to 10 healthy volunteers, and urine samples were collected and analyzed.[17,24] Seven major metabolites were identified, and glucuronidation, oxidation, and *N*-alkylation were the major metabolic pathways. The major component of drug in urine was unchanged indinavir, accounting for 11% of the total dose. In follow-up experiments, single 400-mg oral doses of radiolabeled indinavir were given to six healthy volunteers.[25] The major route of excretion of indinavir was via feces (19% unchanged drug, 64% metabolites); the minor excretory route was via urine (9% unchanged drug, 10% metabolites); and the combined recovery was quantitative. Seven drug metabolites were identified in both plasma and urine: six oxidative metabolites and one glucuronide conjugate. The high level of metabolites in feces is consistent with biliary excretion. The cytochrome P_{450} (CYP) 3A4 hepatic enzyme is the major enzyme responsible for formation of the oxidative metabolites[26]; intestinal CYP3A4 contributes relatively little to its metabolism.[27] Indinavir (like other protease inhibitors) serves as a substrate for the P-glycoprotein efflux membrane transporter, which is distributed in the gastrointestinal tract, liver, kidney, blood-brain barrier, genital tract, and some CD4+ T-lymphocytes.[28] The cellular pump may promote drug secretion into the intestinal lumen, enhance metabolism, or block entry into brain, testes, and some CD4+ T-lymphocytes.

Tissue Penetration

After oral administration in rats, indinavir was distributed rapidly throughout the plasma and lymphatic system, with comparable concentrations.[29] Wong, Gunthard, and colleagues found significant declines in HIV RNA, but not DNA, levels in lymph nodes in a small group of patients on potent indinavir-containing regimens, implying effective lymphoid penetration in humans.[30,31]

Following intravenous administration to rats, the brain plasma indinavir level ratio was 0.18 at steady state, suggesting limited penetration.[29] In vitro and animal experiments showed that indinavir and other protease inhibitors were transported by a P-glycoprotein efflux membrane transporter that is thought to limit brain (and other tissue) penetration.[28] In an intensive clinical study, eight HIV-infected adults who took an indinavir-containing combination regimen underwent sampling of cerebrospinal fluid (CSF) and plasma.[32] The mean values of free indinavir in the CSF were AUC (0 to 8 hours) 1616 nM, C_{max} 294 nM, and C_{min} 122 nM, all exceeding the in vitro IC_{95} for indinavir. Free indinavir accounted for 94% of the drug in CSF and 42% in plasma. The mean ± SD CSF/plasma ratio for free indinavir was 15% ± 3%. Seven of eight subjects had

CSF HIV RNA levels of less than 200 copies/ml. Other population-based pharmacokinetic studies have shown similar results.[33,34]

P-glycoprotein transport may also limit protease inhibitor transport into the testes. Several groups have documented the reduction of HIV RNA in semen in patients taking indinavir-containing regimens,[35,36] though in one study up to 31% of nucleoside-experienced patients had HIV RNA or DNA detected in the semen 6 months after adding indinavir to their regimens.[37]

Enhancement of Indinavir Levels with Ritonavir

By inhibiting hepatic metabolism, ritonavir enhances the levels of other protease inhibitors, including indinavir.[38] Indinavir levels were increased in vitro and in rats, with AUCs in the animal study increased eightfold. Various dose combinations of indinavir/ritonavir have been studied in clinical studies of healthy volunteers,[39,40] allowing twice-daily dosing and administration with food. For indinavir the AUC increased threefold, the C_{max} 30% to 50%, and the C_{min} 15- to 35-fold when combined with ritonavir. In a clinical study in HIV-infected subjects, the combination of indinavir 800 mg/ritonavir 100 mg twice daily also was found to have favorable pharmacokinetic properties.[41] Candidate doses of indinavir/ritonavir of 800/100, 800/200, and 400/400 mg are being further investigated and compared. Once-daily dosing of indinavir/ ritonavir has also been explored but may be limited by tolerability.[42,43]

In a pilot study of 13 HIV-infected patients, the addition of ritonavir to indinavir increased indinavir concentrations in the serum (C_{min} from 65 to 336 ng/ml), CSF (from 39 to 104 ng/ml), and seminal plasma (median 141 to 1634 ng/ml).[44] In six patients with before and after samples, ritonavir increased indinavir levels significantly in CSF 2.4-fold and in seminal plasma by 8.0-fold.

Pharmacokinetics and Antiretroviral Effect

Several groups have related the plasma concentrations of indinavir to its virologic effect.[45–48] Burger and colleagues prospectively followed 65 subjects on an indinavir-containing regimen and observed a virologic failure rate of 37%.[45] In a multivariate analysis, a low plasma concentration of indinavir was an independent predictor of failure. Similarly, Acosta and colleagues studied 43 subjects receiving indinavir combination therapy and found significantly higher indinavir AUC (0 to 8 hours) in treatment-naive subjects with HIV RNA below the limit of detection, compared to those with detectable viral load levels.[46] In another study, higher indinavir C_{min} values using modeling in a naive patient population were significantly associated with virologic suppression to less than 200 copies/ml at week 24.[47] The 90% virologic response rate in this study correlated with an indinavir C_{min} of 110 ng/ml. Anderson and colleagues correlated higher indinavir C_{max} concentrations ($> 7\ \mu g/ml$) with greater CD4+ T-lymphocyte increases in a group of patients with suppressed HIV RNA levels.[48] Another group correlated low indinavir concentrations in hair with lack of virologic response and the development of protease gene mutations[49]; and still others have suggested monitoring saliva levels of indinavir.[50,51] Kakuda et al. showed the feasibility of concentration-controlled therapy in a pilot study of 11 subjects receiving an indinavir-based combination regimen to achieve a target trough indinavir level of 0.15 mg/L.[52] Further investigations will evaluate the virologic response of this approach.

Hepatic or Renal Insufficiency

Twelve patients with clinical evidence of cirrhosis and mild to moderate hepatic insufficiency were administered single doses of 400 mg indinavir.[1] In these patients, a 60% higher mean ± SD AUC and an increased half-life of 2.8 ± 0.5 hours compared to historical controls was demonstrated, indicating decreased metabolism of indinavir. Based on these results, the recommended dose in patients with mild to moderate hepatic insufficiency resulting from cirrhosis is 600 mg q8h. The pharmacokinetics have not been determined in patients with severe hepatic insufficiency or renal insufficiency, but it is assumed that because of the hepatic metabolism of the drug substantial dose reductions for renal insufficiency are not required.[53] It is not known if indinavir is dialyzable by peritoneal dialysis or hemodialysis, though case reports suggest that dosage modification may not be necessary.[54–56]

Gender and Race

The existence of gender differences in indinavir metabolism was investigated in the rat, dog, and monkey and in in vitro studies with human microsomes.[57] Although some metabolic differences between sexes occurred in the rat and dog, no differences occurred in monkeys or in human liver microsome experiments. The effect of gender on indinavir pharmacokinetics was evaluated in a clinical study of 10 HIV-infected women who received standard doses of indinavir (with zidovudine and lamivudine).[1] Compared to pooled historical control data in men, the AUC (0 to 8 hours) and C_{max} were decreased 13%, and the C_{min} was decreased 22%. The clinical significance of these differences is not known. In other clinical studies, comparable pharmacokinetics of indinavir were seen in whites and blacks, both HIV-infected and uninfected volunteers.[1]

Pediatrics

The optimal dosing of indinavir in pediatric patients has not been determined. In a clinical study of 34 pediatric HIV-infected patients (age 4 to 15 years), indinavir dosed at 500 mg/m^2 q8h had an AUC (0 to 8 hours) of 38,742 nM/hr, C_{max} 17,181 nM, and C_{min} 134 nM.[1] Compared to pharmacokinetic results in adults taking indinavir 800 mg q8h, the AUC and C_{max} were higher and the C_{min} lower (50% of pediatric patients had levels of less than 100 nM compared to 10% of adults). A second study of 11 HIV-infected children taking 500 mg/m^2 q8h also showed a lower C_{min}, suggesting that every-6-hours dosing is appropriate.[58] In addition, these investigators showed that subjects with a small body surface area had greater AUC values than adults and suggested that dose reduction is appropriate.

▲ TOXICITY

Early studies showed indinavir to be generally well tolerated. In Phase I trials the only clearly drug-related side effect was a reversible increase in indirect bilirubin.[59] Subsequent studies first documented the occurrence of nephrolithiasis.[22,60] In addition, studies of combination therapy with indinavir and zidovudine first described gastrointestinal side effects.[61,62] In other clinical studies and descriptive series, indinavir has been generally well tolerated in combination regimens[62–65] (Table 14–1). Some comparative studies have demonstrated better or comparable overall tolerance with indinavir than with saquinavir,[66,67] ritonavir,[65,67–69] ritonavir/saquinavir,[65,69] or nelfinavir,[65] whereas others have suggested that saquinavir[65] or nelfinavir[70] is better tolerated.

Crystalluria and Nephrolithiasis

Crystals in the urine, most commonly composed of indinavir base, occur in 32% to 67% of patients,[71–73] particularly in the setting of increased urine pH.[72] In one study, crystalluria occurred most commonly during the first 2 weeks after starting treatment and thereafter could be demonstrated in about 25% of urine sediment samples.[73] Other urinalysis abnormalities that occur commonly in the setting of crystalluria are proteinuria, hemoglobinuria, and pyuria. Case reports have linked indinavir crystalluria to a foreign body giant cell reaction, with acute tubulointerstitial nephritis demonstrated on renal biopsy.[74] It is not clear, however, that crystalluria always leads to nephrolithiasis.

Nephrolithiasis, diagnosed in the setting of flank pain with or without macroscopic or microscopic hematuria, was reported initially in 193 of 2071 patients (9%) from pooled clinical studies of indinavir.[1] A total of 7 of 193 patients (4%) went on to discontinue the drug, whereas others were able to resume therapy. More recently, a higher incidence rate of stone formation has been suggested. In one series of 155 patients, 43% developed nephrolithiasis over 78 weeks.[75] In the ACTG 320 trial, the largest single clinical study of indinavir, with 1156 patients randomized to zidovudine and lamivudine with or without indinavir, 7 patients (1%) experienced renal colic or nephrolithiasis (or both) of severe or greater intensity in the indinavir group compared with no patients in the nucleoside analogue group after a median follow-up of 38 weeks.[64] In a smaller clinical study with 3 years of follow-up, 12 of 33 (36%) patients ultimately experienced clinical signs of nephrolithiasis[76] and additional episodes may occur with continued therapy.[76a]

Specific risks of stone formation that have been suggested include advanced age,[75] female gender,[77] concomitant hepatitis,[78,79] and living in a warm climate or exercising (because of the risk of dehydration).[80,81] Neither a prior or family history of kidney stones nor the concurrent use of acyclovir, sulfa drugs, or vitamin C has been definitively associated with developing nephrolithiasis while taking indinavir.[1] One group compared 15 evaluable patients taking indinavir with urologic complaints and found that 14 of 15 (90%) had a higher indinavir plasma concentration than the mean in a control group of 14 asymptomatic patients taking indinavir.[82] In 6 of these patients, the indinavir dose was reduced to 600 mg q8h; plasma concentrations fell within the 95% confidence interval of the control group, and the patients remained asymptomatic. A higher frequency of nephrolithiasis has been reported in pediatric patients (29%).[1]

Patients may experience one of several other clinical syndromes: back/flank pain with crystalluria without nephrolithiasis or dysuria and urgency with crystalluria.[71] Indinavir nephrolithiasis may be difficult to demonstrate radiologically without the use of intravenous contrast dye because the stones are radiolucent.[83] In general, crystalluria and kidney stones are not associated with changes in renal function, and they can be managed with analgesics, hydration, or interruption of the drug for 1 to 3 days. In one series, 11 (70%) of 18 episodes of indinavir-induced nephrolithiasis were successfully managed with hydration and analgesia over the first 48 hours.[84] However, hypertension, renal atrophy, renal failure, frank obstruction, and anuria have been reported.[71,85–88] In one retrospective analysis of 106 patients, 19% experienced a sustained creatinine elevation of at least 20%, associated with low urinary specific gravity and pyuria, consistent with a crystal nephropathy.[89] All abnormalities were reversible upon discontinuing the drug. In another retrospective analysis of 72 patients, the mean serum creatinine levels increased to more than 1.3 mg/dl in 13 (18%); this increase occurred more commonly in women and was associated with pyuria and microhematuria.[77] Of 193 patients on indinavir who developed nephrolithiasis, 6 (3%) had hydronephrosis and 6 (3%) underwent stent placement.[1]

Daudon and colleagues analyzed kidney stones passed from 29 referred patients taking indinavir-containing regimens for periods of 1 to 20 weeks; they showed the stones to consist of crystals of indinavir base monohydrate.[90] Seven patients had stones also containing small amounts of calcium oxalate or calcium phosphate. It is of interest that the cores of all stones analyzed were made of indinavir, strongly suggesting that indinavir was the promoter of stone formation. Nephrolithiasis occurs more frequently at

▲ **Table 14–1.** COMMON SIDE EFFECTS OF INDINAVIR

Side Effect	Incidence (%)
Gastrointestinal disturbance	
Abdominal pain	9
Diarrhea	5
Nausea	12
Vomiting	4
Headache	6
Hyperbilirubinemia (indirect)	
Total bilirubin >2.5 mg/dl	10
Total bilirubin >5.0 mg/dl	1
Nephrolithiasis (flank pain ± hematuria)	9+

doses of indinavir higher than 2.4 g/day.[91] Nephrolithiasis may be decreased by ensuring adequate hydration (1.5 L of fluids a day).

Bilirubin and Hepatic Transaminase Elevations

Hyperbilirubinemia resulting from elevated indirect bilirubin (higher than 2.5 mg/dl) occurs in about 10% of patients taking indinavir in pooled studies and is dose-related.[1] Most commonly it is subclinical, although occasionally mild scleral icterus occurs. Hyperbilirubinemia may resolve spontaneously and is reversible with discontinuation of the indinavir. Fewer than 1% of patients have associated hepatic enzyme elevations.[1] Patients with preexisting Gilbert's syndrome may experience the highest bilirubin values. It is uncommon for a patient taking indinavir to have a total bilirubin level higher than 5.0 mg/dl. In Merck studies 028 and 033, about 7% to 8% of 302 patients receiving indinavir had total serum bilirubin levels higher than 2.5 mg/dl.[62] In the ACTG 320 trial, 27 of 577 subjects (5%) taking indinavir had total bilirubin more than 2.5 times the upper limit of normal, and 6 others (1%) had total bilirubin more than 5.0 times normal.[64] Laboratory abnormalities other than hyperbilirubinemia are less common. One group described 8 of 117 (7%) patients who developed severe hepatitis (more than 5.0 times normal or 3.5 times baseline transaminase levels) after starting indinavir, although this incidence was similar to that for a group of patients taking nucleoside analogues only; there was a threefold higher risk in patients with chronic viral hepatitis.[92]

Metabolic Disorders

In June 1997 the FDA issued a Public Health Advisory noting 83 cases of hyperglycemia or diabetes mellitus in HIV-positive patients undergoing HIV protease inhibitor therapy.[93] Of the 83 patients, 14 were known to be diabetic at baseline. Altogether, 27 of the 83 required hospitalization, including 6 with problems thought to be life-threatening; 5 cases resulted in diabetic ketoacidosis. The average time of onset was about 76 days after starting an HIV protease inhibitor, although cases occurred in as few as 4 days. In another series, 7 of 117 (6%) patients receiving protease inhibitors developed symptomatic diabetes mellitus.[94] The mechanism is not known, though indinavir has been shown to inhibit one of the glucose transporters involved in insulin-stimulated glucose uptake by adipocytes,[95] or may interfere with insulin signaling, or both.[96]

Indinavir, like other HIV protease inhibitors, has been associated with increased serum lipid levels. One group studied 17 fasted patients taking an indinavir-based combination regimen and found significant increases in mean cholesterol (167 to 206 mg/dl), triglycerides (110 to 158 mg/dl), and low density lipoprotein (LDL) (107 to 136 mg/dl) with no change in high density lipoprotein (HDL) levels.[97] The mechanism remains unknown, although it may be due to changes in serum lipoprotein lipase activity, hepatic lipid metabolism,[97,98] or altered retinoid signaling.[99]

More recently, a fat redistribution or lipodystrophy syndrome characterized by accumulation of abdominal fat and loss of peripheral fat with or without cushingoid features ("buffalo hump"), lipomas, and breast enlargement in women has been associated with HIV protease inhibitors[100–102] (see Chapter 62). The syndrome has been associated with increased serum lipid levels and insulin resistance.[101,102] The abdominal enlargement is characterized by an increase in visceral adipose tissue, typically without an increase in total body weight.[100] During postmarketing surveillance, the FDA reported 62 cases of fat redistribution in patients taking protease inhibitors versus 3 cases among those taking non-protease-inhibitor antiretroviral therapy.[103] During postmarketing surveillance of 282 reports of fat redistribution in patients taking indinavir reported to Merck, 159 (56%) had fat accumulation, 60 (21%) had peripheral wasting, and 63 (22%) had both.[104] Fat accumulation was more common in men and peripheral wasting more common in women. Weight gain was reported in 100% of those with fat accumulation, and weight loss was reported in 83% of those with peripheral wasting.

Long-term sequelae of hyperlipidemia and fat redistribution are not known, although one group found no association between indinavir therapy and myocardial infarction.[105] Henry and colleagues studied 100 randomly selected patients taking an indinavir-based combination regimen and found increased median levels of cholesterol (185 mg/dl, with 39% more than 200 mg/dl), triglycerides (184 mg/dl, with 12% more than 400 mg/dl), decreased median HDL levels (33 mg/dl), and a 56% rate of insulin resistance.[106] They noted that these risk factors have been associated with an increased risk of coronary heart disease and warrant risk factor modification efforts. Morphologic changes typically do not resolve over the short term upon discontinuing indinavir.[101] Current studies are exploring substitution of indinavir with other agents in the setting of fat redistribution. Further investigation into the prevalence, etiology, clinical significance, and management of this syndrome is warranted.

Other Toxicities

Gastrointestinal symptoms may occur with indinavir-containing regimens. In Merck studies 028 and 033 (indinavir versus zidovudine versus the combination) of antiretroviral-naive patients, 4% to 12% of patients randomized to indinavir alone reported abdominal pain, nausea, diarrhea, or vomiting of moderate or greater intensity.[62] In the same studies, 4% to 14% of patients randomized to zidovudine reported these symptoms, as did 4% to 32% of patients randomized to the combination regimen. In studies of zidovudine-experienced patients, there were no differences in gastrointestinal side effects among patients taking a combination of zidovudine and lamivudine with or without indinavir.[63,64]

The FDA issued a warning letter in July 1996 noting 15 case reports of spontaneous bleeding episodes in HIV-positive hemophiliacs taking HIV protease inhibitors. Eleven cases involved hematomas and five involved hemarthroses, with one patient reporting both complications. Most of these patients continued taking protease inhibitor therapy. In a follow-up report using the FDA's postmarketing spontaneous reporting system, 39 of 67 (58%) reports of spontaneous bleeding in patients taking indinavir occurred in hemophiliacs, compared to only 2 of 63 (3%) in hemophiliac patients taking zidovudine.[107] Bleeding episodes tended to resolve upon discontinuation of therapy but recurred in two hemophiliac patients upon rechallenge. The mechanism is not known, though it may involve a direct effect on blood vessels.[108]

Indinavir has also been associated with skin, hair, and nail changes. In one series of 101 patients who started an indinavir-based combination regimen, 48 (57%) developed cheilitis, 34 (40%) dry skin with pruritus, 5 (6%) pyogenic granuloma of the toenails, and 1 (1%) severe alopecia.[109] A localized skin rash was described in 110 patients who started indinavir; these data were in the results of a postmarketing surveillance report, where 67% of the cohort reported onset of the rash within the first 2 weeks of starting therapy, 49 (44%) reported spread that involved the whole body, 86% had associated pruritus, and 81% required symptomatic treatment with antihistamines or corticosteroids.[110] In this case series, 59% continued indinavir therapy despite the presence of the rash. Stevens-Johnson syndrome is a rare complication of indinavir.[111] Paronychia have also been associated with indinavir in case series[112,113] with a fivefold increased risk associated with indinavir treatment in one cohort study.[114] This syndrome, also reported in children, is postulated to be due to interference of indinavir with endogenous retinoid metabolism.[115]

Toxicity of Indinavir in Combination with Ritonavir

In a study of 90 treatment-naive patients who received open-label therapy with two nucleoside analogues and indinavir/ritonavir 400/400 mg twice daily, 7 (8%) patients discontinued treatment over 24 weeks because of an adverse event: increased hepatic transaminases ($n = 1$), nausea ($n = 4$), and diarrhea ($n = 2$).[116] Over the same time, 20% experienced nausea, 10% had circumoral paresthesias, 47% had a cholesterol level higher than 240 mg/dl, and 67% had a triglyceride level high than 200 mg/dl. In a 48-week, open-label randomized study in which 106 patients received a combination regimen containing either the standard dose of indinavir three times daily or indinavir/ritonavir (IDV/RTV) 800/100 mg twice daily, adverse events were evenly distributed except for nausea (48% IDV, 68% IDV/RTV; $P = 0.04$) and dry mouth (24% IDV, 46% IDV/RTV; $P = 0.02$).[117] Further studies are in progress.

▲ EFFICACY

Monotherapy

A 24-week randomized, blinded study (Merck 006) of indinavir at either 200 or 400 mg q6h or zidovudine 200 mg q8h was conducted in 73 p24-antigenemic, mostly zidovudine-experienced HIV-positive patients with CD4+ T-lymphocyte counts less than 500/mm^3 (median 110/mm^3).[60,118] Of the 23 patients in the 400-mg dose cohort, 21 had greater than 1 $\log_{10}$ copies/ml decreases in viral copy number at some point over 24 weeks compared with 12 of 21 in the 200-mg group and 1 of 29 in the zidovudine group. CD4+ T-lymphocyte count changes from baseline at week 24 were +65/mm^3 (400 mg), +43/mm^3 (200 mg), and −11/mm^3 (zidovudine). With variable HIV RNA decreases and documented antiretroviral resistance,[119] indinavir doses later were increased to 600 mg q6h in all patients, but this did not induce further changes in plasma HIV RNA levels or CD4+ T-lymphocyte counts. Sixteen patients originally randomized to zidovudine went on to add open-label indinavir at 600 mg q6h.[118] Median serum HIV RNA levels decreased by 1.98 $\log_{10}$ copies/ml after 8 weeks in this group, with a median CD4+ T-lymphocyte count increase of 126/mm^3 above baseline at 36 weeks. A dose-escalation study (Merck 021) evaluated indinavir at doses of 800 mg q8h, 1000 mg q8h, and 800 mg q6h in 70 HIV-positive patients.[22] Over 24 weeks the viral load decreased about 2 $\log_{10}$ copies/ml and the CD4+ T-lymphocyte count increased about 100 cells/mm^3 from baseline values, without differences among the three treatment groups. After 48 weeks of monotherapy, patients were allowed to add nucleoside analogues and continued to be followed.[91] After 84 to 96 weeks of total therapy, 22% to 36% of patients tested had HIV RNA levels of less than 500 copies/ml and CD4+ T-lymphocyte counts of 145 to 180/mm^3 over baseline.

Two-Drug Combination: Indinavir and Zidovudine

The first reported combination study of indinavir (Merck 019) was a study of 73 antiretroviral-naive patients with serum HIV RNA levels of 20,000 copies/ml or more (median 4.9 $\log_{10}$ copies/ml) and CD4+ T-lymphocyte counts of 500/mm^3 or less (median 221/mm^3) who were randomized to indinavir 600 mg q6h, zidovudine 200 mg q8h, or a combination of the two for 24 weeks.[61] At 24 weeks the change in HIV RNA levels from baseline was −1.5 $\log_{10}$ copies/ml (indinavir), −0.3 $\log_{10}$ copies/ml (zidovudine), and −2.5 $\log_{10}$ copies/ml (combination). The mean absolute CD4+ T-lymphocyte counts increased 50 cells/mm^3 higher in the two indinavir-containing regimens than in the zidovudine monotherapy arm, with sustained increases over 24 weeks. A larger Phase II study (Merck 028) compared similar regimens (indinavir 800 mg q8h, zidovudine 200 mg q8h, or a combination of the two) in 996 antiretroviral therapy-naive patients with baseline CD4+ T-lymphocyte counts of 50 to 250/mm^3.[62] During the study the protocol was amended to add lamivudine to the zidovudine-containing arms. The primary study endpoint was clinical progression to acquired immunodeficiency syndrome (AIDS) or death. A protocol-defined interim analysis of the study found highly significant reductions in clinical progression in the indinavir arms compared to the zidovudine arm; and the study was terminated early. Over a median follow-up of 1 year, reductions in the hazards of clinical progression of 70% (combination group) and 61% (indinavir group) were seen over the hazard rate in the zidovudine group ($P < 0.0001$). In addition, significant changes in HIV RNA and CD4+ T-lymphocyte counts were seen in the indinavir groups compared to the zidovudine group.

Three-Drug Combination: Indinavir and Two Nucleoside Analogues

A three-drug combination study (Merck 035) enrolled 97 patients with zidovudine experience (81% also had taken didanosine, zalcitabine, or stavudine) without prior lamivudine or protease inhibitor experience. They had an HIV RNA level of 20,000 copies/ml or more and CD4+ T-lymphocyte counts of 50 to 400/mm^3. They were randomized to (1) indinavir 800 mg q8h, (2) zidovudine 200 mg q8h/lamivudine 150 mg q12h, or (3) a combination of all three drugs.[63] At baseline, patients had taken zidovudine for a median of 31 months and had a median HIV RNA level of 43,200 copies/ml and a median CD4+ T-lymphocyte count of 144/mm^3. At 24 weeks of follow-up, the median HIV RNA changes were -1.2 $\log_{10}$ copies/ml in the indinavir group, -0.8 $\log_{10}$ copies/ml in the zidovudine/lamivudine group, and -1.8 $\log_{10}$ copies/ml in the triple-combination group. At the same time, 43% of the indinavir group decreased to less than 500 copies/ml compared with 0% of the zidovudine/lamivudine group and 90% of the triple-combination group. Most patients on triple therapy who had viral loads of less than 500 copies/ml also had levels of less than 50 copies/ml using the ultrasensitive viral load assay. Median CD4+ T-lymphocyte count changes from baseline at week 24 were $+101$/mm^3 in the indinavir group, $+46$/mm^3 in the zidovudine/lamivudine group, and $+86$/mm^3 in the triple-combination group. HIV RNA and CD4+ T-lymphocyte changes were sustained at approximately the same levels through 52 weeks of follow-up.

After at least 24 weeks of original therapy, all patients received triple-combination therapy and continue to be followed. The simultaneous introduction of three-drug antiretroviral therapy achieved a virologic effect superior to sequential introduction of the same three drugs.[120] Results with the triple combination were durable through 3 years of follow-up, with 68% and 65% of patients suppressing HIV RNA levels to less than 500 and less than 50 copies/ml, respectively, using an intent-to-treat analysis. At the same time, the CD4+ T-lymphocyte count increased $+230$ cells/mm^3 over baseline[76] (Fig. 14–2). 5-year follow-up results were recently presented and demonstrated durable responses.[76a]

A parallel study (Merck 039) enrolled 320 patients with zidovudine experience without prior lamivudine or protease inhibitor experience and with 50 CD4+ T-lymphocyte cells/mm^3 or less and randomized them to indinavir monotherapy, zidovudine/lamivudine, or the triple combination.[121] At baseline the mean HIV RNA was 74,353 copies/ml and the CD4+ T-lymphocyte count was 18/mm^3. The mean HIV RNA changes from baseline at 24 weeks were -0.36 $\log_{10}$ copies/ml in the indinavir group, -0.25 $\log_{10}$ copies/ml in the zidovudine/lamivudine group, and -1.93 $\log_{10}$ copies/ml in the three-drug combination group. The proportion of patients with viral levels of less than 500 and less than 50 copies/ml were 3% and 2% in the indinavir group, 0% in the zidovudine/lamivudine group, and 56% and 45% in the triple-drug combination group, respectively. Median changes from baseline of the CD4+ T-lymphocyte counts at 24 weeks were $+59$/mm^3 for indinavir, $+7$/mm^3 for zidovudine/lamivudine, and $+61$/mm^3 for the triple combination. These results were updated through 60 weeks of follow-up.[122]

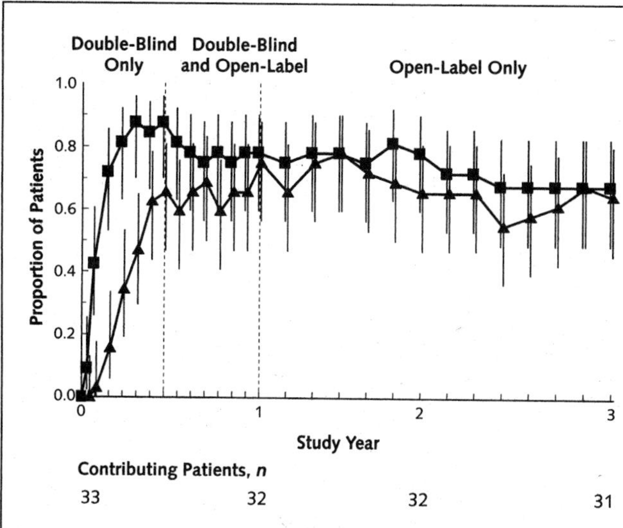

Figure 14–2. Proportions (95% confidence intervals) of subjects randomized to indinavir, zidovudine, and lamivudine, with serum HIV RNA levels <500 copies/ml (*squares*) and <50 copies/ml (*triangles*) by study week in the Merck 035 study. (From Gulick RM, Mellors JW, Havlir D, et al. 3-year suppression of HIV viremia with indinavir, zidovudine, and lamivudine. Ann Intern Med 133:37, 2000, with permission.)

AVANTI 2 was a multinational study of 103 antiretroviral-naive subjects with CD4+ T-lymphocyte counts of 150 to 500/mm^3 who were randomized to receive zidovudine/lamivudine with or without indinavir.[123] At 52 weeks of follow-up, the proportions of subjects with HIV RNA levels of less than 500 and less than 20 were 18% and 4% (zidovudine/lamivudine) versus 60% and 46% (three-drug combination).

A large study of similar combination antiretroviral regimens (ACTG 320) assessed clinical endpoints.[64] In this study 1156 patients with CD4+ T-lymphocyte counts of 200/mm^3 or less (median 86/mm^3) with zidovudine experience but without previous lamivudine or protease inhibitor use were randomized to zidovudine 200 mg q8h/lamivudine 150 mg q12h with or without indinavir 800 mg q8h; they were followed for the occurrence of a new AIDS-defining illness or death. Patients were allowed to substitute stavudine for zidovudine if intolerant. After a median follow-up of 38 weeks, the Data and Safety Monitoring Board (DSMB) of the ACTG recommended stopping the study because of a significant difference between the two treatment arms: 63 patients (11%) taking the two-drug combination had a new AIDS event or death versus 33 patients (6%) on the triple-combination arm (Fig. 14–3). The estimated hazard ratio comparing three drugs to two was 0.5. Thus the three-drug combination of indinavir/zidovudine/lamivudine demonstrated a 50% decrease in the rate of AIDS or death over the zidovudine/lamivudine regimen.

Merck 060 is an ongoing study of 199 antiretroviral-naive patients with a CD4+ T-lymphocyte count of more than 500/mm^3 and an HIV RNA level of more than 1000

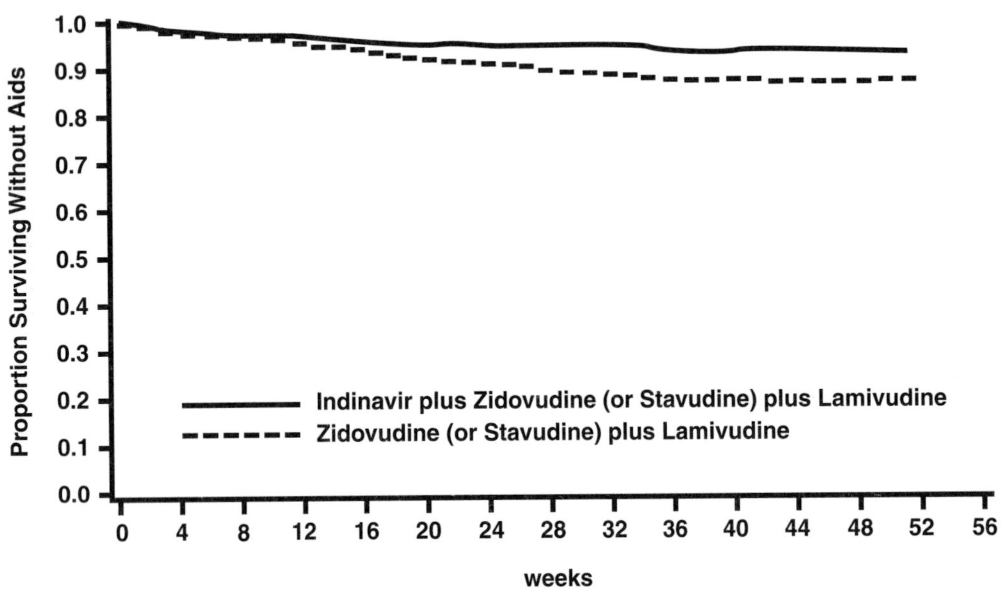

Figure 14–3. Kaplan-Meier estimate of the proportion of subjects not reaching the primary study endpoint of AIDS or death in the ACTG 320 study. (From Hammer SM, Squires KE, Hughes MD, et al. A randomized placebo-controlled trial of indinavir in combination with two nucleoside analogs in human immunodeficiency virus infected persons with CD4 cell counts less than or equal to 200 per cubic millimeter. N Engl J Med 337:725, 1997; Copyright 1997, Massachusetts Medical Society, with permission. All rights reserved.)

copies/ml treated with open-label zidovudine/lamivudine/indinavir.[124] At baseline the mean HIV RNA level was 8227 copies/ml, and the CD4+ T-lymphocyte count was 597/mm^3. In this ongoing study 97% had a serum HIV RNA value of less than 400 copies/ml, and 94% had less than 50 copies/ml at week 96 (on-treatment analysis). In a subset of these patients with sustained viral load levels of less than 50 copies/ml, 12 of 16 had peripheral blood mononuclear cell (PBMC) cultures negative for HIV, and two of these patients had no detectable replication-competent HIV despite examination of large numbers of resting CD4+ T-lymphocyte isolated by leukophoresis.

The OzCombo study randomized 109 treatment-naive subjects with a CD4+ T-lymphocyte level of less than 500/mm^3 and an HIV RNA count of more than 30,000 copies/ml to receive indinavir with zidovudine/lamivudine, stavudine/lamivudine, or stavudine/didanosine.[125] At 12 months of follow-up, 58% had HIV RNA counts of less than 50 copies/ml without significant differences among the three groups. Similar virologic suppression rates were seen with indinavir plus combinations of zidovudine/lamivudine, stavudine/lamivudine, or stavudine/didanosine in the START studies.[126,127]

Other Indinavir Trial Results

Pediatrics

The first reported study of a protease inhibitor-containing regimen in a pediatric population was a pilot study of open-label indinavir 500 mg/m^2 q8h, stavudine 1 mg/kg q12h, and didanosine 90 mg/m^2 q12h in 12 nucleoside-experienced children, 5 of whom had received prior stavudine and didanosine.[128] During the study, the dose of indinavir was increased to 500 mg/m^2 q6h when low trough levels were documented. At 48 weeks the HIV RNA decreased 2.0 $\log_{10}$ copies/ml, and the CD4+ T-lymphocyte count increased 317/mm^3 from baseline. A second pilot study enrolled 15 treatment-experienced children who received indinavir with zidovudine/lamivudine or stavudine/lamivudine and found better virologic outcomes in those who changed at least one nucleoside.[129]

A formal Phase I/II study of indinavir in HIV-infected children has been reported.[130] In this open-label study, 54 mostly treatment-experienced children received indinavir in one of two formulations (free-base liquid suspension or sulfate salt dry-filled capsules) at one of three oral doses (250, 350, or 500 mg/m^2 q8h) for a median of 16 weeks and then added zidovudine/lamivudine. During the study the suspension was found to be less bioavailable, and all children were changed to capsules. Transient decreases in plasma HIV RNA levels were seen in all three dosing groups. Overall, of 48 evaluable patients at 16 weeks, HIV RNA median decreases were -0.01 $\log_{10}$ copies/ml (250 and 350 mg/m^2 groups) and -0.76 $\log_{10}$ copies/ml (500 mg/m^2 group).

A longer-term study enrolled 28 children, about half of whom were treatment-experienced, who took indinavir 400 mg/m^2 q8h/zidovudine/lamivudine.[131] In 70% of patients the indinavir dose was increased to achieve target AUC levels. At 6 months of follow-up, 70% and 48% of subjects had reduced their plasma HIV RNA levels to less than 500 and less than 40 copies/ml, respectively. Another study randomized 25 children to receive open-label indinavir 500 mg/m^2 q8h with stavudine and lamivudine.[132] HIV RNA decreased to less than 400 copies/ml within 1 month in 79% of the children and was sustained through 18 months of follow-up, with concomitant increases in CD4+ T-lymphocyte counts.

Acute HIV Infection

A multinational open-label pilot study (Merck 042) investigated the effects of indinavir, zidovudine, and lamivudine in patients with acute or recent HIV infection.[133] Altogether, 47 patients were enrolled, treated, and followed for up to 1 year. At 3 months of follow-up, 11 of 14 had plasma HIV RNA levels of less than 500 copies/ml, and 2 of 8 had less than 20 copies/ml. From a mean pretreatment baseline plasma HIV RNA level of about 85,000 copies/ml, 89% reduced levels to less than 500 copies/ml; and of the 35 patients with available data, 79% reduced levels to less than 50 copies/ml at 52 weeks of follow-up. Over the same time, CD4+ T-lymphocyte counts increased 210/mm^3 over baseline levels. Notable in this study was a high level of adherence to the medications. Similar results were seen with the same drug regimen in two other studies of primary HIV infection.[134,135]

A different approach was taken in another study that treated 10 patients with acute HIV infection before complete Western blot seroconversion with indinavir/didanosine/hydroxyurea.[136,137] The baseline plasma HIV RNA level was more than 550,000 copies/ml and decreased to less than 50 copies/ml in all subjects. Over 46 weeks of follow-up the CD4+ T-lymphocyte count increased by 154 cells/mm^3 over baseline and CD8 cells decreased, resulting in an increased CD4/CD8 ratio. Seven of eight patients tested on therapy had vigorous CD4+ T-lymphocyte proliferative responses to HIV p24 protein, though a baseline evaluation had not been done. A low frequency of latently infected CD4+ T-lymphocyte was documented in five of six patients tested.

Indinavir and Nonnucleoside Reverse Transcriptase Inhibitors

The use of indinavir and the NNRTI nevirapine has been described in several studies.[138–140] A pilot study of 22 nucleoside-experienced subjects used an open-label regimen of indinavir 800 mg q8h, nevirapine at standard dose, and nucleosides.[138] Despite documenting about a 50% reduction in serum peak and trough indinavir levels, the median decrease in HIV RNA was 3.1 $\log_{10}$ copies/ml at 24 weeks. A second pilot study of 24 subjects treated them with indinavir 800 mg q8h for a week and then added nevirapine at a standard dose.[139] Once again, despite a reduction in indinavir levels by 11% to 48%, about 59% of subjects reduced their HIV RNA levels to 20 copies/ml or less at 58 weeks in a last observation carried forward analysis. A more recent study (ACTG 373) used a combination of indinavir 1000 mg q8h, nevirapine at standard dose, and nucleosides in amprenavir-experienced subjects; it found that 59% had reduced HIV RNA (to <500 copies/ml at week 48).[140]

The combination of indinavir and efavirenz also has been investigated.[141–143] In one study (Dupont-003), 101 subjects were randomized to start indinavir and efavirenz simultaneously or to start indinavir and then add efavirenz and stavudine after 12 weeks.[141] Indinavir was initiated at 800 mg q8h and then later increased to 1000 mg q8h because of the significant drug interaction with efavirenz. Additionally, efavirenz was started at 200 mg qd and then increased to 600 mg qd at 36 weeks. At 60 weeks of follow-up, HIV RNA was decreased -2.5 $\log_{10}$ copies/ml (indinavir/efavirenz) and -1.9 $\log_{10}$ copies/ml (indinavir/efavirenz/stavudine) from baseline levels, with 89% and 68% reducing HIV RNA to less than 400 copies/ml, respectively. The Dupont 006 study was a three-arm study of initial antiretroviral therapy, including one arm with indinavir 1000 mg q8h/efavirenz 600 mg qd.[142] Of 148 initially randomized to this combination, 53% and 47% reduced HIV RNA levels to less than 500 and less than 50 copies/ml, respectively, at 48 weeks in an intent-to-treat analysis. In a nucleoside-experienced group of 184 patients randomized to indinavir 1000 mg q8h/efavirenz or indinavir 800 mg q8h/nucleosides, 68% and 52% had reduced HIV RNA levels (to <400 copies/ml) at 24 weeks.[143]

Indinavir and Ritonavir

Enhancement of indinavir levels by ritonavir allows coadministration on a twice-daily basis, with food.[39,40] An open-label single-armed study of indinavir and ritonavir (both given at 400 mg q12h) with nucleosides explored the virologic activity of this combination in 90 treatment-naive subjects.[116] At 24 weeks, 87% and 71% had reduced HIV RNA levels to less than 500 and less than 80 copies/ml, respectively, in an intent-to-treat analysis. In a randomized study of 104 zidovudine-experienced subjects, patients received zidovudine/lamivudine with open-label indinavir 800 mg q8h or indinavir 800 mg/ritonavir 100 mg bid.[117] The preliminary results at 48 weeks showed no significant differences in HIV RNA changes (-2.0 vs. -1.6 $\log_{10}$ copies/ml), proportions of subjects with HIV RNA of less than 50 copies/ml (70% vs. 66%), or increases in CD4+ T-lymphocyte counts ($+57$ vs. $+70$/mm^3). In preliminary results of a pilot study of indinavir 1200 mg/ritonavir 200 mg given once daily, 80% to 85% of subjects had reduced HIV RNA levels over 16 to 24 weeks in an on-treatment analysis.[144] Further studies are in progress.

Comparisons to Other Protease Inhibitors

Several observational cohort studies have attempted to compare protease inhibitor-based regimens.[67,145–147] In a French cohort of 1402 mostly nucleoside-experienced patients who started indinavir-, ritonavir-, or saquinavir (hard-gel formulation)-based regimens and were followed for a median of 14 months, no differences were found in the rates of clinical progression.[67] Overall, 50% had decreased HIV RNA <1000 copies/ml at 12 months, but the use of saquinavir was associated with a significantly increased risk of virologic failure compared with indinavir [odds ratio (OR) 2.0, $P = 0.001$]; there was no difference observed between indinavir and ritonavir. In a Spanish cohort of 400 mostly nucleoside-experienced patients who started indinavir-, ritonavir-, or saquinavir (hard-gel formulation)-based regimens, overall 45% had reduced HIV RNA to <200 copies/ml at the end of 1 year.[145] However, virologic failure was significantly associated with using a saquinavir-based regimen [relative risk (RR) 1.6, $P = 0.03$]. In a Dutch cohort, 271 treatment-naive and treatment-experienced patients were started on indinavir-, ritonavir-, saquinavir (hard-gel formulation)-based regimens or a saquinavir/ritonavir-based regimen and were followed for 48 weeks; there was no difference in the clinical progression rates among the regimens.[146] Overall, 60% had reduced HIV RNA to <1000 copies/ml at 48 weeks, but the risk for virologic failure was increased significantly with the use of saquinavir-based regimens compared with the other regimens (OR 3.2, $P = 0.001$). In an Italian cohort of 717 treatment-naive patients who started two nucleosides with indinavir, ritonavir, or saquinavir (hard-gel formulation), the use of an indinavir-based regimen was associated with a significantly reduced likelihood of discontinuing therapy for virologic failure compared to the use of a saquinavir-based regimen [relative hazard (RH) 0.24, $P = 0.01$], and there was a trend toward reduced likelihood compared to a ritonavir-based regimen (RH 0.20, $P = 0.07$).[147]

Some randomized comparisons among the protease inhibitors have been completed.[66,68–70] The CHEESE study was an open-label randomized study of 70 antiretroviral-naive patients who received zidovudine/lamivudine with either indinavir 800 mg q8h or saquinavir (soft-gel formulation) 1200 mg tid.[66] At 24 weeks of follow-up, 71% (indinavir group) versus 74% (saquinavir group) had decreased HIV RNA to <50 copies/ml. At the same time, CD4 cells increased significantly more in the saquinavir group than the indinavir group (+89 vs. +162/mm^3, $P = 0.01$), although preliminary data indicated that this difference was not sustained. In the ISS-IP1 study, 1251 nucleoside-experienced patients with CD4 levels of less than 50/mm^3 were randomized to receive either an indinavir- or ritonavir-based regimen and were followed for clinical endpoints.[68] At a mean follow-up of 10 months, 124 deaths and 330 AIDS events had occurred, with no significant difference between the groups ($P = 0.6$). The Danish Protease Inhibitor study enrolled 318 patients, about half of whom were treatment-naive; they were randomized to receive two nucleosides with open-label indinavir, ritonavir, or saquinavir/ritonavir.[69] At 72 weeks of follow-up there was no difference in the proportion of patients who had decreased HIV RNA to 20 copies/ml or less: 51% (indinavir), 41% (ritonavir), 58% (saquinavir/ ritonavir) ($P = 0.08$). Another study randomized 112 treatment-experienced patients to receive stavudine and lamivudine with either indinavir or nelfinavir. After a median follow-up of 9 months, 46% to 47% of subjects in each group reduced their viral load levels to less than 200 copies/ml (on treatment analysis).[70]

Comparisons to Other Antiretroviral Regimens

The Dupont 006 study compared open-label indinavir/zidovudine/lamivudine to efavirenz/zidovudine/lamivudine and indinavir/efavirenz in 450 treatment-naive subjects.[142] At 48 weeks of follow-up, 48% and 43% (indinavir group), 70% and 64% (efavirenz group), and 53% and 47% (indinavir/efavirenz group) had decreased HIV RNA to less than 400 and less than 50 copies/ml, respectively, in an intent-to-treat, missing equals failure analysis. Results were similar at 2 years of follow-up, with 7% to 8% in each group experiencing virologic rebound of more than 50 copies/ml between years 1 and 2.[148] Although the efavirenz-based regimen was statistically superior to the indinavir-based regimen in this analysis, there were excess dropouts in the indinavir group in this open-label study. In a double-blind study of 327 nucleoside-experienced subjects (Dupont 020), patients were randomized to received indinavir and nucleosides with or without efavirenz.[143] At 24 weeks of follow-up, 68% of the indinavir/efavirenz group versus 52% of the indinavir without efavirenz group had decreased HIV RNA to less than 400 copies/ml.

The Glaxo 3005 study enrolled 562 treatment-naive subjects to receive indinavir/zidovudine/lamivudine or abacavir/zidovudine/lamivudine in a double-blind manner.[149] At week 48 about 51% had decreased HIV RNA levels to 400 copies/ml or less in each group in an intent-to-treat, missing equals failure analysis. A statistical difference was seen in the subset of subjects who entered the study with HIV RNA of more than 100,000 copies/ml, where 45% of the indinavir group versus 31% of the abacavir group had reduced plasma HIV RNA levels to less than 50 copies/ml. The CNAA 3014 study had an identical design but administered the drugs in an open-label manner.[150] In this study, 342 antiretroviral-naive subjects received zidovudine/lamivudine in combination with indinavir or abacavir. At 24 weeks, 58% and 61% (indinavir group) and 67% and 73% (abacavir group) had reduced HIV RNA levels to less than 400 and less than 50 copies/ml, respectively. In the subjects with viral load levels of more than 100,000 copies/ml at baseline, 43% (indinavir) and 56% (abacavir) had HIV RNA of less than 50 copies/ml. Self-reported adherence was better in the abacavir group, with 78% of subjects indicating that they had missed less than one dose of medications per week versus 48% in the indinavir group.

The Atlantic study randomized 298 subjects to receive stavudine/didanosine in combination with open-label indinavir, nevirapine, or lamivudine for 48 weeks.[151] At baseline, the HIV RNA was about 18,000 copies/ml, with 13% of subjects having levels of more than 100,000 copies/ml. At 48 weeks, comparable proportions of subjects had reduced viral load levels to less than 50 copies/ml in an intent-to-treat analysis: 49% (indinavir group), 49% (nevirapine), and 40% (lamivudine).

The major indinavir efficacy trials are summarized in Table 14–2.

▲ RESISTANCE

Original attempts to derive HIV resistant to indinavir in vitro by serial passages of wild-type virus in cell culture in the presence of increasing concentrations of the drug were unsuccessful.[9] This led to further studies of resistance involving construction of mutant recombinant protease enzymes and assessment of their susceptibility to indinavir. Using the crystal structure of the HIV protease enzyme complexed with specific protease inhibitors, single amino acid positions in the enzyme were identified as potentially important for drug binding at positions 23, 32, 47, 50, 76, 82, and 84. In the case of each recombinant enzyme with a constructed single amino acid substitution, some loss of sensitivity to the drug occurred, along with an apparent decrease in the efficiency of the enzyme. HIV variants

▲ **Table 14–2.** MAJOR EFFICACY TRIALS OF INDINAVIR

Study	Regimen	No.	Entry Criteria[a]	Results
Two-Drug vs. Three-Drug Combinations				
Gulick et al.[63,76,76a,120] (Merck 035)	IDV/ ZDV + 3TC/ IDV + ZDV + 3TC (double-blind)	97	ZDV-experienced HIV RNA > 20,000 CD4 50–500	Three-drug combination superior: HIV RNA < 50 in 48% at 5 years (ITT analysis)
Hirsch et al.[121,122] (Merck 039)	IDV/ ZDV + 3TC/ IDV + ZDV + 3TC (double-blind)	320	ZDV-experienced CD4 ≤ 50	Three-drug combination superior: HIV RNA < 50 in 45% at week 24 (ITT analysis)
Hammer et al.[64] (ACTG 320)	ZDV + 3TC/ IDV + ZDV + 3TC (open label)	1156	ZDV-experienced CD4 < 200	Three-drug combination superior: 50% decrease in AIDS/death over 38 weeks of follow-up (ITT analysis)
Comparative Studies: Protease Inhibitors				
Floridia et al.[68] (ISS-IP1)	IDV-based regimen RTV-based regimen (open label)	1251	Nucleoside-experienced CD4 < 50	No difference between groups: overall; 124 deaths and 330 AIDS events occurred over 10 months of follow-up
Katzenstein et al.[69] (Danish PI Study)	Two nucleosides + IDV RTV RTV/SQV (open label)	318	46% Treatment-naive 64% Nucleoside-experienced <2 weeks PI	No difference between the groups: HIV RNA ≤ 20 in 51% (IDV), 41% (RTV), 58% (RTV/SQV) at 72 weeks (*P* = 0.08)
Comparative Studies: Protease Inhibitors, NNRTI, Three Nucleosides				
Stazsewski et al.[142,148] (Dupont 006)	EFV + ZDV + 3TC IDV + EFV IDV + ZDV + 3TC (open label)	450	Treatment-naive HIV RNA > 10,000 CD4 > 50	EFV regimen superior: HIV RNA < 50 in 64% (EFV), 47% (IDV/EFV), 43% (IDV) at 48 weeks; increased dropouts in IDV group (ITT analysis)
Stazsewski et al.[149] (Glaxo 3005)	ABC + ZDV + 3TC IDV + ZDV + 3TC (double-blind)	562	Treatment-naive HIV RNA > 10,000 CD4 > 100	HIV RNA < 400 in 51% in both groups at week 48; with baseline HIV RNA > 100,000, IDV regimen superior: HIV RNA < 50 in 45% (IDV) vs. 31% (ABC) (ITT analysis)
Cahn[150] (Glaxo 3014)	ABC + ZDV + 3TC IDV + ZDV + 3TC (open label)	342	Treatment-naive HIV RNA > 5,000	HIV RNA < 400 in 67% (ABC) vs. 58% (IDV) at 24 weeks (ITT analysis)
Squires et al.[151] (Atlantic)	d4T + ddI + NVP d4T + ddI + 3TC d4T + ddI + IDV (open label)	298	Treatment-naive HIV RNA > 500 CD4 > 200	No difference between the groups: HIV RNA < 50 in 49% (NVP), 40% (3TC), 49% (IDV) at 48 weeks (*P* = 0.20) (ITT analysis)
Indinavir and Ritonavir				
Rockstroh et al.[116]	Two nucleosides + IDV/RTV (open label)	90	Treatment-naive HIV RNA > 35,000	HIV RNA < 80 in 71% at 24 weeks (ITT analysis)
Boyd et al.[117]	ZDV + 3TC + IDV ZDV + 3TC + IDV + RTV (open label)	104	ZDV-experienced	No difference between groups: HIV RNA < 50 in 70% (IDV) and 66% (IDV/RTV) at 48 weeks (analysis not specified)

ABC, abacavir; CD4 units, cells mm^3; d4T, stavudine; ddI, didanosine; EFV, efavirenz; HIV RNA units, copies/mL; IDV, indinavir; ITT, intent-to-treat; NVP, nevirapine; OT, on-treatment; RTV, ritonavir; SQV, saquinavir; 3TC, lamivudine; ZDV, zidovudine.
CD4 cells/mm^3; HIV RNA copies/ml.

constructed with multiple mutations had broad cross-resistance to other protease inhibitors.[152]

Clinical Studies

The first study of clinical resistance to protease inhibitors was reported by Condra et al.[119] Early clinical studies of indinavir using suboptimal doses (200 or 400 mg q6h) were associated with transient decreases in viral load levels, followed by subsequent rebounds.[60] In the first well documented case, phenotypic analysis of a viral isolate obtained after 24 weeks of indinavir therapy revealed a fourfold decrease in sensitivity to indinavir and some reduced sensitivity to other protease inhibitors. DNA sequencing of the same isolate revealed seven or eight amino acid changes from the baseline isolate, including three reversions to the HIV protease consensus sequence (not present in the baseline isolate) and five "forward mutations" at positions 10, 46, 63, 82, and 84, during indinavir treatment. Further experiments involved the construction of mutant proviruses using amino acid residue changes at these five positions. None of the single or double amino acid substitutions was associated with a loss of sensitivity

▲ **Table 14–3.** AMINO ACID SUBSTITUTIONS IN THE HIV PROTEASE
▲ ENZYME ASSOCIATED WITH INDINAVIR RESISTANCE[a]

Amino Acid Position	Substitution Type
32, 82, 84, 90	Enzyme active site
10, 20, 24, 36, 46, 54, 63, 64, 71	"Compensatory"

[a]Three or more substitutions required for loss of phenotypic sensitivity.

to indinavir or cross- resistance to other protease inhibitors. Only constructs with three or more mutations resulted in a loss of indinavir sensitivity. Viral isolates in this patient from weeks 40 and 52 revealed numerous additional amino acid substitutions, increasing the resistance to indinavir and inducing high-level cross-resistance to five other protease inhibitors, including saquinavir, A-80987 (a ritonavir analogue), and amprenavir.

In the same study, additional isolates from other patients on prolonged indinavir treatment revealed broad phenotypic resistance to indinavir and high degrees of cross-resistance to other protease inhibitors. Interestingly, the genotypic analyses revealed distinct patterns of multiple mutations in each case. The identified amino acid residues were of two kinds: those close to the active site of the HIV protease enzyme (positions 32, 82, 84, 90) and other "compensatory" changes (at positions 10, 20, 24, 36, 46, 54, 63, 71) (Table 14–3). These compensatory substitutions are thought to represent structural conformational changes or to promote increases in enzymatic activity to compensate for the changes in inhibitor binding.[153]

Condra and colleagues extended their observations using viral isolates from 29 additional patients from early Phase I or II studies of indinavir using suboptimal doses (200 or 400 mg q6h or 600 mg q8h).[154] Development of resistance in 17 of these patients was associated with multiple variable patterns of substitutions of 3 to 11 amino acids in the HIV protease. No repeated pattern of changes was seen among the isolates, although substitutions at positions 46 or 82 (or both) occurred in all resistant isolates. A minimum of three mutations was required for measurable drug resistance. Changes at positions 10, 20, 24, 46, 54, 63, 64, 71, 82, 84, and 90 correlated with phenotypic indinavir resistance selected in vivo.

Continued indinavir therapy was associated with the stepwise accumulation of additional mutations and an associated increase in phenotypic resistance to indinavir. In isolates from 15 patients there was some degree of cross-resistance to other protease inhibitors, including saquinavir (63% cross-resistant), ritonavir (100% cross-resistant), and amprenavir (81% cross-resistant). In a subset of these subjects, the mean proportion of amino acid changes from baseline increased from 4.0% (week 0 to 24) to 7.3% (week 0 to 60), indicating continued evolution of the sequence under continued drug pressure.[155]

A second described mechanism of HIV drug resistance involves mutations in the precursor protein cleavage sites. One group described six patients on indinavir-containing regimens who developed not only amino acid substitutions in the protease enzyme but also a change in the gag p7/p1 cleavage site.[156] In three of these patients the p7/p1 change occurred as early as 6 to 10 weeks after starting therapy. One of the patients developed a second mutation at the gag p1/p6 cleavage site. In vitro, recombinant viruses with protease enzyme mutations at positions 46 and 82 had a 68% reduction in replication rate. The replication rate of viruses with protease mutations was enhanced with the introduction of the gag cleavage site mutations. This compensatory mutation may confer a growth advantage to the virus and serves as an important mechanism of viral resistance.

The way to reduce the development of viral resistance is to use the optimal dose of indinavir (600 mg q6h or 800 mg q8h) and to use the drug in combination with other agents. Emini et al.[157] described resistance results from a Phase I/II study of indinavir monotherapy at doses of less than 2.4 g/day versus the recommended dose of 2.4 g/day.[60,118,157] At 24 weeks, 31 of 37 (84%) patients taking indinavir at doses of less than 2.4 g/day had evidence of indinavir resistance compared to 9 of 21 (43%) patients on 2.4 g/day. Condra et al. described the emergence of resistance mutations in patients on nucleoside analogues, indinavir, or a combination regimen.[158] In one study of patients randomized to indinavir, zidovudine, or both, only 1 of 22 (5%) patients on the combination developed resistance mutations to zidovudine compared to 11 of 17 (65%) of those receiving zidovudine monotherapy.[61] In the same study, 4 of 22 (18%) patients on the combination developed one or more indinavir mutations, compared with 9 of 21 (43%) on indinavir monotherapy.

More potent antiretroviral combinations demonstrate more dramatic results. In a study of patients randomized to indinavir, zidovudine/didanosine, or the triple combination, none of 20 patients on the three-drug combination developed zidovudine or didanosine mutations compared with 10 of 16 (62%) patients on zidovudine/didanosine.[158] Similarly, 2 of 20 (10%) on the triple combination developed indinavir-associated mutations, compared with 13 of 24 (54%) on indinavir monotherapy. In a study of patients randomized to indinavir, zidovudine/lamivudine, or the triple combination,[63,120] 26 of 31 (84%) patients on zidovudine/lamivudine developed lamivudine resistance, and 10 of 31 (32%) patients on indinavir monotherapy developed indinavir resistance. On the triple combination, 26 of 31 (84%) patients had HIV RNA levels that could not be amplified, implying functional drug sensitivity.

Not all patients experiencing virologic failure on indinavir-containing regimens demonstrate resistance to indinavir.[159,160] In the Trilege study, 29 patients who achieved virologic suppression on indinavir-based therapy and then virologic failure after randomization to continue three drugs or change to zidovudine/indinavir were characterized at the time of virologic failure, and no protease inhibitor mutations were found.[159] In the ACTG 343 study, subjects who achieved virologic suppression on an indinavir-based combination regimen were subsequently randomized to continue three drugs or to change to indinavir monotherapy.[160] Of the 26 subjects who experienced virologic rebound (17 on three drugs, 9 on indinavir monotherapy), none showed evidence of indinavir resistance, whereas phenotypic resistance to lamivudine was seen in 14 of 17 (82%). These findings suggest that the development of resistance to indinavir may be delayed after virologic failure. In a pooled study of five indinavir trials,[161] several factors were found to predict the development of resistance to indinavir: a lower baseline CD4+ T-lymphocyte count, using less than a three-drug combination of antiretroviral agents, and HIV RNA levels not suppressed to below the limit of detection.

It may be possible to overcome drug resistance by enhancing drug exposure.[162] Combining ritonavir with indinavir[38–40] leads to an increase in indinavir C_{min} over the protein binding-corrected IC_{95} by 28- to 79-fold. Using a panel of viruses from subjects who had experienced virologic failure on indinavir-containing regimens, Condra and colleagues showed that indinavir/ritonavir combinations of 400/400 mg or 800/100 mg had C_{min} (12 hours) that exceeded the corrected IC_{95} values for half of the isolates tested and the 800/200 mg combination dose for 18 of 20 (90%) of the isolates tested.[162] Even at the 400-mg dose of ritonavir, the C_{min} for ritonavir was less than the IC_{95} value for 19 of 20 isolates, suggesting a minimal contribution by ritonavir to antiretroviral activity. Hsu and colleagues[163] studied 37 patients on an indinavir 800 mg tid regimen with HIV RNA of 50 to 50,000 copies/ml who were changed to open-label indinavir/ritonavir 400/400 mg bid. When given with ritonavir, the indinavir trough concentration was 650% higher, the AUC was unchanged, and the indinavir peak concentration was 51% lower than when indinavir was given alone. At week 36 after the change, 50% of patients had an HIV RNA level of less than 50 copies/ml, and the response correlated with a higher trough indinavir concentration and less virtual phenotypic resistance at baseline.[164] Thus, the indinavir/ritonavir combination may offer benefits for salvage therapy.

Cross-resistance with Other Protease Inhibitors

Hertogs and colleagues characterized 6570 viral isolates from patients referred for resistance testing who had an HIV RNA level of at least 1000 copies/ml.[165] Among them, more than 10-fold phenotypic resistance was demonstrated in 17% to indinavir, in 22% to ritonavir, in 25% to nelfinavir, and in 17% to saquinavir. Cross-resistance among the protease inhibitors occurred in 59% to 80% of the samples and a total of 11% were resistant to all four protease inhibitors. Among the 1117 isolates resistant to indinavir, only 5 (0.4%) were fully sensitive to ritonavir, nelfinavir, and saquinavir. In a subset of viral isolates phenotypically resistant to at least one protease inhibitor, the most frequent amino acid substitutions (>20% frequency) were at protease positions 10, 36, 46, 54, 71, 77, 82, and 90. Among isolates with phenotypic resistance to all four protease inhibitors, these substitutions and changes at positions 48 and 84 were seen. These data imply that despite unique initial mutations a final common pathway exists for these four protease inhibitors.

Serial passage of HIV in the presence of amprenavir yielded virus with reduced sensitivity to the drug, and DNA sequence analysis revealed the sequential accumulation of point mutations with the appearance of substitutions at positions 10, 46, 47, and 50.[166] In other experiments, a single mutation at position 50 conferred a two- to three-fold reduced sensitivity to amprenavir; and a triple mutant at positions 46, 47, and 50 conferred a 14- to 20-fold reduction. The presence of mutations at 10, 46, 47, and 50 conferred a three- to fourfold loss of sensitivity to indinavir.

Results from clinical studies with the sequential use of protease inhibitors are becoming available. The first trial to investigate the sequencing of protease inhibitors (ACTG 333) studied patients who took saquinavir.[167] Patients were randomized to one of two saquinavir arms (hard gel or soft gel capsule) or indinavir. After 72 patients had received 8 weeks of study treatment, an interim analysis of the data was performed. Over the first 8 weeks of study, patients assigned to continue hard gel saquinavir had no change in viral load compared with a 0.3 log_{10} copies/ml decrease in the soft gel saquinavir group and a 0.6 log_{10} copies/ml decrease in the indinavir arm. The plasma HIV RNA response in the indinavir group was more modest than expected. ACTG 359 randomized 277 patients who had taken indinavir and experienced virologic failure to receive saquinavir with ritonavir or nelfinavir together with delavirdine, adefovir, or both.[168] Overall, only 30% of subjects had plasma HIV RNA levels of 500 copies/ml or less at week 16; and there was no difference in response rates between the two dual protease inhibitor regimens. In the ACTG 372b study, indinavir-experienced patients with virologic failure were randomized to receive efavirenz, adefovir, and abacavir or nucleoside analogues, with or without nelfinavir.[169] Overall, at 16 weeks 35% had plasma HIV RNA levels of less than 500 copies/ml, and patients who added nelfinavir had a better virologic response (45% vs. 24% without nelfinavir; $P = 0.046$). In the ACTG 373 trial, 56 subjects who had experienced virologic failure on an amprenavir-containing regimen received open-label indinavir, nevirapine, stavudine, and lamivudine.[140] Overall, 59% had plasma HIV RNA levels of less than 500 copies/ml at week 48, but many subjects received new drugs in addition to indinavir. Further protease inhibitor sequencing studies are in progress.

▲ DRUG INTERACTIONS

All of the HIV protease inhibitors have the potential to cause important drug interactions (Table 14–4) because of their ability to inhibit the cytochrome P_{450} hepatic enzyme system.[2,3,170] Indinavir is a reversible inhibitor of the CYP 3A4 enzyme isoform, a common pathway for hepatic drug metabolism; but it does not inhibit other isoforms, such as CYP1A2, 2C9, or 2E1.[171] Like other inhibitors of 3A4, co-administration of indinavir with terfenadine (Seldane), astemizole (Hismanal), cisapride (Propulsid), or pimozide (Orap) is *contraindicated* because of the potential for cardiac arrhythmias; with midazolam (Versed) or triazolam (Halcion) because of the potential for prolonged sedation; or with ergot derivatives because of the potential for inducing ergotism.[1,2,172] Additionally, indinavir should not be co-administered with rifampin because of an 89% reduction in indinavir AUC[1,173] or St. John's wort because of reductions in indinavir AUC (by 57%) and C_{min} (by 81%).[174] A constituent of St. John's wort, hyperforin, induces CYP3A4, causing increased drug metabolism.[175] Co-administration of

▲ **Table 14–4.** IMPORTANT DRUG INTERACTIONS WITH INDINAVIR

Drug	Interaction/Side Effects (Dose Change)
Contraindicated	
Astemizole (Hismanal)	Cardiac arrhythmias
Cisapride (Propulsid)	Cardiac arrhythmias
Ergot derivatives	Ergotism
Midazolam (Versed)	Extreme sedation
Pimozide (Orap)	Cardiac arrhythmias
Terfenadine (Seldane)	Cardiac arrhythmias
Triazolam (Halcion)	Extreme sedation
Not recommended	
Lovastatin (Mevacor)	Statin levels increased, risk of myopathy
Rifampin	Lowers indinavir levels 90%
Simvastatin (Zocor)	Statin levels increased, risk of myopathy
St. John's Wort	Lowers indinavir levels 57–81%
Use with caution	
Carbamazepine (Tegretol)	Lowers indinavir levels
Dexamethasone	Lowers indinavir levels
Didanosine, original formulation (Videx)	Decreases indinavir absorption (separate drug doses)
Omeprazole (Prilosec)	Decreases indinavir absorption –pH effect
Phenobarbital	Lowers indinavir levels
Phenytoin (Dilantin)	Lowers indinavir levels
Sildenafil (Viagra)	Increases sildenafil levels
Dose Change Required	
Inducers of cytochrome P_{450}	Increase indinavir dose to 1 g q8h
Efavirenz (Sustiva)	
Nevirapine (Viramune)	
Rifabutin (Mycobutin)	Also decrease rifabutin dose to 150 mg qd
Inhibitors of cytochrome P_{450}	Decrease indinavir dose to 600 mg q8h
Delavirdine (Rescriptor)	
Itraconazole (Sporanox)	
Ketoconazole (Nizoral)	
Protease Inhibitor Combinations	
IDV/amprenavir	IDV no change; amprenavir increased 30–65%
IDV/lopinavir/ritonavir	IDV increased (dose reduce to 600 mg bid)
IDV/nelfinavir	IDV increased 50%; nelfinavir increased 83%
IDV/ritonavir	IDV increased 8-fold; ritonavir no change
Indinavir (IDV)/saquinavir	IDV no change; saquinavir increased 5- to 8-fold

indinavir with simvastatin (Zocor) or lovastatin (Mevacor) should also be avoided because their levels would be increased, with the possibility of inducing myopathy.[1,2]

Interactions with Common HIV Medications

The Indinavir Pharmacokinetic Study Group performed a series of crossover studies with three dosing periods: (1) indinavir alone; (2) indinavir in combination with a second drug at standard dose; and (3) the second drug alone.[176] Plasma sampling after 7 to 10 days of drug dosing was performed with 10 to 14 subjects per study, and plasma drug exposures were determined. No clinically significant interactions were seen with indinavir and isoniazid, fluconazole, or trimethoprim-sulfamethoxazole.[177] Another group studied the interaction of indinavir and fluconazole in 13 patients and found a trend toward a decrease in indinavir AUC, without effects on C_{max} or C_{min}, but they questioned the clinical significance of their findings.[178]

In a multidose study, co-administration of ketoconazole once daily with indinavir 600 mg q8h resulted in an 18% increase in indinavir AUC over that seen with indinavir alone at 800 mg q8h; therefore a dose reduction in indinavir is recommended.[1,179] For the same reason, itraconazole use should prompt a dose reduction in indinavir to 600 mg q8h.[1] Co-administration with indinavir increased the AUC of clarithromycin by about 47%, and the indinavir C_{min} by 58% without affecting the indinavir AUC or C_{max}.[180] Indinavir levels were not altered by co-administration with azithromycin[181] or atovaquone.[182]

Co-administration of indinavir and rifabutin increased the plasma concentrations of rifabutin about twofold.[183] This interaction was considered clinically significant, and a dose reduction of rifabutin to 150 mg daily is recommended. Further study of the interaction of indinavir and rifabutin, an inducer of P_{450}, revealed that indinavir levels were reduced about 30% when the drugs were administered concomitantly, suggesting that an indinavir dose increase to 1000 mg q8h may be warranted in addition to the decrease in rifabutin dose. In a study of healthy volunteers involving co-administration of indinavir and rifampin, a highly potent inducer of P_{450}, indinavir levels were reduced about 90%.[173] Because of this marked interaction, indinavir should not be given with rifampin.

Interactions with Nucleoside Analogues

The interaction of indinavir with several nucleoside analogue reverse transcriptase inhibitors has been investigated. The Indinavir PK Study Group tested indinavir in combination with zidovudine or stavudine and found no clinically significant interactions.[176] Another study investigated the combination of zidovudine and lamivudine and found no significant interaction with indinavir.[63] The original formulation of didanosine decreases the absorption of indinavir because of the presence of the buffering agent, which increases gastric pH. Because indinavir requires a normal, acidic pH for optimal absorption, indinavir should be administered at least 1 hour after taking the original formulation of didanosine.[184] The newer enteric coated formulation of didanosine does not interact significantly with indinavir.[185]

Interactions with NNRTIs

The NNRTIs are metabolized by the cytochrome P_{450} system and have interactions with indinavir. Nevirapine is an inducer of P_{450} metabolism and reduces the C_{max} of indinavir 11% and the AUC 28%.[139] Because of this reduction it has been suggested that the indinavir dose be increased to 1000 mg q8h if co-administered with nevirapine.[2] In contrast, delavirdine inhibits the cytochrome P_{450} system and results in an increase in indinavir levels, such that a

600-mg dose of indinavir when co-adminstered with delavirdine achieves an AUC 44% greater than with indinavir 800 mg alone.[186] Therefore it has been suggested that the indinavir dose be reduced to 600 mg tid when the drugs are co-administered.[2] Efavirenz also induces P_{450} metabolism and reduces indinavir levels by about 35%.[187] Increasing the dose of indinavir to 1 g q8h is recommended when co-administering efavirenz[2]; this adjusted dose was superior to using indinavir 1200 mg q12h.[188]

Interactions with Other Protease Inhibitors

Because all the protease inhibitors are metabolized through the cytochrome P_{450} system, they may interact with each other. The interaction of indinavir and saquinavir was investigated in 18 healthy volunteers in a three-panel, dose-escalating, sequential pharmacokinetic study of indinavir and a single dose of either the hard gel or soft gel formulation of saquinavir.[189] Indinavir was administered at 800 mg q8h, and the single dose of saquinavir hard gel was given at 600 mg or the soft gel at 800 mg or 1200 mg. Indinavir increased the mean AUC and C_{max} of saquinavir approximately five- to eightfold. The interaction of indinavir and ritonavir was explored in vitro using human liver microsomes and in vivo in a rat model.[38] Co-administration of the two drugs led to an eightfold increase in the AUC (0 to 8 hours) for indinavir without a change in ritonavir levels. This prompted clinical combination studies of the two agents using 400 mg bid of each drug,[39] and indinavir 800 mg with ritonavir 100 or 200 mg bid.[40]

A clinical study with the combination indinavir/nelfinavir in non-HIV-infected volunteers showed that indinavir raised the AUC of nelfinavir by 83%, and nelfinavir raised the AUC of indinavir by 51%.[190] This favorable interaction led to a clinical trial of twice-daily dosing regimens of the two drugs.[191] At doses of indinavir 1200 mg and nelfinavir 1250 mg given twice daily in nine subjects, the indinavir AUC (0 to 24 hours), C_{max}, and C_{min} were comparable to those seen with standard indinavir dosing without nelfinavir, and the nelfinavir levels were unaffected.

The interaction of indinavir and amprenavir was investigated in a study in HIV-infected volunteers.[192] In a single-dose study, 800 mg of each drug was administered concurrently. Indinavir increased the C_{max} of amprenavir by 31% and the AUC (0 to 8 hours) by 64%; the C_{max} and AUC (0 to 8 hours) of indinavir were not significantly different from historical control values. These data support further investigation of the combination of the two drugs with no dose adjustments.

Interactions with Other Medications

Because indinavir is metabolized extensively by the liver cytochrome P_{450} 3A4 system and this isoform is involved in the metabolism of about 50% of other drugs, certain significant drug interactions may occur. A case report of a patient on a stable indinavir dose who was given carbamazepine for postherpetic neuralgia developed decreased indinavir levels (with therapeutic carbamazepine levels) and experienced virologic failure.[193] Similar concerns have been raised regarding phenytoin, phenobarbital, and dexamethasone.[1] Co-administration of sildenafil and indinavir did not alter the indinavir levels but resulted in a markedly increased sildenafil AUC compared to those of historical controls; thus a dose reduction of sildenafil is appropriate.[194] Methadone[195] and theophylline[196] metabolism were found not to be affected by indinavir co-administration. Similarly, cimetidine, quinidine, and Ortho-Novum 1/35 do not require dose changes when co-administered with indinavir.[1] Co-administration of interleukin-2 increased the indinavir AUC and trough concentrations 88% and 2.5-fold, respectively, which was thought to be due to increased interleukin-6 levels.[197] A small case series found that four of nine subjects taking the proton pump inhibitor omeprazole had markedly decreased indinavir levels, raising concern that the resultant higher pH may have led to decreased absorption of indinavir.[198]

▲ RECOMMENDATIONS FOR USE

Indication

Indinavir is labeled for the treatment of HIV infection in combination with other antiretroviral agents.[1] Current guidelines strongly recommend the use of two nucleoside analogues in combination with a highly active protease inhibitor (indinavir, nelfinavir, or a combination of ritonavir with indinavir, lopinavir, or saquinavir) or the nonnucleoside analogue efavirenz as initial treatment for HIV infection.[2,3] The optimal strategy for initiating therapy with indinavir or indinavir/ritonavir versus other potent protease inhibitors or efavirenz has not been established but is under investigation.

Dosage

Indinavir is formulated as a sulfate salt and is available in 100-, 200-, 333-, and 400-mg capsules; the recommended dose is 800 mg (usually two 400-mg capsules) every 8 hours.[1] Indinavir capsules are sensitive to moisture and should be stored with the desiccant that came in the original container at room temperature. For optimal absorption, indinavir should be administered with water 1 hour before or 2 hours after a meal. Alternatively, indinavir may be taken with juice, coffee, tea, or skim milk or a low-calorie, low-fat small meal. Patients taking indinavir should also ensure adequate hydration by drinking at least 1.5 L (approximately six 8-ounce glasses) of liquids daily to minimize the risk of indinavir-induced kidney stones.

Though not FDA-approved, the combination of indinavir and ritonavir allows once- or twice-daily dosing of both drugs with food. Doses of indinavir/ritonavir that have been investigated are 800/200 mg, 800/100 mg, and 400/400 mg all given twice daily or 1200/200 mg given once daily. As noted, ensuring adequate hydration is important.

Dose Modification

The dose of indinavir should be modified depending on the administration of concurrent medications. When given in conjunction with rifabutin,[183] nevirapine,[139] or efavirenz,[187] (all P_{450} inducers), indinavir should be increased to 1000 mg q8h. When given in conjunction with ketoconazole,[179] itraconazole,[1] or delavirdine,[186] (P_{450} inhibitors), indinavir should be reduced to 600 mg q8h. Similarly, for patients with mild to moderate hepatic insufficiency as a result of cirrhosis, the recommended dose of indinavir is 600 mg q8h.[1]

Special Populations

Pediatric Patients

The optimal dosing regimen has not been established for pediatric patients. Ongoing studies suggest that a dose of 500 mg/m^2 PO q6–8h is well tolerated and has immunologic and virologic activity.[128,130] An investigational oral liquid formulation was compared to standard capsules in 12 healthy volunteers and was shown to be bioequivalent and have an acceptable taste.[199] Further studies are in progress.

Pregnant Women

Current guidelines for the use of antiretroviral therapy in pregnant women emphasize that decisions regarding therapy should be the same as those for women who are not pregnant.[200, 201] Indinavir is rated class C for use in pregnant women: "Risk cannot be ruled out. . . . However, potential benefit may justify potential risk."[1] In studies of rats, indinavir was associated with an increase in the incidence of supernumerary ribs and variations of the vertebral ossification centers; and at postnatal evaluation there was delayed fur development, eye opening, descensus testis, and unilateral ophthalmia.[202] In studies of monkeys, indinavir caused an exacerbation of transient physiologic hyperbilirubinemia.[1]

There are no results available from adequate, well controlled studies in pregnant women. PACTG 358 is an ongoing study that has reported preliminary data on five pregnant women who took indinavir, zidovudine, and lamivudine. It found one episode of nausea and vomiting leading to discontinuation of the drug and one episode each of hyperbilirubinemia and flank pain, both of which resolved spontaneously without drug discontinuation.[203] HIV RNA levels in four women who completed the study were decreased to less than 400 copies/ml, though pharmacokinetic data revealed the indinavir AUC to be reduced compared to postpartum levels in the same subjects and nonpregnant controls. Further preliminary pharmacokinetic data in two women showed the AUC of indinavir to be reduced 63% to 86% compared with postpartum levels.[204] Morris and colleagues reported a retrospective survey of 89 pregnancies in women taking protease inhibitor-containing regimens (26% taking indinavir) at six centers.[205] The HIV perinatal transmission rate was 0 (95% confidence interval 0% to 3%), and adverse maternal, obstetric, and infant events related to protease inhibitors were uncommon.

Postexposure Prophylaxis

Indinavir has been recommended as part of a regimen for occupational postexposure prophylaxis.[206] For most exposures where treatment is indicated, a two-drug regimen of nucleoside analogue reverse transcriptase inhibitors (e.g., zidovudine and lamivudine) is recommended. For exposures with an increased risk for transmission of HIV, it is recommended that a third drug (indinavir, nelfinavir, efavirenz, or abacavir) be added to the regimen. Certain nonoccupational exposures also may warrant postexposure prophylaxis.[207] Postexposure prophylaxes regimens should be taken for 4 weeks. Side effects of prophylaxis regimens are common.[208,209] In one study registry, 340 of 492 (76%) health care workers taking various multiple prophylaxis regimens reported side effects, and 137 (28%) of them discontinued the regimen because of these side effects.[208] Another group described 19 health care workers taking indinavir-containing prophylaxis regimens of whom 7 (37%) discontinued the drugs because of intolerable side effects.[209] The risks and benefits in terms of antiretroviral effects and toxicities are unknown.

REFERENCES

1. Crixivan (indinavir sulfate): prescribing information. West Point, PA, Merck & Co, October 2000.
2. Panel On Clinical Practices for the Treatment of HIV Infection, US Department of Health and Human Services. Guidelines for the use of antiretroviral agents in HIV-infected adults and adolescents. www.hivatis.org (August 13, 2001).
3. Carpenter CJ, Cooper DA, Fischl MA, et al. Antiretroviral therapy in adults: updated recommendations of the International AIDS Society—USA panel. JAMA 283:381, 2000.
4. Palella FJ, Delaney KM, Moorman AC, et al. Declining morbidity and mortality among patients with advanced human immunodeficiency virus infection. N Engl J Med 338:853, 1998.
5. Mocroft A, Vella S, Benfield TL, et al. Changing patterns of mortality across Europe in patients infected with HIV-1: EuroSIDA study group. Lancet 352:1725, 1998.
6. Dorsey BD, Levin RB, McDaniel SL, et al. L-735,524: the design of a potent and orally bioavailable HIV protease inhibitor. J Med Chem 37:3443, 1994.
7. Roberts NA, Martin JA, Kinchington D, et al. Rational design of peptide-based HIV proteinase inhibitors. Science 248:358, 1990.
8. Huff JR. HIV protease: a novel chemotherapeutic target for AIDS. J Med Chem 34:2305, 1991.
9. Vacca JP, Dorsey BD, Schleif WA, et al. L-735,524: an orally bioavailable human immunodeficiency virus type 1 protease inhibitor. Proc Natl Acad Sci USA 91:4096, 1994.
10. Merrill DP, Manion DJ, Chou T-C, Hirsch MS. Antagonism between human immunodeficiency virus type 1 protease inhibitors indinavir and saquinavir in vitro. J Infect Dis 176:265, 1997.
11. St Clair MH, Millard J, Rooney J, et al. In vitro antiviral activity of 141W94 (VX-478) in combination with other antiretroviral agents. Antiviral Res 29:53, 1996.
12. Tremblay C, Merrill DP, Chou T-C, Hirsch MS. Interactions among combinations of two and three protease inhibitors against drug-susceptible and drug-resistant HIV-1 isolates. J AIDS 22:430, 1999.
13. Kohl NE, Emini E, Schleif WA, et al. Active human immunodeficiency virus protease is required for viral infectivity. Proc Natl Acad Sci USA 85:4686, 1988.
14. Chen Z, Li Y, Chen E, et al. Crystal structure at 1.9-Å of human immunodeficiency virus (HIV) II protease complexed with L-735,524, an orally bioavailable inhibitor of the HIV proteases. J Biol Chem 21:26344, 1994.
15. Lin JH, Chen I-W, Vastag KJ, Ostovic D. pH-dependent oral absorption of L-735,524, a potent HIV protease inhibitor, in rats and dogs. Drug Metab Dispos 23:730, 1995.

16. Zhang XQ, Schooley RT, Gerber JG. The effect of increasing alpha$_1$-acid glycoprotein concentration on the antiviral efficacy of human immunodeficiency virus protease inhibitors. J Infect Dis 180:1833, 1999.
17. Yeh KC, Deutsch PJ, Haddix H, et al. Single dose pharmacokinetics of indinavir and the effect of food. Antimicrob Agents Chemother 42:332, 1998.
18. Yeh KC, Stone JA, Carides AD, et al. Simultaneous investigation of indinavir nonlinear pharmacokinetics and bioavailability in healthy volunteers using stable isotope labeling technique: study design and model-independent data analysis. J Pharm Sci 88:568, 1999.
19. Anderson PL, Brundage RC, Bushman L, et al. Indinavir plasma protein binding in HIV-1-infected adults. AIDS 14:2293, 2000.
20. Carver PL, Fleisher D, Zhou SY, et al. Meal composition effects on the oral bioavailability of indinavir in HIV-infected patients. Pharm Res 16:718, 1999.
21. Teppler H, Pomerantz R, Bjornsson T, et al. Pharmacokinetics and tolerability studies of L-735,524, a new HIV protease inhibitor. In: Abstracts of the 1st National Conference on Human Retroviruses and Related Infections. Washington, DC, American Society for Microbiology, 1993, abstract L8.
22. Steigbigel RT, Berry P, Mellors J, et al. Efficacy and safety of the HIV protease inhibitor indinavir sulfate (MK 639) at escalating dose. In: Abstracts of the 3rd Conference on Retroviruses and Opportunistic Infections, Washington, DC. Alexandria, VA, Foundation for Retrovirology and Human Health, 1996, abstract 146.
23. Haas DW, Arathoon E, Thompson MA, et al. Comparative studies of two-times-daily versus three-times-daily indinavir in combination with zidovudine and lamivudine. Protocol 054/069 study teams. AIDS 14:1973, 2000.
24. Balani SK, Arison BH, Mathai L, et al. Metabolites of L-735,524, a potent HIV-1 protease inhibitor, in human urine. Drug Metab Dispos 23:266, 1995.
25. Balani SK, Woolf EJ, Hoagland VL, et al. Disposition of indinavir, a potent HIV-1 protease inhibitor, after an oral dose in humans. Drug Metab Dispos 24:1389, 1996.
26. Chiba M, Hensleigh M, Nishime JA, et al. Role of cytochrome P450 3A4 in human metabolism of MK-639, a potent human immunodeficiency virus protease inhibitor. Drug Metab Dispos 24:307, 1996.
27. Fitzsimmons ME, Collins JM. Selective biotransformation of the human immunodeficiency virus protease inhibitor saquinavir by human small-intestinal cytochrome P4503A4. Drug Metab Dispos 25:256, 1997.
28. Kim RB, Fromm MF, Wandel C, et al. The drug transporter P-glycoprotein limits oral absorption and brain entry of HIV-1 protease inhibitors. J Clin Invest 101:289, 1998.
29. Lin JH, Chiba M, Balani SK, et al. Species differences in the pharmacokinetics and metabolism of indinavir, a potent human immunodeficiency virus protease inhibitor. Drug Metab Dispos 24:1111, 1996.
30. Wong JK, Gunthard F, Havlir DV, et al. Reduction of HIV in blood and lymph nodes following potent antiretroviral therapy and the virologic correlates of treatment failure. Proc Natl Acad Sci USA 94:12574, 1997.
31. Gunthard HF, Wong JK, Ignacio CC, et al. Human immunodeficiency virus replication and genotypic resistance in blood and lymph nodes after a year of potent antiretroviral therapy. J Virol 72:2422, 1998.
32. Haas DW, Stone J, Clough LA, et al. Steady-state pharmacokinetics of indinavir in cerebrospinal fluid and plasma among adults with human immunodeficiency virus type 1 infection. Clin Pharmacol Ther 68:367, 2000.
33. Martin C, Sonnerborg A, Svensson JO, Stahle L. Indinavir-based treatment of HIV-1 infected patients: efficacy in the central nervous system. AIDS 13:1227, 1999.
34. Letendre SL, Capparelli EV, Ellis RJ, McCutchan JA. Indinavir population pharmacokinetics in plasma and cerebrospinal fluid: the HIV Neurobehavioral Research Center Group. Antimicrob Agents Chemother 44:2173, 2000.
35. Gupta P, Mellors J, Kingsley L, et al. High viral load in semen of human immunodeficiency virus type 1-infected men at all stages of disease and its reduction by therapy with protease and nonnucleoside reverse transcriptase inhibitors. J Virol 71:6271, 1997.
36. Gunthard HF, Havlir DV, Fiscus S, et al. Residual human immunodeficiency virus (HIV) type 1 RNA and DNA in lymph nodes and HIV RNA in genital secretions and in cerebrospinal fluid after suppression of viremia for 2 years. J Infect Dis 183:1318, 2001.
37. Mayer KH, Boswell S, Goldstein R, et al. Persistence of human immunodeficiency virus in semen after adding indinavir to combination antiretroviral therapy. Clin Infect Dis 28:1252, 1999.
38. Kempf DJ, Marsh KC, Kumar G, et al. Pharmacokinetic enhancement of inhibitors of the human immunodeficiency virus protease by coadministration with ritonavir. Antimicrob Agents Chemother 41:654, 1997.
39. Hsu A, Granneman GR, Cao G, et al. Pharmacokinetic interaction between ritonavir and indinavir in healthy volunteers. Antimicrob Agents Chemother 42:2784, 1998.
40. Saah AJ, Winchell GA, Nessly ML, et al. Pharmacokinetic profile and tolerability of indinavir-ritonavir combinations in healthy volunteers. Antimicrob Agents Chemother 45:2710, 2001.
41. Van Heeswijk RP, Veldkamp AI, Hoetelmans RM, et al. The steady-state plasma pharmacokinetics of indinavir alone and in combination with a low dose of ritonavir in twice daily dosing regimens in HIV-infected individuals. AIDS 12:F95, 1999.
42. Mallolas J, Blanco JL, Sarasa M, et al. Dose-finding study of once-daily indinavir/ritonavir plus zidovudine and lamivudine in HIV-infected patients. J AIDS 25:229, 2000.
43. Hugen PW, Burger DM, ter Hofstede HJ, et al. Dose-finding study of a once-daily indinavir/ritonavir regimen. J AIDS 25:236, 2000.
44. Van Praag RM, Weverling GJ, Portegies P, et al. Enhanced penetration of indinavir in cerebrospinal fluid and semen after the addition of low-dose ritonavir. AIDS 14:1187, 2000.
45. Burger DM, Hoetelmans RM, Hugen PW, et al. Low plasma concentrations of indinavir are related to virological treatment failure in HIV-1-infected patients on indinavir-containing therapy. Antivir Ther 3:215, 1998.
46. Acosta EP, Henry K, Baken L, et al. Indinavir concentrations and antiviral effect. Pharmacotherapy 19:708, 1999.
47. Acosta EP, Havlir DV, Richman DD, et al. Pharmacodynamics (PD) of indinavir (IDV) in protease-naive HIV-infected patients receiving ZDV and 3TC. In: Abstracts of the 7th Conference on Retroviruses and Opportunistic Infections, San Francisco. Alexandria, VA, Foundation for Retrovirology and Human Health, 2000, abstract 455.
48. Anderson PL, Brundage RC, Kakuda TN, Fletcher CV. Indinavir (IDV) maximum plasma concentration (C_{max}) predicts CD4$^+$ response in persons with highly suppressed HIV RNA. In: Abstracts of the 8th Conference on Retroviruses and Opportunistic Infections, Chicago. Alexandria, VA, Foundation for Retrovirology and Human Health, 2001, abstract 731.
49. Bernard L, Peytavin G, Vuagnat A, et al. Indinavir concentrations in hair from patients receiving highly active antiretroviral therapy. Lancet 352:1757, 1998
50. Hugen PW, Burger DM, de Graff M, et al. Saliva as a specimen for monitoring compliance but not for predicting plasma concentrations in patients with HIV treated with indinavir. Ther Drug Monit 22:437, 2000.
51. Wintergerst U, Kurowski M, Rolinski B, et al. Use of saliva specimens for monitoring indinavir therapy in human immunodeficiency virus-infected patients. Antimicrob Agents Chemother 44:2572, 2000.
52. Kakuda TN, Page LM, Anderson PL, et al. Pharmacological basis for concentration-controlled therapy with zidovudine, lamivudine, and indinavir. Antimicrob Agents Chemother 45:236, 2001.
53. Jayasekara D, Aweeka FT, Rodriguez R, et al. Antiviral therapy for HIV patients with renal insufficiency. J AIDS 21:384, 1999.
54. Fiedler R, Peinhardt R, Deuber HJ, Osten B. Antiviral therapy with lamivudine, stavudine and indinavir in a HIV positive haemodialysis patient. J Am Soc Nephrol 1059A:207, 1998.
55. Guardiola JM, Magues MA, Domingo P, et al. Indinavir pharmacokinetics in haemodialysis-dependent end-stage renal failure. AIDS 12:1395, 1998.
56. Izzedine H, Aymard G, Hamani A, et al. Indinavir pharmacokinetics in haemodialysis. Nephrol Dial Transplant 15:1102, 2000.
57. Lin JH, Chiba M, Chen I-W, et al. Sex-dependent pharmacokinetics of indinavir: in vivo and in vitro evidence. Drug Metab Dispos 24:1298, 1996.
58. Gatti G, Vigano A, Sala N, et al. Indinavir pharmacokinetics and pharmacodynamics in children with human immunodeficiency virus infection. Antimicrob Agents Chemother 44:752, 2000.
59. Deutsch P, Teppler H, Squires K, et al. Antiviral activity of L-735,524, an HIV protease inhibitor, in infected patients. In: Abstracts

of the 34th International Conference on Antimicrobial Agents and Chemotherapy, Orlando. Washington, DC, American Society for Microbiology, 1994, abstract I-59.

60. Mellors J, Steigbigel R, Gulick R, et al. Antiretroviral activity of the oral protease inhibitor, MK-639, in p24 antigenemic, HIV-1 infected patients with <500 CD4/mm^3. In: Abstracts of the 35th International Conference on Antimicrobial Agents and Chemotherapy, San Francisco. Washington, DC, American Society for Microbiology, 1995, abstract I-172.
61. Massari F, Staszewski S, Berry P, et al. A double-blind, randomized trial of indinavir (MK-639) alone or with zidovudine vs. zidovudine alone in zidovudine naive patients. In: Abstracts of the 35th International Conference on Antimicrobial Agents and Chemotherapy, San Francisco. Washington, DC, American Society for Microbiology, 1995, abstract LB6.
62. Lewi DS, Suleiman JM, Uip DE, et al. Randomized, double-blind trial comparing indinavir alone, zidovudine alone and indinavir plus zidovudine in antiretroviral therapy-naive HIV-infected individuals with CD4+ T-lymphocyte counts between 50 and 250/mm^3. Rev Inst Med Trop Sao Paulo 42:27, 2000.
63. Gulick RM, Mellors JW, Havlir D, et al. Treatment with a combination of indinavir, zidovudine, and lamivudine in HIV-infected adults with prior antiretroviral use. N Engl J Med 337:734, 1997.
64. Hammer SM, Squires KE, Hughes MD, et al. A randomized, placebo-controlled trial of indinavir in combination with two nucleoside analogs in human immunodeficiency virus infected persons with CD4+ T-lymphocyte counts less than or equal to 200 per cubic millimeter. N Engl J Med 337:725, 1997.
65. Bonfanti P, Valsecchi L, Parazzini F, et al. Incidence of adverse reactions in HIV patients treated with protease inhibitors: a cohort study. J AIDS 23:236, 2000.
66. Cohen-Stuart JW, Schuurman R, Burger DM, et al. Randomized trial comparing saquinavir soft gelatin capsules versus indinavir as part of triple therapy (CHEESE study). AIDS 13:F53, 1999.
67. Grabar S, Pradier C, Le Corfec E, et al. Factors associated with clinical and virological failure in patients receiving a triple therapy including a protease inhibitor. AIDS 14:141, 2000.
68. Floridia M, Tomino C, Bucciardini R, et al. A randomized trial comparing the introduction of ritonavir or indinavir in 1251 nucleoside-experienced patients with advanced HIV infection: ISS-IP1 clinical investigators. AIDS Res Hum Retroviruses 16:1809, 2000.
69. Katzenstein TL, Kirk O, Pederson C, et al. The Danish Protease Inhibitor Study: a randomized study comparing the virological efficacy of 3 protease inhibitor-containing regimens for the treatment of human immunodeficiency virus type 1 infection. J Infect Dis 182:744, 2000.
70. Roca B, Gomez CJ, Arnedo A. A randomized, comparative study of lamivudine plus stavudine, with indinavir or nelfinavir in treatment-experienced HIV-infected patients. AIDS 14:157, 2000.
71. Kopp JB, Miller KD, Mican JA, et al. Crystalluria and urinary tract abnormalities associated with indinavir. Ann Intern Med 127:119, 1997.
72. Hortin GL, King C, Miller KD, Kopp JB. Detection of indinavir crystals in urine: dependence on method of analysis. Arch Pathol Lab Med 124:246, 2000.
73. Gagnon RF, Tecimer SN, Watters AK, Tsoukas CM. Prospective study of urinalysis abnormalities in HIV-positive individuals treated with indinavir. Am J Kidney Dis 36:507, 2000.
74. Jaradat M, Phillips C, Yum MN, et al. Acute tubulointerstitial nephritis attributable to indinavir therapy. Am J Kidney Dis 35:E16, 2000.
75. Saltel E, Angel JB, Futter NG, et al. Increased prevalence and analysis of risk factors for indinavir nephrolithiasis. J Urol 164:1895, 2000.
76. Gulick RM, Mellors JW, Havlir D, et al. 3-Year suppression of HIV viremia with indinavir, zidovudine and lamivudine. Ann Intern Med 133:35, 2000.
76a. Gulick RM, Mellors J, Havlir D, et al. Indinavir (IDV), zidovudine (ZDV), and lamivudine (3TC): 5-year follow-up. In: Abstracts of the 1st International AIDS Society Conference on HIV Pathogenesis and Treatment, Buenos Aires. Stockholm, Sweden, International AIDS Society, 2001, abstract 215.
77. Sarcletti M, Petter A, Romani N, et al. Pyuria in patients treated with indinavir is associated with renal dysfunction. Clin Nephrol 54:261, 2000.
78. Sarcletti M, Petter A, Romani N, et al. Pyuria in patients treated with indinavir is associated with renal dysfunction. Clin Nephrol 54:261, 2000.
78. Malavaud B, Dinh B, Bonnet E, et al. Increased incidence of indinavir nephrolithiasis in patients with hepatitis B or C infection. Antivir Ther 5:3, 2000.
79. Brodie SB, Keller MJ, Ewenstein BM, Sax PE. Variation in incidence of indinavir-associated nephrolithiasis among HIV-positive patients. AIDS 12:2433, 1998.
80. Bach MC, Godofsky EW. Indinavir nephrolithiasis in warm climates. J Acquir Immune Defic Syndr 14:296, 1997.
81. Martinez E, Leguizamon M, Mallolas J, et al. Influence of environmental temperature on incidence of indinavir-related nephrolithiasis. Clin Infect Dis 29:422, 1999.
82. Dieleman JP, Gyssens IC, van der Ende ME, et al. Urological complaints in relation to indinavir plasma concentrations. AIDS 13:473, 1999.
83. Blake SP, McNicholas MM, Raptopoulous V. Nonopaque crystal deposition causing ureteric obstruction in patients with HIV undergoing indinavir therapy. AJR Am J Roentgenol 171:717, 1998.
84. Kohan AD, Armenakas NA, Fracchia JA. Indinavir nephrolithiasis: an emerging cause of renal colic in patients with human immunodeficiency virus. J Urol 161:1765, 1999.
85. Cattelan AM, Trevenzoli M, Naso A, et al. Severe hypertension and renal atrophy associated with indinavir. Clin Infect Dis 30:619, 2000.
86. Tashima KT, Horowitz JD, Rosen S. Indinavir nephropathy. N Engl J Med 336:138, 1997.
87. Anglicheau D, Duvic C, Nedelec G. Sudden anuria due to indinavir crystalluria. Nephron 86:364, 2000.
88. Hanabusa H, Tagani H, Hataya H. Renal atrophy associated with long-term treatment with indinavir. N Engl J Med 340:392, 1999.
89. Boubaker K, Sudre P, Bally F, et al. Changes in renal function associated with indinavir. AIDS 12:F249, 1998.
90. Daudon M, Estepa L, Viard JP, et al. Urinary stones in HIV-1-positive patients treated with indinavir. Lancet 349:1294, 1997.
91. Stein D, Drusano G, Steigbigel R, et al. Two year follow-up of patients treated with indinavir 800 mg q8h. In: Abstracts of the 4th Conference on Retroviruses and Opportunistic Infections, Washington, DC. Alexandria, VA, Foundation for Retrovirology and Human Health, 1997, abstract 195.
92. Sulkowski MS, Thomas DL, Chaisson RE, Moore RD. Hepatotoxicity associated with antiretroviral therapy in adults infected with human immunodeficiency virus and the role of hepatitis C or B virus infection. JAMA 283:74, 2000.
93. Food and Drug Administration. Public Health Advisory. Rockville, MD, Food and Drug Administration, June 1997.
94. Dever LL, Oruwari PA, Figueroa WE, et al. Hyperglycemia associated with protease inhibitors in an urban HIV-infected minority patient population. Ann Pharmacother 34:580, 2000.
95. Murata H, Hruz PW, Mueckler M. The mechanism of insulin resistance caused by HIV protease inhibitor therapy. J Biol Chem 275:20251, 2000.
96. Schutt M, Meier M, Meyer M, et al. The HIV-1 protease inhibitor indinavir impairs insulin signaling in HepG2 hepatoma cells. Diabetologia 43:1145, 2000.
97. Roberts AD, Muesing RA, Parenti DM, et al. Alterations in serum levels of lipids and lipoproteins with indinavir therapy for human immunodeficiency virus-infected patients. Clin Infect Dis 29:441, 1999.
98. Berthold HK, Parhofer KG, Ritter MM, et al. Influence of protease inhibitor therapy on lipoprotein metabolism. J Intern Med 246:567, 1999.
99. Lenhard JM, Weiel JE, Paulik MA, Furfine ES. Stimulation of vitamin A(1) acid signaling by the HIV protease inhibitor indinavir. Biochem Pharmacol 59:1063, 2000.
100. Miller KD, Jones E, Yanovski JA, et al. Visceral abdominal-fat accumulation associated with use of indinavir. Lancet 351:871, 1998.
101. Viraben R, Aquilina C. Indinavir-associated lipodystrophy. AIDS 12:F37, 1998.
102. Carr A, Samaras K, Burton S, et al. A syndrome of peripheral lipodystrophy, hyperlipidaemia and insulin resistance in patients receiving HIV protease inhibitors. AIDS 12:F51, 1998.
103. Mann M, Piazza-Hepp T, Koller E, et al. Unusual distributions of body fat in AIDS patients: a review of adverse events reported to the Food and Drug Administration. AIDS Patient Care STDs 13:287, 1999.
104. Benson JO, McGhee K, Coplan P, et al. Fat redistribution in indinavir-treated patients with HIV infection: a review of postmarketing cases. J AIDS 25:130, 2000.

105. Coplan PM, Nikas AA, Leavitt RY, etal. Indinavir did not increase the short-term risk of adverse cardiovascular events relative to nucleoside reverse transcriptase inhibitor therapy in four phase III clinical trials. AIDS 15:1584, 2001.
106. Henry K, Zackin R, Dube M, et al. ACTG 5056: metabolic status and cardiovascular disease risk for a cohort of HIV-1-infected persons durably suppressed on an indinavir-containing regimen (ACTG 372A). In: Abstracts of the 8th Conference on Retroviruses and Opportunistic Infections, Chicago. Alexandria, VA, Foundation for Retrovirology and Human Health, 2001, abstract 656.
107. Racoosin JA, Kessler CM. Bleeding episodes in HIV-positive patients taking protease inhibitors: a case series. Haemophilia 5:266, 1999.
108. Wilde JT. Protease inhibitor therapy and bleeding. Haemophilia 6:487, 2000.
109. Calista D, Boschini A. Cutaneous side effects induced by indinavir. Eur J Dermatol 10:292, 2000.
110. Gajewski LK, Grimone AJ, Melbourne KM, Vanscoy GJ. Characterization of rash with indinavir in a national patient cohort. Ann Pharmacother 33:17, 1999.
111. Teira R, Zubero Z, Munoz J, et al. Stevens-Johnson syndrome caused by indinavir. Scand J Infect Dis 30:634, 1998.
112. Bouscarat F, Bouchard C, Bouhour D. Paronychia and pyogenic granuloma of the great toes in patients treated with indinavir. N Engl J Med 338:1776, 1998.
113. Tosti A, Piraccini BM, D'Antuono A, et al. Paronychia associated with antiretroviral therapy. Br J Dermatol 140:1165, 1999.
114. Colson AE, Sax PE, Keller MJ, et al. Paronychia in association with indinavir treatment. Clin Infect Dis 32:140, 2001.
115. Sass JO, Jakob-Solder B, Heitger A, et al. Paronychia with pyogenic granuloma in a child treated with indinavir: the retinoid-mediated side effect theory revisited. Dermatology 200:40, 2000.
116. Rockstroh JK, Bergmann F, Wiesel W, et al. Efficacy and safety of twice daily first-line ritonavir/indinavir plus double nucleoside combination therapy in HIV-infected adults. AIDS 14:1181, 2000.
117. Boyd M, Duncombe C, Newell M, et al. Indinavir/ritonavir vs. indinavir in combination with AZT/3TC for treatment of HIV in nucleoside-experienced patients: a randomized, open-label trial. In: Abstracts of the 8th Conference on Retroviruses and Opportunistic Infections, Chicago. Alexandria, VA, Foundation for Retrovirology and Human Health, 2001, abstract 335.
118. Mellors J, Steigbigel R, Gulick R, et al. A randomized, double blind study of the oral HIV protease inhibitor, L-735,524 vs. zidovudine (ZDV) in p24 antigenemic, HIV-1 infected patients with <500 CD4 cells/mm^3. In: Abstracts of the 2nd National Conference on Human Retroviruses and Related Infections. Washington, DC, American Society for Microbiology, 1995, abstract 183.
119. Condra JH, Schleif WA, Blahy OM, et al. In vivo emergence of HIV-1 variants resistant to multiple protease inhibitors. Nature 374:569, 1995.
120. Gulick R, Mellors J, Havlir D, et al. Simultaneous vs. sequential initiation of therapy with indinavir, zidovudine, and lamivudine for HIV-1 infection: 100-week follow-up. JAMA 280:35, 1998.
121. Hirsch M, Steigbigel R, Staszewski S, et al. A randomized, controlled trial of indinavir, zidovudine, and lamivudine in adults with advanced human immunodeficiency virus type 1 infection and prior antiretroviral therapy. J Infect Dis 180:659, 1999.
122. Hirsch MS, Meibohm A, Rawlins S, et al. Indinavir (IDV) in combination with zidovudine (ZDV) and lamivudine (3TC) in ZDV experienced patients with CD4+ T-lymphocyte counts ≤ 50 cells/mm^3: 60-week follow-up. In: Abstracts of the 5th Conference on Retroviruses and Opportunistic Infections, Chicago. Alexandria, VA, Foundation for Retrovirology and Human Health, 1998, abstract 383.
123. AVANTI Study Group: AVANTI 2: randomized, double-blind trial to evaluate the efficacy and safety of zidovudine plus lamivudine versus zidovudine plus lamivudine plus indinavir in HIV-infected antiretroviral patients. AIDS 14:367, 2000.
124. Chun T-W, McMahon D, Justement JS, et al. Viral reservoirs after two years of sustained serum viral suppression in patients in whom HAART was initiated early: the Merck 060/ICC 004 cohort. In: Abstracts of the 8th Conference on Retroviruses and Opportunistic Infections, Chicago. Alexandria, VA, Foundation for Retrovirology and Human Health, 2001, abstract 396.
125. Carr A, Chuah J, Hudson J, et al. A randomised, open-label comparison of three highly active antiretroviral therapy regimens including two nucleoside analogues and indinavir for previously untreated HIV-1 infection: the OzCombo1 study. AIDS 14:1171, 2000.
126. Squires KE, Gulick R, Tebas P, et al. A comparison of stavudine plus lamivudine versus zidovudine plus lamivudine in combination with indinavir in antiretroviral naive individuals with HIV infection: selection of thymidine analog regimen therapy (START I). AIDS 14:1591, 2000.
127. Eron JJ, Murphy RL, Peterson D, et al. A comparison of stavudine, didanosine and indinavir with zidovudine, lamivudine and indinavir for the initial treatment of HIV-1 infected individuals: selection of thymidine analog regimen therapy (START II). AIDS 14:1601, 2000.
128. Kline MW, Fletcher CV, Harris AT, et al. A pilot study of combination therapy with indinavir, stavudine (d4T), and didanosine (ddI) in children infected with the human immunodeficiency virus. J Pediatr 132:543, 1998.
129. Wintergerst U, Hoffmann F, Solder B, et al. Comparison of two antiretroviral triple combinations including the protease inhibitor indinavir in children infected with human immunodeficiency virus. Pediatr Infect Dis J 17:495, 1998.
130. Mueller BU, Sleasman J, Nelson RP Jr, et al. A phase I/II study of the protease inhibitor indinavir in children with HIV infection. Pediatrics 102:101, 1998.
131. Van Rossum AM, Niesters HG, Geelen SP, et al. Clinical and virologic response to combination treatment with indinavir, zidovudine, and lamivudine in children with human immunodeficiency virus-1 infection: a multicenter study in The Netherlands. J Pediatr 136:780, 2000.
132. Vigano A, Dally L, Bricalli D, et al. Clinical and immuno-virologic characterization of the efficacy of stavudine, lamivudine, and indinavir in human immunodeficiency virus infection. J Pediatr 135:675, 1999.
133. Smith D, Berrey MM, Robertson M, et al. Virological and immunological effects of combination antiretroviral therapy with zidovudine, lamivudine, and indinavir during primary human immunodeficiency virus type 1 infection. J Infect Dis 182:950, 2000.
134. Hecht FM, Chesney MA, Busch MP, et al. Treatment of primary HIV with AZT, 3TC, and indinavir. In: Abstracts of the 5th Conference on Retroviruses and Opportunistic Infections, Chicago. Alexandria, VA, Foundation for Retrovirology and Human Health, 1998, abstract 582.
135. Soravia-Dunand VA, San Millan RD, Yerly S, et al. Viral suppression and CD4-cell recovery in patients with primary HIV-1 infection treated with HAART. In: Abstracts of the 6th Conference on Retroviruses and Opportunistic Infections, Chicago. Alexandria, VA, Foundation for Retrovirology and Human Health, 1999, abstract 637.
136. Lisziewicz J, Jessen H, Finzi D, et al. HIV-1 suppression by early treatment with hydroxyurea, didanosine and a protease inhibitor. Lancet 352:199, 1998.
137. Lori F, Jessen H, Lieberman J, et al. Treatment of human immunodeficiency virus infection with hydroxyurea, didanosine, and a protease inhibitor before seroconversion is associated with normalized immune parameters and limited viral reservoir. J Infect Dis 180:1827, 1999.
138. Harris M, Durakovic C, Rae S, et al. A pilot study of nevirapine, indinavir, and lamivudine among patients with advanced human immunodeficiency virus disease who have had failure of combination nucleoside therapy. J Infect Dis 177:1514, 1998.
139. Murphy RL, Sommadossi JP, Lamson M, et al. Antiviral effect and pharmacokinetic interaction between nevirapine and indinavir in persons infected with human immunodeficiency virus type 1. J Infect Dis 179:1116, 1999.
140. Gulick RM, Smeaton LM, D'Aquila RT, et al. Indinavir, nevirapine, stavudine, and lamivudine for human immunodeficiency virus-infected, amprenavir-experienced subjects: AIDS Clinical Trials Group Protocol 373. J Infect Dis 183:715, 2001.
141. Riddler S, Kahn J, Hicks C, et al. Durable clinical anti-HIV-1 activity (72 weeks) and tolerability for efavirenz (DMP 266) in combination with indinavir (IDV) [DMP 266-003, Cohort IV]. In: Abstracts of the XII World AIDS Conference, Geneva, 1998, abstract 12359.
142. Staszewski S, Morales-Ramirez J, Tashima K, et al. Efavirenz plus zidovudine and lamivudine, efavirenz plus indinavir, and indinavir plus zidovudine and lamivudine in the treatment of HIV infection in adults. N Engl J Med 341:1865, 1999.
143. Haas DW, Fessel WJ, Delapenha RA, et al. Therapy with efavirenz plus indinavir in patients with extensive prior nucleoside reverse-transcriptase inhibitor experience: a randomized, double-blind, placebo-controlled trial. J Infect Dis 183:392, 2001.

144. Suleiman J, Rhodes R, Campo R, et al. Preliminary results from indinavir (IDV) and ritonavir (RTV) in a once-daily regimen (Merck 103/104). In: Abstracts of the 8th Conference on Retroviruses and Opportunistic Infections, Chicago. Alexandria, VA, Foundation for Retrovirology and Human Health, 2001, abstract 336.
145. Casado JL, Perez-Elias MJ, Antela A, et al. Predictors of long-term response to protease inhibitor therapy in a cohort of HIV-infected patients. AIDS 12:F131, 1998.
146. Wit FWN, Van Leeuwen R, Weverling GJ, et al. Outcome and predictors of failure of highly active antiretroviral therapy: one-year follow-up of a cohort of human immunodeficiency virus type 1-infected persons. J Infect Dis 179:790, 1999.
147. Monforte AD, Lepri AC, Rezza G, et al. Insights into the reasons for discontinuation of the first highly active antiretroviral therapy (HAART) regimen in a cohort of antiretroviral naive patients. AIDS 14:499, 2000.
148. Levy R, Labriola D, Ruiz N. Low two-year risk of virologic failure with first regimen HAART. In: Abstracts of the 8th Conference on Retroviruses and Opportunistic Infections, Chicago. Alexandria, VA, Foundation for Retrovirology and Human Health, 2001, abstract 325.
149. Staszewski S, Keiser P, Montaner J, et al. Abacavir-lamivudine-zidovudine vs. indinavir-lamivudine-zidovudine in antiretroviral-naive HIV-infected adults. JAMA 285:1155, 2001.
150. Cahn P. Preliminary efficacy, adherence, and satisfaction with COM/ABC versus COM/IDV, an open-label randomized comparative study (CNAB3014). In: Abstracts of the XIII International Conference on AIDS, Durban, South Africa, 2000, abstract WeOrB606.
151. Squires K, Johnson V, Katlama C, et al. The Atlantic study: A randomized, open-label study to evaluate the efficacy and safety of three triple-combination therapies aimed at different HIV targets in anti-retroviral naive HIV-1 infected patients: final 48 weeks analysis. In: Abstracts of the XIII International Conference on AIDS, Durban, South Africa, 2000, abstract LbPeB7046.
152. Tisdale M, Myers RE, Maschera B, et al. Cross-resistance analysis to human immunodeficiency virus type 1 variants individually selected for resistance to five different protease inhibitors. Antimicrob Agents Chemother 39:1704, 1995.
153. Schock HB, Garsky VM, Kuo LC. Mutational anatomy of an HIV-1 protease variant conferring cross-resistance to protease inhibitors in clinical trials. J Biol Chem 271:31957, 1996.
154. Condra JH, Holder DJ, Schleif WA, et al. Genetic correlates of in vivo resistance to indinavir, a human immunodeficiency virus type 1 protease inhibitor. J Virol 70:8270, 1996.
155. Brown AJL, Korber BT, Condra JH. Associations between amino acids in the evolution of HIV type 1 protease sequences under indinavir therapy. AIDS Res Hum Retroviruses 15:247, 1999.
156. Zhang YM, Imamichi H, Imamichi T, et al. Drug resistance during indinavir therapy is caused by mutations in the protease gene and in its GAG substrate cleavage sites. J Virol 71:6662, 1997.
157. Emini EA, Condra JH, Schleif WA, et al. Maintenance of long-term virus suppression in patients treated with the HIV-1 protease inhibitor Crixivan (indinavir). In: Abstracts of the XIth International Conference on AIDS, Vancouver, 1996, abstract MoB170.
158. Condra JH, Holder DJ, Schleif WA, et al. Bi-directional inhibition of HIV-1 drug resistance selection by combination therapy with indinavir and reverse transcriptase inhibitors. In: Abstracts of the XIth International Conference on AIDS, Vancouver, 1996, abstract ThB932.
159. Descamps D, Flandre P, Calvez V, et al. Mechanisms of virologic failure in previously untreated HIV-infected patients from a trial of induction maintenance therapy. JAMA 283:205, 2000.
160. Havlir DV, Hellmann NS, Petropoulos CJ, et al. Drug susceptibility in HIV infection after viral rebound in patients receiving indinavir-containing regimens. JAMA 283:229, 2000.
161. Drusano GL, Bilello JA, Stein DS, et al. Factors influencing the emergence of resistance to indinavir: role of virologic, immunologic and pharmacologic variables. J Infect Dis 178:360, 1998.
162. Condra JH, Petropoulos CJ, Ziermann R, et al. Drug resistance and predicted virologic responses to human immunodeficiency virus type 1 protease inhibitor therapy. J Infect Dis 182:758, 2000.
163. Hsu A, Zolopa A, Shulman N, et al. Final analysis of ritonavir (RTV) intensification in indinavir (IDV) recipients with detectable HIV RNA levels. In: Abstracts of the 8th Conference on Retroviruses and Opportunistic Infections, Chicago. Alexandria, VA, Foundation for Retrovirology and Human Health, 2001, abstract 337.
164. Kempf D, Hsu A, Jiang P, et al. Response to ritonavir (RTV) intensification in indinavir (IDV) recipients is highly correlated with virtual inhibitory quotient. In: Abstracts of the 8th Conference on Retroviruses and Opportunistic Infections, Chicago. Alexandria, VA, Foundation for Retrovirology and Human Health, 2001, abstract 523.
165. Hertogs K, Bloor S, Kemp SD, et al. Phenotypic and genotypic analysis of clinical HIV-1 isolates reveals extensive protease inhibitor cross resistance: a survey of over 6000 samples. AIDS 14:1203, 2000.
166. Partaledis JA, Yamaguchi K, Tisdale M, et al. In vitro selection and characterization of human immunodeficiency virus type 1 (HIV-1) isolates with reduced sensitivity to hydroxyethylamino sulfonamide inhibitors of HIV-1 aspartyl protease. J Virol 69:5228, 1995.
167. Para MF, Glidden DV, Coombs RW, et al. Baseline human immunodeficiency virus type 1 phenotype, genotype, and RNA response after switching from long-term hard-capsule saquinavir to indinavir or soft-gel-capsule saquinavir in AIDS Clinical Trials Group Protocol 333. J Infect Dis 182:733, 2000.
168. Gulick RM, Hu XJ, Fiscus SA, et al. Randomized study of saquinavir with ritonavir or nelfinavir together with delavirdine, adefovir, or both in human immunodeficiency virus-infected adults with virologic failure on indinavir: AIDS Clinical Trials Group Study 359. J Infect Dis 182:1375, 2000.
169. Hammer S, Squires K, DeGruttola V, et al. Randomized trial of abacavir (ABC) & nelfinavir (NFV) in combination with efavirenz (EFV) & adefovir dipivoxil (ADV) as salvage therapy in patients with virologic failure receiving indinavir (IDV). In: Abstracts of the 6th Conference on Retroviruses and Opportunistic Infections, Chicago. Alexandria, VA, Foundation for Retrovirology and Human Health, 1999, abstract 490.
170. Piscitelli SC, Flexner C, Minor JR, et al. Drug interactions in patients infected with human immunodeficiency virus. Clin Infect Dis 23:685, 1996.
171. Eagling VA, Back DJ, Barry MG. Differential inhibition of cytochrome P450 isoforms by the protease inhibitors, ritonavir, saquinavir, and indinavir. Br J Clin Pharmacol 44:190, 1997.
172. Rosenthal E, Sala F, Chichmanian R-M, Batt M, Cassuto J-P. Ergotism related to concurrent administration of ergotamine tartrate and indinavir. JAMA 281:987, 1999.
173. McCrea J, Wyss D, Stone J, et al. Pharmacokinetic interaction between indinavir and rifampin. Clin Pharmacol Ther 61:152, 1997.
174. Piscitelli SC, Burstein AH, Chaitt D, et al. Indinavir concentrations and St. John's wort. Lancet 355:547, 2000.
175. Moore LB, Goodwin B, Jones SA, et al. St. John's wort induces hepatic drug metabolism through activation of the pregnane X receptor. Proc Natl Acad Sci USA 97:7500, 2000.
176. Indinavir (MK 639) Pharmacokinetic Study Group: Indinavir (MK 639) drug interaction studies. In: Abstracts of the XIth International Conference on AIDS, Vancouver, 1996, abstract MoB174.
177. Sturgill MG, Seibold JR, Boruchoff SE, et al. Trimethoprim/sulfamethoxazole does not affect the steady-state disposition of indinavir. J Clin Pharmacol 39:1077, 1999.
178. De Wit S, Debier M, De Smet M, et al. Effect of fluconazole on indinavir pharmacokinetics in human immunodeficiency virus-infected patients. Antimicrob Agents Chemother 42:223, 1998.
179. McCrea J, Woolf E, Sterrett A, et al. Effects of ketoconazole and other P-450 inhibitors on the pharmacokinetics of indinavir. Pharm Res 13:S485, 1996.
180. Boruchoff SE, Stugill MG, Grasing KW, et al. The steady-state disposition of indinavir is not altered by the concomitant administration of clarithromycin. Clin Pharmacol Ther 67:351, 2000.
181. Foulds G, Laboy-Goral L, Wei GC, Apseloff G. The effect of azithromycin on the pharmacokinetics of indinavir. J Clin Pharmacol 39:842, 1999.
182. Emmanuel A, Gillotin C, Farinotti R, Sadler BM. Atovaquone suspension and indinavir have minimal pharmacokinetic interactions. In: Abstracts of the 12th World AIDS Conference, Geneva, 1998, abstract 12384.
183. Winchell GA, McCrea JB, Carides A, et al. Pharmacokinetic interaction between indinavir and rifabutin. Clin Pharmacol Ther 61:153, 1997.
184. Shelton MJ, Mei H, Hewitt RG, Defrancesco R. If taken 1 hour before indinavir (IDV), didanosine does not affect IDV exposure, despite persistent buffering effects. Antimicrob Agents Chemother 45:298, 2001.

185. Videx EC (didanosine): prescribing information. Princeton, NJ, Bristol-Myers Squibb, December 2000.
186. Ferry JJ, Herman BD, Carel BJ, et al. Pharmacokinetic drug–drug interaction study of delavirdine and indinavir in healthy volunteers. J AIDS 18:252, 1998.
187. Fiske WD, Mayers D, Wagner K, et al. Pharmacokinetics of DMP 266 and indinavir multiple oral doses in HIV-1 infected individuals. In: Abstracts of the 4th Conference on Retroviruses and Opportunistic Infections, Washington, DC. Alexandria, VA, Foundation for Retrovirology and Human Health, 1997, abstract 568.
188. Squires K, Hammer S, DeGruttola V, et al. Randomized trial of abacavir (ABC) in combination with indinavir (IDV) and efavirenz (EFV) in HIV-infected patients (pts) with nucleoside analog experience (NRTI exp). In: Abstracts of the 6th Conference on Retroviruses and Opportunistic Infections, Chicago. Alexandria, VA, Foundation for Retrovirology and Human Health, 1999, abstract LB15.
189. McCrea J, Buss N, Stone J. Indinavir-saquinavir single dose pharmacokinetic study. In: Abstracts of the 4th Conference on Retroviruses and Opportunistic Infections, Washington, DC. Alexandria, VA, Foundation for Retrovirology and Human Health, 1997, abstract 608.
190. Kerr B, Lee C, Yuen G, et al. Overview of in-vitro and in-vivo drug interaction studies of nelfinavir mesylate (NFV), a new HIV-1 protease inhibitor. In: Abstracts of the 4th Conference on Retroviruses and Opportunistic Infections, Washington, DC. Alexandria, VA, Foundation for Retrovirology and Human Health, 1997, abstract 373.
191. Squires K, Riddler S, Havlir D, et al. Coadministration of indinavir (IDV) 1200 mg with nelfinavir (NFV) 1250 mg in a twice daily regimen: preliminary safety, PK activity. In: Abstracts of the 6th Conference on Retroviruses and Opportunistic Infections, Chicago. Alexandria, VA, Foundation for Retrovirology and Human Health, 1999, abstract 364.
192. Sadler BM, Eron J, Wakeford J, et al. Pharmacokinetics of 141W94 and indinavir (IDV) after single-dose coadministration in HIV-positive volunteers. In: Abstracts of the 37th International Conference on Antimicrobial Agents and Chemotherapy, Toronto. Washington, DC, American Society for Microbiology, 1997, abstract A-56.
193. Hugen PW, Burger DM, Brinkman K, et al. Carbamazepine–indinavir interaction causes antiretroviral therapy failure. Ann Pharmacother 34:465, 2000.
194. Merry C, Barry MG, Ryan M, et al. Interaction of sildenafil and indinavir when co-administered to HIV-positive patients. AIDS 13:F101, 1999.
195. Iribarne C, Berthou F, Carlhant D, et al. Inhibition of methadone and buprenorphine N-alkylations by three HIV-1 protease inhibitors. Drug Metab Dispos 26:257, 1998.
196. Mistry GC, Laurent A, Sterrett AT, Deutsch PJ. Effect of indinavir on the single-dose pharmacokinetics of theophylline in healthy subjects. J Clin Pharmacol 39:636, 1999.
197. Piscitelli SC, Vogel S, Figg WD, et al. Alteration in indinavir clearance during interleukin-2 infusions in patients infected with the human immunodeficiency virus. Pharmacotherapy 18:1212, 1998.
198. Burger DM, Hugen PWH, Kroon FP, et al. Pharmokinetic interaction between the proton pump inhibitor omeprazole and the HIV protease inhibitor indinavir. AIDS 12:2080, 1998.
199. Hugen PW, Burger DM, ter Horstede HJ, et al. Development of an indinavir oral liquid for children. Am J Health Syst Pharm 57:1332, 2000.
200. Perinatal HIV Guidelines Working Group Members. Public Health Service Task Force recommendations for the use of antiretroviral drugs in pregnant HIV-1-infected women for maternal health and interventions to reduce perinatal HIV-1 transmission in the United States. www.hivatis.org (May 4, 2001).
201. Perinatal HIV Guidelines Working Group Members. Safety and toxicity of individual aniretroviral agents in pregnancy. www.hivatis.org (February 5, 2001).
202. Riecke K, Schulz TG, Shakibaei M, et al. Developmental toxicity of the HIV-protease inhibitor indinavir in rats. Teratology 62:291, 2000.
203. Wara D, Tuomala R, Bryson Y, et al. PACTG 358—safety, pharmacokinetics and antiretroviral activity of indinavir, zidovudine (ZDV), and lamivudine (3TC) in HIV-1 seropositive pregnant women and infants. In: Abstracts of the 2nd Conference on Global Strategies for the Prevention of HIV Transmission from Mothers to Infants, Montreal, 1999, abstract 447.
204. Hayashi S, Beckerman K, Homma M, et al. Pharmacokinetics of indinavir in HIV-positive pregnant women. AIDS 14:1061, 2000.
205. Morris AB, Cu-Uvin S, Harwell JI, et al. Multicenter review of protease inhibitors in 89 pregnancies. J AIDS 25:306, 2000.
206. Centers for Disease Control and Prevention. Updated U.S. Public Health Service guidelines for the management of occupational exposures to HBV, HCV and HIV and recommendations for postexposure prophylaxis. MMWR Morb Mortal Wkly Rep 50(No. RR-7):11, 2001.
207. Centers for Disease Control and Prevention. Management of possible sexual, injecting-drug use, or other nonoccupational exposure to HIV, including considerations related to antiretroviral therapy. MMWR Morb Mortal Wkly Rep 47(No. RR-17):1, 1998.
208. Wang SA, Panlilio AL, Doi PA, et al. Experience of healthcare workers taking postexposure prophylaxis after occupational HIV exposures: findings of the HIV Postexposure Prophylaxis Registry. Infec Control Hosp Epidemiol 21:780, 2000.
209. Parkin JM, Murphy M, Anderson J, et al. Tolerability and side-effects of post-exposure prophylaxis for HIV infection. Lancet 355:722, 2000.

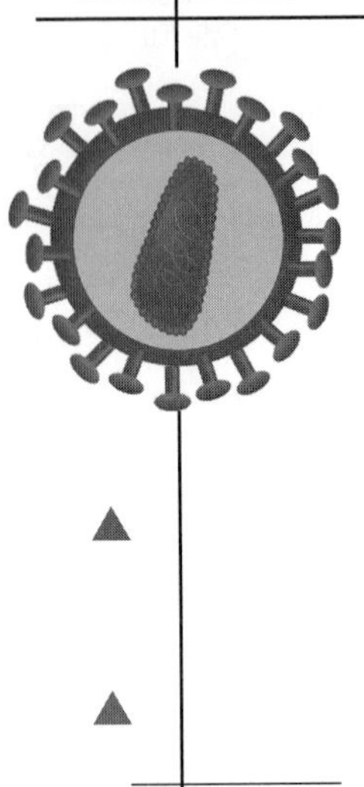

CHAPTER 15

Nelfinavir

Richard H. Haubrich, MD
Diane V. Havlir, MD

Nelfinavir (Viracept) was the fourth protease inhibitor approved by the U.S. Food and Drug Administration (FDA) for the treatment of human immunodeficiency virus (HIV)-infected individuals and the first protease inhibitor to receive concomitant approval in both children and adults. Similar to the other drugs in its class, nelfinavir diminishes HIV replication by inhibiting the HIV-1 protease enzyme required for viral particle maturation. Nelfinavir monotherapy lowers levels of HIV RNA in the plasma by 2 to 3 $\log_{10}$ copies per milliliter in protease-naive patients. Like the other available protease inhibitors, nelfinavir is extensively metabolized by cytochrome P_{450} (CYP) and is an inhibitor of the major hepatic P_{450} CYP3A4 isoform, necessitating careful attention to concomitant medication administration. Gastrointestinal side effects can accompany nelfinavir administration, but overall the drug is well tolerated.

STRUCTURE

The development of nelfinavir is an example of "rational" drug design, wherein computer technology is applied to design compounds based on the crystallographic structure of a target enzyme, circumventing traditional drug development, which relies on mass screening of thousands of potential compounds.[1,2] Nelfinavir is the mesylate salt of a basic amine that was designed to maximize binding and stability of the ligand to the active site of HIV protease. Its molecular weight is 663.90 (567.79 as the free base); and it is slightly soluble in water at pH 2 or lower and freely soluble in methanol, ethanol, isopropanol, and propylene glycol. It is a nonpeptidic protease inhibitor (K_i 2 nM) that is active against HIV-1 and HIV-2. Computer models using evolutionary programming to predict docking of flexible ligands reproduced the structure of nelfinavir in 34 of 100 simulations.[3,4]

IN VITRO ACTIVITY AND MECHANISM OF ACTION

Nelfinavir blocks HIV replication by competitively inhibiting the cleavage of HIV p55 Gag and pl60 GagPol precursor polyproteins to structural proteins and enzymes by the protease enzyme. The target of nelfinavir and other protease inhibitors is the final enzymatic step required to produce mature viral progeny. HIV precursor polyproteins, transcribed and translated from cells with integrated proviral DNA, must be cleaved at eight distinct sites to produce functional, mature virions. The cleavage steps occur at the point in the viral life cycle when virions are released from the infected cell into the plasma or surrounding tissue. Polyproteins are inserted into the cleft of the HIV protease dimer and cleaved into functional proteins. Nelfinavir competitively inhibits this reaction by binding to the substrate-binding region of HIV protease. Virions produced in the presence of nelfinavir and other protease inhibitors are defective particles, which (as seen by electron microscopy) lack the electron-dense core characteristic of mature, infectious HIV. They are unable to infect new cells and are cleared from the circulation by an unknown mechanism.[5]

In vitro, nelfinavir inhibits HIV replication during acute and chronic infection of lymphocyte cell lines and in monocyte cell culture. In acute HIV infection in cell culture, the mean inhibitory concentration is 21 nM (range 9 to 60 nM).[6,7] HIV-1 strains tested in models of acute infection include HIV-1 IIIB, HIV-1 RF, and the clinical isolate HIV-1 RoJo. During infection of a macrophage cell line with HIV-1 strain Ba-L, the inhibitory concentration is similarly low at 23 nM. The therapeutic index was 916 and 526 in experiments using HIV-1 RF in CEM-SS cells and HIV-IIIB in MT-2 cells, respectively. The high therapeutic index of nelfinavir reflects the potent antiviral activity and relatively low cytotoxity present in cell culture systems.[8]

Similar to other protease inhibitors, but distinct from reverse transcriptase inhibitors, nelfinavir is active in vitro in chronically infected cells. Once proviral DNA is formed, reverse transcriptase inhibitors have no effect on production of virus from latently infected cells. Nelfinavir and other protease inhibitors block maturation of viral particles from both acutely and chronically infected cells. When CEM-SS cells chronically infected with HIV-1 IIIB are exposed to nelfinavir, the inhibitory concentration is 40 nM. On radioimmune precipitation analysis of purified virions obtained from these cells, there is dose-related reduced processing of p55 Gag polyprotein to p24 capsid protein. These experiments corroborate that nelfinavir blocks viral production at the final step of viral maturation through inhibition of HIV protease.

The antiviral activity of nelfinavir has also been evaluated against HIV-1 strains resistant to zidovudine and nonnucleoside reverse transcriptase inhibitors (NNRTIs), including pyridinones, nevirapine, and TIBO compounds. In MT-2 cells, the inhibitory concentration is 60 nM for the zidovudine-resistant strain G910-6 HIV-1 and 30 nM for the NNRTI-resistant strain HIV-1 IIIB A17.

In studies conducted to evaluate in vitro activity of nelfinavir against HIV isolates resistant to other protease inhibitors, nelfinavir was active against recombinant HIV-1 strains with amino acid substitution at positions 32 and 82, known to reduce susceptibility to other protease inhibitors. Fourfold to fivefold reductions in nelfinavir sensitivity occurred in the presence of other dual protease inhibitor mutations in the substrate-binding region. High-level resistance to nelfinavir emerged in the presence of isolates with multiple protease inhibitor mutations passed in the presence of other protease inhibitors.[7]

Combination in vitro studies of nelfinavir and reverse transcriptase inhibitors demonstrate synergy for most combinations. Using HIV-1 RF in acute infection of CEM-SS cells and analyzing antiviral activity with a three-dimensional approach, nelfinavir is synergistic with zidovudine (AZT), lamivudine (3TC), and zalcitabine.[9] Nelfinavir is also synergistic with the two-drug combination AZT/3TC. Assays combining nelfinavir/didanosine/stavudine (d4T) demonstrate an additive effect.

▲ PHARMACOKINETICS

Nelfinavir is well absorbed; and the estimated oral bioavailability is 78%. Concomitant administration of food enhances both the maximum plasma concentration (C_{max}) and area under the curve (AUC) plasma concentrations two- to threefold.[10] Fat content of meals does not influence absorption. Nelfinavir is highly bound to serum proteins (> 98%); equilibrium dialysis experiments demonstrate that nelfinavir is highly bound (98%) to human α_1-acid glycoprotein (AAG). In vitro, the inhibitory concentrations in acute HIV infection assays are not affected over the physiologic range of AAG (0.5 to 2.0 mg/ml), except at the highest concentration (2.0 mg/ml).

Peak plasma concentrations of nelfinavir are achieved 2 to 4 hours after dosing. After multiple dosing of 750 mg three times daily, the plasma C_{max} is 3 to 4 μg/ml, with trough levels at 1 to 4 μg/ml. Using the more common schedule of 1250 mg bid, steady-state trough concentrations were 0.7 μg/ml compared to 1.0 μg/ml with 750 mg tid (n = 21).[11] Another study found median trough levels of 1.5 μg/ml, with a wide range (0.3 to 5.9 μg/ml).[12] Peak levels exceed the in vitro inhibitory concentration by more than 100-fold. However, because of the large degree of protein binding, the free drug concentration exceeds the inhibitory concentrations by only several-fold. The average concentration at steady state is 2.3 μg/ml. The concentration of nelfinavir achieved has been shown to be an important predictor of response. In one study the 2-hour postdose nelfinavir concentration was an independent predictor of attaining HIV RNA of less than 400 copies per milliliter after 48 weeks (odds ratio of response 8.1 for those with higher concentrations; $P = 0.005$).[13] The large volume of distribution (2 to 7 L/kg) of nelfinavir suggests that nelfinavir penetrates tissues. Like most protease inhibitors, nelfinavir does not penetrate cerebrospinal fluid (CSF). CSF concentrations were not detectable (< 0.025 μg/ml) in 25 samples from six patients despite average plasma concentrations of 2.4 μg/ml.[14]

Nelfinavir is predominantly metabolized through the hepatic microsome P_{450} isoforms. One major and several minor oxidative metabolites can be found in the plasma after nelfinavir administration. The major oxidative metabolite (M8) has activity comparable to that of the parent compound. Nelfinavir is also an inhibitor of CYP3A4, similar to saquinavir, but is a less potent inhibitor than either indinavir or ritonavir.[15] In vitro, measurements of the drug effect on CYP3A4-mediated testosterone 6-β-hydroxylase indicate K_i values for nelfinavir and saquinavir of 4.8 and 4.0 μM, respectively, compared to 0.7 μM for indinavir and 0.1 μM for ritonavir.[15] In vitro assays for inhibition of other P_{450} isoforms by nelfinavir (CYP2C9, CYP2E1, CYP2C19, CYP2D6, CYP1A2) suggests that in vivo effects are minimal.

The terminal half-life of nelfinavir in the plasma is 3.5 to 5.0 hours. Nelfinavir is excreted unchanged (22%) and as oxidative metabolites (65%) in the stool. Only 1% to 2% of nelfinavir is excreted in the urine. The pharmacokinetics of nelfinavir have not been studied in patients with altered renal function, but clearance for only a small fraction of the drug through the urinary system suggests that effects should be minimal. Nelfinavir kinetics are no different for African American and Caucasian patients.[12] A single 750 mg dose given to HIV-negative patients with liver impairment (Child-Turcotte A–C) demonstrated 49% to 75% increase in AUC due to reduced clearance.[16] The M8 metabolite was reduced. The half-life was longer and maximum concentrations were lower in those with class C liver disease. Multiple-dose studies in patients with hepatitis are in progress.

In children (ages 2 to 13), the clearance is two to three times greater than is observed in adults. A dose of 20 to 30 mg/kg three times daily in children ages 2 to 7 years produces plasma levels similar to those present in adults receiving a 750 mg thrice-daily regimen.[17] Nelfinavir concentrations in infants are variable[18] and are lower than have been seen in older children.

▲ TOXICITY

The most common nelfinavir-associated adverse event described in the early Phase I/II trials was diarrhea or loose stools. This toxicity rarely resulted in treatment discontinuation and often resolved with or without over-the-counter antimotility agents. Data from 696 patients in three randomized, placebo-controlled studies (Nos. 505, 506, and 511; see "Efficacy" for details) support the finding that diarrhea was the most significant toxicity associated with nelfinavir.[19] In these three pivotal Phase II/III studies, patients received nelfinavir alone, 500 or 750 mg tid (Study 505), with d4T (Study 506), or with AZT and 3TC (Study 511). Overall, 77 of 696 of the study participants (11%) stopped nelfinavir by week 16, with 28 (4%) stopping it because of an adverse event. Eleven patients (1.6%) terminated study therapy because of diarrhea. There were no differences in the rate of treatment discontinuation for any reason across the study arms.

Study 505, in which two doses of nelfinavir were compared to placebo, represents the best opportunity to evaluate toxicity, although the placebo phase was only 1 month in duration. Table 15–1 shows the most common moderate to severe adverse events after 1 month (Study 505) and 6 months (Study 511) of follow-up. These events were classified by study investigators as at least possibly related or of unknown relations to nelfinavir. Adverse events caused by concurrent conditions were excluded.

In Study 505, diarrhea was the most common toxicity, occurring only marginally more frequently at the 750 mg dose (21%) than in the placebo group (16%). Twenty percent of patients treated with 750 mg tid of nelfinavir had diarrhea in Study 511, compared to 3% of AZT/3TC-treated patients. The two nelfinavir doses did not differ in terms of the rate of diarrhea (14% vs. 20%; $P = 0.2$). The rate of diarrhea in the d4T/nelfinavir study was modestly higher (about 25%).

Diarrhea due to nelfinavir begins during the first week of therapy and in some patients subsides with continued dosing. Other patients have persistent symptoms that require symptomatic treatment. Most clinicians initiate loperamide for symptomatic treatment and use diphenoxylate-atropine if improvement is not seen. Absorbents (psyllium) have been used. In small trials, pancrelipase (Ultrase MT20, two tablets with each dose of nelfinavir) or calcium tablets have been beneficial.[20]

The overall rate of toxicity with nelfinavir compared favorably to that seen with other protease inhibitor regimens. In one large cohort study, 36.0% of ritonavir patients, 14.0% of indinavir patients, and 8.5% of nelfinavir patients stopped the drug during the first 12 months owing to side effects.[21]

Diabetes, glucose intolerance, elevated triglyceride and cholesterol levels, and lipodystrophy have been reported in patients receiving nelfinavir and other protease inhibitors. The frequency and mechanism to account for these events are poorly characterized at present.[22] An in vitro study of an adipocyte cell line suggested that exposure of the cells to nelfinavir impairs insulin sensitivity and activates lipolysis.[23]

▲ **Table 15–1.** PATIENTS WITH ADVERSE EVENTS OF MODERATE OR SEVERE INTENSITY[a] OR SEVERE LABORATORY TOXICITY REPORTED IN ≥2% OF PATIENTS

	Study 505[b] (%)			Study 511[b] (%)		
Adverse Event	Placebo (n = 32)	Nelfinavir 500 mg tid (n = 32)	Nelfinavir 750 mg tid (n = 29)	Placebo + ZDV/3TC (n = 101)	Nelfinavir 500 mg tid + ZDV/3TC (n = 96)	Nelfinavir 750 mg tid + ZDV/3TC (n = 99)
Clinical						
Asthenia	6	3	3	2	1	1
Headache	0	0	0	2	1	1
Diarrhea	16	13	21	3	14	20
Vomiting	3	3	3	2	1	1
Nausea	3	0	3	4	3	7
Flatulence	0	0	0	0	5	2
Anxiety	0	0	0	0	2	1
Depression	0	0	7	0	0	1
Rash	0	3	0	1	1	3
Laboratory						
Hemoglobin	0	0	0	6	3	2
Neutrophils	0	3	0	4	3	5
ALT (SGPT)	0	0	0	6	1	1
AST (SGOT)	0	0	0	4	1	0
Creatine kinase	0	0	0	7	2	2

ALT, alanine transaminase; AST, aspartate transaminase.

[a]Includes adverse events at least possibly related to the study drug or of unknown relation and excludes concurrent HIV conditions.

[b]Adverse events within 1 month follow-up (Study 505) and 6 months follow-up (Study 511).

The concentration of nelfinavir used in this study was 5- to 20-fold higher than plasma levels.

▲ EFFICACY

Phase I/II Studies

Two small open-label studies of escalating doses of nelfinavir monotherapy were the first to demonstrate the antiviral activity of the drug. At low doses (900 and 1200 mg/day) used in Study 504,[24] 5 of 20 therapy-naive patients had a reduction in HIV RNA levels of 1 $\log_{10}$ copies per milliliter that persisted past 28 days. Thirty patients with CD4+ T-lymphocyte counts of more than 200 cells per cubic millimeter received higher doses (1500, 2250, and 3000 total mg/day divided tid) in Study 503.[25] These patients had median HIV RNA $\log_{10}$ decreases of 1.4, 1.0, and 1.7 copies per milliliter, respectively, after 28 days at the three increasing dose levels. Using the branched-chain DNA HIV RNA quantitative assay with a lower limit of detection of 500 copies per milliliter (Table 15–2), the proportion of patients with undetectable HIV RNA plasma levels at 28 days was 20% for the 1500 mg/day group versus 50% to 60% for the higher dose groups. CD4+ lymphocyte increases ranged from 37 to 100 cells per cubic millimeter. Follow-up of 15 patients for 4 months showed the greatest HIV RNA reduction (1.5 $\log_{10}$ copies per milliliter) in the highest dose group.

Two other small trials examined nelfinavir plus two nucleoside analogues (AZT/3TC or didanosine/d4T) and demonstrated a more than 2 $\log_{10}$ copies per milliliter reduction in HIV RNA levels.[30-32] In one study[30] 10 of 12 patients receiving nelfinavir/AZT/3TC had undetectable viral levels (< 500 HIV RNA copies per milliliter) after 1 year of follow-up. HIV-RNA levels and HIV tissue cultures from semen (n = 4) and gastrointestinal-associated lymphoid tissue (GALT) (n = 9) were evaluated after 1 year of treatment in a subset of these patients. All semen and seven of nine GALT specimens were culture-negative and HIV RNA-negative. Thus a combination regimen of nelfinavir/AZT/3TC reduced HIV replication not only in plasma but also in the lymph tissue and semen.

Phase II/III Studies

Two randomized, double-blind, placebo-controlled studies clarified the magnitude and short-term durability of the antiretroviral activity of nelfinavir used alone or in combination with nucleoside analogues.[26,27] These studies shared several common features: The study patients were naive to protease inhibitors and had HIV RNA levels higher than 15,000 copies per milliliter. Moreover, the trials were randomized, double-blind, and placebo-controlled. Treatment failure—defined by two sequential CD4+ lymphocyte counts or HIV RNA levels that returned to baseline—prompted a blinded switch from placebo to nelfinavir (in patients in a control group) or an open-label change in nucleoside antiretroviral agents (in patients receiving nelfinavir).

Study 505 randomized patients to placebo or nelfinavir (500 mg versus 750 mg tid). Placebo patients crossed over to one of the two doses of nelfinavir after 4 weeks. The 91 patients had a mean HIV RNA level of 4.9 $\log_{10}$ copies per milliliter and a mean CD4+ lymphocyte counts of 275 cells per cubic millimeter at baseline. In the 81% of patients with prior nucleoside therapy, the mean duration of prior treatment was 27 months. At 4 weeks the mean viral load was reduced by 0.1, 0.9, and 1.3 $\log_{10}$ copies per millimeter, and the CD4+ lymphocytes increased 10, 84, and 100 cells per cubic millimeter in the placebo, low-dose nelfinavir, and high-dose nelfinavir groups, respectively. The difference between placebo and nelfinavir was significant ($P < 0.01$). After 16 weeks the mean $\log_{10}$ reduction in HIV RNA was 0.6 copies per milliliter for the 750 mg dose group, which was significantly greater than the reduction for the 500 mg group.

In Study 511 a series of 297 therapy-naive patients with a mean baseline HIV RNA level of 5.2 to 5.3 $\log_{10}$ copies per milliliter and CD4+ lymphocyte count of 276 to 307 cells per cubic millimeter were randomized to nelfinavir (500 or 750 mg tid)/AZT/3TC versus AZT/3TC alone.[27] At week 24 the AZT/3TC patients added nelfinavir. Baseline characteristics were balanced across treatment arms. Larger $\log_{10}$ HIV RNA reductions (using a 50 copy limit assay) were seen in the nelfinavir groups at week 24, with reductions of 3.0 and 2.7 $\log_{10}$ copies per milliliter for the 750- and 500-mg groups, respectively, than for the AZT/3TC group, which decreased 1.4 $\log_{10}$ copies per milliliter. The mean change in HIV RNA (using an area-based measure) was significantly lower in both nelfinavir groups compared to the AZT/3TC group in the intent-to-treat analysis ($P < 0.001$).

The proportions of patients at 24 weeks with HIV RNA of less than 400 copies per milliliter were 81% and 62% for the high-dose and low-dose nelfinavir groups, compared to 8% in the AZT/3TC group (as treated analysis) (Fig. 15–1). The proportion of patients with HIV RNA levels of less than 400 copies per milliliter using the missing equals failure (ITT) analysis were 67% (750 mg), 50% (500 mg), and 7% (placebo). Clearly, both three-drug nelfinavir-containing combinations were superior to dual nucleoside treatment. Follow-up for 12 months confirmed durable suppression; 61% of patients in the 750 mg group had HIV RNA levels of less than 50 copies per milliliter (45% by ITT).[27] The proportion of patients in whom HIV RNA remained undetectable at 12 months was significantly higher in the 750 mg group than in the 500 mg group.

By week 24, patients in the 750- and 500-mg nelfinavir groups had gained a mean of 150 and 138 CD4+ lymphocytes per cubic millimeter, respectively, compared to a 95-cell increase for patients receiving AZT/3TC (P = 0.02 for both nelfinavir doses versus AZT/3TC).

More recently, twice-daily dosing (1250 mg bid) of nelfinavir was compared to 750 mg tid in a study powered to determine equivalency of those regimens.[28] All patients received nelfinavir in combination with d4T and 3TC. An interim analysis of the 283 patients with a mean baseline CD4+ lymphocyte count of 254 to 273 cells per cubic millimeter and an HIV RNA level of 5.0 to 5.1 $\log_{10}$ copies per milliliter demonstrated that both regimens provided equally potent HIV RNA suppression. At 48 weeks approximately

Table 15–2. PHASE II/III CLINICAL STUDIES OF NELFINAVIR

Study	Nelfinavir Dose (mg/d)	Other ARV	Study Duration (mo)	No.	% ARV-Naive	Log_{10} HIV RNA (copies/ml)		CD4+ T Lymphocytes (cells/mm^3)		Percent with HIV RNA < 500 (< 50) Copies/ml[b]
						Baseline	↓ At Last Follow-up	Baseline	↑ At Last Follow-up	
Open-Label Pilot Trials										
504[24]	900–1200	No	1	20	100	4.6	5/20 with 1 log_{10} ↓	351–421	86–216	N/A
503[25]	1500	No	1	10	N/A	4.8	1.4	363	37–100	20
	2250	No	1	10	N/A	5.0	1.9	381	37–100	50–60
	3000	No	1	10	N/A	4.8	1.7	331	37–100	50–60
Randomized Phase III Studies										
505[26]	Placebo	No	1	[a]	19t	N/A	0.1	N/A	10	N/A
	1500 (tid)	No	1	48	19	4.8	0.9	284	84	N/A
	2250 (tid)	No	1	43	19	4.9	1.3	280	100	N/A
511[27]	Placebo	AZT/3TC	12	101	13	5.2	1.4 (wk 24)	276	125–127	7(4) (wk 24) A
	1500 (tid)	AZT/3TC	12	97	13	5.3	2.4	307	192	54 (37) A
	2250 (tid)	AZT/3TC	12	99	13	5.2	2.9	283	198	75 (61) A
542[28]	2250 (tid)	d4T/3TC	12	75	88	5.1	2.1	254	~170	~80 (68) A
	2500 (bid)	d4T/3TC	12	208	90	5.0	2.0	273	~170	~80 (68) A
M98-863[29]	2250 (tid)	d4T/3TC	14	327	100	NR	NR	N/A	224	61 (52) I
	Placebo	LPVr/d4T/3TC	14	326	100	NR	NR	N/A	227	74 (64) I

[a]These patients switched to one of two doses of nelfinavir after 1 month.

[b]Number in parenthesis is % with < 50 copies/ml.

A, as treated; ARV, antiretroviral; ↓, decrease; ↑, increase; I, intent to treat; N/A, not available; NR, not reported; t, percent naive of total cohort.

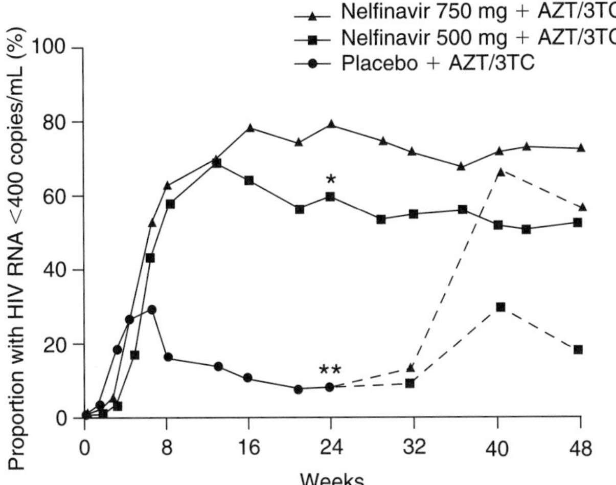

Figure 15–1. Proportion of all patients with HIV RNA < 400 copies per milliliter by standard polymerase chain reaction (PCR) assay (as treated analysis, limit of detection, 400 copies per milliliter). Placebo recipients entering the 24 week extension period were randomized at week 24 to either of the nelfinavir dosages instead of placebo (dashed lines). *P = 0.006 and **P = 0.001, each versus nelfinavir 750 mg at this time point. (Adapted from Saag MS, Tebas P, Sension M, et al. Randomized, double-blind comparison of two nelfinavir doses plus nucleosides in HIV-infected patients [Agouron Study 511]. AIDS 15:1971, 2001, with permission.)

80% of patients in both groups had plasma HIV RNA levels of less than 400 copies per milliliter, and about 68% had less than 50 copies per milliliter. No differences in toxicity were noted. The time to undetectable HIV RNA was similar in the groups. Follow-up to 96 weeks was planned, but the FDA approved the 1250 mg bid schedule during late 1999.

A large double-blind study of nelfinavir dosed at 750 mg tid compared to a ritonavir (100 mg bid)-boosted regimen using lopinavir (400 mg bid) has been presented.[29] The 653 patients received protease inhibitors plus d4T and 3TC for 60 weeks to date. Tolerability of the regimens compared favorably, except for lipid abnormalities, which were more common with lopinavir. At 60 weeks the CD4+ lymphocyte increases were comparable, but more patients on lopinavir/ritonavir had HIV RNA levels of less than 50 copies per milliliter than nelfinavir in an ITT analysis (64% vs. 52%; P = 0.002). Although adherence rates were similar (~65% of patients in both groups had 95% adherence by pill counts), whether missed mid-day doses of nelfinavir could have reduced nelfinavir performance is not clear. The virologic benefit of a boosted protease inhibitor must be weighed against potential long-term lipid toxicities.

A retrospective study (n = 135) compared indinavir (67%) with nelfinavir (33%) in therapy-naive patients with CD4+ lymphocyte counts of 151 to 180 cells per cubic millimeter and HIV RNA levels of 5.1 $\log_{10}$ copies per milliliter. Although baseline characteristics were similar, 80% of nelfinavir versus 68% of indinavir patients had HIV RNA levels of less than 50 copies per milliliter at 12 months (P = 0.15).[33] Differences in adherence may have accounted for the findings.

Dual PI in PI-Naive Studies

The combination of nelfinavir with saquinavir soft gelatin capsules has been examined in a four-arm study: two three-drug, single protease inhibitor (PI) regimens with dual nucleoside analogues; one dual PI alone regimen; and a four-drug regimen with dual PIs and two nucleoside analogues.[34] Of 157 PI-naive patients, 50% were treatment-naive; the mean baseline CD4+ lymphocyte count ranged from 301 to 334 cells per cubic millimeter; and the mean HIV RNA level was 4.7 to 4.8 $\log_{10}$ copies per milliliter (Table 15–3). After 48 weeks of treatment 47% of those on the quadruple regimen versus 26% on dual PI alone had undetectable viral load levels (< 50 copies per milliliter by ITT). Standard triple-drug regimens were intermediate (42% and 38% undetectable for both saquinavir and nelfinavir triple-drug regimens). Subgroup analyses suggested that the quadruple-drug regimen added the greatest benefit to patients with prior treatment experience or high baseline HIV RNA (>4.8 $\log_{10}$ copies per milliliter). The response to saquinavir/nelfinavir without NRTI was suboptimal.

A small study of various dual PIs given without nuclease reverse transcriptase inhibitors (NRTIs) demonstrated a low virologic response at 48 weeks (33% had less than 50 copies per milliliter), but these combinations were safe in PI-naive patients.[35] Another study of nelfinavir/ritonavir demonstrated augmented nelfinavir levels (threefold increase in nelfinavir, eightfold increase in the M8 nelfinavir metabolite) but low virologic success. Only 7 of 20 had HIV RNA levels of less than 400 copies per milliliter at week 48 (ITT).[41] The low responses in these trials were probably due to the fact that the regimens lacked NRTIs. In a study of heavily nucleoside-experienced but PI- and NNRTI-naive patients, the combination of nelfinavir/efavirenz resulted in a superior virologic response compared to nelfinavir alone (74% vs. 35% had less than 500 copies per milliliter at weeks 40 to 48; P < 0.001).[39]

PI-Experienced Studies

Several studies have evaluated nelfinavir alone or in combination with other PIs for PI-experienced patients (Table 15–3). One randomized study compared nelfinavir to indinavir/d4T/3TC.[36] After 9 months 35% of nelfinavir- and 42% of indinavir-treated patients had HIV RNA levels of less than 200 copies per milliliter. A retrospective study of 31 indinavir- or ritonavir-experienced patients evaluated a regimen of d4T/nelfinavir/saquinavir/nevirapine. These nonnucleoside reverse transcriptase inhibitors (NNRTI)-naive patients had mean CD4+ lymphocyte counts of 174 cells per cubic millimeter and HIV RNA levels of less than 4.4 $\log_{10}$ copies per milliliter.[37] The proportions of patients with HIV RNA levels of less than 50 copies per milliliter at 12 months were 56% (10/18 as treated) and 31% (intent to treat).

A large randomized study (n = 277) compared two dual-PI-containing regimens (nelfinavir/saquinavir versus ritonavir/saquinavir) in patients failing previous indinavir therapy.[38] The regimen also included delavirdine, adefovir, or both drugs. All patients were naive to nonnucleoside

▲ **Table 15–3.** DUAL PI AND SALVAGE STUDIES

Study	Nelfinavir Dose (mg/day)	2nd PI Dose (Interval) or NNRTI	Other Agents	Study Duration (mo)	No.	% ARV-Naive (PI-Naive)	HIV RNA (log_{10} copies/ml)		Percent with HIV RNA < 500 (50) Copies/ml at Last Follow-up	CD4+ Lymphocyte Count (cells/mm^3)	
							Baseline	↓ At Last Follow-up		Baseline	↑ At Last Follow-up
SPICE[34]	—	SQV 3600 tid	2 NRTIs	12	26	54 (100)	4.8	2.4	42 (42) I	334	121
	2250 tid	—	2 NRTIs	12	26	54 (100)	4.9	2.6	50 (38) I	305	137
	2250 tid	SQV 2400 tid	2 NRTIs	12	51	53 (100)	4.7	2.5	61 (47) I	300	154
	2250 tid	SQV 2400 tid	—	12	54	50 (100)	4.8	2.4	39 (26) I	301	207
ProA2001[35]	2250 tid	APV 2400 tid	—	12	7	43 (100)	4.9	3.4	N/A (33)[a] I	419	274
	—	APV/IDV tid	—	12	9	33 (100)	4.7	1.7	N/A (33) I	401	119
	—	APV/SQV tid	—	12	8	50 (100)	5.0	2.7	N/A (33) I	295	74
	—	APV 2400 tid	AZT/3TC	12	10	30 (100)	4.2	2.2	N/A (N/A)	393	17
Roca[36]	2250 tid		d4T/3TC	9	56	0 (48)	4.3	N/A	47 (N/A) A	328	35%[b]
	—	IDV 2400 tid	d4T/3TC	9	56	0 (35)	4.6	N/A	46 (N/A) A	312	42%[b]
Casado[37]	2250 tid or 2500 bid	SQV 1800 tid or 2000 bid	d4T/NVP	12	31	0 (0)	4.4	1.95	N/A (31) I N/A (56) A	174	290
ACTG 359[38]	2250 tid	SQV 2400 tid	DLV, ADV[c]	4	138	0 (0)	~4.4	0.1–0.6	33% I	193–258	~19
	—	SQV 800 bid RTV 800 bid	DLV, ADV[c]	4	139	0 (0)	~4.6	0.2–0.4	28% I	228–242	~19
ACTG 364[39]	2250 tid	—	2 NRTIs	12	66	0 (100)	~3.9	N/A	35 (22) I	336	~94[d]
	—	EFV 600	2 NRTIs	12	65	0 (100)	~3.9	N/A	60 (44) I	343	~94[d]
	2250 tid	EFV 600	2 NRTIs	12	64	0 (100)	~3.8	N/A	74 (67) I	379	~94[d]
ACTG 398[40]	2500 bid	APV 2400 bid	EFV, ADV, ABC	6	139	0 (0)	~4.7	1.1	34 I	~202	33
	—	APV 2400 bid SQV 3200 bid	EFV, ADV, ABC	6	116	0 (0)	~4.7	1.2	34 I	~202	53
	—	APV 2400 bid IDV 2400 bid	EFV, ADV, ABC	6	69	0 (0)	~4.7	1.2	36 I	~202	9
	—	APV 2400 bid	EFV, ADV, ABC	6	157	0 (0)	~4.7	0.8	23 I	~202	13

A, as treated; ABC, abacavir; ADV, adefovir; APV, amprenavir; ARV, antiretroviral; d4T, stavudine; DVL, delavirdine; EFV, efavirenz; I, intent to treat; IDV, indinavir; LOD, level of detection; NNRTI, nonnucleoside reverse transcriptase inhibitors; RTV, ritonavir; SQV, saquinavir; 3TC, lamivudine.

[a]Percent of all dual PI LOD = 50 copies per milliliter.

[b]Percent with > a 100-cell increase.

[c]Three arms: DVL, DLV/ADV, ADV.

[d]Increase for all groups combined.

agents. There was no difference between groups in terms of the proportion of patients with HIV RNA levels of less than 500 copies per milliliter at week 16; nelfinavir had 33%, ritonavir had 28% (P = NS). Use of delavirdine in the regimen improved the response. In another large study of patients failing one to three prior PI regimens, dual-PI therapy (nelfinavir, indinavir, or saquinavir plus amprenavir) was superior to amprenavir alone in suppressing the HIV RNA level to less than 200 copies per milliliter at 24 weeks (35% vs. 23%; $P = 0.02$).[40] Although patients with no previous NNRTI treatment had improved success, the choice of the PI to pair with amprenavir did not affect the outcome.

Clinical Efficacy and Ongoing Studies

A major trial has been designed to evaluate the clinical effectiveness of nelfinavir-containing regimens to reduce HIV-related complications. It is a 1300-patient equivalency trial comparing nelfinavir and ritonavir (Community Programs for Clinical Research on AIDS Protocol 042). In this ongoing trial, patients with CD4+ lymphocyte counts of less than 100 cells per cubic millimeter and no prior use of PIs except saquinavir are randomized to receive open-label nelfinavir versus ritonavir plus their current nucleoside analogue antiretroviral therapy.

Another large ongoing study is comparing three regimens: initial nelfinavir, efavirenz, or nelfinavir/efavirenz. All patients also receive two NRTIs. Patients who experience virologic or toxicity failure on the first regimen are randomized to a second regimen: Those initially randomized to nelfinavir move to efavirenz, and those randomized to efavirenz receive nelfinavir. Dual-therapy patients go to a new dual-PI regimen. All switches include new NRTIs. The primary endpoint for the study is failure of the second regimen. Thus the study is evaluating which initial strategy (PI, NNRTI, or combination) leads to long-term success.

Summary

Taken together, results of the clinical trials demonstrate that nelfinavir is a potent antiretroviral agent. There is clear evidence of a dose-response relation, with doses of less than 750 mg tid being suboptimal. Nelfinavir can be used as 1250 mg bid with two nucleoside agents for initial therapy in naive patients. Development of a 625 mg tablet is currently underway to reduce the pill burden for the 1250 mg dosing regimen.

Although a boosted PI regimen (lopinavir/ritonavir) was superior to nelfinavir, the long-term toxicity of boosted regimens is unclear. In nucleoside-experienced patients, efavirenz/nelfinavir (with NRTIs) was superior to nelfinavir (with NRTIs). The role of nelfinavir for PI-experienced patients is unclear. Resistance studies (see below) demonstrated broad cross-resistance to nelfinavir, yet dual-PI studies using nelfinavir have shown comparable virologic responses.

▲ RESISTANCE

Nelfinavir-resistant isolates emerge after multiple passages of HIV in the presence of nelfinavir in vitro and can be isolated from patients exposed to nelfinavir for periods of weeks or more. Similar to other PIs, in the absence of complete viral suppression, resistant virus populations arise with critical mutations at the substrate-binding site that significantly reduce drug activity. Additional compensatory mutations may be selected that enhance viral fitness. The clinical significance of each genetic alteration in the virus genome, selected as a result of nelfinavir exposure and ongoing viral replication, is an area of great importance and of active laboratory and clinical investigation.

Reduced susceptibility to nelfinavir can be induced after 22 passages of HIV-1 in the presence of drug in vitro. The HIV mutant strain was characterized by a D30N substitution. Although this mutant was sevenfold less susceptible to nelfinavir, it remained fully sensitive to indinavir, saquinavir, and ritonavir. The critical nature of this residue is consistent with molecular modeling studies that indicate the formation of a hydrogen bond between residue 30 in the S2 subsite of protease and the P2 phenolic hydroxyl group of nelfinavir.

In vivo, the D30N substitution is the most consistent mutation that emerges in the setting of nelfinavir failure and is associated with reduced phenotypic susceptibility to nelfinavir (5- to 93-fold).[42] Substitutions at other codons develop, including changes at 35, 36, 46, 71, 77, and 88. The resistant mutations commonly associated with other PIs, specifically G48V, V82FT, and I84V, have not been isolated from patients developing nelfinavir resistance, and the L90M was observed in 3 of 55.[42] However, another study found the L90M mutation in 9 of 106 naive patients failing nelfinavir given with d4T and 3TC. In this study there were 31 of 106 with genotypic PI resistance: 22 of 31 with D30N and 9 of 31 with L90M.[43]

The frequency of resistant isolates recovered from patients receiving combination therapy with nelfinavir is less than that in patients receiving nelfinavir monotherapy. This observation predominantly reflects the greater suppression of viral replication achieved with combination nelfinavir regimens and thus less opportunity for nelfinavir-resistant strains to emerge. In 113 randomly selected patients receiving nelfinavir monotherapy or nelfinavir/AZT/3TC, the genotypic substitution at codon 30 was observed in 56% of subjects receiving monotherapy and in 6% receiving triple-combination therapy. As with other PIs, when early viral breakthrough occurs in naive patients treated with nelfinavir/AZT/3TC, the M184V mutation in RT occurs prior to nelfinavir-associated mutations.[44] In one study of 53 naive patients treated with nelfinavir/AZT/3TC, 7 experienced rebound at 28 weeks; 4 of 7 had M184V and only 1 had D30N. No AZT resistance mutations were noted.[45]

Patients treated with other PIs can develop cross-resistance to nelfinavir in the absence of the D30N mutation. The genotypic pattern that predicts lack of clinical response or phenotypic resistance to nelfinavir is varied. In general, the greater the number of substitutions in protease, the less likely is a virologic response to nelfinavir salvage therapy.[46] No single amino acid mutation pattern predicted response, but patients with the L90M had poor responses.[47] The presence of reduced phenotypic susceptibility to nelfinavir after an average of two previous PI regimens was high (33/51, or 65%). Patients with reduced susceptibility (more than fourfold change in IC_{50} by the Virco assay) were unlikely to achieve HIV RNA levels of less than 200 copies per milliliter by 3 months (3%), whereas those with susceptible virus responded 40% of the time.[47]

For patient management strategies, it is important to know if nelfinavir-resistant virus is likely to fail to respond partially or completely to other PI regimens. Determination of phenotypic susceptibility to other PIs from patients failing nelfinavir can help predict future responses. In one cohort of 88 patients, 62% had nelfinavir as the first (and only) PI treatment. Using the ViroLogic assay, 82% of patients failing nelfinavir had reduced susceptibility (more than 2.5-fold change in IC_{50}) to nelfinavir, but fewer than 20% had a more than 2.5-fold change reduced susceptibility to indinavir, ritonavir, saquinavir, or amprenavir.[48] Only 31% had a more than 2.5-fold change in IC_{50} to two or more PIs. Patients in this cohort who had indinavir as their first PI also had a more than 2.5-fold change to indinavir (68%), but 73% had a more than 2.5-fold change to two or more PIs.

The virologic response to a new regimen in patients failing nelfinavir was evaluated in 24 patients who had detectable viremia for a median of 48 weeks. A dual-PI regimen of ritonavir/saquinavir given with d4T and 3TC resulted in an HIV RNA response (less than 500 copies per milliliter at week 24) in 71% of the patients. Another study of 79 patients failing nelfinavir found 65% response at 6 months to ritonavir/saquinavir given with other agents.[49] Thus several studies support the lack of PI cross-resistance from patients who receive nelfinavir as the first PI. Furthermore, responses to dual-PI salvage regimens, after nelfinavir failure, are reasonable.

▲ DRUG INTERACTIONS

Given that nelfinavir is metabolized by several cytochrome P_{450} isoforms, including CYP3A4,[50] the drug has potential interaction with some medications commonly used to treat HIV-infected patients. Drugs that are substrates, inhibitors, or inducers of the CYP3A4 enzymes could potentially interact with nelfinavir. Nucleoside analogues are not metabolized by CYP3A4, and co-administration of nelfinavir with 3TC, AZT, or d4T have no significant ($\leq 35\%$) change in AUC or C_{max} of either the nucleoside analogues or nelfinavir. Buffered didanosine and calcium likewise do not affect nelfinavir concentrations.[51,52]

Inhibition of the CYP3A4 enzymes by nelfinavir can augment blood levels of other drugs metabolized by these enzymes (Table 15–4).[15] Nelfinavir increases terfenadine metabolite levels by almost 50%. This drug and other compounds with similar metabolic properties (e.g., astemizole, cisapride, midazolam, triazolam) should not be given with nelfinavir because of the potential for fatal cardiac arrhythmias or other adverse effects. Nelfinavir also increases rifabutin levels (207% increase in AUC). These increased levels of rifabutin are associated with a higher frequency of toxicities, such as uveitis. A 50% dose reduction of rifabutin is recommended when the drugs are given together. Chronic dosing with nelfinavir leads to reduced (47% lower AUC) levels of ethinyl estradiol with no effect on norethindrone. Thus the dose of ethinyl estradiol may have to be increased with concurrent nelfinavir use, or a different form of contraception should be employed. Nelfinavir can lower phenytoin levels by 20% to 40%, so phenytoin levels must be carefully monitored or alternative agents used.[53] Blood levels of tacrolimus have been increased when nelfinavir is added, with dose adjustment required.[54] Dramatic elevations in simvastatin levels (506% increased AUC) and modest elevations in atorvastatin (74%) occur after nelfinavir dosing.[55] Atorvastatin should be used cautiously with nelfinavir, and simvastatin should not be used at all.

Drugs that induce the CYP3A4 enzyme can reduce plasma nelfinavir concentrations, resulting in subtherapeutic drug levels, less potent and sustained viral suppression, and increased nelfinavir resistance mutations. Rifampin is a potent inducer of CYP3A4, and multiple doses of rifampin lead to an 82% reduction (range 77% to 86%) in plasma nelfinavir concentrations. Rifampin should not be given with nelfinavir. Although not formally studied, it might be expected that carbamazepine, phenobarbital, and phenytoin would lower plasma nelfinavir levels; because lower doses (i.e., 500 mg tid) of nelfinavir have been associated with less complete suppression of HIV RNA levels, these drugs should not be given with nelfinavir.

Inhibitors of CYP3A4 (e.g., ketoconazole) can augment nelfinavir levels. Ketoconazole dosing increases nelfinavir levels by 35% (range 21% to 49%). This interaction is not thought to be clinically important. Azithromycin AUC is increased by 100% by nelfinavir, but nelfinavir levels are not significantly reduced (28% lower AUC).[56] Other drugs with less potent CYP3A4 inhibition would not be expected to alter nelfinavir levels; such drugs include macrolide antibiotics (erythromycin, clarithromycin) and azole antifungals (fluconazole, itraconazole). Finally, dapsone and trimethoprim-sulfamethoxazole should not affect nelfinavir concentrations.

Nelfinavir augments levels of soft gel saquinavir by 392%.[57,58] Based on these data, nelfinavir 750 tid has been used safely with soft gel saquinavir 800 mg tid.[59] Indinavir and nelfinavir dosed together augment levels of both. A study of 1200 and 1250 bid, respectively, showed levels at or above historical three-times-daily regimens with these drugs.[60] Earlier studies of nelfinavir and ritonavir demonstrated a modest increase in the nelfinavir AUC. However, ritonavir at 100 and 200 mg bid given with nelfinavir 1250 mg bid elevates the trough nelfinavir levels by 45% and 90%, respectively.[61] Amprenavir trough levels are also significantly elevated (200%) by co-administration with nelfinavir.[62]

Unlike other PIs, the nonnucleoside agents efavirenz and nevirapine do not significantly alter nelfinavir levels.[63–65] Efavirenz has been given successfully with nelfinavir.[66] Delavirdine augments nelfinavir exposure, but the delavirdine levels are reduced.[67]

▲ **Table 15–4.** PHARMACOLOGIC INTERACTIONS WITH NELFINAVIR

Co-administered Drug	Effect of Nelfinavir on Co-administered Drug AUC	Effect on Nelfinavir AUC	Dose Change	
			Co-administered Drug	Nelfinavir
Documented Interactions[a]				
Terfenadine[b]	↑ 46%[b]	ND	NR	NR
Rifabutin	↑ 207%	↓ 32%	Reduce by 50%	No
Rifampin	ND	↓ 82%	NR	NR
Ketoconazole	ND	↑ 35%	No	No
Ethinyl estradiol	↓ 47%	ND	Yes	No
Azithromycin	↑ 100%	↓ 28%	No	No
Phenytoin	20–40% ↓	↓ (Presumed)	Yes	NR
Tacrolimus	↑ (Presumed)	ND	Yes	No
Simvastatin	↑ 506%	↔	NR	NR
Atorvastatin	↑ 74%	↔	Yes	No
Saquinavir	↑ 392%	↑ 18%	Yes	No
Indinavir	↑ 50%	↑ 83%	Yes	Yes
Ritonavir (500 vs. 200)	↔	↑ 152%/↑ 30%	Yes	Yes
Amprenavir	↑ 160% (trough ↑)	↔	No	No
Delavirdine	↓ 42%	↑ 92%	?	No
Nevirapine	↔	↑ 8%	No	No
Efavirenz	↔	↑ 20%	No	No
Suspected Interactions[c]				
Carbamazipine	ND	↓	—	NR
Phenobarbital	ND	↓	—	NR
No Interaction[d]				
AZT	↓ 35%	↔	No	No
3TC	↑ 10%	↔	No	No
ddI	ND	↔	No	No
d4T	↔	↔	No	No
Dapsone	↔	↔	No	No
Trimethoprim-sulfamethoxazole	↔	↔	No	No
Macrolide antibiotics[e]	↔	↔	No	No
Azole antifungals[f]	↔	↔	No	No
Calcium supplements	ND	↔	No	No

ND, not done; No, no dose change recommended; NR, not recommended for use with nelfinavir; ↑, increase; ↓, decrease; ↔, no change.
[a]Interaction documented by pharmacokinetic study.
[b]Terfenadine carboxylate metabolite. (Note: astemizole, cisapride, triazolam, midazolam, amiodarone, ergot derivatives, and quinidine should not be used with nelfinavir.)
[c]Suspected but not documented by study.
[d]Documented or suspected lack of interaction.
[e]Erythromycin, clarithromycin.
[f]Itraconazole, fluconazole.

▲ RECOMMENDATIONS FOR USE

Nelfinavir, a potent HIV PI, originally recommended for the treatment of HIV-infected adults at a dose of 750 mg (three 250 mg tablets) three times daily, should now be dosed at 1250 mg twice daily. Nelfinavir should be given with a meal or a light snack to maximize bioavailability. Use in treatment-naive patients gives optimal results. As with other PIs, nelfinavir must be given with two NRTIs or combined with an NNRTI and two NRTIs. Data for dual PIs plus two nucleosides is promising, but pill burden and toxicity may limit utility.

Nelfinavir appears to be effective in HIV-infected patients at all disease stages with a broad range of CD4+ lymphocyte counts, including patients with counts of less than 50 cells per cubic millimeter. Clinical trial data suggest that up to 75% to 85% of antiretroviral-naive patients should achieve an undetectable level of HIV RNA (less than 500 copies per milliliter) that persists for 12 months when nelfinavir is given in combination with AZT and 3TC. This should be accompanied by significant increases in CD4+ lymphocytes (more than 100 cells per cubic millimeter).

To date, the clinical efficacy [i.e., reduction of progression of HIV infection to acquired immunodeficiency syndrome (AIDS) and improved survival] of nelfinavir has not been established. However, improved survival and reduced HIV disease progression have been associated with HIV RNA level reductions for other HIV PIs,[68] and a clinical endpoint study comparing combination therapy with nelfinavir versus ritonavir is currently in progress. Whether virologic responses can be further improved by therapeutic drug monitoring, as suggested in one small study, is under investigation.[69]

A nelfinavir pediatric powder containing 50 mg per scoop (1 g) of powder has been used in a small number of children ages 2 to 13. The recommended dose is 20 to 30 mg/kg per dose given three times daily. The powder may be mixed with a variety of diluents (water, milk, formula, soy formula, dietary supplement) but should be consumed within 6 hours. The safety profile in children does not appear different from that in adults. One efficacy study of nelfinavir plus efavirenz demonstrated that 76% of patients had an HIV RNA level of less than 400 copies per milliliter at 48 weeks.[70]

Nelfinavir has an excellent toxicity profile with mild to moderate diarrhea as the most common toxicity. Similar to other PIs, care must be taken to avoid potentially toxic drug interactions with compounds metabolized by CYP34A. Drug interaction and clinical studies conducted to date suggest that combinations of nelfinavir with ritonavir, saquinavir soft gel preparation, and efavirenz can potentially enhance drug activity.

The efficacy of nelfinavir is diminished in patients who have detectable plasma HIV RNA levels despite treatment with other PIs. Patients who failed treatment with one or more previous PIs often have reduced phenotypic susceptibility to nelfinavir (>70%), which may limit the usefulness of this agent in salvage settings. However, randomized trials of dual PIs to date show equal efficacy of nelfinavir/saquinavir compared to ritonavir/saquinavir. Patients who lose virologic suppression during nelfinavir therapy (used as the first PI) have less phenotypic cross-resistance and respond to a new dual-PI regimen in 60% of cases. Whether first-line treatment with nelfinavir allows better responses to a second-line regimen than use of other first-line regimens (another PI, a ritonavir-boosted PI, or an NNRTI) awaits results of randomized studies.

The ability of nelfinavir combined with other agents to maintain suppression of the viral load below detection for up to 12 months has been shown. In the individual patient, therapeutic success at maintaining aviremia requires continued combination therapy and adequate patient adherence to the dose and schedule of the medical regimen. Persistent suppression of HIV replication would afford the best opportunity to prevent the emergence of drug resistance and ultimate failure of the antiviral therapy.

REFERENCES

1. Roberts NA, Martin JA, Kinchington D, et al. Rational design of peptide-based HIV proteinase inhibitors. Science 248:358–361, 1990.
2. Navia MA, Fitzgerald PM, McKeever BM, et al. Three-dimensional structure of aspartyl protease from human immunodeficiency virus HIV-1. Nature 337:615–620, 1989.
3. Gehlhaar DK, Verkhivker GM, Rejto PA, et al. Molecular recognition of the inhibitor AG-1343 by HIV-1 protease: conformationally flexible docking by evolutionary programming. Chem Biol 2:317–324, 1995.
4. Appelt K, Bacquet RJ, Bartlett CA, et al. Design of enzyme inhibitors using iterative protein crystallographic analysis. J Med Chem 34: 1925–1934, 1991.
5. Kohl NE, Emini EA, Schleif WA, et al. Active human immunodeficiency virus protease is required for viral infectivity. Proc Natl Acad Sci USA 85:4686–4690, 1988.
6. Webber S, Khalil D, Kosa M. Preclinical toxicokinetic studies with AG-1343, an orally bioavailable HIV-1 protease inhibitor. In: Program and Abstracts of the 2nd National Conference on Human Retroviruses, Washington, DC, 1995, abstract 93.
7. Patick A, Meimo H, Markowitz M. In vitro antiviral and resistance studies of AG1343, an orally bioavailable inhibitor of HIV-1 protease. In: Program and Abstracts of the 2nd National Conference on Human Retroviruses, Washington, DC, 1995, abstract 184.
8. Agouron. Investigator's brochure Viracept™ (nelfinavir mesylate). La Jolla, CA, Agouron Pharmaceuticals, 1997.
9. Patick A, Boritzki T. Combination of HIV-1 protease inhibitor AG1343 with zidovudine, 2′,3′-dideoxycytidine, or didanosine synergistically inhibits acute HIV-1 infection in vitro. In: Program and Abstracts of the Consensus Symposium on Combined Antiviral Therapy, Lisbon, 1995, abstract P8.
10. Quart B, Chapman S, Peterkin J, et al. Phase I safety, tolerance, pharmacokinetics and food effect studies of AG1343: a novel HIV protease inhibitor. In: Program and Abstracts of the 2nd National Conference on Human Retroviruses and Related Infections, Washington, DC, January–February 1995, abstract LB3.
11. Johnson M, Petersen A, Winslade J, et al. Comparison of bid and tid dosing of Viracept (nelfinavir, NFV) in combination with stavudine (d4T) and lamivudine (3TC). In: Program and Abstracts of the 5th Conference on Retroviruses and Opportunistic Infections, Chicago, February 1998, abstract 373.
12. Scott RC, Greenberg DM, Frye J. Pharmacokinetics (PK) of nelfinavir (NFV) in African American and Caucasian HIV patients. In: Program and Abstracts of the 40th Interscience Conference on Antimicrobial Agents and Chemotherapy, Toronto, September 2000, abstract 1655.
13. Powderly WG, Saag MS, Chapman S, et al. Predictors of optimal virological response to potent antiretroviral therapy. AIDS 13:1873–1880, 1999.
14. Aweeka F, Jayewardene A, Staprans S, et al. Failure to detect nelfinavir in the cerebrospinal fluid of HIV-1 infected patients with and without AIDS dementia complex. J Acquir Immune Defic Syndr Hum Retrovirol 20:39–43, 1999.
15. Kerr B, Lee C, Yuen G, et al. Overview of in-vitro and in-vivo drug interaction studies of nelfinavir mesylate (NFV), a new HIV-1 protease inhibitor. In: Program and Abstracts of the 4th Conference on Retroviruses and Opportunistic Infections, Washington, DC, January 1997, abstract 373.
16. Hsyu PH, Lillibridge JH, Beeby S, et al. Pharmacokinetics (PK) of nelfinavir (NVF) and metabolite M8 in patients with liver impairment after a single oral 750 mg dose of Viracept. In: Program and Abstracts of the 40th Interscience Conference on Antimicrobial Agents and Chemotherapy, Toronto, September 2000, abstract 1657.
17. Krogstad P, Wiznia A, Luzuriaga K, et al. Treatment of human immunodeficiency virus 1-infected infants and children with protease inhibitor nelfinavir mesylate. Clin Infect Dis 28:1109–1118, 1999.
18. Capparelli E, Sullivan J, Mofenson L, et al. Pharmacokinetics of nelfinavir in human immunodeficiency virus-infected infants. Pediatr Infect Dis 20:746–751, 2001.
19. Henry K, Lamarca A, Myers R. The safety of Viracept (nelfinavir mesylate, NFV) in pivotal phase II/III double-blind randomized controlled trials as monotherapy in combination with either d4T or AZT-3TC. In: Program and Abstracts of the 4th Conference on Retroviruses and Opportunistic Infections, Washington, DC, 1997, abstract 240.
20. Ryan A. Pancrelipase for treatment-refractory diarrhea associated with nelfinavir. Am J Health Syst Pharm 57:1177–1178, 2000.
21. Bonfanti P, Valsecchi L, Parazzini F, et al. Incidence of adverse reactions in HIV patients treated with protease inhibitors: a cohort study: Coordinamento Italiano Studio Allergia e Infezione da HIV (CISAI) group. J Acquir Immune Defic Syndr 23:236–245, 2000.
22. Graham N. Metabolic disorders among HIV-infected patients treated with protease inhibitors: a review. J Acquir Immune Defic Syndr 25 (suppl 1):S4–S11, 2000.
23. Rudich A, Vanounou S, Riesenberg K, et al. The HIV protease inhibitor nelfinavir induces insulin resistance and increases basal lipolysis in 3T3-L1 adipocytes. Diabetes 50:1425–1431, 2001.
24. Moyle GJ, Youle M, Higgs C, et al. Safety, pharmacokinetics, and antiretroviral activity of the potent, specific human immunodeficiency virus protease inhibitor nelfinavir: results of a phase I/II trial and extended follow-up in patients infected with human immunodeficiency virus. J Clin Pharmacol 38:736–743, 1998.
25. Markowitz M, Conant M, Hurley A, et al. A preliminary evaluation of nelfinavir mesylate, an inhibitor of human immunodeficiency virus

(HIV)-1 protease, to treat HIV infection. J Infect Dis 177:1533–1540, 1998.

26. Powderly WG, Sension MG, Conant M, et al. The efficacy of Viracept (nelfinavir mesylate, NFV) in pivotal phase II/III double-blind randomized controlled trials as monotherapy and in combination with d4T or AZT/3TC. In: Program and Abstracts of the 4th Conference on Retroviruses and Opportunistic Infections, January 1997, abstract 370.
27. Saag MS, Tebas P, Sension M, et al. Randomized, double-blind comparison of two nelfinavir doses plus nucleosides in HIV-infected patients (Agouron Study 511). AIDS 15:1971–1978, 2001.
28. Johnson M, Nelson M, Peters B, et al. Comparison of bid and tid dosing of nelfinavir when given in combination with stavudine (d4T) and lamivudine (3TC) for up to 48 weeks. In: Program and Abstracts of the 38th Interscience Conference on Antimicrobial Agents and Chemotherapy (ICAAC), San Diego, September 1998, abstract I-216.
29. Ruane P, Mendonca J, Timerman A, et al. Kaletra vs. nelfinavir in antiretroviral-naive subjects: week 60 comparison in a phase III, blinded, randomized clinical trial. In: Program and Abstracts of the 1st IAS Conference on HIV Pathogenesis and Treatment, Buenos Aires, July 2001, abstract 6.
30. Markowitz M, Winslow D, Cao Y. Triple therapy with nelfinavir (Viracept) in combination with AZT an 3TC in 12 antiretroviral-naive subjects chronically infected with HIV-1. In: Program and Abstracts of the 10th International Conference of Antiviral Research, Atlanta, 1997.
31. Pedneault L, Elion R, Adler M. A pilot study of safety and antiviral activity of the combination of stavudine, didanosine and nelfinavir in HIV-infected subjects. AIDS (suppl 2):S17, 1996.
32. Pedneault LER, Adler M. Stavudine (d4T), didanosine (ddI), and nelfinavir combination therapy in HIV-infected subjects: antiviral effect and safety in an ongoing pilot study. In: Program and Abstracts of the 4th Conference on Retroviruses and Opportunistic Infections, Washington, DC, 1997, abstract 241.
33. Moreno R, Perez-Elias MJ, Munoz V, et al. Long-term comparative outcomes of indinavir (IDV) vs. nelfinavir (NFV)-based HAART in naive patients in routine clinical practice. In: Abstracts of the 40th Interscience Conference on Antimicrobial Agents and Chemotherapy, September 2000, abstract 1523.
34. Moyle G, Pozniak A, Opravil M, et al. The SPICE study: 48-week activity of combinations of saquinavir soft gelatin and nelfinavir with and without nucleoside analogues: study of protease inhibitor combinations in Europe. J Acquir Immune Defic Syndr 23:128–137, 2000.
35. Eron JJ, Haubrich R, Lang W, et al. A phase II trial of dual protease inhibitor therapy: amprenavir in combination with indinavir, nelfinavir, or saquinavir. J Acquir Immune Defic Syndr 26:458–461, 2001.
36. Roca B, Gomez C, Arnedo A. A randomized, comparative study of lamivudine plus stavudine, with indinavir or nelfinavir, in treatment experienced HIV-infected patients. AIDS 14:157–161, 2000.
37. Casado J, Dronda F, Hertogs K, et al. Efficacy, tolerance, and pharmacokinetics of the combination of stavudine, nevirapine, nelfinavir, and saquinavir as salvage regimen after ritonavir or indinavir failure. AIDS Res Hum Retroviruses 17:93–98, 2001.
38. Gulick RM, Hu XJ, Fiscus SA, et al. Randomized study of saquinavir with ritonavir or nelfinavir together with delavirdine, adefovir, or both in human immunodeficiency virus-infected adults with virologic failure on indinavir: AIDS Clinical Trials Group study 359. J Infect Dis 182:1375–1384, 2000.
39. Albrecht MA, Bosch RJ, Hammer SM, et al. Nelfinavir, efavirenz, or both after the failure of nucleoside treatment of HIV infection. N Engl J Med 345:398–407, 2001.
40. Hammer S, Mellors J, Vaida F, et al. A randomized, placebo-controlled trial of saquinavir (SQV)sgc, indinavir (IDV) or nelfinavir (NFV) in combination with amprenavir (APV), abacavir (ABC), efavirenz (EFZ) & adefovir (ADV) in patients with protease inhibitor (PI) failure. In: Program and Abstracts of the 7th Conference on Retroviruses and Opportunistic Infections, San Francisco, January–February 2000, abstract LB7.
41. Raines CP, Flexner C, Sun E, et al. Safety, tolerability, and antiretroviral effects of ritonavir-nelfinavir combination therapy administered for 48 weeks. J Acquir Immune Defic Syndr 25:322–328, 2000.
42. Patrick AK, Duran M, Cao Y, et al. Genotypic and phenotypic characterization of human immunodeficiency virus type 1 variants isolated from patients treated with the protease inhibitor nelfinavir. Antimicrob Agents Chemother 42:2637–2644, 1998.
43. Kempf D, Bernstein B, King M, et al. Comparison of the emergence of genotypic resistance over 48 weeks of therapy with ABT-378/R (kaletra) or nelfinavir plus D4T/3TC. In: Program and Abstracts of the 1st IAS Conference on HIV Pathogenesis and Treatment, Buenos Aires, July 2001, abstract 129.
44. Atkinson B, Isaacson J, Knowles M, et al. Correlation between human immunodeficiency virus genotypic resistance and virologic responses in patients receiving nelfinavir monotherapy or nelfinavir with lamivudine and zidovudine. J Infect Dis 182:420–427, 2000.
45. Maguire M, Gartland M, Moore S, et al. Absence of zidovudine resistance in antiretroviral-naive patients following zidovudine/lamivudine/protease inhibitor combination therapy: virologic evaluation of AVANTI 2 and AVANTI 3 studies. AIDS 14:1195–1201, 2000.
46. Walmsley S, Becker M, Zhang M, et al. Predictors of virologic response in HIV-infected patients to salvage antiretroviral therapy that includes nelfinavir. Antivir Ther 6:47–54, 2001.
47. Dronda F, Casado J, Moreno S, et al. Phenotypic cross-resistance to nelfinavir: the role of prior antiretroviral therapy and the number of mutations in the protease gene. AIDS Res Hum Retroviruses 17:211–215, 2001.
48. Kemper CA, Witt MA, Keiser PH, et al. Sequencing of protease inhibitor therapy: insights from an analysis of HIV phenotypic resistance in patients failing protease inhibitors. AIDS 15:609–615, 2001.
49. Zolopa A, Tebas P, Gallant J, et al. The efficacy of ritonavir (RTV)/saquinavir (SQV) antiretroviral therapy (ART) in patients who failed nelfinavir (NFV): a multicenter clinical cohort study. In: Program and Abstracts of the 39th Interscience Conference on Antimicrobial Agents and Chemotherapy, San Francisco, September 1999, abstract 2065.
50. Lillibridge JH, Liang BH, Kerr BM, et al. Characterization of the selectivity and mechanism of human cytochrome P450 inhibition by the human immunodeficiency virus-protease inhibitor nelfinavir mesylate. Drug Metab Dispos 26: 609–616, 1998.
51. Elion R, Kaul S, Knupp C, et al. The safety profile and antiviral activity of the combination of stavudine, didanosine, and nelfinavir in patients with HIV infection. Clin Ther 21:1853–1863, 1999.
52. Kopp Hutzler B, Perez-Rodriguez E, Norton S, et al. Pharmacokinetic (PK) interactions between nelfinavir (NFV) and calcium supplements. AIDS 14(suppl 4):S96, 2000.
53. Shelton MJ, Cloen D, Becker M, et al. Evaluation of the pharmacokinetic (PK) interaction between phenytoin (Phen) and nelfinavir (NFV) in healthy volunteers at steady state. In: Program and Abstracts of the 40th Interscience Conference on Antimicrobial Agents and Chemotherapy, Toronto, September 2000, abstract 426.
54. Schvarcz R, Rudbeck G, Söderdahl G, et al. Interaction between nelfinavir and tacrolimus after orthoptic liver transplantation in a patient coinfected with HIV and hepatitis C virus (HCV). Transplantation 69: 2194–2195, 2000.
55. Hsyu PH, Lewis RH, Schultz MD, et al. Pharmacokinetic interactions between nelfinavir and two HMG-CoA reductase inhibitors simvastatin and atorvastatin. In: 40th Interscience Conference on Antimicrobial Agents and Chemotherapy, Toronto, September 2000, abstract 425.
56. Amsden GW, Nafziger AN, Foulds G, et al. A study of the pharmacokinetics of azithromycin and nelfinavir when coadministered in healthy volunteers. J Clin Pharmacol 40:1522–1527, 2000.
57. Carpenter CC, Fischl MA, Hammer SM, et al. Antiretroviral therapy for HIV infection in 1998: updated recommendations of the International AIDS Society—USA Panel. JAMA 280:78–86, 1998.
58. Kravcik S, Sahai J, Kerr B, et al. Nelfinavir mesylate (NFV) increases saquinavir-soft gel capsule (SQV-SGC) exposure in HIV+ patients. In: Program and Abstracts of the 4th Conference on Retroviruses and Opportunistic Infections, Washington, DC, January 1997, abstract 371.
59. Fletcher CV, Acosta EP, Cheng HL, et al. Competing drug–drug interactions among multidrug antiretroviral regimens used in the treatment of HIV-infected subjects: ACTG 884. AIDS 14:2495–2501, 2000.
60. Squires K, Riddler S, Havlir D, et al. Co-administration of indinavir (IDV) 1200 mg with nelfinavir (NFV) 1250 mg in a twice daily regimen: preliminary safety, PK activity. In: Program and Abstracts of the 6th Conference on Retroviruses and Opportunistic Infections, Chicago, January–February 1999, abstract 364.
61. Kurowski M, Kaeser B, Mroziekiewicz A, et al. The influence of low doses of ritonavir on the pharmacokinetics of nelfinavir 1250 mg bid. In: Program and Abstracts of the 40th Interscience Conference on An-

timicrobial Agents and Chemotherapy, Toronto, September 2000, abstract 1639.
62. Piscitelli S, Bechtel C, Sadler B, et al. The addition of a second protease inhibitor eliminates amprenavir–efavirenz drug interactions and increases plasma amprenavir concentrations. In: Program and Abstracts of the 7th Conference on Retroviruses and Opportunistic Infections, San Francisco, January–February 2000, abstract 78.
63. Skowron G, Leoung G, Dusek A, et al. Stavudine (d4T), nelfinavir (NFV) and nevirapine (NVP): preliminary safety, activity and pharmacokinetics (PK) interactions. In: Program and Abstracts of the 5th Conference on Retroviruses and Opportunistic Infections, Chicago, February 1998, abstract 350.
64. Regazzi MB, Villani P, Maserati R, et al. Clinical pharmacokinetics of nelfinavir combined with efavirenz and stavudine during rescue treatment of heavily pretreated HIV-infected patients. J Antimicrob Chemother 45:343–347, 2000.
65. Villani P, Regazzi MB, Castelli F, et al. Pharmacokinetics of efavirenz (EFV) alone and in combination therapy with nelfinavir (NFV) in HIV-1 infected patients. Br J Clin Pharmacol 48:712–715, 1999.
66. Mildvan D, Martin G, Eyster M. Initial effectiveness and tolerability of nelfinavir (NFV) in combination with efavirenz (EFV, SUSTIVAJ, DMP 266) in antiretroviral therapy naive or nucleoside analogue experienced HIV-1 infected patients: characterization in a phase II, open label, multicenter study at 16 weeks (DMP 266-024). In: Program and Abstracts of the 12th World AIDS Conference, Geneva, June–July 1998, abstract 22386.
67. Cox SR, Schneck DW, Herman BD, et al. Delavirdine (DLV) and nelfinavir (NFV): a pharmacokinetic (PK) drug–drug interaction study in healthy adult volunteers. In: Program and Abstracts of the 5th Conference on Retroviruses and Opportunistic Infections, Chicago, February 1998, abstract 345.
68. Haubrich R, Lalezari J, Follansbee SE, et al. Improved survival and reduced clinical progression in HIV-infected patients with advanced disease treated with saquinavir plus zalcitabine. Antivir Ther 3:33–42, 1998.
69. Burger D, Hugen P, Droste J, et al. Therapeutic drug monitoring (TDM) of nelfinavir (NFV) and indinavir (IDV) in treatment-naive patients improves therapeutic outcome after 1 year: results from Athena. In: Programs and Abstracts of the 1st IAS Conference on HIV Pathogenesis and Treatment, Buenos Aires, July 2001, abstract 30.
70. Starr S, Fletcher C, Spector S, et al. Combination therapy with efavirenz, nelfinavir, and nucleoside reverse transcriptase inhibitors in children infected with human immunodeficiency virus type 1. N Engl J Med 341:1874–1881, 1999.

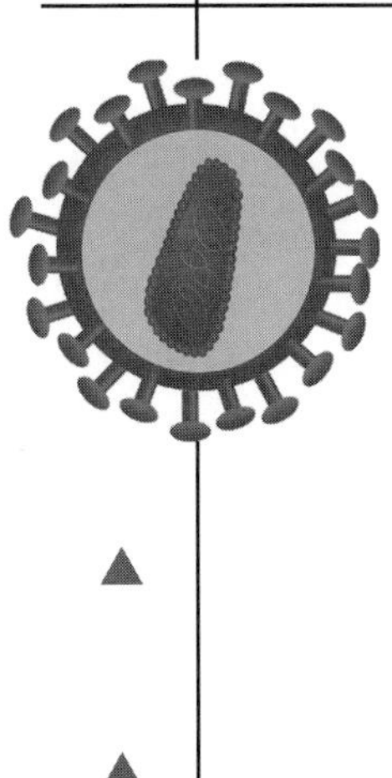

CHAPTER 16

Amprenavir

Robert L. Murphy, MD

Suppression of human immunodeficiency virus type 1 (HIV-1) replication is the primary goal of antiretroviral therapy. Although treatment with reverse transcriptase inhibitors alone and in dual combination is associated with a significant antiviral effect and positive clinical benefit, this response has been limited in duration or suboptimal for most patients.[1–10] Successful treatment of HIV-1 infection requires a regimen that can suppress viral replication maximally, typically to HIV-1 RNA plasma concentrations less than 50 copies per milliliter. This can be easily accomplished with combinations of antiretroviral drugs that include two nucleoside reverse transcriptase inhibitors plus either a protease inhibitor, a nonnucleoside reverse transcriptase inhibitor, or a third nucleoside. The choices involved in selecting an appropriate regimen are many and include presumed or real potency, resistance threshold, prior treatment history, tolerability, long-term toxicities, pharmacokinetic interactions, convenience, pill burden, and the patient's will.

The major impact of highly effective therapies occurred during 1995 and 1996 when potent HIV-1 protease inhibitors were introduced into the clinics. This occurred just 10 years after complete sequencing of the HIV-1 genome in 1985, which revealed the presence of a protease enzyme, subsequently demonstrated to be an aspartyl protease.[11,12] This enzyme has been an attractive target for drug development, as it was reported that a single amino acid substitution in the catalytic site of the HIV-1 protease could lead to the production of immature and noninfectious viral particles.[13] The HIV-1 protease enzyme is a relatively small (99 amino acids), symmetrical homodimer with two aspartyl residues flanking the active site. When the *gag* and *gag-pol* polyprotein precursors interact with the protease enzyme, a catalytic reaction occurs that involves donation of a proton from a water molecule to an aspartyl residue, resulting in a temporary unstable transition state and finally lysis of the substrate molecular peptide bond. In the absence of HIV-1-specific protease activity, viral particles produced by infected cells are immature and noninfectious because the polyprotein precursers have not been appropriately processed into functional viral enzymes and structural proteins. The key to the improvements in potency of antiretroviral regimens was the successful development of inhibitors that bind to the HIV-1 protease substrate site without being cleaved; this was made possible because of the characterization of the crystallized, three-dimensional structure of the HIV-1 protease.[14,15]

Subsequent to this discovery, multiple peptidyl and nonpeptidyl inhibitors of the HIV-1 protease were synthesized and found to be quite potent in vitro.[16–20] Significant antiretroviral effects and clinical benefits have been observed in vivo, particularly when a protease inhibitor has been used in conjunction with two nucleoside reverse transcriptase inhibitors.[21–25] As of 2002, six protease inhibitors—amprenavir, indinavir, lopinavir, nelfinavir, ritonavir, saquinavir—have been approved for use in HIV-1-infected individuals, and numerous others are in development. Because of the observed significant antiretroviral responses and beneficial clinical effects, including a survival advantage in patients with advanced HIV disease, protease inhibitor-containing regimens comprise one of the recommended choices for patients considering treatment for HIV-1 infection.[26,27]

In June 1993, scientists at Vertex Pharmaceuticals (Cambridge, MA, USA), synthesized a potent, low-molecular-weight, orally bioavailable inhibitor of HIV-1 protease referred to as VX-478. Based on encouraging in vitro data, VX-478 was selected for further clinical development. Glaxo Wellcome (Research Triangle Park, NC, USA) and Kissei

Pharmaceutical Co. (Matsumoto City, Japan) entered into licensing agreements with Vertex Pharmaceuticals for the development of this compound. An Investigational New Drug application was filed with the Food and Drug Administration (FDA) in January 1995, and Phase I trials commenced shortly thereafter. Glaxo Wellcome temporarily designated the compound 141W94 and now refers to it by the name amprenavir. Amprenavir was approved for use in patients with HIV-1 infection by the FDA in April 1999. Because of interpatient variable pharmacokinetic characteristics, amprenavir has been reformulated as a calcium phosphate ester prodrug, fos-amprenavir (GW908/VX175), which is currently being studied. Amprenavir and fos-amprenavir have been used or studied with ritonavir to boost overall drug exposure and reduce the pill burden.

▲ STRUCTURE

Amprenavir emerged from a structure-based drug design program that sought to maintain in vitro potency at less than nanomolar concentrations while emphasizing a compact inhibitor size.[28–30] A similar approach was taken in the development of angiotensin-converting enzyme (ACE) inhibitors, such as captopril, where structural information was also used to design smaller, more potent inhibitors.[31] The design strategy of the Vertex program include identification of compounds that had the following characteristics: optimum binding to the catalytic aspartate residues of the protease enzyme and the critical water molecule involved in proteolysis; minimal reorganization of the structure when bound to the enzyme; synthetic accessibility; high antiretroviral potency; low cellular toxicity; and aqueous solubility of the compound without carrying obligate charges.[32] The lead compound in this program was the *N,N*-disubstituted (hydroxyethyl) amino sulfonamide amprenavir (Fig. 16–1). Amprenavir is a peptidomimetic drug containing three asymmetrical centers.

The chemical name of amprenavir is (3*S*)-tetrahydro-3-furyl *N*-[(1*S*,2*R*)-3-(4-amino-*N*-isobutylbenzenesulfonamido)-1-benzyl-2-hydroxypropyl] carbamate. The empiric formula is $C_{25}H_{35}N_3O_6S$. This compound represents one of the smaller, less stereochemically complex of the protease inhibitors under development and one in the sulfonamide class.[33] Amprenavir is compact, has a low molecular weight (506 Da), and is relatively water-soluble (0.19 mg/ml). Its physical appearance is a white to off-white solid. The currently used formulations are 50 and 150 mg soft gel capsules that are stable at room temperature for at least 6 months but must be stored away from direct light and should not be refrigerated. The amprenavir gel capsules contain significant amounts of vitamin E. The total amount of vitamin E in the recommended daily dose of amprenavir is 1744 IU; hence additional supplementation with vitamin E is not advised. The oral solution contains amprenavir 15 mg/ml of solution. The solution contains a large amount of the excipient propylene glycol and therefore is contraindicated in children below the age of 4 years, pregnant women, patients with hepatic or renal insufficiency, and patients treated with disulfiram or metronidazole.

▲ MECHANISM OF ACTION AND IN VITRO ACTIVITY

Figure 16–2 shows a model of amprenavir in the active site of HIV-1 protease. The molecular backbone may minimize the intermolecular strain during binding with the HIV protease and therefore favor tighter, more specific interaction with the catalytic aspartic acid residues and enzyme flaps. Thus amprenavir has a relatively high binding affinity compared to other members of its class. To test amprenavir initially, Cos cells were treated with concentrations of compound ranging from 0.3 to 100.0 nM. The appearance of unprocessed and partially processed *gag* protein (p55, p40, p35) and the disappearance of fully processed cased protein (p24) occurred in response to amprenavir in a dose-dependent fashion. The median inhibitory concentration (IC_{50}) from these initial experiments was 2.2 nM.[32]

Amprenavir is highly lipophilic and rapidly accumulates within CD4+ T lymphocytes in a concentration-dependent manner. Intracellular concentrations are four times higher than extracellular concentrations, attributable to cytosolic protein binding. Amprenavir inhibits the HIV-1 and HIV-2 proteases competitively, with K_i values of 0.60 and 19 nM, respectively. The compound is highly selective (> 5000-fold) for HIV protease versus human aspartic proteases such as renin, pepsin, and cathepsin, which have K_i values of 1750 nM, 3200 nM, and more than 10,000 nM, respectively; and it has low median cytotoxicity (TC_{50} > 50 μM) across a wide panel of human cell lines.

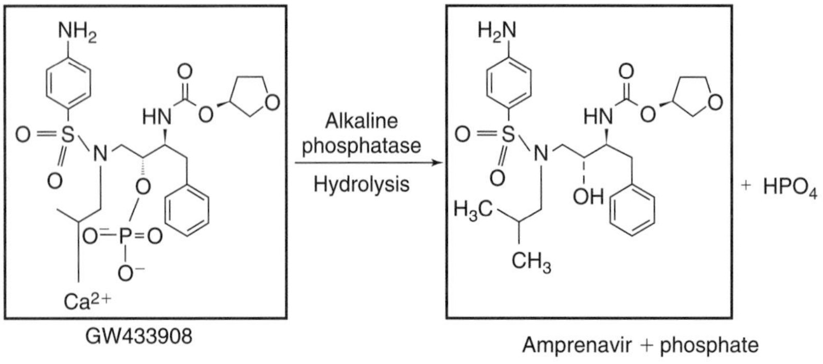

GW433908

Amprenavir + phosphate

Figure 16–1. Chemical structure of amprenavir (141W94, VX-478) and fos-amprenavir, the amprenavir pro-drug (GW908/VX-175). (Courtesy of GlaxoWellcome.)

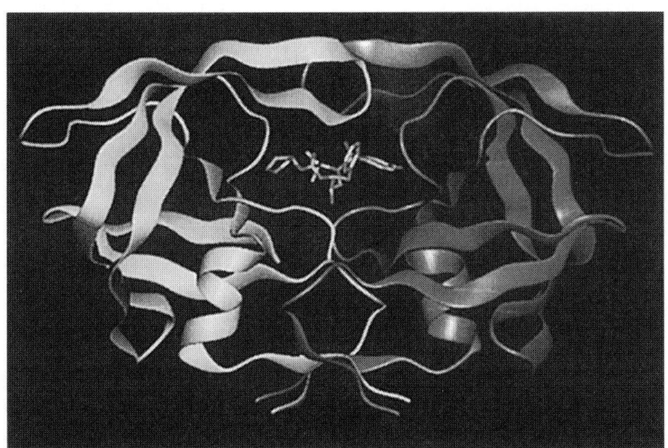

Figure 16–2. Model of amprenavir at the active site of HIV-1 protease. The two subunits of the dimeric enzyme are in different shades.

Amprenavir has highly potent intracellular antiretroviral activity against a number of laboratory strains and low-passaged primary isolates grown in a variety of human cells, including immortalized T cells, monocytic lines, and peripheral blood mononuclear cells. The mean IC_{50} values against a laboratory strain of HIV-1_{IIIB} and against six HIV-1 clinical isolates are 80 and 120 nM, respectively. The typical 90% inhibitory concentration (IC_{90}) obtained against the HIV_{IIIB} in CEM cells is 40 nM as assayed by extracellular p24 antigen. Amprenavir also inhibits the replication of HIV-2 in MT4 cells (IC_{50} 340 nM). *Giardia lamblia* is inhibited at 5 μg/ml, but no activity has been demonstrated against other protozoans, fungi, or bacteria. No activity was observed in vitro against herpes simplex viruses 1 and 2, varcella-zoster virus, human cytomegalovirus, coronavirus, yellow fever virus, respiratory syncytial virus, rotavirus, influenza A virus, or rhinovirus at concentrations up to and including 100 μM. In addition, amprenavir showed no activity against human coronavirus protease or in a human papillomavirus DNA replication assay.[32,33]

The antiretroviral effect of amprenavir is highly synergistic in combination with zidovudine, didanosine, abacavir (1592U89), and the experimental nucleosides 935U83 and 524W91. It is also synergistic with saquinavir and additive with indinavir and ritonavir.[34]

Lack of clinical efficacy in several HIV-1 protease inhibitors has been attributed to avid protein binding, such as what was observed with the Searle compound SC-52151, therefore characterization of plasma protein binding for amprenavir was considered critical.[35–37] However, the degree of protein binding is not necessarily an adequate predictor of the potential for clinical utility. Many of the most familiar pharmaceutical compounds in clinical use (e.g., ibuprofen, warfarin, nortriptyline, ritonavir) are highly protein-bound. There is apparently a complex interplay between the proportion of drug bound to proteins, the types of proteins bound [e.g., albumin versus α_1-acid glycoprotein is relatively weak (K_d 4 μM)] and the dissociation rate ("off-rate") for the drug is fast. Supplementation of cell culture media with additional α_1-acid glycoprotein in an effort to mimic what is proposed to happen in vivo resulted in only a modest twofold increase in IC_{90}.[38] These experiments suggest that protein binding should not significantly affect the clinical activity of amprenavir, and that drug interactions based on protein binding displacement are not anticipated.

▲ PHARMACOKINETICS

Amprenavir is generally well absorbed from the gastrointestinal tract of animals. In single-dose experiments in rats, the bioavailability was estimated to be 25% to 40% using a variety of formulations. In beagle dogs given oral drug, the bioavailability decreased substantially with increases in dose (from 98% at 25 mg/kg to 35% at 175 mg/kg). Comparable to other peptidomimetic protease inhibitors, amprenavir has an early peak absorption in animal models. In rats given a single oral dose, the T_{max} is 0.8 hour. In a multidose study, the elimination half-life (0.9 to 2.9 hours) was similar regardless of the dose or the route of administration. The estimated plasma half-life was 2.9 to 3.5 hours, similar to that calculated in studies involving multiple dosing in dogs. In monkeys administered multiple doses, the mean drug concentrations did not increase proportionally with increases in dose and drug concentration parameters [maximum plasma concentration (C_{max}), and plasma concentration area under the curve (AUC)] decreased during a month on therapy; this was thought to be due to poor absorption as a result of diarrhea associated with the higher dose or the drug vehicle (or both).

Penetration of the drug into the central nervous system in rats resulted in levels 1.7-fold higher than that in blood. In humans, cerebrospinal fluid (CSF) concentrations generally exceeded the expected IC_{90} concentration, and in patients treated for more than 32 weeks with amprenavir, zidovudine, and lamivudine (3TC 8/9) had HIV-1 RNA less than 400 log copies per milliliter in the CSF.[39]

In rats, unchanged drug accounted for small percentages of the administered dose recovered from urine or feces (3% and 8%, respectively). In dogs given oral drug, a higher percentage of the dose was recovered unchanged in feces (39%) but not in urine (< 1%). Multiple metabolites have been seen in these animal models, but no single metabolite appears to predominate.

A total of 78 adult volunteers were enrolled into one of three Phase I clinical pharmacokinetic studies. A single-dose study revealed a plasma half-life of 7.1 to 9.5 hours at doses ranging from 150 to 1200 mg. A single-dose study of amprenavir in combination with zidovudine plus 3TC revealed no significant pharmacokinetic interactions; the most common adverse event was mild to moderate headache. A study comparing a hard gel capsule to a soft gel capsule, with or without food, demonstrated that the soft gel capsule exhibited a 25% higher C_{max} but similar AUC; administration of the soft gel formulation following a standard meal resulted in a 33% reduction in C_{max} and 13% reduction in AUC. Based on these findings, there are no restrictions regarding the timing of dosing in relation to food intake except that amprenavir should not be administered with a high-fat meal.

Amprenavir has a direct effect on HIV-1 concentration in semen. A total of 30 men—19 receiving amprenavir monotherapy and 11 receiving amprenavir/zidovudine/

lamivudine—underwent evaluation of HIV-1 in blood and semen. Most men (77%) had HIV-1 RNA levels in seminal plasma below the limit of quantification during therapy. Amprenavir alone suppressed HIV-1 RNA levels to less than 400 log copies per milliliter in seminal plasma in most cases, a direct demonstration of the antiretroviral effects of amprenavir in the male genital tract. However, eight men had measurable HIV-1 levels in seminal plasma at their last study visit, four with increasing levels, suggesting that replication of HIV-1 in the genital tract may have implications for the selection of resistant virus and sexual transmission of HIV-1.[40]

Amprenavir, like other approved protease inhibitors, is metabolized by the hepatic cytochrome P450 enzyme system, specifically CYP3A4.[41] Significant increases in amprenavir exposure have been reported when it is co-administered with ritonavir, similar to what has been reported when ritonavir is co-administered with indinavir, saquinavir, or nelfinavir.[42,43] Three randomized, two-sequence, mulitdose studies in uninfected volunteers has demonstrated that relative to amprenavir alone, ritonavir co-administration resulted in a 3.3- to 4.0-fold and a 10.84- to 14.25-fold increase in the geometric least-squares mean AUC and minimum concentration, respectively. The ritonavir 100 mg dose twice daily was the best tolerated dose studied. Higher ritonavir doses did not correlate with more amprenavir exposure, whereas higher amprenavir doses were associated with a modest increase in overall exposure.[44] (Fig. 16–3). Clinical studies utilizing the amprenavir/ritonavir combination have emphasized the amprenavir 600 mg/ritonavir 100 mg combined dose administered twice daily. Virologic responses in heavily pretreated patients has met with modest success. In one study of 68 multiple protease inhibitor-experienced patients, the proportion of subjects with HIV-1 RNA less than 200 copies per milliliter at 48 weeks was 36%, and the median decrease in HIV-1 RNA was 1.55 $\log_{10}$ copies per milliliter.[45] When amprenavir is co-administered with other protease inhibitors, plasma pharmacokinetic parameters relative to amprenavir are not consistent among protease inhibitors, nor are the changes consistent with potential interactions in CYP3A4 metabolism or P-glycoprotein transport. Saquinavir lowered the drug exposure, as measured by the AUC; indinavir raised it; and nelfinavir had no appreciable effect.[46] In one retrospective study of amprenavir co-administered with lopinavir/ritonavir, amprenavir concentrations were 49% to 83% lower than expected.[47] These data must be confirmed in a formal pharmacokinetic study; until that time, monitoring of drug concentrations when these agents are co-administered may be warranted.

Conversely, amprenavir exposure is significantly reduced when administered with agents that can induce CYP3A4, such as nevirapine, efavirenz, and rifampin. The effect with efavirenz and presumably with nevirapine is negated in the presence of ritonavir.[48]

▲ TOXICOLOGY

Genetic toxicity has been evaluated in the Ames salmonella/mammalian microsome mutagenicity assay, and no drug-related changes were shown at concentrations up to

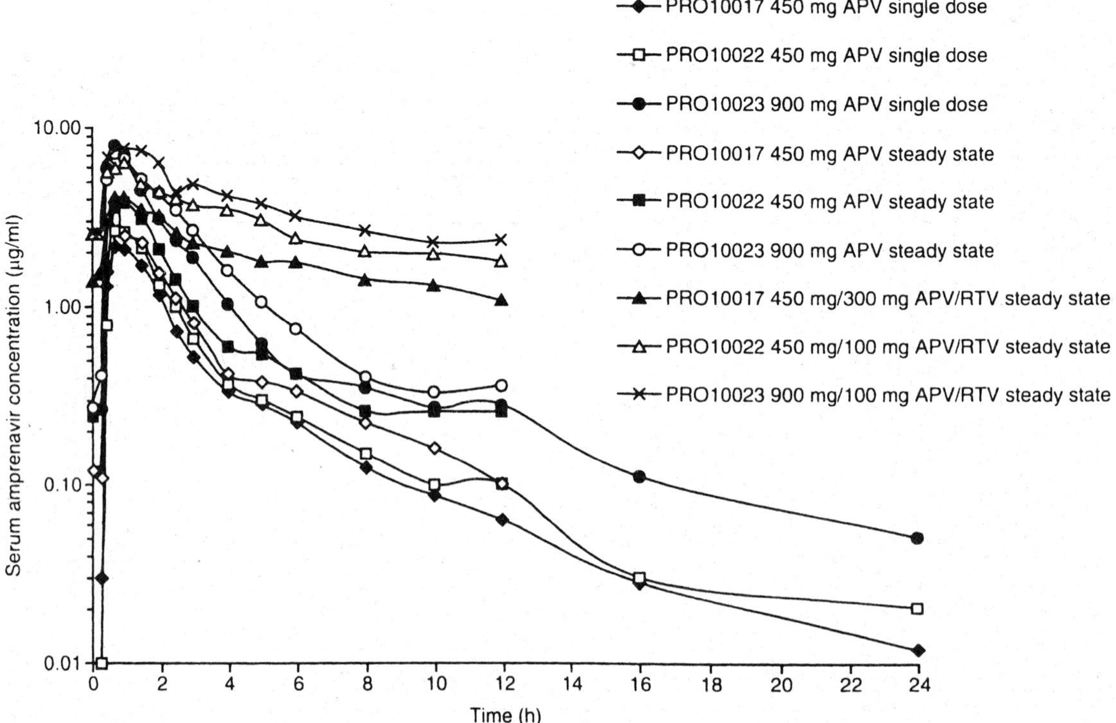

Figure 16–3. Median amprenavir serum concentration-time curves (AUCs) for the dosing regimens used in each study. APV, amprenavir; RTV, ritonavir. (From Sadler BM, Piliero PJ, Preston SL, et al. Pharmacokinetics and safety of amprenavir and ritonavir following multiple dose, co-administration to healthy volunteers. AIDS 15:1009, 2001, with permission.)

5000 g/plate. Animal toxicity studies were performed in mice, rats, cynomolgus monkeys, and beagle dogs. The oral median lethal dose was more than 3000 mg/kg in rats, 2214 mg/kg in male mice, and more than 3000 mg/kg in female mice. Longer-term toxicology studies showed that amprenavir is well tolerated for 6 months at doses up to 750 mg/kg/day in rats and up to 225 mg/kg/day in dogs. The overall results demonstrated a favorable safety profile except for mild gastrointestinal disturbances in the dog and some nonreversible clinical chemistry and microscopic liver changes in the rat, all occurring at adjusted doses considerably higher than what is expected to be achieved in humans.

▲ CLINICAL EFFICACY

The following clinical trials have provided the most clinical experience with amprenavir use.

PROA1002

PROA1002 is a Phase I/II trial established to evaluate the safety, pharmacokinetics, and antiviral activity of multiple doses of amprenavir alone or in combination with abacavir, a nucleoside reverse transcriptase inhibitor (NRTI), in subjects with HIV-1 infection. This is a multicenter, open-label study in protease inhibitor (PI)-naive adults that is being conducted in three phases. In phase A, subjects were enrolled into one of six dosing regimens, and treated for 29 days.

After successfully completing phase A, subjects were allowed to enter phase B, which consisted of combination therapy with zidovudine/3TC with or without abacavir until sufficient animal toxicology cover was generated to allow dosing with amprenavir for more than 4 weeks. At this time subjects were allowed to enter phase C, where amprenavir 1200 mg bid was added to the regimen of zidovudine/3TC with or without abacavir. Phase C is currently ongoing. Amprenavir peak concentrations and AUCs following the first dose and at steady state are similar, indicating that amprenavir does not induce its own metabolism and that the pharmacokinetics of amprenavir remain linear at these doses under steady-state conditions in humans.

In three subjects CSF and plasma samples were obtained 2 hours after the steady-state dose for which plasma pharmacokinetics were determined. The CSF/plasma ratio ranged from 0.45% to 1.30%. In one patient assigned to group III, the CSF concentration was 110.70 ng/ml (220 nM); however, this patient was taking cimetidine and drinking grapefruit juice, both of which are known to inhibit P450 metabolism. The pharmacokinetics of amprenavir and abacavir were unaffected when used in combination.

The baseline median plasma HIV-1 RNA concentrations for the treatment groups ranged from 4.19 to 5.08 $\log_{10}$ copies per milliliter, and the median CD4+ T-lymphocyte counts ranged from 254 to 305 cells per mm^3. As shown in Table 16–1, the response to therapy at 28 days favored patients enrolled in treatment groups III through VI.

In the group of patients receiving amprenavir 900 mg bid/abacavir 300 mg bid, five of six evaluable patients had a reduction in their plasma HIV-1 RNA concentration to below the limits of the assay detection (400 copies per milliliter). The preliminary assessment of this study is that amprenavir is generally well tolerated and, at doses greater than or equal to 900 mg bid with or without the addition of abacavir, there is an impressive surrogate marker response out to 28 days.[49,50]

PROA2001

PROA2001 was a 34-patient Phase II study set up to assess the safety and efficacy of amprenavir in combination with other PIs. Eligible adults with a CD4+ T-lymphocyte count of more than 200 cells per mm^3, an HIV-RNA less of more than 10,000 copies per milliliter, and no prior PI exposure were randomized to receive amprenavir 800 mg tid plus one of the following: saquinavir soft gel capsules 800 mg tid, indinavir 800 mg tid, or nelfinavir 750 mg tid. A fourth cohort received amprenavir alone for 3 weeks followed by the addition of zidovudine 300 mg bid/3TC 150 mg bid. The 4-week results are shown in Table 16–1. The median change from baseline in HIV-1 RNA was −2.57 (amprenavir/indinavir), −1.7 (amprenavir/nelfinavir), −2.53 (amprenavir/saquinavir), and −1.74 (amprenavir/PIs nucleosides) $\log_{10}$ copies per milliliter. Eight patients experienced virologic failure, five on dual PIs and three on the amprenavir/zidovudine/3TC combination. The protease I50V mutation characteristic of amprenavir resistance was not observed, although other key PI mutations were selected in four patients failing therapy.[51]

PROAB2002

PROAB2002 is a Phase II study established to investigate the safety, tolerability, pharmacodynamics, and antiretrovi-

▲ **Table 16–1.** PROA2001: CHANGE IN PLASMA HIV-1 RNA AFTER 4 WEEKS

Group	No. of Patients	Baseline Median HIV-1 RNA ($\log_{10}$ copies/ml)	Median Change from Baseline ($\log_{10}$ copies/ml)[a]
Amprenavir/saquinavir	3	4.45	− 2.53
Amprenavir/indinavir	5	5.14	− 2.57
Amprenavir/nelfinavir	4	4.88	− 3.18
Amprenavir/zidovudine with 3TC added after 3 weeks	4	4.26	− 1.74

[a]Lower limit of detection, < 40 copies per milliliter.

ral activity of multiple dosing of amprenavir in combination with zidovudine/3TC in subjects with HIV infection. A total of 84 subjects previously untreated with 3TC or PIs were enrolled in this multicenter study. Inclusion criteria included plasma HIV-1 RNA concentrations of 10,000 or more copies per milliliter and CD4+ T-lymphocyte counts higher than 150 cells per mm^3. All subjects received zidovudine 300 mg bid/3TC 150 mg bid; and they were randomized to also receive amprenavir at 900 mg bid, 1050 mg bid, or 1200 mg bid. A control group received placebo in place of amprenavir. After 12 weeks, placebo was replaced with amprenavir 1050 mg. The primary analysis was of the antiviral activity at week 12.

The baseline median plasma HIV-1 RNA concentration for the groups ranged from 4.7 to 5.1 $\log_{10}$ copies per milliliter, and the median CD4+ T-lymphocyte counts ranged from 312 to 422 cells per cubic millimeter. The changes in HIV-1 RNA levels were −1.6, −1.8, −1.9 $\log_{10}$ copies per milliliter for the respective amprenavir groups and −1.3 $\log_{10}$ copies per milliliter in the control group. There were no statistical differences noted in the antiviral response or CD4+ T-lymphocyte count changes between the amprenavir dosing groups. At week 60 only 50% of subjects assigned to receive amprenavir remained on amprenavir (owing to premature discontinuation). There were significantly more drug-related rashes ($P = 0.003$) in the highest amprenavir dosing cohorts and more drug discontinuations due to adverse effects in the highest-dose group ($P = 0.022$). Amprenavir-treated subjects experienced an increase in the total nonfasting cholesterol level at week 12 (+28 mg/dl) compared to that of the control group (+2 mg/dl) ($P < 0.001$). The preliminary conclusion of this study is that the triple combination of zidovudine/3TC/amprenavir was generally well tolerated and had excellent antiretroviral activity.[52] In another trial the dual combination of amprenavir/abacavir resulted in a 2.55 $\log_{10}$ copies per milliliter HIV-1 RNA decrease after 24 weeks of therapy with most patients maintaining an HIV-1 RNA level of less than 50 copies per milliliter.[53] In a trial of 39 PI- and 3TC-naive subjects, the combination amprenavir/abacavir/ zidovudine/lamivudine was given. At 48 weeks, 100% of subjects had plasma HIV-1 RNA levels below 400 copies per milliliter and 80% below 50 copies per milliliter.[54]

ACTG 347

ACTG 347 was a 24-week randomized, double-blind Phase II study of amprenavir monotherapy versus amprenavir/zidovudine/3TC in HIV-infected individuals. There were 92 subjects enrolled in the study, none of whom had previously received 3TC or a PI. The median baseline CD4+ T-lymphocyte count was 305 cells per mm^3, and the plasma HIV-1 RNA level was 4.49 $\log_{10}$ copies per milliliter. After a median of 88 days of therapy, it was noted that 15 monotherapy patients and 1 triple-therapy patient had experienced virology rebound or failure ($P = 0.0001$), and the monotherapy treatment arm was stopped. The triple-therapy treatment group continued as originally planned. For patients still receiving triple therapy at 24 weeks, the median decrease in the HIV-1 RNA level was 2.04 $\log_{10}$ copies per milliliter, and 63% of available subjects had HIV-1 RNA levels of less than 500 copies per milliliter. The study drugs were reasonably well tolerated, although a larger number of patients discontinued or modified their therapy in the triple-therapy arm than among those receiving amprenavir alone ($P = 0.04$).[55] Patients who failed the assigned therapy were offered treatment with indinavir/stavudine/3TC/nevirapine in a formal rollover study, ACTG 373. After 48 weeks on the new regimen, 59% of subjects had plasma HIV-1 RNA levels of less than 500 copies per milliliter, and the CD4+ T-lymphocyte counts increased by 94 cells per cubic millimeter. Subjects who had taken the amprenavir combination therapy were more likely to experience virologic failure on the new regimen than those who had taken amprenavir monotherapy (odds ratio 7.7; $P = 0.02$).[56] These data further reinforce the need for combination antiretroviral chemotherapy in all patients considering treatment and highlight the combined toxicities associated with specific therapies.

▲ **Table 16–2.** OUTCOMES OF RANDOMIZED TREATMENT THROUGH WEEK 24 IN STUDY PROAB3006

Outcome	Amprenavir (n = 254)	Indinavir (n = 250)
HIV RNA		
< 400 copies/ml	43%	53%
≥ 400 copies/ml	22%	18%
Discontinued		
Owing to adverse events	16%	8%
Owing to other reasons	14%	12%

PROAB3006

In the largest clinical trial to date involving amprenavir, 504 patients who were treatment-experienced but PI-naive were randomized in an open-label study comparing amprenavir 1200 mg twice daily with indinavir 800 mg three times daily plus at least two NRTIs. The median plasma HIV-1 RNA level was 3.93 $\log_{10}$ copies per milliliter, and the median CD4+ T-lymphocyte count was 399 cells per cubic millimeter. At 24 weeks the CD4+ T-lymphocyte increases were higher in the indinavir group; and in the intent-to-treat analysis, the proportion of patients with HIV-1 RNA levels of less than 400 copies per milliliter were 53% in the indinavir group and 43% in the amprenavir group. Neither difference reached statistical significance (Table 16–2). The responses appeared to be driven by an adverse event profile and discontinuations due to intolerance in the amprenavir arm.[57]

▲ ADVERSE EVENTS

Table 16–3 shows the relative frequency of reported adverse effects among patients receiving amprenavir in the early clinical trials. A common adverse event reported in Phase I pharmacokinetic studies was mild to moderate

▲ **Table 16-3.** FREQUENT TOXICITIES ATTRIBUTED TO
▲ AMPRENAVIR THERAPY

Adverse Event	Expected Rate (Preliminary)
Rash	~ 18% (rate of discontinuation 6%)
Diarrhea, loose stools	7–33%
Nausea, vomiting	10–33%
Asthenia, fatigue	0–10%
Headache	7–44%
Any serious event (grade 3, 4)	0–12%

headache. During the first 4 weeks of therapy in the PROA1002 study, diarrhea, nausea/vomiting, rash, fatigue, and headache were the most commonly reported adverse events potentially associated with amprenavir. Three subjects permanently discontinued the study medication: one with a severe rash requiring hospitalization, one with diarrhea and abdominal pain, and another with an unverified rash. Of the 42 subjects reported, 15 had no clinical adverse events. During the initial 12 weeks of combination therapy in the PROAB2002 study (zidovudine/3TC/amprenavir or placebo), clinical events in more than 10% of patients included gastrointestinal complaints (nausea, diarrhea, flatuence, vomiting), malaise and fatigue, headache, rash, and neuropathy. The most common adverse event reported in this trial was rash, occurring in 22 of 80 subjects. Six patients reported serious adverse events: rash (four), neutropenia (one), and anemia (one). Eight subjects developed hypertriglyceridemia, and one subject had hyperglycemia. The patients discontinued amprenavir treatment before 12 weeks, 9 because of adverse experiences. In the ACTG 347 study, the regimens were reasonably well tolerated. Three patients receiving amprenavir monotherapy and four receiving triple therapy experienced a severe laboratory abnormality, mainly elevations in hepatic transminase levels. Three patients discontinued the study medication because of a related adverse event.[55]

The overall rate of cutaneous adverse events has been approximately 18%. Most rashes have occurred between 7 and 12 days after initiating therapy. At least one case of severe dermatitis has been reported. Anecdotally, some patients have successfully continued to take amprenavir despite a mild rash, and others have been rechallenged after stopping the drug, with no recurrence of rash.

The overall experience in early trials has been that severe (grade 3 or 4) adverse effects potentially attributable to amprenavir have been reported in about 3% of patients. Of 270 patients receiving the drug in nine studies, only 15 (6%) discontinued therapy because of possible side effects.

▲ RESISTANCE

Despite the initial enthusiasm that HIV-1 PIs would be less vulnerable to the development of antiretroviral resistance, in vitro and in vivo evidence clearly demonstrates examples of mutations in the protease gene that confer significant resistance to each of the available PIs. In fact, in vitro viral passages in the presence of multiple PIs have resulted in the selection of isolates cross-resistant to five agents, including amprenavir.[58] However, most viral variants produced in this type of experiment express complex patterns of individual resistance-conferring mutations such that they remain fully or partially susceptible to some PI compounds while being completely resistant to others. When the HIV-1 strains are passaged through T-lymphocyte lines in the presence of increasing concentrations of amprenavir, a sequential accumulation of mutations in the protease gene (L10F, M46I, I47V, I50V) has been characterized that can confer as much as 100-fold reductions in sensitivity.[59]

The I50V mutation appears to be uniquely selected by compounds in the sulfonamide PI class. Unlike the other three mutations listed above, I50V leads to reduced sensitivity to amprenavir when it is the sole substitution in recombinant protease enzyme experiments. This single substitution results in two- to threefold reductions in sensitivity, and triple protease mutants (M46I, I47V, I50V) demonstrate larger reductions in sensitivity (14- to 20-fold).[58] Whereas the single substitution at position 50 reduces the proteolytic efficiency of the enzyme, the addition of mutations at positions 46 and 47 against the background of I50V appears to compensate for this disadvantage, enabling the virus to replicate more easily in the presence of amprenavir. Sulfonamide-resistant variants may remain sensitive to other clinically available PIs.[59] Based on in vitro assays, combinations of PIs including amprenavir in vitro may have the potential to delay the selection of PI-resistant strains.[60] In ACTG 347, viral rebound during monotherapy was associated with protease genotypic mutations, of which 21% were I50V, the mutation unique to amprenavir.[61] Further clinical experience with amprenavir is necessary to determine the significance of these observations.

▲ DRUG INTERACTIONS

One of the major clinical drawbacks with the currently available HIV-1 PIs is the occurrence of potentially dangerous drug interactions related to shared cytochrome P450 enzyme metabolism. Enzyme induction studies in rats and dogs demonstrated nonspecific responses in diverse cytochrome enzymes but no evidence of significant inhibition or induction of CYP3A4, the isoenzyme involved in many clinically relevant drug interactions, such as when certain drugs are co-administered with ritonavir. In experiments involving human liver microsomes, amprenavir has an inhibitory effect on CYP3A4 (K_i 0.6 mM) that is greater than that of saquinavir and slightly less than that of ritonavir. A side-by-side study with other PIs in human liver microsomes showed a rank order of CYP3A4 inhibition of ritonavir >> indinavir = nelfinavir = amprenavir > saquinavir. In vitro studies predict that co-administration of ritonavir and amprenavir can potentiate the concentration of amprenavir, but there is no clinical information about this combination.[62] CYP3A4 is also the primary isozyme responsible for the initial metabolism of amprenavir in human liver microsomes. Because amprenavir inhibits CYP3A4, drugs that are metabolized by that enzyme may have altered pharmacokinetics, and some should be avoided

▲ **Table 16–4.** IMPORTANT DRUG INTERACTIONS WITH
▲ AMPRENAVIR

Drug(s)	Comment
Astemizole, cisapride, midazolam, terfenadine, triazolam	Contraindicated because of potential toxicity resulting from increased plasma concentrations
Ketoconzale	AUC increases 32% for amprenavir and 44% for ketoconazole; no dosage adjustment required
Rifabutin	Rifabutin levels expected to increase and amprenavir to decrease; avoid if possible; dose adjustment may be necessary if used concomitantly
Rifampin	AUC of amprenavir decreases by 81%; the drugs should not be used concomitantly
Zidovudine	AUC increases 31% for zidovudine; no dosage adjustment required
Indinavir	AUC increases 64%, C_{max} 31% for amprenavir; dosage adjustment may not be necessary; well tolerated
Saquinavir	No pharmacokinetic data available but well tolerated
Nelfinavir	No pharmacokinetic data available but well tolerated
Efavirenz	AUC of amprenavir decreases by 30%, efavirenz AUC increases by 15%; no dosage adjustments required

AUC, area under the time-concentration curve.

because of potential serious toxicity, such as terfenadine, astemizile, cisapride, triazolam, and midazolam. Amprenavir also inhibits CYP2C19 but does not inhibit CYP1A2, 2C9, 2D6, or 2E1 activities ($IC_{50} > 200$ mM).

Formal drug interaction studies have examined the pharmacokinetic interaction between amprenavir and ketoconazole, rifabutin, rifampin, clarithromycin, zidovudine/3TC, abacavir, indinavir, saquinavir, nelfinavir, and efavirenz. These findings are summarized below and outlined in Table 16–4.

Ketoconazole

Ketoconazole inhibits CYP3A4. A single-dose, three-period crossover study was designed that examined the pharmacokinetics of both ketoconazole and amprenavir when co-administered. Twelve healthy subjects received amprenavir 1200 mg, ketoconazole 400 mg or both. The AUC and clearance values were different for both amprenavir and ketoconazole following co-administration. The AUC values increased 32% for amprenavir and 44% for ketoconazole. At the doses studied, the two drugs were equally effective in inhibiting CYP3A4, as measured by the erythromycin breath test. These data suggest that the drugs compete for a common metabolic site, most likely CYP3A4 in the liver and possibly the gastrointestinal tract.[63] The magnitude of the change in pharmacokinetic parameters when these drugs are used together does not suggest that a dosage adjustment is required.

Rifampin/Rifabutin

Twelve healthy volunteers were administered amprenavir 1200 mg bid for 4 days followed by rifampin 600 mg or rifabutin 300 mg daily. An erythromycin breath test was performed at baseline, 2 hours after the last dose of amprenavir, and after 1 and 2 weeks of rifampin and rifabutin. The results showed that CYP3A4 is inhibited by amprenavir and induced by rifampin and rifabutin. Eight of twelve subjects taking rifabutin reported flu-like symptoms, an uncommon adverse event when rifamycins are administered alone.[50] If possible, rifabutin and rifampin should not be co-administered with amprenavir. In the event these drugs must be used together, the dosage of rifabutin or rifampin should be reduced, perhaps as much as 50%. Because rifampin reduces the amprenavir AUC by 81%, these drugs should not be administered together.[64]

Clarithromycin

Twelve healthy volunteers were administered amprenavir 1200 mg, clarithromycin 500 mg, or both every 12 hours for a total of seven doses. The erythromycin breath test was used to characterize CYP3A4 activity. The results showed that amprenavir was a more potent inhibitor of CYP3A4 than clarithromycin alone, and that the amprenavir/clarithromycin combination inhibited CYP3A4 no differently than amprenavir alone.[65]

Zidovudine/3TC

Single-dose studies with amprenavir and zidovudine/3TC were performed in 40 HIV-infected volunteers. The pharmacokinetics of amprenavir were not affected by co-administration with zidovudine/3TC. The AUC and C_{max} for zidovudine were increased 31% and 40%, respectively, whereas for 3TC the same parameters decreased 9% and 16%. Because of the only modest increase in exposure to zidovudine, no dosage adjustment appears to be necessary when co-administering amprenavir and zidovudine/3TC.[66]

Abacavir

In patients enrolled in the combination amprenavir/abacavir treatment arm of study PROA1002, both drugs were analyzed pharmacokinetically over a period of 1 month. No significant interactions were noted in the pharmacokinetic parameters.[67]

Indinavir

Single-dose pharmacokinetic analyses were performed on 12 subjects who were co-administered amprenavir 800 mg/indinavir 800 mg. The C_{max} and AUC for amprenavir increased by 31% and 64%, respectively. No appreciable difference from estimates based on historical controls was noted for indinavir esthesias. Three patients complained of circumoral paresthesias. These data support multiple-dose studies of these drugs with no dosage adjustments to either drug.[68] A preliminary analysis of a small cohort treated with amprenavir 800 mg tid/indinavir 800 mg tid revealed a robust antiviral response (HIV-1 RNA level at 4 weeks: $-2.57 \log_{10}$ copies per milliliter) that was well tolerated in five patients.[46]

Saquinavir (Soft Gel Capsules)

No formal pharmacokinetic analyses have taken place regarding saquinavir (soft gel capsules). However, in a preliminary analysis of a small cohort treated with saquinavir 800 mg tid/amprenavir 800 mg tid, there was a $-2.53 \log_{10}$ copies per milliliter change in the HIV-1 RNA level after 4 weeks compared to baseline. It was well tolerated in three patients.[46]

Efavirenz

The nonnucleoside reverse transcriptase inhibitor (NNRTI) efavirenz is a known inducer of P450-mediated metabolism. It reduces the amprenavir AUC by 36%. The effect of amprenavir on efavirenz is negligible. No dosage adjustments are formally recommended at this time.[57] When amprenavir is co-administered with ritonavir, the metabolic induction effect of efavirenz is not observed. Although not formally studied, a similar finding is expected with nevirapine.[48]

▲ RECOMMENDATIONS FOR USE

Amprenavir in combination with other antiretroviral agents is indicated for the treatment of HIV-1 infection in individuals more than 4 years of age. Because of the large pill burden and side effect profile, amprenavir is rarely used as the first drug of choice for mono-PI therapy. Rather, the drug is almost always used as part of a low-dose ritonavir-"boosted" regimen. An amprenavir dose of 1200 mg bid is recommended when administered as a single agent; when co-administered with ritonavir 100 mg, doses as low as 600 mg can be effective and are better tolerated. A prodrug, referred to as fos-amprenavir or GW908/VX175, is in development and offers substantial advantages in terms of pill size and burden. Amprenavir is being used primarily in treatment-experienced patients, in part due to its relatively unique resistance profile. Resistance testing helps identify clinical situations where amprenavir works best. Although amprenavir is potent, it is not as well tolerated as other PIs. However, when co-administered with ritonavir, tolerability may be improved and the induction effect of the NNRTIs nevirapine and efavirenz is negated. Co-administration with other PIs results in unpredictable pharmacokinetic interactions, suggesting that drug concentration monitoring may be indicated. The introduction of fos-amprenavir, expected by 2003, is likely to be useful for individuals infected with HIV-1 that require a PI-based treatment regimen.

REFERENCES

1. Concorde Coordinating Committee. MRC/ANRS randomized double-blind controlled trial of immediate and deferred zidovudine in symptom-free HIV infection. Lancet 343:871, 1994.
2. Volberding PA, Lagakos SW, Grimes JM, et al. A comparison of immediate with deferred zidovudine therapy for asymptomatic HIV-infected adults with CD4 cell counts of 500 or more per cubic millimeter: AIDS Clinical Trials Group. N Engl J Med 333:401, 1995.
3. Hammer SM, Katzenstein DA, Hughes MD, et al. A trial comparing nucleoside monotherapy with combination therapy in HIV-infected adults with CD4 counts from 200-500 per cubic millimeter. N Engl J Med 335:1081, 1996.
4. Katzenstein DA, Hammer SM, Hughes MD, et al. The relation of virologic and immunologic markers to clinical outcomes after nucleoside therapy in HIV-infected adults with 200-500 CD4 cells per cubic millimeter. N Engl J Med 335:1091, 1996.
5. Delta Coordinating Committee. A randomised double-blind controlled trial comparing combinations of zidovudine plus didanosine or zalcitabine with zidovudine alone in HIV-infected individuals. Lancet 348:283, 1996.
6. Sarvolatz LD, Winslow DL, Collins G, et al. Zidovudine alone or in combination with didanosine or zalcitabine in HIV-infected patients with acquired immunodeficiency syndrome or fewer than 200 CD4 cells per cubic millimeter. N Engl J Med 335:1099, 1996.
7. Eron JJ, Benoit SL, Jemsek J, et al. Treatment with lamivudine, zidovudine, or both in HIV-positive patients with 200-500 CD4+ cells per cubic centimeter: North American HIV Working Party. N Engl J Med 333:1662, 1995.
8. Katlama, C, Ingrand D, Loveday C, et al. Safety and efficacy of lamivudine-zidovudine combination therapy in antiretroviral-naive patients: a randomized controlled comparison with zidovudine monotherapy. JAMA 276:111, 1996.
9. Staszewski S, Loveday C, Picazo JJ, et al. Safety and efficacy of lamivudine-zidovudine combination therapy in zidovudine-experienced patients: a randomized controlled comparison with zidovudine monotherapy: Lamivudine European HIV Working Group. JAMA 276:111, 1996.
10. Bartlett JA, Benoit SL, Johnson VA, et al. Lamivudine plus zidovudine compared with zalcitabine plus zidovudine in patients with HIV infection. Ann Intern Med 125:161, 1996.
11. Ratner L, Hasetine W, Patarca R, et al. Complete nucleotide sequencing of the AIDS virus, HTLV-III. Nature 313:277, 1985.
12. Richards AD, Roberts R, Dunn BM, et al. Effective blocking of HIV-1 protease activity by characteristic inhibitors of aspartic protease. FEBS Lett 247:113, 1989.
13. Kohl NE, Emini DA, Schleif LF, et al. Active human immunodeficiency virus protease is required for viral infectivity. Proc Natl Acad Sci USA 85:4686, 1988.
14. Navia MA, Fitzgerald PM, McKeever BM, et al. Three dimensional structure of aspartyl protease from HIV-1. Nature 337:615, 1989.
15. Wlodawer A, Miller M, Jaskolski M, et al. Conserved folding in retroviral proteinases: crystal structure of a synthetic HIV-1 protease. Science 245:616, 1989.
16. De Clercq E. Toward improved anti-HIV chemotherapy: therapeutic strategies for intervention with HIV infections. J Med Chem 38:2491, 1995.
17. Huff JR. HIV protease: a novel chemotherapeutic target for AIDS. J Med Chem 34:2305, 1991.
18. West MI, Farlie DP. Targeting HIV-1 protease: a test of drug-design methodologies. Trends Pharmacol Sci 16:67, 1995.
19. Carr A, Cooper DA. HIV protease inhibitors. AIDS 10(suppl A):S151, 1996.
20. Roberts MM, Martin JA, Kinchington D, et al. Rational design of peptide-base HIV proteinase inhibitors. Science 248:358, 1990.
21. Gulick RM, Mellors JW, Havlir D, et al. Treatment with a combination of indinavir, zidovudine, and lamivudine in HIV infected adults with prior anti-retroviral use. N Engl J Med 337:734, 1997.
22. Cameron DW, Heath-Chiozzi M, Danners S, et al. Randomized placebo-controlled trial of ritonavir in advanced HIV-1 disease. Lancet 351:543, 1998.
23. Collier AC, Coombs RW, Schoenfeld DA, et al. Treatment of human immunodeficiency virus infection with saquinavir, zidovudine, and zalcitabine: AIDS Clinical Trials Group. N Engl J Med 334:1011, 1996.

24. Saag MS, Tebas P, Sension M, et al. Randomized, double-blind comparison of two nelfinavir doses plus nucleosides in HIV-infected patients (Agouron study 511). AIDS 15:1971, 2001.
25. Hammer SM, Squires KE, Hughes MD, et al. A controlled trial of two nucleoside analogues plus indinavir in persons with human immunodeficiency virus infection and CD4 cell counts of 200 per cubic millimeter or less. N Engl J Med 337:725, 1997.
26. Carpenter CC, Fischl MA, Hammer SM, et al. Antiretroviral therapy for HIV infection in 1998: updated recommendations of the International AIDS Society—USA panel. JAMA 280:78,1998.
27. Feinberg MD, Carpenter C, Fauci AS, et al. Guidelines for the use of antiretroviral agents in HIV-infected adults and adolescents. Ann Intern Med 128:1079, 1998.
28. Kim EE, Baker CT, Dwyer MD, et al. Crystal structure of HIV-1 protease in complex with VX-478, a potent and orally bioavailable inhibitor of the enzyme. J Am Chem Soc 117:1181, 1995.
29. Rao BG, Kim EE, Murcko MA. Calculation of solvation and binding free energy differences between VX-478 and its analogs by free energy perturbation and AMSOL methods. J Comput Aided Mol Des 10:23, 1996.
30. Navia MA, Murcko MA. Use of structural information in drug design. Curr Opin Struct Biol 2:202, 1992.
31. Cushman DW, Ondetti MA. History of the design of captopril and related inhibitors of angiotensin. Hypertension 17:589, 1991.
32. Painter GR, St Clair MH, Demiranda P, et al. An overview of the preclinical development of the HIV protease inhibitor VX-478 (141W94). In: Abstracts of the 2nd National Conference on Human Retroviruses and Related Infections, Washington DC, 1995, abstract LB5.
33. Painter GR, Ching S, Reynolds D, et al. 141W94. Drugs Future 21:347, 1996.
34. St Clair MH, Millard J, Rooney J, et al. In vitro antiviral activity of 141W94 (VX-478) in combination with other antretroviral agents. Antiviral Res 29:53, 1996.
35. Arasteh K, Baranowsi K, Knecten H, et al. Preliminary results of antiretroviral activity and pharmacokinetics of three doses of SC-52151 by decreasing its cellular uptake. In: Abstracts of the 2nd European Antiviral Conference, Glasgow, 1994.
36. Sommadossi JP, Schinazi RF, McMillan A, et al. A human serum glycoprotein profoundly affects antiviral activity of the protease inhibitor SC-52151 by decreasing its cellular uptake. In: Abstracts of the 2nd National Conference on Human Retroviruses, Washington, DC, 1995, abstract LB4.
37. Fischl MA, Richman DD, Flexner C, et al. Phase I study of two formulations and dose schedules of SC-52151, a protease inhibitor. In: Abstracts of the 2nd National Conference on Human Retroviruses, Washington, DC, 1995, abstract 186.
38. Livingstone DJ, Pazhanisamy S, Porter DJT, et al. Weak binding of VX-478 to human plasma proteins and implications for anti-human immunodeficiency virus therapy. J Infect Dis 172:1238, 1995.
39. Sereni D. Antiviral activity of amprenavir in combination with zidovudine/3TC in plasma and CSF in patients with HIV infection. J Neurovirol 4:365, 1998.
40. Eron JJ, Smeaton LM, Fiscus SA, et al. The effects of protease inhibitor therapy on human immunodeficiency virus type 1 levels in semen (AIDS Clinical Trials Group Protocol 850). J Infect Dis 181:1622, 1999.
41. Decker C, Laitinen C, Bridson G, et al. Metabolism of amprenavir in liver microsomes: role of CYP3A4 inhibition for drug interaction. J Pharm Sci 87:803, 1998.
42. Merry C, Barry MG, Mulcahy F, et al. Saquinavir pharmacokinetics alone and in combination with ritonavir in HIV-infected patients. AIDS 11:F29, 1997.
43. Van Heswijk RP, Veldkamp AI, Hoetelmans RM, et al. The steady-state plasma pharmacokinetics of indinavir alone and in combination with low dose of ritonavir in twice daily dosing regmens in HIV-1 infected individuals. AIDS 13:F95, 1999.
44. Sadler BM, Piliero PJ, Preston SL, et al. Pharmacokinetics and safety of amprenavir and ritonavir following multiple dose, co-administration to healthy volunteers. AIDS 15:1009, 2001.
45. Katlama C, Schneider L, Agher R, et al. Ritonavir (RTV)/amprenavir (APV) combination therapy in HIV infected patients who failed several protease inhibitor regimens. In: Abstracts of the 1st IAS Conference on HIV Pathogenesis and Treatment, Buenos Aires, 2001, abstract 673.
46. Sadler B, Gillotin C, Lou Y, et al. Pharmacokinetic study of human immunodeficiency virus protease inhibitors used in combination with amprenavir. Antimicros Agents Chemother 45:3663, 2001.
47. Lamotte C, Peytavin G, Duval X, et al. Amprenavir (APV) plasma concentrations are dramatically decreased by the association with ABT378/R in HIV-infected patients (PTS). In: Abstracts of the 1st IAS Conference on HIV Pathogenesis and Treatment, Buenos Aires, 2001, abstract 334.
48. Piscitelli S, Bechtel C, Sadler B, Falloon J. The addition of a second protease inhibitor eliminates amprenavir-efavirenz drug interactions and increases plasma amprenavir concentrations. In: Abstracts of the 7th Conference on Retroviruses and Opportunistic Infections, San Francisco, 2000, abstract 7b.
49. Schooley RT, 141W94 International Study Group. Preliminary data on the safety and antiviral efficacy of the novel protease inhibitor 141W94 in HIV-infected patients with 150-400 CD4+ cells/mm^3. In: Abstracts of the 36th Interscience Conference on Antimicrobial Agents and Chemotherapy, New Orleans, 1996, abstract LB07a.
50. Schooley RT, 141W94 International Study Group: Preliminary data from a phase I/II study on the safety and antiviral efficacy of the combination of 141W94 plus 1592U89 in HIV-infected patients with 150-400 CD4+ cells/mm^3. In: Abstracts of the 4th Conference on Retroviruses and Opportunistic Infections, Washington, DC. Alexandria, VA, Westover Management Group, 1997, abstract LB3.
51. Eron J, Haubrich R, Lang W, et al. A phase II trail of dual protease inhibitor therapy: amprenavir in combination with indinavir, nelfinavir, or saquinavir. J Acquir Immun Defic Syndr 26:458, 2001.
52. Haubrich R, Thompson M, Schooley R, et al. A phase II safety and efficacy study of amprenavir in combination with zidovudine and lamivudine in HIV-infected patients with limited antiretroviral experience. Amprenavir PROAB2002 Study Team. AIDS 13:2411, 1999.
53. Kelleher D, Mellors J, Lederman M, et al. Activity of abacavir combined with protease inhibitors in therapy naive patients. In: Abstracts of the 12th World AIDS Conference, Geneva, 1998, abstract 12210.
54. Kost RG, Hurley A, Zhang L, Vesana M, et al. Open-label phase II trial of amprenavir, abacavir, and fixed-dose zidovudine/lamivudine in newly and chronically infected HIV-1-infected patients. J Acquir Immunodefic Syndr 26:332, 2001.
55. Murphy R, Gulick RM, DeGrottola V, et al. Treatment with amprenavir alone or amprenavir with zidovudine and lamivudine in adults with human immunodeficiency virus infection. J Infect Dis 179:808, 1999.
56. Gulick RM, Smeaton LM, D'Aquila RT, et al. Indinavir, nevirapine, stavudine, and lamivudine for human immunodeficiency virus, amprenavir-experienced subjects: AIDS Clinical Trials Group Protocol 373. J Infect Dis 183:715, 2001.
57. Physicians Desk Reference. Montvale, NJ, Medical Economics, 2001, p. 1338.
58. Tisdale M, Myers RE, Maschera B, et al. Cross-resistance analysis of HIV-1 varients individually selected for resistance to five different protease inhibitors. Antimicrob Agents Chemother 39:1704, 1995.
59. Partaledis JA, Yamagouchi K, Tisdale M, et al. In vitro selection and characterization of HIV-1 isolates with reduced sensitivity to hydroxyethylaminosulfonamide inhibitors of HIV-1 aspartyl protease. J Virol 69:5228, 1995.
60. Pazhanisamy S, Stuver CM, Cullinam AB, et al. Kinetic characterization of HIV-1 protease-resistant variants. J Biol Chem 271:17979, 1996.
61. DePasquale M, Murphy R, Kurtizkes D, et al. Resistance during early virologic rebound on amprenavir plus zidovudine plus lamivudine or amprenavir monotherapy in ACTG protocol 347 [abstract Antiviral Ther 3(suppl 1):50, 1998.
62. Kempf DJ, March KC, Kumar G, et al. Pharmacokinetic enhancement of inhibitors of HIV-1 protease by coadministration with ritonavir. Antimicrob Agents Chemother 41:654, 1997.
63. Polk RE, Israel DS, Pastor A, et al. Pharmacokinetic (PK) interaction between ketoconazole (KCZ) and the HIV protease inhibitor 141W94 after single dose administration to volunteers. In: Abstracts of the 37th Interscience Conference on Antimicrobial Agents and Chemotherapy, Toronto, 1997, abstract A-61.
64. Polk RE, Israel DS, Patron R, et al. Effects of the HIV-1 protease inhibitor, 141W94 and rifampin (RFM) and rifabutin (RFB) on P450 (CYP) 3A4 activity as measured by the erythromycin breath test (ERMBT). In: Abstracts of the 35th Annual Meeting of the Infectious Disease Society of America, San Francisco, 1997, abstract 236.

65. Polk RE, Israel DS, Pastor A, et al. Effects of 141W94 and clarithromycin (CLR) on P450 (CYP) 3A4 activity as measured by the erythromycin breath test. In: Abstracts of the 35th Annual Meeting of the Infectious Disease Society of America, San Francisco, 1997, abstract 237.
66. Sadler BM, Wald JA, Lou Y, et al. The single-dose pharmacokinetics of 141W94, zidovudine, and lamivudine when administered alone and in two- and three-drug combinations. In: Abstracts of the Sixth European Conference on Clinical Aspects and Treatment of HIV Infection, Hamburg, 1997, abstract 257.
67. McDowell JA, Sadler BM, Millard J, et al. Evaluation of potential pharmacokinetic (PK) drug interaction between 141W94 and 1592U89 in HIV+ patients. In: Abstracts of the 37th Interscience Conference on Antimicrobial Agents and Chemotherapy, Toronto, 1997, abstract A-62.
68. Sadler BM, Eron J, Wakeford J, et al. Pharmacokinetics of 141W94 and indinavir (IDV) after single-dose coadministration in HIV-positive volunteers. In: Abstracts of the 37th Interscience Conference on Antimicrobial Agents and Chemotherapy, Toronto, 1997, abstract A-56.

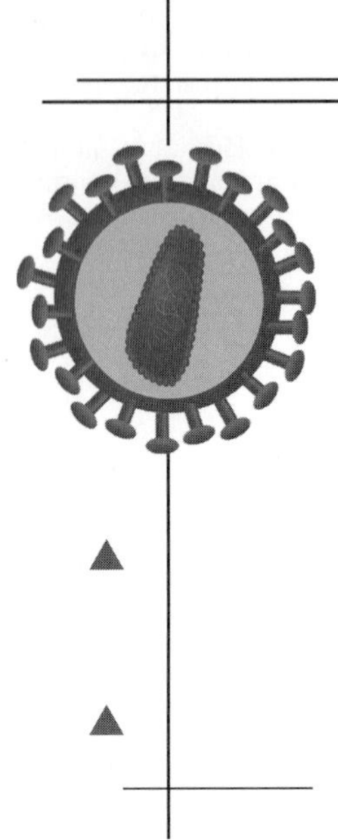

CHAPTER 17

Lopinavir

Steven C. Johnson, MD
Daniel R. Kuritzkes, MD

Lopinavir (formerly known as ABT-378) is the first of the "second-generation" protease inhibitors to be approved for clinical use. Principles of rational drug design and structure-based design were used to select a compound that is active against ritonavir-resistant isolates of human immunodeficiency virus type 1 (HIV-1). In addition, lopinavir is the first approved antiretroviral agent specifically co-formulated with ritonavir, a protease inhibitor that inhibits lopinavir metabolism by the 3A4 isozyme of cytochrome P_{450}. The combination of lopinavir and ritonavir is marketed under the trade name Kaletra. Each Kaletra capsule contains 133.3 mg of lopinavir and 33.3 mg of ritonavir. An oral solution, containing 80 mg of lopinavir and 20 mg of ritonavir per milliliter, is also available. The use of lopinavir/ritonavir in combination with other antiretroviral agents [nucleoside (NRTIs) and nonnucleoside reverse transcriptase inhibitors (NNRTIs)] has produced excellent results in both antiretroviral-naive and antiretroviral-experienced patients.

CHEMICAL STRUCTURE

Lopinavir is a *C2* symmetrical peptidomimetic inhibitor of HIV-1 protease. Chemically, the drug is designated {1S-[1R*, (R*), 3R*, 4R*]}-*N*-(4-{[(2,6 dimethylphenoxy)acetyl] amino}-3-hydroxy-5-phenyl-1-(phenylmethyl)pentyl)tetrahydro-α-(1-methylethyl)-2-oxo-1(2H)-pyrimidineacetamide (Fig. 17–1). It has a molecular weight of 628.80. Development of lopinavir was based on x-ray crystallographic studies of the interaction between the first-generation inhibitor ritonavir and HIV-1 protease.[1] Binding of ritonavir to protease is strongly enhanced by interactions between the isopropylthiazolyl side chain of the P3 peripheral heterocyclic group of the molecule and the substrate-binding pocket of protease. Mutations in HIV-1 protease that lead to substitution of alanine, phenylalanine, or tyrosine for the wild-type valine at amino acid 82 disrupt these interactions, leading to a lower affinity of drug binding. To minimize the effect of resistance mutations on protease inhibitor binding, modifications were introduced to the ritonavir molecule that reduced the importance of hydrophobic interactions with the side chain or Val^{82}. Replacement of the isopropylthiazolyl P3 group with a cyclic urea, and replacement of the P2′ (thiazolyl) methoxycarbonyl moiety with a dimethylphenoxyactyl group produced lopinavir.

IN VITRO ACTIVITY

Lopinavir is a potent inhibitor of HIV-1. The drug inhibits 93% of wild-type protease activity at a concentration of 0.5 nM and binds with a K_i of 1.3 pM.[1] Inhibition of HIV-1 protease by lopinavir is highly specific compared to inhibition of mammalian aspartyl proteases such as renin, cathepsin D, and cathepsin E. Lopinavir is approximately 10 times more potent than ritonavir against wild-type virus. In the absence of human serum, the mean 50% effective concentration (EC_{50}) of lopinavir ranges from 10 to 27 nM (0.006 to 0.017 μg/ml) against HIV-1 laboratory strains and from 4 to 11 nM (0.003 to 0.007 μg/ml) against several clinical strains. The presence of 50% human serum increases the mean EC_{50} of lopinavir against HIV-1 laboratory strains by 7- to 11-

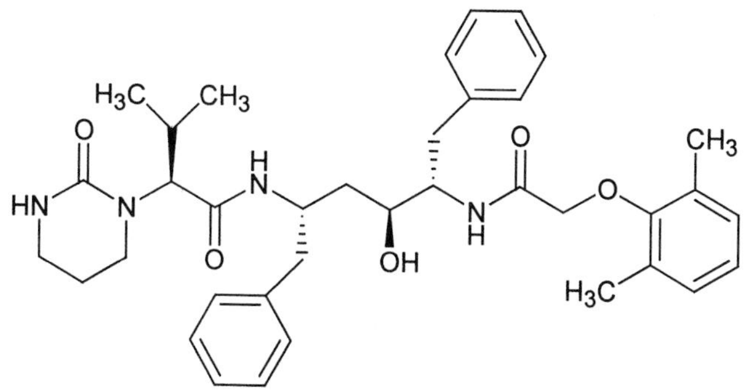

Figure 17–1. Structural formula of lopinavir.

fold, resulting in values that range from 65 to 289 nM (0.04 to 0.18 μg/ml).[2]

▲ PHARMACOKINETICS

When administered by itself, lopinavir achieves relatively modest plasma concentrations due to rapid metabolism by the 3A4 isozyme of cytochrome P_{450} (CYP3A4). The area under the curve (AUC) for lopinavir is greatly increased by concomitant administration of ritonavir, which inhibits the metabolism of lopinavir by CYP3A4 with a K_i of 0.013 μM.[3] In healthy volunteers, simultaneous administration of a 400-mg dose of lopinavir together with 50 mg of ritonavir increases the lopinavir AUC 77-fold over that achieved with lopinavir alone.[1] The AUC of lopinavir varies with the dose of the drug and the dose of concomitant ritonavir. In HIV-infected subjects, the AUC achieved when lopinavir 400 mg bid is administered with ritonavir 100 mg bid is 34% higher than the AUC achieved with lopinavir/ritonavir doses of 200/100 mg bid.[4]

The half-life of lopinavir over a 12-hour dosing interval is approximately 5 to 6 hours when the drug is administered together with ritonavir. A multiple-dose pharmacokinetic study in HIV-seropositive subjects using the 400/100 mg dose of lopinavir/ritonavir determined that at steady state the peak plasma concentration (C_{max}) of lopinavir is 9.6 ± 4.4 μg/ml, and the time to peak concentration (T_{max}) is approximately 4 hours. Administration of a single dose of lopinavir/ritonavir together with a meal with moderate fat content increases the AUC and C_{max} by 48% and 23%, respectively, compared to administration in the fasted state.[2] The mean steady-state trough concentration (C_{trough}) of lopinavir in patients receiving the 400/100 mg dose is 5.5 ± 4.0 μg/ml, which exceeds the protein-binding-adjusted IC_{50} for wild-type isolates of HIV-1 by more than 30-fold.[2,4] The 100 mg bid dose of ritonavir achieves drug levels that are less than 7% of those achieved with the standard dose of ritonavir (600 mg bid). Therefore the observed in vivo activity of the lopinavir/ritonavir co-formulation is attributable almost exclusively to the lopinavir component.

Lopinavir is 98% to 99% bound to plasma proteins, primarily to α_1-acid glycoprotein and albumin. The extent of protein binding, which is constant throughout the therapeutic range, is similar in seronegative volunteers and HIV-infected subjects. The drug is extensively metabolized by CYP3A4. Although ritonavir is a potent inhibitor of CYP3A4, it also induces other P_{450} isozymes, including those responsible for its own metabolism. As a result, lopinavir trough concentrations decline somewhat over time, reaching a steady state within 10 to 16 days. Following a 400/100 mg dose of lopinavir/ritonavir, approximately 10% of administered lopinavir can be recovered from urine and 83% from feces; approximately 22% of the drug is excreted unchanged.[2] After multiple doses less than 3% of lopinavir is excreted unchanged in the urine. Although specific clinical data regarding lopinavir disposition in patients with renal or hepatic impairment are not yet available, the renal clearance of lopinavir is negligible and significant changes in the clearance of the drug in the setting of renal insufficiency are not likely. However, considering the importance of hepatic metabolism in the elimination of this drug, the drug should be administered cautiously to patients with significant liver disease.

The pharmacokinetics of lopinavir/ritonavir have been studied in children aged 6 months to 12 years. A lopinavir dose of 230 mg/m^2 combined with a ritonavir dose of 57.5 mg/m^2 provides lopinavir plasma concentrations similar to those observed in adults receiving the 400/100 mg bid dose of lopinavir/ritonavir, resulting in a mean steady-state AUC of 72.6 ± 31.1 μg/hr/ml, a mean C_{max} of 8.2 ± 2.9 μg/ml, a mean C_{trough} of 4.7 ± 2.9 μg/ml, and a mean C_{min} of 3.4 ± 2.1 μg/ml.[2,5] If co-administered with nevirapine, an inducer of CYP3A4, lopinavir concentrations are reduced. In the presence of nevirapine, a lopinavir/ritonavir dose of 300/75 mg/m^2 provides lopinavir plasma concentrations similar to those observed in adults receiving the 400/100 mg dose without nevirapine.[5]

▲ EFFICACY

The efficacy of lopinavir/ritonavir has been examined in clinical trials in both antiretroviral-naive and antiretroviral-experienced patients. The results of five major clinical trials are reviewed below (Table 17–1).

The antiviral activity of several dosage levels of lopinavir/ritonavir in combination with stavudine (d4T) and lamivudine (3TC) was tested in a study of 100 antiretroviral-naive adults (study M97-720).[6] Subjects initially received (1) one of two dosages of lopinavir/ritonavir (400/100 mg or 200/100 mg) alone followed by the addition of d4T and 3TC at week 3 (group I) or (2) one of two dosages of lopinavir/ritonavir (400/100 mg or 400/200 mg) together with d4T and 3TC beginning at day 0 (group II). Baseline characteristics of the enrolled patients included a median baseline CD4+ T-lymphocyte count of 398 and 310 cells/mm^3 in groups I and II, respectively, and a mean plasma HIV-1 RNA level of 4.9 $\log_{10}$ copies/ml in both groups. According to an intention-to-treat analysis, which counted missing patients as treatment failures, a plasma HIV-1 RNA level of less than 50 copies/ml was achieved in 75% and 79% of patients in groups I and II, respectively, at 48 weeks. Figure 17–2 depicts the antiviral activity over the first 48 weeks of the study.[6] The CD4+ T-lymphocyte

▲ **Table 17–1.** SUMMARY OF MAJOR CLINICAL TRIALS WITH LOPINAVIR/RITONAVIR

Study	Design	Entry criteria	No. of subjects	Antiviral response	Comments
M97-720 (Murphy et al.,[6] Stryker et al.[7])	Randomized, comparison of doses of lopinavir and ritonavir with d4T and 3TC added at 3 wks (group I) or at day 0 (group II)	Antiretroviral-naive; plasma HIV RNA level >5000 copies/ml; no CD4 cell restriction	100	75% and 79% in groups I and II, respectively, reached HIV RNA <50 copies/ml at 48 wks (ITT, M = F)	Illustrates potency and tolerability in antiretroviral-naive subjects
M98-863 (King et al.[8])	Randomized, double-blind comparison of lopinavir/ritonavir versus nelfinavir, both with d4T and 3TC	Antiretroviral-naive (no more than 14 days of any drug and no prior use of d4T or 3TC), plasma HIV RNA level >400 copies/ml; no CD4 cell restriction	653	83% of lopinavir/ritonavir-treated versus 68% of nelfinavir-treated patients reached HIV RNA <50 copies/ml at 48 wks (on treatment analysis)	Lopinavir-ritonavir arm outperformed one of the commonly used regimens in clinical practice
M97-765 (Feinberg et al.[9])	Randomized study of lopinavir with one of two doses of ritonavir, with nevirapine and at least one new NRTI added at day 15	Single PI experience; HIV RNA 1000–100,000 copies/ml	70	Approximately 60% of patients achieved an HIV RNA <400 copies/ml at 96 weeks (ITT, M = F)	Illustrates efficacy of lopinavir/ritonavir with an NNRTI in single PI failures
M98-957 (Clumeck et al.[10])	Randomized trial of lopinavir/ritonavir at one of two doses with efavirenz and NRTIs	Failing PI-based regimen and treated with at least two PIs; NNRTI-naive; HIV RNA level >1000 copies/ml	57	56% of patients achieved an HIV RNA level <50 copies/ml at 48 weeks (ITT, M = F)	Illustrates efficacy of lopinavir/ritonavir with an NNRTI in multiple PI failures
M98-940 (Cahn et al.[11])	Randomized trial of two doses of lopinavir/ritonavir; naive received d4T and 3TC: experienced received nevirapine plus NRTIs	Age 3 mo to 12 yrs; HIV RNA >400 copies/ml; NNRTI-naive	100	At 40 wks, 66% of naive and 63% of experienced subjects achieved HIV RNA <50 copies/ml (ITT analysis)	Illustrates potency and tolerability in children; also indicated effect of nevirapine to lower lopinavir/ritonavir levels

d4T, stavudine; ITT, intention to treat; M = F, missing=failure; NRTI, nucleoside reverse transcriptase inhibitor; PI, protease inhibitor; 3TC, lamivudine; ml, per milliliter.

count increased by approximately 200 to 250 cells/mm^3 over this same time period. After 48 weeks all patients in this study received lopinavir 400 mg bid plus ritonavir 100 mg bid, along with d4T and 3TC at standard doses. Similar levels of viral suppression have been observed after 108 weeks of follow-up.[7]

A randomized, double-blind Phase III study compared the efficacy of lopinavir/ritonavir with that of nelfinavir in treatment-naive patients (study M98-863).[2,8] Both protease inhibitors were used in combination with d4T and 3TC. Lopinavir/ritonavir was dosed at 400/100 mg bid; nelfinavir was dosed at 750 mg tid, but subjects were allowed to change to 1250 mg bid at approximately week 24. At baseline the mean plasma HIV-1 RNA level and CD4+ T-lymphocyte count among the 653 participants were 4.9 $\log_{10}$ copies/ml and 259 cells/mm^3, respectively. At 24 weeks the intention-to-treat analysis showed that a plasma HIV-1 RNA level of less than 400 copies/ml was achieved in 79% of subjects on the lopinavir/ritonavir arm versus 70% in the nelfinavir arm.[2] An on-treatment analysis at 48 weeks confirmed the virologic superiority of the lopinavir/ritonavir arm in this study, with 83% of subjects on the lopinavir/ritonavir arm versus 68% in the nelfinavir arm achieving a plasma HIV-1 RNA level of less than 50 copies/ml.[8] This study illustrates the potency of a lopinavir/ritonavir-containing regimen in antiretroviral-naive patients when compared to one of the antiretroviral treatment regimens commonly used in clinical practice.

The activity of lopinavir/ritonavir in patients failing antiretroviral therapy that included a protease inhibitor plus two nucleoside RT inhibitors was evaluated in study M97-765.[9]

Patients failing their first protease inhibitor (PI)-based regimen with plasma HIV-1 RNA levels between 1000 and 100,000 copies/ml were eligible for study if they were naive to NNRTIs and to at least one NRTI. Patients received lopinavir 400 mg bid plus ritonavir at a dose of either 100 or 200 mg bid for 15 days, after which nevirapine plus at least one new NRTI was added. Seventy patients enrolled in this study. The median baseline CD4+ T-lymphocyte count and plasma HIV-1 RNA level were 349 cells/mm^3 and 4.0 $\log_{10}$ copies/ml, respectively. Prior PI use included indinavir (44%), nelfinavir (36%), saquinavir (13%), ritonavir (6%), and amprenavir (1%). Phenotypic resistance testing

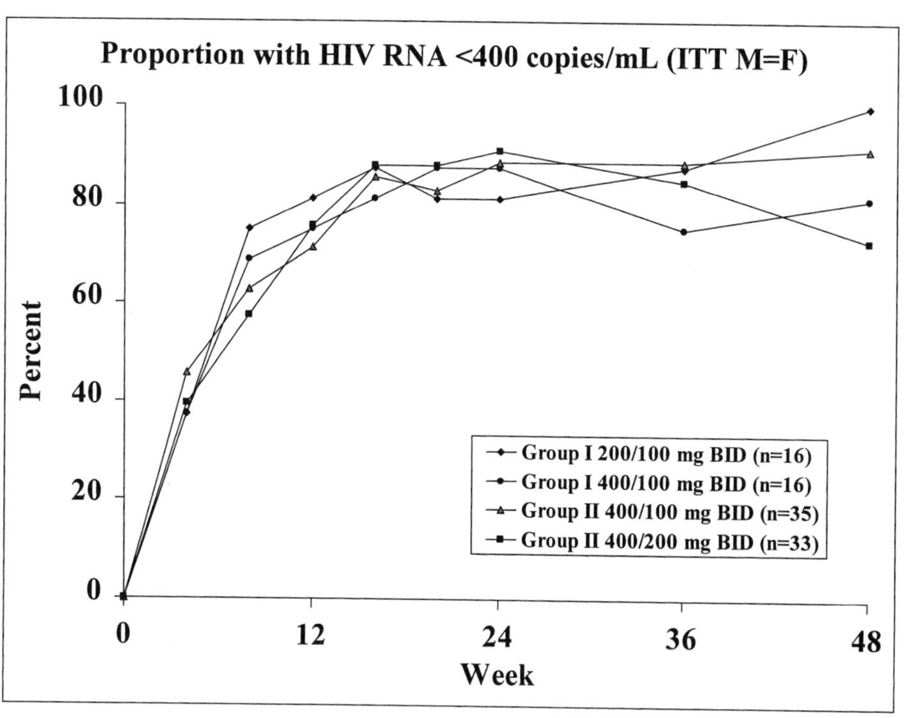

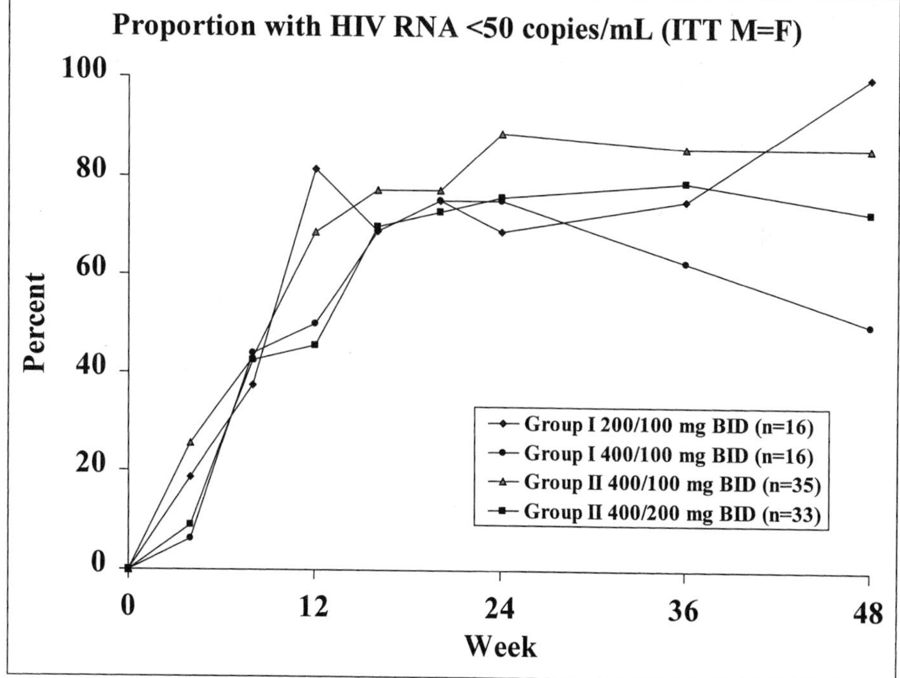

Figure 17–2. Study M97-720. Percentage of patients with plasma HIV-1 RNA below the limit of detection (< 400 and < 50 copies/ml) by treatment group at 48 weeks. *ITT, M = F*: intent-to-treat analysis with missing values considered as treatment failures. (From Murphy R, Brun S, Hicks C, et al. ABT-378/ritonavir plus stavudine and lamivudine for the treatment of antiretroviral-naive adults with HIV-1 infection: 48-week results. AIDS 15:F1, 2001.)

at study entry revealed that viruses from 32% of patients had a fourfold or more loss in susceptibility to three or more PIs. No significant difference in treatment response was observed between the two groups. At week 2, prior to the addition of nevirapine, 80% of patients had either a more than 1 $\log_{10}$ copies/ml decrease in plasma HIV-1 RNA level or achieved a plasma HIV-1 RNA level of less than 400 copies/ml. The intention-to-treat analysis at 96 weeks for the two groups combined showed that approximately 60% of patients achieved a plasma HIV-1 RNA of less than 400 copies/ml. These results demonstrate the efficacy of lopinavir/ritonavir in antiretroviral-experienced patients. However, patients in this study had not received more than one other PI, and other approved PIs have also been effective in this setting.[12] Moreover, activity of the treatment regimen was bolstered by adding two other effective drugs (nevirapine plus a previously unused NRTI).

The use of lopinavir/ritonavir in patients with a greater degree of PI experience was assessed in another study (M98-957).[10] Patients with plasma HIV-1 RNA levels of more than 1000 copies/ml on a failing PI regimen who had been treated with at least two PIs were eligible for study if they were naive to NNRTIs. At baseline, the median plasma HIV-1 RNA level was 4.5 $\log_{10}$ copies/ml. Altogether, 68% of baseline viral isolates demonstrated a fourfold or more loss in susceptibility to three or more other PIs. Patients were randomized to receive lopinavir/ritonavir at a dose of 400/100 mg bid (n = 29) or 400/100 mg bid for 14 days, after which the dose was increased to 533/133 mg bid (four capsules bid, n = 28). All patients also received efavirenz (600 mg daily) beginning at day 0. Twenty-five percent of patients also received at least one new NRTI during the first 8 weeks of the study. After week 24 the dose of lopinavir/ritonavir was changed to 533/133 mg bid in all patients. This change in dosing was prompted by the observation that lopinavir trough levels and the lopinavir AUC were reduced in patients who received lopinavir/ritonavir together with efavirenz, which induces lopinavir/ritonavir metabolism. The intention-to-treat analysis (missing = failure) at 48 weeks demonstrated that 56% of patients achieved a plasma HIV-1 RNA level of less than 50 copies/ml. Successful suppression of plasma HIV-1 RNA was achieved in most patients even though the mean susceptibility of lopinavir among baseline viral isolates was 16-fold higher than that of the wild-type virus. Results of this study strongly suggest that resistance to PIs can be overcome at least in part by increasing drug exposure through ritonavir-mediated inhibition of CYP3A4. Whether comparable results with lopinavir/ritonavir can be achieved in NNRTI-experienced patients remains to be demonstrated.

Two dosage levels of lopinavir/ritonavir have been studied in treatment-naive and treatment-experienced HIV-1-infected children (study M98-940).[11] Lopinavir/ritonavir was administered every 12 hours at a dose of 230/57.5 mg/m^2 or 300/75 mg/m^2 in combination with d4T and 3TC (for antiretroviral-naive children) or together with nevirapine and one or two NRTIs (for antiretroviral-experienced patients). After 12 weeks, all patients received the 300/75 mg/m^2 dose. A total of 100 patients were enrolled in this study. At entry, the median plasma HIV-1 RNA level was 5.1 $\log_{10}$ copies/ml in the antiretroviral-naive group and 4.5 $\log_{10}$ copies/ml in the antiretroviral-experienced group. An intention-to-treat analysis at 40 weeks showed that 84% of naive subjects and 71% of experienced subjects had plasma HIV-1 RNA levels of less than 400 copies/ml; 66% and 63%, respectively, had plasma HIV-1 RNA levels of less than 50 copies/ml.

▲ TOXICITY

Lopinavir/ritonavir has been generally well tolerated in clinical trials. The most commonly observed side effect is diarrhea, which is typically mild to moderate in intensity. The most significant laboratory abnormalities have been elevations in total cholesterol and triglycerides. Table 17–2 lists the most common adverse events and serious or severe (grade 3 or 4) laboratory abnormalities observed in the Phase III efficacy trial that compared lopinavir/ritonavir with nelfinavir.[2,8] Pancreatitis has occurred in some patients receiving lopinavir/ritonavir, including patients who have marked hypertriglyceridemia.

Table 17–2. TREATMENT ASSOCIATED ADVERSE EVENTS OF MODERATE OR SEVERE INTENSITY AND GRADE 3–4 LABORATORY ABNORMALITIES REPORTED IN ≥2% OF ADULT PATIENTS ON STUDY M98-863

Adverse event or grade 3-4 laboratory abnormality	Lopinavir/ritonavir 400/100 mg bid + d4T + 3TC (n = 326) (%)	Nelfinavir 750 mg tid + d4T + 3TC (n = 327) (%)
Abdominal pain	3.1	2.4
Asthenia	3.4	2.8
Headache	2.5	1.8
Diarrhea	13.8	14.4
Nausea	6.4	4.0
Vomiting	2.1	2.4
AST >180 U/L	0.3	2.2
ALT >215 U/L	1.0	2.2
Total cholesterol >300 mg/dl	6.7	2.8
Triglycerides >750 mg/dl	5.1	0.9

ALT, alanine transaminase; AST, aspartate transaminase.
From Kaletra package insert, 2000.

The safety of lopinavir/ritonavir in the subset of patients co-infected with hepatitis B or hepatitis C virus (or both) has also been examined. Not surprisingly, liver enzyme elevations have been observed more commonly in patients with underlying hepatitis.[6,13] In study M97-720, patients with a positive hepatitis B surface antigen or hepatitis C antibody had an eightfold increased relative risk of grade 3 or 4 elevations in aspartate (AST) or alanine (ALT) transaminase on lopinavir/ritonavir.[6]

A number of metabolic complications have been observed in patients receiving PIs and other antiretroviral agents. They include diabetes mellitus, gynecomastia, fat redistribution syndromes (including peripheral and facial wasting, dorsocervical fat pads, truncal obesity), and osteoporosis. The mechanism of these complications and their potential association with individual antiretroviral agents, including lopinavir/ritonavir, remains unclear at this time.

▲ DRUG INTERACTIONS

Lopinavir and ritonavir are inhibitors of CYP3A4, although the combined formulation does not inhibit CYP3A4 as potently as does full-dose ritonavir. Lopinavir/ritonavir also inhibits CYP2D6 in vitro but to a lesser extent than CYP3A4. Consequently, a number of drugs are either contraindicated or require dose adjustment when used with lopinavir/ritonavir. Table 17–3 provides a list of medications that should not be co-administered with lopinavir/ritonavir.[2] Many other drugs are not contraindicated but may require dose adjustment of lopinavir/ritonavir or the concomitant agent.[2,14] Table 17–4 lists some of these important established or potential drug interactions.

Other antiretroviral agents can also have important drug interactions with lopinavir/ritonavir, notably the NNRTIs. Efavirenz induces the hepatic metabolism of lopinavir/

▲ **Table 17–3.** DRUGS THAT SHOULD NOT BE CO-ADMINISTERED
▲ WITH LOPINAVIR/RITONAVIR

Drug class: drug name(s)	Clinical comment
Antiarrhythmics: flecainide, propafenone	Contraindicated due to risk of a life-threatening reaction such as a cardiac arrhythmia
Antihistamines: astemizole, terfenadine	Contraindicated due to risk of a life-threatening reaction such as a cardiac arrhythmia
Antimycobacterial: rifampin	Induction of hepatic metabolism of lopinavir/ritonavir may lead to loss of virologic response or resistance
Ergot derivatives: ergonovine, dihydroergotamine, ergotamine, methylergonovine	Contraindicated due to risk of a life-threatening reaction such as acute ergot toxicity characterized by peripheral vasospasm with ischemia of tissues
GI motility agent: cisapride	Contraindicated due to risk of a life-threatening reaction such as a cardiac arrhythmia
Herbal products: St. John's wort (*Hypericum perforatum*)	Induction of hepatic metabolism of lopinavir/ritonavir may lead to loss of virologic response or resistance
Certain HMG-CoA reductase inhibitors: lovastatin, simvastatin	Potential for serious reactions such as myopathy and rhabdomyolysis
Neuroleptic: pimozide	Contraindicated due to risk of a life-threatening reaction such as a cardiac arrhythmia
Sedative/hypnotics: midazolam, triazolam	Contraindicated due to risk of a life-threatening reaction such as prolonged or increased sedation or respiratory depression

GI, gastrointestinal; HMG-CoA, 3-hydroxy-3-methyl-glutaryl coenzyme A.
From Kaletra package insert, 2000.

ritonavir, resulting in lower concentrations of the PI. Coadministration of efavirenz with lopinavir/ritonavir at the 400/100 mg bid dose reduces C_{min} by 40% to 45%, and the AUC by approximately 20% to 25%.[15] Increasing the dose to 533 mg of lopinavir and 133 mg of the ritonavir component overcomes this effect. Although nevirapine did not have a major effect on steady-state levels of lopinavir in adult patients receiving standard doses of both drugs, coadministration of nevirapine and lopinavir/ritonavir to children aged 6 months to 12 years reduced the C_{min} by 55% and the mean AUC by 22%.[5]

Although lopinavir/ritonavir is not commonly used with other PIs, some clinicians have combined it with other drugs of this class in the setting of extensive drug resistance or when serious nucleoside analogue toxicity (e.g., lactic acidosis) precludes the use of NRTIs. Formal drug interaction studies for other PIs administered together with lopinavir/ritonavir have not yet been reported, but dosage adjustments can be suggested based on the observation that the lopinavir/ritonavir combination increases plasma levels of the other four PIs[2] (Table 17–5).

▲ DRUG RESISTANCE

Lopinavir was designed to be effective against HIV-1 strains resistant to other PIs, particularly ritonavir. It retains activity against many drug-resistant isolates, including ritonavir-resistant viral clones with mutations at position 82 (V82A, V82F, V82S, V82T).[16] However, resistance to lopinavir has been observed both in vitro and in vivo. In vitro, serial passage of HIV-1 in the presence of lopinavir leads to the sequential appearance of the mutations I84V, L10F, M46I, T91S, V32I, and I47V in protease. The EC_{50} for lopinavir of passaged virus was 338-fold higher than that of wild-type virus.[17] The relation of specific mutations in protease to lopinavir susceptibility was explored in a detailed analysis of 112 isolates from patients failing single or multiple PI regimens.[18] Susceptibility to lopinavir was significantly correlated with the number of mutations at 11 sites (protease codons 10, 20, 24, 46, 53, 54, 63, 71, 82, 84, 90). Viruses carrying four or five of these mutations had a median 2.7-fold increase in EC_{50} for lopinavir compared to the wild-type viruses; those with six or seven mutations had a median 13.5-fold increase in EC_{50}; and isolates with eight to ten mutations had a median 44-fold increase. Some isolates that show high-level resistance to lopinavir nevertheless remain susceptible to amprenavir, saquinavir, and the investigational PI tipranavir.[19,20]

Few data are available on patterns of resistance that emerge in HIV-1 isolates from patients failing lopinavir/ritonavir regimens. This relative lack of data reflects the generally high level of virus suppression in patients who received this drug in clinical trials and the relatively recent introduction of lopinavir/ritonavir into general clinical use. Understanding the pattern of mutations selected by lopinavir/ritonavir is important for deciding what drugs might be available for use in patients who fail a lopinavir-containing regimen. No PI-resistance mutations were noted in HIV-1 sequences from 31 PI-naive patients who experienced virologic breakthrough (plasma HIV-1 RNA levels of more than 400 copies/ml) while receiving lopinavir/ritonavir together with d4T and 3TC as part of the Phase III efficacy trial described above.[8,21] By comparison, isolates from 21 of 65 patients experiencing viral breakthrough while taking nelfinavir, d4T, and 3TC carried resistance mutations for nelfinavir (D30N, L90M, or both).

A separate study analyzed the cross resistance to PIs among 56 HIV-1 isolates that were highly resistant to lopinavir.[22] Five of these isolates were obtained from PI-experienced patients who had viral rebound when undergoing salvage therapy with lopinavir/ritonavir. The change in susceptibility to lopinavir was highly correlated with susceptibility to indinavir and ritonavir, but it correlated poorly with susceptibility to amprenavir and saquinavir. For example, viruses with a median 44-fold resistance to lopinavir were only sixfold resistant to amprenavir. Similarly, viruses from PI-experienced patients failing lopinavir/ritonavir-based salvage therapy had 9- to 99-fold resistance to lopinavir but were less than 8.5-fold resistant

Table 17–4. ESTABLISHED OR POTENTIAL DRUG INTERACTIONS BETWEEN LOPINAVIR/RITONAVIR AND NON-HIV DRUGS WITH SUGGESTED ADJUSTMENTS IN DRUG DOSE

Drug class: drug names	Interaction with lopinavir/ritonavir	Adjustment of lopinavir/ritonavir or concomitant drug
Antiarrythmics: amiodarone, bipridil, lidocaine, quinidine	Increased levels of these antiarrhythmics likely	Therapeutic drug monitoring of the antiarhythmic is recommended
Anticonvulsants: cabamazepine, phenobarbital, phenytonin	Potential for reduced level of lopinavir	Dose adjustment unclear. Alternative anticonvulsants are used if possible
Anticoagulant: warfarin	Warfarin levels may be affected	International normalized ratio (INR) is monitored
Antiinfective: clarithromycin	Potential for increased levels of clarithromycin	Clarithromycin dose is reduced in patients with renal impairment
Antimycobacterial: rifabutin	Increased levels of rifabutin	Rifabutin dose is decreased at least 75% from 300 mg/day dose
Antifungals: ketoconazole and itraconazole	Potential for increased levels of both azoles	Dose of itraconazole or ketoconazole not to exceed 200 mg/day
Antiparasitic: atovaquone	Potential for reduced level of atovaquone	Clinical significance unknown
Calcium channel blockers: felodipine, nifedipine, nicardipine	Potential for increased levels of these calcium channel blockers	Caution warranted when using these agents
Colticosteroid: dexamethasone	Potential for reduced level of lopinavir	Limit concomitant use
Disulfiram/metronidazole	Lopinavir/ritonavir oral solution contains alcohol	Concomitant use of lopinavir/ritonavir oral solution with these two agents may lead to a disulfiram-like reaction
Erectile dysfunction agent: sildenafil	Increased level of sildenafil likely	Reduce dose of sildenafil to 25 mg every 48 hours
HMG-CoA reductase inhibitors: atorvastatin, cerivastatin	Increased levels of atorvastatin and cerivastatin likely	Use lowest possible dose or consider pravastain or fluvastatin
Immunosuppressants: cyclosporin, tacrolimus, rapamycin	Increased levels of immunosuppressants likely	Therapeutic drug monitoring with dose adjustment of immunosuppressants
Narcotic analgesics: methadone	Reduced level of methadone	Methadone dose may have to be increased
Oral contraceptive: ethinyl estradiol	Reduced level of ethinyl estradiol	Alternative or additional contraceptive measures should be used

From Kaletra package insert, 2000; and Bertz R, Hsu A, Lam W, et al. Pharmacokinetic interactions between lopinavir/ritonavir (ABT-378r) and other non-HIV drugs [P291]. AIDS 14(suppl 4):S100, 2000.

to amprenavir. Three of these isolates also remained saquinavir-susceptible.

The relation between resistance and clinical response to lopinavir/ritonavir was explored in studies performed in antiretroviral-experienced patients.[23] The response to salvage regimens that included lopinavir/ritonavir was correlated with the number of PI-resistance mutations at baseline. Whereas lopinavir/ritonavir suppressed plasma HIV-1 RNA levels to less than 400 copies/ml through 24 weeks in 91% of patients with isolates that carried none to five resistance mutations, the response rate dropped to 81% in patients with isolates that carried six or seven mutations and was

Table 17–5. DRUG INTERACTIONS BETWEEN LOPINAVIR/RITONAVIR AND OTHER ANTIRETROVIRAL DRUGS AND SUGGESTED ADJUSTMENTS IN DRUG DOSE

Antiretroviral drug	Interaction with lopinavir/ritonavir	Suggested adjustment of lopinavir/ritonavir or concomitant drug[a]
Nevirapine	Lopinavir/ritonavir may be decreased	Lopinavir/ritonavir dose increased to 4 capsules (533/133 mg) bid
Efavirenz	Lopinavir/ritonavir decreased	Lopinavir/ritonavir dose increased to 4 capsules (533/133 mg) bid
Delavirdine	Lopinavir/ritonavir may be increased	Appropriate adjustment not established
Indinavir	Indinavir increased by lopinavir/ritonavir	Indinavir dosed at 600 mg bid
Nelfinavir	Nelfinavir increased by lopinavir/ritonavir	Nelfinavir dosed at 750 mg bid
Saquinavir	Saquinavir increased by lopinavir/ritonavir	Saquinavir dosed at 800 mg bid
Amprenavir	Amprenavir increased by lopinavir/ritonavir	Amprenavir dosed at 750 mg bid

[a]Suggested dosages for protease inhibitors co-administered with lopinavir/ritonavir are based on preliminary pharmacokinetic observations.[2] The safety and efficacy of such combinations have not been established.

From Kaletra package insert, 2000; Hsu A, Bertz R, Renz C, et al. Assessment of the pharmacokinetic interaction between lopinavir/ritonavir (ABT-378/r) and nevirapine (NVP) in HIV-infected pediatric subjects [P292]. AIDS 14(suppl 4):S100, 2000; and Bertz R, Lam W, Hsu A, et al. Assessment of the pharmacokinetic interaction between ABT-378/ritonavir and efavirenz (EFV) in healthy volunteers and HIV$^+$ subjects. Presented at the 40th Interscience Conference on Antimicrobial Agents and Chemotherapy, 2000, Toronto, abstract 424.

only 33% in patients with isolates that carried eight to ten resistance mutations. Similar analyses helped determine the relation between lopinavir susceptibility (as measured in phenotypic tests of drug resistance) and the clinical response at 48 weeks.[10] Virologic suppression (plasma virus load of less than 400 copies/ml) was achieved in 93% of patients with virus that was up to 10-fold resistant to lopinavir and in approximately 73% of patients with virus that was 10- to 40-fold resistant. Higher levels of lopinavir resistance were associated with correspondingly lower response rates. On the basis of these and other data, an IC_{50} more than 10-fold above that of the wild-type virus had been suggested as a "cutoff" for defining clinically significant phenotypic resistance to lopinavir.

Several caveats should be kept in mind when interpreting the results of these studies. First, patients in these studies were naive to NNRTIs and received efavirenz or nevirapine as part of their salvage regimen. Response rates at any given level of lopinavir resistance might be lower in NNRTI-experienced patients. Second, the study population included relatively few patients with high-level (>20-fold) lopinavir resistance. Thus estimates of the response rate at high IC_{50} values must be considered approximate. Third, these data clearly demonstrate that there is a continuous relation between drug susceptibility and treatment response. It is therefore difficult to assign a specific IC_{50} "cutoff" above which lopinavir loses all activity. A more useful approach to interpreting resistance data for this drug (and possibly other pharmacologically enhanced PIs) is to recognize that residual antiviral activity is likely to persist in the setting of partial resistance, and that clinically significant reductions in the plasma HIV-1 RNA level might be obtained by combining several agents with partial activity in patients with few remaining treatment options.

▲ USE DURING PREGNANCY

The lopinavir/ritonavir combination is classified as a category C drug. No treatment-related malformations were noted in studies in pregnant rats or rabbits, but use in pregnant women to date has been limited. If this medication is used during pregnancy, the potential risks and benefits must be considered. Ideally, pregnant patients receiving lopinavir/ritonavir should be included in the Antiretroviral Pregnancy Registry (1-800-258-4263).

▲ INDICATIONS FOR USE

Given the growing number of antiretroviral agents and effective combinations, the precise role of lopinavir/ritonavir in combination therapy for antiretroviral-naive and antiretroviral-experienced patients has not been fully defined. Lopinavir/ritonavir clearly provides a potent option for initial therapy of treatment-naive patients, but a number of other PI-containing and PI-sparing regimens are also highly effective in this patient population. Factors to be considered when choosing antiretroviral regimens in this setting include the inherent potency of the regimen, the results of efficacy trials to date, the ease of administration, the potential for drug toxicity and drug interactions, and the potential for drug resistance with its implications for drug sequencing. Advantages of a lopinavir/ritonavir-containing regimen include its potency and relatively low rate of significant treatment-related side effects. Moreover, the ease of administration (three capsules twice daily) may lead to high degrees of adherence. Potential disadvantages of a lopinavir/ritonavir-containing regimen as initial therapy include the significant incidence of hyperlipidemia (particularly hypertriglyceridemia), the potential for drug interactions due to the ritonavir component, and the relative lack of data regarding the effectiveness of subsequent regimens in patients failing initial therapy with lopinavir/ritonavir. Given its high potency, lopinavir/ritonavir might be particularly useful in the subset of antiretroviral-naive patients with extremely high plasma HIV-1 RNA levels, extremely low CD4+ T-lymphocyte counts, or both.

Lopinavir/ritonavir clearly has a major role in the treatment of antiretroviral-experienced patients. It is useful in patients failing an initial PI-containing regimen and in those with more extensive PI experience. The relative efficacy of this drug compared to other ritonavir-boosted PIs in the setting of salvage therapy is unclear at this time. As noted above, completed studies on the use of lopinavir/ritonavir for salvage therapy have focused on patients naive to NNRTIs. The efficacy of lopinavir/ritonavir in patients who have experienced failure of all three classes of currently available antiretroviral agents remains to be determined. Preliminary data from the lopinavir/ritonavir early access program indicates a diminished virologic response in this setting.[24] As with other antiretroviral agents, the use of this drug in the setting of treatment failure should be guided by the results of resistance testing.

Although lopinavir/ritonavir could have other potential uses, including treatment of primary HIV infection, prevention of mother-to-child transmission of HIV-1, or postexposure prophylaxis following occupational exposure to HIV, there are scant data regarding the safety or efficacy of this medication in these special circumstances.

REFERENCES

1. Sham H, Kempf D, Molla A, et al. ABT-378, a highly potent inhibitor of the human immunodeficiency virus protease. Antimicrob Agents Chemother 42:3218, 1998.
2. Kaletra package insert, 2000.
3. Kumar G, Dykstra J, Roberts E, et al. Potent inhibition of the cytochrome P-450 3A-mediated human liver microsomal metabolism of a novel HIV protease inhibitor by ritonavir: a positive drug–drug interaction. Drug Metab Dispos 27:902, 1999.
4. Bertz R, Lam W, Brun S, et al. Multiple-dose pharmacokinetics (PK) of ABT-378/ritonavir (ABT-378/r) in HIV$^+$ subjects. Presented at the 39th Interscience Conference on Antimicrobial Agents and Chemotherapy, San Francisco, 1999, abstract 327.
5. Hsu A, Bertz R, Renz C, et al. Assessment of the pharmacokinetic interaction between lopinavir/ritonavir (ABT-378/r) and nevirapine (NVP) in HIV-infected pediatric subjects [P292]. AIDS 14(suppl 4): S100, 2000.
6. Murphy R, Brun S, Hicks C, et al. ABT-378/ritonavir plus stavudine and lamivudine for the treatment of antiretroviral-naive adults with HIV-1 infection: 48-week results. AIDS 15:F1, 2001.

7. Stryker R, Brun S, King M, et al. ABT-378/ritonavir (ABT-378/r in antiretroviral naive HIV+ patients: follow-up beyond 2 years and viral load suppression below 3 copies/ml [P46]. AIDS 14(suppl 4):S30, 2000.
8. King M, Bernstein B, Kempf D, et al. Comparison of time to achieve HIV RNA <400 copies/ml and <50 copies/ml in a phase III, blinded, randomized clinical trial of Kaletra vs. NFV in ARV-naive patients. Presented at the 8th Conference on Retroviruses and Opportunistic Infections, Chicago, 2001, abstract 329.
9. Feinberg J, Brun S, Xu Y, et al. Durable suppression of HIV+ RNA after 2 years of therapy with ABT-378/ritonavir (ABT-378/r) treatment in single protease inhibitor experienced patients [P101]. AIDS 14(suppl 4):S46, 2000.
10. Clumeck N, Brun S, Sylte J, et al. Kaletra (ABT-378/r) and efavirenz: one-year safety/efficacy evaluation and phenotypic breakpoints in multiple-PI-experienced patients. Presented at the 8th Conference on Retroviruses and Opportunistic Infections, Chicago, 2001, abstract 525.
11. Cahn P, Renz C, Deetz C, et al. ABT-378/ritonavir (ABT-378/r) in HIV infected children [P225]. AIDS 14(suppl 4):S80, 2000.
12. Tebas P, Patick A, Kane E, et al. Virologic responses to ritonavir-saquinavir-containing regimen in patients who had previously failed nelfinavir. AIDS 13:F23, 1999.
13. Arribas J, Barros C, Gonzalez-Lahoz J, et al. Treatment of HIV+ subjects co-infected with hepatitis B or C: safety and efficacy comparison of ABT-378/ritonavir (ABT-378/r) versus nelfinavir from a phase III blinded randomized clinical trial [P369]. AIDS 14(suppl 4):S124, 2000.
14. Bertz R, Hsu A, Lam W, et al. Pharmacokinetic interactions between lopinavir/ritonavir (ABT-378r) and other non-HIV drugs [P291]. AIDS 14(suppl 4):S100, 2000.
15. Bertz R, Lam W, Hsu A, et al. Assessment of the pharmacokinetic interaction between ABT-378/ritonavir and efavirenz (EFV) in healthy volunteers and HIV+ subjects. Presented at the 40th Interscience Conference on Antimicrobial Agents and Chemotherapy, Toronto, 2000, abstract 424.
16. Chen C, Niu P, Kati W, et al. Activity of ABT-378 against HIV protease containing mutations conferring resistance to ritonavir. Presented at the 4th Conference on Retroviruses and Opportunistic Infections, Washington, DC, 1997, abstract 208.
17. Carrillo A, Stewart K, Sham H, et al. In vitro selection and characterization of human immunodeficiency virus type 1 variants with increased resistance to ABT-378, a novel protease inhibitor. J Virol 72:7532, 1998.
18. Kempf D, Isaacson J, King M, et al. Identification of genotypic changes in human immunodeficiency virus protease that correlate with reduced susceptibility to the protease inhibitor lopinavir among viral isolates from protease inhibitor-experienced patients. J Virol 75:7462, 2001.
19. Molla A, Brun S, Mo H, et al. Genotypic and phenotypic analysis of viral isolates from subjects with detectable viral load on therapy with ABT-378/ritonavir [abstract 39]. Antivir Ther 5(suppl 3):30, 2000.
20. Kemp S, Salim M, Field N, et al. Site-directed mutagenesis and in vitro drug selection studies have failed to reveal a consistent genotypic resistance pattern for tipranavir [abstract 40]. Antivir Ther 5(suppl 3):31, 2000.
21. Bernstein B, Moseley J, Kempf D, et al. Absence of resistance to Kaletra (ABT-378/r) observed through 48 weeks or therapy in antiretroviral naive subjects. Presented at the 8th Conference on Retroviruses and Opportunistic Infections, Chicago, 2001, abstract 453.
22. Brun S, Kempf D, Isaacson J, et al. Patterns of protease inhibitor cross-resistance in viral isolates with reduced susceptibility to ABT-378. Presented at the 8th Conference on Retroviruses and Opportunistic Infections, Chicago, 2001, abstract 452.
23. Kempf D, Isaacson J, King M, et al. Interpretation of genotypic resistance to ABT-378/ritonavir (ABT = 378/r) in protease inhibitor experienced patients using the ABT-378 mutation score[P333]. AIDS 14(suppl 4):S113, 2000.
24. Reitmayer R, Rode R, Bernstein B, et al. Initial efficacy results from the Kaletra (formerly known as ABT-378/r) early access program. Presented at the 8th Conference on Retroviruses and Opportunistic Infections. Chicago, 2001, abstract 328.

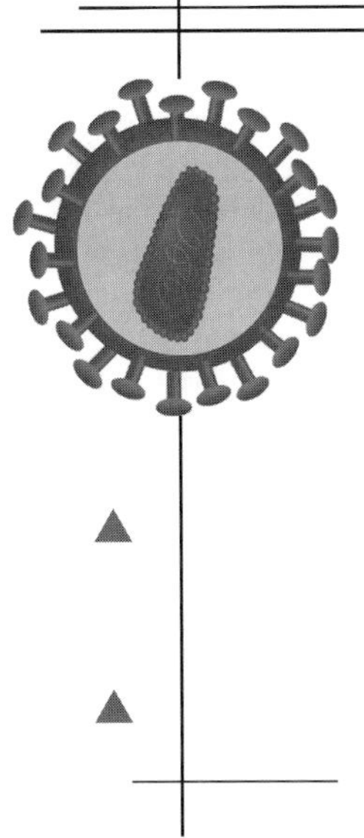

CHAPTER 18

Tenofovir Disoproxil Fumarate

Craig J. Hoesley, MD
Gail Skowron, MD

Tenofovir disoproxil fumarate (tenofovir DF) is the oral prodrug of tenofovir (9-[(R)-(2-phosphonomethoxy)propyl]adenine) (PMPA), a nucleotide (nucleoside monophosphate) analogue with activity against retroviruses and hepadnaviruses. Tenofovir is an acyclic nucleoside phosphonate compound (Fig. 18–1) designed to circumvent the first phosphorylation step necessary for activation of nucleoside analogues, such as zidovudine, didanosine, stavudine, lamivudine, and abacavir.[1] The antiviral activity of unphosphorylated nucleoside analogues may be impeded by their low affinity for cellular nucleoside kinases. Tenofovir differs from the "classic" nucleoside analogues in that it is less dependent on intracellular enzymes for activation.[2] Tenofovir DF received FDA approval in the United States in October 2001, and was approved by the European Medicines Evaluation Agency in February 2002.

MECHANISM OF ACTION AND IN VITRO ACTIVITY

Tenofovir DF is a lipophilic ester derivative of tenofovir designed to improve oral bioavailability. After oral administration and absorption tenofovir DF is rapidly cleaved by nonspecific extracellular carboxyesterases into tenofovir. Once inside cells tenofovir is metabolized by adenylate cyclase and nucleoside diphosphate kinase to tenofovir diphosphate (PMPApp), the active moiety. The antiviral effect of tenofovir is the result of selective interaction of the diphosphate metabolite (PMPApp) with the viral DNA polymerase or reverse transcriptase. Based on the structural resemblance to natural deoxyadenine triphosphates (dATP), PMPApp acts as both a competitive inhibitor and an alternative substrate during the DNA polymerase chain reaction, resulting in DNA chain termination.[1]

Tenofovir has in vitro activity against hepadnaviruses (hepatitis B virus) and retroviruses.[3–5] The dual antiviral activity of tenofovir may prove to be complementary because of the high incidence of co-infection in human immunodeficiency virus (HIV)-infected individuals. In a prospective, non-comparative, open label study, 10 HIV- and hepatitis B virus-infected individuals received tenofovir DF 300 mg once daily in addition to their existing lamivudine-containing regimen. At baseline, all patients were noted to have YMDD mutant hepatitis B virus infection. At 12 weeks the median change in plasma hepatitis B virus DNA concentrations from baseline (8.10 +/− 1.41 $\log_{10}$ copies/ml) was −3.34 +/− 1.31 $\log_{10}$ copies/ml. Further clinical trials of longer duration and larger size will be necessary to fully assess the efficacy of tenofovir DF in co-infected patients.[5a]

The spectrum of antiretroviral activity includes HIV-1 and HIV-2, simian immunodeficiency virus (SIV), feline immunodeficiency virus, visna-maedi virus of sheep, and murine leukemia and sarcoma viruses.[6–9] In vitro activity against non-B HIV-1 subtypes has also been described. The mean 50% inhibitory concentration (IC_{50}) values for tenofovir against HIV-1 subtypes A, C, D, E, F, G, and O in primary peripheral blood mononuclear cell (PBMC) cultures were all within twofold of the HIV subtype B IC_{50} value (range 0.55 to 0.22 μM).[10]

Tenofovir has demonstrated an anti-HIV effect in both lymphocytes and macrophages.[11] The K_i value of PMPApp against HIV-1 reverse transcriptase is 0.022 μM, which is approximately 200-, 3700-, and 2700-fold lower than the K_i value against human DNA polymerases α, β, and γ,

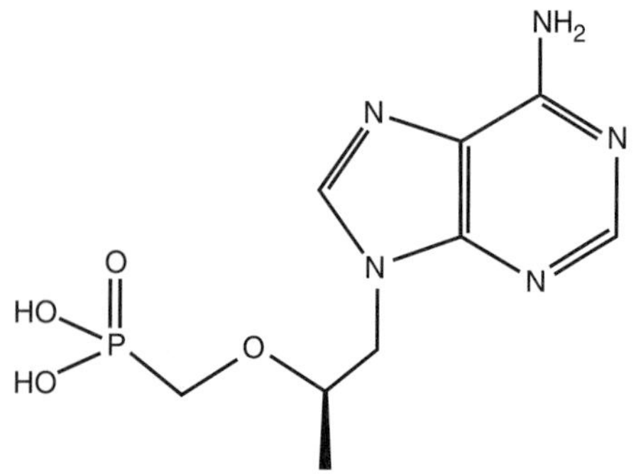

Figure 18–1. Structure of tenofovir disoproxil fumarate, or 9-[(R)-(2-phosphonylmethoxy)propyl]adenine.

respectively.[12] Moreover, tenofovir and tenofovir DF were evaluated in vitro for antiviral activity (IC_{50}) and cytotoxicity (CC_{50}) using both laboratory and clinical HIV-1 strains; they were noted to have favorable selectivity indices (CC_{50}/IC_{50} ratio higher than 2000).[13] The antiviral activity of tenofovir against wild-type laboratory strains of HIV-1 ranges from 0.2 to 6.0 μM.[13] In vitro, PMPApp (K_i 0.022 μM) is slightly more potent than the active phosphorylated metabolite of zidovudine (K_i 0.008 μM).[12] The potency of tenofovir DF monotherapy (300 mg tablet daily) was assessed in 10 antiretroviral-naive HIV-infected individuals who underwent frequent monitoring of plasma HIV-1 RNA levels over 21 days. The individual first phase decay slopes of plasma HIV-1 RNA levels from −0.24 to −0.59 $\log_{10}$ copies/ml (median −0.40 $\log_{10}$ copies/ml) which is similar to the values previously described with ritonavir monotherapy indicating comparable potency between the 2 drugs. The mean reduction in viral load was 1.5 $\log_{10}$ copies/ml by day 21.[12a]

In vitro analysis of MT2 cells infected with the HIV-IIIb strain were utilized to assess the activity of tenofovir in combination with a variety of other antiretroviral agents. The combination of tenofovir with zidovudine, amprenavir, and all nonnucleoside reverse transcriptase inhibitors (NNRTIs) tested demonstrated strong synergistic anti-HIV activity, whereas combinations with didanosine, adefovir, and nelfinavir resulted in minor synergistic inhibition of in vitro HIV replication.[14] Additive HIV inhibition was noted with tenofovir in combination with abacavir, stavudine, lamivudine, zalcitabine, ritonavir, saquinavir, and indinavir.[14,15] No tenofovir-containing combination demonstrated antagonism.

▲ PHARMACOKINETICS

The formulation of tenofovir DF as an oral prodrug for tenofovir has allowed improved oral bioavailability. In vitro metabolic studies using radiolabeled tenofovir and tenofovir disoproxil fumarate in resting and activated peripheral blood lymphocytes demonstrated a more than 1000-fold higher intracellular concentration of the active diphosphorylated metabolite (PMPApp) after incubation with the prodrug compared to tenofovir alone.[13] Owing to its increased cellular permeability, the anti-HIV activity of tenofovir DF is increased by 17- to 90-fold over tenofovir. The diphosphorylation of tenofovir in cells to PMPApp is independent of viral infection, and there is evidence that these active intracellular metabolites persist in cells after the drug is removed, suggesting that an antiviral effect may continue in the absence of repeated tenofovir exposure. Moreover, the long intracellular half-life of PMPApp (~10 to 50 hours) allows once-daily dosing. Animal models have demonstrated that approximately 98% of an intravenous tenofovir dose is eliminated unchanged in the urine after 24 hours.[13] Tenofovir is not a substrate, or inhibitor of the CYP450 enzyme system and does not have significant binding to plasma proteins (Gilead Sciences, Foster City, CA, USA, personal communication).

The pharmacokinetics of tenofovir and tenofovir DF has been studied in HIV-1-infected subjects. An aqueous solution of tenofovir was administered intravenously in single doses of 1 mg/kg and 3 mg/kg, resulting in mean peak serum concentrations of 2.7 and 9.1 μg/ml, respectively.[16] Serum tenofovir concentrations declined in a biexponential manner with a terminal half-life of 7.1 hours. All subjects in the higher dose (3 mg/kg) group had quantifiable serum levels up to 24 hours after the initial dose.

In a randomized, double-blind, placebo-controlled Phase I/II study (GS-97-901) in HIV-infected individuals, the pharmacokinetics of tenofovir DF were studied at doses of 75, 150, 300, and 600 mg given in tablet form. For each dose cohort, fasting patients received a single oral dose; and after a 1-week observation period the same patients received single oral doses after ingesting a high-fat meal for 28 consecutive days. After fasting, the median peak plasma concentrations (C_{max}) of tenofovir DF were 68.6, 111, 240, and 618 ng/ml in the 75, 150, 300, and 600 mg groups, respectively. Tenofovir has a long terminal half-life in serum of approximately 17 hours. At steady state (day 15), median C_{max} values were −80.8, 163, 303, and 633 ng/ml and area under the serum concentration time curve (AUC_{ss}) values of 717, 1,613, 2,937, and 6,073 ng·hr/ml in the same dosing groups when the drug was administered in a fed state.[17] The oral bioavailability of tenofovir DF when administered with food was enhanced (about 40%) and was not affected by repeated dosing.

▲ TOXICITY

The preclinical toxicology studies in animals (rats, dogs, monkeys) administered tenofovir over a minimum of 11 months identified the kidney and bone as potential target organs. Specifically, urinary excretion of calcium and phosphorus was increased in rats and dogs when tenofovir exposure was 11- and 9-fold larger than standard human exposure, respectively; these findings were reversible and not seen when exposure was increased 3- to 5-fold over standard human exposure. Moreover, glucosuria and proteinuria were described in dogs and monkeys at 9- and 12-fold increased exposure but again were reversible and not present when dosing was 3- to 4-fold larger than standard human exposure. Decreased bone marrow density and increased parathyroid hormone secretion were noted in animals when dosing was increased 9- to 50-fold over standard human exposure. These bone toxicities were thought to be secondary to renal toxicity and were reversible with discontinuation of the drug or not seen at all when exposure was only 2- to 4-fold larger than standard human exposure. Other adverse effects noted in animal studies were gastritis, duodenitis, and slight elevations in liver transaminases; these findings were limited to rats in the higher dosing groups (Gilead Sciences, personal communication).

Through February 2001, more than 1600 HIV-infected individuals had received tenofovir DF alone or in combination with other antiretroviral agents in clinical trials, including a number of study participants who had been treated for 3 years or more. In general, tenofovir DF has been well tolerated. In a randomized, double-blind, placebo-controlled Phase II study (GS-98-902), HIV-infected patients received tenofovir DF (75, 150, 300 mg) or placebo once daily for 24 weeks in addition to the patient's existing stable antiretroviral regimen at the time of enrollment. At week 24 placebo patients received tenofovir DF 300 mg once daily, and all treatment groups were followed for a total of 48 weeks (see Efficacy). At week 24 the number of grade 3 or 4 adverse events seen in subjects receiving tenofovir DF was similar to those in subjects receiving placebo (14% to 19%); and the percentage of grade 3 or 4 laboratory abnormalities was similar for the treatment and placebo groups (30% to 34%).[18] There was no evidence of a dose-related increase in adverse events. The reported grade 3 or 4 laboratory abnormalities seen through weeks 24 and 48 in this study are presented in Table 18–1.

Interestingly, there have been no grades 2, 3, or 4 serum creatinine elevations associated with tenofovir DF administration. These findings are particularly significant given the high rate of proximal renal tubular dysfunction described with the structurally similar compound adefovir dipivoxil. In addition, bone mineral density testing was performed in one-third of subjects participating in the above study, and no clinically significant decrease in bone mineral density from baseline was demonstrated in patients receiving tenofovir DF through 48 weeks.[19] In a combined analysis of Phase II and Phase III studies (GS-98-902 and GS-00-907), no increase in fracture rate was seen with tenofovir DF treatment (687 subjects with 778 patients-years of exposure, fracture rate 1.7/100 patient-years) compared to placebo recipients (210 subjects, 99 patient-years of follow-up, fracture rate 3.0/100 patient-years).[20] In contrast to adefovir dipivoxil, serum carnitine deficiency has not been observed with tenofovir DF administration and is not expected because pivolic acid, a component of adefovir dipivoxil, is not present in tenofovir DF. The completion and analysis of ongoing Phase III studies are necessary to formulate a complete toxicity profile for this drug.

▲ EFFICACY

The clinical efficacy of tenofovir DF as measured by absolute CD4 cell count or plasma HIV-1 RNA levels is shown in Table 18–2. Comprehensive data from Phase III clinical trials were not available at the time of this writing, but the 24-week interim analysis of study GS-99-907, an ongoing 48-week Phase III study, is presented.

Tenofovir Disoproxil Fumarate Monotherapy

In a Phase I/II randomized, double-blind, placebo-controlled, dose escalation study (GS-97-901), antiretroviral naive and experienced adults with absolute CD4 cell counts of 200 cells/mm^3 or more and plasma HIV-1 RNA levels of 10,000 copies/ml or higher were administered tenofovir DF at once-daily doses of 75, 150, 300, or 600 mg or placebo for 4 weeks.[17] Antiretroviral-naive patients receiving tenofovir DF had mean HIV-1 RNA level decreases of 0.45, 0.60, 1.57, and 1.40 $\log_{10}$ copies/ml in the 75, 150, 300, and 600 mg groups, respectively. Antiretroviral-experienced patients receiving tenofovir DF had mean HIV-1 RNA level decreases of 0.27, 0.49, 1.06, and 0.66 $\log_{10}$ copies/ml in the 75, 150, 300, and 600 mg groups, respectively. Overall, a dose-related treatment effect was observed, and individuals receiving 300 or 600 mg once daily had an overall mean HIV-1 RNA level reduction of 1.20 and 0.84 $\log_{10}$ copies/ml, respectively, compared to baseline, whereas placebo recipients experienced a 0.03 $\log_{10}$ copies/ml increase over the same period.

Combination Therapy with Tenofovir Disoproxil Fumarate

In a randomized, double-blind, placebo-controlled Phase II study (GS-98-902), 189 HIV-infected patients received tenofovir DF (75, 150, 300 mg) or placebo once daily for 24 weeks in

▲ **Table 18–1.** GRADE 3 OR 4 LABORATORY ABNORMALITIES REPORTED IN GS-98-902

Parameter	Week 24				Week 48		
	Placebo	75 mg	150 mg	300 mg	75 mg	150 mg	300 mg
No. of patients	28	53	51	54	53	51	54
Abnormalities[a] (%)							
Triglyceride elevation	14	17	8	9	21	16	11
Creatinine kinase elevation	14	9	8	11	13	10	11
AST elevation	4	6	6	7	8	6	9
Neutropenia	4	6	2	6	6	4	7
Amylase elevation	4	4	4	0	6	4	6
Serum lipase elevation	4	2	4	2	4	6	4
Serum glucose elevation	0	6	4	0	6	4	0

AST, aspartate aminotransferase.
[a]Abnormalities occurring in five or more patients.
From Gilead Sciences, Foster City, CA, personal communication.

Table 18–2. CLINICAL TRIALS EVALUATING ACTIVITY AND EFFICACY OF TENOFOVIR DISOPROXIL FUMARATE

Trial[a]	Design	Dose (mg)	No. of subjects	Entry criteria	Duration (weeks)	CD4+ T lymphocyte count[b]	HIV RNA[c]	
							Condition 1	Condition 2
GS-97-901	Randomized, double-blind, placebo-controlled	75 150 300 600	59	CD4 ≥ 200 cells/mm^3; HIV RNA ≥ 10,000 copies/ml; ART-naive and experienced	4	Baseline: 356; NA[d]	Naive 75 mg: −0.45 log 150 mg: −0.6 log 300 mg: −1.57 log 600 mg: −1.40 log	Experienced, 75 mg: −0.27 log 150 mg: −0.49 log 300 mg: −1.06 log 600 mg: −0.66 log
GS-98-902	Randomized, double-blind, placebo-controlled	75 150 300	189	HIV RNA 400–100,000 copies/ml; TDF added to stable existing regimen	48	Baseline: 374; NS[d]	Week 24 Placebo: −0.1 log 75 mg: −0.4 log 150 mg: −0.4 log 300 mg: −0.7 log	Week 48 Placebo/300 mg: −0.6 log 75 mg: −0.4 log 150 mg: −0.6 log 300 mg: −0.6 log
GS-99-903	Randomized double-blind placebo-controlled 3TC/EFV + either D_4T or TDF	300	600	HIV RNA > 5000 ART-naive	48	Baseline: 279 cells/μl Week 48 TDF + 169 D_4T + 167		Week 48 <400 cells per milliliters (ITT) D_4T 87% TDF 87% <50 cells per milliliter (ITT) D_4T 81% TDF 82%
GS-00-907	Randomized, double-blind, placebo-controlled	300	552	HIV RNA 400–100,000 copies/ml; TDF added to stable existing regimen	48	Baseline: 427 Week 24 Placebo: −10.6 300 mg: +12.6	Week 24 (interim analysis) Placebo: −0.01 log 300 mg: −0.61 log	Week 48:NA

ART, antiretroviral therapy; NA, not available; NS, no significant difference between placebo and treatment group; TDF, tenofovir disoproxil fumarate; 3TC, lamivudine; EFV, efavirenz, D_4T, stavudine; ITT, intent to treat.

[a]Gilead Sciences, Foster City, CA. Personal communication.

[b]Mean change in absolute CD4+ T-lymphocyte count (cells/mm^3) from baseline.

[c]Mean change in plasma HIV RNA level from baseline (log_{10} copies/ml).

[d]Clinical trial was not powered to assess changes in CD4+ T-lymphocyte counts.

addition to the patient's existing stable antiretroviral regimen (four or fewer drugs) at the time of enrollment. At week 24, placebo patients rolled over in a blinded fashion to tenofovir DF 300 mg once daily, and all treatment groups were followed for a total of 48 weeks.[18,19] Mean baseline plasma HIV RNA levels were 3.8, 3.6, 3.6, and 3.7 $\log_{10}$ copies/ml in the placebo and the 75, 150, and 300 mg treatment groups, respectively. Study participants were highly treatment-experienced with a mean of 4.6 years on antiretroviral therapy and a baseline mean absolute CD4+ T-lymphocyte count of 374 cells/mm^3. In addition, baseline genotyping demonstrated that 94% of patients had nucleoside reverse transcriptase-associated mutations, 57% had protease inhibitor-associated resistant mutations, and 32% had nonnucleoside reverse transcriptase-associated mutations.

Through week 24, the mean change in plasma HIV RNA levels from baseline were − 0.1, − 0.4, − 0.4, and − 0.7 $\log_{10}$ copies/ml in the placebo and 75, 150, and 300 mg groups, respectively. Through week 48, the mean changes in HIV RNA levels from baseline were − 0.4, − 0.6, and − 0.6 $\log_{10}$ copies/ml in the 75, 150, and 300 mg groups, respectively. Placebo recipients were administered tenofovir DF (300 mg) at week 24 resulting in a mean plasma HIV RNA level reduction from baseline of 0.6 $\log_{10}$ copies/ml through week 48.[18,19]

After FDA approval of tenofovir DF, results of a phase III study (903) in antiretroviral naive patients was presented.[21a] Patients were randomized to receive efavirenz, lamivudine with either stavudine (40 mg BID)/stavudine placebo DR or tenofovir DF placebo/tenofovir DF (300 mg qD). Baseline viral load was 81,300 copies/ml and CD4 count was 279 cells/μl. Results at 48 weeks demonstrated equivalence between the two treatment groups, with 87% of patients in each group achieving <400 copies HIV RNA/ml and achievement of <50 copies per milliliter in 82% and 81% of the tenofovir DF and D_4T groups, respectively. CD4 counts increased by 169 cells/μl in the tenofovir group vs. 167 cell/μl in the D_4T group.[21a]

In a randomized, double-blind, placebo-controlled Phase III study (GS-99-907), 552 HIV-infected patients received tenofovir DF (300 mg) once daily or placebo for 24 weeks in addition to their existing antiretroviral regimen. Through week 24, placebo recipients were allowed to receive tenofovir DF for the remainder of the 48-week study period. At baseline, patients had a mean plasma HIV RNA level of 3.36 $\log_{10}$ copies/ml and a mean absolute CD4+ T-lymphocyte count of 427 cells/μl; they had received antiretroviral therapy for a mean 5.4 years. Baseline genotypic analyses in a subset of patients (n = 253) demonstrated that 94% of participants had nucleoside reverse transcriptase-associated mutations, 58% had protease inhibitor-associated resistant mutations, and 48% had nonnucleoside reverse transcriptase-associated mutations.[21]

Through week 24, the mean change in plasma HIV RNA levels from baseline were −0.61 and −0.03 $\log_{10}$ copies/ml in the tenofovir DF and placebo groups, respectively ($P <$ 0.0001). In addition, 45% of tenofovir DF recipients achieved plasma HIV RNA levels less than 400 copies/ml compared to 13% in the placebo group ($P < 0.0001$). Reduction in plasma viral burden to less than 50 copies/ml was seen in 22% of those receiving tenofovir DF compared to 1% of placebo recipients ($P < 0.0001$). The mean change in absolute CD4 cell counts from baseline were + 12.6 and − 10.6 cells/mm^3 in the tenofovir DF and placebo groups, respectively ($P = 0.0008$)[21].

▲ RESISTANCE

The presence and frequency of genotypic mutations related to tenofovir DF exposure has been examined in vitro, and information regarding drug-resistant clinical isolates is accumulating. In the presence of tenofovir, a K65R mutation in HIV reverse transcriptase has arisen during in vitro HIV passage experiments.[22] This single amino acid substitution, shown previously to be selected in vitro in the presence of zalcitabine, results in a three- to fourfold increase in the IC_{50} values for tenofovir compared to wild-type virus.[22,23] Additional HIV reverse transcriptase mutations observed in these in vitro HIV passage experiments include L228R, W25R, and P272S mutations. Recombinant viruses carrying the T69D reverse transcriptase mutation demonstrated a threefold increased IC_{50} for tenofovir compared to wild-type virus.[22] The T69S insertion confers a 23-fold increase in IC_{50} for tenofovir, whereas the T69S insertion plus the M184V mutation confers only a 6-fold increased IC_{50} for tenofovir.[24] In contrast, recombinant viruses expressing alternative reverse transcriptase mutations associated with multi-nucleoside-drug resistance (Q151M, A62V, V75I, F77L, F116Y) showed wild-type susceptibility to tenofovir but reduced susceptibility to zidovudine (38-fold).[22] In addition, recombinant viruses expressing both the M184V (associated with lamivudine resistance) and T215Y (associated with zidovudine resistance) mutations displayed increased susceptibility to tenofovir.[22] In summary, in vitro studies suggest that tenofovir may be active against HIV strains expressing one or more of the common nucleoside reverse transcriptase mutations. A possible explanation for these findings is that tenofovir may be less efficiently removed through pyrophosphorolysis and dinucleotide synthesis in HIV strains with these reverse transcriptase mutations.[25]

In a randomized, double-blind, placebo-controlled Phase II study (GS-98-902), tenofovir DF was added to background therapy in antiretroviral-experienced HIV-infected individuals (see Efficacy). Baseline and postbaseline (week 24, week 48, or early termination) genotypic evaluations were performed in 159 participants, and the development of one or more new reverse transcriptase mutations was noted in approximately 40% of the study population receiving tenofovir DF at 48 weeks. These mutations, however, were consistent with the patient's background antiretroviral therapy and were not associated with loss of HIV RNA suppression.[19] The K65R reverse transcriptase mutation, associated with tenofovir in vitro, developed in only four (2%) patients and was not linked to increasing plasma HIV RNA levels.[19] Baseline and postbaseline phenotypic analyses were performed in subjects randomized to receive tenofovir DF 300 mg once daily (n = 54). At baseline, phenotypes revealed a mean reduced susceptibility of 1.9- and 13.8-

fold over wild-type susceptibility for tenofovir DF and zidovidine, respectively. In regression analyses, plasma HIV RNA suppression was significantly correlated with baseline susceptibility to tenofovir DF ($P = 0.007$) and zidovudine ($P = 0.035$) but not to other nucleoside agents.[19] At week 48 about 50% of evaluable patients demonstrated increased susceptibility to tenofovir DF, and the remaining half displayed reduced susceptibility (2.7- to 4.3-fold) to the drug. Individuals developing the K65R reverse transcriptase mutation ($n = 4$) showed a three- to fourfold reduction in susceptibility to tenofovir DF consistent with prior in vitro studies.[19] As was noted in the genotypic analysis, low-level reduced susceptibility to tenofovir DF was not associated with loss of HIV RNA suppression at 48 weeks. A more detailed genotypic resistance analysis was performed on a larger subset of patients receiving tenofovir DF at 300 mg per day as part of Phase II and III studies (GS-98-902 and GS-99-907). In this analysis, the presence of M4IL or LZIOW as part of at least 3 thymidine-analogue-associated mutations (TAMs) reduced the viral load response to tenofovir DF -0.21 $\log_{10}$ copies/ml, compared TO -0.80 $\log_{10}$ copies/ml when no TAMs were present.[26] In a similar phenotypic resistance analysis, small and incremental reductions in viral load response were noted in patients with reduced tenofovir susceptibility of 1 to 3 and 3 to 4-fold from wild-type, with a greater reduction in viral load response for patients with a greater than 4-fold change.[26] Prior adefovir dipivoxil exposure does not result in the development of reduced susceptibility to tenofovir DF.[27]

▲ DRUG INTERACTIONS

To date, no clinically significant drug interactions have been reported with tenofovir DF therapy. A randomized, open-label, multiple-dose, crossover study (GS-00-909) was performed to assess pharmacologic interactions following co-administration of tenofovir DF with lamivudine, didanosine, indinavir, lopinavir/ritonavir, or efavirenz. Tenofovir steady state exposure (area under the curve [AUC]) were found to be equivalent when co-administered with lamivudine, didanosine, indinavir, or efavirenz. Similarly, indinavir and efavirenz AUC were unaffected in the presence of tenofovir DF therapy. Lamivudine plasma levels were lower in the setting of tenofovir DF co-administration as manifested by a 24% reduction in C_{max} and a 0.9 hour T_{max} delay. These findings are presumably secondary to a slower absorption rate for lamivudine in this setting, but AUC levels were not significantly changed and this interaction is not felt to be clinically significant.[28] Lopinavir and ritonavir area under the curves were lower (15% and 24%, respectively), and the tenofovir AUC was 34% higher during their coadministration.[28] Coadministration of didanosine (buffered tablet formulation) and tenofovir DF resulted in a 44% increase in didanosine AUC; However, a review of Phase II and III trial participants receiving didanosine and tenofovir DF concomitantly for up to 24 weeks showed no apparent increase in didanosine-related adverse events.[29] Further studies are underway with the enteric-coated (Videx EC) formulation to evaluate tenofovir DF and didanosine pharmacokinetics when coadministered with and without food. Further clinical experience and similar pharmacologic analyses are necessary to fully assess the potential for drug interactions with tenofovir DF coadministration.

Of note, tenofovir DF is eliminated through renal excretion, but no formal dosing adjustment recommendations are currently available for patients with acute or chronic renal insufficiency. Clinicians should monitor the prescription of drugs with overlapping toxicities.

▲ RECOMMENDATIONS FOR USE

The efficacy of tenofovir DF in combination with other antiretroviral agents demonstrates the drug's utility in both naive and antiretroviral experienced patients. At this time, the long-term tolerability of tenofovir DF in the treatment of HIV-1-infected individuals as a component of initial combination therapy or in secondary regimens has not been completely elucidated. However, the drug's favorable resistance profile and sustainable anti-HIV activity in patients with documented genotypic resistance to existing nucleoside agents will make it an attractive option for both treatment-naive and treatment-experienced patients.

▲ CONCLUSIONS

At doses of 75 to 600 mg/day tenofovir DF has anti-HIV activity as documented by suppression of plasma HIV RNA levels in antiretroviral-naive patients (range 0.45 to 1.4 $\log_{10}$ copies/ml) and antiretroviral-experienced patients (range 0.3 to 1.1 $\log_{10}$ copies/ml). Sustained antiretroviral activity has been observed up to 48 weeks.

Tenofovir has favorable pharmacokinetics that allow single daily dosing. The oral prodrug tenofovir DF provides improved oral bioavailability, which is further increased when the agent is administered in the fed state. In animal studies, elimination occurred via renal excretion.

The safety of tenofovir DF has been studied in more than 1600 patients in clinical trials, and the drug is generally well tolerated. Elevations in serum triglyceride levels, liver transaminases, and creatine kinase have been observed, but the percentage of study participants with abnormal values was not significantly different than the frequency of these findings observed in patients receiving placebo. Interestingly, nephrotoxicity has not been noted in patients receiving tenofovir DF as was described in individuals receiving the structurally similar compound adefovir dipivoxil. Completion and analysis of Phase III studies are necessary to formulate a complete toxicity profile of this drug.

In vitro genotypic analysis has demonstrated that tenofovir DF maintains activity against most nucleoside-resistant HIV strains but may select for a K65 HIV reverse transcriptase mutation resulting in a three- to fourfold reduction in tenofovir susceptibility. The clinical relevance of the development of genotypic mutations in the setting of tenofovir DF therapy is unclear, but the development of these mutations was rare (fewer than 3% of patients) and not linked to loss of HIV RNA suppression in 48-week clinical trials. Further genotypic and phenotypic analysis of clinical isolates is currently under investigation.

REFERENCES

1. Naesens I, Snocek R, Andrei G, et al. HPMC (cidofovir), PMEA (adefovir), and related acyclic nucleoside phosphonate analogues: a review of their pharmacology and clinical potential in the treatment of viral infections. Antivir Chem Chemother 8:1, 1997.
2. Balzarini J, DeClerq E. 5-Phosphoribosyl 1-pyrophosphate synthetase converts the acyclic nucleoside phosphonates 9-(3-hydroxy-2-phosphonylmethoxypropyl)adenine and 9-(2- phosphonylmethoxyethyl)adenine directly to their antivirally active diphosphate derivatives. J Biol Chem 266:8686, 1991.
3. De Clerq E, Sakium T, Baba M, et al. Antiviral activity of phosphonomethoxyalkyl derivatives of purines and pyrimidines. Antiviral Res 8:261, 1987.
4. Yokota T, Konno K, Shigeta S, et al. Inhibitory effects of acyclic nucleoside phosphonate analogues on hepatitis B virus DNA synthesis in HB1611 cells. Antivir Chem Chemother 5:52, 1994.
5. Srinivas R, Robbins B, Connelly M, et al. Metabolism and in vitro antiretroviral activities of bis(pivaloyloxymethyl) prodrugs of acyclic nucleoside phosphonates. Antimicrob Agents Chemother 37:2247, 1993.

5a. Bochet M, Tubiana R, Benhamov Y, et al. Tenofovir disoproxil fumarate suppresses lamivudine resistant HBV replication in patients co-infected with HIV/HBV. In: Abstracts of the 9th Conference on Betroviruses and Opportunistic Infections, Seattle, 2002, abstract 675.

6. De Clerq E. Acyclic nucleoside phosphonates in the chemotherapy of DNA virus and retrovirus infections. Intervirology 40:295, 1997.
7. Hartmann K, Balzarini J, Higgins J, et al. In vitro activity of acyclic nucleoside phosphonate derivatives against feline immunodeficiency virus in Crandall feline kidney cells and feline peripheral blood lymphocytes. Antivir Chem Chemother 5:13, 1994.
8. Thormar H, Balzarini J, HolyA, et al. Inhibition of visna virus replication by 2′, 3′-dideoxynucleosides and acyclic nucleoside phosphonate analogs. Antimicrob Agents Chemother 37:2540, 1993.
9. Haesens L, Balzarini J, Rosenberg I, et al. 9-(2-Phosphonylmethoxyethyl)-2,6-diaminopurine (PMEDAP): a novel agent with anti-human immunodeficiency virus activity in vitro and potent anti-Moloney murine sarcoma virus activity in vivo. Eur J Clin Microbiol 8:1043, 1989.
10. Palmer S, Buckheit W, Gilbert H, et al. Anti-HIV activity of PMEA, PMPA (9-(2-phosphonylmethoxypropyl)adenine) and AZT against HIV-1 subtypes A, B, C, D, E, F, G, and O. In: Abstracts of the 13th International Conference on Antiviral Research, Baltimore, 2000, abstract 21.
11. Balzarini J, Perno C, Schols D, et al. Activity of acyclic nucleoside phosphonate analogues against human immunodeficiency virus in monocytes/macrophages and peripheral blood lymphocytes. Biochem Biophys Res Commun 178:329, 1991.
12. Cherrington J, Allen S, Bischofberger N, et al. Kinetic interaction of the diphosphates of 9-(2-phosphonylmethoxyethyl)adenine and other anti-HIV active pure congeners with HIV reverse transcriptase and human DNA polymerase α, β, and γ. Antivir Chem Chemother 6:217, 1995.

12a. Lovie M, Hogan C, Hurley A, et al. Determining the relative efficacy of tenofovir DF using frequent measurements of HIV-1 RNA during a short course of monotheraphy in antiretroviral drug naive individuals. In: Abstracts of the 9th Conference on Retroviruses and Opportunistic Infections, Seattle, 2002, abstract 3.

13. Robbins B, Srinivas R, Kim C, et al. Anti-human immunodeficiency virus activity and cellular metabolism of a potential prodrug of the acyclic nucleoside phosphonate 9-R-(2-phosphonomethoxypropyl)adenine (PMPA), bis(isopropyloxymethylcarbonyl)PMPA. Antimicrob Agent Chemother 42:612, 1998.
14. Mulato M, Cherrington J. Anti-HIV activity of adefovir (PMEA) and PMPA in combination with other antiretroviral compounds: in vitro analyses. Antiviral Res 36:91, 1997.
15. Cherrington J, Mulato A. Adefovir (PMEA) and PMPA show synergistic or additive inhibition of HIV replication in vitro in combination with other anti-HIV agents. In: Abstracts of the 12th World AIDS Conference, Geneva, 1998, abstract 4115.
16. Deeks S, Barditch-Crovo P, Lietman P, et al. Safety, pharmacokinetics, and antiretroviral activity of intravenous 9-[2-(R)-(phosphonomethoxy)propyl]adenine, a novel anti-human immunodeficiency virus (HIV) therapy, in HIV-infected adults. Antimicrob Agent Chemother 42: 2380, 1998.
17. Barditch-Crovo P, Deeks S, Collier A, et al. Phase I/II trial of the pharmacokinetics, safety, and antiretroviral activity of tenofovir disoproxil fumarate in human immunodeficiency virus-infected adults. Antimicrob Agents Chemother 45:2773, 2001.
18. Schooley R, Ruane P, Myers R, et al. Tenofovir DF in antiretroviral-experienced patients: results from a 48-week, randomized, double-blind study. AIDS 2002 (in press).
19. Margot N, Isaacson E, McGowan I, et al. Genotypic and phenotypic analyses of HIV-1 in antiretroviral-experienced patients treated with tenofovir DF. AIDS 2002 (in press).
20. Toole J. Tenofovir disoproxil fumarate, NDA 21-356. Presented at United States Food and Drug Administration Antiviral Drugs Advisory Committee, October 3, 2001, Silver Spring, MD.
21. Squires K, Pierone G, Berger D, et al. Tenofovir DF: a 24-week interim analysis from a phase III double blind, placebo controlled study in antiretroviral experienced patients. In: Abstracts of the 41st Interscience Conference on Antimicrobial Agents and Chemotherapy, Chicago, 2001, abstract 666.

21a. Staszewski C, Gallont J, Pozniak AL, et al. Efficacy and safety of tenofovir disopoxil fumarate (TDF) versus stavudine (D_4T) when used in combination with lamivudine (3TC) and efavirenz (EFV) in HIV-1 infected patients, naive to antiretroviral therapy (ART): 48-week interim results. In: Abstracts of the XIV International AIDS Conference, Barcelona, Spain, 2002, abstract LbOr 17.

22. Wainberg M, Miller M, Quan Y, et al. In vitro selection and characterization of HIV-1 with reduced susceptibility to PMPA. Antivir Ther 4:87, 1999.
23. Gu Z, Gao I, Fang H, et al. Identification of a mutation at codon 65 in the JKKK motif of reverse transcriptase that encodes resistance to 2′,3′-dideoxycitidine and 2′,3′-dideoxythiacytidine. Antimicrob Agent Chemother 38:275, 1994.
24. Miller M, Margot N, Hertogs K, et al. Antiviral activity of tenofovir (PMPA) against nucleoside-resistant HIV samples. In: Abstracts of the 40th Interscience Conference on Antimicrobial Agents and Chemotherapy, Toronto, 2000, abstract 2115.
25. Naeger L, Margot N, Miller M. Tenofovir (PMPA) is less efficiently removed through pyrophosphorolysis and dinucleotide synthesis than zidovudine (AZT) by HIV-1 wild-type RT and RT mutants. In: Abstracts of the 40th Interscience Conference on Antimicrobial Agents and Chemotherapy, Toronto, 2000, abstract 1265.
26. Viread (tenofovir DF) prescribing information, Gilead Sciences, Inc., October 2001.
27. Miller M, Margot D, Lamy P, et al. Adefovir and tenofovir susceptibilities of HIV-1 after 24–48 weeks of adefovir dipivoxil therapy: genotypic and phenotypic analyses of study GS-96-408. J AIDS 27:450, 2001.
28. Flaherty J, Kearney B, Wolf J, et al. A multiple-dose, randomized, crossover, drug interaction study between tenofovir DF and lamivudine or didanosine. In: Abstracts of the 1st IAS Conference on HIV Pathogenesis and Treatment, Buenos Aires, 2001, abstract 337 ub.
29. Flaherty J, Kearney B, Wolf J, et al. Coadministration of tenofovir DF (TDF) and didanosine (ddI): A pharmacokinetic and safety evaluation. In: Abstracts of the 41st Interscience Conference on Antimicrobial Agents and Chemotheraphy, Chicago, 2001, abstract I-1729.

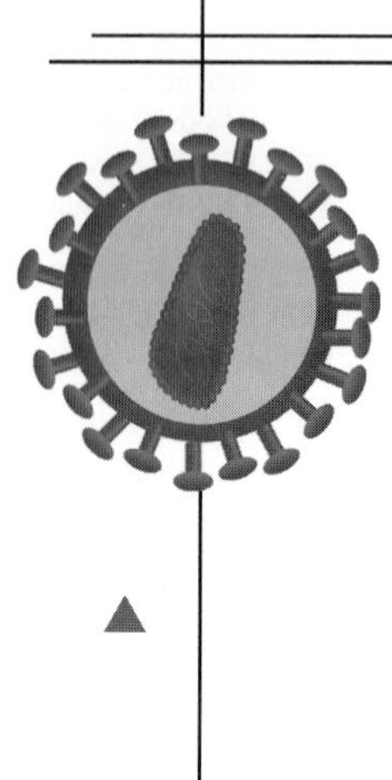

CHAPTER 19

Inhibitors of HIV Attachment and Fusion

J. Michael Kilby, MD

Despite promising results from recent therapeutic advancements, there remains an urgent need to develop new classes of antiretroviral therapy with different mechanisms of action. Currently approved therapies for human immunodeficiency virus (HIV) infection target one of two HIV-specific enzymes: reverse transcriptase (RT) or protease. Each of the currently available agents has the ability to select for less susceptible viral strains both in vitro and in clinical practice. In many cases there is evidence that resistance to one compound confers at least partial resistance to other compounds within that same drug class. Another factor contributing to the need for novel antiretroviral classes is the potential for adverse effects that may be shared to varying degrees by many or all drugs within a class.

Theoretically, the successful inhibition of viral entry into host cells would provide certain advantages over drugs targeting viral enzymes employed in the later steps of the viral life cycle. Blocking cell entry might have potential as a preventive strategy (e.g., as a topical microbicide or systemic "postexposure prophylaxis") or as therapy to limit spread of existing viral infection to other cells and tissues in the body. Because this target is unrelated to RT or protease function, blocking viral entry offers less potential for cross-resistance or shared toxicity with drugs from the currently available therapeutic classes. The process of HIV entry into target cells is complex, involving multiple steps that have been recognized only gradually over many years of research, and it remains incompletely elucidated. The history of investigational attempts to block HIV entry is therefore also complicated, characterized by serendipitous discoveries and occasionally the need for reinterpretation of previous experimental results.

The HIV entry into target cells begins with binding of noncontiguous, folded portions of the viral surface glycoprotein (gp120) to the CD4 molecule expressed on host target cells, particularly T-helper lymphocytes and certain cells in the monocyte/macrophage lineage. The CD4 molecule normally serves to bind major histocompatibility complex (MHC) class II molecules during the process of stabilizing the critical immune response interaction between the T cell receptor and peptide antigens. The initial interaction between the HIV-1 surface glycoproteins and CD4 triggers a conformational change in gp120 to expose an otherwise inaccessible "co-receptor" binding site, which typically has an affinity for chemokines that bind either the CCR5 or CXCR4 class of host receptors.[1,2]

The HIV-1 universally binds to CD4, but the affinity of each individual viral isolate for the chemokine "co-receptors" falls somewhere along a spectrum from selective tropism for CCR5 ("R5" viruses) to dual tropism ("R5X4") to selective tropism for CXCR4 ("X4" viruses). Although almost all HIV isolates infect activated primary CD4+ T-lymphocytes, there are distinct differences in cellular tropism between isolates: R5 viruses are able to replicate efficiently in primary T cells or macrophages (previously called M-tropic viruses), whereas X4 viruses replicate poorly in macrophages but are uniquely pathogenic against established T cell lines in the laboratory (previously called T-tropic). Although there are exceptions to the general rule, most transmitted viruses are CCR5-tropic, whereas CXCR4-tropic viruses more often evolve in the host long after acquisition and are associated with more advanced, progressive disease. HIV-1 isolates, designated syncytium-inducing (SI) because of their ability to induce characteristic "giant cell" formation in laboratory T cell lines, tend to fall into the CXCR4-tropic end of the spectrum, whereas non-syncytium-inducing (NSI) viruses tend to be CKR5-tropic and bind more readily to monocyte/macrophage target cells.

Following attachment at both the CD4 and chemokine receptor sites, the viral transmembrane glycoprotein (gp41) undergoes a conformational change that brings about fusion of the viral and cellular membranes.[2,3] The fusion step allows viral contents to be taken up by the target cell, which ultimately leads to integration into the host nucleus and production of new viral progeny (see Fig. 19–1, later in this chapter). This complex, stepwise process may help explain why the immune system has limited success in controlling HIV replication in that key epitopes are basically protected from antibody access during most of the virus's life cycle.

There are other potential therapeutic targets that could be exploited in the future to alter viral attachment or the trafficking of virally infected cells in the body. For example, host adhesion molecules, such as intracellular (ICAM-1) and vascular cell (VCAM-1) adhesion molecules, contribute to the circulation pattern of HIV-infected T cells,[4] and virion-bound adhesion molecules [ICAM-1, VCAM-1, leukocyte function associated antigen (LFA-1), and very late activation antigen (VLA-4)] may affect viral pathogenicity.[5,6] Strategies to decrease the frequency of activated T cells, although potentially problematic because of the risk of worsening immunosuppression, have been proposed to decrease the risk of spread to new target cells during periods of HIV replication. Examples of experimental therapies that might affect the binding of HIV to T cells at least in part by down-regulating cellular activation include cyclosporine, hydroxyurea, cyclophosphamide, and corticosteroids. Another recognized host target that could play a significant role in the early stages of HIV pathogenesis is the cell surface protein designated DC-SIGN. This protein, expressed in high concentration on dendritic cells, binds avidly to HIV gp120 but does not lead to viral entry. It has been hypothesized that DC-SIGN expression is a critical mediator in the transport of infectious viral particles from mucosal surfaces to the T cells in lymphoid tissues.[7]

Although these and other diverse host targets represent possible areas for future clinical study, this chapter reviews only the status of therapeutic strategies designed to intervene at three fundamental steps of the viral life cycle related to attachment and entry: CD4 binding, chemokine co-receptor binding, and membrane fusion.

▲ BLOCKING THE CD4 RECEPTOR

It has been known since the 1980s that a critical initial step in the viral entry process is the binding of portions of the HIV surface glycoprotein (gp120) to the CD4 receptor, expressed primarily on T-helper lymphocytes.[8,9] The presence of CD4 receptors on cells infected with HIV in vitro was shown to correlate with the formation of syncytia, or multinucleated giant cells, considered characteristic of retroviral infection in the laboratory. Depletion of CD4+ T-lymphocytes has long been recognized as the best characterized immunologic lesion of acquired immunodeficiency syndrome (AIDS) (although the exact pathogenesis of this immunodeficiency remains a point of some controversy). The degree of CD4+ T-lymphocyte deficiency in HIV-infected patients directly correlates with the risk of opportunistic infections and neoplastic conditions. Therefore, a logical therapeutic strategy was to develop inhibitors of CD4 receptor binding.

In 1988 several investigative groups published encouraging in vitro data demonstrating that recombinant, soluble CD4 could competitively inhibit HIV infection and syncytium formation, presumably by acting as a "decoy" by binding to gp120 in place of susceptible CD4-expressing T cells.[10–12] Johnson et al. reported that zidovudine, the only approved HIV therapy at that time, was synergistic with soluble CD4 at suppressing HIV infection in vitro.[13] However, two independent clinical trials, although suggesting there were no severe or frequent toxicities caused by intravenous administration of soluble CD4, did not demonstrate any antiviral effects in vivo.[14,15] These studies represent critical early demonstrations that laboratory-adapted HIV strains may not always reliably predict the behavior of HIV isolates in the clinical setting. The lack of clinical efficacy with soluble CD4 was later explained, at least in part, by the discovery that HIV also utilizes chemokine co-receptors to gain cellular entry. Improved understanding of the multistep viral binding and fusion process has led to a more dynamic, complex viral entry model; therefore the hope for a simple, universal viral entry target may appear less tenable. The question remains, however, about whether these early failures represented a pharmacologic phenomenon in that soluble CD4 may be rapidly metabolized in the body and therefore not achieve sustained effective concentrations in the formulations tested.

One experimental approach to interfering with the gp120–CD4 attachment is to use highly specific antibodies against the CD4 target. A murine monoclonal antibody against a specific sequence of human CD4 was shown to be capable of inhibiting primary HIV isolates from multiple, but not all, clades in an in vitro peripheral blood mononuclear cell infectivity assay.[16] The particular monoclonal antibodies to be utilized for clinical study should be cautiously selected, as anti-CD4 antibody studies involving research subjects with other medical conditions have resulted in long-lasting depletion of the absolute CD4 count in some instances[17] but no apparent adverse effects even at high doses in others.[18]

Another approach is to try to improve the logistics of administering the short-lived soluble CD4 formulations. Early attempts to design a chimeric molecule of CD4 bound to gamma globulin resulted in extending the half-life of the compound, but again no clinically significant antiviral activity was demonstrated in combination with zidovudine.[19] A tetravalent, recombinant antibody-like fusion protein has been developed that has much greater in vitro activity against primary HIV isolates (and not merely laboratory-adapted strains) compared with monovalent CD4-based proteins.[20] This heterotetramer strategy potently inhibited primary HIV isolates from across different clades in in vitro experiments[21] and was protective against infectious HIV challenge in a SCID-hu mouse model.[22]

In a Phase I dose-escalation trial involving HIV-infected adults, a heterotetramer compound designated PRO 542 [CD4–immunoglobulin G2 (IgG2)] had a terminal serum half-life of 3 to 4 days, and single doses were well tolerated.[23] Anti-CD4 antibodies were not detected after single doses. Although the evidence is considered preliminary, statistically significant temporary declines in viral load were observed at the highest-dose group tested (10 mg/kg). The mean HIV RNA change was -0.36 $\log_{10}$ copies/ml 4 hours after dosing, and one subject experienced a an approximately 2 $\log_{10}$ reduction during the 2 weeks following a single dose. A similar trial involving single and recurrent (weekly) intravenous recombinant CD4–IgG2 in HIV-infected children also showed good tolerability and preliminary evidence of dose-related antiviral activity (several children had acute viral load declines of >0.7 $\log_{10}$ copies/ml).[24] Some investigators have speculated that this apparently rapid antiviral effect may relate to more efficient immune clearance of virus when bound to the CD4–IgG2 protein.[23]

▲ "NONSPECIFIC" POLYANION INTERFERENCE

Another series of studies in 1988 suggested the potential for sulfated polyanionic substances to interfere with the initial attachment of HIV to T cells, resulting in potent inhibition of viral replication in vitro.[25–27] One hypothesis was that the highly concentrated negative charges on heparin-like compounds mediate nonspecific interactions with viral glycoproteins. However, oral dextran was not sufficiently bioavailable in clinical studies,[28,29] and attempts to administer dextran intravenously resulted in severe, especially hematologic, adverse events.[30] Some individuals unexpectedly had evidence of increased, rather than decreased, viral load markers on intravenous dextran therapy.[30] In vitro experiments suggest that the particular host cell type studied and the specific sequences of the gp120 binding region in various viral isolates are factors that significantly affect the type and degree of virologic responses to dextran.[31]

An improving understanding of viral entry mechanisms has led to less speculation about "nonspecific interference" and more mechanistic explanations for previous experimental results with polyanionic compounds. There is evidence to suggest that certain polyanions directly interfere with CD4–gp120 binding. Several naphthalene derivatives have been shown to inhibit CD4–gp120 interactions specifically, leading to suppression of HIV replication in the laboratory, but these substances also have the potential for substantial cellular toxicity.[32] Such compounds may have potential as topical microbicides, such as the naphthalene sulfonate polymer "PRO 2000,"[32] which is now in Phase II preventive clinical trials in an intravaginal gel formulation.[33]

A more recent proposal is that some polyanionic compounds actually have an antiviral effect due to interactions at the chemokine receptor level. FP-21399, another naphthalene derivative related to chemical photography dyes, has been under development because it may specifically target gp120–CXCR4 binding. This compound blocked HIV replication in SCID-hu mice and effectively concentrated in lymphoid tissues in this animal model.[34] A Phase I study of intravenous FP-21399 involving 34 HIV-infected adults suggested that the compound is relatively well tolerated, although the agent or its metabolites result in a bluish discoloration of the urine and skin.[35] Further clinical data are necessary to determine whether a significant in vivo antiviral effect is possible and practically achievable. More detailed knowledge of the tertiary structure of the HIV-1 surface glycoproteins and mapping experiments utilizing monoclonal antibodies has suggested that other polynanions (e.g., heparin and dextran sulfate) specifically interfere with the CXCR4 co-receptor region, in contrast to CD4 or CCR5 binding.[36]

▲ BLOCKING THE "CHEMOKINE CO-RECEPTOR" NEXUS

Between 1995 and 1997 a number of investigative groups reported that beta chemokines and their derivatives had a significant inhibitory effect on viral replication in vitro.[37–39] The initial observations occurred at a time when the CD4 receptor was the only well characterized cell entry mechanism for HIV, so the implications of these findings were not fully understood. As already summarized, NSI viruses typically require the presence of the beta chemokine receptor CCR5 in addition to CD4.[40,41] CCR5 is the major receptor for RANTES, macrophage inflammatory protein-α (MIP-1α), and MIP-β, which are natural mediators of inflammatory reactions and chemotaxis already known to have HIV suppressive effects in vitro. SI or "T-tropic" viral isolates, often associated with more rapid disease progression in the setting of advanced HIV infection and AIDS, tend to utilize the alpha chemokine receptor CXCR4 (also called fusin).[42] The natural ligand for CXCR4 is stromal-derived factor (SDF-1), a protein constitutively expressed in many tissues that may mediate cellular trafficking such as the homing of lymphocytes to inflamed tissues or the repopulation of transplanted stem cells into bone marrow.[43,44] There are extensive databases on agents potentially relevant to the HIV/chemokine nexus at multiple pharmaceutical companies because the seven transmembrane G-coupled protein structure of the chemokine receptors is common in many other biologic processes important to medicine.

Strategies for inhibiting the chemokine co-receptor step might be broadly divided into two categories: (1) manipulation of chemokine receptor expression and function; and (2) administration of ligands or their derivatives to serve as competitive inhibitors. However, this distinction may not always be clear-cut. The suppressive effects of both CXCR4 and CCR5 ligands in vitro may be mediated by receptor internalization into vesicles or early endosomes, not merely by competitive inhibition of binding.[45] The potency of the beta chemokines (RANTES>>MIP-1β >MIP 1α) for preventing HIV infection of primary CD4+ T-lymphocyte correlates with the degree of receptor down-regulation in one experimental model.[46]

Novel approaches to the therapeutic manipulation of chemokine receptor expression have also been explored. A gene therapy strategy involving expression of a modified CXCR4 molecule (an "intrakine") demonstrated antiviral effects against T-tropic HIV in vitro, possibly because the altered CXCR4 was effectively trapped in the endoplasmic reticulum and not appropriately expressed on the cell surface for HIV binding.[47] In a different approach, Carroll et al. performed a series of clinical trials in which leukopheresis is performed on HIV-infected individuals, isolated CD4+ T-lymphocyte are co-stimulated ex vivo with CD3/CD28, and then the amplified CD4+ T-lymphocyte population is reinfused into the host. In addition to the potential benefits of increased absolute CD4+ T-lymphocyte counts, these reinfused CD4+ T-lymphocyte may result in less susceptibility to M-tropic virus disease progression because the co-stimulation process down-regulates cellular CCR5 expression.[48] The possibility of using antibodies, actively induced or passively administered, against chemokine receptors as a therapeutic approach has also been proposed.[49]

The most straightforward approach to blocking chemokine receptors is to administer natural ligands or other small molecules that may serve as competitive inhibitors. Several investigative groups continue to explore the potential of the beta chemokines as agents targeting CCR5 binding. Although there is little or no experience with these compounds in clinical trials, the results from cell culture experiments[50,51] and an "intact lymphoid tissue" model[52] provide further evidence for antiviral effectiveness of several of the RANTES derivatives. These agents have limited bioavailability and would require parenteral administration. There is limited information regarding the safety of infusing an inflammatory mediator and signaling molecule such as RANTES with the potential for myriad nonspecific effects.

Several small molecules targeting the CCR5 receptor are in preclinical development. A nonpeptide designated TAK-779 has the potential advantage of inhibiting RANTES/CCR5 binding without interfering with RANTES binding to other chemokine receptors. TAK-779 is a highly selective, potent agent in vitro, but clinical studies have not been completed at this time.[53,54] Another small nonpeptide molecule selective antagonist of CCR5, called Schering C, has potent activity in the SCID-hu mouse model in preliminary studies and has pharmacokinetic characteristics suggesting that oral administration may be plausible; moreover, there is no rapid selection for drug resistance during rounds of in vitro infection.[55]

There is no clinical information available about administering SDF-1, the alpha chemokine ligand for CXCR4, as a competitive inhibitor in humans. Laboratory studies to characterize SDF structure and function better have been completed.[56] Poor bioavailability and low potency inhibition may limit the clinical feasibility of this approach.

Several injectable small peptides that specifically block HIV binding to the CXCR4 receptor appear promising, but they are still in preclinical or early clinical development. In comparison to derivatives of the natural ligands of CCR5, which represent large complex chemical structures with limited bioavailability, several of these smaller molecules show potential for distinct advantages in terms of the prospects for bulk synthesis and predictable pharmacokinetics. T22 is a synthesized 18-amino acid CXCR4 blocker with limited bioavailability.[57] A smaller derivative, T134 (14 amino acids), exhibited greater potency and less cytotoxicity in vitro.[58] A polycationic compound called ALX40-4C also has demonstrated CXCR4 blocker effects in vitro.[59] The antiviral effect of ALX40-4C may be nonspecifically charge-mediated rather than related to down-regulation of receptors.

Bicyclam agents are another example of small-molecule CXCR4 inhibitors with clinical potential, including one agent that has entered Phase II trials. Several studies by De Clercq and colleagues described the in vitro antiretroviral effects of bicyclam compounds years before the role of the chemokine "co-receptors" was understood.[60–62] More recent in vitro investigations involving one of these compounds, AMD3100, provided convincing data to support the feasibility of blocking HIV-1 entry via the CXCR4 co-receptor.[63] AMD3100 interferes with receptor binding to the natural ligand SDF-1 and to a monoclonal antibody specific for CXCR4 (12G5). Although "time of addition" and cell fusion/entry assays demonstrate that AMD3100 interacts specifically with CXCR4, the mechanism of action may involve altering the tertiary structure of the receptor rather than directly signaling the receptor.[63] In vitro experiments demonstrate that this bicyclam compound provides sufficient selective pressure on X4 viruses to induce the emergence of R5 isolates, which theoretically could provide a clinical advantage.[64] A clinical trial of AMD3100 in healthy volunteers demonstrated that oral bioavailability was inadequate, but intravenous dosing resulted in reasonably sustained (about 8 to 12 hours) drug levels that correlate with potent antiviral effects in vitro.[65]

A single amino acid substitution in the viral envelope sequence that results in loss of a positive electrostatic charge can confer significant drug resistance to AMD3100.[66] On the other hand, it is noteworthy that unrelated small-molecule inhibitors of CXCR4 binding, such as T134, may have no cross-drug resistance with the bicyclams, which suggests that binding sites and resistance mechanisms are certainly not identical for all CXCR4 inhibitors.[58] Utilizing small molecules, entry inhibitor combinations to help avoid or overcome drug resistance is also a conceivable therapeutic strategy, as discussed later.

Several uncertainties remain that have limited rapid clinical development of inhibitors of the chemokine co-receptor nexus. There appears to be significant variability in the inhibitory effects of chemokines against specific viral strains, and these differences are more complex than just the SI and NSI distinctions.[67] There is insufficient information regarding the normal role chemokines play in inflammatory responses and other physiologic processes. It is clear, however, that it is possible to design agents that specifically block HIV binding without triggering the functional activity of the chemokine receptor. The discovery of the role of CCR5 receptors in HIV was due in part to the recognition of mutations affecting CCR5 expression among individuals who were "multiply exposed" to HIV yet not infected with the virus.[68–70] Thus there is solid evidence from nature that individuals with altered CCR5 expression may have relative protection from HIV infection without suffering any apparent consequences to their overall health. However, evidence related to the effects of alterations in the CXCR4 pathway raises theoretical concerns. Knockout mice that cannot express SDF-1, the ligand for CXCR4, undergo abnormal fetal development (cardiac and B cell lymphopoiesis defects) and die perinatally.[71] Another theoretical concern is that effectively blocking one of the chemokine receptors may merely provide selection pressure for the outgrowth of viruses utilizing alternative receptors. One undesirable scenario is that selectively inhibiting NSI viruses by administering one of the CCR5 receptor antagonists for example, may ultimately drive the evolution of viral strains within an individual to SI CXCR4-utilizing viruses[51] associated with more rapid clinical progression and CD4 depletion.[72] Therefore a multimodal attack against several receptors may be necessary, which could mean that challenges lie ahead in verifying the safety and efficacy of this approach.

▲ BLOCKING MEMBRANE FUSION

The strategies outlined so far have focused on the interactions between HIV and the surface glycoprotein gp120. The subsequent step in the viral entry process, gp-41-mediated membrane fusion, has potential as a more universal therapeutic target because it may be utilized by all HIV isolates regardless of cellular tropism or antigenic variations, although this is debatable, as discussed later.

Early studies of the gp41 molecular sequence revealed "heptad repeat" sequences in two regions that give the protein periodic hydrophobicity. These consensus motifs ("leucine zippers") were predictive of an alpha-helical structure within the transmembrane glycoprotein.[73,74] Synthetic peptides, originally called DP107 and DP178, corresponding to these heptad repeat sequences were found to inhibit HIV infection in vitro.[75,76] A series of experiments over the next several years suggested that these regions of gp41 form a helical bundle, or "coiled coil" structure, that is critical for membrane fusion to occur. Mutations in these leucine zipper regions of gp41 were found to disrupt the "coiled coil" structure and thereby interfere with membrane fusion and infectivity. It was proposed that synthetic peptides corresponding to these alpha helical regions had antiretroviral activity mediated by disruption of the tertiary protein structure of the protein.[77–81]

A model of gp-41-mediated membrane fusion was proposed that was analogous to the "spring-loaded" mechanism described for influenza virus.[82] When influenza virus first binds to a target cell, hemaglutinin goes through a conformational change, extending from a loop structure to an extended "coiled coil." This allows a "fusion peptide" to shift to a favorable position so membrane fusion can occur. The corresponding model proposed for HIV gp41 (Fig. 19–1) is that the fusion peptide is in an unexposed position when gp41 is in its native, "nonfusogenic" state. After gp120 binds to a target cell, gp41 changes conformation, unfolding by a molecular hinge mechanism. The fusion peptide is then extended away from the virus surface and therefore better able to insert into the cell membrane. If the transmembrane glycoprotein (gp41) then returns to its native, folded ("hairpin") conformation, the result would be to pull the viral and cell membranes into close proximity for fusion and viral entry to occur. Based on this model, the

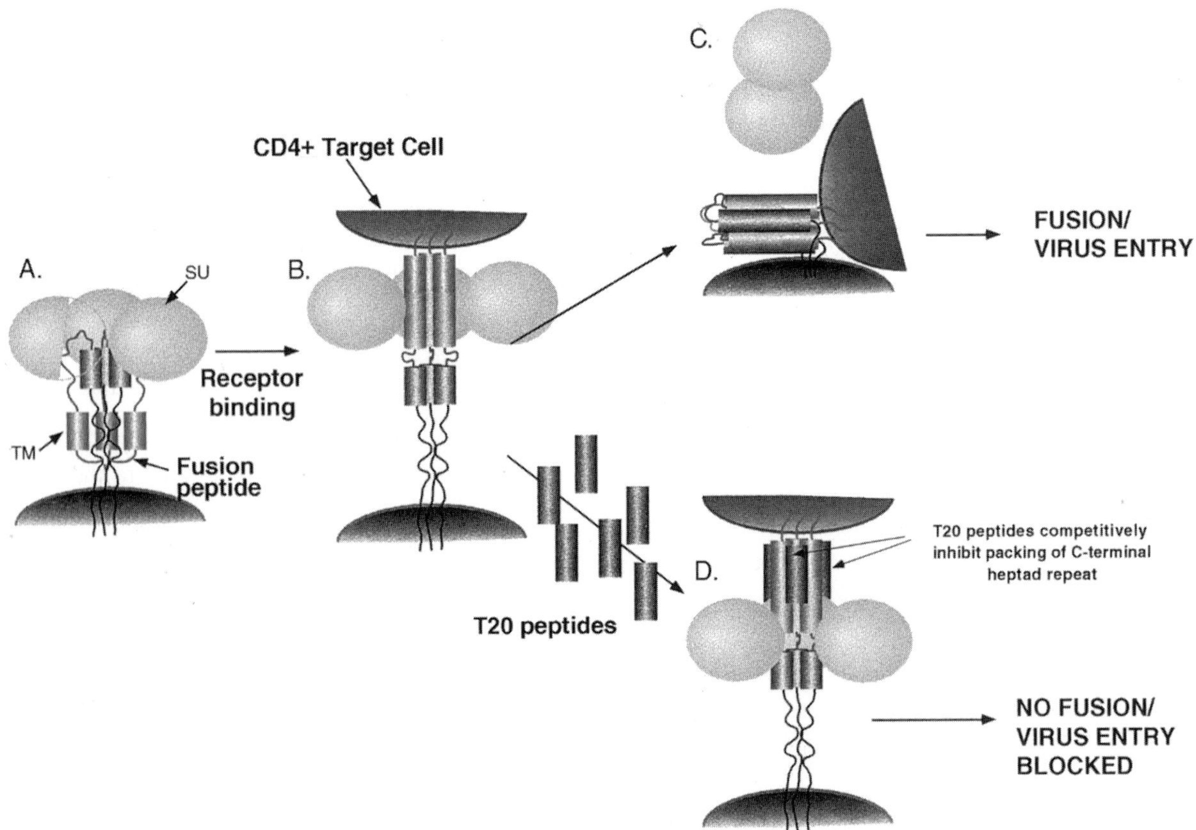

Figure 19–1. Steps involved in HIV attachment to target cells, membrane fusion, and entry. The *boxes* denote the proposed mechanism of action for investigational agents described throughout this chapter. (From D'Souza MP, Cairns JS, Plaeger SF. Current evidence and future directions for targeting HIV entry: therapeutic and prophylactic strategies. JAMA 284:215, 2000.)

mechanism of action for synthetic peptides mimicking these heptad repeat regions might be that they competitively bind to one of the heptad repeat regions when gp41 is in its extended conformation and prevent the structure from folding back onto itself.

A 36-amino-acid peptide, corresponding to DP178 and renamed "T-20," was found to be a potent inhibitor of HIV-1 in vitro, demonstrating a 50% inhibitory concentration (IC_{50}) of 1.7 ng/ml in T cell lines.[75] It remains controversial how much the T20 peptide sequence represents a "universal target" against HIV clinical isolates. One investigation[83] suggested that both the gp41 N-terminal heptad repeat region and the gp120/chemokine co-receptor interactions contribute to the degree of T20 sensitivity. These in vitro experiments point to a higher IC_{50} for R5 than for X4 viral isolates; and chimeras containing different gp120 V3 loop sequences suggest envelope mutations that affect co-receptor usage and also modulate T-20 sensitivity. This observation might be extrapolated to suggest that patients with more advanced or progressive HIV disease would be more likely to experience a potent antiviral response to T20. However, another group of investigators screened more than 100 clinical HIV isolates and found no difference in the fusion inhibitor (T-20 or T-1249) IC_{50} for R5, X4, or dual tropic viral isolates.[84] Some of these same researchers were involved in studies demonstrating that changes in the gp41 heptad repeat sequences are key determinants of fusion inhibitor sensitivity.[85,86] Obviously, more studies are needed to resolve this controversy. It remains possible that, as seems to be the case with RT and protease inhibitors, some aspects of drug susceptibility may be determined by amino acid sequences far removed from the target site but linked by function or complex folding of viral proteins.

In the first clinical trial of a membrane fusion inhibitor,[87] the T20 peptide was administered intravenously for 14 days to 16 HIV-infected adults. Patients received T-20 monotherapy in a dose-escalation protocol, in which four patients each received 3, 10, 30, and finally 100 mg IV twice daily. No serious adverse effects were noted during short-term administration. The median half-life of the drug was 1.83 hours. The nadir drug concentrations in the highest-dose group were substantially higher than the IC_{50} of the drug, and the overall pharmacokinetic profile suggested that intermittent or continuous subcutaneous T-20 administration might be feasible.

The plasma HIV RNA level results demonstrated significant, dose-related declines in plasma HIV RNA levels during intravenous T-20 treatment. There was a significant decline in plasma HIV RNA when all 16 subjects were considered together (-0.39 $\log_{10}$ copies/ml; $P < 0.05$). The median change in plasma viral load in the 100-mg dose group was -1.96 $\log_{10}$ copies/ml by day 15 (Fig. 19–2). An analysis of viral dynamics showed that the initial slope of virus decline, a measure of antiretroviral potency, was comparable to that achieved with other approved HIV therapies including three- and four-drug combinations of RT and protease inhibitors. These findings provided "proof-of-concept" that therapeutics targeting a viral entry event could result in safe, clinically meaningful inhibition of viral replication.

The second clinical trial of T-20 (TRI-003), involved 78 subjects enrolled at multiple sites around the United States.[88] This trial allowed patients to add T-20 therapy to their preexisting oral antiretroviral regimens. This was a dose-ranging study designed to compare escalating doses of continuous subcutaneous infusion (CSI) with intermittent subcutaneous injections of T-20. Thus the phase II trial added critical information to the initial clinical study: experience with more practical routes of administration in an outpatient setting; concurrent administration with other antiretroviral therapies; and a longer (28-day) administration period. Patients were eligible for the study if they had viral loads of more than 5000 copies/ml and were either on no other therapy or had not changed their antiretroviral regimen over the previous 6 weeks.

This trial was remarkable because of the extensive prior antiretroviral treatment experience of the subjects. The mean number of antiretroviral drugs previously used by each subject was between nine and ten. Subjects had experienced clinical failure on a median of three protease inhibitors in the past, and more than 40% had been exposed to all clinically available protease inhibitors. Although this trial answers important questions about the safety of combining T-20 with other therapies, it is essentially measuring virologic responses to T-20 "functional monotherapy" in many cases. The mean baseline HIV RNA level of the subjects was approximately 5.0 $\log_{10}$ copies/ml (100,000 copies/ml), and the mean CD4 count was 130 cells/μl.

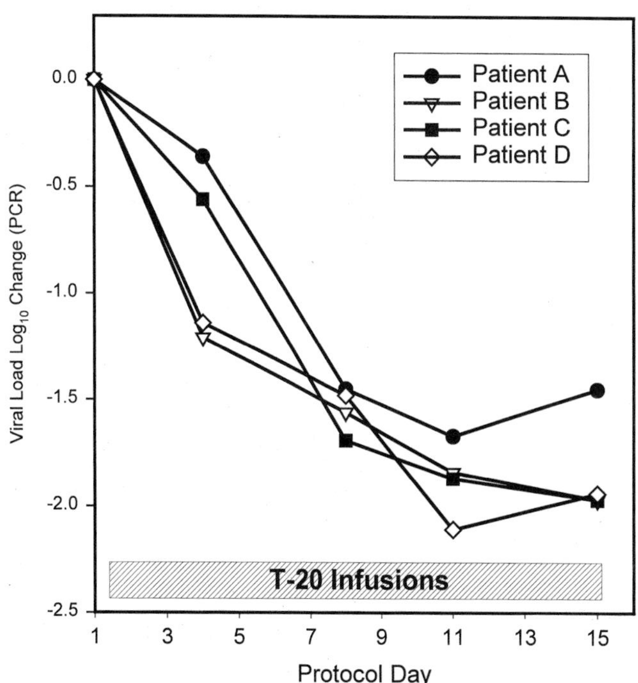

Figure 19–2. Plasma viral load changes from baseline for the four subjects in the 100-mg dose group. *Shaded bar* denotes the T-20 treatment period. (From Kilby JM, Hopkins S, Venetta TM, et al. Potent suppression of HIV-1 replication in humans by T-20, a peptide inhibitor of gp41-mediated virus entry. Nat Med 4:1302, 1998.)

The primary adverse events observed during the trial were infusion-related problems on the arms receiving CSI. Subcutaneous infusion devices used as "insulin pumps" in diabetic patients were evaluated in this study as a way to make administration less cumbersome compared with maintaining long-term intravenous access. Unfortunately, many of the subjects experienced frequent "alarms" from the infusion pump signifying that the drug was not flowing appropriately under the skin. Concurrent with these disruptive alarms, many individuals noted tender nodules under the skin at the infusion site, suggesting that the drug was accumulating locally rather than being absorbed rapidly into the circulation. Fourteen of the CSI subjects (37%) switched over to intermittent subcutaneous administration, and one patient in the highest-dose group (100 mg/day CSI) withdrew from the study because of infusion site pain. Two subjects developed an infusion site abscess or other signs of infection. Patients receiving intermittent injections had less severe local reactions, although tender nodules were still common. Only one intermittent subcutaneous arm subject withdrew from the study because of toxicity, which was a disseminated rash.

The concerns about the CSI administration route were partially alleviated by the pharmacokinetic results in the study. The trough concentrations were higher in the intermittent injection groups than in any of the CSI groups. The group receiving 50 mg twice daily had trough levels of approximately 1 μg/ml, whereas the 100 mg twice daily group had trough levels in the 1 to 3 μg/ml range (all higher than the in vitro IC_{50} for the drug). Preliminary analysis of T-20 plasma kinetics in these intermittent injection subjects showed relatively stable drug levels for more than 12 hours after administration. Evidence of a "depot effect" with subcutaneous administration suggested that continuous subcutaneous or intravenous administration is unnecessary.

Over a 28-day administration period, dose-related reductions in plasma HIV RNA levels were demonstrated that confirmed the findings in the Phase I trial (Fig. 19–3). In an intent-to-treat analysis, the median nadir of the viral load was 0.5 to 1.0 $\log_{10}$ copies/ml lower than baseline in the lower-dose groups. The 100-mg CSI group experienced nearly a full order of magnitude (90%) decline, and the 50-mg twice daily and the 100-mg twice daily intermittent therapy groups had more than 90% declines. The overall trend in the higher-dose groups, however, was an initial decline followed by a more gradual return toward baseline viral loads. Clinically significant changes in absolute CD4+ T-lymphocyte counts were generally not observed during this brief dose-finding study, although there was a statistically significant increase from baseline to day 28 in the 100-mg SC group (mean change of +26 cells/μl, $P < 0.05$).

The temporary antiviral effect of T-20 single-agent therapy in some individuals raised the important question of selection for resistance to fusion inhibitors. Although the gp41 sequences were desirable as therapeutic targets in part because they are highly conserved, point mutations associated with decreased susceptibility have been selected for in cell cultures in the presence of fusion inhibitor peptides.[85] Point mutations in these same regions of the fusion protein appeared to evolve under drug pressure for at least one patient from the Phase I study,[89] and were detected at some point in about half of the patients treated with higher T-20 doses in the TRI-003 trial.[88] In some cases these point mutations are concurrent with phenotypic T20 resistance of more than 10-fold increases in IC_{50} and a few cases of more than 100-fold increases. Formal analysis using site-directed mutagenesis is ongoing to evaluate single and multiple novel amino acid substitutions with respect to their impact on T-20 susceptibility.

Altogether, 61 of the initial Phase II subjects plus 10 other subjects who had received prior T-20 therapy were later enrolled in a 48-week rollover protocol. This protocol (T20-205) evaluated the long-term effects of administering open-label T-20 at 50 mg q12h SC in addition to conventional, oral, highly active antiretroviral therapy (HAART) regimens.[90] Investigators were provided with a genotypic analysis of each subject's HIV isolate at baseline to help determine an "optimized background" HAART regimen for each individual. Overall, a mean plasma HIV RNA level decline of 1.33 $\log_{10}$ copies/ml was achieved within 14 days of T-20 plus HAART, and this degree of response was maintained throughout the remainder of the 48-week period ($P < 0.001$ for change from baseline at 48 weeks) (Fig.

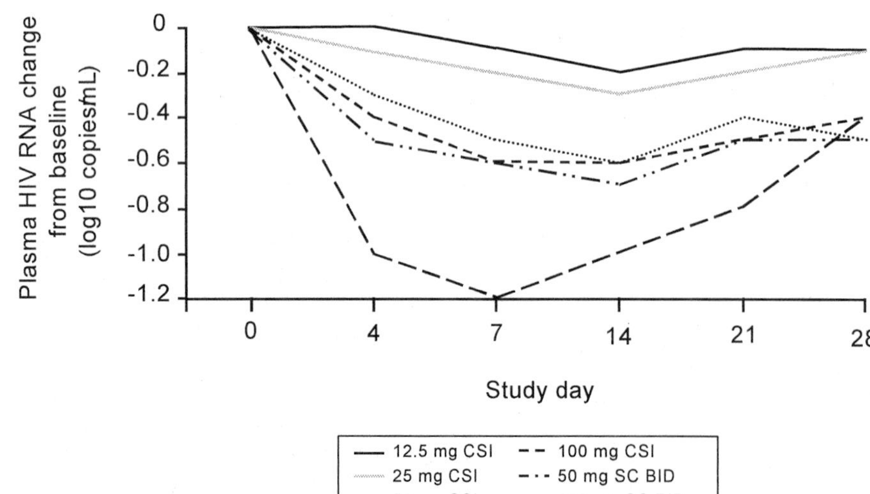

Figure 19–3. Viral load changes observed when subcutaneous T-20 was added to preexisting, failing regimens among heavily pretreated patients in an open label Phase II study (T20-003). CSI, continuous subcutaneous infusion via an "insulin pump" device; SC, intermittent subcutaneous dosing. (From Kilby JM, Lalezan JP, Eron JJ, et al. The safety, plasma pharmacokinetics, and antiviral activity of subcutaneous enfuvirtide (T-20), a peptide inhibitor of gp41-mediated virus fusion, in HIV-infected adults. AIDS Res Hum Retrovirus 18:685, 2002.)

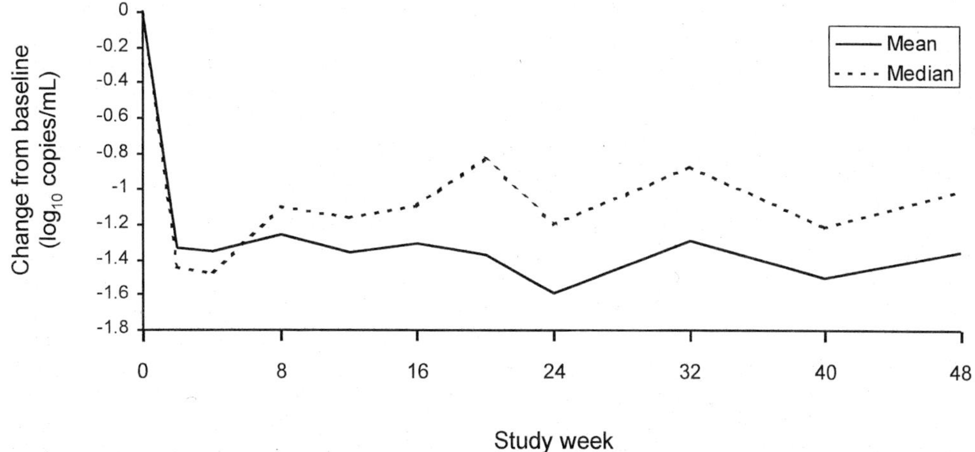

Figure 19–4. Mean and median change from baseline viral load over the 48-week open-label T20 205 study. (From Cohen C, Eron J, Kilby M, et al. 48 week analysis of patients receiving T-20 as a component of multi-drug salvage therapy. Abstract LB 116 XIII International AIDS Conference, Durban, South Africa, 2000.)

19–4). The mean gain in absolute CD4+ T-lymphocyte count at 48 weeks was 84.9 cells/μl ($P < 0.001$ for change from baseline). Potent responses were seen with comparable frequency regardless of the presence of multidrug-resistant isolates, suggesting the possibility of a substantial fusion inhibitor contribution to the durability of response to the multiagent "salvage regimens." Approximately one-third of the treated subjects experienced virologic failure (returned to within 0.5 log_{10} copies/ml of baseline viral load), and 14 subjects discontinued the study owing to treatment failure. Only three subjects discontinued the study because of adverse events. The most common adverse events were mild local reactions, typically tender or pruritic, erythematous nodules at the injection sites.

Sixteen-week data have been presented from another Phase II randomized trial involving 71 patients who were protease-experienced but nonnuclearse reverse transcriptase inhibitor (NNRTI)-naive at entry. These subjects were randomized to a salvage antiretroviral regimen (abacavir/amprenavir/low-dose ritonavir/efavirenz) alone versus the same regimen plus one of three doses of subcutaneous T20 (50, 75, or 100 mg twice daily). There was a consistent dose-related trend toward additional virologic and immunologic benefit on T20 plus HAART. The pooled T20 arms achieved a median change of -2.27 log_{10} copies/ml compared with -1.65 log_{10} copies/ml in the control group. Interestingly, the differential response was greater among subjects with high viral loads (>20,000 copies/ml) at baseline. The gain in CD4+ T-lymphocyte counts over 16 weeks was +10 in the control group versus +64 and +74 in the 75- and 100-mg T20 arms, respectively.[91]

Pediatric protocols evaluating the safety and activity of T20 are in progress. A preliminary report[92] has been presented on 12 children ages 3 to 12 years who initially added T20 to a stable background regimen and then were allowed to continue T20 and change the background antiretroviral regimen if desired. The subjects receiving the 60 mg/m^2 dose had already achieved about 1.0 log_{10} copies/ml viral load declines on the seventh day after adding T20.

In two large Phase III randomized trials evaluating the fusion inhibitor plus "optimized background" (OB) versus "optimized background" alone among patients with prior "triple class" (nucleoside RT inhibitors, NNRTIs, protease inhibitors) treatment experience, T-20 demonstrated remarkable activity. In the clinical trial (T20-301; TORO-1) involving 491 subjects from the Americas (United States, Canada, Brazil), randomized 2:1 to T20 + OB versus OB alone. The T-20 ARM achieved 0.934 log_{10} more reduction in HIV RNA than OB at 24 weeks (-1.697 vs. -0.763 log_{10} copies/ml; $P < 0.0001$).[92a] In a comparable trial design (T20-302; TORO-2) involving another 504 subjects in Europe and Australia showed similar results.[92b] In this trial, the T-20 recipients had 0.78 log_{10} copies/ml more reduction in viral load than the OB group (-1.43 vs. -0.65 log_{10} copies/ml; $P < 0.0001$). Adverse events were similar to those observed in earlier studies. These data firmly established T-20 as an effective agent for ART experienced patients with advanced HIV infection. FDA approval is expected by January, 2003.

Another peptide fusion inhibitor compound with the same proposed mechanism of action, T-1249, is under development. T-1249 has demonstrated potency against a diversity of HIV-1 and HIV-2 isolates in vitro, including those with T-20 resistance-conferring mutations; and it has pharmacokinetics to support once-daily dosing. Phase I results of a 14-day dose-escalation trial of T-1249 monotherapy among 72 HIV-infected, treatment-experienced patients have been reported.[93] Two episodes of possible drug-related serious adverse events were encountered: a hypersensitivity reaction (oral ulcers, rash, fever) and severe neutropenia. Local injection site reactions occurred in 40% and tended to be mild. The plasma half-life and bioavailability of T-1249 supported once-daily subcutaneous dosing. The viral load response was dose-related, with the patients given the highest dose experiencing a -1.40 log_{10} copies/ml decline at 14 days. Because no dose-limiting adverse events were encountered, further evaluations of higher doses appear warranted.

▲ PROSPECTS FOR ENTRY INHIBITOR COMBINATIONS

Based on the experiences with currently available antiretroviral drugs, there is interest in whether viral entry inhibitors could have additive or even synergistic effects in terms of antiviral activity. A marked degree of in vitro synergy has been demonstrated, for example, when the peptide fusion inhibitor T-20 is combined with the small-molecule CXCR4 inhibitor AMD3100. There was no additive cellular toxicity, and the degree of synergy increased with increasing dosages of the two compounds.[94] Synergy has also been shown when T-20 is combined with TAK-779, one of the CCR5 attachment inhibitors. Laboratory investigations support the idea that multiple receptor-binding events are required prior to the fusion step,[95] which leads to the prediction that blocking fusion while also blocking the rate-limiting step of co-receptor binding would be a highly synergistic strategy.

Combinations of CXCR4 and CCR5 inhibitors have shown promise in vitro as a potently effective way to suppress mixed viral populations.[96] Some other combinations of entry inhibitor agents have shown mixed effects depending on the individual isolate (TAK-779 plus RANTES derivatives) or outright antagonism (CXCR4 attachment inhibitors AMD-3100 and Met-SDF-1β). Although these interactions are complex in some circumstances, overall there is hope that carefully selected entry inhibitor combinations may ultimately be successful at decreasing the emergence of resistance and increasing the breadth of antiviral responses.

▲ FUTURE CONSIDERATIONS

Major areas of entry inhibitor development requiring further study include the following.

1. *Designing inhibitors and administration routes that are "user-friendly" and cost-effective for long-term use.* The ideal solution, of course, would be the ability to target entry steps using an oral drug formulation. This process initially seemed possible with small molecules in development such as AMD3100 and Schering C, but clinical data regarding significant antiviral activity with these compounds have not yet been reported.

Oral formulations are not likely to be developed for peptides such as T-20 and T-1249, but the prospects for once-daily or even less frequent subcutaneous administration appear reasonable. This raises the possibility of intermittent administration and directly observed therapy using this class of therapy in the future.

Although parenteral administration is not feasible for most HIV-infected patients worldwide, in the United States many patients are already accustomed to self-administered subcutaneous injections (erythropoietin, filgrastim, interleukin-2) or intravenous therapy (antibacterials, ganciclovir, foscarnet). Particularly in the setting of salvage therapy, when there are little or no effective treatment alternatives, subcutaneous injections may be a viable option for many individuals in the developed world. As an obvious example, patients with diabetes mellitus have been managing home insulin therapy for this chronic illness for many years. Although the process of manufacturing synthetic peptides runs the risk of becoming prohibitively expensive, technologic improvements and increasing demand encourage streamlining the production costs. Again, commercial preparations of insulin serve as examples of proteins that have been synthesized inexpensively for widespread parenteral use.

2. *Characterizing and quantifying the risks for entry inhibitor-resistant virus selection.* If currently approved classes of antiretroviral therapy serve as any guide, drug resistance is an important area on which to concentrate our attention when designing entry and fusion inhibitors. There are already reports about variable viral isolate responses to fusion inhibitors, potential for selection pressures to induce population viral phenotype shifts with chemokine co-receptor inhibition, and HIV point mutations occurring under drug pressure that appear to confer drug resistance. More information will be available in the near future about the risks of fusion inhibitor resistance when peptides such as T-20 are combined strategically with conventional antiretroviral agents. The rapidly evolving knowledge base regarding the complex steps involved in virus binding and entry should help optimize the development of agents targeting these steps while avoiding problems with resistance. In addition, a greater understanding of these factors may help in the design of effective therapeutic regimens, including multiagent entry inhibitor combinations.

3. *Working out the ideal role for entry inhibitors in combination with other therapies and in the "sequencing" of initial and salvage antiretroviral regimens.* Most clinicians today cannot agree on how to sequence currently approved drugs, so arriving at a consensus regarding the role of an investigational agent at this stage of development may be unrealistic. One logical strategy for the use of agents that successfully block viral fusion or entry is for postexposure prophylaxis or intervention early in the course of acute infection. Although evaluating entry inhibitors in the clinical setting of needlestick injuries or during pregnancy to prevent maternal-fetal transmission seems to be a high priority, designing trials to target these special circumstances has been extremely challenging for other agents for a variety of ethical and logistical reasons. One could envision utilizing viral entry inhibitors at a point early in an established infection with the strategy of driving the viral load to low levels and then initiating oral HAART. Theoretically, this tactic could help prevent initial, irreversible immunologic sequelae of acute infection while minimizing the chances of selection for resistance to potent RT and protease inhibitors.

The most urgent niche for entry and fusion inhibitors in clinical practice at present, of course, is using these agents as salvage therapy for patients who have failed conventional combination therapy. Clinical trials of fusion inhibitors have been designed thus far with this priority in mind; and as would be predicted, there is no evidence to suggest overlap between resistance to viral entry inhibitors and conventional antiretroviral classes.

REFERENCES

1. Kwong PD, Wyatt R, Robinson J, et al. Structure of an HIV gp120 envelope glycoprotein in complex with the CD4 receptor and a neutralizing antibody. Nature 393:648, 1998.
2. Wyatt R, Sodroski J. The HIV-1 envelope glycoproteins: fusogens, antigens, and immunogens. Science 280:1884, 1998.

3. Matthews T, Wild C, Chen CH, et al. Structural rearrangements in the transmembrane glycoprotein after receptor binding. Immunol Rev 140:93, 1994.
4. Bucy RP, Hockett RD, Derdeyn CA, et al. Initial increase in blood CD4(+) lymphocytes after HIV antiretroviral therapy reflects redistribution from lymphoid tissues. J Clin Invest 103:1391, 1999.
5. Fortin JF, Cantin R, Bergeron MG, Tremblay MJ. Interaction between virion-bound host ICAM-1 and the high-affinity state of LFA-1 on target cells renders R5 and X4 isolates of HIV-1 more refractory to neutralization. Virology 268:493, 2000.
6. Liao Z, Roos JW, Hildreth JE. Increased infectivity of HIV-1 particles bound to cell surface and solid-phase ICAM-1 and VCAM-1 through acquired adhesion molecules LFA-1 and VLA-4. AIDS Res Hum Retroviruses 16:355, 2000.
7. Geijtenbeek TBH, Kwon DS, Torensma R, et al. DC-SIGN, a dendritic cell-specific HIV-1-binding protein that enhances trans-infection of T cells. Cell 100:587, 2000.
8. Dalgleish AG, Beverley PCL, Clapham PR, et al. The CD4 antigen is an essential component of the receptor for the AIDS retrovirus. Nature 312:763, 1984.
9. Klatzmann D, Champagne E, Chamaret S, et al. T-lymphocyte T4 molecule behaves as the receptor for human retrovirus LAV. Nature 312: 767, 1984.
10. Fisher RA, Bertonis JM, Meier W. HIV infection is blocked in vitro by recombinant soluble CD4. Nature 331:76, 1988.
11. Hussey RE, Richardson NE, Kowalski M. A soluble CD4 protein selectively inhibits HIV replication and syncytium formation. Nature 331:78, 1988.
12. Deen KC, McDougal JS, Inacker R. A soluble form of CD4 (T4) protein inhibits AIDS virus infection. Nature 331:82, 1988.
13. Johnson VA, Barlow MA, Chou TC. Synergistic inhibition of HIV-1 replication in vitro by recombinant soluble CD4 and 3-azido-3-deoxythymidine. J Infect Dis 159:837, 1989.
14. Kahn JO, Allan JD, Hodges TL. The safety and pharmacokinetics of recombinant soluble CD4 (rCD4) in subjects with AIDS and AIDS-related complex. Ann Intern Med 112:254, 1990.
15. Schooley RT, Merigan TC, Gaut P. Recombinant soluble CD4 therapy in patients with AIDS and AIDS-related complex. Ann Intern Med 112:247, 1990.
16. Shearer MH, Timanus DK, Benton PA, et al. Cross-clade inhibition of HIV-1 primary isolates by monoclonal anti-CD4. J Infect Dis 177:1727, 1998.
17. Moreland LW, Bucy RP, Koopman WJ. Regeneration of T cells after chemotherapy. N Engl J Med 332:1651, 1995.
18. Knox S, Levy R, Hodgkinson S, et al. Observations of the effect of chimeric anti-CD4 monoclonal antibody in patients with mycosis fungoides. Blood 77:20, 1991.
19. Meng T-C, Fischl MA, Cheeseman SH, et al. Combination therapy with recombinant human soluble CD4-immunoglobulin G and zidovudine in patients with HIV infection: a phase I study. J Acquir Immun Defic Syndr Hum Retrovirol 8:152, 1998.
20. Allaway GP, Davis-Bruno KL, Beaudry GA, et al. Expression and characterization of CD4-IgG2, a novel heterotetramer that neutralizes primary HIV type 1 isolates. AIDS Res Hum Retroviruses 11:533, 1995.
21. Trkola A, Pomales AB, Yuan H, et al. Cross-clade neutralization of primary isolates of HIV-1 by human monoclonal antibodies and tetrameric CD4-IgG. Virol 69:6609, 1995.
22. Gauduin MC, Allaway GP, Olson WC, et al. CD4-immunoglobulin G2 protects Hu-PBL-SCID mice against challenge by primary HIV-1 isolates. J Virol 72:3475, 1998.
23. Jacobson JM, Lowy I, Fletcher CV, et al. Single-dose safety, pharmacology, and antiviral activity of the HIV-1 entry inhibitor PRO 542 in HIV-infected adults. J Infect Dis 182:326, 2000.
24. Shearer WT, Israel RJ, Starr S, et al. Recombinant CD4-IgG2 in HIV-1-infected children: phase 1/2 study: the Pediatrics AIDS Clinical Trials Group Protocol 351 Study Team. J Infect Dis 182:1774, 2000.
25. Baba M, Pauwels R, Balzarini J. Mechanisms of inhibitory effect of dextran sulfate and heparin on replication of HIV in vitro. Proc Natl Acad Sci USA 85:6132, 1988.
26. Baba M, Snoeck R, Pauwels R. Sulfated polysaccharides are potent and selective inhibitors of various enveloped viruses, including HSV, CMV, VSV, and HIV. Antimicrob Agents Chemother 32:1742, 1988.
27. Mitsuya H, Looney DJ, Kuno S. Dextran sulfate suppression of viruses in the HIV family: inhibition of virion binding to $CD4^+$ cells. Science 240:646, 1988.
28. Abrams DI, Kuno S, Wong R. Oral dextran sulfate (UA001) in the treatment of the acquired immunodeficiency syndrome (AIDS) and AIDS-related complex. Ann Intern Med 110:183, 1989.
29. Lorentsen KJ, Hendrix CW, Collins JM. Dextran sulfate is poorly absorbed after oral administration. Ann Intern Med 111:561, 1989.
30. Flexnor C. HIV-protease inhibitors. N Engl J Med 338:1281, 1998.
31. Meylan P, Kornbluth RS, Zbinden I, Richman DD. Influence of host cell type and V3 loop of the surface glycoprotein on susceptibility of HIV-1 to polyanion compounds. Antimicrob Agents Chemother 38:2910, 1994.
32. Rusconi S, Moonis M, Merrill D, et al. Naphthalene sulfonate polymers with CD4-blocking and anti-HIV-1 activities. Antimicrob Agents Chemother 40:234, 1996.
33. Van Damme L, Wright A, Depraetere K, et al. A phase I study of a novel potential intravaginal microbicide, PRO 2000, in healthy sexually inactive women. Sex Transm Infect 76:126, 2000.
34. Ono M, Wada Y, Wu Y, et al. FP-21399 blocks HIV envelope protein-mediated membrane fusion and concentrates in lymph nodes. Nat Biotechnol 15:343, 1997.
35. Dezube BJ, Dahl TA, Wong TK, et al. A fusion inhibitor (FP-21399) for the treatment of HIV infection: a phase I study. J Infect Dis 182:607, 2000.
36. Moulard M, Lortat-Jacob H, Mondor I, et al. Selective interactions of polyanions with basic surfaces on HIV-1 gp120. J Virol 74:1948, 2000.
37. Cocchi F, Devico AL, Garzino-Demo A, et al. Identification of RANTES, MIP-1 alpha, and MIP-1 beta as the major HIV-suppressive factors produced by $CD8^+$ T cells. Science 270:1811, 1995.
38. Pal R, Garzino-Demo A, Markham PD, et al. Inhibition of HIV-1 infection by the beta chemokine MDC. Science 278:695, 1997.
39. Arenzana-Seisedos F, Virelizier JL, Rousset D. HIV blocked by chemokine antagonist. Nature 383:400, 1996.
40. Dragic T, Litwin V, Allaway GP, et al. HIV-1 entry into $CD4^+$ cells is mediated by the chemokine receptor CC-CKR-5. Nature 381:667, 1996.
41. Deng H, Liu R, Ellmeier W, et al. Identification of a major co-receptor for primary isolates of HIV-1. Nature 381:661, 1996.
42. Feng Y, Broder CC, Kennedy PE, Berger EA. HIV-1 entry cofactor: functional cDNA cloning of a seven-transmembrane, G protein-coupled receptor. Science 272:872, 1996.
43. Bleul CC, Farzan M, Choe H, et al. The lymphocyte chemoattractant SDF-1 is a ligand for LESTR/fusin and blocks HIV-1 entry. Nature 382:829, 1996.
44. Oberlin E, Amara A, Bachelerie F, et al. The CXC chemokine SDF-1 is the ligand for LESTR/fusin and prevents infection by T-cell-line-adapted HIV-1. Nature 382:833, 1996.
45. Amara A, Gall SL, Schwartz O, et al. HIV coreceptor down-regulation as antiviral principle: SDF-1 alpha-dependent internalization of the chemokine receptor CXCR4 contributes to inhibition of HIV replication. J Exp Med 186:139, 1997.
46. Trkola A, Paxton WA, Monard SP, et al. Genetic subtype-independent inhibition of HIV-1 replication by CC and CXC chemokines. J Viro 72:396, 1998.
47. Chen JD, Bai X, Yang AG. Inactivation of HIV-1 chemokine co-receptor CXCR-4 by a novel intrakine strategy. Nat Med 3:1110, 1997.
48. Carroll RG, Riley JL, Levine BL, et al. Differential regulation of HIV-1 fusion cofactor expression by CD28 costimulation of $CD4^+$T cells. Science 276:273, 1997.
49. Wu L, Larosa G, Kassam N, et al. Interaction of chemokine receptor CCR5 with its ligands: multiple domains for HIV-1 gp120 binding and a single domain for chemokine binding. J Exp Med 186:1373, 1997.
50. Simmons G, Clapham PR, Picard L. Potent inhibition of HIV-1 infectivity in macrophages and lymphocytes by a novel CCR5 antagonist. Science 276:276, 1997.
51. Mosier DE, Picchio GR, Gulizia RJ, et al. Highly potent RANTES analogues either prevent CCR5-using HIV-1 in vivo or rapidly select for CXCR4-using variants. J Virol 73:3544, 1999.
52. Margolis L, Glushakova S, Grivel JC, et al. Blockade of CCR5-tropic HIV-1 replication in human lymphoid tissue by CC chemokines. J Clin Invest 101:1876, 1998.
53. Baba M, Nishimura O, Kanzaki N, et al. A small-molecule, nonpeptide CCR5 antagonist with highly potent and selective anti-HIV-1 activity. Proc Natl Acad Sci USA 96:5698, 1999.
54. Dragic T, Trkola A, Thompson DA, et al. A binding pocket for a small

molecule inhibitor of HIV-1 entry within the transmembrane helices of CCR5. Proc Natl Acad Sci USA 97:5639, 2000.
55. Baroudy BM. A small molecule antagonist of CCR5 that effectively inhibits HIV-1: potential as a novel antiretroviral agent. Presented at the 7th CROI, San Francisco, 2000, abstract S17.
56. Crump MP, Gong JH, Loetscher P, et al. Solution structure and basis for functional activity of SDF-1. EMBO J 16:6996, 1997.
57. Murakami T, Nakajima T, Koyanagi Y. A small molecule CXCR4 inhibitor that blocks T cell line-tropic HIV-1 infection. J Exp Med 186:1389, 1997.
58. Arakaki R, Tamamaura H, Premanathan M. T134, a small-molecule CXCR4 inhibitor, has no cross-drug resistance with AMD3100, a CXCR4 antagonist with a different structure. J Virol 73:1719, 1999.
59. Doranz BJ, Grovit-Ferbas K, Sharron MP, et al. A small molecule inhibitor directed against the chemokine receptor CXCR4 prevents its use as an HIV coreceptor. J Exp Med 186:1395, 1997.
60. De Clercq E, Yamamoto N, Pauwels R, et al. Potent and selective inhibition of HIV-1 and HIV-2 replication by a class of bicyclams interacting with a viral uncoating event. Proc Nat Acad Sci USA 89:5286, 1992.
61. De Clercq E, Yamamoto N, Pauwels R, et al. Highly potent and selective inhibition of HIV by the bicyclam derivative JM3100. Antimicrob Agents Chemother 38:668, 1994.
62. De Vreese K, Van Nerum I, Vermeire K, et al. Sensitivity of HIV to bicyclam derivatives is influenced by the three-dimensional structure of gp120. Antimicrob Agents Chemother 41:2616, 1997.
63. Donzella G, Schols D, Lin S. AMD3100, a small molecule inhibitor of HIV-1 entry via the CXCR4 co-receptor. Nat Med 4:72, 1998.
64. Este JA, Cabrera C, Blanco J, et al. Shift of clinical HIV-1 isolates from X4 to R5 and prevention of emergence of the syncytium-inducing phenotype by blockade of CXCR4. J Virol 73:5577, 1999.
65. Hendrix CW, Flexner C, MacFarland RT, et al. Pharmacokinetics and safety of AMD-3100, a novel antagonist of the CXCR4 chemokine receptor, in human volunteers. Antimicrob Agents Chemother 44:1667, 2000.
66. Labrosse B, Brelota A, Heveker N, et al. Determinants for sensitivity of HIV coreceptor CXCR4 to the bicyclam AMD3100. J Virol 72:6381, 1998.
67. Mackewicz CE, Barker E, Levy JA. Role of beta-chemokines in suppressing HIV replication. Science 174:1393, 1996.
68. Paxton WA, Martin SR, Tse D, et al. Relative resistance to HIV-1 infection of CD4 lymphocytes from persons who remain uninfected despite multiple high-risk sexual exposure. Nat Med 2:412, 1996.
69. Dean M, Carrington M, Winkler C, et al. Genetic restriction of HIV-1 infection and progression to AIDS by a deletion allele of the CKR5 structural gene. Science 273:1856, 1996.
70. Liu R, Paxton WA, Choe S, et al. Homozygous defect in HIV-1 coreceptor accounts for resistance of some multiply-exposed individuals to HIV-1 infection. Cell 86:367, 1996.
71. Nagasawa T, Hirota S, Tachibana K, et al. Defects of B-cell lymphopoiesis and bone-marrow myelopoiesis in mice lacking the CXC chemokine PBSF/SDF-1. Nature 382:635, 1996.
72. Scarlatti G, Tresoldi E, Bjorndal A, et al. In vivo evolution of HIV-1 co-receptor usage and sensitivity to chemokine-mediated suppression. Nat Med 3:1259, 1997.
73. Gallaher W, Ball J, Garry R, et al. A general model of the transmembrane proteins of HIV and other retroviruses. AIDS Res Hum Retroviruses 5:431, 1989.
74. Delwart E, Mosialos G, Gilmore T. Retroviral envelope glycoproteins contain a "leucine zipper"-like repeat. AIDS Res Hum Retroviruses 6:703, 1989.
75. Wild C, Greenwell T, Matthews T. A synthetic peptide from HIV-1 gp41 is a potent inhibitor of virus-mediated cell-cell fusion. AIDS Res Hum Retroviruses 9:1051, 1993.
76. Wild CT, Shugars DC, Greenwell TK, et al. Peptides corresponding to a predictive alpha-helical domain of HIV-1 gp41 are potent inhibitors of virus infection. Proc Natl Acad Sci USA 91: 9770, 1994.
77. Chen CH, Matthews T, McDanal C, et al. A molecular clasp in HIV-1 TM protein determines the anti-HIV activity of gp41 derivatives: implication for viral fusion. J Virol 69:3771, 1995.
78. Wild C, Greenwell T, Shugars D, et al. The inhibitory activity of an HIV-1 peptide correlates with its ability to interact with a leucine zipper structure. AIDS Res Hum Retroviruses 11:323, 1995.
79. Wild C, Oas T, McDanal C, et al. A synthetic peptide inhibitor of HIV replication: correlation between solution structure and viral inhibition. Proc Natl Acad Sci USA 89:10537, 1992.
80. Dubay J, Roberts S, Brody B, et al. Mutations in the leucine zipper of HIV-1 transmembrane glycoprotein affect fusion and infectivity. J Virol 65:4748, 1992.
81. Wild C, Dubay JW, Greenwell T, et al. Propensity for a leucine zipper-like domain of HIV-1 gp41 to form oligomers correlates with a role in virus-induced fusion rather than assembly of the glycoprotein complex. Proc Natl Acad Sci USA 91:12676, 1994.
82. Carr C, Kim PS. A spring-loaded mechanism for the conformational change of influenza hemaglutinin. Cell 73:823, 1993.
83. Derdeyn CA, Decker JM, Sfakianos JN, et al. Sensitivity of HIV-1 to the fusion inhibitor T-20 is modulated by coreceptor specificity defined by the V3 loop of gp120. J Virol 74:8358, 2000.
84. Greenberg ML, McDanal CB, Stanfield-Oakley SA, et al. Virus sensitivity to T-20 and T-1249 is independent of coreceptor usage. presented at the 8th Conference on Retroviruses and Opportunistic Infections, Chicago, 2001, abstract 473.
85. Rimsky LT, Shugar DC, Matthews T. Determinants of HIV-1 resistance to gp41-derived inhibitory peptides. J Virol 72:986, 1998.
86. Mink MA, Janumpalli S, Davison DK, et al. Correlation of gp41 binding and antiviral potencies of the T-20 fusion inhibitor using clinical trial isolate-derived sequences. Presented at the 8th Conference on Retroviruses and Opportunistic Infections, Chicago, 2001, abstract 474.
87. Kilby JM, Hopkins S, Venetta TM, et al. Potent suppression of HIV-1 replication in humans by T-20, a peptide inhibitor of gp41-mediated virus entry. Nat Med 4:1302, 1998.
88. Kilby JM, Lalezan JP, Eron JJ, et al. The safety, plasma pharmacokinetics, and antiviral activity of subcutaneous enfuvirtide (T-20), a peptide inhibitor of gp41-mediated virus fusion, in HIV-infected adults. AIDS Res Hum Retrovirus 18:685, 2002.
89. Wei X, Kilby M, Hopkins S, et al. HIV-1 selection in response to inhibition of virus fusion and entry. Presented at the 6th Conference on Retroviruses and Opportunistic Infections, Chicago, 1999, abstract 611.
90. Cohen C, Eron J, Kilby M, et al. 48 week analysis of patients receiving T-20 as a component of multi-drug salvage therapy. Abstract LB 116 XIII International AIDS Conference, Durban, South Africa, 2000.
91. Lalezari J, Drucker J, Demasi R, et al. A controlled phase II trial assessing three doses of T-20 in combination with abacavir, amprenavir, low dose ritonavir, and efavirenz in non-nucleoside naive, protease inhibitor-experienced, HIV-1-infected adults. Presented at the 8th Conference on Retroviruses and Opportunistic Infections, Chicago, 2001, abstract LB5.
92. Church J, Cunningham C, Palumbo P, et al. Safety and antiviral activity of chronic subcutaneous administration of T-20 in HIV-1-infected children. Presented at the 8th Conference on Retroviruses and Opportunistic Infections, Chicago, 2001, abstract 681.
92a. Henry K, Lalezari J, O'Hearn M, et al. Enfuvirtide (T-20) in combination with an optimized background (OB) regimen vs. OB alone in patients with prior experience or resistance to each of three classes of approved antiretroviral (ARVs) in North America and Brazil. Presented at XIV International AIDS Conference, Barcelona, 2002, abstract LBOr19B
92b. Clotet B, Lazzarin A, Cooper D, et al. Enfuvirtide (T-20) in combination with an optimized background (OB) regimen vs. OB alone in patients with prior experience or resistance to each of three classes of approved antiretrovirals (ARVs) in Europe and Australia. Presented at XIV International AIDS Conference, Barcelona, 2002, abstract LBOr19A
93. Eron J, Merigan T, Kilby M, et al. A 14-day assessment of the safety, pharmacokinetics, and antiviral activity of T-1249, a peptide inhibitor of membrane fusion. Presented at the 8th Conference on Retroviruses and Opportunistic Infections, Chicago, 2001, abstract 14.
94. Tremblay C, Kollman C, Giguel F, et al. Strong in vitro synergy observed between the fusion inhibitor T-20 and a CXCR4 blocker, AMD3100. Presented at the 7th Conference on Retroviruses and Opportunistic Infections, San Francisco, 2000, abstract 500.
95. Edwards T, McManus C, Richardson T, et al. Multimeric CD4 and coreceptor binding is required to activate HIV-1 envelope protein trimers. Presented at the 8th Conference on Retroviruses and Opportunistic Infections, Chicago, 2001, abstract 105.
96. Rusconi S, La Seta-Catamancio S, Citterio P, et al. Combined effect of AOP-RANTES and Met-SDF-1beta in inhibiting infections by PHI viral isolates in vitro. Presented at the 7th Conference on Retroviruses and Opportunistic Infections. San Francisco, 2000, abstract 501.

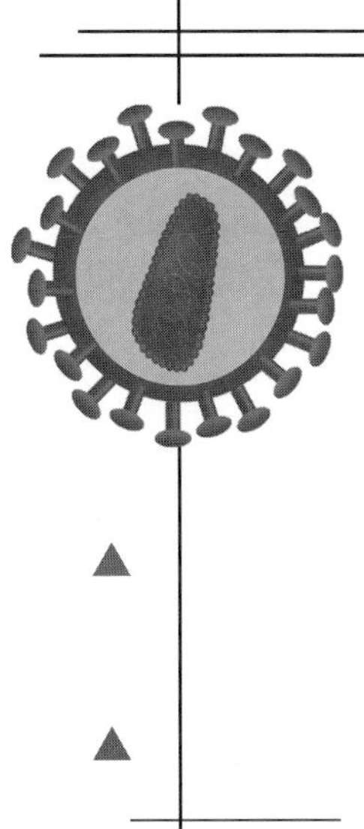

CHAPTER 20
New Drugs in Development

George J. Hanna, MD
Martin S. Hirsch, MD

Despite the seemingly large number of drugs approved for treating human immunodeficiency virus type 1 (HIV-1) infection, there is an ongoing need for new antiretroviral agents for several reasons. Patients may have poor tolerance to, or experience significant adverse effects from, several of the currently available drugs. Agents with improved tolerability and safety profiles are needed. Because complicated antiretroviral regimens continue to challenge patients, new drugs with favorable pharmacokinetic profiles (e.g., long half-lives and lack of interaction with food) should improve adherence to the regimens. Moreover, breakthrough of viral replication can occur on current regimens, even if adherence is good, indicating that more potent regimens may be required for durable virus suppression. Finally, antiretroviral drug resistance to any of the currently used drugs may emerge and cause therapeutic failure. Virus with resistance to one drug is often cross-resistant to other drugs in the same class, making the selection of salvage regimens difficult. New agents or classes of drugs with activity against virus resistant to currently available drugs are urgently needed.

Antiretroviral agents may target various steps in the replicative cycle of HIV-1, though all currently approved anti-HIV-1 drugs inhibit either the viral reverse transcriptase (RT) or protease enzyme. Other steps in the replicative cycle are promising targets of antiretroviral therapy and are being increasingly studied. They include viral attachment to susceptible cells; virus entry and uncoating; ribonuclease H activity of the viral polymerase required for efficient reverse transcription; integration of the viral genome into a host chromosome; transcription and translation of viral nucleotide sequences; and virus assembly, maturation, and budding.

Predicting which compounds will ultimately prove clinically useful or the speed of their development is difficult. These issues are influenced by intrinsic properties of the drug (e.g., potency, pharmacokinetics, adverse effects) as well as the development strategies of individual pharmaceutical companies and regulatory processes of individual countries.

Many anti-HIV-1 drugs are currently in development. The amount and quality of information on such drugs vary. Some pharmaceutical companies report widely on their compounds throughout the development process, whereas others report little before drug approval. Much of the information presented here has been presented in abstract form only or has been provided directly by pharmaceutical companies. The information reported here summarizes available information on many drugs that are in clinical trials and on some promising novel classes of drugs that are in preclinical development; the information is not intended to be encyclopedic. Some agents in development are covered more comprehensively in other chapters [e.g., emtricitabine or FTC (see Chapter 7), co-receptor binding and fusion inhibitors (see Chapter 19), and immune-based therapies (see Chapter 21)]. The drugs discussed in the chapter are listed in Table 20–1.

NUCLEOSIDE ANALOGUE REVERSE TRANSCRIPTASE INHIBITORS

Diaminopurine Dioxolane

(−)-β-D-2,6-Diaminopurine dioxolane (DAPD) is a purine nucleoside analogue that, without further metabolism, has only moderate potency against HIV-1. After absorption,

▲ **Table 20–1.** SELECTED ANTIRETROVIRAL AGENTS IN DEVELOPMENT

Agent	Manufacturer
Nucleoside Reverse Transcriptase Inhibitors	
Emtricitabine [(−)-2′,3′-dideoxy-5-fluoro-3′-thiacytidine (FTC)]	Triangle Pharmaceuticals
(−)-β-D-2,6-Diaminopurine dioxolane (DAPD)	Triangle Pharmaceuticals
(−)-2′-Deoxy-3′-oxa-4′-thiocytidine ((−)-dOTC, BCH-10618)	Biochem Pharma
ACH-126,443 [2′,3′-dideoxy-2′,3′-didehydro-β-L(−)-5-fluorocytidine (β-L-Fd4C)]	Achillion Pharmaceuticals
Nonnucleoside Reverse Transcriptase Inhibitors	
Emivirine (MKC-442)	Triangle Pharmaceuticals
Capravirine (AG-1549, S-1153)	Agouron Pharmaceuticals
DPC-083	DuPont Pharmaceuticals
DPC-961	DuPont Pharmaceuticals
(+)-Calanolide A (NSC-650886)	Sarawak MediChem Pharmaceuticals
Costatolide [(−)-calanolide B (NSC-661122)]	Sarawak MediChem Pharmaceuticals
Dihydrocostatolide [(−)/-dihydrocalanolide B (NSC-661123)]	Sarawak MediChem Pharmaceuticals
TMC120 (R147681)	Tibotec
TMC125 (R165335)	Tibotec
SJ-3366	Samjin Pharmaceuticals Company
Protease Inhibitors	
Atazanavir	Bristol-Myers Squibb
Tipranavir (PNU-140690)	Boehringer Ingelheim
Mozenavir (DMP-450)	Triangle Pharmaceuticals
GW433908	GlaxoSmithKline
DPC-681	DuPont Pharmaceuticals
DPC-684	DuPont Pharmaceuticals
TMC126	Tibotec
CD4 Binding Inhibitors	
PRO-542	Progenics Pharmaceuticals
CCR5 Co-receptor Binding Inhibitors	
Schering C	Schering-Plough
Schering D	Schering-Plough
Fusion Inhibitors	
Pentafuside (T-20)	Trimeris
T-1249	Trimeris

however, it is readily deaminated to dioxolane guanosine (DXG) by adenosine deaminase, an enzyme found throughout human tissue, including blood plasma. DXG, which undergoes phosphorylation to its biologically active triphosphate intracellularly, is a guanosine analogue with at least 10-fold increased potency against HIV-1 compared to DAPD. However, DXG has limited aqueous solubility, prompting the development of the orally bioavailable DAPD as a prodrug that is converted to DXG. DAPD and DXG are also active against hepatitis B virus.

In vitro the DXG median effective concentration (EC_{50}) for wild-type HIV-1 is typically in the range 0.03 to 0.30 μM. Virus with resistance to zidovudine, lamivudine, abacavir, or nonnucleoside reverse transcriptase inhibitors (NNRTIs) shows little cross resistance to DXG in vitro.[1,2] In fact, virus with NNRTI resistance mutations may be hypersusceptible to DXG in vitro.[3] Virus with multinucleoside resistance conferred by the Q151M complex shows decreased susceptibility to DXG, but multinucleoside-resistant virus with insertion mutations around codon 69 may remain susceptible to DXG.[3] In vitro passage of HIV-1 in the presence of DXG selects virus with reduced susceptibility to DXG.[2] Resistant virus has the RT mutation K65R or L74V and has approximately four- to ninefold decreased susceptibility to DXG. Each of these mutations also confers decreased susceptibility to didanosine. DXG is synergistic against HIV-1 in vitro in combination with several other nucleoside RT inhibitors, NNRTIs, and protease inhibitors.

DAPD is rapidly absorbed and converted to DXG, and plasma DXG levels are higher than those for DAPD.[4] The plasma half-life of DAPD is approximately 1 hour, and that of DXG is about 7 hours, supporting dosing every 12 to 24 hours.

A dose-range monotherapy study examined the safety and antiviral efficacy of oral DAPD in HIV-1-infected adults treated for 15 days.[5] In antiretroviral-naive subjects, the two highest doses (300 or 500 mg twice daily) resulted in a maximum median reduction in plasma HIV-1 RNA of 1.5 $\log_{10}$ copies/ml. However, in patients heavily pretreated with multiple other nucleoside RT inhibitors (NRTIs), virologic responses to DAPD monotherapy were attenuated. There were no genetic changes in the RT coding region suggestive of acquisition of new resistance mutations during the 15-day study. DAPD was well tolerated at all doses tested, and the most frequently reported adverse effects included headache, nausea, and diarrhea.

DAPD appears to be a potent NRTI with favorable pharmacokinetics and good short-term patient tolerance. However, its long-term activity and safety and its clinical efficacy against virus resistant to didanosine or to multiple nucleosides remain to be defined.

Other NRTIs

2′-Deoxy-3′-oxa-4′-thiocytidine (dOTC; BCH-10652) consists of the racemic mixture of (+)-dOTC and (−)-dOTC, cytosine analogues structurally related to lamivudine. Although clinical development of the racemic mixture of dOTC was stopped because of toxicity [apparently related to the (+)-dOTC enantiomer], preclinical development of (−)-dOTC (BCH-10618) is continuing. In vitro, wild-type clinical isolates of HIV-1 display (−)-dOTC EC_{50} in the range of 0.2 to 4.8 μM.[6,7] The (−)-dOTC EC_{50} remains relatively unchanged against virus isolates with resistance mutations to zidovudine or NNRTIs but increases three- to fivefold against viruses with the lamivudine resistance mutation M184V.[7] In vitro passage of HIV-1 under (−)-dOTC selection selects for virus with the K65R, V75I, or M184V mutation.[8] However, selected viruses have only two- to fourfold reduced susceptibility to (−)-dOTC. (−)-dOTC displays additive to slightly synergistic activity against HIV-1 when combined with several other NRTIs, NNRTIs, or protease inhibitors (PIs). Extrapolating from studies in which the racemic mixture was administered, (−)-dOTC is likely to prove to be well absorbed orally, to allow once- or twice-daily dosing, and to be eliminated renally.[9,10]

ACH-126,443 [2′,3′-dideoxy-2′,3′-didehydro-β-L(−)-5-fluorocytidine, β-L-Fd4C] is a cytosine analogue with an L-configuration designed to minimize mitochondrial toxicity.[11] In vitro, the ACH-126,443 EC_{50} of wild-type HIV-1 is 0.1 to 0.5 μM, and the drug is also active against hepatitis B virus. Preliminary studies suggest that HIV-1 resistant to other NRTIs (including ones with M41L/T215Y, Q151M complex, or insertion mutations around codon 69) had no significant change in susceptibility to ACH-126,443.[12] However, the lamivudine resistance-associated M184V increased the EC_{50} to 1 to 4 μM. Whether drug levels high enough to suppress virus with M184V can be achieved in vivo remains unknown. In vitro, synergistic antiviral activity was noted when ACH-126,443 was combined with zidovudine or stavudine; and ACH-126,443 appeared to protect cells against other NRTI-induced mitochondrial toxicity.[11] The intracellular half-life of the triphosphate form of ACH-126,443 is more than 8 hours, potentially allowing for once-daily dosing.

A series of 4′-ethynyl-substituted nucleosides have been designed to be active against viruses with resistance to currently available NRTIs.[13] Several were potent HIV-1 inhibitors and suppressed viruses with nucleoside resistance mutations (including viruses with M41L/T215Y, L74V, K65R, Q151M complex, or insertion mutations around codon 69) with an EC_{50} of 0.0004 to 0.0100 μM. These compounds were acid-resistant, suggesting that stomach acidity should not interfere with their bioavailability.

▲ NONNUCLEOSIDE REVERSE TRANSCRIPTASE INHIBITORS

Emivirine

Emivirine [6-benzyl-1-(ethoxymethyl)-5-isopropyl-uracil; MKC-442] is a member of the hydroxyethyl phenyl thymine (HEPT) class. Although it is structurally a nucleoside analogue, it functions as an NNRTI, causing noncompetitive inhibition of RT. Emivirine appears to be equally active against various group M clades of HIV-1, but it has poor activity against HIV-2.

The emivirine EC_{50} of wild-type clinical HIV-1 isolates typically ranges from 0.002 to 0.040 μM. Virus with reduced susceptibility to nucleoside RT inhibitors remains susceptible to emivirine, although virus with NNRTI resistance mutations (including K103N and Y181C) often demonstrates markedly reduced susceptibility. Emivirine interacts additively to synergistically in vitro with certain other NNRTIs, NRTIs, and PIs.

Emivirine is rapidly absorbed after oral administration, and food has little effect on its oral bioavailability. It is highly bound to human serum proteins (> 75%). Emivirine distributes widely in human tissue, including cerebrospinal fluid. It crosses the placenta readily, and newborn infant drug levels are 70% to 80% of those seen in the mother.[14] Its plasma half-life is 8 to 10 hours, allowing twice-daily dosing. Emivirine is metabolized primarily by human cytochrome P_{450} CYP3A4 and CYP3A5, with CYP1A2 also playing a role.[15] Drugs that induce these enzymes, such as rifampin, can decrease emivirine blood levels significantly. Drugs that inhibit these enzymes, such as ritonavir, indinavir, and nelfinavir, can increase emivirine blood levels markedly, which may necessitate dose reductions of emivirine to avoid toxicity. Emivirine is also an inducer of the cytochrome P_{450} enzymes that metabolize it. This can decrease the blood levels of other drugs metabolized by these enzymes substantially, including nevirapine, delavirdine, efavirenz, indinavir, nelfinavir, ketoconazole, and clarithromycin.

In NNRTI-naive adults, monotherapy with emivirine (750 mg twice daily) causes a decrease in plasma HIV-1 RNA of 1.4 $\log_{10}$ copies/ml at day 8. Subsequently, plasma HIV-1 RNA levels rise, accompanied by the development of NNRTI-resistance mutations. In antiretroviral-naive adults with median plasma HIV-1 RNA of 4.3 $\log_{10}$ copies/ml, the combination of emivirine with stavudine and lamivudine decreased plasma HIV-1 RNA to 400 copies/ml (or less) in 63% of subjects and 50 copies/ml (or less) in 47% at 24 weeks, shown by an intention-to-treat analysis.[16] In a similar analysis, the combination of emivirine with stavudine and didanosine in antiretroviral-naive adults with higher viral loads (median baseline plasma HIV-1 RNA of 5.0 $\log_{10}$ copies/ml) decreased plasma HIV-1 RNA to 400 copies/ml or less in 42% of subjects and 50 copies/ml or less in 25% at 24 weeks.[17] Preliminary results in antiretroviral-experienced but NNRTI-naive adults suggest good activity of emivirine in combination with efavirenz plus at least one NRTI.[18] Virologic failure to emivirine-containing regimens has been associated with the development of NNRTI-resistance mutations in most subjects, most commonly RT K103N, which confers cross resistance to all currently approved NNRTIs.[19,20] Viruses from a minority of treated individuals develop other mutations (including RT K101E, V108I, Y181C, and G190A); the clinical susceptibility of these viruses to regimens that include other NNRTIs is currently unclear.

The most frequent adverse effects during treatment with emivirine have included headache, dizziness, nausea, diarrhea, and rash. The rash, seen in up to 17% of subjects, is generally mild to moderate in severity and usually resolves even with continued treatment. Rarely, the rash is associated with systemic symptoms (e.g., fever, oral ulceration, elevated hepatic enzyme levels), and in these cases emivirine should be stopped and not reintroduced because of concerns over a possible hypersensitivity reaction. Asymptomatic elevations in hepatic enzymes are seen in some patients.

Emivirine is a potent NNRTI that may possibly offer options to patients who are intolerant of other NNRTIs, though this area has not been studied. However, its shared cross-resistance patterns with currently available NNRTIs compromises its likely efficacy in patients with virologic failure to currently approved NNRTIs.

Capravirine

Capravirine (AG-1549, S-1153) is an imidazole compound that was selected as the result of a screening effort to identify drugs with activity against HIV-1 resistant to other NNRTIs.[21] It appears to lack antiviral activity against HIV-2.

Capravirine is a potent antiretroviral agent with an EC_{50} against wild-type HIV-1 in the range of 0.002 to 0.010 μM.[21] Virus resistant to zidovudine or lamivudine remains susceptible to capravirine. In vitro, HIV-1 with common single NNRTI resistance mutations often retains full susceptibility (as with K103N, Y188C, and G190A) or has only minimal (less than fivefold) reductions in sensitivity (L100I and V106A) to capravirine.[21] However, some viruses with single amino acid mutations in RT have moderate decreases in susceptibility (Y181C with 14-fold reduction, L234I with 22-fold reduction), and double mutations sometimes confer considerable decreases in sensitivity (L100I/K103N with approximately 40-fold reduction). In vitro passage of HIV-1 in the presence of capravirine selects viruses with reduced susceptibility to the drug. However, high-level capravirine resistance in these viruses appears to require more than one mutation in RT (V106A/F227L or K103T/V106A/L234I, each with >100-fold decreased susceptibility). Capravarine displays in vitro synergism with several NRTIs and PIs.

Capravirine has good oral bioavailability. Administration with meals increases its bioavailability approximately twofold.[22] It has an elimination half-life of 2 to 3 hours, requiring at least twice-daily dosing, and it is metabolized primarily by human cytochrome P_{450} CYP3A4. Inhibitors of these enzymes (including some protease inhibitors) increase capravirine blood levels. Capravarine can also induce cytochrome P_{450} enzymes and may inhibit CYP3A4, but the significance of these observations on clinical pharmacokinetic interactions requires further study.

Monotherapy with capravirine (2100 mg twice daily) in NNRTI-naive adults resulted in a mean decrease in plasma HIV-1 RNA of 1.69 $\log_{10}$ copies/ml at day 10 of therapy.[23] This was comparable to a mean decrease of 1.65 $\log_{10}$ copies/ml seen in subjects taking the combination of zidovudine/lamivudine/nelfinavir in the same study. Capravirine is usually well tolerated. The most frequent adverse events have been mild (transient nausea, vomiting, diarrhea), occurring more often with higher doses. Taking capravirine with food may ameliorate the nausea.[24] The clinical development of capravirine has been slowed by the finding of vasculitis in dogs receiving high doses of capravirine in toxicology studies. To date, no humans have been reported to develop vasculitis resulting from capravirine. The clinical significance of the toxicology studies in dogs remains to be determined.

In summary, capravirine is a potent NNRTI that appears to have a resistance profile considerably different from that of currently approved NNRTIs. If it proves to be safe, it may be useful in NNRTI-naive patients. It may also be useful in those with early failure to currently available NNRTIs when limited genotypic resistance is present. However its efficacy against HIV-1 with multiple NNRTI resistance mutations, as seen in patients who continue a failing NNRTI-containing regimen, is unclear.

Quinazolinone Compounds

A search for compounds structurally related to efavirenz but with increased potency against HIV-1 with efavirenz resistance mutations has identified several active compounds including DPC-083 and DPC-961.[25,26] These agents have potency against wild-type HIV-1 equivalent to that of efavirenz (in the range 0.001 to 0.005 μM) but have increased potency against virus containing the single NNRTI resistance mutations K103N or the double mutations L100I/K103N, K103N/V108I, or K103N/P225H. They do not have activity against HIV-2. Although these mutation patterns are the most common ones conferring efavirenz resistance, all also confer decreased susceptibility to the other currently available NNRTIs. These compounds appear to retain activity against virus with other NNRTI resistance mutations as well, including V106A and Y181C. They show less plasma serum protein binding than efavirenz, which may result in significantly greater biologically active free drug levels.

Both DPC-083 and DPC-961 have good oral bioavailability.[27,28] The terminal half-life of DPC-961 is approximately 50 hours, and that for DPC-083 is more than 140 hours, allowing for once-daily (or possibly less frequent) dosing. After 9 days treatment with either compound at 100 mg/day, the trough levels of free drug were significantly higher than the EC_{90} of several NNRTI-resistant viruses (>10-fold for virus with K103N, and >1.5 fold for virus with the double NNRTI resistance mutations K103N/V108I, K103N/Y181C, and K103N/P225H).

If well tolerated, these compounds may be useful components of salvage regimens against virus resistant to currently used NNRTIs, although the effects of multiple NNRTI resistance mutations on their clinical activity remain to be determined.

Calanolide Compounds

(+)-Calanolide A (NSC-650886) is a compound originally isolated from the rain forest tree *Calophyllum lanigerum*.[29] It is active against wild type HIV-1 isolates with an EC_{50} of approximately 0.1 μM but not against HIV-2. It is also active against virus with the NNRTI resistance mutation RT Y181C. However, viruses with other NNRTI resistance mutations (including the commonly seen K103N) are often resistant to it. (+)-Calanolide A has good oral bioavailability, and food has little effect on its absorption.[30] Its half-life is 15 to 20 hours. Two weeks of monotherapy with 600 mg twice daily resulted in a mean reduction in plasma HIV-1 RNA of 0.8 $\log_{10}$ copies/ml.[31] The most common adverse effects have been taste perversion, dizziness, headache, and gastrointestinal effects (nausea, dyspepsia, eructation).

Two structurally related compounds have also been studied in vitro: costatolide [(−)-calanolide B, NSC-661122] and dihydrocostatolide [(−)-dihydrocalanolide B, NSC-661123].[32] They are active against wild-type HIV-1 with an EC_{50} of 0.06 to 1.40 μM for costatolide and 0.1 to 0.8 μM for dihydrocostatolide. Both are active against different clades of HIV-1 but have no activity against HIV-2. They also share (+)-calanolide A's activity against HIV-1 with RT Y181C, but all three show poor efficacy against virus with K103N and varying efficacy against virus with other NNRTI resistance mutations.

Other NNRTIs

In an effort to identify compounds with activity against HIV-1 resistant to currently approved NNRTIs, candidate triazene and pyrimidine compounds were screened against both wild-type and NNRTI-resistant strains. A dianilinopyrimidine derivative, TMC120 (R147681) has been selected for further clinical development.[33] TMC120 shows potent antiviral activity, with an EC_{50} of 0.0009 μM against wild-type HIV-1 and less than 10-fold decreased susceptibility (with EC_{50} remaining at < 0.01 μM) against HIV-1 with the NNRTI resistance mutations K103N, V106A, Y181C, or G190A/S. However, virus with L100I has TMC120 EC_{50} of 0.016 μM, and virus with Y188L (which requires two nucleotide changes from the wild type) has an EC_{50} of 0.042 μM. A small clinical trial compared two doses of TMC120 (50 or 100 mg twice daily) to placebo in treatment-naive HIV-1-infected adults.[34] TMC120 caused a reduction in plasma HIV-1 RNA of approximately 1.5 $\log_{10}$ copies/ml and a rise in CD4+ T-lymphocyte count of approximately 120 cells/mm^3 at 8 days of monotherapy. The drug appeared safe and well tolerated over this short period.

Using a similar screening strategy, a diaminopyrimidine derivative, TMC125 (R165335), was also found to have excellent activity against both wild-type HIV-1 and HIV-1 with resistance mutations to currently approved NNRTIs.[35] Wild-type virus had a TMC125 EC_{50} of 0.0014 μM, whereas virus with NNRTI resistance mutations (including K103N, Y181C, Y188L, and the double mutations L100I/K103N and K103N/Y181C) had an EC_{50} of less than 0.02 μM. When tested against more than 1000 HIV-1 clinical isolates with phenotypic resistance to at least one NNRTI, TMC125 inhibited 77% of them at 0.01 μM and 97% at 0.1 μM.[36] Early clinical trials are underway.

SJ-3366 belongs to the HEPT class of NNRTIs (similar to emivirine). SJ-3366 is highly potent against wild-type HIV-1, with the EC_{50} usually in the range of 0.0002 to 0.0030 μM.[37] It is active against various clades of HIV-1; and unlike most other NNRTIs tested to date, it has significant activity against HIV-2 although at a much higher EC_{50}. At low concentrations (< 0.005 μM), SJ-3366 inhibits HIV-1 RT specifically but has no activity against HIV-2 RT. At higher concentrations (0.1 to 0.2 μM), it appears to inhibit virus attachment of both HIV-1 and HIV-2. SJ3366 exhibits additive interactions with several other NNRTIs, NRTIs, and PIs. Although SJ-3366 retains activity against some viruses with single NNRTI resistance mutations, its activity is significantly reduced against viruses with other NNRTI resistance mutations (including K101E, K103N, and Y181C).

The activity of foscarnet (phosphonoformic acid, PFA) against HIV-1 has been recognized for more than 15 years.[38] However, its potency is modest (EC_{50} of approximately 15 μM), it is not orally bioavailable, and it has significant toxicities. Alkylglycerol analogues of foscarnet have been developed with significant improvement in potency.[39] The two leading candidates, methyl batyl-PFA (MB-PFA) and ethyl batyl-PFA (EB-PFA), have EC_{50} values of 0.28 and 0.39 μM, respectively. These compounds were equally active against viruses with resistance to zidovudine, lamivudine, multiple nucleosides, and currently approved NNRTIs.[40] However the zalcitabine and didanosine resistance mutation K65R conferred three- to eightfold decreased susceptibility to these analogues. In vitro selection with the foscarnet analogues resulted in virus with more than 10-fold decreased susceptibility.[40] However, the patterns of mutations (including RT W88G, S117T, M164I, and L214F) conferring resistance were different from those seen with nucleosides or other NNRTIs, and several of these mutations reversed zidovudine resistance when introduced on a background of zidovudine resistance mutations.

▲ PROTEASE INHIBITORS

Atazanavir

Atazanavir (BMS-232632) is an azapeptide inhibitor of HIV-1 protease. With an EC_{50} of 0.002 to 0.005 μM against wild-type virus, it appears to be more potent in vitro than currently available protease inhibitors.[41] It also has in vitro activity against many virus isolates with decreased susceptibility to other protease inhibitors. One study suggested that although virus with resistance to saquinavir, nelfinavir, or amprenavir may remain fully susceptible to atazanavir virus resistant to ritonavir or indinavir demonstrates moderately decreased susceptibility (six- to ninefold).[42] A larger study of more than 60 clinical isolates with varying resistance profiles to currently used PIs suggested that atazanavir often retains activity against virus with resistance to one or two other PIs.[43] However, viruses with high level resistance to multiple PIs and carrying large numbers of resistance mutations often had loss of susceptibility to atazanavir.[43,44] In vitro selection with atazanavir resulted in the acquisition of mutations at several codons in protease, accompanied by approximately 100-fold decreased susceptibility.[42] Several mutational pathways appeared and overlapped with the resistance profile of some current PIs. These atazanavir-resistant isolates had variable levels of phenotypic cross resistance to other PIs, although saquinavir retained the best activity against them. In vitro, atazanavir shows additive antiviral effects when combined with nucleoside RT inhibitors or with other PIs.[41]

Atazanavir has good oral bioavailability, and its absorption is increased with a light meal.[45] Co-administration with didanosine and stavudine decreases its blood levels, but administration of these nucleosides an hour before atazanavir does not affect those blood levels. The half-life of atazanavir is approximately 6 hours, and its concentration in plasma is above the serum protein binding-corrected EC_{90} for 24 hours after a single dose of 600 mg, allowing once-daily dosing. Atazanavir undergoes metabolism primarily by hepatic cytochrome P_{450} CYP3A4. Administering atazanavir with ritonavir (an inhibitor of CYP3A4) increases levels of atazanavir severalfold.[46] When co-administered with saquinavir, atazanavir blood levels remain unchanged, but saquinavir levels increase severalfolds.[45]

Two weeks of monotherapy with atazanavir in antiretroviral-naive adults reduced plasma HIV-1 RNA levels by a median 1.5 $\log_{10}$ copies/ml.[47] Subsequent treatment with didanosine, stavudine, and atazanavir (at 200, 400, or 500 mg daily) for 24 weeks resulted in virologic suppression similar to that seen with didanosine, stavudine, and nelfinavir.[48] The median decrease in plasma HIV-1 RNA levels was approximately 2.5 $\log_{10}$ copies/ml; approximately 60% of subjects had less than 400 copies/ml, and 30% had less than 50 copies/ml. The most frequent adverse effects have been diarrhea and nausea. The most common laboratory abnormality associated with treatment has been elevation of serum unconjugated bilirubin, seen in 28% of subjects treated with 400 mg daily.[48] Although usually mild and transient, unconjugated hyperbilirubinemia has caused jaundice in a few subjects. Hyperbilirubinemia has not been associated with elevations of hepatic transaminase levels, and it has been successfully managed with dose reductions of atazanavir in several patients. Unlike other protease inhibitors, atazanavir has caused little adverse change in blood lipids to date.[48]

Atazanavir is a potent PI with the potential for once-daily administration. Its activity against some PI-resistant viruses may make it a reasonable salvage component in patients with early failure to a PI-containing regimen. It may also become useful as initial therapy, particularly because of its lipid-sparing properties when compared with other PIs.

Tipranavir

Tipranavir (PNU-140690) belongs to a new class of non-peptidic inhibitors of HIV-1 protease (the dihydropyrones) discovered by structure-based design efforts.[49,50] It has good activity in vitro against wild-type laboratory and clinical HIV-1 strains, with the IC_{90} typically less than 0.2 μM.[51] Tipranavir also has good in vitro activity against HIV-1 isolates with high-level resistance to currently available PIs.[52,53] One study examined 134 viruses with varying degrees of resistance to currently available PIs, with 105 clinical isolates having more than 10-fold resistance to at least three of the PIs (indinavir, ritonavir, nelfinavir, saquinavir).[54] Only two of these isolates had high-level resistance ($>$ 10-fold) to tipranavir, and 8 had intermediate resistance (4- to 10-fold). In vitro, tipranavir exhibits additive to synergistic antiviral effects when combined with some RT inhibitors or with ritonavir.[51,55] Tipranavir has good oral bioavailability, although its absorption is substantially increased when taken with meals and is reduced when taken with antacids.[56] Blood trough levels averaged higher than 1 μM (above the predicted protein binding-corrected IC_{90} of wild-type HIV-1) in dose regimens of 900 mg three times daily and higher.[57] Tipranavir is a substrate and an inducer of cytochrome P_{450} CYP3A4. When it is combined with ritonavir, tipranavir concentrations are significantly increased, whereas ritonavir concentrations are decreased.[58] This may allow adequate tipranavir blood levels with less frequent dosing if tipranavir is administered with ritonavir.

In PI-naive patients on stable dual NRTI therapy with plasma HIV-1 RNA more than 4000 copies/ml, addition of tipranavir (900 to 1500 mg three times daily) caused a mean reduction in plasma HIV-1 RNA of 1.0 to 1.3 $\log_{10}$ copies/ml at week 4.[59] By week 12 the viral load decreases were attenuated (0.6 to 0.7 $\log_{10}$ copies/ml), but no PI resistance mutations or any consistent patterns of new mutations were seen. A study of combination tipranavir (300 to 1200 mg) with ritonavir (200 mg) given twice daily in PI-naive patients resulted in a median plasma HIV-1 RNA decrease of 1.4 to 1.6 $\log_{10}$ copies/ml at 2 weeks.[60] The most common adverse effects of tipranavir have been mild to moderate diarrhea, nausea, vomiting, and abdominal discomfort.

Mozenavir

Mozenavir (DMP-450) is a member of a novel class of non-peptidic protease inhibitors, the cyclic urea compounds.[61] It has potent activity against wild-type HIV-1 in vitro with EC_{90} of approximately 0.1 to 0.2 μM.[62] Mozenavir also has activity against HIV-2. In vitro studies have shown it to have synergistic activity with several other protease inhibitors and RT inhibitors. HIV-1 with the primary PI resistance mutations at codons 82 or 84 shows three- to ninefold decreased susceptibility to mozenavir.[62] Combinations of resistance mutations in protease (e.g., V82F/I84V) can confer up to 100-fold decreased susceptibility. Passage of HIV-1 under mozenavir selection has resulted in mozenavir-resistant virus with mutations V82I, I84V, and L90M in protease.[62]

Mozenavir appears to have good oral bioavailability, with no significant food effects. Its terminal half-life is approximately 9 hours. It is an inhibitor of cytochrome P_{450} 3A4 and therefore increases the blood levels of drugs metabolized by these enzymes, including saquinavir and indinavir.[63]

Preliminary studies have shown that, in combination with stavudine and lamivudine, mozenavir administration (at 1250 mg twice a day or three times a day) resulted in a mean decrease in plasma HIV-1 RNA of 2.2 to 2.3 $\log_{10}$ copies/ml at 4 weeks of therapy.[64] This was similar to the suppression of viral load seen with indinavir in the same study. Mozenavir appears to be well tolerated in limited studies. The most frequent adverse effects have been mild to moderate gastrointestinal symptoms.[65] Mozenavir has been associated with increases in bilirubin and hepatic transaminases but appears to cause significantly less elevation in total and low density lipoprotein (LDL) cholesterol than indinavir.

Other Protease Inhibitors

GW433908 is the calcium phosphate ester prodrug of amprenavir. It is more water-soluble than amprenavir and appears to be hydrolyzed to amprenavir as it is absorbed through the gut epithelium. The resulting properties of the prodrug allow decreased daily pill count and smaller pill size than amprenavir, which may enhance adherence. In a clinical trial involving antiretroviral-naive HIV-1-infected subjects, GW433908 [1395 mg (3 tablets) or 1865 mg (4 tablets) twice daily] was rapidly converted to amprenavir in vivo.[66] In combination with abacavir and lamivudine, GW433908 caused similar plasma HIV-1 RNA decreases and CD4+ T-lymphocyte count increases to amprenavir at 4 weeks. Subjects treated with GW433908 had a higher incidence of headaches and sleep disorders but a lower incidence of gastrointestinal complaints (nausea, diarrhea, abdominal pain) than subjects treated with amprenavir.

DPC 681 and DPC 684 belong to a new class of nonpeptidic PIs, the substituted sulfonamides. They are highly active against wild-type HIV-1, with and EC_{90} of 0.004 to 0.008 μM; and they retain activity against nonclade B HIV-1 isolates.[67] They are fully active in vitro against virus with the nelfinavir resistance mutations D30N and have fivefold or less decreased activity against laboratory variants with three to five PI resistance mutations. When tested against 30 clinical HIV-1 isolates with several PI resistance mutations (including mutations at protease codons 82, 84, and 90), DPC 681 and DPC 684 typically showed less than ten-fold decrease in activity, and average EC_{50} remained less than 0.02 μM.[67]

In an effort to design PIs with activity against both wild-type HIV-1 and virus with resistance to currently available PIs, a series of PIs (exemplified by TMC126) has been developed.[68] These compounds inhibit wild-type and some PI-resistant virus isolates with an EC_{50} of 0.0001 μM. Most (95%) tested HIV-1 clinical isolates with decreased susceptibility to currently available protease inhibitors remained susceptible to TMC126 (EC_{50} $\leq$0.01 μM). In selection experiments, drug resistant strains appeared to emerge slowly and used genetic pathways different from viruses resistant to currently available protease inhibitors.

▲ ATTACHMENT AND ENTRY INHIBITORS

The process of attachment and entry of HIV-1 into host cells is an important target for antiretroviral drugs.[69–71] Advances in our knowledge of this process are reviewed in Chapter 19 along with a discussion of recently developed compounds that interfere with binding to CD4,[72–75] binding to CXCR4;[76–82] and binding to CCR5.[83–85] Inhibitors of fusion are also under development,[86–90] and they are also reviewed in Chapter 19. Combinations of attachment and fusion inhibitors have been shown to have synergistic or additive effects against HIV-1 in vitro.[91–93]

▲ FUTURE PROSPECTS

Integrase Inhibitors

After viral entry into the host cell, the viral RT synthesizes a linear double-stranded DNA copy of the viral genomic RNA. The HIV-1 integrase then mediates the integration of the HIV-1 DNA into the host chromosome. HIV-1 integrase is a rational target for antiretroviral therapy, as it is essential for replication and there is no cellular equivalent of the enzyme.[94] Integration consists of at least two distinct steps. First, the integrase processes the 3′ ends of the linear viral DNA by removing two nucleotides from each 3′ end (terminal cleavage step). Second, the integrase cleaves the target host DNA and mediates ligation of the viral DNA into the cellular DNA (strand transfer step). Several compounds have been promoted as integrase inhibitors, but their specificity for integrase and their mode of antiviral activity are unclear.[95] The development of in vitro assays that specifically evaluate these functions of integrase may speed the development of integrase inhibitors.[95,96] Two diketo acids (L-731,988 and L-708,906) have been identified that inhibit the strand transfer step.[96] Both inhibited HIV-1 replication in vitro with EC_{50} of 1 to 2 μM. Passage of HIV-1 in the presence of these compounds resulted in virus resistant to them. Specific mutations in integrase were found to cause in vitro resistance to these inhibitors. Other compounds in this class are under development.

Inhibitors of Nucleocapsid Protein Zinc Fingers

The HIV-1 p7 nucleocapsid (p7NC) protein contains two structural motifs, termed zinc fingers, each of which consists of a peptide segment [sequence C-X_2-C-X_4-H-X_4-C, where X is any amino acid and C (cysteine) and H (histidine) act as chelators] coordinated to zinc. These motifs are highly conserved in retroviruses and are important when packaging the genomic RNA into progeny virions. Electrophilic agents that attack the sulfur atoms in cysteine can lead to ejection of zinc and disruption of p7NC.[97,98] Several of these agents are active in vitro against HIV-1 with an EC_{50} in the range of 1 to 20 μM, and they have additive to synergistic antiviral activity when combined with several currently available antiretroviral drugs. Preclinical and early clinical development of this class of antiretroviral agents is continuing.[99]

Other Strategies

Other steps in viral replication may also offer suitable targets for antiretroviral therapy, including HIV-1 genomic RNA degradation (mediated by the ribonuclease H activity of the viral polymerase) during reverse transcription and modulation of HIV-1 transcription and translation mediated by the viral proteins Tat and Rev. Gene therapy may also offer alternative strategies in the future.[100,101] For example, antisense oligonucleotides may be useful for preventing translation of viral mRNA, and ribozymes (enzymatic RNA molecules designed to recognize and cleave specific other RNAs) could be used to cleave HIV-1-specific RNA intracellularly.

REFERENCES

1. Rando RF, Wainberg MA, Nguyen-Ba N, et al. Study of in vitro anti HIV-1 activities of (−)-β-D-1,3-dioxolane guanine and (−)-β-D-2,6-diaminopurine dioxolane. In: Program and Abstracts of the 40th Interscience Conference on Antimicrobial Agents and Chemotherapy Addendum, San Francisco. Washington DC, American Society for Microbiology, 1999, abstract 932.
2. Bazmi HZ, Hammond JL, Cavalcanti SC, et al. In vitro selection of mutations in the human immunodeficiency virus type 1 reverse transcriptase that decrease susceptibility to (−)-beta-D-dioxolane-guanosine and suppress resistance to 3′-azido-3′-deoxythymidine. Antimicrob Agents Chemother 44:1783, 2000.
3. Borroto-Esoda K, Mewshaw J, Wakefield D, et al. The nucleoside reverse transcriptase inhibitor DAPD is active against resistant HIV-1 isolates from patients failing standard nucleoside therapy. In: Abstracts of the 3rd International Workshop on HIV Drug Resistance and Treatment Strategies, San Diego. London, International Medical Press, 1999, abstract 3.
4. Wang LH, Bigley JW, St Claire RL, et al. Preliminary assessments of the pharmacokinetics of DAPD and its active metabolite DXG in HIV-infected subjects. In: Program and Abstracts of the 7th Conference on Retroviruses and Opportunistic Infections, San Francisco. Alexandria, VA, Foundation for Retrovirology and Human Health, 2000, abstract 103.
5. Eron JJ, Kessler H, Thompson M, et al. Clinical HIV suppression after short term monotherapy with DAPD. In: Program and Abstracts of the 40th Interscience Conference on Antimicrobial Agents and Chemotherapy, Toronto. Washington DC, American Society for Microbiology, 2000, abstract 690.
6. De Muys JM, Gourdeau H, Nguyen-Ba N, et al. Anti-human immunodeficiency virus type 1 activity, intracellular metabolism, and pharmacokinetic evaluation of 2′-deoxy-3′-oxa-4′-thiocytidine. Antimicrob Agents Chemother 43:1835, 1999.
7. Gu Z, Nguyen-Ba N, Ren C, et al. BCH-10618, a new potent anti-HIV-1 NRTI. In: Frontiers in Drug Development for Antiretroviral Therapies, Puerto Rico. New York, Elsevier Science, 2000, abstract 15.
8. Gu Z, Nguyen-Ba N, Mellors J, et al. In vitro selection and characterization of HIV-1 resistance to BCH-10618. In: Program and Abstracts of the 8th Conference on Retroviruses and Opportunistic Infections, Chicago. Alexandria, VA, Foundation for Retrovirology and Human Health, 2001, abstract 472.
9. Smith PF, Forrest A, Ballow CH, et al. Absolute bioavailability and disposition of (−) and (+) 2′-deoxy- 3′-oxa-4′-thiocytidine (dOTC) following single intravenous and oral doses of racemic dOTC in humans. Antimicrob Agents Chemother 44:1609, 2000.
10. Smith PF, Forrest A, Ballow CH, et al. Safety, tolerability, and pharmacokinetics of single oral doses of BCH-10652 in healthy adult males. Antimicrob Agents Chemother 44:2816, 2000.
11. Dutschman GE, Bridges EG, Liu SH, et al. Metabolism of 2′,3′-dideoxy-2′,3′-didehydro-beta-L(−)-5-fluorocytidine and its activity in combination with clinically approved anti-human immunodeficiency virus beta-D(+)nucleoside analogs in vitro. Antimicrob Agents Chemother 42:1799, 1998.
12. Dunkle LM, Oshana SC, Cheng YC, et al. ACH-126,443: a new nucleoside analog with potent activity against wild-type and resistant HIV-1 and a promising pharmacokinetic and mitochondrial safety profile. In: Program and Abstracts of the 8th Conference on Retroviruses and Opportunistic Infections, Chicago. Alexandria, VA, Foundation for Retrovirology and Human Health, 2001, abstract 303.
13. Kodama EI, Kohgo S, Kitano K, et al. 4′-Ethynyl nucleoside analogs: potent inhibitors of multidrug-resistant human immunodeficiency virus variants in vitro. Antimicrob Agents Chemother 45:1539, 2001.
14. Gray G, Volaris A, McIntyre J, et al. Pharmacokinetics (PK) and safety of emivirine (EMV, MKC-442) in HIV-1-infected pregnant women and their offspring. In: Program and Abstracts of the 39th Interscience Conference on Antimicrobial Agents and Chemotherapy, San Francisco. Washington DC, American Society for Microbiology, 1999, abstract 334.
15. Szczech GM, Furman P, Painter GR, et al. Safety assessment, in vitro and in vivo, and pharmacokinetics of emivirine, a potent and selective nonnucleoside reverse transcriptase inhibitor of human immunodeficiency virus type 1. Antimicrob Agents Chemother 44:123, 2000.
16. Sereni D, Arasteh K, Gathiram V, et al. Antiviral activity, safety, and tolerability of emivirine (EMV, Coactinon) + stavudine (d4T, Zerit) + lamivudine (3TC, Epivir) in treatment-naive HIV-infected volunteers (MKC-301). In: Program and Abstracts of the 37th Annual Meeting of the Infectious Diseases Society of America, Philadelphia. Alexandria, VA, Infectious Diseases Society of America, 1999, abstract 364.
17. Raffi F, Arasteh K, Gathiram V, et al. 24-Week results of the antiviral activity, safety, and tolerability of emivirine (EMD, Coactinon) + stavudine (d4T, Zerit) + didanosine (ddI, Videx) in treatment-naive HIV-infected patients (MKC-302). In: Program and Abstracts of the 7th Conference on Retroviruses and Opportunistic Infections, San Francisco. Alexandria, VA, Foundation for Retrovirology and Human Health, 2000, abstract 514.
18. Hicks C, Harmon J, Anderson J, et al. Dual NNRTI therapy [MKC-442, emivirine (EMV) + efavirenz (EFV)] for patients failing PI regimens: pharmacokinetics and short-term efficacy. In: Program and Abstracts of the 7th Conference on Retroviruses and Opportunistic Infections, San Francisco. Alexandria, VA, Foundation for Retrovirology and Human Health, 2000, abstract 670.
19. McCreedy B, Borroto-Esoda K, Harris J, et al. Genotypic and phenotypic analysis of HIV-1 from patients receiving combination therapy containing two nucleoside reverse transcriptase inhibitors (NRTIs) and the non-NRTI, emivirine (MKC-442). In: Abstracts of the 3rd International Workshop on HIV Drug Resistance and Treatment Strategies, San Diego. London, International Medical Press, 1999, abstract 13.
20. Borroto-Esoda K, Harris J, Klish C, et al. Genotypic and phenotypic analysis of HIV-1 from patients receiving combination therapy containing two nucleoside reverse transcriptase inhibitors (NRTI), a protease inhibitor, and emivirine (EMV, Coactinon). In: Program and Abstracts of the 7th Conference on Retroviruses and Opportunistic Infections, San Francisco. Alexandria, VA, Foundation for Retrovirology and Human Health, 2000, abstract 751.
21. Fujiwara T, Sato A, el-Farrash M, et al. S-1153 inhibits replication of known drug-resistant strains of human immunodeficiency virus type 1. Antimicrob Agents Chemother 42:1340, 1998.
22. Hayashi S, Amantea M, Hawley P, et al. Effects of fasting (F), high fat (H) and low fat (L) meals on the pharmacokinetics (PK) of a single oral dose of capravirine (CPV), a nonnucleoside reverse transcriptase inhibitor (NNRTI), in healthy volunteers. In: Program and Abstracts of the 40th Interscience Conference on Antimicrobial Agents and Chemotherapy, Toronto. Washington DC, American Society for Microbiology, 2000, abstract 1667.
23. Hernandez J, Amador L, Amantea M, et al. Short-course monotherapy with AG1549, a novel nonnucleoside reverse transcriptase inhibitor (NNRTI), in antiretroviral-naive patients. In: Program and Abstracts of the 7th Conference on Retroviruses and Opportunistic Infections, San Francisco. Alexandria, VA, Foundation for Retrovirology and Human Health, 2000, abstract 669.
24. Dezube BJ, Jacobs MS, Leoung G, et al. A second generation non-nucleoside reverse transcriptase inhibitor (S-1153) for the treatment of HIV infection: a phase I study. In: Conference Record of the 12th International Conference on AIDS, Geneva. Stockholm, International AIDS Society, 1998, abstract 12214.
25. Corbett JW, Ko SS, Rodgers JD, et al. Expanded-spectrum nonnucleoside reverse transcriptase inhibitors inhibit clinically relevant mutant variants of human immunodeficiency virus type 1. Antimicrob Agents Chemother 43:2893, 1999.
26. Corbett JW, Ko SS, Rodgers JD, et al. Inhibition of clinically relevant mutant variants of HIV-1 by quinazolinone non-nucleoside reverse transcriptase inhibitors. J Med Chem 43:2019, 2000.
27. Fiske WD, Brennan JM, Harrison RR, et al. Pharmacokinetics of a second-generation NNRTI, DPC 083, after multiple oral doses in healthy volunteers. In: Program and Abstracts of the 7th Conference on Retroviruses and Opportunistic Infections, San Francisco. Alexandria, VA, Foundation for Retrovirology and Human Health, 2000, abstract 99.
28. Joshi AS, Jiao QT, Waggett DS, et al. Pharmacokinetics of a second-generation NNRTI, DPC 961, after multiple oral doses in healthy

volunteers. In: Program and Abstracts of the 7th Conference on Retroviruses and Opportunistic Infections, San Francisco. Alexandria, VA, Foundation for Retrovirology and Human Health, 2000, abstract 102.

29. Kashman Y, Gustafson KR, Fuller RW, et al. The calanolides, a novel HIV-inhibitory class of coumarin derivatives from the tropical rainforest tree, Calophyllum lanigerum. J Med Chem 35:2735, 1992.
30. Creagh T, Ruckle JL, Tolbert DT, et al. Safety and pharmacokinetics of single doses of (+)-calanolide a, a novel, naturally occurring nonnucleoside reverse transcriptase inhibitor, in healthy, human immunodeficiency virus-negative human subjects. Antimicrob Agents Chemother 45:1379, 2001.
31. Sherer R, Dutta B, Anderson R, et al. A phase IB study of (+)-calanolide A in HIV-1-infected, antiretroviral-therapy-naive patients. In: Program and Abstracts of the 7th Conference on Retroviruses and Opportunistic Infections, San Francisco. Alexandria, VA, Foundation for Retrovirology and Human Health, 2000, abstract 508.
32. Buckheit RW Jr, White EL, Fliakas-Boltz V, et al. Unique anti-human immunodeficiency virus activities of the nonnucleoside reverse transcriptase inhibitors calanolide A, costatolide, and dihydrocostatolide. Antimicrob Agents Chemother 43:1827, 1999.
33. De Bethune MP, Andries K, Ludovici D, et al. TMC120 (R147681), a next-generation NNRTI, has potent in vitro activity against NNRTI-resistant HIV variants. In: Program and Abstracts of the 8th Conference on Retroviruses and Opportunistic Infections, Chicago. Alexandria, VA, Foundation for Retrovirology and Human Health, 2001, abstract 304.
34. Gruzdev B, Horban A, Boron-Kaczmarska A, et al. TMC120, a new nonnucleoside reverse transcriptase inhibitor, is a potent antiretroviral in treatment naive, HIV-1 infected subjects. In: Program and Abstracts of the 8th Conference on Retroviruses and Opportunistic Infections, Chicago. Alexandria, VA, Foundation for Retrovirology and Human Health, 2001, abstract 13.
35. Andries K, de Bethune MP, Kukla MJ, et al. R165335-TMC125, a novel nonnucleoside reverse transcriptase inhibitor (NNRTI) with nanomolar activity against NNRTI resistant HIV strains. In: Program and Abstracts of the 40th Interscience Conference on Antimicrobial Agents and Chemotherapy, Toronto. Washington DC, American Society for Microbiology, 2000, abstract 1840.
36. De Bethune MP, Hertogs K, Azijn H, et al. R165335-TMC125, a third generation non nucleoside reverse transcriptase inhibitor (NNRTI), inhibits 98% of more than 2,000 recombinant HIV clinical isolates at 100 nM. In: Program and Abstracts of the 40th Interscience Conference on Antimicrobial Agents and Chemotherapy, Toronto. Washington DC, American Society for Microbiology, 2000, abstract 1841.
37. Buckheit RW, Watson K, Fliakas-Boltz V, et al. SJ-3366, a unique and highly potent nonnucleoside reverse transcriptase inhibitor of human immunodeficiency virus type 1 (HIV-1) that also inhibits HIV-2. Antimicrob Agents Chemother 45:393, 2001.
38. Sandstrom EG, Kaplan JC, Byington RE, et al. Inhibition of human T-cell lymphotropic virus type III in vitro by phosphonoformate. Lancet 1:1480, 1985.
39. Hostetler KY, Hammond JL, Kini GD, et al. In vitro anti-HIV-1 activity of sn-2-substituted 1-O-octadecyl-sn-glycero-3-phosphonoformate analogues and synergy with zidovudine. Antivir Chem Chemother 11:213, 2000.
40. Hammond JL, Koontz DL, Bazmi HZ, et al. Alkylglycerol prodrugs of phosphonoformate are potent in vitro inhibitors of nucleoside-resistant human immunodeficiency virus type 1 and select for resistance mutations that suppress zidovudine resistance. Antimicrob Agents Chemother 45:1621, 2001.
41. Robinson BS, Riccardi KA, Gong YF, et al. BMS-232632, a highly potent human immunodeficiency virus protease inhibitor that can be used in combination with other available antiretroviral agents. Antimicrob Agents Chemother 44:2093, 2000.
42. Gong YF, Robinson BS, Rose RE, et al. In vitro resistance profile of the human immunodeficiency virus type 1 protease inhibitor BMS-232632. Antimicrob Agents Chemother 44:2319, 2000.
43. Colonno RJ, Hertogs K, Larder BA, et al. BMS-232632 sensitivity of a panel of HIV-1 clinical isolates resistant to one or more approved protease inhibitors. In: Abstracts of the 4th International Workshop on HIV Drug Resistance and Treatment Strategies, Stitges, Spain. London, International Medical Press, 2000, abstract 8.
44. Palmer S, Shafer RW, Merigan TC. Highly drug-resistant HIV-1 clinical isolates are cross-resistant to many antiretroviral compounds in current clinical development. AIDS 13:661, 1999.
45. O'Mara E, Mummaneni V, Randall D, et al. BMS-232632: a summary of multiple-dose pharmacokinetic, food effect, and drug interaction studies in healthy subjects. In: Program and Abstracts of the 7th Conference on Retroviruses and Opportunistic Infections, San Francisco. Alexandria, VA, Foundation for Retrovirology and Human Health, 2000, abstract 504.
46. O'Mara E, Mummaneni V, Bifano M, et al. Steady-state pharmacokinetic interaction study between BMS-232632 and ritonavir in healthy subjects. In: Program and Abstracts of the 8th Conference on Retroviruses and Opportunistic Infections, Chicago. Alexandria, VA, Foundation for Retrovirology and Human Health, 2001, abstract 740.
47. Sanne I, Piliero P, Wood R, et al. Safety and antiviral efficacy of a once-daily HIV-1 protease inhibitor BMS-232632: 24 week results from a phase II clinical trial. In: Program and Abstracts of the 40th Interscience Conference on Antimicrobial Agents and Chemotherapy, Toronto. Washington DC, American Society for Microbiology, 2000, abstract 691.
48. Squires K, Gatell J, Piliero P, et al. AI424-007: 48-week safety and efficacy results from a phase II study of a once-daily HIV-1 protease inhibitor (PI), BMS-232632. In: Program and Abstracts of the 8th Conference on Retroviruses and Opportunistic Infections, Chicago. Alexandria, VA, Foundation for Retrovirology and Human Health, 2001, abstract 15.
49. Thaisrivongs S, Skulnick HI, Turner SR, et al. Structure-based design of HIV protease inhibitors: sulfonamide-containing 5,6-dihydro-4-hydroxy-2-pyrones as non-peptidic inhibitors. J Med Chem 39:4349, 1996.
50. Turner SR, Strohbach JW, Tommasi RA, et al. Tipranavir (PNU-140690): a potent, orally bioavailable nonpeptidic HIV protease inhibitor of the 5,6-dihydro-4-hydroxy-2-pyrone sulfonamide class. J Med Chem 41:3467, 1998.
51. Poppe SM, Slade DE, Chong KT, et al. Antiviral activity of the dihydropyrone PNU-140690, a new nonpeptidic human immunodeficiency virus protease inhibitor. Antimicrob Agents Chemother 41:1058, 1997.
52. Back NK, van Wijk A, Remmerswaal D, et al. In-vitro tipranavir susceptibility of HIV-1 isolates with reduced susceptibility to other protease inhibitors. AIDS 14:101, 2000.
53. Rusconi S, La Seta Catamancio S, Citterio P, et al. Susceptibility to PNU-140690 (tipranavir) of human immunodeficiency virus type 1 isolates derived from patients with multidrug resistance to other protease inhibitors. Antimicrob Agents Chemother 44:1328, 2000.
54. Larder BA, Hertogs K, Bloor S, et al. Tipranavir inhibits broadly protease inhibitor-resistant HIV-1 clinical samples. AIDS 14:1943, 2000.
55. Chong KT, Pagano PJ. In vitro combination of PNU-140690, a human immunodeficiency virus type 1 protease inhibitor, with ritonavir against ritonavir-sensitive and -resistant clinical isolates. Antimicrob Agents Chemother 41:2367, 1997.
56. Baldwin JR, Borin MT, Wang Y, et al. Effects of food and antacid on bioavailability of the protease inhibitor PNU-140690 in healthy volunteers. In: Program and Abstracts of the 5th Conference on Retroviruses and Opportunistic Infections, Chicago. Alexandria, VA, Foundation for Retrovirology and Human Health, 1998, abstract 649.
57. Borin MT, Wang Y, Schneck DW, et al. Multiple-dose safety, tolerance, and pharmacokinetics of the protease inhibitor PNU-140690 in healthy volunteers. In: Program and Abstracts of the 5th Conference on Retroviruses and Opportunistic Infections, Chicago. Alexandria, VA, Foundation for Retrovirology and Human Health, 1998, abstract 648.
58. Baldwin JR, Borin MT, Ferry JJ, et al. Pharmacokinetic (PK) interaction between the HIV protease inhibitors tipranavir and ritonavir. In: Program and Abstracts of the 39th Interscience Conference on Antimicrobial Agents and Chemotherapy, San Francisco. Washington DC, American Society for Microbiology, 1999, abstract 657.
59. Wang Y, Freimuth WW, Daenzer CL, et al. Safety and efficacy of PNU-140690, a new non-peptidic HIV protease inhibitor, and HIV genotypic changes in patients in a phase II study. In: Abstracts of the 2nd International Workshop on HIV Drug Resistance and Treatment Strategies, Lake Maggiore, Italy. London, International Medical Press, 1998, abstract 5.
60. Wang Y, Daenzer C, Wood R, et al. The safety, efficacy, and viral dynamics analysis of tipranavir, a new-generation protease inhibitor, in a phase II study in antiretroviral-naive HIV-1-infected patients. In: Program and Abstracts of the 7th Conference on Retroviruses and Opportunistic Infections, San Francisco. Alexandria, VA, Foundation for Retrovirology and Human Health, 2000, abstract 673.
61. Ala PJ, Huston EE, Klabe RM, et al. Molecular basis of HIV-1 protease drug resistance: structural analysis of mutant proteases complexed

with cyclic urea inhibitors. Biochemistry 36:1573, 1997; Erratum. Biochemistry 36:6556, 1997.
62. Hodge CN, Aldrich PE, Bacheler LT, et al. Improved cyclic urea inhibitors of the HIV-1 protease: synthesis, potency, resistance profile, human pharmacokinetics and X-ray crystal structure of DMP 450. Chem Biol 3:301, 1996.
63. Wang LH, Chittick GE, Patanella JE, et al. Effects of a novel HIV-1 protease inhibitor (PI), DMP450, on the pharmacokinetics (PK) of indinavir (IDV) and saquinavir (SQV). In: Program and Abstracts of the 40th Interscience Conference on Antimicrobial Agents and Chemotherapy, Toronto. Washington DC, American Society for Microbiology, 2000, abstract 1647.
64. Sierra J, Nino S, Volkow P, et al. Preliminary profile of the antiviral activity, metabolic effects, safety, and pharmacokinetics of DMP450, a novel cyclic urea protease inhibitor. In: Program and Abstracts of the 40th Interscience Conference on Antimicrobial Agents and Chemotherapy, Toronto. Washington DC, American Society for Microbiology, 2000, abstract 540.
65. Chittick GE, Wang LH, Demasi RA, et al. Effects of a novel HIV-1 protease inhibitor (PI), DMP450, on cardiac tracing, serum lipids and glucose tolerance, as compared to indinavir (IDV). In: Program and Abstracts of the 40th Interscience Conference on Antimicrobial Agents and Chemotherapy, Toronto. Washington DC, American Society for Microbiology, 2000, abstract 1648.
66. Wood R, Arasteh K, Pollard R, et al. GW433908, a novel prodrug of the HIV protease inhibitor (PI) amprenavir (APV): safety, efficacy, and pharmacokinetics (PK) (APV20001). In: Program and Abstracts of the 8th Conference on Retroviruses and Opportunistic Infections, Chicago. Alexandria, VA, Foundation for Retrovirology and Human Health, 2001, abstract 333.
67. Kaltenbach RF 3rd, Trainor G, Getman D, et al. DPC 681 and DPC 684: potent, selective inhibitors of human immunodeficiency virus protease active against clinically relevant mutant variants. Antimicrob Agents Chemother 45:3021, 2001.
68. Erickson J, Gulnik S, Suvorov L, et al. A femtomolar HIV-1 protease inhibitor with subnanomolar activity against multidrug resistant HIV-1 strains. In: Program and Abstracts of the 8th Conference on Retroviruses and Opportunistic Infections, Chicago. Alexandria, VA, Foundation for Retrovirology and Human Health, 2001, abstract 12.
69. Baribaud F, Pohlmann S, Doms RW. The role of DC-SIGN and DC-SIGNR in HIV and SIV attachment, infection, and transmission. Virology 286:1, 2001.
70. D'Souza MP, Cairns JS, Plaeger SF. Current evidence and future directions for targeting HIV entry: therapeutic and prophylactic strategies. JAMA 284:215, 2000.
71. Cairns JS, D'Souza MP. Chemokines and HIV-1 second receptors: the therapeutic connection. Nat Med 4:563, 1998.
72. Allaway GP, Davis-Bruno KL, Beaudry GA, et al. Expression and characterization of CD4-IgG2, a novel heterotetramer that neutralizes primary HIV type 1 isolates. AIDS Res Hum Retroviruses 11:533, 1995.
73. Trkola A, Pomales AB, Yuan H, et al. Cross-clade neutralization of primary isolates of human immunodeficiency virus type 1 by human monoclonal antibodies and tetrameric CD4-IgG. J Virol 69:6609, 1995.
74. Jacobson JM, Lowy I, Fletcher CV, et al. Single-dose safety, pharmacology, and antiviral activity of the human immunodeficiency virus (HIV) type 1 entry inhibitor PRO 542 in HIV-infected adults. J Infect Dis 182:326, 2000.
75. Shearer WT, Israel RJ, Starr S, et al. Recombinant CD4-IgG2 in human immunodeficiency virus type 1-infected children: phase 1/2 study. J Infect Dis 182:1774, 2000.
76. Donzella GA, Schols D, Lin SW, et al. AMD3100, a small molecule inhibitor of HIV-1 entry via the CXCR4 co-receptor. Nat Med 4:72, 1998.
77. Schols D, Este JA, Henson G, et al. Bicyclams, a class of potent anti-HIV agents, are targeted at the HIV coreceptor fusin/CXCR-4. Antivir Res 35:147, 1997.
78. Este JA, Cabrera C, Blanco J, et al. Shift of clinical human immunodeficiency virus type 1 isolates from X4 to R5 and prevention of emergence of the syncytium-inducing phenotype by blockade of CXCR4. J Virol 73:5577, 1999.
79. Hendrix CW, Flexner C, MacFarland RT, et al. Pharmacokinetics and safety of AMD-3100, a novel antagonist of the CXCR-4 chemokine receptor, in human volunteers. Antimicrob Agents Chemother 44:1667, 2000.
80. Murakami T, Nakajima T, Koyanagi Y, et al. A small molecule CXCR4 inhibitor that blocks T cell line-tropic HIV-1 infection. J Exp Med 186:1389, 1997.
81. Doranz BJ, Grovit-Ferbas K, Sharron MP, et al. A small-molecule inhibitor directed against the chemokine receptor CXCR4 prevents its use as an HIV-1 coreceptor. J Exp Med 186:1395, 1997.
82. MacFarland RT, Yasuda N, Witvrouw M, et al. An orally bioavailable CXCR4 antagonist for inhibition of HIV replication. In: Program and Abstracts of the 40th Interscience Conference on Antimicrobial Agents and Chemotherapy, Toronto. Washington DC, American Society for Microbiology, 2000, abstract 1845.
83. Trkola A, Ketas TJ, Nagashima KA, et al. Potent, broad-spectrum inhibition of human immunodeficiency virus type 1 by the CCR5 monoclonal antibody PRO 140. J Virol 75:579, 2001.
84. Baba M, Nishimura O, Kanzaki N, et al. A small-molecule, nonpeptide CCR5 antagonist with highly potent and selective anti-HIV-1 activity. Proc Natl Acad Sci USA 96:5698, 1999.
85. Strizki JM, Xu S, Wagner NE, et al. SCH-C (SCH 351125), an orally bioavailable, small molecule antagonist of the chemokine receptor CCR5, is a potent inhibitor of HIV-1 infection in vitro and in vivo. Proc Natl Acad Sci USA 98:12718, 2001.
86. Kilby JM, Hopkins S, Venetta TM, et al. Potent suppression of HIV-1 replication in humans by T-20, a peptide inhibitor of gp41-mediated virus entry. Nat Med 4:1302, 1998.
87. Eron J, Merigan T, Kilby M, et al. A 14-day assessment of the safety, pharmacokinetics, and antiviral activity of T-1249, a peptide inhibitor of membrane fusion. In: Program and Abstracts of the 8th Conference on Retroviruses and Opportunistic Infections, Chicago. Alexandria, VA, Foundation for Retrovirology and Human Health, 2001, abstract 14.
88. Eckert DM, Malashkevich VN, Hong LH, et al. Inhibiting HIV-1 entry: discovery of D-peptide inhibitors that target the gp41 coiled-coil pocket. Cell 99:103, 1999.
89. Jin BS, Ryu JR, Ahn K, et al. Design of a peptide inhibitor that blocks the cell fusion mediated by glycoprotein 41 of human immunodeficiency virus type 1. AIDS Res Hum Retroviruses 16:1797, 2000.
90. Root MJ, Kay MS, Kim PS. Protein design of an HIV-1 entry inhibitor. Science 291:884, 2001.
91. Tremblay CL, Kollmann C, Giguel F, et al. Strong in vitro synergy between the fusion inhibitor T-20 and the CXCR4 blocker AMD-3100. J Acquir Immune Defic Syndr 25:99, 2000.
92. Tremblay CL, Kollmann C, Giguel F, et al. In vitro synergy observed between the fusion inhibitor T-20 and a CCR5 inhibitor TAK-779. In: Program and Abstracts of the 40th Interscience Conference on Antimicrobial Agents and Chemotherapy, Toronto. Washington DC, American Society for Microbiology, 2000, abstract 1164.
93. Rusconi S, La Seta Catamancio S, Citterio P, et al. Combination of CCR5 and CXCR4 inhibitors in therapy of human immunodeficiency virus type 1 infection: in vitro studies of mixed virus infections. J Virol 74:9328, 2000.
94. Pommier Y, Marchand C, Neamati N. Retroviral integrase inhibitors year 2000: update and perspectives. Antivir Res 47:139, 2000.
95. Farnet CM, Wang B, Hansen M, et al. Human immunodeficiency virus type 1 cDNA integration: new aromatic hydroxylated inhibitors and studies of the inhibition mechanism. Antimicrob Agents Chemother 42:2245, 1998.
96. Hazuda DJ, Felock P, Witmer M, et al. Inhibitors of strand transfer that prevent integration and inhibit HIV-1 replication in cells. Science 287:646, 2000.
97. Rice WG, Supko JG, Malspeis L, et al. Inhibitors of HIV nucleocapsid protein zinc fingers as candidates for the treatment of AIDS. Science 270:1194, 1995.
98. Rice WG, Baker DC, Schaeffer CA, et al. Inhibition of multiple phases of human immunodeficiency virus type 1 replication by a dithiane compound that attacks the conserved zinc fingers of retroviral nucleocapsid proteins. Antimicrob Agents Chemother 41:419, 1997.
99. Goebel F-D, Hemmer R, Schmit JC, et al. Phase I/II dose escalation and randomized withdrawal study with add-on azodicarbonamide in patients failing on current antiretroviral therapy. AIDS 15:33, 2001.
100. Buchschacher GL Jr. Molecular targets of gene transfer therapy for HIV infection. JAMA 269:2880, 1993.
101. Kaplan JC, Hirsch MS. Therapy other than reverse transcriptase inhibitors for HIV infection. Clin Lab Med 14:367, 1994.

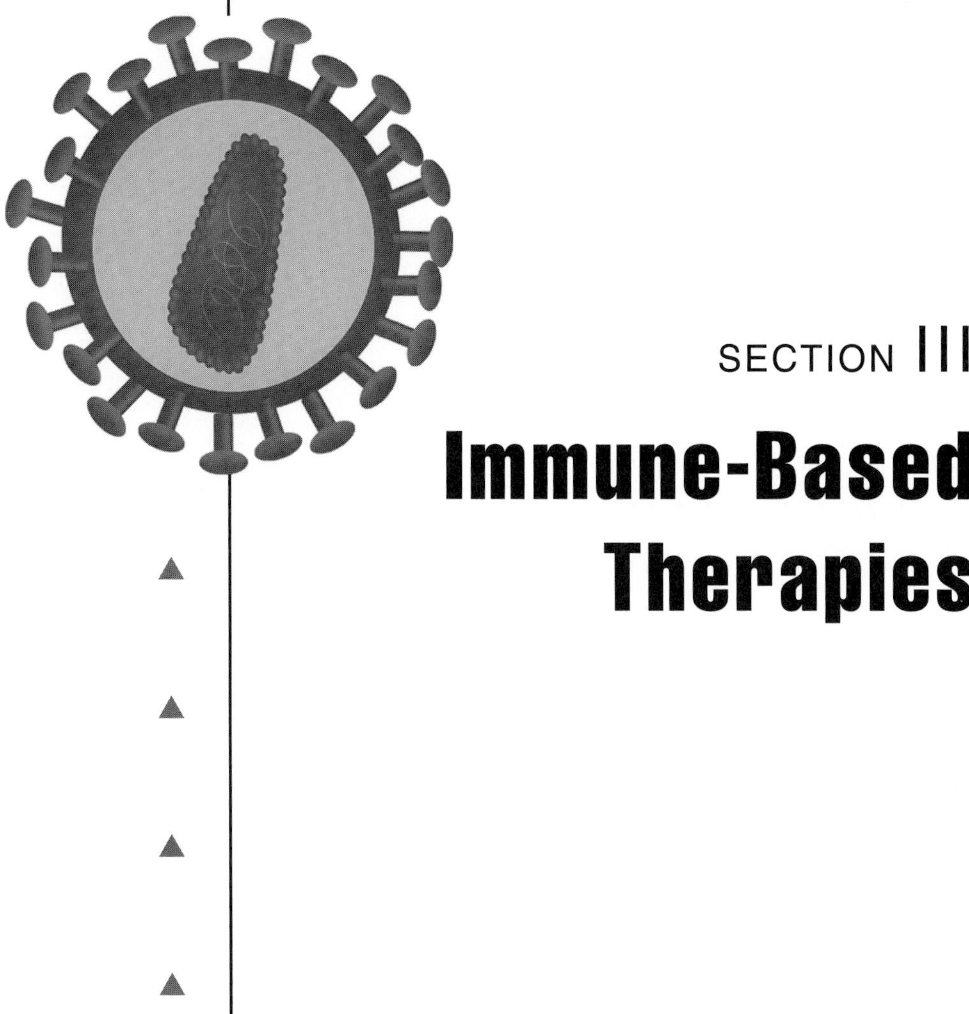

SECTION III

Immune-Based Therapies

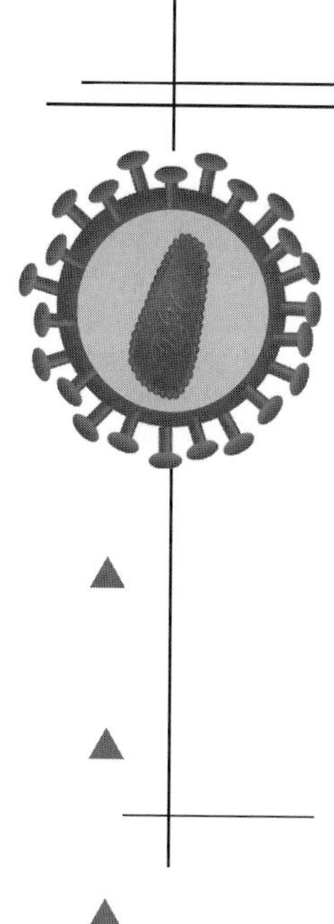

CHAPTER 21

General Immune-Based Therapies in the Management of HIV-Infected Patients

Joseph A. Kovacs, MD

The development of highly active antiretroviral drugs, especially protease inhibitors or nonnucleoside reverse transcriptase inhibitors, has resulted in the identification of potent combination regimens that have markedly improved survival and clearly serve as the mainstay of current therapy for human immunodeficiency virus (HIV)-infected patients. However, despite the profound suppression of viral replication that can be seen, the level of immune restoration and the duration of viral suppression associated with such therapies appears to be limited in many patients.[1,2] Furthermore, in many additional patients adverse effects, difficulty adhering to the rigorous medication regimens, or both decrease the feasibility of long-term therapy with these drugs. Thus identification of effective alternative therapeutic approaches for the treatment of HIV-infected patients is essential.

Given that most HIV-related complications, including opportunistic infections and malignancies, are a result of the immunosuppression induced by HIV, rather than being directly mediated by HIV itself, an alternative approach to complement antiretroviral therapy is to target the immune system directly in an effort to expand immune function, prevent further immunologic deterioration, or improve the host immune response to HIV.[3,4]

A variety of immune-based approaches to the management of HIV infection have been evaluated, but to date no immunotherapy has been documented to have a consistent clinical benefit in controlled trials. Many approaches have been evaluated in a preliminary fashion in uncontrolled trials and thus have only limited applicability to the management of HIV-infected patients at present. This chapter briefly summarizes approaches currently being investigated and then focuses on studies with interleukin-2 (IL-2), interferon-α, and granulocyte/macrophage colony-stimulating factor (GM-CSF). These three cytokines, which have been more extensively studied than other therapies, have demonstrable effects on surrogate markers and are U.S. Food and Drug Administration (FDA)-approved for other indications.

Approaches to immune restoration have included therapy with a variety of cytokines, including IL-2,[5] IL-12,[6] interferon-α,[7,8] interferon-γ,[9] and GM-CSF[10]; adoptive immunotherapy using peripheral blood lymphocytes or bone marrow transplants[11-15]; and passive immunization with hyperimmune globulin.[16-18] Studies with IL-12 in HIV-infected patients have been limited, and the potential for immunologic enhancement has not been well delineated.[6] In limited trials conducted during the 1980s, interferon-γ was not associated with benefit, although reevaluation of its role in the management of certain opportunistic infections may be warranted.[9,19] Adoptive immunotherapy studies with small numbers of patients have to date shown no consistent benefit.[11-13,15] Passive immunization also failed to demonstrate consistent benefit.[16-18]

Gene therapy approaches utilizing both CD4 and CD8 cells transduced with a variety of constructs that attempt to improve targeting of HIV-infected cells or protect cells from HIV infection are also underway but are at a preliminary stage.[14,20,21]

▲ INTERLEUKIN-2

Interleukin-2 is a cytokine secreted primarily by activated CD4 helper cells.[22] It plays a crucial role in the proliferation and differentiation of a variety of cells important to host immune responses, including CD4 helper cells, CD8 cytotoxic cells, antibody-producing B cells, natural killer (NK) cells, and monocytes/macrophages. Early in vitro studies demonstrated that IL-2 could restore deficient NK cell activity and cytomegalovirus (CMV) specific cytotoxicity to cells from patients with acquired immunodeficiency syndrome (AIDS), providing a rationale for clinical trials of IL-2 in this setting.[23,24]

Early clinical trials of IL-2, which used a variety of doses and durations of treatment and routes of administration but did not provide long-term therapy, did not demonstrate any long-term immunologic or clinical benefit.[25–27] Given that IL-2 can activate lymphocytes, which may facilitate replication of HIV, investigators began studies combining IL-2 with antiretroviral therapies.[28–30] These studies, which initially focused on patients with relatively intact immune systems, demonstrated that IL-2, when administered intermittently for 5-day cycles approximately every 2 months at a dose 12 million to 18 million international units (IU) per day by continuous intravenous infusion (CIV), resulted in substantial, sustained increases in CD4+ T-lymphocyte counts with no concomitant effect on CD8 cells. Based on V-beta analysis, this CD4+ T-lymphocyte count increase was polyclonal and was associated with an increase in the number of CD4+ T-lymphocyte count expressing the high-affinity IL-2 receptor (CD25).[28] Plasma HIV load measured by the branched DNA assay demonstrated a transient increase in some patients that peaked at the end of IL-2 therapy and returned to baseline within a week of discontinuing IL-2.[28,31] Other similar studies noted an increase in NK cell activity, or lymphokine activated killer (LAK) cell activity, during IL-2 therapy.[32] Patients with lower CD4+ T-lymphocyte counts (who were being treated exclusively with nucleoside analogues), especially those with CD4+ T-lymphocyte counts less than 100 cells/mm^3, did not demonstrate similar CD4+ T-lymphocyte count responses but did exhibit more frequent increases in plasma HIV levels that were often sustained.[28]

A randomized trial undertaken to evaluate these preliminary observations clearly demonstrated that intermittent IL-2 therapy can lead to a substantial, sustained increase in CD4+ T-lymphocyte counts without inducing increases in plasma viral load.[5] Sixty patients with CD4+ T-lymphocyte counts higher than 200 cells/mm^3 were randomized to receive either licensed antiretroviral drugs combined with intermittent CIV IL-2 or antiretroviral therapy alone. The control group showed a gradual decline in CD4+ T-lymphocyte count number during the 14 months of the study (−5 cells/month), whereas the IL-2 group showed a mean increase of 37 cells/month ($P < 0.001$) (Fig. 21–1) with a concomitant increase in the CD4+ T-lymphocyte count percentage. There was no difference in the CD8 cell number over time. Additionally, there was a substantial increase in CD4+ T-lymphocyte that were CD25 (high-affinity IL-2 receptor)-positive and a preferential expansion of naive CD4+ T-lymphocyte (Fig. 21–2). Importantly, no differences in plasma HIV levels were seen between the two groups over time (Fig. 21–1). During an extension phase in which dosing of IL-2 was individualized, the mean CD4+ T-lymphocyte count for

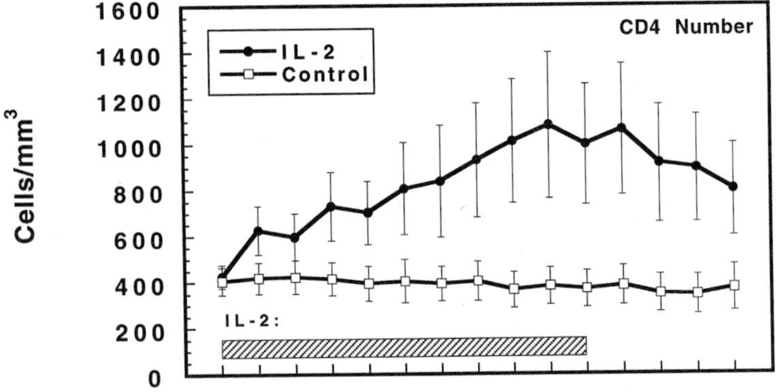

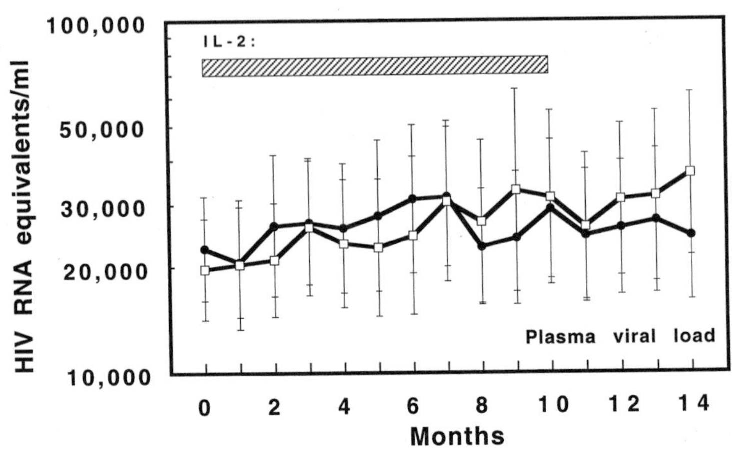

Figure 21–1. Changes in mean CD4+ T-lymphocyte count (*top*) and viral load, as measured by the branched DNA assay (*bottom*), during a randomized, controlled trial of intermittent interleukin-2 (IL-2) therapy in HIV-infected patients with baseline CD4 counts of > 200 cells/mm^3. Although the CD4+ T-lymphocyte count more than doubled in the IL-2 group (*closed circles*) compared to the control group (*open squares*), the plasma HIV RNA level changes did not differ significantly between the groups. *Error bars* are 2 SE, which approximate the 95% confidence intervals. *Shaded bars* indicate the period during which IL-2 was administered (approximately every 2 months, from months 0 to 10). (Modified from Kovacs JA, Vogel S, Albert JM, et al. Controlled trial of interleukin-2 infusions in patients infected with the human immunodeficiency virus. N Engl J Med 335:1350, 1996. Copyright 1996, Massachusetts Medical Society.)

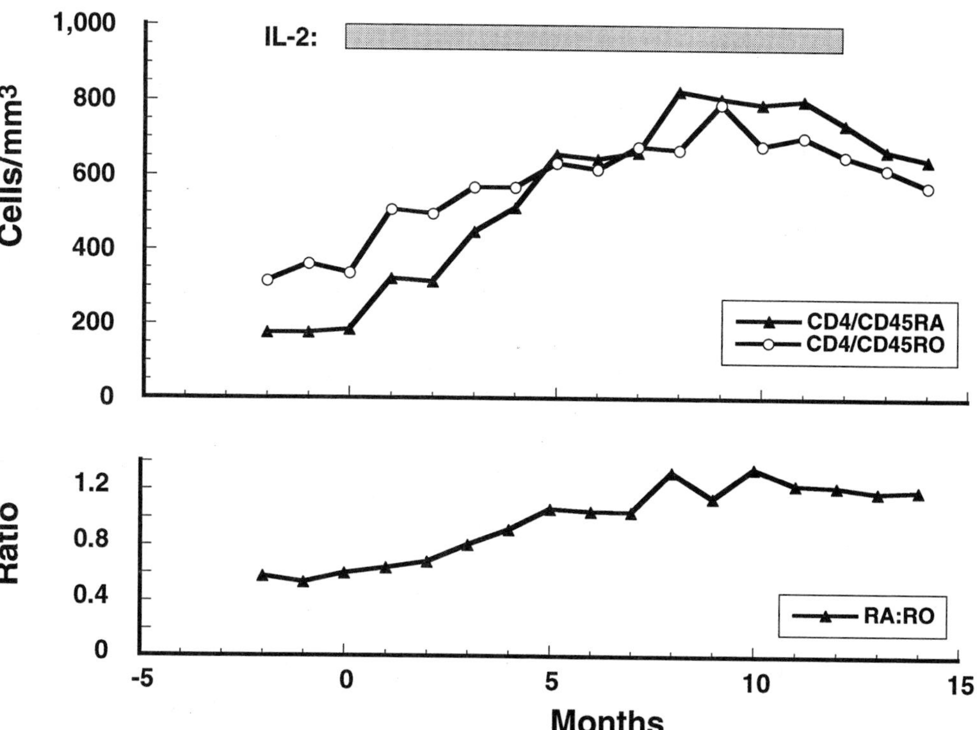

Figure 21–2. Changes in naive and memory CD4+ T-lymphocyte count in 11 patients whose CD4+ T-lymphocyte counts increased to more than 1000 cells/mm^3 during a year of IL-2 therapy. *Top panel* shows the mean naive (*closed triangles*) and memory (*open circles*) CD4+ T-lymphocyte count during the year of IL-2 therapy; *bottom panel* shows the ratio of naive to memory cells during that period. During IL-2 therapy there is an increase in both naive and memory cells, but naive cells expand preferentially, leading to an increase in the naive to memory ratio over time. Memory cells were defined as all cells that were CD45RO$^+$; naive cells were the CD45RO$^-$ cells, which are also CD45RA$^+$.

the IL-2 group was maintained at approximately double the baseline value through the follow-up period (Fig. 21–3).[5] For the control group the mean CD4+ T-lymphocyte count approached that of the IL-2 group during the extension phase.

Two additional randomized trials utilizing intermittent intravenous IL-2 regimens found similar results. One study examined the relative efficacy of polyethylene glycol-modified IL-2 (PEG IL-2) compared to CIV IL-2 or to antiretroviral therapy alone in 115 patients with CD4+ T-lymphocyte counts of 200 to 500 cells/mm^3.[33] Median CD4+ T-lymphocyte count increases of 44 (PEG), 359 (CIV), and −46 (control) cells/mm^3 were seen. Both IL-2 groups showed increased delayed-type hypersensitivity responses compared to a decrease in the control group. Another randomized trial examining the relative efficacy of 3-, 4-, or 5-day infusions in 81 patients with more severe CD4 depletion (baseline CD4+ T-lymphocyte counts of 100 to 300 cells/mm^3) found a trend toward better responses with longer therapy.[34]

Although CIV IL-2 therapy is associated with substantial immunologic effects, the need for continuous infusions, with the associated high cost, inconvenience, drug toxicities, and catheter-related complications, has led to a focus on alternative routes of administration. Studies using

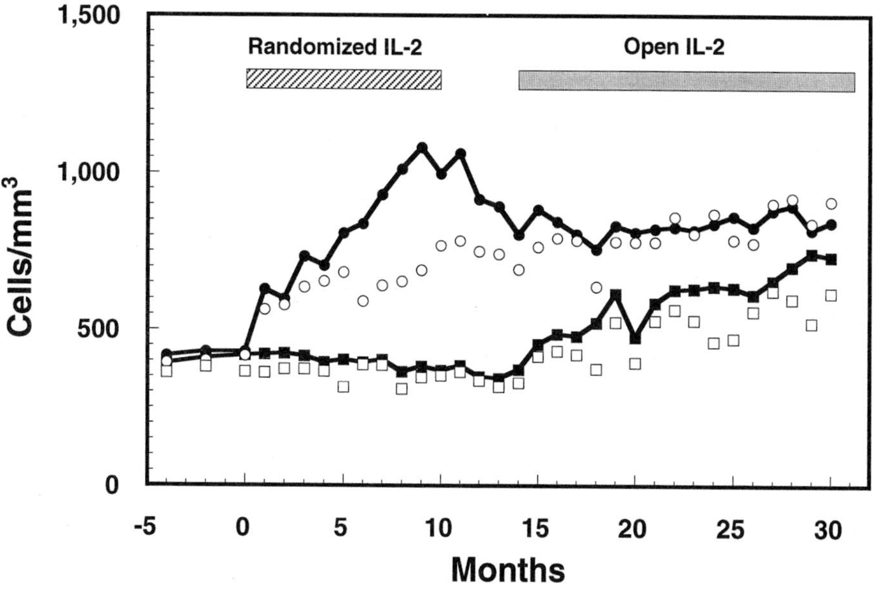

Figure 21–3. Long-term changes in mean (*closed symbols*) and median (*open symbols*) CD4+ T-lymphocyte counts during a randomized, controlled trial of IL-2 in HIV-infected patients with baseline CD4 counts of more than 200 cells/mm^3. During the open phase of the study, both groups were eligible to receive IL-2. In the IL-2 group (*circles*), the CD4+ T-lymphocyte count was maintained at approximately double the baseline value for 30 months; and in the control group (*squares*) the CD4+ T-lymphocyte count approached the IL-2 group values during the open, extension phase of the study. (Modified from Kovacs JA, Vogel S, Albert JM, et al. Controlled trial of interleukin-2 infusions in patients infected with the human immunodeficiency virus. N Engl J Med 335:1350, 1996. Copyright 1996, Massachusetts Medical Society.)

subcutaneous (SC) PEG IL-2 (which is no longer being manufactured) found inadequate immunologic enhancement.[33,35–37] However, standard IL-2 administered subcutaneously twice daily (usual starting dose was 4.5 to 7.5 million IU bid) has activity similar to that of CIV IL-2 but is more convenient and better tolerated.[37–39]

A number of randomized trials have focused on optimizing the administration of SC IL-2. One study in which patients were randomized to monthly or every other month cycles and to two doses (1.5 million or 7.5 million IU SC twice a day) of IL-2 found that the higher dose induced significantly greater CD4+ T-lymphocyte count responses, and that monthly therapy led to more rapid responses.[40] The inconvenience of monthly therapy probably does not warrant the more frequent dosing schedule, however. Three studies comparing three doses (1.5 million, 4.5 million, and 7.5 million IU twice a day) to antiretrovirals alone found a dose-dependent increase in CD4+ T-lymphocyte count number, though each of the two higher doses induced substantial CD4+ T-lymphocyte count increases.[41–43] No harmful long-term effect of IL-2 on viral load was seen in any of these randomized trials; transient increases in plasma HIV RNA levels can be seen at day 5 in fewer than 5% of the SC IL-2 cycles.[37]

Most studies have found no evidence of enhanced viral suppression in patients receiving IL-2. However, a meta-analysis of long-term follow-up of three CIV studies suggested that IL-2 therapy led to a diminished plasma HIV RNA level; and a controlled trial of 82 patients, more than 50% of whom were receiving protease inhibitor (PI) therapy, similarly suggested improved viral control in IL-2 recipients.[44,45] In the largest controlled trial conducted to date (511 patients), however, IL-2 therapy did not have a significant impact on viral load after 12 months.[46]

The development of highly active antiretroviral therapy (HAART) has provided the opportunity to examine the potential role of IL-2 in patients in whom a high level of viral suppression is achieved. ACTG 328 examined the effect of IL-2 in a randomized trial of PI-naive patients with baseline CD4+ T-lymphocyte counts between 50 and 350 cells/mm^3 who received 12 weeks of HAART and had suppressed plasma HIV RNA levels to less than 5000 copies/ml.[39] Median CD4+ T-lymphocyte counts were significantly higher in the IL-2 recipients (614 cells/mm^3 for SC IL-2 and 800 cells/mm^3 for initial CIV IL-2 vs. 396 cells/mm^3 for controls) in the setting of good viral control (about 80% of patients had < 50 HIV RNA copies/ml).

Because a substantial proportion of patients receiving HAART are immunologic nonresponders (minimal or no increase in CD4+ T-lymphocyte count), the ability of IL-2 to increase the CD4+ T-lymphocyte count number in this setting has also been studied. In three randomized studies of patients with CD4+ T-lymphocyte counts less than 200 to 250 cells/mm^3 and viral loads of less than 50 to 1000 copies/ml following 6 to 9 months of HAART therapy, intermittent IL-2 SC therapy induced a significant increase in CD4+ T-lymphocyte counts within 12 to 24 weeks.[47–49]

An alternative approach to intermittent IL-2 therapy has been the continuous administration of lower doses of SC IL-2, either daily using IL-2 or twice-weekly using PEG IL-2. Preliminary studies with such continuous therapy demonstrated increases in eosinophils, NK number, and NK and LAK cell activity; but most studies have not demonstrated an increase in CD4 or CD8 cell number.[35,36,50] A small study (11 patients) observed transient increases in CD4+ T-lymphocyte count number with continuous three times per week therapy, with tachyphylaxis developing as therapy was continued.[51] One recent randomized, controlled study compared the effects of daily SC IL-2 (1.2 million IU/m^2/day) administered for 6 months to antiretroviral therapy alone in 115 patients (CD4+ T-lymphocyte count < 300 cells/mm^3).[52] Significant increases in NK and eosinophil cell number were seen in the IL-2 group. Although an early (weeks 4 and 8) increase in CD4+ T-lymphocyte count number was seen, significant differences between the two groups were not sustained. A significant increase in the CD4+ T-lymphocyte count percent and the CD4/CD8 ratio was driven in part by a significant decline in the CD8 cell number in the IL-2 group.

Administration of IL-2 is associated with a large number of side effects that are usually dose-related and that tend to be less frequent and less severe with subcutaneous therapy.[5,33,37,39] The most common dose-limiting toxicities are related to the constitutional symptoms that invariably occur at doses higher than 3 million IU/day: Fever, chills, rigors, sweats, muscle and joint pains, nausea, and vomiting are common.[5,38] Additional toxicities include fluid retention due to a capillary leak syndrome; elevations in hepatic enzymes and bilirubin; acalculous cholecystitis; diarrhea; renal dysfunction due in part to the intravascular volume depletion resulting from the capillary leak and to the use of nonsteroidal antiinflammatory drugs; metabolic abnormalities including hyponatremia, hypocalcemia, hypomagnesemia, hypoalbuminemia, and phosphate abnormalities; hypothyroidism; cardiomyopathy and congestive heart failure; neurologic abnormalities; mucositis; rash that is occasionally desquamative; and hypotension. Some of these toxicities are potentially life-threatening, but such severe toxicities are rarely seen at the doses used in HIV-infected patients. Many side effects that occur can be diminished by administering adjunctive medications (Table 21–1). Prednisone can blunt some of the toxicities [and tumor necrosis factor-α (TNF-α) production], but it also simultaneously blunts the CD4+ T-lymphocyte count increase.[53] Most of the side effects that develop during IL-2 therapy are alleviated quickly, within a few days of discontinuing IL-2.

Among those who have demonstrated an immunologic benefit from IL-2 therapy, patient inconvenience and discomfort can be decreased by individualizing the dosing regimen.[54] A strategy designed to maintain the CD4+ T-lymphocyte count above a threshold level (e.g., double the baseline value, or a count of 800 or 1000 cells/mm^3) often results in decreasing the frequency of an IL-2 cycle to yearly or less often.[5,54]

Although substantial CD4+ T-lymphocyte count increases can be induced by intermittent IL-2, the clinical benefit of these immunologic changes has not yet been demonstrated. Studies examining the function of CD4+ T-lymphocyte count in patients receiving IL-2 suggest that the functionality of CD4+ T-lymphocyte count before and after IL-2 are similar.[55,56] Two studies, one a meta-analysis of three trials, found a trend toward fewer opportunistic infections in

▲ **Table 21–1.** CYTOKINES THAT ARE POTENTIAL IMMUNOMODULATORS FOR THE TREATMENT OF HIV INFECTION

Cytokine	Trade name	FDA-approved Indication	Potential additional role for HIV infection
Interleukin-2			
Aldesleukin	Proleukin (Chiron)	Treatment of metastatic renal cell cancer or metastatic malignant melanoma	Intermittent therapy: increase in CD4+ T cell number Continuous therapy: increase in natural killer (NK) cell number
Interferon-alfa			
Interferon alfa-2a	Roferon-A (Roche)	Treatment of hairy cell leukemia, AIDS-related Kaposi's sarcoma, chronic myelogenous leukemia, chronic hepatitis C	Antiretroviral agent in patients with limited alternatives
Interferon alfa-2b	Intron A (Schering)	Treatment of hair cell leukemia, malignant melanoma, follicular lymphoma, condylomata acuminata, AIDS-related Kaposi's sarcoma, chronic hepatitis B, chronic hepatitis C	Antiretroviral agent in patients with limited alternatives
GM-CSF			
Sargramostim	Leukine (Immunex)	Adjunctive therapy following chemotherapy or bone marrow transplantation in a variety of conditions; mobilization of hematopoietic progenitor cells	Increase in CD4+ T cell number Decrease in infections
Filgrastim	Neupogen (Amgen)	Adjunctive therapy following chemotherapy or bone marrow transplantation in a variety of conditions; mobilization of hematopoietic progenitor cells; severe chronic neutropenia	Increase in CD4+ and CD8+ T cell numbers

patients receiving IL-2, suggesting clinical benefit.[39,44] The true clinical efficacy of IL-2 therapy (i.e., the ability of IL-2 to prevent opportunistic infections and death) must be addressed in Phase 3 studies with clinical endpoints; two such studies are currently underway, one in patients with more than 300 CD4 cells/mm^3[57] and the other in patients with fewer than 300 CD4 cells/mm^3 at baseline.[58] Evidence of clinical benefit is needed before IL-2 can be broadly recommended for the management of HIV-infected patients.

In addition to its ability to increase CD4+ T-lymphocyte counts, the potential for IL-2 to accelerate clearance of latent reservoirs of HIV has also been studied. Although initial studies suggested that it was difficult to culture HIV in a proportion of patients who had received IL-2 together with HAART therapy,[59] studies examining viral rebound following discontinuation of antiretroviral therapy found that plasma HIV levels increased in all patients, with no difference in the kinetics of rebound in the IL-2 and non-IL-2 recipients.[60]

At present, IL-2 should primarily be administered during clinical trials designed to understand better the role of IL-2 in managing HIV-infected patients. If clinical benefit is documented by ongoing trials, IL-2 can potentially play a role in patients who are immunologic nonresponders to HAART therapy and in patients with ongoing viral replication and declining CD4+ T-lymphocyte numbers. IL-2 therapy may allow periods off antiretroviral therapy or decrease the exposure to antiretroviral therapy. Early utilization of IL-2 (with antiretroviral therapy only during IL-2 cycles) might permit deferral of the initiation of ongoing antiretroviral therapy.

For physicians who administer IL-2 outside a clinical trial setting, an awareness of the toxicities and management of these toxicities is essential (Table 21–2). Because of the transient viral activation that can occur, antiviral therapy should be co-administered with IL-2, although a 24-week controlled trial of 36 patients with CD4+ T-lymphocyte counts of more than 350 cells/mm^3 who were not receiving antiretroviral therapy found no difference in plasma HIV RNA levels and a significant (though perhaps blunted) increase in CD4+ T-lymphocyte count number in IL-2 recipients compared to controls.[61] Because IL-2 results in trafficking effects on lymphocytes, with a potentially dramatic and rapid decline in lymphocytes (including CD4 cells) in the blood during IL-2 therapy and a marked, rapid rebound increase in lymphocytes immediately after discontinuing IL-2,[62] it is not helpful to check CD4+ T-lymphocyte counts during or immediately after IL-2 therapy. For moderate toxicities the IL-2 dose should be reduced by 3 million to 6 million IU/day. Discontinuation of IL-2 usually results in rapid alleviation of most adverse effects. Initially, cycles should probably be administered approximately every other month; but once a CD4+ T-lymphocyte count increase has been achieved, decreasing the frequency based on CD4+ T-lymphocyte counts can improve patient tolerability without loss of immunologic benefit.[54]

▲ INTERFERON-α

Interferon-α is a cytokine produced by a variety of cells that has antiviral as well as antiproliferative and immunomodulating effects.[63] Interferon-α is currently approved for the treatment of AIDS-related Kaposi's sarcoma (discussed elsewhere) and hepatitis B and hepatitis C; it has antiretroviral effects in vitro as well as in vivo.[64] Studies in

▲ **Table 21–2.** MANAGEMENT OF INTERLEUKIN-2-RELATED TOXICITIES

Adverse effect	Management
Constitutional symptoms (fever, chills, muscle and joint aches, fatigue)	Ibuprofen (300–600 mg q6h) alternating with acetaminophen (650 mg q6h); should be started prior to interleukin-2 (IL-2)
Nausea/vomiting	Prochlorperazine (10 mg PO or 25 mg PR q4–6h) or ondansetron [0.15 mg/kg IV (10 mg for 70 kg) or 8–16 mg PO q6–8h]
Diarrhea	Loperamide (2 mg q4–6h PO) or Lomotil (1–2 tablets qid)
Hypotension	Increase oral fluid intake, or administer fluid bolus (e.g., 500 cc normal saline)
Mucositis	2% Solution of kaolin pectate, xylocaine, and benadryl (swish prn)
Anxiety/insomnia	Lorazepam (1 mg PO q6–8h prn); flurazepam and diphenhydramine are alternatives; avoid in patients with any mental status changes
Rash or itching	Diphenhydramine (25–50 mg PO q6h prn) or hydroxyzine (25 mg PO tid prn)
Injection site reaction	Apply heat prn; rotate sites
Creatinine elevation	Fluids as above; discontinue meds that may be contributing, especially non steroidals
Hyponatremia	Follow closely for values < 130 mEq/L Normal saline supplementation (50–100 ml/hr) for values < 128 mEq/L Discontinue IL-2 for values < 125 mEq/L
Hypomagnesemia	Oral magnesium supplementation
Hypocalcemia	Oral calcium supplementation (may be due to low albumin)
Dyspepsia	Ranitidine (150 mg PO q12h) or cimetidine 300 mg PO q6h)
Other significant toxicities or if above toxicities do not respond to therapy	Discontinue IL-2

patients with Kaposi's sarcoma demonstrated higher tumor regression rates in those with high baseline CD4+ T-lymphocyte counts, suggesting that this activity was related at least in part to immunomodulating effects rather than direct antiproliferative effects.[7,8] These studies similarly suggested that antiretroviral activity was also related to the level of immunocompetence. A randomized, placebo-controlled trial of interferon-α (starting dose, 35 million U/day SC) in 34 asymptomatic patients with more than 400 cells/mm^3 and positive HIV cultures of peripheral blood mononuclear cells demonstrated antiretroviral activity, with 41% of the interferon-α group compared to 13% of the control group developing persistently negative HIV cultures ($P = 0.05$).[65] Toxicities in the interferon-α group were common and included flu-like symptoms, granulocytopenia, and elevated liver function tests; 35% of the interferon-α group withdrew because of toxicities.

Subsequent uncontrolled and controlled studies of interferon-α in combination with a nucleoside analogue (zidovudine, zalcitabine, or didanosine) have suggested modest enhancement of anti-HIV activities (< 0.5 $\log_{10}$ copies/ml decline in plasma HIV RNA levels) with regimens that included interferon-α, but with more frequent toxicities.[66–70] Moreover, the CD4+ T-lymphocyte count response to antiretroviral therapy appears to be blunted in patients receiving interferon-α presumably as a consequence of the antilymphoproliferative effect of this agent.[71] None of these studies has demonstrated that interferon-α therapy has any effect on clinical progression.[69,71,72]

Currently, the role of interferon-α in HIV-infected patients is largely limited to treatment of patients with Kaposi's sarcoma or those with chronic hepatitis B or hepatitis C infection. During the era of HAART it appears to have a limited role when used exclusively as an antiretroviral drug, although it may be considered for patients who have failed available drug regimens. Anecdotal reports suggest that the combination of interferon-α and ribavirin, which is FDA-approved for treating hepatitis C infection, also may have anti-HIV activity.[73] It is important to assess the anti-HIV activity of polyethylene glycol-conjugated interferon-α, which appears to have greater antihepatitis C activity than the unmodified drug and thus may become the treatment of choice for this infection.[74,75] An intriguing retrospective study of patients diagnosed with progressive multifocal leukoencephalopathy during the mid-1980s suggests that interferon-α may be active against this disease.[76]

Dosing regimens of interferon-α for the treatment of HIV infection have not been optimally defined, but the higher doses used in initial studies are poorly tolerated. A reasonable approach is to start at a lower dose, in the range of 1 million to 5 million units administered daily or three times a week and increase as tolerated, usually to a maximum of 5 million to 10 million units. Acetaminophen or ibuprofen may lead to improved tolerance of the constitutional symptoms, which also tend to diminish with time. Administration of the drug at night may improve tolerance, as the peak of the symptoms then occur during sleep.

Immunization in an attempt to induce anti-interferon-α antibodies (to counteract overproduction of interferon-α) is also being studied in HIV-infected patients, though a recent controlled trial showed no benefit to this approach.[77]

▲ GRANULOCYTE/MACROPHAGE COLONY-STIMULATING FACTOR

Granulocyte/macrophage colony-stimulating factor is a cytokine that induces proliferation and differentiation of progenitor cells of the granulocyte/macrophage pathways and activation of mature cells.[78] Initial in vitro studies suggested that GM-CSF enhanced HIV infection, although under differing conditions viral suppression was seen. Initial clinical trials with GM-CSF were undertaken to help increase neutrophil counts but were subsequently expanded to examine potential beneficial immunologic and antiretroviral effects. Whereas a small uncontrolled trial (12 patients, 4 weeks of therapy)[79] found no effect on viral load or CD4 or CD8 cell number, a randomized open-label trial (244 patients, 12 weeks of therapy) found no change in p24 antigen levels but a 53% increase in CD4+ T-lymphocyte count number, with a similar increase in CD8 cell number and consequently no change in the CD4/CD8 ratio at week 12.[80] Following discontinuation of therapy, these values were not sustained but rapidly returned to baseline. No significant difference in infections was seen between the two groups.

A subsequent randomized, placebo-controlled study (105 patients, 24 weeks of therapy) in relatively antiretroviral-naive patients (< 6 months of zidovudine) with CD4+ T-lymphocyte counts less than 300 cells/mm^3 or a history of an opportunistic infection found no significant difference in the incidence of opportunistic infections or survival between groups receiving GM-CSF (125 μg/m^2) or placebo.[81] A statistically significant decrease in plasma HIV levels (-0.60 $\log_{10}$ copies/ml vs. -0.07 $\log_{10}$ copies/ml) was seen at 6 months in the GM-CSF group; with subgroup analysis, statistical significance was seen only in patients receiving nucleoside analogue monotherapy. An additional small placebo-controlled study of 20 patients found a suggestion of decreasing viral load and increasing CD4+ T-lymphocyte counts in those receiving GM-CSF.[82]

A phase III placebo-controlled trial in 309 patients with advanced disease (CD4+ T-lymphocyte counts less than 50 cells/mm^3 or less than 100 cells/mm^3 with a history of prior opportunistic infection) examined the effects of GM-CSF (250 μg three times a week for 24 weeks) on clinical endpoints (AIDS-defining opportunistic infections, bacterial pneumonia, or death).[10] No significant difference was seen in these protocol-defined endpoints, though the incidence of any infection (including skin, oropharyngeal, urinary tract) or death was significantly less in the GM-CSF group (120 vs. 104 events, $P = 0.03$). A significant increase in CD4+ T-lymphocyte count number but not percent was also seen.

Thus the potential benefit of GM-CSF as an immunomodulator in HIV-infected patients remains to be demonstrated. Studies examining the effects on AIDS-related endpoints have not shown GM-CSF therapy to have any benefit. CD4+ T-lymphocyte count increases have been seen, but whether it represents expansion of CD4+ T-lymphocyte or effects related to changes in trafficking remains unclear. Furthermore, whereas some studies suggest modest antiretroviral activity, others have not found this or have seen decreases in viral load only in subsets.

A randomized, placebo-controlled trial of granulocyte colony-stimulating factor (G-CSF) in 30 HIV-infected patients with CD4+ T-lymphocyte counts of less than 350 cells/mm^3 demonstrated a transient increase in CD4 cells, CD8 cells, and NK cells; no change in NK activity or plasma HIV RNA levels; and a decrease in phytohemagglutinin (PHA)- and *Candida* antigen-stimulated proliferation.[83] The CD4+ T-lymphocyte and CD8 increases resulted from an increase in memory and activated cells. Additional studies are clearly needed before either GM-CSF or G-CSF is utilized clinically in HIV-infected patients as an immunomodulator for targeting nonmyeloid cells.

▲ IMMUNOSUPPRESSIVE THERAPY

Because immune activation may lead to an increase in HIV replication or more efficient replication, an alternative approach to immune enhancement has been to suppress the immune system in an attempt to slow HIV replication. Agents used for this purpose include cyclosporin A, corticosteroids, and IL-10. Cyclosporin A did not seem to provide benefit in trials conducted during the 1980s,[84,85] but an open 1-year trial of prednisolone (0.3 to 0.5 mg/kg/day PO) in 44 patients with CD4+ T-lymphocyte counts of 200 to 800 cells/mm^3 found evidence of decreased CD4+ T-lymphocyte activation and CD4+ T-lymphocyte count increases (mean pretherapy, 421 cells/mm^3; mean 1 year posttherapy, 523 cells/mm^3) without concomitant CD8 count increases.[86] This increase occurred primarily during the first 3 months, following which the CD4+ T-lymphocyte counts decreased somewhat and remained stable during the rest of the year. Plasma HIV RNA level remained unchanged during the year. Given the potential immunosuppressive effects of corticosteroids, controlled trials are needed to evaluate better the immunologic and clinical benefits of such therapy in HIV-infected patients.[87] Adverse effects of corticosteroids, including an association with the development of avascular necrosis, must be considered when assessing the risk/benefit ratio of such therapy.[88]

Interleukin-10 is an anti-inflammatory cytokine that in single-dose studies in HIV-infected patients was shown to lead to a transient decline in plasma HIV RNA level.[89] However, a randomized, placebo-controlled 39-patient trial of three doses of subcutaneously administered IL-10 found no significant change in plasma HIV RNA levels or CD4+ T-lymphocyte count number during 4 weeks of therapy.[90]

Acknowledgment. The U.S. government has been issued a patent for immunologic enhancement with intermittent IL-2 therapy, listing J.A.K. as one of the inventors.

REFERENCES

1. Connors M, Kovacs JA, Krevat S, et al. HIV infection induces changes in CD4$^+$ T-cell phenotype and depletions within the CD4$^+$ T-cell repertoire that are not immediately restored by antiviral or immune-based therapies. Nat Med 3:533, 1997.
2. Grabar S, Le Moing V, Goujard C, et al. Clinical outcome of patients with HIV-1 infection according to immunologic and virologic response after 6 months of highly active antiretroviral therapy. Ann Intern Med 133:401, 2000.
3. Lederman MM. Host-directed and immune-based therapies for human immunodeficiency virus infection. Ann Intern Med 122:218, 1995.
4. Sneller MC, Lane HC. Immunologic approaches to the therapy of HIV-1 infection. Ann NY Acad Sci 685:687, 1993.
5. Kovacs JA, Vogel S, Albert JM, et al. Controlled trial of interleukin-2 infusions in patients infected with the human immunodeficiency virus. N Engl J Med 335:1350, 1996.
6. Jacobson MA, Hardy D, Connick E, et al. Phase 1 trial of a single dose of recombinant human interleukin-12 in human immunodeficiency virus-infected patients with 100–500 CD4 cells/μL. J Infect Dis 182:1070, 2000.
7. Lane HC, Kovacs JA, Feinberg J, et al. Anti-retroviral effects of interferon-alpha in AIDS-associated Kaposi's sarcoma. Lancet 2:1218, 1988.

8. De Wit R, Schattenkerk JK, Boucher CA, et al. Clinical and virological effects of high-dose recombinant interferon-alpha in disseminated AIDS-related Kaposi's sarcoma. Lancet 2:1214, 1988.
9. Lane HC, Davey RT Jr, Sherwin SA, et al. A phase I trial of recombinant human interferon-gamma in patients with Kaposi's sarcoma and the acquired immunodeficiency syndrome (AIDS). J Clin Immunol 9:351, 1989.
10. Angel JB, High K, Rhame F, et al. Phase III study of granulocyte-macrophage colony-stimulating factor in advanced HIV disease: effect on infections, CD4+ T-lymphocyte counts and HIV suppression. Leukine/HIV Study Group. AIDS 14:387, 2000.
11. Lane HC, Masur H, Longo DL, et al. Partial immune reconstitution in a patient with the acquired immunodeficiency syndrome. N Engl J Med 311:1099, 1984.
12. Lane HC, Zunich KM, Wilson W, et al. Syngeneic bone marrow transplantations and adoptive transfer of peripheral blood lymphocytes combined with zidovudine in human immunodeficiency virus (HIV) infection. Ann Intern Med 113:512, 1990.
13. Klimas N, Patarca R, Walling J, et al. Clinical and immunological changes in AIDS patients following adoptive therapy with activated autologous CD8 T cells and interleukin-2 infusion. AIDS 8:1073, 1994.
14. Walker RE, Bechtel CM, Natarajan V, et al. Long-term in vivo survival of receptor-modified syngeneic T cells in patients with human immunodeficiency virus infection. Blood 96:467, 2000.
15. Zunich KM, Lane HC, Davey RT, et al. Phase I/II studies of the toxicity and immunogenicity of recombinant gp160 and p24 vaccines in HIV-infected individuals. AIDS Res Hum Retroviruses 8:1335, 1992.
16. Jacobson JM, Colman N, Ostrow NA, et al. Passive immunotherapy in the treatment of advanced human immunodeficiency virus infection. J Infect Dis 168:298, 1993.
17. Vittecoq D, Chevret S, Morand JL, et al. Passive immunotherapy in AIDS: a double-blind randomized study based on transfusions of plasma rich in anti-human immunodeficiency virus 1 antibodies vs. transfusions of seronegative plasma. Proc Natl Acad Sci USA 92:1195, 1995.
18. Levy J, Youvan T, Lee ML. Passive hyperimmune plasma therapy in the treatment of acquired immunodeficiency syndrome: results of a 12-month multicenter double-blind controlled trial: the Passive Hyperimmune Therapy Study Group. Blood 84:2130, 1994.
19. Agosti JM, Coombs RW, Collier AC, et al. A randomized, double-blind, phase I/II trial of tumor necrosis factor and interferon-gamma for treatment of AIDS-related complex (protocol 025 from the AIDS Clinical Trials Group). AIDS Res Hum Retroviruses 8:581, 1992.
20. Morgan RA. Genetic strategies to inhibit HIV. Mol Med Today 5:454, 1999.
21. Dornburg R, Pomerantz RJ. HIV-1 gene therapy: promise for the future. Adv Pharmacol 49:229, 2000.
22. Smith KA. Interleukin-2: inception, impact, and implications. Science 240:1169, 1988.
23. Siegel JP, Rook AH, Djeu JY, Quinnan GV Jr. Interleukin 2 therapy in infectious diseases: rationale and prospects. Infection 12:298, 1984.
24. Rook AH, Masur H, Lane HC, et al. Interleukin-2 enhances the depressed natural killer and cytomegalovirus-specific cytotoxic activities of lymphocytes from patients with the acquired immune deficiency syndrome. J Clin Invest 72:398, 1983.
25. Lane HC, Siegel JP, Rook AH, et al. Use of interleukin-2 in patients with acquired immunodeficiency syndrome. J Biol Response Mod 3:512, 1984.
26. Volberding P, Moody DJ, Beardslee D, et al. Therapy of acquired immune deficiency syndrome with recombinant interleukin-2. AIDS Res Hum Retroviruses 3:115, 1987.
27. Ernst M, Kern P, Flad HD, Ulmer AJ. Effects of systemic in vivo interleukin-2 (IL-2) reconstitution in patients with acquired immune deficiency syndrome (AIDS) and AIDS-related complex (ARC) on phenotypes and functions of peripheral blood mononuclear cells (PBMC). J Clin Immunol 6:170, 1986.
28. Kovacs JA, Baseler M, Dewar R, et al. Increases in CD4 T lymphocytes with intermittent courses of interleukin-2 in patients with human immunodeficiency virus infection: a preliminary study. N Engl J Med 332:567, 1995.
29. Schwartz DH, Skowron G, Merigan TC. Safety and effects of interleukin-2 plus zidovudine in asymptomatic individuals infected with human immunodeficiency virus. J Acquir Immune Defic Syndr 4:11, 1991.
30. Ramachandran RV, Katzenstein D, Merigan TC. Long-term effects of interleukin-2 on CD4 cell counts in human immunodeficiency virus-infected patients [letter]. J Infect Dis 170:1044, 1994.
31. Kovacs JA, Imamichi H, Vogel S, et al. Effects of intermittent interleukin-2 therapy on plasma and tissue human immunodeficiency virus levels and quasispecies expression. J Infect Dis 182:1063, 2000.
32. Mazza P, Bocchia M, Tumietto F, et al. Recombinant interleukin-2 (rIL-2) in acquired immune deficiency syndrome (AIDS): preliminary report in patients with lymphoma associated with HIV infection. Eur J Haematol 49:1, 1992.
33. Carr A, Emery S, Lloyd A, et al. Outpatient continuous intravenous interleukin-2 or subcutaneous, polyethylene glycol-modified interleukin-2 in human immunodeficiency virus-infected patients: a randomized, controlled, multicenter study. J Infect Dis 178:992, 1998.
34. Saravolatz L, Mitsuyasu R, Sneller M, et al. Duration of Proleukin IL-2 therapy is more important than total dose in achieving CD4 expansion. In: Abstracts of the 36th Interscience Conference on Antimicrobial Agents and Chemotherapy, New Orleans, 1996, abstract I149.
35. Teppler H, Kaplan G, Smith KA, et al. Prolonged immunostimulatory effect of low-dose polyethylene glycol interleukin 2 in patients with human immunodeficiency virus type 1 infection. J Exp Med 177:483, 1993.
36. Teppler H, Kaplan G, Smith K, et al. Efficacy of low doses of the polyethylene glycol derivative of interleukin-2 in modulating the immune response of patients with human immunodeficiency virus type 1 infection. J Infect Dis 167:291, 1993.
37. Levy Y, Capitant C, Houhou S, et al. Comparison of subcutaneous and intravenous interleukin-2 in asymptomatic HIV-1 infection: a randomised controlled trial: ANRS 048 study group. Lancet 353:1923, 1999.
38. Davey RT Jr, Chaitt DG, Piscitelli SC, et al. Subcutaneous administration of interleukin-2 in human immunodeficiency virus type 1-infected persons. J Infect Dis 175:781, 1997.
39. Mitsuyasu R, Pollard R, Gelman R, Weng D. Prospective, randomized, controlled phase II study of highly active antiretroviral therapy (HAART) with continuous IV (CIV) or subcutaneous (SC) interleukin-2 (IL-2) in HIV-infected patients with $CD4^+$ counts of 50–350 cells/mm^3: ACTG 328—final results at 84 weeks. In: Abstracts of the 8th Conference on Retroviruses and Opportunistic Infections, Chicago, 2001, abstract 17.
40. Davey RT Jr, Chaitt DG, Albert JM, et al. A randomized trial of high- versus low-dose subcutaneous interleukin-2 outpatient therapy for early human immunodeficiency virus type 1 infection. J Infect Dis 179:849, 1999.
41. Losso MH, Belloso WH, Emery S, et al. A randomized, controlled, phase II trial comparing escalating doses of subcutaneous interleukin-2 plus antiretrovirals versus antiretrovirals alone in human immunodeficiency virus-infected patients with $CD4^+$ cell counts $\geq 350/mm^3$. J Infect Dis 181:1614, 2000.
42. Ruxrungtham K, Suwanagool S, Tavel JA, et al. A randomized, controlled 24-week study of intermittent subcutaneous interleukin-2 in HIV-1 infected patients in Thailand: Vanguard Study Group. AIDS 14:2509, 2000.
43. Arduino R, Nannini E, Rodriguez-Barradas M, et al. Meta-analysis of the CD4 cell response to 3 doses of subcutaneous interleukin-2 (scIL-2) across 3 Vanguard studies. In: Abstracts of the 8th Conference on Retroviruses and Opportunistic Infections, Chicago, 2001, abstract 346.
44. Emery S, Capra WB, Cooper DA, et al. Pooled analysis of 3 randomized, controlled trials of interleukin-2 therapy in adult human immunodeficiency virus type 1 disease. J Infect Dis 182:428, 2000.
45. Davey RT Jr, Murphy RL, Graziano FM, et al. Immunologic and virologic effects of subcutaneous interleukin 2 in combination with antiretroviral therapy: a randomized controlled trial. JAMA 284:183, 2000.
46. Abrams DI, Bebchuk JD, Denning ET, Markowitz NP. IL-2 therapy produces no change in HIV RNA after one year. In: Abstracts of the 40th Interscience Conference on Antimicrobial Agents and Chemotherapy, Toronto, 2000, abstract L11.
47. Katlama C, Duvivier C, Chouquet C, et al. ILSTIM (ANRS 082): a randomized comparative open-label study of interleukin-2 (IL2) in patients with CD4 $< 200/mm^3$ despite effective HAART. In: Abstracts of the 7th Conference on Retroviruses and Opportunistic Infections, San Francisco, 2000, abstract 543.
48. Arno A, Ruiz L, Juan M, et al. Efficacy of low-dose subcutaneous interleukin-2 to treat advanced human immunodeficiency virus type 1 in

persons with ≤ 250/μl CD4 T cells and undetectable plasma virus load. J Infect Dis 180:56, 1999.
49. David D, Naït-Ighil L, Dupont B, et al. Rapid effect of interleukin-2 therapy in human immunodeficiency virus infected patients whose CD4 cell counts increase only slightly in response to combined antiretroviral treatment. J Infect Dis 183:730, 2001.
50. Jacobson EL, Pilaro F, Smith KA. Rational interleukin 2 therapy for HIV positive individuals: daily low doses enhance immune function without toxicity. Proc Natl Acad Sci USA 93:10405, 1996.
51. Larsen CS, Ostergard L, Moller BK, Buhl MR. Subcutaneous interleukin-2 in combination with anti-retroviral therapy for treatment of HIV-1-infected subjects. Scand J Infect Dis 32:153, 2000.
52. Lalezari JP, Beal JA, Ruane PJ, et al. Low-dose daily subcutaneous interleukin-2 in combination with highly active antiretroviral therapy in HIV^+ patients: a randomized controlled trial. HIV Clin Trials 1:1, 2000.
53. Tavel JA, Walker RE, Hahn B, et al. Prednisone decreases rIL-2-related toxicities but also blunts the rIL-2-related $CD4^+$ cell response in HIV^+ patients. In: Abstracts of the 8th Conference on Retroviruses and Opportunistic Infections, Chicago, 2001, abstract 348.
54. Chaitt D, Metcalf J, Kovacs J, et al. Extended therapy with subcutaneous interleukin-2 (scIL-2) in HIV-infection: long-term follow-up of 3 trials. In: Abstracts of the 8th Conference on Retroviruses and Opportunistic Infections, Chicago, 2001, abstract 347.
55. Kelleher AD, Roggensack M, Emery S, et al. Effects of IL-2 therapy in asymptomatic HIV-infected individuals on proliferative responses to mitogens, recall antigens and HIV-related antigens. Clin Exp Immunol 113:85, 1998.
56. Giedlin M, McGrath M, Gascon R, et al. Immunological characterization of HIV seropositive patients treated with subcutaneous Proleukin (aldesleukin) recombinant Interleukin-2. Int Conf AIDS 11:282, 1996.
57. www.espritstudy.org
58. www.silcaat.com
59. Chun TW, Engel D, Mizell SB, et al. Effect of interleukin-2 on the pool of latently infected, resting $CD4^+$ T cells in HIV-1-infected patients receiving highly active anti-retroviral therapy. Nat Med 5:651, 1999.
60. Davey RT Jr, Bhat N, Yoder C, et al. HIV-1 and T cell dynamics after interruption of highly active antiretroviral therapy (HAART) in patients with a history of sustained viral suppression. Proc Natl Acad Sci USA 96:15109, 1999.
61. Fisher M, Nelson M, Dykhoff A, et al. Randomised study of intermittent subcutaneous interleukin-2 (IL-2) therapy without anti-retrovirals versus no treatment. Presented at the 13th International Conference on AIDS 2000, abstract LbOr28.
62. Kovacs JA, Vogel S, Metcalf JA, et al. Interleukin-2 induced immune effects in human immunodeficiency virus-infected patients receiving intermittent interleukin-2 immunotherapy. Eur J Immunol 31:1351, 2001.
63. Baron S, Tyring SK, Fleischmann WJ, et al. The interferons: mechanisms of action and clinical applications. JAMA 266:1375, 1991.
64. Ho DD, Hartshorn KL, Rota TR, et al. Recombinant human interferon alfa-A suppresses HTLV-III replication in vitro. Lancet 1:602, 1985.
65. Lane HC, Davey V, Kovacs JA, et al. Interferon-alpha in patients with asymptomatic human immunodeficiency virus (HIV) infection: a randomized, placebo-controlled trial. Ann Intern Med 112:805, 1990.
66. Fischl MA, Uttamchandani RB, Resnick L, et al. A phase I study of recombinant human interferon-alpha 2a or human lymphoblastoid interferon-alpha n1 and concomitant zidovudine in patients with AIDS-related Kaposi's sarcoma. J Acquir Immune Defic Syndr 4:1, 1991.
67. Krown SE, Gold JW, Niedzwiecki D, et al. Interferon-alpha with zidovudine: safety, tolerance, and clinical and virologic effects in patients with Kaposi sarcoma associated with the acquired immunodeficiency syndrome (AIDS). Ann Intern Med 112:812, 1990.
68. Kovacs JA, Bechtel C, Davey RT Jr, et al. Combination therapy with didanosine and interferon-alpha in human immunodeficiency virus-infected patients: results of a phase I/II trial. J Infect Dis 173:840, 1996.
69. Lane HC, Herpin B, Banks S, et al. Zidovudine vs. alpha interferon vs. the combination in patients with early HIV infection. Presented at the 8th International Conference on AIDS, abstract 1992, Mo15.
70. Fischl MA, Richman DD, Saag M, et al. Safety and antiviral activity of combination therapy with zidovudine, zalcitabine, and two doses of interferon-alpha2a in patients with HIV: AIDS Clinical Trials Group Study 197. J Acquir Immune Defic Syndr Hum Retrovirol 16:247, 1997.
71. Haas DW, Lavelle J, Nadler JP, et al. A randomized trial of interferon alpha therapy for HIV type 1 infection. AIDS Res Hum Retroviruses 16:183, 2000.
72. Krown SE, Aeppli D, Balfour HH Jr. Phase II, randomized, open-label, community-based trial to compare the safety and activity of combination therapy with recombinant interferon-alpha2b and zidovudine versus zidovudine alone in patients with asymptomatic to mildly symptomatic HIV infection: HIV protocol C91-253 study team. J Acquir Immune Defic Syndr Hum Retrovirol 20:245, 1999.
73. Landau A, Batisse D, Piketty C, Kazatchkine MD. Effect of interferon and ribavirin on HIV viral load [letter]. AIDS 14:96, 2000.
74. Zeuzem S, Feinman SV, Rasenack J, et al. Peginterferon alfa-2a in patients with chronic hepatitis C. N Engl J Med 343:1666, 2000.
75. Heathcote EJ, Shiffman ML, Cooksley WG, et al. Peginterferon alfa-2a in patients with chronic hepatitis C and cirrhosis. N Engl J Med 343:1673, 2000.
76. Huang SS, Skolasky RL, Dal Pan GJ, et al. Survival prolongation in HIV-associated progressive multifocal leukoencephalopathy treated with alpha-interferon: an observational study. J Neurovirol 4:324, 1998.
77. Gringeri A, Musicco M, Hermans P, et al. Active anti-interferon-alpha immunization: a European-Israeli, randomized, double-blind, placebo-controlled clinical trial in 242 HIV-1-infected patients (the EURIS study). J Acquir Immune Defic Syndr Hum Retrovirol 20:358, 1999.
78. Deresinski SC. Granulocyte-macrophage colony-stimulating factor: potential therapeutic, immunological and antiretroviral effects in HIV infection. AIDS 13:633, 1999.
79. Scadden DT, Pickus O, Hammer SM, et al. Lack of in vivo effect of granulocyte-macrophage colony-stimulating factor on human immunodeficiency virus type 1. AIDS Res Hum Retroviruses 12:1151, 1996.
80. Barbaro G, Di Lorenzo G, Grisorio B, et al. Effect of recombinant human granulocyte-macrophage colony-stimulating factor on HIV-related leukopenia: a randomized, controlled clinical study. AIDS 11:1453, 1997.
81. Brites C, Gilbert MJ, Pedral-Sampaio D, et al. A randomized, placebo-controlled trial of granulocyte-macrophage colony-stimulating factor and nucleoside analogue therapy in AIDS. J Infect Dis 182:1531, 2000.
82. Skowron G, Stein D, Drusano G, et al. The safety and efficacy of granulocyte-macrophage colony-stimulating factor (sargramostim) added to indinavir- or ritonavir-based antiretroviral therapy: a randomized double-blind, placebo-controlled trial. J Infect Dis 180:1064, 1999.
83. Aladdin H, Ullum H, Dam Nielsen S, et al. Granulocyte colony-stimulating factor increases $CD4^+$ T cell counts of human immunodeficiency virus-infected patients receiving stable, highly active antiretroviral therapy: results from a randomized, placebo-controlled trial. J Infect Dis 181:1148, 2000.
84. Andrieu J, Even P, Venet A. Effects of cyclosporin on T-cell subsets in human immunodeficiency virus disease. Clin Immunol Immunopathol 46:181, 1988.
85. Phillips A, Wainberg MA, Coates R, et al. Cyclosporine-induced deterioration in patients with AIDS. Can Med Assoc J 140:1456, 1989.
86. Andrieu JM, Lu W, Levy R. Sustained increases in CD4 cell counts in asymptomatic human immunodeficiency virus type 1-seropositive patients treated with prednisolone for 1 year. J Infect Dis 171:523, 1995.
87. Corey L. Reducing T cell activation as a therapy for human immunodeficiency virus infection. J Infect Dis 171:521, 1995.
88. Masur H, Miller KD, Jones EC, et al. High prevalence of avascular necrosis (AVN) of the hip in HIV infection: magnetic resonance imaging of 339 asymptomatic patients. In: Abstracts of the IDSA 38th Annual Meeting, New Orleans, 2000, 214 (abstract 15).
89. Weissman D, Ostrowski M, Daucher JA, et al. Interleukin-10 decreases HIV plasma viral load: results of a phase 1 clinical trial. In: Abstracts of the 4th Conference on Retroviruses and Opportunistic Infections, 1997, abstract 37.
90. Angel JB, Jacobson MA, Skolnik PR, et al. A multicenter, randomized, double-blind, placebo-controlled trial of recombinant human interleukin-10 in HIV-infected subjects. AIDS 14:2503, 2000.

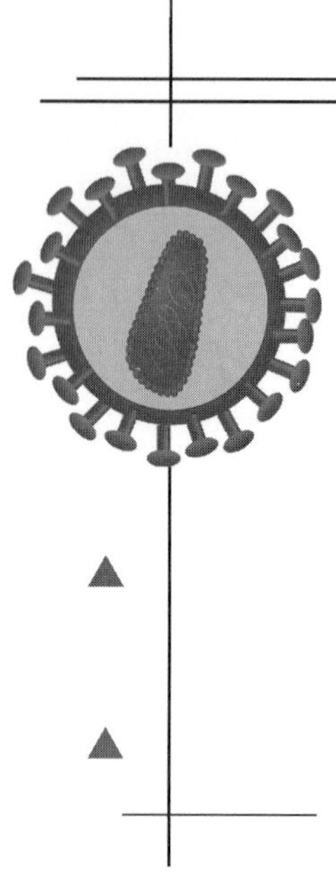

CHAPTER 22

Approach to HIV Antigen-Specific Immune Enhancement

R. Pat Bucy, MD, PhD

This chapter focuses on new strategies that may enhance the endogenous antiviral immune response. Although there is no current regimen utilizing these strategies that has established clinical utility, there is significant renewed interest in this form of immune-based therapy. This renewed interest is motivated by several factors. First, there is the recognition that even the most potent combination antiretroviral agents available do not lead to viral eradication. Second, the realization that any antiretroviral regimen can lead to clinically important toxicities has increased the interest in pursuing alternatives to a strictly antiretroviral drug strategy, particularly structured therapy interruptions (STIs). Third, there is a growing body of data indicating that some individuals can mount an immune response that can efficiently control viral replication at levels associated with minimal disease progression. This chapter provides a conceptual overview of the available information on therapeutic immunization and the use of therapy interruptions as both an intervention to stimulate anti-human immunodeficiency virus (HIV) immunity and an analytical tool to determine directly the capability of in vivo immune responses to control viral replication.

▲ EVIDENCE OF IMMUNE CONTROL OF VIRAL REPLICATION

A growing body of evidence supports the hypothesis that an active immune response is the primary control mechanism of in vivo viral replication.[1] Individuals who have maintained an extremely low viral load without significant disease progression over many years, termed long-term nonprogressors (LT-NPs), have evidence of both CD4+ and CD8+ T-lymphocyte-mediated immune responses to HIV. In contrast, typical patients who progress to more advanced HIV disease over time have evidence of active CD8+ T-lymphocyte responses but lack HIV-specific CD4+ T-lymphocyte responses.[2] In support of the role of HIV-specific CD4+ T-lymphocyte activity, studies have documented preservation of strong immune responses among patients who started highly active antiretroviral therapy (HAART) early after initial infection and then had therapy withdrawn.[3–5] Upon withdrawal of therapy, their viral loads remained low for extended periods of time. In other studies, HIV-antigen-specific CD8+ T-lymphocyte responses stimulated during early infection were associated with a significant decrease in viremia, and these responses could be detected throughout the asymptomatic "clinically latent" phase of chronic infection.[6–8]

Animal model studies provide the most compelling evidence of the role of the immune system in controlling viral replication. In models of rhesus macaques infected with simian immunodeficiency virus (SIV), two groups have independently shown that viral replication is dependent on continual effector immune responses.[9,10] These studies demonstrated in vivo that depletion of CD8+ T-lymphocytes with cytotoxic anti-CD8 monoclonal antibodies resulted in rapid increases in the plasma viral load. SIV antigen-specific CD8+ T-lymphocytes identified from these depleted animals with specific peptide/major histocompatibility complex type I (MCH-I) tetramer reagents, grown out, and reinfused into the animals, regain control of SIV replication at levels similar to the prior set point in the individual animal after several months (Fig. 22–1). Even in SIV-infected animals with undetectable plasma HIV RNA, depletion of CD8+ T-lymphocytes (without an appreciable change in the number of target CD4+ T-lymphocytes) results in a two- to four-fold log rise in viral load within

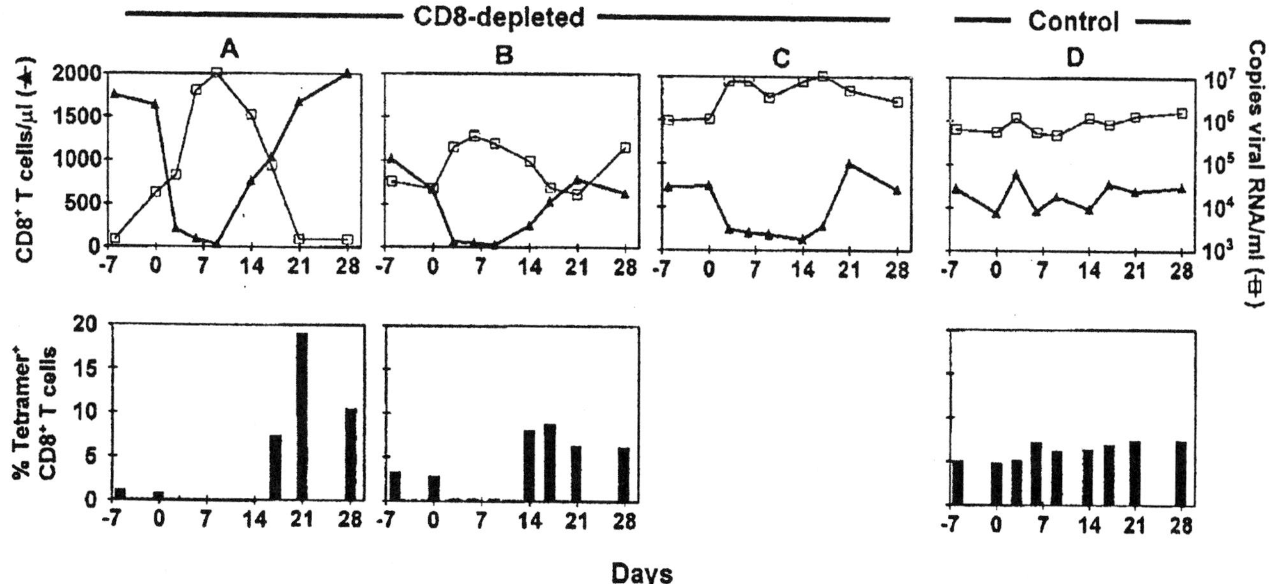

Figure 22–1. Effect of CD8+ lymphocyte depletion on control of virus replication in rhesus monkeys during chronic simian immunodeficiency virus in macaques (SIVmac) infection. *A-D, top panels,* Monkeys infected with SIVmac for more than 9 months were depleted of CD8+ lymphocytes with cM-T807, or they received a control monoclonal antibody. CD8+ lymphocyte enumeration and plasma viral RNA levels were measured. *A–C,* CD8+ lymphocyte-depleted monkeys. *D* Control monoclonal antibody-treated monkey. *A,B,D, bottom panels,* Mamu A*01/p11C, C-M tetramer-binding cytolytic T lymphocytes (CTLs) were assessed. *A,B,* CD8+ lymphocyte-depleted monkeys. *D,* Control monoclonal antibody-treated monkey. (From Schmitz JE, Kuroda MJ, Santra S, et al. Control of viremia in simian immunodeficiency virus infection by CD8(+) lymphocytes. Science 283:857, 1999. Copyright 1999 American Association for the Advancement of Science, with permission.)

several days. Thus, the presence of CD8+ T-lymphocytes is required to maintain the steady-state level of viral replication.

Other studies using the SIV infection model in rhesus macaques provide further support for the critical role of effective cellular immunity in controlling retrovirus infection. As in human infection with HIV, strong cytotoxic T-lymphocyte (CTL) responses have been associated with control of the initial viremia of SIV infection.[11–13] In vaccine studies, infection with a live attenuated SIV strain is associated with induction of a vigorous immune response[14] and protection from subsequent infection with a virulent strain.[15,16] In studies evaluating the kinetics of viremia in rhesus macaques with acute SIV infection, a clear relation was demonstrated between the extent of early viremia (7 days after infection) and the subsequent viremia level well into chronic infection.[17] Faster, stronger immune responses during the early phase of infection were associated with improved control of replication. Other vaccine studies designed to block the initial infection demonstrated that although vaccination failed to block infection in animals challenged with an infectious dose of virus, the level of viral replication during chronic infection was lower than in control animals and substantially fewer vaccinated macaques progressed to acquired immunodeficiency syndrome (AIDS).[18] Subsequent studies showed that immunization with SIV vaccines of several types, including live viral vectors based on vaccinia viruses[19] or DNA vaccines with either protein boosts[20] or exogenous interleukin-2 (IL-2) adjuvants[21] also failed to block infection but resulted in significantly lower viral loads and decreased mortality in chronically infected animals (Fig. 22–2). The basic observation that immunization prior to infection can fail to provide "sterilizing immunity" but have a significant impact on the level of viremia in chronic disease (and hence disease progression) supports the role of the immune system as a potent antiviral mechanism. Numerous groups of investigators have confirmed and extended this concept using several SIV strains and various vaccines.[22–28]

Following up on the key observation that the level of viremia 7 days after primary infection was correlated with the eventual set point of the viral load,[17] a group of rhesus macaques were infected with pathogenic SIV; antiretroviral treatment (tenofovir) was started after 3 days and discontinued after 28 days.[29,30] All animals maintained an extremely low viremia after therapy was stopped and were resistant to homologous high-dose viral challenge with only a transient viremic episode. Furthermore, three animals challenged with a widely divergent heterologous pathogenic strain of SIV were also resistant to viral challenge, but treatment with depleting anti-CD8 monoclonal antibody caused a rapid rise in viremia of both the heterologous and homologous challenge strains. The viremia was brought back to low levels after the regrown CD8+ T-lymphocytes were reinfused. These data emphasize the critical kinetic competition between antigen activation of the immune response and viral growth rate, particularly during the first several weeks of the infection.

These insights into immune control of SIV infection have been extended to immunization after infection, when animals were started on antiretroviral therapy (tenofovir, stavudine, and didanosine) 2 weeks after infection and immunized while on antiretroviral therapy.[31] After three injections of a poxvirus-based SIV vaccine (NYVAC-SIV-

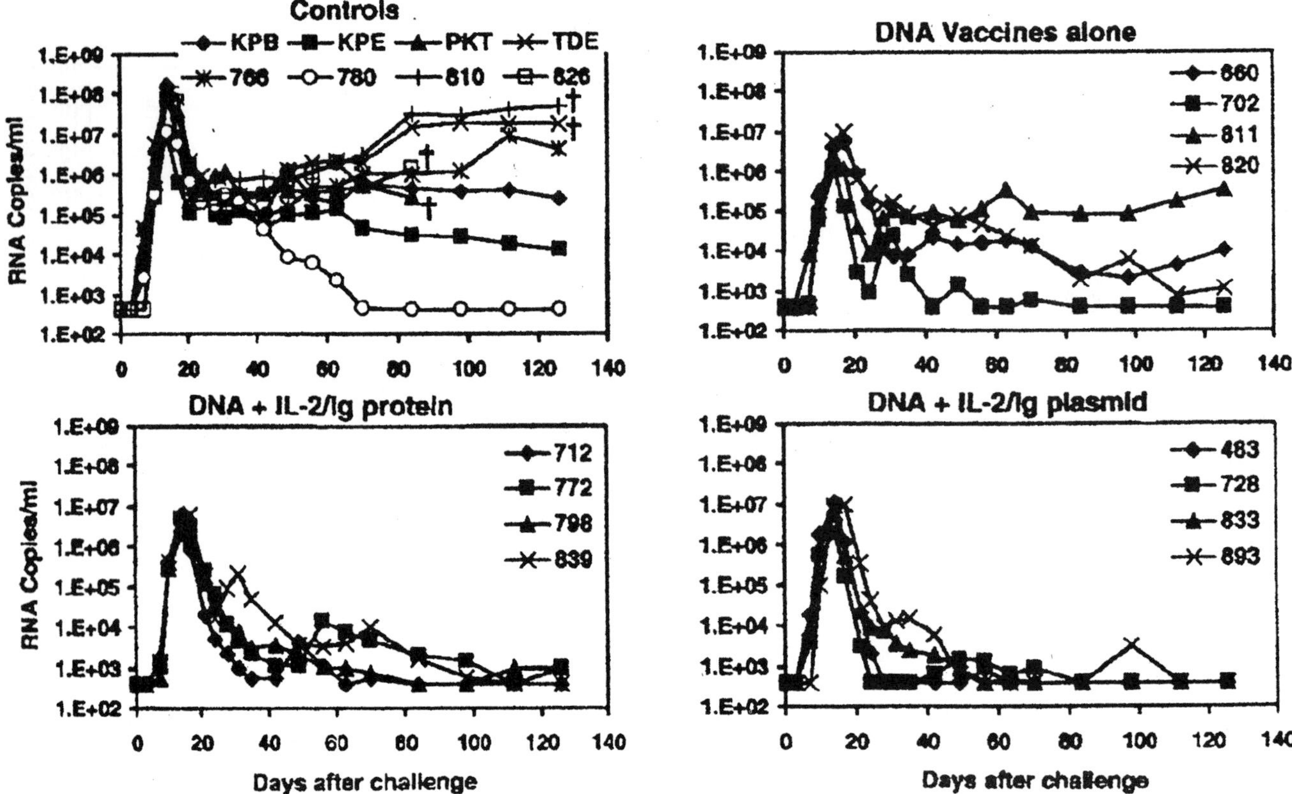

Figure 22–2. Viral loads after immunization of SIV exogenous interleukin-2 (IL-2) adjuvants. (From Barouch DH, Santra S, Schmitz JE, et al. Control of viremia and prevention of clinical AIDS in rhesus monkeys by cytokine-augmented DNA vaccination. Science 290:486, 2000. Copyright 2000 American Association for the Advancement of Science, with permission.)

gag-pol-env), therapy was stopped 6 months after infection, and immune responses and viral loads were assessed. Six of eight animals experienced transient rebounds and maintained a viral load of less than 5000 copies per milliliter for an extended time. The two failures had incomplete suppression of viral replication on the antiretroviral therapy (ART) regimen (> 10,000 copies per milliliter). In contrast only one of eight animals given neither ART nor the SIV vaccine maintained low viral loads during chronic infection, but four of seven animals showed good control of infection after ART plus a "mock vaccine" containing no SIV sequences.

Although the results obtained in the SIV infection models are not completely analogous to the typical course of HIV-1 infection in humans, these data provide a substantial impetus to study enhancement of HIV-specific immunity in humans. As conceptualized by Shen and Siliciano (Fig. 22–3),[32] the pattern of plasma viral vRNA and CD4+ T-lymphocytes can be maintained by either immunization (at least in some circumstances) or continual ART. Deletion of CD8+ T-lymphocytes allows extremely high viral replication, and the rate of disease progression is directly related to the viral replication rate.[33] The applicability of the macaque models to human HIV infection has been questioned because of the rapid course of the disease in macaques and the substantial CD4+ T-lymphocyte depletion, which occurs during the first 3 weeks of the infection. Furthermore, the use of early initiation of ART in studies that demonstrate substantial immune responses raises questions regarding the clinical applicability of these model regimens. How quickly HIV replication damages the immune system beyond its ability to mount an efficient response to control levels of viral replication, which permits an extended time off therapy with minimal disease progression, remains to be determined.

The nature of the defect that allows coexistence of an active immune response with continued viral replication during chronic infection is unclear. The CD8+ T-lymphocyte response appears to be inefficient due to a deficiency of HIV-specific helper CD4+ T-helper lymphocyte activity[2] intrinsic defects in the CD8+ T-lymphocyte response,[34,35] or both. The provision of viral antigen alone in the absence of ART therefore is unlikely to induce efficient immune control of HIV replication, as significant viral antigen exposure is already present. With the rare exception of long-term nonprogressors, humans do not develop immunologic control of replication without the help of therapeutic intervention. Hence some form of immune enhancement therapy is necessary if patients are to be able to control viral replication immunologically.

▲ THERAPEUTIC IMMUNIZATION PRIOR TO THE HAART ERA

The idea that administration of specific exogenous antigen could boost the immune response beyond that stimulated by the presence of the infectious virus itself was

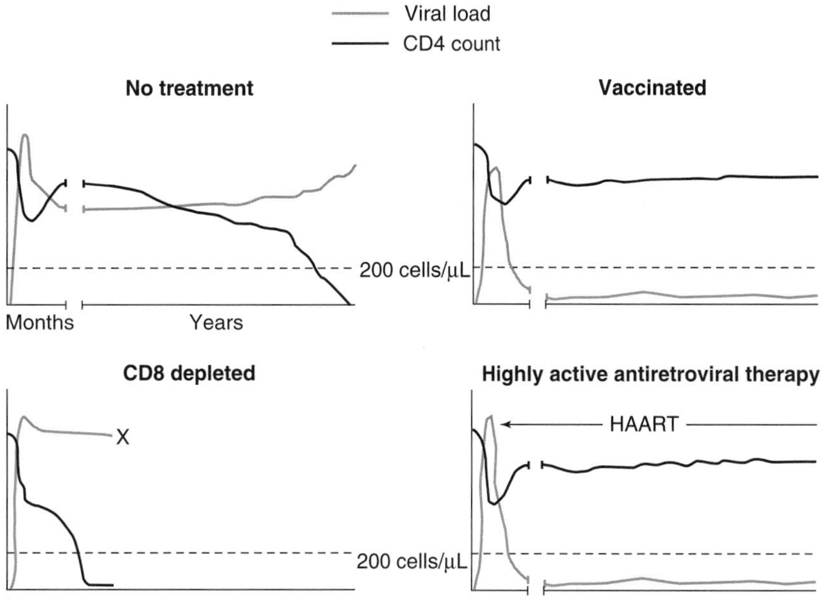

Figure 22–3. Plasma vRNA and CD4+ T-lymphocytes maintained by immunization or continuous antiretroviral therapy. (Redrawn from Shen X, Siliciano RF. Preventing AIDS but not HIV-1 infection with a DNA vaccine. Science 290:463, 2000. Copyright 2000 American Association for the Advancement of Science, with permission.)

investigated prior to the widespread use of HAART. During the early 1990s the dynamic nature of HIV infection in the asymptomatic phase was not fully understood, but it was considered to be a latent infection, primarily in lymphoid tissues. In retrospect, immunization with exogenous antigen during periods of ongoing viral replication may not be expected to achieve an optimal effect. However, there are lessons to be learned from studies of therapeutic immunization completed during this time (Table 22–1).

Most of these trials used proteins from the viral envelope (gp120 and gp160) in asymptomatic patients with high CD4+ T-lymphocyte counts. The study endpoints were primarily indices of disease progression, such as decreasing CD4+ T-lymphocyte counts, changes in plasma viral load, or the incidence of clinical endpoints (AIDS-defining events or death). In addition, many of these studies measured various in vitro indices of immunogenicity, such as antibody responses and lymphocyte proliferation assays (LPAs), which is an index primarily dependent on antigen-specific CD4+ T-lymphocyte function.

One of the earliest reports[36] compared recombinant $gp120_{MN}$ to adjuvant alone in 573 patients. All subjects assigned to the active intervention arm received a 300 μg dose of vaccine in alum each month for 6 months. and then continued on a bimonthly schedule with a 600 μg dose. The control group received only the alum. Patients with previous antiretroviral therapy for more than 2 months or any ART during the previous 9 months were excluded. The median viral load in this trial was 9250 copies per milliliter with an interquartile range of 2670 to 26960 copies per milliliter. After 15 months there were no differences in the rate of disease progression as assessed by the CD4+ T-lymphocyte count, plasma HIV RNA, or frequency of clinical endpoints. Although the vaccine regimen was safe, no specific measures of immunogenicity were determined.

A smaller trial examined[37] various doses of a recombinant gp160 vaccine. The control used was the standard recombinant hepatitis B vaccine, rather than the alum adjuvant. A total of 57 subjects with more than 400 CD4+ T lymphocytes per cubic millimeter were enrolled: 12 subjects received hepatitis B vaccine alone, and 45 subjects received either 20, 80, 320, or 1280 μg of the recombinant gp160. There was no difference in the rates of CD4+ T-lymphocyte decline among the control or any of the vaccine groups. All doses of gp160 stimulated cell-mediated immunity as measured by LPA or by IL-2 or interferon-γ (IFNγ) production. An extremely high fraction (44 of 45 subjects) had an LPA SI of more than 5 when stimulated with gp160, and most increased the amount of IL-2 and IFNγ production after specific antigen stimulation. The plasma viral load was not reported for these subjects. This study concluded that immunization of HIV-positive subjects with recombinant envelope proteins is immunogenic but does not alter the CD4+ T-lymphocyte decline, plasma vRNA levels, or the development of clinical endpoints. These findings have been confirmed in several other studies of the gp160 vaccines, including an ACTG trial in HIV-infected children,[38] a large Canadian study with a 3-year follow-up,[39] a Scandinavian study with subjects who enrolled with more than 200 CD4+ T-lymphocytes per cubic millimeter,[40] a European study with a 2-year follow-up of 208 subjects some of whom received some ART,[41] a 5-year follow-up study of 608 patients in a Phase II trial in the United States,[42] and two concurrent ACTG trials using several antigen preparations[43,44] (Table 22–1).

Several studies have also been conducted with a whole virus vaccine preparation depleted of gp120 (Remune). The particles are immunogenic, as measured by induction of LPA, delayed-type hypersensitivity (DTH) responses, and cytokine production.[45–48] One study reported a significant difference in CD4+ T-lymphocyte count in subjects immunized with Remune[49] but no change in the plasma vRNA. A large trial of Remune in the United States confirmed that this antigen preparation was immunogenic and resulted in a statistically

▲ **Table 22–1.** RANDOMIZED, DOUBLE-BLIND, PLACEBO-CONTROLLED TRIALS OF THERAPEUTIC IMMUNIZATION CONDUCTED PRIOR TO HAART

Study	Patients Studied			Antigen Used: Dose and Schedule	Endpoints	Clinical Results/ Immunogencity/Safety
	No.	ART Status	CD4 Count[a]			
Eron[36]	573	Excluded: asymptomatic HIV+ adults	>600	$rgp120_{MN}$: none vs. 300 μg × 6, 600 μg q2mo	Rate of CD4 decline, plasma vRNA clinical EP and safety	No effect vs. placebo/no measure of Immunogenicity/no adverse events
Valentine[37] (ACTG 137)	57	Excluded: asymptomatic HIV+ adults	>400	rgp160 (IIIB): none vs. 20, 80, 320 1280 μg	Ab and LPA, plasma vRNA, CD4 count, clinical EP and safety	No effect vs. placebo/ ↑ Ab and LPA at higher Ag doses/no adverse events
Lambert[38] (ACTG 218)		Excluded: asymptomatic HIV+ infants and children		rgp 120 (SF-2), rgp 160 (IIIB), rgp 120 (MN): alum vs. doses of 50–320 μg	Ab and LPA, plasma vRNA, CD4 count	No effect vs. placebo/30–56% (LPA) 65% (Ab) responses/no adverse events
Tsoukas[39]	278	Excluded at entry: asymptomatic HIV+ adults	>500	rgp 160 (IIIB): alum vs. 320 μg × 6/yr	Rate of CD4 decline, plasma vRNA, clinical EP and safety	No effects vs. placebo/no measure of immunogenicity/no adverse events
Sandstrom[40] (Nordic VAC-04)	835	Not excluded: asymptomatic HIV+ adults	>200	rgp 160 (LAI): alum vs. 160 μg × 6, then q3mo	Rate of CD4 decline, plasma vRNA, clinical EP and safety	No effects vs. placebo/no measure of immunogenicity/no adverse events
Goebel[41]	208	Not excluded: asymptomatic HIV+ adults	>200 & >500	rgp 160 (IIIB), rgp 120 (MN): alum vs. rgp 160 × 6, then rgp 120 × 3	Rate of CD4 decline, plasma vRNA, LPA to gp 160, clinical EP and safety	No effects vs. placebo/ ↑ LPA to new epitopes in rgp 160/no adverse events
Birx[42,44] (rgp 160 Phase II)	608	Not excluded: asymptomatic HIV+ adults	>400	rgp 160 (NL4-3): alum vs. 160 μg × 6 then q2mo for 5 yr	Rate of CD4 decline, plasma vRNA, LPA to gp 160, clinical EP and safety	No effect vs. placebo/ ↑ Ab and LPA to rgp 160/no adverse events
Schooley[43] (ACTG 209 & 214)	128 164	Not excluded: asymptomatic HIV+ adults	>500 50-499	Multiple recombinant HIV rgp 120s: alum vs. 300 μg × 6 q1mo	CD4 count, plasma vRNA, LPA to gp 120 variants, clinical EP and safety	No effect vs. placebo/ ↑ LPA strain-specific rgp 120 epitopes/no adverse events
Kahn[50] (IRC 806)	2527	Not excluded: asymptomatic HIV+ adults	300-549	gp 120 depleted whole virus (HZ321): IFA vs 10 μg p24 in preparation	Clinical EP and CD4 count, LPA to p24, safety	10 copies/ml increase in CD4 count/ ↑ LPA to p24/no adverse events

ART, antiretroviral therapy; CD4 count, CD4+ T-lymphocyte count; EP, endpoint; HAART, highly active, antiretroviral therapy; IFA, immunofluorescence assay; LPA, lymphocyte proliperation assay; rgp, recombinant gene product.
[a]Cells/mm^3.

significant, though modest, increase in CD4+ T-lymphocytes but showed no difference in the frequency of clinical endpoints.[50] Complete analysis of the plasma viral load from this trial was not completed, but no clear-cut differences were reported. Other types of HIV immunization have also been attempted in infected subjects, including trials with a DNA vaccine[51] and a lipopeptide conjugate vaccine.[52] ALVAC (canarypox virus with inserted HIV genes) has shown immunogenicity in uninfected human volunteers[53,54] and is currently being examined in several clinical trials; but no results have yet appeared regarding its efficacy in HIV-infected subjects. In summary, immunization with several candidate HIV vaccines can stimulate evidence of HIV-specific cell-mediated immunity in vitro but do not result in changes in viral load or disease progression.

▲ THERAPY INTERRUPTION: STRATEGY TO INDUCE AND MEASURE ANTI-HIV IMMUNITY

Despite the poor outcome of therapeutic immunization during the pre-HAART era, the possibility remains that therapeutic immunization used in conjunction with more potent antiretroviral drug regimens may prove more efficacious. A key feature of current investigations of therapeutic immunization is the withdrawal of ART as a measure of the efficacy of the intervention. Because the dynamics of viral replication unmodified by antiretroviral drugs is thought to reflect the efficiency of the antiviral immune response, withdrawal of therapy at the end of a series of interventions to increase anti-HIV immunity can serve as a "read-out" for trial endpoints, which is called analytical therapy interruption (ATI). The withdrawal of HAART therapy is better known, however, as an STI, where the "S" stands for various adjectives, including "structured," "strategic," "scheduled," and "supervised".

There are several uses of STIs in clinical trials. First, there is the concept that a short withdrawal of all therapy allows rebound of viral replication and thereby stimulates the immune system as a form of "endogenous" immunization. A second rationale is that in patients who are failing an antiretroviral regimen withdrawal of all therapy may result in the return of wild-type variants because of the selective growth advantage of wild-type virus in the absence of drug selective pressure. A third rationale is that combination antiretroviral regimens are complex and toxic, and intermittent therapy may be able to delay disease progression as effectively as continuous therapy. Because disease progression is slow in many individuals, this strategy may produce equivalent benefit but with less drug toxicity. The latter two reasons to withdraw therapy are not primarily directed toward enhancement of HIV-specific immunity and are not reviewed further in this chapter.

Initial investigations using therapy interruption were small exploratory studies that demonstrated that viral rebound occurred despite prolonged periods of previously undetectable levels.[55–57] The time lag between withdrawal of HAART and detection of viral rebound was variable,[56,58] with a median time to detection of viral load of around 1 weeks. Significant T-lymphocyte activation accompanied the rebound in viral replication and was coincident with a fall in CD4+ T-lymphocyte counts.[59] CD4+ T-lymphocyte counts rise fairly quickly after ART is restarted, suggesting that these changes are associated with redistribution of T lymphocytes from tissue sites, rather than CD4+ T-lymphocyte destruction and regrowth. Increased CD8+ T-lymphocyte activation is associated with increased frequency of HIV specific CD8+ T-lymphocytes [60,61] as well as increases in HIV-specific CD4+ T-lymphocytes function in some subjects.[58,62] There have been several reports of an acute illness similar to the primary infection syndrome after therapy withdrawal in chronically infected subjects.[63,64] These symptoms rapidly resolved with the reinstitution of HAART. In all of the reported studies, viral replication has been suppressed again by the same HAART regimen that was used prior to the interruption. As demonstrated in subjects withdrawn from therapy during antiretroviral failure, wild-type variants have a preferential growth advantage when therapy is withdrawn, and so the development of resistance is rare.[65,66] Given the above potential complications and the lack of clearly demonstrated benefit in chronic infection, STI should be performed with the "S" indicating "supervised" in the setting of a clinical trial.

The concept of induction of a more efficient immune response by a short withdrawal of therapy was strengthened by observations that some subjects maintained prolonged low viral replication after therapy withdrawal. "Berlin patient," who was started on antiretroviral therapy early in disease, briefly discontinued therapy due to an episode of hepatitis A, and then completely stopped therapy, was able to maintain undetectable plasma HIV RNA.[3] Other subjects were subsequently reported who also started HAART early after infection, had histories of intermittent therapy, subsequently stopped therapy, and demonstrated persistently low viral loads associated with heighten indices of a specific, ongoing anti-HIV immune response.[4]

In a prospective trial of eight subjects treated with HAART prior to seroconversion,[5] nearly complete control of viral replication was observed after therapy withdrawal. These eight subjects maintained in vitro evidence of strong HIV-specific immune responses while on therapy. In three of the eight patients, efficient immune control of HIV replication was present after the first withdrawal of therapy. Two of five other subjects who underwent a second STI were able to maintain viral loads below 5000 copies per milliliter for a median follow-up of 6.5 months (Fig. 22–4). Overall, five of the eight patients were able to control viral replication efficiently off therapy, which is a substantially higher proportion than has been observed in natural history cohorts. These findings complement the results observed in studies of rhesus macaques that underwent early initiation of intermittent therapy described above.[67]

A few trials have been initiated to examine cycles of STI, with the rationale that repeated brief exposure to viral antigen heightens the HIV-specific immune response and results in a delayed and reduced viral rebound. In one study, eight subjects underwent three consecutive STIs, the first two of which lasted 30 days.[62,68] After the third STI the viral load rebounded in all subjects; however, the magnitude of viral load rebound after 32 weeks off therapy was significantly lower than the baseline viral load in six of the eight subjects. Four of the responders had HIV RNA levels below 10,000 copies per milliliter. CD4+ and CD8+ T-lymphocyte immune responses after STI were more pronounced in the subjects who maintained low viral loads after the third STI. In addition, the doubling time of viral rebound was lengthened after the second and third withdrawals.

In another trial, 12 subjects underwent three successive STIs.[69] The rate of the initial rise in viremia was delayed during the second and third STIs compared to during the first STI, but the long-term effect on viral replication off therapy was not examined. Transient increases in both CD4+ and CD8+ T-lymphocyte immune responses were noted. Increases in laboratory indices of both CD4+ and CD8+ T-lymphocyte immune responses were also demonstrated in a report of three patients who underwent STIs of varying lengths, but these increased responses were not sufficient to prevent viral rebound with subsequent withdrawals.[70]

In a significantly larger study of 128 patients with chronic infection, the Swiss-Spanish Intermittent Therapy Trial (SSITT),[71] no clear decrease in the magnitude of viral rebound was demonstrated after the third STI compared to the first. In this trial the therapy interruptions were of 2 weeks' duration, similar to the median time to detection in other studies. After the first withdrawal 24% of patients had undetectable viral loads, whereas 2 weeks after the fourth withdrawal 17% of patients had undetectable viral loads. Most of the subjects were unable to maintain viral loads below 10,000 copies per milliliter after a prolonged final therapy withdrawal. After the STI, an increase in HIV-specific proliferative responses were detected, but no clear

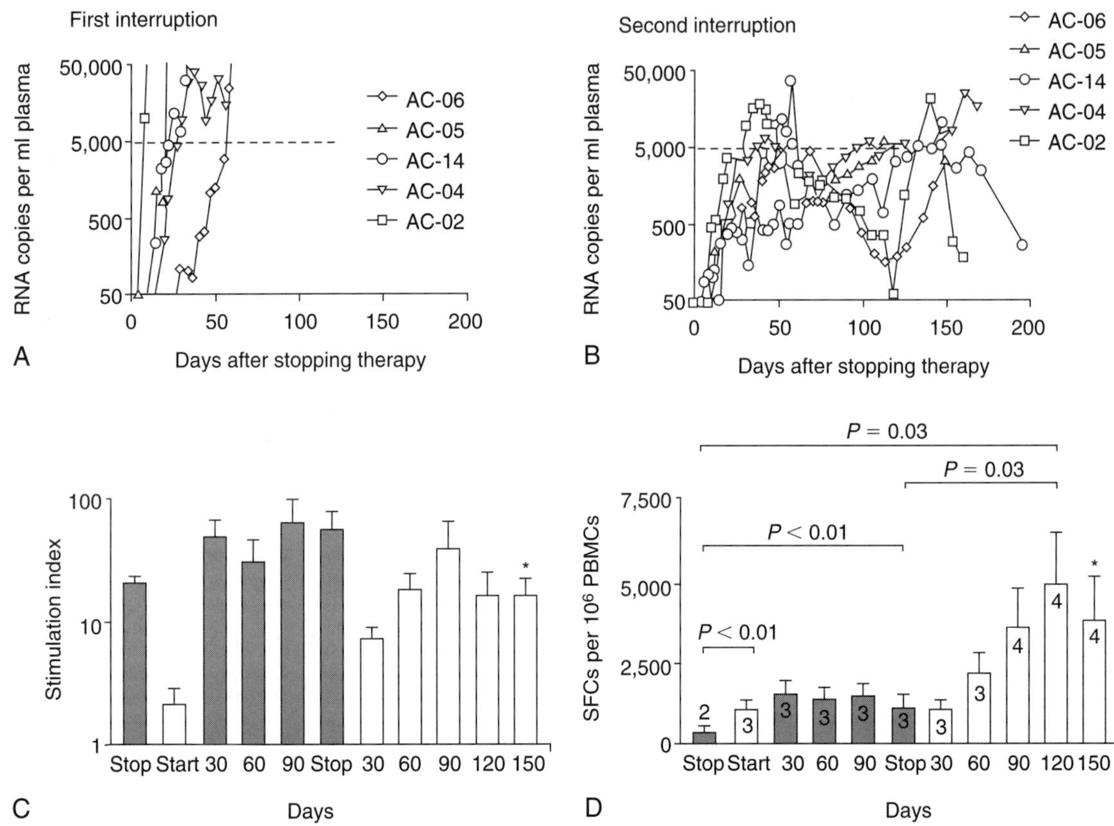

Figure 22–4. Virology and immunology in subjects requiring repeated treatment interruption. *A,* Five subjects met viremia criteria to reinstitute therapy during the first treatment interruption. Viral load (RNA copies per milliliter of plasma) at the time of therapy resumption was as follows: AC-02, 187,000; AC-04, 14,800; AC-05, 116,000; AC-06, 139,000; AC-14, 111.000. Upon reinitiation of therapy, the HIV-1 load declined below limits of detection in all individuals within 35–130 days (data not shown). *B,* After a median of 16 weeks of additional therapy (range 13–30 weeks), therapy was again interrupted. *C, D,* Gag-specific T-helper lymphocyte responses *(C)* and HIV-1-specific CTL responses *(D)* were assessed at the time therapy was stopped (stop), at the time of protocol-mandated reinstitution of therapy (start), and at designated days in between. *Shaded bars* indicate assays performed when subjects were on HAART. CTL magnitudes are given as the mean of total CTL responses per individual, calculated as the sum of responses against optimal CTL epitopes. The median number of CTL epitopes recognized per individual, indicated within the bars, reached a median of four per individual after the last interruption (range two to nine). CTL responses were confirmed by cloning and testing in cytolytic assays. p values are calculated for changes in CTL magnitude. *Asterisk* indicates that analysis was limited to four subjects. (Redrawn from Rosenberg ES, Altfield M, Poon SH, et al. Immune control of HIV-1 following early treatment of acute infection. Nature 407:523, 2000, with permission.)

trends were detected in an HIV-specific CD8+ T-lymphocyte Elispot assay. Thus the initial experience with brief STI cycles in chronically infected patients have not yielded the same positive results associated with STIs in subjects who started HAART early after acute infection.

▲ MECHANISM OF THE DEFECT IN IMMUNITY DURING STEADY-STATE CHRONIC INFECTION

Ongoing replication of HIV results in damage to the immune system, particularly the CD4+ T-lymphocyte pool, and reconstitution of the system develops slowly with HAART alone.[72] Because subjects who began HAART early can sustain efficient immune control, HIV appears to delete preferentially the HIV-specific subpopulation of CD4+ T-lymphocytes early during infection. Although the thymus is not completely inactive in adult humans,[73,74] production of T-lymphocytes with newly rearranged T-lymphocyte receptors is slow. The strategy of waiting until a new repertoire of HIV-specific CD4+ T-lymphocytes is produced from the thymus most likely would require many years of continuous HAART therapy. However, the lack of a measurable immune response using proliferation assays does not provide complete evidence of the deletion of all antigen-reactive cells. It is possible that some HIV-specific CD4+ T-lymphocytes are rendered anergic because of the products produced by HIV replication. For example, gp120 has been proposed to induce anergy by direct interaction with CD4[75–80] in the context of prolonged low-intensity stimulation of the T-lymphocyte receptor. Another possible contributor is the HIV tat protein, which has been shown to have inhibitory properties on both T-lymphocytes and antigen-presenting cells.[81–83] Exogenous co-stimulation of CD4+ T-lymphocytes with HIV antigens results in some degree of activity among cells derived from chronically infected subjects.[84–86] In addition, several groups have shown the presence of CD4+ T-lymphocytes that can be induced to express IFNγ by different HIV-1 antigens,[84,87–89] indicating that these viral antigen-specific cells have not been completely deleted. If clonal deletion of HIV-specific CD4+ T-lymphocytes is the primary mechanism for the relative absence of antiviral CD4+ T-lymphocyte activity in chronic disease, the success of therapeutic immunization during the HAART era is likely to be ineffective. If, on the other hand, viral products render such cells anergic during chronic infection, attempts to reverse this anergic phenotype may be successful.

Therefore the goal of therapeutic immunization for HIV disease is distinct from the goal of standard vaccination of antigen-naive subjects. The assessment of effective immunization is not merely whether in vitro responses have been stimulated but whether an immune-based intervention can stimulate a more efficient immune response in vivo than was present during chronic infection prior to ART. This assessment is complicated, as viral replication may stimulate the immune response via antigen production, but it may also produce viral products that induce anergy in CD4+ T-lymphocytes, as before. Thus therapy interruption alone may not work because of the production of inhibitory proteins associated with viral growth.

▲ CONCLUSIONS

Specific therapeutic immunization or interruption from antiretroviral therapy under optimal conditions may allow induction of an efficient immune response that could control HIV replication at a level low enough to block significant disease progression. However, neither of these approaches has yet shown clear therapeutic benefit; and whether such strategies will ultimately prove effective remains speculative. Several clinical trials are underway that are designed to boost HIV-specific immune responses while subjects are on HAART. These trials utilize analytical therapy interruption to assess the characteristics of the immune response, rather than rely on in vitro immune response surrogates as primary endpoints for the trial. Modulation of both the immunization effect while on HAART and the initial stage of viral rebound during the analytic therapy interruption by the use of various cytokines or other adjuvants is an area of active investigation.

REFERENCES

1. Bucy RP. Viral and cellular dynamics in HIV disease. Curr Infect Dis Rep 3:295, 2001.
2. Rosenberg ES, Billingsley JM, Caliendo AM, et al. Vigorous HIV-1-specific CD4+ T cell responses associated with control of viremia. Science 278:1447, 1997.
3. Lisziewicz J, Rosenberg E, Lieberman J, et al. Control of HIV despite the discontinuation of antiretroviral therapy. N Engl J Med 340:1683, 1999.
4. Ortiz GM, Nixon DF, Trkola A, et al. HIV-1-specific immune responses in subjects who temporarily contain virus replication after discontinuation of highly active antiretroviral therapy. J Clin Invest 104:R13, 1999.
5. Rosenberg ES, Altfield M, Poon SH, et al. Immune control of HIV-1 following early treatment of acute infection. Nature 407:523, 2000.
6. Brander C,Walker BD. T lymphocyte responses in HIV-1 infection: implications for vaccine development. Curr Opin Immunol 11:451, 1999.
7. McMichael AJ, Ogg G, Wilson J, et al. Memory CD8+ T cells in HIV infection. Philos Trans R Soc Lond B Biol Sci 355:363, 2000.
8. Bucy RP, Kilby JM. Perspectives on inducing efficient immune control of HIV-1 replication: a new goal for HIV therapeutics? AIDS 15:S36, 2001.
9. Schmitz JE, Kuroda MJ, Santra S, et al. Control of viremia in simian immunodeficiency virus infection by CD8(+) lymphocytes. Science 283: 857, 1999.
10. Jin X, Bauer DE, Tuttleton SE, et al. Dramatic rise in plasma viremia after CD8(+) T cell depletion in simian immunodeficiency virus-infected macaques. J Exp Med 189: 991, 1999.
11. Reimann KA, Snyder GB, Chalifoux LV, et al. An activated CD8+ lymphocyte appears in lymph nodes of rhesus monkeys early after infection with simian immunodeficiency virus. J Clin Invest 88:1113, 1991.
12. Shen L, Chen ZW, Letvin NL. The repertoire of cytotoxic T lymphocytes in the recognition of mutant simian immunodeficiency virus variants. J Immunol 153:5849, 1994.
13. Kuroda MJ, Schmitz JE, Barouch DH, et al. Analysis of Gag-specific cytotoxic T lymphocytes in simian immunodeficiency virus-infected rhesus monkeys by cell staining with a tetrameric major histocompatibility complex class I- peptide complex. J Exp Med 187:1373, 1998.
14. Johnson RP, Glickman RL, Yang JQ, et al. Induction of vigorous cytotoxic T-lymphocyte responses by live attenuated simian immunodeficiency virus. J Virol 71:7711, 1997.
15. Shibata R, Siemon C, Czajak SC, et al. Live, attenuated simian immunodeficiency virus vaccines elicit potent resistance against a challenge with a human immunodeficiency virus type 1 chimeric virus. J Virol 71:8141, 1997.
16. Miller CJ, McChesney MB, Lu X, et al. Rhesus macaques previously infected with simian/human immunodeficiency virus are protected from vaginal challenge with pathogenic SIVmac239. J Virol 71:1911, 1997.
17. Lifson JD, Nowak MA, Goldstein S, et al. The extent of early viral replication is a critical determinant of the natural history of simian immunodeficiency virus infection. J Virol 71:9508, 1997.
18. Hirsch VM, Goldstein S, Hynes NA, et al. Prolonged clinical latency and survival of macaques given a whole inactivated simian immunodeficiency virus vaccine. J Infect Dis 170:51, 1994.
19. Hirsch VM, Fuerst TR, Sutter G, et al. Patterns of viral replication correlate with outcome in simian immunodeficiency virus (SIV)-infected macaques: effect of prior immunization with a trivalent SIV vaccine in modified vaccinia virus Ankara. J Virol 70:3741, 1996.
20. Robinson HL, Montefiori DC, Johnson RP, et al. Neutralizing antibody-independent containment of immunodeficiency virus challenges by DNA priming and recombinant pox virus booster immunizations. Nat Med 5:526, 1999.
21. Barouch DH, Santra S, Schmitz JE, et al. Control of viremia and prevention of clinical AIDS in rhesus monkeys by cytokine-augmented DNA vaccination. Science 290:486, 2000.
22. Seth A, Ourmanov I, Schmitz JE, et al. Immunization with a modified vaccinia virus expressing simian immunodeficiency virus (SIV) Gag-Pol primes for an anamnestic Gag-specific cytotoxic T-lymphocyte response and is associated with reduction of viremia after SIV challenge. J Virol 74:2502, 2000.
23. Barouch DH, Craiu A, Kuroda MJ, et al. Augmentation of immune responses to HIV-1 and simian immunodeficiency virus DNA vaccines by IL-2/Ig plasmid administration in rhesus monkeys. Proc Natl Acad Sci USA 97:4192, 2000.
24. Egan MA, Charini WA, Kuroda MJ, et al. Simian immunodeficiency virus (SIV) gag DNA-vaccinated rhesus monkeys develop secondary cytotoxic T-lymphocyte responses and control viral replication after pathogenic SIV infection. J Virol 74:7485, 2000.
25. Kumar A, Lifson JD, Li Z, et al. Sequential immunization of macaques with two differentially attenuated vaccines induced long-term virus-specific immune responses and conferred protection against AIDS caused by heterologous simian human immunodeficiency virus [SHIV(89.6)P]. Virology 279:241, 2001.
26. Barouch DH, Santra S, Kuroda MJ, et al. Reduction of simian-human immunodeficiency virus 89.6P viremia in rhesus monkeys by recombinant modified vaccinia virus Ankara vaccination. J Virol 75:5151, 2001.
27. Amara RR, Villinger F, Altman JD, et al. Control of a mucosal challenge and prevention of AIDS by a multiprotein DNA/MVA vaccine. Science 292:69, 2001.

28. Chen X, Scala G, Quinto I, et al. Protection of rhesus macaques against disease progression from pathogenic SHIV-89.6PD by vaccination with phage-displayed HIV-1 epitopes. Nat Med 7:1225, 2001.
29. Lifson JD, Rossio JL, Arnaout R, et al. Containment of simian immunodeficiency virus infection: cellular immune responses and protection from rechallenge following transient postinoculation antiretroviral treatment. J Virol 74:2584, 2000.
30. Lifson JD, Rossio JL, Piatak M, Jr, et al. Role of CD8(+) lymphocytes in control of simian immunodeficiency virus infection and resistance to rechallenge after transient early antiretroviral treatment. J Virol 75:10187, 2001.
31. Hel Z, Venzon D, Poudyal M,et al. Viremia control following antiretroviral treatment and therapeutic immunization during primary SIV251 infection of macaques. Nat Med 6:1140, 2000.
32. Shen X, Siliciano RF. Preventing AIDS but not HIV-1 infection with a DNA vaccine. Science 290:463, 2000.
33. Lyles RH, Munoz A, Yamashita TE, et al. Natural history of human immunodeficiency virus type 1 viremia after seroconversion and proximal to AIDS in a large cohort of homosexual men: multicenter AIDS Cohort Study. J Infect Dis 181:872, 2000.
34. Shankar P, Russo M, Harnisch B, et al. Impaired function of circulating HIV-specific CD8(+) T cells in chronic human immunodeficiency virus infection. Blood 96:3094, 2000.
35. Trimble LA, Shankar P, Patterson M, et al. Human immunodeficiency virus-specific circulating CD8 T lymphocytes have down-modulated CD3zeta and CD28, key signaling molecules for T-cell activation. J Virol 74:7320, 2000.
36. Eron JJJr, Ashby MA, Giordano MF, et al. Randomised trial of MN-rgp120 HIV-1 vaccine in symptomless HIV-1 infection. Lancet 348:1547, 1996.
37. Valentine FT, Kundu S, Haslett PA, et al. A randomized, placebo-controlled study of the immunogenicity of human immunodeficiency virus (HIV) rgp160 vaccine in HIV-infected subjects with > or = 400/mm^3 CD4 T lymphocytes (AIDS Clinical Trials Group Protocol 137). J Infect Dis 173:1336, 1996.
38. Lambert JS, McNamara J, Katz SL, et al. Safety and immunogenicity of HIV recombinant envelope vaccines in HIV-infected infants and children: National Institutes of Health-sponsored Pediatric AIDS Clinical Trials Group (ACTG-218). J Acquir Immune Defic Syndr Hum Retrovirol 19:451, 1998.
39. Tsoukas CM, Raboud J, Bernard NF, et al. Active immunization of patients with HIV infection: a study of the effect of VaxSyn, a recombinant HIV envelope subunit vaccine, on progression of immunodeficiency. AIDS Res Hum Retroviruses 14:483, 1998.
40. Sandstrom E, Wahren B. Therapeutic immunisation with recombinant gp160 in HIV-1 infection: a randomised double-blind placebo-controlled trial: Nordic VAC-04 Study Group. Lancet 353:1735, 1999.
41. Goebel FD, Mannhalter JW, Belshe RB, et al. W. Recombinant gp160 as a therapeutic vaccine for HIV-infection: results of a large randomized, controlled trial: European Multinational IMMUNO AIDS Vaccine Study Group. AIDS 13:1461, 1999.
42. Birx DL, Loomis-Price LD, Aronson N, et al. Efficacy testing of recombinant human immunodeficiency virus (HIV) gp160 as a therapeutic vaccine in early-stage HIV-1-infected volunteers: rgp160 phase II vaccine investigators. J Infect Dis 181:881, 2000.
43. Schooley RT, Spino C, Kuritzkes D, et al. Two double-blinded, randomized, comparative trials of 4 human immunodeficiency virus type 1 (HIV-1) envelope vaccines in HIV-1-infected individuals across a spectrum of disease severity: AIDS clinical trials groups 209 and 214. J Infect Dis 182:1357, 2000.
44. Ratto-Kim S, Sitz KV, Garner RP, et al. Repeated immunization with recombinant gp160 human immunodeficiency virus (HIV) envelope protein in early HIV-1 infection: evaluation of the T cell proliferative response. J Infect Dis 179:337, 1999.
45. Trauger RJ, Ferre F, Daigle AE, et al. Effect of immunization with inactivated gp120-depleted human immunodeficiency virus type 1 (HIV-1) immunogen on HIV-1 immunity, viral DNA, and percentage of CD4 cells. J Infect Dis 169:1256, 1994.
46. Turner JL, Trauger RJ, Daigle AE, Carlo DJ. HIV-1 immunogen induction of HIV-1-specific delayed-type hypersensitivity: results of a double-blind, adjuvant-controlled, dose-ranging trial. AIDS 8:1429, 1994.
47. Moss RB, Trauger RJ, Giermakowska WK, et al. Effect of immunization with an inactivated gp120-depleted HIV-1 immunogen on beta-chemokine and cytokine production in subjects with HIV-1 infection. J Acquir Immune Defic Syndr Hum Retrovirol 14:343, 1997.
48. Maino VC, Suni MA, Wormsley SB, et al. Enhancement of HIV type 1 antigen-specific CD4+ T cell memory in subjects with chronic HIV type 1 infection receiving an HIV type 1 immunogen. AIDS Res Hum Retroviruses 16:539, 2000.
49. Churdboonchart V, Moss RB, Sirawaraporn W, et al. Effect of HIV-specific immune-based therapy in subjects infected with HIV-1 subtype E in Thailand. AIDS 12:1521, 1998.
50. Kahn JO, Cherng DW, Mayer K, et al. Evaluation of HIV-1 immunogen, an immunologic modifier, administered to patients infected with HIV having 300 to 549 × 106/L CD4 cell counts: a randomized controlled trial. JAMA 284:2193, 2000.
51. MacGregor RR, Boyer JD, Ugen KE, et al. First human trial of a DNA-based vaccine for treatment of human immunodeficiency virus type 1 infection: safety and host response. J Infect Dis 178:92, 1998.
52. Seth A, Yasutomi Y, Jacoby H, et al. Evaluation of a lipopeptide immunogen as a therapeutic in HIV type 1-seropositive individuals. AIDS Res Hum Retroviruses 16:337, 2000.
53. Clements-Mann ML, Weinhold K, Matthews TJ, et al. Immune responses to human immunodeficiency virus (HIV) type 1 induced by canarypox expressing HIV-1MN gp120, HIV-1SF2 recombinant gp120, or both vaccines in seronegative adults: NIAID AIDS Vaccine Evaluation Group. J Infect Dis 177:1230, 1998.
54. Evans TG, Keefer MC, Weinhold KJ, et al. A canarypox vaccine expressing multiple human immunodeficiency virus type 1 genes given alone or with rgp120 elicits broad and durable CD8+ cytotoxic T lymphocyte responses in seronegative volunteers. J Infect Dis 180:290, 1999.
55. Jubault V, Burgard M, Le Corfec E, et al. High rebound of plasma and cellular HIV load after discontinuation of triple combination therapy [letter]. AIDS 12:2358, 1998.
56. Harrigan PR, Whaley M, Montaner JS. Rate of HIV-1 RNA rebound upon stopping antiretroviral therapy. AIDS 13:F59, 1999.
57. Garcia F, Plana M, Vidal C, et al. Quick viral load rebound after one year of successful HAART in chronic HIV-1 infected patients in very early stages. Presented at the 6th Conference on Retroviruses and Opportunistic Infections, 1999, abstract 629.
58. Ruiz L, Martinez-Picado J, Romeu J, et al. Structured treatment interruption in chronically HIV-1 infected patients after long-term viral suppression. AIDS 14:397, 2000.
59. Davey RT Jr, Bhat N, Yoder C, et al. HIV-1 and T cell dynamics after interruption of highly active antiretroviral therapy (HAART) in patients with a history of sustained viral suppression. Proc Natl Acad Sci USA 96:15109, 1999.
60. Haslett PA, Nixon DF, Shen Z, et al. Strong human immunodeficiency virus (HIV)-specific CD4+ T cell responses in a cohort of chronically infected patients are associated with interruptions in anti-HIV chemotherapy. J Infect Dis 181:1264, 2000.
61. Papasavvas E, Ortiz GM, Gross R, et al. Enhancement of human immunodeficiency virus type 1-specific CD4 and CD8 T cell responses in chronically infected persons after temporary treatment interruption. J Infect Dis 182:766, 2000.
62. Garcia F, Plana M, Vidal C, et al. Dynamics of viral load rebound and immunological changes after stopping effective antiretroviral therapy. AIDS 13:F79, 1999.
63. Kilby JM, Goepfert PA, Miller AP, et al. Recurrence of the acute HIV syndrome after interruption of antiretroviral therapy in a patient with chronic HIV infection: a case report. Ann Intern Med 133:435, 2000.
64. Colven R, Harrington RD, Spach DH, et al. Retroviral rebound syndrome after cessation of suppressive antiretroviral therapy in three patients with chronic HIV infection. Ann Intern Med 133:430, 2000.
65. Miller V, Sabin C, Hertogs K, et al. Virological and immunological effects of treatment interruptions in HIV-1 infected patients with treatment failure. AIDS 14:2857, 2000.
66. Deeks SG, Wrin T, Liegler T, et al. Virologic and immunologic consequences of discontinuing combination antiretroviral-drug therapy in HIV-infected patients with detectable viremia. N Engl J Med 344:472, 2001.
67. Lori F, Lewis MG, Xu J, et al. Control of SIV rebound through structured treatment interruptions during early infection. Science 290:1591, 2000.
68. Garcia F, Plana M, Ortiz GM, et al. The virological and immunological consequences of structured treatment interruptions in chronic HIV-1 infection. AIDS 15:F29, 2001.

69. Ruiz L, Carcelain G, Martinez-Picado J, et al. HIV dynamics and T-cell immunity after three structured treatment interruptions in chronic HIV-1 infection. AIDS 15:F19, 2001.
70. Carcelain G, Tubiana R, Samri A, et al. Transient mobilization of human immunodeficiency virus (HIV)-specific CD4 T-helper cells fails to control virus rebounds during intermittent antiretroviral therapy in chronic HIV type 1 infection. J Virol 75:234, 2001.
71. Fagard C, Lebraz M, Gunthard H, et al. SSITT: a prospective trial of strategic treatment interruptions in 128 patients. Presented at the 8th Conference on Retroviruses and Opportunistic Infections, 2001, abstract 357.
72. Lederman MM, Valdez H. Immune restoration with antiretroviral therapies: implications for clinical management. JAMA 284:223, 2000.
73. Douek DC, McFarland RD, Keiser PH, et al. Changes in thymic function with age and during the treatment of HIV infection. Nature 396:690, 1998.
74. McCune JM. Thymic function in HIV-1 disease. Semin Immunol 9:397,1997.
75. Diamond DC, Sleckman BP, Gregory T, et al. Inhibition of CD4+ T cell function by the HIV envelope protein, gp120. J Immunol 141:3715, 1988.
76. Oyaizu N, Chirmule N, Kalyanaraman VS, et al. Human immunodeficiency virus type 1 envelope glycoprotein gp120 produces immune defects in CD4+ T lymphocytes by inhibiting interleukin 2 mRNA. Proc Natl Acad Sci USA 87:2379, 1990.
77. Banda NK, Bernier J, Kurahara DK, et al. Crosslinking CD4 by human immunodeficiency virus gp120 primes T cells for activation-induced apoptosis. J Exp Med 176:1099, 1992.
78. Meyaard L, Schuitemaker H, Miedema F. T-cell dysfunction in HIV infection: anergy due to defective antigen- presenting cell function? Immunol Today 14:161, 1993.
79. Foster S, Beverley P, Aspinall, R. gp120-Induced programmed cell death in recently activated T cells without subsequent ligation of the T cell receptor. Eur J Immunol 25:1778, 1995.
80. Chirmule N, Avots A, LakshmiTamma SM, et al. CD4-mediated signals induce T cell dysfunction in vivo. J Immunol 163:644, 1999.
81. Chirmule N, Than S, Khan SA, Pahwa S. Human immunodeficiency virus Tat induces functional unresponsiveness in T cells. J Virol 69:492, 1995.
82. Wu MX, Schlossman SF. Decreased ability of HIV-1 tat protein-treated accessory cells to organize cellular clusters is associated with partial activation of T cells. Proc Natl Acad Sci USA 94:13832, 1997.
83. Cohen SS, Li, C, Ding L, et al. Pronounced acute immunosuppression in vivo mediated by HIV Tat challenge. Proc Natl Acad Sci USA 96:10842, 1999.
84. Pitcher CJ, Quittner C, Peterson DM, et al. HIV-1-specific CD4+ T cells are detectable in most individuals with active HIV-1 infection, but decline with prolonged viral suppression. Nat Med 5:518, 1999.
85. Chougnet C, Thomas E, Landay AL, et al. CD40 ligand and IFN-gamma synergistically restore IL-12 production in HIV-infected patients. Eur J Immunol 28:646, 1998.
86. Dybul M, Mercier G, Belson M, et al. CD40 ligand trimer and IL-12 enhance peripheral blood mononuclear cells and CD4+ T cell proliferation and production of IFN-gamma in response to p24 antigen in HIV-infected individuals: potential contribution of anergy to HIV-specific unresponsiveness. J Immunol 165:1685, 2000.
87. Wilson JD, Imami N, Watkins A, et al. Loss of CD4+ T cell proliferative ability but not loss of human immunodeficiency virus type 1 specificity equates with progression to disease. J Infect Dis 182:792, 2000.
88. Betts MR, Ambrozak DR, Douek DC, et al. Analysis of total human immunodeficiency virus (HIV)-specific CD4(+) and CD8(+) T-cell responses: relationship to viral load in untreated HIV infection. J Virol 75:11983, 2001.
89. McNeil AC, Shupert WL, Iyasere CA, et al. High-level HIV-1 viremia suppresses viral antigen-specific CD4+ T cell proliferation. Proc Natl Acad Sci USA 98:13878, 2001.

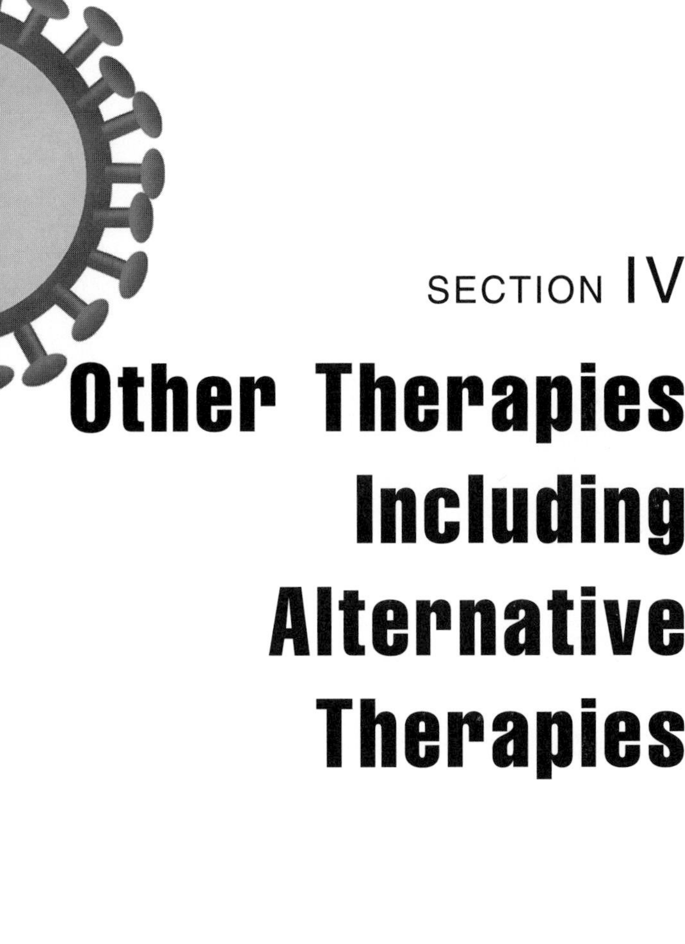

SECTION IV

Other Therapies Including Alternative Therapies

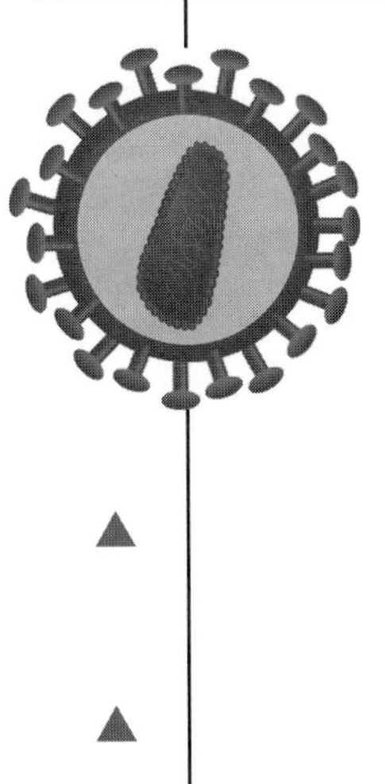

CHAPTER 23

Complementary and Alternative Therapies

Donald I. Abrams, MD
Charles Steinberg, MD

Complementary and alternative medicine (CAM) therapies are defined as "interventions neither widely taught in medical schools nor generally available in U.S. hospitals."[1] In view of the fact that information on human immunodeficiency virus/acquired immunodeficiency syndrome (HIV-AIDS) itself was not taught in medical schools until the 1980s, it should come as no surprise that the use of CAM interventions for treatment dates back to the onset of the outbreak of the disease. At the beginning of the HIV-AIDS epidemic, prior to identification of the etiologic agent, early alternative therapies included high-dose intravenous or oral vitamin C and topical application of the sensitizer dinitrochlorobenzene.[2–11] While immunomodulators and antivirals such as isoprinosine and ribavirin were commencing clinical trials as possible therapies at the research centers, they were also obtained over the counter in easily accessed foreign markets. In the absence of a standard treatment during the first 5 years of the epidemic, alternative use and acquisitions of therapies filled the gap.

When zidovudine was approved in late 1986, an orthodox treatment became available by prescription to patients for the first time.[12] This led to a brief slowdown in the interest in alternative agents. It was hoped that additional antiretroviral agents would soon be released. When none quickly appeared, however, there was another surge in the alternative movement from 1987 through 1989. In 1989 results of large clinical trials demonstrated that zidovudine was useful in patients with early stages of HIV infection.[13,14] At the same time, expanded access programs for additional nucleoside analogues were established, giving patients for whom zidovudine failed or whose disease progressed access to other potentially beneficial therapeutic agents.[15,16] This again ushered in a period of decreased interest in alternative interventions.

Some individuals, despite the availability of prescribed antiretroviral therapies, continued to use alternative treatments. Often these interventions were described as "complementary" to their prescribed antiretroviral medication. In 1993 the alternative therapy movement blossomed again following discouraging reports of the results of the large collaborative Concorde trial, which evaluated early versus deferred zidovudine therapy in patients with asymptomatic HIV infection.[17,18] These disappointing results, coupled with the discouraging news from other clinical trials reported at the 1993 International Conference on AIDS, combined to foster a sentiment of disenchantment over available treatments. Increasing numbers of patients again sought therapy for their HIV infection from alternative sources.

The current era of highly active antiretroviral therapy (HAART) was inaugurated in 1995 with promising surrogate marker information emanating from trials combining zidovudine and lamivudine followed by even more impressive responses when adding a protease inhibitor.[19–23] With the rapid licensure and approval of the first four protease inhibitors and two non-nucleoside reverse transcriptase inhibitors (NNRTIs), the anti-HIV arsenal dramatically increased. The excitement and hope generated by the possibility of prolonged viral suppression utilizing prescribed medication virtually supplanted the need to obtain potential alternative antiretroviral interventions from the buyer's clubs. Although alternative agents aimed specifically at the retrovirus are utilized less frequently, therapies are still sought for some of the manifestations of HIV disease where orthodox medicine has little to offer. Immune reconstitution and management of treatment-related complications are current areas where the highest interest in complementary and alternative intervention remains. In addition, as effectively treated patients with HIV are living longer lives with a greater semblance of normalcy than their predecessors, many turn to CAM for health maintenance and for an increased sense of well-being.

Discussing factors that prompt patients to explore alternative therapies, Eisenberg, of the Center for Alternative Medicine and Research at the Beth Israel Deaconess Medical Center in Boston, enumerated five possible reasons[24]: (1) for health promotion and disease prevention; (2) when conventional therapies have been exhausted; (3) when conventional therapies have questionable efficacy or are associated with significant adverse effects; (4) when no conventional therapy exists to relieve the patient's condition; and (5) when the conventional approach is held to be emotionally or spiritually without benefit. Regardless of why a patient may seek alternative therapies, Eisenberg suggested that the primary care provider be cognizant of the possibility and approach the patient with a line of direct questioning to establish a sense of shared decision-making in the process of utilizing alternative therapies. Particularly with the current protease inhibitors and NNRTIs, which are so intricately linked to hepatic metabolism via the cytochrome P_{450} system, it becomes even more important that providers with patients on these complex regimens are aware of all the additional substances patients are ingesting. Whether the alternatives utilize hepatic metabolism is largely unknown because of a lack of study in most instances; however, if a protease-containing regimen appears to be less effective or more toxic than expected, one might consider the possibility of a drug–drug interaction between the conventional therapy and the CAM agent.

Embarking on a line of questioning with regard to alternative therapies does take time during the patient interview session. It also requires the awareness of the provider that patients may be seeking alternative treatments. Eisenberg outlined the best mechanism for integrating questions regarding the use of alternatives into the standard medical interview. The neutrality with which the question regarding the use of CAM therapies is asked influences the honesty of the response. Eisenberg advised that it is not necessary to use a label that may be perceived as judgmental, such as "alternative," "complementary," or "unorthodox." He recommended that the alternative regimens be documented in the patient's medical record.

In 1990 Eisenberg conducted a telephone survey of 1539 adults in the United States and found that 34% reported using at least one unconventional therapy.[24] Nearly three-fourths of those using unconventional therapies did not inform their primary care provider. The greatest use of alternative agents was found among non-Blacks ages 25 to 49 years with higher education and income levels. The out-of-pocket expenditures for visits to providers of alternative interventions surpassed the out-of-pocket cost of visits to traditional primary care providers in this 1990 survey. These findings were corroborated by a subsequent similar trial.[25] A more recent telephone survey suggested that use of CAM interventions has become increasingly widespread in the United States over the past 50 years; and that once individuals commence an alternative intervention they tend to maintain the practice for years.[26] It is of note that another assessment comparing utilization of alternative therapies to conventional treatments reports a much lower percentage of Americans who actually utilize these interventions as either complementary or alternative to orthodox health care.[27] In the 1996 Medical Expenditure Panel Survey, a probability sampling of more than 16,000 adults found that an estimated 6.5% of the population made visits to both practitioners of unconventional therapies and conventional medical care: 1.8% used only unconventional services, 59.5% used only conventional care, and 32.2% used neither.[27] This study underestimated the use of CAM therapies, as it collected information only about visits to the various providers.

Numerous studies have investigated the use of alternative therapies by patients with HIV infection.[28–31] Most of this research was conducted prior to the wide availability of HAART regimens, including protease inhibitors in combination with other agents. These studies have estimated that 40% to 70% of patients with HIV infection in the United States and Europe utilize alternative therapies. In an evaluation of determinants of alternative therapy use in British Columbia, where the government pays for licensed drugs, 34% of 1019 participants noted that they had used complementary treatments.[32] Of these individuals, 53% used dietary supplements and vitamins. The users were more likely to have an AIDS diagnosis, moderate or severe pain, more educational degrees, and were not currently on antiretroviral therapies. A survey of 1049 HIV-positive women enrolled in the Women's Interagency HIV Study found that use of complementary and alternative medicine was similar in the HIV-infected women and a group of 236 HIV-negative controls.[33] Similar to findings among men, the women using alternative agents tended to be older, have higher levels of education and income, and less frequently be women of color. Chinese herbs were the most frequent drugs reported. Seventy percent of those women did not disclose their alternative drug use to their health provider.

Information obtained since the onset of the HAART era suggests that the use of CAM therapies has not declined significantly. In a study from Toronto, 100 HIV patients receiving treatment in a tertiary care hospital were asked to enumerate their current use of CAM therapies and recall their use of such agents prior to the protease inhibitor era.[34] The study was conducted in early 1998 and participants were mainly homosexual white men with a mean CD4+ T-lymphocyte count of 285 cells per cubic millimeter and an HIV RNA level of 3.5 $\log_{10}$ copies per milliliter, 85% of whom were on a protease-containing regimen at the time. Interestingly, 87% reported now using an average of 6.0 CAM therapies (range 1 to 25) compared with 67% using an average of 4.8 therapies (range 1 to 14) prior to the HAART era. Whereas in the past most reported using products to "boost immunity" (β-carotene 22%, *N*-acetylcysteine 21%, and echinacea, garlic, and ginseng 19% each), now agents are used predominantly to promote "general well-being" (vitamins 72%, marijuana 25%, zinc 24%, garlic 23%).

▲ NATIONAL CENTER FOR COMPLEMENTARY AND ALTERNATIVE MEDICINE

In 1993 the National Institutes of Health established the Office of Alternative Medicine (OAM).[35] In 1995 the office granted its first funds to investigate alternative therapies in HIV infection. Bastyr University in Seattle, a naturopathic institution, received funding to become the center for HIV alternative studies. The university established a national database cohort of HIV-infected individuals using alternative therapies.[36] They collected prevalence and follow-up information on outcome measures of patients employing a wide variety of complementary interventions. In addition, they provided seed funding to investigators conducting small pilot interventional trials in patients with HIV.

In 1998 the OAM was upgraded to the National Center for Complementary and Alternative Medicine (NCCAM).[37] The establishment of NCCAM allowed more funds to be available for the study of CAM therapies in patients with HIV. Although there is not currently an NCCAM-funded Center of Excellence for the study of CAM in HIV, the Center has awarded a number of grants to investigate promising or widely used interventions. Recognizing a growing concern, the Center has recently issued a request for proposals to investigate potential interactions between botanicals and HIV therapies. As there have already been a number of reports of possible CAM–drug interactions affecting plasma levels of antiretroviral drugs, such studies are urgently needed. The existence of this program reflects the acceptance that use of complementary therapies will continue in patients with HIV despite excellent viral suppression and evidence of immune reconstitution.

Care providers for HIV-infected individuals should be familiar with some of the common complementary and alternative agents in current use. Physicians who care for HIV- infected individuals must be familiar with these approaches for several reasons. First, about half of any HIV patient group uses them. Second, some treatments interact with standard therapies in significant ways. Third, some specific therapies have clearly been shown to do harm, whereas others could conceivably show benefit. The line between standard and alternative therapies itself has blurred. When an alternative's therapeutic value is documented, it becomes standard therapy rapidly.[38] Fourth, some "complementary" approaches, such as nutrition, exercise, and stress reduction, are logical adjuncts to therapy. Finally, because care of the HIV patient is a long-term proposal, the physician–patient relationship is paramount. When patients see that their physician is interested in the healing approaches they are pursuing, trust and rapport deepen. There is still truth to an observation made a dozen years earlier that "when health care providers take the time to get involved and learn about the panoply of alternative therapy options—including the rationales for prescribing alternative treatments, their most frequent toxicities, and the reasons patients are optimistic about their use—the resulting compassionate understanding, confidence, and trust could conceivably provide a significant therapeutic benefit itself for the individual with HIV infection."[4]

The NCCAM has provided a more concrete framework for the discussion of CAM therapies. The Center has divided the interventions into five major domains: (1) alternative medical systems; (2) mind–body interventions, (3) biologic-based therapies (herbs); (4) manipulative and body-based systems (massage); and (5) energy therapies (magnets).[39] The NCCAM categorization provides a useful framework for review of available information that currently exists on the use of these various CAM interventions in the HIV population. When data from controlled clinical trials is unavailable, a description of some widely used modalities in each category is offered.

▲ ALTERNATIVE MEDICAL SYSTEMS

Traditional Chinese Medicine (TCM) is a system of healing that has been developed over thousands of years. It is used by more than 20% of the people on our planet. It uses acupuncture, herbs, diet, and associated therapies, with an emphasis on treating the whole person rather than the disease.[40] Two individuals, each suffering with the same "disease" in Western terms, might receive different Chinese medical treatments. Each individual has unique strengths, weaknesses, imbalances, and lifelong patterns that affect how their body deals with HIV. The idea is to understand all of this and then effect changes in the underlying constitution of the individual by altering the flow of energy, or *qi*. TCM has been mysterious and ill-comprehended by Western health care practitioners until recently, when more have shown interest and received training in these approaches.

Despite this highly individualized approach of Chinese medicine, standard clinical trials have been designed to test herbal formulations and acupuncture treatments for HIV-related illness. Especially in the San Francisco Bay Area, where much traditional Chinese medicine is practiced by the large local Asian community, patients with HIV infection often seek herbal therapies or acupuncture, not as specific antiretroviral or immunomodulating interventions but most frequently to treat certain symptomatic manifestations, such as wasting, nausea, sleep disturbances, and pain. In one clinical trial, a 31-herb combination based on two preparations, Enhance and Clear Heat, was administered to patients with two or more AIDS-related symptoms. Participants were randomized to receive either 28 pills of the Chinese herbal preparation or placebo daily for 12 weeks.[41] No significant changes were seen in any of the major outcome variables studied, but there was a greater change in median life satisfaction in the herbal group. Another subsequent randomized double-blind, placebo-controlled study of standard Chinese herbs showed no difference in symptoms, quality of life, viral load, or CD4+ T-lymphocyte counts between the herb group and the placebo group.[42] The Chinese herb group had twice the frequency of gastrointestinal disturbances.

In several uncontrolled studies and anecdotal reports, formulas containing TCM ingredients such as astragalus, lingustrum, ginseng, licorice, and other Chinese herbs have shown some effectiveness against various symptoms such as fatigue, night sweats, weight loss, diarrhea, and skin rashes. In general, they did not appear to improve immune parameters or the viral load. In one pilot evaluation of an herbal formula called Source Qi, HIV patients with chronic pathogen-negative diarrhea experienced a modest, nonstatistically significant decrease in the average number of stools per day for each week of the 8-week open-label study.[43] Surprisingly, patients who were receiving nelfinavir therapy fared slightly worse than patients on other protease inhibitors. It was postulated that the increase in the known nelfinavir side effect of diarrhea could have resulted from an increased nelfinavir effect overall, perhaps due to increased nelfinavir blood levels via an herb–drug interaction. This underscores the need to obtain data on interactions of the most widely used Chinese herbs with antiretroviral agents.

Aware that acupuncture was being widely used for painful peripheral neuropathy in patients refractory to analgesics, the Community Programs for Clinical Research on AIDS designed a factorial trial of a standard acupuncture regimen and amitriptyline.[44] A total of 250 persons with HIV-related neuropathy were enrolled in the nationwide trial. There was no statistically significant difference between the two interventions with regard to the reduction of neuropathic pain, making conclusions about efficacy (or the lack thereof) of either regimen problematic. The fact that the study was conducted in the setting of a federally funded HIV clinical trials group, however, speaks for the viability of evaluating alternative therapies in the mainstream clinical research infrastructure.

▲ MIND–BODY INTERVENTIONS

Meditation and certain uses of hypnosis, prayer, and some forms of art, dance, or music therapy are considered CAM mind–body interventions. Evidence of clinical benefit has moved some of these practices from the CAM realm into mainstream medicine. Among them are cognitive-behavioral therapies and various means of stress reduction. Integration of previously alternative practices into the overall health care program is a goal of careful investigation of CAM therapies.

In a survey of CAM use in the United States during the 1990s, 7% of the survey population reported having tried some form of spiritual healing, making it the fifth most frequently used treatment.[25] Among the large survey of 1016 participants in Bastyr University's Alternative Medical Care Outcomes in AIDS (AMCOA) study, 56% reported utilizing prayer and 33% spiritual activities as alternative interventions.[36] Data from other surveys suggest that most patients have a spiritual life and regard their spiritual health as important as their physical health.[45] A number of studies have shown a direct relation between religious involvement and spirituality and positive health outcomes such as mortality, physical and mental illness, quality of life, and coping.[46] Prayer itself was shown to have a positive effect on the outcome of patients in the coronary care unit (CCU).[47] In this blinded controlled trial involving 393 subjects, hospitalized patients who were prayed for by prayer groups had outcomes superior to those who were not. A recent study of 799 coronary care patients failed to demonstrate a clinical benefit for intercessory prayer, although it differs from the earlier trial in that patients were randomized at the time of hospital discharge rather than during their CCU stay.[48] An editorial accompanying the current trial mentions "the weakness of the study is that the effect explored has no basis within the current scientific paradigm. If found to be true, such an effect would indeed challenge our understanding of the universe and perhaps even overturn much accumulated scientific knowledge to date."[49]

Despite some healthy skepticism, a systemic review of available data from randomized trials of "distant healing" found that about 57% of the 23 trials involving nearly 3000 patients did show a positive treatment effect.[50] The authors proposed that such evidence merits further study. An accepted definition of distant healing is "a conscious, dedicated act of mentation attempting to benefit another person's physical or emotional well-being at a distance."[51] A double-blind randomized trial of distant healing was conducted in 40 patients with advanced AIDS at the beginning of the HAART era.[51] Pair-matched subjects were assigned to either 10 weeks of distant healing treatment or a control group. Healers included practitioners from Christian, Jewish, Buddhist, Native American, and shamanic traditions as well as those practicing secular methods. Each subject in the distant healing group was treated by a total of 10 practitioners, and each of the 40 practitioners treated a total of five patients. Baseline CD4+ T-lymphocyte counts were less than 100 cells per cubic millimeter in both arms of the study. All patients were receiving prophylaxis for *Pneumocystis carinii* pneumonia (PCP) and 90% to 95% were on protease inhibitor-containing antiretroviral therapy regimens. At 6 months a blinded chart review found that the treatment subjects had significantly fewer AIDS-defining illnesses and required less medical attention in the form of doctor visits and hospitalizations. There was no effect on the CD4+ T-lymphocyte counts. Participants who had been in the treatment group had significantly improved mood compared with controls. The NCCAM is now funding an expanded controlled distant healing study involving 150 participants. One-third of the patients in this trial will be "healed" by nurses who have been trained as healers to assess whether the technology can be transferred.

Meditation is the practice of focusing and quieting the mind and remaining in a state of inner awareness for a period of time. It appears to be effective for lowering stress. Some use meditation or other relaxation exercises as the first step in imagery and healing visualizations.[52] Creating inner mental pictures that are focused on healing, such as imagining stronger, more numerous CD4+ T lymphocytes, infections clearing, or rashes disappearing may be a way the mind can lead the body toward healing. Work with cancer patients has suggested that such imagery has value.[53] For example, people learn to picture mentally that their tumors are shrinking or their immune cells are destroying their cancer cells. People can visualize their body growing stronger and their immune system winning out over their disease. At a minimum, these positive images help create a more hopeful attitude. Researchers in psychoneuroimmunology are trying to demonstrate a physical benefit from visualization.

▲ BIOLOGICALLY BASED THERAPIES

Herbal remedies, special diets, and food products used therapeutically (nutraceuticals) are considered biologically based in the NCCAM classification. The medicinal potential of plants and herbs cannot be ignored by even those most skeptical of alternative therapies. Many of the drugs in common use, as well as a number of potent cytotoxic chemotherapy agents, are derived from the world's flora. In a comprehensive review, 63 ingredients listed in the Chinese Materia Medica were found to have in vitro activity against HIV.[54] Such compounds included terpenes, flavinoids, polysaccharides, coumarins, tannins, lectins, quinolones, peptides, and other alkaloids. The natural substances were reported to have activity inhibiting reverse transcriptase and protease enzymes as well as interfering with infection at the viral cell entry level. In addition, the dicaffeolyquinic acids derived from Bolivian medicinal plant extracts are currently being evaluated as possible inhibitors of HIV integrase.[55]

Herbal Preparations

Hypericin is an extract from St. John's wort with reputed broad-spectrum antiviral effects against HIV, herpes, cytomegalovirus (CMV), and Epstein-Barr virus (EBV).[56] Initially, people with HIV used St. John's wort as an antiretroviral agent because of in vitro evidence that hypericin inhibits HIV replication. However, hypericin blood levels from the oral herb were less than 1/100th of the test tube levels that showed antiviral effects. A study of high intravenous doses of hypericin was terminated because participants developed hepatotoxicity and photodermatitis.[57] Although interest in St. John's wort dwindled as an antiviral agent, it skyrocketed again as an antidepressant and became widely used. Clinical trials have demonstrated effectiveness against mild to moderate depression. St. John's wort is believed to exert its effect by inhibiting reuptake of serotonin, norepinephrine, and dopamine by neurons.[58,59] Studies have shown that St. John's wort induces cytochrome P_{450} 3A4 isoform and can dramatically lower indinavir levels in healthy volunteers.[60] The indinavir area under the curve was reduced by a mean of 57%, and the extrapolated 8-hour indinavir trough was reduced by 81%. Another study demonstrated that St. John's wort lowered nevirapine levels by 20%.[61] This has led to a recommendation that anyone on protease inhibitors or NNRTIs avoid using St. John's wort. These reports serve to caution doctors and patients about unknown drug–herb interactions and heighten the need to study interactions of other frequently ingested CAM agents.

Allicin is a high-dose garlic concentrate from China, used there mainly to treat refractory diarrhea. It is generally well tolerated but does produce a strong garlic taste and smell in those who utilize it. A 6-week pilot study of intractable *Cryptosporidium parvum* diarrhea demonstrated decreased stool frequency with stable or increased weight.[62] Stools became negative for *Cryptosporidium* organisms in four of the eight patients who were on treatment for longer than 8 weeks. Garlic preparations are now also being utilized for their lipid-lowering effect in the treatment of HAART-associated hyperlidipemia. NIH researchers reported that garlic supplements sharply reduced the blood concentrations of the protease inhibitor saquinavir by 50%.[63] In a classic pharmacokinetic study, nine HIV-negative volunteers received 3 days of saquinavir and then took garlic capsules twice daily for 3 weeks. At the ensuing analysis it was found that the saquinavir levels had decreased 51%, and the average maximum concentrations had fallen 54%. Even after a 10-day washout without any further garlic supplementation, the blood levels of saquinavir still averaged 35% lower than baseline values. These findings have wide- reaching implications and again emphasize the need to evaluate carefully the potential impact of widely used CAM therapies on levels of antiretroviral agents and other conventional treatments used by patients with HIV.

There are several herbal products used by people living with HIV that are thought to stimulate the immune system, such as echinacea, viscum album (mistletoe), goldenseal, shitake and reishi mushrooms, acemannen (aloe), and garlic. Although each has a theoretical basis, with evidence of active ingredients and groups of vocal users and supporters, each still needs to be researched further in people with HIV.[64] The interactions between HIV and the immune system are so intricate that the idea of "stimulating the immune system" is an obvious oversimplification. A stimulus to CD4+ T lymphocytes might help the body fight infections or, instead, might lead to increased viral replication. Boosting certain cytokines, such as interleukin-2 (IL-2) or IL-12 may help the host, whereas boosting other cytokines, such as tumor necrosis factor-α (TNFα), may lead to disease progression. Some of these "immune-boosting" herbs may have herb–drug interactions, such as the ones mentioned above for St. John's wort and garlic, and may be contraindicated in patients on protease inhibitors and NNRTIs. Echinacea, a member of the daisy family, is widely utilized in short-term pulses as prophylaxis and treatment for upper respiratory tract infection.[58,59] Whereas immunostimulatory effects have been demonstrated with short-term use, there is concern that long-term use (> 8 weeks) may be associated with the potential for immunosuppression.[65] This theoretical concern has led some to recommend that chronic use of echinacea is contraindicated in patients with HIV infection, although no data from controlled clinical trials are available.[59] Others are concerned that the immune activation prompted by echinacea ingestion may stimulate HIV replication, although, again, data are absent.

In addition to immunomodulatory effects, some mushroom extracts may also have benefit as lipid-lowering agents.[66] The reishi mushroom (*Ganoderma lucidum*) appears to be a natural source of 3-hydroxy-3-methylglutaryl coenzyme A (HMG CoA) reductase inhibitor.[67] Cholestin, produced by red yeast fermented on rice, was briefly sold in health food stores.[68] Red yeast products have long served as dietary staples and medicines in Asia. Cholestin was found to be a natural source of the statin, mevinolin, and other compounds that inhibit HMG CoA reductase. A placebo-controlled trial of Cholestin 1.2 g twice daily led to reductions in cholesterol, low density lipoprotein (LDL)-cholesterol, and triglycerides.[69] Oyster mushrooms are also a natural source of mevinolin. Shiitake mushrooms may also have lipid-lowering and immune modulating effects. However, a clinical trial of intravenous lentinan, a shiitake mushroom extract used as an immunomodulator in Japan, had no discernible benefit in a small pilot study in HIV patients.[70] Some proponents suggest that the beneficial effects of these products are best realized when ingested by mouth as nature intended rather than being offered as parenteral pharmaceutical products.

Tea tree oil is an extract from an Australian bush (melaleuca). Melaleuca extracts are used as natural remedies and are appreciated for their broad antibiotic activities.[71] Excellent in vitro activity has been demonstrated against isolates of *Candida* species. Malaleuca products, including soaps, impregnated dental floss, toothpicks, and mouthwashes, are available over the counter in natural foods stores. Investigators reported on the results of using a malaleuca oral solution (Breathaway) in patients with refractory oral *Candida*.[72] After 4 weeks of treatment, five patients were cured, five were improved, and two had no response. A mycologic response with clearing of *Candida* was documented in 8 of 12 evaluable patients; all 8 have been clinical responders. There were no relapses perceived at 4 weeks off treatment.

Silymarin, extracted from the seeds of the milk thistle plant, has repeatedly been shown in a number of studies to help with the regeneration of liver cells damaged by exposure to chemical agents.[73] It is used to treat poisoning by *Amanita phalloides* mushrooms and has helped protect the liver from injury due to other chemicals.[74] It is being used increasingly by the CAM community to accelerate the healing of hepatitis and to lower elevated hepatic transaminases. In one study silymarin use doubled the survival rate from cirrhosis.[75] Milk thistle is particularly attractive to HIV patients co-infected with hepatitis B, hepatitis C, or both who may be at increased risk to develop transaminase elevations in response to initiation of HAART. It is usually dosed to provide the active constituent at 400 to 500 mg/day. Although patients use it to prevent antiretroviral therapy-associated hepatotoxicity, there are scant data about its potential interactions with these drugs. Animal studies show that it may have cytochrome P_{450} effects, but an older study showed it had no effect on levels of aminopyrine and phenylbutazone in humans.[76] Drug interaction data with antiretroviral agents is clearly needed.

Vitamins

Vitamin C, one of the first interventions proposed as a potential alternative therapy, continues to be consumed by a significant segment of the HIV-infected population for its potential antiviral and antioxidant activities.[4,77] During the early days of the epidemic, prior to the availability of any conventional antiviral therapies, high doses of vitamin C (up to 50 g/day) were administered by either the oral routes or intravenous infusion. The rationale was based on anecdotal observation of broad antiviral activity as well as in vitro activity demonstrated against a human retrovirus.[7,8] Patients were advised to escalate their vitamin C intake to "bowel tolerance," that is, to ingest as much ascorbate as possible, titrating the dose to intolerability of the resultant diarrhea. Enthusiasm for this intervention in the community waned when many of the early proponents of high-dose vitamin C therapy died secondary to the progression of their AIDS-related illness.

A resurgence of interest in the potential therapeutic utility of antioxidants in general and vitamin C in particular ensued following the National Institutes of Health-sponsored conference in 1990, where the biologic and clinical actions of vitamin C were reviewed.[77] Oxidative stress is postulated to be toxic to lymphocytes, potentiating the destructive effect of HIV in infected patients. Vitamin C is thought to be one of the first-line defenses against free radical damage, as well as having a potential role in preserving immune function. In vitro studies support the notion of antiretroviral activity.[7] Another potential beneficial pathway of vitamin C's activity is its ability to raise intracellular glutathione levels.[8] These data generated a new wave of ascorbate enthusiasm, reminiscent of that during the early 1980s. Community interest and further investigation of the antiretroviral potency of vitamin C has subsequently waned again, however, in the presence of new, more effective conventional antiviral treatments.

Use of vitamins and supplements is a highly individualized choice, with some patients using none and others taking literally dozens a day. In other areas of HIV medicine, consensus panels of experts have issued guidelines to assist the HIV practitioner. There is no such consensus and no expert guidelines about vitamins and supplements. Some HIV caregivers never mention these substances, whereas others devote extensive energy to them. In the absence of data from well controlled clinical trials, HIV patients are likely to benefit from a daily multivitamin, as has been recommended for the general adult population.[78] The use of supplemental vitamin E at a dose of 400 IU daily may also be offered to older patients despite a report that it offered no apparent effect on cardiovascular outcomes in 9541 high risk subjects followed for 4 to 6 years.[79]

Vitamin B deficiencies are common in individuals with HIV infection because of both poor absorption and increased need.[80] A daily multiple vitamin or vitamin B-complex dose usually has 50 mg of each of the basic B vitamins; two of these a day is a good way to overcome potential absorption problems. An observational study showed improved survival for those with increased vitamin B intake.[81] Vitamin B_{12} is unique in its poor oral uptake in patients with gastric atrophy or terminal ileum problems and can be given by injection or as a nasal gel. Studies show that up to one-third of HIV-positive people may be vitamin B_{12}-deficient.[81] There is a significant relation between high vitamin B_{12} levels in HIV-positive individuals and improved mental functioning.[82] Vitamin B_{12} replacement has been reported to help with fatigue, anemia, and central and peripheral neurologic problems. Some physicians begin treating a vitamin B_{12}-deficient person with a daily dose of 1000 μg IM, decreasing the dose to three times a week, once a week, and finally to once a month.

Anabolic Agents and Antiwasting Therapies

Testosterone and its derivatives have been used increasingly in an attempt to increase lean body mass.[83] In addition to using testosterone supplementation in the subset of patients with HIV infection who are also hypogonadal, eugonadal men have turned to supplementary testosterone to counteract wasting.[84] Intramuscular or transdermal testosterone preparations require prescription and cooperation of a primary care provider.[85] However, individuals who seek a testosterone-like benefit have been turning to dehydroepiandrosterone (DHEA), a naturally occurring adrenal steroid. DHEA was previously studied for its possible immunomodulatory and antiretroviral activity when early reports discovered that AIDS patients had depleted stores.[86] Dyner et al. enrolled 31 subjects in a 16-week Phase I dose-escalating trial.[87] No changes were seen in lymphocyte subsets or p24 antigen levels; a transient increase in serum neopterin levels was noted. Whereas these less than impressive findings in the initial Phase I study may have thwarted future clinical trials, DHEA nonetheless became a popular buyer's club item. Although the side effects observed with DHEA in the clinical trial were rare, including insomnia, fatigue, and nasal congestion, it has subsequently been noted anecdotally that women taking the preparation may develop hirsutism and deepening of the voice. A placebo-controlled trial in women with HIV, however, showed no evidence of adverse effects.[88] Half of the group of 29 women on HAART were randomly assigned to receive DHEA 50 mg/day for 6 months. They gained a mean 1.4 kg of weight compared to the placebo group participants who lost 1.2 kg and had improvement on multiple quality of life parameters. It is of note that the DHEA group experienced a CD4+ T-lymphocyte increase of 107 cells per cubic millimeter compared to a drop of 11 cells per cubic millimeter in the control group. An ongoing NCCAM-funded randomized placebo-controlled trial is currently investigating the antiviral, immunomodulatory, and body composition effects of DHEA in individuals with undetectable HIV RNA levels at baseline.

Carnitine is an amino acid that helps bring energy to muscle cells and to store calories in the body as weight. Its deficiency is thought to be part of the cause of wasting, fatigue, and increased blood triglyceride levels found with advanced HIV illness. These high triglyceride levels imply that fat is being circulated in the bloodstream but not being used as energy or stored in adipose cells. Giving 1500 mg of carnitine four times a day on an empty stomach reduced elevated triglyceride levels,[89] and symptoms of wasting and fatigue were alleviated. TNF levels were lowered in some patients, and it is thought that lowering TNF levels can slow viral replication. Carnitine reportedly helps both skeletal and heart muscle, and it is being tried for various cardiac muscle problems as well as AIDS-related and azidothymidine (AZT)-related myositis. It is available over the counter or by prescription. Carnitine and B vitamins have also been suggested as treatments for lactic acidosis and mitochondrial toxicity. An uncontrolled Dutch trial in six patients with lactic acidosis suggested benefit.[90] Prospective controlled trials are needed. L-Acetyl-carnitine has been found to be deficient in patients with peripheral neuropathy related to the dideoxy nucleoside analogue drugs.[91] A small trial of 1500 mg twice a day showed benefit with diminished symptoms and cutaneous peripheral nerve regeneration.[92]

Creatine and glutamine are other amino acid supplements utilized by patients for HIV-related manifestations. Creatine, taken in doses up to 25 g/day by weight lifters, is thought to build muscle by increasing muscle phosphocreatine, an energy source.[93] Creatine has been combined with resistance exercise as a therapy for the wasting syndrome. An NCCAM-funded randomized, placebo-controlled clinical trial is currently examining the impact of creatine supplementation on lean body mass and other viral and immune parameters in patients with HIV infection. Glutamine, also used in large doses to treat wasting, may help heal gut mucosa in chronic diarrheal states. In one randomized, placebo-controlled trial, glutamine 40 g/day plus antioxidants caused a significant increase in weight and body cell mass in wasted AIDS patients.[94]

Δ^a-Tetrahydrocannabinol (dronabinol), synthetic version of the active component of marijuana, is one of the licensed therapies available for the anorexia associated with HIV-related wasting.[95,96] Some individuals, however, prefer to inhale their cannabinoids rather than ingest them.[97] In the San Francisco Bay Area, cannabis buyer's clubs increased in number following the passage of legislation in 1996 that allowed the use of marijuana as medicine.[98] On producing a physician's letter confirming the diagnosis of one of the indicated conditions, which includes AIDS and wasting, an individual can select from a variety of vintages of marijuana to purchase for medical use. The mechanism of action of cannabinoids on appetite stimulation remains unclear. The effect may be related to increasing the sensory appeal of food or decreasing satiety.[99] It has also been suggested that the endocannabinoids may be involved in increasing the reward effects of eating.[100] Clinical trials have demonstrated that, in a controlled residential setting, individuals inhaling marijuana increased their caloric intake and weight over time.[101]

A recently completed safety trial of smoked marijuana, oral dronabinol, and dronabinol placebo in nonwasting HIV patients demonstrated significant weight gain in both cannabinoid arms compared to placebo recipients, although the study was not powered for efficacy.[102] The weight gained, however, was predominantly adipose tissue and not lean body mass.[103] Cannabinoids are metabolized by the hepatic cytochrome P_{450} system. The potential for a cannabis–antiretroviral drug interaction or a direct effect of cannabis on the immune system was the impetus for the 21-day inpatient safety study. No adverse pharmacokinetic interaction was observed in patients on a stable regimen that included indinavir or nelfinavir when they smoked marijuana cigarettes or received dronabinol 2.5 mg three times a day.[104] Nor was there evidence of an adverse effect on HIV RNA levels or immune parameters in the trial.[102] These safety results have supported plans to move forward with studies investigating the potential effectiveness of cannabis for HIV-associated peripheral neuropathy. Animal models and anecdotal data suggest that cannabinoids may provide relief from neuropathic pain when opioids have been generally ineffective.[105] The University of California Center for Medicinal Cannabis Research is currently funding a number of trials investigating the effects of smoked marijuana on HIV neuropathy.[106]

▲ MANIPULATIVE AND BODY-BASED METHODS

Chiropractic manipulation and massage are two examples of interventions in the NCCAM-delineated category of manipulative and body-based methods. Massage was cited as the third most frequently used intervention: by 54% of the 1016 first eligible participants in the AMCOA study.[36] Although many patients with HIV visit practitioners of these therapies for maintenance of general well-being or treatment of particular underlying musculoskeletal problems, few controlled studies are available. In one trial, 42 HIV-infected individuals with no active medical symptoms were evaluated in a study to access the effects of massage therapy alone or massage therapy combined with either exercise training or stress management counseling on immune function and quality of life.[107] The investigators hypothesized that immune function may become further suppressed by chronic anxiety and depression.

Patients were randomized into four groups including massage only, massage and exercise, massage and stress management, and a control group. Only the control group demonstrated an increase in CD4+ T-lymphocytes following the 12-week intervention, with the massage and exercise and massage and stress management cohorts sustaining a drop in CD4+ T-lymphocyte counts. No significant differences were found among the groups on any of the quality-of-life measures comparing pre- and poststudy values. The authors concluded that short-term massage therapy alone or combined with either exercise training or stress management counseling did not have a significant impact on immune function or quality of life measures and that "these alternative therapies, while not harmful, should not be used as substitutes for more conventional therapies for HIV infected persons."[107]

As with any attempt to investigate alternative interventions scientifically, proponents of massage therapy may question the power of the study based on the sample number enrolled, whether the appropriate massage techniques were employed, whether the appropriate patient population was investigated, and whether the correct immune parameters to monitor were chosen. Hence, as with most of the other alternatives in current widespread use, clinical results are not likely to influence those who strongly adhere to their favorite alternative intervention.

▲ ENERGY THERAPIES

Energy therapies are described as those based on activation or generation of energy fields either originating in the body or acting externally on the body. *Qi gong*, a component of Traditional Chinese Medicine, is an example of an energy therapy. Combining movement, meditation, and breathing control, the practice enhances the flow of vital energy (*qi*) with the intent to improve circulation and enhance immune function. As yet, no clinical trials evaluating energy therapies for HIV and their manifestations have been reported.

▲ CAUTIONS

Many who utilize CAM therapies automatically equate the "naturalness" of the interventions with safety. Unfortunately, in addition to the CAM–antiretroviral drug interactions described above, there are other reports of adverse effects from ingestion of a number of apparently benign CAM therapies. In addition to the protease inhibitor interaction, excessive garlic ingestion (four cloves daily) was implicated in the inhibition of platelet aggregation in an 87-year-old man with a resultant spontaneous spinal epidural hematoma.[108] A platelet aggregation defect was also thought to be responsible for bilateral spontaneous subdural hematomas in a 37-year-old woman with a 2-year history of ingesting of 120 mg of gingko biloba daily.[109] This patient's prolonged bleeding time corrected upon discontinuation of the herbal supplement. Ginsenosides are also known to inhibit platelet aggregation in vitro and prolong both prothrombin and partial thromboplastin times in rats.[59] These effects are important preoperatively in patients who may experience excessive bleeding if they do not report and discontinue their CAM interventions before surgery. Specifically, agents known to induce qualitative platelet defects—garlic, gingko, ginseng—should be discontinued at least 7 days prior to surgery.

Dietary supplements that contain ephedra alkaloids (also known as *ma huang*) are widely available and utilized for weight loss and energy enhancement.[110,111] These agents may cause significant cardiovascular side effects including hypertension, palpitations, and tachycardia. Strokes and seizures have also been reported. Ephedrine, the predominant active compound, is a noncatecholamine sympathomimetic agent that indirectly releases endogenous norepinephrine. These sympathomimetic effects are the cause of the adverse cardiovascular and central nervous system effects as well as a number of reported fatalities. The preoperative recommendation is to discontinue ephedra compounds at least 24 hours prior to surgery.[59] Other frequently used preparations that are of concern in patients undergoing surgical procedures are kava and valerian, antianxiety agents, that may potentiate the sedative effects of anesthetics by an herb–drug interaction. St. John's wort, through induction of cytochrome P_{450} 3A4 isoforms, can significantly increase the metabolism of many concomitantly administered drugs, including many that are integral to perioperative care. In addition to the surgical concerns, a comprehensive, well referenced risk–benefit profile of commonly used herbal therapies has recently been reported.[60]

▲ EVALUATING CAM THERAPIES

Ideally, it would be desirable to be able to investigate each widely used CAM therapy for its safety and effectiveness. Establishment of the NCCAM allows increased guidance and funding in this domain, but it remains a challenge to determine what CAM therapies should be investigated and how to go about studying them. Certainly agents in widespread use in the community that have biologic plausibility should be studied to determine if they truly have clinical benefit. Substances with a potential for a CAM–drug interaction with the patient's prescribed regimen should also be investigated to rule out detrimental pharmacokinetics. Although it seems that agents should be assayed to demonstrate that they have no benefit or may in fact be harmful, the history of the alternative therapies movement suggests that there are always strong proponents of the intervention who do not accept the results of a trial. They might suggest that the preparation used in the study was the wrong one, the patient population was incorrect, or there were flaws in the trial design that interfered with the interpretation of the results. The lack of standardized preparations of many CAM products does present a challenge when attempting to study the agent or reproduce the results of another investigator. One commentator lamented "how can an herb be standardized if its active ingredients are not known and there is no suitable bioassay?"[38]

NCCAM offered a Methodological Manifesto to assist investigators interested in conducting clinical trials to investigate CAM therapies.[112] The document asserts that different studies may require different methodologic and analytic approaches. It suggests that one use the strongest possible design and most appropriate statistical procedures. It does concede that clinical trials may not be the only route to take and that observational studies may provide useful information to inform the design of subsequent controlled studies. Although alternative therapies are being tested, NCCAM warns against alternative outcomes and suggests that investigators utilize standard recognized clinical trial endpoints. They believe that existing quantitative procedures should be robust enough to analyze data generated in trials of CAM interventions and that other statistical systems are generally not required. Although they claim that complex complementary medical systems could be studied as "gestalts," operationally this is a challenge to study sections used to reviewing more orthodox proposals. When asked to evaluate a proposed traditional Chinese medicine intervention for patients co-infected with HIV and hepatitis C, for example, reviewers were stymied by how to untangle the effects of the herbs from those of acupuncture or *qi gong* and how to determine which moiety of the herbal preparation was, in fact, the active part of the whole. Hence, despite all good intentions, orthodox values and mind sets of review panels may hamper rapid, increased investigation of CAM therapies. One essay suggested that even if conducted under the most rigid circumstances, results of clinical trials of CAM agents may be difficult for many conventional scientist/clinicians to embrace. The authors noted that physicians adherent to the traditions of conventional medicine, when evaluating results of studies of homeopathic interventions, for example, "reject seemingly solid evidence because it is not compatible with theory."[113]

▲ INTEGRATIVE CLINICAL APPROACH

Despite the lack of evidence-based data from controlled clinical trials, some lifestyle modification recommendations can be suggested for patients grappling with ongoing HIV infection. With all of the difficulties inherent in assaying CAM therapies, these interventions may never be supported by hard data but may emanate from common sense and clinical experience. The astute primary care provider will attempt to integrate some of these recommendations into the patient's overall therapeutic plan. The patient, in turn, may benefit from being empowered by easily being able to make these potentially salubrious lifestyle modifications.

Nutrition

Helping a patient eat an optimum diet is not easy. There is perhaps no area in lifestyle choices more complex than nutrition. Changing nutritional habits can be difficult. People living with HIV are believed to benefit from a high-protein, low-fat, nutrient-rich diet with frequent, regular meals that include fresh fruits and vegetables, rich complete proteins, and whole grains, with less sweets and less highly refined foods. A good diet for someone with HIV would have multiple protein sources such as lean meat, cheese, fish, chicken, nuts, and yogurt. A vegetarian diet, if well thought out, can also provide adequate and complete proteins to the HIV-infected individual. Strict macrobiotic diets, however, are extremely low in protein and may not be ideal for HIV-positive individuals. Several servings daily of fresh fruits, grains such as rice, whole wheat, or barley, and a variety of vegetables are also important. Small, frequent meals are generally easier to digest than a single large portion and are encouraged for this patient population.

High blood lipid levels and fat accumulation abnormalities have recently been the focus of attention, with increased focus on long-term metabolic side effects of HIV infection and its treatment. Along with inherited tendencies, the fat content and caloric excesses of what patients eat are obviously important. When patients eliminate the high-fat "fast foods" such as cheeseburgers, fries, and milk shakes and reduce the other obvious fat sources such as ice cream, butter, cream, eggs, red meat, and high-fat cheeses, significant improvement in the blood lipid level occurs.[114] Elimination of dairy products may also decrease sinus congestion, flatulence, and loose stools.

Food and beverages must also be free of pathogens. All animal products must be thoroughly cooked or pasteurized. "Safe kitchen" behavior means avoiding contact between uncooked animal products and foods that are not cooked. For example, cutting up a raw chicken on a cutting board later used for salad or fresh vegetables is not safe. "Health" foods such as raw calves' liver and raw goats' milk can carry pathogens that can be a source of significant morbidity or mortality to someone with advanced HIV disease. Gourmet delights such as sushi, rare or raw meats, raw oysters, raw egg in a caesar salad, and unpasteurized aged cheeses may be contaminated with helminths, *Yersinia*, *Salmonella*, *Escherichia coli*, *Listeria*, and other organisms. Many municipal water treatment systems do not filter appropriately to remove *Cryptosporidium parvum*. Thus knowledge about local water processing procedures can help patients, especially those with low CD4+ T-lymphocyte counts, decide on the utility of replacing tap water with bottled or filtered water.[115]

Exercise

Routine physical exercise has demonstrated value for people with HIV. For those without symptoms, vigorous regular aerobic workouts, 30 to 45 minutes three or four times per week, are excellent ways to maintain health. In the AMCOA study, 64% of the first 1016 eligible participants reported that they regularly did aerobic exercise, making it the most frequently mentioned activity.[36] Aerobic exercise conditions the heart and lungs, helps combat depression by raising endorphin levels, and in several studies actually raised the CD4+ T-lymphocyte counts slightly.[116,117] One pre-HAART study showed slower progression to AIDS and a 170% increase in CD4+ T-lymphocyte counts in a group of regular exercisers compared to controls.[118] In contrast, extreme endurance workouts, such as marathons, may be associated with a transient reduction in immune system function and reduced CD4+ T-lymphocyte counts.[119]

Resistance exercises with weights or machines help build muscle and preserve lean body mass. One study showed that regular resistance exercise also lowered elevated triglyceride levels.[120] A helpful, detailed workbook on exercise for HIV-positive patients is available.[121] Written collaboratively by AIDS activists and physicians, it discusses in detail nutrition and anabolic steroids as well. Exercise, with or without anabolic supplements, has been used to combat the HAART-associated fat redistribution syndrome.[114,122]

Substance Abuse Cessation

A central lifestyle choice for any person living with HIV is to consider dealing with any form of substance abuse. Overall health and the health of the immune system can be significantly improved when certain substances are avoided. Dealing with these substances may be the most difficult challenge an individual can face. Addiction is its own life-threatening illness.

Cigarette smoking has been correlated in HIV-positive patients with an increased incidence of low body weight, *Pneumocystis* pneumonia, bronchitis, bacterial pneumonia, thrush, and more frequent cases of cryptococcal meningitis.[123] Smoking increases the risk of cardiovascular disease, which is already high in the HIV patient, with metabolic complications such as hyperlipidemia, hypertension, and diabetes. Smoking cessation restores the lungs' ability to cleanse themselves within just a few weeks, and lung function continues to improve over months. Cardiovascular risk is reduced more slowly.

Abuse of alcohol and hard drugs leads to riskier sexual behaviors and injures the very organs (brain and liver) that are vulnerable to HIV and antiretroviral drug toxicity. Researchers at the University of Miami studied 220 HIV-positive drug abusers and found that heavy alcohol users were four times less likely to achieve a positive virologic response to HAART.[124] CD4+ T-lymphocyte counts were also lower in heavy drinkers. The use of alcohol among hepatitis C co-infected patients greatly amplifies the progression of liver disease. In vitro studies showed that cocaine use increases viral replication.[125] In practice, when patients have quit alcohol or illicit drugs, the improvement in their sense of well-being and their health has been obvious to themselves and their doctors and is reflected in improved laboratory values, including liver function tests and CD4+ T-lymphocyte counts.

Addressing Emotional and Spiritual Needs

The HIV-positive individual is challenged by emotional and spiritual issues from the time of first being tested. All the aspects of dealing with a life-threatening disease as well as all the ongoing issues of life, including career, love, sexuality, relationships, and self-worth, require attention. People living with HIV often compress decades of emotional and spiritual issues into a few short months or years. Getting involved in counseling for these issues is one of the best things an HIV-positive individual can do.

Metaphysical approaches that look for meaning and encourage self-love and self-responsibility are popular. They provide a context for looking at all these crucial issues, with emphasis on the value of positive thinking and "attitudinal healing." They may also lead to confusion between accepting responsibility for one's health and feeling guilty for being ill. The risk is to think that if what one believes can affect outcome when one is sick it must mean he or she did not "do it" right. People can come to believe that it is their fault they are sick. Attitude and belief may have power, but HIV illness is much more complex.

The books and tapes of Ram Dass, Stephen Levine, Elizabeth Kubler-Ross, Gerald Jampolsky, Bernie Siegel, and others have been widely read in the AIDS community. These authors offer possible answers in the search for inner peace, deeper meaning, and connectedness. Whether these approaches provide simply greater peace through understanding and faith or more directly affect the immune system awaits further study by psychoneuroimmunologists.

▲ CONCLUSIONS

Despite an apparent lull in the utilization of alternative therapies for HIV infection, the history of the CAM movement over the past 20 years suggests that the current phase may in fact be transient. Even with the availability of potent combination antiretroviral drug regimens, individuals with HIV infection are still interested in the use of treatments complementary to their orthodox therapies, especially for treating manifestations of HIV infection for which effective agents are not prescribed by their physicians. Obviously, pharmacokinetic interaction studies cannot be undertaken for every alternative treatment a patient with HIV infection might adopt. This increases the responsibility of the care provider to have an open, honest conversation with each patient with regard to the use of CAM agents in addition to those that have been prescribed. Careful documentation in the patient's medical record also supplies this useful information to others who may need to provide care for their patients. The possibility of hepatic damage or drug–CAM therapy interactions that may alter the concentration of antiretroviral agents, particularly protease inhibitors, increases the stakes during the current era of HIV therapeutics.

Providers should question their patients regarding the use of alternative and complementary interventions and counsel them as completely as possible regarding possible concerns. To do so effectively, caregivers must stay informed about agents in widespread use, consulting available references and resources to ensure, as much as possible, the continued well-being of patients utilizing alternative and complementary therapies for their HIV infection. There are several basic principles used when combining these alternative and complementary approaches with standard medical care in a comprehensive model.

1. *Individualize*. Each patient is unique. Each health care provider is unique. Each provider–patient relationship is unique. Both individuals need to be true to their knowledge, beliefs, experiences, and intentions. Physicians must help patients avoid treatment envy. (Look what "they" are doing, let's try that.) Both must avoid treatment bashing. (It didn't work for "them," so why waste time and money?)

2. *Relationship*. Help create with your patients a trusting, mutually respectful, collaborative relationship. Facilitate honest communication both ways. Together, clarify goals, plans, and revisions frequently. Imagine a scenario in which the doctor focuses just on the goal of making the viral load undetectable for the long term and the patient focuses just on the goal of improving quality of life today. This is a setup for misunderstanding, distrust, and disagreement, all spelling "poor adherence."

3. *Consumer beware*. Educate patients about for the red flags of fraud: the use of the word "cure," phrases such as "it's only available outside the country," "its contents are secret," "it heals different things such as AIDS, cancer, aging, and arthritis," "there is only one source of this treatment," and "there is a conspiracy to suppress this therapy." The Federal Task Force on AIDS Fraud warns that "when something sounds too good to be true, it usually is."

4. *Nonexclusivity*. There is no a priori reason modern medical care must exclude CAM. It is not an either/or situation. It can be both. A recent men's exercise magazine headline read "Exercise rivals AZT." They are not rivals, they are complementary. Physicians without knowledge of an alternative modality may discourage its use simply because it is unfamiliar. An alternative practitioner might down play the value of standard medical care as not holistic or discourage the use of Western medications by labeling them "toxic" or "unnatural." Health care providers' egos and defensiveness should not create such barriers. The practitioner in any field, alternative or mainstream, who says, "For this to work you have to stop all your other therapies" is robbing his or her patients of a comprehensive approach. Many individuals combine different modalities into an optimal health plan.

5. *Hopefulness*. Years ago pioneer AIDS activist Michael Callen described the one common link in the long-term survivors he interviewed. It was hope. At the news from one particularly pessimistic International AIDS Conference a decade ago, the death rate in San Francisco jumped significantly. Today in the epidemic, with rapidly expanding knowledge of pathogenesis, improved technology to measure viral load and drug resistance, potent and more user-friendly antiretroviral regimens, and complementary medical approaches, there are indeed many reasons to truly be hopeful.

REFERENCES

1. Eisenberg DM, Kessler RC, Foster C, et al. Unconventional medicine in the United States: prevalence, costs and patterns of use. N Engl J Med 328:246, 1993.
2. Abrams DI. Dealing with alternative therapies for HIV. In: Sande MA, Volberding P (eds) The Medical Management of AIDS, 5th ed. Philadelphia, WB Saunders, 1997, p 143.
3. Abrams DI. Alternative therapies. In: Repoza NP (ed) HIV Infection and Disease: Monographs for Physicians and Other Health Care Workers. Chicago, AMA Press, 1989, p 163.
4. Abrams DI. Alternative therapies in HIV infection. AIDS 4:1179, 1990.
5. Abrams DI. Dealing with alternative therapies for HIV. In: Sande MA, Volberding P (eds) The Medical Management of AIDS, 4th ed. Philadelphia, WB Saunders, 1995, p 183.
6. Abrams DI. Alternative therapies. In: Wormser G (ed) A Clinical Guide to AIDS and HIV. Philadelphia, Lippincott-Raven, 1996, p 379.
7. Harakeh S, Jariwalla RJ, Pauling L. Suppression of human immunodeficiency virus replication by ascorbate in chronically and acutely infected cells. Proc Natl Acad Sci USA 87:7245, 1990.
8. Jariwalla RJ, Harakeh S. HIV suppression by ascorbate and its enhancement by glutathione precursor (PO-B-3697). In: Abstracts of the Eight International Conference on AIDS, Amsterdam, 1992, vol 2, p B207.
9. Mills BL. Stimulation of T-cellular immunity by cutaneous application of dinitrochlorobenzene. J Am Acad Dermatol 6:1089, 1986.
10. Stricker RB, Elswood BF, Abrams DI. Dendritic cells and dinitrochlorobenzene (DNCB): a new treatment approach to AIDS. Immunol Lett 29:191, 1991.
11. Stricker RB, Elswood BF. Topical dinitrochlorobenzene in HIV disease. J Am Acad Dermatol 28:796, 1993.
12. Fischl MA, Richman DD, Hansen N, et al. Azidothymidine (AZT) in the treatment of patients with AIDS and AIDS-related complex: a double-blind, placebo-controlled trial. N Engl J Med 317:185, 1987.
13. Fischl MA, Richman DD, Hansen N, et al. The safety and efficacy of zidovudine (AZT) in the treatment of subjects with mildly symptomatic human immunodeficiency virus type 1 (HIV) infection: a double-blind, placebo trial. Ann Intern Med 112:727, 1990.
14. Volberding PA, Lagakos SW, Koch MA, et al. Zidovudine in asymptomatic human immunodeficiency virus infection: a controlled trial in persons with fewer than 500 CD4-positive cells per cubic millimeter. N Engl J Med 322:941, 1990.
15. Cooley TP, Kunches LM, Saunders CA, et al. Once-daily administration of 2,3-dideoxyinosine (ddl) in patients with acquired immunodeficiency syndrome or AIDS-related complex: results of a phase I trial. N Engl J Med 322:1340, 1990.
16. Lambert JS, Seidlin N, Reichman RC, et al. 2, 3-Dideoxyinosine (ddl) in patients with the acquired immunodeficiency syndrome or AIDS-related complex: a phase I trial. N Engl J Med 322:1333, 1990.
17. Aboulker JR, Swart AM. Preliminary analysis of the Concorde trial. Lancet 341:889, 1993.
18. Concorde Coordinating Committee. Concorde: MRC/ANRS randomised double-blind controlled trial of immediate and deferred zidovudine in symptom-free HIV infection. Lancet 343:871, 1994.
19. Eron JJ, Benoit SL, Jemsek J, et al. Treatment with lamivudine, zidovudine, or both in HIV-infected patients with 200 to 500 CD4+ cells per cubic millimeter. N Engl J Med 333:1662, 1995.
20. Kitchen VS, Skinner C, Ariyoshi K, et al. Safety and efficacy of saquinavir in HIV infection. Lancet 345:952, 1995.
21. Markowitz M, Saag M, Powderly WG, et al. A preliminary study of retonavir, an inhibitor of HIV-1 protease, to treat HIV-1 infection. N Engl J Med 333:1534, 1995.
22. Danner SA, Carr A, Leonard JM, et al. A short term study of the safety, pharmacokinetics, and efficacy of ritonavir, an inhibitor of HIV-1 protease. N Engl J Med 333:1528, 1995.
23. Gulick R, Mellors J, Havlir D, et al. Potent and sustained antiretroviral activity of indinavir in combination with zidovudine and lamivudine. N Engl J Med 337:734, 1997.
24. Eisenberg DM. Advising patients who seek alternative medical therapies. Ann Intern Med 127:61, 1997.
25. Eisenberg DM, Davis RB, Ettner SL, et al. Trends in alternative medicine use in the United States, 1990–1997: results of a follow-up national survey. JAMA 280:1569, 1998.
26. Kessler RC, Davis RB, Foster DF, et al. Long-term trends in the use of complementary and alternative medical therapies in the United States. Ann Intern Med 135:262, 2001.
27. Druss BG, Rosenheck RA. Association between use of unconventional therapies and conventional medical services. JAMA 282:651, 1999.
28. Greenblatt RM, Hollander H, McMaster JR, et al. Polypharmacy among patients attending an AIDS clinic: utilization of prescribed, unorthodox, and investigational treatments. J Acquir Immune Defic Syndr 4:136, 1991.
29. Anderson WH. Patient use and assessment of conventional and alternative therapies for HIV infection and AIDS. AIDS 74:561, 1993.

30. Dwyer JT, Salvato-Schille AM, Coulston A, et al. The use of unconventional remedies among HIV-positive men living in California. J Assoc Nurses AIDS Care 6:17, 1995.
31. De Visser R, Ezzy D, Bartos M. Alternative or complementary? Nonallopathic therapies for HIV/AIDS. Altern Ther 6:44, 2000.
32. Ostrow M, Cornelisse PGA, Hogg RS, et al. Determinants of complementary therapy use in HIV-infected individuals receiving antiretroviral or anti-opportunistic agents. J Aquir Immune Defic Syndr 15:115, 1997.
33. Berrier J, Young M, Barkan S, et al. Use of complementary/alternative therapies by HIV+ women: the Women's Interagency HIV Study (WIHS). In: Abstracts of the International Conference on AIDS, Vancouver, 1996, vol 2, p 424.
34. Waring V, Tseng A, Salit IE. Complementary therapy: changes in patterns of use among HIV clinic patients. In: Abstracts of the XIIth International Conference on AIDS, Geneva, 1998, p 849, abstract 42379.
35. Marwick C. Alternative medicine office urged to act rapidly. JAMA 270:1409, 1993.
36. Greene KB, Berger J, Reeves C, et al. Most frequently used alternative and complementary therapies and activities by participants in the AMCOA study. J Assoc Nurses AIDS Care 10:60, 1999.
37. http://nccam.nih.gov.
38. Goldman P. Herbal medicines today and the roots of modern pharmacology. Ann Intern Med 135:594, 2001.
39. Gertz MA, Bauer BA. Caring (really) for patients who use alternative therapies for cancer. J Clin Oncol 19:4346, 2001.
40. Cohen MR. Review of HIV-related traditional chinese medicine research. In: Standish LJ, Galantino ML, Calabrese C (eds) AIDS and Complementary and Alternative Medicine: Current Science and Practice. Edinburgh, Churchill-Livingstone, 2002.
41. Burack JH, Cohen MR, Hahn JA, et al. A pilot randomized controlled trial of Chinese herbal treatment for HIV-associated symptoms. J Acquir Immune Defic Syndr 12:386, 1996.
42. Weber R, Christen L, Loy M, et al. Randomized, placebo controlled trial of Chinese herb therapy for HIV-1 infected individuals. J Acquir Immune Defic Syndr 22:56, 1999.
43. Cohen MR, Mitchell TF, Bacchetti P, et al. Use of a Chinese herbal medicine for treatment of HIV-associated pathogen-negative diarrhea. Integrative Med 2:79, 1999.
44. Shlay JC, Chaloner K, Max MB, et al. Acupuncture and amitriptylene for pain due to HIV related peripheral neuropathy. JAMA 280:1590, 1998.
45. Mueller PS, Plevak DJ, Rummans TA. Religious involvement, spirituality and medicine: implications for clinical practice. Mayo Clin Proc 76:1225, 2001.
46. Gunderson L. Faith and healing. Ann Intern Med 132:169, 2000.
47. Byrd RC. Positive therapeutic effects of intercessory prayer in a coronary care unit population. South Med J 81:826, 1988.
48. Aviles JM, Whelan E Sr, Hernke DA, et al. Intercessory prayer and cardiovascular disease progression in a coronary care population: a randomized controlled trial. Mayo Clin Proc 76:1192, 2001.
49. Koenig HG. Religion, spirituality and medicine: how are they related and what does it mean? Mayo Clin Proc 76:1189, 2001.
50. Astin JA, Harkness E, Ernst E. The efficacy of "distant healing": a systemic review of randomized trials. Ann Intern Med 132:903, 2000.
51. Sicher F, Targ E, Moore D, Smith HS. A randomized double-blind study of the effect of distant healing in a population with advanced AIDS: report of a small scale study. West J Med 169:356, 1998.
52. Rossman ML, Bressler DE. Imagery and guided imagery. In: A Textbook of Complementary and Alternative Medicine. Baltimore, Williams & Wilkins, 1999.
53. Simonton OC, Mathews-Simonton S, Creighton J. Getting Well Again. Los Angeles, JP Tarcher, 1978.
54. Chang RY, Kong XB. Meta-survey of plant and herb material as treatment for HIV. In: Abstracts of the XIth International Conference on AIDS, Vancouver, 1996, vol 1, p 22, abstract Mo.B.303.
55. Hazuda D, Blau C, Felock P, et al. Isolation and characterization of a novel class of human immunodeficiency virus integrase inhibitors from natural produce screening . In: Abstracts of the XIth International Conference on AIDS, Vancouver, 1996, vol 1, p 58, abstract Mo.A.1020.
56. Lavie G, Valentine F, Levin B, et al. Studies of the mechanisms of action of the antiretroviral agents hypericin and pseudohypericin. Proc Natl Acad Sci USA 86:5963, 1989.
57. Gulick RM, McAuliffe V, Holden-Wiltse J, et al. Phase I studies of hypericin, the active compound in St. John's wort, as an antiretroviral agent in HIV-infected adults: AIDS Clinical Trials Group Protocols 150 and 258. Ann Intern Med 130:510, 1999.
58. Ang-Lee MK, Moss J, Yuan C-S. Herbal medicines and perioperative care. JAMA 286:208, 2001.
59. Ernst E. The risk-benefit of commonly used herbal therapies: ginkgo, St. John's wort, ginseng, echinacea, saw palmetto and kava. Ann Intern Med 136:42, 2002.
60. Piscitelli SC, Burstein AH, Chaitt D, et al. Indinavir concentrations and St. John's wort. Lancet 355:547, 2000.
61. De Maat MMR, Hoetelmans RMW, van Gorp ECM, et al. A potential interaction between St. John's wort and nevirapine? Presented at the First International Workshop on Clinical Pharmacology of HIV Therapy, The Netherlands, 2000, abstract 2.8.
62. Searchlight Alliance. Allicin in *Cryptosporidium* Diarrhea. Searchlight, Los Angeles, Spring 1994.
63. Piscatelli SC, Burwtein AH, Welden N, et al. The effect of garlic supplements on the pharmacokinetics of saquinavir. Clin Infect Dis 34:234, 2001.
64. Barrett B, Kiefer D, Rabago D. Assessing the risks and benefits of herbal medicine: an overview of scientific evidence. Altern Ther 5:40, 1999.
65. Boullata JI, Nace AM. Safety issues with herbal medicine. Pharmacotherapy 20:257, 2000.
66. http://www.fungiperfecti.com.
67. Komodo Y, Shimizu M, Sonoda Y, Sato Y. Ganodermic acid and its derivatives as cholesterol synthesis inhibitors. Chem Pharm Bull (Tokyo) 37:531, 1989.
68. Havel RJ. Dietary supplement or drug? The case of cholestin. Am J Clin Nutr 69:175, 1999.
69. Heber D, Yip I, Ashley JM, et al. Cholesterol-lowering effects of a proprietary Chinese red-yeast-rice dietary supplement. Am J Clin Nutr 69:231, 1999.
70. Abrams DI, Greco M, Wong R, et al. Results of a phase I/II placebo-controlled dose finding pilot study of lentinan in patients with HIV infection. Presented at the Sixth International Conference on AIDS, San Francisco, vol 3, 1990, p 207.
71. Allen P. Tea tree oil: the science behind the antimicrobial hype. Lancet 358:1245, 2001.
72. Vasquez JA, Vaishampayan J, Arganoza MT, et al. Use of an over-the-counter product, Breathaway AE (Melaleuca oral solution) as an alternative agent for refractory oropharyngeal candidiasis in AIDS patients. In: Abstracts of the XIth International Conference on AIDS, Vancouver, 1996, vol 2, p 109, abstract We.B.3305.
73. Saller R, Meier R, Brignoli R. The use of silymarin in the treatment of liver diseases. Drugs 61:2035, 2001.
74. Palasciano G, Portincasa P, Palmieri V, et al. The effect of silymarin on plasma levels of malondialdehydein in patients receiving long-term treatment with psychotropic drugs. Curr Ther Res 55:537, 1994.
75. Ferenci P, Dragosics B, Dittrich H, et al. Randomized controlled trial of silymarin treatment in patients with cirrhosis of the liver. J Hepatol 9:105, 1989.
76. Leber HW, Knauff S. Influence of silymarin on drug metabolizing enzymes in rats and man. Arzneimittelforshung 26:1603, 1976.
77. Block G, Henson DE, Levine M. Vitamin C: a new look. Ann Intern Med 114:909, 1991.
78. Willett WC, Stampfer MJ. What vitamins should I be taking, doctor? N Engl J Med 345:1819, 2001.
79. Heart Outcomes Prevention Evaluation Study Investigators. Vitamin E supplementation and cardiovascular events in high-risk patients. N Engl J Med 342:154, 2000.
80. Tang AM, Smit E. Selected vitamins in HIV infection.: a review. AIDS Patient Care STDS 12:263, 1998.
81. Piscitelli SC. Use of complementary medicines by patients with HIV: Full sail into uncharted waters. Medscape HIV/AIDS 6(3), 2000. (www.medscape.com/Medscape?HIV/journal/2000/v06.n03/mha0605.pisc/mhao6o5.pisc-01.html).
82. Shor-Posner G, Campa A, Wilkie F, et al. Increased cobalamin levels are associated with better cognitive function in HIV disease. In: Abstracts of the XIIth International Conference on AIDS, Geneva, 1998, p 865, abstract 42359.
83. Bhasin S, Storer T, Strakova J, et al. Testosterone increases lean body mass, muscle size and strength in hypogonadal men. Clin Res 42:74A, 1991.

84. Dobs AS, Dempsy MA, Landenson PW, et al. Endocrine disorders in men infected with HIV. Am J Med 84:611, 1988.
85. Place VA, Atkinson L, Prather DA, et al. Transdermal testosterone replacement through genital skin. In: Nieschlag E, Behre HM (eds) Testosterone: Action, Deficiency, Substitution. Berlin, Springer-Verlag, 1990, p 165.
86. Merril CR, Harrington MG. Plasma dehydroepiandrosterone levels in HIV infection. JAMA 261:1149, 1989.
87. Dyner TS, Lang W, Geaga J, et al. An open-label dose-escalation trial of oral dehydroepiandrosterone tolerance and pharmacokinetics in patients with HIV disease. J Acquir Immune Defic Syndr 6:459, 1993.
88. Ulmar S, Feleke G, Roginsky MS. Effect of dehydroepiandrosterone (DHEA) on clinical and laboratory parameters in female patients with AIDS. In: Abstracts of the XIIth International Conference on AIDS, Geneva, 1998, p 848, abstract 42373.
89. Di Simone C, Tzantzoglu S, Famularo G, et al. High dose L-carnitine improves immunologic and metabolic parameters in AIDS patients. Immunopharmacol Immunotoxicol 15:1, 1993.
90. Brinkman K, Vrouenraets SME, van der Meer J, et al. Treatment of lactic acidosis. Presented at the 2nd International Workshop on Adverse Drug Reactions and Lipodystrophy in HIV, Toronto, 2000, abstract P15.
91. Famularo G, Moretti S, Marcellini S, et al. Acetyl-carnitine deficiency in AIDS patients with neurotoxocity on treatment with antiretroviral nucleoside analogs. AIDS 11:185, 1997.
92. Hart AM, Terenghi G, Johnson M. L-Acetyl carnitine therapy in HIV associated peripheral neuropathy: a quantitative immunohistochemical study of cutaneous innervation. Presented at the 2nd International Workshop on Adverse Drug Reactions and Lipodystrophy in HIV, Toronto, 2000, abstract P45.
93. Casey A, Constantin-Teodosiu D, Howell S, et al. Creatine ingestion favorably affects performance and muscle metabolism during maximal exercise in humans. Am J Physiol 271:E31, 1996.
94. Shabert J, Winslow C, Shabert JK. Glutamine/antioxidant supplementation promotes gain in body cell mass in HIV patients with weight loss. In: Abstracts of the XIIth International Conference on AIDS, Geneva, 1998, p 841, abstract 42336.
95. Gorter R, Seefried M, Volberding P. Dronabinol effects on weight in patients with HIV infection. AIDS 6:127, 1992.
96. Struwe M, Kaemfper SH, Geiger CF, et al. Effect of dronabinol on nutritional status in HIV infection. Ann Pharmacol 27:827, 1993.
97. Grinspoon L, Bakalar JB, Doblin R. Marijuana as medicine: a plea for reconsideration. JAMA 273:1875, 1995.
98. Kassirer JP. Federal foolishness and marijuana. N Engl J Med 336:366, 1997.
99. Hollister LE. Hunger and appetite and single doses of marijuana, alcohol, and dextroamphetamine. Clin Pharmacol Ther 12:44, 1971.
100. Mechoulam R. Role of Endocannabinoid Receptors in Health. Presented at the NIDA Workshop on Clinical Consequences of Marijuana, Rockville, MD, 2001, p 17.
101. Greenberg I, Kuenhle J, Mendelson JH, et al. Effects of marijuana use on body weight and caloric intake in humans. Psychopharmacology 49:79, 1976.
102. Abrams D, Leiser R, Shade S, et al. Short-term safety of cannabinoids in HIV patients. In: Abstracts of the 8th Conference on Retroviruses and Opportunistic Infections, Chicago, 2001, p 269, abstract 744.
103. Mulligan K, Abrams DI, Leiser RL, Schambelan M. Body composition changes in HIV-infected men consuming self-selected diets during a placebo-controlled inpatient study of cannabinoids. In: Abstracts of the 8th Conference on Retroviruses and Opportunistic Infections, Chicago, 2001, p 238, abstract 647.
104. Kosel BW, Aweeka FT, Benowitz NL, et al. The effects of cannabinoids on the pharmacokinetics of indinavir and nelfinavir. AIDS 16:543, 2002.
105. National Institutes of Health (NIH) Workshop on the Medical Utility of Marijuana. Report to the Director. Washington, DC. http://www.medmjscience.org/Pages/reports/nihpt3.html, 1997.
106. http://www.cmcr.ucsd.edu.
107. Birk TJ, MacArthur RD, McGrady A, et al. Lack of effect of 12 weeks of massage therapy on immune function and quality of life in HIV-infected persons. In: Abstracts of the XIth International Conference on AIDS, Vancouver, 1996, vol 2, p 270, abstract Th.B.4105.
108. Rose KD, Croissant PD, Parliament CF, Levin MB. Spontaneous spinal epidural hematoma with associated platelet dysfunction from excessive garlic ingestion: a case report. Neurosurgery 26:880, 1990.
109. Rowin J, Lewis SL. Spontaneous bilateral subdural hematomas associated with chronic *Ginkgo biloba* ingestion. Neurology 46:1775, 1996.
110. Haller CA, Benowitz NL. Adverse cardiovascular and central nervous system events associated with dietary supplements containing ephedra alkaloids. N Engl J Med 343:1833, 2000.
111. Samenuk D, Link MS, Homoud MK, et al. Adverse cardiovascular events temporally associated with ma huang, an herbal source of ephedrine. Mayo Clin Proc 77:12, 2002.
112. Levin JS, Glass TA, Kushi LH, et al. Quantitative methods in research on complementary and alternative medicine: a methodological manifesto; NIH Office of Alternative Medicine. Med Care 35:1079, 1997.
113. Vandenbroucke JP, de Craen AJM. Alternative medicine: a "mirror image" for scientific reasoning in conventional medicine. Ann Intern Med 135:507, 2001.
114. Bellos N. HIV lipodystrophy with exercise works best, AIDS Alert 15:10, 126, 2000.
115. Eisenberg JNS, Wade TJ, Charles S, et al. Risk factors in HIV-associated diarrhoeal disease: the role of drinking water, medication and immune status. Epidemiol Infect 128:73, 2001.
116. LaPerriere A. Klimas N, Fletcher M, et al. Changes in CD4+ cell enumeration following aerobic exercise training in HIV-1 disease: possible mechanisms and practical applications. Int J Sports Med 18(suppl 1):S56, 1997.
117. Stringer WW, Berezovskaya M, O'Brien WA, et al. The effect of exercise training on aerobic fitness, immune indices and quality of life in HIV+ patients. Med Sci Sports Exerc 30:11, 1998.
118. Mustafa T. Association between exercise and HIV disease progression on a cohort of homosexual men. Ann Epidemiol 9:127, 1999.
119. Pizza FX, Flynn MG, Sawyer T, et al. Run training versus cross-training: effect of increased training on circulating leukocyte subsets. Med Sci Sports Exerc 27:355, 1995.
120. Yarasheski K, Tebas P, Stanerson B, et al. Resistance exercise training reduces hypertriglyceridemia in HIV infected men treated with antiviral treatment. Presented at the 7th Conference on Retroviruses and Opportunistic Infections, San Francisco, 2000, abstract 54.
121. Mooney M , Nelson V. Built to Survive: A Comprehensive Guide to the Medical Use of Anabolic Steroids, Nutrition and Exercise for HIV(+) Men and Women. PoWeR: Program for Wellness Restoration, Houston, 2000.
122. Roubenoff R. A pilot study of exercise training to reduce truncal fat in adults with HIV-associated fat redistribution. AIDS 13:1373, 1999.
123. Nemecheck PM, Stolifer J. A retrospective study on the effect of smoking on total body weight and body cell mass. Presented at the XII International Conference on AIDS, Geneva, 1998, abstract 42340.
124. Miguez MJ, Burbano X, Morales G, Shor-Posner G. Alcohol use and HIV infection in the HAART era. Am Clin Lab 20:20, 2001.
125. Roth MD, Tashkin DP, Choi R, et al. Cocaine enhances human immunodeficiency virus replication in a model of severe combined immunodeficient mice implanted with human peripheral blood leukocytes. J Infect Dis 185:701, 2002.

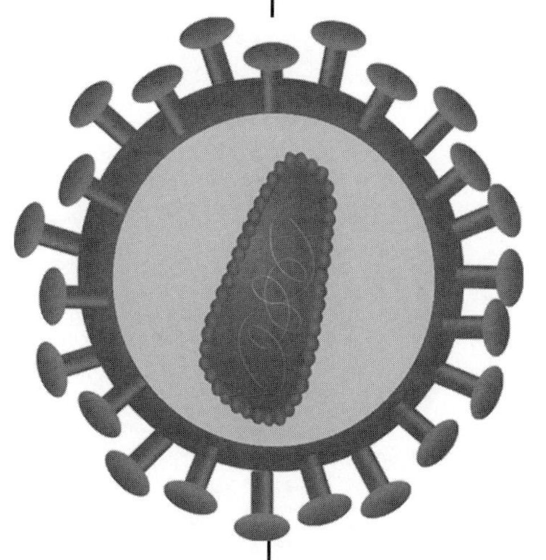

SECTION V

Strategies for Managing Antiretroviral Therapies

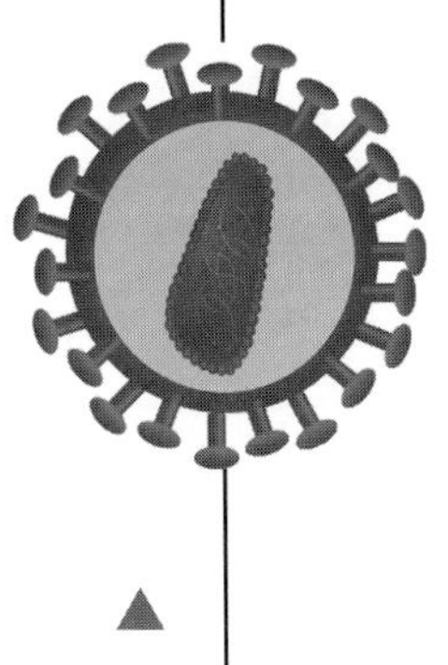

CHAPTER 24

Acute HIV Infection

Gregory K. Robbins, MD, MPH
Bruce D. Walker, MD

Acute human immunodeficiency virus (HIV) infection is associated with a transient symptomatic viral syndrome that occurs at the time of the initial high level of HIV replication following exposure to the virus. Most newly infected individuals develop this syndrome, and as a result most seek medical care, but only a small fraction are appropriately diagnosed. As with many other acute viral illnesses, the symptoms are nonspecific and mimic acute mononucleosis syndrome or acute influenza infection.[1] Recognition and treatment of HIV infection at this early stage of infection appears to have important implications not only in terms of potential reduction of viral transmission at the time when viral load is at its highest[2] but also because an increasing body of data suggests that early lowering of the viral load may augment HIV-specific immune function[3–5] and lead to enhanced immune control of viremia.[6] This chapter reviews the pathogenesis of the acute HIV syndrome and discusses issues related to the timely diagnosis of this illness, including data regarding the effects of treatment at this early stage of infection.

▲ EPIDEMIOLOGY OF ACUTE INFECTION

The expanding HIV pandemic has resulted in more than 50 million infections worldwide, with more than 16,000 new cases occurring every day.[7] In the United States there are more than 40,000 new infections each year, and most of these persons are ill enough to seek consultation with a health care provider.[8] Present trends in the epidemic in the United States suggest that new infections occur disproportionately in persons of color and, increasingly, among women as a result of both heterosexual transmission and injection drug use. Unfortunately, the failure to consider this diagnosis and the nonspecific nature of the presenting symptoms result in an appropriate diagnosis in only a fraction of such cases. In developing countries, the challenge of recognizing acute HIV infection is further confounded by poor access to medical care and to appropriate diagnostic tests and by a broader differential diagnosis for associated symptoms. The importance of recognizing persons with acute infection is underscored by data that newly infected individuals, in whom the viral load is extremely high, may be responsible for up to half of all new infections[9,10] and by data suggesting that early therapy can augment HIV-specific immune function.[3,6] Rising rates of sexually transmitted diseases other than HIV in recent years are likely to contribute to the increase in new HIV infections.[11–14]

▲ TRANSMISSION

Most HIV transmissions worldwide occur across a genital mucosal surface,[15] although acute infection has also been documented following oral sex,[8,16] and injection drug use continues to be responsible for large numbers of new cases. Soon after HIV was identified as the cause of acquired immunodeficiency syndrome (AIDS), virus was isolated from the semen of a man with asymptomatic HIV infection,[17] and it shortly thereafter was shown to be present in the female genital tract of infected persons.[18,19] Even after prolonged treatment with highly active antiretroviral therapy (HAART), virus remains detectable in the blood as well as in the male and female genital tracts.[20,21]

Detailed studies in animal models of AIDS virus infections have provided insights into the earliest events of transmission, including the earliest target cells.[22] Virus is transmitted either as free virus or as cell-associated virus, and the risk of transmission is closely linked to the viral load, for both sexual transmission and mother-to-child transmission.[2,23–26] The earliest target cell for the virus is thought to be the tissue Langerhans cell.[22] This dendritic cell (DC) expresses a recently described integrin termed DC-SIGN, which is a dendritic cell-specific C-type lectin.[27,28] It is thought that DC-SIGN stabilizes the virus and protects it from proteolytic degradation,[29] and the DC traffics with the virus to the regional lymph node. DC-SIGN is not a receptor for the virus; instead, it promotes efficient infection of cells that express CD4 and chemokine co-receptors. Within a few days, virus replicates in the regional lymph nodes, and within 4 to 11 days of mucosal entry it is widely disseminated to the brain, spleen, and gut associated lymphoid tissue (GALT). This leads to a period of intense viral replication that is likely responsible for the symptomatic phase of acute infection, as the immune system begins to contain the viremia. Viral loads in the plasma in excess of 90 million RNA molecules per milliliter of plasma have been documented during this stage of infection,[6] a number far in excess of what is typically reported during the chronic phase of infection.[30] Despite the particularly robust virus replication at this time in acute infection, standard antibody tests are usually still negative.

Acquisition of acute HIV infection is facilitated by breaks in the mucosal barrier or inflammation, such as occur with genital ulcer disease, urethritis, and cervicitis.[31–34] These conditions likely contribute to the more widespread epidemics in populations with a high incidence of genital ulcer disease, such as Sub-Saharan Africa. Drug treatment, such as the use of progesterone, can cause thinning of the vaginal epithelium and promote transmission in animal models of acute AIDS virus infection.[35] Nonoxynol 9 has also been shown paradoxically to increase the risk of HIV transmission, and this is thought to be due to vaginal irritation and ulceration.[36] Furthermore, nonoxynol 9 may increase epithelial production of the proinflammatory mediators, interleukin-1 (IL-1) and nuclear factor κB (NF-κB). These cytokines in turn trigger macrophage production of macrophage inflammatory protein-1α/β (MIP-1α/β) and tumor necrosis factor-α (TNF-α), which recruit additional neutrophils and macrophages and may lead to more efficient HIV transmission.[37]

An increased incidence of mastitis may result in increased transmission of virus in breast milk, which promotes acute infection in newborns.[38,39] On the other hand, male circumcision may diminish transmission.[2,40] Genetic factors also influence transmission (e.g., genetic polymorphisms in cell surface co-receptors that affect the ability to become infected) and the type of virus transmitted.[41] Viral entry requires binding of the envelope glycoprotein to the CD4 molecule as well as a chemokine co-receptor.[42] Studies of clade B virus, the dominant viral strain in the United States and Europe, indicate that most acute infections are mediated by R5 viruses (so designated because they prefer CCR5 as the co-receptor[43]). A homozygous 32-basepair deletion in the CCR5 molecule results in a markedly impaired ability of cells to be infected by R5 viruses and in a decreased rate of progression of the disease. In contrast, these persons can still be infected with X4 strains of virus that use the CXCR4 chemokine receptor to gain entry into cells.[44] However, these persons typically remain uninfected even after repeated exposures, as R5 strains of virus seem to be the most important infecting strains, and X4 viruses are rarely transmitted. Heterozygosity for the 32-basepair deletion in CCR5 results in retardation of disease progression but still allows the initial infection to be established.[45] Whether these co-receptor polymorphisms result in different peak levels of initial viremia or modulation of symptoms during the acute syndrome is not yet clear. However, recently increased production of RANTES has been shown to correlate with initially more explosive viral replication followed by a slower disease progression.[46]

The level of viremia in the transmitter is also a factor in transmission. Epidemiologic tracing suggests that HIV transmission can occur a few days before the onset of clinical symptoms in persons with acute HIV infection, at a time when the viral load is usually rapidly increasing.[47,48] The importance of the viral load for transmission is also underscored by studies showing that acquisition of HIV infection during pregnancy,[49] with resultant high-level viremia in the mother, results in the highest risk of perinatal transmission.[50] Cesarean delivery in women with viral loads of more than 1000 copies per milliliter may decrease the risk of transmission.[51,52] HIV transmission through breastfeeding also occurs,[38,39,53] and the risk may be higher in women who acquire HIV infection while breastfeeding. Viral load has an incremental impact on transmission, and individuals with viral loads of more than 50,000 copies per milliliter have a more than 50-fold increased risk per sex act of transmitting the virus.[2] However, transmission has also been documented prior to detectable HIV RNA in the serum.[164,164a]

Persons who have been highly exposed to HIV and yet remain seronegative suggest the possibility that transmission can lead to abortive infection in some cases,[54] but this remains highly controversial. Clearance has been reported in children who have had documented HIV-1 perinatal transmission.[55] HIV-specific immune responses in the absence of detectable virus have been found in some situations, particularly in cohorts of highly exposed sex workers.[56–58] However, there are no convincing data to indicate that the observed immune responses are a result of transient infection.[59] It is possible that exposure to noninfectious viral proteins in these cases leads to induction of immune responses, perhaps through cross-presentation by dendritic cells.[60] It has been shown in vitro that noninfectious HIV can be processed and presented within uninfected cells to induce cytotoxic T-lymphocytes,[61] which supports a model of immunologic priming in these persons. However, longitudinal studies now show that these exposed but uninfected persons are still susceptible to subsequent infection.[62] Understanding early events in persons who are clearly exposed but do not become infected and in those who are able to clear early infection is important for vaccine design.

▲ IMMUNOPATHOGENESIS OF ACUTE INFECTION

The dramatic increase in plasma viremia that occurs during the acute infection is likely the cause of the acute symptomatic illness, and it is associated with induction of both innate and adaptive immune responses to the virus. Little is known at this point regarding innate immunity (e.g., natural killer cells) during acute infection. In contrast, studies of adaptive immunity in persons with acute HIV infection have led to significant new insights into HIV pathogenesis and to prospects for immune-based therapies for HIV infection.

Early Viral Events of Acute HIV Infection

The most comprehensive data regarding early events following transmission come from animal studies in the simian immunodeficiency virus (SIV) model of AIDS pathogenesis. Following contact with tissue dendritic cells, the AIDS virus is presented to dermal/mucosal lymphocytes; it then rapidly migrates to local and regional lymph nodes associated with these cells, where it infects CD4+ T-lymphocytes and leads to a phase of exponential viral growth. Within lymph nodes, viral replication is initially confined to germinal centers; but as replication continues, the entire parenchyma is affected.[63] Virus then breaks into the circulation and is disseminated to susceptible targets in the rest of the body, including brain, spleen, and GALT.[64] Of these areas, GALT may be the most important site of virus production, leading to the extremely high levels of viremia characteristic of acute infection.[64] Rapid HIV replication is associated with release of local cytokines and can be associated with mucosal ulceration and intestinal symptoms (diarrhea, nausea) that can occur during the acute infection syndrome.[65] Free virions released during the acute phase of infection are trapped in the follicular dendritic cell (FDC) network in lymph nodes,[66] which serves as a major reservoir for virus from the time of acute symptomatic illness onward.[67]

The early events of acute HIV infection are associated with extremely high levels of plasma viremia. Although some published studies suggest that acute infection might be associated with viral loads of only a few hundred thousand RNA copies per milliliter of plasma or less, it is now clear that levels are typically 10- to 100-fold higher than that.[6] In fact, published data regarding acute HIV infection should always be compared in light of the relative viral loads in different cohorts. Those reporting average viral loads of less than one million viral particles per milliliter of plasma are unlikely to represent acute infection but, rather, early infection that is already approaching a virologic set point.

Genetic analysis of acute infection reveals that the initial viremia is due to rapid replication of a highly homogeneous virus population.[68] As the immune system responds to the infecting virus, selection pressure is associated with enhanced viral diversification. It is this virus population that infects activated CD4+ T-lymphocytes, of which a small fraction then revert to resting memory cells, establishing a latent reservoir of infected cells.[69] Even extremely early therapy does not prevent the establishment of this reservoir, which then becomes a major obstacle to virus eradication.[70]

Cytotoxic T-Lymphocytes

Following the peak viral load associated with dissemination of virus throughout the body, viremia typically drops precipitously in adults. This drop in viremia is associated with the induction of virus-specific immune responses. The best temporal association between the drop in peak viral load is the appearance of virus-specific cytotoxic T lymphocytes (CTLs), which correlates with the onset of symptoms.[71,72] These cells are generated in response to viral infection and serve to contain virus replication by killing infected cells, thereby limiting the production of progeny virions by direct lysis of infected cells and secretion of antiviral cytokines.[73] The antiviral effectiveness of these cells stems in part from the fact that they can target virus during the most vulnerable phase of the viral life cycle (i.e., when virus is intracellular and lacks its protective outer envelope).[73]

The ability of CTLs to recognize infected cells depends on the presentation of processed viral proteins at the cell surface in the context of a class I molecule.[74] There is a diverse but limited number of class I molecules expressed in the human population; they fall into three groups (A, B, C) and are genetically determined and inherited. Each person expresses, at most, two A alleles, two B alleles, and two C alleles, which provides, at most, six cell surface molecules that can present viral antigens to alert the immune system to the presence of infection. It is now clear that specific class I alleles are associated with better outcomes, whereas others are associated with worse outcomes.[75–77] Moreover, CTLs restricted by some alleles, such as HLA A2, do not appear until after the viral set point has been achieved during the early stages of infection.[78] This suggests that the role of these cells in containing the initial viremia is likely limited. In contrast, CTLs restricted by other alleles (e.g., B27 and B57) are generated earlier in infection, prior to the drop in viremia; and persons expressing these alleles are statistically more likely to have nonprogressing HIV infection.[79–81] Moreover, HIV-uninfected persons with these alleles are more likely to respond to candidate HIV vaccines, suggesting that these alleles may be better at presenting antigen to the immune system.[82] Homozygosity for A, B, or C alleles (or a combination) is associated with more rapid disease progression,[76] likely because this limits the total number of viral proteins (epitopes) that can be presented to the immune system. The extent to which these alleles and polymorphisms affect acute infection remains to be determined.[83]

T-Helper Cell Responses

The ability of CTLs to function properly is critically dependent on the presence of virus-specific T-helper cells.[84] These cells, which recognize viral protein presented in the context of a class II molecule, are generated after initial antigen expression by dendritic cells that serve to initiate this immune response.[85,86] The most dramatic hole in the immune repertoire in chronic progressive HIV infection, compared to what is expected to be present in a controlled viral infection, is the absence of HIV-specific T-helper cells.[87] It appears that the ability of HIV to infect activated CD4+ T-lymphocytes selectively likely accounts for the lack of generation of substantial HIV-specific T-helper cell responses in most persons. This may occur through direct cytopathic effects[88] or through activation-induced cell death (apoptosis)[89,90] with TNF and other cytokines,[91] which appear after overstimulation of these cells at the time of extremely high viral loads during acute infection. Whatever the cause, these cells are typically undetectable during the acute phase of infection and are deficient in most infected persons during the chronic phase of infection as well. There are now numerous animal and human studies indicating that lowering the viral load during acute infection, through antiretroviral therapy or immunization, is associated with the generation of strong virus-specific T-helper cell responses.[3–5,92,93] Early treatment of acute infection thus changes the way the immune system reacts to the virus[3] and results in strong T-helper cell responses, which may have important implications for long-term control (see below). The dominant target of these responses is the viral Gag protein,[3–5] although only limited studies have examined other proteins for their contribution to this response.

Neutralizing Antibodies

Many acute viral infections are contained by the early development of neutralizing antibodies, which directly neutralize free virus. This is not the case with HIV. Antibodies are produced but they appear after the period of high viremia[71]; in fact, the lack of antibody response during the acute symptomatic phase of infection makes serologic diagnosis at this critical early period unreliable. Most of the antibodies that are ultimately produced are directed against virion debris and are thus nonneutralizing.[94] Although the virus is capable of inducing neutralizing antibodies, they typically appear long after the viral set point is achieved and so appear to have little to do with the initial drop in viremia.[71] When these antibodies do finally appear some months after the acute infection, they tend to have limited ability to cross-recognize the many quasi-species that are typically generated; and they have a limited impact on the viral set point during chronic infection.[95] However, studies of persons with treated acute infection have now demonstrated the generation of a strong neutralizing antibody response to their own virus, which appears to contribute to immune control in some individuals.[96] This may be the result of early therapy preventing viral diversification, allowing maturation of effective neutralizing antibodies to a homogeneous virus population.[68]

Importance of the Early Level of Viremia to Subsequent Disease Progression

The landmark studies of Mellors and colleagues in persons from the Multicenter AIDS Cohort Study (MACS) were the first to show that the level of viremia was a predictor of subsequent disease progression.[97] More recent longitudinal studies of seroincidence cases in the MACS trial show that the viral set point achieved within 6 months of acute infection is also highly predictive of disease progression.[30] The potential link between these findings and enhanced functional immunity is provided by a number of studies indicating that lowering the viral load during the acute phase of infection augments virus-specific T-helper cell responses.[3–5] Although multiple factors, including host genetic factors, differences in viral pathogenic potential, and virus-specific immune responses affect the rate of viral replication, increasingly more data indicate that the cellular immune response plays a dominant role in determining the viral set point.[98,99]

▲ CLINICAL MANIFESTATIONS

The first cases of a clinical syndrome associated with acute HIV infection were reported in 1985.[100,101] They provided evidence that the signs and symptoms of acute HIV infection mimic those of other acute viral illnesses, such as influenza and infectious mononucleosis, and thus present a diagnostic challenge to practitioners. These signs and symptoms appear within days to weeks of the initial exposure (estimated to range from 6 to 56 days).[101–104] They are thought to correspond to the emergence of virus-specific immune responses rather than to the level of viremia.[105]

The most common signs and symptoms of acute infection are fever, severe fatigue, rash, headache, lymphadenopathy, and pharyngitis (Table 24–1).[1] Most studies have found that a rare proportion of patients are symptomatic, whether they acquire infection by the sexual route or through blood products, and symptomatic infection is independent of virus clade and geographic locale.[108–110] In prospective studies, the percentage of persons who develop symptomatic infection has been as high as 87%.[8] In one U.S. study, 95% of these patients sought consultation with a health care provider, but only one in four was appropriately diagnosed with acute HIV infection.[8] The magnitude and duration of symptoms varies widely among infected persons, with some studies suggesting that more symptomatic illnesses are associated with a worse prognosis.[111–115] Most persons are ill enough to miss work, and in some the symptoms last a number of weeks.[109,113–117] Failure to recognize acute HIV infection indicates a strong need for educational efforts to inform both health care providers and

Table 24–1. SYMPTOMS ASSOCIATED WITH ACUTE HIV INFECTION

Symptom	Incidence (%)
Fever	96
Lymphadenopathy	74
Pharyngitis	70
Rash[a]	70
Myalgias or arthralgias	54
Diarrhea	32
Headache	32
Nausea and vomiting	27
Hepatosplenomegaly	14
Weight loss	13
Thrush	12
Neurologic disorders[b]	12

[a]Including erythematous maculopapular, vesiculopapular, vasculitis, and oral/genital ulcers.

[b]Including meningoencephalitis, aseptic meningitis, peripheral neuropathy, facial palsy, Guillain-Barré syndrome, brachial neuritis, cognitive impairment, and psychosis.

Adapted from Guidelines for Antiretroviral Therapy[106] and Nui.[107]

persons at risk for acquiring the infection about the signs and symptoms of acute HIV infection.

Some of the clinical manifestations of acute HIV infection are suggestive enough in the proper epidemiologic setting that health care providers should be definitely familiar with them. Dermatologic manifestations can be particularly helpful. Rash, which is frequent, is most commonly described as papular, morbilliform, or maculopapular and may be transient (Fig. 24–1). Biopsies of skin lesions reveal perivascular and interstitial inflammatory infiltrates in the upper and mid-reticular dermis and in some cases in isolated areas of epidermal necrosis.[118,119] Lesions vary in size from a few millimeters to 1 cm; they tend to be distributed to the upper thorax but may involve the head and arms. In a detailed assessment of 22 patients with acute HIV infection, 17 were found to have rashes, which were most profuse around the collar region.[120] Biopsies of the acute skin rash reveal lymphocytic infiltrates of CD4+ and CD8+ T-lymphocytes,[120] possibly indicating a virus-specific immune response.[121] Dermatologic manifestations also include oral ulcers (Fig. 24–2) and genital ulcers (Fig. 24–3),[122,123] which should always prompt consideration of acute HIV infection.[1]

In addition to the dermatologic problems, other disorders have been reported. Prominent among them are the manifestations of central nervous system (CNS) infection, which can accompany acute HIV infection and present as aseptic meningitis, acute encephalitis, Guillain-Barré syndrome, or Bell's palsy.[124] Transient immunosuppression associated with acute infection can lead to opportunistic infections, particularly oral candidiasis. *Pneumocystis carinii* pneumonia, tuberculosis, and reactivation of other infections have been reported to occur with the initial transient depletion of CD4+ T-lymphocytes. Other, less frequent manifestations include heparin-like anticoagulant vasculitis,[125] ulcerative esophagitis,[126–128] nonspecific gastroenteritis,[129] acute hepatitis,[130,131] pancreatitis,[132,133] pneumonitis,[134–136] myositis,[137] acute myeloradiculoneuritis,[138] acute psychosis,[139] transient neurologic deficits,[140–142] meningoradiculitis,[143] myocarditis,[144] hemophagocytic syndrome with severe systemic involvement,[145] and Stevens-Johnson syndrome.[146]

Although laboratory abnormalities can be seen during acute HIV infection, such as general leukopenia, thrombocytopenia,[122] mild increase in neutrophils, early transient CD4+ T-lymphocyte depletion, expansion of CD8+ T-lymphocytes,[147] and inversion of the CD4+ /CD8+ ratio,[117,148] the sensitivity and specificity of these abnormalities is so poor as to be not helpful for establishing

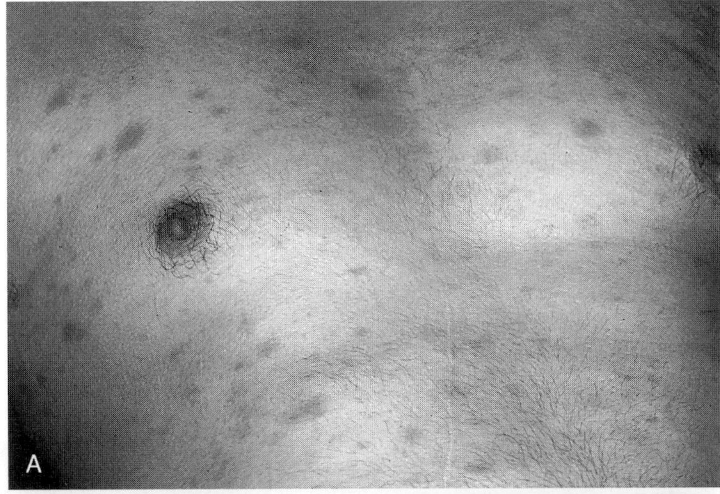

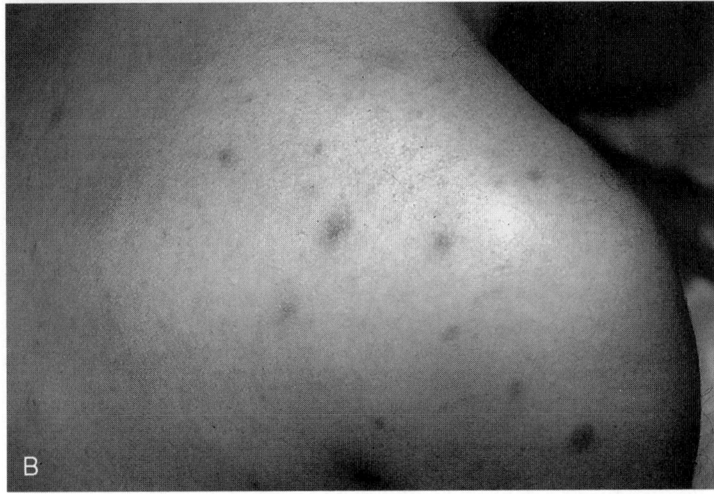

Figure 24–1. *A*, Maculopapular skin eruption in acute HIV infection. *B*, Vesiculopapular eruption during acute HIV infection.

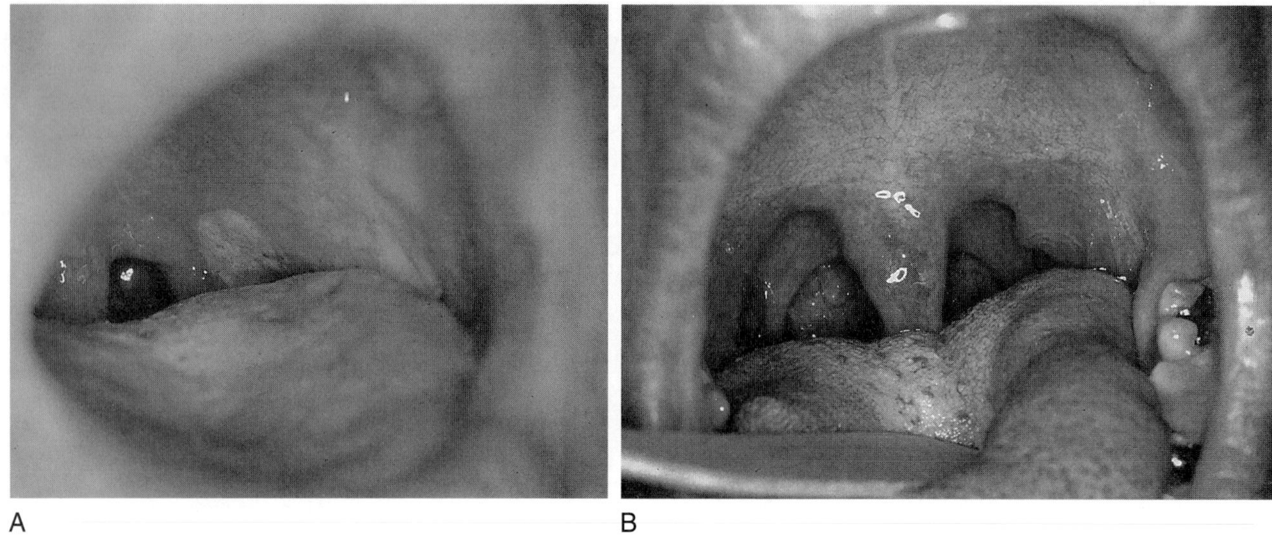

Figure 24–2. *A*, Oropharyngeal ulcer in acute HIV infection. *B*, Thrush, diffuse oropharyngeal edema, and tonsillar erosion during acute HIV infection.

the diagnosis.[1,149] The speed of progression has been associated with the degree of symptoms at the time of acute infection,[111–115,150,151] but extremely symptomatic acute illness can also be seen in persons who go on to maintain nonprogressing illness.[3] Individuals with symptomatic acute HIV infection are more likely to have CD4+ T-lymphocyte counts of less than 500 cells per cubic millimeter (75% vs. 42%) at a 3-year follow-up.[115] One study showed that patients with a week or more of fever are twice as likely to develop AIDS within the next 6 years compared to those with less than 7 days of fever.[152] Lower nadir CD4+ T-lymphocyte counts and smaller spontaneous drops in HIV RNA within the first 30 days of follow-up also correlate with faster disease progression.[153] Among 1046 seroconverters in the U.S. Navy and Marine Corps known to have seroconverted within the previous 2 years, almost half had CD4+ T-lymphocyte counts of less than 500 cells per cubic millimeter.[154]

Clinical manifestations in children deserve special comment. Infants who acquire infection in utero are often asymptomatic or present with nonspecific signs and symptoms. Most commonly they include fever, low birth weight, delayed growth, diarrhea, and candidiasis. A DiGeorge-like syndrome of thymic deficiency has also been described, and the presence of lower CD4+ and CD8+ T-lymphocyte counts correlated with a worse prognosis.[155] The presence of HIV antibodies in the neonate may reflect either maternal antibody or true infection; as a result, this test is unreliable until maternal antibody has waned (usually 6 to 12 months of life). HIV polymerase chain reaction (PCR) assays can diagnose most perinatal transmissions at 1 month.[156] Many centers test at delivery and at weeks 4, 12, and 24. HIV viremia rapidly increases in the neonate, and higher viral titers also appear to correlate with faster disease progression.[49] Unlike adults, infants continue to have high-level viremia for months without depleting the circu-

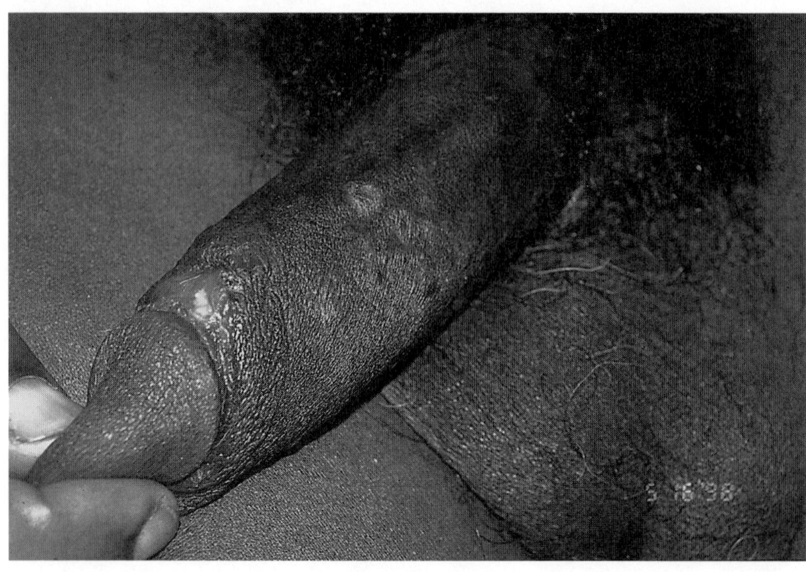

Figure 24–3. Penile ulcer during HIV infection.

lating CD4+ T-lymphocyte population.[157] In untreated women the risk of perinatal transmission has been estimated to be 14% to 42%. Most HIV transmission is believed to occur during delivery, and up to one-third of all transmissions occur with breastfeeding. Treatment of both the mother and neonate with antiretroviral agents has been shown to decrease dramatically the risk of transmission.[52,158] Cesarean delivery may further decrease the risk of HIV transmission in women with high HIV viral loads or those with prolonged rupture of membranes[51] (reviewed by Kourtis et al.[159]).

▲ DIAGNOSIS OF ACUTE HIV INFECTIONS SEE ALSO CHAPTER 1.

There is no single algorithm that allows an accurate clinical diagnosis of acute HIV infection.[149] Furthermore, acute HIV infection cannot be diagnosed with a standard enzyme-linked immunosorbent assay (ELISA) and Western blot tests for evidence of antibody responses, as these responses typically are not generated during the early stages of acute symptomatic illness. Serologic tests typically first become positive 22 to 27 days after acute infection, usually after the symptoms of acute infection have resolved and well after the time of peak viremia.[1] The diagnosis of acute infection must be based on detection of virus rather than on the basis of an immune response to the virus. Although direct culture of virus is possible, it remains a research tool and is not approved for diagnosis of acute HIV infection; rather, the diagnosis is based on detection of viral HIV RNA or HIV protein (p24 antigen).

The only test currently licensed for detection of HIV infection before antibodies have been generated is the p24 antigen test, which detects the presence of the viral core protein in either serum or plasma.[160] This test is used to screen all blood donations in the United States to detect contaminated blood during the "window" period before the development of detectable antibodies and thus is widely available in blood banks. The p24 antigen remains detectable for approximately 40 days and is usually negative in chronically infected individuals. This test is based on an ELISA format; it can be rapidly performed with same-day results and is considered inexpensive (under $20).

The presence of HIV can also be detected by viral RNA assays using either target amplification (Amplicor-PCR) system or signal amplification techniques [b-DNA or nucleic acid sequence-based amplifications (NASBA)]. A positive viral load in the absence of detectable antibodies establishes the presumptive diagnosis of acute HIV infection. False-positive results have been reported and may be higher when using the b-DNA assay.[161] These viral RNA assays have not been approved for the diagnosis of infection, and positive RNA assays must be confirmed by documentation of subsequent seroconversion to secure a diagnosis of acute HIV infection. The RNA tests become positive 5 days before the p24 antigen assay and 1 to 3 weeks prior to the detection of antibodies.[162] The average viral load at the time of symptomatic acute HIV infection is higher than 10 million viral particles per milliliter of plasma; and, in our experience, viral loads of less than 100,000 copies per milliliter of plasma are unlikely to represent acute infection.[6] Persons with lower levels of viremia are likely to have been infected longer and are thus approaching the relative viral set point that is achieved during the months following acute infection. Although the presently available commercial assays for viral RNA have high sensitivity and specificity, there have been reports of false-positive results, usually less than 3000 HIV RNA copies per milliliter of plasma. Because these low levels are below the levels seen with acute infection, false-positive results are unlikely to be a problem when diagnosing acute infection but require additional tests to rule out established HIV infection. Overall, although assays for viral RNA are slightly more sensitive than p24 antigen detection, they also have a slightly higher false-positive rate and significantly higher cost.[149] The sensitivity and specificity of p24 antigen detection (89% and 100%) and RNA assay (100% and 97%) mean that confirmation of these assays with follow-up tests is essential.[149] Our current testing algorithm is depicted in Figure 24–4.

Modified serologic assays that detect antibodies to major HIV proteins are useful for establishing the diagnosis of recent infection. The "detuned enzyme-linked immunosorbent assay" (ELISA) has been widely used in the research setting to establish that infection has occurred within the past 180 days.[163] This assay involves the use of a standard ELISA for HIV that has been made less sensitive. Thus during early infection, after full seroconversion by Western blot assay, persons score negative by this assay and positive on the standard ELISA, whereas months after acute infection they become positive on both (Fig. 24–5). Busch and Satten offered a more detailed proposal for stag-

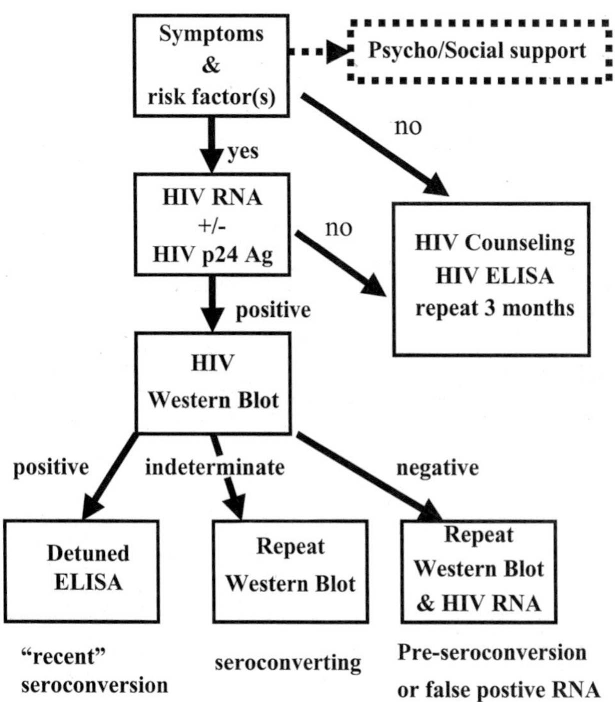

Figure 24–4. Algorithm for laboratory testing for acute HIV infection.

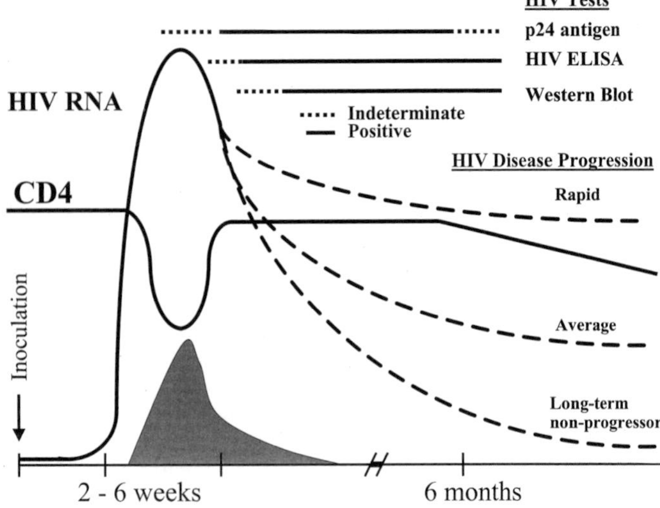

Figure 24–5. Dynamics of laboratory tests during early HIV infection. The shaded area represents the symptomatic illness.

ing early HIV infection after reviewing 43 blood donors who were retrospectively identified as seroconverters. Six stages of early HIV infection were described: stage 0, intermittent viremia; stage 1, definite viremia; stage 2, viremia and p24 antigenemia; stage 3, HIV ELISA-reactive; stage 4, HIV Western blot-indeterminate; stage 5, Western blot-positive without p31 band; and stage 6, Western blot positive with p31 band.[162] One additional stage of early HIV should be considered—detuned ELISA-unreactive—as noted above.[163,165]

Because the clinical signs and symptoms of acute HIV infection are nonspecific, the diagnosis is often overlooked. The classic presentation is a mononucleosis-like presentation; the differential diagnosis is extensive, but many potential infections can be ruled out with laboratory testing. The major elements in the differential diagnosis are infections due to acute viral illnesses including the Epstein-Barr virus (EBV),[166] herpes simplex virus, measles, rubella, varicella, cytomegalovirus (CMV), influenza, adenovirus, enteroviruses, dengue,[167] rocky mountain spotted fever, ehrlichiosis, Lyme disease, leptospirosis,[168] syphilis, typhus, typhoid fever, viral hepatitis, esophagitis,[128,169–171] toxoplasmosis,[172] and cryptosporidiosis.[173] One must also be aware that other infections may be transmitted with HIV, such as hepatitis (A, B, C), syphilis, CMV, EBV, *Chlamydia*, gonorrhea, human papilloma virus (HPV), Kaposi sarcoma-associated *herpesvirus* (KSHV), herpes simplex virus type 6 (HSV-6), GB virus type C (GBV-C), *bacterial*, and others. Practitioners should consider which diagnoses are likely based on the clinical and epidemiologic observations and request appropriate laboratory tests for those diagnoses, rather than attempt to conduct extensive tests to screen for all possibilities.

▲ TIMING OF SEROCONVERSION

The first-generation HIV assays were able to detect HIV infection approximately 2 to 3 months after infection, and the newer second- and third-generation assays are able to detect HIV even earlier.[174] A study of 41 health care workers (HCWs) with occupational acquisition found that 95% developed detectable HIV-1 antibodies by 2 months.[175] Markov modeling of these cases estimated an average time to seroconversion of 2.4 months, somewhat longer than the Centers for Disease Control and Prevention (CDC) estimate of a median time to seroconversion of 46 days (mean 65 days).[176] The longest time from exposure to seroconversion remains somewhat controversial, as it is difficult to exclude with any confidence subsequent exposures as the infection source. However, in one study, two HCWs (5%) had late seroconversion (6 to 12 months) after the alleged sole exposure; and in one of these cases genetic analysis of the HCW and source patient confirmed that this was in fact delayed seroconversion from the occupational exposure.[177] Studies of transfusion-associated transmission have also provided more definitive timing from exposure to seroconversion and helped define the window period (infectious but HIV ELISA-negative) to approximately 42 days with older assays. Other studies have reported the onset of clinical symptoms 2 to 6 weeks after presumed transmission, and newer HIV antibody ELISA tests can detect HIV infection as early as 30 days after symptoms.[176,178] As a result, some public health HIV testing guidelines have reduced the recommended interval for repeat HIV testing to exclude this negative HIV antibody window period from 6 months to 3 months.[178]

▲ TREATMENT OF ACUTE INFECTION

The optimal medical management of acute HIV infection remains to be determined and is presently largely driven by anecdotal reports and small pilot studies with relatively brief follow-up. Although there are compelling reasons to consider early therapy, they must be weighed in light of increasing evidence of drug-related toxicities over time. There is now little hope that early therapy will result in viral eradication,[70] but emerging data suggest that it might lead to enhanced immune responses to the virus.[3–5] Whether there is a clinical benefit to early treatment has not yet been answered and can be determined only by large clinical trials. Nevertheless, emerging data highlight both the benefits and risks of early treatment of acute infection.

To date, there have been only two randomized, controlled clinical trials of antiviral therapy for acute infection that studied involved persons with a medical history and symptoms consistent with acute infection and laboratory evidence of recent infection.[179,180] Because both studies were conducted some years ago, persons received what would now be considered substandard antiviral therapy. In the first study, 77 patients within a mean of 25 days of symptomatic acute HIV infection were randomized to zidovudine monotherapy (250 mg bid) or placebo, which was continued for 6 months. At the end of 6 months of treatment, those receiving zidovudine had a mean increase in the CD4+ T-lymphocyte count of 8.9 cells per cubic millimeter, whereas those in the placebo group had a decrease of 12 cells per cubic millimeter. Disease progression was significantly lower in the zidovudine group. Subjects were followed for an additional 28 months, and the two groups received a similar amount of zidovudine. At the end of this follow-up, the zidovudine group continued to have a lower incidence of disease progression, but the difference was no longer significant. Differences in CD4+ T-lymphocyte counts were also no longer significant (5.0 vs. 3.2 cells per cubic millimeter).[181] In the second study, 28 patients with symptomatic acute HIV infection were randomized to zidovudine (1000 mg/day) or placebo for 24 weeks. Zidovudine recipients had significantly higher CD4+ T-lymphocyte counts at week 48 (666 vs. 362 cells per cubic millimeter) (P = 0.004) but no difference in HIV RNA levels or disease progression.[180] Because these studies were not designed as clinical endpoint studies and utilized what is considered substandard therapy by today's standards, they did not provide a definitive answer as to whether there is clinical benefit to early intervention with antiretroviral therapy.

Other nonrandomized studies of early treatment have included multidrug combination therapy, and they are beginning to suggest a benefit in terms of clinical outcome.[182–185] Treatment with triple-drug therapy, including a protease inhibitor (PI), in a cohort of 41 subjects with primary HIV infection led to a profound, sustained decrease in viral load, with 80% of evaluable subjects having viral loads of less than 50 copies per milliliter at 52 weeks; and all experienced sustained increases in their CD4+ T-lymphocyte counts.[5] Moreover, further follow-up of these patients (n = 47) demonstrated that treatment with HAART during the primary infection led to a decrease in disease progression at 3 years of follow-up, compared to persons who were not treated.[186] Such studies show that current combination regimens can effectively lower the viral load even when initial levels of viremia are quite high, but they do not address the clinical benefit compared to that seen with delayed therapy. Studies have not yet clearly addressed whether early therapy is beneficial compared to delayed therapy based on the present guidelines.

An important consideration when treating acute infection is whether tests for the presence of antiviral drug-resistant viruses should be carried out immediately. Surveillance studies in persons with acute infection have documented transmission of multidrug-resistant virus,[187] but it is unclear whether these cases are increasing. Brenner found that the primary resistance to nucleoside (NRTIs) and nonnucleoside (NNRTIs) reverse transcriptase inhibitors and to PIs during 1997 to 1999 was 21% and 15%, respectively. Ten percent of persons with new infections were found to have genotypic evidence of multidrug resistance, which was confirmed with phenotypic testing.[188] In another study, among 80 persons with early HIV infection diagnosed between 1995 and 1999, there was primary resistance to at least one antiretroviral agent in 16.3%, and 3.8% had multidrug resistance.[189] Several other studies have found similar incidences and evidence for growing resistance among patients with acute HIV infection.[190,191] In addition, naturally occurring polymorphisms in reverse transcriptase (RT) and PI genes not normally selected for by antiretroviral therapy commonly occur during acute or early infection and may increase the risk of drug failure.[192,193] Genotypic and phenotypic resistance testing may permit optimal use of available antiretroviral agents. Current guidelines recommend genotypic testing, and others have advocated phenotypic testing as well in the setting of primary HIV infection.[193–195] Strategies for optimal selection of antiretroviral therapy in the setting of emerging resistance must be explored. Despite growing resistance, computer modeling of resistance patterns observed in San Francisco since 1996 suggests that resistance may not dramatically increase the spread of HIV or of resistant HIV strains among persons with primary HIV infection.[196]

Our own approach is to treat persons with acute infection immediately with HAART and perform genotypic resistance testing on the initial isolate. When possible, we also perform genotypic testing on the source patient and review that individual's antiretroviral history. Almost all patients have opted to initiate combination antiretroviral therapy, generally two NRTIs and a PI (although several have chosen two NRTIs and efavirenz or a four-drug regimen. HIV RNA has dropped to undetectable levels in all patients, except two who had evidence of genotypic resistance and another with medication nonadherence.

▲ EFFECTS OF EARLY THERAPY ON IMMUNE CONTROL OF HIV

An argument for early therapy is the hypothesis that lowering the viral load during acute infection lessens impairment of the development of virus-specific T-helper lymphocyte responses and allows maturation of immune responses that will subsequently be able to control the viremia, possibly in the absence of ongoing therapy. This hypothesis is based in part on animal model data. Using a pathogenic strain of HIV, it was shown that early treatment of experimental infection (in this case just 16 weeks of didanosine monotherapy) resulted in a markedly better outcome. The untreated animals were all dead within 6 months, which is typical for this model, whereas five of the six animals that received just 16 weeks of a suboptimal therapy were alive and well 3 years later. Numerous studies have now documented that early treatment leads to the generation of strong virus-specific T-helper lymphocyte responses, which are analogous to those that are otherwise seen only in persons who spontaneously control viremia without the need for drug therapy.[3–5] Such observations have led to two hypotheses: (1) early treatment results in maturation of effective immune responses that allow control of viremia; or (2) early treatment followed by transient treatment interruption leads to exposure to a regulated amount of virus, which leads to further enhancement of immunity and control of viremia after subsequent treatment interruptions.

Although data regarding early treatment as a means of enhancing effective immunity are still limited, it has now been shown that this approach leads to at least transient control of viremia in some patients. In the initial study using this approach, five of eight persons with treated acute infection were able to control their viremia to levels lower than 500 viral RNA copies per milliliter of plasma after a median of 6 months off therapy. Three of the eight were able to control the viremia with simple treatment cessation and never met criteria to restart therapy (i.e., a viral load higher than 50,000 copies per milliliter of plasma on a single occasion, or a viral load of more than 5000 RNA copies per milliliter of plasma for three consecutive weeks); the other two patients controlled their viremia after a third interruption.[6] Control here is a relative term, in that all patients experienced a viral rebound but were then able to contain their viremia below the parameters noted above. For those controlling viremia after the first treatment interruption (essentially treatment cessation), follow-up was more than 400 days in two of the subjects, both of whom maintained viral loads of less than 1000 copies per milliliter. The individuals who met the criteria to restart therapy had an excellent virologic response to HAART resumption; and the exposure to autologous virus was noted to increase the breadth and diversity of the CTL response. With a second stop of therapy, all but one of the patients were able to extend the period before meeting criteria to restart therapy. This ongoing study clearly indicates that at least transient immune control can be achieved in most persons with treated acute infection who undergo a complicated interruption regimen in which retreatment is linked to the magnitude and duration of the viral load increase.[6] However, the potential clinical benefit of early initiation of antiretroviral therapy in terms of delay in disease progression and death compared to the added risk of long-term metabolic toxicities and emergence of drug resistance must be tested in large clinical trials.[197] Other important questions remain unanswered: What is the durability of control in these persons? What predicts control? How long after acute infection can one still obtain augmented immune control with supervised treatment interruption? Are there other more effective approaches, such as therapeutic immunization or administration of cytokines (e.g., IL-2) to augment effective immunity? Expanded clinical trials are needed to answer these questions.[197] It is important to point out that treatment of chronic infection has not led to similar levels of enhanced control of viremia following treatment interruption,[198–200] the reasons for which are not known. It is likely that other means to augment immunity must be pursued for chronic infection.[197]

▲ CONCLUSIONS

Acute HIV infection is accompanied by a recognizable clinical syndrome with most new cases. With new infections on the rise, it is imperative that persons presenting with compatible clinical illness be evaluated for risk factors and then appropriately screened. Increasing evidence indicates that early treatment not only may decrease the chance of transmission but also change the way in which the immune system interacts with the virus. Although studies of treatment of acute infection indicate that it leads to at least transient immune control in most infected persons, the numbers of subjects studied remains small. There is a need for controlled clinical trials in this setting to determine whether treatment of the acute infection confers a clinical benefit. As the HIV epidemic enters its third decade, expanded studies of acutely infected persons is likely to provide novel insights into HIV pathogenesis and into new approaches for effective treatment and prevention.

REFERENCES

1. Kahn JO, Walker BD. Acute human immunodeficiency virus type 1 infection. N Engl J Med 339:33, 1998.
2. Quinn TC, Wawer MJ, Sewankambo N, et al. Viral load and heterosexual transmission of human immunodeficiency virus type 1. Rakai Project Study Group. N Engl J Med 342:921, 2000.
3. Rosenberg ES, Billingsley JM, Caliendo AM, et al. Vigorous HIV-1-specific CD4+ T cell responses associated with control of viremia. Science 278:1447, 1997.
4. Oxenius A, Price DA, Easterbrook PJ, et al. Early highly active antiretroviral therapy for acute HIV-1 infection preserves immune function of CD8+ and CD4+ T lymphocytes. Proc Natl Acad Sci USA 97:3382, 2000.
5. Malhotra U, Berrey MM, Huang Y, et al. Effect of combination antiretroviral therapy on T-cell immunity in acute human immunodeficiency virus type 1 infection. J Infect Dis 181:121, 2000.
6. Rosenberg ES, Altfeld M, Poon SH, et al. Immune control of HIV-1 after early treatment of acute infection. Nature 407:523, 2000.
7. UNAIDS. Global Summary of the HIV/AIDS Epidemic, December 2000. Geneva, UN, 2000.
8. Schacker T, Collier AC, Hughes J, et al. Clinical and epidemiologic features of primary HIV infection. Ann Intern Med 125:257, 1996. Erratum. Ann Intern Med 126:174, 1997.
9. Ahlgren DJ. Role of primary infection in epidemics of HIV in gay cohorts. J Acquir Immune Defic Syndr Hum Retrovirol 11:204, 1996.
10. Cates W Jr, Chesney MA, Cohen MS. Primary HIV infection—a public health opportunity. Am J Public Health 87:1928, 1997.
11. St Louis ME, Wasserheit JN, Gayle HD. Janus considers the HIV pandemic—harnessing recent advances to enhance AIDS prevention. Am J Public Health 87:10, 1997.
12. Weinstock H, Sweeney S, Satten GA, Gwinn M. HIV seroincidence and risk factors among patients repeatedly tested for HIV attending sexually transmitted disease clinics in the United States, 1991 to 1996: STD Clinic HIV Seroincidence Study Group. J Acquir Immune Defic Syndr Hum Retrovirol 19:506, 1998.
13. Valleroy LA, MacKellar DA, Karon JM, et al. HIV prevalence and associated risks in young men who have sex with men. Young Men's Survey Study Group. JAMA 284:198, 2000.
14. McFarland WM, Katz MH. HIV incidence among young men who have sex with men—seven U.S. cities, 1994–2000. MMWR Morbid Mortal Wkly Rep 50:440, 2001.
15. Royce RA, Sena A, Cates W, Cohen MS. Sexual transmission of HIV. N Engl J Med 336:1072, 1997.
16. Padian NP, Glass S. Transmission of HIV possibly associated with exposure of mucous membrane to contaminated blood. MMWR Morb Mortal Wkly Rep 46:620, 1997.
17. Ho DD, Schooley RT, Rota TR, et al. HTLV-III in the semen and blood of a healthy homosexual man. Science 226:451, 1984.
18. Vogt MW, Witt DJ, Craven DE, et al. Isolation patterns of the human immunodeficiency virus from cervical secretions during the menstrual cycle of women at risk for the acquired immunodeficiency syndrome. Ann Intern Med 106:380, 1987.
19. Pomerantz RJ, de la Monte SM, Donegan SP, et al. Human immunodeficiency virus (HIV) infection of the uterine cervix. Ann Intern Med 108:321, 1988.
20. Dornadula G, Zhang H, VanUitert B, et al. Residual HIV-1 RNA in blood plasma of patients taking suppressive highly active antiretroviral therapy. JAMA 282:1627, 1999.

21. Zhang H, Dornadula G, Beumont M, et al. Human immunodeficiency virus type 1 in the semen of men receiving highly active antiretroviral therapy. N Engl J Med 339:1803, 1998.
22. Spira AI, Marx PA, Patterson BK, et al. Cellular targets of infection and route of viral dissemination after an intravaginal inoculation of simian immunodeficiency virus into rhesus macaques. J Exp Med 183:215, 1996.
23. Khouri YF, McIntosh K, Cavacini L, et al. Vertical transmission of HIV-1. Correlation with maternal viral load and plasma levels of CD4 binding site anti-gp120 antibodies. J Clin Invest 95:732, 1995.
24. Thea DM, Steketee RW, Pliner V, et al. The effect of maternal viral load on the risk of perinatal transmission of HIV-1: New York City Perinatal HIV Transmission Collaborative Study Group. AIDS 11:437, 1997.
25. Dickover RE, Garratty EM, Herman SA, et al. Identification of levels of maternal HIV-1 RNA associated with risk of perinatal transmission. Effect of maternal zidovudine treatment on viral load. JAMA 275:599, 1996.
26. Cao Y, Krogstad B, Korber BT, et al. Maternal HIV-1 viral load and vertical transmission of infection: the Ariel Project for the prevention of HIV transmission from mother to infant. Nat Med 3:549, 1997.
27. Geijtenbeek TB, Torensma R, van Vliet SJ, et al. Identification of DC-SIGN, a novel dendritic cell-specific ICAM-3 receptor that supports primary immune responses. Cell 100:575, 2000.
28. Geijtenbeek TB, Kwon DS, Torensma R, et al. DC-SIGN, a dendritic cell-specific HIV-1-binding protein that enhances trans-infection of T cells. Cell 100:587, 2000.
29. Geijtenbeek TB, van Vliet SJ, van Duijnhoven GC, et al. DC-sign, a dentritic cell-specific HIV-1 receptor present in placenta that infects T cells in trans–a review. Placenta 22(suppl A):S19, 2001.
30. Lyles RH, Munoz A, Yamashita TE, et al. Natural history of human immunodeficiency virus type 1 viremia after seroconversion and proximal to AIDS in a large cohort of homosexual men. Multicenter AIDS Cohort Study. J Infect Dis 181:872, 2000.
31. Schacker T, Ryncarz AJ, Goddard J, et al. Frequent recovery of HIV-1 from genital herpes simplex virus lesions in HIV-1-infected men. JAMA 280:61, 1998.
32. Lawn SD, Subbarao S, Wright TC Jr, et al. Correlation between human immunodeficiency virus type 1 RNA levels in the female genital tract and immune activation associated with ulceration of the cervix. J Infect Dis 181:1950, 2000.
33. Posavad CM, Koelle DM, Shaughnessy MF, Corey L. Severe genital herpes infections in HIV-infected individuals with impaired herpes simplex virus-specific CD8+ cytotoxic T lymphocyte responses. Proc Natl Acad Sci USA 94:10289, 1997.
34. Cohen MS, Hoffman IF, Royce RA, et al. Reduction of concentration of HIV-1 in semen after treatment of urethritis: implications for prevention of sexual transmission of HIV-1. AIDSCAP Malawi Research Group. Lancet 349:1868, 1997.
35. Marx PA, Spira AI, Gettie A, et al. Progesterone implants enhance SIV vaginal transmission and early virus load. Nat Med 2:1084, 1996.
36. Stephenson J. Widely used spermicide may increase, not decrease, risk of HIV transmission. JAMA 284:949, 2000.
37. Fichorova RN, Tucker LD, Anderson DJ. The molecular basis of nonoxynol-9-induced vaginal inflammation and its possible relevance to human immunodeficiency virus type 1 transmission. J Infect Dis 184:418, 2001.
38. Semba RD, Kumwenda N, Hoover DR, et al. Human immunodeficiency virus load in breast milk, mastitis, and mother-to-child transmission of human immunodeficiency virus type 1. J Infect Dis 180:93, 1999.
39. John GC, Nduati RW, Mbori-Ngacha DA, et al. Correlates of mother-to-child human immunodeficiency virus type 1 (HIV-1) transmission: association with maternal plasma HIV-1 RNA load, genital HIV-1 DNA shedding, and breast infections. J Infect Dis 183:206, 2001.
40. Gray RH, Kiwanuka N, Quinn TC, et al. Male circumcision and HIV acquisition and transmission: cohort studies in Rakai, Uganda: Rakai Project Team. AIDS 14:2371, 2000.
41. Hogan CM, Hammer SM. Host determinants in HIV infection and disease. Part 1: Cellular and humoral immune responses. Ann Intern Med 134:761, 2001.
42. Feng Y, Broder CC, Kennedy PE, Berger EA. HIV-1 entry cofactor: functional cDNA cloning of a seven-transmembrane, G protein-coupled receptor. Science 272:872, 1996.
43. Berger EA, Doms RW, Fenyo EM, et al. A new classification for HIV-1 [letter]. Nature 391:240, 1998.
44. O'Brien TR, Winkler C, Dean M, et al. HIV-1 infection in a man homozygous for CCR5 delta 32 [letter]. Lancet 349:1219, 1997.
45. Dean M, Carrington M, Winkler C, et al. Genetic restriction of HIV-1 infection and progression to AIDS by a deletion allele of the CKR5 structural gene. Hemophilia Growth and Development Study, Multicenter AIDS Cohort Study, Multicenter Hemophilia Cohort Study, San Francisco City Cohort, ALIVE Study. Science 273:1856, 1996. Erratum. Science 274:1069, 1996.
46. Murphy PM. Viral exploitation and subversion of the immune system through chemokine mimicry. Nat Immunol 2:116, 2001.
47. Pilcher CD, Shugars DC, Fiscus SA, et al. HIV in body fluids during primary HIV infection: implications for pathogenesis, treatment and public health. AIDS 15:837, 2001.
48. Pilcher CD, Vernazza P, Battegay M, et al. Sexual transmission can precede symptoms in primary HIV-1 infection. Presented at the 8th Conference on Retroviruses and Opportunistic Infections, 2001, abstract 411.
49. Dickover RE, Dillon M, Leung KM, et al. Early prognostic indicators in primary perinatal human immunodeficiency virus type 1 infection: importance of viral RNA and the timing of transmission on long-term outcome. J Infect Dis 178:375, 1998.
50. Keerasuntonpong A, Pitt J, Gaut PL, Daar ES. Primary human immunodeficiency virus type 1 infection in pregnancy. Obstet Gynecol 94:844, 1999.
51. Read JS, Tuomala R, Kpamegan E, et al. Mode of delivery and postpartum morbidity among HIV-infected women: the women and infants transmission study. J Acquir Immune Defic Syndr 26:236, 2001.
52. Landers DV, Duarte G. Mode of delivery and the risk of vertical transmission of HIV-1. N Engl J Med 341:205, 1999.
53. Semba RD, Kumwenda N, Taha TE, et al. Mastitis and immunological factors in breast milk of human immunodeficiency virus-infected women. J Hum Lact 15:301, 1999.
54. Sahu GK, Chen JJ, Huang JC, et al. Transient or occult HIV-1 infection in high-risk adults. AIDS 15:1175, 2001.
55. Bryson YJ, Pang S, Wei LS, et al. Clearance of HIV infection in a perinatally infected infant. N Engl J Med 332:833, 1995.
56. Rowland-Jones S, Sutton J, Ariyoshi K, et al. HIV-specific cytotoxic T-cells in HIV-exposed but uninfected Gambian women. Nat Med 1:59, 1995. Erratum. Nat Med 1:598, 1995.
57. Rowland-Jones SL, Dong T, Fowke KR, et al. Cytotoxic T cell responses to multiple conserved HIV epitopes in HIV-resistant prostitutes in Nairobi. J Clin Invest 102:1758, 1998.
58. Rowland-Jones SL, Dong T, Dorrell L, et al. Broadly cross-reactive HIV-specific cytotoxic T-lymphocytes in highly-exposed persistently seronegative donors. Immunol Lett 66:9, 1999.
59. Letvin NL, Walker BD. HIV versus the immune system: another apparent victory for the virus. J Clin Invest 107:273, 2001.
60. Albert ML, Sauter B, Bhardwaj N. Dendritic cells acquire antigen from apoptotic cells and induce class I-restricted CTLs. Nature 392:86, 1998.
61. Buseyne F, Le Gall S, Boccaccio C, et al. MHC-I-restricted presentation of HIV-1 virion antigens without viral replication. Nat Med 7:344, 2001.
62. Kaul R, Rowland-Jones SL, Kimani J, et al. Late seroconversion in HIV-resistant Nairobi prostitutes despite pre-existing HIV-specific CD8+ responses. J Clin Invest 107:341, 2001.
63. Couedel-Courteille A, Butor C, Juillard V, et al. Dissemination of SIV after rectal infection preferentially involves paracolic germinal centers. Virology 260:277, 1999.
64. Veazey RS, DeMaria M, Chalifoux LV, et al. Gastrointestinal tract as a major site of CD4+ T cell depletion and viral replication in SIV infection. Science 280:427, 1998.
65. Ullrich R, Schmidt W, Zippel T, et al. Mucosal HIV infection. Pathobiology 66:145, 1998.
66. Smith BA, Gartner S, Liu Y, et al. Persistence of infectious HIV on follicular dendritic cells. J Immunol 166:690, 2001.
67. Schacker T, Little S, Connick E, et al. Rapid accumulation of human immunodeficiency virus (HIV) in lymphatic tissue reservoirs during acute and early HIV infection: implications for timing of antiretroviral therapy. J Infect Dis 181:354, 2000.
68. Altfeld M, Rosenberg ES, Shankarappa R, et al. Cellular immune re-

sponses and viral diversity in individuals treated during acute and early HIV-1 infection. J Exp Med 193:169, 2001.
69. Finzi D, Hermankova M, Pierson T, et al. Identification of a reservoir for HIV-1 in patients on highly active antiretroviral therapy. Science 278:1295, 1997.
70. Finzi D, Blankson J, Siliciano JD, et al. Latent infection of CD4+ T cells provides a mechanism for lifelong persistence of HIV-1, even in patients on effective combination therapy. Nat Med 5:512, 1999.
71. Koup RA, Safrit JT, Cao Y, et al. Temporal association of cellular immune responses with the initial control of viremia in primary human immunodeficiency virus type 1 syndrome. J Virol 68:4650, 1994.
72. Borrow P, Lewicki H, Hahn BH, et al. Virus-specific CD8+ cytotoxic T-lymphocyte activity associated with control of viremia in primary human immunodeficiency virus type 1 infection. J Virol 68:6103, 1994.
73. Yang OO, Kalams SA, Trocha A, et al. Suppression of human immunodeficiency virus type 1 replication by CD8+ cells: evidence for HLA class I-restricted triggering of cytolytic and noncytolytic mechanisms. J Virol 71:3120, 1997.
74. Goulder PJR, Rowland SL, McMichael AJ, Walker BD. Anti-HIV cellular immunity: recent advances towards vaccine design. AIDS 13:s121, 1999.
75. Kaslow RA, Carrington M, Apple R, et al. Influence of combinations of human major histocompatibility complex genes on the course of HIV-1 infection. Nat Med 2:405, 1996.
76. Carrington M, Nelson GW, Martin MP, et al. HLA and HIV-1: heterozygote advantage and B*35-Cw*04 disadvantage. Science 283:1748, 1999.
77. Saah AJ, Hoover DR, Weng S, et al. Association of HLA profiles with early plasma viral load, CD4+ cell count and rate of progression to AIDS following acute HIV-1 infection. Multicenter AIDS Cohort Study. AIDS 12:2107, 1998.
78. Goulder PJ, Altfeld MA, Rosenberg ES, et al. Substantial differences in specificity of HIV-specific cytotoxic T cells in acute and chronic HIV infection. J Exp Med 193:181, 2001.
79. Migueles SA, Sabbaghian MS, Shupert WL, et al. HLA B*5701 is highly associated with restriction of virus replication in a subgroup of HIV-infected long term nonprogressors. Proc Natl Acad Sci USA 97:2709, 2000.
80. Goulder PJ, Brander C, Tang Y, et al. Evolution and transmission of stable CTL escape mutations in HIV infection. Nature 412:334, 2001.
81. Flores-Villanueva PO, Yunis EJ, Delgado JC, et al. Control of HIV-1 viremia and protection from AIDS are associated with HLA-Bw4 homozygosity. Proc Natl Acad Sci USA 98:5140, 2001.
82. Kaslow RA, Rivers C, Tang J, et al. Polymorphisms in HLA class I genes associated with both favorable prognosis of human immunodeficiency virus (HIV) type 1 infection and positive cytotoxic T-lymphocyte responses to ALVAC-HIV recombinant canarypox vaccines. J Virol 75:8681, 2001.
83. Walker BD, Korber BT. Immune control of HIV: the obstacles of HLA and viral diversity. Nat Immunol 2:473, 2001.
84. Kalams SA, Walker BD. The critical need for CD4 help in maintaining effective cytotoxic T lymphocyte responses. J Exp Med 188:2199, 1998.
85. Bennett SR, Carbone FR, Karamalis F, et al. Help for cytotoxic-T-cell responses is mediated by CD40 signalling. Nature 393:478, 1998.
86. Schoenberger SP, Toes RE, van der Voort EI, et al. T-cell help for cytotoxic T lymphocytes is mediated by CD40-CD40L interactions. Nature 393:480, 1998.
87. Miedema F, Meyaard L, Koot M, et al. Changing virus-host interactions in the course of HIV-1 infection. Immunol Rev 140:35, 1994.
88. Gandhi RT, Chen BK, Straus SE, et al. HIV-1 directly kills CD4+ T cells by a Fas-independent mechanism. J Exp Med 187:1113, 1998.
89. Abbas AK. Die and let live: eliminating dangerous lymphocytes. Cell 84:655, 1996.
90. Pantaleo G, Fauci AS. Apoptosis in HIV infection. Nat Med 1:118, 1995.
91. Barcellini W, Rizzardi GP, Poli G, et al. Cytokines and soluble receptor changes in the transition from primary to early chronic HIV type 1 infection. AIDS Res Hum Retroviruses 12:325, 1996.
92. Barouch DH, Craiu A, Kuroda MJ, et al. Augmentation of immune responses to HIV-1 and simian immunodeficiency virus DNA vaccines by IL-2/Ig plasmid administration in rhesus monkeys. Proc Natl Acad Sci USA 97:4192, 2000.
93. Hel Z, Venzon D, Poudyal M, et al. Viremia control following antiretroviral treatment and therapeutic immunization during primary SIV251 infection of macaques. Nat Med 6:1140, 2000.
94. Parren PW, Burton DR, Sattentau QJ. HIV-1 antibody—debris or virion? Nat Med 3:366, 1997.
95. Poignard P, Sabbe R, Picchio GR, et al. Neutralizing antibodies have limited effects on the control of established HIV-1 infection in vivo. Immunity 10:431, 1999.
96. Montefiore D, Hill TS, Vo HT, et al. Neutralizing antibodies associated with viremia control in a subset of individuals after treatment of acute human immunodeficiency virus type 1 infection. J Virol 75:10200, 2001.
97. Mellors JW, Rinaldo CR Jr, Gupta P, et al. Prognosis in HIV-1 infection predicted by the quantity of virus in plasma. Science 272:1167, 1996.
98. Schmitz JE, Kuroda MJ, Santra S, et al. Control of viremia in simian immunodeficiency virus infection by CD8+ lymphocytes. Science 283:857, 1999.
99. Jin X, Bauer DE, Tuttleton SE, et al. Dramatic rise in plasma viremia after CD8(+) T cell depletion in simian immunodeficiency virus-infected macaques. J Exp Med 189:991, 1999.
100. Ho DD, Sarngadharan MG, Resnick L, et al. Primary human T-lymphotropic virus type III infection. Ann Intern Med 103:880, 1985.
101. Cooper DA, Gold J, Maclean P, et al. Acute AIDS retrovirus infection. Definition of a clinical illness associated with seroconversion. Lancet 1:537, 1985.
102. Tindall B, Barker S, Donovan B, et al. Characterization of the acute clinical illness associated with human immunodeficiency virus infection. Arch Intern Med 148:945, 1988.
103. Clark SJ, Saag MS, Decker WD, et al. High titers of cytopathic virus in patients with symptomatic primary HIV-1 infection. N Engl J Med 324:954, 1991.
104. Daar ES, Moudgil T, Meyer RD, Ho DD. Transient high levels of viremia in patients with primary human immunodeficiency virus type 1 infection. N Engl J Med 324:961, 1991.
105. Cossarizza A, Ortolani C, Mussini C, et al. Massive activation of immune cells with an intact T cell repertoire in acute human immunodeficiency virus syndrome. J Infect Dis 172:105, 1995.
106. DHHS. Guidelines for the Use of Antiretroviral Agents in HIV-Infected Adults and Adolescents. Washington, DC, 2001.
107. Niu MT, Stein DS, Schnittman SM. Primary human immunodeficiency virus type 1 infection: review of pathogenesis and early treatment intervention in humans and animal retrovirus infections. J Infect Dis 168:1490, 1993.
108. Bollinger RC, Brookmeyer RS, Mehendale SM, et al. Risk factors and clinical presentation of acute primary HIV infection in India. JAMA, 278:2085, 1997.
109. Montessori V, Rouleau D, Raboud J, et al. Clinical characteristics of primary HIV infection in injection drug users. AIDS 14:1868, 2000.
110. Lavreys L, Thompson ML, Martin HL Jr, et al. Primary human immunodeficiency virus type 1 infection: clinical manifestations among women in Mombasa, Kenya. Clin Infect Dis 30:486, 2000.
111. Schacker TW, Hughes JP, Shea T, et al. Biological and virologic characteristics of primary HIV infection. Ann Intern Med 128:613, 1998.
112. Lindback S, Brostrom C, Karlsson A, Gaines H. Does symptomatic primary HIV-1 infection accelerate progression to CDC stage IV disease, CD4 count below 200 × 10(6)l, AIDS, and death from AIDS? BMJ 309:1535, 1994.
113. Clark SJ, Shaw GM. The acute retroviral syndrome and the pathogenesis of HIV-1 infection. Semin Immunol 5:149, 1993.
114. Keet IP, Krijnen P, Koot M, et al. Predictors of rapid progression to AIDS in HIV-1 seroconverters. AIDS 7:51, 1993.
115. Pedersen C, Lindhardt BO, Jensen BL, et al. Clinical course of primary HIV infection: consequences for subsequent course of infection. BMJ 299:154, 1989.
116. Vanhems P, Allard R, Cooper DA, et al. Acute human immunodeficiency virus type 1 disease as a mononucleosis-like illness: is the diagnosis too restrictive? Clin Infect Dis 24:965, 1997. Erratum. Clin Infect Dis 25:352, 1997.
117. Gaines H, von Sydow M, Pehrson PO, Lundbegh P. Clinical picture of primary HIV infection presenting as a glandular-fever-like illness. BMJ 297:1363, 1988.
118. Barnadas MA, Alegre M, Baselga E, et al. Histopathological changes of primary HIV infection. Description of three cases and review of the literature. J Cutan Pathol 24:507, 1997.

119. Brehmer-Andersson E, Torssander J. The exanthema of acute (primary) HIV infection. identification of a characteristic histopathological picture? Acta Derm Venereol 70:85, 1990.
120. Lapins J, Lindback S, Lidbrink P, et al. Mucocutaneous manifestations in 22 consecutive cases of primary HIV-1 infection. Br J Dermatol 134:257, 1996.
121. Ringler DJ, Hancock WW, King NW, et al. Immunophenotypic characterization of the cutaneous exanthem of SIV-infected rhesus monkeys. Apposition of degenerative Langerhans cells and cytotoxic lymphocytes during the development of acquired immunodeficiency syndrome. Am J Pathol 126:199, 1987.
122. Kinloch-de Loes S, de Saussure P, Saurat JH, et al. Symptomatic primary infection due to human immunodeficiency virus type 1: review of 31 cases. Clin Infect Dis 17:59, 1993.
123. Felten A, Lecompte T, Ferchal F, Agbalika F. Primary HIV-1 infection associated with prominent genital ulcers [letter]. Genitourin Med 69:78, 1993.
124. Krasner CG, Cohen SH. Bilateral Bell's palsy and aseptic meningitis in a patient with acute human immunodeficiency virus seroconversion. West J Med 159:604, 1993.
125. Bernard E, Dellamonica P, Michiels JF, et al. Heparine-like anticoagulant vasculitis associated with severe primary infection by HIV [letter]. AIDS 4:932, 1990.
126. Ruiz-Laiglesia FJ, Torrubia-Perez CB, Perez-Calvo JI. Ulcerative esophagitis during primary HIV infection [letter]. Arch Intern Med 156:1115, 1996.
127. Fusade T, Liony C, Joly P, et al. Ulcerative esophagitis during primary HIV infection [letter]. Am J Gastroenterol 87:1523, 1992.
128. Lafeuillade A, Chaffanjon P, Pellegrino P, et al. Oesophageal candidiasis in primary HIV infection [letter]. Eur J Med 1:126, 1992.
129. Jolles S, Kinloch de Loes S, Johnson MA, Janossy G. Primary HIV-1 infection: a new medical emergency [editorial]?. BMJ 312:1243, 1996.
130. Casseb JS, Caterino-de-Araujo A. [Difficulties in diagnosing atypical primary HIV-1 infection: report of a case.] Rev Inst Med Trop Sao Paulo 36:287, 1994.
131. Molina JM, Welker Y, Ferchal F, et al. Hepatitis associated with primary HIV infection [letter]. Gastroenterology 102:739, 1992.
132. Cuenca Carvajal C, Ortiz Vega M, Gomez Antunez M, et al. [Acute pancreatitis complicating primary HIV-1 infection.] An Med Interna 15:324, 1998.
133. Sinicco A, Sciandra M, Di Garbo A, et al. Primary HIV infection presenting with acute pancreatitis [letter]. Scand J Infect Dis 31:423, 1999.
134. Herrero JA, Gil R, Pastor C, Sanchez D. [Pneumonitis associated with primary infection by HIV (letter).] Enferm Infecc Microbiol Clin 9:385, 1991.
135. Ong EL, Mandal BK. Primary HIV-I infection associated with pneumonitis. Postgrad Med J 67:579, 1991.
136. Jouveshomme S, Couderc LJ, Ferchal F, et al. Lymphocytic alveolitis after primary HIV infection with CMV coinfection. Chest 112:1127, 1997.
137. Combes R, Amouyal G, Rene E. [Pancreatitis, hypocalcemia and myositis associated with primary HIV infection (letter).] Gastroenterol Clin Biol 15:860, 1991.
138. Yasuoka C, Kikuchi Y, Yasuoka A, et al. Successful treatment of acute myeloradiculoneuritis with high-dose corticosteroids in a patient with primary HIV-1 infection. Jpn J Infect Dis 53:171, 2000.
139. Martel JW. [Encephalitis in connection with primary HIV infection as a differential diagnosis in acute psychosis.] Lakartidningen 86:1701, 1989.
140. Card T, Wathen CG, Luzzi GA. Primary HIV-1 infection presenting with transient neurological deficit [letter]. J Neurol Neurosurg Psychiatry 64:281, 1998.
141. Hardy WD, Daar ES, Sokolov RT Jr, Ho DD. Acute neurologic deterioration in a young man [clinical conference]. Rev Infect Dis 13:745, 1991.
142. Ho DD, Rota TR, Schooley RT, et al. Isolation of HTLV-III from cerebrospinal fluid and neural tissues of patients with neurologic syndromes related to the acquired immunodeficiency syndrome. N Engl J Med 313:1493, 1985.
143. Beytout J, Llory JF, Clavelou P, et al. [Meningoradiculitis in the primary phase of HIV infection: value of plasmapheresis (letter).] Presse Med 18:1031, 1989.
144. Eerens F, Van Cleemput J, Peetermans WE. A probable primary HIV infection associated with acute non-specific myocarditis causing severe dilated cardiomyopathy. Acta Clin Belg 54:220, 1999.
145. Martinez-Escribano JA, Pedro F, Sabater V, et al. Acute exanthem and pancreatic panniculitis in a patient with primary HIV infection and haemophagocytic syndrome. Br J Dermatol 134:804, 1996.
146. Mortier E, Zahar JR, Gros I, et al. Primary infection with human immunodeficiency virus that presented as Stevens-Johnson syndrome [letter]. Clin Infect Dis 19:798, 1994.
147. Biggs B, Newton-John HF. Acute HTLV-III infection. A case followed from onset to seroconversion. Med J Aust 144:545, 1986.
148. Gaines H, Albert J, von Sydow M, et al. HIV antigenaemia and virus isolation from plasma during primary HIV infection. Lancet 1:1317, 1987.
149. Daar ES, Little S, Pitt J, et al. Diagnosis of primary HIV-1 infection. Los Angeles County Primary HIV Infection Recruitment Network. Ann Intern Med 134:25, 2001.
150. Pedersen C, Nielsen JO, Dickmeis E, Jordal R. Early progression to AIDS following primary HIV infection [letter]. AIDS 3:45, 1989.
151. Henrard DR, Daar E, Farzadegan H, et al. Virologic and immunologic characterization of symptomatic and asymptomatic primary HIV-1 infection. J Acquir Immune Defic Syndr Hum Retrovirol 9:305, 1995.
152. Veugelers PJ, Kaldor JM, Strathdee SA, et al. Incidence and prognostic significance of symptomatic primary human immunodeficiency virus type 1 infection in homosexual men. J Infect Dis 176:112, 1997.
153. Kaufmann GR, Cunningham P, Zaunders J, et al. Impact of early HIV-1 RNA and T-lymphocyte dynamics during primary HIV-1 infection on the subsequent course of HIV-1 RNA levels and CD4+ T-lymphocyte counts in the first year of HIV-1 infection. Sydney Primary HIV Infection Study Group. J Acquir Immune Defic Syndr 22:437, 1999.
154. Gorham ED, Garland FC, Mayers DL, et al. CD4 lymphocyte counts within 24 months of human immunodeficiency virus seroconversion. Findings in the US Navy and Marine Corps. The Navy Retroviral Working Group. Arch Intern Med 153:869, 1993.
155. Kourtis AP, Ibegbu C, Nahmias AJ, et al. Early progression of disease in HIV-infected infants with thymus dysfunction. N Engl J Med 335:1431, 1996. Erratum. N Engl J Med 336:595, 1997.
156. Rogers MF, Ou CY, Rayfield M, et al. Use of the polymerase chain reaction for early detection of the proviral sequences of human immunodeficiency virus in infants born to seropositive mothers. New York City Collaborative Study of Maternal HIV Transmission and Montefiore Medical Center HIV Perinatal Transmission Study Group. N Engl J Med 320:1649, 1989.
157. Krogstad P, Uittenbogaart CH, Dickover R, et al. Primary HIV infection of infants: the effects of somatic growth on lymphocyte and virus dynamics. Clin Immunol 92:25, 1999.
158. Connor EM, Sperling RS, Gelber R, et al. Reduction of maternal-infant transmission of human immunodeficiency virus type 1 with zidovudine treatment. Pediatric AIDS Clinical Trials Group Protocol 076 Study Group. N Engl J Med 331:1173, 1994.
159. Kourtis AP, Bulterys M, Nesheim SR, Lee FK. Understanding the timing of HIV transmission from mother to infant. JAMA 285:709, 2001.
160. Galetto-Lacour A, Kinloch-de Lous S, Hirschel B, Perrin L. [Primary HIV infection: an often suspected diagnosis but confirmed late.] Schweiz Med Wochenschr 125:341, 1995.
161. Hirsch MS, Brun-Vezinet F, D'Aquilia RT, et al. Antiretroviral drug resistance testing in adult HIV-1 infection: recommendations of an international AIDS Society—USA panel. JAMA 283:2417, 2000.
162. Busch MP, Satten GA. Time course of viremia and antibody seroconversion following human immunodeficiency virus exposure. Am J Med 102:117, 1997.
163. Janssen RS, Satten GA, Stramer SL, et al. New testing strategy to detect early HIV-1 infection for use in incidence estimates and for clinical and prevention purposes. JAMA. 280:42, 1998.
164. Fiebig E, Heldebrant C, Peddada L, et al. Dynamics of HIV viremia preceding antibody seroconversion in plasma donors: implications for detection of primary infection by p24 antigen and nucleic acid amplification screening assays. Presented at the 8th Conference on Retroviruses and Opportunistic Infections, 2001, abstract 415.
164a. Delwart E, Kalmin N, Jones S, et al. First case of HIV transmission by an RNA-screened blood donation. 9th Conference of Retroviruses and Opportunistic Infections 2001, abstract 768W.
165. McFarland W, Busch M, Kellogg TA, et al. Detection of early HIV in-

fection and estimation of incidence using a sensitive/less-sensitive enzyme immunoassay testing strategy at anonymous counseling and testing sites in San Francisco. J Acquir Immune Defic Syndr 2:484, 1999.

166. Rosenberg E, Cotton D. Primary HIV infection and the acute retroviral syndrome. AIDS Clin Care 9:19, 1997.
167. Cabie A, Abel S, Lafaye JM, et al. [Dengue or acute retroviral syndrome?] Presse Med 29:1173, 2000.
168. Hudson CP, Levett PN, Edwards CN, et al. Severe primary HIV-1 infection among black persons in Barbados. Int J STD AIDS 8:393, 1997.
169. Chaffanjon P, Lafeuillade A, Quilichini R, Aubert L. [Primary HIV infection with severe and unusual manifestations (letter).] Presse Med 21:536, 1992.
170. Clotet B. Oesophageal candidiasis in people with primary HIV infection [letter]. AIDS 5:1034, 1991.
171. Tindall B, Hing M, Edwards P, et al. Severe clinical manifestations of primary HIV infection. AIDS 3:747, 1989.
172. Mateos Rodriguez F, Fuertes Martin A, MarcosToledano M, Jiminez Lopez A. [Primary HIV infection with esophageal candidiasis and acute toxoplasmosis (letter).] An Med Interna 15:50, 1998.
173. Moss PJ, Read RC, Kudesia G, McKendrick MW, Prolonged cryptosporidiosis during primary HIV infection. J Infect 30:1, 1995.
174. Busch MP, Kleinman SH, Jackson B, et al. Committee report. Nucleic acid amplification testing of blood donors for transfusion-transmitted infectious diseases: report of the Interorganizational Task Force on Nucleic Acid Amplification Testing of Blood Donors. Transfusion 40:143, 2000.
175. Cardo DM, Culver DH, Ciesielski CA, et al. A case-control study of HIV seroconversion in health care workers after percutaneous exposure: Centers for Disease Control and Prevention Needlestick Surveillance Group. N Engl J Med 337:1485, 1997.
176. Busch MP, Satten GA. Time course of viremia and antibody seroconversion following HIV exposure. Transfusion 102:117, 1997.
177. Ciesielski CA, Metler RP. Duration of time between exposure and seroconversion in healthcare workers with occupationally acquired infection with human immunodeficiency virus. Am J Med 102:115, 1997.
178. Lindback S, Thorstensson R, Karlsson AC, et al. Diagnosis of primary HIV-1 infection and duration of follow-up after HIV exposure. Karolinska Institute Primary HIV Infection Study Group. AIDS 14:2333, 2000.
179. Kinloch-De Loes S, Hirschel BJ, Hoen B, et al. A controlled trial of zidovudine in primary human immunodeficiency virus infection. N Engl J Med 333:408, 1995. Erratum. N Engl J Med 333:408, 1995.
180. Niu MT, Bethel TJ, Holodniy M, et al. Zidovudine treatment in patients with primary (acute) human immunodeficiency virus type 1 infection: a randomized, double-blind, placebo-controlled trial. DATRI 002 Study Group. Division of AIDS Treatment Research Initiative. J Infect Dis 178:80, 1998.
181. Kinloch-de Loes S, Perneger TV. Primary HIV infection: follow-up of patients initially randomized to zidovudine or placebo. J Infect 35:111, 1997.
182. Luzuriaga K, Bryson Y, Krogstad P, et al. Combination treatment with zidovudine, didanosine, and nevirapine in infants with human immunodeficiency virus type 1 infection. N Engl J Med 336:1343, 1997.
183. Perrin L, Rakik A, Yerly S, et al. Combined therapy with zidovudine and L-697,661 in primary HIV infection. AIDS 10:1233, 1996.
184. Perrin L, Hirschel B. Combination therapy in primary HIV infection. Antiviral Res 29:87, 1996.
185. Perrin L, Yerly S, Charvier A, et al. Zidovudine plus didanosine in primary HIV-1 infection. Antivir Ther 2:5, 1997.
186. Berrey MM, Schacker T, Collier AC, et al. Treatment of primary human immunodeficiency virus type 1 infection with potent antiretroviral therapy reduces frequency of rapid progression to AIDS. J Infect Dis 183:1466, 2001.
187. Alexander CS, Dong W, Schechter MT, et al. Prevalence of primary HIV drug resistance among seroconverters during an explosive outbreak of HIV infection among injecting drug users. AIDS 13:981, 1999.
188. Brenner B, Wainberg MA, Salomon H, et al. Resistance to antiretroviral drugs in patients with primary HIV-1 infection. Investigators of the Quebec Primary Infection Study. Int J Antimicrob Agents 16:429, 2000.
189. Boden D, Hurley A, Zhang L, et al. HIV-1 drug resistance in newly infected individuals. JAMA 282:1135, 1999.
190. Little SJ. Is transmitted drug resistance in HIV on the rise? It seems so. BMJ 322:1074, 2001.
191. Yerly S, Kaiser L, Race E, et al. Transmission of antiretroviral-drug-resistant HIV-1 variants. Lancet 354:729, 1999.
192. Brown AJ, Precious HM, Whitcomb JM, et al. Reduced susceptibility of human immunodeficiency virus type 1 (HIV-1) from patients with primary HIV infection to non nucleoside reverse transcriptase inhibitors is associated with variation at novel amino acid sites. J Virol 74:10269, 2000.
193. Balotta C, Berlusconi A, Pan A, et al. Prevalence of transmitted nucleoside analogue-resistant HIV-1 strains and pre-existing mutations in pol reverse transcriptase and protease region: outcome after treatment in recently infected individuals. Antivir Ther 5:7, 2000.
194. Hirsch MS, Conway B, D'Aquilia RT, et al. Antiretroviral drug resistance testing in HIV Infection of adults: implications for clinical management. JAMA 279:1984, 1998.
195. Carpenter CC, Cooper DA, Fischl MA, et al. Antiretroviral therapy in adults: updated recommendations of the International AIDS Society—USA Panel. JAMA 283:381, 2000.
196. Blower SM, Aschenbach AN, Gershengorn HB, Kahn JO. Predicting the unpredictable: transmission of drug-resistant HIV. Nat Med 7:1016, 2001.
197. Altfeld M, Walker BD. Less is more? STI in acute and chronic HIV-1 infection. Nat Med 7:881, 2001.
198. Carcelain G, Tubiana R, Samri A, et al. Transient mobilization of human immunodeficiency virus (HIV)-specific CD4 T-helper cells fails to control virus rebounds during intermittent antiretroviral therapy in chronic HIV type 1 infection. J Virol 75:234, 2001.
199. Ruiz L, Martinez-Picardo J, Romeu J, et al. Structured treatment interruption in chronically HIV-1 infected patients after long-term viral suppression. AIDS 14:397, 2000.
200. Garcia F, Plana M, Ortiz GM, et al. The virological and immunological consequences of structured treatment interruptions in chronic HIV-1 infection. AIDS 15:F29, 2001.

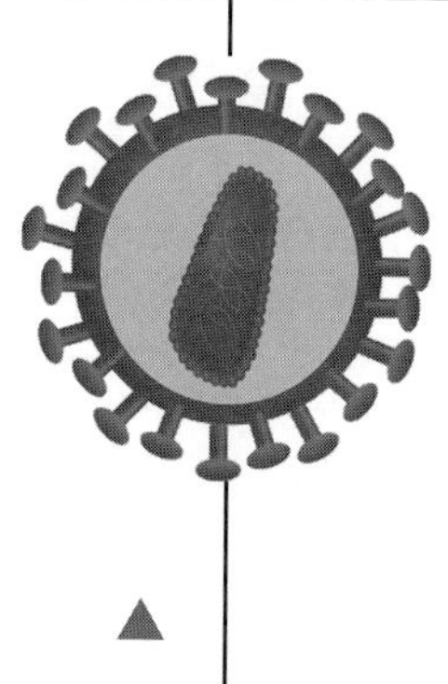

CHAPTER 25

Occupational and Nonoccupational Exposure Management

David K. Henderson, MD
Julie Louise Gerberding, MD, MPH

Primary prevention—that is, preventing exposure to human immunodeficiency virus (HIV)—is by far the most effective mechanism of preventing infection in both community and occupational settings. When exposure does occur, administration of antiretroviral agents for secondary prevention may be appropriate. The strongest evidence to support the efficacy of postexposure prophylaxis is derived from experience with occupational exposures to HIV in health care settings. Nonetheless, these data are likely to apply to the management of community exposures as well. Although we learned a great deal about occupational risks and the management of occupational exposures during the first two decades of experience with HIV infection in the health care setting, several issues relating to the management of HIV infection in health care remain to be solved. This chapter reviews our current understanding of the epidemiology, pathogenesis, and management of occupational and nonoccupational exposures to HIV and discusses the complex issues relating to the management of HIV-infected health care providers.

▲ PATHOGENESIS OF HIV INFECTION

The rationale for postexposure prophylaxis is based on the assumption that antiretroviral agents can be administered and delivered in pharmacologically active form to target cells in time to interrupt one or more of the crucial steps of the initial infection. The pathogenesis of the initial infection has not been defined, but dendritic cells in the skin or mucous membranes appear to be the first cells to interact with HIV.[1–7] Dendritic cells can trap HIV through surface ligands and then transfer virus to susceptible CD4+ T-lymphocytes.[8,9] HIV remains highly infectious when bound to the surface of dendritic cells, even in the presence of neutralizing antibody.[10] Some data suggest that dendritic cells also can be infected with HIV and may represent a hidden reservoir.[11] The factors that determine the cellular outcome of HIV transfer to CD4+ T-lymphocytes are the subject of intense investigation but are still not fully defined. In theory, interventions that block the successful transfer of HIV from dendritic cells to susceptible CD4+ T-lymphocytes or can, in some way, prevent the earliest rounds of productive infection would likely prevent acute infection.

▲ IMMUNOLOGIC DEFENSES AGAINST ACUTE HIV INFECTION

The cellular immune system appears to play a key role in determining the outcome of exposure to HIV. Studies of lymphocytes from seronegative sexual partners of HIV-infected individuals have demonstrated the presence of HIV-specific cellular cytotoxic responses.[12,13] Similarly, some health care workers who sustained percutaneous exposures to blood from HIV-infected patients but did not become infected developed lymphocyte reactivity that was specific for HIV antigens.[14] Puro and coworkers reported a single instance of an individual who sustained an occupational exposure to HIV and subsequently had HIV sequences detected transiently from circulating blood by nucleic acid amplification during combination antiretroviral prophylaxis.[15] The health care worker remained HIV antibody-negative but did develop HIV-specific T-helper responses, as assessed by interleukin-2 production, 13 months

All material in this chapter is in the public domain, with the exception of any borrowed figures or tables.

following the exposure.[15] Animal studies also provide indirect support for the role of cell-mediated immunity in early defense against acute HIV infection. For example, as early as 1994 Ruprecht and her coworkers demonstrated that intact cellular immunity is required for successful postexposure prophylaxis.[16] More recently, the studies of Putkonen and coworkers demonstrated that simian immunodeficiency virus (SIV)-challenged macaques in which infection was prevented by postexposure prophylaxis developed cell-mediated immunity that either prevented or substantially limited infection from a second challenge.[17] Thus based on our current understanding of the early events in the pathogenesis of, and host defense against, acute HIV infection, initiation of antiretroviral chemoprophylaxis soon after exposure, in combination with a cellular immune response, may prevent or inhibit systemic HIV infection. This preventive effect theoretically occurs by limiting the proliferation of virus in the dendritic cells or regional lymph nodes during a "window of opportunity" during which the virus remains localized.

▲ EXPOSURES PRESENTING A RISK FOR TRANSMISSION

Most occupational infections have resulted from parenteral or percutaneous exposures to blood from a patient known to be infected with HIV. Of the 56 cases of occupational infection reported to the U.S. Centers for Disease Control and Prevention (CDC), 48 resulted from parenteral exposures and 5 from mucosal exposures.[18] Of these 56 infections, 2 occurred in individuals who sustained both mucous membrane and parenteral exposures; one had an unknown route of exposure.[18] Whereas parenteral exposures are associated with the highest risk (i.e., the risk for infection associated with transfusion of a unit of contaminated blood approaches 100%[19]), the risk associated with mucous membrane exposures is not trivial. Mucosal exposures are presumably responsible for most instances of sexual transmission. The risk for infection associated with a parenteral occupational exposure is approximately 0.3% per exposure,[20] and the risk for a single sexual encounter is estimated to be of the same magnitude as the parenteral exposure risk (i.e., 0.1% to 0.5%).[21–25] Although not measured with precision, the risk associated with mucosal exposures is likely to be of the same magnitude. Cutaneous exposures are associated with substantially less risk.[26] Needlestick injuries with hollow-bore injection needles have been responsible for most occupational infections among health care providers. To our knowledge, to date no infections have been documented to result from a needlestick with a solid surgical needle. The reasons for this discrepancy are unclear but may include the fact that such needles carry a smaller inoculum of blood and exposures to such needles are less likely to be reported (because they occur most often among surgeons, and members of the surgical team and operating room staff are notorious for underreporting occupational exposures). In addition, infections have resulted from scalpel accidents, laboratory accidents, and other, more unusual exposures. We advocate treating all documented parenteral or mucosal exposures to blood from an infected individual as exposures and recommend offering postexposure antiretroviral prophylaxis to individuals sustaining such exposures. When information is available that influences the magnitude of risk, we advocate sharing this information with the exposed individual to allow him or her to use the data when deciding about further treatment. Such data may also be of use when determining the prophylaxis regimen to be offered to the exposed individual. Exposures to blood (and blood cells) represent the primary risk for transmission. Fluids such as saliva and tears, unless they contain blood, have not been implicated in HIV transmission. The CDC has been tracking occupational infections since the beginning of the epidemic. Nurses and laboratory technicians have sustained the most frequent occupational infections. The professions of those sustaining documented occupational infections that have been reported to the CDC are summarized in Table 25–1.[18] The CDC has also collected data on 138 health

▲ **Table 25–1.** U.S. HEALTH CARE WORKERS WITH DOCUMENTED AND POSSIBLE OCCUPATIONALLY ACQUIRED HIV INFECTION, BY OCCUPATION, THROUGH JUNE 30, 2000

Occupation	Documented occupational transmission[a]	Possible occupational transmission[b]
Dental workers, Including dentists	0	6
Embalmer/morgue technician	1	2
Emergency medical technician/paramedic	0	12
Health aide/attendant	1	15
Housekeeper/maintenance worker	2	13
Laboratory technician		
Clinical	16	17
Nonclinical	3	0
Nurse	23	35
Physician		
Nonsurgical	6	12
Surgical	0	6
Respiratory therapist	1	2
Technician		
Dialysis	1	3
Surgical	2	2
Technician/therapist *(other than those listed above)*	0	9
Other health care occupations	0	4
Total	56	138

Health care workers are defined as persons, including students and trainees, who have worked in a health care, clinical, or HIV laboratory setting at any time since 1978.

[a]Health care workers who had documented HIV seroconversion after occupational exposure or had other laboratory evidence of occupational infection.

[b]These health care workers have been investigated and are without identifiable behavioral or transfusion risks; each reported percutaneous or mucocutaneous occupational exposures to blood, body fluids, or laboratory solutions containing HIV. Seroconversion specifically resulting from an occupational exposure was not documented.

From Centers for Disease Control and Prevention. Surveillance of Health Care Workers with HIV/AIDS. Atlanta, CDC, 2001.

care workers who fit in a category called "possible occupational transmission."[18] Information about their occupations is provided in Table 25–1.[18]

▲ RATIONALE FOR ADMINISTERING ANTIRETROVIRAL CHEMOPROPHYLAXIS

Epidemiologic Studies

Investigators working at the CDC designed a retrospective case–control study to attempt to identify specific factors associated with occupational risk for HIV infection. This study matched health care workers with occupational infection (i.e., documented HIV seroconversions following occupational exposures) detected through well documented anecdotal case reports with health care workers who: (1) had sustained occupational exposures to HIV; (2) had reported the exposures to the CDC; and (3) did not subsequently become infected.[27] This study identified four exposure-related factors as being associated with infection following occupational exposure: the depth or severity of the exposure; the presence of visible blood on the device causing the injury; the fact that the device causing the injury had been in the source patient's veins or arteries; and exposures to blood from a source patient who died within 60 days of the exposure.[28] All four of these factors likely operate as surrogates for inoculum size. The fifth factor associated with increased risk for occupational infection in this case–control study was "not taking zidovudine as postexposure prophylaxis," suggesting an approximately 80% protective effect for zidovudine postexposure prophylaxis. The retrospective study design has limitations[29] but provides indirect support for the concept that postexposure prophylaxis may be effective.

Clinical Studies

Studies of antiretroviral treatment efficacy for preventing vertical transmission of HIV provide additional rationale for using these drugs for postexposure prophylaxis. Lindegren and coworkers demonstrated that the incidence of perinatally transmitted HIV infection in the United States declined by two-thirds from 1992 to 1997 and ascribed this decrease primarily to the efficacy of peripartum treatment.[30] In the AIDS Clinical Treatment Group (ACTG) protocol 076 investigators administered zidovudine to mothers before birth and during labor and delivery and to the infant for 6 weeks after birth.[31] Administration of zidovudine was associated with a 67% reduction in vertical HIV transmission.[31] Subsequent studies have confirmed these findings.[30,32–46] A study from a large, metropolitan hospital demonstrated that administration of antiretroviral agents to the newborn within the first 48 hours of life significantly reduces the risk for perinatal HIV transmission, even when the mother was not treated before or during labor.[38] This was the first prospective clinical trial to demonstrate the efficacy of postexposure antiretroviral prophylaxis in humans.[38]

Animal Studies

Early studies using animal models of postexposure prophylaxis demonstrated limited if any treatment effect. For example, the initial studies of the safety and efficacy of chemoprophylaxis in mice[47] and cats[48] demonstrated minimal treatment benefit. The specific characteristics of these models (e.g., size of viral inocula, routes of administration) have caused some investigators to question their relevance to HIV prophylaxis in humans.[49] A series of studies conducted in a nude mouse model (i.e., an athymic mouse into which human hematolymphoid organs had been engrafted) provided some encouragement for the use of postexposure prophylaxis.[50–53] Subsequent studies in the mouse-Rauscher murine leukemia virus model demonstrated that zidovudine can be efficacious in preventing infection and that chemoprophylactic efficacy in the model required intact cellular immunity.[16] Studies in what may well be a more relevant macaque model have produced mixed results. The earliest studies[54–56] again demonstrated limited effect from the antiretroviral agents.

More recent studies in the SIV or HIV-2 macaque models, generally employing lower viral inocula, have demonstrated a clearly protective effect of postexposure prophylaxis in these models. One of the first studies to demonstrate a treatment benefit was that of Van Rompay and colleagues.[57] Böttiger and coworkers demonstrated that a 3-day course of the nucleoside analogue BEA-005 (2,3′-dideoxy-3′-hydroxymethylcytidine) could abrogate either SIV or HIV-2 infection following an intravenous or intrarectal inoculation of these viruses.[58] Tsai et al. demonstrated that phosphonylmethoxypropyladenine (PMPA) (Tenofovir; Gilead Sciences, Foster City, CA, USA) was highly efficacious in preventing infection in a macaque SIV model.[59] In further studies using the macaque SIV tenofovir model, these investigators found that all macaques that received postinoculation treatment for 28 days were protected, whereas only half of the macaques treated for 10 days and none treated for only 3 days remained infection-free.[60] Delaying treatment also was found to be detrimental in this model. Whereas 100% of macaques that received tenofovir within 24 hours of intravenous SIV infection remained uninfected, only 50% of the animals that received the first dose of the agent 48 hours following infection and only 25% of the animals that received the first dose of treatment at 72 hours after inoculation remained uninfected.[60] In a study of similar design evaluating prophylaxis following vaginal inoculation of macaques with HIV-2, Otten and coworkers found similar results, with all of the animals treated within 48 hours remaining uninfected. Breakthrough infections occurred in animals receiving tenofovir at 72 hours following inoculation.[61]

Additional Experience with HIV Postexposure Prophylaxis in Humans

The fact that occupational HIV infections in health care workers are occurring at a stable or reduced frequency in the United States is consistent with the hypothesis that antiretroviral prophylaxis may be efficacious. Figure 25–1 stratifies

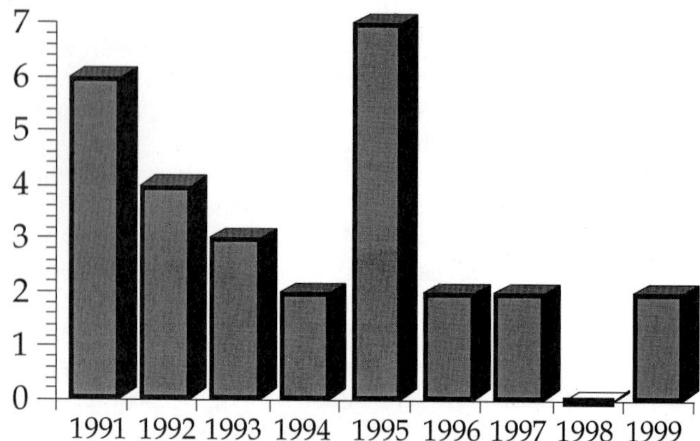

Figure 25–1. Documented occupational HIV infections reported to the CDC, 1991–1999. (Data courtesy of Elise Beltrami, MD.)

the cases of occupational infections reported to the CDC from 1992 through 1999 (E. Beltrami, CDC, personal communication) and demonstrates a decrease in the number of cases of occupational HIV infections reported to the CDC. Although there are several possible explanations for this decrease (e.g., decreased reporting to CDC, less aggressive case-finding, fewer exposures due to increased use of primary exposure prevention, efficacy of highly active antiretroviral therapy), widespread use of postexposure antiretroviral therapy could be an important factor contributing to the observed decrease.

Two anecdotal case reports are relevant to a discussion of postexposure treatment efficacy. In the first case report, a child who had received a transfusion of HIV-infected blood (a situation that produces infection in nearly 100% of such cases[19]) remained uninfected following a protracted postexposure prophylaxis regimen.[62] In the second, a health care worker who had sustained an occupational HIV exposure, HIV DNA was detected in the plasma during three-drug postexposure prophylaxis. The worker remained uninfected (as assessed by serial nucleic acid tests and antibody determinations) but did produce an HIV-specific cellular immune response.[15]

Anecdotal reports of postexposure treatment failure have also accumulated. According to the CDC, prophylaxis failures have been documented in at least 21 instances.[63] In most (n = 16) of these cases, zidovudine was used as a single agent. Two instances of failure of a two-nucleoside analogue regimen and three instances in which a three-drug regimen failed have been documented. For 62% of these instances of failure, the source patient had antiretroviral "experience" (i.e., had been receiving one or more antiretroviral agents) prior to the exposure, raising the concern that antiretroviral resistance may be contributing to chemoprophylaxis failure.[63]

▲ MANAGEMENT OF OCCUPATIONAL EXPOSURES TO HIV

Immediate Management

Recommendations for the immediate management of HIV exposures are based on logic or intuition, rather than data. Nonetheless, it is reasonable to recommend that exposure sites be decontaminated as soon as possible (i.e., whenever patient safety permits). Puncture wounds and other cutaneous injuries should be washed with soap and water. When the injury results in a visible defect, the wound should be irrigated with sterile saline, a disinfectant, or other suitable solution. Mucosal exposures involving the mouth and nose should be flushed with water. Following an ocular exposure, eyes should be irrigated with clean water, saline, or sterile irrigants designed for this purpose.[64] Decontaminating with bleach, iodophors, peroxide, or other hospital disinfectants as an immediate measure for wound care is not contraindicated, but at least one anecdotal report clearly documents failure of bleach to prevent transmission in an exposure setting.[64]

Exposure Reporting

Ensuring accurate reporting of exposures is a key first step in managing exposures. Institutional procedures for reporting exposures should be simple, user-friendly, and widely publicized. Underreporting of occupational exposures to blood is a long-standing problem.[65–75] Institutions must educate staff about the risks prevalent in the workplace and must ensure that all staff members perceive these risks. Institutions should also develop mechanisms to facilitate reporting of exposures and to streamline the provision of follow-up care. Institutional occupational medical systems must protect the confidentiality of the exposed worker. If health care worker confidentiality is not preserved, institutional programs are doomed to failure.

Staff Education

Education is important to both primary and secondary prevention efforts. Employees should be apprised about the epidemiology of blood-borne pathogen infection, risks for infection, primary and secondary prevention interventions, importance of reporting exposures, and the availability of and mechanisms to gain access to postexposure management programs. Annual training is now required by the Occupational Health and Safety Administration (OSHA), mandating that institutions: (1) provide periodic training for health care workers about blood-borne infectious occupational risks prevalent in the hospital environment; (2) provide workers with information about the effective use of infection control procedures to reduce the risk of occupational exposures; (3) provide barriers to health care workers to reduce the risk of occupational exposures to blood and blood-containing fluids; (4) require employees to follow certain work practices and procedures in the processes of health care delivery; (5) immunize at-risk, susceptible health care workers who are in their employ with hepatitis B vaccine; and (6) follow certain protocols when managing health care workers who have sustained occupational exposures to blood-borne pathogens.[76]

Clinical Evaluation

Assessment of the Potential Exposure and the Source Patient

An extremely important step in postexposure management is for the practitioner involved in the care of the individual reporting the exposure to evaluate the circumstances of exposure to make certain an exposure has in fact occurred. This assessment includes detailed evaluation of the exposure event and thorough evaluation of the source patient. The source patient's medical record should be reviewed for pertinent historical or serologic information. If the source patient's status with respect to blood-borne pathogen infection is not known, the source patient should be informed of the incident and tested for serologic evidence of blood-borne virus infection consonant with applicable state and local laws. Because of the evidence suggesting that the timing of prophylaxis is an important variable,[60,61] serologic testing of the source patient, preferably by enzyme immunoassay, should be carried out as soon as is practical. The rapid test currently marketed in the United States provides an alternative to the enzyme immunoassay but, in our opinion, must be used with circumspection, at least in part because of its subjective endpoint. When a skilled operator performs the test, a negative result is highly reliable. If the test is used to decide whether prophylaxis should be administered, an enzyme immunoassay should be performed as soon as possible to confirm the result of the rapid test. We believe that in settings in which testing is not immediately available and the provider is certain an exposure has occurred, the best strategy is to begin prophylaxis immediately and then either discontinue or modify the regimen when testing results or additional information is obtained.

In instances in which the source is known to be HIV-infected, the practitioner should collect all the readily available information about the source patient's status, including whether the individual has received (or is currently receiving) antiretroviral therapy, current immunologic and virologic parameters (e.g., viral burden, CD4+ T-lymphocyte count), and length of time the patient has been diagnosed with HIV infection. If information about the source patient's viral isolates is available (i.e., information concerning phenotypic or genotypic resistance of the isolates), this information should be considered as well. In many instances none of this information is available, so protocols must be developed to manage exposed individuals in the absence of such data.

If the source patient's blood-borne infection status is unknown and cannot be learned, the practitioner providing care for the exposed individual should make an epidemiologic assessment about the likelihood of exposure and proceed accordingly. Types of information that can likely assist the provider in this setting include the severity of the exposure, the precise circumstances of the exposure, the demographics of the source patient (if known), and the presence of other epidemiologically linked infection markers (e.g., hepatitis B virus, hepatitis C virus). Each of these "source-unknown" instances must be managed on a case-by-case basis.

Because antiretroviral agents are associated with substantial risks for side effects and occasionally severe toxicities, these agents must not be prescribed casually. The U.S. Public Health Service has established a National Clinicians' Post-Exposure Prophylaxis Hotline (PEPLINE) at the University of California at San Francisco to provide expert advice to practitioners about the management of exposures to HIV. Summary data from the PEPLINE experience suggest that postexposure prophylaxis is being prescribed far too often. For example, in 1997 about 58% of the calls to the PEPLINE were for instances in which the staff of the PEPLINE recommended either stopping or not starting postexposure prophylaxis.[77] The data from 1998 were equally as concerning. Overall, 59% of calls in 1998 were for similar circumstances, prompting a similar recommendation from the PEPLINE staff.[78] One reason for the problem of overtreatment may be that the individuals who are asked to manage occupational exposures are not familiar with the risks associated with treatment and are easily (and understandably) swayed by the anxiety of the health care provider who has reported the exposure. Hopefully, ready access to and use of expert consultants such as those supported by the PEPLINE will reduce the number of unnecessary courses prescribed. The PEPLINE can be accessed at 888-448-4911 and via the World Wide Web at http://pepline.ucsf.edu/pepline.

Initial Assessment

The initial evaluation of the exposed individual should take place as soon as possible after the exposure. The clinician should obtain blood for both hepatitis and HIV-1 serologic tests and baseline blood chemistries. A careful history should be obtained from the exposed individual about her or his medical status (e.g., possibility of pregnancy, underlying illnesses, current medications). The medication history is particularly relevant because virtually all of the available antiretroviral agents have the potential for serious drug interactions. Protease inhibitors are especially prone to this problem and have major interactions with virtually all drugs that are metabolized through hepatic oxidative phosphorylation. Certain dietary supplements (e.g., St. John's wort) may also influence the metabolism of the protease inhibitors.[79] Managing situations in which the exposed individual is taking other medications is another scenario where expert consultation is advisable. Information about drug interactions also can be found in the manufacturer's product insert. The treating clinician should be able to provide detailed, supportive counseling to the exposed individual about the risks associated with the exposure and with the postexposure management. Employees requiring follow-up should be counseled regarding: (1) the epidemiology and transmissibility of HIV; (2) the magnitude of risk for occupational infection associated with similar exposures; (3) the importance of returning for follow-up evaluations and care; (4) techniques that effectively minimize the risk of secondary transmission; (5) the planned postexposure management program, including the side effects associated with postexposure antiretroviral chemoprophylaxis and the strategies used to manage the side effects; and (6) the procedures used to protect the medical privacy and confidentiality of the exposed worker. Additional blood samples should be obtained for HIV antibody testing at 6 weeks, 12 weeks, and 6 months following the exposure. Some centers obtain an additional sample at 1 year after the exposure, but this is not routine. Simultaneous exposure to hepatitis C virus and HIV represents a special circumstance for which the 1-year follow-up assessment is recommended (discussed in more detail later in the chapter).

Selecting a Chemoprophylaxis Regimen

Although a number of antiretroviral agents have been used for postexposure prophylaxis, the largest reported experience describes the use of zidovudine used alone. Currently, two-drug regimens (e.g., zidovudine plus lamivudine) and three-drug regimens (e.g., zidovudine, lamivudine, and a protease inhibitor) are recommended for postexposure prophylaxis for certain types of exposures.[63,80] The most recently reported CDC guidelines recommend a two-drug regimen (zidovudine plus lamivudine) as the "basic" regimen but offer alternative "basic" regimens (e.g., lamivudine plus stavudine, didanosine plus stavudine).[63] For exposures associated with an increased risk for infection (i.e., large-bore hollow needle exposures, deep puncture wounds, exposures to devices on which blood was clearly visible, exposures to needles that had been in an artery or vein, and exposures to blood from source patients who have symptomatic HIV infection, AIDS, the acute seroconversion illness, or known high viral loads), CDC recommends a three-drug regimen. Although this approach (i.e., two drugs for some exposures and three for others) is not universally endorsed by all experts in the field, these recommendations do represent a consensus of most expert consultants' views. The three-drug regimen recommended is a combination of the basic regimen plus one of the following agents: indinavir, nelfinavir, efavirenz, abacavir.[63] A variety of other regimens have been used, particularly in settings in which the source patient for an exposure has extensive antiretroviral experience and in instances in which antiretroviral resistance is known or highly suspected. Current U.S. Public Health Service recommendations for prophylaxis are summarized in Tables 25–2 and 25–3.[63] Certain special problems relating to the choice of regimen (e.g., selecting drugs for individuals who are or may be pregnant; selecting a regimen in instances in which the source patient has significant antiretroviral experience; selecting a regimen for individuals exposed to blood from a source patient known to harbor resistant isolates) are discussed in more detail later in the chapter.

Side Effects/Toxicity

Because most prophylaxis regimens involve short-term antiretroviral treatment (i.e., a 4-week course), side effects might be less of a problem than in the case of chronic therapy of HIV infection with these agents. Unfortunately, this assumption is incorrect. As many as three-fourths of health care workers who take postexposure prophylaxis experience substantive treatment-associated side effects.[81] In almost all reported studies at least 50% of individuals taking postexposure prophylaxis experience reportable side effects.[63,82] As a class, antiretroviral agents are by no means easily tolerated by those taking them, and each has a potential to produce substantial toxicity.[83] Common side effects of nucleoside analogues used for postexposure prophylaxis include bone marrow suppression, nausea, vomiting, diarrhea, abdominal pain, headache, neuropathies, myalgias, lassitude, malaise, and insomnia. Whereas most of these adverse reactions have been relatively mild and reversible, more severe toxicity has occasionally been reported.[84,85] In addition, administration of didanosine has been associated with fatal and nonfatal pancreatitis among HIV-infected patients treated for longer than 4 weeks; how-

Table 25–2. CENTERS FOR DISEASE CONTROL AND PREVENTION RECOMMENDATIONS FOR POSTEXPOSURE PROPHYLAXIS FOR PERCUTANEOUS EXPOSURES TO HIV

Exposure type	HIV-positive, class 1[a]	HIV-positive, class 2[b]	HIV status or source unknown	HIV-negative
Less severe (e.g., solid needle, superficial injury)	Recommend basic PEP	Recommend expanded PEP	Generally, no PEP warranted; however, consider basic PEP[c] for source with HIV risk factors[d]	No PEP warranted
More severe (e.g., large-bore hollow needle, deep puncture, visible blood on device, or needle used in patient's artery or vein)	Recommend expanded PEP	Recommend basic PEP	Generally, no PEP warranted; however, consider basic PEP[c] for source with HIV risk factors[d]	No PEP warranted

[a]Asymptomatic HIV infection or known low viral load (e.g., < 1500). If drug resistance is a concern, obtain expert consultation. Initiation of postexposure prophylaxis (PEP) should not be delayed pending expert consultation; and because expert consultation alone cannot substitute for face-to-face counseling, resources should be available to provide immediate evaluation and follow-up care for all exposures.

[b]Symptomatic HIV infection, AIDS, acute seroconversion, or known high viral load. See also footnote *a*.

[c]The designation "consider PEP" indicates that PEP is optional and should be based on an individualized decision between the exposed health care worker and the treating clinician.

[d]If PEP is offered and taken and the source is later determined to be HIV-negative, PEP should be discontinued.

From Centers for Disease Control and Prevention. Updated U.S. Public Health Service guidelines for the management of occupational exposures to HBV, HCV, and HIV and recommendations for postexposure prophylaxis. MMWR Morb Mortal Wkly Rep 50(RR-11):1, 2001.

Table 25–3. CENTERS FOR DISEASE CONTROL AND PREVENTION RECOMMENDATIONS FOR POSTEXPOSURE PROPHYLAXIS FOR MUCOUS MEMBRANE AND NONINTACT SKIN EXPOSURES TO HIV

Exposure type	HIV-positive, class 1[a]	HIV-positive, class 2[b]	HIV status or source unknown	HIV-negative
Small volume (e.g., few drops or brief contact)	Consider basic PEP[c]	Recommend basic PEP	Generally, no PEP warranted; however, consider basic PEP[c] for source with HIV risk factors[d]	No PEP warranted
Large volume (e.g., major blood splash or prolonged contact)	Recommend basic PEP	Recommend expanded PEP	Generally, no PEP warranted; however, consider basic PEP[c] for source with HIV risk factors[d]	No PEP warranted

For a discussion of "basic" and "expanded," see text.
[a]Asymptomatic HIV infection or known low viral load (e.g., < 1500). If drug resistance is a concern, obtain expert consultation. Initiation of postexposure prophylaxis (PEP) should not be delayed pending expert consultation; and because expert consultation alone cannot substitute for face-to-face counseling, resources should be available to provide immediate evaluation and follow-up care for all exposures.
[b]Symptomatic HIV infection, AIDS, acute seroconversion, or known high viral load. See also footnote *a*.
[c]The designation "consider PEP" indicates that PEP is optional and should be based on an individualized decision between the exposed healthcare worker and the treating clinician.
[d]If PEP is offered and taken and the source is later determined to be HIV-negative, PEP should be discontinued.
From Centers for Disease Control and Prevention. Updated U.S. Public Health Service guidelines for the management of occupational exposures to HBV, HCV, and HIV and recommendations for postexposure prophylaxis. MMWR Morb Mortal Wkly Rep 50(RR-11):1, 2001.

ever, this complication has not yet been observed in patients taking the 4-week course of prophylaxis. The combination of zidovudine plus lamivudine in the doses recommended by the CDC is perhaps the best-tolerated of the current options.

Addition of a protease inhibitor to the postexposure prophylaxis regimen is associated with an increase in some of the side effects noted for the nucleoside analogues (e.g., nausea, vomiting, diarrhea, headache, abdominal pain) as well as hyperglycemia, diabetes mellitus, worsening of preexisting diabetes (including cases of ketoacidosis), hyperlipidemia, anorexia, dysgeusia, and paresthesias. In addition, a few cases of nephrolithiasis have been associated with the administration of indinavir as part of a prophylaxis regimen,[86,87] and one instance of lipodystrophy associated with prophylaxis administration has been reported.[88] The risk for nephrolithiasis associated with indinavir administration can be reduced substantially by encouraging the individual to consume at least 48 ounces of water per day (i.e., six 8-ounce glasses distributed throughout the day).[63]

Despite some success administering nonnucleoside reverse transcriptase inhibitors (NNRTIs) to prevent vertical transmission of HIV,[41] agents of this class have not been primary choices for prophylaxis in most published guidelines for preventing infection through other routes.[63,80,89,90] Rash occurs commonly with the nonnucleoside drugs; this rash and its typical accompanying fever may be confused with the acute HIV seroconversion illness. Occasionally the skin-related side effects associated with the NNRTIs are severe. Fever and gastrointestinal symptoms are also common with the NNRTIs. Two cases of severe hepatic dysfunction (one requiring liver transplantation) have been reported in health care workers taking nevirapine as part of a prophylaxis regimen.[91] In addition, 10 more cases of hepatic dysfunction have been reported in association with nevirapine-containing prophylaxis regimens. Finally, the U.S. Food and Drug Administration (FDA) has received two reports of "possible" Stevens-Johnson syndrome in health care workers taking nevirapine as a component of a prophylaxis regimen.[91]

Because many of the common side effects associated with postexposure chemoprophylaxis can be anticipated (i.e., nausea, headache, diarrhea), the clinician who provides postexposure chemoprophylaxis can counsel the exposed individual about these side effects and can preemptively prescribe treatment for the common mild side effects. Treatment with antiemetics, analgesics, and antimotility agents can substantially increase the comfort of the individual receiving postexposure prophylaxis and, more importantly, promote completion of the prescribed treatment course.

Adherence to Prophylaxis Regimens

Additional strategies to increase adherence to the prophylaxis regimen are extremely important. Early experience with high-dose zidovudine prophylaxis [i.e., 1200 mg/day in six divided doses for the first 3 days, then 1000 mg/day in five doses (skipping the 4 a.m. dose) for the next 28 days] can be summarized as follows. Approximately 51% of the health care workers offered the full 28-day course of zidovudine completed the therapy at the full dose, and an additional 13% completed at a reduced dose of zidovudine; thus 64% of those initiating chemoprophylaxis completed the regimen.[81,92–95] The remaining 36% did not complete the course for a variety of reasons, including side effects/subjective symptoms (10%); subjective, unspecified discomfort with (or concerns about) taking the drugs (15%); and "personal" reasons (10%) (e.g., family vacations). Excluding the latter group from the analysis, approximately 25% discontinued the agents at least in part because of side effects the worker ascribed to the regimen. During this early experience with chemoprophylaxis, the strategy of preemptive symptom management was not emphasized.

The experience with adherence to multiple drug prophylaxis regimens is similar.[86,96,97] In one large series two-thirds of the exposed workers who were prescribed multiple-drug prophylaxis regimens received two agents (primarily zidovudine and lamivudine) and one-third received three drugs (with a protease inhibitor most commonly added as the third agent). For those receiving multiple-drug prophylaxis, 64% completed the regimen, with slightly fewer completing the three-drug regimen than those who took only two drugs. Side effects/subjective symptoms were the primary reason cited for discontinuing therapy.[96]

The likelihood of an individual health care worker adhering to a prophylaxis regimen appears to depend on several variables, among them: (1) the perceived seriousness of the exposure; (2) the individual's understanding of the risks of infection; (3) the individual's perception of the efficacy of prophylaxis; (4) effective counseling about what is known (and what the exposed individual should anticipate) about the side effects associated with the agents prescribed for the course of antiretroviral chemoprophylaxis; (5) the specific regimen chosen for prophylaxis (i.e., two versus three drugs, the duration of therapy, the specific agents selected); and (6) the quality of follow-up care, including the extent to which truly anticipated side effects are treated preemptively, the extent to which unanticipated regimen-related side effects can be treated effectively, and the treating clinician's willingness to reduce the dose or modify the regimen.

Follow-Up

Baseline serologies and chemistries should be obtained from the exposed individual at the time the exposure is reported. Individuals should return for follow-up at least every other week while receiving postexposure chemoprophylaxis (more frequently if side effects of therapy warrant more intensive follow-up). Serologic studies should be done at 6 weeks, 3 months, 6 months, and (optionally) 1 year following exposure. The value of the 1-year follow-up visit remains controversial; however, some case reports of late seroconversion (i.e., more than 6 months following exposure) have now been reported.[98] Whereas we do not routinely recommend aggressive diagnostic evaluation (e.g., viral burden/load evaluation or polymerase chain reaction testing) such testing may be of value in instances in which the diagnosis of acute infection (i.e., acute retroviral illness) is being considered.

Most infections are detected within the first 3 months of the exposure. Only a few have been detected later than 6 months following the exposure, and fewer than five have been detected later than 6 months following exposure.

Management of Sexual, Drug Use, and Atypical Exposures

Despite the fact that the data assembled to date about postexposure management primarily have been derived from occupational exposures in the health care setting, they may be relevant to some exposures in the community as well.[99–102] However, just as in cases of occupational HIV exposures, antiretroviral agents should not be prescribed casually. Postexposure chemoprophylaxis for community exposures should be provided in the context of a program that includes careful evaluation of the circumstances of exposure; evaluation of the exposed individual; and provision of counseling about the exposure, the risks for infection, and secondary transmission and the risks and benefits of postexposure antiretroviral treatment. Often the risk for transmission associated with the community exposure may be quite small, and the physician's role is primarily one of reassurance. As already noted, exposure to blood or cells represents the primary risk. Exposures to saliva or emesis or other body fluids (unless they contain blood) are associated with minimal risk. Transmission of HIV has been associated with bite exposures,[103–106] an unfortunately common occurrence for police and correctional officials; we consider these exposures significant. Evaluation of the exposed individual should include baseline testing for preexisting HIV infection and a commitment to careful follow-up, with monitoring for HIV infection and the development and management of toxicity from the therapy provided.

Counseling is a critical component of any postexposure management program. Just as health care workers who sustain occupational exposures are counseled about primary prevention in the setting of occupational exposures, individuals who have sustained community exposures are an attentive, captive audience for counseling about primary prevention.[99,100,107] The postexposure setting provides the clinician with a clear opportunity to counsel these individuals about risk-reduction strategies that can assist in decreasing the likelihood of subsequent exposure. Counseling for victims of sexual assault must take into account the considerable physical and psychosocial trauma that has been experienced by these individuals.[102]

Investigators working at the University of California at San Francisco conducted a pilot project evaluating the potential for administering postexposure antiretroviral chemoprophylaxis for sexual or drug use exposures to HIV.[108] This project clearly demonstrated the feasibility of such a program. One interesting finding from this study that contrasts strikingly with data from studies of exposure management in the health care setting is that, whereas similar rates of side effects were seen among persons who took antiretroviral agents following sexual or drug use exposures to HIV, four-fifths of the study population completed the full 28-day course of postexposure prophylaxis.[108] Although the reasons for the increased level of adherence were not investigated in the study, the study design included mandatory adherence counseling with skilled, experienced counselors.

Special Problems or Circumstances for Selecting a Chemoprophylaxis Regimen

Advisability of Expert Consultation

Because of the manner in which postexposure prophylaxis programs are administered at many institutions throughout the United States, frequently individuals who prescribe chemoprophylaxis are often only peripherally familiar with the subject. Many of these programs are managed by emergency room or occupational health personnel who have limited experience managing patients who are receiving antiretroviral agents. Examples of situations for which expert guidance is usually indicated include (but are not limited to) instances in which the source patient is known or highly suspected to harbor antiretroviral-resistant HIV isolates, management of exposures in pregnant or breastfeeding women, management of "source-unknown" exposures, and instances in which the regimen must be modified (i.e., dose reductions or regimen changes) owing to side effects or toxicities. An experienced consultant is often best situated to select the number of agents to be administered and to help tailor a regimen specifically for a unique situation. Postexposure management represents a circumstance for which some conservatism may be most appropriate. If one prescribes a multiple-drug regimen so toxic the individual cannot take it, the purpose of prophylaxis is defeated. Clinicians skilled in providing care to HIV-infected patients serve as a ready source of this expertise. If local expertise is not readily available, the already mentioned PEPLINE is an excellent resource.

Pregnancy

Offering postexposure prophylaxis to an individual who is or might be pregnant is associated with another obvious set of issues. The risk to the fetus of administering antiretroviral agents—even for the 28-day course of postexposure prophylaxis—is undefined. Based primarily on experience gleaned from other settings (e.g., animal studies and studies attempting to prevent vertical HIV transmission), several principles have been developed to guide treatment decisions. First, the exposed woman must be the person who decides whether to take postexposure prophylaxis for an exposure; the treating clinician should not impose a decision. Second, the exposed woman must have access to accurate, thorough, unbiased counseling that emphasizes what is known (and not known) about: (1) the risks for infection associated with the type of exposure sustained; (2) the efficacy of postexposure prophylaxis; (3) the adverse drug effects that can be reasonably anticipated; and (4) the potential for short- and long-term toxicities for her offspring (including carcinogenicity and teratogenicity). Third, the regimen selected for a pregnant health care worker should be an optimal regimen (i.e., one that has the best chance of preventing infection), but regimen selection should be balanced by what is known concerning potential adverse effects on the fetus. Fourth, pregnant workers electing to take postexposure chemoprophylaxis should be carefully followed prospectively and advised to seek consultation at the earliest appearance of signs of adverse drug-related events.

Almost all antiretroviral agents have at least some potential for carcinogenicity, teratogenicity, and mutagenicity. Many of the agents have been shown to be mutagenic in premarketing studies in animals. With respect to zidovudine, for example, carcinogenicity studies of rats and mice receiving zidovudine for 18 to 22 months demonstrated an increased risk for certain hepatic tumors.[90] In these studies, however, the animals received up to 35 times the label-indication dosage for humans.[90] Obviously, the relevance of these data to the clinical setting in humans is unclear. Animal studies of a more recently marketed NNRTI, efavirenz, may have more relevance. In these studies, teratogenic effects were observed in cynomolgus monkeys at drug levels similar to those produced with human dosing. Malformations observed in these studies included anencephaly, unilateral anophthalmia, microphthalmia, and cleft palate. Because of the potential relevance of these studies, most authorities do not recommend the use of efavirenz during pregnancy.

We have little information about the safety of administering postexposure prophylaxis to HIV-negative pregnant women; furthermore, we have virtually no information about the pharmacokinetics of antiretroviral agents during pregnancy. The most relevant experience with the use of these agents during pregnancy comes from studies attempting to prevent vertical transmission of HIV from infected mothers to their offspring. For example, several years' follow-up is now available for the participants in the ACTG protocol 076 study. The available evidence suggests that zidovudine administration in this study was apparently safe and well tolerated. In addition, the Antiretroviral Pregnancy Registry is available for individuals who voluntarily report that they are taking antiretroviral agents during pregnancy. This registry has systematically evaluated registrants for evidence of an increased risk for birth defects among children who had in utero exposures to antiretroviral agents.[109–111] Investigators in France have identified fetal toxicity associated with antiretroviral administration during gestation (discussed later in the chapter); however, the U.S. registry has not yet identified serious toxicities related to in utero exposure to antiretroviral agents. Whereas substantial data are available concerning the use of zidovudine during pregnancy, only limited data are available concerning the use of lamivudine (or other antiretrovirals) in this setting. These limited data suggest that lamivudine appears relatively safe during pregnancy for both mother and fetus.[112,113] Even less is known about the safety of protease inhibitors and NNRTIs during pregnancy. Because of certain toxicities linked to indinavir (i.e., hyperbilirubinemia and nephrolithiasis), some experts have discouraged its use during pregnancy.[63]

Blanche and coworkers reported two infant deaths (among children who remained HIV-uninfected) in a large trial in France comparing zidovudine alone with zidovudine plus lamivudine used to prevent vertical HIV transmission.[114] Both of these deaths were caused by progressive neurologic disease thought to be related to mitochondrial toxicity of the nucleoside analogues administered during the study. When this cohort was examined in detail for fetal toxicity, an additional six cases of potential mitochondrial toxicity were identified.[114] These results stand in contrast to data from several large cohorts in the United States, including CDC surveillance data, and data sets from CDC studies of maternal-fetal transmission, the National Institutes of Health's AIDS Clinical Trials Group Studies, and the Women and Infants Transmission Study. No fetal deaths attributable to antiretroviral-induced mitochondrial toxicity have been identified in these studies or in the Antiretroviral Pregnancy Registry. In addition, postmarketing data from the manufacturers of nucleoside analogues have not identified additional deaths attributable to mitochondrial toxicity. The reason for the differences in outcome in the French and U.S. trials remains unexplained.

Management of Exposures When the Source Patient Has Experience with Antiretroviral Agents

One of the most challenging issues facing individuals who manage HIV exposures is the management of exposures to blood from a patient who has extensive experience with antiretroviral agents. Several reports document exposures to antiretroviral-resistant isolates.[115,116] In a few instances, prophylaxis failure has been associated with genotypic or phenotypic resistance to the agent(s) selected for therapy.[80] In addition, failures of prophylaxis have been associated with HIV isolates that were resistant to one or more of the three drugs included in the standard three-drug regimen.[115,117,118] Conversely, genotypic resistance has not necessarily predicted treatment failure. Zidovudine monotherapy appeared to be effective in the ACTG 076 trial even though 25% to 30% of the women had HIV isolates that demonstrated genotypic zidovudine resistance.[33] Thus we simply do not know the extent to which drug resistance influences transmission risk. Nonetheless, tailoring regimens to include agents to which the source patient's HIV isolates are not likely to be resistant makes intuitive sense, particularly in situations in which a patient is known or highly suspected to harbor resistant isolates.[78] Tailoring these regimens with the advice of experts in HIV therapy is the best recourse in these cases. Even though many of the drugs exhibit cross-resistance among agents in a single class, using "salvage-like" regimens for all health care workers who have exposures to blood from antiretroviral-experienced patients is both unnecessary and unnecessarily risky. Such a strategy would result in the administration of newer, less well tested agents to the exposed health care workers. One suggestion has been to employ resistance testing to manage HIV exposures; however, because of the difficulty of obtaining results in a timely fashion, in most institutions such a suggestion is simply not practical and of no proven benefit.

Management of Exposures for Which Reporting Was Delayed

Occasionally, exposures are not reported in a timely fashion. In most of the relevant animal models, initiation of postexposure prophylaxis within 24 hours of exposure provides results that are similar to treatment before virus inoculation. On the other hand, the longer treatment is delayed, the less likely it is to be beneficial.[60,61] Nonetheless, treatment for an exposure associated with a higher-risk exposure is not contraindicated and may confer some benefit.

Management of Simultaneous Exposures to HIV and HCV

Simultaneous exposure to HIV and hepatitis C virus (HCV) merits special consideration. Two of the three well documented instances of delayed HIV seroconversions after occupational exposure have occurred in individuals who acquired both HIV and HCV from one exposure. In both of these cases the progression of HCV illness was unusually rapid and the course of infection unusually severe.[119] In two other instances simultaneous infection with HIV and HCV was associated with a highly aggressive course of HIV disease.[120,121] These cases represent anecdotal reports, and there is no definitive evidence that simultaneous infection influences the progression of either disease. Nonetheless, for those simultaneously exposed to HIV and HCV and who then develop HCV infection, many experts recommend following the individuals for at least a year to detect delayed HIV seroconversion.

▲ MANAGEMENT OF HIV-INFECTED PROVIDERS

Historical Perspective

During the two decades since the acquired immunodeficiency syndrome (AIDS) epidemic began, only three providers have been reported to have transmitted HIV to patients.[122–128] Nonetheless, there is substantial concern about the management of health care workers who are infected with this blood-borne pathogen.

A theoretical risk for provider-to-patient transmission of HIV was reported early in the epidemic, primarily because of the striking epidemiologic similarities between AIDS/HIV infection and hepatitis B. As early as 1985 the CDC[129,130] and others[131] suggested that provider-to-patient transmission of the agent responsible for AIDS was at least a theoretical possibility. In the October 1985 recommendations the CDC noted that the difficult issues related to the management of HIV-infected health care workers who perform invasive procedures (including recommendations regarding the serologic testing of these health care providers) would be addressed in a subsequent guideline.[129] These "invasive procedure" guidelines, issued in April 1986, concluded that "routine serologic testing for evidence of [HIV] infection is not necessary for health care workers who perform or assist in invasive procedures or for patients undergoing invasive procedures, since the risk of transmission in this setting is so low."[132] The guidelines also advocated that health care workers who have illnesses that might compromise their ability to perform invasive procedures adequately and safely be evaluated medically to determine their physical and mental competence for performing invasive procedures.[132] Thus the "case-by-case" management strategy for HIV-infected health care workers was born.

The initial case cluster of provider-to-patient transmission of HIV that occurred in a Florida dentist's practice[122–125] received national publicity and created substantial anxiety among both patients and providers. This highly unusual cluster has engendered a great deal of controversy.[115,122,123,125,133–188] How transmission of HIV in this dentist's practice occurred at the frequency with which it was detected remains unexplained. The transmission rate in his practice far exceeded (by several orders of magnitude) every published estimate of the theoretical rate of transmission. Twenty years into the HIV epidemic in the

United States, this case cluster remains the only one detected. The additional 11 years' experience since this first case cluster was identified has yielded only two additional potential cases of provider-to-patient HIV transmission.[126–128] In one instance, an HIV-infected orthopedic surgeon in France apparently transmitted infection to one of his patients. Unlike the cluster in the Florida dentist's practice in which no clear correlation existed between the invasiveness of the procedures performed and the occurrence of HIV transmission, in the French case the patient who became infected had undergone a particularly complex, prolonged operative procedure.[126] A third instance of putative transmission from a health care provider (a nurse in this instance) to a patient was reported,[128] but no likely mechanism for transmission could be identified.

Look-Back Studies

Substantial resources have been expended in a number of retrospective, "look-back" studies, evaluating patients of practitioners identified as being HIV-infected.[126,172,189–200] Thousands of patients have been evaluated in these studies, with the only case identified as putatively iatrogenic transmission being the French case already cited. Several authors of these studies have argued that such studies are a waste of time, effort, and substantial resources.[191,193,200–202]

U.S. Public Health Service Recommendations

Shortly after the case cluster in the Florida dentist's practice was identified, the CDC issued guidelines (July 1991)[136] recommending that:

> *Health-care workers who perform exposure-prone procedures should know their HIV antibody statuses. Health-care workers who perform exposure-prone procedures and who do not have serologic evidence of immunity to HBV from vaccination or from previous infection should know their HBsAg statuses, and, if positive, should also know their HBeAg statuses. Health-care workers who are infected with HIV or HBV (and are HBeAg positive) should not perform exposure-prone invasive procedures unless they have sought counsel from an expert review panel and have been advised under what circumstances, if any, they may continue to perform these procedures. Such circumstances would include notifying prospective patients of the health-care worker's seropositivity before they undergo [an] exposure-prone invasive procedure.*

These guidelines fell short of defining exposure-prone procedures. They did however, provide characteristics of procedures that might be categorized as exposure-prone.[136]

> *Characteristics of exposure-prone procedures include digital palpation of a needle tip in a body cavity or the simultaneous presence of a health-care worker's fingers and a needle or other sharp instrument or object in a poorly visualized or highly confined anatomical site. Performance of exposure-prone procedures presents a recognized risk of percutaneous injury to the health care worker, and—if such an injury occurs—the health-care worker's blood is likely to contact the patient's body cavity, subcutaneous tissues, and/or mucous membranes.*

These guidelines were met with substantial resistance from the medical community[203] at least in part due to lack of any consensus about which procedures should be classified as "exposure-prone."[204] Subsequently, the Director of the CDC concluded that this matter should be the province of individual state health departments and issued a recommendation that states develop their own strategies to determine which procedures were "exposure-prone."[205] A federal law passed the following year required states either to adopt the CDC guidelines or develop individual state guidelines that the states could certify as being equivalent to the 1991 CDC guidelines.[206] Several states created their own guidelines, resulting in a patchwork of guidelines across the United States. The CDC Director's letter to state health departments emphasized the potential for considering each case as unique and listed factors that might be considered, such as the procedure itself, the skill and technical expertise of the practitioner, and the stage of the practitioner's illness (including the potential that she or he might be impaired).

The 1991 CDC guidelines were criticized in the medical literature for a variety of reasons. Some experts in the field argued that the risk was too small to justify this kind of intervention.[143,146,161,164,179,207] Surgeons thought that the concept of "exposure-prone" procedures was not appropriate, with some experts arguing that the biggest variable in exposure risk might be the technical abilities of the surgeon rather than the specific procedure.[204] Nonetheless, the 1991 guidelines remain in effect and have not yet been revised.

The issue of providers who are infected with bloodborne pathogens remains one of the most problematic and controversial issues in clinical medicine. Virtually all experts in this field believe that the risk of provider-to-patient transmission is extremely small;[115,135,145,155,208] however, the consequences of iatrogenic infection (for the patient, the provider, and the health care institution) are substantial. When crafting policy, one must be walk a fine line between patients' rights and the rights of infected health care workers.

Several pieces of information are needed to address the management of infected providers.

- Can the risk of provider-to-patient transmission of HIV be accurately quantified?
- What factors influence the risk of patient exposure to the blood of the practitioner, and can these factors be modified with technology or new prevention strategies?

- What ethical issues are associated with the management of infected providers?
- What are the legal and sociopolitical implications of restricting or not restricting infected providers from practice?

Magnitude of the Risk of Provider-to-Patient Transmission

None of these questions is easy to answer. Despite the fact that several estimates of the magnitude of the risk of provider-to-patient transmission have been reported,[135,209–215] the risk is so small it likely cannot be measured with precision. Reported estimates for the risk of provider-to-patient transmission of HIV include the 1 in 42,000 to 1 in 420,000 procedures the CDC estimated,[135,214] the 1 in 1 million procedures estimated in two studies;[211,213] the 7.5 infections per million invasive radiologic procedures estimated based on a computer model,[209] the one infection estimated for every 83,000 hours of surgery by an HIV-infected surgeon,[212] and the one infection for every 26 million dental procedures performed by an HIV-infected dentist.[215] What is clear to most individuals who have studied this issue is that the risk of an infected provider transmitting HIV to a patient is extremely low but not zero.

Primary Prevention: Preventing Occupational Exposures

During the 20 years since recognition of the HIV epidemic in the United States substantial progress has been achieved in decreasing the risk of occupational exposures (thereby decreasing the risk of transmitting blood-borne pathogens to providers and to patients).[26,115,145,216–245] The best strategy, by far, for preventing transmission of blood-borne infections is to prevent health care worker injuries.[145] Numerous strategies have been shown to be effective for reducing occupational injuries, including educating the staff concerning implementation and then monitoring their adherence to appropriate infection control practices and precautions.[216] In addition to effective staff education, retraining them about occupational risks, modifying procedures and work practices that are intrinsically risky, using technologic advancements shown to be safe and effective, and using effective vaccines (e.g., hepatitis B vaccine) have been clearly linked to risk reduction in the health care setting.[246] Another mechanism through which infected providers may decrease the risk of iatrogenic transmission of HIV is through appropriate therapy, of their illnesses. Combination therapy (highly active antiretroviral therapy or HAART) effectively lowers the viral burden in the bloodstreams of infected patients and may decrease the risk associated with exposure.[247–258] Whereas this tenet has not been (and likely cannot ever be) tested in the setting of the HIV-infected provider, the principle has been shown to be operative in the setting of heterosexual transmission[248,249,252,257,258] and vertical/perinatal transmission.[247,253–256]

The fact that most of these successful prevention interventions were not available at the time the risk estimates were constructed is also worthy of additional emphasis. Their implementation should further reduce what was already an extremely small risk of provider-to-patient transmission.

Ethical, Legal, and Sociopolitical Issues

The ethical, legal, and sociopolitical issues associated with managing HIV-infected providers have been discussed intensively in the medical literature; nonetheless, they remain the source of a great deal of disagreement and controversy. The substance of most of these arguments relates to the direct competition between the rights of the individual (i.e., the health care provider) and the rights of society (the patient). Compelling arguments have been proffered on both sides of these issues. A major argument of those who lean toward restriction of infected providers is the doctrine of informed consent.[152,153,183,184,259–262] From this perspective, because the risk of transmitting HIV to patients would likely be viewed as "significant" by many if not most patients, informed consent would be required.[260,263] Conversely, other authorities believe that the magnitude of risk for provider-to-patient transmission is so small it is "negligible" and therefore would not require informed consent.[144,146,168,264] Some experts have argued that a double standard exists; (that is, in many states health care workers are not permitted to test patients for blood-borne pathogen infections, whereas infected practitioners are required to notify patients of their infection status before performing "exposure-prone invasive procedures" on patients).[154,188] Others suggest that the relationship between patients and their health care providers differs substantively from the relationship between providers and their patients, thereby negating the double-standard argument.[265] Providers are independent of their patients' decision-making, whereas patients are dependent on their providers. Novick has argued that the risks associated with HIV-infected providers are dwarfed by risks that we choose not to consider (e.g., surgeon's comparative mortality rates, surgeons' postoperative infection rates, surgeons' use of alcohol).[171]

Another component to the argument proffered against restrictions is that HIV-infected providers have been viewed as disabled in the courts. The Americans with Disabilities Act, initially passed in 1990, was interpreted by the U.S. Supreme Court during the late 1990s to define HIV infection as a disability.[266,267] An important issue addressed in the Court's opinion was that a patient with asymptomatic HIV infection did not pose "a direct threat to the health or safety of others." The term "direct threat" is defined as "a significant risk to the health or safety of others."[268] The Court relied on the definition of "significant risk" that was provided by an amicus curiae brief from the American Medical Association to the Court in the case of Arline v. the Board of Education[269] that characterized "significant risk" associated with transmission of an infectious disease (in the Arline case, tuberculosis) as being a conjoint assessment of the route of transmission, the risk for transmission associated with an exposure, the severity of the harm that might be produced by infection, and the duration of infectiousness.[269] Because the assessment of "significant risk" is the product of four factors, courts have wide latitude in interpretation. Whereas cases of discrimination against HIV-infected patients have generally been found in favor of the patient,[267] cases of discrimination against infected providers have most often not favored the provider.[261,264,270] Some have argued that restricting the practices of infected providers should be viewed as discrimination under the Americans with Disabilities Act,[146,188,268] pointing out that the courts have found that a dentist could not refuse to provide office-based care to an HIV-infected patient.[267] Some authorities in the field have suggested that this apparent double standard is due in great measure to the positions medical professional organizations have taken.[188] Still others have argued that the practitioner's responsibility to the patient and the requirement for informed consent makes this issue moot.[265]

The public's perceptions of risks in society are uneven at best. For example, members of society are willing to accept substantial risks they perceive as "voluntary" (i.e., someone "elects" to drive a car, smoke cigarettes, consume alcohol).[271] Conversely, society is much less willing to accept what its members perceive to be "involuntary" risks, almost irrespective of their magnitude. Thus the same society that annually tolerates an extraordinary number of tobacco- or alcohol-related deaths may be less willing to accept any level of risk for provider-to-patient transmission of HIV. Similarly, the same health care professionals who have blithely dismissed or ignored the 200 annual health care worker deaths related to occupational infections with hepatitis B and who were slow to accept hepatitis B vaccines were literally terrified by identification of the substantially smaller risk for occupational infection with HIV. Thus society's lack of willingness to accept some level of risk for provider-to-patient transmission of blood-borne pathogens remains a major obstacle to the development of any policy relative to the management of providers infected with blood-borne pathogens. A decade ago 94% of a national sample of adults in a public opinion poll expressed the opinion that HIV-infected providers should be required to inform their patients of their infection status, and more than 60% believed that HIV-infected surgeons should be barred from practicing.[271] Most distressingly, more than 50% of the respondents in this survey believed that all HIV-infected physicians should not be allowed to practice medicine.[271]

A fundamental principle underlying health care is that providers, wherever and to whatever extent possible, do not cause harm to their patients. This principle is at the heart of the issue relating to infected providers and is, in many respects, totally unrealistic when expressed devoid of clinical context. All who practice medicine invariably do involuntary harm at some point in their careers. Virtually every medication has side effects, and virtually every intervention is associated with risk. Nonetheless, as an ideal, each of us aspires to "primum non nocere" as a standard. Conversely, restricting the practices of infected providers for risks of a magnitude that may be considered negligible in the context of our lives[259] deprives practitioners of their livelihood and may, in a broader sense, deprive some patients access to health care.

Current Status and Prospects for the Future

Because the primary risk of transmitting blood-borne pathogens is through exposure of the patient's bloodstream to blood from the infected provider, invasive procedures represent the major risk for provider-to-patient transmission of blood-borne pathogens, and routine patient care activities pose no measurable risk of transmission.[129,131,272] Some professional societies or organizations established positions regarding the management of HIV-infected health care providers prior to documentation of the first instance of provider-to-patient HIV transmission.[273–280] Each of these proposals acknowledged the presence of a theoretical risk for provider-to-patient transmission of HIV. A few recommended that HIV-infected providers voluntarily restrict themselves from the practice of invasive procedures.[276,278,279] Others advocated the "case-by-case" management strategy.[275,277] Documentation that HIV transmission had, in fact, occurred in a practice setting prompted the American Medical Association, the American Dental Association, and ultimately the CDC to modify their positions and to recommend that HIV-infected health care providers who perform invasive procedures voluntarily restrict their practices.[136] Still other organizations, such as the Society for Healthcare Epidemiology in America took an intermediate position, arguing that voluntary restrictions be recommended for only the small subset of invasive procedures that have been epidemiologically implicated in the transmission of blood-borne pathogens.[281]

Several individuals and organizations have advocated revising the existing U.S. Public Health Service guidelines. The complex issue of the management of HIV-infected providers will likely continue to engender a great deal of discussion and controversy over the next decade. As noted elsewhere, "The central issue is . . . whether those who are [HIV-] infected should be deprived of the right to practice medicine. In confronting that question, it is essential that we ask whether the rights of patients to refuse to subject themselves to the remotest of risks should trump the rights of doctors who are confronting their own AIDS related mortality to care for patients as long as their skills remain unimpaired. Quiet and careful deliberation, not noisy clamor, is what is needed."[282]

We live in a democracy in which the public, guided by political leaders who express the will of the public, exert control over final decisions about such issues. The role of science in this situation, in our view, is to continue to characterize the factors that influence the risk for transmission of blood-borne pathogens and to understand the early events in the pathogenesis of infection, to present a rational, balanced, science-based discussion of the risks on all sides of the issue, to make the best effort possible to educate the populace about these competing risks, to make sentient recommendations to our political leaders based in science, and then to abide by the will of the people as expressed though our political process.

Potential for Occupational Infection with Secondary Pathogens

Often HIV-infected providers are motivated to work with other immunosuppressed patients. In this situation, medical and administrative concerns may be generated because these relatively immunosuppressed individuals may be in environments in which exposure to other opportunistic pathogens may occur. Fortunately, most of the HIV-associated opportunistic pathogens (e.g., *Toxoplasma gondii, Mycobacterium avium* complex, *Cryptococcus neoformans*) are not transmitted from person to person. Other common opportunistic pathogens can be transmitted from person to person, but most individuals have been exposed during infancy or early in childhood (e.g., *Pneumocystis carinii*). A third group of these pathogens can be transmitted from person to person but require fecal-oral exposure (e.g., *Salmonella, Cryptosporidium*) or a violation of basic infection control precautions (e.g., cytomegalovirus, herpes simplex virus) for transmission to occur. Only a few of the more common opportunistic pathogens present a substantive risk to immunocompromised health care workers, among them varicella-zoster virus (VZV), rubella virus, measles virus, and *Mycobacterium tuberculosis*.

Some authorities have expressed concern about the potential for bidirectional transmission of these organisms as a result of immunocompromised health care workers participating in direct patient care. In our view, institutional policy should prohibit *any* health care worker who is susceptible to VZV, rubella, or measles (irrespective of her or his immunologic status) from providing care to any patient with any of these infections.[281]

A special problem relates to the care of patients who are infected with isolates of multiple drug-resistant *Mycobacterium tuberculosis* (MDR-TB), which can be a significant, life-threatening problem for any patient but particularly for those who have compromised cellular immunity. *Any* health care worker (again, irrespective of her or his immunologic status) who develops signs or symptoms consistent with pulmonary tuberculosis should be immediately assessed for the presence of that disease. For individuals who have compromised immunity, irrespective of the underlying cause, and institutional occupational medicine personnel should maintain an increased index of suspicion for opportunistic infections and especially for tuberculosis and MDR-TB in settings in which these infections are known to be present.[281] Occupational medicine staff should work with supervisors and with the affected health care worker to assist in the assignment of duties to health care providers who have compromised cellular immunity.[281] The health care provider must be full apprised of the risks but should be allowed to have input into her or his assignment. In an instance in which clinical assignments must be modified, any such modification must provide "reasonable accommodation" for the affected provider as outlined in the Americans With Disabilities Act.

REFERENCES

1. Blauvelt A, Katz SI. The skin as target, vector, and effector organ in human immunodeficiency virus disease. J Invest Dermatol 105(suppl 1):122S, 1995.
2. Blauvelt A. The role of skin dendritic cells in the initiation of human immunodeficiency virus infection. Am J Med 102:16, 1997.
3. Spira AI, Marx PA, Patterson BK, et al. Cellular targets of infection and route of viral dissemination after an intravaginal inoculation of simian immunodeficiency virus into rhesus macaques. J Exp Med 183:215, 1996.
4. Martin JC, Bandres JC. Cells of the monocyte-macrophage lineage and pathogenesis of HIV-1 infection. J Acquir Immune Defic Syndr 22:413, 1999.
5. Pope M. SIV replication and the dendritic cell. AIDS Res Hum Retroviruses 14(suppl 1):S71, 1998.
6. Pope M. Mucosal dendritic cells and immunodeficiency viruses. J Infect Dis 179(suppl 3):S427, 1999.
7. Rowland-Jones SL. HIV: the deadly passenger in dendritic cells. Curr Biol 9:R248, 1999.
8. Pope M, Gezelter S, Gallo N, et al. Low levels of HIV-1 infection in cutaneous dendritic cells promote extensive viral replication upon binding to memory CD4$^+$ T cells. J Exp Med 182:2045, 1995.
9. Ayehunie S, Groves RW, Bruzzese AM, et al. Acutely infected Langerhans cells are more efficient than T cells in disseminating HIV type 1 to activated T cells following a short cell-cell contact. AIDS Res Hum Retroviruses 11:877, 1995.
10. Heath SL, Tew JG, Tew JG, et al. Follicular dendritic cells and human immunodeficiency virus infectivity. Nature 377:740, 1995.
11. Tacchetti C, Favre A, Moresco L, et al. HIV is trapped and masked in the cytoplasm of lymph node follicular dendritic cells. Am J Pathol 150:533, 1997.
12. Mazzoli S, Trabattoni D, Lo Caputo S, et al. HIV-specific mucosal and cellular immunity in HIV-seronegative partners of HIV-seropositive individuals. Nat Med 3:1250, 1997.
13. Kelker HC, Seidlin M, Vogler M, et al. Lymphocytes from some long-term seronegative heterosexual partners of HIV-infected individuals proliferate in response to HIV antigens. AIDS Res Hum Retroviruses 8:1355, 1992.
14. Clerici M, Levin JM, Kessler HA, et al. HIV-specific T-helper activity in seronegative health care workers exposed to contaminated blood. JAMA 271:42, 1994.
15. Puro V, Calcagno G, Anselmo M, et al. Transient detection of plasma HIV-1 RNA during postexposure prophylaxis. Infect Control Hosp Epidemiol 21:529, 2000.
16. Ruprecht RM, Bronson R. Chemoprevention of retroviral infection: success is determined by virus inoculum strength and cellular immunity. DNA Cell Biol 13:59, 1994.
17. Putkonen P, Makitalo B, Bottiger D, et al. Protection of human immunodeficiency virus type 2-exposed seronegative macaques from mucosal simian immunodeficiency virus transmission. J Virol 71:4981, 1997.
18. Centers for Disease Control and Prevention. Surveillance of Health Care Workers with HIV/AIDS. Atlanta, CDC, 2001.
19. Ward JW, Deppe DA, Samson S, et al. Human immunodeficiency virus infection from blood donors who later developed the acquired immunodeficiency syndrome. Ann Intern Med 106:61, 1987.
20. Henderson DK, Saah AJ, Zak BJ, et al. Risk of nosocomial infection with human T-cell lymphotropic virus type III/lymphadenopathy-associated virus in a large cohort of intensively exposed health care workers. Ann Intern Med 104:644, 1986.
21. Mayer KH, Anderson DJ. Heterosexual HIV transmission. Infect Agents Dis 4:273, 1995.
22. Seidlin M, Vogler M, Lee E, et al. Heterosexual transmission of HIV in a cohort of couples in New York City. AIDS 7:1247, 1993.
23. Mastro TD, de Vincenzi I. Probabilities of sexual HIV-1 transmission. AIDS 10(suppl A):S75, 1996.
24. Lurie P, Miller S, Hecht F, et al. Postexposure prophylaxis after nonoccupational HIV exposure: clinical, ethical, and policy considerations. JAMA 280:1769, 1998.
25. DeGruttola V, Seage GR III, Mayer KH, et al. Infectiousness of HIV between male homosexual partners. J Clin Epidemiol 42:849, 1989.
26. Fahey BJ, Koziol DE, Banks SM, et al. Frequency of nonparenteral occupational exposures to blood and body fluids before and after universal precautions training. Am J Med 90:145, 1991.

27. Centers for Disease Control and Prevention. Case-control study of HIV seroconversion in health-care workers after percutaneous exposure to HIV-infected blood—France, United Kingdom, and United States, January 1988–August 1994. MMWR Morb Mortal Wkly Rep 44:929, 1995.
28. Cardo DM, Culver DH, Ciesielski CA, et al. A case-control study of HIV seroconversion in health care workers after percutaneous exposure. N Engl J Med 337:1485, 1997.
29. Henderson DK. Postexposure treatment of HIV—taking some risks for safety's sake. N Engl J Med 337:1542, 1997.
30. Lindegren ML, Byers RH, Jr, Thomas P, et al. Trends in perinatal transmission of HIV/AIDS in the United States. JAMA 282:531, 1999.
31. Connor EM, Sperling RS, Gelber R, et al. Reduction of maternal-infant transmission of human immunodeficiency virus type 1 with zidovudine treatment. Pediatric AIDS Clinical Trials Group Protocol 076 Study Group. N Engl J Med 331:1173, 1994.
32. Sperling RS, Shapiro DE, Coombs RW, et al. Maternal viral load, zidovudine treatment, and the risk of transmission of human immunodeficiency virus type 1 from mother to infant: Pediatric AIDS Clinical Trials Group Protocol 076 Study Group. N Engl J Med 335:1621, 1996.
33. Eastman PS, Shapiro DE, Coombs RW, et al. Maternal viral genotypic zidovudine resistance and infrequent failure of zidovudine therapy to prevent perinatal transmission of human immunodeficiency virus type 1 in Pediatric AIDS Clinical Trials Group Protocol 076. J Infect Dis 177:557, 1998.
34. Frenkel LM, Cowles MK, Shapiro DE, et al. Analysis of the maternal components of the AIDS clinical trial group 076 zidovudine regimen in the prevention of mother-to-infant transmission of human immunodeficiency virus type 1. J Infect Dis 175:971, 1997.
35. Kind C, Rudin C, Siegrist CA, et al. Prevention of vertical HIV transmission: additive protective effect of elective cesarean section and zidovudine prophylaxis: Swiss Neonatal HIV Study Group. AIDS 12:205, 1998.
36. Kind C. Mother-to-child transmission of human immunodeficiency virus type 1: influence of parity and mode of delivery: Paediatric AIDS Group of Switzerland. Eur J Pediatr 154:542, 1995.
37. Simpson BJ, Shapiro ED, Andiman WA. Reduction in the risk of vertical transmission of HIV-1 associated with treatment of pregnant women with orally administered zidovudine alone. J Acquir Immune Defic Syndr Hum Retrovirol 14:145, 1997.
38. Bulterys M, Orloff S, Abrams E, et al. Impact of zidovudine post-perinatal exposure prophylaxis on vertical HIV-1 transmission: a prospective cohort study in four US cities. In: Global Strategies for the Prevention of HIV Transmission from Mothers to Infants, Toronto, 1999, abstract 15.
39. Saba J, PETRA Trial Study Team. Interim analysis of early efficacy of three short ZDV/3TC combinations regimens to prevent mother-to-child transmission of HIV-1: the PETRA trial. In: 6th Annual Conference on Retroviruses and Opportunistic Infections, Chicago, 1999, abstract S7.
40. Blanche S, et al. Zidovudine-lamivudine for prevention of mother to child HIV-1 transmission. In: 6th Annual Conference on Retroviruses and Opportunistic Infections, Chicago, 1999, abstract 267.
41. Guay LA, Musoke P, Fleming T, et al. Intrapartum and neonatal single-dose nevirapine compared with zidovudine for prevention of mother-to-child transmission of HIV-1 in Kampala, Uganda: HIVNET 012 randomised trial. Lancet 354:795, 1999.
42. Marseille E, Kahn JG, Mmiro F, et al. Cost effectiveness of single-dose nevirapine regimen for mothers and babies to decrease vertical HIV-1 transmission in sub-Saharan Africa. Lancet 354:803, 1999.
43. Lorenzi P, Spicher VM, Laubereau B, et al. Antiretroviral therapies in pregnancy: maternal, fetal and neonatal effects: Swiss HIV Cohort Study, the Swiss Collaborative HIV and Pregnancy Study, and the Swiss Neonatal HIV Study. AIDS 12:F241, 1998.
44. Shaffer N, Chuachoowong R, Mock PA, et al. Short-course zidovudine for perinatal HIV-1 transmission in Bangkok, Thailand: a randomised controlled trial: Bangkok Collaborative Perinatal HIV Transmission Study Group. Lancet 353:773, 1999.
45. Wiktor SZ, Ekpini E, Karon JM, et al. Short-course oral zidovudine for prevention of mother-to-child transmission of HIV-1 in Abidjan, Cote d'Ivoire: a randomised trial. Lancet 353:781, 1999.
46. Dabis F, Msellati P, Meda N, et al. 6-Month efficacy, tolerance, and acceptability of a short regimen of oral zidovudine to reduce vertical transmission of HIV in breastfed children in Cote d'Ivoire and Burkina Faso: a double-blind placebo-controlled multicentre trial. DITRAME Study Group; Diminution de la Transmission Mere-Enfant. Lancet 353:786, 1999.
47. Ruprecht RM, O'Brien LG, Rossoni LD, et al. Suppression of mouse viraemia and retroviral disease by 3′-azido-3′deoxythymidine. Nature 323:467, 1986.
48. Tavares L, Roneker C, Johnston K, et al. 3′-Azido-3′deoxythymidine in feline leukemia virus-infected cats: a model for therapy and prophylaxis of AIDS. Cancer Res 47:3190, 1987.
49. Black RJ. Animal studies of prophylaxis. Am J Med 102(suppl 5B):39, 1997.
50. Kaneshima H, Shih CC, Namikawa R, et al. Human immunodeficiency virus infection of human lymph nodes in the SCID-hu mouse. Proc Natl Acad Sci USA 88:4523, 1991.
51. McCune JM, Namikawa R, Shih CC, et al. Suppression of HIV infection in AZT-treated SCID-hu mice. Science 247:564, 1990.
52. Rabin L, Hincenbergs M, Moreno MB, et al. Use of standardized SCID-hu Thy/Liv mouse model for preclinical efficacy testing of anti-human immunodeficiency virus type 1 compounds. Antimicrob Agents Chemother 40:755, 1996.
53. Shih CC, Kaneshima H, Rabin L, et al. Postexposure prophylaxis with zidovudine suppresses human immunodeficiency virus type 1 infection in SCID-hu mice in a time-dependent manner. J Infect Dis 163:625, 1991.
54. Fazely F, Haseltine WA, Rodger RF, et al. Postexposure chemoprophylaxis with ZDV or ZDV combined with interferon-alpha: failure after inoculating rhesus monkeys with a high dose of SIV. J Acquir Immune Defic Syndr 4:1093, 1991.
55. Martin LN, Murphey CM, Soike KF, et al. Effects of initiation of 3′-azido,3′-deoxythymidine (zidovudine) treatment at different times after infection of rhesus monkeys with simian immunodeficiency virus. J Infect Dis 168:825, 1993.
56. McClure HM, Anderson DC, Fultz P, et al. Prophylactic effects of AZT following exposure of macaques to an acutely lethal variant of SIV (SIV/SMM/PBj-14) [abstract]. In: 5th International Conference on AIDS, Ottawa, 1989.
57. Van Rompay KK, Marthas ML, Ramos RA, et al. Simian immunodeficiency virus (SIV) infection of infant rhesus macaques as a model to test antiretroviral drug prophylaxis and therapy: oral 3′-azido-3′-deoxythymidine prevents SIV infection. Antimicrob Agents Chemother 36:2381, 1992.
58. Böttiger D, Johansson NG, Samuelsson B, et al. Prevention of simian immunodeficiency virus, SIVsm, or HIV-2 infection in cynomolgus monkeys by pre- and postexposure administration of BEA-005. AIDS 11:157, 1997.
59. Tsai CC, Follis KE, Sabo A, et al. Prevention of SIV infection in macaques by (R)-9-(2-phosphonylmethoxypropyl)adenine. Science 270:1197, 1995.
60. Tsai CC, Emau P, Follis KE, et al. Effectiveness of postinoculation (R)-9-(2-phosphonylmethoxypropyl) adenine treatment for prevention of persistent simian immunodeficiency virus SIVmne infection depends critically on timing of initiation and duration of treatment. J Virol 72:4265, 1998.
61. Otten RA, Smith DK, Adams DR, et al. Efficacy of postexposure prophylaxis after intravaginal exposure of pig-tailed macaques to a human-derived retrovirus (human immunodeficiency virus type 2). J Virol 74:9771, 2000.
62. Katzenstein TL, Dickmeiss E, Aladdin H, et al. Failure to develop HIV infection after receipt of HIV-contaminated blood and postexposure prophylaxis. Ann Intern Med 133:31, 2000.
63. Centers for Disease Control and Prevention. Updated U.S. Public Health Service guidelines for the management of occupational exposures to HBV, HCV, and HIV and recommendations for postexposure prophylaxis. MMWR Morb Mortal Wkly Rep 50(RR-11):1, 2001.
64. Gerberding JL, Henderson DK. Management of occupational exposures to bloodborne pathogens: hepatitis B virus, hepatitis C virus, and human immunodeficiency virus. Clin Infect Dis 14:1179, 1992.
65. Hamory BH. Underreporting of needlestick injuries in a university hospital. Am J Infect Control 11:174, 1983.
66. Mangione CM, Gerberding JL, Cummings SR. Occupational exposure to HIV: frequency and rates of underreporting of percutaneous and mucocutaneous exposures by medical housestaff. Am J Med 90:85, 1991.

67. Schechter MT, Marion SA, Elmslie KD, et al. How many persons in Canada have been infected with human immunodeficiency virus? An exploration using backcalculation methods. Clin Invest Med 15:331, 1992.
68. Henry K, Campbell S. Needlestick/sharps injuries and HIV exposure among health care workers: national estimates based on a survey of U.S. hospitals. Minn Med 78(11):41, 1995.
69. Resnic FS, Noerdlinger MA. Occupational exposure among medical students and house staff at a New York City Medical Center. Arch Intern Med 155:75, 1995.
70. Benitez Rodriguez E, Ruiz Moruno AJ, Cordoba Dona JA, et al. Underreporting of percutaneous exposure accidents in a teaching hospital in Spain. Clin Perform Qual Health Care 7(2):88, 1999.
71. Haiduven DJ, Simpkins SM, Phillips ES, et al. A survey of percutaneous/mucocutaneous injury reporting in a public teaching hospital. J Hosp Infect 41:151, 1999.
72. Lee CH, Carter WA, Chiang WK, et al. Occupational exposures to blood among emergency medicine residents. Acad Emerg Med 6:1036, 1999.
73. MacDonald MA, Elford J, Kaldor JM. Reporting of occupational exposures to blood-borne pathogens in Australian teaching hospitals. Med J Aust 163:121, 1995.
74. Manian FA. Blood and body fluid exposures among surgeons: a survey of attitudes and perceptions five years following Universal Precautions. Infect Control Hosp Epidemiol 17:172, 1996.
75. Shiao JS, McLaws ML, Huang KY, et al. Prevalence of nonreporting behavior of sharps injuries in Taiwanese health care workers. Am J Infect Control 27:254, 1999.
76. Department of Labor OSHA. Occupational exposure to bloodborne pathogens; final rule. Fed Reg 56:64175, 1991.
77. Bangsberg D, Goldschmidt RH. Postexposure prophylaxis for occupational exposure to HIV. JAMA 282:1623, 1999.
78. Henderson DK. Postexposure chemoprophylaxis for occupational exposures to the human immunodeficiency virus. JAMA 281:931, 1999.
79. Piscitelli SC, Burstein AH, Chaitt D, et al. Indinavir concentrations and St. John's wort. Lancet 355:547, 2000.
80. Centers for Disease Control and Prevention. Public Health Service guidelines for the management of health-care worker exposures to HIV and recommendations for postexposure prophylaxis. MMWR Morb Mortal Wkly Rep 47(RR-7):1, 1998.
81. Beekmann SE, Fahrner R, Henderson DK, et al. Zidovudine safety and tolerance among uninfected healthcare workers: a brief update. Am J Med 102:63, 1997.
82. Ippolito G, Puro V, Italian Registry of Antiretroviral Prophylaxis. Zidovudine toxicity in uninfected healthcare workers. Am J Med 102:58, 1997.
83. Struble KA, Pratt RD, Gitterman SR. Toxicity of antiretroviral agents. Am J Med 102:65, 1997.
84. Henry K, Acosta EP, Jochimsen E. Hepatotoxicity and rash associated with zidovudine and zalcitabine chemoprophylaxis. Ann Intern Med 124:855, 1996.
85. D'Silva M, Leibowitz D, Flaherty JP. Seizure associated with zidovudine. Lancet 346:452, 1995.
86. Swotinsky RB, Steger KA, Sulis C, et al. Occupational exposure to HIV: experience at a tertiary care center. J Occup Environ Med 40:1102, 1998.
87. Wang SA, Puro V. Toxicity of post-exposure prophylaxis for human immunodeficiency virus. In: Panlilio L (ed) Ballière's Clinical Infectious Diseases. London, Ballière-Tindall, 1999, p 349.
88. Spenatto N, Viraben R. Early lipodystrophy occurring during post-exposure prophylaxis. Sex Transm Infect 74:455, 1998.
89. Centers for Disease Control and Prevention. Update: provisional Public Health Service recommendations for chemoprophylaxis after occupational exposure to HIV. MMWR Morb Mortal Wkly Rep 45:468, 1996.
90. Centers for Disease Control. Public Health Service statement on management of occupational exposure to human immunodeficiency virus, including considerations regarding zidovudine postexposure use. MMWR Morb Mortal Wkly Rep 39(RR):1, 1990.
91. Centers for Disease Control and Prevention. Serious adverse events attributed to nevirapine regimens for postexposure prophylaxis after HIV exposures—worldwide, 1997–2000. MMWR Morb Mortal Wkly Rep 49:1153, 2001.
92. Fahrner R, Beekmann S, Koziol D, et al. Safety of zidovudine administered as postexposure chemoprophylaxis to healthcare workers sustaining HIV-related occupational exposures. Presented at the 34th Interscience Conference on Antimicrobial Agents and Chemotherapy, Orlando, 1994.
93. Fahrner R, Beekmann S, Koziol D, et al. Safety of zidovudine (ZDV) administered as post-exposure chemoprophylaxis to healthcare workers (HCW) after occupational exposures to HIV. In: VIIIth International Conference on AIDS, Amsterdam, 1992.
94. Beekmann SE, Fahrner R, Koziol DE, et al. Safety of zidovudine (AZT) administered as post-exposure chemoprophylaxis to healthcare workers (HCW) sustaining occupational exposures (OE) to HIV [abstract]. In: 30th Annual Meeting of the Infectious Diseases Society of America, Anaheim, CA, 1992.
95. Beekmann SE, Fahrner R, Koziol DE, et al. Safety of zidovudine (AZT) administered as postexposure chemoprophylaxis to healthcare workers (HCW) sustaining occupational exposures (OE) to HIV. In: 33rd Interscience Conference on Antimicrobial Agents and Chemotherapy, New Orleans, Washington, DC, American Society for Microbiology, 1993, abstract 1121.
96. Fahrner R, Beekmann SE, Nelson L, et al. Combination post-exposure prophylaxis (PEP): a prospective study of HIV-exposed health care workers (HCW). In: 12th International Conference on AIDS, Geneva, 1998.
97. Sepkowitz KA, Rivera P, Louther J, et al. Postexposure prophylaxis for human immunodeficiency virus: frequency of initiation and completion of newly recommended regimen. Infect Control Hosp Epidemiol 19:506, 1998.
98. Ciesielski CA, Metler RP. Duration of time between exposure and seroconversion in healthcare workers with occupationally acquired infection with human immunodeficiency virus. Am J Med 102:115, 1997.
99. Katz MH, Gerberding JL. The care of persons with recent sexual exposure to HIV. Ann Intern Med 128:306, 1998.
100. Katz MH, Gerberding JL. Postexposure treatment of people exposed to the human immunodeficiency virus through sexual contact or injection-drug use. N Engl J Med 336:1097, 1997.
101. Kahn JO. Post-exposure prevention of HIV-1 infection. Antivir Ther 3(suppl 4):45, 1998.
102. Bamberger JD, Waldo CR, Gerberding JL, et al. Postexposure prophylaxis for human immunodeficiency virus (HIV) infection following sexual assault. Am J Med 106:323, 1999.
103. Richman KM, Rickman LS. The potential for transmission of human immunodeficiency virus through human bites. J Acquir Immune Defic Syndr 6:402, 1993.
104. Khajotia RR, Lee E. Transmission of human immunodeficiency virus through saliva after a lip bite. Arch Intern Med 157:1901, 1997.
105. Vidmar L, Poljak M, Tomazic J, et al. Transmission of HIV-1 by human bite. Lancet 347:1762, 1996.
106. Pretty IA, Anderson GS, Sweet DJ. Human bites and the risk of human immunodeficiency virus transmission. Am J Forensic Med Pathol 20:232, 1999.
107. Gerberding JL, Katz MH. Post-exposure prophylaxis for HIV. Adv Exp Med Biol 458:213, 1999.
108. Martin JN, Roland ME, Bamberger JD, et al. Postexposure prophylaxis after sexual or drug use exposure to HIV: final results from the San Francisco Post Exposure Prevention Project. In: 7th Conference on Retroviruses and Opportunistic Infections, San Francisco, 2000, abstract 196.
109. Centers for Disease Control. Birth outcomes following zidovudine therapy in pregnant women. MMWR Morb Mortal Wkly Rep 43:415, 1994.
110. Anonymous. Antiretroviral Pregnancy Registry for didanosine (VIDEX, ddI), lamivudine (EPIVIRTM, 3tc), saquinavir (INVIRASE, SAQ), stavudine (ZERIT, d4T), zalcitabine (HIVID, ddC) zidovudine (RETROVIR, ZDV). Interim report, 1 January 1989 through December 1996. Research Triangle Park, NC, Bristol Myers Squibb, Glaxo Wellcome, Hoffman-LaRoche, and Merck, 1997.
111. Culnane M, Fowler MG, Lee S, et al. Evaluation for late effects of in utero (IU) ZDV exposure among uninfected infants born to HIV^+ women enrolled in ACTG 076 and 210 [abstract 485]. Clin Infect Dis 25:445, 1997.
112. Moodley J, Moodley D, Pillay K, et al. Antiviral effect of lamivudine alone and in combination with zidovudine in HIV-infected pregnant women. In: Abstracts of the 4th Conference on Retroviruses and Opportunistic Infections, Washington, DC, 1997, p 176, abstract 607.

113. Johnson MA, Goodwin C, Yuen GJ, et al. The pharmacokinetics of 3TC administered to HIV-1 infected women (pre-partum, during labor and post-partum) and their offspring. In: Proceedings from the XI International Conference on AIDS, Vancouver, 1996, p 249, abstract Tu.C.445.
114. Blanche S, Tardieu M, Rustin P, et al. Persistent mitochondrial dysfunction and perinatal exposure to antiretroviral nucleoside analogues. Lancet 354:1084, 1999.
115. Beltrami EM, Williams IT, Shapiro CN, et al. Risk and management of blood-borne infections in health care workers. Clin Microbiol Rev 13:385, 2000.
116. Tack PC, Bremer JW, Harris AA, et al. Genotypic analysis of HIV-1 isolates to identify antiretroviral resistance mutations from source patients involved in health care worker occupational exposures. JAMA 281:1085, 1999.
117. Beltrami E, Luo C-C, DelaTorre N, et al. HIV transmission after an occupational exposure despite prophylaxis with a combination drug regimen. In: 4th Decennial Conference on Nosocomial and Healthcare-Associated Infections, 2000. Atlanta, Centers for Disease Control and Prevention, 2000, p 125, abstract P-S2-62.
118. Beltrami E. Occupational HIV infection due to isolates resistant to antiretrovirals chosen for postexposure prophylaxis. In: 6th Annual Conference on Retroviruses and Opportunistic Infections, Chicago, 1999.
119. Chiarello LA, Gerberding JL. Human immunodeficiency virus in health care settings. In: Mandell GL, Bennett JE, Dolin R (eds) Principles and Practice of Infectious Diseases. Philadelphia, Churchill Livingstone, 2000, p 3052.
120. Ippolito G, Puro P, De Carli G, et al. The risk of occupational HIV infection in health care workers: Italian multicentre study. Arch Intern Med 153:1451, 1993.
121. Ippolito G, Puro V, Petrosillo N, et al. Simultaneous infection with HIV and hepatitis C virus following occupational conjunctival blood exposure. JAMA 280:28, 1998.
122. Centers for Disease Control. Possible transmission of human immunodeficiency virus to a patient during an invasive dental procedure. MMWR Morb Mortal Wkly Rep 39:489, 1990.
123. Centers for Disease Control. Update: transmission of HIV infection during an invasive dental procedure—Florida. MMWR Morb Mortal Wkly Rep 40:21, 1991.
124. Ou CY, Ciesielski CA, Myers G, et al. Molecular epidemiology of HIV transmission in a dental practice. Science 256:1165, 1992.
125. Ciesielski CA, Bell DM, Marianos DW. Transmission of HIV from infected health-care workers to patients. AIDS 5(suppl 2):S93, 1991.
126. Lot F, Seguier JC, Fegueux S, et al. Probable transmission of HIV from an orthopedic surgeon to a patient in France. Ann Intern Med 130:1, 1999.
127. Blanchard A, Ferris S, Chamaret S, et al. Molecular evidence for nosocomial transmission of human immunodeficiency virus from a surgeon to one of his patients. J Virol 72:4537, 1998.
128. Goujon CP, Schneider VM, Grofti J, et al. Phylogenetic analyses indicate an atypical nurse-to-patient transmission of human immunodeficiency virus type 1. J Virol 74:2525, 2000.
129. Centers for Disease Control. Summary and recommendations for preventing transmission of infection with human T-lymphotropic virus type III/lymphadenopathy-associated virus in the workplace. MMWR Morb Mortal Wkly Rep 34:681, 1985.
130. Centers for Disease Control. Update: evaluation of human T-lymphotropic virus type III/lymphadenopathy-associated virus infection in health-care personnel—United States. MMWR Morb Mortal Wkly Rep 34:575, 1985.
131. Gerberding JL, Henderson DK. Design of rational infection control policies for human immunodeficiency virus infection. J Infect Dis 156:861, 1987.
132. Centers for Disease Control. Recommendations for preventing transmission of infection with human T-lymphotropic virus type III/lymphadenopathy-associated virus during invasive procedures. MMWR Morb Mortal Wkly Rep 35:221, 1986.
133. Brown J, Chapman S, Lupton D. Infinitesimal risk as public health crisis: news media coverage of a doctor-patient HIV contact tracing investigation. Soc Sci Med 43:1685, 1996.
134. Bell DM, Shapiro CN, Gooch BF. Preventing HIV transmission to patients during invasive procedures. J Public Health Dent 53:170, 1993.
135. Bell DM, Shapiro CN, Culver DH, et al. Risk of hepatitis B and human immunodeficiency virus transmission to a patient from an infected surgeon due to percutaneous injury during an invasive procedure: estimates based on a model. Infect Agents Dis 1:263, 1992.
136. Centers for Disease Control. Recommendations for preventing transmission of human immunodeficiency virus and hepatitis B virus to patients during exposure-prone invasive procedures. MMWR Morb Mortal Wkly Rep 40(RR-8):1, 1991.
137. Centers for Disease Control. Update: investigations of persons treated by HIV-infected health-care workers—United States. MMWR Morb Mortal Wkly Rep 42:329, 1993.
138. Ciesielski C, Marianos D, Ou C-Y, et al. Transmission of human immunodeficiency virus in a dental practice. Ann Intern Med 116:798, 1992.
139. Ciesielski CA, Marianos DW, Schochetman G, et al. The 1990 Florida dental investigation: the press and the science. Ann Intern Med 121:886, 1994.
140. Collignon P. Infection risks to patients from HIV-infected health care workers. Ann Intern Med 124:277, 1996.
141. Doran K. When a physician is HIV positive: an examination of legal and practical aspects. QRC Advis 14:4, 1998.
142. Ecker JL. Mandatory disclosure of human immunodeficiency virus status by surgeons is philosophically and practically counterproductive. Am J Obstet Gynecol 172:1647, 1995.
143. Erridge P. The rights of HIV infected healthcare workers. BMJ 312:1625, 1996.
144. Gardam MA, Flanagan WF, Salit IE. The HIV-positive dentist: balancing the rights of the health care worker and the patient. Can Med Assoc J 164:1715, 2001.
145. Gerberding JL. Provider-to-patient HIV transmission: how to keep it exceedingly rare. Ann Intern Med 130:64, 1999.
146. Gostin LO. A proposed national policy on health care workers living with HIV/AIDS and other blood-borne pathogens. JAMA 284:1965, 2000.
147. Gostin LO. Infected physicians: what are the ethical and legal standards? Internist 32:9, 1991.
148. Gostin L. HIV-infected physicians and the practice of seriously invasive procedures. Hastings Center Rep 19(1):32, 1989.
149. Gostin L. The HIV-infected health care professional: public policy, discrimination, and patient safety. Arch Intern Med 151:663, 1991.
150. Hardie J. Current infection control policies must be challenged. Quintessence Int 26:751, 1995.
151. Hardie J. AIDS and dentistry: a retrospective analysis of the Florida case. J Can Dent Assoc 59:987, 1993.
152. Harris J, Holm S. Is there a moral obligation not to infect others? BMJ 311:1215, 1995.
153. Harris J, Holm S. Risk-taking and professional responsibility. J R Soc Med 90:625, 1997.
154. Heilman RS. Doctors and AIDS: double standard and double jeopardy. Radiographics 11:382, 1991.
155. Henderson DK. The HIV- or HBV-infected healthcare provider and society's perception of risk: science, nonscience, and nonsense. Ann Allergy 68:197, 1992.
156. Henderson DK. Human immunodeficiency virus infection in patients and providers. In: Wenzel R (ed) Prevention and Control of Nosocomial Infections, 2nd ed. Baltimore, Williams & Wilkins, 1992, p 42.
157. Heptonstall J, Gill ON, Porter K, et al. Health care workers and HIV. Commun Dis Rep 3:147, 1993.
158. Heptonstall J, Gill ON. HIV, occupational exposure, and medical responsibilities. Lancet 346:578, 1995.
159. Horowitz LG. Murder and cover-up could explain the Florida dental AIDS mystery. Br Dent J 177:423, 1994.
160. Horowitz LG. Sexual homicide with HIV in a Florida dental office? J Clin Pediatr Dent 19:61, 1994.
161. Karrel AI. HIV-infected physicians: how best to protect the public? Can Med Assoc J 152:1059, 1995.
162. Koelbl JJ. HIV-positive health-care professionals: perspectives and recommendations. Compendium 14:1458, 1993.
163. Koelbl JJ. The HIV-positive dental student. Dentistry 14(2):4, 1994.
164. Landesman SH. The HIV-positive health professional: policy options for individuals, institutions, and states: public policy and the public—observations from the front line. Arch Intern Med 151:655, 1991.
165. Le Leu LA, Jezukaitis PT. Restrictions on HIV-infected health care workers. Med J Aust 162:498, 1995.
166. Molinari JA. Infected health-care professionals: healers or modern day lepers? Part 2. Approaches and recommendations. Compendium 14:966, 1993.

167. Molinari JA. Infected health-care professionals: healers or modern day lepers? Part 1. Issues and considerations. Compendium 14:706, 1993.
168. Murphy TF. Health care workers with HIV and a patient's right to know. J Med Philos 19:553, 1994.
169. Neiburger EJ. Fuzzy science: a look at CDC's analysis of the Acer case. CDS Rev 89(2):22, 1996.
170. Neidle EA. Forging policy in the eye of the storm. J Public Health Dent 52:317, 1992.
171. Novick A. Human immunodeficiency virus guidelines should be based on science, not hysteria. Am J Obstet Gynecol 172:1647, 1995.
172. Robert LM, Chamberland ME, Cleveland JL, et al. Investigations of patients of health care workers infected with HIV: the Centers for Disease Control and Prevention database. Ann Intern Med 122:653, 1995.
173. Robinson P, Challacombe S. Transmission of HIV in a dental practice—the facts. Br Dent J 175:383, 1993.
174. Robinson EN Jr, de Bliek R. The college student, the dentist, and the North Carolina senator: risk analysis and risk management of HIV transmission from health care worker to patient. Med Decis Making 16(1):86, 1996.
175. Rohlfsen RJ. HIV-infected surgical personnel under the ADA: do they pose a direct threat or are reasonable accommodations possible? J Contemp Health Law Policy 16:127, 1999.
176. Rosner F, Sordillo PP, Wolpaw JR, et al. Ethical considerations concerning the HIV-positive physician. N Y State J Med 92:151, 1992.
177. Schaffner W. Surgeons with HIV infection: the risk to patients. J Hosp Infect 18(suppl A):191, 1991.
178. Schaffner W, Mishu-Allos B. Protecting patients when their surgeon or dentist is infected with a blood-borne virus. J Hosp Infect 30(suppl):156, 1995.
179. Schatz B. Supporting and advocating for HIV-positive health care workers. Bull NY Acad Med 72(suppl 1):263, 1995.
180. Schoeffel A. Discrimination: exposure-prone procedures and HIV-infected health care professionals—Estate of Mauro v. Borgess Medical Center. Am J Law Med 24:127, 1998.
181. Scott HD. The HIV-infected health care worker: another AIDS policy conundrum. Ann Intern Med 116:341, 1992.
182. Scully C, Porter SR. Can HIV be transmitted from dental personnel to patients by dentistry? Br Dent J 175:381, 1993.
183. Singh D. Health care workers with AIDS: the patient's right to know. Med Law 20(1):49, 2001.
184. Tereskerz PM, Pearson RD, Jagger J. Infected physicians and invasive procedures: national policy and legal reality. Milbank Q 77:511, 1999.
185. Vlahakis EG, Brieger GM, MacGibbon AL. Restrictions on HIV-infected health care workers. Med J Aust 162:109, 1995.
186. Wiseman F. Mandatory screening for physicians performing seriously invasive procedures: an ethical analysis. Plast Surg Nurs 19:167, 1999.
187. Zazzali ME. HIV-infected health care workers who perform invasive, exposure-prone procedures: defining the risk and balancing the interests of health care workers and patients. Seton Hall Law Rev 28:1000, 1998.
188. Zinberg JM. Under the ADA: double standards for HIV-positive patients and providers. Bull Am Coll Surg 85(4):8, 2000.
189. Armstrong FP, Miner JC, Wolfe WH. Investigation of a health care worker with symptomatic human immunodeficiency virus infection: an epidemiological approach. Milit Med 152:414, 1987.
190. Babinchak TJ, Renner C. Patients treated by a thoracic surgeon with HIV: a review. Chest 106:681, 1994.
191. Danila RN, MacDonald KL, Rhame FS, et al. A look-back investigation of patients of an HIV-infected physician: public health implications. N Engl J Med 325:1406, 1991.
192. Dickinson GM, Morhart RE, Klimas NG, et al. Absence of HIV transmission from an infected dentist to his patients: an epidemiologic and DNA sequence analysis. JAMA 269:1802, 1993.
193. Donnelly M, Duckworth G, Nelson S, et al. Are HIV lookbacks worthwhile? Outcome of an exercise to notify patients treated by an HIV infected health care worker; incident management teams. Commun Dis Public Health 2:126, 1999.
194. Gooch B, Marianos D, Ciesielski C, et al. Lack of evidence for patient-to-patient transmission of HIV in a dental practice. J Am Dent Assoc 124:38, 1993.
195. Jaffe HW, McCurdy JM, Kalish ML, et al. Lack of HIV transmission in the practice of a dentist with AIDS. Ann Intern Med 121:855, 1994.
196. Longfield JN, Brundage J, Badger G, et al. Look-back investigation after human immunodeficiency virus seroconversion in a pediatric dentist. J Infect Dis 169:1, 1994.
197. Mishu B, Schaffner W, Horan JM, et al. A surgeon with AIDS: lack of evidence of transmission to patients. JAMA 264:467, 1990.
198. Rogers AS, Froggatt JW, Townsend T, et al. Investigation of potential HIV transmission to the patients of an HIV-infected surgeon. JAMA 269:1795, 1993.
199. Stephens BJ, Sinden PG, Ketcham RH, et al. The consequences of disclosure: one hospital's response to the presence of an HIV-positive physician. Hosp Health Serv Adm 40:457, 1995.
200. Von Reyn CF, Gilbert TT, Shaw FE Jr, et al. Absence of HIV transmission from an infected orthopedic surgeon: a 13-year look-back study. JAMA 269:1807, 1993.
201. Robinson E, Joce R, O'Donovan D, et al. Lookbacks for HIV infected health care workers. Commun Dis Public Health 3:143, 2000.
202. Tapper ML, Dickinson GL, Gerberding JL, et al. "Look-back" notifications for HIV/HBV-positive healthcare workers. Infect Control Hosp Epidemiol 13(8):82, 1992.
203. Hermann DHJ. Commentary: a call for authoritative CDC guidelines for HIV-infected health care workers. J Law Med Ethics 22:176, 1994.
204. American College of Surgeons. Statement on the surgeon and HIV infection: American College of Surgeons. Bull Am Coll Surg 83(2):27, 1998.
205. Strama BT. HIV-infected health care workers: the legal perspective. Bull NY Acad Med 72(suppl 1):240, 1995.
206. Public Health and Welfare Act. USC, 1994.
207. Burris S. Human immunodeficiency virus-infected health care workers: the restoration of professional authority. Arch Fam Med 5:102, 1996.
208. Henderson DK. Management of health-care workers who are infected with the human immunodeficiency virus or other bloodborne pathogens. In: DeVita V, Hellman S, Rosenberg S (eds) AIDS: Etiology, Diagnosis, Treatment, and Prevention, 3rd ed. Philadelphia, Lippincott, 1993.
209. Hansen ME, McIntire DD. HIV transmission during invasive radiologic procedures: estimate based on computer modeling. AJR Am J Roentgenol 166:263, 1996.
210. Neidle E, American Dental Association. Estimates of the risk of endemic transmission of hepatitis B virus and human immunodeficiency virus to patients by the percutaneous route during invasive surgical and dental procedures. In: Open Meeting on the Risks of Transmission of Bloodborne Pathogens to Patients During Invasive Procedures, Atlanta, 1991.
211. Rhame FS. The HIV-infected surgeon. JAMA 264:507, 1990.
212. Lowenfels AB, Wormser G. Risk of transmission of HIV from surgeon to patient. N Engl J Med 325:888, 1991.
213. Schulman KA, McDonald RC, Lynn LA, et al. Screening surgeons for HIV infection: assessment of a potential public health program. Infect Control Hosp Epidemiol 15:147, 1994.
214. Chamberland ME. HIV transmission from health care worker to patient: what is the risk? Ann Intern Med 116:871, 1992.
215. Siew C, Chang SB, Gruninger SE, et al. Self-reported percutaneous injuries in dentists: implications for HBV, HIV, transmission risk. J Am Dent Assoc 123:36, 1992.
216. Beekmann SE, Vlahov D, Koziol DE, et al. Temporal association between implementation of universal precautions and a sustained, progressive decrease in percutaneous exposures to blood. Clin Infect Dis 18:562, 1994.
217. Chiarello LA, Cardo DM. Comprehensive prevention of occupational blood exposures: lessons from other countries. Infect Control Hosp Epidemiol 21:562, 2000.
218. Cohen MS, Do JT, Tahery DP, et al. Efficacy of double gloving as a protection against blood exposure in dermatologic surgery. J Dermatol Surg Oncol 18:873, 1992.
219. Cohn GM, Seifer DB. Blood exposure in single versus double gloving during pelvic surgery. Am J Obstet Gynecol 162:715, 1990.
220. Culver J. Preventing transmission of blood-borne pathogens: a compelling argument for effective device-selection strategies. Am J Infect Control 25:430, 1997.
221. Gerberding JL, Ramiro N, Perlman J, et al. Intraoperative blood exposures at San Francisco General Hospital: provider injuries and patient recontacts. Presented at the 31st Annual Meeting of the Infectious Diseases Society of America, New Orleans, 1993.

222. Greco RJ, Garza JR. Use of double gloves to protect the surgeon from blood contact during aesthetic procedures. Aesthetic Plast Surg 19:265, 1995.
223. Ippolito G, De Carli G, Puro V, et al. Device-specific risk of needlestick injury in Italian health care workers. JAMA 272:607, 1994.
224. Jagger J. Reducing occupational exposure to bloodborne pathogens: where do we stand a decade later? Infect Control Hosp Epidemiol 17:573, 1996.
225. Kovavisarach E, Jaravechson S. Comparison of perforation between single and double-gloving in perineorrhaphy after vaginal delivery: a randomized controlled trial. Aust NZJ Obstet Gynaecol 38:58, 1998.
226. McPherson DC, Parris NB. Reducing occupational exposure to blood in the OR. Todays OR Nurse 14(10):23, 1992.
227. Mendias EP, Ross AM. Health professional students' occupational exposures to blood-borne pathogens: primary and secondary prevention strategies. J Am Coll Health 49:193, 2001.
228. O'Connor RE, Krall SP, Megargel RE, et al. Reducing the rate of paramedic needlesticks in emergency medical services: the role of self-capping intravenous catheters. Acad Emerg Med 3:668, 1996.
229. Pietrabissa A, Merigliano S, Montorsi M, et al. Reducing the occupational risk of infections for the surgeon: multicentric national survey on more than 15,000 surgical procedures. World J Surg 21:573, 1997.
230. Sistrom MG, Coyner BJ, Gwaltney JM, et al. Frequency of percutaneous injuries requiring postexposure prophylaxis for occupational exposure to human immunodeficiency virus. Infect Control Hosp Epidemiol 19:504, 1998.
231. Smoot EC. Practical precautions for avoiding sharp injuries and blood exposure. Plast Reconstr Surg 101:528, 1998.
232. Bebbington MW, Treissman MJ. The use of a surgical assist device to reduce glove perforations in postdelivery vaginal repair: a randomized controlled trial. Am J Obstet Gynecol 175:862, 1996.
233. Centers for Disease Control and Prevention. Evaluation of blunt suture needles in preventing percutaneous injuries among health-care workers during gynecologic surgical procedures—New York City, March 1993–June 1994. MMWR Morb Mortal Wkly Rep 46(2):25, 1997.
234. Hartley JE, Ahmed S, Milkins R, et al. Randomized trial of blunt-tipped versus cutting needles to reduce glove puncture during mass closure of the abdomen. Br J Surg 83:1156, 1996.
235. Chiu KY, Fung B, Lau SK, et al. The use of double latex gloves during hip fracture operations. J Orthop Trauma 7:354, 1993.
236. Jensen SL, Kristensen B, Fabrin K. Double gloving as self protection in abdominal surgery. Eur J Surg 163:163, 1997.
237. Kuo YH, Fabiani JN, Mohamed AS, et al. Decreasing occupational risk related to blood-borne viruses in cardiovascular surgery in Paris, France. Ann Thorac Surg 68:2267, 1999.
238. Lewis FR Jr, Short LJ, Howard RJ, et al. Epidemiology of injuries by needles and other sharp instruments: minimizing sharp injuries in gynecologic and obstetric operations. Surg Clin North Am 75:1105, 1995.
239. Lowenfels AB, Mehta V, Levi DA, et al. Reduced frequency of percutaneous injuries in surgeons: 1993 versus 1988. AIDS 9:199, 1995.
240. Mingoli A, Sapienza P, Sgarzini G, et al. Influence of blunt needles on surgical glove perforation and safety for the surgeon. Am J Surg 172:512, 1996.
241. Quebbeman EJ, Telford GL, Wadsworth K, et al. Double gloving: protecting surgeons from blood contamination in the operating room. Arch Surg 127:213, 1992.
242. Salkin JA, Stuchin SA, Kummer FJ, et al. The effectiveness of cut-proof glove liners: cut and puncture resistance, dexterity, and sensibility. Orthopedics 18:1067, 1995.
243. Schwimmer A, Massoumi M, Barr CE. Efficacy of double gloving to prevent inner glove perforation during outpatient oral surgical procedures. J Am Dent Assoc 125:196, 1994.
244. Upton LG, Barber HD. Double-gloving and the incidence of perforations during specific oral and maxillofacial surgical procedures. J Oral Maxillofac Surg 51:261, 1993.
245. Hester RA, Nelson CL. Methods to reduce intraoperative transmission of blood-borne disease. J Bone Joint Surg Am 73:1108, 1991.
246. Henderson DK. Preventing occupational infection with the human immunodeficiency virus in the healthcare environment. In: Armstrong D, Cohen J (eds) Infectious Diseases. Vol. 2. London, Mosby, 1999, p 1–7.
247. Mofenson LM, Lambert JS, Stiehm ER, et al. Risk factors for perinatal transmission of human immunodeficiency virus type 1 in women treated with zidovudine: Pediatric AIDS Clinical Trials Group study 185 team. N Engl J Med 341:385, 1999.
248. Operskalski EA, Stram DO, Busch MP, et al. Role of viral load in heterosexual transmission of human immunodeficiency virus type 1 by blood transfusion recipients: Transfusion Safety Study Group. Am J Epidemiol 146:655, 1997.
249. Fiore JR, Zhang YJ, Bjorndal A, et al. Biological correlates of HIV-1 heterosexual transmission. AIDS 11:1089, 1997.
250. Popper SJ, Sarr AD, Travers KU, et al. Lower human immunodeficiency virus (HIV) type 2 viral load reflects the difference in pathogenicity of HIV-1 and HIV-2. J Infect Dis 180:1116, 1999.
251. Vella S, Galluzzo MC, Giannini G, et al. Plasma HIV-1 copy number and in vitro infectivity of plasma prior to and during combination antiretroviral treatment. Antiviral Res 47:189, 2000.
252. Hisada M, O'Brien TR, Rosenberg PS, et al. Virus load and risk of heterosexual transmission of human immunodeficiency virus and hepatitis C virus by men with hemophilia: the Multicenter Hemophilia Cohort Study. J Infect Dis 181:1475, 2000.
253. Gabiano C, Tovo PA, de Martino M, et al. Mother-to-child transmission of human immunodeficiency virus type 1: risk of infection and correlates of transmission. Pediatrics 90:369, 1992.
254. O'Donovan D, Ariyoshi K, Milligan P, et al. Maternal plasma viral RNA levels determine marked differences in mother-to-child transmission rates of HIV-1 and HIV-2 in The Gambia: MRC/Gambia Government/University College London Medical School working group on mother-child transmission of HIV. AIDS 14:441, 2000.
255. Shaffer N, Roongpisuthipong A, Siriwasin W, et al. Maternal virus load and perinatal human immunodeficiency virus type 1 subtype E transmission, Thailand: Bangkok Collaborative Perinatal HIV Transmission Study Group. J Infect Dis 179:590, 1999.
256. Leroy V, Montcho C, Manigart O, et al. Maternal plasma viral load, zidovudine and mother-to-child transmission of HIV-1 in Africa: DITRAME ANRS 049a trial. AIDS 15:517, 2001.
257. Quinn TC, Wawer MJ, Sewankambo N, et al. Viral load and heterosexual transmission of human immunodeficiency virus type 1: Rakai Project Study Group. N Engl J Med 342:921, 2000.
258. Ragni MV, Faruki H, Kingsley LA. Heterosexual HIV-1 transmission and viral load in hemophilic patients. J Acquir Immune Defic Syndr Hum Retrovirol 17:42, 1998.
259. Blatchford O, O'Brien SJ, Blatchford M, et al. Infectious health care workers: should patients be told? J Med Ethics 26:27, 2000.
260. Strong C. Should physicians infected with human immunodeficiency virus be allowed to perform surgery? Am J Obstet Gynecol 168:1344, 1993.
261. Orentlicher D. From the Office of the General Counsel: HIV-infected surgeons: Behringer v Medical Center. JAMA 266:1134, 1991.
262. De Ville KA. Nothing to fear but fear itself: HIV-infected physicians and the law of informed consent. J Law Med Ethics 22:163, 1994.
263. Daniels N. HIV-infected professionals, patient rights, and the "switching dilemma." JAMA 267:1368, 1992.
264. Shuster E. A surgeon with acquired immunodeficiency syndrome: a threat to patient safety? The case of William H. Behringer. Am J Med 94:93, 1993.
265. Fost N. Patient access to information on clinicians infected with blood-borne pathogens. JAMA 284:1975, 2000.
266. Americans with Disabilities Act. USC, 1997.
267. Abbott v. Bragdon. 1st Circuit; 1998, p. F3d 87.
268. Gostin LO, Feldblum C, Webber DW. Disability discrimination in America: HIV/AIDS and other health conditions. JAMA 281:745, 1999.
269. *School Board vs. Arline*. 480 U.S. 273, 1987.
270. Van Detta JA. Typhoid Mary meets the ADA: a case study of the direct threat standard under the Americans with Disabilities Act. Harv J Law Public Policy 22:853, 1999.
271. Lo B, Steinbrook R. Health care workers infected with the human immunodeficiency virus: the next steps. JAMA 267:1100, 1992.
272. Centers for Disease Control. Recommendations for prevention of HIV transmission in health-care settings. MMWR Morb Mortal Wkly Rep 36(suppl 2S):1S, 1987.
273. AMA Council on Ethical and Judicial Affairs. Ethical issues involved in the growing AIDS crisis. JAMA 259:1360, 1988.
274. AMA Council on Ethical and Judicial Affairs. Ethical issues in the growing AIDS crisis: the HIV-positive practitioner. JAMA 260:790, 1988.

275. American Academy of Pediatrics, Task Force on Pediatric AIDS. Pediatric guidelines for infection control of human immunodeficiency virus (acquired immunodeficiency virus) in hospitals, medical offices, schools, and other settings. Pediatrics 82:801, 1988.
276. American Academy of Orthopedic Surgeons Task Force on AIDS and Orthopedic Surgery. Recommendations for the Prevention of Human Immunodeficiency Virus (HIV) Transmission in the Practice of Orthopedic Surgery. Park Ridge, IL, AAOS, 1989.
277. American Hospital Association. Management of HIV Infection in the Hospital, 3rd ed. Chicago, AHA, 1988.
278. Committee on Ethics, The American College of Obstetricians and Gynecologists. Human immunodeficiency virus infection: physicians' responsibilities. Obstet Gynecol 75:1043, 1990.
279. Department of Health and Social Security. AIDS: HIV-infected health care workers—report of the recommendations of the Expert Advisory Group on AIDS. London, Her Majesty's Stationery Office, 1988.
280. Speller DC, Shanson DC, Ayliffe GA, et al. Acquired immunodeficiency syndrome: recommendations of a working party of the Hospital Infection Society. J Hosp Infect 15:7, 1990.
281. AIDS/Tuberculosis Subcommittee of the Society for Healthcare Epidemiology of America. Management of healthcare workers infected with hepatitis B virus, hepatitis C virus, human immunodeficiency virus, or other bloodborne pathogens: AIDS/TB Committee of the Society for Healthcare Epidemiology of America. Infect Control Hosp Epidemiol 18:349, 1997.
282. Bayer R. Discrimination, informed consent, and the HIV infected clinician. BMJ 314:915, 1997.

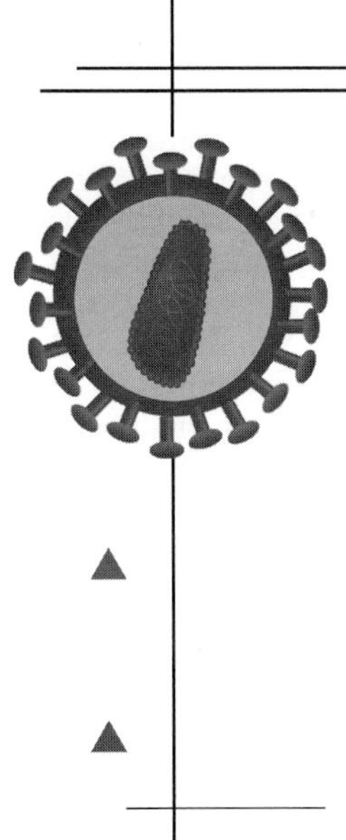

CHAPTER 26

HIV Resistance Testing in Clinical Practice

Andrew R. Zolopa, MD
Richard T. D'Aquila, MD

The rapid introduction of antiretroviral drug resistance testing into clinical practice is an example of how cutting edge technologies, developed because of advances in molecular genetics, can quickly alter the day-to-day management of human immunodeficiency virus (HIV)-infected patients. Information about HIV genetics and drug susceptibility is now commonly used to help make treatment decisions for HIV-infected patients. The biology of drug failure, the resistance assays available to clinicians, the clinical trial data underlying current guidelines for the use of resistance testing in the clinic, and some promising new directions for managing antiretroviral drug failure are summarized in this chapter. This field will undoubtedly continue to change and advance, so the reader is encouraged to use the information here as a starting point for reviewing even more current literature.

▲ WHY MEASURE RESISTANCE?

Antiretroviral drug-resistant HIV-1 is important to assess because many HIV-infected patients still experience drug failure.[1–3] Insufficient chemotherapeutic suppression of drug-resistant virus mutants probably accounts for a large proportion of these treatment failures. Indeed, HIV can escape the inhibitory effects of every drug developed to date through emergence of resistant mutants. Selection of HIV mutants in vitro when virus is grown in subinhibitory levels of the agent is an important criterion for determining whether a putative new inhibitor specifically targets HIV, rather than impairing virus replication only because it causes cellular toxicity. It is likely that each HIV-specific inhibitor is able to select resistant mutants, regardless of its target virus gene product. This is due to the error-prone nature of the HIV reverse transcription at each replication cycle[4] coupled with the large number of replication events per day.[5,6] Current, more effective combination regimens help minimize, but do not eliminate, emergence of drug-resistant mutants.

A second factor likely involved in drug failure is inadequate drug exposure. This factor is likely to contribute to the limits of current combination regimens in preventing emergence of drug-resistant mutants. Subinhibitory drug levels are common in vivo, at least transiently, because of poor adherence or other reasons for insufficient drug exposure at sites of replication in vivo. Moreover, low drug levels may, in turn, allow selection of either a preexisting or a newly generated drug-resistant mutant. Drug failure may therefore involve a cascade of subinhibitory drug levels and the outgrowth of resistant virus.

Resistance is most relevant to clinical management because the chance for successful virus suppression decreases with each combination antiretroviral regimen failure. This remains true despite the rapid growth in the availability of U.S. Food and Drug Administration (FDA)-approved antiretroviral agents and the best clinical practice. This is due at least in part to the emergence of viral mutants with cross resistance to antiretroviral drugs never used before by that patient. This cross resistance occurs within the same class as drugs that have been used and failed and varies by drug class and by drugs within each class.[7] This problem limits the utility of the growing drug armamentarium, making it more important than ever to utilize these drugs in ways that maximize effectiveness and minimize the development of cross resistance. There is accumulating evidence from clinical trials and observational cohort studies that resistance testing is a valuable tool for the clinician in the strategic management of antiretroviral therapy. These tests allow more informed and individualized choices of the next set of new drugs, called a *rescue regimen*, so that each new drug is as active as possible. It is important to individualize the choices of drugs in rescue regimens using resistance tests for two reasons: (1) A drug may fail by a mechanism other than resistance (e.g., inadequate exposure of wild type virus to the drug); and (2) the degree of cross resistance to as yet unused drugs varies depending on which of several possible mutations may have been selected during failure of an individual drug. Individualized decision-making may lead to more optimal sequencing of antiretroviral regimens over the long term. To minimize toxicity and maximize the benefit of therapy, information about potential cross resistance must not be used in isolation but in conjunction with the patient's antiretroviral treatment history, immunologic status, and pharmacologic data and the clinician's knowledge of antiretroviral drugs. Resistance testing maybe a less useful adjunct in patients with extensive drug experience who harbor virus with extensive cross resistance in each drug class. Yet even in this setting, resistance testing may allow the practitioner to optimize a regimen with the fewest antiretroviral agents and thereby limit potential toxicities and cost. Nonetheless, such patients need new drugs with novel mechanisms of inhibition to suppress the replication of viruses resistant to all current drug classes.

▲ RESISTANCE ASSAYS

There are currently two types of antiretroviral drug-resistance assays commercially available to the clinician: genotypic assays and phenotypic assays. Several genotypic assays are available, one of which is the TRUEGENE kit (Visible Genetics, Toronto, Canada), which has been given FDA approval. The availability of FDA-approved genotype kits enables testing to be done in local laboratories as well as larger reference laboratories. There are two major commercially available phenotype assays, and a third assay that has been available in France has recently become available in the United States. Phenotypic tests are likely to remain limited to a small number of reference laboratories because they are biohazardous and require more sophisticated, expensive technology.

All of the available assays, both phenotypic and genotypic, start with a polymerase chain reaction (PCR) step. Cross-contamination is therefore a potential problem, and rigorous quality control standards are required for the testing laboratory. Clinicians also must remember this possibility when results do not make sense for a specific situation; the result may inadvertently be a report on another patient's virus.

Genotype assays detect changes in the DNA sequence of the relevant HIV genes. DNA in the coding regions of genes is organized into nucleotide triplets, or codons. Each triplet encodes a single amino acid of the gene product (protein). Genotypic tests indirectly measure resistance by detecting mutations in the HIV-1 genome that lead to one or more specific amino acid substitutions in HIV protease or reverse transcriptase, which are the gene products targeted by current inhibitors. These specific changes in the protein cause drug resistance and are selected by drug pressure from the randomly occurring background of HIV genetic variability. ("Silent mutations" are nucleic acid changes that do not alter the amino acid sequence because of the redundance of the genetic code.) Mutations are designated in a shorthand format. The HIV gene is indicated first, followed by a single letter abbreviation for the wild-type amino acid present at a particular location in a protein (and encoded by a particular triplet of nucleotides, or codon). The number of the amino acid (and codon) follows. The single letter code for the new, mutant amino acid that has replaced the wild-type amino acid is given next. The designation PR L90M, for example, indicates that the wild-type amino acid leucine at position 90 of the protease has been replaced with a methionine.

Specific mutations are sought in genotypic assays. These changes have been previously associated with drug resistance. The mutation(s) may have been correlated with a change in a phenotypic assay in vitro. In some cases these mutations may have been associated with a lack of clinical response in vivo, as measured by a decrease in the plasma HIV RNA levels; this is more conclusive evidence that specific mutation(s) predict a lack of drug effect. The best evidence that a mutation causes drug resistance would involve both in vitro phenotypic data and viral load response data from several independent studies. Genotypes can be difficult to interpret. The number of resistance mutations, as well as the complexity of the patterns of such mutations, is large and continues to grow (http://www.iasusa.org/resistance mutations/revisedmutafigures-11.30.01.pdf, accessed March 10, 2002) (Fig. 26–1).[8] In addition, multiple mutations in a single gene sequence may produce interactive effects. Such interactions may be additive or synergistic, such that when present together the mutations increase resistance. Negative interactions also occur, in which one mutation decreases the resistance caused by another mutation. (These authors thought that such resistance-suppressing interactions were likely to have minimal, transient effects on viral load responses in vivo and were not to be relied on to maintain the effectiveness of the drug whose resistance is suppressed in vitro. Few in vivo studies haved tested this concept, though.)

Despite this complexity, many clinicians are learning how to incorporate genotypic information into their treatment plans. In addition, there are systems under development to help interpret the genotype information for the clinician (discussed later). Genotype tests are less expensive than phenotype tests, have a more rapid turnaround time to a result, and are more widely available, as many reference and hospital laboratories are now providing this service. Limited surveys suggest that performance of these tests has improved, and the earlier concern that many laboratories may have unacceptable false-negative rates for detection of mutations may no longer be warranted.[9,10]

The resistance mutations characterized to date all render the virus less susceptible to the drug to varying degrees. None leads to complete, absolute resistance in vitro,

MUTATIONS IN THE REVERSE TRANSCRIPTASE GENE ASSOCIATED WITH RESISTANCE TO REVERSE TRANSCRIPTASE INHIBITORS

A. Nucleoside and Nucleotide Reverse Transcriptase Inhibitors

	Mutations
Multi-nRTI Resistance: 151 Complex	A62V, V75I, F77L, F116Y, Q151M
Multi-nRTI Resistance: 69 Insertion Complex[1]	M41L, A62V, D67N, 69 insert, K70R, L210W, T215Y/F, K219Q/E
Multi-nRTI Resistance[2] (NAMs)	M41L, D67N, K70R, L210W, T215Y/F, K219Q/E
Zidovudine[3–5]	M41L, D67N, K70R, L210W, T215Y/F, K219Q/E
Didanosine[6]	K65R, L74V, M184V
Zalcitabine	K65R, T69D, L74V, M184V
Stavudine[3,7]	M41L, D67N, K70R, K75T/M/S/A, L210W, T215Y/F, K219Q/E
Abacavir[8]	M41L, K65R, D67N, K70R, L74V, Y115F, M184V, L210W, T215Y/F, K219Q/E
Lamivudine[9]	E44D, V118I, M184V/I
Tenofovir DF[3,10]	K65R

B. Nonnucleoside Reverse Transcriptase Inhibitors

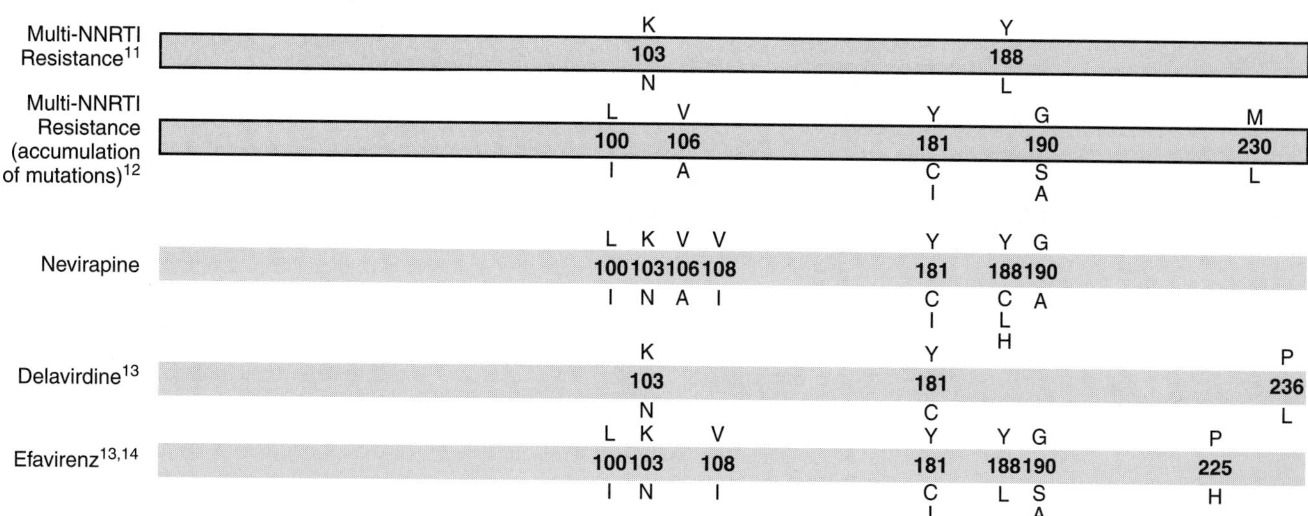

Figure 26–1.

Illustration continued on following page

MUTATIONS IN THE PROTEASE GENE ASSOCIATED WITH RESISTANCE TO PROTEASE INHIBITORS

C. Protease Inhibitors[15]

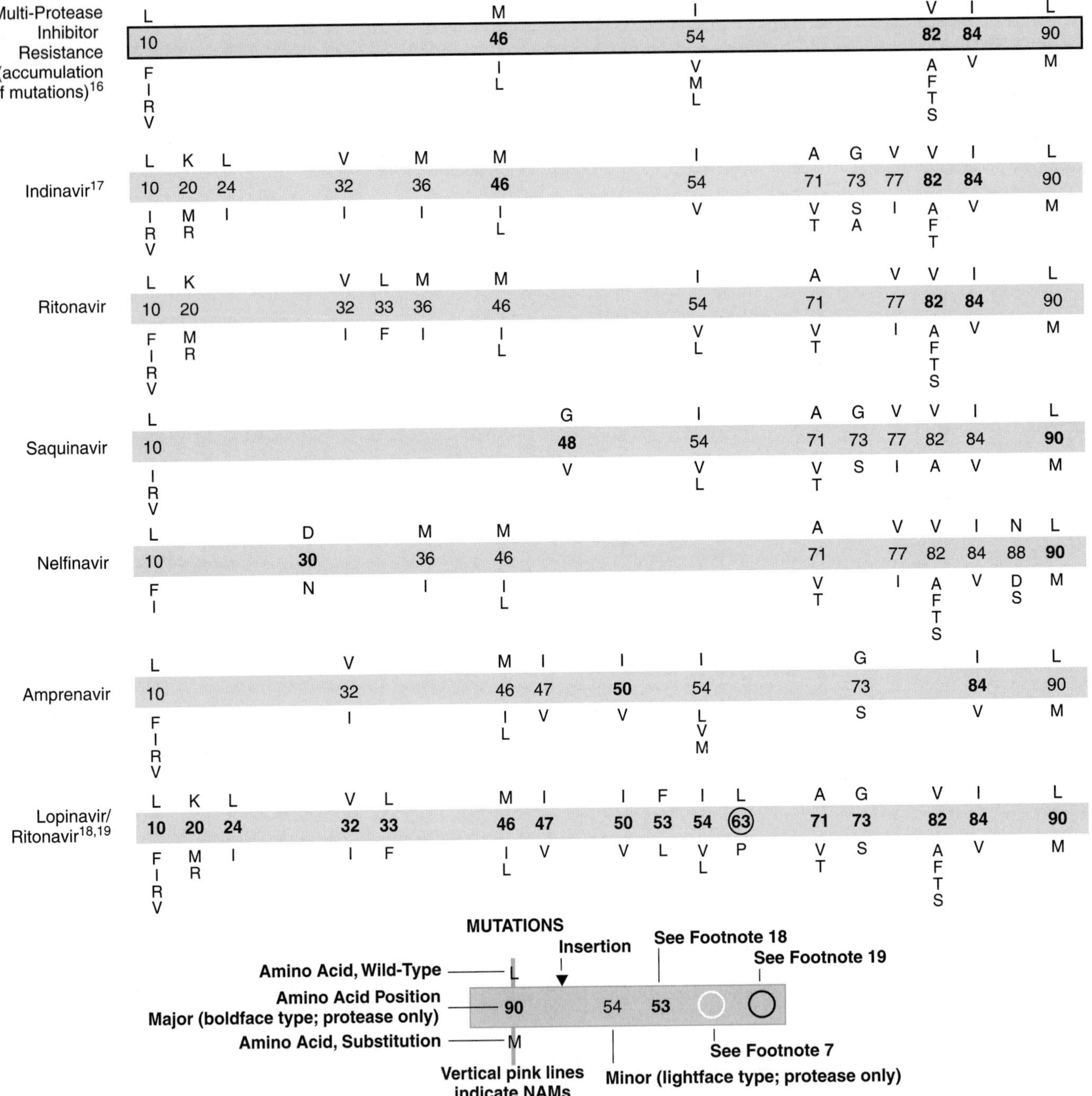

Figure 26–1. Resistance mutations. *A*, RT mutations associated with reduced susceptibility to nucleoside reverse transcriptase inhibitors. *B*, RT mutations associated with reduced susceptibility to nonnucleoside reverse transcriptase inhibitors. *C*, mutations associated with decreased susceptibility to protease inhibitors. For each amino acid residue, the letter above the bar indicates the amino acid associated with wild-type virus and the letter(s) below indicates the substitution(s) that confer viral resistance. The number shows the position of the mutation in the protein. Mutations selected by protease inhibitors in Gag cleavage sites are not listed because their contribution to resistance is not yet fully defined. NAMs, multi-nRTI-associated mutations; nRTI, nucleoside reverse transcriptase inhibitor; NNRTI, nonnucleoside reverse transcriptase inhibitor. Amino acids: A, alanine; C, cysteine; D, aspartate; E, glutamate; F, phenylalanine; G, glycine; H, histidine; I, isoleucine; K, lysine; L, leucine; M, methionine; N, asparagine; P, proline; Q, glutamine; R, arginine; S, serine; T, threonine; V, valine; W, tryptophan; Y, tyrosine. For full details of footnotes refer to article. (From International AIDS Society–USA. D'Aquila RT, Schapiro JM, Brun-Vézinet F, Clotet B, Conway B, Demeter LM, Grant RM, Johnson VA, Kuritzkes DR, Loveday C, Shafer RW, Richman DD. Drug resistance mutations in HIV-1. Topics HIV Med 2002; 10:11–15, with permission. Updates available at: *www.iasusa.org*)

although it is not yet clear for most drugs how much resistance is necessary to lose their inhibitory effect in vivo. In many cases, such substitutions in the amino acid sequence lead to diminished binding of the pertinent antiretroviral drug to the target protein. However, there are also more complex mechanisms for resistance. For example, several common mutations conferring resistance to nucleoside reverse transcriptase (RT) inhibitors—originally identified as accumulating during zidovudine failure and causing zidovudine resistance[11]—do not diminish drug-binding substantially. They seem, instead, to improve the enzymatic efficiency of the RT[12] and allow the RT to remove the terminal nucleoside triphosphate incorporated into a growing strand of newly synthesized HIV DNA.[13,14] The broad cross resistance caused by this set of mutations now seems to be caused by the removal, to varying degrees, of each of the nucleoside reverse transcriptase inhibitor (NRTI) triphosphate terminators.

Although most resistance mutations impair virus replicative capacity in the absence of drug,[15] there can also be compensatory mutations that accumulate and at least partially reverse the deleterious effects of other mutations on replicative capacity. The study of resistance mutation effects on virus replicative capacity is an active area of investigation.[16–18] Although these effects seem to be associated with the duration of mutant persistence off-drug and the pace of the decline of CD4 + T-lymphocytes on the failing drug, it is not yet possible to factor such effects into clinical decision-making about drug therapy reliably. Evaluation of the virus's replicative capacity phenotype requires methods different from those used to determine a drug susceptibility phenotype (described later); such techniques are still under development and have only recently become available clinically.

The commercially available phenotypic assays are recombinant virus assays that amplify the RT and protease genes from the predominant quasispecies in the patient's plasma virus RNA. These amplicons are inserted into a laboratory virus strain lacking these genes. Virus is then produced in the laboratory, and its ability to replicate in cell culture in the presence of various drug concentrations is measured (Fig. 26–2). Results are expressed as the concentration of drug required to inhibit 50% of growth (IC_{50}) and as the fold change in IC_{50} relative to a wild-type control strain. From the example given in Figure 26–2, the patient's isolate shows a 10-fold change for zidovudine; in this case, the wild-type control laboratory virus requires 0.5 μM concentration of zidovudine compared to the patient's virus, which requires 5 μM concentration, to inhibit 50% of the replication of HIV in cell culture. Compared with a genotype test, a phenotype test is considered to be a more direct measure of resistance (or, more accurately, of reduced viral susceptibility to a given drug); thus the results may be easier to interpret by clinicians familiar with antimicrobial susceptibility testing for other nonviral pathogens. However, phenotypic assays are more expensive than genotypic assays, have a slower turnaround time to a result, and are available commercially through only a small number of centralized reference laboratories worldwide. Furthermore, the IC_{50} values, or "cutpoints," that define resistance phenotypically have been based on the technical

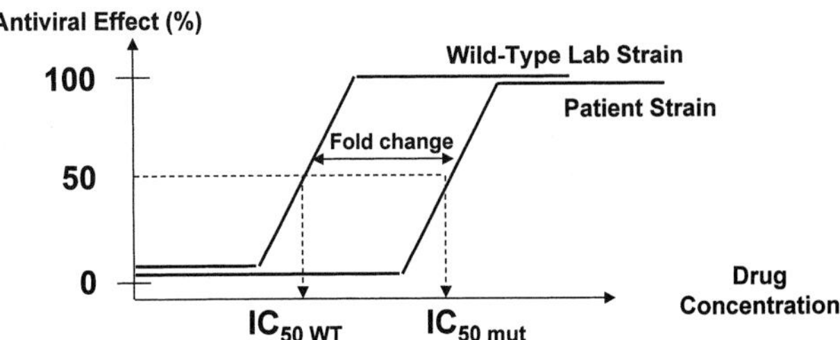

Figure 26–2. Resistance (phenotype) definitions. IC_{50}, 50% inhibitory concentration; IC_{50} mut/$IC_{50\ WT}$, fold change (e.g., $IC_{50\ mu}$ 5 μM/$IC_{50\ WT}$ 0.5 μM is a 10-fold change).

variability of the assay or, more recently, the biologic variability of wild-type strains. The clinical cutpoints, which define when a particular agent has reduced activity in vivo, have yet to be defined for most available antiretroviral agents (discussed later). Moreover, the reliability of phenotype testing has been subject to only one survey that compared results from two major reference laboratories and concluded that the results were similar; that study was limited in that primarily drug-susceptible viruses were tested.[19]

At this point it is not clear whether the genotype or phenotype test for drug susceptibility is better for patient management or under what circumstances one test would be superior to the other. The selection of one over the other depends on specific factors, such as access, cost, turnaround time, and the availability of expert interpretation. It is thought that in certain situations (e.g., highly experienced patients with complex resistance patterns) employing both phenotype and genotype tests may provide the best information for crafting a rescue regimen. However, currently there are no data to support this idea.

▲ EVIDENCE FOR RESISTANCE TESTING FROM CLINICAL TRIALS: SELECTIVE REVIEW

The clinical trial data underlying the new recommendations for resistance testing have accumulated rapidly during the past few years. To date, numerous retrospective studies and a growing number of randomized, controlled prospective trials have demonstrated the clinical utility of resistance testing. In this section we highlight some of the most important evidence prior to presenting current guidelines based on these data and on expert opinions.

Retrospective analyses of monotherapy studies first indicated that resistance was associated with more rapid progression during antiretroviral therapy, including some studies that controlled for other prognostic factors in addition to results of either genotypic or phenotypic tests.[20,21] The prognostic value of genotypic resistance testing was also illustrated in a retrospective analysis of a clinical cohort of protease inhibitor (PI)-experienced patients who received saquinavir/ritonavir dual PI-based therapy.[22] Response to saquinavir/ritonavir combination therapy was best predicted by protease-resistance mutations as determined by a baseline genotype. The resistance profile explained nearly two-thirds of the variation in virologic outcomes at 12 weeks compared with an explained variance (R^2) of less than 50% based on standard clinical parameters alone. In multivariate models, the resistance predictors were found to be independent of clinical parameters. This study illustrated that genotypic resistance information provided prognostic information about a patient's response to dual PI therapy that could not be obtained through standard clinical assessment, including antiretroviral treatment history, baseline CD4+ T-lymphocyte counts, viral load, and clinical status.

The long-term prognostic value of phenotypic resistance testing was demonstrated in a retrospective analysis of treatment-experienced patients.[23] In this clinical cohort study, the baseline phenotype provided prognostic information on virologic response at 1 year and beyond. The prognostic value of the phenotype was not limited to a particular salvage regimen and was shown to be independent of other clinical and antiretroviral drug history variables. Virologic response was predicted by the number of drugs to which the patient's isolate was sensitive at baseline, and the phenotype was better able to discriminate in vitro drug susceptibility than was the patient's antiretroviral drug history.

There have been dozens of retrospective analyses that demonstrate the prognostic value of genotype and phenotype information in experienced patients switching to new antiretroviral regimens. These studies have been conducted in a wide variety of patient groups and with many treatment regimens. The Resistance Collaborative Group used a standardized methodology and has summarized many of the early retrospective trials.[24] The uniform finding of this review was that resistance tests, whether genotypic or phenotypic, provided prognostic information independent of other known prognostic factors, such as baseline viral load or receipt of a drug from a new antiretroviral class. Based on these and many other studies, it is now clear that resistance testing has important prognostic value that cannot be obtained by standard clinical assessment alone.

Although retrospective studies demonstrate the prognostic value of resistance testing, it does not prove that resistance testing can improve outcomes when applied prospectively. In addition to retrospective studies, there are now reports from eight prospective, randomized, controlled trials of resistance testing that delineate the effect of resistance testing on the virologic response (Table 26–1). Some,[25–30] but not all, of these studies demonstrated a benefit in terms of virologic outcome: Patients whose therapy changes were guided by resistance testing had better viral load responses than patients receiving usual care without testing. Follow-up in the GART and VIRA3001 studies was only 12 to 16 weeks; however, in the VIRADAPT study a persistent benefit was seen through 24 weeks and, in an open-label phase, through 48 weeks.

In the HAVANA study, 326 heavily pretreated patients on failing antiretroviral therapy were randomized to one of four groups: genotyping with expert advice, genotyping without expert advice, no genotypic testing with expert advice, and no genotypic testing without advice (standard of care).[29] In an intent-to-treat analysis, the group with both genotyping and advice had the best results: 69% achieved HIV viral loads of less than 400 copies per milliliter at week 24, compared with 47% of patients with expert advice, 49% of patients with genotypic testing, and 36% for those in the standard-of-care group. Interestingly, the differences in outcomes seemed to be driven by the most heavily pretreated patients. This study is an important step forward in our understanding of the relative effects of resistance testing and expert advice. In earlier prospective trials, such as the GART study,[25] it was not clear how much of the benefit in virologic response was due to the benefit of the resistance test and how much was due to the expert advice given with the test results. It appears from the HAVANA study that expert advice and genotype tests provide independent, additive benefits for antiretroviral management of treatment-experienced patients.

▲ **Table 26–1.** PROSPECTIVE STUDIES OF HIV-1 RESISTANCE TESTING

Study	Design	Duration (weeks)	No. of Patients	First PI Failure (%)	Change in VL (log_{10} copies/ml)	Percent of patients with VL < 400 copies/ml
VIRADAPT[12]	GT vs. SOC	12	108	~40	−1.04 vs. −0.46[a]	29% vs. 14%[b]
		24		−1.15 vs. −0.67	32% vs. 14%[b]	
GART[11]	GT vs. SOC[c]	48	153	~50	−1.19 vs. −0.61[a]	34% vs. 22%
		24			−0.94 vs. −0.47	
VIRA3001[13]	PT vs. SOC	16	274	100	−1.23 vs. −0.87	45% vs. 34%
Kaiser[17]	PT vs. SC	16	40	25	−0.25 vs. −0.4	N/A
NARVAL[18]	GT vs. PT vs. SOC[c]	12	541	<30	−1.1 vs. −1.0 vs. −0.7	44% vs. 35% vs. 36%[b]
ARGENTA[15]	GT vs. SOC	12	174	~50	N/A	27% vs. 12% 21%
		24				vs. 17% (P = ns)
HAVANA[14]	GT vs. SOC	12	274	23	−1.3 vs. −1.1	66% vs. 53%
		24			−1.1 vs. −0.8	57% vs. 42%
CCTG575[16]	PT vs. SOC	24	256	~80	−0.71 vs. −0.69	48% vs. 48%[d]
		48			(P = NS)	46% vs. 46%[d]

GT, genotype; NS, not significant; PI, protease inhibitor; PT, phenotype; SOC, standard of care; VL, viral load.
[a]Adapted from Demeter 2000. (8th Retrovirus Conference)
[b]Limit of detection: 200 copies/ml.
[c]Resistance-test results included expert interpretation.
[d]Limit of detection: 500 copies/ml.
From Rice HL, Zolopa AR. HIV drug resistance testing: an update for the clinician. AIDS Clin Care 13:89, 2001.

In another randomized, prospective trial, ARGENTA, genotypic testing was compared with standard-of-care treatment in 174 heavily pretreated patients.[30] Adherence was assessed by patient self-reporting. In an intent-to-treat analysis at 3 months, 27% of the patients who underwent genotypic testing had viral loads of less than 500 copies per milliliter compared with 12% of patients who were randomized to no testing (standard of care) ($P = 0.02$). At 6 months, however, the difference was no longer statistically significant (17% vs. 21%, respectively). Not surprisingly, patient adherence strongly influenced the longer-term virologic responses. This study illustrates the important fact that resistance testing can help provide an antiretroviral regimen with more virologic activity as measured by initial response, but long-term success is still primarily determined by patient adherence to the regimen.

Not all prospective trials of resistance testing have demonstrated an improvement in virologic outcomes. In the California Collaborative Treatment Group study 575 (CCTG 575), 256 PI-experienced patients who had experienced treatment failure [80% had experienced first PI failure, and 76% were nonnucleoside reverse transcriptase inhibitor (NNRTI)-naive] were randomized to undergo phenotypic testing or no testing (standard of care).[31] The investigators found no significant differences in virologic response between the groups in terms of change in viral load from baseline or in the proportion of patients with viral loads of less than 400 copies per milliliter (or 50 copies per milliliter) measured at 6 months and 12 months. For example, at 6 months, 48% had less than 400 copies per milliliter in both the phenotype testing group and the standard-of-care group. In a post hoc subgroup analysis of patients with high degrees of baseline resistance (i.e., those with resistance to three or more PIs), the proportion of patients who achieved viral loads of less than 400 copies per milliliter at 6 months was significantly higher in the phenotype-testing group (50% vs. 17%; $P = 0.02$). One reason for the "negative results" in this trial overall was that the virologic response in the standard-of-care group, including subjects with any degree of resistance, was surprisingly good. This likely reflects at least two factors. First, most of the patients in this trial entered when failing a nelfinavir-based first regimen. In other studies investigators have shown that nelfinavir-selected, nelfinavir-resistant viruses almost always lack cross resistance to other PIs and that salvage therapy following nelfinavir failure tends to be relatively successful in achieving a good virologic response even without a resistance test.[32,33] This is relatively unique for nelfinavir versus other drugs. Moreover, the results of CCTG 575 reflect the fact that practitioners who routinely employ resistance tests in the management of their patients begin to learn what patterns of resistance are likely for a particular history of antiretroviral treatments.

A smaller trial from the Kaiser group[34] and the NARVAL trial[35] also showed no benefit from resistance assays in terms of initial viral load response. However, these studies were characterized by a much more heavily pretreated population who had limited new drug options. Resistance testing may, however, have other benefits in heavily pretreated patients. For example, eliminating drugs that are unlikely to be beneficial limits unnecessary drug exposure, toxicity, and expense. In the NARVAL study, patients in the standard-of-care arm received new drugs and triple-class therapy in their new regimens at twice the rate of patients who underwent resistance tests. Despite this difference, the levels of virologic suppression in response to salvage therapy were similar across the arms of the study. This pattern of antiretroviral use suggests that resistance testing may allow the clinician the ability to be more selective and more effective at recycling antiretroviral agents to better preserve treatment options over the long term.

▲ INTERPRETATION OF RESISTANCE TEST RESULTS

The complexity of genotype results at times leaves even experienced clinicians confused. This complexity results from the large number of mutations associated with drug resistance, variable cross resistance, and difficulty of predicting mutational interactions. In most cases, clinicians rely on the interpretation that comes as part of the genotype report rather than trying to directly interpret the list of mutational changes themselves. Results from the HAVANA trial demonstrate the importance of expert interpretation in genotype testing; however, a consultation with an expert is not always practical. For phenotypic assays, interpretation is a matter of defining the values that indicate when a virus is resistant, the so-called cutpoints, as discussed below. For genotypic assays, there are three possible methods or systems of interpretation currently available: expert advice, "rules-based" algorithms, and "virtual phenotyping."

Genotypic Test Interpretation

Expert advice is the best tested interpretation method. An expert may not be readily available, however, and there is still variation in the interpretation of genotypes between experts. In a European study Schmidt and colleagues[36] showed that frequently there were differences of opinion among a panel of experts interpreting genotypes. In a similar study, Call and colleagues[37] found better levels of agreement among a small panel of experts at a single institution. Overall, it appears that experts in the field are rapidly coming to a general consensus on genotype results. Efforts to develop, update, and disseminate such a consensus via the worldwide web are ongoing (http://www.iasusa.org, accessed March 8, 2002).

A rules-based algorithm is an interpretative system that can be computerized. These computer-generated interpretations are given has part of the genotype report in a standardized fashion. However, it should be noted that the "rules" that make up the algorithms are derived from expert panels according to current knowledge, and therefore these algorithms require regular updating. Some of these algorithms are publicly available (e.g., http://hivdb.stanford.edu/hiv/, accessed March 8, 2002), and others are proprietary (e.g., Visible Genetics GuideLines, rules that are part of the kit recently approved by the FDA). Discrepancies have been found among these still-evolving systems in preliminary reports of a few comparison studies.[38]

Another approach to interpreting complex genotype information uses relational genotype-phenotype databases. One proprietary example of such an approach to interpretation is available commercially (the so-called virtual phenotype). In this system the patient's genotype is matched with similar genotypes in the database that have previously determined matching phenotypes. The interpretive report includes a probabilistic estimate of a phenotype based on genotypes that match the patient's isolate at the important drug-resistant codons. It is important to note that the matches are not to a complete protease and RT sequence but only to important mutations associated with resistance for each drug as determined, again, by experts. The clinical role of such an interpretation scheme has not yet been fully validated, and studies are ongoing. One potential advantage of this approach may be to provide better quantification of the magnitude of resistance.

Phenotypic Test Interpretation

The interpretation of phenotype test results appears to be more straightforward than that of genotype test results. There is also an advantage in the direct report of the magnitude of resistance inherent in an IC_{50} that is often used by clinicians to help identify drugs to which the patient's virus is less resistant when no drugs remain to which the virus is susceptible. However, interpretation is still essential for phenotype test results. The level of reduced susceptibility, the so-called cutpoint, for a given antiretroviral drug is still being determined for most of the drugs used in practice. The criterion for such a cutpoint is also changing. Recently, commercial phenotype reports have moved from using cutpoints defined by the technical aspects of the assay (reproducibility) to cutpoints defined by the variation seen in wild-type virus. These "biologic cutpoints" are derived by testing many clinical isolates from drug-naive subjects, then using the resulting distribution of phenotypes to define the normal variation as the basis for defining the "normal range" (median value plus 2 SD) of drug susceptibility. This move has led to different cutpoints for different drugs. From the clinician's point of view, however, it is more desirable if the "cutpoints" could distinguish a virus that would respond to a given drug from a virus that would not respond—a "clinical cutpoint." For example, having phenotypic cutpoints defined as "fully active," "partially active," or "not active" for each of the antiretroviral drugs would likely be the most useful values for the clinician, as recycling partially active drugs in treatment regimens of experienced patients is often the only option. To date, however, clinical cutpoints have been only tentatively defined for a small number of the available drugs.[38,39]

▲ GUIDELINES FOR RESISTANCE TESTING: WHO SHOULD BE TESTED?

The role of resistance testing in clinical practice is still evolving. Guidelines for the use of resistance testing have been updated by expert panels and will continue to evolve with our knowledge base. The International AIDS Society—USA,[40] the U.S. Department of Health and Human Services, with the Henry J. Kaiser Family Foundation (http://www.hivatis.org., April 23, 2001), and the EuroGuidelines Group for HIV Resistance[41] have all recently issued guidelines, which are summarized in Table 26–2. These guidelines currently recommend resistance testing in certain clinical situations. It is important to keep in mind that resistance test results do not stand alone. The clinician is strongly encouraged to place the results of resistance tests into the broader clinical context of the patient, including the patient's antiretroviral history, CD4+ T-lymphocyte count, and viral load longitudinal profiles, clinical status, significant prior drug toxicities, and adherence behavior (Fig. 26–3).

Acute and Recent Infection

All of the guidelines suggest that the provider at least consider resistance testing, and the EuroGuidelines recommend testing for patients who present with acute infection in whom antiretroviral therapy is being initiated. The rationale for resistance testing in this setting is to treat a drug-resistant virus, if present, appropriately to maximize preservation of HIV-specific immune responses. However, therapy in this situation should not be delayed while waiting for test results, as it can be modified quickly after drug initiation if necessary. The decision to test should depend on the local risk of drug-resistance transmission, the specific likelihood of transmission from

▲ **Table 26–2.** SUMMARY OF EXPERT PANEL RECOMMENDATIONS FOR RESISTANCE TESTING

Clinical Setting	IAS-USA	DHHS	EuroGuidelines
Primary/recent HIV infection	Consider	Consider	Recommended if (1) treatment to be initiated; (2) high local transmission rate of resistance; (3) transmission suspected from a treated individual Consider in other situations (or store specimen)
Chronic HIV infection	Consider	Generally not recommended	Consider, or store specimen
First regimen failure	Recommended	Recommended	Recommended
Multiple regimen failure	Recommended	Recommended	Recommended
Pregnancy	Recommended	Recommended	Recommended

From Rice HL, Zolopa AR. HIV drug resistance testing: an update for the clinician. AIDS Clin Care 13:89, 2001.

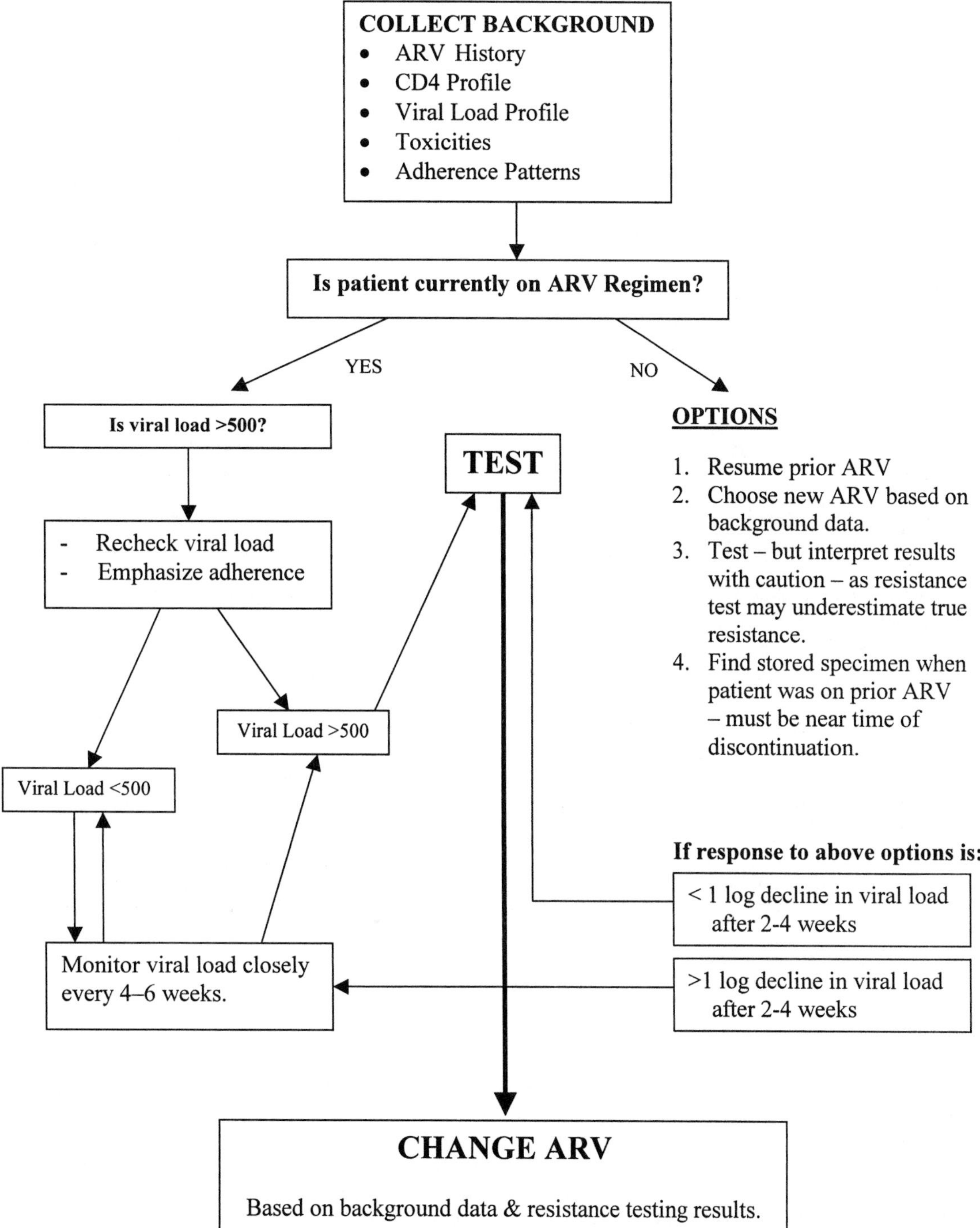

Figure 26–3. Optimal use of resistance testing in antiretroviral (ARV)-experienced patients.

a treated individual in whom resistance is known or suspected, and test availability and cost considerations. The exact distinction between an acute infection and recent infection is not well established, but preservation of anti-HIV immune responses has been demonstrated only in subjects treated effectively at presentation with symptomatic primary infection within a few weeks of putative acquisition.[42]

Chronic Infection

In the absence of a history of known exposure or symptomatic primary infection, the duration of HIV infection prior to initial presentation is difficult to date. Most newly presenting, drug-naive patients therefore are said to have chronic or established infection of indeterminate duration. Current recommendations call for resistance testing to be considered as an option in this setting,[40] again based on the same factors discussed for acute infection. Resistance testing has not been recommended more strongly in antiretroviral-naive patients who have such chronic infection[40] because of a concern that tests will most likely be negative for two reasons. First, until recently it seemed likely that the prevalence of resistance would be low among those infected in the past. Second, without the selective pressure of antiretroviral therapy resistant mutants that may have been transmitted would be expected to become "minority subpopulations." Wild-type HIV-1 should predominate in the virus population over time off-drug. Wild-type virus has been observed to outgrow resistant mutants at a variable rate when drugs are stopped in treatment-experienced patients. However, resistant virus may remain archived in long-lived cells, only to reemerge later if drug selection pressure returns. Detection of a small percentage (< 20%) of resistant virus, expected to be common if drugs were not started for a prolonged period (> 1 year) after the initial infection, may not be possible with the current genotypic or phenotypic assays; thus there may be a high pretest probability of a false-negative result.

Studies have cast some new light on these issues. There may be a temporal trend of increasing prevalence of newly acquired resistant virus over time. There has been a preliminary report of an increasing prevalence of resistance in newly infected patients from nine North American cities from 1995 to 2000.[43] For patients enrolled from 1995 to 1998, the overall prevalence of resistance (measured by phenotype with a >10-fold change in IC_{50}) was 3.8%, compared with 14.0% in the group enrolled between 1999 and 2000. Most concerning is that 6% of newly infected patients enrolled between 1999 and 2000 had multidrug-resistant virus (i.e., resistance to two or more antiretroviral classes). The second assumption, that resistant virus would be present only as undetectable subpopulations, has been questioned by other preliminary reports. A Boston cohort of 88 consecutive, chronically infected, antiretroviral-naive patients who presented for initial antiretroviral treatment in 1999 identified at least one mutation associated with drug resistance in 18% using a commercially available genotype test kit.[44] All those with resistance were documented by laboratory testing to have been infected for more than about 6 months.[44] This suggests that resistant mutants may persist off-drug longer than expected after the initial infection; either relatively fit transmitted mutants or lack of a competing wild-type virus can be hypothesized. Another report documented persistence of mutations acquired at initial infection in several subjects.[45] Although the detection of mutations in chronically infected, drug-naive subjects may underestimate the prevalence of resistance, it may be high enough to consider a screening resistance test as a cost-effective strategy.[46] Another study of drug-resistance patterns in more than 700 antiretroviral-naive subjects from 10 U.S. cities between 1997 and 2000 identified nearly 8% with a least one major drug-resistance mutation.[47] Interestingly, no difference was detected in that study in terms of the prevalence of drug-resistant mutations in recently infected patients compared with those who were chronically infected.[47] A large-scale population survey also reported a high prevalence of drug-resistant virus among patients who denied prior antiretroviral drug exposure.[48] There are not yet adequate data to document that drug-naive patients with resistant virus have better virologic outcomes with resistance test-guided drug choices.

Treatment Failure

All three guidelines recommend resistance testing for patients on antiretroviral therapy who are experiencing suboptimal viral suppression (i.e., detectable viremia) (Table 26–2; Fig. 26–3). Ideally, the plasma specimen for resistance testing should be obtained while the patient is still on the failing regimen, so selection pressure is maintained; as little as 2 weeks off-drug allows some mutants to escape detection.[49] All tests currently require that the plasma viral load be higher than 500 to 1000 copies per milliliter at the time of testing. In general, results are likely to be most reliable for agents in the patient's current regimen; however, resistance that developed from prior antiretroviral regimens is likely to be maintained and detectable if some selection pressure remains. It is important to note that resistance testing is recommended for all patients experiencing antiretroviral (ARV) failure when changing the ARV regimen is being considered. The goals and outcomes of resistance testing, however, are different for patients on their first failing ARV drug compared to those who have experienced multiregimen failure. With virologic failure of the first regimen, documentation of drugs to which the patient's virus is resistant at this stage may prove to be useful when choosing later salvage regimens, at which time recycling antiretroviral drugs not used for a prolonged duration may be considered. Randomized controlled trials have demonstrated that resistance testing in the setting of the first regimen failure can improve outcomes, with more likelihood of achieving a complete virologic response to the second regimen. In some cases, virologic failure (particularly early failure) can result from the development of resistance to only one or some of the drugs in the treatment regimen. Knowing which drugs in the failing regimen remain active could theoretically allow the clinician to later "recycle" the other drugs in an effort to preserve treatment options for the long term. The concept of switching only a single drug to which the virus is resistant has not been tested in clinical trials, although some clinicians do consider it in some settings.

The usefulness of resistance testing is likely to be different with multiple-regimen failure than with first-regimen failure. In the setting of multiple-regimen failure, resistance testing should help optimize the number of at least partially active drugs in the new regimen while avoiding the potential toxicity, inconvenience, and cost of drugs that are not likely to be even partially active. Although finding a new regimen that provides complete virologic control is unlikely in patients who have experienced multiple regimen failure, limiting the toxicities and side effects from drugs not likely to add to the virologic activity of the regimen is an important clinical goal.

Pregnancy and Postexposure Prophylaxis

The IAS-USA and EuroGuidelines explicitly recommend the use of resistance testing in pregnant women with detectable viral loads to optimize therapy for the mother and reduce the risk of perinatal transmission. Postexposure prophylaxis regimens may also be optimized through resistance testing if a sample from the source patient is available, although initiation of prophylaxis obviously should not be delayed while awaiting results.

▲ CONCLUSIONS AND PROMISING NEW DIRECTIONS

Drug resistance testing has rapidly been adopted for antiretroviral management. Despite the relative expense of resistance tests, studies suggest that testing is cost-effective in certain situations.[26,46] Both genotype and phenotype tests have been shown to improve virologic outcome of a rescue regimen, at least in the short term. Interpretations of genotypic tests are improving but require further validation. Phenotype testing is most likely to be useful when clinical cutpoints have been defined for all drugs used in practice. Measures of the replication capacity phenotype may be useful in some settings in the future. Situations in which testing is recommended may expand, particularly if recent preliminary data from drug-naive patients with chronic infection are confirmed. However, new directions of research are likely to be important when used in combination with resistance testing to fulfill the promise of individualized drug failure management by determining the degree of drug exposure and of virus resistance.

There are various degrees of reduced susceptibility, and in some cases "boosting" the plasma concentrations of a PI through addition of low-dose ritonavir can overcome some degree of resistance. Hence a prognostic tool that incorporates drug levels and a measure of HIV resistance may allow practitioners to better craft antiretroviral regimens. Data from the VIRADAPT trial and others suggest that adequate drug levels and resistance testing improve outcomes.[50] The inhibitory quotient (IQ) refers to a value that includes information about a drug's actual concentration at the trough of the dosing interval (i.e., plasma C_{MIN}) divided by a measure of the pathogen's susceptibility to that drug (i.e., IC_{50} or IC_{90}). Theoretically, the IQ should be a better predictor of virologic response because, for most drugs, the level of viral resistance is relative to the drug concentration. Preliminary data support the use of IQ and virtual IQ for ritonavir-boosted PI regimens, although more clinical validation is required. In a study of indinavir-experienced patients who underwent boosting with ritonavir, Kempf and colleagues demonstrated that the virtual IQ better discriminated virologic response over 48 weeks than measuring only virus resistance. Current challenges to this approach include the availability and standardization of therapeutic drug monitoring. Virus exposure to ARV drugs may also be limited by cellular proteins that efflux ARV drugs out of cells (e.g., P-glycoprotein and other proteins in the ATP-binding cassettetransporter family). Research on the detection of individual differences during such processes is at an even earlier stage. The future does hold the prospect of continued improvement in ARV drug management based on better understanding and detection of the biologic mechanisms of drug failure.

REFERENCES

1. Deeks SG, Hecht F, Swanson M, et al. HIV RNA and CD4 cell count response to protease inhibitor therapy in an urban AIDS clinic: response to both initial and salvage therapy. AIDS 13:F35, 1999.
2. Ledergerber B, Egger M, Opravil M, et al. Clinical progression and virological failure on highly active antiretroviral therapy in HIV-1 patients: a prospective cohort study: Swiss HIV Cohort Study. Lancet 353:863, 1999.
3. Lucas GM, Chaisson RE, Moore RD. Highly active antiretroviral therapy in a large urban clinic: risk factors for virologic failure and adverse drug reactions. Ann Intern Med 131:81, 1999.
4. Mansky LM, Temin HM. Lower in vivo mutation rate of human immunodeficiency virus type 1 than that predicted from the fidelity of purified reverse transcriptase. J Virol 69:5087, 1995.
5. Wei X, Ghosh SK, Taylor ME, et al. Viral dynamics in human immunodeficiency virus type 1 infection. Nature 373:117, 1995.
6. Ho DD, Neumann AU, Perelson AS, et al. Rapid turnover of plasma virions and CD4 lymphocytes in HIV-1 infection. Nature 373:123, 1995.
7. Hanna GJ, D'Aquila RT. Antiretroviral drug resistance in HIV-1. Curr Infect Dis Rep 1:289, 1999.
8. Drug Resistance Mutations Group. Update on drug resistance mutations in HIV-1. Top HIV Med 9(6):21, 2001.
9. Schuurman R, Brambilla D, de Groot T, et al. Underestimation of HIV type 1 drug resistance mutations: results from the ENVA-2 genotyping proficiency program. AIDS Res Hum Retroviruses 18:243, 2002.
10. Shafer RW, Hertogs K, Zolopa AR, et al. High degree of interlaboratory reproducibility of human immunodeficiency virus type 1 protease and reverse transcriptase sequencing of plasma samples from heavily treated patients. J Clin Microbiol 39:1522, 2001.
11. Larder BA, Kemp SD. Multiple mutations in HIV-1 reverse transcriptase confer high-level resistance to zidovudine (AZT). Science 246:1155, 1989.
12. Caliendo AM, Savara A, An D, et al. Effects of zidovudine-selected human immunodeficiency virus type 1 reverse transcriptase amino acid substitutions on processive DNA synthesis and viral replication. J Virol 70:2146, 1996.
13. Arion D, Kaushik N, McCormick S, et al. Phenotypic mechanism of HIV-1 resistance to 3′-azido-3′-deoxythymidine (AZT): increased polymerization processivity and enhanced sensitivity to pyrophosphate of the mutant viral reverse transcriptase. Biochemistry 37:15908, 1998.
14. Meyer PR, Matsuura S, Moshin Mian A, et al. A mechanism of AZT resistance: an increase in nucleotide-dependent primer unblocking by mutant HIV-1 reverse transcriptase. Mol Cell 4:35, 1999.
15. Coffin JM. HIV population dynamics in vivo: implications for genetic variation, pathogenesis, and therapy. Science 267:483, 1995.
16. Martinez-Picado J, Savara AV, Sutton L, D'Aquila RT. Replicative fitness of protease inhibitor-resistant mutants of human immunodeficiency virus type 1. J Virol 73:3744, 1999.
17. Mammano F, Trouplin V, Zennou V, Clavel F. Retracing the evolutionary pathways of human immunodeficiency virus type 1 resistance to protease inhibitors: virus fitness in the absence and in the presence of drug. J Virol 74:8524, 2000.
18. Deeks SG, Wrin T, Hoh R, et al. Virologic and immunologic consequences of discontinuing combination antiretroviral-drug therapy in HIV-infected patients with detectable viremia. N Engl J Med 344:472, 2001.
19. Qari SH, Respress R, Weinstock H, et al. Comparative analysis of two commercial phenotypic assays for drug susceptibility testing of human immunodeficiency virus type 1. J Clin Microbiol 40:31, 2002.
20. D'Aquila RT, Johnson V, Welles S, et al. Zidovudine resistance and human immunodeficiency virus type 1 disease progression during antiretroviral therapy. Ann Intern Med 122:401, 1995.
21. Japour AJ, Welles S, D'Aquila RT, et al. Prevalence and clinical significance of zidovudine resistance mutations in human immunodeficiency virus isolated from patients following long-term zidovudine treatment. J Infect Dis 171:1172, 1995.

22. Zolopa AR, Warford A, Montoya JG, et al. HIV-1 genotypic resistance patterns predict response to saquinavir-ritonavir therapy in patients in whom previous previous protease inhibitor therapy had failed. Ann Intern Med 131:813, 1999.
23. Call SA, Saag M, Westfall A, et al. Phenotypic drug susceptibility testing predicts long-term virologic suppression better than treatment history in patients with human immunodeficiency virus infection. J Infect Dis 183:401, 2001.
24. DeGruttola V, Dix V, D'Aguila R, et al. The relation between baseline HIV drug resistance and response to antiretroviral therapy: re-analysis of retrospective and prospective studies using a standardized data analysis plan. Antivir Ther 5:41, 2000.
25. Baxter JD, Meyers DL, Wentworth DN, et al. A randomized study of antiretroviral management based on plasma genotypic antiretroviral resistance testing in patients failing therapy: CPCRA 046 Study Team for the Terry Beirn Community Programs for Clinical Research on AIDS. AIDS 14:F83, 2000.
26. Durant J, Clevenberg P, Halfon P, et al. Drug-resistance genotyping in HIV-1 therapy: the VIRADAPT randomised controlled trial. Lancet 353:2195, 1999.
27. Clevenbergh P, Durant J, Halfon P, et al. Persisting long-term benefit of genotype-guided treatment for HIV-infected patients failing HAART; the Viradapt Study: week 48 follow-up. Antivir Ther 5:65, 2000.
28. Cohen C, Hunt S, Sension M, et al. Phenotypic resistance testing significantly improves response to therapy: final analysis of a randomized trial (VIRA3001). Antivir Ther 5(suppl 3): abstract 84, 2000.
29. Tural C, Ruiz L, Holtzer C, et al. Clinical utility of HIV-1 genotyping and expert advice: the Havana Trial. AIDS 16:209, 2002.
30. De Luca A, Antinori A, Cingolani A, et al. A prospective, randomized study on the usefulness of genotypic resistance testing and the assessment of patient-reported adherence in unselected patients failing potent HIV therapy (ARGENTA): final 6-month results. In: 8th Conference on Retroviruses and Opportunistic Infections, Chicago, 2001.
31. Haubrich R, Keiser P, Kemper C, et al. CCTG575: a randomized, prospective study of phenotype testing versus standard of care for patients failing antiretroviral therapy. In: 1st IAS Conference on HIV Pathogenesis and Treatment. Buenos Aires, 2001.
32. Tebas P, Patick AK, Kane EM, et al. Virologic responses to a ritonavir-saquinavir-containing regimen in patients who had previously failed nelfinavir. AIDS 13:F23, 1999.
33. Zolopa A, Tebas P, Gallant J, et al. The efficacy of ritonavir (RTV)/saquinavir (SQV) antiretroviral therapy (ART) in patients who failed nelfinavir (NFV): a multi-center clinical cohort study. Presented at the 39th Interscience Conference on Antimicrobial Agents and Chemotherapy: 1999, San Francisco, abstract 2065.
34. Melnick D, Rosenthal J, Cameron M, et al. Impact of phenotypic antiretroviral drug resistance testing on the response to salvage antiretroviral therapy in heavily experienced patients. In: 7th Conference on Retroviruses and Opportunistic Infections, San Francisco, 2000.
35. Meynard J, Vray M, Morand-Joubert L, et al. Impact of treatment guided by phenotypic or genotypic resistance tests on the response to antiretroviral therapy: a randomized trial (NARVAL, ANRS 088). Antivir Ther 5(suppl 3):67, 2000.
36. Schmidt JC, Robert I, Fontaine E, et al. Inter-person variable in interpreting sequencing results for HIV-1 resistance testing. Antivir Ther 5(suppl 3), 2000.
37. Call S, Johnson VA, Westfall AO, et al. Degree of agreement among interpretations of genotypic resistance testing results in a cohort of ART-experienced individuals. In: 40th Interscience Conference on Antimicrobial Agents and Chemotherapy, Toronto, 2000.
38. Lanier E, Hellmann N, Scott J, et al. Determination of a clinically relevant phenotypic resistance "cutoff" for abacavir using the PhenoSense Assay. In: 8th Conference on Retroviruses and Opportunistic Infections, Chicago, 2001.
39. Kempf D, Hsu A, Jiang P, et al. Identification of clinically relevant phenotypic and genotypic breakpoints for ABT-378/r in multiple PI-experienced, NNRTI naive patients. Antivir Ther 5(suppl 3):70, 2001, abstract 89.
40. Hirsch MS, Brun-Vézinet F, D'Aquilia RT, et al. Antiretroviral drug resistance testing in adult HIV-1 infection: recommendations of an international AIDS society—USA panel. JAMA 283:2417, 2000.
41. Miller V, Vandamme AM, Loveday C, et al. Clinical and laboratory guidelines for the use of HIV-1 drug resistance testing as part of treatment management: recommendations for the European setting. AIDS 15:309, 2001.
42. Rosenberg ES, Altfeld M, Poon S, et al. Immune control of HIV-1 after early treatment of acute infection. Nature 407:523, 2000.
43. Little S, Holte S, Routy JP, et al. Antiretroviral resistance and response to initial therapy among recently HIV-infected subjects in North America. Antivir Ther 6(suppl 1):21, 2001, abstract 25.
44. Hanna G, Balaguera H, Steger K, et al. Drug-selected and non-clade B pol genotypes in chronically HIV-1-infected antiretroviral-naive adults in Boston. In: 8th Conference on Retroviruses and Opportunistic Infection, Chicago, 2001.
45. Little SJ, Daar ES, Holte S, et al. Persistence of transmitted drug resistance among subjects with primary HIV infection not receiving antiretroviral therapy. In: 9th Conference on Human Retroviruses and Opportunistic Infections, Seattle, 2002.
46. Weinstein MC, Goldie S, Losina E, et al. Use of genotypic resistance testing to guide hiv therapy: clinical impact and cost-effectiveness. Ann Intern Med 134:440, 2001.
47. Zaidi I, Weinstock T, Woods J, et al. Prevalence of mutations associated with antiretroviral drug resistance among HIV-1-infected persons in 10 US cities, 1997–2000. Antivir Ther 6(suppl 1):118, 2001, abstract 155.
48. Richman DD. The prevalence of antiretorivral drug resistance in the US. Presented at the 41st Interscience Conference on Amtimicrobial Agents and Chemotherapy, Chicago, 2001, abstract LB-17.
49. Devereux HL, Youle M, Johnson M, et al. Rapid decline in detectability of HIV-1 drug resistance mutations after stopping therapy. AIDS 13:F123, 1999.
50. Durant J, Glevenbergh P, Garraffo R, et al. Importance of protease inhibitor plasma levels in HIV-infected patients treated with genotypic-guided therapy: pharmacological data from the Viradapt Study. AIDS 14:1333, 2000.

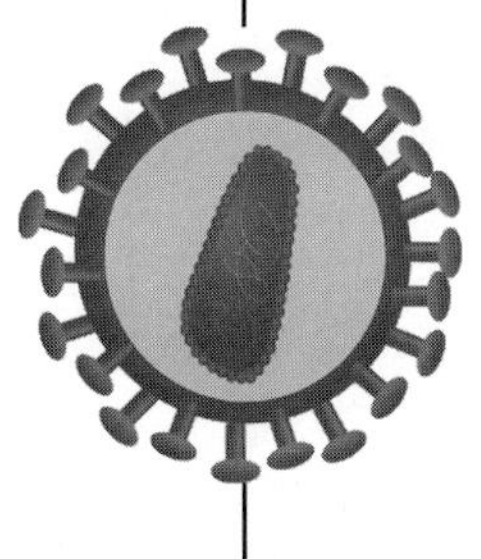

CHAPTER 27

Strategic Use of Antiretroviral Therapy

Michael S. Saag, MD

Advances in the understanding of human immunodeficiency virus (HIV) pathogenesis, the use of viral load in clinical practice, and the availability of 16 Food and Drug Administration (FDA)-approved antiretroviral agents have led to a revolution in the care of HIV-infected patients.[1–5] Persistent, high-level viral replication is now established as the driving force of HIV pathogenesis, with up to 10 billion virions produced in an infected individual each day.[6–9] Viral load measurements, as determined by either signal amplification (branched-chain DNA) or nucleic acid amplification [reverse transcription-polymerase chain reaction, (RT-PCR) or nucleic acid sequence-based assay (NASBA)] techniques enable the clinician to determine the degree to which an antiretroviral therapeutic regimen is working and, more importantly, when the regimen is failing.[10–14] This allows therapy to be switched at the time of antiretroviral failure rather than at the time of clinical failure. Once a regimen begins to fail, clinicians can choose from dozens of potential alternative regimens, utilizing both existing approved drugs and experimental therapeutic agents. The ability to choose the most effective next regimen has been greatly enhanced by resistance testing technologies.[15] Taken together, clinicians have the potential to achieve long-term clinical benefits by keeping the viral load as low as possible for as long as possible.

Through the appropriate use of antiretroviral therapies, a striking reduction in HIV-associated mortality has been demonstrated over the last several years.[16–18] Despite these advances, newly recognized toxicities of antiretroviral treatment have begun to limit the long-term benefits of chronic therapy.[19–24] Moreover, the durability of the antiretroviral effect is quite variable. Many factors influence the ability to sustain suppression of viral replication, including pharmacokinetic properties of the regimen, tissue penetration, cellular penetration, appropriate intracellular processing, antiretroviral drug history, tolerability of the regimen, adherence, potency of the regimen, and the development of resistance.[15,25–31] To achieve the most durable effect of antiretroviral therapy, clinicians must develop a strategic approach that minimizes the risk of failure of a given regimen and maximizes the number of future potential options. This is best achieved by establishing a thorough understanding of the biology of HIV disease and the principles of antiretroviral therapy.

THE BIOLOGY OF HIV INFECTION

Since HIV was identified in 1983, several landmark discoveries have helped elucidate the mechanisms by which HIV causes the immune system dysfunction associated with the acquired immunodeficiency syndrome (AIDS). These discoveries are usually linked to the application of newly developed technology in the laboratory. Soon after discovery of the virus, investigators demonstrated the presence of HIV in virtually all tissues of the body, including the brain.[32,33] Utilizing p24 antigen assays, an association was made between the level of p24 antigen in plasma and the stage of disease, with higher levels of viremia observed during the time of acute seroconversion and again in the later stages of advanced HIV disease.[34–36] Most of the individuals who were asymptomatic with high CD4+ T-lymphocyte counts had no appreciable p24 antigenemia detected. During the late 1980s, utilizing tissue culture techniques investigators were able to titrate the amount of infectious virus in plasma.[34,37,38] Much like p24 antigenemia, higher levels of infectious virus in plasma was noted at the time of acute seroconversion and again in later stages of disease.[35,36,39] Although the plasma culture technique was more sensitive than the p24 antigen technique, substantial numbers of patients with asymptomatic disease, as well as those on antiretroviral therapy, had undetectable levels of infectious virus.[34,37,38]

Utilizing this information, a picture of HIV pathogenesis emerged whereby the virus established widespread infection early in the course of disease (at the time of seroconversion), stimulating a potent immune system response. During the period of clinical latency, which lasts up to 10 to 12 years, initial models of pathogenesis suggested that viral replication was under effective control by the immune system, only to reappear as high-level viremia during later stages of disease (Fig. 27–1).[35,36,39] This model, however, could not explain the slow, yet progressive decline in CD4+ T-lymphocyte counts and immune system function that occurs during the period of clinical latency. With the advent of quantitative PCR technology during the early 1990s, the association of HIV replication and immune system destruction was more completely described. Piatak and colleagues were the first to describe the presence of detectable virus at *all* stages of HIV infection, including the period of clinical latency.[12,13] As was demonstrated with p24 antigen and quantitative plasma culture techniques, the highest levels of viral RNA were detected at the time of acute seroconversion and during later stages of disease.[12,40] However, lower levels of virus were detected even at the early, asymptomatic stages of the disease, implying that viral replication is a continuous, ongoing process even during the period of clinical latency.

The application of viral load testing to determine the activity of antiretroviral therapeutic regimens led to the opportunity to define further the nature of HIV replication in vivo. Even with the use of relatively weak antiretroviral regimens, such as zidovudine monotherapy, an 80% (0.9 log) reduction in viral load was noted within 1 week of the initiation of therapy, with a relatively symmetrical return to baseline within 1 week after discontinuing treatment.[41] Based on these observations, it was apparent that viral replication was not only continuous but also quite rapid.[42] However, it was not until the dramatic responses to HIV protease and nonnucleoside reverse transcriptase inhibitors were observed that the magnitude of the rate of viral replication in vivo was fully appreciated.

In separate reports, Wei et al. and Ho et al. quantitated the rapid turnover of HIV in vivo, demonstrating the production and clearance of up to 10 billion virions each day (approximately 400 million virions per hour).[6,7] The half-life of virions in the circulation is estimated to be 1 to 2 hours or less. When new rounds of viral replication are blocked by antiretroviral therapy, the amount of measurable virus drops by more than 99% within 2 to 7 days of initiating therapy. The estimated life cycle (or generation time) of HIV, which represents the time from release of a virion until it infects another cell resulting in the release of new progeny, is estimated to be 2 days (Fig. 27–2).[8,43,44] These data were generated by observing the rapid decay in viral load over the first few weeks of potent therapy and represent the contribution of the acutely infected cells in the host, which have a half-life of 1 to 2 days. These cells represent more than 99% of the daily virus production. The remaining production of virus comes from a longer-lived population of cells that contribute to the slower, "second phase" decay of plasma viremia (Fig. 27–3).[44,45] Therefore within 8 to 12 weeks after initiation of potent therapy, plasma HIV RNA levels generally fall below 400 copies per milliliter of plasma. It usually takes several weeks longer to reach undetectable levels when utilizing ultrasensitive

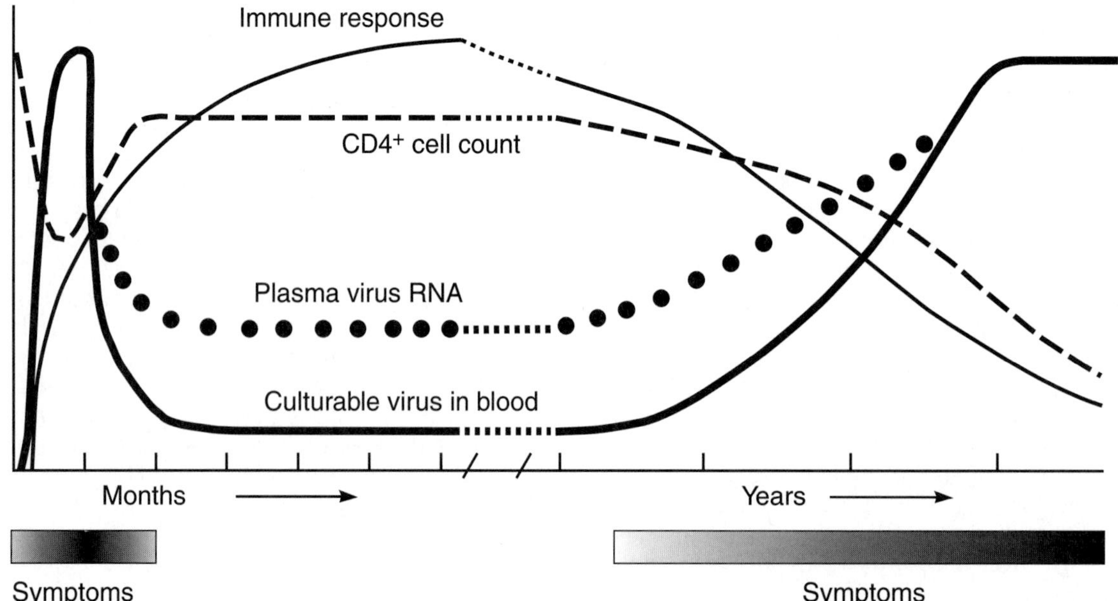

Figure 27–1. Natural history of HIV-1 infection over time. (Modified from Saag MA, Holodniy M, Kuritzkes DR, et al. HIV viral load markers in clinical practice. Nature Med 2:625, 1996. Copyright 1996 Macmillan Magazines Limited, with permission.)

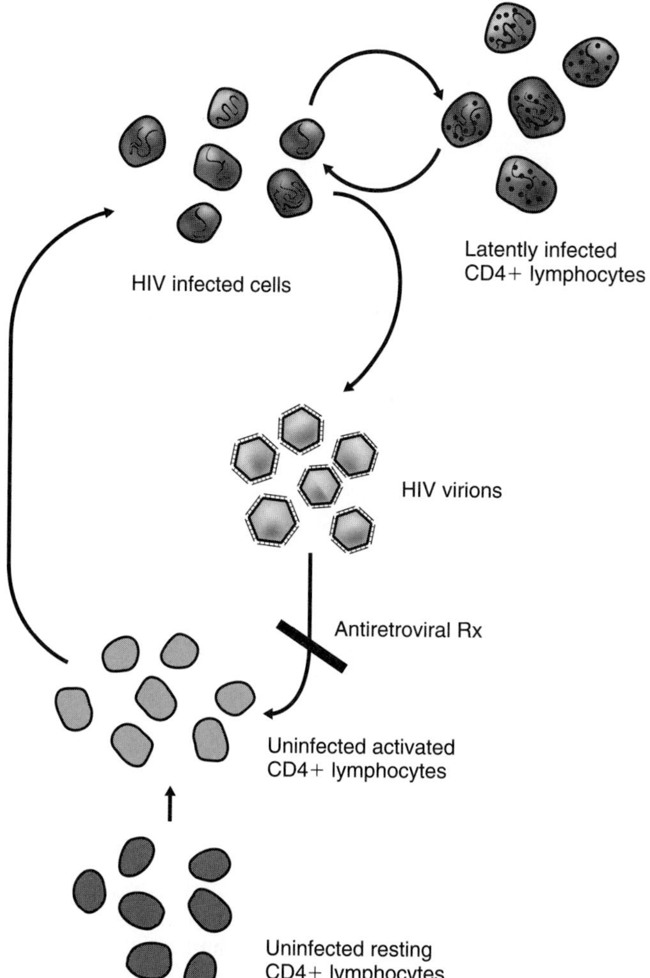

Figure 27–2. HIV-1 replication is rapid in vivo. Plasma HIV-1 viremia, depicted here as HIV-1 results from spillover of recently produced virus from infected cells in lymphatic tissue. Uninfected, activated CD4+ T-lymphocytes are the predominant target of HIV-1 infection. Once infected, these cells produce virus within 1 to 2 days and continue producing virus for an estimated 1 to 3 days. More than 99% of the virus detected in the bloodstream comes from recently infected CD4+ T-lymphocytes. The remaining less than 1% of virus comes from chronically infected CD4+ T-lymphocytes or macrophages, which have life spans ranging from a few days to several years. (Redrawn with modification from Perelson et al. HIV-1 dynamics in vivo: virion clearance rate, infected cell life-span, and viral generation time. Science 271:1582, 1996.) Copyright 1996 American Association for the Advancement of Science, with permission.)

virologic techniques (limit of detection approximately 5 to 50 copies per milliliter). Most viral replication takes place in lymphoid organs, where most of the CD4+ T-lymphocytes reside.[25,46–51] The detection of virus in plasma, as measured for example by the plasma "viral load," represents spillover of virus from the site of production (lymphatic tissue) into the bloodstream where it can be readily detected. In addition to the gradual reduction in absolute CD4+ T lymphocytes over time, loss of lymphoid architecture within lymph nodes also occurs and is believed to contribute to the relative lack of immune system efficiency at later stages of the disease.[46,47] Although most newly formed virions do not result in infection of a neighboring cell, on average several million new CD4+ T-lymphocytes are infected each day.[7,43] This high-level, continuous production of virus and subsequent infection of new CD4+ T-lymphocytes helps explain how the CD4+ cells' decline and immune system destruction occur during the time of clinical latency.

Activated CD4+ T-lymphocytes are the principal targets of HIV replication. The estimated life span of an infected CD4+ T-lymphocyte is 1 to 2 days.[52] Each infected cell has an instantaneous burst size of approximately 4000 copies per cell.[25] The calculated burst size per cell is remarkably constant and is independent of stage of disease, plasma viral load, and antiretroviral treatment status.[25] Thus the plasma viral load is a direct reflection of the number of infected cells in the body producing virus at any moment in time.

Whereas the *instantaneous* burst size, defined as the number of measurable virions produced by an infected cell at any given moment, is ~4000 copies per cell, the *effective* burst size, defined as the number of viruses produced that result in productive infection of a neighboring cell, at steady state is approximately 1 virion per cell (Fig. 27–4). At steady state, each patient establishes an equilibrium between the production and destruction of virus-producing cells such that as each productive cell is destroyed or stops producing virus it is replaced by another newly infected, productive cell. Clinically, this equilibrium establishes a relatively stable viral load value over time, defined as the viral "set point."[8,53] Mellors and colleagues have demonstrated a direct relation between the viral load, or set point, and the rate of CD4+ T-lymphocyte count decline.[54] When viewed in the context of the direct relation between plasma viral load and the number of productively infected cells at any moment in time, these findings are not surprising.

Much attention has focused on how actively producing cells are eliminated.[55,56] The leading possibilities are the direct cytopathic effect of the virus (or deleterious effects of virions budding from the cell membrane), virus-induced cell apoptosis, or direct destruction via an effective immune system response. Initial experience with tissue culture growth of the virus supported the concept of a direct cytopathic effect.[57] Under the stimulation of phytohemagglutinin and interleukin-2 (IL-2), most virus-infected cells died within several days of becoming infected in tissue culture, often through the development of large syncytia. Syncytia have never been demonstrated in vivo, and so the concept of death of cells via this mechanism remains uncertain. Apoptosis, or programmed cell death, is a natural mechanism for eliminating lymphocytes of the immune system. Viral proteins, or cytokines released in response to viral infection, may trigger the apoptotic pathway in actively producing cells, although the degree to which this occurs is not known.

More recently, there is a growing appreciation for the role of HIV-specific immune system responses to eliminate virus-producing cells.[58–62] Rosenberg et al. reported a study of eight seroconverters, each of whom was treated within days to a couple of weeks after the onset of symptoms of their initial HIV infection.[63] After at least 10 months of highly active antiretroviral therapy (HAART), each patient

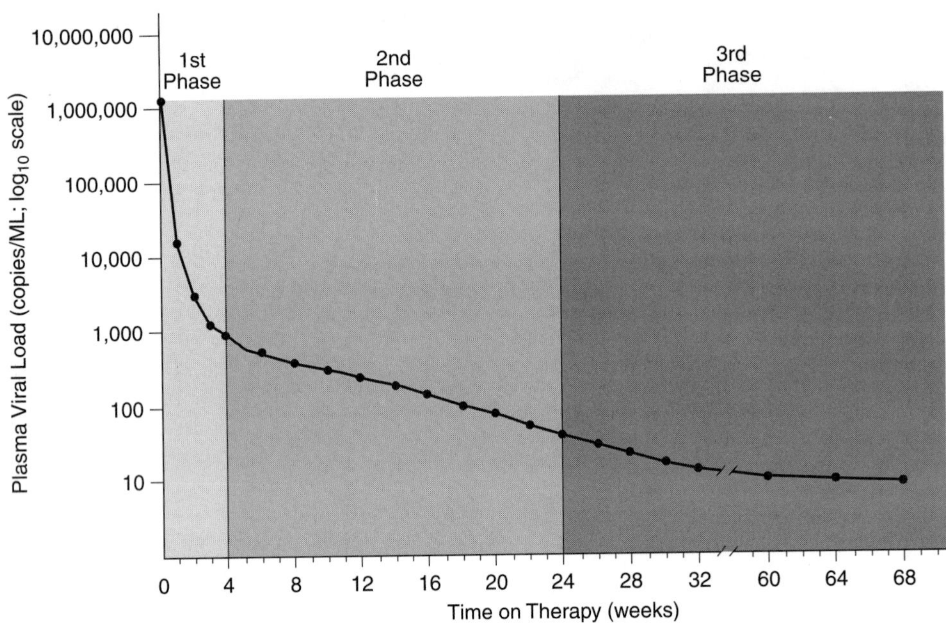

Figure 27–3. Typical plasma HIV RNA response to potent antiretroviral therapy. After initiation of treatment, a sharp decrease in viral load is observed over the first 2 to 4 weeks of therapy. Thereafter a steady, less steep decline in plasma viral load is observed. These differential rates of decline have been arbitrarily divided into "phases" for purposes of mathematic modeling. In reality, they represent a continuum of viral decay as the life span of productively infected cells is exhausted. If all further new infection is completely blocked for a sufficient period of time (new estimates: many years) to allow all existing infected cells to die, a cure is theoretically possible.

had therapy withdrawn. Three of the patients had stabilization of the viral load at less than 1000 copies per milliliter that has persisted for more than 1 year; the remaining patients were restarted on therapy for several weeks and underwent a second withdrawal of therapy. Following the second treatment interruption, all patients established at least transient low levels of plasma viral load, indicating establishment of an effective immune response. Five of the eight patients remained off therapy at the time of publication. High levels of anti-HIV-specific CD4+ T-lymphocyte activity were demonstrated in association with control of replication. This level of CD4+ T-lymphocyte help is typical in "long-term nonprogressor" patients, who naturally control viral infection and do not suffer CD4+T lymphopenia despite chronic HIV infection. In contrast, when therapeutic withdrawal of treatment is performed in patients with chronic, well established HIV infection who were not treated within 12 to 20 weeks of acute infection, viral load values tend to rebound back to high levels.[64,65] These patients have extremely low or absent HIV-specific CD4+ T-helper lymphocyte responses. Profound depletion of the total number of CD4+ T lymphocytes, which develops over a period of years, leads to the development of the typical clinical syndrome of AIDS.

Taken together, HIV pathogenesis is best depicted as a vicious cycle of production of large numbers of HIV virions that infect activated CD4+ target cells, which in turn produce more viruses that infect additional cells (Fig. 27–5).[9] The function of the targeted CD4+ cells, ironically, is to create an HIV-specific, coordinated response against the virus that is attacking them. Current thinking supports the concept that cytotoxic CD8+ T-lymphocytes, under the support of an HIV-specific CD4+ T-lymphocyte response, are responsible, at least in part, for eliminating the active virus-producing HIV-infected cells.[61–63,66–69] The HIV-specific CD4+ T-helper lymphocyte responses appear to be lost early (within the first few weeks after infection), perhaps never to return. The continuous infection of other activated CD4+ cells is believed to lead to impairment of the immune responses to other antigens/pathogens, thereby creating potential deficits in the immune system's response to opportunistic processes. The goal of effective antiretroviral therapy therefore is to block, as completely as possible, the ability of the virus to infect uninfected CD4+ T-lymphocytes, thereby inhibiting de novo production of virus and, at the same time, preserving immune system competence.[57]

▲ STRATEGIC USE OF ANTIRETROVIRAL THERAPY

Simply stated, the goal of antiretroviral therapy is to inhibit completely viral replication in vivo and sustain the effect for as long as possible. Theoretically, if complete suppression is sustained for a long enough time to allow the population of chronically infected of cells to decay to extinction, eradication of HIV (or a true cure) is possible. Whether a cure is truly achievable is critical to establishing the foundation of a antiretroviral therapeutic strategy. If cure is indeed possible, all patients should be treated with the most potent agents early and aggressively during the course of their infection, much like the treatment of acute

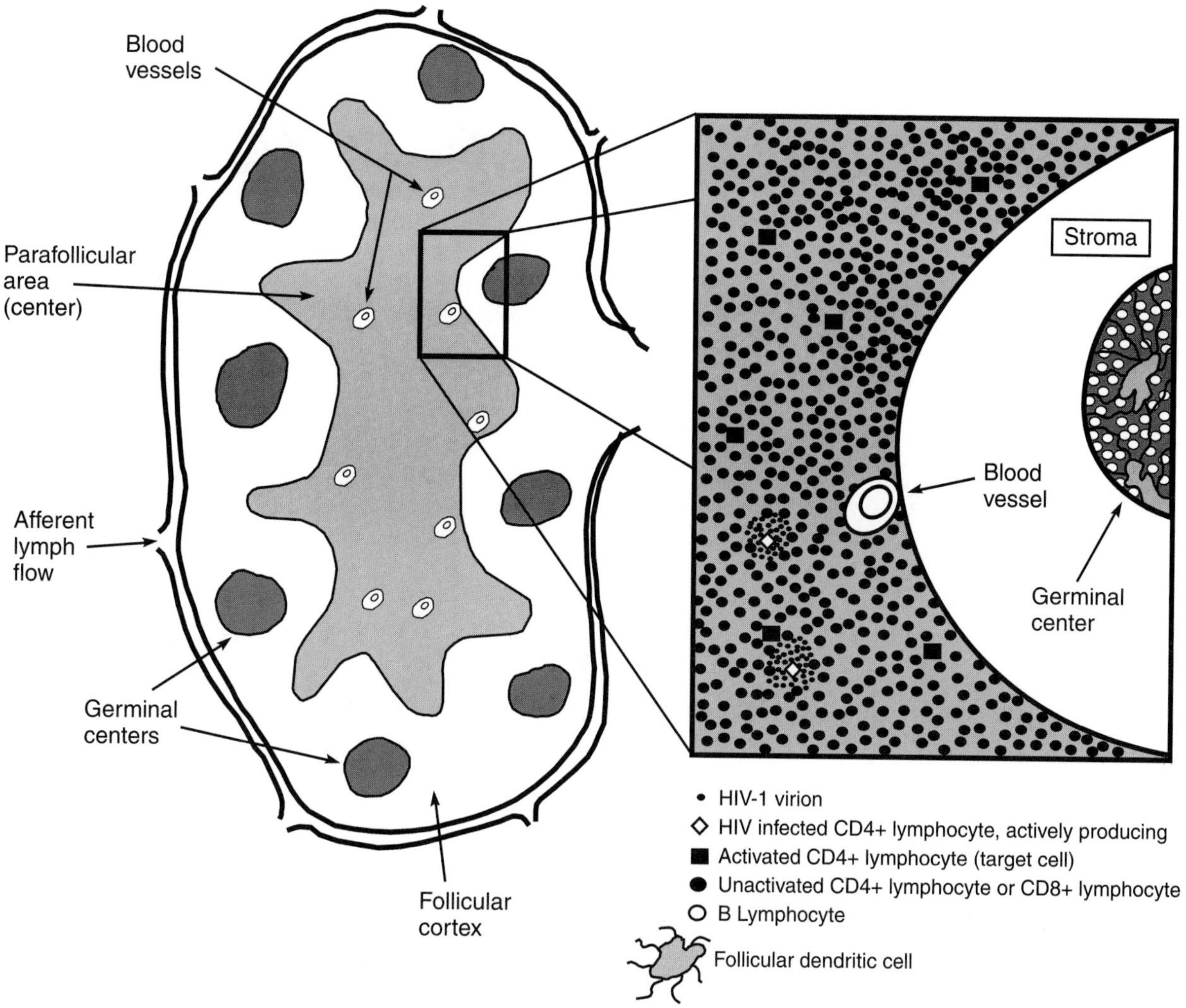

Figure 27–4. Lymph node from a patient with established HIV infection. The actively producing cells (diamonds) excrete high levels of HIV virions (black dots), with an average instantaneous burst size of 4000 copies per cell. These newly produced virions are trapped by follicular dendritic cells (large cells in germinal center), are absorbed onto circulating resting CD4+ T-lymphocytes (black closed circles) or activated CD4+ T-lymphocytes (black squares) passing by, or spill into the circulation. The actual number of target (activated) cells infected by virus produced by any actively producing cell is small: about one new cell infected over the lifespan of each actively producing cell at steady state.

lymphocytic leukemia. If a cure with antiretroviral therapy alone is not a realistic possibility, other strategic approaches must be considered, more like the treatment of chronic lymphocytic leukemia.

Whether eradication is possible depends in large part on the life span of longer-lived, chronically infected cells and whether complete (or relatively complete) suppression of viral replication is achievable. About 99+% of the plasma viremia is generated by actively producing CD4+ T-lymphocytes with a relatively short half-life (1 to 2 days), the remaining 1% or less of plasma viremia is produced by longer-lived cells that previously were predicted to have an estimated *average* half-life of 14 to 28 days, although some of the cells could have a life span as short as 2 to 4 days or as long as more than 400 days (Fig. 27–2).[43,45,70] If the life span of these long-lived cells is 28 days or less and all de novo infection is completely blocked, eradication may be achieved as early as 3 to 5 years after initiation of therapy;[43,44] however, if the life span of the longer-lived chronically infected cells is substantially longer (on the order of 400 days) or if latently infected cells (that contain proviral DNA) are able to circulate and express virus at a later time, the time required for complete eradication of HIV could be on the order of decades and may not be achievable, even with complete block of de novo rounds of replication sustained over a long period of time.[47,60] Data generated during the latter portion of the 1990s demonstrated that the half-life of the chronically infected population of cells was not 14 to 28 days as originally assumed but, rather, 6 months at the shortest or 44 months at the longest.[26,56,71–73] Thus the time to eradication under the assumption of complete arrest of all de novo infection now ranges from 12 to 60 years of continuous antiretroviral therapy.

As indicated above, the concept of eradicating HIV from an infected individual requires chronically infected cells to

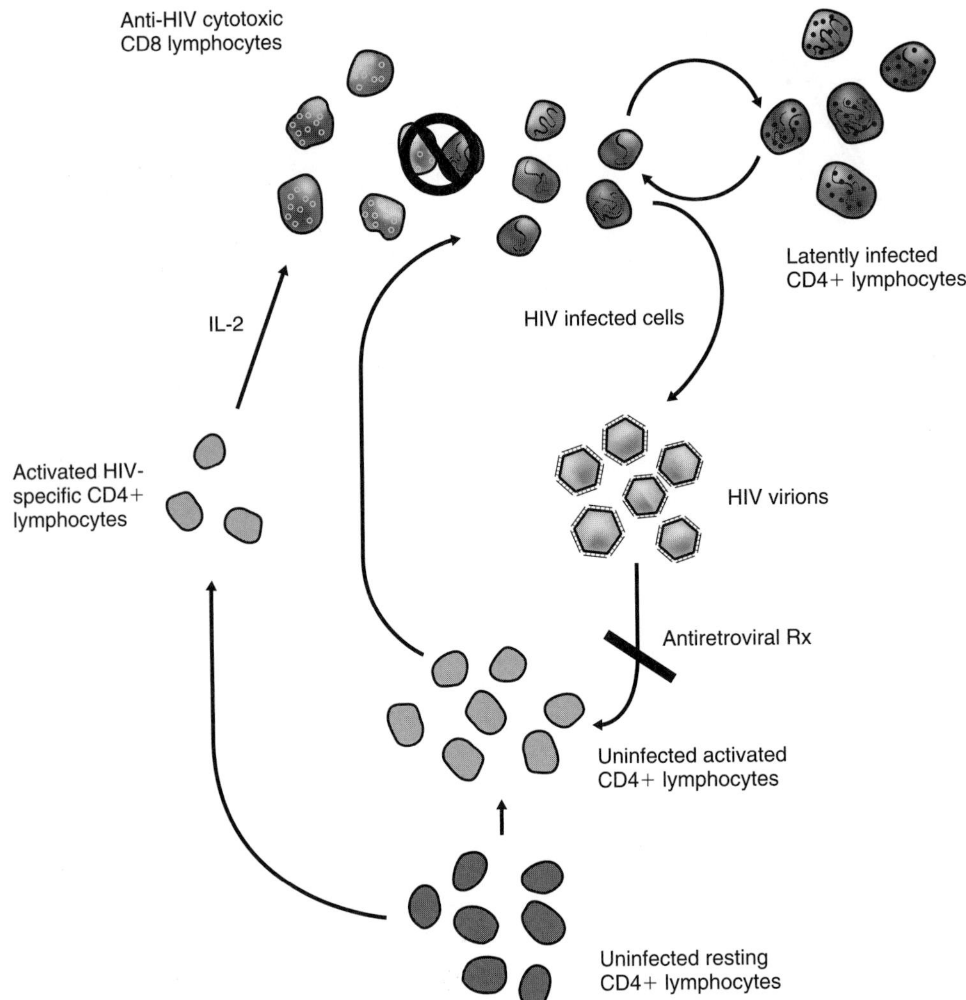

Figure 27–5. More complete picture of HIV pathogenesis. Actively producing CD4+ lymphocytes are killed, at least in part, by HIV-specific CD8+ cytotoxic lymphocytes. These cytotoxic cells are stimulated by cytokines (e.g., interleukin-2) produced by HIV-specific CD4+ lymphocytes. In the presence of functioning CD4+ T-lymphocytes, the inherent anti-HIV immune response is capable of controlling viral replication in an efficient manner. Unfortunately, early during the course of infection (soon after the time of seroconversion), most of the HIV-specific CD4+ activity is lost, and the immune response is much less efficient. Early treatment, prior to the time of seroconversion, helps preserve the HIV-specific immune response, potentially abrogating the need for antiretroviral therapy.

have a relatively short half-life but also requires *complete* block of all new rounds of de novo infection and this block must be sustained for a long enough time to allow all chronically infected, productive cells within the body to be destroyed or die off. To achieve eradication, inhibitory levels of antiretroviral therapy must be maintained above inhibitory concentrations within all body compartments and within all susceptible target cells, ideally on a continuous basis. Thus a "cure" for HIV infection assumes complete penetration of antiretroviral drugs into the cells in all compartments of the body where the virus is replicating and strict adherence to the regimen for a period long enough to allow the infected cells to die off. An important issue in the discussion of a potential "cure" relates to the relation of "undetectable" levels of plasma virus to complete suppression of viral replication. "Undetectable" levels of HIV in plasma are a function of a laboratory assay; complete suppression is a biologic phenomenon. All too often patients and clinicians assume that achieving an undetectable level of virus is synonymous with complete suppression. Even when plasma viral load values are less than a theoretical 1 $\log_{10}$ copy per milliliter, an estimated 75,000 to 150,000 cells are still producing virus in lymphoid tissue (Fig. 27–6).[25] Zhang et al. reported evidence of genetic drift in the envelope region in virus isolated from a patient who was treated at the time of seroconversion and sustained levels of less than 50 copies per milliliter for more than 20 months, supporting the notion of ongoing low-level replication when plasma viral load values are undetectable.[26] Therefore low-level viral replication appears to be ongoing even in the face of potent, yet incomplete viral suppression.[55] This implies that breakthrough viremia will ultimately occur; it is simply a question of when. Inevitably, more sensitive virologic assays will

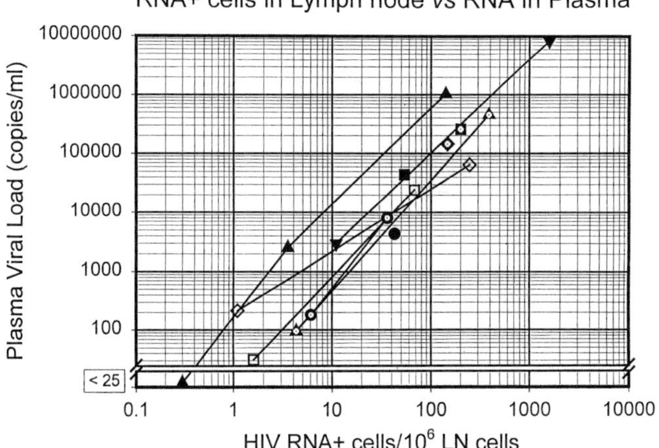

Figure 27–6. A log–log plot of the relation between plasma viral load (copies per milliliter) and the number of cells actively producing virus in lymphatic tissue. Each point represents a separate biopsy time point paired with the plasma viral load obtained at the time of biopsy. The lines connecting points with the same symbol represent values obtained from the same patient before and after initiation of potent antiretroviral therapy. The slope of this line is 1.6, and the Pearson correlation coefficient (R) is 0.95, indicating a strong relation between the number of cells producing virus in the body and the plasma viral load. (Modified from Hockett RD, Kilby JM, Derdeyn CA, et al. Constant mean viral copy number per infected cell in tissues regardless of high, low, or undetectable plasma HIV RNA. J Exp Med 189:1545, 1999.)

become commercially available and help narrow the gap between "undetectable" and "complete suppression." At the present time, however, it does not appear that currently available antiretroviral agents, even when used in combination, are potent enough to achieve and maintain truly complete suppression. Thus a gap continues to exist between the ideal goal of antiretroviral therapy (defined as complete suppression of de novo infection) and the achievable goal of antiretroviral therapy (defined as achieving undetectable levels of virus by available viral load techniques). Although many patients are able to achieve undetectable levels of virus, other patients are able to get only to a level of 5000 to 10,000 copies per milliliter.[74–76] The ability to achieve undetectable levels of virus is heavily dependent on the baseline viral load and the treatment history of the patient: the higher the baseline viral load and the more heavily treated the patient, the more difficult it is to achieve undetectable levels of virus.[77–83] Once undetectability is achieved, however, especially using assays that can detect 25 copies of virus per milliliter or less, the original baseline viral load is no longer a factor with regard to the durability of the antiviral effect, although treatment history may still be a factor in the relative ease of resistance development.

Taken together, evidence of chronically infected cells living for extended periods of time combined with evidence of ongoing, low-level replication in the face of "undetectable" levels of plasma viremia indicates that eradication of HIV is not likely to occur with potent antiretroviral therapy alone. Although eradication of HIV remains the ultimate goal of therapy, a more realistic goal at the present time would be to sustain suppression as completely as possible for as long as possible utilizing existing therapy in a strategic fashion over time.

Initiation of Therapy

The ultimate success of antiretroviral therapy is total eradication, or cure, as discussed above. In the case of health care workers who have been exposed to infected blood through percutaneous needlestick exposure, the use of antiretroviral therapy appears to help abort early infection and, in this regard, is the best example of eradication occurring as a result of antiretroviral therapy.[84,85] Similarly, prevention of perinatal infection through the use of prepartum and peripartum treatment of the mother and postpartum treatment of the neonate is another example where early infection is either prevented or aborted after exposure through the use of antiretroviral therapy.[86] Other than these two situations, successful antiretroviral therapy (cure) has not been achieved. Rather, antiretroviral "success" is defined more as the absence of antiretroviral failure rather than as success per se. Therefore prevention of antiretroviral failure becomes the principal goal of antiretroviral therapy.

Advanced planning is essential for long-term success of antiretroviral therapy. With the development of a large number of more potent antiretroviral agents, there has been a paradigm shift in the approach to therapy: The goal of therapy has changed from keeping patients alive from this year to the next to keeping patients alive from this decade to the next. To achieve the best long-term suppression of viral replication, clinicians must approach therapeutic decision-making in the same way a chess master approaches a match, thinking several moves ahead. The choice of initial therapy has profound implications on the effectiveness of subsequent regimens and the availability of viable choices of therapy in the future (Table 27–1).

The goals of chronic administration of antiretroviral therapy can be seen as twofold: to prevent clinical progression and to prevent or delay development of resistance. Over the last several years the guidelines for treatment of HIV infection have appeared to vacillate, owing in large part to the emerging realization that a cure was not readily achievable with antiretroviral therapy alone.[87] The "treat early, treat hard" approach to therapy was initially linked with the idea that complete, maintained viral suppression could result in the eradication of HIV from the body within a short time.[57] In addition, confusion regarding the goals of therapy at different stages of disease contributes to the apparent "change" in guidelines. To prevent the emergence of viral resistance, relatively complete viral suppression is required. Therefore, in all newly treated patients the principal goal of treatment should be to achieve virologic suppression to undetectable levels. However, clinical benefit can still be realized with less than maximal suppression of viral load.[74,80,88,89] A reduction in HIV RNA levels of 0.5 $\log_{10}$ copies per milliliter below baseline is associated with relative maintenance of the CD4+ T-lymphocyte count over time, provided this degree of viral suppression is sustained.[74,80,89] Therefore for patients who have experienced

▲ **Table 27–1.** VARIOUS DEFINITIONS OF SUCCESS, FAILURE, AND SUBSEQUENT REGIMENS BASED ON INITIAL REGIMEN

Initial Regimen	Definition of Success ($\log_{10}$ copies/ml)	Definition of Failure ($\log_{10}$ copies/ml)	Subsequent Regimens
$NRTI_1/NRTI_2/NRTI_3$	< 50	$> 1{,}000$	$NRTI_4/NRTI_5/PI_1$
$NRTI_1/NRTI_2/NNRTI_1$	< 50	$> 1{,}000$	$NRTI_3/NRTI_4/PI_1$
$NRTI_1/NRTI_2/PI_1$	< 50	$> 500–1{,}000$	$NRTI_3/NNRTI_1/PI_2(-PI_3)$
$NRTI_1/NNRTI_1/PI_1$	< 50	$> 500–1{,}000$	$NRTI_2/NNRTI_2/PI_2(-PI_3)$

$NNRTI_1$, $NNRTI_2$, first and second nonnucleoside reverse transcriptase inhibitors; $NRTI_1$, $NRTI_2$, $NRTI_3$, $NRTI_4$, first, second, third, and fourth nucleoside reverse transcriptase inhibitors; PI_1, PI_2, PI_3, first, second, and third protease inhibitors.

multiple regimens and already have multidrug resistance, the goal of therapy changes to prevention of clinical progression. In this setting, a reasonable target is to achieve and sustain viral load values at least 0.5 $\log_{10}$ copies per milliliter below baseline.

The "treat early, treat hard" approach to therapy is grounded in concepts other than eradication.[57,87] Most clinical trials confirm that the first treatment represents the "best shot" at achieving profound suppression of viral replication. Based on current knowledge of HIV pathogenesis, early and profound suppression also prevents the development of resistance by limiting replication, preserving immune system integrity (before there is loss of critical clones of responsive cells), and creating a higher virologic hurdle for emergence of viral resistance.[90–92] Although this rationale is clearly sound, the approach rests on assumptions concerning adherence, toxicity, pharmacokinetics/pharmacodynamics, absence of meaningful immune system recovery, and antiretroviral effects that have proven difficult to realize or to be untrue. First, complete adherence to complex antiretroviral regimens is difficult for most patients to maintain.[31,93,94] Multiple studies demonstrate a striking relation between adherence and success of antiretroviral therapeutic regimens. Second, although serious toxicity is relatively uncommon with initial treatment for early disease, prolonged exposure to treatment is associated with an increasing number of metabolic and hepatic complications.[20,21,95–101] Third, drug pharmacokinetics and pharmacodynamics are subject to variability that can reduce the effectiveness of treatment.[28,102] Not all patients are able to achieve and sustain similar levels of intracellular concentrations of drug.[29,103] Fourth, although treatment that is initiated late in the course of disease (e.g., at CD4+ T-lymphocyte counts of less than 100 cells per microliter) is associated with a worse outcome, treatment started at moderate CD4+ T-lymphocyte counts (e.g., 350 cells per microliter) can be accompanied by preservation of immune competence that does not seem to be clinically distinguishable from that seen when starting therapy at earlier stages (e.g., CD4+ T-lymphocyte count of 600 cells per microliter).[78,104]

There are additional considerations that argue against universal application of early treatment, including failure of therapy to achieve "undetectable" viral load levels in a substantial proportion of patients and the limitations of subsequent treatment options for patients in whom treatment is failing.[105] Moreover, much of the data on progression of HIV disease from the Multicenter AIDS Cohort Study (MACS), which has been used to support earlier intervention, is derived from untreated individuals.[53] The use of data from untreated cohorts, although providing information on the natural history of disease prior to the influence of antiretroviral therapy, is anachronistic during the treatment era. Because the impact of treatment on the viral load determinants of progression is immediate, its predictive value is negated once potent treatment is initiated. Moreover, most clinicians do not idly observe progression of disease in their patients without introducing some intervention prior to the onset of profound CD4+ T-lymphocyte decline or the development of clinical disease. More recent data sets derived from clinical cohorts of treated individuals are more valuable for the "treatment era." Although longer-term follow up is lacking, these data indicate little disease progression among patients who initiated therapy with more moderate CD4+ T-lymphocyte counts (e.g., 350 cells per microliter), even if their viral load values at the time of treatment initiation are high (e.g., $> 100{,}000$ copies per milliliter).[78,104]

Based on such considerations, along with the increased frequency of long-term adverse events of treatment, a more conservative approach is advocated. Among asymptomatic patients, treatment may be initiated relatively early (e.g., at CD4+ T-lymphocyte counts of 350 to 500 cells per microliter) rather than very early using antiretroviral combinations that are likely to reduce the viral load below 50 copies per milliliter.[1,4,5] Selection of the specific regimen is based on the predicted likelihood of patient tolerance and adherence, with consideration of short- and long-term toxicities. Other considerations include the availability of the treatments and, indirectly, their costs as well as the objective of keeping open the options for subsequent treatment with the concept that virtually all regimens fail eventually. Most importantly, to ensure the best chance for success, patients should understand the rationale for treatment initiation and genuinely be "ready to start" therapy.

The potency of the initial regimen is critical to the long-term success of the initial regimen. Regimens for initial treatment should be of sufficient potency to ensure a high likelihood of achieving viral load levels below the limit of detection (< 50 copies per milliliter). In a general sense, the intensity of the regimen is proportional to the stage of infection and the baseline viral load level. For example, for patients with relatively low viral load values (e.g., $< 70{,}000$ to 100,000 copies per milliliter), triple nucleoside reverse (NRTI) therapy may be used. For patients with more advanced disease and higher viral load values, a four-drug 'boosted' (using the pharmacokinetic properties of low-dose ritonavir) protease inhibitor (PI)-containing regimen may be optimal. Most studies of efavirenz plus two NRTIs demonstrate activity comparable to that of non-boosted PI-containing regimens.[106] Studies comparing efavirenz to boosted PI regimens have not been done. A common question concerns the relative potency of various nonnucleoside reverse transcriptase inhibitor (NNRTI) containing regimens, yet the relative potencies of efavirenz- and nevirapine-containing initial regimens can be clarified only in head-to-head comparative trials, which are ongoing.

Minimizing the risk of short- and long-term toxicities is also critical when selecting the initial treatment regimen. Although PI/dual nRTI regimens are potent options with the longest experience for viral suppression, the possibilities of long-term metabolic toxicities are potential deterrents to their use. Owing to the high interindividual pharmacokinetic variability for most PIs when used by themselves with two NRTIs, ritonavir boosting is often essential for optimal benefit.[27,107–111] However, ritonavir-boosted regimens are more likely to be associated with hypertriglyceridemia and possibly insulin resistance and lipodystrophy. As a result, interest in PI-sparing regimens as initial therapy has increased, along with the desire to reserve the class for subsequent therapy.

Drugs cannot work if they are not taken. Creating a regimen that is relatively easy for the patient to take therefore is essential when designing initial treatment. Moreover, frequently missed doses not only decreases the ability of the drugs to work, it is a recipe for the development of antiretroviral resistance. A meta-analysis was performed that included intent-to-treat results of clinical trials of triple-drug antiretroviral therapy (defined as dual NRTIs plus a PI, an NNRTI, or another NRTI) in groups of 30 or more patients with 2 weeks or more of prior drug exposure who were treated at least 24 weeks.[112] Analysis of 48-week results indicate remarkable comparability among the regimens in reducing viral load to levels less than 400 copies per milliliter or 50 copies per milliliter along with comparable degrees of CD4+ T-lymphocyte count increases (Table 27–2). Multivariate linear regression analysis indicated that among variables commonly associated with prediction of drug effect, including drug class, baseline CD4+ T-lymphocyte count, and baseline viral load, the only significant variable that predicted the ability to reduce the viral load to 400 copies per milliliter or less or to 50 copies per milliliter or less or that predicted increases in CD4+ T lymphocytes was the daily pill count. In another study comparing identical regimens as part of clinical trials involving prisoners versus patients seen in routine clinical practice, the prisoners, who had drugs administered under conditions of directly observed therapy, had substantially better virologic outcomes (90% vs. 75% achieved viral load values of less than 400 copies per milliliter).[113] These data underscore the importance of drug-taking behavior, commitment to the regimen, simplicity of regimens, and overall adherence to the success of the initial regimen.

Strategies for keeping subsequent treatment options open require consideration of which of the remaining available drugs are likely to be active after the initial regimen fails based on what is known about class cross-resistance. Resistance to all of the drugs in the failing regimen often does not occur simultaneously. For example, in the ACTG 343 trial, among patients failing a regimen consisting of a PI and a lamivudine-containing dual NRTI combination, solitary resistance to lamivudine (M184V) was demonstrated in most of the failing cases with demonstrated resistance. (Parenthetically, a substantial number of patients with virologic failure had no evidence of resistance mutations at all, indicating the value of resistance testing for patients with first failure.)[114] Another initial strategy using triple-class regimens that included a PI, an NNRTI, and an NRTI should generally be avoided for initial treatment, as their use may result in few subsequent treatment options at the time of failure.

Notwithstanding all of the considerations listed above, perhaps the most important issue related to the long-term success of antiretroviral therapy is the degree to which the patient desires to start therapy. Patients' "buy in" is based in large part on their understanding of the rationale of treatment (i.e., why should they start) and the degree to

Table 27–2. META-ANALYSIS OF RANDOMIZED CONTROLLED CLINICAL TRIALS INVOLVING TWO NUCLEOSIDE AGENTS COMBINED WITH EITHER A PI, AN NNRTI, OR ANOTHER NUCLEOSIDE: 48-WEEK OUTCOMES

Parameter	Change in CD+ T-Lymphocyte Count % < 400 copies/ml	% < 50 HIV RNA	Mean Increase (cells/μl)
PI regimens			
No. treatment groups	11	11	10
Average estimate (95% CI)	52% (49, 55)	44% (41, 47)	166 cells/μl (142, 190)
NNRTI regimens			
No. treatment groups	7	6	8
Average estimate (95% CI)	61% (57, 59)	51% (47, 56)	152 cells/μl (111, 193)
Three nRTI regimens			
No. treatment groups	3	3	3
Average estimate (95% CI)	54% (50, 59)	45% (40, 49)	147 cells/μl (126, 168)
Total			
No. treatment groups	21	20	21
Average estimate (95% CI)	55% (53, 57)	46% (44, 48)	158 cells/μl (142, 174)

Adapted from Bartlett JA, DeMasi R, Quinn J, et al. Overview of the effectiveness of triple combination therapy in antiretroviral-naive HIV-1 infected adults. AIDS 15: 1369, 2001.

Table 27–3. STRATEGIC PLANNING: ISSUES TO BE ADDRESSED AT THE TIME ANTIRETROVIRAL THERAPY IS INITIATED OR CHANGED

Define initial (or new) regimen
Delineate parameters of success (virologic target of new therapy; e.g., < 50 copies/ml)
Define parameters of failure (viral load value that will initiate a change in the new regimen)
Define the next regimen: specifically list the regimen(s) to be used should the new regimen fail
Explain/discuss with the patient the new regimen, parameters of success and failure, and subsequent regimens to be considered should the new regimen fail

which they believe they have a role to play when selecting of the regimen. The "best" choice of therapy must encompass not just potency, appropriate pharmacokinetics, minimal toxicity, and relative ease of administration, it must include strong consideration of how the regimen fits into the patients' day-to-day activities and their beliefs regarding the likelihood that the regimen will work.

Taken together, the timing of therapy initiation is a complex decision process that requires an understanding of HIV biology, pathogenesis, natural history, pharmacology, toxicology, psychology, and behavior. In this regard, therapy is genuinely "tailored" for each patient, making guidelines for the initiation of therapy entirely relative rather than absolute. The use of antiretroviral therapy is comparable to running a marathon, rather than a sprint, and should be viewed as a long-term process, employing strategies appropriate to this perspective. The parameters of success and the definition of failure for the individual regimen should be defined at the time the initial antiretroviral regimen is chosen (Table 27–3). In addition, the regimen(s) to be used subsequently when the original regimen fails should be clearly defined at the time the initial regimen is initiated. Therapeutic parameters must be individualized, with definitions of success and failure depending on the regimen chosen and the clinical setting of the patient. Although the ideal goal of therapy is to suppress viral replication below the level of detection, some patients, especially those with high initial viral load levels, may not be able to achieve this level of success. In such cases multidrug regimens may be required to achieve optimal suppression but at the cost of more regimen complexity and increased chance of nonadherence.

Management of Antiretroviral Failure

Antiretroviral therapy "failure" is a relative term that can be defined in terms of both clinical and virologic parameters. Clinical failure is the easiest to define: progression of clinical symptomatology or the development of a new opportunistic infection or death in the face of antiretroviral therapy. From a virologic standpoint, antiretroviral failure simply means the loss of control of viral replication; however, this loss of control is often incremental and in most cases is only partially lost. When viral load testing was first used in clinical practice, virologic failure was originally defined as a return toward (within 0.3 to 0.5 $\log_{10}$ copies/ml) the original baseline viral load.[10] Soon thereafter the definition was more stringently defined as a confirmed return to detectable levels of virus (for those who had previously achieved undetectable levels) or a persistance of viral load of more than 1000 to 10,000 copies per milliliter for those unable to achieve undetectable levels of circulating virus.[115] This definition of failure is most appropriate for a patient's first regimen, with the goal of therapy being driven predominantly by the desire to avoid the development of resistance. For patients who have experienced multiple regimen failures, the development of clinical progression (clinical failure) is infrequent provided the viral load level is maintained below 0.5 $\log_{10}$ copies/ml (threefold) of the original viral load set point.[80,88] Therefore the definition of virologic "failure" is totally dependent on the clinical setting and must be individualized for each patient, taking into account the history of antiretroviral therapy, baseline viral load, response to therapy, and availability of options for treatment once "failure" has occurred. Once the definitions of success and failure have been delineated, the choice of subsequent regimens depends on the prior exposure to antiretroviral agents, previous adverse experiences, potential drug–drug interactions, underlying disease, CD4+ T-lymphocyte count/viral load status, and the perspective of the patient regarding the ability to adhere to a complex drug regimen. As is done when selecting the initial regimen, selection of the first and subsequent failure regimens should include consideration of potential options available at the time the next regimen fails. Although it is understood that the alternative choices of available agents and the perspective of the patient may change substantially by the time the next therapeutic regimen fails, the conceptual approach of defining subsequent regimens in advance emphasizes the impact that regimen decisions have on future treatment options and establishes a pattern of long-term strategic thinking that is required for optimal long-term outcome.

The reasons for antiretroviral therapy failure are multifactorial. The four primary reasons for failure include toxicity/intolerance, development of resistance, pharmacodynamics, and nonadherence. Each of these factors is discussed individually below.

Toxicity/Intolerance

Each pharmaceutical agent is associated with a unique set of toxicities. The degree to which a given toxicity is tolerated by the patient depends on a number of factors, including the nature and severity of the toxicity, the degree to which the toxicity interferes with day-to-day living, and the willingness of the patient to live with the toxicity. Generally, a patient who is totally asymptomatic is less willing to tolerate an adverse experience from a medication than a patient who has more advanced, symptomatic disease or has previously experienced disease progression. In addition, the degree to which a patient believes the regimen will provide benefit is proportional to the patient's willingness to tolerate an adverse experience.

With the use of combination therapy, the individual adverse experience profile for a given agent is compounded by drug–drug interactions, altered pharmacokinetic profiles, and synergistic toxicities of the drugs. Some adverse experiences develop soon after initiation of therapy, and the symptoms may wane after several weeks (tachyphylaxis). Depending on the nature of the toxicity, its severity, the tendency of the toxicity to develop tachyphylaxis, and the willingness of the patient to tolerate the toxicity, the decision to discontinue a specific agent (or not) must be individualized. In general, dose reduction or withholding a single agent for even a short period of time is generally not an option based on concern of inducing resistant virus to the agent while using a suboptimal dose or exposing the virus to a partially suppressive regimen with inadequate potency from the remaining agents in the regimen.

Development of Resistance

Resistance is a function of two principal conditions: (1) innate susceptibility of the virus [typically expressed in terms of 50% (IC_{50}) or 90% (IC_{90}) inhibitory concentration from an in vitro assay]; and (2) the achievable level of drug in susceptible target cells, where viral replication takes place. In the case of antibacterial therapy, the difference between the in vitro susceptibility and the tissue concentration of drug is often as much as 100- to 1000-fold; however, in the case of antiviral therapy, the therapeutic window is generally much smaller. The maximum tolerated dose of most antiretroviral agents limits tissue levels of drug to single-digit multiples of the IC_{90} (e.g., three- to seven-fold) at trough levels. Therefore any genetic mutation that reduces the susceptibility of the virus to even a modest degree may have significant clinical implications.

To manage resistance clinically, the biology of how resistance develops should be understood. HIV exists in vivo as a quasi-species.[116] After initial infection with a predominant genotype, viral replication ensues at an extraordinary rate, resulting in the production of progenitor viruses that are highly related yet genetically distinct. The major reason for the generation of such enormous diversity is the relative infidelity of the reverse transcriptase (RT) enzyme. RT is a relatively sloppy enzyme, creating a transcriptional error every 3000 to 4000 basepairs (bp) transcribed.[117,118] Because HIV is a 9000-bp virus, on average one to two transcriptional errors occur with each replication cycle. With the generation of 10 billion virions per day, a wide variety of genetic mutants are theoretically produced on a daily basis. Most of these transcriptional errors are believed to lead to stop codons and defective virions, although critical point mutations that confer resistance to antiviral therapy may be generated. Under the conditions of selective pressure, these mutated viruses become the predominant genotype. Although most of these errors are neutral or lead to stop codons, several mutations may lead to the development of new virions with altered fitness or selective advantage.[119] When the mutation results in reduced fitness, the mutant virus grows less well and becomes a minor component of the quasi-species. However, when the mutant virus is more fit and has a selective growth advantage, it may dominate the quasi-species rapidly (within days).[6] Therefore a major difference between antibacterial susceptibility testing and antiretroviral testing becomes immediately obvious: Antibacterial tests are performed against a single clone of bacteria isolated from an infected source, whereas antiretroviral tests are performed on a swarm of viruses that coexist in different frequencies and change in rapid fashion upon challenge with a new selective pressure (e.g., initiation of a new antiretroviral regimen).

The likelihood of the development of resistance mutations in vivo is a function of two factors: the relative potency of the antiretroviral regimen and the degree of ongoing replication occurring while the regimen is being administered. A regimen that has relatively poor potency creates little selective pressure on the virus to mutate; in such cases, resistance mutations are unlikely to develop (Fig. 27–7). In contrast, a highly active regimen generates substantial selected pressure for the virus to mutate. The likelihood of resistance development then becomes a function of the degree of replication allowed to occur while the regimen is being administered: the more replication allowed to occur under strong selective pressure, the faster resistance develops. Theoretically, if a regimen is completely suppressive, no resistance develops because no replication is taking place and resistance mutations do not have the chance to develop.

The two primary targets of most antiretroviral therapies—virally encoded RT and protease enzymes—are highly plastic molecules. Some of the mutations induced by one agent may lead to reduced susceptibility of the virus to other agents (cross-resistance), especially to agents with the same mechanism of action (e.g., NNRTIs and PIs). Although most resistance-conferring mutations reduce the susceptibility of the virus to a significant degree, some mutations also cause substantially less efficient function

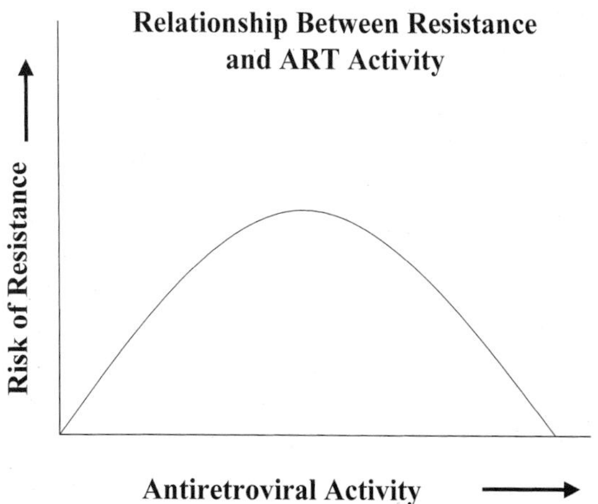

Figure 27–7. Likelihood of developing resistance is directly related to the relative activity of antiretroviral therapy (ART). In the absence of meaningful activity (far left-hand side) there is no selective pressure exerted that can lead to resistance. Similarly, in the absence of viral replication (complete suppression of virus; far right-hand side), no resistance can develop because there is no ongoing replication. However, when regimens are only partially suppressive (middle portion of figure), there is ongoing replication in the presence of ample selective pressure, creating a higher likelihood of resistance. (Modified from presentations by Doug Richman and Emilio Emini.)

than wild-type virus, resulting in a virus with decreased replication capacity (i.e., less "fit").[119]

Common mutations selected by NRTIs, NNRTIs, and PIs are shown in Figure 27–8.[120] Although there is general concordance between laboratory-selected mutations induced by serial passage of the virus in the presence of drug and those mutations observed in clinical isolates, some mutations selected in vitro have not been demonstrated from clinical specimens among patients receiving drug.[15] In either case, mutations can be viewed as primary or secondary. Primary mutations are defined as those that have a demonstrable effect on the degree of resistance to the given agent. Secondary mutations often have no discernible effect on the susceptibility of the virus to the drug but are likely selected on the basis of their ability to improve the fitness of the virus, usually as a compensatory mutation that allows more effective viral replication or enzyme function.

Variable degrees of resistance are conferred by single point mutations, depending on the specific agent and the ease of resistance development. For example, a single point mutation at amino acid position 181 of the RT enzyme can lead to profound reduction in susceptibility to most NNRTIs, whereas single amino acid changes in RT may lead to only partial reduction in susceptibility to zidovudine.[121,122] Upon development of subsequent mutations, the degree of resistance increases incrementally, ultimately resulting in high-level resistance when four or five resistance-conferring mutations are present.[123,124] A similar pattern of sequential mutation acquisition within the protease gene product region is required for the development of high-level PI resistance.[125,126] To complicate matters, although the sequential acquisition of mutations may be common among agents within a particular class, the precise mutation responsible for conferring resistance is generally agent-specific but with varying degrees of cross-reactivity (depending on the drugs and the mutation in question). As an example, a single point mutation at amino acid position 30 (D30N) of the protease gene product leads to a severalfold reduction in susceptibility of the virus to nelfinavir but not other PIs.[127,128] Subsequent acquisition of other mutations, at amino acid positions 82 or 84 of the protease gene product leads to high-level resistance to nelfinavir and other PIs as well. To complicate matters further, some point mutations create secondary changes in the functional gene product, leading to improved fitness or some degree of reversal of resistance.[119] In the case of lamivudine, an M184V mutation results in substantial reduction of lamivudine susceptibility while partially reversing zidovudine resistance or delaying the emergence of zidovudine resistance when the two agents are used together in a regimen.[129] Taken together, drug-induced mutations occur under the influence of multiple factors, often resulting in variable phenotypic expression and clinical consequences.

In addition to de novo development of resistance, some viral variants with resistance-conferring mutations may preexist as subpopulations within infected T lymphocytes and macrophages.[82,130] Under the conditions of strong selective pressure, these preexistent mutants may rapidly become the predominant species expressed in vivo. The best example of this phenomenon is the development of rapid resistance observed when NNRTIs are administered as monotherapy.[6,130] Resistant viral variants have been observed as early as 5 days after the initiation of NNRTI monotherapy, with complete conversion of the predominant genotype in plasma from wild-type to resistant within 14 to 28 days after initiation of therapy.[6]

The concept of preexistent viral mutants plays a critical role in the strategic sequencing of antiretroviral regimens and the ability of a new regimen to succeed after a previous regimen has failed. At the time a regimen fails because of the development of resistance, resistant genotypes predominate in the plasma. As the regimen is changed, if these virions are susceptible to the new regimen, a shift in the population generally occurs, with suppression of the previous resistant viruses (ideally to undetectable levels).[6,130] If the new regimen is not completely suppressive, some degree of replication continues, potentially utilizing the preexisting resistant mutants as substrates for the ongoing production of virus. This may lead to the creation of individual virions with multiple resistance mutations. This scenario is most likely to occur in the context of so-called sequential monotherapy, whereby a single agent is added to an existing failing regimen. A common example of sequential monotherapy is the addition of indinavir to a failing regimen of zidovudine/lamivudine. In this case, resistance mutations to zidovudine and lamivudine already exist at the time indinavir is added. If the new regimen is only partially suppressive, mutations that confer resistance to indinavir begin to appear sequentially on the background of zidovudine and lamivudine resistance mutations, potentially leading to multidrug-resistant virions.[125]

The development of resistance is often an incremental process, perhaps best thought of as a function of chance; that is, the likelihood of resistance development is directly related to the degree of ongoing replication and the chance that a resistance mutant may be precisely the virus that infects a susceptible, activated CD4+ lymphocyte passing by at that moment in time. Even with regimens that are highly potent, yet not completely suppressive, a single point mutation may occur that confers partial reduction in susceptibility.[125,131] This results in a slightly higher degree of viral replication, thereby increasing the likelihood of the development of a second resistance-conferring mutation, leading to even further reduction in susceptibility and increased replication in the face of high selective pressure. Therefore mutations occurring after the first mutation often appear more rapidly because of the higher degree of replication that occurs after development of the first mutation. The resultant end-product is a highly resistant mutant that has multiple coexisting resistance mutations. From a clinical perspective, the more rapid acquisition of subsequent mutations suggests that regimens should be changed early in the course of virologic failure to avoid the development of higher-level resistance, assuming that viable therapeutic options exist for the patient in question.

Pharmacologic Aspects

For antiretroviral drugs to have activity in vivo, the drugs must be absorbed and delivered to the site where viral replication is occurring (e.g., CD4+ T-lymphocytes) and be appropriately processed by the target cell into an active

MUTATIONS IN THE REVERSE TRANSCRIPTASE GENE ASSOCIATED WITH RESISTANCE TO REVERSE TRANSCRIPTASE INHIBITORS

A. Nucleoside and Nucleotide Reverse Transcriptase Inhibitors

Agent	Codon	Wild type	Mutant
Multi-nRTI Resistance: 151 Complex	62	A	V
	75	V	I
	77	F	L
	116	F	Y
	151	Q	M
Multi-nRTI Resistance: 69 Insertion Complex[1]	41	M	L
	62	A	V
	67	D	N
	69	▼	insert
	70	K	R
	210	L	W
	215	T	Y, F
	219	K	Q, E
Multi-nRTI Resistance (NAMs)	41	M	L
	67	D	N
	70	K	R
	210	L	W
	215	T	Y, F
	219	K	Q, E
Zidovudine	41	M	L
	67	D	N
	70	K	R
	210	L	W
	215	T	Y, F
	219	K	Q, E
Didanosine	65	K	R
	74	L	V
	184	M	V
Zalcitabine	65	K	R
	69	T	D
	74	L	V
	184	M	V
Stavudine	41	M	L
	67	D	N
	70	K	R
	75	K	T, M, S, A
	210	L	W
	215	T	Y, F
	219	K	Q, E
Abacavir	41	M	L
	65	K	R
	67	D	N
	70	K	R
	74	L	V
	115	Y	F
	184	M	V
	210	L	W
	215	T	Y, F
	219	K	Q, E
Lamivudine	44	E	D
	118	V	I
	184	M	V, I
Tenofovir DF	65	K	R

B. Nonnucleoside Reverse Transcriptase Inhibitors

Agent	Codon	Wild type	Mutant
Multi-NNRTI Resistance	103	K	N
	188	Y	L
Multi-NNRTI Resistance (accumulation of mutations)	100	L	I
	106	V	A
	181	Y	C, I
	190	G	S, A
	230	M	L
Nevirapine	100	L	I
	103	K	N
	106	V	A
	108	V	I
	181	Y	C, I
	188	Y	C, L, H
	190	G	A
Delavirdine	103	K	N
	181	Y	C
	236	P	L
Efavirenz	100	L	I
	103	K	N
	108	V	I
	181	Y	C
	188	Y	L
	190	G	S
	225	P	H

Figure 27-8.

Illustration continued on following page

MUTATIONS IN THE PROTEASE GENE ASSOCIATED WITH RESISTANCE TO PROTEASE INHIBITORS

C. Protease Inhibitors

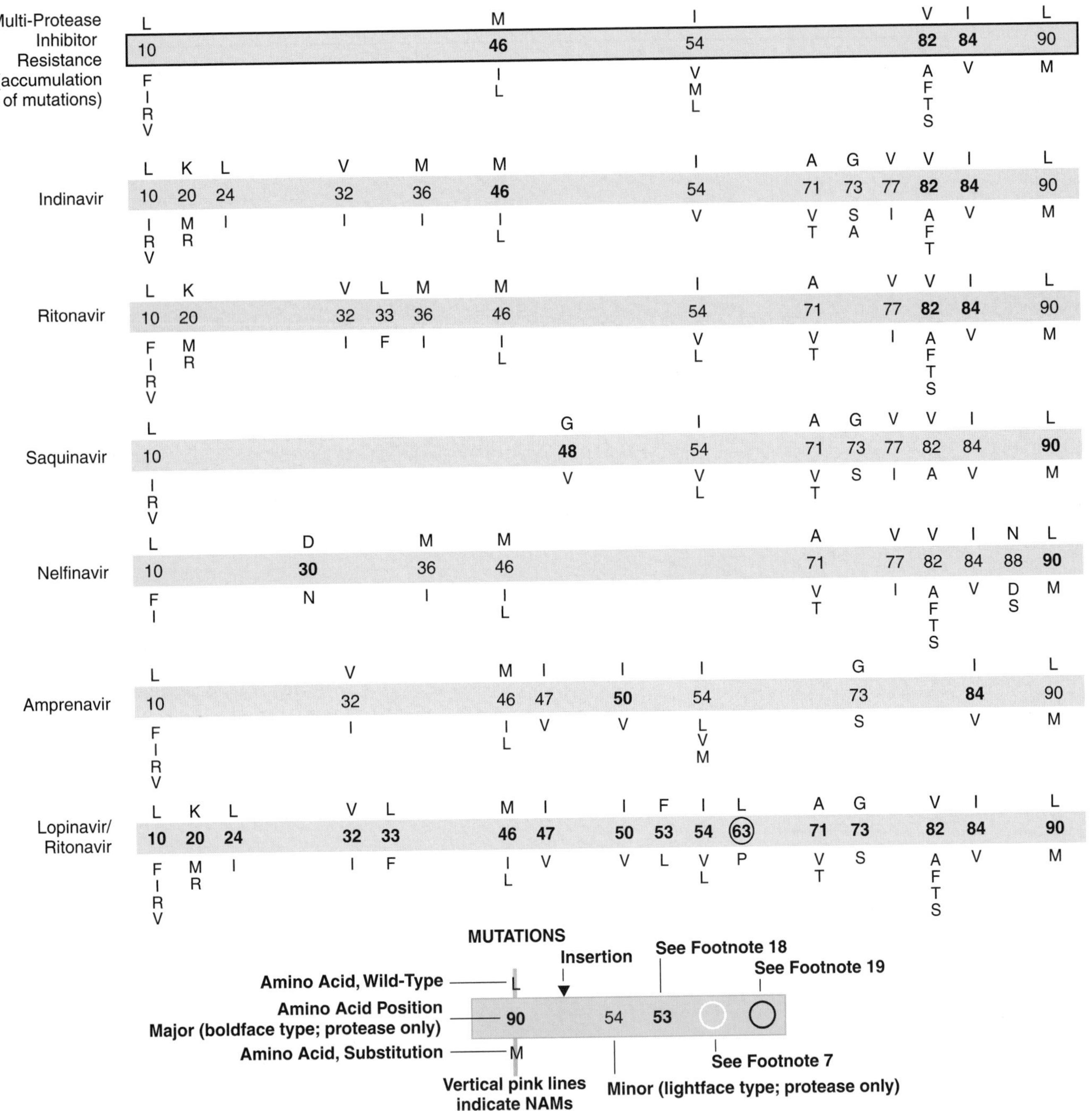

Figure 27–8. Common point mutations conferred by use of protease inhibitors (*A*), nucleoside reverse transcriptase inhibitors (*B*), and nonnucleoside reverse transcriptase inhibitors (*C*), mutations associated with decreased susceptibility to protease inhibitors. For each amino acid residue listed, the letter above the listing represents the wild-type virus, and the letter below the listing represents the mutation. Amino acids: A, alanine; C, cysteine; D, aspartate; E, glutamate; F, phenylalanine; G, glycine; H, histidine; I, isoleucine; K, lysine; L, leucine; M, methionine; N, asparagine; P, proline; Q, glutamine; R, arginine; S, serine; T, theronine; V, valine; W, tryptophan; Y, tyrosine. For full details of footnotes refer to article. (From International AIDS Society–USA. D'Aquila RT, Schapiro JM, Brun-Vézinet F, Clotet B, Conway B, Demeter LM, Grant RM, Johnson VA, Kuritzkes DR, Loveday C, Shafer RW, Richman DD. Drug resistance mutations in HIV-1. Topics HIV Med 2002; 10:11–15, with permission. Updates available at *www.iasusa.org*)

moiety (e.g., the triphosphate derivative of nucleosides). The relative amount of drug in plasma may or may not reflect the amount of drug at the active, intracellular site of replication; therefore measuring plasma levels may only partially describe the relative activity of an agent. Just like toxicity profiles and resistance patterns, each drug has its own unique characteristics of absorption, metabolism, tissue penetration (including penetration into various body compartments, such as the central nervous system), intracellular processing, intracellular half-life, and mechanism of elimination (including the first-pass effect; see Chapter 67). Not only is the pharmacologic profile unique for each agent, but the absorption and metabolic processing may vary from patient to patient. This interpatient variability becomes critical when interpreting data from studies that involve large populations of patients receiving combination antiretroviral regimens. Even when patients within a given population adhere completely to the regimen, a fixed-dose regimen of a drug given every 8 hours may lead to adequate concentrations at the target site for most individuals but be too low to sustain complete suppression in some or too high in others, resulting in early drug failure or excess toxicity, respectively.[132] Because most antiretroviral agents have narrow therapeutic windows, these issues become critical when trying to implement a strategy of complete suppression of viral replication for all patients. Thus many current studies focus on measuring drug levels as part of a strategy to achieve improved virologic outcome with less toxicity. To date, not enough data have been generated to recommend this approach in clinical practice.

Adherence

To achieve and *maintain* complete suppression of viral replication as a goal of therapy, patients must take all of the agents comprising a combination regimen at the prescribed time and under the proper conditions. Because of drug–drug interactions and the interference of food with the absorption of some agents, many patients must adhere to complicated regimens that require careful planning of meals, sometimes in conjunction with taking up to 20 to 30 tablets at different times during the day. Even the most dedicated and committed patients find it difficult to remember to take each pill as prescribed every day over several months to years. Based on experience with other chronic diseases, such as hypertension, up to one-third of patients are able to adhere to their regimen 90% of the time, but most patients adhere poorly or intermittently.[133–135] For diseases in which the consequences of nonadherence result in some degree of morbidity, such as the use of insulin in brittle diabetics, the adherence is much better but still not 100%. In most instances, HIV infection is more like hypertension than diabetes; that is, most individuals with HIV infection are relatively asymptomatic and even those with symptoms usually do not experience the consequences of missed doses of their medicines. Because the objective of therapy is to maintain complete suppression and to achieve this objective drug levels must remain above the IC_{90} at the target site throughout the entire viral life cycle, intermittent dosing that allows some degree of replication to occur in the face of high selective pressure becomes a recipe for the development of resistance and ultimate antiretroviral failure.

Several factors may contribute to poor or intermittent adherence. The most common factor is poor instructions given to the patient regarding the regimen and its possible adverse experiences.[135] The development of side effects and their severity have a significant impact on a patient's willingness to take medications as prescribed or to continue a given regimen. The degree to which a patient is willing to tolerate adverse effects of medications is related to several factors, including the nature of the side effect, how much it interferes with the patient's ability to carry on daily activities, the severity of the patient's underlying condition (the more serious the disease, the higher the rate of adherence), and the patient's belief that the regimen is likely to be effective.[136] Regimens given once or twice daily have a higher degree of adherence than three or four time a day regimens or those that require strict timing of drug administration in relation to meals. Other factors, such as level of education, socioeconomic status, and underlying substance abuse, generally do not predict adherence.[31]

▲ STRATEGIES FOR CHANGING THERAPY

Failure of antiretroviral therapy can generally be divided into two categories: failure resulting from toxicity and that resulting from virologic escape. The strategies for managing toxicity and virologic escape are quite different and are discussed separately.

Strategies for Changing Therapy Because of Toxicity

Toxicity may be due to a single agent in a regimen or to multiple agents. Adverse events may manifest either through the inherent toxicity of the offending agent(s), through additive toxicity between two or more agents, or through adverse drug–drug interactions. Even though most of the approved agents have been in widespread use for only a few years, the most common adverse experiences are well established and fairly distinctive for each drug. In cases where a side effect occurs that is commonly associated with a particular drug in the regimen, it is relatively easy to ascribe the toxicity to the most likely offending agent and adjust the regimen appropriately. However, in other cases, overlapping toxicities or uncommon side effects occur that are difficult to ascribe to a particular drug. In such cases it is best to stop all antiretroviral therapy, wait for the adverse effect to abate or decrease in severity, and reinstate therapy with a new regimen that substitutes one or more new drugs for the most likely offending agent(s).

When adjusting regimens because of toxic effects, several guidelines should be followed. When toxicities are noted within 2 to 4 weeks after initiating a new regimen, the most likely offending agent can be removed and a new drug without overlapping toxicity added to the remaining drugs in the regimen. For example, the development of rash from nevirapine usually occurs 14 to 28 days after initiating the regimen, in which case another agent of similar potency can be substituted into the regimen without changing the nucleoside backbone. Similarly, early manifestations of distal symmetric peripheral neuropathy (DSPN) in patients who are taking didanosine or stavudine or anemia among patients taking zidovudine should prompt the substitution of another NRTI for the offending agent. When toxicity to an agent develops weeks to months after the regimen had been initiated and the virologic response has achieved and maintained undetectable levels of virus, substitution of a new drug for the most likely offending agent is still an appropriate approach. In this case it is assumed that the existing regimen has suppressed viral replication sufficiently to prevent the development of resis-

▲ **Table 27–4.** REVIEW OF SWITCH STUDIES

Study	No.	Follow-Up (week)	TGs	Chol	Glu/IR	Body Change	Comments
2NRTI + PI → 2NRTI + efavirenz[139]	33	40	NC	NC	NC	NC	Subset analysis of a cohort of 624 patients evaluated for body fat, lipid, and glucose abnormalities
2NRTI + PI → 2NRTI + efavirenz[140]	39	24	~↑	NC	NC	NC	Virologic control maintained. Modest increase in HDL-cholesterol
2NRTI + PI → 2NRTI + efavirenz[141]	43	24	~↑	NC	—	NC	Viral load remained < 50 copies/ml in all patients. HDL-cholesterol unchanged
2NRTI + PI → 2NRTI + efavirenz[142]	25	24	~↓	NC	—	NC	Randomized to NVP, EFV, or control. Only 1 patient had rebound VL in NEV group vs. 2 EFV vs. 1 PI
2NRTI + PI → 2NRTI + efavirenz[143]	25	24	~↑	~↑	↓	~↓ VAT	All patients remained at < 500 copies/ml
2NRTI + PI → 2NRTI + efavirenz[144]	165	24	—	NC	—	—	Improvement in HDL-cholesterol in EFV group
2NRTI + PI → 2NRTI (+ ABC) + efavirenz[145]	27	36	~↓	~↓	~↓	NC	Some overall fat loss by BIA (2.5 kg), but no change in symptoms of fat redistribution. Virologic failure in 1 patient
2NRTI + PI → 2NRTI[146]	56	24	↓	↑ HDL	—	NC	No virologic failure. Some increase in lipoatrophy (5 patients)
2NRTI + PI → 2NRTI + efavirenz[147]	45	48	↓	~↓	—	—	Virologic failure in 2 patients
2NRTI + PI → 2NRTI + efavirenz[148]	20	24	NC	NC	NC	NC	No virologic failures. Subjective improvement in morphologic appearance but no change in anthropometric studies
2NRTI + PI → 2NRTI + efavirenz[149]	93	52	↓	NC	↓	↓ WHR ↓ VAT	Switch (46) vs. controls (47). Moderate increase in HDL with EFV; no difference in VL outcome. SQ fat loss no different
2NRTI + PI → 2NRTI + efavirenz[150]	41	52	—	—	NC	—	Patients with lipodystrophy syndrome; only IR and Glu tolerance evaluated
2NRTI + PI → 2NRTI + EFV or NVP[151]	100	52	↓	↓	—	NC	VL suppression maintained in 80%. No difference between EFV and NVP groups

tance-conferring mutations to the drugs remaining in the regimen as the regimen is changed. Perhaps the best example of this is the development of metabolic disturbances among patients taking a PI-containing regimen who replace the PI with an NNRTI agent or abacavir while maintaining the nucleoside backbone. Multiple small studies have been reported demonstrating successful maintenance of virologic control with improvement in lipid profiles but variable success in correcting insulin resistance or body composition abnormalities (Table 27–4). Conversely, when side effects are noted weeks to months after starting a regimen that has not successfully achieved an optimal virologic response, it is best to change at least two, and possibly all, of the agents in the regimen (including the drug most likely responsible for the adverse effect) based on resistance testing results because of concerns regarding rapid development of resistance to a new drug when it is added as "sequential monotherapy."

Strategies for Changing Therapy Because of Virologic Failure

Virologic failure may result from an inability to achieve the desired level of viral suppression initially defined or the return of plasma HIV RNA to unacceptable levels after having achieved and sustained the targeted degree of viral suppression for months or years previously. In either case, the existence of the undesirable plasma HIV RNA value should be confirmed with repeat testing before any change in therapy is initiated. This point has been emphasized with results from ACTG study 343, where solitary increases in viral load ("blips") up to 1000 copies per milliliter were noted among several patients who had otherwise maintained undetectable levels of virus.[137,138] The blips were not associated with an increased risk of long-term virologic failure or with an increased risk of developing resistance. Even patients who experienced several blips during the course of the study had no apparent long-term adverse consequences.

Once an elevated plasma HIV RNA level has been confirmed, resistance testing can help identify which drugs, if any, may be contributing to the rebounding viral load (Table 27–5) (see Chapter 26).[15] The absence of resistance mutations in the face of rising viral load implies problems with adherence or potential pharmacologic difficulties, such as poor absorption, increased metabolism (possibly due to a drug–drug interaction), decreased intracellular processing, or increased extrusion of drug from the intracellular compartment (e.g., as occurs with induction of P-glycopeptide pumps). When only one of the drugs in the regimen has induced detectable resistance mutations, changing more

Table 27–4. REVIEW OF SWITCH STUDIES *Continued*

Study	No.	Follow-Up (week)	TGs	Chol	Glu/IR	Body Change	Comments
2NRTI + PI → 2NRTI + nevirapine[152]	23	24	↓	↓	↓	↓ WHR	Diet not reported
2NRTI + PI → 2NRTI + nevirapine[153]	138	24	~↓	~↓	—	~↓	Rebound in HIV RNA occurred more often in PI group than NVP group (29% vs. 11%; $P < 0.5$)
2NRTI + PI → 2NRTI + nevirapine[154]	60	36	↓	↓	NC	NC	Randomized study. Virologic failure: 4 NVP, 3 PI
2NRTI + PI → 2NRTI + NVP + adefovir + OH-urea[155]	80	24	↓	↓	NC	↓ VAT	Randomized (2:3) study. No effect on HDL-cholesterol. Virologic failure: 3 (6%) exp, 6 (19%) PI. Intolerance in 15 exp. patients
2NRTI + PI → 2NRTI + NVP or 2NRTI + EFV[156]	116	12	~↓	NC	↓	NC	Offered switch to NNRTI due to intolerance of PI; 67% < 200 copies/ml at switch. No change in viral load
2NRTI + PI → 2NRTI + nevirapine[157]	40	48	↓	NC	↓	NC	Severe rash in 6 patients; therapy changed to EFV. One patient with virologic failure
2NRTI + PI → 2NRTI + nevirapine[142]	26	24	↓	↓	—	NC	Randomized to NVP, EFV, or control. Only 1 patient had rebound VL in NVP group vs. 2 EFV and 1 control
2NRTI + PI → 2NRTI + nevirapine[158]	63	60	↓	NC	—	NC	Nonrandomized; 10 patients received EFZ, 63 NVP. Infrequent virologic failure. CD4+ T-lymphocyte count increase of 82 cells/μl
2NRTI + PI → 2NRTI + nevirapine[159]	68	24	~↓	NC	—	—	Virologic failure in 4 cases. Modest CD4+ T-lymphocyte increase
d4T → ZDV or ABC[160]	59	36	↓	NC	NC	↓ SAT VAT NC	Some patients (n = 18) on dual NRTI; remainder (n = 41) on PI/NRTI. Lactate declined significantly
2NRTI + PI → 2NRTI + ABC[161]	211	24	~↓	↓	↓	—	Randomized to continue PI or not. Failures: ABC (9; 3 virologic); PI (14; 2 virologic)
2NRTI + PI → 2NRTI + ABC[162]	163	52	↓	↓	—	—	Randomized to continue PI or not. Virologic failures: ABC (11), PI (5)
2NRTI + PI → 2NRTI + ABC[163]	105	45	~↓	~↓	—	—	Randomized to continue PI (106) or not (105). Virologic failures: ABC (4) vs. PI (2)

ABC, abacavir; BIA, bioelectrical impedence analysis; Chol, cholesterol; d4T, stavudine; EFV, efavirenz; exp, experimental; Glu/IR, glucose/insulin resistance; HDL, high density lipoprotein; NC, no change; NNRTI, nonnucleoside reverse transcriptase inhibitor; NR, not reported; NRTI, nucleoside reverse transcriptase inhibitor; NVP, nevirapine; PI, protease inhibitor; VL, viral load; SAT, subcutaneous adipose tissue; 3TC, lamivudine; TGs, triglycerides; VAT, visceral adipose tissue; WHR, waist hip ratio; ZDV, zidovudine; —, not done; ↑ or ↓, significant increase or decrease; ~↑ or ~↓, nonsignificant trend of increase or decrease.

than the single drug should be considered because there may be low-level resistance to the other agents in the form of subpopulations. The activity of the next regimen should be at least as potent as the original regimen and ideally of more potency. In the absence of resistance testing, failure should be associated with the entire regimen rather than attempting to ascribe the failure to a particular drug in the regimen. In general, intensification with the addition of a single agent added to a failing regimen should be avoided except in circumstances where a substantial reduction in viral load has been achieved but not to undetectable levels within 16 to 20 weeks of initiating therapy. Even when these conditions are met, great care should be used to ensure that the persistent detectable viral load is not due to problems with adherence, which would be aggravated with the addition of yet another pill to take. The addition of single new drugs, "sequential monotherapy," is less likely to achieve either the targeted virologic effect or a durable response and more likely to lead to the development of multidrug-resistant isolates. Conversely, in cases where adherence is judged to be the reason for failure, the substitution of ritonavir-boosted PIs (e.g., low-dose ritonavir added to saquinavir, indinavir, amprenavir, or lopinavir) for single PIs enable the regimen to be given less frequently. Several studies with regimens of dual PIs given twice daily have reported comparable virologic results, lower total drug costs, greater tolerability, and improved adherence.

Selection of the next regimen must be individualized based, in relatively equal parts, on the last regimen, the resistance test results obtained while the patient is still taking the failing regimen, and prior exposure to other agents, with emphasis on tolerability and potential residual resistant (archived) viruses that are being harbored in latently infected cells. As when selecting the initial regimen, consideration must be given to what the patient is willing to take and likely to tolerate. In situations where options are limited because of previous toxicity or prior failure of available agents, it may be necessary to "recycle" an antiretroviral drug back into a new regimen. When this is necessary, it is best to use agents that have not been utilized in the last two or three regimens and to avoid recycling two or three agents from a single previous regimen back together. Ideally, the new regimen should consist of two or more agents deemed to be active, preferably with drugs that have not been used together in previous regimens. Pharmacokinetic enhancement, such as boosting

▲ **Table 27–5.** COMPARISON OF GENOTYPIC AND PHENOTYPIC
▲ RESISTANCE ASSAYS

Issues	Genotypic Assays	Phenotypic Assays
Availability	Generally available	Restricted availability
Time to results	Days	Weeks
Technical issues	Straightforward	Demanding
Susceptibility measurement	Indirect	Direct
Sensitivity (minor species)	Poor	Poor
Interpretation	Complex	Straightforward
Cost	Moderately expensive	Expensive
Major limitations	May not correlate with phenotype	Cutoff values poorly defined

PI levels with low-dose ritonavir, should be exploited whenever possible in the setting of multiple-regimen failure. The use of multidrug (six or more drugs) rescue therapy has shown variable antiretroviral activity.[164–166] However, this approach often leads to substantial toxicity and problems with adherence, drug–drug interactions, and cost.

Use of a "supervised" treatment interruption (STI) may be of clinical benefit among patients with multidrug-resistant mutations in an attempt to exploit the rapid reversion to wild-type viruses in this setting.[167–169] Such a strategy should be undertaken with great caution owing to the rapid increase in viral load and marked reduction in CD4+ T-lymphocyte count in association with reversion to wild-type virus around week 8 of the STI.[167] Therefore frequent assessments should be performed during the STI with early resumption of treatment with any sign of plummeting CD4+ T-lymphocyte count.

On occasion, patients present with a "discordant" response, whereby the viral load is successfully suppressed but the CD4+ T-lymphocyte count fails to increase. Several options exist for managing a "discordant" response, but because the reasons for the discordant responses are not well understood there is no clearly defined or optimal approach to management. Drug-related toxic effects, inhibition of de novo CD4+ T-lymphocyte synthesis, sequestration of cells within lymphoid tissue, and interference with clonal expansion of memory CD4+ T-lymphocytes have been proposed as potential mechanisms. The approach to management depends on the suspected reason for the discordant response. For example, substituting specific drugs in the regimen, removing potentially cytotoxic drugs, and eliminating hydroxyurea-containing regimens are valid options when bone marrow toxicity is suspected. Alternatively, the use of cytokines, such as IL-2 or granulocyte- and granulocyte/macrophage colony-stimulating factors, are potential approaches to expand the cell populations directly. Although there are not enough data to recommend cytokine therapy at this time, many clinicians are using trials of IL-2 (3.0 to 4.5 million units twice daily for 5 days every 2 months) in an attempt to raise the CD4+ T-lymphocyte counts among patients who have achieved successful suppression of HIV but have persistently low CD4+ T-lymphocyte counts (e.g., < 100 cells per microliter). Prior to attempting to use IL-2, clinicians must be thoroughly familiar with the use of IL-2 and the management of its complications (see Chapter 21).

The use of therapeutic drug monitoring (TDM) has been proposed as a means of enhancing virologic outcomes and assessing reasons for virologic failure or toxicity (see Chapter 67). TDM is a process whereby drug levels are measured at fixed time intervals after a dose of medicine has been ingested. The PK curve of a given drug can be modeled with as few as one or two measurements. Once determined, the peak and trough levels can be calculated and used to assess the likelihood of virologic suppression or development of toxicity. Although the concept is attractive on face value, multiple assumptions limit the usefulness of TDM in practice. For example, to model accurately, the time of dosing must be known precisely. Relying on verbal reports of dosing is inaccurate. Moreover, the modeling assumes that the patient is at steady state, which means that all previous doses were taken correctly and on time, which may not be the case. The modeling is inaccurate if it utilizes levels determined on samples obtained within the first 2 hours (absorption/distribution phase) of dosing; therefore, only levels for samples obtained "post-peak" can be used. Because TDM is based solely on plasma levels, there is no consideration for intracellular drug concentrations or intracellular processing, creating further limitations of the technique. Nonetheless, TDM can be a useful adjunct to therapy when assessing the possibility of nonadherence or poor absorption (e.g., absence of drug in the bloodstream) or in cases of extremely advanced disease where higher doses of drug are being considered to maximize antiretroviral benefit. Outside of these two circumstances, TDM remains a research tool.

Except in cases of toxicity, it is preferable to continue even "failing" drug regimens that maintain selective pressure on the viruses rather than permanently discontinuing all antiretroviral therapy, especially in settings in which the CD4+ T-lymphocyte counts are maintained despite a rebound in viral replication. In cases where the regimen is changed, the same concepts of defining the target plasma RNA values that define success and failure of the regimen in the current clinical setting still apply and should be discussed with the patient.

REFERENCES

1. Carpenter CCJ, Cooper DA, Fischl MA, et al. Antiretroviral therapy for HIV infection in adults: updated recommendations of the International AIDS Society—USA panel. JAMA 283:381–390, 2000.
2. National Institutes of Health Panel to Define Principles of Therapy of HIV Infection. Guidelines for the use of antiretroviral agents in HIV-infected adults and adolescents. Ann Intern Med 128: 1079–1100, 1998.
3. Gazzard B, Moyle G, BHIVA Guidelines Writing Committee. 1998. Revision to the British HIV Association guidelines for antiretroviral treatment of HIV seropositive individuals. Lancet 352:314–316, 1998.
4. US Department of Health and Human Services Panel on Clinical Practices for Treatment of HIV Infection. Guidelines for the Use of Antiretroviral Agents in HIV-1 Infected Adults and Adolescents. Washington, DC, DHHS, 2001, www.hivatis.org/trtgdlns.html.
5. US Department of Health and Human Services Panel on Clinical Practices for Treatment of HIV Infection. Guidelines for the Use of Antiretroviral Agents in HIV-1 Infected Adults and Adolescents. MMWR Morb Mortal Wkly Rep 47(RR-5):1–41, 1998.

6. Wei X, Ghosh SK, Taylor ME, et al. Viral dynamics in HIV-1 infection. Nature 373:117–122, 1995.
7. Ho DD, Neumann AU, Perelson AS, et al. Rapid turnover of plasma virions and CD4+ lymphocytes in HIV-1 infection. Nature 373: 123–126, 1995.
8. Coffin JM. HIV population dynamics in vivo: implications for genetic variation, pathogenesis, and therapy. Science 267:483–489, 1995.
9. Wain-Hobson S. AIDS: virological mayhem. Nature 373:102, 1995.
10. Saag MS, Holodniy M, Kuritzkes DR, et al. HIV viral load markers in clinical practice. Nat Med 2:625–629, 1996.
11. Holodniy M, Katzenstein DA, Sengupta S. Detection and quantification of human immunodeficiency virus RNA in patient serum by use of the polymerase chain reaction. J Infect Dis 163:862–866, 1991.
12. Piatak M, Saag MS, Yang LC, et al. High levels of HIV-1 in plasma during all stages of infection determined by competitive PCR. Science 259:1749–1754, 1993.
13. Piatak M Jr, Saag MS, Yang LC, et al. Determination of plasma viral load in HIV-1 infection by quantitative competitive polymerase chain reaction. AIDS 7 (suppl 2):S65–S71, 1993.
14. Cao Y, Ho DD, Todd J, et al. Clinical evaluation of branched DNA signal amplification for quantifying HIV type 1 in human plasma. AIDS Res Hum Retroviruses 11:353–361, 1995.
15. Hirsch MS, Conway B, D'Aquila RT, et al. Antiretroviral drug resistance testing in adult HIV-1 infection: recommendations of an International AIDS Society—USA panel. JAMA 283:2417–2426, 2000.
16. Hogg RS, Heath KV, Yip B, et al. Improved survival among HIV-infected individuals following initiation of antiretroviral therapy. JAMA 279:450–454, 1998.
17. Palella FJ, Delaney KM, Moorman AC, et al. Declining morbidity and mortality among patients with advanced human immunodeficiency virus infection. N Engl J Med 338:853–860, 1998.
18. Palella F, Moorman A, Chmiel J, et al. Continued low morbidity and mortality among patients with advanced HIV infection and their patterns of highly active antiretroviral therapy (HAART) usage. Presented at the 7th Conference on Retroviruses and Opportunistic Infections, 2000, p 216.
19. Carr A, Samaras K, Burton S, et al. A syndrome of peripheral lipodystrophy, hyperlipidaemia and insulin resistance in patients receiving HIV protease inhibitors. AIDS 12:F51–F58, 1998.
20. Carr A, Miller J, Law M, Cooper DA. A syndrome of lipoatrophy, lactic acidaemia and liver dysfunction associated with HIV nucleoside analogue therapy: contribution to protease inhibitor-related lipodystrophy syndrome. AIDS 14:F25–F32, 2000.
21. Carr A, Samaras K, Chisholm DJ, Cooper DA. Pathogenesis of HIV-1-protease inhibitor-associated peripheral lipodystrophy, hyperlipidaemia, and insulin resistance. Lancet 351:1881–1883, 1998.
22. Yarasheski KE, Tebas P, Sigmund C, et al. Insulin resistance in HIV protease inhibitor-associated diabetes. J Acquir Immune Defic Syndr 21:209–216, 1999.
23. Schambelan M, Benson C, Carpenter CCJ, et al. Metabolic complications guidelines: recommendation of the International AIDS Society—USA panel. J AIDS (in press).
24. Masur H, Miller KD, Jones EC, et al. High prevalence of avascular necrosis (AVN) of the hip in HIV infection: magnetic resonance imaging of 339 asymptomatic patients. Presented at the 38th Annual Meeting of the Infectious Diseases Society of America, 2000.
25. Hockett RD, Kilby JM, Derdeyn CA, et al. Constant mean viral copy number per infected cell in tissues regardless of high, low, or undetectable plasma HIV RNA. J Exp Med 189:1545–1559, 1999.
26. Zhang L, Ramratnam B, Tenner-Racz K, et al. Quantifying residual HIV-1 replication in patients receiving combination antiretroviral therapy. N Engl J Med 340:1605–1613, 1999.
27. Acosta EP, Henry K, Baken L, et al. Indinavir concentrations and antiviral effect. Pharmacotherapy 19:708–712, 1999.
28. Acosta EP, Kakuda TN, Brundage RC, et al. Pharmacodynamics of human immunodeficiency virus type 1 protease inhibitors. Clin Infect Dis 30(suppl 2):S151–S159, 2000.
29. Sommadossi JP, Zhou XJ, Moore J, et al. Impairment of stavudine phosphorylation in patients receiving a combination of zidovudine and stavudine. Presented at the 5th Conference on Retroviruses and Opportunistic Infections, 1998.
30. Hsu A, Granneman GR, Bertz RJ. Ritonavir-clinical pharmacokinetics and interactions with other anti-HIV agents. Clin Pharmacokinet 35: 275–291, 1998.
31. Chesney MA, Morin M, Sherr L. Adherence to HIV combination therapy. Soc Sci Med 50:1599–1605, 2000.
32. Shaw GM, Harper ME, Hahn BH, et al. HTLV-III infection in brains of children and adults with AIDS encephalopathy. Science 227: 177–181, 1985.
33. Bagasra O, Lavi E, Bobroski L. Cellular reservoirs of HIV-1 in the central nervous system of infected individuals: identification by the combination of in situ polymerase chain reaction and immunohistochemistry. AIDS 10:573–585, 1996.
34. Coombs RW, Welles SL, Hooper C. Association of plasma human immunodeficiency virus type-1 RNA level with risk of clinical progression in patients with advanced infection. J Infect Dis 174:704–712, 1996.
35. Daar ES, Moudgil T, Meyer RD, Ho DD. Transient high levels of viremia in patients with primary human immunodeficiency virus type 1 infection. N Engl J Med 324:961–964, 1991.
36. Clark SJ, Saag MS, Decker WD, et al. High titers of cytopathic virus in plasma of patients with symptomatic primary HIV-1 infection. N Engl J Med 324:954–960, 1991.
37. Ho DD, Moudgil T, Alam M. Quantitation of human immunodeficiency virus type 1 in the blood of infected persons. N Engl J Med 321:1621–1625, 1989.
38. Saag MS, Crain MJ, Decker WD. High-level viremia in adults and children infected with human immunodeficiency virus: relation to disease stage and CD4+ lymphocyte levels. J Infect Dis 164:72–80, 1991.
39. Clark SJ, Shaw GM. Acute retroviral syndrome and the pathogenesis of HIV-1 infection. Semin Immunol 5:149–155, 1993.
40. Schacker T, Hughes JP, Shea T, et al. Biological and virologic characteristics of primary HIV infection. Ann Intern Med 128:613–620, 1998.
41. Kappes JC, Saag MS, Shaw GM, et al. Assessment of antiretroviral therapy by plasma viral load testing: standard and ICD HIV-1 p24 antigen and viral RNA (QC-PCR) assays compared. Acquir Immune Defic Syndr Hum Retrovir 10:139–149, 1995.
42. Saag MS, Emini EA, Laskin OL. Short-term clinical evaluation of L-697,661, a nonnucleoside inhibitor of HIV-1 reverse transcriptase. N Engl J Med 329:1065–1072, 1993.
43. Perelson AS, Neumann AU, Markowitz M, et al. HIV-1 dynamics in vivo: virion clearance rate, infected cell life-span, and viral generation time. Science 271:1582–1586, 1996.
44. Perelson AS, Essunger P, Cao Y, et al. Decay characteristics of HIV-1 infected compartments during combination therapy. Nature 387: 188–191, 1997.
45. Perelson AS, Essunger P, Ho DD. Dynamics of HIV-1 and CD4 lymphocytes in vivo. AIDS 11(suppl A):517–524, 1997.
46. Fauci AS. Host factors and the pathogenesis of HIV-induced disease. Nature 384:529–534, 1996.
47. Chun TW, Fauci AS. Latent reservoirs of HIV: obstacles to the eradication of virus. Proc Natl Acad Sci USA 96:10958–10961, 1999.
48. Wong JK, Gunthard HF, Havlir DV, et al. Reduction of HIV in blood and lymph nodes after potent antiretroviral therapy and the virologic correlates of treatment failure. Proc Natl Acad Sci USA 94: 12574–12579, 1997.
49. Dybul M, Chun TW, Ward DJ, et al. Evaluation of lymph node virus burden in human immunodeficiency virus-infected patients receiving efavirenz-based protease inhibitor–sparing highly active antiretroviral therapy. J Infect Dis 181:1273–1279, 2000.
50. Boucher C, Nijhuis M, Schipper P, et al. Reduction of HIV in blood and lymph nodes after potent antiretroviral therapy. Presented at the 4th Conference on Retroviruses and Opportunistic Infections, 1997.
51. Cavert W, Notermans DW, Staskus K, et al. Kinetics of response in lymphoid tissues to antiretroviral therapy of HIV-1 infection. Science 276:960–964, 1997.
52. Nelson PW, Mittler JE, Perelson A. Effect of drug efficacy and the eclipse phase of the viral life cycle on estimates of HIV viral dynamic parameters. J Acquir Defic Syndr Hum Retrovir 26:405–412, 2001.
53. Mellors JW, Rinaldo CR Jr, Gupta P, et al. Prognosis in HIV-1 infection predicted by the quantity of virus in plasma. Science 272: 1167–1170, 1996.
54. Mellors JW, Munoz AM, Giorgi JV, et al. Plasma viral load and CD4+ lymphocytes as prognostic markers of HIV-1 infection. Ann Intern Med 126:946–954, 1997.
55. Ferguson NM, deWolf F, Ghani AC, et al. Antigen-driven CD4+ T cell and HIV-1 dynamics: residual viral replication under highly ac-

tive antiretroviral therapy. Proc Natl Acad Sci USA 96:15167–15172, 1999.

56. Finzi D, Siliciano RF. Viral dynamics in HIV-1 infection. Cell 93: 665–671, 1998.
57. Ho DD. Time to hit HIV, early and hard. N Engl J Med 333:450–451, 1995.
58. Autran B, Carcelain G, Li TS, et al. Positive effects of combined antiretroviral therapy on CD4+ T cell homeostasis and function in advanced HIV disease. Science 277:112–116, 1997.
59. Bucy RP. Immune clearance of HIV type 1 replication-active cells: a model of two patterns of steady state HIV infection. AIDS Res Hum Retroviruses 15:223–227, 1999.
60. Saag MS, Kilby JM. HIV-1 and HAART: a time to cure, a time to kill. Nat Med 5:609–611, 1999.
61. Rosenberg ES, Billingsley JM, Caliendo AM, et al. Vigorous HIV-1-specific CD4+ T cell responses associated with control of viremia. Science 278:1447–1450, 1997.
62. Rosenberg ES, Walker BD. HIV type 1-specific helper T cells: a critical host defense. AIDS Res Hum Retroviruses 14(suppl 2): S143–S147, 1998.
63. Rosenberg ES, Altfeld M, Poon SH, et al. Immune control of HIV-1 after early treatment of acute infection. Nature 407:523–526, 2000.
64. Davey RT Jr, Bhat N, Yoder C, et al. HIV-1 and T cell dynamics after interruption of highly active antiretroviral therapy (HAART) in patients with a history of sustained viral suppression. Proc Natl Acad Sci USA 96:15109–15114, 1999.
65. Ruiz L, Martinez-Picado J, Romeu J, et al. Structured treatment interruption in chronically HIV-1 infected patients after long-term viral suppression. AIDS 14:397–403, 2000.
66. Borrow P, Lewicki H, Wei X, et al. Antiviral pressure exerted by HIV-1-specific cytotoxic T lymphocytes (CTLs) during primary infection demonstrated by rapid selection of CTL escape virus. Nat Med 3: 205–211, 1997.
67. Borrow P, Lewicki H, Hahn BH, et al. Virus-specific CD8+ cytotoxic T-lymphocyte activity associated with control of viremia in primary human immunodeficiency virus type 1 infection. J Virol 68: 6103–6110, 1994.
68. Altfeld M, Rosenberg ES, Mukherjee J, et al. Enhancement of HIV-1 specific CTL responses during structured treatment interuptions (STI) following treated acute HIV-1-infection is associated with control of HIV-1 viremia. Presented at the XIII International AIDS Conference, 2000.
69. Walker CM, Moody DJ, Stites DP, Levy JA. CD8+ lymphocytes can control HIV infection in vitro by suppressing virus replication. Science 234:1563–1566, 1986.
70. Mclean AR, Michie CA. In vivo estimates of division and death rates of human T-lymphocytes. Proc Natl Acad Sci USA 92:3707–3711, 1995.
71. Chun TW, Carruth L, Finzi D, et al. Quantification of latent tissue reservoirs and total body fat viral load in HIV-1 infection. Nature 387: 183–188, 1997.
72. Wong JK, Hezareh M, Gunthard HF, et al. Recovery of replication-competent HIV despite prolonged suppression of plasma viremia. Science 278:1291–1295, 1997.
73. Finzi D, Hermankova M, Pierson T, et al. Identification of a reservoir for HIV-1 in patients on highly active antiretroviral therapy. Science 278:1295–1300, 1997.
74. Deeks SG, Hecht FM, Swanson M, et al. HIV RNA and CD4 cell count response to protease inhibitor therapy in an urban AIDS clinic: response to both initial and salvage therapy. AIDS 13:F35–F43, 1999.
75. Hammer SM, Squires KE, Hughes MD, et al. A controlled trial of two nucleoside analogues plus indinavir in persons with human immunodeficiency virus infection and CD4 cell counts of 200/μl or less. N Engl J Med 337:725–733, 1997.
76. Gulick RM, Mellors JW, Havlir D, et al. Treatment with indinavir, zidovudine, and lamivudine in adults with human immunodeficiency virus infection and prior antiretroviral therapy. N Engl J Med 337: 734–739, 1997.
77. Chaisson RE, Keruly JC, Moore RD. Association of initial CD4 cell count and viral load with response to highly active antiretroviral therapy. JAMA 284:3128–3129, 2000.
78. Hogg RS, Yip B, Wood E, et al. Diminished effectiveness of antiretroviral therapy among patients initiating therapy with CD4+ cell counts below 200/mm^3. Presented at the 8th Conference on Retroviruses and Opportunistic Infections, 2001.
79. Moore R, Keruly J, Bartlett J, Chaisson R. Start HAART early (CD4 > 350 cells/μl) or later? Evidence for greater effectiveness if started early. Presented at the 7th Conference on Retroviruses and Opportunistic Infections, 2000, p 174.
80. Marschner IC, Collier AC, Coombs RW, et al. Use of changes in plasma levels of human immunodeficiency virus type 1 RNA to assess clinical benefit to antiretroviral therapy. J Infect Dis 177:40–47, 1998.
81. Yerly S, Kaiser L, Perneger TV, et al. Time of initiation of antiretroviral therapy: impact on HIV-1 viraemia: the Swiss HIV Cohort Study. AIDS 14:243–249, 2000.
82. Chun TW, Davey RT Jr, Ostrowski M, et al. Relationship between pre-existing viral reservoirs and the re-emergence of plasma viremia after discontinuation of highly active anti-retroviral therapy. Nat Med 6:757–761, 2000.
83. Kempf DJ, Rode RA, Xu Y, et al. The duration of viral suppression during protease inhibitor therapy for HIV-1 infection is predicted by plasma HIV-1 RNA at the nadir. AIDS 12:F9–F14, 1998.
84. Clerici M, Levin JM, Kessler HA. HIV-specific T-helper activity in seronegative health care workers exposed to contaminated blood. JAMA 271:42–46, 1994.
85. Centers for Disease Control and Prevention. Public health service guidelines for the management of health-care worker exposures to HIV and recommendations for post-exposure prophylaxis. MMWR Morb Mortal Wkly Rep 47(RR-7):1–33, 1998.
86. Connor EM, Sperling RS, Gelber R, et al. Reduction of maternal-infant transmission of human immunodeficiency virus type 1 with zidovudine treatment: Pediatric AIDS Clinical Trials Group Protocol 076 Study Group. N Engl J Med 331:1173–1180, 1994.
87. Saag MS, Schooley RT. Initiation of antiretroviral therapy: current controversies in when and with what to start. Top HIV Med 8(4): 8–13, 2000.
88. Deeks S, Barbour J, Martin JN, et al. Sustained CD4+ T cell response after virologic failure of protease inhibitor-based regimens in patients with human immunodeficiency virus infection. J Infect Dis 181: 946–953, 2000.
89. Deeks SG, Barbour JD, Martin JN, Grant RM. Delayed immunologic deterioration among patients who virologically fail protease inhibitor-based therapy. Presented at the 7th Conference on Retroviruses and Opportunistic Infections, 2000, p 120.
90. Emini EA, Graham DJ, Gotlib L. HIV and multidrug resistance. Nature 364:679, 1993.
91. Richman DD. Resistance of clinical isolates of human immunodeficiency virus to antiretroviral agents. Antimicrob Agents Chemother 37:1207–1213, 1993.
92. Richman DD, Havlir D, Corbeil J, et al. Nevirapine resistance mutations of human immunodeficiency virus type 1 selected during therapy. J Virol 68:1660–1666, 1994.
93. Bangsberg DR, Hecht FM, Charlebois ED, et al. Adherence to protease inhibitors, HIV-1 viral load, and development of drug resistance in an indigent population. AIDS 14:357–366, 2000.
94. Arnsten J, Demas P, Gourevitch M, et al. Adherence and viral load in HIV-infected drug users: comparison of self-report and medication event monitors (MEMS). Presented at the 7th Conference on Retroviruses and Opportunistic Infections, 2000, p 88.
95. Carr A, Samaras K, Thorisdottir A, et al. Diagnosis, prediction, and natural course of HIV-1 protease inhibitor-associated lipodystrophy, hyperlipidaemia, and diabetes mellitus: a cohort study. Lancet 353: 2093–2099, 1999.
96. Hadigan C, Meigs JB, Corcoran C, et al. Metabolic abnormalities and cardiovascular disease risk factors in adults with human immunodeficiency virus infection and lipodystrophy. Clin Infect Dis 32: 130–139, 2001.
97. Blacksin MF, Kloser PC, Simon J. Avascular necrosis of bone in human immunodeficiency virus infected patients. Clin Imaging 23: 314–318, 1999.
98. Brinkman K, Smeitink JA, Romijn JA, Reiss P. Mitochondrial toxicity induced by nucleoside-analogue reverse-transcriptase inhibitors is a key factor in the pathogenesis of antiretroviral-therapy-related lipodystrophy. Lancet 354:1112–1115, 1999.
99. Tebas P, Powderly WG, Claxton S, et al. Accelerated bone mineral loss in HIV-infected patients receiving potent antiretroviral therapy. AIDS 14:F63–F67, 2000.

100. Hoy J, Hudson J, Law M, Cooper DA. Osteopenia in a randomized multicenter study of protease inhibitor (PI) substitution in patients with the lipodystrophy syndrome and well-controlled HIV viremia. Presented at the 7th Conference on Retroviruses and Opportunistic Infections, 2000, p 114.
101. Glesby MJ, Hoover PR, Vaamonde CM. Osteonecrosis in patients infected with HIV: A case-control study. J Infect Dis 184:519–523, 2001.
102. Fletcher CV, Anderson PL, Kakuda TN, et al. A novel approach to integrate pharmacologic and virologic characteristics: an in vivo potency (IVP) index for antiretroviral agents. Presented at the 8th Conference on Retroviruses and Opportunistic Infections, 2001.
103. Flexner C, Speck RR. Role of multidrug transporters in HIV pathogenesis. Presented at the 8th Conference on Retroviruses and Opportunistic Infections, 2001, p 281.
104. Chen R, Westfall A, Cloud G, et al. Long-term survival after initiation of antiretroviral therapy. Presented at the 8th Conference on Retroviruses and Opportunistic Infections, 2001.
105. Henry K. The case for more cautious, patient-focused antiretroviral therapy. Ann Intern Med 132:306–322, 2000.
106. Staszewski S, Morales-Ramirez J, Tashima KT, et al. Efavirenz plus zidovudine and lamivudine, efavirenz plus indinavir, and indinavir plus zidovudine and lamivudine in the treatment of HIV-1 infection in adults: study 006 team. N Engl J Med 341:1865–1873, 1999.
107. Acosta EP, Gulick R, Katzenstein D, et al. Pharmacokinetic (PK) evaluation of saquinavir soft gel capsules (SQV)/ritonavir (RTV) or SQV/nelfinavir (NFV) in combination with delavirdine (DLV) and/or adefovir dipivoxil (ADV)—ACTG 359. Presented at the 6th Conference on Retroviruses and Opportunistic Infections, 1999.
108. Andrade A, Flexner C. HIV-related drug metabolism and cytochrome P450 enzymes. AIDS Clin Care 12:91–95, 2000.
109. Benson C, Brun S, King M, et al. Two year follow-up of ABT378/ritonavir (ABT-378/r) in antiretroviral naive HIV+ patients. Presented at the 40th Interscience Conference on Antimicrobial Agents and Chemotherapy, 2000, p 282.
110. Cameron DW, Japour AJ, Xu Y, et al. Ritonavir and saquinavir combination therapy for the treatment of HIV infection. AIDS 13: 213–224, 1999.
111. Casado JL, Moreno A, Marti-Belda P, et al. Increased indinavir levels using twice daily ritonavir/indinavir at 100/800 mg improves virological response even after multiple failure. Presented at the 40th Interscience Conference on Antimicrobial Agents and Chemotherapy, 2000, p 301.
112. Bartlett JA, DeMasi R, Quinn J, et al. Overview of the effectiveness of triple combination therapy in antiretroviral-naive HIV-1 infected adults. AIDS 15:1369–1377, 2001.
113. Kirkland LR, Fischl MA, Tashira KT, et al. Response to lamivudine-zidovudine plus abacavir twice daily in ART-NAIVE, incarcerated patients with HIV taking directly observed treatment. Clin Infect Dis 34: 511–518, 2002.
114. Havlir DV, Hellmann NS, Petropoulos CJ, et al. Drug susceptibility in HIV infection after viral rebound in patients receiving indinavir-containing regimens. JAMA 283:229–234, 2000.
115. Carpenter CCJ, Fischl MA, Hammer SM, et al. Antiretroviral therapy for HIV infection in 1998: updated recommendations of the International AIDS Society—USA panel. JAMA 280:78–86, 1998.
116. Saag MS, Hahn BH, Gibbons J, et al. Extensive variation of human immunodeficiency virus type-1 in vivo. Nature 334:440–444, 1988.
117. Drake JW. Rates of spontaneous mutation among RNA viruses. Proc Natl Acad Sci USA 90:4171–4175, 1993.
118. Mansky LM, Temin HM. Lower in vivo mutation rate of human immunodeficiency virus type 1 than that predicted from the fidelity of purified reverse transcriptase. J Virol 69:5087–5094, 1995.
119. Deeks SG, Wrin T, Duecy E, et al. Decreased HIV-1 fitness after long-term virologic failure of protease inhibitor-based therapy: relationship to immunologic response. Presented at the 7th Conference on Retroviruses and Opportunistic Infections, 2000, p 104.
120. International AIDS Society—USA Resistance Mutations Project Panel. Update on drug resistance mutations in HIV-1. Top HIV Med 9:31–33, 2001.
121. Kuritzkes DR, Bell S, Shugarts D, Abrams D. Development of resistance to lamivudine (3TC) in NUCA 3001, a phase II comparative study of 3TC versus zidovudine versus 3TC plus zidovudine. Presented at the 2nd National Conference on Human Retroviruses and Related Infections, 1995.
122. Saag MS, Emini EA, Laskin OL, et al. A short-term clinical evaluation of L-697,661, a non-nucleoside inhibitor of HIV-1 reverse transcriptase: L-697,661 working group. N Engl J Med 329:1065–1072, 1993.
123. Larder BA, Darby G, Richman DD. HIV with reduced sensitivity to zidovudine (AZT) isolated during prolonged therapy. Science 243: 1731–1734, 1989.
124. Larder BA, Chesebro B, Richman DD. Susceptibilities of zidovudine-susceptible and -resistant human immunodeficiency virus isolates to antiviral agents determined by using a quantitative plaque reduction assay. Antimicrob Agents Chemother 34:436–441, 1990.
125. Condra JH, Schleif WA, Blahy OM. In vivo emergence of HIV-1 variants resistant to multiple protease inhibitors. Nature 374:569–571, 1995.
126. Condra JH, Holder DJ, Schleif WA, et al. Genetic correlates of in vivo viral resistance to indinavir, a human immunodeficiency virus type 1 protease inhibitor. J Virol 70:8270–8276, 1996.
127. Patrick A, Mo H, Markowitz M. Antiviral and resistance studies of AG1343, an orally bioavailable inhibitor of human immunodeficiency virus protease. Antimicrob Agents Chemother 40:292–297, 1996.
128. Kravcik S, Farnsworth A, Patick A, et al. Long-term follow-up of combination protease inhibitor therapy with nelfinavir and saquinavir (soft gel) in HIV infection. Presented at the 5th Conference on Retroviruses and Opportunistic Infections, 1998.
129. Larder BA, Kemp SD, Harrigan PR. Antiviral potency of AZT + 3TC combination therapy supports virological observations. Presented at the 2nd National Conference on Human Retroviruses and Related Infections, 1995.
130. Havlir DV, Gamst A, Eastman S, Richman DD. Nevirapine-resistant human immunodeficiency virus: kinetics of replication and estimated prevalence in untreated patients. J Virol 70:7894–7899, 1996.
131. Larder BA, Kellam P, Kemp SD. Convergent combination therapy can select viable multidrug-resistant HIV-1 in vitro. Nature 365:451–453, 1993.
132. Murphy RL, Sommadossi JP, Lamson M, et al. Antiviral effect and pharmacokinetic interaction between nevirapine and indinavir in persons infected with human immunodeficiency virus type 1. J Infect Dis 179:1116–1123, 1999.
133. Urquhart J. Partial compliance in cardiovascular disease: risk implications. Br J Clin Pract 73(suppl):2, 1994.
134. Greenberg RN. Overview of patient compliance with medication dosing: a literature review. Clin Ther 65:590, 1984.
135. Wright EC. Non-compliance: or how many aunts has Matilda? Lancet 342:909, 1993.
136. Urquhart J. Patient non-compliance with drug regimens: measurement, clinical correlates, economic impact. Eur Heart J 17(suppl A):8, 1996.
137. Havlir D, Levitan D, Bassett R, et al. Prevalence and predictive value of intermittent viraemia in patients with viral suppression. Antiviral Ther 5(suppl 3):89, 2000.
138. Havlir DV, Marschner IC, Hirsch MS, et al. Maintenance antiretroviral therapies in HIV infected patients with undetectable plasma HIV RNA after triple-drug therapy: AIDS Clinical Trials Group Study 343 team. N Engl J Med 339:1261–1268, 1998.
139. Gharakhanian S, Salhi Y, Adda N, et al. Identification of fat redistribution/metabolic anomalies in a cohort treated by 2 NRTIs + 1 PI, and absence of significant modification following PI substitution. Presented at the 7th Conference on Retroviruses and Opportunistic Infections, 2000, p 84.
140. Viciana P, Alarcon A, Martin D, et al. Partial improvement of lipodystrophy after switching from HIV-1 protease inhibitors (PI) to efavirenz (EFV). Presented at the 7th Conference on Retroviruses and Opportunistic Infections, 2000, p 84.
141. Bonnet E, Lepec R, Bluteau M, et al. Evolution of lipodystrophy syndrome and lipidic profile in HIV patients after switching from protease inhibitors to efavirenz. Presented at the 7th Conference on Retroviruses and Opportunistic Infections, 2000, p 84.
142. Negredo E, Cruz L, Ruiz L, et al. Impact of switching from protease inhibitors (PI) to nevirapine (NVP) or efavirenz (EFV) in patients with viral suppression. Presented at the 40th Interscience Conference on Antimicrobial Agents and Chemotherapy, 2000, p 277.
143. Moyle GJ, Baldwin C, Dent N, et al. Management of protease inhibitor (PI)-associated lipodystrophy by substitution with efavirenz

(EFV) in virologically controlled HIV-infected persons. Presented at the 39th Interscience Conference on Antimicrobial Agents and Chemotherapy, 1999, p 526.

144. Katlama C. Successful substitution of protease inhibitors with Sustiva (efavirenz) in patients with undetectable plasma HIV-1 RNA levels: results of a prospective, randomized, multicenter, open-label study (DMP 266-027). Presented at the XIII International AIDS Conference, 2000.
145. Bickel M, Rickerts V, Klauke S, et al. The Protra study: switch from PI to abacavir (ABC) and efavirenz (EFV) in HIV-1 infected adults previously treated with 2 NRTIs and a PI with undetectable HIV-RNA levels (vRNA). Presented at the 40th Interscience Conference on Antimicrobial Agents and Chemotherapy, 2000, p 324.
146. Knechten H, Sturner KH, Hohn C, Braun P. 24-Week follow-up of patients switching from a protease inhibitor (PI) containing regimen with lamivudine (3TC) and stavudine (d4T) or zidovudine (AZT) to an efavirenz (EFV) based therapy. Presented at the 40th Interscience Conference on Antimicrobial Agents and Chemotherapy, 2000, p 324.
147. Maggiolo F, Migliorino M, Pravettoni G, et al. Management of PI-associated metabolic changes by substitution with efavirenz in virologically controlled HIV+ persons. Presented at the 40th Interscience Conference on Antimicrobial Agents and Chemotherapy, 2000, p 325.
148. Lafon E, Bani Sadr F, Chandemerle C, et al. LIPSTOP study: evolution of clinical lipodystrophy (LD), blood lipids, visceral (VAT) and subcutaneous (SAT) adipose tissue after switching from protease inhibitor (PI) to efavirenz (EFV) in HIV-1 infected patients. Presented at the 40th Interscience Conference on Antimicrobial Agents and Chemotherapy, 2000, p 325.
149. Martinez E, Romeu J, Garcia-Viejo MA, et al. An open randomized study on the replacement of HIV-1 protease inhibitors by efavirenz in chronically suppressed HIV-1-infected patients with lipodystrophy. Presented at the 8th Conference on Retroviruses and Opportunistic Infections, 2001.
150. Estrada V, De Villar NGP, Martinez-Larrad T, et al. Switching to efavirenz from protease inhibitor-based therapy does not improve insulin resistance after one year in HIV patients with lipodystrophy syndrome. Presented at the 8th Conference on Retroviruses and Opportunistic Infections, 2001.
151. Casado JL, Arrizabalaga J, Antela A, et al. Long-term efficacy and tolerance of switching the protease inhibitor for nonnucleoside reverse transcriptase inhibitors: a 52-week, multicenter, prospective study. Presented at the 8th Conference on Retroviruses and Opportunistic Infections, 2001.
152. Martinez E, Conget I, Lozano L, et al. Reversion of metabolic abnormalities after switching from HIV-1 protease inhibitors to nevirapine. AIDS 13:805–810, 1999.
153. Barreiro P, Soriano V, Blanco F, et al. Risks and benefits of replacing protease inhibitors by nevirapine in HIV-infected subjects under long-term successful triple combination therapy. AIDS 14:807–812, 2000.
154. Ruiz L, Negredo E, Domingo P, et al. Clinical, virological, and immunological benefit of switching the protease inhibitor (PI) by nevirapine (NVP) in HAART-experienced patients suffering lipodystrophy (LD): 36-week follow-up. Presented at the 7th Conference on Retroviruses and Opportunistic Infections, 2000, p 114.
155. Carr A, Hudson J, Chuah J, et al. HIV protease inhibitor substitution in patients with lipodystrophy: a randomised, multicentre, open-label study. AIDS 15:1811–1815, 2001.
156. Munoz V, Casado JL, Moreno A, et al. Persistent viral suppression after switching a protease inhibitor (PI)-containing regimen to a non-nucleoside reverse transcriptase inhibitor (NNRTI)-based therapy (BEGIN study). Presented at the 39th Interscience Conference on Antimicrobial Agents and Chemotherapy, 1999, p 524.
157. Tebas P, Yarasheski K, Powderly WG, et al. A prospective open-label pilot trial of a maintenance nevirapine (NVP)-containing regimen in patients with undetectable viral loads (VL) on protease inhibitor (PI) regimens for at least 6 months. Presented at the 7th Conference on Retroviruses and Opportunistic Infections, 2000, p 83.
158. Raffi F, Esnault JL, Reliquet V, et al. The maintavir study, substitution of a nonnucleoside reverse transcriptase inhibitor (NNRTI) for a protease inhibitor (PI) in patients with undetectable plasma HIV-1 RNA: 18 months follow-up. Presented at the 40th Interscience Conference on Antimicrobial Agents and Chemotherapy, 2000, p 277.
159. Buisson M, Grappin M, Piroth L, et al. Simplified maintenance therapy with NNRTI (nevirapine) in patients with long-term suppression of HIV-1 RNA: first results of a cohort study. Presented at the 40th Interscience Conference on Antimicrobial Agents and Chemotherapy, 2000, p 327.
160. Saint-Marc T, Partisani M, Poizot-Martin I, Touraine JL. Reversibility of peripheral fat wasting (lipoatrophy) on stopping stavudine therapy. Presented at the 7th Conference on Retroviruses and Opportunistic Infections, 2000, p 85.
161. Goebel FD, Walli RK. A novel use of abacavir to simplify therapy in PI-experienced patients successfully treated with HAART: CNA30017. Presented at the 7th Conference on Retroviruses and Opportunistic Infections, 2000, p 84.
162. Opravil M, Hirschel B, Lazzarin A, et al. Simplified maintenance therapy with abacavir + lamivudine + zidovudine in patients with HAART-induced long-term suppression of HIV-1 RNA: final results. Presented at the 40th Interscience Conference on Antimicrobial Agents and Chemotherapy, 2000, p 278.
163. Montaner JSG. A novel use of abacavir to simplify therapy and reduce toxicity in PI experienced patients successfully treated with HAART: 48-week results (CNA30017). Presented at the 40th Interscience Conference on Antimicrobial Agents and Chemotherapy, 2000, p 278.
164. Miller V, Gute P, Carlebach A, et al. Baseline resistance and virological response to mega-HAART salvage therapies. Presented at the 6th Conference on Retroviruses and Opportunistic Infections, 1999.
165. Workman C, Mussen R, Sullivan J. Salvage therapy using six drugs in heavily pretreated patients. Presented at the 5th Conference on Retroviruses and Opportunistic Infections, 1998.
166. Montaner JSG, Harrigan R, Jahnke N, et al. Multi-drug rescue therapy (MDRT) following failure to multiple regimens: preliminary results. Antiviral Ther 3(suppl 2):80(abstract 76c), 1998.
167. Deeks SG, Wrin T, Liegler T, et al. Virologic and immunologic consequences of discontinuing combination antiretroviral-drug therapy in HIV-infected patients with detectable viremia. N Engl J Med 344: 472–480, 2001.
168. Miller V, Sabin C, Hertogs K, et al. Virological and immunological effects of treatment interruptions in HIV-1 infected patients with treatment failure. AIDS 14:2857–2867, 2000.
169. Miller V, Sabin C, Hertogs K, et al. Antiretroviral treatment interruptions in patients with treatment failure: analyses from the Frankfurt HIV cohort. Antivir Ther 5(suppl 2):22(abstract 25), 2000.

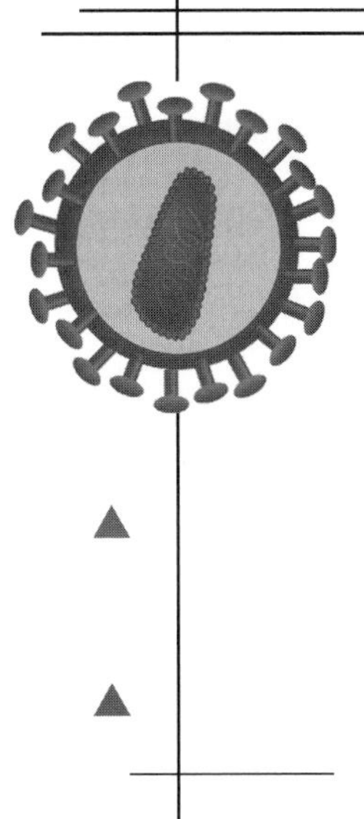

CHAPTER 28

Managing Pregnant Patients

D. Heather Watts, MD
Howard Minkoff, MD

Women with heterosexually acquired human immunodeficiency virus (HIV) infection are the most rapidly increasing group of HIV-infected individuals in the United States. Women now account for 21% of persons living with HIV reported to the U.S. Centers for Disease Control and Prevention (CDC).[1] Because the predominant mode of HIV transmission worldwide is heterosexual, women account for more than half of the HIV-infected population.[2] More than 85% of women with acquired immunodeficiency syndrome (AIDS) are in their reproductive years, and an estimated 6000 HIV-positive women deliver annually in the United States.[3] Identification of HIV-positive pregnant women has increased because of the availability of antiretroviral therapy and other interventions to prevent perinatal transmission, recommendations by the U.S. Public Health Service (USPHS) and others encouraging HIV testing of all pregnant women in the United States, and linkage of federal funding of AIDS programs to effective prevention of perinatal transmission of HIV.

When counseling women with coexistent HIV infection and pregnancy, issues to be discussed include the impact of the pregnancy on maternal health and choice of therapy, and the effect of HIV on pregnancy outcome and the woman's life expectancy. Additionally, the long-term care needs of the child, the risk of perinatal transmission, interventions to minimize that risk, and follow-up testing of the infant and the course of pediatric HIV infection if it occurs should be considered. Recommendations for specific antiretroviral therapy during pregnancy must take into account the gestational age at which pregnancy and HIV infection were diagnosed, previous or current antiretroviral therapy, maternal CD4+ T-lymphocyte count and HIV RNA level, potential toxicities, and maternal wishes. Treatment regimens for HIV and strategies to prevent perinatal transmission have become complex. When caring for the HIV-infected pregnant woman, providers are urged to consult online treatment guidelines referenced here for the most current information.

HIV TESTING DURING PREGNANCY

Initially, HIV testing during pregnancy was offered only to "at risk" women. As the rate of heterosexual transmission increased and as interventions to reduce perinatal transmission were identified, recommendations were made for "routine" counseling of all pregnant women about HIV infection and the benefits of testing.[4] Despite those recommendations, up to 10% of HIV-infected pregnant women in the United States did not receive zidovudine in 1997, suggesting a need for a broader approach to detection and treatment.[3] In an effort to increase the rate of HIV testing during pregnancy and to destigmatize the process, in 1999 the Institute of Medicine recommended universal HIV testing with patient notification as a routine component of prenatal care.[5] HIV testing would be done on all pregnant women unless they specifically refused after being notified that the test was to be done. These recommendations have been endorsed by the American College of Obstetricians and Gynecologists (ACOG) and the American Academy of Pediatrics (AAP).[6] Revised testing guidelines from the USPHS were expected to be released in 2001 and were to be posted on the CDC website at www.cdc.gov when finalized.

Women initially presenting for care late during pregnancy or when they are in labor have a two- to fourfold increased risk of HIV seropositivity than do women presenting earlier for prenatal care.[7–9] Risk factors for late care such as drug abuse are also risk factors for HIV seropositivity. Antiretroviral therapy, even if initiated during labor, may decrease the risk of perinatal transmission of HIV,[10,11] or if given to the infant within 48 hours of delivery may reduce perinatal transmission. HIV testing should be offered as soon as possible to women presenting in labor who were not previously tested, and results should be available rapidly. Offering rapid HIV testing during labor and the early postpartum period is complex, with many ethical and logistical issues involved.[12] Each institution should develop its own procedures, perhaps combining intrapartum testing with rapid testing programs for health care worker exposures for efficiency.

▲ IMPACT OF PREGNANCY ON MATERNAL HEALTH AND ON THERAPY OF HIV

Studies from the United States and Europe have not indicated accelerated progression to AIDS or death among women with an intervening pregnancy.[13–15] In both HIV-positive and HIV-negative pregnant women, CD4+ T-lymphocyte counts have been noted to decrease, with rebound after birth. CD4 percentages appear to be more stable over time.[16] No benefit to maternal health from pregnancy termination has been demonstrated. In developing countries, pregnancy may lead to more rapid progression to AIDS or death, although data are limited.[17,18]

As with other serious medical conditions during pregnancy, therapy for the HIV-positive pregnant woman should be essentially the same as if she were not pregnant unless clear fetal or maternal contraindications to standard therapy exist. In addition, antiretroviral therapy during pregnancy is indicated for prevention of perinatal transmission of HIV. Experience with most antiretroviral therapy during pregnancy is limited. Available data on currently approved antiretroviral drugs are shown in Table 28–1.

Pregnant women receiving antiretroviral drugs or other HIV therapy with limited past use during pregnancy should be monitored in the same way as other high-risk pregnant women. Specifically, a detailed sonogram at approximately 18 to 20 weeks' gestation for fetal anatomy and confirmation of gestational age should be obtained. Frequent prenatal visits during the third trimester to measure fundal height, blood pressure, and other parameters to assess maternal status are indicated. In addition, for women receiving agents with recommended limited clinical use during pregnancy, sonograms for fetal growth and fluid volume at approximately 32 and 36 weeks' gestation should be done. All pregnant women should be instructed in daily assessment of fetal movement during the third trimester and urged to report any significant decrease to their health care provider. If any concerns regarding fetal growth or health are identified on clinical examination or ultrasonography, antepartum testing should be initiated and continued until delivery. Maternal laboratory studies such as complete blood counts, electrolytes, and liver function testing should be done on a regular basis to monitor for toxicity as indicated for specific drugs. In addition to routine cord blood studies, complete blood count, electrolyte and creatinine assays, and liver function tests should be obtained from the cord blood when possible.

Nucleoside Reverse Transcriptase Inhibitors

The antiretroviral drug with which there is the most experience during pregnancy is zidovudine (ZDV), which was also the first drug with demonstrated efficacy in the prevention of perinatal transmission of HIV. ZDV, as administered in the Pediatric AIDS Clinical Trials Group (PACTG) trial 076 (Table 28–2) was well tolerated by mothers and infants.[19] Maternal side effects and toxicities were similar for the ZDV and placebo groups. Anemia was more common at 6 weeks of age among ZDV-treated infants but resolved after ZDV was stopped, and no infant required transfusion. Because of the proven value of ZDV for preventing perinatal transmission, when choosing a therapeutic regimen for a pregnant woman for her own health, if possible, ZDV should be included in this regimen. If the woman is intolerant of oral ZDV, inclusion of intravenous ZDV during labor (Table 28–2) and oral ZDV for the infant should be considered.

Limited pharmacokinetic and safety data are available for lamivudine (3TC) and didanosine (ddI) as well. In a study of 18 pregnant women receiving 3TC, pharmacokinetic results were similar in pregnant women and nonpregnant individuals, and no major safety issues were identified.[20] Similarly, among 11 women studied, the pharmacokinetics of oral ddI were not significantly different during the third trimester of pregnancy and 6 weeks postpartum.[21] A study of the combination of stavudine (d4T) and 3TC during pregnancy is in progress in the PACTG. The use of zalcitabine (ddC) and abacavir during human pregnancy has not been studied. Because of maternal toxicity, developmental toxicity, and hydrocephalus in animal studies and low placental passage in primate studies, ddC is not recommended for use during pregnancy. Use of abacavir is limited by the risk of potentially fatal hypersensitivity reactions.

All nucleoside analogues appear to cross the placenta in primates, but ZDV, d4T, and 3TC cross with fetal/maternal drug ratios higher than 0.7 compared to ddI and ddC, which have ratios of 0.3 to 0.5.[22] Because placental transfer and pretreatment of the infant prior to HIV exposure during labor may be responsible for a portion of the beneficial effect of ZDV in PACTG 076, consideration should be given to including either d4T or 3TC in the regimen for enhanced placental transfer if a woman is unable to take ZDV.

Animal studies suggest that all nucleosides except ddI (category B) pose potential fetal risk (although often at high, maternally toxic doses) and are therefore classified by the U.S. Food and Drug Administration (FDA) as pregnancy category C.[22] Among cases of ZDV exposure during pregnancy prospectively reported to the Antiretroviral Pregnancy Registry, no increased risk of birth defects or specific pattern of defects was seen.[23] Too few cases of the use of other antiretroviral agents during continuing pregnancies have been reported to allow assessment of potential maternal or fetal risks. All cases of antiretroviral

▲ **Table 28–1.** PRECLINICAL AND CLINICAL DATA RELEVANT TO THE USE OF ANTIRETROVIRAL AGENTS DURING PREGNANCY

Antiretroviral drug	FDA pregnancy category	Newborn/maternal drug ratio	Long-term animal carcinogenicity studies	Animal reproduction studies	Major toxicities	Concerns specific to pregnancy
Nucleoside reverse transcriptase inhibitors						
Zidovudine (AZT,ZDV)	C	0.85 (human)	Increase in rodent noninvasive vaginal tumors, possible transplacental carcinogenesis (see text)	Increased resorption in rats and rabbits. No teratogenicity in rats, rabbits at usual dose. Increased malformations at near-lethal dose in rats	Bone marrow suppression, myopathy	Most well studied ARV agent, safe for short term. See discussion of mitochondrial toxicity, rodent tumors
Zalcitibine (ddC)	C	0.3–0.5 (rhesus monkey)	Thymic lymphomas in rats at 1000× human dose	Hydrocephalus in rats at 2000× human dose, skeletal defects and decreased weight at moderate doses	Neuropathy	No studies
Didanosine (ddI)	B	0.5 (human)	Negative in rodents	No impaired fertility or teratogenicity in rats, rabbits	Pancreatitis, neuropathy	PK study (n = 14) shows no need for dose modification. Possible increased risk of lactic acidosis during pregnancy with long-term ddI/d4T
Stavudine (d4T)	C	0.76 (rhesus monkey)	Not completed	Increased resorptions at >200 × human doses, decreased sternal ossification at >400 × human doses	Peripheral neuropathy	Phase I/II study in progress. No change in PK in pregnant primates. Possible increased risk of lactic acidosis in pregnancy with long-term ddI/d4T
Lamivudine (3TC)	C	~1.0 (human)	Negative in rodents	Increased resorptions in rabbits but not rats. No increase in malformations	Pancreatitis increased in children	PK study (n = 20) shows no need for dose modification, well tolerated No studies
Abacavir (ABC)	C	Passage in rats	Not completed	Anasarca, skeletal abnormalities at 35× human dose in rodents, not seen in rabbits	Potentially fatal hypersensitivity reactions with symptoms of fever, skin rash, fatigue, nausea, vomiting, diarrhea, abdominal pain	No studies
Nonnucleoside reverse transcriptase inhibitors						
Nevirapine	C	~1.0 (human)	Not completed	Impaired fertility in female rats, decreased fetal weight. No increase in malformations in rats, rabbits	Rash, drug interactions, potentially fatal hepatotoxicity	Phase I study during late pregnancy, well tolerated. Phase III studies discussed in section on perinatal transmission
Delavirdine	C	Unknown	Not completed	Increased resorptions, fetal deaths in rats, rabbits at high doses. Increased ASD/VSD in rats at high doses	Rash, drug interactions	No studies

Table continued on following page

Table 28–1. PRECLINICAL AND CLINICAL DATA RELEVANT TO THE USE OF ANTIRETROVIRAL AGENTS DURING PREGNANCY *Continued*

Antiretroviral drug	FDA pregnancy category	Newborn/maternal drug ratio	Long-term animal carcinogenicity studies	Animal reproduction studies	Major toxicities	Concerns specific to pregnancy
Efavirenz	C	~1.0 (cynomolgous monkey	Not completed	Increased fetal resorptions in rats. Anencephaly, anophthalmia, microphthalmia, cleft palate in cynomolgous monkeys at doses similar to human doses	Rash, drug interactions	None planned. Pregnancy should be avoided because of primate teratogenicity
Protease inhibitors				Class effects: hyperglycemia, possible fat redistribution and lipid abnormalities, increased bleeding episodes in hemophiliacs		
Indinavir	C	Yes in rats, low in rabbits	Not completed	No effect on fertility in rodents. No teratogenicity in rats, rabbits, dogs. Developmental abnormality (extra ribs) in rats	Kidney stones, hyperbilirubinemia, drug interactions	Phase I/II study in progress. Theoretical concerns are kidney stones, hyperbilirubinemia in neonate from maternal exposure
Ritonavir	B	Yes in rats	Positive in male but not female rats at 4× human dose	Increased resorptions, decreased fetal weight in rats, rabbits at maternal toxic doses. No teratogenicity in rats, rabbits	Nausea, vomiting, diarrhea; increased triglycerides, transaminases; drug interactions	Phase I/II study in progress, preliminary data suggest little placental transfer
Saquinavir	B	Minimal in rats, rabbits	Not completed	No effect on fertility, no teratogenicity in rats, rabbits	Nausea, diarrhea	Phase I/II study in progress with saquinavir/low-dose ritonavir
Nelfinavir	B	Unknown	Not completed	No effect on fertility, no teratogenicity in rats, rabbits	Diarrhea, drug interactions	Phase I/II study in progress
Amprenavir	C	Unknown	Not completed	Increased resorptions in rabbits, developmental skeletal abnormalities in rabbits, rats. No teratogenicity	Nausea, vomiting, diarrhea, rash, oral paresthesias, increased liver function tests	No studies
Lopinavir	C	Unknown	Not completed	Increased resorptions, developmental abnormalities at toxic maternal doses in rats. No effects in rabbits. No teratogenicity	Nausea, vomiting, diarrhea, pancreatitis, drug interactions	No studies
Other agents						
Hydroxyurea	D	Crosses in animals	Carcinogenic in rats, potentially in humans	Testicular atrophy and decreased spermatogenesis in rats. Teratogenic with multiple defects seen in rats, rabbits, hamsters, cats, monkeys		Reported use in 16 women, 13 during first trimester. No anomalies seen. Because of unclear efficacy in HIV therapy and potential teratogenicity based on animal studies, use should be avoided during pregnancy

A, adequate, well controlled studies of pregnant women fail to demonstrate a risk to the fetus during the first trimester of pregnancy (and there is no evidence of risk during the later trimesters). B, animal reproduction studies fail to demonstrate a risk to the fetus; adequate, well controlled studies of pregnant women have not been conducted. C, safety in human pregnancy has not been determined; animal studies are either positive for fetal risk or have not been conducted; and the drug should not be used unless the potential benefit outweighs the potential risk to the fetus. D, positive evidence of human fetal risk based on adverse reaction data from investigational or marketing experiences, but the potential benefits from the use of the drug in pregnant women may be acceptable despite its potential risks.

ARV, antiretroviral; ASD/VSD, atrial septal defect/ventricular septal defect; FDA, Food and Drug Administration; PK, pharmacokinetic; X, studies in animals or reports of adverse reactions have indicated that the risk associated with the use of the drug for pregnant women clearly outweighs any possible benefit.

Table 28–2. RECOMMENDATIONS FOR ZIDOVUDINE USE IN PREGNANT WOMEN AND THEIR INFANTS TO REDUCE VERTICAL TRANSMISSION OF HIV

Antepartum	ZDV 100 mg PO five times daily or 200 mg PO three times daily to start as soon as possible after 13 weeks' gestation
Intrapartum	Loading dose: ZDV 2 mg/kg IV over 1 hours followed by 1 mg/kg/hr until delivery
Infant	2 mg/kg PO every 6 hours (total 8 mg/kg/day) for 6 weeks, beginning within 8–12 hours after birth

ZDV, zidovudine.

use in pregnancy should be reported to the Antiretroviral Pregnancy Registry (PO Box 13398, Research Triangle Park, NC 27709-9976; telephone 1-800-722-9292, ext. 38465; www.APRegistry.com).

An additional concern regarding the use of nucleoside analogue drugs is the potential for mitochondrial toxicity in both mother and infant. Nucleoside analogue drugs can induce mitochondrial dysfunction by binding to mitochondrial gamma DNA polymerase and interfering with replication.[24] The greatest inhibition of mitochondrial gamma DNA polymerase is seen with ddC, followed in order by ddI, d4T, 3TC, ZDV, and abacavir. Clinical disorders associated with mitochondrial toxicity include neuropathy, myopathy, cardiomyopathy, pancreatitis, hepatic steatosis, and lactic acidosis.

Three cases of fatal lactic acidosis, two accompanied by pancreatitis, were reported among pregnant or recently delivered women who had been on ddI and d4T therapy along with a third agent (one nelfinavir, one an investigational protease inhibitor, one nevirapine) since before conception.[25] Several additional nonfatal cases of lactic acidosis in pregnant women on ddI and d4T were also identified. Two cases of fatal liver failure in pregnant women on zidovudine, lamivudine, and nelfinavir have also been reported. Cases developed during late pregnancy; and in several cases the presentation was similar to that seen with acute fatty liver of pregnancy, a rare, life-threatening condition that has been linked to mitochondrial fatty oxidation disorders in the fetus (homozygotic) and mother (heterozygotic).[26] Although the frequency of lactic acidosis and related mitochondrial disorders in HIV-infected pregnant women is unknown, it is possible that the metabolic changes of late pregnancy may enhance susceptibility to complications of nucleoside agents, especially those with greater inhibition of mitochondrial gamma DNA polymerase. Enhanced susceptibility is suggested also by the syndrome of acute fatty liver of pregnancy and animal data that demonstrate reduced mitochondrial fatty acid oxidation during late pregnancy and in animals treated with exogenous estradiol and progesterone to mimic pregnancy levels.[27,28] Given the potential for increased toxicity and the nonspecific nature of symptoms due to conditions such as lactic acidosis that may overlap with normal pregnancy symptoms, providers caring for HIV-infected women receiving nucleoside analogues must be vigilant for subtle signs and symptoms suggestive of mitochondrial toxicity. Hepatic enzyme levels and electrolytes should be assessed frequently during the last trimester and new symptoms evaluated thoroughly. One reasonable approach would be to monitor hepatic function and other laboratory values monthly during the third trimester and with the onset of any new symptoms. Women with substantial elevations in transaminase levels above baseline or other new abnormalities should have the studies repeated immediately. In the absence of other explanations such as preeclampsia for the persistent laboratory abnormalities, consideration should be given to discontinuing nucleoside agents, either with substitution of agents from another class of antiretrovirals or discontinuation of all antiretrovirals. This decision must be made after carefully considering all possible causes for the laboratory abnormalities, taking into account the clinical circumstances and balancing the risk of transmission with viral rebound from stopping therapy versus the infrequent but potentially fatal risk of continuing therapy if the abnormalities are related to mitochondrial toxicity. In view of the reports of maternal deaths and toxicity associated with prolonged use of d4T and ddI during pregnancy, this combination should be used during pregnancy with caution and only if other nucleoside agents cannot be given because of resistance or toxicity.

Concerns regarding potential mitochondrial toxicity in infants exposed to nucleoside agents in utero and during the neonatal period were raised by a French group who reported eight cases of HIV-uninfected infants with abnormalities potentially related to mitochondrial dysfunction developing several months after discontinuing prophylactic nucleoside therapy among 1754 exposed fetuses.[29] Two infants had progressive neurologic symptoms and died several months after completing in utero and neonatal courses of ZDV/3TC. Three other infants had mild to moderate symptoms, and three had asymptomatic laboratory abnormalities. Mitochondrial abnormalities were not proven to be the cause of the abnormalities, and the relation between these findings and in utero and neonatal nucleoside exposure has not been established. In response to these concerns, investigators from several large cohort studies in the United States reviewed all 353 deaths among more than 20,000 children born to HIV-infected women and found no deaths similar to those in the French cohort, although only 6% of the children had been exposed to the combination of ZDV/3TC.[30] Review of data on living children from these cohorts for diagnoses or conditions suggestive of mitochondrial dysfunction is ongoing.

Comparing uninfected children exposed to ZDV with those exposed to placebo in the PACTG 076 trial and in the Thai short-course trial, no differences have been seen in growth, immunologic, or cognitive parameters with up to 5.6 years and 18 months of follow-up respectively; and no deaths related to mitochondrial toxicity or tumors have occurred.[31,32] Neurologic adverse events have also been reviewed among 1798 children in the PETRA study, a randomized trial that included a placebo arm and three ZDV/3TC treatment arms with therapy for the mother, neonate, or both for prevention of perinatal transmission of HIV.[33] No increase in the risk of neurologic events was seen with ZDV/3TC exposure compared to placebo, regardless of the intensity of treatment. Current data suggest that if in utero and neonatal exposure to nucleosides causes mitochondrial dysfunction the risk must be low and the risk of severe or fatal disease must be rare. This potential risk must be compared to the clear benefit of nucleoside therapy in reducing perinatal transmission of HIV, an ultimately fatal infection, but emphasizes the need for long-term follow-up of children exposed to antiretroviral agents.

An additional concern raised regarding the use of ZDV during pregnancy has been the possibility of transplacental carcinogenesis. ZDV causes vaginal epithelial neoplasms in adult mice that are believed to be a topical effect from reflux of urine containing high concentrations of ZDV onto highly metaplastic vaginal epithelium. No increase in the incidence of tumors in other organs has been seen in adult mice or rats receiving ZDV. Data from two studies in mice treated during pregnancy with ZDV have raised the concern of a transplacental carcinogenic effect in the offspring. In a study at the National Cancer Institute using doses of ZDV up to 30 times those used in human pregnancy, mice in the highest dose group had an increased rate of liver, lung, and female reproductive tumors compared to controls.[34] No increased risk of tumors was seen in a similar study using doses approximately three times those used in humans; the study was conducted by Glaxo Wellcome, manufacturer of ZDV.[35] Little is known about the sensitivity or reliability of the mouse model used in these studies for predicting transplacental carcinogenicity in humans. No tumors have been observed in studies following more than 1000 children exposed to ZDV in utero for an average of 3 years.[31,32,36] Currently, the known benefits of ZDV in preventing perinatal transmission of HIV far outweigh the hypothetical risks of transplacental carcinogenesis suggested by a single study.[37] However, these concerns further emphasize the need for long-term follow-up of children exposed to ZDV and other drugs during pregnancy.

Nonnucleoside Reverse Transcriptase Inhibitors

Among the approved nonnucleoside reverse transcriptase inhibitors (NNRTIs) nevirapine, delavirdine, and efavirenz, pharmacokinetic data are available only for nevirapine in pregnant women.[38,39] The drug was well tolerated when given as a single dose to women in labor. The drug crossed the placenta, and blood concentrations in the neonates were similar to those in the mother. Use of nevirapine for preventing perinatal transmission is discussed in more detail later in the chapter. Earlier use during pregnancy and use of multiple doses have not been studied. Although severe, even fatal hepatotoxicity and skin reactions have occurred among HIV-infected persons receiving nevirapine, toxicity with single-dose therapy during pregnancy has been minimal. Whether longer-term use during pregnancy is associated with enhanced toxicity is unknown.

All NNRTIs are FDA category C. Animal teratogenicity studies of nevirapine have not indicated specific problems except increased low birth weight in rats at 1.5 times the human dose. Studies in rodents have indicated an increased risk of ventricular septal defect with delavirdine exposure. Particularly concerning is a recent report of birth defects among 3 (18%) of 20 monkeys treated with efavirenz at doses similar to human dosing. Defects included cleft palate (one monkey), microphthalmia (one monkey), and anencephaly and unilateral anophthalmia (one monkey) (Safety AlertCDupont Merck). Women taking efavirenz should be counseled regarding the potential risks during pregnancy and provided with appropriate contraception. If a woman conceives on efavirenz, she should notify her provider at once for a discussion of risks and options. If the woman is less than 10 weeks past her last menstrual period, most clinicians would recommend that she switch from efavirenz to either a protease inhibitor or nevirapine because of the concerning data from monkeys. Decisions regarding switching must be individualized based on gestational age and remaining antiretroviral options for the woman. Women should be informed of the data in monkeys, the limited data in humans (no defects among the 24 first-trimester exposures to efavirenz reported to the Antiretroviral Pregnancy Registry[23]), and the less than 100% sensitivity of prenatal ultrasonography for detecting birth defects, especially defects such as cleft palate and anophthalmia. Options for the woman include termination of pregnancy or continuation with detailed ultrasonography at 18 to 20 weeks' gestation.

Protease Inhibitors

The data on protease inhibitor use during pregnancy are limited. Preliminary pharmacokinetic and safety data are available from ongoing PACTG studies of various protease inhibitors in combination with ZDV and 3TC. Among five pregnant women receiving indinavir 800 mg tid in combination with ZDV and 3TC, one woman discontinued therapy because of nausea and vomiting. One woman had transient hyperbilirubinemia, and one had flank pain without confirmed renal stones; both continued on therapy. Among three women with complete data, indinavir levels as measured by area under the curve (AUC) were lower during pregnancy than postpartum or in previous studies of nonpregnant persons, but all of the women had a decreased to undetectable viral load on therapy.[40] A second report of two women on the same dose of indinavir found reductions in AUC of 63% to 86% during pregnancy compared to postpartum levels.[41] In the PACTG study of nelfinavir 750 mg tid, levels in nine pregnant women were lower than those reported in nonpregnant adults; and the dose has been modified to 1250 mg bid. Likewise, in the study of saquinavir soft gel capsules 1200 mg tid, levels were inadequate in pregnant women; and the study has been modified to evaluate the pharmacokinetics of saquinavir 800 mg bid with ritonavir 100 mg bid. Studies of amprenavir or lopinavir/ritonavir during pregnancy have not yet been done. The limited data thus far indicating decreased AUC of protease inhibitors during pregnancy underscores the need for rapid completion of pharmacokinetic studies during pregnancy and for careful monitoring of the response of HIV RNA levels for pregnant women on antiretroviral therapy in case suboptimal drug levels lead to an incomplete virologic response. Whether these suboptimal levels are associated with more frequent development of resistance remains to be determined.

Animal studies have indicated variable placental transfer. For example, in mice indinavir and ritonavir both achieved higher concentrations in the fetus than in the mother after maternal dosing. However, in rabbits there was little placental transfer of indinavir. Limited data from the studies discussed above have suggested little placental transfer of indinavir, ritonavir, and nelfinavir in humans (cord blood levels 0% to 12% of maternal levels), but more data are needed.

Some toxicities of protease inhibitors such as nausea and vomiting may be exacerbated by pregnancy, whereas others such as the diarrhea associated with nelfinavir may be mitigated by the decrease in gastrointestinal motility. Reports of an increased risk of diabetes in nonpregnant individuals receiving protease inhibitors are concerning for pregnant women given the increased insulin requirements of pregnancy and the significant rate of gestational diabetes in healthy pregnant women. An increased risk of gestational diabetes with protease inhibitors may be anticipated. All women receiving protease inhibitors should have a 1-hour 50-g glucose screen at the usual 24- to 28-week intervals. Consideration should be given also to regular assessment of fasting and postprandial blood glucose levels in pregnant women on protease inhibitors during the third trimester until more experience is gained. In addition, the side effects of indinavir (kidney stones and hyperbilirubinemia) may be a special problem during late pregnancy. Women receiving indinavir should undergo amniotic fluid volume surveillance during late pregnancy, and the infant's caregiver should be aware of the potential increased risk of hyperbilirubinemia and renal stones in the infant.

No adverse fetal effects or abnormalities have been seen in rodents or rabbits exposed to saquinavir or nelfinavir.[42] Increased rates of resorption and spontaneous abortion, low birth weight, and skeletal developmental abnormalities have been seen in rats or rabbits with indinavir, ritonavir, amprenavir, and lopinavir, usually at doses that were toxic to the pregnant animals. No specific defects have been associated with protease inhibitor use in humans, although experience with first trimester exposure is limited.[23]

When offering therapy with the limited pharmacokinetic data available, the physiologic changes of pregnancy must be considered. Maternal plasma volume increases by 45%, whereas red blood cell mass increases only 20% to 30%, leading to dilutional anemia. Cardiac output and glomerular filtration rate increase by 30% to 50%, potentially increasing clearance of drugs with renal metabolism. Absorption of inhaled medications may be increased because the tidal volume during pregnancy increases by 200 ml; pulmonary blood flow is increased as well. Albumin levels decrease by 20%, leading to potentially decreased protein binding of drugs. The effects of pregnancy on levels of a specific drug vary depending on the type of clearance and metabolism of the drug and the method of administration. The adequacy of antiretroviral drug levels during pregnancy can be monitored indirectly by regular assessment of HIV RNA levels after initiation of therapy.

Decisions about therapy and pregnancy must be individualized based on the woman's clinical, virologic, and immunologic status and the gestational age of the pregnancy. If women are first diagnosed as being HIV-positive during pregnancy, they should undergo a thorough history and physical examination, CD4+ T-lymphocyte determination, and assessment of HIV RNA levels. Therapeutic options, as indicated based on the CD4+ T-lymphocyte count and plasma HIV RNA level in a nonpregnant state, should be discussed, as should the options for preventing perinatal transmission. According to the most recent adult treatment guidelines, therapy for maternal health would not be indicated currently with a CD4+ T-lymphocyte count higher than 350 cells/μl and an HIV RNA level less than 30,000 cop/ml by bDNA assay and less than 55,000 copies/ml by reverse transcriptase-polymerase chain reaction (RT-PCR) assay,[42] but combination antiretroviral therapy should be offered for prophylaxis against transmission. Based on data presented below, highly active combination antiretroviral therapy should be offered to all pregnant women with HIV RNA levels higher than 1000 copies/ml to decrease the risk of perinatal transmission and the indications for scheduled cesarean delivery.[22] If the woman is in the first trimester of pregnancy, waiting to start therapy until 12 weeks or later, when organogenesis is complete, may be considered. If HIV positivity is detected late in pregnancy (more than 36 weeks), initiation of the PACTG 076 ZDV regimen may be considered, with institution of therapy based on the CD4+ T-lymphocyte count and HIV RNA levels when available.

Women who are on antiretroviral therapy and become pregnant must have therapeutic options discussed with them. In many women the pregnancy is diagnosed after the period of maximal organogenesis, and there would be little potential benefit from discontinuing therapy. In addition, when pregnancy is diagnosed early in women on combination therapy, the risk of a rebound in HIV RNA levels and potentially enhanced perinatal transmission with interruption of therapy must be balanced against the risk of teratogenesis. In general, unless clear data suggest a risk of teratogenicity in humans, it is reasonable to continue a woman's stable antiretroviral regimen during the first trimester of pregnancy. If the choice is made to stop antiretroviral therapy during the first trimester, all agents should be stopped simultaneously and then reinstated simultaneously when a reasonable period has passed to ensure that therapy is tolerated. If the patient's regimen during pregnancy does not include ZDV, intravenous ZDV during labor and oral ZDV for the infant should be added in an effort to prevent perinatal transmission of HIV. Women on combination antiretroviral therapy for their own health should receive the routine care and follow-up they would on these agents if they were not pregnant. In addition, the high-risk obstetric surveillance discussed above should be included. If women choose not to go on combination antiretroviral therapy during pregnancy, they should continue to be monitored with regular CD4+ T-lymphocyte counts and HIV RNA testing every 3 to 4 months in case indications for therapy should change. In addition, they should be encouraged to take the PACTG 076 ZDV regimen to reduce perinatal transmission.

▲ PREVENTION OF PERINATAL TRANSMISSION

The rate of perinatal transmission of HIV in developed countries had fallen dramatically from rates of 15% to 33% before the availability of antiretroviral therapy[3,43–46] to 3% to 8% with maternal ZVD therapy,[10,19,47–51] and now to 3% or less with maternal ZVD therapy and scheduled cesarean delivery or combination antiretroviral therapy and undetectable maternal HIV RNA levels.[52–57] Unfortunately, transmission rates remain high in countries without antiretroviral therapy or available breastfeeding alternatives.[58–60]

Transmission of HIV may occur during the antepartum, intrapartum, or postpartum period. In nonbreastfeeding populations, about one-third (20% to 60%) of transmissions appear to occur in utero, with the remaining two-thirds (40% to 80%) occurring during labor and delivery.[61–65] Evidence suggestive of intrapartum transmission includes delayed detection of HIV by culture, antigen detection, or DNA in the neonate[63–65]; later onset of clinical symptoms[62]; detection of HIV in cervicovaginal secretions of infected women that is reduced after antiretroviral therapy that has been shown to reduce transmission[66–68]; significantly higher transmission rates in the first-born twin compared to the second-born twin[69]; the association of higher transmission rates with increasing duration of ruptured membranes during labor[70–72]; and reduced transmission among women delivered by cesarean section before labor and membrane rupture.[53,54] Thus because much of the perinatal transmission of HIV appears to occur late in pregnancy or during delivery, interventions directed at late pregnancy, delivery, and the neonate would be expected to reduce transmission significantly. Transmission of HIV through breastfeeding, both with primary infection during breastfeeding (mean about 29%, range 16% to 42%) and with HIV infection antedating pregnancy (median about 14%, range 9% to 32%) has been well documented.[43,58,73–76]

Factors consistently associated with an increased risk of perinatal transmission of HIV before widespread use of antiretroviral therapy during pregnancy include advanced maternal HIV infection as determined by clinical diagnosis of AIDS, low CD4+ T-lymphocyte count or percent, maternal p24 antigenemia or high plasma HIV RNA levels, longer duration of ruptured membranes before delivery, placental inflammation, and sexually transmitted diseases.[44,46,58–60,70–72,74,77–85] Factors less consistently associated with an increased risk of transmission include preterm birth, maternal illicit drug use, vitamin A deficiency, female gender of the infant, and mode of delivery.[43,60,70,80–82,86–94] The impact of mode of delivery on transmission is discussed in more detail later.

Studies from untreated and treated cohorts of pregnant women have consistently demonstrated an association between maternal HIV RNA levels and the risk of transmission.[46,83,86,95–106] In untreated women, transmission rates increased from about 10% (range 0% to 22%) among women with HIV RNA levels near delivery of fewer than 1000 copies/ml, to 17% (range 0% to 67%) with levels of 1000 to 10,000 copies/ml, to 33% (range 22% to 64%) with levels of more than 10,000 copies/ml. Among women receiving antiretroviral therapy, predominantly zidovudine monotherapy, transmission rates increased from 1% (range 0% to 7%) with HIV RNA levels less than 1000 copies/ml, to 6% (range 0% to 12%) with levels of 1000 to 10,000 copies/ml, and to 13% (range 9% to 29%) with levels higher than 10,000 copies/ml. Treatment lowered the transmission rate among women in each viral load group, even among women with low or undetectable HIV RNA levels, suggesting that the effects of treatment are not all related to decreasing maternal plasma HIV RNA levels but may also be related to decreasing genital tract HIV levels and pre- and postexposure prophylaxis of the infant. Not all infants born to treated women in these studies received neonatal antiretroviral therapy. Transmission rates are low among women with HIV RNA levels below 1000 copies/ml, but there is not a threshold below which the absence of transmission can be ensured.

Given the relation of maternal plasma HIV RNA levels to perinatal transmission, maternal antiretroviral therapy would be expected to reduce transmission. ZVD was the first drug with a demonstrated impact on perinatal transmission of HIV. In the PACTG 076 study, use of ZDV, as outlined in Table 28–2, begun between 14 and 34 weeks' gestation, resulted in reduced transmission, from 25.5% in the placebo-treated group to 8.3% in the ZDV-treated group.[19] Subsequent follow-up of a larger number of infants born in this study has shown slightly lower rates of transmission in the treated group.[98] Several subsequent reports from nonrandomized cohorts confirmed the benefits of ZDV therapy among women with characteristics similar to those in the PACTG 076 study (CD4+ T-lymphocyte count more than 200/μl) and women with more advanced disease[47,48,107–109] and when only maternal therapy was given.[110,111] The exact mechanism of action of ZDV for perinatal transmission is unclear. Among women with low HIV RNA levels at the start of therapy, such as those in the PACTG 076 study, reduction of HIV RNA levels appears to account for only a small portion of the prevention of transmission,[98] whereas among groups with higher starting HIV RNA levels reduction of plasma HIV RNA levels appears to be a more important factor.[65,86]

Trials evaluating shorter regimens of single or double antiretroviral agents to prevent perinatal transmission are summarized in Table 28–3.[11,19,105,112–118] Significant reductions in transmission were seen even among breastfeeding populations with antepartum/intrapartum, intrapartum/postpartum, intrapartum/neonatal, and antepartum/intrapartum/postpartum regimens. No reduction in transmission compared to placebo was seen when only intrapartum ZDV/3TC was given. Adding neonatal ZDV to antepartum/intrapartum regimens begun by 36 weeks' gestation did not appear to decrease transmission further. The efficacy of intrapartum/neonatal ZDV/3TC was similar to that of intrapartum/neonatal nevirapine in the SAINT trial using the same nevirapine regimen as in the HIVNET 012 trial. In contrast to its use in women and infants without other antiretroviral therapy, adding nevirapine to existing antiretroviral therapy did not further reduce the already low transmission rate of 1.5% seen in the placebo arm.[118] For short-course therapy, the nevirapine regimen is the simplest, least expensive option; and both maternal and infant doses can be directly observed at the time of hospitalization for delivery. Development of genotypic resistance after single-dose nevirapine therapy in women and infants has been reported in previously untreated pregnant women and women on additional antiretroviral therapy, and it is of concern.[119,120] The persistence and clinical significance of

Table 28–3. PHASE III RANDOMIZED TRIALS OF ANTIRETROVIRAL DRUGS TO REDUCE PERINATAL TRANSMISSION OF HIV

Country	Drugs	Breast feeding	Maternal therapy			Infant therapy	Duration of follow-up	Transmission rate	
			Antepartum (AP)	Intrapartum (IP)	Postpartum (PP)			Placebo or control	Active drug
USA, France[19]	Placebo-controlled, zidovudine (ZDV)	No	100 mg PO 5× /day, start 14–34 weeks	2 mg/kg IV over 1 hour, then 1 mg/kg/hr infusion	None	2 mg/kg PO qid for 6 weeks	18 months	25.5%	8.3% ZDV
Thailand[105]	Placebo-controlled, ZDV	No	300 mg PO bid, start at 36 weeks	300 mg PO every 3 hours	None	None	6 months	18.9%	9.4%
Thailand[112]	Factorial design (long-long, long-short, short-short, short-long), ZDV	No	300 mg PO bid, start at 28 or 36 weeks	300 mg PO every 3 hours	None	2 mg/kg PO qid for 6 weeks or 3 days	6 months	Short-short 10.5%; this arm dropped at interim analysis	Short-long 8.6%, long-short 4.7%, long-long 6.5%
Ivory Coast[113]	Placebo-controlled, ZDV	Yes	300 mg PO bid, start at 36 weeks	300 mg PO every 3 hours	None	None	3 months 24 months	24.9% 30.0%	15.7% 22.0%
Ivory Coast, Burkina Faso[114,115]	Placebo-controlled, ZDV	Yes	300 mg PO bid, start at 36–38 weeks	600 mg PO at onset of labor	300 mg PO bid for 1 week	None	6 months 15 months	27.5% 30.6%	18.0% 21.5%
S. Africa, Uganda, Tanzania, (PETRA)[116]	Placebo-controlled ZDV/3TC; four arms (AP/IP/PP vs. IP/PP vs. IP vs. placebo)	69%	300 mg ZDV + 150 mg 3TC PO bid, start at 36 weeks	300 mg ZDV PO every 3 hours + 150 mg 3TC PO every 12 hours	300 mg ZDV + 150 mg 3TC PO bid for 1 week	ZDV 4 mg/kg + 3TC 2 mg/kg PO bid for 1 week	6 weeks 18 months	17.2% 27.0%	8.6% 3 parts 10.8% 2 parts 17.7% IP only 21% 3 parts 25% 2 parts, 28% IP only
Uganda[11]	Nevirapine (NVP) vs. ZDV	Yes	None	Single 200 mg NVP PO or ZDV 600 mg PO then 300 mg every 3 hours	None	Single NVP 2 mg/kg at 48 hours or ZDV 4 mg/kg bid for 1 week	14–16 weeks 12 months	ZDV 25.1% ZDV 24.0%	NVP 13.1% NVP 16.0%
S. Africa (Saint)[117]	ZDV/3TC vs. NVP	40%	None	Single 200 mg NVP or ZDV 300 mg PO every 3 hours + 150 mg 3TC PO every 12 hours	None	Single NVP 2 mg/kg at 48 hours or ZDV 4 mg/kg + 3TC 2 mg/kg PO bid for 1 week	8 weeks	ZDV/3TC 10.9%	NVP 13.3%
US, Europe, Brazil, Bahamas (PACTG 316)[118]	NVP vs. placebo, in addition to existing maternal antiretroviral therapy, at least ZDV	No	No study therapy	Single dose 200 mg NVP PO	No study therapy	Single NVP 2 mg/kg at 48 hours	3 months	Placebo 1.4%	NVP 1.5%

the resistance mutations after single-dose nevirapine remains to be determined. Most studies, with the exception of the PETRA trial, have shown sustained benefit of the peripartum therapy through 15 months of age even in breastfeeding groups. Trials of continued therapy for the mother or infant during breastfeeding, as well as exclusive breastfeeding with early weaning, are underway to try to further reduce transmission in women without safe alternatives to breastfeeding.

More recent observational data suggest that transmission rates are reduced even further, to 2% or lower, by the use of maternal combination antiretroviral therapy or the PACTG 076 ZDV regimen along with scheduled cesarean delivery. Four small studies reported one transmission (0.6%) among a total of 160 infants born to women on two or more antiretroviral agents during pregnancy.[55,56,121,122] Similarly low transmission rates have been reported, most notably from the Women and Infants Transmission Study (WITS), which found a transmission rate of 1.1% among 187 women on combination antiretroviral therapy that included a protease inhibitor.[57,123,124] In WITS, this effect remained significant in the multivariate analysis adjusting for maternal HIV RNA level and other factors associated with transmission, although most women on highly active antiretroviral therapy (HAART) had HIV RNA levels of less than 40,000 copies/ml. These data suggest that highly active antiretroviral regimens indicated for HIV-infected women for their own health are also beneficial in reducing the risk of perinatal transmission.

Early studies of the impact of mode of delivery on the risk of HIV transmission yielded conflicting results because of the lack of differentiation of cesarean delivery before labor and membrane rupture from those done after often prolonged labor and rupture and because of their inability to differentiate antepartum from intrapartum transmission.[52,80,90–94] As discussed above, several lines of evidence suggested that a large proportion of transmission occurred during the labor and delivery process, implying that planned cesarean delivery, avoiding labor and membrane rupture, could reduce transmission. This hypothesis was confirmed by two studies of different design. An individual patient data meta-analysis including data from 15 prospective cohorts demonstrated a significantly lower infection rate among infants delivered by scheduled cesarean section compared to other modes (urgent cesarean or vaginal delivery), with an unadjusted odds ratio (OR) of 0.45 [95% confidence interval (CI) of 0.35 to 0.58] and an OR of 0.43 (95% CI 0.33 to 0.56) adjusted for ZVD use, maternal disease stage, and birth weight.[53] Among more than 1400 women who received ZDV, most on the PACTG 076 schedule, the rate of transmission was 2% with scheduled cesarean delivery and 7% with other modes of delivery. An international randomized trial produced similar results, with a transmission rate of 1.8% among women assigned to scheduled cesarean delivery and 10.5% in those assigned to deliver vaginally (OR 0.2, 95% CI 0.1 to 0.6).[54] In an analysis stratified by ZDV use, the transmission rate was 4% with scheduled cesarean delivery and 20% with vaginal delivery among those not on antiretroviral agents (adjusted OR 0.2, 95% CI 0 to 0.8), 1% with scheduled cesarean delivery, and 4% with vaginal delivery for those receiving ZDV (adjusted OR 0.2, 95% CI 0 to 1.7). The magnitude of the reduced transmission was similar in the two groups; but because of the small number of transmissions (six total) in the ZDV group, the difference was not statistically significant. In both studies the risk of transmission was not reduced by cesarean section performed after labor or if rupture of membranes had occurred. Neither of these studies included HIV RNA determinations or women on highly active antiretroviral therapy, making it impossible to determine the potential benefit of scheduled cesarean section among women with undetectable HIV RNA or on combination therapy. More recent studies suggest the benefit of scheduled cesarean section even when adjusting for the maternal HIV RNA level at delivery among women receiving no treatment or ZDV, but most of these women had HIV RNA levels above 1000 copies/ml.[86,102] In women not receiving antiretroviral therapy in Thailand, vaginal delivery was associated with an increased risk of transmission even when adjusting for quintile of maternal HIV RNA, but only 10 women had HIV RNA levels below 1000 copies/ml. In the European Collaborative Study, the adjusted OR with 95% CI for the reduction in transmission with elective cesarean section was 0.15 (0.03 to 0.64) for those with HIV RNA above the median of 5500 copies/ml and 0.37 (0.08 to 1.71) for those with HIV RNA below the median. Seventy-nine percent of the women received no antiretroviral therapy. However, the increased risks of cesarean section compared to vaginal delivery to the mother (discussed further later) and potentially the neonate must be weighed carefully against the potential benefit among women with extremely low HIV RNA levels or on HAART who would be expected to have a risk of transmission of 2% or less regardless of delivery mode. Based on current data, ACOG and the USPHS recommend discussing scheduled cesarean delivery with all pregnant women, emphasizing the potential benefits for women with HIV RNA levels above 1000 copies/ml and indicating the lower probability of benefit for women with lower HIV RNA levels.[22,125]

For HIV-infected women who present in labor who have not previously received antiretroviral therapy during pregnancy, several options are available to try to reduce the risk of transmission.[22] Based on the data discussed above, intrapartum and neonatal ZDV/3TC or nevirapine have similar efficacy. Other options for therapy in the current USPHS guidelines include intravenous ZDV intrapartum for the mother and 6 weeks of oral ZDV for the infant (Table 28–2), which is recommended based on observational data, and the combination of this ZDV regimen and the two-dose nevirapine regimen, recommended on theoretical grounds. A New York State-wide study of more than 900 infants found transmission rates of 6% with ZDV begun during pregnancy, 10% with ZDV begun during labor and given to the neonate, 9% with neonatal ZDV only begun by 48 hours of age and usually within 24 hours of age, and 18% with neonatal ZDV begun after 48 hours of age, which was not significantly different from the 27% seen if no ZDV was given to the woman or infant.[10] A smaller study from North Carolina observed a transmission rate of 3% with the full PACTG 076 regimen, 11% with intrapartum and neonatal ZDV, 27% with neonatal ZDV only with time of initiation not specified, and 31% with no maternal or infant antiretroviral therapy.[49] No randomized trials of infant therapy-only have been reported, but the data discussed here suggest that ZDV therapy for the infant may be beneficial in reducing transmission if given as soon as possible after birth and definitely within 48 hours. Although infants born to untreated women might be considered eligible for post-exposure prophylaxis with two or three drugs, similar to health care workers exposed to needlestick injury, no data are available regarding combination therapy given only to the newborn to prevent transmission.

With the availability of current antiretroviral therapy and an ever-growing pool of HIV-infected women in their reproductive years, women many enter pregnancy with complex treatment histories. The impact of viral resistance on the efficacy of therapy for preventing perinatal transmission and for maternal health is unknown. Use of maximally suppressive antiretroviral regimens, rather than ZDV or dual combination therapy, should minimize the chance of resistance developing during pregnancy. In the PACTG 076 study, ZDV resistance mutations were present in one treatment-naive woman at enrollment and developed in 1 (2.6%) of 39 women with paired enrollment and delivery specimens.[126] Resistance mutations were not associated with an increased risk of transmission. Any ZDV resistance mutation was detected in 25% of 142 isolates from women treated early in the WITS trial with ZDV for their own health, and 14 had codon 215 mutations or more than one mutation, suggesting higher level resistance.[127] On univariate analysis the presence of a resistance mutation was not associated with an increased risk of perinatal transmission; but on multivariate analysis, adjusting for the duration of ruptured membranes and total lymphocyte count, resistance mutations were associated with an increased risk of transmission. This finding could be related to the increased risk of viral resistance among women with high HIV RNA levels not adjusted for in the analysis. Codon 215 ZDV resistance mutations were detected in 9.6% of 62 consecutive women in the Swiss HIV in Pregnancy Study, but perinatal transmission did not occur among any of the women with the resistance mutation despite receipt of ZDV only.[128] Although perinatal transmission of HIV with genotypic resistance has been reported,[129,130] it is not clear that the presence of the mutations increases the risk of transmission. No data currently suggest that pregnancy per se should be an indication for HIV resistance testing despite an advisory panel recommendation suggesting that this expensive, complex testing be done in all pregnant women with detectable HIV.[131] Until further data are available, resistance testing for HIV-infected pregnant women should be done for the same indications as in nonpregnant persons, specifically for those who do not respond to an initial HAART regimen, those who have persistently detectable HIV RNA levels with a history of multiple therapeutic regimens, or where the prevalence of resistant HIV in the community is high.[22]

The impact of short-term (less than 6 months) ZDV monotherapy on maternal health, viral load, and long-term prognosis remains a concern. Given the expanded indications for combination antiretroviral therapy in the mother to prevent perinatal transmission in addition to indications for therapy for their own health, only women with high CD4+ T-lymphocyte counts and extremely low HIV RNA levels would be receiving ZDV monotherapy, and the rate of development of resistance mutations would be expected to be low. In a small study following viral load and infectivity by culture among women with low viral levels, HIV-1 plasma RNA and infectivity remained stable during and after gestation.[132] Among women treated with ZDV only during pregnancy, there was a trend toward an increase in viral load measured by peripheral blood mononuclear cell infectivity 6 months postpartum compared with levels before initiation of ZDV. However, most of these women had indications for combination therapy based on current guidelines. Preliminary data from ACTG 288, the follow-up study of women enrolled in PACTG 076, do not suggest a difference in clinical progression between ZDV- and placebo-treated women.[133] Thus there does not seem to be a significant negative impact of short-term ZDV therapy of the mother on the development of resistance, maternal health, or long-term prognosis among women without current indications for combination antiretroviral therapy.

Antiretroviral therapy for women after pregnancy should be based on maternal HIV RNA, CD4+ T-lymphocyte count, and maternal wishes. For women who have been on combination therapy during pregnancy for their own health, these regimens should be continued with postpartum reassessment of adherence and response to therapy. Among women treated prophylactically for perinatal transmission, therapy can be discontinued at delivery with reassessment at the 6-week postpartum visit for indications for therapy, or therapy can be continued if the mother chooses. Plans for therapy after delivery should be discussed before initiation of therapy during pregnancy for women who are being treated only to prevent transmission who do not have other indications for therapy for their own health. Continued care, assessment, and antiretroviral therapy as indicated after pregnancy must be ensured for the HIV-positive woman.

▲ TREATMENT AND PROPHYLAXIS OF OPPORTUNISTIC INFECTIONS DURING PREGNANCY

As with antiretroviral therapy, treatment and prophylaxis of opportunistic infections during pregnancy should follow guidelines similar to those for nonpregnant women.[134] Drugs frequently used for treatment or prophylaxis of opportunistic infections are summarized in Table 28–4. Primary prophylaxis for *Pneumocystis carinii* pneumonia should be offered to women with CD4+ T lymphocyte counts below 200/μl, unexplained fever (higher than 100°F) for 2 weeks or more, or a history of oropharyngeal candidiasis; secondary prophylaxis should be offered to all women with previous *P. carinii* pneumonia. Primary, and probably secondary, prophylaxis may be discontinued for women on highly active antiretroviral therapy with sustained elevations in their CD4+ T lymphocyte count above 200/μl.[135–137] Trimethoprim-sulfamethoxazole (TMP-SMZ), one double-strength tablet daily, is the first choice for prophylaxis during pregnancy. Alternatives include aerosolized pentamidine, 300 mg monthly via Respirgard II nebulizer, or oral dapsone 100 mg daily. Therapy may be continued

Table 28–4. USE OF DRUGS FOR TREATMENT OR PROPHYLAXIS OF OPPORTUNISTIC INFECTIONS DURING PREGNANCY

Drug	Pregnancy category	Concerns regarding use during pregnancy	Recommended use during pregnancy
Acyclovir	C	Well tolerated	Treatment of frequent or severe symptomatic herpes outbreaks, use for prevention of recurrences at term still investigational
Amphotericin B	B	None identified	Documented invasive fungal disease
Azithromycin	B	None identified	MAC prophylaxis or treatment, *Chlamydia trachomatis* infection
Cidofovir	C	Embryotoxic and teratogenic in animals	Treatment or secondary prophylaxis of life-threatening or sight-threatening CMV
Ciprofloxacin, other quinolones	C	Arthropathy in immature animals; not teratogenic in animal studies	None
Clarithromycin	C	Teratogenic in rodents	Treatment of secondary prophylaxis of MAC ony if other choices exhausted
Clindamycin	B	None identified	Secondary prophylaxis of *Toxoplasma* encephalitis; treatment of anaerobic bacterial infections
Dapsone	C	None identified	Alternative choice for primary or secondary PCP prophylaxis
Doxycycline, other tetracyclines	D	Incorporated into fetal bones, teeth with staining; maternal fatty liver	None
Erythromycin	B	Hepatotoxicity with erythromycin estolate, other forms acceptable	Bacterial and chlamydial infections
Ethambutol	B	Teratogenic in animals	Active tuberculosis, treatment of MAC
Fluconazole	C	Abnormal ossification, structural defects in rats, case reports of craniofacial, skeletal abnormalities in humans with prolonged in utero exposure	Only for documented systemic disease, not prophylaxis; not for treatment of vaginal or oral *Candida*
Foscarnet	C	Teratogenic in rats, rabbits	Treatment or secondary prophylaxis of life-threatening or sight-threatening CMV
Ganciclovir	C	Teratogenic in rabbits, mice	Treatment or secondary prophylaxis of life-threatening or sight-threatening CMV
Isoniazid	C	Prophylactic vitamin K recommended at birth to prevent hemorrhagic disease. Possible increase in hepatotoxicity	Active tuberculosis or prophylaxis for exposure, skin test conversion
Itraconazole	C	Teratogenic in rats, mice	Documented systemic disease
Ketoconazole	C	Teratogenic in rats, rabbits	None
Leucovorin	C/A	Not teratogenic at recommended doses	Use with pyrimethamine
Pentamidine, aerosolized	C	Embryocidal but not teratogenic in rats with systemic use; limited systemic absorption with aerosol use	Alternative primary or secondary PCP prophylaxis
Pyrimethamine	C	Teratogenic in mice, rats, hamsters; folate antagonist, use with leucovorin	Secondary prophylaxis of *Toxoplasma* encephalitis; alternative primary or secondary PCP prophylaxis if unable to use TMP-SMZ, dapsone, or aerosolized pentamidine
Rifabutin	B	None identified	Treatment or prophylaxis of MAC, active tuberculosis
Rifampin	C	Teratogenic in mice, rats, not rabbits; no clear teratogenicity in humans; vitamin K recommended at birth to prevent hemorrhagic disease of the newborn	Active tuberculosis
Sulfadiazine	B	Increased jaundice, theoretical increased risk of kernicterus if used near delivery	Secondary prophylaxis of toxoplasmic encephalitis
Trimethoprim-sulfamethoxazole	C	Possible increase in congenital cardiac defects with first trimester use; increased jaundice, theoretical increased risk of kernicterus if used near delivery	Primary and secondary PCP prophylaxis
Vaccines			
Hepatitis B		Inactivated or recombinant; safe during pregnancy	All susceptible
Pneumococcal		Safe during pregnancy	Consider if not given within past 5 years, as per recommendations in nonpregnant adults
Influenza		Inactivated vaccine, safe during pregnancy	Give before flu season to women who will be in the second or third trimester during peak flu season
Varicella		Live virus vaccine, contraindicated for pregnancy	None
MMR (measles, mumps, rubella)		Live virus vaccine, contraindicated for pregnancy	None

CMV, cytomegalovirus; MAC, *Mycobacterium avium* complex; PCP, *Pneumocystis carinii* pneumonia; TMP-SMZ, trimethoprim-sulfamethoxazole.

up to delivery, with the infant's caregivers informed of maternal sulfa therapy so they can institute careful monitoring of bilirubin levels in the infant. Prophylaxis for *Mycobacterium avium* complex (MAC) should be offered for CD4+ T-lymphocyte counts lower than 50/μl or previous documented MAC infection. Azithromycin, 1200 mg once weekly, is the first choice for therapy during pregnancy, as in nonpregnant individuals. Clarithromycin should be avoided during pregnancy because of teratogenicity in animals. TMP-SMZ also provides prophylaxis against *Toxoplasma* encephalitis in women who are seropositive for antibodies to *Toxoplasma gondii*. For women with previous toxoplasma encephalitis, an appropriate prophylaxis regimen should be offered throughout pregnancy. Women with a positive tuberculin skin test without prior treatment or who have had contact with active tuberculosis with no evidence of active disease themselves may be given isoniazid or rifampin prophylaxis during pregnancy although they should be monitored closely, as pregnant women may have an increased risk of liver toxicity with isoniazid.[138] For women with no evidence of active tuberculosis but exposure to multidrug-resistant tuberculosis, prophylactic therapy may best be deferred until after delivery. For treatment of active tuberculosis during pregnancy, especially for multidrug-resistant tuberculosis, the regimen should be developed in consultation with obstetric and infectious disease specialists.

Primary prophylaxis for other conditions, including mucosal candidiasis and other fungal infections, is best avoided during pregnancy. Treatment of invasive fungal disease should be provided as it would be for a nonpregnant individual. Likewise, prophylaxis for cytomegalovirus (CMV) disease is not recommended during pregnancy because of the potential toxicity of the drugs and limited experience with their use during pregnancy. However, for women with life-threatening or sight-threatening CMV infections during pregnancy, treatment should be provided in consultation with obstetric and infectious disease specialists. Pneumococcal, hepatitis B, and influenza vaccines may be administered to pregnant women with the same indications as for nonpregnant individuals. Live virus vaccines such as rubella, measles, mumps, and varicella are contraindicated during pregnancy.

▲ MANAGEMENT OF THE HIV-POSITIVE PREGNANT WOMAN

The HIV-positive pregnant woman should undergo a thorough history and physical examination to document baseline findings and to allow early identification and treatment of any complications (Table 28–5). Included in the baseline studies are funduscopic, neurologic, and pelvic examinations, including cervical cytology and, if indicated, testing for *Neisseria gonorrhoeae* and *Chlamydia trachomatis*. If not done within the past year, all HIV-positive women should be tested for tuberculosis with a skin test using intermediate strength (5-TU) purified protein derivative (PPD). Platelet count and lymphocyte subset determinations and plasma HIV RNA testing should be added to routine prenatal laboratory studies. The baseline antibody level for *T. gondii* should be determined if not done previously; and liver function testing should be undertaken.

Options for therapy including potential benefits and risks should be discussed (Fig. 28–1). Women who meet current criteria for antiretroviral therapy for their own health should be offered an appropriate combination regimen, generally including two nucleoside agents and one or more protease inhibitors or two nucleoside agents and one NNRTI. In general, pregnant women tend to receive antiretroviral therapy at a frequency similar to that of nonpregnant women, with similar virologic and immunologic results.[139]

Women who would not generally have therapy recommended for their own health but who have HIV RNA levels higher than 1000 copies/ml should be offered a HAART regimen to attempt to decrease their HIV RNA to undetectable levels, thereby minimizing the risk of perinatal transmission and the need for scheduled cesarean delivery. The potential benefits of a combination regimen in this setting, including maximizing antiretroviral activity and minimizing the chance of developing of viral resistance, should be discussed along with potential maternal and infant short- and long-term toxicity, the complexity of the regimen, and the need for strict adherence and impact on future therapeutic options. If a woman who otherwise would

Table 28–5. EVALUATION OF THE HIV-INFECTED PREGNANT WOMAN

1. History, with special attention to a history suggestive of seroconversion illness, hospitalizations, immunizations, previous liveborn children who may require testing for HIV
2. Physical examination, with special attention to opthalmologic, neurologic, and pelvic examination
3. Tuberculin skin testing if not done within past year
4. Laboratory testing
   a. *Toxoplasma gondii* and cytomegalovirus antibody status
   b. Complete blood count, including differential and platelet count, repeat every 4–12 weeks, depending on current antiretroviral therapy
   c. Hepatitis B panel, including surface antigen, surface antibody, and core antibody
   d. Blood type, Rh, and indirect Coombs' test
   e. Serologic test for syphilis; repeat during third trimester if continuing risk of exposure
   f. Rubella antibody
   g. Hemoglobin electrophoresis if of African, Asian, or Mediterranean descent
   h. Serum creatinine, electrolytes; repeat every 4–12 weeks depending on therapy and trimester
   i. Liver transaminases and bilirubin at baseline and every 4–12 weeks depending on therapy and trimester
   j. Lymphocyte subsets
   k. Plasma HIV RNA level at baseline and 4 weeks after change in therapy, then every 4–8 weeks until undetectable; repeat at 32–36 weeks for counseling regarding mode of delivery
5. Discuss option of maternal serum marker screening (α-fetoprotein, estriol, human chorionic gonadotropin) for neural tube defects and Down syndrome at 16–18 weeks
6. Ultrasonography at 18–20 weeks for confirmation of dates and detection of anomalies. Consider follow-up ultrasonography for growth and fluid volume at 32–36 weeks if receiving antiretroviral therapy with limited previous use during pregnancy
7. Glucola (50 g) testing for gestational diabetes at 24–28 weeks' gestation

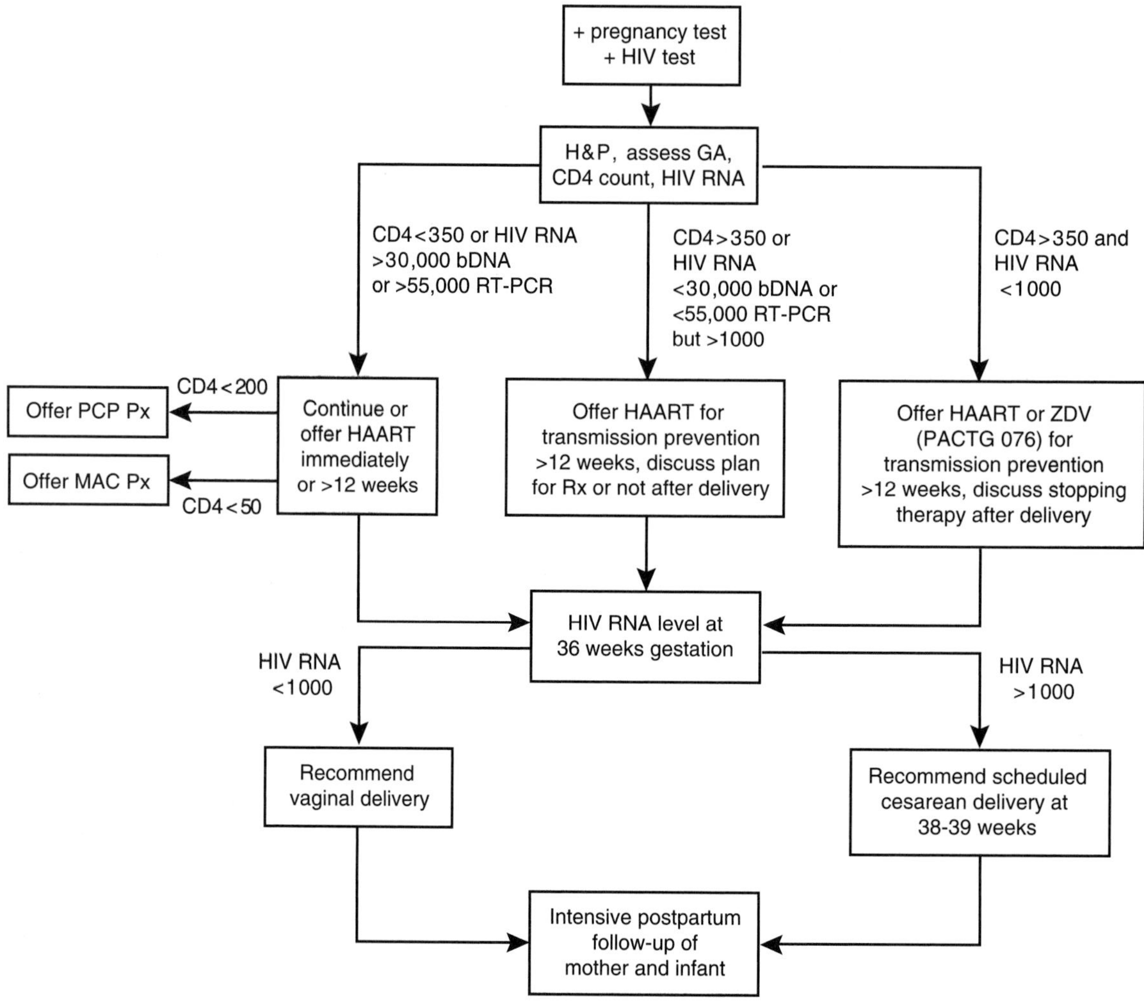

Figure 28–1. Algorithm for managing the pregnant HIV-infected woman. See text for complete discussion. bDNA, plasma HIV RNA level determined by the branched-chain DNA assay in copies/ml; CD4+ T-lymphocyte count in cells/μl; GA, gestational age; HAART, highly active antiretroviral therapy; H & P, history and physical examination; PX, prophylaxis; RT-PCR, plasma HIV RNA level determined by the reverse transcription–polymerase chain reaction assay (in copies/ml).

not be given combination antiretroviral therapy outside of pregnancy chooses to start a combination regimen to prevent transmission, the option of continuing the therapy postpartum versus stopping all therapy at delivery until indications for therapy occur should be discussed in detail before starting therapy. If a woman elects not to take combination therapy during pregnancy or has an undetectable HIV RNA level before therapy, she should be encouraged to take the PACTG 076 regimen as outlined in Table 28–2. HIV RNA testing should be done approximately 4 weeks after any change in therapy. Pregnant women should be monitored on a regular basis for toxicity due to the current therapeutic regimen. Serum lactate testing is difficult to perform, and normal values during pregnancy have not been established. Thus routine lactate testing is not recommended but may be helpful if symptoms suggestive of lactic acidosis are present. In addition, a baseline sonogram should be offered at 18 weeks for all women and follow-up sonograms for women on therapy other than ZDV should be considered during the third trimester.

Maternal serum testing between 16 and 20 weeks of pregnancy using α-fetoprotein, estriol, and human chorionic gonadotropin is the current method of screening women at low risk for carrying fetuses with neural tube defects, several other birth defects, and certain chromosomal abnormalities including Down syndrome. Approximately 60% of cases of Down syndrome and most neural tube defects can be detected with a screening positive rate of 5%.[140] The option of this testing should be discussed with all pregnant women at the appropriate gestational age window; a more complex discussion is required for HIV-infected women. Serum testing to detect chromosomal and other defects is a screening test, with the diagnostic tests for the 5% with positive screens being ultrasonography and amniocentesis. Although some abnormal results may be explained by ultrasound detection of a birth defect, multiple gestation, or erroneous pregnancy dating, about half of the women with positive screens require amniocentesis for a definitive diagnosis. Amniocentesis carries with it a complication rate of approximately 5/1000, ranging from transient fluid leakage to pregnancy loss. The risk of HIV transmission related to amniocentesis has not been well quantified, as amniocentesis is generally avoided in HIV-infected women. Thus HIV-infected women must understand that serum testing is a screening method that may require invasive testing for definitive diagnosis of a defect or a normal result. If they are unwilling to undergo amniocentesis, serum screening should not be done, as an abnormal result is nondiagnostic and causes significant anxiety. If full testing is desired and amniocentesis is indicated, it should be done only after optimization of the maternal antiretroviral therapy and under direct ultrasound guidance to avoid traversing the placenta or contacting the fetus.

Studies from the United States and Europe have not suggested any difference in birth weight or gestational age for untreated HIV-positive women and similar controls.[77,141,142] In developing countries, the rates of low birth weight and preterm birth appear to be increased among HIV-positive women, possibly related to nutritional differences or concurrent infections.[143] Data from Europe suggest a potential beneficial effect of ZDV on birth weight and gestational age but a potential increase in preterm births among women receiving long-term protease inhibitor therapy.[121,144,145] U.S. data have not confirmed an increased risk of preterm birth with combination therapy.[57] Women who are HIV-positive should have high-risk obstetric care with increased surveillance for infections and preterm labor; they should undergo targeted studies based on any specific antiretroviral agents or opportunistic infection prophylaxis they are receiving and on their anticipated side effects.

Discussions on the mode of delivery should be begun with the woman as early during pregnancy as possible. As already discussed, scheduled cesarean delivery appears to reduce the risk of intrapartum transmission of HIV among women on no antiretroviral therapy or ZDV monotherapy. Whether scheduled cesarean delivery offers additional benefit to women on HAART regimens or with undetectable HIV RNA is unknown. In HIV-negative populations, cesarean section done after labor or membrane rupture is associated with a five- to sevenfold increased risk of morbidity, especially postpartum infection, and mortality compared to that seen with vaginal delivery, with scheduled cesarean delivery being associated with an intermediate risk.[146–148] Early case-control studies suggested an increased risk of postpartum complications among HIV-infected women undergoing cesarean section, often after labor or membrane rupture, compared to HIV-negative women.[149–152] Several of the studies suggest an increased risk of postpartum pneumonia among HIV-infected women, but the rate was low. Cohort studies, including data from the randomized trial, do not suggest that risks to HIV-infected women are greater than among HIV-negative women with similar characteristics.[54,153,154] Current data suggest that the magnitude of increased risk with cesarean delivery compared to vaginal delivery is similar for HIV-infected women and HIV-negative women. The risk of postpartum infections may be minimized by diagnosis and treatment of genital infections, including bacterial vaginosis during pregnancy, and use of prophylactic antibiotics at cesarean section, although data specific to HIV-infected women are unavailable.

Current practice guidelines from ACOG recommend scheduled cesarean delivery for HIV-infected women with HIV RNA levels higher than 1000 copies/ml near delivery and provision of scheduled cesarean delivery for any HIV-infected woman who elects it.[125] The woman's decision regarding mode of delivery should be respected regardless of her choice. If scheduled cesarean section is chosen, ACOG guidelines allow scheduling at 38 weeks' gestation based on clinical and ultrasonography parameters to minimize the chance of labor or membrane rupture before the procedure, rather than the 39 weeks gestational age usually recommended to minimize the chance of infant respiratory distress.

Women should continue their oral antiretroviral therapy as much as possible, receive the loading dose of intravenous ZDV, and be placed on a continuous infusion of ZDV before scheduled cesarean delivery or during labor. Pregnant women on regimens that include stavudine (d4T) may be given oral d4T during labor without intravenous ZDV, or the d4T can be discontinued intrapartum and intravenous ZDV given instead. If vaginal delivery is chosen, scalp electrodes and other invasive fetal procedures should be avoided, and the duration of ruptured membranes should be minimized by avoiding artificial rupture of membranes but inducing labor if rupture occurs before active labor. Infants should be washed thoroughly before receiving injections or having any blood withdrawn.

The HIV-positive women and their infants require intensive follow-up during the postpartum period (Table 28–6). Women require intensive psychosocial follow-up to deal with concerns regarding potential HIV infection in the infant and to ensure continued adherence to antiretroviral therapy if medication is continued. When safe alternatives exist, breast-feeding is not recommended for HIV-positive pregnant women. The relative risks and benefits of breastfeeding versus bottle feeding in developing countries remain to be determined. Lactation suppression is not recommended for women who choose not to breastfeed because of the limited efficacy and potential complications of bromocriptine, including seizures and strokes.

Table 28–6. ISSUES CONSIDERED DURING THE PERIPARTUM/POSTPARTUM PERIOD

1. Continuation versus discontinuation of antiretroviral therapy, depending on initial indications for therapy and maternal wishes
2. Need for additional support for adherence to antiretroviral medications given the demands for newborn care and loss of incentive of decreasing perinatal transmission
3. Need for enhanced psychosocial support during determination of infant infection status
4. Recommendation for HIV-infected women not to breastfeed
5. Contraceptive counseling, taking into consideration potential interactions of hormonal contraceptives and other maternal therapy
6. Review maternal status regarding the need for opportunistic infection prophylaxis, immunizations, other health maintenance such as mammograms, cervical cytology
7. Determination of infant infection status; provision of antiretroviral prophylaxis of treatment as indicated
8. Provision of infant *Pneumocystis carinii* prophylaxis beginning at 4–6 weeks of age
9. Infant immunizations as recommended according to HIV status

As for all postpartum women, contraceptive counseling should be undertaken and contraceptives provided before hospital discharge. Condom use is routinely recommended, but other options, including hormonal contraceptive agents, can be offered to HIV-infected women taking into account the usual contraindications and potential interactions with other medications. Nucleoside reverse transcriptase inhibitors do not seem to have significant interactions with hormonal contraceptives. Ritonavir, nelfinavir, rifampin, rifabutin, and possibly amprenavir decrease ethinyl estradiol levels, which may affect the contraceptive efficacy of combination oral contraceptives. Estradiol levels increase with indinavir and efavirenz, although the significance of this increase is unclear. Potential interactions of other antiretrovirals with oral contraceptives have not been studied. A study is in progress in the Adult ACTG to evaluate interactions of depot medroxyprogesterone acetate with several antiretroviral agents. Intrauterine devices or tubal ligation can be offered to carefully selected women, regardless of HIV status.[155] As discussed above, antiretroviral therapy after delivery must be individualized depending on maternal preferences, CD4+ T-lymphocyte count, and HIV RNA level.

The infant should be followed with studies to detect HIV through the PCR or cultures to allow detection of infant infection, if it is present, as early as possible.[156] Infants should be continued on ZDV until 6 weeks of age unless infection is documented before this point. If infection is documented in the infant, combination antiretroviral therapy and follow-up by pediatric infectious disease specialists is recommended. All infants should be started on primary prophylaxis against *P. carinii* pneumonia at 4 to 6 weeks of age until they are determined to be HIV-negative by viral testing after 3 months of age.[134] If serial negative tests are obtained through 3 months of age, prophylaxis may be stopped, but infants should continue to be tested periodically. Childhood immunizations should be started on schedule as recommended for HIV-positive children, with recommendations followed depending on the infectious status once it is determined.

REFERENCES

1. Centers for Disease Control and Prevention. HIV/AIDS Surveillance Rep 11:1, 1999.
2. World Health Report 1999, Making a Difference. World Health Organization, Geneva, 1999, pp 19–22.
3. Lindegren ML, Byers RH, Thomas P, et al. Trends in perinatal transmission of HIV/AIDS in the United States. JAMA 282:531, 1999.
4. Centers for Disease Control USPHS recommendations for human immunodeficiency virus counseling and voluntary testing for pregnant women. MMWR Morb Mortal Wkly Rep 44:1, 1995.
5. Stoto MA, Almario DA, McCormick MC. Reducing the Odds: Preventing Perinatal Transmission of HIV in the United States. National Academy Press, Washington, DC, 1999.
6. American College of Obstetricians and Gynecologists. American Academy of Pediatrics and American College of Obstetricians and Gynecologists Joint Statement on Human Immunodeficiency Virus Screening. ACOG, Washington, DC, 1999.
7. Lindsay MK, Feng TI, Peterson HB, et al. Routine human immunodeficiency virus infection screening in unregistered and registered inner-city parturients. Obstet Gynecol 77:599, 1991.
8. Donegan SP, Steger KA, Recla L, et al. Seroprevalence of human immunodeficiency virus in parturients at Boston City Hospital: implications for public health and obstetric practice. Am J Obstet Gynecol 167:622, 1992.
9. Minkoff HL, McCalla S, Feldman J. The relationship of cocaine use to syphilis and HIV infection among inner city parturient women. Am J Obstet Gynecol 163:521, 1990.
10. Wade NA, Birkhead GS, Warren BL, et al. Abbreviated regimens of zidovudine prophylaxis and perinatal transmission of the human immunodeficiency virus. N Engl J Med 339:1409, 1998.
11. Guay LA, Musoke P, Fleming T, et al. Intrapartum and neonatal single-dose nevirapine compared with zidovudine for prevention of mother-child transmission of HIV-1 in Kampala, Uganda: HIVNET 012 randomised trial. Lancet 354:795, 1999.
12. Minkoff H, O'Sullivan MJ. The case for rapid HIV testing during labor. JAMA 279:1743, 1998.
13. Burns DN, Landesman S, Minkoff H, et al. The influence of pregnancy on human immunodeficiency virus type 1 infection: antepartum and postpartum changes in human immunodeficiency virus type 1 viral load. Am J Obstet Gynecol 178:355, 1998.
14. Weisser M, Rudin C, Battegay M, et al. Does pregnancy influence the course of HIV infection? Evidence from two large Swiss cohort studies. J Acquir Immune Defic Syndr Hum Retrovirol 17:404, 1998.
15. Saada M, Le Chenadec J, Berrebi A, et al. Pregnancy and progression to AIDS: results of the French prospective cohorts. AIDS 14:2355, 2000.
16. Biggar RJ, Pahwa S, Minkoff H, et al. Immunosuppression in pregnant women infected with human immunodeficiency virus. Am J Obstet Gynecol 161:1239, 1989.
17. Deschamps MM, Pape JW, Desvarieux M, et al. A prospective study of HIV-seropositive asymptomatic women of childbearing age in a developing country. J Acquir Immune Defic Syndr 6:446, 1993.
18. Kumar RM, Uduman SA, Khurrana AK. Impact of pregnancy on maternal AIDS. J Reprod Med 42:429, 1993.
19. Connor EM, Sperling RS, Gelber R, et al. Reduction of maternal-infant transmission of human immunodeficiency virus type 1 with zidovudine treatment: pediatric AIDS Clinical Trials Group Protocol 076 Study Group. N Engl J Med 331:1173, 1994.
20. Moodley J, Moodley D, Pillay K, et al. Pharmacokinetics and antiretroviral activity of lamivudine alone or when co-administered with zidovudine in human immunodeficiency virus type 1-infected pregnant women and their offspring. J Infect Dis 178:1327, 1998.
21. Wang Y, Livingston E, Patil S, et al. Pharmacokinetics of didanosine in antepartum and postpartum human immunodeficiency virus-infected pregnant women and their neonates: an AIDS Clinical Trials Group study. J Infect Dis 180:1536, 1999.
22. Centers for Disease Control and Prevention. USPHS task force recommendations for the use of antiretroviral drugs in pregnant women infected with HIV-1 for maternal health and for reducing perinatal HIV-1 transmission in the United States. MMWR Morb Mortal Wkly Rep 47(RR-2):1, 1998. Updated February 2001. Available at www.hivatis.org.
23. Antiretroviral Pregnancy Registry. Interim report. 1/1/89–7/31/00; issued 12/01.
24. Brinkman K, Ter Hofstede HJM, Burger DM, et al. Adverse effects of reverse transcriptase inhibitors: mitochondrial toxicity as common pathway. AIDS 12:1735, 1998.
25. Bristol-Myers Squibb. Dear health care provider letter, January 5, 2001. Available at www.fda.gov/medwatch/safety/2001/zerit&videx_letter.htm.
26. Ibday JA, Yang Z, Bennett MJ. Liver disease in pregnancy and fetal fatty acid oxidation defects. Mol Genet Metab 71:182, 2000.
27. Grimbert S, Fisch C, Deschamps D, et al. Decreased mitochondrial oxidation of fatty acids in pregnant mice: possible relevance to development of acute fatty liver of pregnancy. Hepatology 17:628, 1993.
28. Grimbert S, Fisch C, Deschamps D, et al. Effects of female sex hormones on mitochondria: possible role of acute fatty liver of pregnancy. Am J Physiol 268:G107, 1995.
29. Blanche S, Tardieu M, Rustin P, et al. Persistent mitochondrial dysfunction and perinatal exposure to antiretroviral nucleoside analogues. Lancet 354:1084, 1999.
30. Perinatal Safety Review Working Group. Nucleoside exposure in the children of HIV-infected women receiving antiretroviral drugs: absence of clear evidence for mitochondrial disease in children who died before 5 years of age in five United States cohorts. J Acquir Immune Defic Syndr 25:261, 2000.

31. Culnane M, Fowler MG, Lee SS, et al. Lack of long-term effects of in utero exposure to zidovudine among uninfected children born to HIV-infected women. JAMA 281:151, 1999.
32. Chotpitayasunondh T, Vanprapar N, Simonds RJ, et al. Safety of late in utero exposure to zidovudine in infants born to human immunodeficiency virus-infected mothers: Bangkok. Pediatrics 107:1, 2001.
33. Lange J, Stellato R, Brinkman K, et al. Review of neurological adverse events in relation to mitochondrial dysfunction in the prevention of mother to child transmission of HIV: PETRA study. Presented at the Second Conference on Global Strategies for the Prevention of HIV Transmission from Mothers to Infants, September 1999, Montreal, abstract 250.
34. Olivero OA, Anderson LM, Diwan BA, et al. Transplacental effects of 3′-azido-2′3′-dideoxythymidine(AZT): tumorigenicity in mice and genotoxicity in mice and monkeys. J Natl Cancer Inst 89:1602, 1997.
35. Ayers KM, Torrey CE, Reynolds DJ. A transplacental carcinogenicity bioassay in CD-1 mice with zidovudine. Fundam Appl Toxicol 38:195, 1997.
36. Hanson IC, Antonelli TA, Sperling RS, et al. Lack of tumors in infants with perinatal HIV-1 exposure and fetal/neonatal exposure to zidovudine. J Acquir Immune Defic Syndr Hum Retrovirol 20:463, 1999.
37. Reggy AA, Rogers MF, Simonds RJ. Using 3′-azido′2′3′-dideoxythymidine (AZT) to prevent perinatal human immunodeficiency virus transmission and risk of transplacental carcinogenesis. J Natl Cancer Inst 89:1566, 1997.
38. Mirochnik M, Fenton T, Gagnier P, et al. Pharmacokinetics (Pk) of nevirapine (NVP) in human immunodeficiency virus-infected pregnant women and their neonates Pediatric AIDS Clinical Trials Group Protocol 250 team. J Infect Dis 178:368, 1998.
39. Musoke P, Guay LA, Bagenda D, et al. A phase I/II study of the safety and pharmacokinetics of nevirapine in HIV-1-infected pregnant Ugandan women and their neonates (HIVNET 006). AIDS 13:479, 1999.
40. Wara D, Tuomala R, Bryson Y, et al. PACTG 358: safety, pharmacokinetics and antiretroviral activity of indinavir, zidovudine (ZDV), and lamivudine (3TC) in HIV-1 seropositive pregnant women and infants. Presented at the Second Conference on Global Strategies for the Prevention of HIV Transmission from Mothers to Infants. Montreal, September 1999, abstract 447.
41. Hayashi S, Beckerman K, Homma M, et al. Pharmacokinetics of indinavir in HIV-positive pregnant women. AIDS 14:1061, 2000.
42. Centers for Disease Control and Prevention. Report of the NIH panel to define principles of therapy of HIV infection and guidelines for the use of antiretroviral agents in HIV-infected adults and adolescents. MMWR Morb Mortal Wkly Rep 47(RR-5):1, 1998. Updated February 2001. Available at www.hivatis.org.
43. Hutto C, Parks WP, Lai S, et al. A hospital-based prospective study of perinatal infection with human immunodeficiency virus type 1. J Pediatr 118:347, 1991.
44. European Collaborative Study. Risk factors for mother-to-child transmission of HIV-1. Lancet 339:1007, 1992.
45. Thomas PA, Weedon J, Krasinski K, et al. Maternal predictors of perinatal human immunodeficiency virus transmission: the New York City Perinatal HIV Transmission Collaborative Study Group. Pediatr Infect Dis J 13:489, 1994.
46. Mayaux M-J, Dussaix E, Isopet J, et al. Maternal virus load during pregnancy and mother-to-child transmission of human immunodeficiency virus type 1: the French perinatal cohort studies. J Infect Dis 175:172, 1997.
47. Boyer PJ, Dillon M, Navaie M, et al. Factors predictive of maternal-fetal transmission of HIV-1: preliminary analysis of zidovudine given during pregnancy and/or delivery. JAMA 271:1925, 1994.
48. Frenkel LM, Wagner LE II, Demeter LM, et al. Effects of zidovudine use during pregnancy on resistance and vertical transmission of human immunodeficiency virus type 1. Clin Infect Dis 20:1321, 1995.
49. Fiscus SA, Adimora AA, Schoenbach VJ, et al. Trends in human immunodeficiency virus (HIV) counseling, testing, and antiretroviral treatment of HIV-infected women and perinatal transmission in North Carolina. J Infect Dis 180:99, 1999.
50. Wiznia AA, Crane M, Lanbert G, et al. Zidovudine use to reduce perinatal HIV type 1 transmission in an urban medical center. JAMA 275:1504, 1996.
51. Mayaux M-J, Teglas JP, Mandelbrot L, et al. Acceptability and impact of zidovudine for prevention of mother-to-child human immunodeficiency virus transmission in France. J Pediatr 131:857, 1997.
52. Mandelbrot L, Le Chenadec J, Berrebi A, et al. Perinatal HIV-1 transmission: interaction between zidovudine prophylaxis and mode of delivery in the French perinatal cohort. JAMA 280:55, 1998.
53. International Perinatal HIV Group. The mode of delivery and the risk of vertical transmission of human immunodeficiency virus type 1: a meta-analysis of 15 prospective cohort studies. N Engl J Med 340:977, 1999.
54. European Mode of Delivery Collaboration. Elective caesarean-section versus vaginal delivery in prevention of vertical HIV-1 transmission: a randomised clinical trial. Lancet 353:1035, 1999.
55. McGowan JP, Crane M, Wiznia AA, et al. Combination antiretroviral therapy in human immunodeficiency virus-infected pregnant women. Obstet Gynecol 94:641, 1999.
56. Clarke SM, Mulcahy F, Healy CM, et al. The efficacy and tolerability of combination antiretroviral therapy in pregnancy: infant and maternal outcome. Int J STD AIDS 11:220, 2000.
57. Women and Infants Transmission Study Investigators. Trends in mother-to-infant transmission of HIV in the WITS cohort: impact of 076 and HAART therapy. Presented at the XIII International AIDS Conference, Durban, South Africa, July 2000, abstract LBOr4.
58. Ryder RN, Nsa W, Hassy SE, et al. Perinatal transmission of the human immunodeficiency virus type 1 to infants of seropositive women in Zaire. N Engl J Med 320:1637, 1989.
59. St Louis ME, Kamenga M, Brown C, et al. Risk for perinatal HIV-1 transmission according to maternal immunologic, virologic, and placental factors. JAMA 269:2853, 1993.
60. Temmerman M, Nyong'o A, Bwayo J, et al. Risk factors for mother-to-child transmission of human immunodeficiency virus-1 infection. Am J Obstet Gynecol 172:700, 1995.
61. Blanche S, Tardieu M, Duliege A-M, et al. Longitudinal study of 94 symptomatic infants with perinatally acquired human immunodeficiency virus infection: evidence for a bimodal expression of clinical and biological symptoms. Am J Dis Child 144:1210, 1990.
62. European Collaborative Study. Children born to women with HIV-1 infection: natural history and risk of transmission. Lancet 337:253, 1991.
63. Luzuriaga K, McQuilken P, Alimenti A, et al. Early viremia and immune responses in vertical human immunodeficiency virus type 1 infection. J Infect Dis 167:1008, 1993.
64. McIntosh K, Pitt J, Brambilla D, et al. Blood culture in the first 6 months of life for the diagnosis of vertically transmitted human immunodeficiency virus infection. J Infect Dis 170:996, 1994.
65. Mock PA, Shaffer N, Bhadrakom C, et al. Maternal viral load and timing of mother-to-child HIV transmission, Bangkok, Thailand. AIDS 13:407, 1999.
66. Clemetson DB, Moss GB, Willerford DM, et al. Detection of HIV DNA in cervical and vaginal secretions: prevalence and correlates among women in Nairobi, Kenya. JAMA 269:2860, 1993.
67. Henin Y, Mandelbrot L, Henrion R, et al. Virus excretion in the cervicovaginal secretions of pregnant and nonpregnant HIV-infected women. J Acquir Immune Defic Syndr 6:72, 1993.
68. Chuachoowong R, Shaffer N, Siriwasin W, et al. Short-course antenatal zidovudine reduces both cervicovaginal human immunodeficiency virus type 1 RNA levels and risk of perinatal transmission. J Infect Dis 181:99, 2000.
69. Duliege A-M, Amos CI, Felton S, et al. Birth order, delivery route, and concordance in the transmission of human immunodeficiency virus type 1 from mothers to twins. J Pediatr 126:625, 1995.
70. Burns DN, Landesman S, Muenz LR, et al. Cigarette smoking, premature rupture of membranes and vertical transmission of HIV-1 among women with low CD4+ levels. J Acquir Immune Defic Syndr 7:718, 1994.
71. Minkoff H, Burns DN, Landesman S, et al. The relationship of the duration of ruptured membranes to vertical transmission of human immunodeficiency virus. Am J Obstet Gynecol 173:585, 1995.
72. Landesman SH, Kalish LA, Burns DN, et al. Obstetrical factors and the transmission of human immunodeficiency virus type 1 from mother to child. N Engl J Med 334:1617, 1996.
73. Kind C, Brandle B, Wyler C-A, et al. Epidemiology of vertically transmitted HIV-1 infection in Switzerland: results of a nationwide prospective study. Eur J Pediatr 151:442, 1992.

74. Ryder RN, Nsa W, Hassy SE, et al. Perinatal transmission of the human immunodeficiency virus type 1 to infants of seropositive women in Zaire. N Engl J Med 320:1637, 1989.
75. Palasanthrian P, Ziegler JB, Stewart GJ, et al. Breast-feeding during primary maternal human immunodeficiency virus infection and risk of transmission from mother to infant. J Infect Dis 167:441, 1993.
76. VanderPerre P, Lepage P, Homsy J, et al. Mother-to-infant transmission of human immunodeficiency virus by breast milk: presumed innocent or presumed guilty? Clin Infect Dis 15:502, 1992.
77. Minkoff HL, Henderson C, Mendez H. Pregnancy outcomes among mothers infected with human immunodeficiency virus and uninfected control subjects. Am J Obstet Gynecol 163:1598, 1990.
78. European Collaborative Study. Perinatal findings in children born to HIV-infected mothers. Br J Obstet Gynaecol 101:136, 1994.
79. Abrams EJ, Matheson PB, Thomas PA, et al. Neonatal predictors of infection status and early death among 332 infants at risk of HIV-1 infection monitored prospectively from birth. Pediatrics 96:451, 1995.
80. Tovo P-A, de Martino M, Gabiano C, et al. Mode of delivery and gestational age influence perinatal HIV-1 transmission. J Acquir Immune Defic Syndr Hum Retrovirol 11:88, 1996.
81. Kumar RM, Uduman SA, Khurranna AK. Impact of maternal HIV-1 infection on perinatal outcome. Int J Gynaecol Obstet 49:137, 1995.
82. Nair P, Alger L, Hines S, et al. Maternal and neonatal characteristics associated with HIV infection in infants of seropositive women. J Acquir Immun Defic Syndr 6:298, 1993.
83. Van Dyke RB, Korber BT, Popek E, et al. The Ariel project: a prospective cohort study of maternal-child transmission of human immunodeficiency virus type 1 in the era of maternal antiretroviral therapy. J Infect Dis 179:319, 1999.
84. Wabwire-Mangen F, Gray RH, Mmiro FA, et al. Placental membrane inflammation and risks of maternal-to-child transmission of HIV-1 in Uganda. J Acquir Immune Defic Syndr 22:379, 1999.
85. Sutton MY, Sternberg M, Nsuami M, et al. Trichomoniasis in pregnant human immunodeficiency virus-infected and human immunodeficiency virus-uninfected women: prevalence, risk factors, and association with low birth weight. Am J Obstet Gynecol 181:656, 1999.
86. Shaffer N, Roongpisuthipong A, Siriwasin W, et al. Maternal virus load and perinatal human immunodeficiency virus type 1 subtype E transmission, Thailand. J Infect Dis 179:590, 1999.
87. Rodriguez EM, Mofenson LM, Chang B-H, et al. Association of maternal drug use during pregnancy with maternal HIV culture positivity and perinatal HIV transmission. AIDS 10:273, 1996.
88. Semba RD, Miotti PG, Chiphangwi JD, et al. Maternal vitamin A deficiency and mother-to-child transmission of HIV-1. Lancet 343:1593, 1994.
89. Burns DN, Fitzgerald G, Semba R, et al. Vitamin A deficiency and other nutritional indices during pregnancy in human immunodeficiency virus infection: prevalence, clinical correlates, and outcome. Women and Infants Transmission Study Group. Clin Infect Dis 29:328, 1999.
90. Dunn DT, Newell ML, Mayaux MJ, et al. Mode of delivery and vertical transmission of HIV-1: a review of prospective studies. J Acquir Immune Defic Syndr 7:1064, 1994.
91. Maguire A, Sanchez E, Fortuny C, et al. Potential risk factors for vertical HIV-1 transmission in Catalonia, Spain: the protective role of cesarean section. AIDS 11:1851, 1997.
92. Kuhn L, Bobat R, Coutsoudis A, et al. Cesarean deliveries and maternal-infant HIV transmission: results from a prospective study in South Africa. J Acquir Immune Defic Syndr Hum Retrovirol 11:478, 1996.
93. Mandelbrot L, Mayaux M-J, Bongain A, et al. Obstetric factors and mother-to-child transmission of human immunodeficiency virus type 1: the French perinatal cohorts. Am J Obstet Gynecol 175:661, 1996.
94. Kind C, Rudin C, Siegrist CA, et al. Prevention of vertical transmission: additive protective effect of elective cesarean section and zidovudine prophylaxis. AIDS 12:205, 1998.
95. Thea DM, Steketee RW, Pliner V, et al. The effect of maternal viral load on the risk of perinatal transmission of HIV-1. AIDS 11:437, 1997.
96. Mofenson LM, Lambert JS, Stiehm ER, et al. Risk factors for perinatal transmission of human immunodeficiency virus type 1 in women treated with zidovudine. N Engl J Med 341:385, 1999.
97. Dickover RE, Garratty EM, Herman SA, et al. Identification of levels of maternal HIV-1 RNA associated with risk of perinatal transmission: effect of maternal zidovudine treatment on viral load. JAMA 275:599, 1996.
98. Sperling RS, Shapiro DE, Coombs RW, et al. Maternal viral load, zidovudine treatment, and the risk of transmission of human immunodeficiency virus type 1 from mother to infant. N Engl J Med 335:1621, 1996.
99. Coll O, Hernandez M, Boucher CAB, et al. Vertical HIV-1 transmission correlates with a high maternal viral load at delivery. J Acquir Immune Defic Syndr Hum Retrovirol 14:26, 1997.
100. Burns DN, Landesman S, Wright DJ, et al. Influence of other maternal variables on the relationship between maternal virus load and mother-to-infant transmission of human immunodeficiency virus type 1. J Infect Dis 175:1206, 1997.
101. Fang G, Burger H, Grimson R, et al. Maternal plasma human immunodeficiency virus type 1 RNA level: a determinant and projected threshold for mother-to-child transmission. Proc Natl Acad Sci USA 92:12100, 1995.
102. European Collaborative Study. Maternal viral load and vertical transmission of HIV-1: an important factor but not the only one. AIDS 13:1377, 1999.
103. Garcia PM, Kalish LA, Pitt J, et al. Maternal levels of plasma human immunodeficiency virus type 1 RNA and the risk of perinatal transmission. N Engl J Med 341:394, 1999.
104. Mazza C, Ravaggi A, Rodella A, et al. Influence of maternal CD4 levels on the predictive value of virus load over mother-to-child transmission of human immunodeficiency virus type 1 (HIV-1). J Med Virol 58:59, 1999.
105. Shaffer N, Chuachoowong R, Mock PA, et al. Short-course zidovudine for perinatal HIV-1 transmission in Bangkok, Thailand: a randomized controlled trial. Lancet 353:773, 1999.
106. Ioannidis JPA, Abrams EJ, Ammann A, et al. Perinatal transmission of human immunodeficiency virus type 1 by pregnant women with RNA virus loads < 1,000 copies/ml. J Infect Dis 183:539, 2001.
107. Matheson PB, Thomas PA, Abrams EJ, et al. Efficacy of antenatal zidovudine in reducing perinatal transmission of human immunodeficiency virus type 1 (HIV). J Infect Dis 172:353, 1995.
108. Fiscus SA, Adimora AA, Schoenbach VJ, et al. Perinatal HIV infection and the effect of zidovudine therapy on transmission in rural and urban counties. JAMA 275:1483, 1996.
109. Cooper ER, Nugent RP, Diaz C, et al. After AIDS Clinical Trial 076: the changing pattern of zidovudine use during pregnancy, and the subsequent reduction in the vertical transmission of human immunodeficiency virus in a cohort of infected women and their infants. J Infect Dis 174:1207, 1996.
110. Simpson GJ, Shapiro ED, Andiman WA. Reduction in the risk of vertical transmission of HIV-1 associated with treatment of pregnant women with orally administered zidovudine alone. J Acquir Immune Defic Syndr 14:145, 1997.
111. Frenkel LM, Cowless MK, Shapiro DE, et al. Analysis of the maternal components of the AIDS Clinical Trial Group 076 zidovudine regimen in the prevention of mother-to-infant transmission of human immunodeficiency virus type 1. J Infect Dis 175:971, 1997.
112. Lallemant M, Jourdain G, Le Coeur S, et al. A trial of shortened zidovudine regimens to prevent mother-to-child transmission of human immunodeficiency virus type 1: perinatal HIV Prevention Trial (Thailand) investigators. N Engl J Med 343:982, 2000.
113. Wiktor SZ, Ekpini E, Karon J, et al. Short-course zidovudine for prevention of mother-to-child transmission of HIV-1 in Abidjan, Cote d'Ivoire: a randomised trial. Lancet 353:781, 1999.
114. Dabis F, Msellati P, Meda N, et al. 6-Month efficacy, tolerance and acceptability of a short regimen of oral zidovudine to reduce vertical transmission of HIV in breastfed children in Cote d'Ivoire and Burkina Faso: a double-blind placebo-controlled multicentre trial. Lancet 353:786, 1999.
115. DITRAME ANRS 049 Study Group. 15-Month efficacy of maternal oral zidovudine to decrease vertical transmission of HIV-1 in breastfed African children. Lancet 354:2050, 1999.
116. Gray G, PETRA Trial Management Committee. The PETRA study: early and late efficacy of three short ZDV/3TC combination regimens to prevent mother-to-child transmission of HIV-1. Presented to the 13th International AIDS Conference, Durban, South Africa, July 2000, abstract LbOr5.
117. Moodley D, SAINT Investigators Team. The SAINT trial: nevirapine (NVP) versus zidovudine (ZVD) + lamivudine (3TC) in prevention of

peripartum HIV transmission. Presented at the 13th International AIDS Conference, Durban, South Africa, July 2000, abstract LbOr2.
118. Dorenbaum A, PACTG 316 Study Team. Report of results of PACTG 316: an international phase III trial of standard antiretroviral (ARV) prophylaxis plus nevirapine (NVP) for prevention of perinatal HIV transmission. Presented at the Eighth Conference on Retroviruses and Opportunistic Infections, Chicago, February 2001, abstract LB7.
119. Jackson JB, Mracna M, Guay L, et al. Selection of nevirapine (NVP) resistance mutations in Ugandan women and infants receiving NVP prophylaxis to prevent HIV-1 vertical transmission (HIVNET-012). Presented at the 13th International AIDS Conference, Durban, South Africa, July 2000, abstract LbOr13.
120. Cunningham CK, Britto P, Gelber R, et al. Genotypic resistance analysis in women participating in PACTG 316 with HIV-1 RNA > 400 copies/ml. Poster presentation at the Eighth Conference on Retroviruses and Opportunistic Infections, Chicago, February 2001, abstract 712.
121. Lorenzi P, Spicher VM, Laubereau B, et al. Antiretroviral therapies in pregnancy: maternal, fetal and neonatal effects: Swiss HIV Cohort Study, the Swiss Collaborative HIV and Pregnancy Study, and the Swiss Neonatal HIV Study. AIDS 12:241, 1998.
122. Morris AB, Cu-Uvin S, Harwell JI, et al. Multicenter review of protease inhibitors in 89 pregnancies. J Acquir Immune Defic Syndr 25:306, 2000.
123. Helfgott A, Eriksen N, Lewis S, et al. Highly active antiretroviral therapy for the prevention of perinatal HIV. Poster presentation at the Society for Maternal Fetal Medicine annual meeting, Miami Beach, January 2000, abstract 289.
124. Beckerman KP, Morris AB, Stek A. Mode of delivery and the risk of vertical transmission of HIV-1 [letter]. N Engl J Med 341:205, 1999.
125. American College of Obstetricians and Gynecologists Committee Opinion: Scheduled Cesarean Delivery and the Prevention of Vertical Transmission of HIV Infection. No. 234. Washington, Dc, ACOG, May 2000.
126. Eastman PS, Shapiro DE, Coombs RW, et al. Maternal viral genotypic zidovudine resistance and infrequent failure of zidovudine therapy to prevent perinatal transmission of human immunodeficiency virus type 1 in Pediatric AIDS Clinical Trials Group Protocol 076. J Infect Dis 177:557, 1998.
127. Welles SL, Pitt J, Colgrove R, et al. HIV-1 genotypic zidovudine drug resistance and the risk of maternal–infant transmission in the women and infants transmission study: the Women and Infants Transmission Study Group. AIDS 14:263, 2000.
128. Kully C, Yerly S, Erb P, et al. Codon 215 mutations in human immunodeficiency virus-infected pregnant women. J Infect Dis 179:705, 1999.
129. Colgrove RC, Pitt J, Chung PH, et al. Selective vertical transmission of HIV-1 antiretroviral resistance mutations. AIDS 12:2281, 1998.
130. Johnson VA, Woods C, Hamilton CD, et al. Vertical transmission of an HIV-1 variant resistant to multiple reverse transcriptase and protease inhibitors. In: Abstracts of the 6th Conference on Retroviruses and Opportunistic Infections, Chicago, January-February 1999, abstract 266.
131. Hirsch MS, Brun-Vezinet F, D'Aquila RT, et al. Antiretroviral drug resistance testing in adult HIV-1 infection: recommendations of an international AIDS Society-USA panel. JAMA 283:2417, 2000.
132. Melvin AJ, Burchett SK, Watts DH, et al. Effect of pregnancy and zidovudine therapy on viral load in HIV-1 infected women. J Acquir Immune Defic Syndr Hum Retrovirol 14:232, 1997.
133. Bardeguez A, Mofenson LM, Fowler MG, et al. Lack of clinical or immunologic disease progression with transient use of zidovudine (ZDV) to reduce perinatal HIV transmission in PACTG 076. Presented at the 12th World AIDS Conference, Geneva, June-July 1998, abstract 12233.
134. Centers for Disease Control and Prevention. 1999 USPHS/IDSA guidelines for the prevention of opportunistic infection in persons infected with human immunodeficiency virus: US Public Health Service (USPHS) and Infectious Diseases Society of America (IDSA). MMWR Morb Mortal Wkly Rep 48:1, 1999 (available at www.hivatis.org). 2001 Update available at www.hivatis.org.
135. Weverling GJ, Mocroft A, Ledergerber B, et al. Discontinuation of Pneumocystis carinii pneumonia prophylaxis after start of highly active antiretroviral therapy in HIV-1 infection: EuroSIDA Study Group. Lancet 353:1293, 1999.
136. Kirk O, Lundgren JD, Pedersen C, et al. Can chemoprophylaxis against opportunistic infections be discontinued after an increase in CD4 cells induced by highly active antiretroviral therapy? AIDS 13:1647, 1999.
137. Dworkin MS, Hanson DL, Kaplan JE, et al. Risk for preventable opportunistic infections in persons with AIDS after antiretroviral therapy increases CD4+ T lymphocyte counts above prophylaxis thresholds. J Infect Dis 182:611, 2000.
138. Franks AL, Binkin NJ, Snider DE, et al. Isoniazid hepatitis among pregnant and postpartum Hispanic patients. Public Health Rep 104:151, 1989.
139. Minkoff H, Ahdieh L, Watts DH, et al. The relationship of pregnancy to the use of highly active antiretroviral therapy. Am J Obstet Gynecol 184:1221, 2001.
140. Haddow JE, Palomki GE, Knight GJ, et al. Prenatal screening for Down's syndrome with use of maternal serum markers. N Engl J Med 327:588, 1992.
141. Johnstone FD, MacCallum L, Brettle R. Does infection with HIV affect the outcome of pregnancy? BMJ 296:467, 1988.
142. Selwyn PA, Schoenbaum EE, Davenny K, et al. Prospective study of human immunodeficiency virus infection and pregnancy outcomes in intravenous drug users. JAMA 261:1289, 1989.
143. Temmerman M, Chomba EN, Ndinya-Achola J, et al. Maternal human immunodeficiency virus-1 infection and pregnancy outcome. Obstet Gynecol 83:495, 1994.
144. European Collaborative Study. Is zidovudine therapy in pregnant HIV-infected women associated with gestational age and birthweight? AIDS 13:119, 1999.
145. European Collaborative Study and the Swiss Mother + Child HIV Cohort Study: combination antiretroviral therapy and duration of pregnancy. AIDS 14:2913; 2000.
146. Nielsen TF, Hakegaard KH. Postoperative cesarean section morbidity: a prospective study. Am J Obstet Gynecol 146:911; 1983.
147. Van Ham MAPC, van Dongen PWJ, Mulder J. Maternal consequences of cesarean section: a retrospective study of intra-operative and post-operative maternal complications of cesarean section during a 10-year period. Eur J Obstet Gynecol Reprod Biol 74:1, 1997.
148. McMahon MJ, Luther ER, Bowes WA Jr, et al. Comparison of a trial of labor with an elective second cesarean section. N Engl J Med 335:689, 1996.
149. Semprini AE, Castagna C, Ravizza M, et al. The incidence of complications after cesarean section in 156 HIV-positive women. AIDS 9:913, 1996.
150. Grubert TA, Reindell D, Kastner R, et al. Complications after cesarean section in HIV-1-infected women not taking antiretroviral treatment. Lancet 354:1612, 1999.
151. Maiques-Montesinos V, Cervera-Sanchez J, Bellver-Pradas J, et al. Post-cesarean section morbidity in HIV-positive women. Acta Obstet Gynecol Scand 78:789, 1999.
152. Vimercati A, Greco P, Loverro G, et al. Maternal complications after caesarean section in HIV infected women. Eur J Obstet Gynecol Reprod Biol 90:73, 2000.
153. Watts DH, Lambert JS, Stiehm ER, et al. Complications according to mode of delivery among HIV-infected women with CD4+ T-lymphocyte counts of 500 or less. Am J Obstet Gynecol 173:100, 2000.
154. Read J, Kpamegan E, Tuomala R, et al. Mode of delivery and postpartum morbidity among HIV-infected women: the Women and Infants Transmission Study (WITS). J Acquir Immun Defic Syndr 26:236, 2001.
155. Sinei SK, Morrison CS, Sekadde-Kigondu C, et al. Complications of use of intrauterine devices among HIV-1-infected women. Lancet 351:1238, 1998.
156. Centers for Disease Control and Prevention. Guidelines for the use of antiretroviral agents in pediatric HIV infection. MMWR Morb Mortal Wkly Rep 47(RR-4):1, 1998. Updated January 2000. Available at www.hivatis.org.

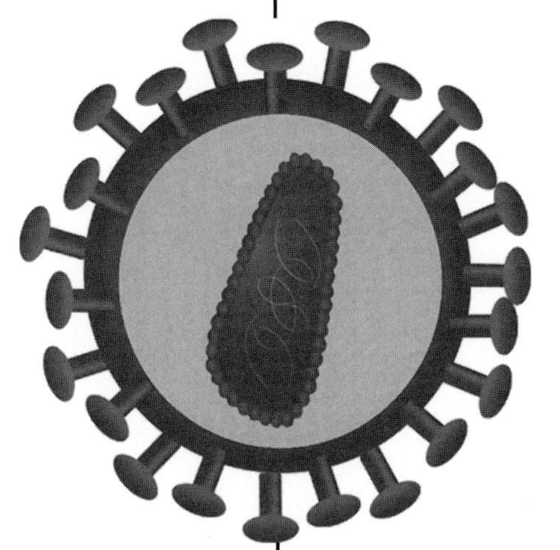

SECTION VI

Diagnosis, Therapy, and Prevention of Opportunistic Processes

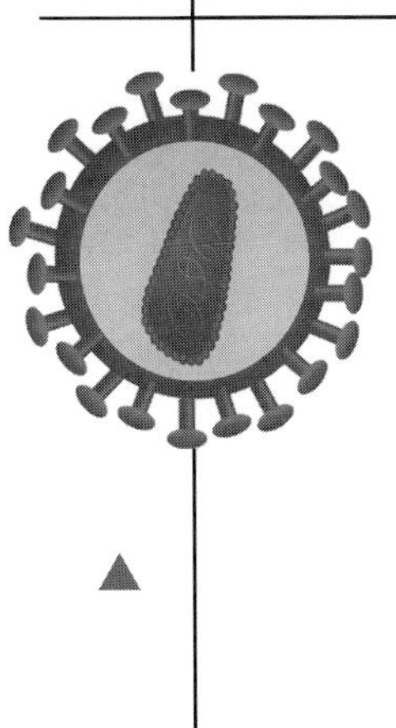

CHAPTER 29
Pneumocystosis

Henry Masur, MD

During the first decade of the acquired immunodeficiency syndrome (AIDS) epidemic, *Pneumocystis carinii* pneumonia (PCP) became widely recognized as the most common presenting clinical manifestation of AIDS in North America and western Europe.[1–7] Clinicians became quite adept at monitoring CD4+ T-lymphocyte counts to determine when patients were most likely to develop PCP, and they became familiar with recognizing the initial manifestations, establishing the diagnosis, instituting therapy, and prescribing prophylaxis.[8–12]

Since the mid-1990s the AIDS epidemic has witnessed dramatic changes in the epidemiology and management of PCP. In patients with access to medical care, PCP has become a much less common disease as a result of early diagnosis of human immunodeficiency virus (HIV) disease, widespread use of anti-*Pneumocystis* prophylaxis, and early intervention with highly active antiretroviral therapy.[3,12–22] PCP continues to be common, however, in those who do not have access to medical care, do not get tested for HIV infection early in the course of their disease, elect not to treat their HIV disease consistently and aggressively, or do not respond optimally to available regimens.[18–22] Thus PCP continues to occur in North America and western Europe, but its incidence differs among patient populations depending on the availability and quality of their long-term medical management.[18–22] PCP also occurs in patients in developing countries, but it may not be as frequent in certain areas, such as sub-Saharan Africa, as it is in North America or Europe for reasons that are not well understood.[23–26]

TAXONOMY

Pneumocystis can be found in a wide variety of animals, including rodents, horses, nonhuman primates, and humans. The organism is difficult to culture: murine *Pneumocystis* can be grown with difficulty, achieving only a modest increase in number. Human *Pneumocystis* has never been cultivated successfully. Antigenic analysis indicates that each species of animal is infected by a distinct form of *Pneumocystis*.[27] The environmental reservoir of *Pneumocystis* is unknown, but humans do not appear to acquire it from other animals. Many humans appear to be infected early in life and can probably be reinfected by different human strains later in life.

Pneumocystis occurs in three distinct forms: cyst, tachyzoite, and sporozoite. Its morphology and its response to the antiparasitic agent pentamidine led to its original classification as a protozoon. However, evaluation of mRNA sequences, enzyme structure, and the cell wall suggest that it is taxonomically closer to fungi such as *Saccharomyces*, although it shares some characteristics of protozoa.

CLINICAL PRESENTATION

Pneumocystis carinii pneumonia almost always presents as pulmonary dysfunction. Although extrapulmonary or disseminated disease has been repeatedly reported in the literature, it is a curiosity that is infrequent regardless of the type of prophylaxis a patient is receiving.[11,12,28–30] When patients come to medical attention early in the course of their PCP, they typically have minimal symptoms. They often complain of a mild cough, exertional dyspnea, or a substernal “catching.” They may have a normal chest radiograph and normal arterial blood gases with no fever at this juncture, although a thin-section computed tomography (CT) scan might show pulmonary infiltrates, and a bronchoalveolar lavage or induced sputum specimen could contain many organisms.[11,12,28–30] Diagnosis and initiation of therapy at this stage clearly is associated with the best prognosis for avoiding hospitalization, complications, and death.[31–38] Patients may also present with more advanced disease, first coming to medical attention when they are on the brink of respiratory failure. Another presentation of which clinicians should be aware is pneumothorax. Finding a pneumothorax in a patient with no other precipitating cause should raise the diagnostic possibility of HIV-related PCP.

This disease most often presents with clinical and radiologic features consistent with bilateral pneumonia, manifesting with fever, nonproductive cough, shortness of breath, and the characteristic diffuse interstitial pulmonary infiltrates on chest radiography. Almost every conceivable radiographic pattern has been reported with PCP, including diffuse alveolar infiltrates, lobar infiltrates, nodules, cavities, upper lobe predominance, and asymmetrical patterns.[28–30,39–42] Thus clinicians must suspect PCP when pulmonary symptoms occur in any patient with HIV, regardless of radiologic appearance, especially if the patient has a low CD4+ T-lymphocyte count.

Today, patients continue to develop PCP despite the efficacy of prophylactic regimens and antiretroviral agents (Table 29–1).[19–21,43] One issue that has been apparent since before the era of antiretroviral therapy is that PCP occurs over a fairly wide range of CD4+ T-lymphocyte counts: although most cases occur at CD4+ T-lymphocyte counts of less than 100 cells/μl, and 85% to 90% occur at CD4+ T-lymphocyte counts of less than 200 cells/μl, some occur at counts of 200 to 300/μl and a few at CD4+ T-lymphocyte counts of more than 300/μl.[5,10] A substantial fraction of these patients presenting with PCP at CD4+ T-lymphocyte counts of more than 200/μl have not manifested either unexplained fever or oropharyngeal candidiasis.[10] Thus more sensitive laboratory or clinical indicators of disease would be useful. The HIV viral load is an independent predictor of AIDS-defining events,[44,45] but how precisely to use this factor to indicate the utility of initiating PCP prophylaxis is currently unclear. A high viral load (e.g., > 100,000 copies/ml) in a patient with a CD4 count of 200 to 300 cells/μl would be a logical reason to consider prophylaxis. Clinical markers, including wasting, the occurrence of a previous AIDS-defining event, or the occurrence of a previous episode of pneumonia of any type, also are risk factors for PCP independent of the CD4+ T-lymphocyte count. It may be reasonable to use these indicators to initiate PCP prophylaxis before the CD4+ T-lymphocyte count falls to 200/mm^3, especially in patients whose HIV viral load is high or whose CD4+ T-lymphocyte counts are declining rapidly. In addition, if another opportunistic infection occurred at an unusually high CD4+ T-lymphocyte count or if a prior episode of PCP occurred at a CD4+ T-lymphocyte count of more than 200 cells/μl, it is probably prudent to recommend prophylaxis despite a "high" CD4+ T-lymphocyte count.

Considerable evidence supports the concept that the CD4+ T-lymphocyte count is an accurate indicator of susceptibility to PCP even in patients receiving highly active antiviral therapy (HAART) or interleukin-2 (IL-2).[46–49] The nadir of the CD4+ T-lymphocyte fall prior to the institution of HAART or IL-2 does not influence the predictive value of counts substantially.[49]

▲ **Table 29–1.** REASONS PATIENTS DEVELOP PCP DURING THE ERA OF HAART

Failure to Take Prophylaxis
Lack of awareness of HIV infection
Failure of health care provider to prescribe prophylaxis
Lack of access to health care
Lack of compliance
Development of PCP before recommended indicators occur
Breakthrough of Prophylaxis
Immunologic failure
Less than complete efficacy of prophylactic regimen
Drug resistance (?)

HAART, highly active antiviral therapy; PCP, *Pneumocystis carinii* pneumonia.

▲ DIAGNOSIS

A definitive diagnosis of PCP depends on recognition of organisms in pulmonary secretions or tissue. *Pneumocystis* from humans has never been convincingly grown in culture despite extensive efforts using various culture media, cell types, and special conditions. Detection of serum antibodies by highly specific Western blot techniques or other serologic approaches has yielded interesting epidemiologic data but has not yet been shown to be useful for diagnosing acute disease or monitoring the response to therapy or the prognosis.[50–52]

An approach to the diagnosis and management of PCP is outlined in Figure 29–1, and sensitivities of diagnostic procedures for PCP are summarized in Table 29–2. At most medical centers, PCP is diagnosed by detecting organisms in bronchoalveolar lavage fluid or induced sputum. Prior to the early 1980s, open lung biopsy was conventionally used to diagnose PCP.[53,54] When bronchoscopy was introduced, it became clear that bronchial washings and brushings could detect *Pneumocystis* in 30% to 70% of cases.[53,55,56] Washings or brushings do not sample as many alveoli as bronchoalveolar lavage, however. When bronchoalveolar lavage is properly performed (i.e., the bronchoscope is wedged in a terminal bronchiole and 10- to 20-ml aliquots of normal saline are instilled until 30 to 40 ml has been collected), this technique rarely misses cases of AIDS-associated PCP; the sensitivity of the procedure is 95% to 99%. Some laboratories report that aerosolized pentamidine-treated patients may be more difficult to diagnose.[57–59] Some reports suggest that site-specific lavage (i.e., performing lavage in a radiologically affected area of the lung), preferentially lavaging the upper lobes, or performing bilateral lavage may increase the diagnostic yield.[60,61] Bilateral lavage or upper lobe lavage is not, however, performed routinely at most centers.

Bronchoalveolar lavage is safe and well tolerated when performed by an experienced operator. Even in patients who are thrombocytopenic or neutropenic, complications are rare. Clinically significant hemorrhage is unusual, even if patients are thrombocytopenic. Many patients have a temperature elevation and perhaps a chill or rigor during

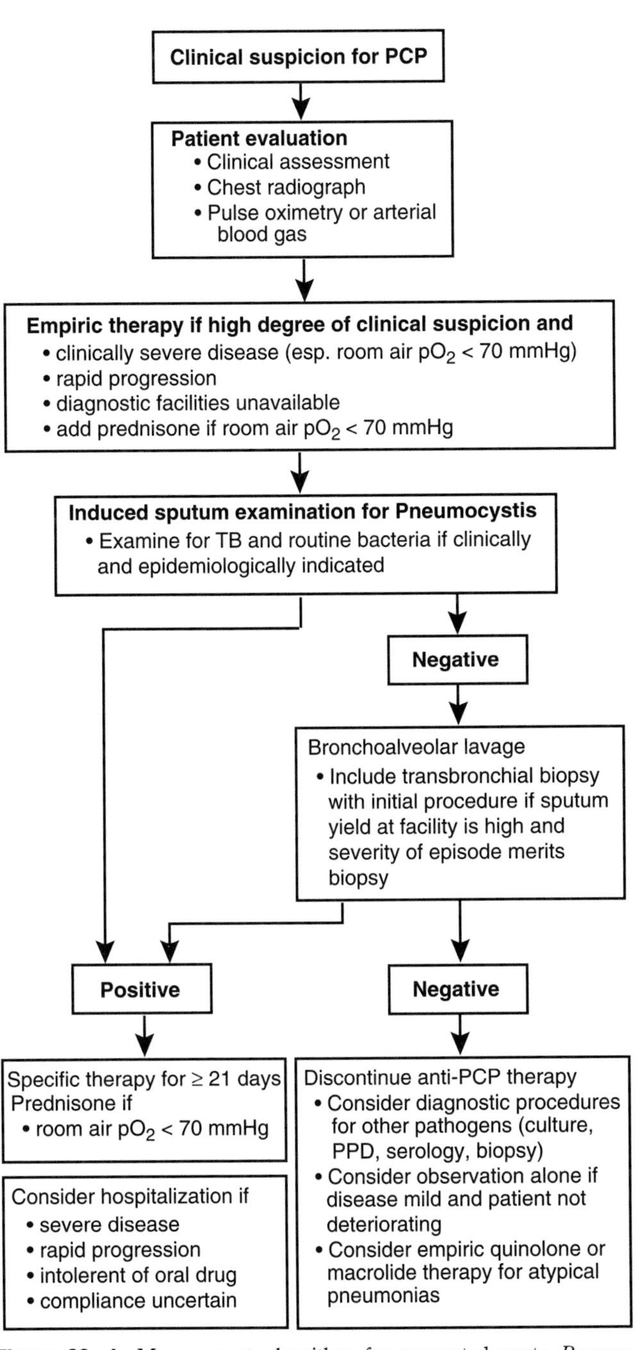

Figure 29–1. Management algorithm for suspected acute *Pneumocystis carinii* pneumonia (PCP). PPD, purified protein derivative; TB, tuberculosis.

the first 2 to 12 hours following bronchoalveolar lavage. Immediately following lavage, the chest radiograph may reveal new infiltration at the site of the lavage, but such infiltrates should disappear within 24 hours.

Transbronchial biopsy is rarely necessary to diagnose PCP, so it is often not performed as an initial diagnostic procedure. If bronchoalveolar lavage does not reveal PCP or any other likely pathogen, bronchoscopy is often repeated, especially if the patient fails to improve on empiric therapy; and transbronchial biopsy is performed to search for processes other than PCP, such as infection with cytomegalovirus, mycobacteria, or fungi. The diagnostic yield of transbronchial biopsy for any of these processes is subject to sampling artifact because characteristically only a few small pieces of tissue are obtained. The more severe the PCP and the more tissue obtained, the higher is the diagnostic yield. At most centers it is unusual to detect PCP by transbronchoscopic biopsy if bronchoalveolar lavage has been negative because of the high sensitivity of the procedure.

Table 29–2. SENSITIVITY OF PROCEDURES TO DIAGNOSE PCP BY VISUALIZATION OF THE ORGANISM

Technique	Sensitivity (%)	Comment
Expectorated sputum	10–30	Rarely used
Induced sputum	10–97	Many medical centers have >80% sensitivity and 99% specificity
Nonbronchoscopic lavage	Variable	At a few centers more readily available than bronchoscopy
Bronchoscopy		
Washings	30–70	Rarely used
Brushings	30–70	Rarely used
Lavage	95–99	Procedure of choice
Biopsy	70–90	Rarely necessary to diagnose PCP
Open lung biopsy	99	Rarely necessary

Open lung biopsy has a high yield of PCP detection if a large piece of tissue from an affected lobe is obtained. However, the diagnostic sensitivity of bronchoalveolar lavage and transbronchoscopic biopsy for virtually all pathogens makes open lung biopsy rarely necessary. Few medical centers perform more than a few open lung biopsies on AIDS patients per year. Patients with suspected extensive pulmonary Kaposi's sarcoma comprise one of the few populations in whom open lung biopsy is likely to be useful, although even here CT scans and endobronchial examination may suffice.

Percutaneous needle aspiration is occasionally useful for obtaining tissue from focal lesions if bronchoalveolar lavage is nondiagnostic. Although *Pneumocystis* occasionally is documented to cause such focal disease, in most circumstances another causative process is identified.

Bronchoscopy, an obviously invasive procedure, although safe, is uncomfortable, expensive, time-consuming, and not always readily available. Several alternative approaches to the diagnosis have been assessed.

Nonbronchoscopic alveolar lavage has been reported to have a higher diagnostic yield than induced sputum at one center.[62] This technique does not require an expensive bronchoscope but instead uses a disposable plastic catheter. It has been proposed that nonpulmonologists could use this technique in their offices. However, the yield of this technique is not as high as bronchoalveolar lavage in the best of circumstances; at some centers the yield has been considerably lower. Moreover, any catheter passed through the epiglottis has the potential to induce bronchospasm or vomiting and aspiration. Thus operators must be prepared to deal with airway emergencies and to be trained in conscious sedation procedures. For many nonpulmonologists, such potential complications, although rare, make this procedure imprudent for use in settings where full anesthesia or critical care support is not available.

Video-assisted thoracoscopy (VATS) with biopsy is rarely used to diagnose PCP unless an unusual manifestation such as a nodule is being evaluated. VATS can be quite helpful, however, for diagnosing other types of HIV-associated pulmonary pathology.

Detection of organisms in sputum offers the advantage of a noninvasive procedure that can be easily scheduled and is less expensive to perform. Expectorated sputum has a low yield and is usually not worthwhile. For patients who are intubated, tracheal aspirates also have a low diagnostic yield. Saline induction of sputum produces samples that provide far superior results compared to expectorated samples. Many institutions report a diagnostic yield from induced sputum of 75% to 95%.[63–67] Such high sensitivity requires that patients be encouraged to cough up material after nebulization with normal saline and should be performed using a high-flow nebulization delivery device. High sensitivity also requires scrupulous laboratory processing of the specimen, including digestion of mucoid material, centrifugation of cellular material into a pellet, and thorough direct microscopy by an experienced observer using an appropriate stain on the microscopic slide. Many laboratories prefer a direct immunofluorescent stain that permits easy visualization of cysts or trophozoites. However, Giemsa, Diff-Quick, toluidine blue-O, and methenamine silver have been used successfully. The methenamine silver and toluidine blue-O techniques stain only cysts, whereas the Giemsa, Diff-Quick, and immunofluorescent techniques allow detection of both cysts and trophozoites.

There has been considerable interest in using the polymerase chain reaction (PCR) to detect *Pneumocystis* in blood, sputum, bronchoalveolar lavage fluid, urine, or oral washings.[68–78] Several laboratories have reported that PCR can detect *Pneumocystis* in the serum or urine of a small fraction of patients with PCP, but the sensitivity appears to be low in these specimens.[68–70] PCR has been used more successfully to detect *Pneumocystis* in bronchoalveolar lavage fluid, sputum, and oral washes. Detection of *Pneumocystis* in an oral wash would be advantageous for diagnostic or epidemiologic studies, as such a specimen is easier to obtain than induced sputum.[72,76,78] For these specimens, PCR provides more sensitivity than staining, but false-positive results have diminished the clinical utility of currently available assays. A highly specific PCR assay might be easier to perform than tinctorial methods for some laboratories if they have already established a rigorously organized PCR laboratory for a wide variety of pathogens. However, more work is needed to develop approaches that can distinguish patients who have active pneumonitis due to *Pneumocystis* from patients who are colonized. Quantitative assays are currently being developed that show promise for effectively distinguishing such patients.[77] The use of PCR assays, especially with oral washes, is currently a research procedure and is not available for diagnostic purposes in most laboratories.

Nonspecific tests have been described for inclusion in the diagnostic evaluation of pulmonary dysfunction. Oxygen saturation evaluation during rest and exercise,[79,80] gallium scanning, and serum enzymes such as lactate dehydrogenase[81–83] have been studied for their ability to predict the presence of PCP. None of these tests appears to be specific and sensitive enough to warrant diagnostic use in clinical settings.

▲ THERAPY

To treat PCP effectively, there are three principles of cardinal importance. (1) Prompt initiation of therapy can improve prognosis. (2) Trimethoprim-sulfamethoxazole is the drug of choice for mild, moderate, or severe disease. (3) Prednisone therapy improves survival for patients with moderate or severe disease.

Initial Therapy

Because the best indicator of prognosis is the alveolar-arterial gradient at the time specific therapy is initiated,[31–38] it is logical to make prompt initiation of appropriate therapy a high priority. This obviously requires that patients be trained to come to their health care provider when they have any suggestive symptoms, even if such symptoms are mild, and that health care providers expeditiously initiate management by obtaining diagnostic tests, starting empiric therapy, or both.

Therapeutic regimens[84–91] for acute PCP are listed in Tables 29–3 and 29–4. In some situations, empirical therapy prior to confirming the diagnosis may be appropriate: Patients with room air PO_2 above 80 mm Hg, patients who are clinically stable, and patients who do not have prompt access to diagnostic facilities are reasonable candidates for empirical therapy.[92–94] Therapy can be administered orally if there is no evidence of gastrointestinal dysfunction and the patient adheres to the regimen. If therapy is empirical, a macrolide (e.g., azithromycin) or quinolone (e.g., levofloxacin, gatifloxacin or moxifloxaciin) is often added to treat other processes that are likely to present with manifestations similar to PCP.

Trimethoprim-sulfamethoxazole is always the drug of choice unless the patient has a history of life-threatening intolerance.[84–91] In every study performed to date, including HIV-infected and HIV-uninfected patients, trimethoprim-sulfamethoxazole has been as effective as alternative drugs or more effective. Specifically, there are few patients who have a poorer clinical response to trimethoprim-sulfamethoxazole than to other drugs, except perhaps intravenous pentamidine, which has equivalent efficacy but is more toxic.[89–91] Trimethoprim-sulfamethoxazole is well absorbed orally and can be given by mouth to compliant patients who have no major gastrointestinal dysfunction and who have only mild disease. A dose of two double-strength (DS) tablets (each DS tablet contains 160 mg trimethoprim plus 800 mg sulfamethoxazole) or intravenous trimethoprim

▲ **Table 29–3.** THERAPY FOR *PNEUMOCYSTIS CARINII* PNEUMONIA

Drug	Route	Dose	Comments
First Choice			
Trimethoprim-sulfamethoxazole (TMP-SMX)	PO	2 DS tablets q8h	Six tablets qd preferred over eight tablets qd to reduce toxicity. For patients <60 kg or >100 kg, adjust dose to equivalent of trimethoprim 5 mg/kg q8h
	IV	TMP 5 mg/kg plus SMX 25 mg/kg q8h	As above; q8h regimen preferred over q6h regimen; leucovorin not indicated unless substantial cytopenia
Second Choices			
Trimethoprim/dapsone	PO/PO	320 mg q8h/100 mg qd	Less convenient than TMP-SMX
Atovaquone	PO	750 mg bid or 1500 mg qd	For mild disease, well tolerated
Clindamycin plus	PO/IV	300–450 mg q6h	Rash, diarrhea, hepatitis, methemoglobinemia occur
Primaquine	PO	15–30 mg qd	
Pentamidine	IV	300 mg qd	Pancreatitis, nephrotoxicity, hypoglycemia occur
Trimetrexate/leucovorin	IV/IV	45 mg/m^2 qd/25 mg q6h	Bone marrow suppression, rash
Adjunctive Therapy	PO, IV	40 mg q12h × 5 days	If room air PO_2 <70 mm Hg within 72 hours of initiating therapy
Prednisone/solomedrol	PO, IV	40 mg qd × 5 days 20 mg qd × 11 days	

5 mg/kg with sulfamethoxazole 25 mg/kg is preferred every 8 hours rather than every 6 hours to reduce toxicity. There is no need to give concurrent leucovorin (there may be some reduction in efficacy, although this point is controversial and not conclusively established) unless cytopenias occur that appear to be drug-related.[95] Patients may be managed on oral therapy as outpatients if they have mild disease (room air PO_2 > 80 mm Hg), their clinical disease is not progressing rapidly, they are reliable, and they have no major gastrointestinal dysfunction.

There is evidence that *Pneumocystis* can develop resistance to sulfamethoxazole, the more active component of the trimethoprim-sulfamethoxazole combination.[96–103] This resistance has been demonstrated by sequencing the target enzyme for sulfamethoxazole, dihydropteroate synthase. Resistance occurs especially in patients who have been exposed to sulfonamides or sulfones in the past (Table 29–5). Whether such resistance is of a magnitude to be clinically important remains to be determined. Current reports are contradictory.[98,101,102] Helweg-Larsen et al. reported that *DHPS* mutations were an independent predictor of mortality in a retrospective analyses of a Danish cohort.[98] Some data support this observation,[101] but a large trial coordinated by the CDC did not.[102]

Toxicities of trimethoprim-sulfamethoxazole and other drugs are listed in Chapter 66.[8,28,84,85,87,88,90,91,104–107] A complete blood count, electrolytes, liver function tests, and creatinine should be monitored two or three times weekly to assess toxicity, as should symptoms and signs. Repeat chest radiographs and arterial blood gases are not necessary unless the patient is deteriorating or is clinically tenuous (i.e., the initial PO_2 on room air was less than 70 to 80 mm Hg). A chest radiograph at the end of the therapeutic course is useful for future comparison. Monitoring sulfonamide levels is unnecessary except in unusual patients with unstable renal function or patients receiving renal replacement therapy.[107] A 21-day course is standard, although there is no compelling evidence that 21 days of therapy is more effective than 14 days. Trimethoprim-sulfamethoxazole pharmacokinetics are not influenced significantly by other drugs, although the dose should be adjusted if there is significant renal dysfunction.

The efficacy of trimethoprim plus dapsone is comparable to that of trimethoprim-sulfamethoxazole, and the former may be somewhat better tolerated than the latter.[84,108] This regimen is less convenient than trimethoprim-sulfamethoxazole because the dapsone must be taken once per day and the trimethoprim three times daily. Occasional patients develop clinically important methemoglobinemia while on dapsone or hemolyze as a result of glucose-6-phosphate deydrogenase (G6PD) deficiency. It is rarely necessary to screen for G6PD deficiency prior to therapy unless there is a strong suspicion of deficiency, as might be the case for patients of Mediterranean ancestry. It is not clear how many patients who are truly intolerant of trimethoprim-sulfamethoxazole can tolerate this regimen. A history of life-threatening trimethoprim-sulfamethoxazole intolerance should preclude the use of dapsone plus trimethoprim. For patients who do not tolerate trimethoprim-sulfamethoxazole owing to non-life-threatening complications, dapsone-trimethoprim is a reasonable option.

Intravenous pentamidine appears to have efficacy equivalent to that of trimethoprim-sulfamethoxazole.[8,28,89,90,109–111] When given in a daily dose of 4 mg/kg or perhaps 3 mg/kg (the latter is less well studied[111]), the response to therapy is excellent. However, nephrotoxicity,[112] dysglycemia,[113] pancreatitis, and cardiac arrhythmias[114] (torsade de pointes; see Chapter 66) make this drug complicated to administer.[90–92] A baseline electrocardiogram to assess the QT interval (see Chapter 66) is useful but not mandatory: If the QT interval is more than 0.48 second and cannot be corrected by normalizing electrolytes or if other drugs that substantially prolong the QT interval are used concurrently (e.g., amiodarone, sotalol, perhaps certain quinolones), a cardiologist might be consulted before administering the drug. The use of monitoring to follow QT intervals and rhythm is controversial. Patients may become hypoglycemic during therapy or even during the several weeks after

▲ **Table 29–4.** SELECTED TRIALS FOR THERAPY OF ACUTE PCP

Study	Eligibility	Design	No.	Drug Regimens	Failure at day 21 (%)			Comments
					Failure of Response	Failure due to Toxicity	Death	
Safrin (ACTG 108)[84]	Confirmed PCP Symptomatic PAO_2-PaO_2 at 45 mm Hg	Randomized, double-blind, 21 day course	181	TMP-SMX 2 DS PO tid (weight adjusted)	9.4	35.9	6.2	Underpowered. No statistical difference in efficacy, toxicity, mortality
				Dapsone 100 mg PO qd plus TMP 300 mg PO tid	11.9	23.7	3.4	
				Clindamycin 600 mg PO tid plus primaquine 30 mg PO qd	6.9	32.8	3.4	
Hughes[85]	Confirmed IsCP Symptomatic PAO_2-PaO_2 at 45 mm Hg	Randomized, double-blind, 21 day course	322	TMP-SMX 2 DS PO tid	7.0	20.0	6.0	More failures to respond with atovaquone ($P = 0.002$) but less treatment-limiting toxicity ($P = 0.001$)
				Atovaquone 750 mg (tablets) PO tid	20.0	7.0	7.0	
Dohn[86]	Confirmed PCP Symptomatic PAO_2-PaO_2 at 45 mm Hg	Randomized, open label, 21 day course	109	Pentamidine 3–4 mg IV qd	17.0	36.0	17.0	More failures to respond with atovaquone ($P = 0.18$) but less treatment-limiting toxicity ($P < 0001$)
				Atovaquone 750 mg (tablets) PO tid	20.0	4.0	16.0	
Sattler (ACTG 029/031)[87]	Confirmed PCP PAO_2-PaO_2 at >30 mm Hg	Randomized, double-blind × 10 days, 21 day course	215	TMP-SMX 5 mg/kg and 25 mg/kg IV q6h	20.0	28.0	16.0	Trimetrexate associated with higher failure-to-respond rate ($P = 0.008$) higher death rate ($P = 0.088$), but less serious toxicity ($P < 0.001$)
				Trimetrexate 45 mg/m^2 IV qd with leucovorin 20 mg/m^2 q6h	38.0	9.0	31.0	
Bozzette (CCTC)[88]	Confirmed PCP	Randomized, stratified by oxygenation, confirmed and presumed PCP	328	Standard PCP therapy				
				Prednisone	0.13[a]	—	12.0	Corticosteroids reduce risk of respiratory failure at 21 days ($P = 0.004$) and death by day 84 ($P = 0.026$)
				No prednisone	0.28[a]	—	23.0	

ACTG, AIDS Clinical Trial Group; CCTG, California Clinical Trials Group; CPCRA, Community Program for Clinical Research in AIDS; DS, double-strength tablets; SS, single-strength tablets; TMP-SMX, trimethoprim-sulfamethoxazole.

[a]Relative risk.

▲ **Table 29–5.** DHPS MUTATIONS ASSOCIATED WITH
▲ SULFORAMIDE OR SULFONE EXPOSURE

Study	Year	*DHPS* mutations (%) Prophylaxis	No Prophylaxis	*P*
Ma[100]	1999	69	20	0.01
Helweg-Larsen[98]	1999	62	11	0.0001
Huang[99]	2000	80	48	<0.001
Kazanjian[101]	2000	76	23	0.001

therapy. This hypoglycemia may be profound and symptomatic; and it can rarely result in death.[112,113] Following acute therapy, the effects of pentamidine on the pancreas may lead to decreased insulin production and hyperglycemia, requiring chronic insulin therapy. Renal dysfunction may manifest as azotemia or tubular dysfunction. Renal dysfunction appears to be a risk factor for dysglycemia. The pancreatitis associated with pentamidine can be severe: There is some evidence that patients who have been given didanosine or zalcitabine (and perhaps stavudine) may be predisposed to pentamidine-induced pancreatitis, but this remains to be confirmed.

Aerosolized pentamidine has been used for therapy of acute PCP.[110] Although it is somewhat effective, especially for patients with mild disease, the relatively low response rate and high relapse rate makes it a poor option for therapy. It should almost never be used for therapy of acute disease.

Atovaquone has few life-threatening toxicities and a high degree of efficacy.[85,86,115] It is not, however, as potent as trimethoprim-sulfamethoxazole or intravenous pentamidine. In addition, steady-state levels are not reached for several days, absorption can be unpredictable, and some patients find the current liquid formulation to be unpleasant. Atovaquone absorption is improved by ingestion with a high-fat meal. Thus atovaquone has a therapeutic role for patients with mild, stable disease who have no evidence of gastrointestinal dysfunction. For this population, if neither trimethoprim-sulfamethoxazole nor trimethoprim-dapsone is tolerable, atovaquone is a good option. An intravenous preparation is not commercially available. Mutations in cytochrome b, the target for atovaquone, have been described.[116] Their clinical importance is unknown.

Trimetrexate, a dihydrofolate reductase inhibitor, is available as a parenteral agent.[87] Despite its similarity to methotrexate, this drug is extremely well tolerated when given with appropriate doses of leucovorin. Trimetrexate has a mechanism of action different from that of the active moiety of trimethoprim-sulfamethoxazole, but it is not as potent as either trimethoprim-sulfamethoxazole or intravenous pentamidine, although it is better tolerated. This drug represents a parenteral option for patients who cannot tolerate or who fail trimethoprim-sulfamethoxazole and intravenous pentamidine.

Clindamycin plus primaquine is an effective regimen that appeared comparable to trimethoprim-sulfamethoxazole and dapsone-trimethoprim in large but underpowered studies.[84,117,118] Clindamycin can be given orally or parenterally; primaquine is available only as an oral preparation. The regimen is inconvenient in that two drugs are involved. In addition, clindamycin causes a substantial amount of rash, diarrhea, and hepatic dys-function in this population, and primaquine can be associated with G6PD deficiency-related hemolysis. This regimen is a reasonable alternative for patients with mild disease who can absorb an oral regimen and who cannot tolerate trimethoprim-sulfamethoxazole.[117,118]

Prednisone is part of standard therapy for patients whose initial room air PO_2 is less than 70 mm Hg.[88,119–122] Studies show that mortality is reduced substantially in HIV-infected patients with room air PO_2 below 70 mm Hg when prednisone is added to specific chemotherapy within 72 hours of initial therapy. Symptomatically and in terms of oxygenation, PCP also disappears faster with prednisone than without. Whether there is an important survival benefit when prednisone is added to specific therapy for patients with initial PO_2 values higher than 70 mm Hg is unclear because the mortality in this population is low without prednisone therapy.

There has been considerable concern about the safety of prednisone. There is, however, no convincing evidence that a 21-day course using the regimen in Table 29–6 increases the likelihood that another opportunistic infection, Kaposi's sarcoma, or tuberculosis will appear or, if present, will be exacerbated. Metabolic abnormalities induced by prednisone are usually readily managed.

Acute PCP can be complicated by electrolyte abnormalities (especially syndromes of inappropriate antidiuretic hormone) or pneumothorax.[123,124] These complications can be managed using standard principles.

Should antiretroviral therapy be initiated or continued when patients have acute PCP? There is little information to indicate whether initiating HAART in the face of acute PCP can improve outcome. It is conceivable that such therapy could exacerbate pulmonary dysfunction by causing a more intense inflammatory response. In general, it is probably preferable not to initiate HAART during an episode of PCP; absorption of drugs and adherence may be erratic and could thus lead to rapid development of retroviral resistance to the HAART regimen. In addition, if multiple drugs (trimethoprim-sulfamethoxazole plus HAART) are

▲ **Table 29–6.** APPROACH TO PATIENTS FAILING PCP THERAPY

Days 4–6
- Repeat chest radiograph
  - Assess possibility of new process
- Perform or repeat bronchoscopy
  - Confirm PCP
  - Rule out concurrent infection or tumor
- Consider Swan-Ganz catheter or lung scan
  - Rule out congestive heart failure
  - Consider pulmonary emboli
- Consider empirical therapy for bacterial processes
  - Consider quinolone for community-acquired pneumonia
- Add prednisone if not already part of regimen

Days 6–8
- Consider switching to
  - First choice: trimethoprim-sulfamethoxazole (IV)
  - Second choice: pentamidine (IV)
  - Third choice: trimetrexate (IV)
- Combinations of these drugs are used by some clinicians

started simultaneously it may be difficult to know to what to attribute toxicity. For patients who have been receiving HAART it may be preferable to suspend HAART therapy until the patient is stable.

Salvage Therapy

A frequent issue is how to manage patients who are not improving on their initial regimen (Table 29–6). Clinicians must understand that the median time to clinical or physiologic improvement is 4 to 8 days, and that the natural history of PCP is to get worse during the initial 72 hours following institution of therapy unless prednisone is part of the regimen.[11,120] Thus a change in therapy before a 4- to 8-day course of therapy is premature; it is preferable to wait 6 to 8 days before changing agents rather than changing earlier. If a patient is deteriorating and the PO_2 on room air approaches or falls below 70 mm Hg at any point, prednisone should be added to the regimen.

There have been no trials to determine the best time to switch therapy, the most effective salvage regimen, or if combination therapy (e.g., trimethoprim-sulfamethoxazole plus intravenous pentamidine) is preferable to a single-drug regimen. Many clinicians carefully assess the patient for concurrent pulmonary processes (i.e., bronchoscopy should be repeated after 4 days of therapy looking for pathogens other than *Pneumocystis*, and the patient should be carefully assessed for concurrent noninfectious processes such as heart failure, bronchospasm, or emboli); if there is no response after 6 to 8 days of therapy, they switch from trimethoprim-sulfamethoxazole to pentamidine first and then to trimetrexate. (Some clinicians add subsequent drugs in preference to switching.) Some clinicians prefer not to use pentamidine in patients who have been heavily exposed to didanosine, zalcitabine, or stavudine. If a patient is deteriorating or failing to improve prior to days 6 to 8 on a regimen other than trimethoprim-sulfamethoxazole, strong consideration should be given to using this regimen, even if desensitization is required in the intensive care unit.

In terms of alternatives to trimethoprim-sulfamethoxazole or intravenous pentamidine, a clindamycin plus primaquine combination has been used successfully to salvage some patients failing their initial therapy.[118] Because primaquine is available only as an oral agent, and because clindamycin alone is ineffective in animal models, many clinicians are reluctant to use clindamycin-primaquine as a salvage regimen if other options such as trimetrexate are available. Some clinicians have used aerosolized pentamidine in addition to intravenous therapy, but there are no data to indicate if this is useful or safe.

Mechanical ventilation is an appropriate option for many patients with PCP. Patients who had a good quality of life prior to the onset of PCP and who have not received at least 6 to 8 days of therapy, have not received corticosteroids, or have reversible processes such as congestive heart failure or pneumothorax are reasonable candidates for mechanical ventilation if they are willing to try this mode of support and if their functional status was reasonable prior to PCP. The goals of mechanical ventilation and a realistic assessment of the prognosis must be carefully reevaluated daily. A summary of an approach to a patient who appears to be failing therapy is presented in Table 29–6.

▲ PREVENTION

Chemoprophylaxis

Chemoprophylaxis for PCP is considered to be the standard of care for patients with CD4+ T-lymphocyte counts of less than 200/μl and for patients with oropharyngeal thrush regardless of the CD4+ T-lymphocyte count.[8–10,13–16,125–159] Trimethoprim-sulfamethoxazole is the agent of choice; dapsone, dapsone-pyrimethamine, aerosolized pentamidine, and atovaquone can be recommended for patients who do not tolerate trimethoprim-sulfamethoxazole. Figure 29–2 summarizes an approach to prevention.

During the era prior to HAART, lifelong PCP prophylaxis was recommended; that is, once the patient's CD4+ T-lymphocyte count fell to less than 200 cells/μl or the patient had an episode of PCP, the anti-PCP prophylaxis should be instituted for life.[8–10,13–16] Because HAART regimens have been used extensively, numerous studies have documented that neither primary nor secondary prophylaxis need be continued in patients whose CD4+ T-lymphocyte counts rise to more than 200 cells/μl as a consequence of HAART. Tables 29–7 and 29–8 summarize the reported trials that have provided extensive evidence supporting discontinuation of primary and secondary prophylaxis for patients whose CD4+ T-lymphocytes rise to at least 200 cells/μl.

Are all patients with CD4+ T-lymphocyte counts higher than 200 cells/μl protected from PCP without prophylaxis?[156] As suggested above, the recommendation that prophylaxis can be safely stopped is a statistical assessment. As in the era prior to antiretroviral therapy, some patients with CD4+ T-lymphocyte counts well above 200 cells/μl develop PCP, but such cases are unusual and still support the advantage of stopping prophylaxis in terms of convenience, toxicity, ecologic pressure on microbial flora,[145–158] and cost (the latter advantage is admittedly small in most cases). There may, however, be some patients in whom prophylaxis should not be stopped. Although there are no data to support such recommendations, clinicians might consider continuing prophylaxis in patients with high viral loads (i.e., >50,000 to 100,000 copies/ml), rapidly declining CD4+ T-lymphocyte counts, wasting, candidiasis, or a prior episode of PCP at CD4+ T-lymphocyte counts of more than 200 cells/μl.

Trimethoprim-Sulfamethoxazole

Trimethoprim-sulfamethoxazole is clearly the drug of choice for prophylaxis because it is more effective in preventing PCP than other alternatives; moreover, it is well tolerated and inexpensive. Table 29–9 shows the results of selected trials that compared the efficacy of trimethoprim-sulfamethoxazole to aerosolized pentamidine or to dapsone, dapsone plus pyrimethamine, or atovaquone. In every large

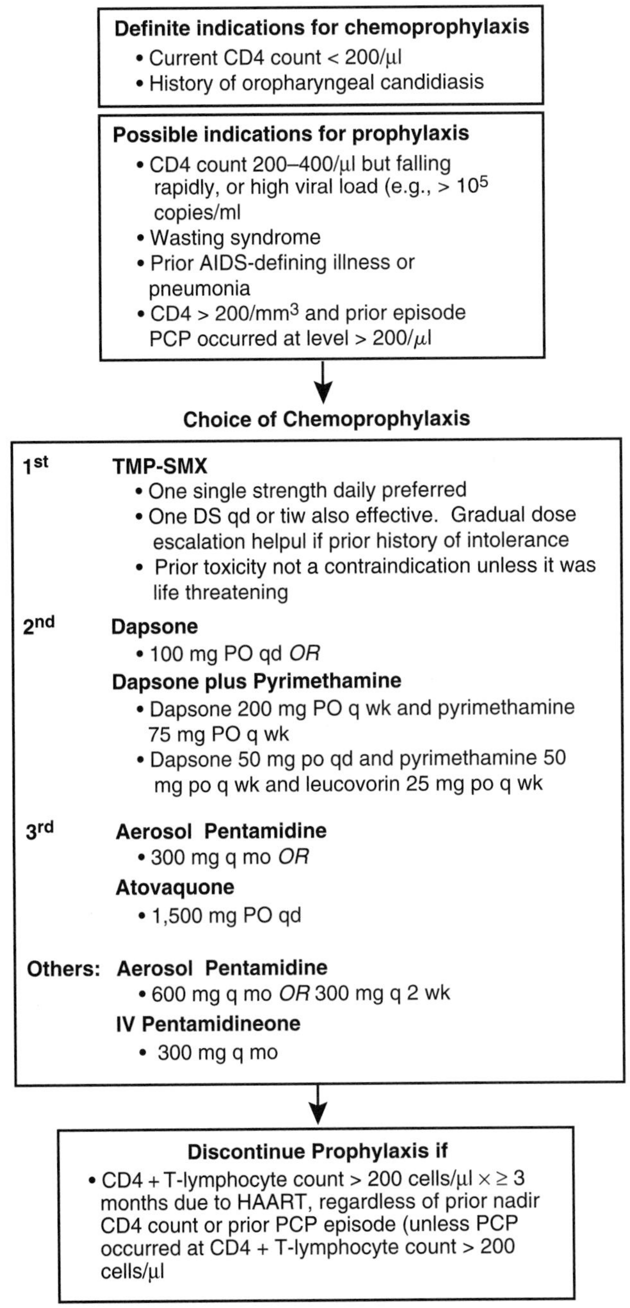

Definite indications for chemoprophylaxis
- Current CD4 count < 200/μl
- History of oropharyngeal candidiasis

Possible indications for prophylaxis
- CD4 count 200–400/μl but falling rapidly, or high viral load (e.g., > 10^5 copies/ml
- Wasting syndrome
- Prior AIDS-defining illness or pneumonia
- CD4 > 200/mm^3 and prior episode PCP occurred at level > 200/μl

Choice of Chemoprophylaxis

1st **TMP-SMX**
- One single strength daily preferred
- One DS qd or tiw also effective. Gradual dose escalation helpul if prior history of intolerance
- Prior toxicity not a contraindication unless it was life threatening

2nd **Dapsone**
- 100 mg PO qd *OR*

Dapsone plus Pyrimethamine
- Dapsone 200 mg PO q wk and pyrimethamine 75 mg PO q wk
- Dapsone 50 mg po qd and pyrimethamine 50 mg po q wk and leucovorin 25 mg po q wk

3rd **Aerosol Pentamidine**
- 300 mg q mo *OR*

Atovaquone
- 1,500 mg PO qd

Others: **Aerosol Pentamidine**
- 600 mg q mo *OR* 300 mg q 2 wk

IV Pentamidineone
- 300 mg q mo

Discontinue Prophylaxis if
- CD4 + T-lymphocyte count > 200 cells/μl × ≥ 3 months due to HAART, regardless of prior nadir CD4 count or prior PCP episode (unless PCP occurred at CD4 + T-lymphocyte count > 200 cells/μl

Figure 29–2. Algorithm for prevention of PCP. TMP-SMX, trimethoprim-sulfamethoxazole.

trial trimethoprim-sulfamethoxazole has demonstrated efficacy equal or superior to that of other regimens for primary or secondary prophylaxis. There are also data demonstrating that trimethoprim-sulfamethoxazole reduces the frequency of bacterial respiratory infections[133] and toxoplasmosis.[159,160] True breakthroughs of PCP are highly unusual for patients who are adherent to any of the recommended regimens of trimethoprim-sulfamethoxazole. Most breakthroughs occur in patients with CD4 counts of less than 50 cells/μl and are probably due to a poor host immune response rather than drug resistance. Logically, drug resistance if likely to occur eventually if prophylactic regimens are used widely. Until recently, as already noted (see Therapy), resistance had been impossible to detect because the human-derived organism cannot be grown in vitro. However, studies of dihydropteroate synthase genes from human isolates suggest that mutations do occur that could confer resistance.[96–103] Whether such isolates are in fact clinically resistant to trimethoprim-sulfamethoxazole prophylaxis remains to be proven.

Table 29–7. SAFETY OF DISCONTINUING PRIMARY PCP PROPHYLAXIS IN PATIENTS WITH A HAART-INDUCED RISE IN CD4 COUNT TO > 200 μl

Study	No. of Patients	Nadir CD4 (cells/μl)	Mean Follow-up (months)	PCP Cases (no.)
Utrecht[145]	62	85	14.0	0
Swiss[146]	262	110	11.3	0
Eurosida[147]	319	123	5.0	0
ASD[96]	1112	146	—	5
HOPS[148]	131	113	18.2	0
Hividore[149]	193	117	9.6	1
GESIDA[150]				
Stop	233	113	20	0 (0–4.6)[c]
Continue	230	98	19	0 (0–4.3)[c]
CIOP[151]				
Stop	355	—	6.3	0 (0–2.5)[c]
Continue	353	—	6.1	0 (0–2.5)[c]

[a]Adult spectrum of disease.
[b]HIV outpatient study.
[c]95% Confidence interval.

Trimethoprim-sulfamethoxazole is associated with well recognized toxicities (see Chapter 67), including fever, rash, pruritus, neutropenia, anemia, thrombocytopenia, hepatitis, pancreatitis, aseptic meningitis, interstitial nephritis, and crystalluria.[8,104–106,125,127] These toxicities are more likely to occur with high-dose prophylactic regimens.[8,125,127,129] A substantial number of patients must discontinue this prophylaxis because of toxicities, although minor laboratory abnormalities are not necessarily an indication to switch to less effective alternatives. Trimethoprim-sulfamethoxazole use is also associated with increased trimethoprim-sulfamethoxazole-resistant enteric bacilli and *Streptococcus pneumoniae*.[161]

Analyses of trials using various doses of trimethoprim-sulfamethoxazole suggest that low doses are better tolerated than high doses, although only three studies comparing various trimethoprim-sulfamethoxazole regimens have been completed in patients with HIV infection.[129,131,139] There is no evidence that a single-strength (SS) tablet daily is less effective than a DS daily tablet, although there have been no studies adequately powered to prove equivalence. Thus it is reasonable to consider using an SS tablet once daily in preference to a DS tablet once or twice daily. There has been considerable enthusiasm for intermittent regimens, such as one DS tablet three times a week. One study compared one DS tablet per day to one DS tablet three times a week for a mixed population of patients undergoing primary and secondary prophylaxis.[139] When evaluated by intention-to-treat analysis, there was no difference in efficacy or tolerability of the two regimens. However, when evaluated by the regimen the patient was following at the time PCP developed, there

▲ **Table 29–8.** SAFETY OF DISCONTINUATING OF SECONDARY PCP PROPHYLAXIS IN PATIENTS WITH HAART-INDUCED RISE
▲ IN CD4 COUNT TO >200 μl

Study	No.	Nadir CD4 (cells/μl) (median)	Time CD4 >200 cells/μl	%VL <50 copies/ml	Mean Follow-up (months)	Cases of PCP
Utrecht[145]	16	53	7.3	69	7.8	0
Eurosida[153]	69	60	5	49	—	0
European[154]	325	50	11	76	13	0
INSERM[155]	51	—	—	—	30	0
Stop Cox 2[156]	55	25	—	91	10	0
Madrid[157]	29	—	—	—	—	1
GESIDA[150]	99					
Stop	60	32	9	52	12	0
Continue	33	26	7	46	11	0
CIOP[158]	124					
Stop	40	—	—	—	9.1	0
Continue	35	—	—	—	7.3	0

VL, viral load.

were significantly more breakthroughs for patients with the intermittent regimen. This suggests that intermittent regimens may be less effective than daily regimens, but there are alternative interpretations of this trial as well.

Whether trimethoprim-sulfamethoxazole regimens that employ doses of less than one DS tablet daily provide as much efficacy for preventing toxoplasmosis or bacterial respiratory infections is uncertain. Thus it is not clear what trimethoprim-sulfamethoxazole regimen provides the best option in terms of both efficacy for all targeted pathogens and tolerability. All regimens in Figure 29–2 are reasonable. Part of the consideration of which regimen to choose involves compliance; a daily regimen may be easier for some patients than a three times per week regimen. There is no evidence that daily or even intermittent leucovorin therapy is useful for preventing cytopenias.

The utility of "desensitization" regimens or gradual dose escalation of trimethoprim-sulfamethoxazole has been controversial. Two trials have been completed that compare gradual dose escalation of trimethoprim-sulfamethoxazole to immediate introduction of the full-strength dose. In both trials, gradual dose escalation resulted in a higher number of patients being able to tolerate prophylaxis at the study endpoint (12 weeks in one study and 6 months in the other).[143,144] Table 29–10 summarizes two regimens that have been studied.

An issue that frequently confronts a clinician is whether it is safe to rechallenge a patient who has previously been intolerant to trimethoprim-sulfamethoxazole. Data from the ACTG 021 study indicate that patients who have a history of non-life-threatening toxicity are just as likely to tolerate another challenge with trimethoprim-sulfamethoxazole as are patients with no history of intolerance.[133] Thus unless a patient has a history of a life-threatening toxicity such as anaphylaxis or a desquamative skin reaction, it is reasonable to attempt to maintain that patient on trimethoprim-sulfamethoxazole again, perhaps initiating therapy with a gradual dose escalation regimen.

Dapsone

Dapsone prophylaxis is considered the best alternative for patients who cannot tolerate trimethoprim-sulfamethoxazole.[8,125–128] A daily dose of 100 mg PO may be associated with rash, fever, methemoglobinemia, or hemolysis. Patients with significant G6PD deficiency are likely to have substantial hemolysis. There is no uniform opinion as to the need to test all intended recipients of dapsone for G6PD deficiency before instituting prophylaxis or for monitoring methemoglobinemia. Many centers do not routinely do such testing unless the patient has a high probability of deficiency (i.e., Mediterranean descent).

How many trimethoprim-sulfamethoxazole-intolerant patients can tolerate dapsone is unclear; 80% is a reasonable estimate.[162] Dose reduction of dapsone to improve tolerability is not recommended because doses less than 100 mg/day are considerably less effective than the full-dose regimen.

Dapsone alone has no antibacterial activity, and it is not clear if it has substantial anti-*Toxoplasma* activity when used without pyrimethamine. Dapsone plus pyrimethamine is effective for reducing the frequency of both PCP and toxoplasmosis using either regimen listed in Figure 29–2.[125,130,138,163]

Dapsone may not be well absorbed when administered concurrently with a buffer such as is contained in some didanosine preparations. There are conflicting pharmacokinetic data about the importance of this potential interaction (see Chapter 3).

Pentamidine

Aerosolized pentamidine delivered by the Respirgard nebulizer (Marquest, Englewood, CO, USA) is effectively prevents PCP, especially in patients with CD4+ T-lymphocyte counts of more than 100/μl[3,8,125–128,132,133,141] but it was not as effective as trimethoprim-sulfamethoxazole or dapsone. Aerosolized pentamidine has no activity against other pathogens. It is well tolerated, although a few patients experience bronchospasm that may require pretreatment with albuterol. A few cases of pancreatitis have been reported to be associated with aerosolized pentamidine, but whether this association is causal or coincidental is uncertain. Uncontrolled or poorly controlled reports suggest that a monthly dose of 600 mg or biweekly doses of 300 mg may be more effective than 300 mg once per month.[134,164] Such a

▲ **TABLE 29–9.** SELECTED TRIALS ASSESSING EFFICACY AND SAFETY FOR PCP PROPHYLAXIS

Study	Eligibility	Design	No.	Drug Regimen	Failure (%) PCP Breakthrough	Failure (%) Rx-limiting Toxicity	Comments
Primary Prophylaxis							
Bozzette (ACTG 081)[128]	CD4 <200/μl No prior PCP or toxo AZT 1 month	Randomized, open label	843	TMP-SMX 1 DS PO bid Dapsone 50 mg PO bid AP 300 mg q mo	18 17 21	27 20 4	TMP-SMX or dapsone superior to AP for CD4 <100/mm (P = 0.4) but not for group as whole
Schneider[129]	CD4 <200/μl No prior PCP	Randomized, open label	260	TMP-SMX 1 SSPO qd TMP-SMX 1 DS PO qd	0 0	30 40	Both highly effective lower dose better tolerated (P = 0.007)
Podzamczer[130]	CD4 <200/μl No prior PCP	Randomized	230	TMP-SMX 1 DS bid, tiw Dapsone 100 mg PO qd plus pyrimethamine 50 mg PO biw	0 6.3	9.6 9.3	TMP-SMX more effective for PCP (P < 0.0001) by intent to treat but only one episode occurred on study drug similar toxicity (P = 0.95)
Bozzette[131]	CD4 <200/μl No prior PCP	Randomized, open label	107	TMP-SMX 1 DS bid qd TMP-SMX 1 DS bid tiw	0 0	42 24	Three times weekly is better tolerated than daily with AZT
Schneider[132]	CD4 <200/μl No prior PCP	Controlled	215	TMP-SMX 1 DS qd TMP-SMX 1 SS qd AP 300 mg q mo	0 0 11	21 26 0	TMP-SMX is more effective than AP but also more toxic
Secondary Prophylaxis							
Hardy (ACTG 021)[133]	Prior PCP	Randomized, open label	310	TMP-SMX 1 DS PO qd AP 300 mg q mo	9.1 23.1	27 4	TMP-SMX superior response rate (P < 0.001)
Rizzardi[134]	Prior PCP	Randomized, open label	205	AP 300 mg q mo 300 mg twice/mo	 13.1 5.1	 1 1	Efficacy difference not statistically significant
Mixed Primary and Secondary Prophylaxis							
Murphy (GW 213)[135]	TMP-SMX intolerant Prior PCP CD4 <200/mm	Randomized, open label	150	Atovaquone 1500 mg PO qd Atovaquone 750 mg PO qd AP 300 mg q mo	21 19 16	14 20 6	Preliminary analysis Preliminary analysis; atovaquone and dapsone have similar efficacy but different toxicity profiles
El-Sadr (ACTG 277/CPCRA 034)[136]	TMP-SMX intolerant Prior PCP	Randomized, open label	1057	Dapsone Atovaquone 1500 mg PO qd	18.3 15.5	27.5 26.8	Suggests clindamycin plus primaquine not highly effective at doses used
Barber[137]	CD4 <200/μl ± Prior PCP	Retrospective	262	TMP-SMX—any Dapsone—any Clindamycin plus primaquine	3.4 11.0 30.7	35 13 28	
Opravil[138]	"High risk" Prior PCP CD4 <200/μl	Randomized, open label	53	Dapsone 200 mg PO q wk plus pyrimethamine 75 mg PO q wk plus leucovorin PRN AP 300 mg q mo	4	30	Dapsone-pyrimethamine is more effective for preventing toxoplasmosis while patients receiving drug (not by intent to treat); but no difference for PCP
El Sadr[139]	CD4 <200/μl CD4% <15 Prior PCP	Randomized, open label	2625	TMP-SMX DS qd TMP-SMX DS 3/wk	3.5 4.1	8.5 6.1	Trends favor daily TMP-SMX but differences not statistically significant
Dunne[140]	CD4 <100/μl Prior PCP in 27%	Randomized, double-blind	724	Standard PCP prophylaxis plus azithromycin 1200 mg PO q wk or rifabutin 300 mg qd or both	8.2 13.1 8.5	— — —	Azithromycin associated with 50% reduction in PCP for patients who were also receiving other prophylaxis

ACTG, AIDS Clinical Trials Group; AP, aerosolized pentamidine; AZT, zidovudine; CPCRA, Community Program for Clinical Research AIDS; DS, double-strength tablets; Rx, therapy; SS, single-strength tablets; TMP-SMX, trimethoprim-sulfamethoxazole; toxo, toxoplasmosis; GW, Glaxo Wellcome.

▲ **Table 29–10.** GRADUAL INITIATION OF TRIMETHOPRIM-SULFAMETHOXAZOLE PROPHYLAXIS

Day of Regimen	Trimethoprim-Sulfamethoxazole Suspension (TMP 8 mg/ml, SMX 40 mg/ml)
Procedure one[143]	Dose
1–3	1 ml PO qd
4–6	2 ml PO qd
7–9	5 ml PO qd
10–12	10 ml PO qd
13–14	20 ml PO qd
Procedure two[144]	Dose with antihistamine pretherapy days 1–6
1	1.25 ml qd
2	1.25 ml qd
3	1.25 ml qd
4	2.5 ml qd
5	2.5 ml qd
≥6	1 SS tablet qd

regimen could be tried in patients who break through the standard dose and who cannot tolerate or fail the oral regimen. Data exist for other regimens, particularly a well studied regimen that used an ultrasonic Fisons nebulizer.[135] This nebulizer is not currently available in the United States.

When patients use a nebulizer that induces coughing, there is potential for the transmission of respiratory pathogens to staff and other patients if appropriate environmental ventilation and personal protection systems (i.e., masks) are not utilized. Outbreaks of tuberculosis associated with aerosolized pentamidine facilities have been reported. Aerosol pentamidine has the potential to be teratogenic, so pregnant patients and health care workers should avoid exposure.

Atovaquone

Two trials indicate that a daily atovaquone dose of 1500 mg of the liquid suspension has efficacy comparable to that of aerosolized pentamidine[141] or oral dapsone.[136] Atovaquone has efficacy for treating *Toxoplasma* disease, but the effectiveness of this regimen for preventing toxoplasmosis is unknown. Atovaquone has no antibacterial activity. Atovaquone is metabolized by the cytochrome P_{450} system, and levels can be reduced by ritonavir-containing HAART regimens.

Atovaquone suspension has the disadvantage of a consistency that some patients find unpleasant. A regimen of 1500 mg/day is also much more expensive than other drug regimens.

Other Drugs

A variety of other drugs have some activity for preventing PCP. In a study of azithromycin prophylaxis for *Mycobacterium avium-intracellulare*, a post hoc analysis showed that patients (all of whom received standard PCP prophylaxis) receiving azithromycin had a 50% reduction in the risk of developing PCP compared to those who received no azithromycin.[140] Intravenous pentamidine has appeared to provide protection against PCP in some observational studies but not in others. Long-term intravenous administration may be associated with substantial toxicity, especially in patients heavily exposed to didanosine, zalcitabine, or stavudine. Results with clindamycin plus primaquine have been disappointing.[137]

Respiratory Isolation

Rodent studies demonstrate unequivocally that *Pneumocystis* is an airborne pathogen that is transmissible from healthy animals or animals with PCP to members of the same species.[165–168] Human *Pneumocystis* is immunologically distinct from the organisms that infect other species.[169,170] Environmental sampling suggests that human *Pneumocystis* is present in random air samples, especially adjacent to humans with active PCP.[171,172] Thus it might be logical to isolate patients with active PCP from other susceptible patients. This might be especially reasonable because there is mounting evidence that some patients with multiple episodes of PCP are infected with different strains of *Pneumocystis* during sequential episodes, suggesting that the disease may be due to acquisition of a new strain from the environment rather than reactivation of latent infection.[173,174]

Current Centers for Disease Control and Prevention guidelines do not recommend respiratory isolation for patients with PCP. However, some institutions do attempt to isolate patients with PCP from other susceptible patients and do not place patients with PCP in hospital rooms with an immunologically susceptible roommate. This is a logical approach.

REFERENCES

1. Gottlieb MS, Schroff R, Schanker HM, et al. Pneumocystis carinii pneumonia and mucosal candidiasis in previously healthy homosexual men: evidence of a new acquired cellular immunodeficiency. N Engl J Med 305:1425, 1981.
2. Masur H, Michelis MA, Greene JB, et al. An outbreak of community-acquired Pneumocystis carinii pneumonia: initial manifestation of cellular immune dysfunction. N Engl J Med 305:1431, 1981.
3. Moore RD, Chaisson RE. Natural history of opportunistic disease in an HIV-infected urban clinical cohort. Ann Intern Med 124:663, 1996.
4. Hoover DR, Graham NMH, Bacellar H, et al. Epidemiologic patterns of upper respiratory illness and Pneumocystis carinii pneumonia in homosexual men. Am Rev Respir Dis 144:756, 1991.
5. Masur H, Ognibene FP, Yarchoan R, et al. CD4 counts as predictors of opportunistic pneumonias in human immunodeficiency virus (HIV) infection. Ann Intern Med 111:223, 1989.
6. Hoover DR, Saah AJ, Bacellar H, et al. Clinical manifestations of AIDS in the era of Pneumocystis prophylaxis. N Engl J Med 329:1922, 1993.
7. Munoz A, Schrager LK, Bacellar H, et al. Trends in the incidence of outcomes defining acquired immunodeficiency syndrome in the Multicenter AIDS Cohort Studies: 1985–1991. Am J Epidemiol 137:423, 1993.
8. Masur H. Drug therapy: prevention and treatment of Pneumocystis pneumonia. N Engl J Med 327:1853, 1992.
9. USPHS guidelines for prophylaxis against Pneumocystis carinii pneumonia for persons infected with HIV. MMWR Morb Mortal Wkly Rep 38:1, 1989.
10. Phair J, Munoz A, Detels R, et al. The risk of Pneumocystis carinii pneumonia among men infected with HIV-1. N Engl J Med 322:1607, 1990.
11. Kovacs JA, Hiemenz JW, Macher AM, et al. Pneumocystis carinii pneumonia: a comparison between patients with the acquired immunodeficiency syndrome and patients with other immunodeficiencies. Ann Intern Med 100:663, 1984.

12. Stover DE, White DA, Romano PA, et al. Spectrum of pulmonary diseases associated with the acquired immune deficiency syndrome. Am J Med 78:429, 1985.
13. Centers for Disease Control. Recommendations for prophylaxis against Pneumocystis carinii pneumonia for adults and adolescents infected with human immunodeficiency virus. MMWR Morb Mortal Wkly Rep 41(RR-4):1, 1992.
14. Centers for Disease Control. 1995 Revised guidelines for prophylaxis against Pneumocystis carinii pneumonia for children infected with or perinatally exposed to human immunodeficiency virus. MMWR Morb Mortal Wkly Rep 44(RR-4):1, 1995.
15. USPHS/IDSA guidelines for the prevention of opportunistic infections in persons infected with human immunodeficiency virus: a summary. MMWR Morb Mortal Wkly Rep 44(RR-8):1, 1995.
16. US Public Health Service (USPHS) and the Infectious Diseases Society of America (IDSA) guidelines for the prevention of opportunistic infections in persons infected with the human immunodeficiency virus: a summary. MMWR Morb Mortal Wkly Rep 46(RR):1, 1997.
17. Montaner JSG, Le T, Hogg R, et al. The changing spectrum of AIDS index diseases in Canada. AIDS 8:693, 1994.
18. Stansell JD, Osmond DH, Charlebois E, et al. Predictors of Pneumocystis carinii pneumonia in HIV-infected persons. Am J Respir Crit Care Med 155:60, 1997.
19. Kaplan JE, Hanson D, Navin TR, Jones JL. Risk factors for primary Pneumocystis carinii pneumonia in HIV infected adolescents and adults in the United States: reassessment of indications for chemoprophylaxis. J Infect Dis 178:1126, 1998.
20. Kaplan JE, Hanson D, Dworkin MS, et al. Epidemiology of human immunodeficiency virus associated opportunistic infections in the United States in the era of highly active antiretroviral therapy. Clin Infect Dis 30(suppl 1):S5, 2000.
21. Lundgren JD, Barton SE, Lazzarin A, et al. Factors associated with the development of Pneumocystis carinii pneumonia in 5,025 European patients with AIDS. Clin Infect Dis 21:106, 1995.
22. Saah AJ, Hoover DR, Peng Y, et al. Predictors for failure of Pneumocystis carinii pneumonia prophylaxis. JAMA 273:1197, 1995.
23. Russian DA, Kovacs J. Pneumocystis carinii in Africa: an emerging pathogen? Lancet 346:1242, 1995.
24. Malin AS, Gwanzura LKZ, Klein S, et al. Pneumocystis carinii pneumonia in Zimbabwe. Lancet 346:1258, 1995.
25. Zar HJ, Maarteus G, Wood R, Hussey G. Pneumocystis carinii pneumonia in HIV infected patients in Africa—an important pathogen? S Afr Med J 90:684, 2000.
26. Graham SM, Mtitimila EI, Kamanga HS, et al. Clinical presentation and outcome of Pneumocystis pneumonia in Malawian children. Lancet 355:369, 2000.
27. Beard CB, Carter JL, Keely SP, et al. Genetic variation in Pneumocystis carinii isolates from different geographic regions: implications for transmission. Emerg Infect Dis 6:265, 2000.
28. Sattler FR, Walzer PD. Pneumocystis carinii. Baillieres Clin Infect Dis 2:409, 1995.
29. Telzak EE, Cote RJ, Gold JWM, et al. Extrapulmonary Pneumocystis carinii infections. Rev Infect Dis 12:380, 1990.
30. Suster B, Akerman M, Orenstein M, et al. Pulmonary manifestations of AIDS: review of 106 episodes. Radiology 161:87, 1986.
31. Bennett CL, Weinstein RA, Shapiro MF, et al. A rapid preadmission method for predicting inpatient course of disease for patients with HIV-related Pneumocystis carinii pneumonia. Am J Respir Crit Care Med 150:1503, 1994.
32. Benfield TL, Helweg-Larsen J, Bang D, et al. Prognostic markers of short-term mortality in AIDS-associated Pneumocystis carinii pneumonia. Chest 119:844, 2001.
33. Brenner M, Ognibene FP, Lack EE, et al. Prognostic factors and life expectancy of patients with acquired immunodeficiency syndrome and Pneumocystis carinii pneumonia. Am Rev Respir Dis 136:1199, 1987.
34. Hawley PH, Ronco JJ, Guillemi SA, et al. Decreasing frequency but worsening mortality of acute respiratory failure secondary to AIDS-related Pneumocystis carinii pneumonia. Chest 106:1456, 1994.
35. Rosen MJ, Clayton K, Schnieder RF, et al. Intensive care of patients with HIV infection. Am J Respir Crit Care Med 155:67, 1997.
36. Wachter RM, Russi MB, Block DA, et al. Pneumocystis carinii pneumonia and respiratory failure in AIDS: improved outcomes and increased use of intensive care units. Am Rev Respir Dis 143:251, 1991.
37. Curtis JR, Yarnold PR, Schartz DN, et al. Improvements in outcomes of acute respiratory failure for patients with human immunodeficiency virus related Pneumocystis carinii pneumonia. Am J Resir Crit Care Med 162:393, 2000.
38. Mansharani NG, Garland R, Delaney D, Koziel H. Management and outcomes of patients of adult Pneumocystis carinii pneumonia 1985–1995: comparison of HIV associated cases to other immunocompromised states. Chest 118:704, 2000.
39. Moskovic E, Miller R, Pearson M. High resolution computed tomography of Pneumocystis carinii pneumonia in AIDS. Clin Radiol 42:239, 1990.
40. DeLorenzo LJ, Huang CT, Maguire G, et al. Roentgenographic patterns of Pneumocystis carinii pneumonia in 104 patients with AIDS. Chest 91:323, 1987.
41. Kennedy CA, Goetz MB. Atypical roentgenographic manifestations of Pneumocystis carinii pneumonia. Arch Intern Med 152:1390, 1992.
42. Boiselle PM, Crans CA, Kaplan MA. The changing face of Pneumocystis carinii pneumonia in AIDS patients. AJR Am J Roentgenol 172:1301, 1999.
43. Masur H. Emerging issues in HIV therapeutics. 41st Interscience Conference on Antimicrobial Agents and Chemotherapy (ICAAC), Chicago, 2001, abstract 586.
44. Mellors JW, Rinaldo CR, Gupta P, et al. Prognosis in HIV-1 infection predicted by the quantity of virus in plasma. Science 272:1167, 1996.
45. Lyles RH, Munoz A, Yamashita TE, et al. Natural history of human immunodeficiency virus type 1 viremia after seroconversion and proximal to AIDS in a large cohort of homosexual men: multicenter AIDS cohort study. J Infect Dis 181:872, 2000.
46. Dworkin MS, Williamson J, Jones JL, Kaplan JE. Prophylaxis with trimethoprim-sulfamethoxazole for human immunodeficiency virus-infected patients: impact on risk for infectious diseases. Clin Infect Dis 33:393, 2001.
47. Dworkin MS, Hanson DL, Navin TR. Survival of patients with AIDS, after diagnosis of Pneumocystis carinii pneumonia, in the United States. J Infect Dis 183:1409, 2001.
48. Dworkin MS, Hanson DL, Kaplan JE, et al. Risk for preventable opportunistic infections in persons with AIDS after antiretroviral therapy increases $CD4^+$ T lymphocyte counts above prophylaxis thresholds. J Infect Dis 182:611, 2000.
49. Miller V, Mocroft A, Reiss P, et al. Natural history of human immunodeficiency virus type 1 viremia after seroconversion and proximal to AIDS in a large cohort of homosexual men: multicenter AIDS cohort study. J Infect Dis 181:872, 2000.
50. Lundgren B, Lundgren JD, Nielsen T, et al. Antibody responses to a major Pneumocystis carinii antigen in human immunodeficiency virus-infected patients with and without P. carinii pneumonia. J Infect Dis 165:1151, 1992.
51. Peglow SL, Smulian AG, Linke MJ, et al. Serologic responses to Pneumocystis carinii antigens in health and disease. J Infect Dis 161:296, 1990.
52. Walzer PD. Immunologic features of Pneumocystis carinii infection in humans. Clin Diagn Lab Immunol 6:149, 1999.
53. Stover DE, White DA, Romano PA, et al. Diagnosis of pulmonary disease in acquired immune deficiency syndrome (AIDS): role of bronchoscopy and bronchoalveolar lavage. Am Rev Respir Dis 180:659, 1984.
54. Hughes WT. Current status of laboratory diagnosis of Pneumocystis carinii pneumonitis. CRC Crit Rev Clin Lab Sci 6:145, 1975.
55. Ognibene FP, Shelhamer J, Gill V, et al. The diagnosis of Pneumocystis carinii pneumonia in patients with the acquired immunodeficiency syndrome using subsegmental bronchoalveolar lavage. Am Rev Respir Dis 129:929, 1984.
56. Baughman RP. Current methods of diagnosis. In: Walzer PD (ed) Pneumocystis carinii Pneumonia. New York, Marcel Dekker, 1994, p 381.
57. Levine SJ, Masur H, Gill VJ, et al. Effect of aerosolized pentamidine prophylaxis on the diagnosis of Pneumocystis carinii pneumonia by induced sputum examination in patients infected with the human immunodeficiency virus. Am Rev Respir Dis 144:760, 1991.
58. Jules-Elysee KM, Stover DE, Zaman MB, et al. Aerosolized pentamidine: effect on diagnosis and presentation of Pneumocystis carinii pneumonia. Ann Intern Med 112:750, 1990.
59. Metersky ML, Catanzaro A. Diagnostic approach to Pneumocystis carinii pneumonia in the setting of prophylactic aerosolized pentamidine. Chest 100:1345, 1991.

60. Levine SJ, Kennedy D, Shelhamer JH, et al. Diagnosis of Pneumocystis carinii pneumonia by multiple lobe, site-directed bronchoalveolar lavage with immunofluorescent monoclonal antibody staining in human immunodeficiency virus-infected patients receiving aerosolized pentamidine chemoprophylaxis. Am Rev Respir Dis 146:838, 1992.
61. Meduri GU, Stover DE, Greeno RA, et al. Bilateral bronchoalveolar lavage in the diagnosis of opportunistic pulmonary infections. Chest 100:1272, 1991.
62. Bustamante EA, Levy H. Sputum induction compared with bronchoalveolar lavage by Ballard catheter to diagnose Pneumocystis carinii pneumonia. Chest 105:816, 1994.
63. Pitchenik AE, Ganjei P, Torres A, et al. Sputum examination for the diagnosis of Pneumocystis carinii pneumonia in the acquired immunodeficiency syndrome. Am Rev Respir Dis 33:226, 1986.
64. Bigby TO, Margolskiii D, Curtis JL, et al. The usefulness of induced sputum in the diagnosis of Pneumocystis carinii pneumonia in patients with the acquired immunodeficiency syndrome. Am Rev Respir Dis 133:515, 1986.
65. Kovacs JA, Ng VL, Masur H, et al. Diagnosis of Pneumocystis carinii pneumonia: improved detection in sputum with use of monoclonal antibodies. N Engl J Med 318:589, 1988.
66. Zaman MK, Wootan OJ, Suprahmanya B, et al. Rapid noninvasive diagnosis of Pneumocystis carinii from the induced liquefied sputum. Ann Intern Med 107:7, 1988.
67. Ng VL, Garner I, Weymouth LA, et al. The use of mucolysed induced sputum for the identification of pulmonary pathogens associated with human immunodeficiency virus infection. Arch Pathol Lab Med 113:488, 1989.
68. Schluger N, Godwin T, Sepkowitz K, et al. Application of DNA amplification to pneumocystosis: presence of serum Pneumocystis carinii DNA during human and experimentally induced Pneumocystis carinii pneumonia. J Exp Med 176:1327, 1992.
69. Lipschik GY, Gill VJ, Lundgren JD, et al. Improved diagnosis of Pneumocystis carinii infection by polymerase chain reaction on induced sputum and blood. Lancet 340:203, 1992.
70. Sepkowitz K, Schluger N, Godwin T, et al. DNA amplification in experimental pneumocystosis: characterization of serum Pneumocystis carinii DNA and potential P. carinii carrier states. J Infect Dis 168:421, 1993.
71. Chouaid C, Roux P, Lavard I, et al. Use of polymerase chain reaction technique on induced-sputum samples for the diagnosis of Pneumocystis carinii pneumonia in HIV-infected patients. Am J Clin Pathol 104:72, 1995.
72. Fischer S, Gill VJ, Kovacs J, et al. The use of oral washes to diagnose Pneumocystis carinii pneumonia: a blinded prospective study using a PCR based detection system. J Infect Dis 184:1485, 2001.
73. Sign A, Trebesius K, Roggenkamp A, et al. Evaluation of diagnostic value and epidemiological implications of PCR for Pneumocystis carinii in different immunosuppressed and immunocompetent patients groups. J Clin Microbiol 38:1461, 2000.
74. Torres J, Goldman M, Wheat LJ, et al. diagnosis of Pneumocystis carinii pneumonia in human immunodeficiency virus infected patients with polymerase chain reaction: a blinded comparison to standard methods. Clin Infect Dis 30:141, 2000.
75. Huang SN, Fischer SH, O'Shaughnessy E, et al. Development of PCR assay for diagnosis of Pneumocystis carinii pneumonia based on amplification of the multicopy major surface glycoprotein gene family. Diagn Microbiol Infect Dis 35:27, 1999.
76. Wakefield AE, Miller RF, Guiver LA, Hopkins JM. Oropharyngeal samples for detection of Pneumocystis carinii by DNA amplification. Q J Med 86:401, 1993.
77. Larsen HH, Masur H, Kovacs JA, et al. A rapid and quantitative real time PCR assay for Pneumocystis carinii. In: Program and Abstracts of the 38th Annual Meeting of the Infectious Disease Society of America, New Orleans, 2000, p 87, abstract 272.
78. Helwig-Larson J, Jensen JS, Benfield T, et al. Diagnostic use of PCR for detection of Pnemocystis carinii in oral wash samples. J Clin Microbiol 36:2068, 1996.
79. Kvale PA, Rosen MJ, Hopewell PC, et al. A decline in the diffusing capacity does not indicate opportunistic lung disease in asymptomatic persons infected with the human immunodeficiency virus. Am Rev Respir Dis 148:390, 1993.
80. Chouaid C, Maillard D, Housset B, et al. Cost effectiveness of noninvasive oxygen saturation measurement during exercise for the diagnosis of Pneumocystis carinii pneumonia. Am Rev Respir Dis 147:1360, 1993.
81. Zaman MK, White DA. Serum lactate dehydrogenase and Pneumocystis carinii pneumonia: diagnostic and prognostic significance. Am Rev Respir Dis 137:796, 1988.
82. Quist J, Hill AR. Serum lactate dehydrogenase (LDH) in Pneumocystis carinii pneumonia, tuberculosis, and bacterial pneumonia. Chest 108:415, 1995.
83. Bentsen KD, Nielsen TL, Eaftinck Schattenkerk JKM, et al. Serum type III procollagen peptide in patients with Pneumocystis carinii infection. Am Rev Respir Dis 148:1558, 1993.
84. Safrin S, Finkelstein DM, Feinberg J, et al. Comparison of three regimens for treatment of mild to moderate Pneumocystis carinii pneumonia in patients with AIDS: a double-blind, randomized, trial of oral trimethoprim-sulfamethoxazole, dapsone-trimethoprim, and clindamycin-primaquine: ACTG 108. Ann Intern Med 124:792, 1996.
85. Hughes WT, Leoung G, Kramer F, et al. Comparison of atovaquone (566C80) with trimethoprim-sulfamethoxazole to treat Pneumocystis carinii pneumonia in patients with AIDS. N Engl J Med 328:1521, 1993.
86. Dohn MN, Weinberg WG, Torres RA, et al. Oral atovaquone compared with intravenous pentamidine for Pneumocystis carinii pneumonia in patients with AIDS. Ann Intern Med 121:174, 1994.
87. Sattler FR, Frame P, Davis R, et al. Comparison of trimetrexate with leucovorin versus trimethoprim-sulfamethoxazole for moderate to severe episodes of Pneumocystis carinii pneumonia in patients with AIDS. J Infect Dis 170:165, 1994.
88. Bozzette SA, Sattler FR, Chiu J, et al. A controlled trial of early adjunctive treatment with corticosteroids for Pneumocystis carinii pneumonia in acquired immunodeficiency syndrome. N Engl J Med 323:1451, 1990.
89. Sattler FR, Cowan R, Nielsen DM, et al. Trimethoprim sulfamethoxazole compared with pentamidine for treatment of Pneumocystis carinii pneumonia in the acquired immunodeficiency syndrome: a prospective, noncrossover study. Ann Intern Med 109:280, 1988.
90. Wharton JM, Coleman DL, Wofsy CB, et al. Trimethoprim-sulfamethoxazole or pentamidine for Pneumocystis carinii pneumonia in the acquired immunodeficiency syndrome: a prospective randomized trial. Ann Intern Med 105:37, 1986.
91. Hughes WT. Pneumocystis carinii Pneumonitis. Boca Raton, FL, CRC Press, 1987.
92. Miller RF, Millar AB, Weller D IV, et al. Empirical treatment without bronchoscopy for Pneumocystis carinii pneumonia in the acquired immunodeficiency syndrome. Thorax 44:559, 1989.
93. Tu JV, Biem J, Detsky AS. Bronchoscopy versus empirical therapy in HIV-infected patients with presumptive Pneumocystis carinii pneumonia. Am Rev Respir Dis 148:370, 1993.
94. Masur H, Shelhamer JS. Empiric outpatient management of HIV related pneumonia: economical or unwise [editorial]? Ann Intern Med 124:451, 1996.
95. Safrin S, Lee BL, Sande MA. Adjunctive folinic acid with trimethoprim-sulfamethoxazole for Pneumocystis carinii pneumonia in AIDS patients is associated with an increased risk of therapeutic failure and death. J Infect Dis 170:912, 1994.
96. Kazanjian P, Locke AB, Hossler PA. Pneumocystis carinii mutations associated with sulfa and sulfone prophylaxis failures in AIDS patients. AIDS 12:873, 1998.
97. Mei Q, Gurunathan S, Masur A, Kovacs J. Failure of co-trimoxazole in Pneumocystis carinii infection and the mutations in dihydropteroate synthase gene. Lancet 351:1631, 1998.
98. Helweg-Larsen J, Benfield TL, Eugen-Olsen J, et al. Effects of mutations in Pneumocystis carinii dihydropteroate synthase gene on outcome of AIDS-associated P. carinii pneumonia. Lancet 354:1318, 1999.
99. Huang L, Beard CB, Creasman J, et al. Related articles sulfa or sulfone prophylaxis and geographic region predict mutations in the Pneumocystis carinii dihydropteroate synthase gene. J Infect Dis 182:1192, 2000.
100. Ma L, Borio L, Masur H, Kovacs JA. Pneumocystis carinii dihydropteroate synthase but not dihydrofolate reductase gene mutations correlate with prior trimethoprim-sulfamethoxazole or dapsone use. J Infect Dis Dec 180:1969, 1999.
101. Kazanjian P, Armstrong W, Hossler PA, et al. Pneumocystis carinii mutations are associated with duration of sulfa or sulfone prophylaxis exposure in AIDS patients. J Infect Dis 182:551, 2001.

102. Navin TR, Beard CB, Huang L, et al. Effect of mutations in Pneumocystis carinii dihydropteroate synthase gene on outcome of P. carinii pneumonia in patients with HIV-1: a prospective study. Lancet 358:545, 2001.
103. Takahashi T, Hosoya N, Endo T, et al. Relationship between mutations in dihydropteroate synthase of Pneumocystis carinii f. sp. Hominis isolates in Japan and resistance to sulfonamide therapy. J Clin Microbiol 38:3161, 2000.
104. Greenberg S, Reiser IW, Chou SY, et al. Trimethoprim-sulfamethoxazole induces reversible hyperkalemia. Ann Intern Med 119:291, 1993.
105. Martin GJ, Paparello SF, Decker CF. A severe systemic reaction to trimethoprim-sulfamethoxazole in a patient infected with the human immunodeficiency virus. Clin Infect Dis 16:175, 1992.
106. Jung AC, Paauw DS. Management of adverse reactions to trimethoprim-sulfamethoxazole in human immunodeficiency virus-infected patients. Arch Intern Med 154:2402, 1994.
107. Joos B, Blaser J, Opravil M, et al. Monitoring of co-trimoxazole concentrations in serum during treatment of Pneumocystis carinii pneumonia. Antimicrob Agents Chemother 39:2661, 1995.
108. Medina I, Mills J, Leoung G, et al. Oral therapy for Pneumocystis carinii pneumonia in the acquired immunodeficiency syndrome: a controlled trial of trimethoprim-sulfamethoxazole versus trimethoprim-dapsone. N Engl J Med 323:776, 1990.
109. Conte JE Jr, Chernoff D, Feigel DW Jr, et al. Intravenous or inhaled pentamidine for treating Pneumocystis carinii pneumonia in AIDS. Ann Intern Med 113:203, 1990.
110. Montgomery AB, Feigal DW Jr, Sattler F, et al. Pentamidine aerosol versus trimethoprim-sulfamethoxazole for Pneumocystis carinii in acquired immune deficiency syndrome. Am J Respir Crit Care Med 151:1068, 1995.
111. Conte JE Jr, Hollander H, Golden JA. Inhaled pentamidine or reduced dose intravenous pentamidine for Pneumocystis carinii pneumonia: a pilot study. Ann Intern Med 107:495, 1987.
112. O'Brien JG, Dong BJ, Coleman RL, et al. A 5-year retrospective review of adverse drug reactions and their risk factors in human immunodeficiency virus-infected patients who were receiving intravenous pentamidine therapy for Pneumocystis carinii pneumonia. Clin Infect Dis 24:854, 1997.
113. Stahl Bayliss CM, Kalman CM, Laskin OL. Pentamidine-induced hypoglycemia in patients with the acquired immune deficiency syndrome. Clin Pharmacol Ther 39:271, 1986.
114. Taylor AJ, Hull RW, Coyne PE, et al. Pentamidine-induced torsades de pointes: safe completion of therapy with inhaled pentamidine. Clin Pharmacol Ther 49:698, 1991.
115. Falloon J, Kovacs J, Hughes W, et al. A preliminary evaluation of 566C80 for the treatment of Pneumocystis carinii pneumonia in patients with the acquired immunodeficiency syndrome. N Engl J Med 325:1534, 1991.
116. Kazanjian P, Armstrong W, Hossler PA, et al. Pneumocystis carinii cytochrome b mutations are associated with atovaquone exposure in patients with AIDS. J Infect Dis 183:819, 2001.
117. Toma E, Fournier S, Dumont M, et al. Clindamycin/primaquine versus trimethoprim-sulfamethoxazole as primary therapy for Pneumocystis carinii pneumonia in AIDS: a randomized, double-blind pilot trial. Clin Infect Dis 17:178, 1993.
118. Noskin GA, Murphy R, Black JR, et al. Salvage therapy with clindamycin/primaquine for Pneumocystis carinii pneumonia. Clin Infect Dis 14:183, 1992.
119. Gagnon S, Botta AM, Fischl MA, et al. Corticosteroids as adjunctive therapy for severe Pneumocystis carinii pneumonia in the acquired immunodeficiency syndrome: a double blind, placebo-controlled trial. N Engl J Med 323:1444, 1990.
120. Montaner JSG, Lawson LM, Levitt N, et al. Corticosteroids prevent early deterioration in patients with moderately severe Pneumocystis carinii pneumonia and the acquired immunodeficiency syndrome (AIDS). Ann Intern Med 113:14, 1990.
121. Nielsen TL, Eeftinck Schattenkerk JK, Jensen BN, et al. Adjunctive corticosteroid therapy for Pneumocystis carinii pneumonia in AIDS: a randomized European multicenter open label study. J Acquir Immune Defic Syndr 5:726, 1992.
122. National Institutes of Health–University of California Expert Panel for Corticosteroids as Adjunctive Therapy for Pneumocystis Pneumonia: consensus statement on the use of corticosteroids as adjunctive therapy for Pneumocystis pneumonia in the acquired immunodeficiency syndrome. N Engl J Med 323:1500, 1990.
123. Renzi PM, Corbeil C, Chass M, et al. Bilateral pneumothoraces hasten mortality in AIDS patients receiving secondary prophylaxis with aerosolized pentamidine: association with a lower DL_{co} prior to receiving aerosolized pentamidine. Chest 102:491, 1992.
124. Tunon-de-Lara JM, Constans J, Vincent MP, et al. Spontaneous pneumothorax associated with Pneumocystis carinii pneumonia: successful treatment with talc pleurodesis. Chest 101:1177, 1993.
125. Ioannidis JPA, Cappelleri JC, Skolnik PR, et al. A meta-analysis of the relative efficacy and toxicity of Pneumocystis carinii prophylactic regimens. Arch Intern Med 156:177, 1996.
126. 2001 United States Public Health Service–Infectious Disease Society of America Guidelines for Prevention of Opportunistic Infections in Persons Infected with Human Immunodeficiency Virus. www.hivatis.org.
127. Kovacs JA, Masur H. Prophylaxis against opportunistic infections in patients with human immunodeficiency virus. N Engl J Med 342:1416, 2000.
128. Bozzette SA, Finkelstein DM, Spector SA, et al. A randomized trial of three anti-Pneumocystis agents in patients with advanced human immunodeficiency infection. N Engl J Med 332:693, 1995.
129. Schneider MME, Nielsen TL, Nelsing S, et al. Efficacy and toxicity of two doses of trimethoprim-sulfamethoxazole as primary prophylaxis against Pneumocystis carinii pneumonia in patients with human immunodeficiency virus. J Infect Dis 171:1632, 1995.
130. Podzamczer D, Salazar A, Jiminez J, et al. Intermittent trimethoprim-sulfamethoxazole compared with dapsone-pyrimethamine for the simultaneous primary prophylaxis of Pneumocysti pneumonia and toxoplasmosis in patients infected with HIV. Ann Intern Med 122:755, 1995.
131. Bozzette SA, Forthal D, Sattler FR, et al. The tolerance for zidovudine plus thrice weekly or daily trimethoprim-sulfamethoxazole with and without leucovorin for primary prophylaxis in advanced HIV disease. Am J Med 98:177, 1995.
132. Schneider MME, Hoepelman AIM, Eertlnck Schattenkerk JKM, et al. A controlled trial of aerosolized pentamidine or trimethoprim-sulfamethoxazole as primary prophylaxis against Pneumocystis carinii pneumonias in patients with human immunodeficiency virus infection. N Engl J Med 327:1836, 1992.
133. Hardy WD, Feinberg J, Finkelstein DM, et al. A controlled trial of trimethoprim-sulfamethoxazole or aerosolized pentamidine for secondary prophylaxis of Pneumocystis carinii pneumonia in patients with the acquired immunodeficiency syndrome: AIDS Clinical Trials Group 021. N Engl J Med 327:1842, 1992.
134. Rizzardi GP, Lazzarin A, Musicco M, et al. Better efficacy of twice monthly than monthly aerosolized pentamidine for secondary prophylaxis of Pneumocystis carinii pneumonia in patients with AIDS: an Italian multicenter randomized controlled trial. J Infect 31:99, 1995.
135. Murphy RL, Lavelle JF, Allan JD, et al. Aerosol pentamidine prophylaxis following Pneumocystis carinii pneumonia in AIDS patients: results of blinded dose-comparsion study using an ultrasonic nebulizer. Am J Med 90:782, 1985.
136. El-Sadr W, Murphy RL, Yurik RM, et al. Atovaquone compared with dapsone for the prevention of Pneumocystis carinii pneumonia in patients with HIV infection who cannot tolerate trimethoprim, sulfonamides, or both. N Engl J Med 339:1889, 1998.
137. Barber BA, Pegram S, High KP. Clindamycin/primaquine as prophylaaxis for Pneumocystis carinii pneumonia. Clin Infect Dis 23:718, 1996.
138. Opravil M, Hirschel B, Lazzarin A, et al. Once-weekly administration of dapsone/pyrimethamine vs. aerosolized pentamidine as combined prophylaxis for Pneumocystis carinii pneumonia and toxoplasmic encephalitis in human immunodeficiency virus-infected patients. Clin Infect Dis 20:531, 1995.
139. El-Sadr W, Luskin-Hawk R, Yurik TM, et al. A randomized trial of daily and thrice weekly trimethoprim-sulfamethoxazole for the prevention of Pneumocystis carinii pneumonia in HIV infected individuals. Clin Infect Dis 29:775, 1999.
140. Dunne MW, Bozzette S, McCutchan JA, et al. Efficacy of azithromycin in prevention of Pnemocystis carinii pneumonia: a randomised trial: California Collaborative Treatment Group. Lancet 354:891, 1999.
141. Chan C, Montaner J, LeFebvre EA, et al. Atovaquone suspension compared with aerosolized pentamidicine for prevention of Pneumocystis carinii pneumonia in human immunodeficiency virus infected subsets intolerant of trimethoprim or sulfamethoxazole. J Infect Dis 180:369, 1999.

142. Chu Sy, Hanson DL, Ciesielski C, et al. Prophylaxis against Pneumocystis carinii pneumonia at higher CD^+ T-cell counts [letter]. JAMA 273:848, 1995.
143. Para MF, Dohn M, Fram P, et al. ACTG 268 Trial: gradual initiation of trimethoprim/sulfamethoxazole (T/S) as primary prophylaxis for Pneumocystis carinii pneumonia (PCP). In: Abstracts of the 4th Conference on Retroviruses and Opportunistic Infections, Washington, DC. Alexandria, VA, Westover Management Group, 1997, abstract 2.
144. Leoung G, Stanford J, Giordano M, et al. A randomized, double-blind trial of TMP/SMX dose escalation vs. direct rechallenge in HIV^+ persons at risk for PCP and with prior treatment-limiting rash or fever. In: Abstracts of the 37th Interscience Conference on Antimicrobial Agents and Chemotherapy, Toronto, 1997, abstract LB10.
145. Schneider MME, Borleffs JCC, Stolk RP, et al. Discontinuation of Pneumocystis carinii pneumonia prophylaxis in HIV-1 infected patients treated with highly active antiretroviral therapy. Lancet 353:201, 1999.
146. Furrer H, Egger M, Opravil M, et al. Discontinuation of primary prophylaxis against Pneumocystis carinii pneumonia in HIV-1-infected adults treated with combination antiretroviral therapy. N Engl J Med 340:1301, 1999.
147. Weverling GJ, Mocroft A, Ledergerber B, et al. Discontinuation of Pneumocystis carinii pneumonia prophylaxis after start of highly active antiretroviral therapy in HIV-1 infection. Lancet 353:1293, 1999.
148. Yangco BF, VonBargen JC, Moorman AC, Holmberg SD. Discontinuation of chemoprophylaxis for Pneumocystis carinii pneumonia in patients with HIV infection. Ann Intern Med 132:201, 2000.
149. Kirk O, Lundgren JD, Pederson C, et al. Can chemoprophylaxis against opportunistic infections be discontinued after an increase in CD4 cells induced by highly active antiretroviral therapy? AIDS 13:1647, 1999.
150. Lopez JC, Miro JM, Pena JM, et al. A randomized trial of the discontinuation of primary and secondary prophylaxis against Pneumocystis carinii pneumonia after HAART in patients with HIV infection. N Engl J Med 344:159, 2001.
151. Mussini C, Pezzotti P, Govoni A, et al. Discontinuation of primary prophylaxis for Pneumocystis carinii pneumonia and toxoplasmic encephalitis in human immunodeficiency virus type I-infected patients: the changes in opportunistic prophylaxis study. J Infect Dis 181:1635, 2000.
152. Furrer H, Opravil M, Rossi M, et al. Discontinuation of primary prophylaxis in HIV infected patients at high risk of Pneumocystis pneumonia: a prospective multicentre study. AIDS 15:501, 2001.
153. Ledergerber B, Mocroft A, Reiss P, et al. Discontinuation of secondary prophylaxis against Pneumocystis carinii pneumonia in patients with HIV infection who have a response to antiretroviral therapy. N Engl J Med 344:168, 2001.
154. Abgrail S, Matheron S, LaMoing V, et al. Can secondary Pneumocystis carinii prophylaxis be discontinued in HIV infected patients treated with HAART? Presented at the 7th Conference on Retroviruses and Opportunistic Infections, San Francisco, 2000, abstract Tuorb360.
155. Jubault V, Pacanowski J, Rabian C, Viard J-P. Interruption of prophylaxis for major opportunistic infections in HIV-infected patients receiving triple combination antiretroviral therapy. Ann Med Interne (Paris) 151:163, 2000.
156. Furrer H, Opravil M, Rossi M, et al. Stop Cox 2: is it safe to discontinue secondary PCP prophylaxis? Experience of the Swiss Cohort Study. Presented at the Conference on Retroviral Disease and Opportunistic Infection, San Francisco, 2001.
157. Soriano V, Dona C, Rodriguez-Rosado, et al. Discontinuation of secondary prophylaxis for opportunistic infections in HIV-infected patients receiving highly active antiretroviral therapy AIDS 14:383, 2000.
158. Mussini C, Pazzoti P, Borghi V. An open, controlled, randomized study of discontinuation of prophylaxis for PCP in patients with AIDS. Presented at the 7th Conference on Retroviruses and Opportunistic Infections, San Francisco, 2000, abstract MOPeB2275.
159. Zeller V, Joulian M, Truffaut C, et al. Discontinuing maintenance treatment for Pneumocystis pneumonia, toxoplasmic encephalitis, and disseminated Mycobacterium avium complex infection. In: Program and Abstracts of the 1st IAS Conference on HIV Pathogenesis and Treatment, Buenos Aires, 2001, abstract 737.
160. Carr A, Tindall B, Brew BJ, et al. Low-dose trimethoprim-sulfamethoxazole prophylaxis for toxoplasmic encephalitis in patients with AIDS. Ann Intern Med 117:106, 1992.
161. Martin JN, Rose DA, Hadley WK, et al. Emergence of trimethoprim-sulfamethoxazole resistance in the AIDS era. J Infect Dis 1880:809, 1999.
162. Holtzer CD, Flaherty JF Jr, Coleman RL. Cross-reactivity in HIV-infected patients switched from trimethoprim-sulfamethoxazole to dapsone. Pharmacotherapy 18:831, 1998.
163. Girard PM, Landman R, Gaudebout C, et al. Dapsone-pyrimethamine compared with aerosolized pentamidine as primary prophylaxis against Pneumocystis carinii pneumonia and toxoplasmosis in HIV infection. N Engl J Med 328:1514, 1993.
164. Golden JA, Katz MH, Chernoff DN, et al. A randomized comparison of once monthly or twice monthly high dose aerosolized pentamidine prophylaxis. Chest 104:743, 1993.
165. Cushion MT. Transmission and epidemiology. In: Walzer PD (ed) Pneumocystis carinii Pneumonia, 2nd ed. New York, Marcel Dekker, 1994, p 123.
166. Hughes WT. Natural mode of acquisition for de novo infection with Pneumocystis carinii. J Infect Dis 145:842, 1982.
167. Hendley JO, Weller TH. Activation and transmission in rats of infection with Pneumocystis. Proc Soc Exp Biol Med 137:1401, 1971.
168. Walzer PD, Schnelle V, Armstrong D, et al. Nude mouse: a new experimental model for Pneumocystis carinii infection. Science 197:177, 1977.
169. Demanche C, Berthelemy M, Petit T, et al. Phylogeny of Pneumocystis carinii from 18 primate species confirms host specificity and suggests coevolution. J Clin Microbiol 39:2126, 2001.
170. Denis CM, Mazars E, Guyot K, et al. Genetic divergence at the SODA locus of six different formae species of Pneumocystis carinii. Med Mycol 38:289, 2000.
171. Wakefield AE. Detection of DNA sequences identical to Pneumocystis carinii in samples of ambient air. J Eukaryot Microbiol 41:116S, 1994.
172. Bartlett MS, Lee CH, Lu JJ. Pneumocystis carinii detected in air. J Eukaryot Microbiol 41:75S, 1994.
173. Keely SP, Stringer JR, Baughman RP, et al. Genetic variation among Pneumocystis carinii hominis isolates in recurrent pneumocystosis. J Infect Dis 172:595, 1995.
174. Hauser PM, Blanc DS, Sudre P, et al. Genetic diversity of Pneumocystis carinii in HIV-positive and -negative patients as revealed by PCR-SSCP typing. AIDS 15:461, 2001.

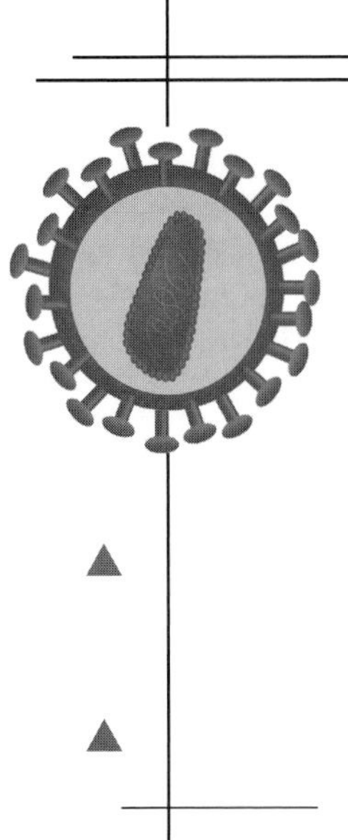

CHAPTER 30
Toxoplasmosis

Henry W. Murray, MD
Christine Katlama, MD

Prior to the advent of acquired immunodeficiency syndrome (AIDS), toxoplasmosis was largely recognized as a common, worldwide protozoal infection that produced few if any clinical manifestations in otherwise healthy, immunocompetent children and adults; at best, 20% to 25% of such individuals developed cervical lymphadenitis, a self-limited flu-like illness, or both. In addition, although lifelong infection was known to persist in all infected persons, it typically remained quiescent and of little consequence in the presence of intact cellular immunity.[1,2]

In three particular settings, however, toxoplasmosis did cause important clinical disease and destruction of vital tissues: in infants born to women infected with *Toxoplasma gondii* during pregnancy; in a small fraction of individuals who, when infected as children or adults, develop retinochoroiditis; and in patients with an underlying T cell disorder (primarily AIDS) who develop a life-threatening syndrome with cerebral or disseminated disease, or both. Regarding the latter disorders, patients treated with corticosteroids or cytotoxic agents, transplant recipients, and those with immunocompromising neoplastic disorders (e.g., Hodgkin's disease) were recognized to be at risk for reactivation of previously acquired toxoplasmosis and severe, progressive infection if initially exposed when already immunosuppressed.[1-3]

Despite the relatively high prevalence of latent *T. gondii* infection in the general population[2] and its capacity to behave as an opportunistic pathogen,[1-4] toxoplasmosis was seldom recognized in immunocompromised hosts prior to 1980. The emergence of the profound immunodeficiency of advanced human immunodeficiency virus (HIV) infection predictably and strikingly altered the clinical relevance of toxoplasmosis, especially as it relates to central nervous system disease in patients with fully established AIDS.[5-20]

BIOLOGY, EPIDEMIOLOGY, TRANSMISSION

Biology

Toxoplasma gondii, an obligate intracellular protozoan, exists in three forms: oocyst, tissue cyst, and tachyzoite. After inadvertent oral ingestion of oocysts or tissue cysts, both of which contain tachyzoites, the latter are released, enter the bloodstream, and disseminate to the tissues. Tachyzoites, responsible for acute toxoplasmosis, replicate intracellularly and parasitize and destroy new cells until an effective immune response develops. Surviving parasites then encyst in various tissues, including brain, retina, skeletal muscle, myocardium, and lung and thereafter usually remain quiescent for life. Years later, especially if T cell-dependent immune mechanisms fail, tachyzoites may be liberated by cyst rupture, leading to reactivated infection.[1,2]

Oocysts develop in the intestinal mucosal cells of the cat, the definite host. Cats become infected after ingesting cysts in raw animal tissue or poorly cooked meat, or they take in oocysts shed by other felines. After 1 to 2 weeks, initial shedding of oocysts ceases and seldom resumes.[21] Oocysts sporulate before becoming infectious, a process favored by warm, moist conditions typical of those found in dampened soil or litter boxes. Sporulated oocysts may persist in an infectious state for a year or more.[1,2]

Tissue cysts arise in host cells in virtually any organ. Maintaining cysts in a quiescent state and controlling tachyzoites potentially liberated by periodic cyst breakdown requires mechanisms mediated by antigen-sensitized T cells and activating cytokines. Thus in previously infected individuals who subsequently become immunosuppressed or T cell-deficient, residual tissue cysts represent a ready endogenous source of tachyzoites poised to escape. Because immunologically intact and deficient individuals may develop retinochoroiditis as a manifestation of reactivated infection,[2] prevention of retinal cyst breakdown presumably requires additional mechanisms.

The tachyzoite, which can invade any nucleated cell (Fig. 30–1), is the obligate intracellular form and requires a host cell for growth and multiplication. Uncontrolled, proliferating tachyzoites rupture free from the infected host cell and probably repeatedly escape into the circulation. Replication at systemic sites then continues until immune responses develop.[1,2,4,22,23]

Epidemiology and Transmission

Although cats, small mammals, and birds serve as natural reservoirs, virtually any animal that ingests material contaminated by oocysts or cyst-containing tissue can become infected. Undercooked pork and lamb (and less commonly venison or beef) are frequently implicated in transmission to humans. If meat is not heated to 60°C or frozen to below −20°C, cysts remain viable.[2,21]

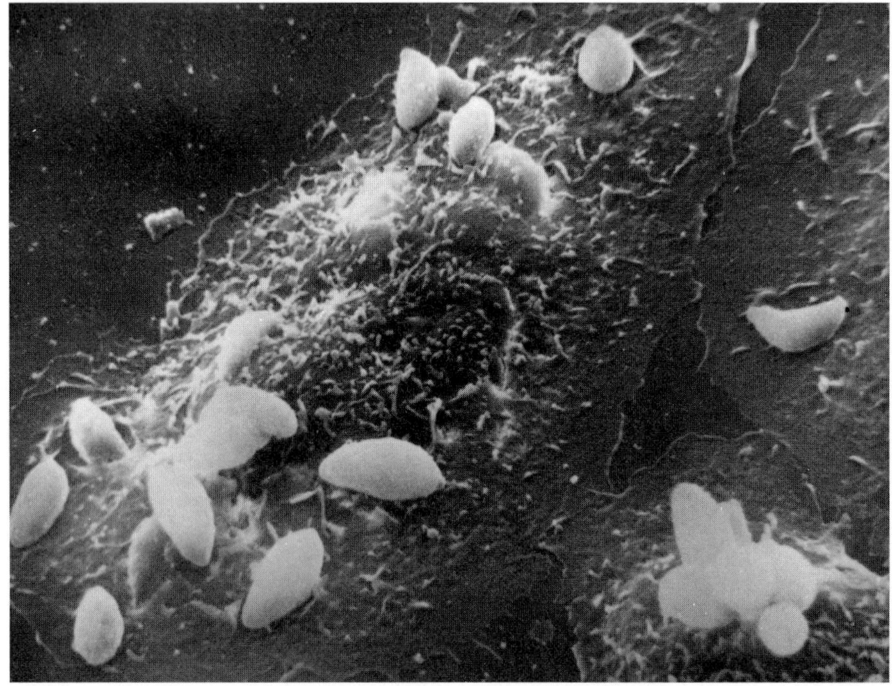

A

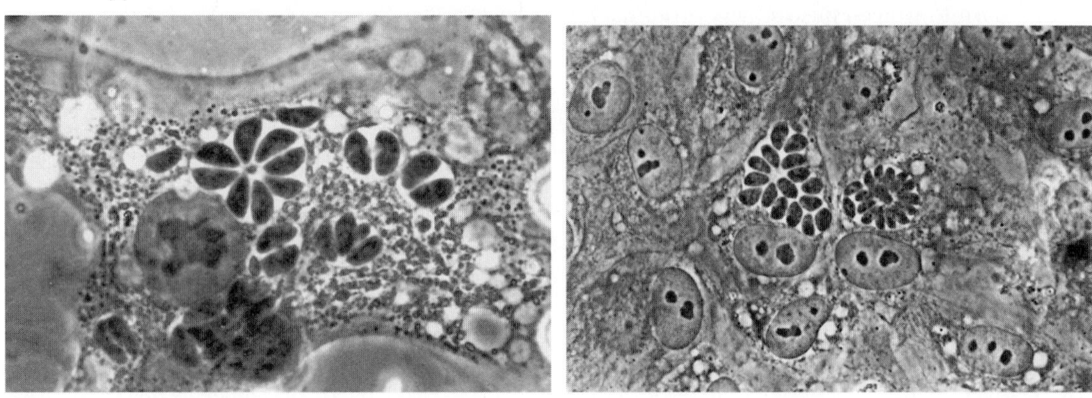

B

Figure 30–1. *A*, Scanning electron micrograph showing *Toxoplasma gondii* tachyzoites attaching to and being ingested by cultivated human monocyte-derived macrophages during in vitro infection. Photograph taken by Dr. Gilla Kaplan, The Rockefeller University. (From Murray HW. Immunotherapy for AIDS-associated toxoplasmosis. In: Sande MA, Root RK [eds]. Contemporary Issues in Infectious Diseases, vol 9: Treatment of Serious Infections in the 1990s. New York, Churchill Livingstone, 1992, p 205.) *B*, Photomicrographs of unstimulated human macrophages (*left*) and fibroblasts (*right*) 20 hours after in vitro infection with tachyzoites showing overt intracellular replication with up to 8 to 16 organisms per vacuole. At the initiation of in vitro infection, there had been one tachyzoite per vacuole. (From Murray HW. Survival of intracellular pathogens within human mononuclear phagocytes. Semin Hematol 25:101, 1988.)

The frequency and prevalence of human *T. gondii* infection varies depending on age, dietary habits, climate, and proximity to cats. In the United States serologic evidence of prior infection is present in 10% to 40% of healthy adults.[7] Seropositivity to *T. gondii* [specific immunoglobulin G(IgG) antibody, evidence of prior infection] in HIV-infected adults and children in the United States is reported to range from 8% to more than 25%.[18,24,25] In other countries, seroprevalence rates in the general and HIV-infected populations are also variable, ranging up to 70% to 90% (e.g., Central America, Brazil, South Pacific, France, Germany, Austria).[2,18,19] All HIV-infected individuals who are seropositive to *T. gondii* have latent infection and are at risk for developing reactivated toxoplasmosis once they become T cell-deficient. In addition, seroconversion data from countries of high *T. gondii* prevalence indicate that newly acquired infection may occur in up to 1% to 2% of HIV-infected persons per year.[11,18,19,21] In such a setting, primary infection may be clinically severe, with diffuse, multiorgan involvement that is difficult to control despite treatment. Avoiding exposure to *T. gondii* is particularly important for all HIV-infected individuals who are *Toxoplasma*-seronegative (see below).[21]

The three principal modes of human transmission of *T. gondii* are (1) ingestion of cat-derived oocysts or undercooked food containing tissue cysts; (2) transplacental spread; and (3) inadvertent direct administration.[1,2] Cats confined indoors and fed processed foods are unlikely to be a source of infection. Congenital infection, which is uncommon,[26] occurs if the mother acquires acute infection during pregnancy. Although congenital infection has been documented in infants born to HIV-infected women who themselves had had previously controlled latent toxoplasmosis,[27,28] the risk of this complication is low.[29,30] *T. gondii* may rarely be transmitted by needlestick, transplantation of infected organs into seronegative recipients, transfusion of whole blood, leukocytes or platelets, or contaminated drinking water.[1,2]

▲ IMMUNE RESPONSE TO INFECTION AND HOST DEFENSE

In healthy individuals, tachyzoites induce humoral and cellular immune responses, reflected in IgM and then IgG antibodies followed by T cell reactivity to *T. gondii* antigen.[31–33] Both responses initially control proliferating parasites. Specific antibody opsonizes tachyzoites, enhancing killing by cytokine-stimulated cells (e.g., mononuclear phagocytes); acting with the alternative complement pathway, it also lyses the organism.[1,2,4,22]

Once CD4 cell counts decline to below 100 to 150/mm^3, as many as one-third of HIV-infected patients with latent toxoplasmosis develop clinically apparent, reactivated disease within 24 months.[34] The 12-month risk of reactivation also correlates with CD4+ T-lymphocyte number: The risk is 20% with fewer than 150 cells/mm^3,[34] 25% with fewer than 100 cells/mm^3,[35] and 48% with fewer than 50 cells/mm^3.[36] Given the irreversible damage present when some patients initially present for therapy, it is clearly important to test all HIV-infected individuals for IgG antibody to *T. gondii* and to provide primary prophylaxis for all seropositive patients by the time CD4+ T-lymphocyte counts have reached 100 cells/mm^3.[18,34]

▲ CLINICAL MANIFESTATIONS IN HIV-INFECTED PATIENTS

Acute Infection

Reactivation of latent *Toxoplasma* infection is the pathogenetic mechanism usually thought to be responsible for clinically apparent disease. There is little clinical experience with primary *T. gondii* infection in this patient population; whether an HIV-infected individual with adequate CD4 cells (e.g., >200 cells/mm^3) behaves normally and controls the initial infection is not clear.[11,18,21] If infection is satisfactorily controlled and the inflammatory response is intact, one would expect that 7 to 21 days after initial exposure about 20% of patients would develop cervical lymphadenopathy, either asymptomatic or accompanied by a flu-like illness lasting 1 to 3 weeks. Additional responses (e.g., those expressed in 20% to 40% of otherwise healthy patients) include generalized lymphadenopathy, splenomegaly, or hepatomegaly. Transient complaints of low-grade fever, arthralgias, myalgias, headache, fatigue, sore throat, abdominal pain, or rash. Retinochoroiditis can also complicate acute infection.[1,2]

Primary toxoplasmosis acquired by patients already CD4 cell-deficient would likely be more widely disseminated and progressive and perhaps respond less well to treatment then reactivated disease.[2] In such a setting, serious visceral manifestations, including pneumonitis, myositis, myocarditis, orchitis, and encephalitis (manifesting as intracerebral mass lesions), would be expected.[1,2]

Reactivated Infection

Most cases of AIDS-associated toxoplasmosis appear to represent reactivation of latent infection.[18] Clinical manifestations therefore depend on where infection reactivates anatomically and the intensity of the local inflammatory response, which may vary according to the CD4+ T-lymphocyte number.[37]

The central nervous system (CNS) (encephalitis, abscess), lung (pneumonitis), and eye (retinochoroiditis) are favored sites of symptomatic reactivated infection. CNS disease is by far the most common. Because parasites encyst in any organ and recurrent parasitemia associated with reactivation may also lead to new organ seeding, clinically apparent manifestations of extracerebral toxoplasmosis may be diverse. Indeed, autopsy studies often demonstrate multiorgan involvement not recognized antemortem; as many as 50% of patients with extracerebral disease do not have concurrent CNS lesions.[38–40]

Extracerebral Infection

Along with pneumonitis and retinochoroiditis, the following extracerebral manifestations have been reported but are not common: endocrinopathies with pituitary or adrenal lesions (or both) and various symptoms and signs related to focal involvement of skin, peritoneum, testes, stomach, pancreas, bladder, skeletal muscle, liver, myocardium, lymph nodes, and duodenum and colon.[11,18,38–40] Occult infection can be demonstrated at autopsy in still other sites, including bone marrow, pharynx, and pericardium.[38–40] A syndrome resembling septic shock, with high fever, hypotension, respiratory symptoms or overt pneumonitis, and multiorgan failure, can also develop in response to disseminated reactivated infection.[41–43] This syndrome may be associated with thrombocytopenia and striking elevations in serum lactate dehydrogenase (LDH) levels.[41–43]

Neurologic Disease

Headache, confusion, altered mental status, and fever are presenting complaints in about 50% of patients with intracerebral infection (encephalitis with or without overt abscess). The onset of illness can be insidious or abrupt. As many as 30% have seizures as an initial manifestation, and 50% to 60% demonstrate focal neurologic signs.[6–11,13,18,19] Nuchal rigidity or other meningeal signs are unusual. High fevers and shaking chills are also unusual. Because intracerebral toxoplasmosis is typically multifocal with destructive, inflammatory mass lesions, virtually any neurologic syndrome may develop and yield motor or sensory deficits; brain stem, basal ganglia, or cerebellar dysfunction; movement disorders; an array of neuropsychiatric findings; and varying effects on the level of consciousness, including coma. Hemiparesis is the most common focal deficit among a long list of others, including cranial nerve lesions, focal seizures, aphasia, visual field losses, ataxia, dysmetria, tremor, and hemiballismus and extrapyramidal signs.[6–11,13,18,19] Spinal cord involvement can produce transverse myelitis or a conus medullaris syndrome.[44] Hydrocephalus, choroid plexitis, and cerebral hemorrhage may also occur.[45,46]

Eye Involvement

Ocular disease is probably the most common clinical manifestation of HIV-associated extracerebral toxoplasmosis.[47–52] In 30% to 60% of cases of retinochoroiditis, encephalitis is also present.[47–52] (Conversely, however, relatively few patients presenting with cerebritis also have retinochoroiditis.) Visual symptoms due to *Toxoplasma* retinitis include loss of visual acuity, "floaters," and red, inflamed sclera. Ophthalmologic examination reveals yellow-white areas of full-thickness necrotizing retinitis, occasionally with hemorrhage and vascular sheathing. Lesions are predominantly unilateral. The presence of inflammation in the anterior or posterior segment, or both (hyalitis), is highly suggestive of *Toxoplasma* retinitis and occurs in 60% to 70% of cases. Fluorescein angiography reveals hyperfluorescence starting from the periphery and progressing toward the center of the lesions. This distinguishes *Toxoplasma* retinitis from cytomegalovirus (CMV) retinitis.[50,52] *Toxoplasma* retinitis should also be differentiated from retinitis due to varicella-zoster virus, syphilis, and fungi including *Pneumocystis carinii*.

Pneumonitis

Pulmonary manifestations of toxoplasmosis have accounted for up to 35% of extraneurologic *Toxoplasma* disease.[53–57] Fever and dyspnea are the most frequent symptoms, whereas cough and sputum may be absent. Chest radiographs usually show diffuse bilateral pulmonary infiltrates.[53–61] Multiple nodular densities have been reported. A rise in LDH levels has been reported to be suggestive of the diagnosis.[60] A diagnosis of pulmonary toxoplasmosis can be established by direct examination of bronchoalveolar lavage, which reveals *T. gondii* trophozoites when stained by a Giemsa or immunofluorescence technique.[61] Lung histology may also reveal tachyzoites with Giemsa staining. Disseminated *Toxoplasma* infection may manifest as acute respiratory distress syndrome associated with septic shock and thrombocytopenia.[41–44,62]

▲ DIAGNOSIS

Routine Laboratory Test Results

Routine laboratory tests seldom yield specific information pointing to toxoplasmosis. The white blood cell (WBC) count is not characteristically abnormal, nor is the neutrophil count. CD4+ T-lymphocyte counts are rarely more than 200/mm^3. Most patients have counts less than 100/mm^3 and often less than 50 cells/mm^3.[18,21] The chest film and electrocardiogram may indicate pneumonitis or rarely myocarditis. Thrombocytopenia and elevated serum LDH values suggest the septic form of infection often associated with pneumonitis. Although not common, other routine laboratory results can reflect extracerebral involvement of the pituitary, pancreas, liver, and bladder.

Definitive Diagnosis

The definitive diagnosis of toxoplasmosis as the cause of encephalitis or extraneurologic disease requires direct demonstration of the tachyzoite form in involved tissues or in blood or other fluids. Because obtaining an appropriate sample and visualizing or isolating this organism may require invasive procedures and considerable technical expertise, few centers are prepared to cultivate *Toxoplasma* by animal inoculation or tissue culture. Standard practice has evolved to allow a presumptive diagnosis of *Toxoplasma* encephalitis acceptable in most instances (see later).[11,63,64] Establishing an empiric diagnosis of *Toxoplasma* encephalitis is considered particularly appropriate for patients with compatible neurologic disease who are not receiving prophylaxis with trimethoprim-sulfamethoxazole (TMP-SMX) or pyrimethamine plus dapsone and who have (1) less than 200 CD4+ T-lymphocyte cells/mm^3; (2) anti-*Toxoplasma* immunoglobulin G (IgG) antibody in the serum, and (3) a clear-cut response to empiric anti-*Toxoplasma* therapy.

Establishing a diagnosis of *Toxoplasma* retinitis is usually done by expert funduscopic examination performed by a retinal specialist. Some syndromes are sufficiently similar to processes caused by other pathogens, so a specific diagnosis is necessary. This usually requires visualizing the organism by histology.

Serology

Cases of AIDS-related toxoplasmosis have been described in patients whose serum was reported to lack anti-*Toxoplasma* IgG.[20,63] However, in the United States and western Europe, an undetectable IgG level is unusual if the test is performed in a reliable reference laboratory. Serum anti-*Toxoplasma* IgM antibodies are seldom detected. Explanations for IgG seronegativity include a recent primary infection (IgM antibody testing is occasionally useful in such patients[7]), laboratory error including failure to test the serum at low dilutions or undiluted, and the theoretical notion of loss of preexisting antibody in advanced AIDS. Nevertheless, if toxoplasmosis is presumptively diagnosed in an AIDS patient who is IgG-seronegative, the chances of being incorrect are certainly more than 90% and probably closer to 97% to 100%.

Although anti-*Toxoplasma* IgG is also found in cerebrospinal fluid (CSF) in 30% to 70% of patients with encephalitis,[6–8] its presence alone does not permit a diagnosis of intracerebral disease.[7,65] Measuring intrathecal production of IgG has been suggested to be diagnostically useful.[65] However, CSF is not routinely available because (1) many patients with intracerebral toxoplasmosis do not undergo lumbar puncture because of concern for herniation, and (2) standard CSF testing infrequently yields specific diagnostic information. It is not part of a routine diagnostic evaluation at most centers.

Histopathologic Findings and Culture

Free and intracellular tachyzoites can be directly visualized in Giemsa-stained cytocentrifuged preparations of CSF, bronchoalveolar lavage material, induced sputum, and peritoneal fluid as well as in bone marrow aspirates, peripheral blood or buffy coat smears, and tissue imprints (touch preparations).[1,2,11,13,19,66–69] Tachyzoites can also be detected in these materials by immunofluorescence.[68]

Peripheral blood, CSF, or any body fluid or properly obtained tissue can be used to attempt parasite isolation by intraperitoneal inoculation of mice or in vitro addition to cell (e.g., fibroblasts) cultures that support intracellular replication (Fig. 30–1).[1,2,18] The latter method may document the organism by microscopic examination within 2 to 3 days.[18,68–72] In contrast, mouse inoculation may not yield diagnostic results for up to 4 to 6 weeks and thus may be confirmatory but of little other clinical usefulness. Using the cell culture method (which appears to be more sensitive than microscopic examination of standard cytocentrifuge preparations),[66] parasitemia has been demonstrated in 14% to 38% of patients (79% in one study)[68] with intracerebral or extracerebral toxoplasmosis (or both).[18] Few centers perform cultures for *Toxoplasma*, however.

Even though biopsy of involved tissues (e.g., brain or lung) is no longer common diagnostic practice, some patients do come to organ biopsy, especially those who have failed to respond to empiric anti-*Toxoplasma* therapy. Cerebral lesions are most often approached by needle biopsy. Open excisional brain biopsy yields more satisfactory material than does needle biopsy or aspiration, but it is usually performed only if needle biopsies fail to reveal a causative process.[18]

The histologic reaction to infection may vary among organs; in the brain it ranges from granulomatous-type changes to a modest, focal inflammatory response to evidence of severe tissue destruction with widespread necrosis.[1,2,6,8,10,18,19] Because all individuals seropositive to *T. gondii* are presumed to harbor at least some cyst forms deep in their tissues, observing a few scattered cysts in histologically quiescent sites does not necessarily establish the diagnosis of active toxoplasmosis. In contrast, finding intra- or extracellular tachyzoites (implying cyst rupture) or numerous cysts that have provoked an inflammatory reaction is considered evidence of disease (Fig. 30–2). The sensitive peroxidase-antiperoxidase technique, which stains cysts, liberated tachyzoites, and free parasite

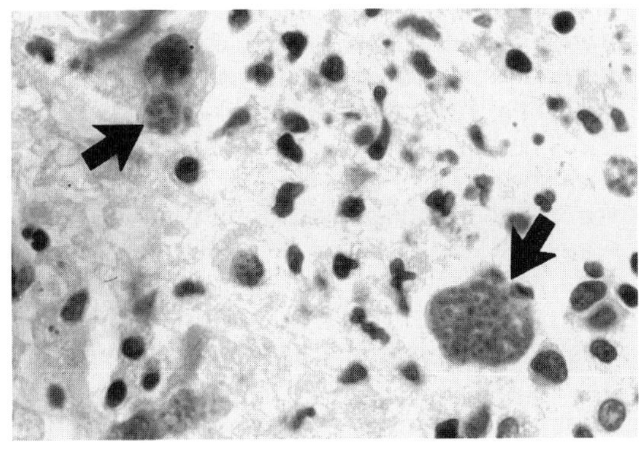
A

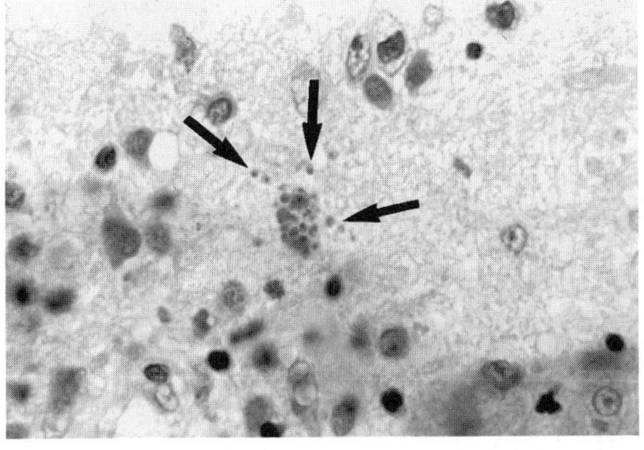
B

Figure 30–2. Histologic appearance of reactivated intracerebral toxoplasmosis in a patient with advanced AIDS who underwent brain biopsy. *A*, Section shows inflammatory response and one large and one small brain cyst (*arrows*). *B*, Cyst breakdown with released tachyzoites (*arrows*). (H&E) (From Murray HW: Immunotherapy for AIDS-associated toxoplasmosis. In Sande MA, Root RK [eds] Contemporary Issues in Infectious Diseases, vol 9: Treatment of Serious Infections in the 1990s. New York, Churchill Livingstone, 1992, p 205.)

antigen,[18] should be applied to fixed tissues that are apparently negative by routine staining.

Neuroimaging Studies

Standard Testing

Reportedly, 10% to 43% of patients with encephalitis have only a solitary parenchymal lesion demonstrated by computed tomography (CT)[6,8,12,13,71,72]; rarely, the CT scan is negative (3% to 10%).[6,8,63,73] However, multiple focal intracerebral lesions are most typical of toxoplasmosis, especially if more sensitive magnetic resonance imaging (MRI) is used (Fig. 30–3).[18] On MRI testing, more than 80% of patients have multiple lesions.[71–80] Therefore if a single lesion is found on CT and confirmed to be solitary by MRI, lymphoma or another cause of focal brain lesions associated with AIDS should be a primary consideration, even if there is contrast enhancement.[71–80] With intracerebral toxoplasmosis, lesions are most often bilateral and contrast (ring)-enhancing (80% to 90%), induce a mass effect with edema, and frequently develop in the basal ganglia, thalamus, or hemispheres at the corticomedullary junction.[6,8,10,11,13,18,71–80] There is, however, no specific CT or MRI result that is accepted as absolutely diagnostic of intracerebral toxoplasmosis. For example, multifocal disease and ring-enhancing lesions can be seen in 40% to 50% of AIDS patients with CNS lymphoma.[74]

Functional Imaging

In an effort to sharpen the noninvasive (but still presumptive) diagnosis of toxoplasmosis, other imaging techniques have been evaluated, especially to help differentiate infection from lymphoma. There has been some experience with MR spectroscopy. Both single-photon emission computed tomography (SPECT) using thallium 201(^{201}Tl) and positron emission tomography (PET)[81–95] using labeled substrates such as 2-fluorodeoxyglucose appear useful. In patients with mass lesions on CT or MRI, the *absence* of increased uptake on ^{201}Tl SPECT scanning (Fig. 30–4) and *decreased* activity on PET scans ("cold" or hypometabolic lesions) are characteristic of infection (e.g., toxoplasmosis or other infections); lymphoma is almost invariably associated with increased uptake using these two scanning techniques.[85–91]

Small lesions (< 8 mm) may be difficult to resolve with SPECT or PET scans; and although uncommon, both false-positive and false-negative results may occur. These noninvasive tests have been proposed to be especially useful, for example, in patients who heretofore would have been candidates for brain biopsy: (1) those suspected of having toxoplasmosis but in whom MRI demonstrates only a solitary intracerebral lesion; (2) *Toxoplasma*-seronegative patients with multifocal enhancing lesions; (3) the unusual individual with intracerebral disease and more than 200 CD4 cells/mm^3.[71] From a practical perspective, however, most such patients have an empiric trial of antitoxoplasma therapy for 10 to 14 days. If they then do not demonstrate radiologic improvement, a biopsy is performed.

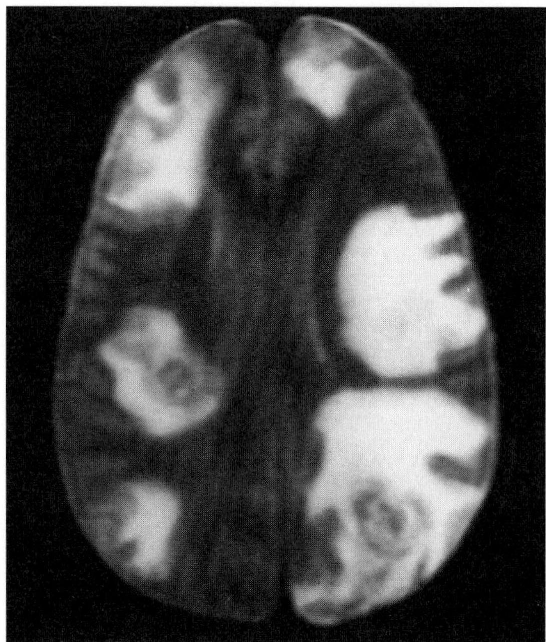

Figure 30–3. Magnatic resonance image (MRI) showing multifocal brain lesions with pronounced edema in an AIDS patient with toxoplasmosis. (Courtesy of Dr. Henry Masur, National Institutes of Health.)

Detection of *Toxoplasma* Antigen and DNA

Antigen can be detected by conventional assays in serum or urine in 25% to 30% patients with AIDS-related toxoplasmosis.[18,96–104] In contrast, depending on the material tested (CSF, blood, buffy coat, bronchoalveolar lavage fluid, aqueous humor, brain tissue), parasite DNA can be detected by the polymerase chain reaction (PCR) in an appreciably larger proportion of patients. In those with documented or presumed encephalitis, positive PCR results using CSF have been reported in about 50% (range 12% to 100%) with essentially no false-negative reactions (100% specificity).[18,71,97–103] Sensitivity may be increased by simultaneously testing CSF and blood or testing CSF prior to initiating therapy. PCR testing using blood or buffy coat from patients with intracerebral infection is an attractive approach to consider. In two studies, positive reactions were reported in 16% to 68% with occasional false-positive results.[18,103] In patients with parasitemia alone without encephalitis, PCR results using blood were positive in 84%.[63] Thus despite limitations in sensitivity and availability, the high specificity of PCR testing for *Toxoplasma* DNA makes this method of diagnosis useful if a positive result is generated.

Response to Empiric Treatment

Most patients with cerebral toxoplasmosis (65% to 90%) respond rapidly to two-drug treatment with pyrimethamine plus either sulfadiazine or clindamycin.[2,11–13,18,20,63,71] Thus a clear-cut clinical and neuroradiographic response to empiric therapy is now considered essentially diagnostic of toxoplasmosis.[18,71] In one study, neurologic improvement was

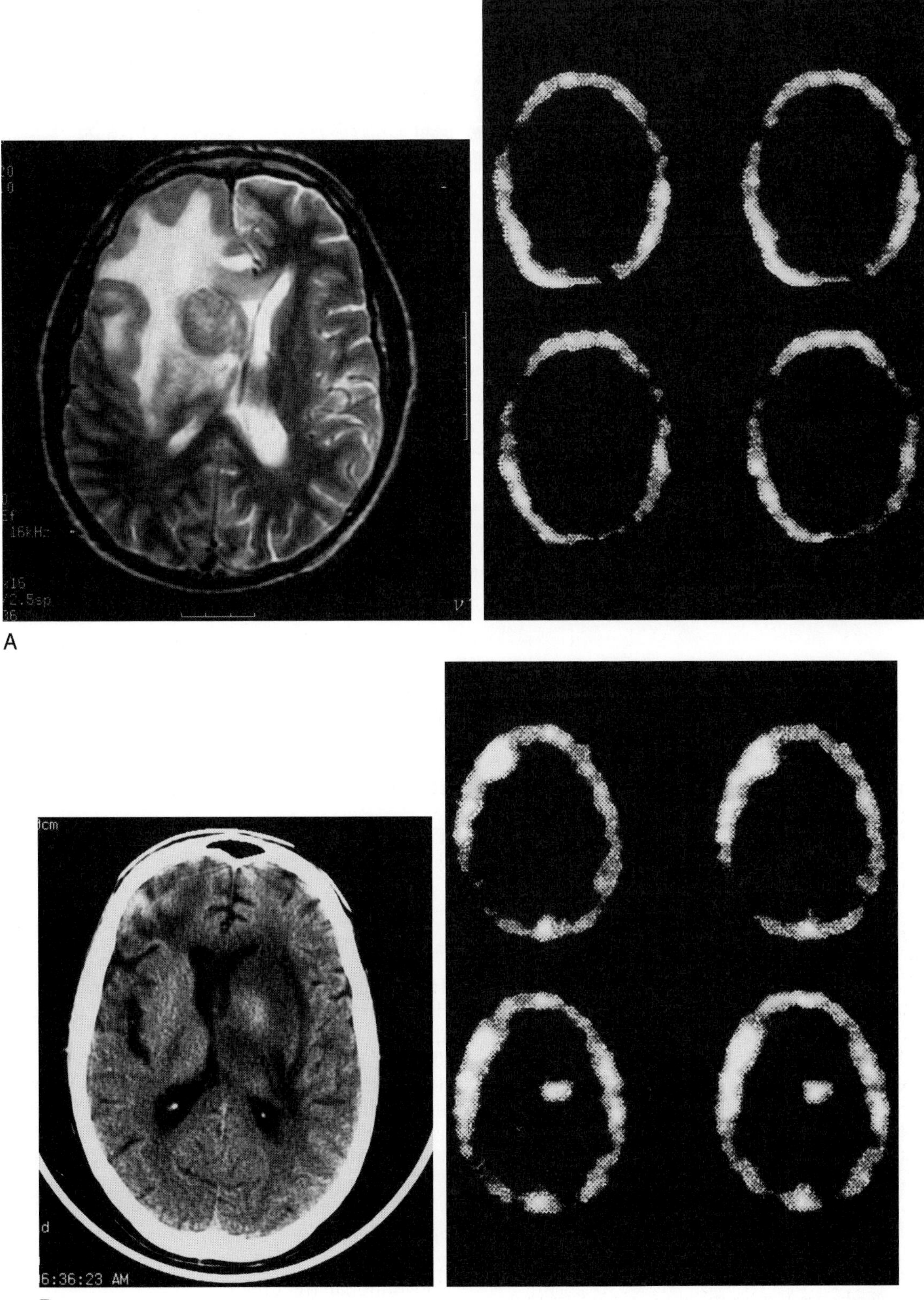

Figure 30–4. Appearance of thallium-201 single-photon emission competed tomography (SPECT) scans in AIDS-related toxoplasmosis (*A*) versus lymphoma (*B*). *A*, MRI showing large right-sided lesion with edema in a *Toxoplasma*-seropositive patient who responded to empiric anti-*Toxoplasma* therapy (*left*). SPECT scan shows no uptake at the site of the lesion (*right*). *B*, CT scan in an AIDS patient with biopsy-documented lymphoma showing contrast-enhancing right frontal and left thalamic lesions (*left*), both of which demonstrate increased uptake on the SPECT scan (*right*). (Courtesy of Drs. David Warren, James Hurley, and Josephine Rini, The New York Hospital–Cornell Medical Center.)

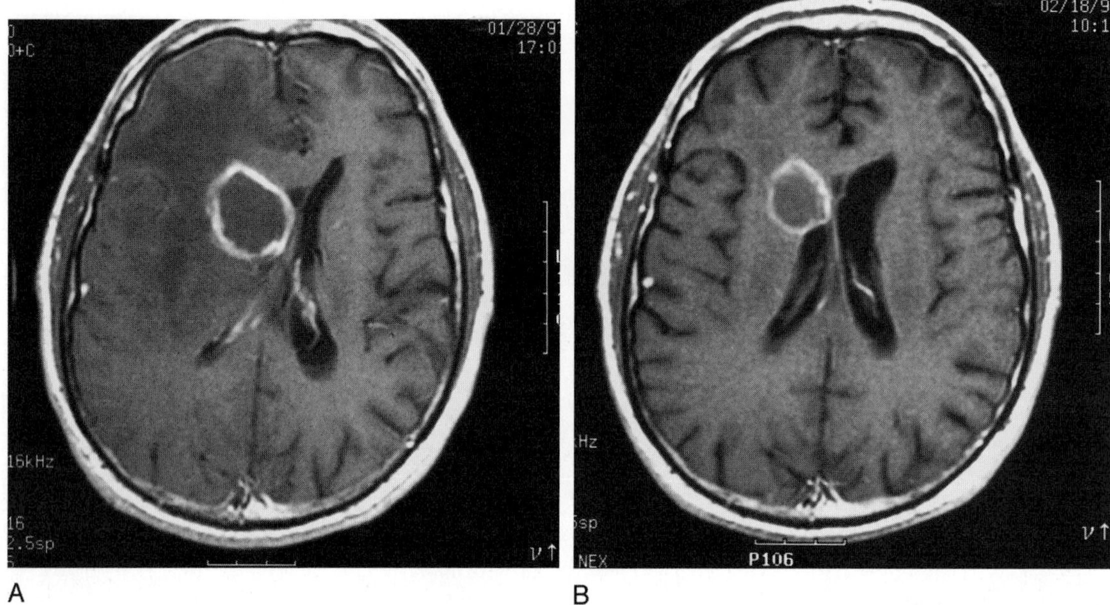

Figure 30–5. Neuroradiographic response to empiric anti-*Toxoplasma* therapy in a patient with AIDS. *A*, Pretreatment MRI demonstrates a solitary ring-enhancing lesion, adjacent large hypodense area of edema, and mass effect with ventricular compression and shift. *Toxoplasma* serology was positive, and lesion showed no uptake on thallium-201 SPECT scan. *B*, After 3 weeks of pyrimethamine-sulfadiazine treatment, the extent of edema, mass effect, and lesion size have clearly diminished. (Courtesy of Dr. David Warren, The New York Hospital–Cornell Medical Center.)

seen in 50% of patients by day 5 and in 86% by day 7; altogether, 91% showed clear evidence of a response by day 14 of treatment.[17,71] In the same study, 57% demonstrated neuroradiographic improvement at week 3.[71] Figure 30–5 illustrates such a response to empiric therapy. Therefore patients who demonstrate clinical progression or new signs during the first week of therapy and those who show no apparent improvement after 10 to 14 days of treatment should undergo brain biopsy.[71,105–107] Patients who fail to respond to 14 to 21 days of therapy most often have lymphoma, but as many as 25% of biopsied treatment nonresponders are still found to have toxoplasmosis as the cause of their CNS mass lesions.

Corticosteroids, which have no clearly positive or negative effect on either the kinetics or extent of the overall response,[2,11] are frequently used to help manage associated increased intracranial pressure. If corticosteroids are employed, some caution should still be exercised when interpreting clinical and radiologic responses because of nonspecific antiinflammatory effects.

Role of Brain Biopsy

For diagnosis of AIDS-associated CNS toxoplasmosis, brain biopsy has evolved over the years into a secondary procedure now reserved for only a limited number of clinical situations in carefully selected patients. In a decision analysis model of management strategies, similar outcomes for *Toxoplasma*-seropositive patients were assigned to early biopsy versus empiric therapy with delayed biopsy in nonresponders.[108] For *Toxoplasma*-seronegative patients with cerebral mass lesions, results from this model favored the use of early brain biopsy.[108]

Summary of Diagnosis and Initial Management

The algorithm in Figure 30–6 summarizes an overall approach to the patient with suspected cerebral toxoplasmosis.

▲ TREATMENT

Treatment for toxoplasmosis includes primary therapy for clinically active infection followed by maintenance therapy to suppress recurrent disease for patients whose CD4+ T-lymphocyte counts do not rise above 200 cells/mm^3. Recommendations for treatment, which almost always involve combination agents, and summaries of selected treatment trials are shown in Tables 30–1 through 30–4 in the following sections.

Primary Therapy

Conventional Treatment

Standard therapy for intracerebral toxoplasmosis consists of pyrimethamine plus sulfadiazine (Table 30–1).[108,115,116] For patients intolerant to sulfonamides, pyrimethamine plus clindamycin has been as effective in most[11–13,71] (but not all[115]) studies. Patients with pneumonitis, retinochoroiditis, other focal organ involvement, or disseminated infection

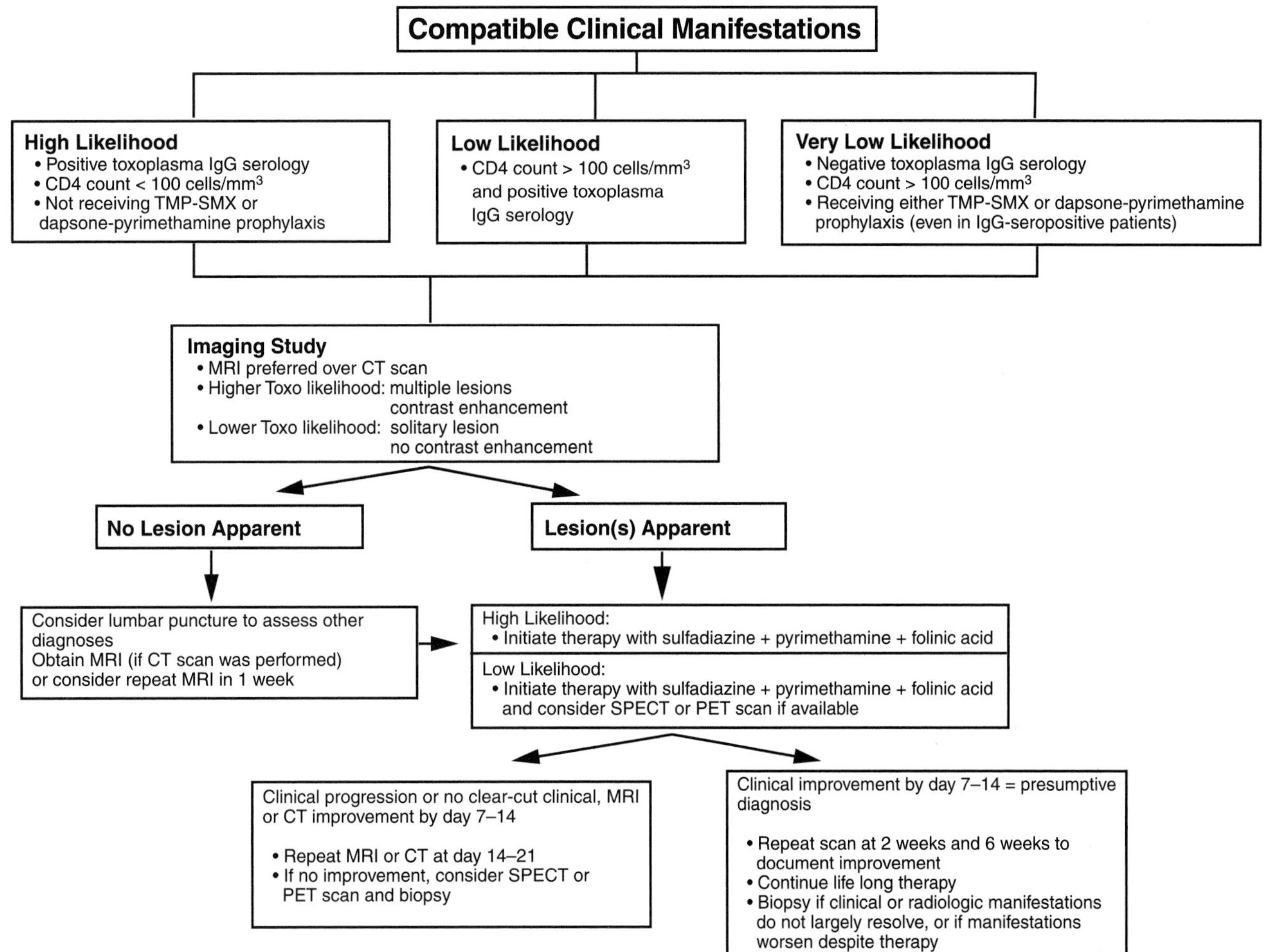

Figure 30–6. Algorithm indicating an approach to the diagnosis and initial management of suspected toxoplasmosis.

receive the same combination regimens. Folinic acid (leucovorin calcium) is routinely included with any pyrimethamine-containing regimen to reduce bone marrow toxicity.[18]

Initial responses to primary therapy are seen in 65% to 90% of patients with documented or presumed neurotoxoplasmosis who do not have far-advanced infection (Table 30–2).[2,11–13,71,108,115,116] Most patients with retinochoroiditis also respond and show improved visual acuity within 6 weeks.[52] Patients with pneumonitis or disseminated infection may not respond as well as those with encephalitis alone.[58,59] There are no firm guidelines for patients with *documented* toxoplasmosis at any anatomic site who fail to respond promptly or develop new signs of progression during treatment and who have no evidence of an additional pathogenic process. Therapeutic choices are largely limited to using higher doses of the drugs initially selected or empirically adding one or more additional anti-*Toxoplasma* agents to the regimen.

Initial treatment is given to responding patients for at least 4 to 6 weeks before considering a reduction in drug dosages and maintenance therapy. For patients with CNS infection, the imaging study originally employed (CT or MRI) should be repeated at the end of the first month of treatment[18,71] to provide additional confirmation that the extent of neurologic disease (mass effect, enhancement, lesion size and number) is receding. Although serial scans over subsequent months can demonstrate complete or near-complete resolution of an impressive amount of localized and multifocal disease (Fig. 30–7), repeated studies in a steadily improving patient who is receiving standard therapy are not required.

Rash and other adverse inflammatory-type reactions to sulfonamides are well recognized in HIV-infected patients. In addition, sulfadiazine-treated patients may develop crystalluria, hematuria, renal colic with sludge or stones, and occasionally some degree of renal insufficiency.[117,118] A high daily fluid intake should be part of the regimen in any patient receiving sulfadiazine. The most relevant toxicity of pyrimethamine is bone marrow suppression (megaloblastic anemia, leukopenia, thrombocytopenia). Overall, as many as 40% to 60% of patients cannot tolerate the combination of pyrimethamine plus sulfadiazine.[108] Clindamycin is well known for inducing gastrointestinal complaints and diarrhea, but it also produces rash.[12,119,120] Indeed, unacceptably high rates of diarrhea (31%) and rash (21%) developed in

Table 30–1. SELECTED PRIMARY PROPHYLAXIS TRIALS IN *T. GONDII*–SEROPOSITIVE PATIENTS AT DEFINITE RISK FOR REACTIVATED TOXOPLASMOSIS

Trial	Eligibility[a]	Design	No. of Patients[a]	Oral Regimen	Median Follow-up	TOXO[b] (%)	Toxicity (%)	Comments and Control
Carr[109]	Secondary prophylaxis for PCP	Retrospective	22	TMP-SMX 2 DS biwkly	290 d	0	5	12/36 (33%) Seropositive pentamidine-treated controls developed TOXO
Girard[110]	CDC stage IV, <200 CD4 cells	Randomized, open label	135	Dapsone 50 mg qd plus pyrimethamine 50 mg q plus folinic acid 25 mg q wk	539 d	4	24	28/127 (22%) Seropositive pentamidine-treated controls developed TOXO
Jacobson[111c]	Seropositive, <200 CD4 or prior OI	Double blind, randomized, placebo-controlled	264	Pyrimethamine 25 mg tiw; no folinic acid	254 d	5	27	4% Seropositive placebo-treated controls developed TOXO; 21% had toxicity. PCP prophylaxis also allowed: TMP-SMX (in 54%) and dapsone-pyrimethamine (in 12%). Increased death rate with pyrimethamine (29% vs. 16%)
Opravil[112]	Advanced HIV or prior OI; median CD4 105–116	Randomized, open label	120	Dapsone 200 mg q wk plus pyrimethamine 75 mg q wk; folinic acid not given routinely	543 d	3	30	Subgroup analysis vs. 120 seropositive pentamidine-treated controls of whom 12% developed TOXO
Podzamcer[113]	<200 CD4	Randomized, open label	131	TMP-SMX 2 DS tiw vs. dapsone 100 mg biwkly plus pyrimethamine 50 mg biwkly; no folinic acid	430 d 430 d	2 3	10 9	Groups included 65 and 66 patients. Similar efficacy and toxicity
Leport[114c]	Seropositive, <200 CD4	Double blind, randomized, placebo-controlled	274	Pyrimethamine 50 mg tiw plus folinic acid 15 mg tiw	12 mo[d]	4	20	Placebo controls (m = 280): 12% developed TOXO; 7% had toxicity

CDC, Centers for Disease Control and Prevention; DS, double strength; OI, opportunistic infection; PCP, *Pneumocystis carinii* pneumonia; tiw, three times a week; TMP-SMX, trimethoprim-sulfamethoxazole; TOXO, toxoplasmosis:

[a]Number of patients who were seropositive at study entry (and therefore at high risk for reactivated toxoplasmosis); does not necessarily indicate the total number of patients entered.

[b]Patients who developed toxoplasmosis using "on-treatment" rather than intention-to-treat analysis. In some trials, intention-to-treat analysis did not show benefit from prophylaxis primarily because of drug adverse reactions that resulted in crossover to the other arm or discontinuation of treatment.

[c]In this trial, seropositivity to *T. gondii* was a required entry criterion.

[d]Mean follow-up period.

[a]CD4 cells/mm^3

Table 30–2. SELECTED TREATMENT TRIALS IN AIDS-RELATED TOXOPLASMOSIS[a]

Trial	Design	No. of Patients	Regimen	Complete/Partial Response by day 42 (%)	Toxicity (%)	Comments
Leport[114]	Open label	35	Pyrimethamine 100–200 mg PO × 1–2, then 50–100 mg PO qd plus sulfadiazine 2–6 g PO qd plus folinic acid 5–50 mg IM qd	89[b]	71	18/24 Responders maintained relapse-free on reduced doses; 10/35 stopped at least one drug (toxicity)
Danneman[12]	Randomized, open label	59	Pyrimethamine 200 mg PO × 1, then 75 mg PO qd plus sulfadiazine 25 mg/kg q6h plus folinic acid ≥ 10 mg PO qd	70	32	Similar efficacy and toxicity in both arms
			Pyrimethamine as above plus clindamycin 1200 mg IV q6h × 21 d, then 300 mg PO q6h or 800 mg PO q8h plus folinic acid as above	65	23	
Luft[71]	Open label	49	Pyrimethamine 200 mg PO × 1, then 75 mg PO qd plus clindamycin 600 mg PO q6h plus folinic acid 10 mg PO qd	75	17	86% Responders improved by day 7 of therapy.
Katlama et al.[115]	Randomized, open label	299	Pyrimethamine 50 mg PO qd × 42 d, then 25 mg PO qd plus sulfadiazine 1 g PO q6h × 42 d, then 0.5 g PO q6h plus folinic acid > 50 mg PO q wk	76	30	Initial efficacy similar. Relapse during maintenance phase was 2× higher for clindamycin arm, although less toxicity and fewer drug discontinuations
			Pyrimethamine as above plus clindamycin 600 mg PO q6h × 42 d, then 300 mg PO q6h plus folinic acid as above	68	11	

[a]Eligibility for each of these trials included clinical, neurologic, and CT or MRI resutls consistent with toxoplasmosis.
[b]Responses within first 8 weeks of therapy.

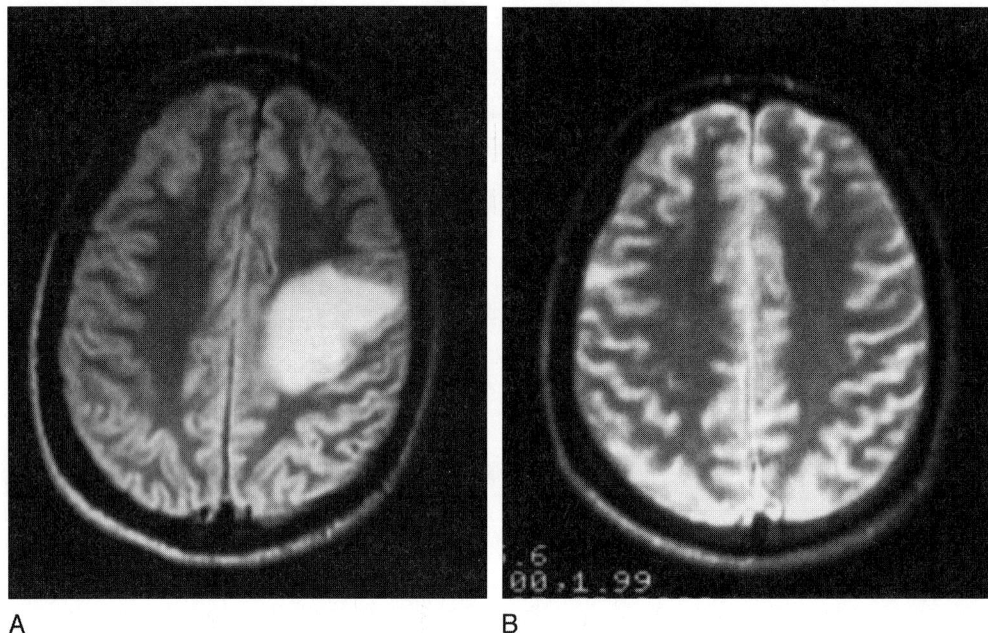

Figure 30–7. Neuroradiographic (MRI) response to treatment with pyrimethamine plus clindamycin in an AIDS patient with biopsy-documented intracerebral toxoplasmosis. *A*, Pretreatment scan. *B*, Essentially normal MRI after 11 weeks of combination therapy. (*A*: From Murray HW. Immunotherapy for AIDS-associated toxoplasmosis. In: Sande MA, Root RK [eds]. Contemporary Issues in Infectious Diseases, vol 9: Treatment of Serious Infections in the 1990s. New York, Churchill Livingstone, 1992, p 205.)

patients who received clindamycin alone (300 mg twice daily) in a trial of primary prophylaxis.[119] Other adverse reactions and potential drug interactions in patients receiving sulfonamides, pyrimethamine, clindamycin, dapsone, or one of the alternative agents discussed here are detailed in Chapter 66.

Other Regimens

Atovaquone

Hydroxynaphthoquinones are potent in vitro inhibitors of parasitic protozoa including *Plasmodium* and *T. gondii.* Atovaquone has been demonstrated to have good protective activity against acute murine toxoplasmosis and to reduce the viability and number of cysts in brains of chronically infected mice.[121] Atovaquone acts as an inhibitor of the mitochondrial electron transport chain of parasitic protozoa, resulting in inhibition of pyrimidine synthesis.

Several properties of atovaquone had appeared attractive particularly in patients with advanced HIV infection: a mechanism of action unrelated to folate antagonism, activity against the two most frequent opportunistic agents (*Pneumocytis carinii* and *T. gondii*), and a prolonged half-life (4 to 6 days) with a potential dosing advantage for long-term prophylaxis. There have been surprisingly few published data to evaluate atovaquone.[122–124] In a pilot study of atovaquone (750 mg four times per day) as first-line therapy for acute *Toxoplasma* encephalitis (TE) in 24 patients, 7 patients failed to respond to pyrimethamine/sulfadiazine combination.[122] A wide range of plasma drug concentration was observed. The main side effects were a slight increase in liver enzymes in 13 patients, cutaneous rash in 6, gastrointestinal disturbances in 3. Only one patient had to stop therapy (because of liver toxicity).[122]

Atovaquone has been evaluated as salvage therapy in 93 patients with AIDS-related TE who were intolerant to or failing standard therapy with either pyrimethamine-sulfodiazine or pyrimethamine-clindamycin.[124] At the end of the 6-week acute therapy phase (750 mg four times per day), clinical improvement was noted in 52% of patients and radiologic improvement in 37%. The median survival for all patients was 189 days (Kaplan-Meier estimate). A posthoc analysis revealed a correlation between clinical and radiologic responses and median atovaquone plasma concentrations.

Although these studies have confirmed the efficacy of atovaquone for acute TE therapy, there have been insufficient data to recommend atovaquone as first-line treatment for TE owing to the uncertainty of the clinical response. Therefore currently atovaquone (750 mg four times per day) should be considered as salvage therapy for TE only in patients intolerant to standard regimens with pyrimethamine combined with sulfadiazine or clindamycin. Trimetrexate has been used successfully to treat a few patients with cerebral toxoplasmosis.

Macrolides

Clarithromycin has shown activity against *T. gondii* in vitro and in murine models. In a pilot study, clarithromycin (2 g/day) combined with pyrimethamine (75 mg/day) was given to 13 AIDS patients with TE.[125] A complete clinical response was noted in six of eight evaluable patients and a partial response in two. Five patients were withdrawn prematurely, mainly because of toxicity. Whether clarithromycin itself had a beneficial effect is questionable, as it was used in combination with higher doses of pyrimethamine than were normally used in combination with sulfadiazine or clindamycin. No further studies have evaluated prospectively the role of clarithromycin in *T. gondii* infection.

Azithromycin has been reported to be active in vitro and in animal models. In a murine model of toxoplasmosis, prophylactic azithromycin administered alone at a high dosage was found to be only partially effective.[126] Complete protection was not seen even at a dosage of 300 mg/kg/day. In contrast, the combination of azithromycin with either sulfadiazine or pyrimethamine was synergistic; 100% and 93% survival of mice, respectively, after 30 days was observed. These findings are consistent with preliminary data in humans.[127,128] Adverse events have been observed (leading to discontinuation of therapy in 50% of cases) and consisted mainly of fever, rash, and increased liver enzymes.[128] In the absence of robust controlled studies comparing combination therapy with macrolides with standard therapy, macrolides should be used only in patients who do not respond, or are intolerant, to conventional therapy with sulfadiazine-pyrimethamine, clindamycin-pyrimethamine, or atovaquone-pyrimethamine.

Other Drugs

Sulfamethoxazole-trimethoprim,[129,130] doxycycline,[131] sulfadoxine-pyrimethamine,[132] and trimetrexate have been used with success in some patients.[129–131, 133]

Corticosteroids and Antiseizure Drugs

Glucocorticoids are recommended for patients with symptoms of raised intracranial pressure or moderately severe intracranial hypertension with displacement of median brain structures, although data supporting their use in this context are virtually nonexistent. Many neurologists recommend Decadron 4 mg IV q6h, although other regimens may be used.

Patients with seizures at presentation should be given anticonvulsant therapy during the acute phase of anti-*Toxoplasma* therapy. Phenobarbital, phenytoin sodium, or diphenylhydantoin are not recommended because of potential drug interactions. Sodium valproate is preferred.

Maintenance (Suppressive) Therapy

Relapse rates are as high as 80% in CD4 cell-deficient patients with treated intracerebral toxoplasmosis who are not given secondary prophylaxis.[7] Thus prior to the era of highly active retroviral therapy (HAART), there was no debate about the requirement for lifelong suppressive treatment once primary therapy had satisfactorily induced remission. A number of agents have been used alone or in combination with varying degrees of success as secondary prophylaxis (Table 30–3).[13,18,120–140] Breakthrough relapses rates of 10% to 40% have occurred for each maintenance regimen despite different treatment protocols, including pyrimethamine plus sulfadiazine.[13,135] In patients with treatment-responsive ocular involvement, for example, 20% may develop recurrent retinochoroiditis (relapse) within 24 months despite continuing on pyrimethamine plus either sulfadiazine or clindamycin.[52,115] Failure of secondary (and primary) prophylaxis may result from noncompliance, drug intolerance, poor gastrointestinal absorption, or lack of efficacy due to a poor host immune response, lack of drug potency, or conceivably drug resistance.

Table 30–3. MAINTENANCE REGIMENS (SECONDARY PROPHYLAXIS) FOR AIDS-RELATED TOXOPLASMOSIS

Oral Drug	Suggested Regimens
Preferred combinations[a]	
Daily treatment	
Pyrimethamine *plus*	25–75 mg qd
Sulfadiazine *or*	500–1000 mg q6h or 1 g q12h
Clindamycin	300–600 q6h or 450 mg q8h
Intermittent treatment	
Pyrimethamine *plus*	50 mg thrice weekly
Sulfadiazine	1 g q12h thrice weekly
Other regimens[a]	
Atovaquone alone	750 mg q6h
Pyrimethamine *plus*	25 mg qd
Atovaquone *or*	750 mg q6h
Clarithromycin *or*	1000 mg qd
Dapsone *or*	100 mg twice weekly
Azithromycin	600–1800 mg qd
Pyrimethamine-sulfadoxine (Fansidar)	25 mg/500 mg (1 tablet) twice weekly

[a]Folinic acid (10–25 mg/day) should be used with all pyrimethamine-containing regimens.

The most straightforward approach to maintenance therapy is to continue the agents to which the patient with active toxoplasmosis has already responded and shown tolerance. For pyrimethamine plus sulfadiazine, decreasing the doses of each drug is the typical practice to reduce drug toxicity while preventing reactivation. Abundant clinical experience supports high-level suppressive efficacy in patients able to continue receiving this particular combination indefinitely.[11,18] Treatment with pyrimethamine plus sulfadiazine and leucovorin should probably be given daily. However, thrice-weekly administration also appears effective.[139] In patients who respond to pyrimethamine plus clindamycin as primary therapy, reducing the dose of pyrimethamine to 25 mg/day but keeping clindamycin at full doses is a standard approach.[18]

The ENTA study compared maintenance therapy comprised of pyrimethamine 25 mg daily with either sulfadiazine 2 g daily or oral clindamycin 1.2 g daily in 175 patients, with a mean follow-up of 13 months.[115] The pyrimethamine-sulfadiazine combination appeared to be significantly more effective than the pyrimethamine-clindamycin combination, with relapse rates of 7% and 28%, respectively. The toxicity of these two combinations was lower than with acute therapy: 28% in the pyrimethamine/sulfadiazine-treated patients and 20% in the pyrimethamine/clindamycin-treated patients. Rash and fever were more frequent (12%) among pyrimethamine/sulfadiazine-treated patients, and diarrhea was more frequent

▲ **Table 30–4.** DISCONTINUATION OF MAINTENANCE ANTI-*TOXOPLASMA* THERAPY IN PATIENTS WHO COMPLETED AN INITIAL COURSE OF THERAPY AND HAD A CD4+ T-LYMPHOCYTE INCREASE DUE TO HAART

Study	No.	Relapses	Patient-years
Denmark[148]	8	0	11
Madrid[146]	9	0	18
GESIDA[143]	27	0	12
France[149]	19	0	—

HAART, highly active antiretroviral therapy.

(14%) in those receiving pyrimethamine/clindamycin. It is of interest that hematologic toxicity with either combination was uncommon (<5%).

Table 30–3 also lists other regimens (including atovaquone with or without pyrimethamine) that decrease (but certainly do not prevent all) recurrences. Among these secondary prophylactic regimens is a particularly convenient one if patients are sulfa-tolerant: a single tablet of Fansidar (pyrimethamine 25 mg plus sulfadoxine 500 mg) twice weekly. Although associated with frequent (41%) but mild to moderate allergic reactions, twice-weekly Fansidar maintained 90% of patients relapse-free at 12 months and 80% at 24 months; the probability of remaining free of *Pneumocystis carinii* pneumonia (PCP) was also about 90% at 24 months.[134] Patients maintained on pyrimethamine-sulfadiazine or dapsone (but not pyrimethamine-clindamycin) also appear to be protected against PCP.[18,140]

Discontinuation of Maintenance Therapy

If a patient's CD4+ T-lymphocyte count has risen to more than 200 cells/mm^3 for 3 months or more as a result of HAART, the patient has completed an entire course of therapy, and the patient is asymptomatic with regard to toxoplasmosis, it appears safe to discontinue maintenance therapy so long as the CD4+ T-lymphocyte count remains over 200 cells/mm^3 (Table 30–4).[140–148,148a] Some experts perform a CT scan or MRI scan to provide additional information supporting the safety of discontinuing secondary prophylaxis for toxoplasmosis. U.S. Public Health Service–Infectious Disease Society of America guidelines were revised in 2001 to endorse discontinuation of maintenance therapy for toxoplasmosis (Tables 30–4 and 30–5).[140] Although data about toxoplasmosis have not been extensive, available data are consistent with experience regarding pneumocystosis, CMV disease, *Mycobacterium avium* complex disease, and cryptococcosis.

▲ PRIMARY PREVENTION

Primary Prevention

It is standard practice to provide primary prophylaxis to all *Toxoplasma*-seropositive patients who are immunodeficient (Tables 30–4 and 30–5).[18,21,140,146] A CD4 cell count of less than 100 cells/mm^3 is widely accepted as the latest time at which prophylaxis should be initiated.[140] At this stage, 25% to 40% of untreated patients develop intracerebral disease within a 1- or 2-year period.[18,146,147] In contrast, the 12-month incidence of cerebral toxoplasmosis in seropositive patients with less than 100 CD4 cells/mm^3 was reduced from 34% to 8% if one of the following agents was used: TMP-SMX, dapsone, pyrimethamine, pyrimethamine-sulfadoxine (Fansidar), or sulfadiazine.[146]

Numerous studies of primary prophylaxis had been carried out by 1995,[21] each with certain limitations and varying degrees of completeness and success, using one of three regimens: TMP-SMX, dapsone-pyrimethamine, or pyrimethamine alone. In addition to variable drug dosages and administration schedules (ranging from daily to once-weekly), data interpretation has also been difficult because of disparate results generated by patient intolerance to the assigned drug and the use of intention-to-treat versus on-therapy analyses.[21] Additional trials have also been reported (Tables 30–3 and 30–4). Neither spiramycin nor clarithromycin alone is active as a primary prophylactic agent,[11,18] and current data also do not support the routine use of monotherapy with dapsone, pyrimethamine, or azithromycin.[109–114,150–155]

The doses and administration schedules of TMP-SMX and pyrimethamine-dapsone that are recommended for PCP prophylaxis appear adequate for prevention of toxoplasmosis (Tables 30–3 and 30–4).[21] Aerosolized pentamidine does

▲ **Table 30–5.** DISCONTINUATION OF PRIMARY ANTI-*TOXOPLASMA* PROPHYLAXIS IN PATIENTS SEROPOSITIVE FOR *TOXOPLASMA* AND WITH CD4 > 200 CELLS μl

Study	No.	Mean Follow-up (months)	Patient-years	Incidence/100 Patient-years (95% CI)
Swiss[142]				
Stop	199	17.0	272	0 (0–1.1)
Continue	121	11.0	110	0 (0–4.2)
CIOP[141]				
Stop	115	7.2	72	0 (0–7.3)
Continue	128	6.0	72	0 (0–7.3)
GESIDA[143]				
Stop	155	9.6	—	0
Continue	147	9.6	—	0
EUROSIDA[144]	319	5.0	247	0 (0–23)
HOPS[145]	146	18.2	402	0
Paris[147]	34	16.0	—	0

not protect against toxoplasmosis.[113,151] The optimal prophylactic regimen to prevent reactivation, using either TMP-SMX or dapsone-pyrimethamine, has not been fully defined regarding either drug doses or daily versus intermittent administration.

Although TMP-SMX and dapsone-pyrimethamine are quite active as primary prophylaxis in *Toxoplasma*-seropositive patients with less than 100 CD4 cells/mm^3,[132] failures do occur. Atovaquone, with or without pyrimethamine, is thought to be a reasonable regimen in patients intolerant to the preferred treatments (Table 30–6).[132]

Discontinuing Primary Prophylaxis

In *Toxoplasma*-seropositive patients who respond to HAART with sustained increases (>3 months) in CD4 cell counts to more than 200 cells/mm^3, experience in more than 500 patients indicates that primary prophylaxis can be safely discontinued (Table 30–5).[140–145] Susceptibility is best determined by the current CD4+ T-lymphocyte count. Following a CD4+ T-lymphocyte rise due to HAART, the absolute CD4+ T-lymphocyte count (or the percent of lymphocytes that are CD4+) is substantially more important than the prior nadir CD4+ T-lymphocyte count or the viral load. Although an occasional case of toxoplasmosis occurs at CD4+ T-lymphocyte counts of more than 100 cells/μl, such cases are unusual. If CD4+ T-lymphocyte counts subsequently decline to levels below 200 cells/mm^3, prophylaxis should be reinstituted.

Pregnant Women and Children

Case reports demonstrate that *Toxoplasma*-seropositive pregnant women with an apparently quiescent infection, once they develop advanced HIV disease, can transmit infection to the fetus.[27,28] Detailed studies, however, indicate that this occurrence is unusual in pregnant women who are

Table 30–6. PRIMARY PROPHYLAXIS TO PREVENT FIRST EPISODE OF AIDS-RELATED TOXOPLASMOSIS

Oral Drug[a]	Suggested Regimens
Preferred treatment	
TMP-SMX[b]	1 DS tablet qd. Alternatives: 1 SS tablet qd, 1 DS tablet q12h tiw, or 1 DS tablet tiw
Pyrimethamine-dapsone	50 mg q wk/50 mg qd. Alternatives: 25 mg + 100 mg qd biw, or 75 mg + 200 mg q wk
Other treatments	
Pyrimethamine-sulfadoxine (Fansidar)	25 mg/500 mg (1 tablet) biw or 3 tablets once q 2 wk
Atovaquone	1500 mg qd
Atovaquone-pyrimethamine	1500 mg qd/25 mg qd

biw, twice-weekly; q wk, once weekly; q 2 wk, every 2 weeks; tiw, three times per week.

[a]Folinic acid (10–25 mg/d) should be given with any pyrimethamine-containing regimen.

[b]DS, double-strength tablet (160 mg TMP + 800 mg SMX); SS, single-strength tablet (80 mg TMP + 400 mg SMZ).

at an early stage of their HIV disease.[29,30] Nevertheless, if clinically warranted, pediatricians should consider congenital toxoplasmosis in infants born to any HIV-infected woman with serologic evidence of prior exposure to *T. gondii*. Such consideration would be even stronger, of course, if during pregnancy the mother showed evidence of recently acquired or clinically active toxoplasmosis.

Because TMP-SMX is thought by most experts to be reasonably safe during pregnancy, *Toxoplasma*-seropositive pregnant women with less than 100 CD4 cells/mm^3 should also receive primary prophylaxis to prevent reactivation. One recent study of 195 mother-infant pairs suggested that the combination of antiretroviral agents plus folate antagonists was associated with a higher risk of congenital abnormalities.[140a] Other data bases need to be queried to determine if these results can be substantiated. Because of concern over teratogenic effects of pyrimethamine, options during the first trimester for women unable to tolerate TMP-SMX include no prophylaxis or perhaps dapsone alone (not thought by some experts to be teratogenic). After the first trimester, pyrimethamine (plus dapsone) is believed to be safe, but possible risks to the fetus have led some experts to suggest deferring all prophylaxis in TMP-SMX-intolerant women until after delivery.[140] It is presumed but as yet unproven that continuing primary prophylaxis during pregnancy not only protects the mother but reduces fetal transmission.

Pregnant women with active toxoplasmosis (e.g., encephalitis) and those who become pregnant while undergoing standard maintenance therapy (secondary prophylaxis) pose a therapeutic problem that fortunately is not frequent. The dilemma is whether to use the most effective regimen for the mother, which would include pyrimethamine (posing a risk to the fetus), or opt during the first trimester for an alternative regimen without pyrimethamine (Tables 30–1, 30–3 and 30–4). Appropriate consultation with specialists should be sought in these unusual situations.

Toxoplasmosis is not a common opportunistic infection in HIV-infected children. Nevertheless, children who are older than 1 year of age, who qualify for prophylaxis for PCP, and who are at risk (*Toxoplasma*-seropositive) are candidates for primary anti-*Toxoplasma* prophylaxis.[140] In practice, such children would likely already be receiving TMP-SMX for PCP prophylaxis and, in contrast to HIV-infected adults, usually tolerate this treatment well. Alternatives to TMP-SMX include dapsone-pyrimethamine-leucovorin or atovaquone alone.[140] Primary prophylaxis for younger children who may be immunodeficient despite high absolute CD4+ T-lymphocyte counts can also be considered if *Toxoplasma* serology is positive.

Other Preventive Measures

All HIV-infected persons should be tested for IgG antibody to *T. gondii*. Those found to be seronegative should be retested for anti-*Toxoplasma* IgG if and when the CD4+ T-lymphocyte count declines to 100/mm^3 to determine if interval infection has been acquired and primary prophylaxis is warranted.

Irrespective of the CD4+ T-lymphocyte count, seronegative individuals should also undertake measures to reduce future oral exposure to *T. gondii*.[156–159] All undercooked meat should be avoided, especially pork and lamb. Previously frozen meats (to −20°C for 24 hours) are considered safe because tissue cysts are killed by freezing. Fruits and vegetables (potentially contaminated with oocysts from outdoor cats or other felines) should be carefully washed before being eaten uncooked. Hand washing is necessary after contact with fresh raw meat, after gardening, or after contact with soil where oocysts might have been deposited. Kitchen surfaces should also be washed after contact with raw meat. Toxoplasmosis has rarely been acquired via drinking apparently contaminated (unfiltered) water in both rural and urban settings.[156,157] Although there is no recommendation to boil filtered water to prevent transmission of *Toxoplasma*, it would be prudent to take such precautions if, for example, one must drink stream water to which felines have access.

Cat ownership per se does not appear to increase the risk of infection in HIV-positive persons,[158,159] so cat owners need not give up their pets. However, they should keep their current pets indoors to reduce the likelihood of the cat acquiring new infection, and cats should be fed processed or cooked foods for the same reason. Personal contact with stray cats or new cat adoption should also be avoided lest these animals (especially kittens) be recently infected and actively shedding oocysts. Ideally, litter boxes should be changed daily by an HIV-negative person to prevent any excreted oocysts from having time to sporulate. Alternatively, disposable gloves followed by hand washing can be used by whoever carefully empties the litter box; some have also recommended disinfecting the litter box with boiling water after each litter change.[18,21] Because only recently infected cats excrete oocysts and usually for a limited period (less than 14 days), most long-term indoor cats do not pose a hazard to their HIV-infected owners; therefore there is no reason to test a cat's stool or serum for evidence of *T. gondii* infection. However, cats are occasionally reinfected and resume self-limited oocyst shedding—hence the importance of the preceding recommendations for all cats living in the household of an HIV-infected person.

REFERENCES

1. Kasper LH. Toxoplasma infection. In: Harrison's Textbook of Medicine. New York, McGraw-Hill, 1998, pp 1197–1202.
2. Montoya JG, Remington JS. Toxoplasma gondii. In: Mandell GL, Bennett JE, Dolin R (eds) Principles and Practice of Infectious Diseases, 5th ed, Philadelphia, Churchill Livingstone, 2000, p 2858.
3. Ruskin J, Remington JS. Toxoplasmosis in the compromised host. Ann Intern Med 84:193, 1976.
4. Hunter CA, Remington JS. Immunopathogenesis of toxoplasmic encephalitis. J Infect Dis 170:1057, 1994.
5. Murray HW, Rubin BY, Masur H, et al. Impaired production of lymphokines and immune (gamma) interferon in the acquired immunodeficiency syndrome. N Engl J Med 310:883, 1984.
6. Navia BA, Petito CK, Gold JWM, et al. Cerebral toxoplasmosis complicating the acquired immune deficiency syndrome: clinical and neuropathological findings in 27 patients. Ann Neurol 19:224, 1986.
7. Luft BJ, Remington JS. Toxoplasmic encephalitis. J Infect Dis 157:1, 1988.
8. Carrazana EJ, Rossitch E, Samuels MA. Cerebral toxoplasmosis in the acquired immune deficiency syndrome. Clin Neurol Neurosurg 91:291, 1989.
9. Luft BJ, Hafner R. Toxoplasmic encephalitis. AIDS 4:593, 1990.
10. Strittmatter C, Lang W, Wiestler OD, et al. The changing pattern of human immunodeficiency virus-associated cerebral toxoplasmosis: a study of 46 postmortem cases. Acta Neuropathol (Berl) 83:475, 1992.
11. Luft BJ, Remington JS. Toxoplasmic encephalitis in AIDS. Clin Infect Dis 15:211, 1992.
12. Dannemann B, McCutchan JA, Israelski D, et al. Treatment of toxoplasmic encephalitis in patients with AIDS: a randomized trial comparing pyrimethamine plus clindamycin to pyrimethamine plus sulfadiazine. Ann Intern Med 116:33, 1992.
13. Renold C, Sugar A, Chave J-P, et al. Toxoplasma encephalitis in patients with the acquired immunodeficiency syndrome. Medicine 71:224, 1992.
14. Decker CF, Tuazon CU. Toxoplasmosis: an update on clinical and therapeutic aspects. Prog Clin Parasitol 3:21, 1993.
15. Mariuz P, Bosler EM, Luft BJ. Toxoplasmosis in individuals with AIDS. Infect Dis Clin North Am 8:365, 1994.
16. New LC, Holliman RE. Toxoplasmosis and human immunodeficiency virus (HIV) disease. J Antimicrob Chemother 33:1079, 1994.
17. Wong SY, Remington JS. Toxoplasmosis in the setting of AIDS. In: Broder S, Merigan TC, Bolognesi D (eds) Textbook of AIDS Medicine. Baltimore, Williams & Wilkins, 1994, p 223.
18. Wong SY, Israeliski DM, Remington JS. AIDS-associated toxoplasmosis. In: Sande MA, Volberding PA (eds) The Medical Management of AIDS, 4th ed. Philadelphia, WB Saunders, 1995, p 460.
19. Cohen BA. Neurologic manifestations of toxoplasmosis in AIDS. Semin Neurol 19:201, 1999.
20. Luft BJ, Chua A. Central nervous system toxoplasmosis in HIV pathogenesis, diagnosis, and therapy. Curr Infect Dis Rep 2:358, 2000.
21. Richards FO, Kovacs JA, Luft BJ. Preventing toxoplasmic encephalitis in persons infected with human immunodeficiency virus. Clin Infect Dis 21(suppl 1):S49, 1995.
22. Murray HW. Immunotherapy for AIDS-associated toxoplasmosis. In: Sande MA, Root RK (eds) Contemporary Issues in Infectious Diseases, vol 9: Treatment of Serious Infections in the 1990s. New York, Churchill Livingstone, 1992, p 205.
23. Murray HW. Survival of intracellular pathogens within human mononuclear phagocytes. Semin Hematol 25:101, 1988.
24. Israelski DM, Chmiel JS, Poggensee L, et al. Prevalence of Toxoplasma infection in a cohort of men at risk of AIDS and toxoplasmic encephalitis. J Acquir Immun Defic Syndr 6:414, 1993.
25. Hell KJ, Church JA, Ross L. Toxoplasma gondii seroprevalence in HIV-infected children. In: Abstracts of the 4th Conference on Retroviruses and Opportunistic Infections, Washington, DC, January 1996, abstract 344.
26. Hohfeld P, Daffos F, Costa J-M, et al. Prenatal diagnosis of congenital toxoplasmosis with a polymerase chain reaction test on amniotic fluid. N Engl J Med 331:695, 1994.
27. Mitchell CD, Erlich SS, Mastrucci MT, et al. Congenital toxoplasmosis occurring in infants perinatally infected with human immunodeficiency virus-1. Pediatr Infect Dis J 9:512, 1990.
28. Marty P, Bongain A, Rahal A, Prenatal diagnosis of severe fetal toxoplasmosis as a result of toxoplasmic reactivation in an HIV-positive woman. Prenat Diagn 14:414, 1994.
29. Anonymous. Low incidence of congenital toxoplasmosis in children born to women infected with human immunodeficiency virus: European Collaborative Study and Research Network on Congenital Toxoplasmosis. Eur J Obstet Gynecol Reprod Biol 68:93, 1996.
30. Lefevre-Elbert V, Ciraru-Vigneron N, Garin JF, et al. Toxoplasmosis serological reactivation and parasitemia in a cohort of HIV positive pregnant women. In: Abstracts of the XIth International Conference on AIDS, Vancouver, July 7–12, 1996, abstract We.B.3228.
31. Yap G, Pesin M, Sher A. Cutting edge: IL-12 is required for the maintenance of IFN-gamma production in T cells mediating chronic resistance to the intracellular pathogen, Toxoplasma gondii. J Immunol 165:628, 2000.
32. Murray HW, Gellene RA, Libby DM, et al. Activation of tissue macrophages from AIDS patients: in vitro responses of AIDS alveolar macrophages to lymphokines and gamma interferon. J Immunol 135:2374, 1985.
33. Murray HW, Rubin BY, Carriero SM, et al. Human mononuclear phagocyte antiprotozoal mechanisms: oxygen-dependent vs. oxygen-independent activity against intracellular Toxoplasma gondii. J Immunol 134:1982, 1985.

34. Stellbrink HJ, Fuhrer-Burow R, Raedler A, et al. Risk factors for severe disease due to Toxoplasma gondii in HIV-positive patients. Eur J Epidemiol 9:633, 1993.
35. Oksenhendler E, Charreau I, Tournerie C, et al. Toxoplasma gondii infection in advanced HIV infection. AIDS 8:483, 1994.
36. Laing RB, Flegg PJ, Brettle RP, et al. Clinical features, outcome and survival from cerebral toxoplasmosis in Edinburgh AIDS patients. Int J STD AIDS 7:258, 1996.
37. Falangola MF, Reichler BS, Petito CK. Histopathology of cerebral toxoplasmosis in human immunodeficiency virus infection: a comparison between patients with early-onset and late-onset acquired immunodeficiency syndrome. Hum Pathol 25:1091, 1994.
38. Rabaud C, May T, Amiel C, et al. Extracerebral toxoplasmosis in patients infected with HIV: a French national survey. Medicine 73:306, 1994.
39. Hofman P, Bernard E, Michiels JF, et al. Extracerebral toxoplasmosis in the acquired immunodeficiency syndrome (AIDS). Pathol Res Pract 189:894, 1993.
40. Jautzke G, Sell M, Thalmann U, et al. Extracerebral toxoplasmosis in AIDS: histological and immunohistological findings based upon 80 autopsy cases. Pathol Res Pract 189:428, 1993.
41. Albrecht H, Skorde J, Arasteh K, et al. Disseminated toxoplasmosis in AIDS patients: report of 16 cases. Scand J Infect Dis 27:71, 1995.
42. Gandhi S, Lyubsky S, Jimenez-Lucho V. Adult respiratory distress syndrome associated with disseminated toxoplasmosis. Clin Infect Dis 19:169, 1994.
43. Lucet JC, Bailly MP, Bedos JP, et al. Septic shock due to toxoplasmosis in patients infected with the human immunodeficiency virus. Chest 104:1054, 1993.
44. Vyas R, Ebright JR. Toxoplasmosis of the spinal cord in a patient with AIDS: case report and review. Clin Infect Dis 23:1061, 1996.
45. Berlit P, Popescu O, Wend Y, et al. Disseminated cerebral hemorrhages as unusual manifestation of toxoplasmic encephalitis in AIDS. J Neurol Sci 143:187, 1996.
46. Falangola MF, Petito CK. Choroid plexus infection in cerebral toxoplasmosis in AIDS patients. Neurology 43:2035, 1993.
47. Weiss A, Margo CE, Ledford DK, et al. Toxoplasmic retinochoroiditis as an initial manifestation of the acquired immune deficiency syndrome. Am J Ophthalmol 101:248, 1986.
48. Friedman D. Neuro-ophthalmic manifestations of human immunodeficiency virus infection. Neurol Clin 9:55, 1991.
49. Gagliuso DJ, Teich SA, Friedman AH, et al. Ocular toxoplasmosis in AIDS patients. Trans Am Ophthalmol Soc 88:63, 1990.
50. Holland GN, Engstrom RE, Glasgow BJ, et al. Ocular toxoplasmosis in patients with the acquired immunodeficiency syndrome. Am J Ophthalmol 106:653, 1988.
51. Pivetti-Pezzi P, Accorinti M, Tamburi S, et al. Clinical features of toxoplasmic retinochoroiditis in patients with the acquired immunodeficiency syndrome. Ann Ophthalmol 26:73, 1994.
52. Cochereau-Massin I, LeHoang P, Lautier-Frau M, et al. Ocular toxoplasmosis in human immunodeficiency virus-infected patients. Am J Ophthalmol 114:130, 1992.
53. Oksenhendler E, Cadranel J, Sarfati C, et al. Toxoplasma gondii pneumonia in patients with the acquired immunodeficiency syndrome. Am J Med 88:18, 1990.
54. Schnapp L, Geaghan S, Campagna A, et al. Toxoplasma gondii pneumonitis in patients infected with the human immunodeficiency virus. Arch Intern Med 152:1073, 1992.
55. Rabaud C, May T, Lucet JC, et al. Pulmonary toxoplasmosis in patients infected with the human immunodeficiency virus: a French national survey. Clin Infect Dis 23:1249, 1996.
56. Bonilla CA, Rosa UW. Toxoplasma gondii pneumonia in patients with the acquired immunodeficiency syndrome: diagnosis by bronchoalveolar lavage. South Med J 87:659, 1994.
57. Nash G, Kerschmann RL, Nerndier B, et al. The pathological manifestations of pulmonary toxoplasmosis in the acquired immunodeficiency syndrome. Hum Pathol 25:652, 1994.
58. May T, Rabaud C, Katlama C, et al. Toxoplasmose extracerebrale au cours du SIDA: resultats d'une enquete nationale. Med Mal Infect 23:190, 1993.
59. Pomeroy C, Filice GA. Pulmonary toxoplasmosis: a review. Clin Infect Dis 14:863, 1992.
60. Pugin J, Vanhems P, Hirschel B, et al. Extreme elevations of serum lactic dehydrogenase differentiating pulmonary toxoplasmosis from Pneumocystis pneumoniae. N Engl J Med 327:1643, 1992.
61. Derouin F, Sarfati CI, Beauvais B, et al. Laboratory diagnosis of pulmonary toxoplasmosis in patients wit acquired immunodeficiency syndrome. J Clin Microbiol 7:1661, 1989.
62. Buhr M, Heise W, Aarsteh K, et al. Disseminated toxoplasmosis with sepsis in AIDS. Clin Invest 70:1079, 1992.
63. Porter SS, Sande MA. Toxoplasmosis of the central nervous system in the acquired immunodeficiency syndrome. N Engl J Med 327:1643, 1992.
64. Cohn JA, McMeeking A, Cohen W, et al. Evaluation of the policy of empiric treatment of suspected Toxoplasma encephalitis in patients with the acquired immunodeficiency syndrome. Am J Med 86:521, 1989.
65. Potasman I, Resnick L, Luft BJ, et al. Intrathecal production of antibodies against Toxoplasma gondii in patients with toxoplasmic encephalitis and AIDS. Ann Intern Med 108:49, 1988.
66. Cintini C, Romani R, Magno S, et al. Diagnosis of Toxoplasma gondii infection in AIDS patients by a tissue culture technique. Eur J Clin Microbiol Infect Dis 14:434, 1995.
67. Albrecht H, Sobottka I, Stellbrink HJ, et al. Diagnosis of disseminated toxoplasmosis using a peripheral blood smear. AIDS 10:799, 1996.
68. Brouland JP, Audouin J, Hofman P, et al. Bone marrow involvement by disseminated toxoplasmosis in acquired immunodeficiency syndrome: the value of bone marrow trephine biopsy and immunohistochemistry for the diagnosis. Hum Pathol 27:302, 1996.
69. Eggers C, Gross U, Klinker H, et al. Limited value of cerebrospinal fluid for direct detection of Toxoplasma gondii in toxoplasmic encephalitis associated with AIDS. J Neurol 242:644, 1995.
70. Gadea I, Cuenca M, Benito N, et al. Bronchoalveolar lavage for the diagnosis of disseminated toxoplasmosis in AIDS patients. Diagn Microbiol Infect Dis 22:339, 1995.
71. Luft BJ, Hafner R, Korzun AH, et al. Toxoplasmic encephalitis in patients with the acquired immunodeficiency syndrome. N Engl J Med 329:995, 1993.
72. Jarvik JG, Hesselink JR, Kennedy C, et al. Acquired immunodeficiency syndrome: magnetic resonance patterns of brain involvement with pathologic correlation. Arch Neurol 45:731, 1998.
73. Levy RM, Mills CM, Posin JP, et al. The efficacy and clinical impact of brain imaging in neurologically symptomatic AIDS patients: a prospective CT/MRI study. J Acquir Immune Defic Syndr 3:461, 1990.
74. Kupfer MC, Zee CS, Colletti PM, et al. MRI evaluation of AIDS-related encephalopathy: toxoplasmosis vs. lymphoma. Magn Reson Imaging 8:51, 1990.
75. Ciricillo SF, Rosenblum ML. Use of CT and MR imaging to distinguish intracranial lesions and to define the need for biopsy in AIDS patients. J Neurosurg 73:720, 1990.
76. Ciricillo SF, Rosenblum ML. Imaging of solitary lesions in AIDS. J Neurosurg 74:1029, 1991.
77. Steinmetz H, Arendt G, Hefter H, et al. Focal brain lesions in patients with AIDS: aetiologies and corresponding radiological patterns in a prospective study. J Neurol 242:69, 1995.
78. Weisberg LA, Greenbereg J, Stazio A. Computed tomographic findings in cerebral toxoplasmosis in adults. Comput Med Imaging Graph 12:379, 1988.
79. Chinn RJ, Wilkinson ID, Hall-Crasggs MA, et al. Toxoplasmosis and primary central nervous system lymphoma in HIV infection: diagnosis with MR spectroscopy. Radiology 197:649, 1995.
80. Chang L, Miller BL, McBride D, et al. Brain lesions in patients with AIDS: H-1 MR spectroscopy. Radiology 197:525, 1995.
81. Gianotti N, Marenzi R, Messa C, et al. Thallium-201 single photon emission computed tomography in the management of contrast-enhancing brain lesions in a patient with AIDS. Clin Infect Dis 23:185, 1996.
82. Ruiz A, Ganz WI, Post MJD, et al. Use of thallium-201 brain SPECT to differentiate cerebral lymphoma from Toxoplasma encephalitis in AIDS patients. Am J Neuroradiol 15:1885, 1994.
83. O'Malley JP, Ziessman HA, Kumar PN, et al. Diagnosis of intracranial lymphoma in patients with AIDS: value of ^{201}Tl single-photon emission computed tomography. AJR Am J Roentgenol 163:417, 1994.
84. Naddaf SY, Akisik MF, Aziz M, et al. Comparison between ^{201}Tl-chloride and ^{99}Tc(m)-sestambi SPECT brain imaging for differentiating

intracranial lymphoma from non-malignant lesions in AIDS patients. Nucl Med Commun 19:47, 1998.

85. Ghesani M, DeRogatis A, Burns SM, et al. Thallium-201 brain SPECT to differentiate lymphoma from infectious intracranial lesions in patients with AIDS. In: Abstracts of the 43rd Annual Meeting of the Society of Nuclear Medicine, Denver, 1996, abstract 1236.
86. D'Amico A, Messa C, Castagna A, et al. Diagnostic accuracy and predictive value of ^{201}Tl SPET for the differential diagnosis of cerebral lesions in AIDS patients. Nucl Med Commun 18:741, 1997.
87. Lorberboym M, Estok L, Machac J, et al. Rapid differential diagnosis of cerebral toxoplasmosis and primary central nervous system lymphoma by thallium-201 SPECT. J Nucl Med 37:1150, 1996.
88. Barker DE, Trepashko D, DeMarais P, et al. Utility of thallium brain SPECT in the exclusion of CNS lymphoma in AIDS. In: Abstracts of the 4th Conference on Retroviruses and Opportunistic Infections, Washington, DC, January 1996, abstract 708.
89. Pintado V, Navas E, Mitjavila M, et al. Thallium-201 SPECT in differentiating lymphomas from nonmalignant CNS lesions in AIDS patients. In: Abstracts of the 36th Interscience Conference on Antimicrobial Agents and Chemotherapy, New Orleans, 1996, abstract I123.
90. Skiest DJ, Erdman W, Change WE, et al. SPECT thallium-201 combined with Toxoplasma serology for the presumptive diagnosis of focal central nervous system mass lesions in patients with AIDS. J Infect 40:274, 2000.
91. Pierce MA, Johnson MD, Maciunas RJ, et al. Evaluating contrast-enhancing brain lesions in patients with AIDS using positron emission tomography. Ann Intern Med 123:594, 1995.
92. Villriuger K, Jager H, Dichhgans M, et al. Differential diagnosis of CNS lesions in AIDS patients by FDG-PET. J Comput Assist Tomogr 19:532, 1995.
93. Campbell M, O'Doherty MJ, Barrington SF, et al. FDG and methionine positron emission tomography (PET) scanning in patients with HIV disease and cerebral pathology. In: Abstracts of the XIth International Conference on AIDS, Vancouver, July 1996, abstract Tu.B.2264.
94. Hoffman JM, Waskin HA, Schifter T, et al. FDG-PET in differentiating lymphoma from nonmalignant central nervous system lesions in patients with AIDS. J Nucl Med 34:567, 1993.
95. Hawkins R, Hoh C, Glaspy J, et al. Positron emission tomography scanning in cancer. Cancer Invest 12:74, 1994.
96. Letillois MF, Laigle V, Santoro F, et al. Toxoplasma gondii surface antigen-1 in sera of HIV-infected patients as an indicator of reactivated toxoplasmosis. Eur J Clin Microbiol Infect Dis 14:899, 1995.
97. Lavard I, Chouaid C, Poux P, et al. Pulmonary toxoplasmosis in HIV-infected patients: usefulness of polymerase chain reaction and cell culture. Eur Respir J 8:697, 1995.
98. Lamoril J, Molina JM, de Gouvello A, et al. Detection by PCR of Toxoplasma gondii in blood in the diagnosis of cerebral toxoplasmosis in patients with AIDS. J Clin Pathol 49:89, 1996.
99. Cingolani A, De Luca A, Ammassari A, et al. PCR detection of Toxoplasma gondii DNA in CSF for the differential diagnosis of AIDS-related focal brain lesions. J Med Microbiol 45:472, 1996.
100. Dupon M, Cazenave J, Pellegrin JL, et al. Detection of Toxoplasma gondii by PCR and tissue culture in cerebrospinal fluid and blood of human immunodeficiency virus-seropositive patients. J Clin Microbiol 33:2421, 1995.
101. Novati R, Castagna A, Morsica G, et al. Polymerase chain reaction for Toxoplasma gondii DNA in the cerebrospinal fluid of AIDS patients with focal brain lesions. AIDS 8:1691, 1994.
102. Schoondermark-van de Ven E, Galama J, Kraaijeveld C, et al. Value of the polymerase chain reaction for the detection of Toxoplasma gondii in cerebrospinal fluid from patients with AIDS. Clin Infect Dis 16:661, 1993.
103. Rodriguez JC, Martinez MM, Martinez AR, Royo G. Evaluation of different techniques in the diagnosis of Toxoplasma encephalitis. J Med Microbiol 46:597, 1997.
104. Cosin J, Miralles P, Moreno S, et al. Stereotactic brain biopsy of focal intracerebral lesions in AIDS patients. Int Conf AIDS 10:195, 1994.
105. Chappell ET, Guthrie BL, Orestein J. The role of stereotactic biopsy in the management of HIV-related focal brain lesions. Neurosurgery 30:82, 1992.
106. MacArthur RD, Nandi P, McMillen L, et al. CT guided brain biopsy findings in HIV-infected persons: a retrospective review of 44 cases at an urban medical center. In: Abstracts of the XIth International Conference on AIDS, Vancouver, July 1996, abstract we.B.3286.
107. Mathews C, Barba D, Fullerton SC. Early biopsy versus empiric treatment with delayed biopsy of non-responders in suspected HIV-associated cerebral toxoplasmosis: a decision analysis. AIDS 9:1243, 1995.
108. Haverkos HW. Assessment of therapy of Toxoplasma encephalitis: the TE Study Group. Am J Med 82:907, 1987.
109. Carr AC, Tindall B, Brew BJ, et al. Low-dose trimethoprim-sulfamethoxazole prophylaxis for toxoplasmic encephalitis in patients with AIDS. Ann Intern Med 117:106, 1992.
110. Girard P-M, Landman R, Gaudebout C, et al. Dapsone-pyrimethamine compared with aerosolized pentamidine as primary prophylaxis against Pneumocystis carinii pneumonia and toxoplasmosis in HIV infection. N Engl J Med 328:1514, 1993.
111. Jacobson MA, Besch CL, Chikd C, et al. Primary prophylaxis with pyrimethamine for toxoplasmic encephalitis in patients with advanced human immunodeficiency virus disease: results of a randomized trial. J Infect Dis 169:384, 1994.
112. Opravil M, Hirschel B, Lazzarin A, et al. Once-weekly administration of dapsone/pyrimethamine vs. aerosolized pentamidine as combined prophylaxis for Pneumocystis carinii pneumonia and toxoplasmic encephalitis in human immunodeficiency virus-infected patients. Clin Infect Dis 20:531, 1995.
113. Podzamczer D, Salazar A, Jimenez J, et al. Intermittent trimethoprim-sulfamethoxazole compared with dapsone-pyrimethamine for the simultaneous primary prophylaxis of Pneumocystis pneumonia and toxoplasmosis in patients infected with HIV. Ann Intern Med 122:755, 1995.
114. Leport C, Chene G, Morlat P, et al. Pyrimethamine for primary prophylaxis of toxoplasmic encephalitis in patients with human immunodeficiency virus infection: a double-blind, randomized trial. J Infect Dis 173:91, 1996.
115. Katlama C, De Wit S, O'Doherty E, et al. Pyrmiethamine-clindamycin vs. pyrimethamine-sulfadiazine as acute and long-term therapy for toxoplasmic encephalitis in patients with AIDS. Clin Infect Dis 22:368, 1996.
116. Leport C, Raffi F, Matheron S, et al. Treatment of central nervous system toxoplasmosis with pyrimethamine/sulfadiazine combination in 35 patients with the acquired immunodeficiency syndrome. Am J Med 84:94, 1988.
117. Simon DI, Brosius FC, Rothstein DM. Sulfadiazine crystalluria revisited: the treatment of Toxoplasma encephalitis in patients with acquired immunodeficiency syndrome. Arch Intern Med 150:2379, 1990.
118. Bachmeyer C, Gorin I, Deleuze J, et al. Pyrimethamine as primary prophylaxis of toxoplasmic encephalitis in patients infected with human immunodeficiency virus: open study. Clin Infect Dis 18:479, 1994.
119. Jacobson MA, Besch CL, Child C, et al. Toxicity of clindamycin as prophylaxis for AIDS-associated toxoplasmic encephalitis. Lancet 339:333, 1992.
120. Katlama C. Evaluation of the efficacy and safety of clindamycin plus pyrimethamine for induction and maintenance therapy of toxoplasmic encephalitis in AIDS. Eur J Clin Microbiol Infect Dis 10:189, 1991.
121. Garaujo F, Huskingon J, Remington JS. Remarkable in vitro and in vivo activities of the hydroxynaphthoquinone, 566C80, against tachyzoites and tissue cysts of Toxoplasma gondii. Antimicrob Agents Chemother 35:293, 1991.
122. Kovacs JA, NIAID-Clinical Center Intramural AIDS Program. Efficacy of atovaquone in treatment of toxoplasmosis in patients with AIDS. Lancet 340:637, 1992.
123. Katlama C, Mouthon B, Gourdon D, et al. Atovaquone as long-term suppressive therapy for toxoplasmic encephalitis in patients with AIDS and multiple drug intolerance. AIDS 10:1107, 1996.
124. Torres RA, Weinberg W, Stansell J, et al. Atovaquone for salvage treatment and suppression of toxoplasmic encephalitis in patients with AIDS. Clin Infect Dis 24:422, 1997.
125. Fernandes-Martin J, Leport C, Morlat P, et al. Pyrimethamine-clarithromycin combination for therapy of acute toxoplasma encephalitis in patients with AIDS. Antimicrob Agents Chemother 10:2049, 1991.
126. Remington JS. Macrolides, azalides, and streptogramins in treatment of opportunistic infections in immunocompromised patients. In: Zin-

ner SH, Young LS, Acar JF, et al (eds) Expanding Indications for the New Macrolides, Azalides, and Streptogramins. New York, Marcel Dekker, 1997, p 189.

127. Dunne MW, Williams DJ, Young LS. Azithromycin and the treatment of opportunistic infections. Rev Contemp Pharmacother 5:373, 1994.
128. Farthing C, Rendel M, Currie B, et al. Azithromycin for cerebral toxoplasmosis. Lancet 339:437, 1992.
129. Canessa A, Del Bono V, De Leo P, et al. Cotrimoxazole therapy for Toxoplasma gondii encephalitis in AIDS patients. Eur J Clin Microbiol Infect Dis 11:125, 1992.
130. Masur H, Polis MA, Tuazon CU, et al. Salvage trial of trimetrexate-leucovorin for the treatment of cerebral toxoplasmosis in patients with AIDS. J Infect Dis 167:1422, 1993.
131. Ruf B, Schurmann D, Bergmann F, et al. Efficacy of pyrimethamine-sulfadoxine in the prevention of toxoplasmic encephalitis relapses and Pneumocystis carinii pneumonia in HIV-infected patients. Eur J Clin Microbiol Infect Dis 12:325, 1991.
132. Pedrol E, Gonzalez-Clemente J, Gatell JM, et al. Central nervous system toxoplasmosis in AIDS patients: efficacy of an intermittent maintenance therapy. AIDS 4:511, 1990.
133. Morris JT, Kelly JW. Effective treatment of cerebral toxoplasmosis with doxycycline. Am J Med 93:107, 1992.
134. Torre D, Casari S, Speranza F, et al. Randomized trial of trimethoprim-sulfamethoxazole versus pyrimethamine-sulfadiazine for therapy of toxoplasmic encephalitis in patients with AIDS. Antimicrob Agents Chemother 42:1346, 1998.
135. Leport C, Tournerie C, Raguin G, et al. Long-term followup of patients with AIDS on maintenance therapy for toxoplasmosis. Eur J Clin Microbiol Infect Dis 10:191, 1991.
136. Girard PM, Lepretre A, Detruchis P, et al. Failure of pyrimethamine-clindamycin combination for prophylaxis of Pneumocystis carinii pneumonia and toxoplasmosis. Lancet 1:1459, 1989.
137. De Gans J, Portegies P, Reiss P, et al. Pyrimethamine alone as maintenance therapy for central nervous system toxoplasmosis in 38 patients with AIDS. J Acquir Immune Defic Syndr 5:137, 1992.
138. Foppa CU, Bibi T, Gregis G, et al. A retrospective study of primary and maintenance therapy of toxoplasmic encephalitis with oral clindamycin and pyrimethamine. Eur J Clin Microbiol Infect Dis 10:187, 1991.
139. Podzamczer D, Miro JM, Ferrer E, et al. Thrice-weekly sulfadiazine-pyrimethamine in HIV-infected patients. Eur J Microbiol Infect Dis 19:89, 2000.
140. USPHS/IDSA 2001 Prevention of Opportunistic Infections Working Group: 1999 USPHS/IDSA guidelines for the prevention of opportunistic infections in persons infected with human immunodeficiency virus. http//:www.hivatis.org. and Anals Intern Med 2002; 137: in press.
140a. Jungmann EM, Mercey D, DeRuiter A, et al. Is first trimester exposure to the combination of antiretroviral therapy and folate antagonists a risk factor for congenital abnormalities? Sex Transm Inf 77:441, 2001.
141. Mussini C, Pezzotti P, Govoni A, et al. Discontinuation of primary prophylaxis for Pneumocystis carinii pneumonia and toxoplasmic encephalitis in human immunodeficiency virus type 1-infected patients: the changes in opportunistic prophylaxis study. J Infect Dis 181:1635, 2000.
142. Furrer H, Opravil M, Bernasconi E, et al. Stopping primary prophylaxis in HIV-1-infected patients at high risk of toxoplasma encephalitis. Lancet 355:2217, 2000.
143. Miro JM, Lopez J, Podzamczer D, et al. Discontinuation of primary or secondary Toxoplasma gondii prophylaxis is safe in HIV-1-infected patients after immunological recovery with HAART: final results of the GESIDA 04/98-B study. In: Abstracts of the 39th Interscience Conference on Antimicrobial Agents and Chemotherapy, Toronto, 2000, abstract L-16.
144. Ledergerber B, Mocroft A, Reiss P, et al. Discontinuation of secondary prophylaxis against Pneumocystis carinii pneumonia in patients with HIV infection who have a response to antiretroviral therapy: eight European study groups. N Engl J Med 18:168, 2001.
145. Yangco BG, Von Bargen JC, Moorman AC, Holmberg SD. Discontinuation of chemoprophylaxis against Pneumocystis carinii pneumonia in patients with HIV infection: HIV Outpatient Study (HOPS) Investigators. Ann Intern Med 132:201, 2000.
146. Soriano V, Dona C, Rodriguez-Rosado R, et al. Discontinuation of secondary prophylaxis for opportunistic infections in HIV-infected patients receiving highly active antiretroviral therapy. AIDS 4:383, 2000.
147. Jubault V, Pacanowski J, Rabian C, Viard J-P. Interruption of prophylaxis for major opportunistic infections in HIV-infected patients receiving triple combination antiretroviral therapy. Ann Med Interne 151:163, 2000.
148. Kirk O, Lunmdgren JD, Pederson C, et al. Can chemoprophylaxis against opportunistic infections be discontinued after an increase in CD4 cells induced by highly active antiretroviral therapy? AIDS 13:1647, 1999.
148a. Kirk O, Reis P, Ubert-Foppa C, et al. Safe interruption of maintenance therapy against previous infection with four common HIV-associated opportunistic pathogens during potent antiretroviral therapy. Ann Intern Med 2002; 137: in press.
149. Zeller V, Joulian M, Truffaut C, et al. Discontinuing maintenance treatment for pneumonia, toxoplasmic encephalitis, and disseminated Mycobacterium avium complex infection. In: Program and Abstracts of the 1st IAS Conference on HIV Pathogen Treatment, Buenos Aires, July 2001, abstract 737.
150. Oksenhendler E, Charreau I, Tournerie C, et al. Toxoplasma gondii infection in advanced AIDS. AIDS 8:483, 1994.
151. Klinker H, Langmann P, Richter E. Pyrimethamine alone as prophylaxis for cerebral toxoplasmosis in patients with advanced HIV infection. Infection 24:324, 1996.
152. Torres RA, Barr M, Thorn M, et al. Randomized trial of dapsone and aerosolized pentamidine for the prophylaxis of Pneumocystis carinii pneumonia and toxoplasmic encephalitis. Am J Med 95:573, 1993.
153. Durant J, Hazime F, Carles M, et al. Prevention of Pneumocystis carinii pneumonia and of cerebral toxoplasmosis by roxithromycin in HIV-infected patients. Infection 23(suppl 1):S33, 1995.
154. Rizzardi GP, Lazzarin A, Musicco M, et al. Risks and benefits of aerosolized pentamidine and cotrimoxazole in primary prophylaxis of Pneumocystis carinii pneumonia in HIV-1 infected patients: a two-year Italian multicentric randomized trial. J Infect 32:123, 1991.
155. Mallolas J, Zamora L, Gatell JM, et al. Primary prophylaxis for Pneumocystis carinii pneumonia: a randomized trial comparing cotrimoxazole, aerosolized pentamidine and dapsone plus pyrimethamine. AIDS 7:59, 1993.
156. Benenson MW, Takafuji ET, Lemon SM, et al. Oocyst-transmitted toxoplasmosis associated with ingestion of contaminated water. N Engl J Med 307:666, 1982.
157. Bowie WR, King AS, Werker DH, et al. Outbreak of toxoplasmosis associated with municipal drinking water. Lancet 350:173, 1997.
158. Wallace MR, Rossetti, Olson PE. Cats and toxoplasmosis risk in HIV-infected adults. JAMA 269:76, 1993.
159. Glaser CA, Angulo FJ, Rooney JA. Animal-associated opportunistic infections among persons infected with the human immunodeficiency virus. Clin Infect Dis 18:14, 1994.

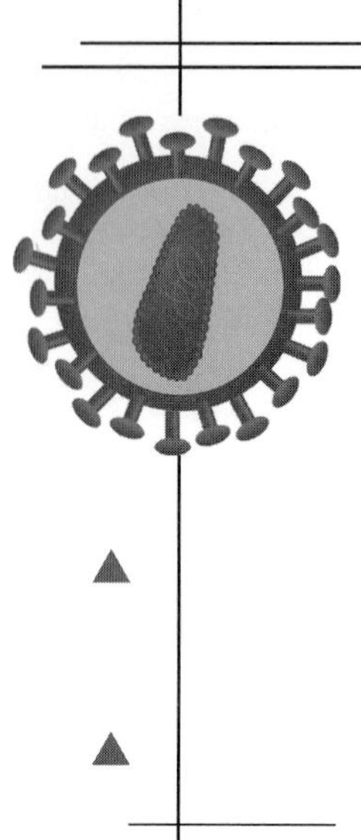

CHAPTER 31

Cryptosporidium, Isospora, and *Cyclospora* Infections

Timothy P. Flanigan, MD
Christine A. Wanke, MD

It has only been since the advent of the acquired immunodeficiency syndrome (AIDS) epidemic that the spore-forming protozoa that infect the gastrointestinal tract (*Cryptosporidium, Microsporidium, Isospora,* and *Cyclospora*) have been identified as significant, ubiquitous human pathogens. Initially, these pathogens were thought to cause only rare or esoteric infections; but it is now recognized that they infect both immunocompetent and immunodeficient hosts worldwide.[1-3] In many communities, infection with these parasites is the leading cause of chronic diarrheal illness. In the developing world, where more than 90% of human immunodeficiency virus (HIV)-infected patients live, diarrheal illness usually due to these protozoa is the most common opportunistic infection after tuberculosis.

The spectrum of illness caused by these enigmatic parasites is broad and is closely linked to host immunocompetence.[4] This explains why infections by these pathogens were first recognized in severely immunocompromised individuals with AIDS who presented with chronic diarrhea and wasting illness. Clearance of these intestinal pathogens is directly related to the ability to mount an effective immune response at the site of the infection, the intestinal mucosa. For example, among patients with cryptosporidiosis, the course of disease is directly related to the stage of immunodeficiency as measured by the CD4+ T-lymphocyte count.[4,5] What has become clear, with the advent of highly active antiretroviral therapy (HAART), is that the best therapy for some of these pathogens, such as that causing cryptosporidiosis, is augmentation of immune responses through direct suppression of HIV replication with antiretroviral agents.[6-9] The severity of illness with the two most common of these protozoal parasites, *Cryptosporidium* and *Microsporidium*, appears to be linked to improvement or deterioration of immune function related to suppression or activation of HIV. We have come full circle in that the HIV epidemic has uncovered many of the biologic, epidemiologic, and immunologic secrets of these protozoan infections among humans; and now better therapy for HIV is leading directly to curative treatment for patients with these protozoal parasites through immune restoration. This chapter deals with *Cryptosporidium, Isospora,* and *Cyclospora*. *Microsporidium* is addressed in Chapter 32. Table 31–1 highlights many of the similarities and differences among these three parasites.

CRYPTOSPORIDIUM

Clinical Presentation

Typically, acute infection with *Cryptosporidium* is characterized by watery diarrhea, crampy epigastric abdominal pain, weight loss, anorexia, malaise, and flatulence.[3,5] Diarrhea, the most noteworthy symptom, can range from a few loose bowel movements a day to more than 50 stools (more than 15 L) per day. Nausea and vomiting are common. Diarrhea and abdominal pain are usually exacerbated by eating, particularly with difficult-to-digest foods such as milk and dairy products or fatty foods. The spectrum of symptoms from infection varies widely; in fact, there are reports of asymptomatic shedding of *Cryptosporidium* for months after the primary infection.

In patients with severe immunodeficiency characterized by a CD4+ T-lymphocyte count well under 200 cells/mm^3, symptoms may begin insidiously with only mild diarrhea but then increase in severity over time. Many of these

▲ **Table 31-1.** COMPARISON OF *CRYPTOSPORIDIUM, ISOSPORA,* AND *CYCLOSPORA*

Similarities			
Biology	Protozoa Intracellular location in epithelial cells of the intestine Spororozoite infects the mucosa Spore or oocyst is shed in stool and transmits infection		
Epidemiology	Frequent cause of diarrhea in tropical regions and places with poor sanitation Acute diarrhea in children and immunocompetent hosts; chronic diarrhea in patients with AIDS		
Diagnosis	Microscopic stool examination Detection of cysts or spores requires expertise and proper stains		
	Cryptosporidium	***Isospora***	***Cyclospora***
Differences			
Morphology and fecal isolates	Oocysts: 4–6 μm, seen well with modified acid-fast stains	Oocysts: 20–30 μm, seen well on modified acid-fast stain and wet preparation	Oocysts: 8–10 μm, seen well on acid-fast stain and wet preparation
Morphology and small bowel biopsy specimens	Easily seen on light microscopy as 4 μm round blue dots on the apical membrane of the enterocyte	Easily seen on light microscopy as 20 μm oval blue enterocyte inclusions	Not seen well with light microscopy; reported with electron microscopy
Transmission	Fecal-oral, person to person, food- and water-borne	Presumably food- and water-borne	Food- and water-borne
Antibiotic treatment Acute disease	No consistently effective therapy; initiate HAART Consider paromomycin 500–750 mg PO tid × 14–21 days	Trimethoprim-sulfamethoxazole, one double-strength tablet twice daily × 7–10 days Alternative: Ciprofloxacin 500 mg PO bid × 7–10 days	Trimethoprim-sulfamethoxazole, one double-strength tablet twice daily × 7–10 days Alternative: Ciprofloxacin 500 mg PO bid × 7–10 days
Chronic maintenance	None (consider continuing paromomycin if response)	Trimethoprim-sulfamethoxazole, one double-strength tablet tiw or qd Alternative: Ciprofloxacin 500 mg PO qd	Trimethoprim-sulfamethoxazole, one double-strength tablet PO qd or tiw Alternative: Ciprofloxacin 500 mg PO qd

patients experience voluminous watery diarrhea, with a loss of more than 10% of total body weight. Severe malabsorption is the rule, and many patients avoid eating because it worsens the diarrhea and abdominal pain. Symptoms often remit for periods of time, but these respites are usually brief. Before the advent of HAART, most patients with AIDS never cleared the infection and so died with cryptosporidial diarrhea.

Cryptosporidial enteritis occurs in HIV-infected individuals who are immunologically competent, as determined by a normal CD4+ T-lymphocyte count. Those individuals have a clinical course similar to HIV-seronegative persons; they are able to clear the infection over a few days to a few weeks.[4,5] The median CD4+ T-lymphocyte count of individuals who develop chronic severe disease is well under 50 cells/mm^3,[5] whereas it appears that all patients with CD4+ T-lymphocyte counts higher than 200 cells/mm^3 are able to clear cryptosporidial enteritis.[4]

A subset of patients with AIDS and cryptosporidiosis develop biliary tract involvement associated with right upper quadrant pain, nausea, and vomiting.[5,10] Laboratory examination is significant for elevated serum alkaline phosphatase and γ-glutamyl transferase levels. This is a difficult-to-treat complication in individuals with exceedingly low CD4+ T-lymphocyte counts and long-standing chronic cryptosporidial enteritis.[5,11] Endoscopic retrograde cholangiopancreatography (ERCP) may reveal dilatation of bile ducts with multiple luminal irregularities and distal duct strictures consistent with partial obstruction or sclerosing cholangitis.

Physical examination of individuals with cryptosporidial enteritis is usually unrevealing. Patients may have orthostatic hypotension and other signs of dehydration. Low-grade fever and mild leukocytosis are common. The abdomen is soft, with mild tenderness to palpation. Laboratory examination often reveals electrolyte disturbances consistent with diarrhea and dehydration. Fecal examination may reveal mucus, but blood and leukocytes are rarely seen. Charcot-Leyden crystals are characteristic of *Isospora belli* infection and amebiasis but not cryptosporidiosis.[2] Lactose intolerance and fat malabsorption are well documented, and the D-xylose test is abnormal. An abnormal D-xylose test correlates strongly with small intestinal infection with *Cryptosporidium* and *Microsporidium.*[12,13]

Biology

Cryptosporidium, Isospora belli, and *Cyclospora* are spore-forming sporozoa in the class of human protozoal pathogens.[1,3] Sporozoites are seen within oocysts and are the infectious form of the parasite.[14] *Cryptosporidium* infection has been identified in numerous species of animals, including mammals, fish, turkeys, and even reptiles such as rattlesnakes.[1]

Although the parasite was first described in 1907,[15] it received no clinical attention until it was recognized as a significant cause of diarrhea in domestic animals (e.g., cows, horses, pigs). The first human case was described in 1976,[16] but cryptosporidiosis was thought to be an esoteric illness until 1982, when the Centers for Disease Control reported 21 homosexual men with severe diarrhea caused by *Cryptosporidium.*[17] It is now recognized that *Cryptosporidium* is the number one cause of protozoal diarrhea worldwide in both immunocompetent and immunodeficient persons.

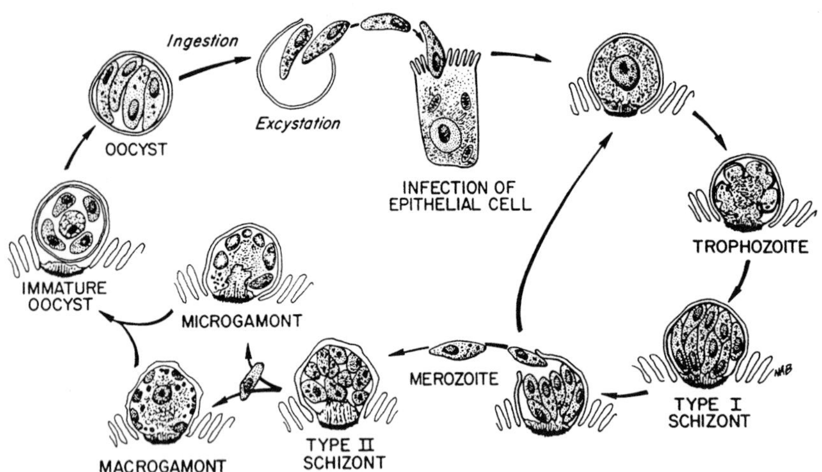

Figure 31–1. Life cycle of *Cryptosporidium* species. (From Flanigan TP, Soave R. Cryptosporidiosis. Prog Clin Parasitol 3:1, 1993, with permission.)

Intestinal infection is initiated by ingestion of the oocysts, with subsequent excystation and release of four sporozoites from each oocyst in the gastrointestinal tract. Sporozoites implant immediately in the host epithelial cells and begin a cycle of autoinfection at the luminal surface of the epithelium. The sexual stage of the parasite results in oocysts, which are excreted in the stool and are immediately infectious to other hosts and can reinfect the same host, even without reingestion. Figure 31–1 shows the life cycle of *Cryptosporidium*. An infectious dose of *Cryptosporidium* is as low as 10 oocysts, thereby facilitating transmission.[18]

The most common site of *Cryptosporidium* infection is the small intestine, although it is frequently present in the colon and the biliary tract of persons with immunodeficiency.[2,12,13] *Cryptosporidium* infects only the epithelial surface of the mucosa; it does not invade the submucosal layer or cause ulcerations. Infection of the epithelial lining of the respiratory tract with associated cough has been reported, although it is uncommon.[1]

Cryptosporidium is a ubiquitous parasite; and transmission has been documented from animals to humans, from humans to humans (particularly in day-care centers), and from environmental sources such as water reservoirs.[1,19,20] Person-to-person transmission of *Cryptosporidium* is often underappreciated; outbreaks have been well documented in the hospital setting and in families. In Michigan, for example, 71% of families with a symptomatic child had other infected family members.[21,22] All individuals in the hospital setting with cryptosporidial diarrhea should follow enteric precautions, although isolation is not necessary to prevent roommate-to-roommate transmission.[23]

Cryptosporidium has been identified as the etiologic agent of several extensive water-borne outbreaks usually caused by surface-infected groundwater sources, often involving farm animals.[11] The oocyst is only 4 μm in diameter, making it difficult to clear through filtration, and it is resistant to routine chlorination.[19] The first documented water-borne outbreak (in San Antonio, Texas) had a 34% attack rate and was linked to sewage contamination of the well water supply, which was chlorinated but not filtered.[24] In 1987 an outbreak in Georgia resulted in an estimated 13,000 cases of cryptosporidial enteritis despite the filtered and chlorinated public supply that met the established Environmental Protection Agency guidelines.[20] Improved filtering of the water supply ultimately helped terminate the outbreak. An outbreak in Milwaukee, Wisconsin in 1993 afflicted some 375,000 residents when the spring runoff from grazing lands was not adequately filtered in the public water supply.[11,25] This massive environmental contamination led to severe illness with both small intestinal disease and biliary tract infection in HIV-infected patients with CD4+ T-lymphocyte counts under 50 cells/mm^3, and it resulted in a marked increase in morbidity and mortality in these patients.[11]

Diagnosis

The diagnosis of *Cryptosporidium* is primarily based on identifying the oocysts in stool.[26] Oocysts stain red with varying intensities with a modified acid-fast technique; this technique allows differentiation of the *Cryptosporidium* oocysts from yeasts that are similar in size and shape but not acid-fast. Oocysts can also be detected by direct immunofluorescence assays that are commercially available utilizing monoclonal antibodies raised to *Cryptosporidium* antigens.[27] In addition, an enzyme-linked immunosorbent assay may be used to detect *Cryptosporidium* in fecal specimens and tissues.[28,29] There is no consensus on the optimal oocyst detection method in fecal samples, although one comparison of a modified acid-fast stain and a fluorescein-labeled monoclonal antibody technique showed comparability for diarrheal samples but improved detection with the immunofluorescence method for formed specimens.[26,30] Cryptosporidial enteritis can also be diagnosed on small intestinal biopsy sections by identifying developmental stages, found individually or in clusters, on the brush border of the mucosal epithelial surfaces.[30] Organisms project into the lumen because of their intracellular but extracytoplasmic nature, and they appear basophilic with hematoxylin and eosin staining. Electron microscopy allows resolution of cellular detail.

In individuals with profuse diarrheal illness, a single stool specimen is usually adequate for the diagnosis. In individuals with less severe disease, repeat stool sampling is recommended, although there have been no controlled studies showing the utility of three consecutive stool samples as is the case for *Giardia* infection.

Treatment

Standard dogma is that there is no reliable palliative or curative treatment for severe cryptosporidiosis in immunodeficient hosts. Until the advent of HAART, patients with severe immunodeficiency characterized by CD4+ T-lymphocyte counts under 50 cells/mm^3 and chronic cryptosporidial diarrhea had little hope of ever eradicating the infection and living a normal life. Many of these patients were treated with intravenous hyperalimentation for life to reverse the severe wasting and chronic dehydration resulting from massive cryptosporidial infection of the small intestine.

With the availability of HAART, it is now commonplace for patients with severe diarrhea who can take combination antiretroviral agents and achieve viral suppression to clear *Cryptosporidium* infection.[6–9] HAART can result in complete, sustained clinical, microbiologic, and histologic resolution of HIV-associated cryptosporidiosis and microsporidiosis. Presumably, this is due to arresting HIV replication with subsequent rises in CD4+ T-lymphocyte count and restoration of immunocompetence.

Interestingly enough, it is not clear what specific elements of the immune system are required for control of cryptosporidiosis, although clinical and experimental data implicate both humoral and cellular immunity.[31] The importance of antibody-mediated immunity is suggested by the fact that immunocompromised patients with congenital hypogammaglobulinemia may develop severe chronic disease.[32] Clinical and experimental data indicate that antibodies at the mucosal surface play an important role. For example, hyperimmune cow colostrum obtained from cows hyperimmunized with *Cryptosporidium* has been used successfully to treat individual cases of chronic disease.[33,34] In the murine model of infection, both monoclonal and polyclonal antibodies directed against sporozoite surface antigens have been successful in preventing infection.[35] In addition, experimental data in Balb-c mice infected with cryptosporidia indicate that both systemic CD4 cells and interferon-α are important in protective immune responses.[36]

Initial treatment of individuals with *Cryptosporidium* infection should be directed toward symptomatic treatment of diarrhea. Rehydration and repletion of electrolyte losses orally or intravenously is of paramount importance. Severe diarrhea, which may be more than 10 L/day in patients with AIDS, often requires intensive support. Aggressive efforts at oral rehydration should be made with Gatorade, bouillon, or oral rehydration solution that contains glucose, sodium bicarbonate, and potassium. Often intravenous repletion of fluids and electrolytes is essential to correct losses of bicarbonate, potassium, magnesium, and phosphorus. Treatment with antimotility agents often provides temporary relief and may play an important adjunctive role in therapy, but these agents are not consistently effective. Treatment with loperamide or tincture of opium often palliates symptoms of severe illness. Octreotide, a synthetic octapeptide analogue of naturally occurring somatostatin that is approved for the treatment of secreting tumor-induced diarrhea, is no more effective than other oral antidiarrheal agents.[37] More than 95 interventional agents have been tried for the treatment of cryptosporidiosis with no consistent success, including drugs effective against other parasites and protozoa.

Paromomycin, a nonabsorbable aminoglycoside with in vitro activity against *Cryptosporidium*,[38,39] is indicated for the treatment of intestinal amebiasis. At extremely high doses paromomycin is effective in the treatment of animal models of cryptosporidiosis. The commonly used human dose (500 mg qid) is a fraction of this amount. A meta-analysis of 11 paromomycin studies reported a response rate of 67%. Relapse data are sparse, however, and the long-term success rates dropped to 33%.[40] A randomized study of paromomycin (500 mg qid × 21 days) in patients with AIDS showed it to be no more effective than placebo.[40] The high incidence of death in this trial is a clear reminder of the life-threatening nature of this infection in patients with advanced HIV disease in which immunosuppression cannot be reversed by HAART. At present there is no consistently effective pharmacologic or immunologic therapy directed specifically against *Cryptosporidium*.[2]

In HIV-positive patients who present with *Cryptosporidium*, initial efforts should be directed at restoring fluid and electrolyte balance and controlling symptoms with antidiarrheal agents. Infections with other pathogens must be ruled out because co-infection with *Clostridium difficile*, other bacterial pathogens, or some protozoa is not uncommon. Many of these co-infections respond to specific therapies. Once patients are rehydrated and electrolyte balance is restored, efforts should be directed at obtaining optimal HIV suppression with HAART.[6–9] This is certainly challenging because the symptoms of *Cryptosporidium* (including nausea, vomiting, abdominal pain, and diarrhea) may discourage all but the hardiest and most highly motivated patients from taking many pills a day. Close coaching by the physician and the patient's understanding of the importance of viral suppression, with resultant immune restoration and resolution of symptoms, is critical.

Prevention

Infection control measures are limited by resistance of the *Cryptosporidium* oocysts to common disinfectants. Ammonia, sodium hypochlorite, and formalin have been used in the laboratory setting.[1] In households, washing infected surfaces with bleach provides effective decontamination. Enteric precautions with good hygiene (e.g., hand washing) and proper disposal of contaminated materials (e.g., diapers) are important. Boiled or bottled drinking water should be considered by HIV-infected persons with CD4+ T-lymphocyte counts of less than 200 cells/mm^3 because the present drinking water purification standards do not uniformly destroy viable oocysts, and the infectious dose is small.[41] This is particularly important when surface contamination may occur in water sources such as during spring runoff or in households using well water. If personal-use water filters are utilized, they should be capable of removing particles

1 μm in diameter.[41] HIV-infected persons who travel in developing countries should meticulously avoid drinking tap water and contaminated water resources. At-risk persons should avoid contact with obvious sources of *Cryptosporidium* oocysts, such as other infected humans (especially regarding sexual practices that involve oral exposure to feces), farm animals (particularly cattle), and domestic pets that are extremely young (<6 months), have diarrhea, or have been strays.

Interestingly, in a large outpatient HIV study, patients who were receiving therapy or chemoprophylaxis for mycobacterial disease with rifabutin or clarithromycin were significantly protected against developing cryptosporidiosis. The prophylactic efficacy of either drug was 75% or more.[42] Another study, however, found rifabutin but not clarithromycin to be protective[43]; therefore the data are conflicting on this point.

▲ ISOSPORA

In normal hosts, symptomatic illness caused by *Isospora* is usually characterized by 3 days to 3 weeks of diarrhea, abdominal pain, and occasionally nausea, vomiting, and fever.[3] The pattern of clinical illness resulting from *Isospora* infection depends on the host's immunocompetence. It is impossible to differentiate isosporiasis from cryptosporidiosis clinically. Symptomatic illness in immunocompromised hosts, including patients with AIDS, results in protracted, severe diarrhea associated with malabsorption and dehydration.[44] Microscopic examination of the small bowel in patients infected with *Isospora* demonstrates shortened villi and infiltration of the lamina propria with inflammatory cells, particularly eosinophils.[45]

Isospora is rarely identified as a cause of AIDS-associated diarrhea in the United States and Europe (fewer than 1% of cases), whereas in Africa, Asia, Haiti, and Latin America it is a frequent cause of AIDS-related diarrhea.[3] The environmental reservoirs of *Isospora* are not well understood. There is no evidence that human *Isospora* can infect animals other than humans. All phases of the life cycle occur within the human small intestine, with the release of immature, unsporulated oocysts in the feces that are initially noninfective and then, within a few days, become infective as sporulation occurs. Transmission therefore is presumed to be via food and water contamination with human feces.

The diagnosis is made by identifying oocysts in stool by examining of a wet mount or by acid-fast staining of stool concentrates. *Isospora* is easily distinguished from *Cryptosporidium* and *Cyclospora* by its large size. Multiple stool samples may be necessary because shedding can be intermittent. Peripheral blood eosinophils and Charcot-Leyden crystals have been reported in the stool of patients with *Isospora* infection.

Treatment for *Isospora* infection (Table 31–1) is easily accomplished with a 7- to 10-day course of trimethoprim-sulfamethoxazole (one double-strength tablet twice daily), which is effective in both immunocompetent and immunodeficient hosts, including patients with AIDS.[44–46] Ciprofloxacin 500 mg PO bid is an effective alternative.[47] Most patients with AIDS relapse within 1 to 2 months of stopping therapy; and suppressive therapy with daily trimethoprim-sulfamethoxazole (1 double-strength tablet qd or tiw) or ciprofloxacin (500 mg PO qd) is recommended.

▲ CYCLOSPORA

The first case of human *Cyclospora* infection was reported in 1979 from Papua, New Guinea, but this protozoan did not garner much attention until 1993, when it was recognized that an acid-fast stain of stool could identify the oocysts, and therefore made the diagnosis significantly easier.[48,49] In 1996 and 1997 there was an explosive increase in cases caused by multiple outbreaks primarily from food-borne contamination.[49] Prior to 1996 there were only three reported outbreaks in the United States. From May through August of 1996, more than 1400 cases of cyclosporiasis had been reported throughout the United States and Canada, of which more than 60% were laboratory-confirmed.[50] No deaths have been reported. Outbreaks in 1996 and 1997 were due, most notably, to fresh raspberries imported from Central America, mesclun lettuce, and basil. In all probability, *Cyclospora* has been a cause of diarrheal outbreaks in the past but was unrecognized.

The parasite was not named until 1993, and many of its hosts are still unknown.[48,51] Previous underdiagnosis of *Cyclospora* has probably been due to the following factors: It is an unknown infection to many physicians; clinical laboratories do not routinely screen for *Cyclospora* unless it is requested; shedding of *Cyclospora* is intermittent; and acid-fast staining may be relatively insensitive for detecting the oocysts because of variable uptake of stains.

After ingestion of *Cyclospora*, diarrhea occurs in 1 to 11 days.[48,49] Diarrhea due to *Cyclospora* is similar to that induced by *Cryptosporidium* and *Isospora*, although upper gastrointestinal symptoms may initially predominate. Patients have reported watery diarrhea alternating with constipation. Nausea, abdominal cramping, anorexia, weight loss, and vomiting are frequent. The illness is self-limiting in immunocompetent individuals, although it may last for weeks. In immunocompromised hosts, particularly patients with AIDS, diarrhea is prolonged, severe, and associated with a high rate of recurrence.[51] *Cyclospora* may infect the biliary tract much like *Cryptosporidium*. The small intestine is the primary site of infection. Villous atrophy and crypt hyperplasia are found in the infected jejunum, as is common with *Cryptosporidium* and *Isospora*.

Cyclospora resembles *Isospora* in that its oocysts are excreted unsporulated and require days to weeks outside the intestinal tract for maturation and to gain infective potential.[52] The oocyst of *Cyclospora* is round, much like that of *Cryptosporidium*, and is 8 to 10 μm in diameter.[48,49] Early on, *Cyclospora* was called *Cryptosporidium grande*, or large *Cryptosporidium*, because of its *Cryptosporidium*-like appearance and its approximately doubled size. It may be necessary to use a micrometer to make the correct diagnosis. Like the oocysts of *Cryptosporidium* and *Isospora*, the oocysts of *Cyclospora* can be seen using one of many acid-fast staining techniques, including the modified Ziehl-Nielsen or the Kinyoun acid-fast stain. Stool specimens

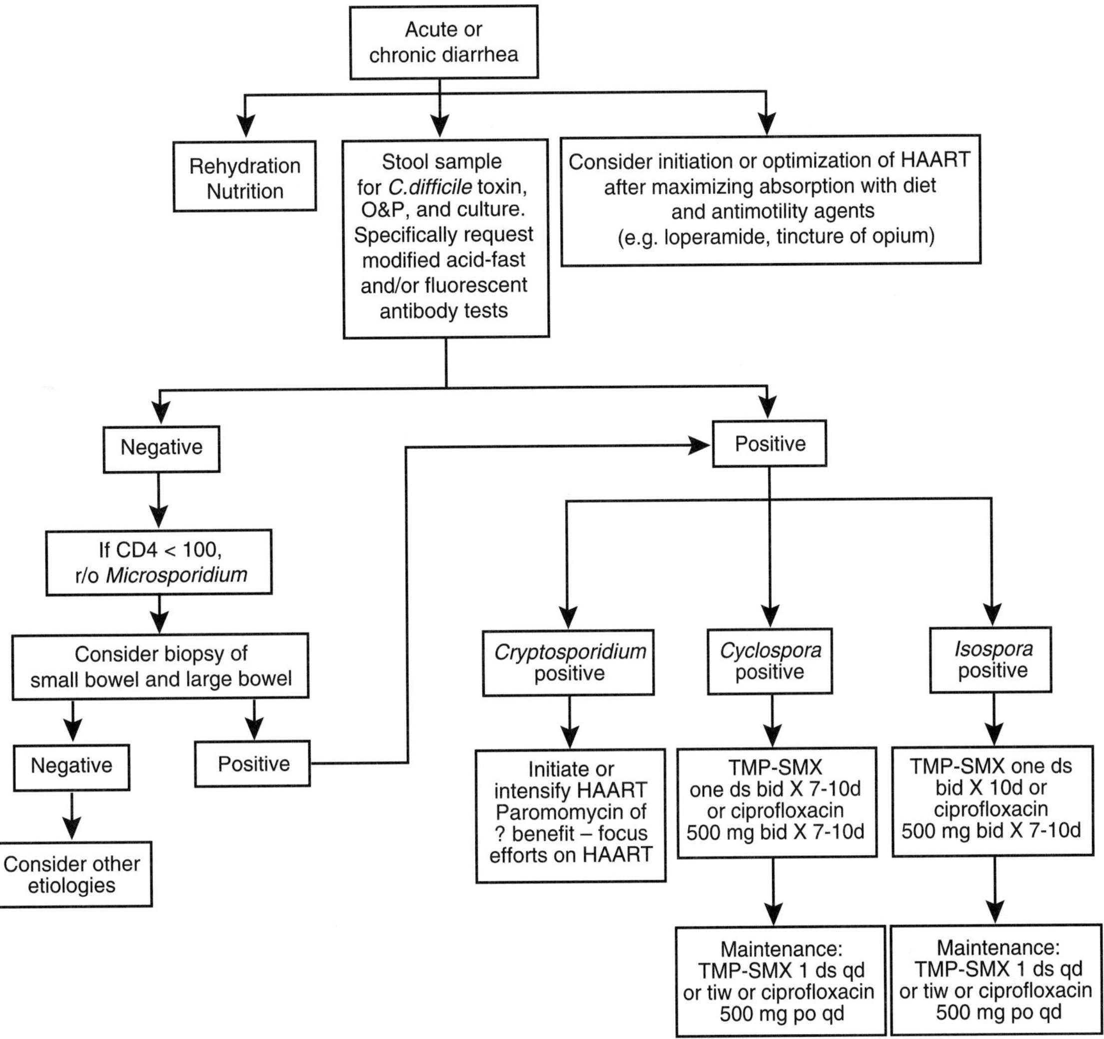

Figure 31–2. Algorithm for managing cryptosporidiosis, isosporidosis, and cyclosporiasis. TMP-SMX, trimethoprin-sulfamethoxazole; DS, double strength; HAART, highly active antiretroviral therapy.

examined for ova and parasites usually are not examined for *Cyclospora* unless it is specifically requested. Alternatively, stool specimens can be fixed in 10% formalin and examined with an epifluorescence microscope, and oocytes are easily discernible by autofluorescence.[53]

Cyclospora has been implicated in water-borne outbreaks in the United States and the developing world. The methods used to prevent water-borne transmission of cryptosporidiosis should be followed to prevent *Cyclospora* infection. Transmission via contaminated raw food as well as raw beef has been reported. Raw fruits and vegetables should be washed thoroughly. In the developing world, infection may increase during the rainy season, as was documented in Nepal.[54] This would not be surprising because seasonal variation is common among other environmental protozoal infections. In Haiti, more than 10% of HIV-infected adults with chronic diarrhea have *Cyclospora* infection.[51] Much like *Isospora,* it appears to be an uncommon cause of diarrhea in adults with AIDS in the United States and Europe.

Treatment of patients with *Cyclospora* (Table 31–1) is effective using trimethoprim-sulfamethoxazole double-strength twice daily for immunocompetent and immunodeficient hosts.[51,54] Ciprofloxacin 500 mg PO bid for 10 days is an effective alternative.[47] Secondary prophylaxis with trimethoprim-sulfamethoxazole (1 double-strength tablet qd or tiw) or ciprofloxacin (500 mg PO qd) is effective for preventing relapse.

An algorithm for the management of infections with *Cryptosporidium, Isospora,* and *Cyclospora* is presented in Figure 31–2.

REFERENCES

1. Fayer E (ed). Cryptosporidium and Cryptosporidiosis, 2nd ed. Boca Raton, FL, CRC Press, 1997.
2. Flanigan TP, Soave R. Cryptosporidiosis. Prog Clin Parasitol 3:1, 1993.
3. Goodgame RW. Understanding intestinal spore-forming protozoa: cryptosporidia, microsporidia, Isospora, and Cyclospora. Ann Intern Med 124:429, 1996.
4. Flanigan TP, Whalen C, Toerner J, et al. Cryptosporidium infection and CD4+ T-lymphocyte counts. Ann Intern Med 116:840, 1992.
5. Hashmey R, Smith NH, Cron S, et al. Cryptosporidiosis in Houston, Texas: a report of 95 cases. Medicine 76:118, 1997.
6. Grube H, Ramratnam B, Ley C, et al. Resolution of AIDS associated cryptosporidiosis after treatment with indinavir. Am J Gastroenterol 92:726, 1997.

7. Milono MD, Tashima KT, Farrar D, et al. Resolution of AIDS-related opportunistic infections with EAART. AIDS Reader Winter:21, 1998.
8. Miao YM, Avad-El-Kariem FM, Franzen C, et al. Eradication of cryptosporidia and microsporidia following successful antiretroviral therapy. J AIDS 25:124, 2000.
9. Carr A, Marriott D, Field A, et al. Treatment of HIV-associated microsporidiosis and cryptosporidiosis with combination antiretroviral therapy. Lancet 351:256, 1998.
10. Ducreux M, Buffet C, Lamy P, et al. Diagnosis and prognosis of AIDS related cholangitis. AIDS 9:875, 1995.
11. Vakil NB, Schwartz SM, Buggy BP, et al. Biliary cryptosporidiosis in HIV-infected people after the waterborne outbreak of cryptosporidiosis in Milwaukee. N Engl J Med 334:19, 1996.
12. Kotler D, Francisco A, Clayton F, et al. Small intestinal injury and parasitic diseases in AIDS. Ann Intern Med 113:444, 1990.
13. Kotler D, Francisco A, Clayton F, et al. Effects of enteric parasitoses and HIV infection upon small intestinal structure and function in patients with AIDS. J Clin Gastroenterol 16:10, 1993.
14. Clark DP, Sears CL. The pathogenesis of cryptosporidiosis. Parasitol Today 12:221, 1996.
15. Tyzzer EF. A sporozoan found in the peptic glands of the common mouse. Proc Soc Exp Biol Med 5:12, 1907.
16. Nime FA, Burek JD, Page DL, et al. Acute enterocolitis in a human being infected with the protozoan Cryptosporidium. Gastroenterology 70:592, 1976.
17. Anonymous. Cryptosporidiosis: assessment of chemotherapy of males with acquired immunodeficiency syndrome (AIDS). MMWR Morb Mortal Wkly Rep 31:589, 1982.
18. DuPont HL, Chappell CL, Sterling CR, et al. The infectivity of Cryptosporidium parvum in healthy volunteers. N Engl J Med 332:855, 1995.
19. Widmer G, Carraway M, Tzipori S. Water-borne Cryptosporidium: a perspective from the U.S.A. Parasitol Today 12:109, 1996.
20. Hayes EB, Matte TD, O'Brien TR, et al. Large community outbreak of cryptosporidiosis due to contamination of a filtered public water supply. N Engl J Med 320:1372, 1989.
21. Anonymous. Cryptosporidiosis among children attending day-care centers Georgia, Pennsylvania, Michigan, California, New Mexico. MMWR Morb Mortal Wkly Rep 33:599, 1984.
22. Combee CL, Collinge ML, Britt EM. Cryptosporidiosis in a hospital-associated day care center. Pediatr Infect Dis J 5:528, 1986.
23. Bruce BB, Blass MA, Blumberg HM, et al. Risk of Cryptosporidium parvum transmission between hospital roommates. Clin Infect Dis 31:947, 2000.
24. D'Antonio RG, Winn RE, Taylor JP, et al. A waterborne outbreak of cryptosporidiosis in normal hosts. Ann Intern Med 103:886, 1985.
25. MacKenzie WR, Hoxie NJ, Proctor ME, et al. A massive outbreak in Milwaukee of Cryptosporidium infection transmitted through the public water supply. N Engl J Med 331:161, 1994.
26. Ungar BLP. Cryptosporidium. In: Mandell GL, Bennett JE, Dolin R (eds) Principals and Practice of Infectious Diseases, 4th ed, vol 1. New York, Churchill Livingstone, 1995, p 2500.
27. Sterling CR, Arrowood MD. Detection of Cryptosporidium sp. infection using a direct immunofluorescence assay. Pediatr Infect Dis J 5(suppl):S139, 1986.
28. Ungar BLP. Enzyme-linked immunoassay for detection for Cryptosporidium antigens in fecal specimens. J Clin Microbiol 28:2491, 1990.
29. Bonnin A, Petrella T, Dubremetz JF, et al. Histopathological method for diagnosis of cryptosporidiosis using monoclonal antibodies. Eur J Clin Microbiol Infect Dis 9:664, 1990.
30. Weber R, Bryan RT, Bishop HS, et al. Threshold of detection of Cryptosporidium oocysts in human stool specimens: evidence for low sensitivity of current diagnostic methods. J Clin Microbiol 29:1323, 1991.
31. Flanigan TP. HIV infection and cryptosporidiosis: protective immune responses. Am J Trop Med Hyg 50(suppl):29, 1994.
32. Lasser KH, Lewin KJ, Ryning FW. Cryptosporidial diarrhea in a patient with congenital hypogammaglobulinemia. Hum Pathol 10:234, 1979.
33. Ungar BLP, Ward DJ, Fayer R, et al. Cessation of Cryptosporidium associated diarrhea in an acquired immunodeficiency syndrome patient after treatment with hyperimmune bovine colostrum. Gastroenterology 98:486, 1990.
34. Tzipori S, Robertson D, Chapman C. Remission of diarrhea due to cryptosporidiosis in an immunodeficient child treated with hyperimmune bovine colostrum. BMJ 293:2283, 1986.
35. Arrowood MJ, Mead J, Mahrt JL, et al. Effects of immune colostrum and orally administered antisporozoite monoclonal antibodies on the outcome of Cryptosporidium parvum in neonatal mice. Infect Immun 57:2283, 1989.
36. Ungar BLP, Kao TC, Burris JA, et al. Independent roles for IFN-gamma and CD4 lymphocytes in protective immunity. J Immunol 147:1014, 1991.
37. Simon DM, Cello JP, Valenzuela J, et al. Multicenter trial of octreotide in patients with refractory acquired immunodeficiency syndrome-associated diarrhea. Gastroenterology 108:1753, 1995.
38. Marshall MS, Flanigan TP. Paromomycin inhibits Cryptosporidium infection of a human enterocyte cell line. J Infect Dis 165:772, 1992.
39. White AC Jr, Chappell CL, Hayat CS, et al. Paromomycin for cryptosporidiosis in AIDS: a prospective, double-blind trial. J Infect Dis 170:419, 1994.
40. Hewitt RG, Yiannoutsos CT, Higgs ES, et al. Paromomycin: no more effective than placebo for treatment of cryptosporidiosis in patients with advanced human immunodeficiency virus infection. Clin Infect Dis 31:1084, 2000.
41. Centers for Disease Control and Prevention. 1997 USPHS/IDSA guidelines for prevention of opportunistic infections in persons infected with human immunodeficiency virus. MMWR Morb Mortal Wkly Rep 46(RR-12):5, 1997.
42. Holmberg SD, Moorman AC, Von Bargen JC, et al. Possible effectiveness of clarithromycin and rifabutin for cryptosporidiosis chemoprophylaxis in HIV diseases. JAMA 279:384, 1998.
43. Fichtenbaum CJ, Zactin R, Feinberg J, et al. Rifabutin but not clarithromycin prevents cryptosporidiosis in persons with advanced HIV infection. AIDS 14:2889, 2000.
44. DeHovitz JA, Pape JW, Boncy M, et al. Clinical manifestations and therapy of Isospora belli infection in patients with the acquired immunodeficiency syndrome. N Engl J Med 315:87, 1986.
45. Keystone JS, Kozarsky P. Isospora belli, Sarcocystis species, Blastocystis hominis, and Cyclospora. In: Mandell GL, Bennett JE, Dolin R (eds) Principles and Practice of Infectious Diseases, 5th ed, vol 2. New York, Churchill Livingstone, 2000, p 2915.
46. Pape JW, Verdier RI, Johnson WD Jr. Treatment and prophylaxis of Isospora belli infection in patients with the acquired immunodeficiency syndrome. N Engl J Med 320:1044, 1989.
47. Verdier RI, Fitzgerald DW, Johnson WD Jr, Pape JW. Trimethoprim/sulfamethoxazole compared with ciprofloxacin for treatment and prophylaxis of Isospora belli and Cyclospora cayetanensis infection in HIV-infected patients: a randomized, controlled trial: brief communication. Ann Intern Med 132:885, 2000.
48. Soave R. Cyclospora: an overview. Clin Infect Dis 23:429, 1996.
49. Ortega Y, Sterling CR, Gilman RH, et al. Cyclospora species, a new protozoan pathogen of humans. N Engl J Med 328:1308, 1996.
50. Massachusetts Medical Society. Outbreak of cyclosporiasis—Northern Virginia, Washington, D.C., Baltimore, Maryland, metropolitan area. MMWR Morb Mortal Wkly Rep 46:689, 1997.
51. Pape JW, Verdier RI, Boncy M, et al. Cyclospora infection in adults infected with HIV: clinical manifestations, treatment, and prophylaxis. Ann Intern Med 121:654, 1994.
52. Herwaldt BL. Cyclospora cayetanensis: a review, focusing on the outbreaks of cyclosporiasis in the 1990s: emerging infections. Clin Infect Dis 31:1040, 2000.
53. Berlin OGW, Peter JB, Gagne C, et al. Autofluorescence and the detection of Cyclospora oocysts. Emerg Infect Dis 4:127, 1998.
54. Hoge CW, Shlim DR, Ghmire M, et al. Placebo-controlled trial of clotrimoxazole for Cyclospora infections among travelers and foreign residents in Nepal. Lancet 345:691, 1990.

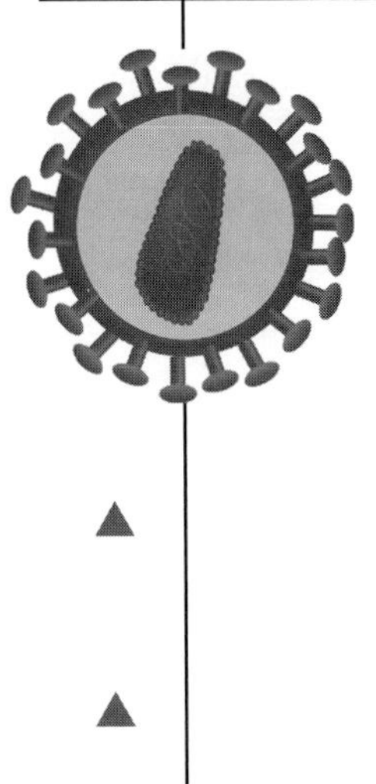

CHAPTER 32

Microsporidiosis

Louis M. Weiss, MD, MPH

Microsporidia is a nontaxonomic designation used to refer to a group of obligate, intracellular parasites belonging to the phylum Microspora. The Microsporidia are ubiquitous organisms that are emerging pathogens in humans. They are most likely zoonotic or waterborne infections (or both). In the immunosuppressed host [e.g., those treated with immunosuppressive drugs or infected with human immunodeficiency virus (HIV), particularly at advanced stages of these diseases] microsporidia can produce a wide range of clinical diseases. The most common manifestation is gastrointestinal tract infection; encephalitis, ocular infection, sinusitis, myositis, and disseminated infection have also been described. These organisms have also been reported in immunocompetent individuals.

In 1857 *Nosema bombycis*, a parasite of silkworms, was the first organism identified as belonging to the order Microsporidia,[1,2] and in 1959 Microsporidia were identified as etiologic in human infection.[3] The Microsporidia are important agricultural parasites in insects, fish, laboratory rodents, rabbits, fur-bearing animals, and primates.[1,2,4] They have been described in dogs and birds kept as household pets.[4,5] In their hosts most infect the digestive tract, although reproductive, respiratory, muscle, excretory, and nervous system infections have been documented.[2,4,6,7]

The phylum Microspora contains more than 1000 species distributed into 144 genera, of which the following have been demonstrated to cause human disease (Table 32–1)[2,4,6,7]: *Nosema* (*N. corneum* renamed *Vittaforma corneae*[8] and *N. algerae* renamed *Bracheola algerae*)[9] *Pleistophora*, *Encephalitozoon*, *Enterocytozoon*[10], *Septata*[11] (reclassified as *Encephalitozoon*[12]), *Trachipleistophora*[13,14] and *Brachiola*.[9] In addition, the genus *Microsporidium* has been used to designate Microsporidia of uncertain taxonomic status.[4] *Vittaforma corneae*,[15] *Enc. cuniculi*,[2] *Enc. hellem*,[16] *T. hominis*,[13] and *Enc. intestinalis*[17,18] have been cultivated in tissue culture systems in vitro. *Enterocytozoon bieneusi* has not been cultivated continuously in vitro, although limited in vitro cultivation of *Ent. bieneusi* has been reported.[19] Adenovirus can mimic the cytopathologic effect of Microsporidia.[20] *N. salmonis*, an organism related to *Ent. bieneusi*, can be grown in vitro.[21,22] Experimental infection of simian immunodeficiency virus (SIV)-infected rhesus monkeys with *Ent. bieneusi* from human tissue has been demonstrated.[23]

Encephalitozoon hellem has been associated with superficial keratoconjunctivitis, sinusitis, respiratory disease, prostatic abscesses, and disseminated infection.[4,6,7] *Encephalitozoon cuniculi* has been associated with hepatitis, encephalitis, and disseminated disease.[24–27] *Encephalitozoon (Septata) intestinalis* is associated with diarrhea, disseminated infection, and superfical keratoconjunctivitis.[4,11,28] *Nosema*, *Vittaforma*, and *Microsporidium* have been associated with stromal keratitis associated with trauma in immunocompetent hosts.[7,15] *Pleistophora*, *Brachiola*, and *Trachipleistophora* have been associated with myositis.[4,9,13,29,30] *Trachipleistophora* has been associated with encephalitis and disseminated disease.[13,14,31] *Enterocytozoon bieneusi*, originally described in humans,[10] is associated with malabsorption, diarrhea, and cholangitis.[4,32]

▲ GENERAL CHARACTERISTICS

The Microsporidia are true eukaryotes, containing a nucleus with a nuclear envelope, an intracytoplasmic membrane system, chromosome separation on mitotic spindles,[33]

▲ **Table 32–1.** MICROSPORIDIA IDENTIFIED AS PATHOGENIC TO
▲ HUMANS

Identified in Patients with AIDS
Encephalitozoon
Enc. cuniculi
Enc. hellem
Enc. intestinalis
Enterocytozoon bieneusi
Trachipleistophora
T. hominis
T. anthropopthera
Pleistophora sp.
Brachiola
B. vesicularum
B. (Nosema) algerae
B. (Nosema) connori
Identified in other Patients
Encephalitzoon
Enc. cuniculi
Enc. hellem
Enc. intestinalis
Enterocytozoon bieneusi
Pleistophora sp.
Brachiola
B. (Nosema) algerae
Nosema
N. ocularum
Vittaforma cornea
Microsporidium
M. africanus
M. ceylonesis

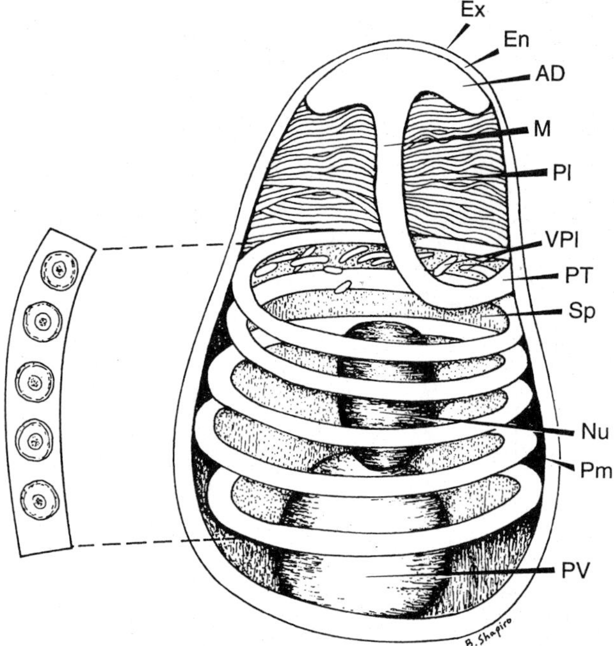

Figure 32–1. Structure of a microsporidian spore. Depending on the species, the size of the spore can vary from 1 to 10 μm, and the number of polar tubule coils can vary from a few to 30 or more. Extrusion apparatus consists of the polar tube (PT), vesiculotubular polaroplast (Vpl), lamellar polaroplast (Pl), anchoring disk (AD), and manubrium (M). This organelle is characteristic of the Microsporidia. A cross section of the coiled polar tube is illustrated. The nucleus (Nu) may be single (e.g., in *Encephalitozoon* and *Enterocytozoon*) or a pair of abutted nuclei termed a diplokaryon (e.g., in *Nosema*). The plasma membrane (Pm) separates the spore coat from the sporoplasm (Sp), which contains ribosomes in a coiled helical array. En, endospore, an inner thicker electron-lucent region; Ex, exospore, an outer electron-dense region; PV, posterior vacuole, a membrane-bound structure. (From Wittner M, Weiss LM [eds]. The Microsporidia and Microsporidiosis. Washington, DC, ASM Press, 1999, with permission.)

and a Golgi apparatus.[34] Microsporidia lack mitochondria and centrioles and have prokaryote-size ribosomes[35,36] lacking a 5.8S ribosome subunit but having sequences homologous to the 5.8S region in the 23S subunit.[37] The small subunit rRNA of several Microsporidia have been sequenced and found to be significantly shorter than both eukaryotic and prokaryotic small subunit rRNA.[36,38] These rRNA genes are in a subtelomeric location on each chromosome of *Enc. cuniculi*[39,40] and lack the paromomycin binding site.[41] Sequence data of rRNA from the Microsporidia have been used to develop diagnostic polymerase chain reaction (PCR) primers and in the study of phylogenetic relations (reviewed by Weiss and Vossbrinck[38] and Weiss[42]). The karyotype of several members of the phylum Microspora has been determined by pulsed field electrophoresis. The genome size of the Microsporidia varies from 2.3 to 19.5 Mb.[4] The genomic size of the Encephalitizoonidae is less than 3.0 Mb, making them the smallest eukaryotic nuclear genomes so far identified.[39,43,44]

Microsporidia are currently classified on the basis of ultrastructural features, including the size and morphology of the spores, number of coils of the polar tube, developmental life cycle, and the host–parasite relationship.[1,45,46] Molecular analysis of rRNA genes has begun to alter this classification system.[38,47] Antigenic differences between Microsporidia demonstrable by sodium dodecyl sulfate-polyacrylamide gel electrophoresis (SDS-PAGE) and Western blot analysis[48,49] have been used as adjunctive evidence when determining phylogenetic relationships among the Microsporidia infecting humans.[12,49] Molecular phylogenetic data indicates that the Microsporidia are related to fungi and are not "primitive eukaryotes."[50–52]

Microsporidia form characteristic unicellular spores (Fig. 32–1) that are environmentally resistant. *Enc. cuniculi* spores remain viable for 6 days when in water and 4 weeks when dry at 22°C.[53] *Nosema bombycis* spores may remain viable for 10 years in distilled water. Spores may be killed by exposure for 30 minutes to 70% ethanol, 1% formaldehyde, or 2% Lysol or by autoclaving at 120°C for 10 minutes.[53] Whereas Microsporidia spores can be as large as 12 μm, the Microsporidia infecting humans have spores that range from 1 to 4 μm. The spore coat consists of an electron-dense, proteinaceous exospore, an electron-lucent endospore composed of chitin and protein, and an inner membrane or plasmalemma.[54] A defining characteristic of all Microsporidia is an extrusion apparatus that consists of a polar tube attached to the inside of the anterior end of the spore by an anchoring disc; depending on the species, it forms 4 to approximately 30 coils around the sporoplasm in the spore. During germination the polar tube rapidly everts, forming a hollow tube that brings the sporoplasm into intimate contact with the host cell. The polar tube provides a bridge to deliver the sporoplasm to the host cell.

The mechanism by which the polar tube interacts with the host cell membrane is not known, but it may require the participation of host cell proteins such as actin.[55] It is possible that the sporoplasm interacts with the host cell membrane as it emerges from the polar tube. If a spore is phagocytosed by a host cell, germination occurs and the polar tube can pierce the phagocytic vacuole, delivering sporoplasm into the host cell cytoplasm. The overall process of germination and formation of the polar tube inoculates the sporoplasm directly into a host cell, functioning essentially like a hypodermic needle.[56–58]

Conditions that promote germination vary widely among species, presumably reflecting the organism's adaptation to its host and external environment[59,60] (reviewed in Wittner and Weiss[4]). Conditions that promote spore discharge include pH shifts,[61] dehydration followed by rehydration,[62] various cations[63] and anions,[64] mucin or polyanions,[65] hydrogen peroxide,[60,66] ultraviolet radiation, and the calcium ionophore A 23187.[67] Inhibitors of spore discharge include magnesium chloride, ammonium chloride, low salt concentrations, sodium fluoride, ultraviolet light, temperatures higher than 40°C, calcium channel antagonists, calmodulin inhibitors,[66] cytochalasin D, demecolcine, and itraconazole.[66] Regardless of the stimuli required for activation, all Microsporidia appear to exhibit the same response to the stimuli (i.e., increased intrasporal osmotic pressure). This results in an influx of water into the spore accompanied by swelling of the polaroplasts and posterior vacuole prior to spore discharge. In *Brachiola (Nosema) algerae*, it has been proposed that activation brings trehalose in contact with the enzyme trehalase, causing increased osmotic pressure.[68–71] The polar tube then discharges from the anterior pole of the spore in an explosive reaction, occurring in less than 2 seconds. It has been suggested that the hollow tube is formed by a process of eversion, similar to everting the finger of a glove.[56]

▲ EPIDEMIOLOGY

Although intitially regarded as rare, Microsporidia are now believed to be common enteric pathogens that are self-limited or asymptomatic in normal hosts.[72–74] Reported prevalence rates among those with acquired immunodeficiency syndrome (AIDS) have varied between 2% and 70% depending on the symptoms of the population studied and the diagnostic technique employed.[6,7,43,54] Co-infection with different Microsporidia or other enteric pathogens can occur. Asymptomatic carriage can occur in immunocompromised patients. *Enc. cuniculi* isolates from various animal species have been identified and separated based on the number of tetranucleotide repeats (5′GTTT3′) in the intergenic spacer region of their rRNA genes.[75] Differences have also been found in the intergenic spacer region of rRNA genes of *Ent. bieneusi*.[76,77] Such differences may prove useful for epidemiologic identification of the environmental source of Microsporidia isolated from humans.

Serosurveys in humans have demonstrated a high prevalence of antibodies to *Enc. cuniculi* and *Enc. hellem*, suggesting that asymptomatic infection may be common.[78,79] Serologic cross-reactivity among Microsporidia has been demonstrated by immunofluorescence[80] and Western blotting.[81] Singh et al.[82] found positive titers in 6 of 69 healthy adults in England, 38 of 89 Nigerians with tuberculosis, 13 of 70 Malaysians with filariasis, and 33 of 92 Ghanians with malaria. In another study 14 of 115 travelers returning from the tropics and 0 of 48 nontravelers were seropositive.[83] In a study of HIV-positive male subjects, 10 of 30 were seropositive and all had traveled to the tropics.[84] These data suggest that Microsporidia are common in humans and, similar to other gastrointestinal pathogens, are associated with travel or residence in the tropics or developing nations.

It is likley that many of the Microsporidia infections are zoonotic. *Encephalitozoon* is a widely distributed parasite of mammals and birds, and the onset of microsporidiosis has been associated with exposure to livestock, fowl, and pets.[74] *Encephalitozoon* has been described in lovebirds and budgerigars (parakeets),[5] and one case of *Enc. hellem* has been reported in a patient who had two pet lovebirds.[85] Up to 30% of dogs in animal shelters may excrete microsporidia in their stools, and *Enc. cuniculi* was etiologic in the death of Maltese puppies in a recent outbreak.[74,86] *Encephalitozoon* was found in the stools of many animals in a survey in an epidemiologic survery in Mexico. *Ent. bieneusi* has been reported in pigs,[87] dogs, and SIV-infected rhesus monkeys.[88] *Nosema* and *Vittaforma* infections are believed to be due to traumatic inoculation of environmental spores of insect pathogens into the cornea.

It has been possible to transmit *Encephalitozoon* via rectal infection in rabbits, suggesting that sexual transmission may also occur.[89] *Enc. hellem* has been demonstrated in respiratory tract mucosa as well as the prostate and urogenital tract of patients, raising the possibility of respiratory and sexual transmission in humans. Although congenital transmission of *Enc. cuniculi* has been demonstrated in rabbits, mice, dogs, horses, foxes, and squirrel monkeys, no such congenital transmission has been demonstrated in humans.[90–92] It is possible that many of the microsporidia are also water-borne pathogens. Enterocytozoonidae such as *Nucleospora* (previously *Enterocytozoon*) *salmonis*[93] have been found in fish,[94] and many of the human pathogenic Microsporidia have been detected in surface water supplies.[95–99]

▲ MICROSPORIDIAN INFECTION IN NON-AIDS PATIENTS

Levaditi et al. suggested in 1923 that microsporidians could be associated with human disease.[100] This was proven in 1973 when a 4-month-old athymic male infant died with severe diarrhea and malabsorption; at autopsy microsporidia (*N. connori*) were discovered in the lungs, stomach, small and large bowel, kidneys, adrenal glands, myocardium, liver, and diaphragm.[101] Disease due to *Encephalitozoon* was suggested by positive immunoglobulin G (IgG) and IgM indirect immunofluorescence assays (using *Enc. cuniculi*) in a 3-year-old boy with seizures and hepatomegaly.[78,83] *Encephalitozoon sp.* was also reported[3] in a 9-year-old Japanese boy with headache, vomiting, spastic convulsions, and recurrent fever infection. *Encephalitozoon sp*. have been found in the stools of patients in surveys for the etiology of diarrhea in less developed countries.[102] *Ent. bieneusi* has been identified as a cause of self-limited diarrhea in immunocompetent hosts,[72,103–105] in 1% of African children with diarrhea in an epidemiologic study,[106,107] and in patients undergoing liver and bone marrow transplantation.[108–113] A *Pleistophora* sp. was identified in 1985 in skeletal muscle of an HIV-negative patient with myositis and has also been described in the skeletal muscle of HIV-positive patients.[6,29,30] *Brachiola algerae* infection of the skin with dissemination has been seen in a patient with leukemia.[114]

Two cases of corneal microsporidiosis due to *Microsporidium africanus*[115] in Botswana and *Microsporidium ceylonesis*[91] in Sri Lanka were described in 1973 and 1981, respectively. Additional cases of microsporidian keratitis have been identified in immunocompetent hosts.[4] One of these organisms was classified as *N. ocularum*,[116,117] and the other, which was successfully propagated in vitro, was named *N. corneum*[118] (now *V. cornea*[8]). Among immunologically normal patients with corneal infections, one patient required enucleation,[115] one underwent unsuccessful penetrating keratoplasty,[119] one was successfully treated with a corneal transplant,[116] and the last was maintained on a variety of topical agents without effect until keratoplasty.[118]

▲ MICROSPORIDIAN INFECTION IN AIDS PATIENTS

Microsporidia were recognized as opportunistic pathogens causing diarrhea and wasting in AIDS patients in 1985.[10] Since then, although most reported cases have still involved diarrhea, the spectrum of diseases caused by these organisms has expanded to include keratoconjunctivitis, disseminated disease, hepatitis, myositis, sinusitis, kidney and urogenital infection, ascites, cholangitis, and asymptomatic carriage.[4,6,74]

In patients with HIV infection evaluated for diarrhea the prevalence of microsporidiosis has ranged from 7% to 50%.[120–127] Weber et al. examined 1271 stool specimens from 845 HIV-infected patients in Switzerland and found Microsporidia in 8 of 88 patients with chronic diarrhea, 3 of 57 patients with self-limited diarrhea, and 0 of 700 asymptomatic patients.[6] Rabeneck et al., in a prospective study, found microsporidia in 29% of patients seen at an HIV primary care clinic, but there was no association with the presence of diarrhea (18/55 with diarrhea and 13/51 without diarrhea had microsporidia on duodenal biopsy).[128,129] Patients with microsporidiosis in this study had a mean CD4+ T-lymphocyte count of 113 cells/mm^3. It is thus likely, as is true for other gastrointestinal protozoa, that asymptomatic carrier states exist. During a 15-month follow-up of this study, diarrhea developed in 2 of the 13 asymptomatic patients and continued in the 18 symptomatic patients.[130] Kotler and Orenstein, in a study of patients presenting to a gastroenterology clinic, found that 39% of patients with HIV and diarrhea (55/141) had microsporidiosis and that the presence of microsporidia was associated with wasting, a mean CD4+ T-lymphocyte count of 28 cells/mm^3, and abnormal D-xylose tests.[131] In contrast, only 2.6% of HIV patients without diarrhea (1/38) had microsporidiosis, and this patient subsequently developed diarrhea on follow-up. Coyle et al.,[132] using the polymerase chain reaction (PCR) employing primers to rRNA gene of *Ent. bieneusi*, found that 37% (25/68) of HIV patients with diarrhea and 2.3% (1/43) of HIV patients without diarrhea had microsporidiosis. The one asymptomatic patient had an abnormal D-xylose test. Based on these studies microsporidia appear to demonstrate strength of association, coherence, and reproducibility with respect to being etiologic for a diarrheal syndrome. Further evidence of the association of microsporidia with diarrhea is provided by the utility of albendazole in the treatment of microsporidian infection. Therapy with albendazole results in cure of diarrhea associated with the elimination of *Enc. intestinalis* from the stools of infected patients[133]; treatment with fumagillin has a similar effect in patients with *Ent. bieneusi* infection.[134]

Enterocytozoon sp.

The major syndrome associated with microsporidiosis is diarrhea and wasting. This is usually due to *Ent. bieneusi* (more than 90% of cases in the United States) and occasionally *Enc. intestinalis* (in Europe this organism may be a more frequent cause of diarrhea[18]). *Ent. bieneusi* occurs most commonly when CD4+ T-lymphocyte counts are less than 50 cells/mm^3; it presents with chronic nonbloody diarrhea, anorexia, weight loss, and bloating without associated fever. Although originally thought to invade only enterocytes, it has been demonstrated that *Ent. bieneusi* can also invade cholangioepithelium.[32] When present in the cholangioepithelium this organism has been associated with sclerosing cholangitis, AIDS cholangiopathy, and cholecystitis. Interestingly, an *Ent. bieneusi*-like organism has been identified in SIV-infected rhesus monkeys as the etiologic agent of cholangitis and hepatitis.[88,135] Systemic dissemination does not appear to occur with *Ent. bieneusi*. One case report described this organism in nasal mucosa, which likely resulted from direct inoculation of spores from gastrointestinal secretions.[136] Reports indicate that *Ent. bieneusi* may cause self-limited infections in immunocompetent patients.[72] Other intestinal pathogens may occur simultaneously or sequentially with this or any other microsporidian.

This parasite has a unique intracellular developmental life cycle.[137] A characteristic feature of this organism is the presence of electron-lucent inclusions demonstrating a lamellar structure. These inclusions are closely associated with the nuclear envelope or endoplasmic reticulum (or both). The earliest intraepithelial stages of the parasite are rounded proliferative cells limited by a typical unit membrane in direct contact with the host cell cytoplasm. In these cells nuclear division is not immediately followed by cytokinesis, thus resulting in the production of multinucleate proliferative plasmodia. After the production of multiple nuclei the parasites form electron-dense disk-like structures that cluster in stacks of three to six, eventually forming the coiled portion of the polar tube. When these multinucleated sporagonial plasmodia divide by invagination of the plasmalemma, multiple spores are formed. In mature spores the polar tubule has five to seven coils that appear in two rows when seen in cross sections by transmission electron microscopy.

Encephalitozoon sp.

Encephalitozoon sp. are widely distributed in many animals.[74] Three members of the family Encephalitozoonidae have been associated with disease in humans: *Enc. cuniculi*, *Enc. hellem*, and *Enc. intestinalis* (previously known as *Septata intestinalis*). It appears that these microsporidia have the capacity to disseminate widely in their hosts, and involvement of most organs by these organisms has now been documented.[4,6,74,138]

Encephalitozoon intestinalis has been associated with diarrheal disease,[11] cholangitis,[139] keratoconjunctivitis, osteomyelitis of the mandible,[140] and disseminated infection[133,141] in AIDS patients. The ability of this parasite to disseminate correlates with its ability to grow in many cell types both in vivo and in vitro. Elimination of this parasite from patients with diarrhea treated with albendazole correlates with the resolution of symptoms.[133,142] The parasite develops in the cytoplasm of intestinal enterocytes, macrophages, fibroblasts, and endothelial cells of the lamina propria and in epithelial cells of the kidney and gallbladder.[11] Sporogony is tetrasporous, and tubular appendages originate from the sporont surface and terminate in an enlarged bulb-like structure. Unlike other Encephalitizoonidae, *Enc. intestinalis*-infected cells have a unique parasite-secreted fibrillar network surrounding the developing organisms, so the parasitophorous vacuole appears septate. Mature spores in cross section have a single row of four to seven coils of polar tubules.

Encephalitozoon cuniculi has been associated with hepatitis,[143] peritonitis,[144] hepatic failure,[25] disseminated disease with fever,[24,25,138] renal insufficiency, and intractable cough.[145] These infections have been reported to respond to albendazole.[24,138,145] Granulomatous encephalitis due to *Enc. cuniculi* was first described in rabbits in 1922, and cases of encephalitis and seizures due to *Enc. cuniculi* have been reported in AIDS patients.[26] *Enc. cuniculi* was identified in cerebrospinal fluid, sputum, urine, and stool specimens from a 29-year-old man with a CD4+ T-lymphocyte count of 0 cells/mm^3, and he had enhancing lesions demonstrable by both computed tomography (CT) and magnetic resonance imaging (MRI) of the brain that diminished when albendazole was administered.[26]

Encephalitozoon hellem has been reported to cause disseminated disease associated with renal failure, nephritis, pneumonia, bronchitis, and keratoconjunctivitis.[146–148] This organism is also recognized to cause infection of the nasal epithelium and is an important etiologic agent in cases of sinusitis in patients with HIV infection. Among the ocular infections due to Encephalitozoonidae reported in the literature, most have been attributed to *Enc. hellem*, including three cases originally classified as due to *Enc. cuniculi*.[7,149] The remaining cases have been due to *Encephalitozoon sp.* or *Enc. intestinalis*.[150] Ocular microsporidian infection in HIV-1-infected patients has been restricted to the superficial epithelium of the cornea and conjunctiva (i.e., superficial keratoconjunctivitis) and has rarely progressed to corneal ulceration. Patients present with bilateral punctate epithelial keratopathy and conjunctival inflammation resulting in redness, foreign body sensation, photophobia, and changes in visual acuity. Slit-lamp examination usually demonstrates punctate epithelial opacities, granular epithelial cells with irregular fluorescein uptake, conjunctival injection, superficial corneal infiltrates, and a noninflamed anterior chamber.

Encephalitozoon hellem has been cultured in vitro from the urine of patients with disseminated microsporidiosis[151] and those with keratoconjunctivitis.[49] As this organism has been found in the lung, it has been suggested that respiratory spread of this microsporidian may occur.[147] Due to the presence of this organism in the urogenital tract including the prostate, and the ability to transmit this organism by rectal inoculation in rabbits, it is possible that *Enc. hellem* may be acquired as a sexually transmitted disease.[152] *Enc. hellem* and *Enc. cuniculi* have similar developmental life cycles.[33] The genus is characterized by the presence of a phagosome-like parasitophorous vacuole. Nuclei of all stages are unpaired. Meronts divide repeatedly by binary fission. Sporonts divide into two sporoblasts that mature into spores. No tubular appendages or fibrillar networks are produced, as is seen in *Enc. intestinalis*. In cross section the mature spore has five to seven coils in single rows (Fig. 32–2).

Other Microsporidia

Trachipleistophora hominis is a pansporoblastic microsporidian that has been described in several patients with disseminated disease in the setting of AIDS.[13] The organism has been cultivated in vitro. *Trachipleistophora anthropophthera* infection has presented as encephalitis, myositis, and keratoconjunctivitis.[14,31] Several of these patients responded clinically to albendazole. *Brachiola vesicularum* caused myositis in an HIV-1-infected patient and

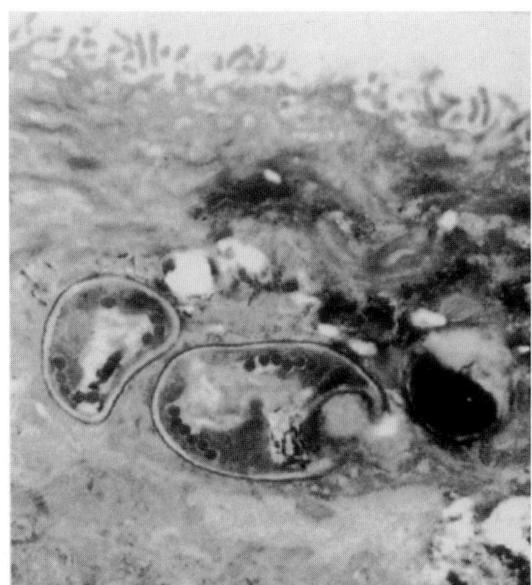

Figure 32–2. Electron micrograph of conjunctival scraping demonstrating Microsporidia (*Encephalitozoon hellem*). Thick-walled spores with single nuclei and five or six coils of polar tubes are demonstrated. (Courtesy of A. Cali and P.M. Takvorian, Rutgers University. From Weiss LM, Keohane EM. The uncommon gastrointestinal protozoa: microsporidia, Blastocystis, Isospora, Dientamoeba and Balantidium. Curr Clin Top Infect Dis 17:147, 1997, with permission.)

▲ **Table 32–2.** DIAGNOSIS OF MICROSPORIDIOSIS

Test	Utility
Urine examination	This is often positive in cases of microsporidiosis due to microsporidia other than *Enterocytozoon* and should be done in all suspected microsporidia cases.
Stool examination	This is useful for gastrointestinal presentations. At least three stools should be examined. The combination of chromotrope and chemofluorescent stains provides the highest sensitivity and specificity.
Endoscopy	This should be considered for all patients with chronic diarrhea of more than 2 months' duration and negative stool and urine examinations. In this group endoscopy has yielded a diagnosis of microsporidia presence in up to 30% of patients. Tissue should be examined by a microsporidial stain. Touch preparations are useful for rapid diagnosis (within 24 hours). If microsporidia are demonstrated to invade the lamina propria, the urine examination should be repeated, as *Encephalitozoon* is are the most likely etiologic agent. In this setting albendazole has high efficacy.
Polymerase chain reaction (PCR)	This test is available as a research technique. Species identification can be performed on stool, urine, and tissue samples.
Electron microscopy	This identifies the species of microsporidia involved and is crucial for identification of new species. It is essential for the characterization of microsporidia in unusual or new locations.
Conjunctival scrapings	This has a high diagnostic yield in microsporidian keratoconjunctivitis. Urine examination should also be performed in suspected cases to screen for disseminated microsporidiosis.
Nasal scrapings	This can be useful for the diagnosis of microsporidian sinusitis. As most of the microsporidia associated with sinusitis are present in the kidneys, urine examination should be routine for suspected sinusitis cases. If these tests are negative, biopsy of nasal mucosa may be useful for diagnosis.
Serology	This is not useful for diagnosis but may be useful for epidemiologic surveys.

responded to a regimen of albendazole and itraconazole.[9] Cases of myositis due to *Pleistophora* sp. have also been reported in AIDS patients.[29,30,153]

▲ DIAGNOSIS

Diagnostic tests for patients with suspected microsporidiosis are described in Table 32–2. In general, a urine examination should be done whenever microsporidiosis is considered, as microsporidia associated with disseminated disease such as *Encephalitozoon* and *Trachipleistophora* have invariably been present in such specimens when examined. As gastrointestinal disease with *Ent. bieneusi* is not associated with disseminated disease, this organism is not seen in the urine. For gastrointestinal disease, examination of three stools with chromotrope and chemofluorescent stains is often sufficient for diagnosis. If the stool examination is negative and the diarrhea is chronic (more than 2 months' duration), endoscopy should be performed.

Effective morphologic demonstration of microsporidia by light microscopy can be accomplished by staining methods that produce differential contrast between the spores of the microsporidia and the cells and debris in clinical samples (e.g., stool) in which they are found. In addition, given the small size of the spores (1 to 5 μm) adequate magnification (i.e., 1000×) is required for visualization. Chromotrope 2R,[127] calcofluor white (fluorescent brightener 28),[154] and Uvitex 2B[126] have been reported to be useful as selective stains for microsporidia in stool specimens and other body fluids (Fig. 32–3). The chromotrope 2R-based method of Weber et al.[127] is similar to a standard trichrome stain, but the chromotrope 2R concentration is 10-fold higher and the staining time is longer. Further modifications of this method by Ryan et al.,[155] using aniline blue in place of fast green, and Kokoskin et al.,[156] using an elevated temperature, are preferred by some laboratories. Using this stain, spores appear as 1 to 3-μm ovoid light pink structures with a belt-like stripe girding them diagonally and equatorially against a green or blue background. Spores can also be visualized by ultraviolet (UV) microscopy using chemofluorescent optical brightening agents such as Calcofluor

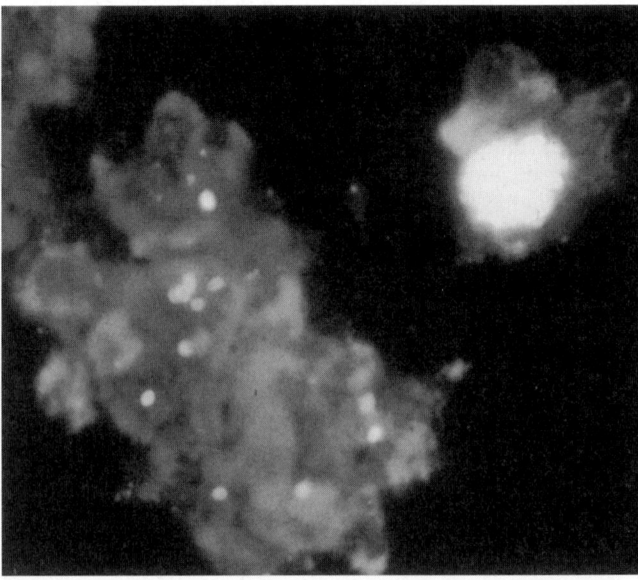

Figure 32–3. Calcofluor white stain demonstrating fluorescent *Encephalitozoon hellem* spores in the urine of a patient with disseminated infection. (Courtesy of E. Didier, Tulane Regional Primate Research Center. From Weiss LM, Keohane EM. The uncommon gastrointestinal protozoa: microsporidia, Blastocystis, Isospora, Dientamoeba and Balantidium. Curr Clin Top Infect Dis 17:147, 1997, with permission.)

white M2R (fluorescent brightener 28, Fungi-Fluor) and Uvitex 2B (Fungiqual A; Dieter Reinehr and Manfred Rembold, Spezialchemikalien fur die Medizinische Diagnostik, Kandern, Germany), which stain chitin in the spore wall (endospore layer).

Microsporidia in body fluids other than stool have been visualized with Chromotrope 2R, optical brightening agents, Giemsa, Brown-Hopps Gram stain, acid-fast staining, or Warthin-Starry silver staining. Microsporidiosis can be also be diagnosed by examining biopsy material or touch preparations. In paraffin-embedded sections, microsporidial spores are discernible to experienced observers with hematoxylin and eosin and can also be seen with Chromotrope 2A or Gram (Brown-Hopps) stain. Microscopic examination of corneal tissue, obtained by gentle rubbing over the conjunctiva and cornea with a tissue swab, has revealed multiple gram-positive, oval organisms in epithelial cells. These organisms often contain a periodic acid-Schiff (PAS)-positive anterior granule. Fresh tissue may also be examined by phase-contrast microscopy, and because of their thick walls unstained spores are refractile, appearing green and possibly birefringent.

Using 50 stool specimens positive for microsporidia by transmission electron microscopy (TEM), both the chromotrope 2R and chemofluorescent brightening stains identified 100% of specimens when at least 50 high power (i.e., 1000×) fields were examined.[157] In a study employing Uvitex 2B, all of the 186 stool samples examined from 19 patients with biopsy-proven *Ent. bieneusi* infection were positive, and none of the 55 stool samples from 16 biopsy-negative patients were positive.[126] In another study Uvitex 2B staining detected microsporidia in all chromotrope 2R stain-positive samples and identified several additional samples (from three patients) as positive.[158] On reexamination, stool samples from these patients were also positive with the chromotrope 2R stain. All patients with positive duodenal biopsies were positive on stool examination by chromotrope or chemofluorescence methods. Of the six patients with negative duodenal biopsies who were identified as positive by chromotrope or chemofluorescence staining, four had confirmation of microsporidia in the stool by TEM. In infections with low numbers of spores it is likely that these noninvasive methods have a higher sensitivity than biopsy techniques. The limit of detecting microsporidia by these techniques appears to be 5×10^4 organisms/ml (500 organisms/10 μl).[157] Overall, the sensitivity of the chemofluorescent brightener-based stains is slightly higher than chromotrope-based stains (especially when low numbers of spores are present in a sample); however, the specificity of the chemofluorescent stains is lower (90% vs. 100% in one study).[157] Based on an analysis of the performance characteristics of these smears, it has been suggested that chemofluorescent stains should be utilized for screening stool specimens and that all positive specimens be confirmed by a chromotrope 2R stain before being considered truely positive. Neither the chromotrope nor the chemofluorescent stains provide information on the species of microsporidia being identified. Another report notes that these stains may give false positive results due to insect microsporidia contaminating ingested food.

Polyclonal serum prepared to other microsporidia (*Enc. cuniculi*) has been reported to react with *Ent. bieneusi*.[81,159] Monoclonal antibodies to *Enc. hellem*,[160] *Enc. intestinalis*,[161] and *Ent. bieneusi*[162,163] have been described but are not commercially available. Diagnosis of microsporidiosis by detecting IgM antibody was reported in a case of disseminated *Enc. cuniculi* infection with encephalitis in an immunocompetent 2-year-old boy.[3] Enzyme-linked immunosorbent assay (ELISA) titers to *Enc. hellem*, *Enc. cuniculi*, and *Vit. corneae* were not useful for diagnosis in a study of 12 AIDS patients with *Ent. bieneusi*, 2 AIDS patients with *Enc. intestinalis*, and 2 immunocompetent patients with *Vit. corneae*.[164] False-negative titers were present in seven of the patients with microsporidiosis, and half of the control patients (without clinical microsporidiosis) had positive serology to Microsporidia. This is consistent with other AIDS-associated infections in which serology has not proven useful.

Homology PCR cloning of the rRNA genes of many of the microsporidia pathogenic in humans has been accomplished and are in the GenBank database.[38,42] It has been possible to design PCR primers to these small subunit rRNA genes to identify microsporidia at the species level in clinical samples without the need for ultrastructural examination. Two main approaches have been employed in the construction of PCR primers for microsporidia: the design of universal pan-microsporidia primers and the design of species-specific primer pairs. These PCR techniques have been applied to biospy specimens, urine, cultures, and more recently stool specimens and should greatly facilitate both diagnosis and epidemiologic studies.[165–167] See Weiss and Vossbrinck[38] for a review of the PCR tests for microsporidiosis.

▲ TREATMENT

Two agents, fumagillin and albendazole, have demonstrated consistent activity against Microsporidia in vitro and in vivo.[133,134,141,142,168–178] Despite initial reports of favorable treatment with metronidazole for intestinal infection with *Ent. bieneusi*, this drug has not been effective in other studies,[32,121,141,178,179] nor is there is in vitro activity of metronidazole against *Enc. cuniculi*.[172] Other medications used without success in the treatment of gastrointestinal microsporidiosis are azithromycin, paromomycin (microsporidia lack the binding site for this drug), and quinacrine. Atovaquone has been anecdotally reported to have limited efficacy in microsporidiosis,[178,180] but there is no in vitro activity.[172] Sparfloxacin and chloroquine have demonstrated in vitro activity against microsporidia but have not been used clinically.[172] Prophylaxis with trimethoprim-sulfamethoxazole is not effective for preventing microsporidiosis, and this drug combination has no in vitro or in vivo activity against these organisms.[181] Thalidomide[182,183] and octreotide have been reported to decrease diarrhea in patients with microsporidiosis probably secondary to their effects on enterocytes. For a review of drugs used in microsporidiosis in animals see Costa and Weiss.[184]

▲ **Table 32–3.** THERAPY FOR MICROSPORIDIOSIS

Organism	Drug	Dosage[a]
Enterocytozoon bieneusi	No effective commercial treatment. Oral fumagillin 60 mg/day appears effective. Albendazole[b] has resulted in clinical improvement in up to 50% of patients.	
Encephalitzoon infection (e.g., systemic, sinusitis, encephalitis, hepatitis)		
Enc. cuniculi	Albendazole	400 mg bid
Enc. hellem	Albendazole	400 mg bid
Enc. intestinalis	Albendazole	400 mg bid
Encephalitozoon keratoconjunctivitis	Fumagillin solution[c] (Fumadil B 3 mg/ml)	2 drops every 2 hours for 4 days, then 2 drops 4 times a day[d]
	Patients may also need albendazole if systemic infection is present	
Trachipleistophora hominis	Albendazole	400 mg bid
Brachiola vesicularum	Albendazole ± Itraconozole	400 mg bid 400 mg qd

[a]The duration of treatment for microsporidiosis has not been established. Relapse of infection has occurred upon stopping treatment. Patients should be maintained on treatment for at least 4 weeks, and most patients should be on treatment indefinitely.
[b]Albendazole 400 mg bid.
[c]Fumidil B (fumagillin bicylohexylammonium; Mid-Continent Agrimarketing, Overland Park, KS, USA).
[d]Eyedrops should be continued indefinitely; relapse is common on stopping treatment.

Albendazole, a benzimidazole that binds to β-tubulin, has activity against microsporidiosis (Tables 32–3 and 32–4). Albendazole is effective in inhibiting the growth of *Nosema bombycis* in vitro in *Spodoptera frugiperda* cells and in vivo in *Heliocoverpa zea* larvae and pupae.[171] In vitro albendazole has activity against all of the Encephalitozoonidae (*Enc. hellem, Enc. cuniculi, Enc. intestinalis*) at concentrations of less than 0.1 mg/ml, and this is true in vivo as well in animal models.[185,188,202] Data on the sequence of the Encephalitzoonidae β-tubulin genes demonstrates an amino acid sequence associated with sensitivity to benzimidazoles (e.g., albendazole) in these microsporidia.[203,204] Albendazole is poorly absorbed: Peak serum levels 2 hours after an oral dose are 0.20 to 0.94 μg/ml, but absorption is increased if the medication is taken with food containing relatively high concentrations of fat. This drug is protein-bound (70%); is distributed in the blood, bile, and cerebrospinal fluid; and is eliminated by the kidneys. After oral administration hepatic metabolism converts albendazole to albendazole sulfoxide, which is detectable in the systemic circulation. Although side effects are rare, the following have been reported: hypersensitivity (rash, pruritus, fever), neutropenia (reversible), central nervous system (CNS) effects (dizziness, headache), gastrointestinal disturbances (abdominal pain, diarrhea, nausea, vomiting), hair loss (reversible), and elevated hepatic enzymes (reversible). Albendazole is not carcinogenic or mutagenic. In animals (rats and rabbits), at dosages of 30 mg/kg it was embryotoxic and teratogenic. Thus albendazole is not recommended for use in pregnant women. There have been no well controlled studies during human pregnancy. There is a report of pseudomembranous colitis following albendazole treatment.[205]

In AIDS patients with diarrhea due to *Enc. intestinalis*, treatment with albendazole results in resolution of the diarrhea and elimination of the organism.[133,169] In cases of chronic sinusitis and disseminated infection due to *Enc. hellem*, treatment with 400 mg of albendazole twice daily resulted in resolution of symptoms and clearance of the organism.[148,206] Clinical improvement was demonstrated after albendazole treatment in a patient with disseminated *Enc. cuniculi* infection involving the CNS, conjunctiva, sinuses, kidney, and lungs.[26,145] Albendazole (400 mg bid) also resulted in clinical improvement in patients with disseminated infection with myositis due to *T. hominis* and a patient with myositis due to a *Bachiola vesicularum*.[9,13]

Albendazole treatment has not been as successful against *Ent. bieneusi* infection. Although in some patients treatment with albendazole resulted in symptomatic improvement, the organism persisted during treatment in all patients with no improvement in D-xylose absorption tests.[168,175] In addition, relapse occurred rapidly upon discontinuation of albendazole therapy. In a study of 29 patients with *Ent. bieneusi* infection 50% had symptomatic improvement after albendazole treatment.[168] An additonal 37 patients (66 patients in total) have been treated on this protocol with similar results. Other studies have found that albendazole had no efficacy in *Ent. bieneusi* infection.[186]

Fumagillin was isolated in 1949 from *Aspergillus fumigatus*. Amebicidal effects were first noted in vitro against *Entamoeba histolytica*, and fumagillin was used during the 1950s to treat humans afflicted with amebiasis. Fumagillin has been used to treat honeybees infected with the microsporidian *Nosema apis*, resulting in a reduction in infected bees.[189] Fumagillin has been used to treat infections by both mi-

▲ **Table 32–4.** DRUGS USED FOR ANIMAL AND HUMAN MICROSPORIDIOSIS

Drug	Organism	Disease	References
Albendazole	*Encephalitozoon cuniculi*	GI, CNS, HEP, EYE, GU	26, 133, 142, 168, 169, 175, 177, 185–187
	Encephalitozoon hellem	EYE, GI, SYS, ENT	
	Encephalitozoon intestinalis	GI, EYE, SYS, GU, ENT	
	Enterocytozoon bieneusi	GI[a], BIL[a]	
	Trachipleistophora hominis	MYO	
	Nosema bombycis	SYS (insect host)	
Fumagillin	*Encephalitozoon hellem*	EYE	134, 174, 178, 188–194
	Encephalitozoon cuniculi	EYE, SYS (murine host)	
	Encephalitozoon intestinalis	EYE	
	Enterocytozoon bieneusi	GI	
	Nosema apis	SYS (insect host)	
	Nosema kingi	SYS (insect host)	
	Octosporea muscaedomesticae	SYS (insect host)	
	Pleistophora anguillarum	Beko (fish host)	
	Loma salmonae	Gill infection (fish host)	
	Nucleospora salmonis	SYS (fish host)	
Metronidazole	*Enterocytozoon bieneusi*	GI[a]	32, 121, 141, 178, 179
	Encephalitozoon intestinalis	GI[b]	
Itraconazole	*Encephalitozoon cuniculi*	EYE[a]	9, 85, 195, 196
	Brachiola vesicularum	MYO[a]	
Trimethoprim-sulfamethoxazole	Enterocytozoon bieneusi	GI[c]	181
Atovaquone	*Enterocytozoon bieneusi*	GI[c]	178, 180
	Encephalitozoon cuniculi[b]		
Furazolidone	*Enterozytozoon bieneusi*	GI[a]	178, 197, 198
Nitazoxanide	*Enterocytozoon bieneusi*	GI[a]	199
Benomyl	*Nosema* sp.	SYS (insect host)	200
Toltrazuril	*Nucleospora salmonis*	SYS[c]	201
	Glugea anomala	SYS (fish host)	

Infections are in human hosts unless indicated in parentheses (i.e., insect, fish, or murine host).
BIL, cholangitis; CNS, encephalitis; ENT, sinus infections; EYE, ocular infections; GI, gastrointestinal disease (diarrhea); GU, genitourinary infections; HEP, hepatitis; MYO, myositis; SYS, systemic infection.
[a]Limited efficacy in vivo.
[b]No efficacy in vitro.
[c]No efficacy in vivo.
Adapted from Costa S, Weiss LM. Drug treatment of microsporidiosis. Drug Resistance Updates 3:1, 2000.

crosporidians and myxosporeans in various types of fish.[190–192] Toxicity has been described with the use of fumagillin in fish. Fumagillin at 0.25 and 1.0 g/kg in food for 60 days administered to rainbow trout resulted in a reduction of the hematopoietic tissue of the kidney and spleen on histologic examination and a reduction of the hematocrit in treated fish. Fumagillin and its semisynthetic analogue TNP-470 have been found to have activity in vitro and in vivo against microsporidians pathogenic for humans including *Enc. cuniculi*, *Enc. hellem*, *Enc. intestinalis*, *V. corneae*, and *Ent. bieneusi*.[134,174,178,188,193,194] It is of concern that this agent is “static” and not “cidal.” When fumagillin is discontinued in vitro, organisms start to grow and return to pretreatment levels. In one study, which demonstrated that fumagillin was active in cases of *Ent. bieneusi* infection, thrombocytopenia occurred in all four patients receiving fumagillin, with one patient having a grade 4 thrombocytopenia with epistaxis.[178] A dose-escalation trial of fumagillin was subsequently performed on HIV patients infected with *Ent. bieneusi*.[134] This study employed doses of 10 mg/day for 14 days, 20 mg/day for 14 days, 40 mg/day for 14 days, and 60 mg/day for 14 days, with the patients being seen at weeks 1, 2, 4, and 6. Efficacy was assessed by the clearance of microsporidia from stool and duodenal biopsies. Of 29 patients, 21 exhibited transient clearing of parasites from their stools. These patients were in the first three dosage groups. In the 60 mg/day group, 8 of 11 patients did not have spores in their stools at week 6 and remained free of them in stool specimens for a mean follow-up of 11 months. Duodenal biopsies on the same eight patients did not demonstrate microsporidia by either light or electron microscopy. A recent study of 12 patients also revealed efficacy.[134a]

Fumagillin binds in a selective, covalent fashion to the metalloprotease methionine aminopeptidase 2

(MetAP2).[207,208] MetAP2 has been demonstrated to be the common target for other fumagillin analogues (e.g., TNP470/AGM-1470) and ovalicin. Crystallization studies have demonstrated that the specific binding site of the reactive epoxide of fumagillin and MetAP2 is a histidine residue at position 231.[208] Methionine aminopeptidase activity is essential for eukaryotic cell survival, as removal of the terminal methionine of a protein is often essential for its function and posttranslational modification (e.g., myrislyation). In microsporidia, homology PCR with sequencing of the amplicons has demonstrated the presence of MetAP2 genes in several microsporidia (L.M. Weiss, unpublished data).

Solutions of the soluble salt Fumidil B (fumagillin bicylohexylammonium, Mid-Continent Agrimarketing, Overland Park, KS, USA) applied topically have been demonstrated to be nontoxic to the cornea. Treatment of ocular microsporidiosis can be accomplished using a solution of Fumidil B (3 mg/ml) in saline (fumagillin 70 mg/ml)[170,174]; the treatment should be continued indefinitely, as recurrence is known to occur upon stopping these drops. It is of note that although clearance of microsporidia from the eye can be demonstrated, the organism is often still present systemically and can be demonstrated in the urine or in nasal smears. In such cases the use of albendazole as a systemic agent is reasonable and effective. Topical treatment with thiabendazole (0.4% suspension), a related benzimidazole, was infective in one case of keratitis due to *Enc. hellem*.[174]

Two patients with *Encephalitozoon*-like organisms have been reported to respond to imidazole (fluconazole and itraconazole) administration.[209] Yee et al. described complete improvement of a patient with *Enc. hellem* infection over a 6-week period who was given oral itraconazole (200 mg bid) after debulking the cornea.[85] Disenhouse et al., in contrast, saw no improvement in a patient with *Enc. hellem* treated with itraconazole 100 mg tid.[174] In vitro data have not confirmed antimicrosporidian activity for imidazole compounds. Sulfa drugs have had variable results in vitro and in vivo and are not recommended for treatment. Polymyxin B, propamidine isethionate 0.1% (Brolene), gramicidin, neomycin sulfate, and tetracycline appear to have limited efficacy for the treatment of microsporidia and should not be used except to treat secondary bacterial infections. Keratoplasty appears to provide temporary improvement in some cases, and debulking by corneal scrapping may be useful in cases not responding to medical treatment. Steroids may be useful for decreasing the associated inflammatory response but have no direct action on microsporidia.

▲ PREVENTION

Patients have developed microsporidiosis while on trimethoprim-sulfamethoxazole prophylaxis.[181] Currently, no prophylactic antiparasitic agents have been identified for these organisms. Although the epidemiology of the microsporidia that infect humans is unknown, it is likely that these are food- or waterborne pathogens; and the usual sanitary measures that prevent contamination of food and water with the urine and feces of animals should decrease the chance for infection. In addition, hand washing and general good hygienic habits probably reduce the chance for contamination of the conjunctiva and cornea. The importance and prevalence of these organisms in our water supplies is an open question.

▲ CONCLUSIONS

Since the original description of microsporidiosis in patients with AIDS in 1985, there has been a geometric increase in the number of reports describing a variety of disease entities caused by these protozoan parasites. *Enterocytozoon bieneusi* has been reported as an important cause of diarrhea and wasting syndrome as well as biliary system disease, and microsporidia of the family Encephalitozoonidae have been associated with disseminated disease, diarrhea, sinusitis, and ocular infections. There has been a dramatic increase in our ability to culture in vitro, treat, and diagnose the Encephalitozoonidae. Therapy for *Ent. bieneusi* infection is still problematic and is limited by the lack of an in vitro culture system for this organism. It is clear that microsporidia are found in immunocompetent and immunocompromised hosts; and as our diagnostic acumen and testing improve, new disease syndromes will likely be attributed to these organisms.

REFERENCES

1. Sprague V. Systematics of the Microsporidia. In: Bulla LA, Cheng TC (eds) Comparative Pathobiology, vol 2. New York, Plenum Press, 1977, pp 1–510.
2. Canning EU, Lom J. The Microsporidia of Vertebrates. London, Academic press, 1986.
3. Matsubayashi H, Koike T, Mikata T, Hagiwara S. A case of Encephalitozoon-like body infection in man. Arch Pathol 67:181, 1959.
4. Wittner M, Weiss L (eds). The Microsporidia and Microsporidiosis. Washington, DC, ASM Press, 1999, p 553.
5. Black SS, Steinohrt LA, Bertucci DC, Rogers LB, Didier ES. Encephalitozoon hellem in budgerigars (Melopsittacus undulatus). Vet Pathol 34:189, 1997.
6. Weber R, Bryan RT, Schwartz DA, Owen RL. Human microsporidial infections. Clin Microbiol Rev 7:426, 1994.
7. Rastrelli P, Didier E, Yee R. Microsporidial keratitis. Opthalmol Clin North Am 7:614, 1994.
8. Silveira H, Canning EU. Vittaforma corneae n. comb. for the human microsporidium Nosema corneum Shadduck, Meccoli, Davis & Font, 1990, based on its ultrastructure in the liver of experimentally infected athymic mice. J Eukaryot Microbiol 42:158, 1995.
9. Cali A, Takvorian PM, Lewin S, et al. Brachiola vesicularum, n. g., n. sp., a new microsporidium associated with AIDS and myositis. J Eukaryot Microbiol 45:240, 1998.
10. Desportes I, Le Charpentier Y, Galian A, et al. Occurrence of a new microsporidian: Enterocytozoon bieneusi n. g., n. sp., in the enterocytes of a human patient with AIDS. J Protozool 32:250, 1985.
11. Cali A, Kotler DP, Orenstein JM. Septata intestinalis n. g., n. sp., an intestinal microsporidian associated with chronic diarrhea and dissemination in AIDS patients. J Eukaryot Microbiol 40:101, 1993.
12. Hartskeerl RA, Van Gool T, Schuitema AR, et al. Genetic and immunological characterization of the microsporidian Septata intestinalis Cali, Kotler and Orenstein, 1993: reclassification to Encephalitozoon intestinalis. Parasitology 110(Pt 3):277, 1995.
13. Field AS, Marriott DJ, Milliken ST, et al. Myositis associated with a newly described microsporidian, Trachipleistophora hominis, in a patient with AIDS. J Clin Microbiol 34:2803, 1996.

14. Yachnis AT, Berg J, Martinez-Salazar A, et al. Disseminated microsporidiosis especially infecting the brain, heart, and kidneys. report of a newly recognized pansporoblastic species in two symptomatic AIDS patients. Am J Clin Pathol 106:535, 1996.
15. Shadduck JA, Meccoli RA, Davis R, Font RL. Isolation of a microsporidian from a human patient. J Infect Dis 162:773, 1990.
16. Didier PJ, Didier ES, Orenstein JM, Shadduck JA. Fine structure of a new human microsporidian, Encephalitozoon hellem, in culture. J Protozool 38:502, 1991.
17. Visvesvara GS, da Silva AJ, Croppo GP, et al. In vitro culture and serologic and molecular identification of Septata intestinalis isolated from urine of a patient with AIDS. J Clin Microbiol 33:930, 1995.
18. Van Gool T, Canning EU, Gilis H, et al. Septata intestinalis frequently isolated from stool of AIDS patients with a new cultivation method. Parasitology 109(Pt 3):281, 1994.
19. Visvesvara G, Leitch GJ, Pieniazek NJ, et al. Short-term in vitro culture and molecular analysis of the microsporidian, Enterocytozoon bieneusi. J Eukaryot Microbiol 42:506, 1995.
20. Visvesvara GS, Leitch GJ, Wallace S, et al. Adenovirus masquerading as microsporidia. J Parasitol 82:316, 1996.
21. Wongtavatchai J, Conrad PA, Hedrick RP. In vitro characteristics of the microsporidian: Enterocytozoon salmonis. J Eukaryot Microbiol 42:401, 1995.
22. Docker MF, Kent ML, Hervio DML, et al. Ribosomal DNA sequence of Nucleospora salmonis Hedrick, Groff and Baxa, 1991 (Microsporea: Enterocytozoonidae): implications for phylogeny and nomenclature. J Eukaryot Microbiol 44:55, 1997.
23. Tzipori S, Carville A, Widmer G, et al. Transmission and establishment of a persistent infection of Enterocytozoon bieneusi, derived from a human with AIDS, in simian immunodeficiency virus-infected rhesus monkeys. J Infect Dis 175:1016, 1997.
24. Orenstein JM, Gaetz HP, Yachnis AT, et al. Disseminated microsporidiosis in AIDS: are any organs spared [letter]? AIDS 11:385, 1997.
25. Sheth SG, Bates C, Federman M, Chopra S. Fulminant hepatic failure caused by microsporidial infection in a patient with AIDS [letter]. AIDS 11:553, 1997.
26. Weber R, Deplazes P, Flepp M, et al. Cerebral microsporidiosis due to Encephalitozoon cuniculi in a patient with human immunodeficiency virus infection. N Engl J Med 336:474, 1997.
27. Croppo GP, Visvesvara GS, Leitch GJ, et al. Western blot and immunofluorescence analysis of a human isolate of Encephalitozoon cuniculi established in culture from the urine of a patient with AIDS. J Parasitol 83:66, 1997.
28. Sheikh RA, Prindiville TP, Yenamandra S, et al. Microsporidial AIDS cholangiopathy due to Encephalitozoon intestinalis: case report and review. Am J Gastroenterol 95:2364, 2000.
29. Grau A, Valls ME, Williams JE, et al. [Myositis caused by Pleistophora in a patient with AIDS.] Med Clin (Barc) 107:779, 1996.
30. Chupp GL, Alroy J, Adelman LS, et al. Myositis due to Pleistophora (Microsporidia) in a patient with AIDS. Clin Infect Dis 16:15, 1993.
31. Vavra J, Yachnis AT, Shadduck JA, Orenstein JM. Microsporidia of the genus Trachipleistophora—causative agents of human microsporidiosis: description of Trachipleistophora anthropophthera n. sp. (Protozoa: Microsporidia). J Eukaryot Microbiol 45:273, 1998.
32. Pol S, Romana CA, Richard S, et al. Microsporidia infection in patients with the human immunodeficiency virus and unexplained cholangitis. N Engl J Med 328:95, 1993.
33. Desportes-Livage I. Biology of microsporidia [in process citation]. Contrib Microbiol 6:140, 2000.
34. Takvorian PM, Cali A. Enzyme histochemical identification of the Golgi apparatus in the microsporidian, Glugea stephani. J Eukaryot Microbiol 41:63S, 1994.
35. Curgy JJ, Vavra J, Vivares C. Presence of ribosomal RNAs with prokaryotic properties in Microsporidia, eukaryotic organisms. Biol Cell 38:49, 1980.
36. Vossbrinck CR, Maddox JV, Friedman S, et al. Ribosomal RNA sequence suggests microsporidia are extremely ancient eukaryotes. Nature 326:411, 1987.
37. Vossbrinck CR, Woese CR. Eukaryotic ribosomes that lack a 5.8S RNA. Nature 320:287, 1986.
38. Weiss LM, Vossbrinck CR. Microsporidiosis: molecular and diagnostic aspects. Adv Parasitol 40:351, 1998.
39. Vivares CP, Metenier G. Towards the minimal eukaryotic parasitic genome [in process citation]. Curr Opin Microbiol 3:463, 2000.
40. Brugere JF, Cornillot E, Metenier G, et al. Encephalitozoon cuniculi (Microspora) genome: physical map and evidence for telomere-associated rDNA units on all chromosomes. Nucleic Acids Res 28:2026, 2000.
41. Katiyar SK, Visvesvara GS, Edlind TD. Comparisons of ribosomal RNA sequences from amitochondrial protozoa: implications for processing mRNA binding and paromomycin susceptibility. Gene 152:27, 1995.
42. Weiss LM. Molecular phylogeny and diagnostic approaches to microsporidia [in process citation]. Contrib Microbiol 6:209, 2000.
43. Biderre C, Pages M, Metenier G, et al. On small genomes in eukaryotic organisms: molecular karyotypes of two microsporidian species (Protozoa) parasites of vertebrates. C R Acad Sci III 317:399, 1994.
44. Biderre C, Pages M, Metenier G, et al. Evidence for the smallest nuclear genome (2.9 Mb) in the microsporidium Encephalitozoon cuniculi. Mol Biochem Parasitol 74:229, 1995.
45. Sprague V, Becnel JJ, Hazard EL. Taxonomy of phylum Microspora. Crit Rev Microbiol 18:285, 1992.
46. Levine ND, Corliss JO, Cox FEG, et al. A newly revised classification of the protozoa. J Protozool 27:37, 1980.
47. Baker MD, Vossbrinck CR, Didier ES, et al. Small subunit ribosomal DNA phylogeny of various microsporidia with emphasis on AIDS related forms. J Eukaryot Microbiol 42:564, 1995.
48. Langley RC, Cali A, Somberg EW. Two-dimensional electrophoretic analysis of spore proteins of the microsporida. J Parasitol 73:910, 1987.
49. Didier ES, Didier PJ, Friedberg DN, et al. Isolation and characterization of a new human microsporidian, Encephalitozoon hellem (n. sp.) from three AIDS patients with keratoconjunctivitis. J Infect Dis 163:617, 1991.
50. Keeling PJ, McFadden GI. Origins of microsporidia. Trends Microbiol 6:19, 1998.
51. Weiss LM, Edlind TD, Vossbrinck CR, Hashimoto T. Microsporidian molecular phylogeny: the fungal connection. J Eukaryot Microbiol 46:17S, 1999.
52. Hirt RP, Logsdon JM Jr, Healy B, et al. Microsporidia are related to fungi: evidence from the largest subunit of RNA polymerase II and other proteins. Proc Natl Acad Sci USA 96:580, 1999.
53. Waller T. Sensitivity of Encephalitozoon cuniculi to various temperatures, disinfectants and drugs. Lab Anim 13(227), 1979.
54. Vavra J. Structure of the Microsporidia. In: Bulla LA Jr, Cheng TC (eds) Comparative Pathobiology, vol 1. New York, Plenum Press, 1976, pp 1–85.
55. Foucault C, Drancourt M. Actin mediates Encephalitozoon intestinalis entry into the human enterocyte-like cell line, Caco-2. Microb Pathog 28:51, 2000.
56. Loin J. On the structure of the extruded microsporidian polar filament. Z Parasitenkd 38:200, 1972.
57. Weidner E. Cell invasion by microsporidian spores: an ultrastructural study. J Protozool 18(suppl):13, 1971.
58. Weidner E. Ultrastructural study of microsporidian invasion into cells. Z Parasitenkd 40:227, 1972.
59. Undeen AH. A proposed mechanism for the germination of microsporidian (Protozoa, Microspora) spores. J Theor Biol 142:223, 1990.
60. Loin J, Vavra J. The mode of sporoplasm extrusion in microsporidian spores. Acta Protozool 1:81, 1963.
61. Undeen AH, Epsky ND. In vitro and vivo germination of Nosema locustae (Microspora: Nosematidae) spores. J Invertebr Pathol 56:371, 1990.
62. Whitlock V, Johnson S. Stimuli for the in vitro germination of Nosema locustae (Microspora: Nosematidae) spores. J Invert Pathol 56:57, 1990.
63. Frixione E, Ruiz L, Undeen AH. Monovalent cations induce microsporidian spore germination in vitro. J Eukaryot Microbiol 41:464, 1994.
64. Undeen AH, Avery SW. Effect of anions on the germination of Nosema algerae (Microspora: Nosematidae) spores. J Invertebr Pathol 52:84, 1988.
65. Pleshinger J, Weidner E. The microsporidian spore invasion tube. IV. Discharge activation begins with pH-triggered Ca^{2+} influx. J Cell Biol 100:1934, 1985.

66. Leitch GJ, He Q, Wallace S, Visvesvara GS. Inhibition of the spore polar filament extrusion of the microsporidium, Encephalitozoon hellem, isolated from an AIDS patient. J Eukaryot Microbiol 40:711, 1993.
67. Weidner E, Byrd W. The microsporidian spore invasion tube. II. Role of calcium in the activation of invasion tube discharge. J Cell Biol 93:970, 1982.
68. Undeen AH, Vandermeer RK. The effect of ultraviolet radiation on the germination of Nosema algerae Vávra and Undeen (Microsporida: Nosematidae) spores. J Protozool 37:194, 1990.
69. Undeen AH, Frixione E. The role of osmotic pressure in the germination of Nosema algerae spores. J Protozool 37:561, 1990.
70. Undeen AH, Vandermeer RK. Conversion of intrasporal trehalose into reducing sugars during germination of Nosema algerae (Protista: Microspora) spores: a quantitative study. J Eukaryot Microbiol 41:129, 1994.
71. Undeen AH, ElGazzar LM, Vandermeer RK, Narang S. Trehalose levels and trehalase activity in germinated and ungerminated spores of Nosema algerae (Microspora: Nosematidae). J Invertebr Pathol 50:230, 1987.
72. Weber R, Bryan RT. Microsporidial infections in immunodeficient and immunocompetent patients. Clin Infect Dis 19:517, 1994.
73. Mathis A. Microsporidia: emerging advances in understanding the basic biology of these unique organisms [in process citation]. Int J Parasitol 30:795, 2000.
74. Deplazes P, Mathis A, Weber R. Epidemiology and zoonotic aspects of microsporidia of mammals and birds [in process citation]. Contrib Microbiol 6:236, 2000.
75. Didier ES, Vossbrinck CR, Baker MD, et al. Identification and characterization of three Encephalitozoon cuniculi strains. Parasitology 111(Pt 4):411, 1995.
76. Rinder H, Katzwinkel-Wladarsch S, Loscher T. Evidence for the existence of genetically distinct strains of Enterocytozoon bieneusi. Parasitol Res 83:670, 1997.
77. Rinder H, Katzwinkel-Wladarsch S, Thomschke A, Loscher T. Strain differentiation in microsporidia. Tokai J Exp Clin Med 23:433, 1998.
78. Bergquist NR, Stintzing G, Smedman L, et al. Diagnosis of encephalitozoonosis in man by serological tests. BMJ 288:902, 1984.
79. Van Gool T, Vetter JC, Weinmayr B, et al. High seroprevalence of Encephalitozoon species in immunocompetent subjects. J Infect Dis 175:1020, 1997.
80. Niederkorn J, Shadduck J, Weidner E. Antigenic cross-reactivity among different microsporidian spores as determined by immunofluorescence. J Parasitol 66:675, 1980.
81. Weiss LM, Cali A, Levee E, et al. Diagnosis of Encephalitozoon cuniculi infection by western blot and the use of cross-reactive antigens for the possible detection of microsporidiosis in humans. Am J Trop Med Hyg 47:456, 1992.
82. Singh M, Kane GJ, Mackinlay L, et al. Detection of antibodies to Nosema cuniculi (Protozoa: Microscoporidia) in human and animal sera by the indirect fluorescent antibody technique. Southeast Asian J Trop Med Public Health 13:110, 1982.
83. WHO parasitic diseases surveillance, antibody to Encephalitozoon cuniculi in man. WHO Wkly Epidemiol Rec 58:30, 1983.
84. Bergquist R, Morfeldt-Mansson L, Pehrson PO, et al. Antibody against Encephalitozoon cuniculi in Swedish homosexual men. Scand J Infect Dis 16:389, 1984.
85. Yee RW, Tio FO, Martinez JA, et al. Resolution of microsporidial epithelial keratopathy in a patient with AIDS. Ophthalmology 98:196, 1991.
86. Snowden K, Logan K, Didier ES. Encephalitozoon cuniculi strain III is a cause of encephalitozoonosis in both humans and dogs. J Infect Dis 180:2086, 1999.
87. Deplazes P, Mathis A, Muller C, Weber R. Molecular epidemiology of Encephalitozoon cuniculi and first detection of Enterocytozoon bieneusi in faecal samples of pigs. J Eukaryot Microbiol 43:93S, 1996.
88. Mansfield KG, Carville A, Shvetz D, et al. Identification of an Enterocytozoon bieneusi-like microsporidian parasite in simian-immunodeficiency-virus-inoculated macaques with hepatobiliary disease. Am J Pathol 150:1395, 1997.
89. Fuentealba IC, Mahoney NT, Shadduck JA, et al. Hepatic lesions in rabbits infected with Encephalitozoon cuniculi administered per rectum. Vet Pathol 29:536, 1992.
90. Zeman DH, Baskin GB. Encephalitozoonosis in squirrel monkeys (Saimiri sciureus). Vet Pathol 22:24, 1985.
91. Ashton N, Cook C, Clegg R. Encephalitozoonosis (Nosematosis) causing bilaterial cataract in a rabbit. Fr J Opthalmol 60:618, 1976.
92. Hunt R, King N, Foster H. Encephalitozoonosis: evidence for vertical transmission. J Infect Dis 126:221, 1972.
93. Desportes-Livage I, Chilmonczyk S, Hedrick R, et al. Comparative development of two microsporidian species: Enterocytozoon bieneusi and Enterocytozoon salmonis, reported in AIDS patients and salmonid fish, respectively. J Eukaryot Microbiol 43:49, 1996.
94. Chilmonczyk S, Cox WT, Hedrick RP. Enterocytozoon salmonis n. sp.: an intranuclear microsporidium from salmonid fish. J Protozool 38:264, 1991.
95. Avery SW, Undeen AH. The isolation of microsporidia and other pathogens from concentrated ditch water. J Am Mosq Control Assoc 3:54, 1987.
96. Cotte L, Rabodonirina M, Chapuis F, et al. Waterborne outbreak of intestinal microsporidiosis in persons with and without human immunodeficiency virus infection. J Infect Dis 180:2003, 1999.
97. Franzen C, Muller A. Cryptosporidia and microsporidia: waterborne diseases in the immunocompromised host. Diagn Microbiol Infect Dis 34:245, 1999.
98. Fournier S, Liguory O, Santillana-Hayat M, et al. Detection of microsporidia in surface water: a one-year follow-up study [in process citation]. FEMS Immunol Med Microbiol 29:95, 2000.
99. Hunter PR. Waterborne outbreak of microsporidiosis [letter]. J Infect Dis 182:380, 2000.
100. Levaditi C, Nicolau S, Schoen R. Nouvelles donnees sur l'Encephalitozoon cuniculi. C R Soc Biol 89:1157, 1923.
101. Margileth A, Strano A, Chandra R, et al. Disseminated nosematosis in an immunologically compromised infant. Arch Pathol 95:145, 1973.
102. Enriquez FJ, Taren D, Cruz-Lopez A, et al. Prevalence of intestinal encephalitozoonosis in Mexico. Clin Infect Dis 26:1227, 1998.
103. Albrecht H, Sobottka I. Enterocytozoon bieneusi infection in patients who are not infected with human immunodeficiency virus [letter]. Clin Infect Dis 25:344, 1997.
104. Lopez-Velez R, Turrientes MC, Garron C, et al. Microsporidiosis in travelers with diarrhea from the tropics. J Travel Med 6:223, 1999.
105. Fournier S, Liguory O, Garrait V, et al. Microsporidiosis due to Enterocytozoon bieneusi infection as a possible cause of traveller's diarrhea. Eur J Clin Microbiol Infect Dis 17:743, 1998.
106. Bretagne S, Foulet F, Alkassoum W, et al. [Prevalence of Enterocytozoon bieneusi spores in the stool of AIDS patients and African children not infected by HIV.] Bull Soc Pathol Exot 86:351, 1993.
107. Drobniewski F, Kelly P, Carew A, et al. Human microsporidiosis in African AIDS patients with chronic diarrhea [letter]. J Infect Dis 171:515, 1995.
108. Sax PE, Rich JD, Pieciak WS, Trnka YM. Intestinal microsporidiosis occurring in a liver transplant recipient. Transplantation 60:617, 1995.
109. Gumbo T, Hobbs RE, Carlyn C, et al. Microsporidia infection in transplant patients. Transplantation 67:482, 1999.
110. Metge S, Van Nhieu JT, Dahmane D, et al. A case of Enterocytozoon bieneusi infection in an HIV-negative renal transplant recipient. Eur J Clin Microbiol Infect Dis 19:221, 2000.
111. Rabodonirina M, Bertocchi M, Desportes-Livage I, et al. Enterocytozoon bieneusi as a cause of chronic diarrhea in a heart-lung transplant recipient who was seronegative for human immunodeficiency virus. Clin Infect Dis 23:114, 1996.
112. Kelkar R, Sastry PS, Kulkarni SS, et al. Pulmonary microsporidial infection in a patient with CML undergoing allogeneic marrow transplant. Bone Marrow Transplant 19:179, 1997.
113. Guerard A, Rabodonirina M, Cotte L, et al. Intestinal microsporidiosis occurring in two renal transplant recipients treated with mycophenolate mofetil. Transplantation 68:699, 1999.
114. Visvesvara GS, Belloso M, Moura H, et al. Isolation of Nosema algerae from the cornea of an immunocompetent patient. J Eukaryot Microbiol 46:10S, 1999.
115. Pinnolis M, Egbert PR, Font RL, Winter FC. Nosematosis of the cornea: case report, including electron microscopic studies. Arch Ophthalmol 99:1044, 1981.
116. Cali A, Meisler DM, Lowder CY, et al. Corneal microsporidioses: characterization and identification. J Protozool 38:215S, 1991.
117. Cali A, Meisler DM, Rutherford I, et al. Corneal microsporidiosis in a patient with AIDS. Am J Trop Med Hyg 44:463, 1991.

118. Davis R, Font R, Keisler M, Shadduck J. Corneal microsporidiosis: a case report including ultrastructural observations. Ophthalmology 97:953, 1990.
119. Ashton N, Wirasinha P. Encephalitozoonosis (nosematosis) of the cornea. Br J Ophthalmol 57:669, 1973.
120. Deluol AM, Poirot JL, Heyer F, et al. Intestinal microsporidiosis: about clinical characteristics and laboratory diagnosis. J Eukaryot Microbiol 41:33S, 1994.
121. Eeftinck Schattenkerk JK, van Gool T, van Ketel RJ, et al. Clinical significance of small-intestinal microsporidiosis in HIV-1-infected individuals. Lancet 337:895, 1991.
122. Field AS, Hing MC, Milliken ST, Marriott DJ. Microsporidia in the small intestine of HIV-infected patients: a new diagnostic technique and a new species. Med J Aust 158:390, 1993.
123. Greenson JK, Belitsos PC, Yardley JH, Bartlett JG. AIDS enteropathy: occult enteric infections and duodenal mucosal alterations in chronic diarrhea. Ann Intern Med 114:366, 1991.
124. Molina JM, Sarfati C, Beauvais B, et al. Intestinal microsporidiosis in human immunodeficiency virus-infected patients with chronic unexplained diarrhea: prevalence and clinical and biologic features. J Infect Dis 167:217, 1993.
125. Michiels JF, Hofman P, Saint Paul MC, et al. Pathological features of intestinal microsporidiosis in HIV positive patients: a report of 13 new cases. Pathol Res Pract 189:377, 1993.
126. Van Gool T, Snijders F, Reiss P, et al. Diagnosis of intestinal and disseminated microsporidial infections in patients with HIV by a new rapid fluorescence technique. J Clin Pathol 46:694, 1993.
127. Weber R, Bryan RT, Owen RL, et al. Improved light-microscopical detection of microsporidia spores in stool and duodenal aspirates: the Enteric Opportunistic Infections Working Group. N Engl J Med 326:161, 1992.
128. Orenstein JM, Dieterich DT, Kotler DP. Systemic dissemination by a newly recognized intestinal microsporidia species in AIDS. AIDS 6:1143, 1992.
129. Rabeneck L, Gyorkey F, Genta RM, et al. The role of Microsporidia in the pathogenesis of HIV-related chronic diarrhea. Ann Intern Med 119:895, 1993.
130. Rabeneck L, Genta RM, Gyorkey F, et al. Observations on the pathological spectrum and clinical course of microsporidiosis in men infected with the human immunodeficiency virus: follow-up study. Clin Infect Dis 20:1229, 1995.
131. Kotler DP, Orenstein JM. Prevalence of intestinal microsporidiosis in HIV-infected individuals referred for gastroenterological evaluation. Am J Gastroenterol 89:1998, 1994.
132. Coyle CM, Wittner M, Kotler DP, et al. Prevalence of microsporidiosis due to Enterocytozoon bieneusi and Encephalitozoon (Septata) intestinalis among patients with AIDS-related diarrhea: determination by polymerase chain reaction to the microsporidian small-subunit rRNA gene. Clin Infect Dis 23:1002, 1996.
133. Molina JM, Oksenhendler E, Beauvais B, et al. Disseminated microsporidiosis due to Septata intestinalis in patients with AIDS: clinical features and response to albendazole therapy. J Infect Dis 171:245, 1995.
134. Molina JM, Goguel J, Sarfati C, et al. Trial of oral fumagillin for the treatment of intestinal microsporidiosis in patients with HIV infection: ANRS 054 Study Group. Agence Nationale de Recherche sur le SIDA [in process citation]. AIDS 14:1341, 2000.
134a. Molina JM, Tourneur M, Sarfati C, et al. Fumagillin treatment of intestinal microsporidiosis. N Engl J Med 346:1963, 2002.
135. Mansfield KG, Carville A, Hebert D, et al. Localization of persistent Enterocytozoon bieneusi infection in normal rhesus macaques (Macaca mulatta) to the hepatobiliary tree. J Clin Microbiol 36:2336, 1998.
136. Hartskeerl RA, Schuitema AR, van Gool T, Terpstra WJ. Genetic evidence for the occurrence of extraintestinal Enterocytozoon bieneusi infections. Nucleic Acids Res 21:4150, 1993.
137. Cali A, Owen RL. Intracellular development of Enterocytozoon, a unique microsporidian found in the intestines of AIDS patients. J Protozool 37:145, 1990.
138. Mertens RB, Didier ES, Fishbein MC, et al. Encephalitozoon cuniculi microsporidiosis: infection of the brain, heart, kidneys, trachea, adrenal glands, and urinary bladder in a patient with AIDS. Mod Pathol 10:68, 1997.
139. Willson R, Harrington R, Stewart B, Fritsche T. Human immunodeficiency virus 1-associated necrotizing cholangitis caused by infection with Septata intestinalis. Gastroenterology 108:247, 1995.
140. Belcher JW Jr, Guttenberg SA, Schmookler BM. Microsporidiosis of the mandible in a patient with acquired immunodeficiency syndrome. J Oral Maxillofac Surg 55:424, 1997.
141. Gunnarsson G, Hurlbut D, DeGirolami PC, et al. Multiorgan microsporidiosis: report of five cases and review. Clin Infect Dis 21:37, 1995.
142. Weber R, Sauer B, Spycher MA, et al. Detection of Septata intestinalis in stool specimens and coprodiagnostic monitoring of successful treatment with albendazole. Clin Infect Dis 19:342, 1994.
143. Terada S, Reddy KR, Jeffers LJ, et al. Microsporidan hepatitis in the acquired immunodeficiency syndrome. Ann Intern Med 107:61, 1987.
144. Gordon S, Reddy K, Gould E, et al. The spectrum of liver disease in the acquired immunodeficiency syndrome. J Hepatol 2:475, 1986.
145. De Groote MA, Visvesvara G, Wilson ML, et al. Polymerase chain reaction and culture confirmation of disseminated Encephalitozoon cuniculi in a patient with AIDS: successful therapy with albendazole. J Infect Dis 171:1375, 1995.
146. Schwartz DA, Bryan RT, Hewan-Lowe KO, et al. Disseminated microsporidiosis (Encephalitozoon hellem) and acquired immunodeficiency syndrome: autopsy evidence for respiratory acquisition. Arch Pathol Lab Med 116:660, 1992.
147. Weber R, Kuster H, Visvesvara GS, et al. Disseminated microsporidiosis due to Encephalitozoon hellem: pulmonary colonization, microhematuria, and mild conjunctivitis in a patient with AIDS. Clin Infect Dis 17:415, 1993.
148. Visvesvara GS, Leitch GJ, da Silva AJ, et al. Polyclonal and monoclonal antibody and PCR-amplified small-subunit rRNA identification of a microsporidian, Encephalitozoon hellem, isolated from an AIDS patient with disseminated infection. J Clin Microbiol 32:2760, 1994.
149. Lowder CY, Meisler DM, McMahon JT, et al. Microsporidia infection of the cornea in a man seropositive for human immunodeficiency virus. Am J Ophthalmol 109:242, 1990.
150. Lowder CY, McMahon JT, Meisler DM, et al. Microsporidial keratoconjunctivitis caused by Septata intestinalis in a patient with acquired immunodeficiency syndrome. Am J Ophthalmol 121:715, 1996.
151. Visvesvara GS, Leitch GJ, Moura H, et al. Culture, electron microscopy, and immunoblot studies on a microsporidian parasite isolated from the urine of a patient with AIDS. J Protozool 38:105s, 1991.
152. Birthistle K, Moore P, Hay P. Microsporidia: a new sexually transmissible cause of urethritis [letter]. Genitourin Med 72:445, 1996.
153. Macher A, Neafie R, Angritt P, Tuur S. Microsporidia myositis and the acquired immunodeficiency syndrome (AIDS): a four year followup. Ann Intern Med 109:343, 1988.
154. Vavra J, Dahbiova R, Hollister WS, Canning EU. Staining of microsporidian spores by optical brighteners with remarks on the use of brighteners for the diagnosis of AIDS-associated human microsporidioses. Folia Parasitol 40:267, 1993.
155. Ryan NJ, Sutherland G, Coughlan K, et al. A new trichrome-blue stain for detection of microsporidial species in urine, stool, and nasopharyngeal specimens. J Clin Microbiol 31:3264, 1993.
156. Kokoskin E, Gyorkos TW, Camus A, et al. Modified technique for efficient detection of microsporidia. J Clin Microbiol 32:1074, 1994.
157. Didier ES, Orenstein JM, Aldras A, et al. Comparison of three staining methods for detecting microsporidia in fluids. J Clin Microbiol 33:3138, 1995.
158. DeGirolami PC, Ezratty CR, Desai G, et al. Diagnosis of intestinal microsporidiosis by examination of stool and duodenal aspirate with Weber's modified trichrome and Uvitex 2B strains. J Clin Microbiol 33:805, 1995.
159. Zierdt CH, Gill VJ, Zierdt WS. Detection of microsporidian spores in clinical samples by indirect fluorescent-antibody assay using whole-cell antisera to Encephalitozoon cuniculi and Encephalitozoon hellem. J Clin Microbiol 31:3071, 1993.
160. Croppo GP, Visvesvara GS, Leitch GJ, et al. Identification of the microsporidian Encephalitozoon hellem using immunoglobulin G monoclonal antibodies. Arch Pathol Lab Med 122:182, 1998.
161. Beckers PJ, Derks GJ, Gool T, et al. Encephalotozoon intestinalis-specific monoclonal antibodies for laboratory diagnosis of microsporidiosis. J Clin Microbiol 34:282, 1996.
162. Achbarou A, Thellier M, Accoceberry I, et al. Production of immunological probes raised against Enterocytozoon bieneusi and Encephalitozoon intestinalis, two microsporidian species causing intestinal infections in man. J Eukaryot Microbiol 46:32S, 1999.

163. Accoceberry I, Thellier M, Desportes-Livage I, et al. Production of monoclonal antibodies directed against the microsporidium Enterocytozoon bieneusi. J Clin Microbiol 37:4107, 1999.
164. Didier E, Kotler D, Dietrich D, et al. Serologic studies in human microsporidiosis. AIDS 7:S8, 1993.
165. Katzwinkel-Wladarsch S, Lieb M, Helse W, et al. Direct amplification and species determination of microsporidian DNA from stool specimens. Trop Med Int Health 1:373, 1996.
166. Ombrouck C, Ciceron L, Biligui S, et al. Specific PCR assay for direct detection of intestinal microsporidia Enterocytozoon bieneusi and Encephalitozoon intestinalis in fecal specimens from human immunodeficiency virus-infected patients. J Clin Microbiol 35:652, 1997.
167. Fedorko DP, Hijazi YM. Application of molecular techniques to the diagnosis of microsporidial infection. Emerg Infect Dis 2:183, 1996.
168. Dieterich DT, Lew EA, Kotler DP, et al. Treatment with albendazole for intestinal disease due to Enterocytozoon bieneusi in patients with AIDS. J Infect Dis 169:178, 1994.
169. Dore GJ, Marriott DJ, Hing MC, et al. Disseminated microsporidiosis due to Septata intestinalis in nine patients infected with the human immunodeficiency virus: response to therapy with albendazole. Clin Infect Dis 21:70, 1995.
170. Rosberger DF, Serdarevic ON, Erlandson RA, et al. Successful treatment of microsporidial keratoconjunctivitis with topical fumagillin in a patient with AIDS. Cornea 12:261, 1993.
171. Haque A, Hollister WS, Willcox A, Canning EU. The antimicrosporidial activity of albendazole. J Invertebr Pathol 62:171, 1993.
172. Beauvais B, Sarfati C, Challier S, Derouin F. In vitro model to assess effect of antimicrobial agents on Encephalitozoon cuniculi. Antimicrob Agents Chemother 38:2440, 1994.
173. Ditrich O, Kucerova Z, Koudela B. In vitro sensitivity of Encephalitozoon cuniculi and E. hellem to albendazole. J Eukaryot Microbiol 41:37S, 1994.
174. Diesenhouse MC, Wilson LA, Corrent GF, et al. Treatment of microsporidial keratoconjunctivitis with topical fumagillin. Am J Ophthalmol 115:293, 1993.
175. Blanshard C, Ellis DS, Tovey DG, et al. Treatment of intestinal microsporidiosis with albendazole in patients with AIDS. AIDS 6:311, 1992.
176. Franssen FF, Lumeij JT, van Knapen F. Susceptibility of Encephalitozoon cuniculi to several drugs in vitro. Antimicrob Agents Chemother 39:1265, 1995.
177. Molina JM, Chastang C, Goguel J, et al. Albendazole for treatment and prophylaxis of microsporidiosis due to Encephalitozoon intestinalis in patients with AIDS: a randomized double-blind controlled trial. J Infect Dis 177:1373, 1998.
178. Molina JM, Goguel J, Sarfati C, et al. Potential efficacy of fumagillin in intestinal microsporidiosis due to Enterocytozoon bieneusi in patients with HIV infection: results of a drug screening study: the French Microsporidiosis Study Group. AIDS 11:1603, 1997.
179. Asmuth DM, DeGirolami PC, Federman M, et al. Clinical features of microsporidiosis in patients with AIDS. Clin Infect Dis 18:819, 1994.
180. Anwar-Bruni DM, Hogan SE, Schwartz DA, et al. Atovaquone is effective treatment for the symptoms of gastrointestinal microsporidiosis in HIV-1-infected patients. AIDS 10:619, 1996.
181. Albrecht H, Sobottka I, Stellbrink HJ, Greten H. Does the choice of Pneumocystis carinii prophylaxis influence the prevalence of Enterocytozoon bieneusi microsporidiosis in AIDS patients [letter]? AIDS 9:302, 1995.
182. Sharpstone D, Rowbottom A, Nelson M, Gazzard B. The treatment of microsporidial diarrhoea with thalidomide [letter]. AIDS 9:658, 1995.
183. Sharpstone D, Rowbottom A, Francis N, et al. Thalidomide: a novel therapy for microsporidiosis. Gastroenterology 112:1823, 1997. Erratum. Gastroenterology 113:1054, 1997.
184. Costa S, Weiss LM. Drug treatment of microsporidiosis. Drug Resistance Updates 3:1, 2000.
185. Weiss LM, Michalakakis E, Coyle CM, et al. The in vitro activity of albendazole against Encephalitozoon cuniculi. J Eukaryot Microbiol 41:65S, 1994.
186. Leder K, Ryan N, Spelman D, Crowe SM. Microsporidial disease in HIV-infected patients: a report of 42 patients and review of the literature. Scand J Infect Dis 30:331, 1998.
187. Blanshard C, Ellis DS, Dowell SP, et al. Electron microscopic changes in Enterocytozoon bieneusi following treatment with albendazole. J Clin Pathol 46:898, 1993.
188. Didier ES. Effects of albendazole, fumagillin, and TNP-470 on microsporidial replication in vitro. Antimicrob Agents Chemother 41:1541, 1997.
189. Katsnelson H, Jamieson C. Control of Nosema disease of honeybees with fumagillin. Science 115:70, 1952.
190. Kano T, Fukui H. Studies on Pleistophora infection in eel, Anguilla japonica I. Experimental induction of microsporidiosis and fumagillin efficacy. Fish Pathol 16:193, 1982.
191. Kent M, Dawe S. Efficacy of fumagillin DCH against experimentally induced Loma salmonae (Microsporea) infections in chinnok salmon Oncorhynchus tsawytscha. Dis Aquat Org 20:231, 1994.
192. Higgins M, Dent M, Moran J, et al. Efficacy of the fumagillin analog TNP-470 for Nucleospora salmonis and Loma salmonae infection in chinook salmon Oncorhynchus tsawytscha. Dis Aquat Org 11:45, 1998.
193. Shadduck J. Effect of fumagillin on in vitro multiplication of Encephalitozoon cuniculi. J Protozool 27:202, 1980.
194. Coyle C, Kent M, Tanowitz HB, et al. TNP-470 is an effective antimicrosporidial agent. J Infect Dis 177:515, 1998.
195. Rossi P, Urbani C, Donelli G, Pozio E. Resolution of microsporidial sinusitis and keratoconjunctivitis by itraconazole treatment. Am J Ophthalmol 127:210, 1999.
196. Gritz DC, Hoisciaw DS, Neger RE, et al. Ocular and sinus microsporidial infection cured with systemic albendazole. Am J Ophthalmol 124:241, 1997.
197. Dionisio D, Manneschi LI, Di Lollo S, et al. Enterocytozoon bieneusi in AIDS: symptomatic relief and parasite changes after furazolidone. J Gun Pathol 50:472, 1997.
198. Dionisio D, Sterrantino G, Meli M, et al. Use of furazolidone for the treatment of microsporidiosis due to Enterocytozoon bieneusi in patients with AIDS. Recent Prog Med 86:394, 1995.
199. Bicart-See A, Massip P, Linas MD, Datry A. Successful treatment with nitazoxanide of Enterocytozoon bieneusi microsporidiosis in a patient with AIDS. Antimicrob Agents Chemother 44:167, 2000.
200. Hsiao T. Benomyl: a novel drug for controlling a microsporidian disease of the alfalfa weevil. J Invertebr Pathol 22:303, 1973.
201. Schmahl G, el Toukhy A, Ghaffar FA. Transmission electron microscopic studies on the effects of toltrazuril on Glugea anomala, Moniez, 1887 (Microsporidia) infecting the three-spined stickleback Gasterosteus aculeatus. Parasitol Res 76:700, 1990.
202. Didier ES, Maddry JA, Kwong CD, et al. Screening of compounds for antimicrosporidial activity in vitro. Folia Parasitol 45:129, 1998.
203. Edlind T, Visvesvara G, Li J, Katiyar S. Cryptosporidium and microsporidial beta-tubulin sequences: predictions of benzimidazole sensitivity and phylogeny. J Eukaryot Microbiol 41:38S, 1994.
204. Li J, Katiyar SK, Hamelin A, et al. Tubulin genes from AIDS-associated microsporidia and implications for phylogeny and benzimidazole sensitivity. Mol Biochem Parasitol 78:289, 1996.
205. Shah V, Marino C, Altice F. Albendazole-induced pseudomembranous colitis. Am J Gastroenterol 91:1453, 1996.
206. Lecuit M, Oksenhendler E, Sarfati C. Use of albendazole for disseminated microsporidian infection in a patient with AIDS. J Infect Dis 19:332, 1994.
207. Griffith E, Su Z, Niwayama S, et al. Molecular recognition of angiogenesis inhibitors fumagillin and ovalicin by methionine aminopeptidase 2. Proc Natl Acad Sci USA 95:15183, 1998.
208. Liu S, Widom J, Kemp C, et al. Structure of human methionine aminopeptidase-2 complexed with fumagillin. Science 282:1324, 1998.
209. Orenstein JM, Seedor J, Friedberg DN, et al. Microsporidian keratoconjunctivitis in patients with AIDS. MMWR Morbid Mortal Wkly Rep 188, 1990.

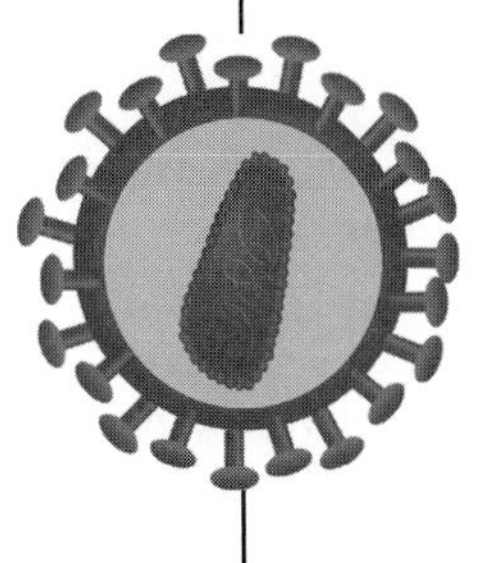

CHAPTER 33

Mycobacterium Tuberculosis Infection

Fred Gordin, MD

EPIDEMIOLOGY AND NATURAL HISTORY

Impact of HIV Infection on Tuberculosis

Tuberculosis is the leading cause of death worldwide among persons infected with the human immunodeficiency virus (HIV). Approximately one-third of all acquired immunodeficiency syndrome (AIDS)-related deaths are due to tuberculosis.[1] By mid-1994 it was estimated that 5 million to 6 million people across the globe were infected with both *Mycobacterium tuberculosis* and HIV.[2] By 1997 almost 8% of the more than 8 million tuberculosis cases were attributable to HIV infection, with most of these individuals living in Africa, South Asia, and Southeast Asia.[3,4] In Africa almost one-third of all persons with tuberculosis are HIV infected. Areas of the world with access to highly active antiretroviral therapy have reported decreasing rates of tuberculosis, such as those reported by the EuroSIDA Study.[5] More common, however, is the situation in Kenya, where increasing HIV infection has been followed by an increase in both active tuberculosis and latent infection.[6]

The impact of HIV infection on tuberculosis in the United States was first noted during the mid to late 1980s.[7] Case rates of tuberculosis steadily declined from the 1950s to a nadir of 22,201 new cases in 1985, then increased from 1986 until 1992 when 26,673 cases were reported.[7,8] Epidemiologic data showed that excessive numbers of cases of tuberculosis were being reported from the same demographic groups that had high rates of HIV infection: men, racial and ethnic minorities, and persons 25 to 44 years of age.[8] In addition to the impact of HIV infection, other factors accounting for the increase in the number of tuberculosis cases included changes in immigration patterns; an increase in persons living in group settings such as nursing homes, shelters, and prisons; and decreased funding of the public health infrastructure.[8,9]

The profoundly increased occurrence of tuberculosis in HIV-infected persons is due to increased reactivation of tuberculosis in persons with latent tuberculosis infection, as well as higher rates of primary tuberculosis after recent exposure to *M. tuberculosis*.[10] In normal, immunocompetent persons approximately 10% of individuals infected with *M. tuberculosis* develop clinically active disease: 5% during the first 2 years after infection, and the other 5% sometime during the remainder of their lives.[11] The diminution of cellular immunity in persons infected with HIV results in an inability to contain *M. tuberculosis* in a dormant state. In a study of injecting drug users, all of whom were purified protein derivative (PPD)-positive and were followed for 2 years without prophylaxis, none of 62 HIV-negative patients developed active tuberculosis compared to 7 of 49 persons who were HIV-positive.[12] Other studies have demonstrated that, without intervention, persons dually infected with HIV and *M. tuberculosis* develop active tuberculosis at rates of 5 to 16/100 person-years.[13–15]

It had been assumed that in low-prevalence countries such as the United States more than 90% of tuberculosis in adults was due to reactivation of latent disease. Studies using DNA fingerprinting, however, demonstrated that up to 40% of all new cases of tuberculosis in San Francisco and New York City appear to be due to recent infection.[16,17] Furthermore, among HIV-infected persons, up to two-thirds appeared to have new infection. Outbreaks of tuberculosis caused by recent transmission in HIV-infected persons have been well documented in a variety of settings, including hospitals, residential facilities, prisons, shelters, and social networks.[18–23] The increased susceptibility to new infection with *M. tuberculosis* is emphasized by the documented occurrence of exogenous reinfection following successful therapy for clinical tuberculosis in HIV-infected patients.[24]

Extent of the Problem in the United States

In 1999 tuberculosis cases in the United States declined to 17,531, the lowest number yet recorded.[25] Because HIV testing is recommended but not mandatory for persons with tuberculosis, the impact of HIV on tuberculosis in the United States cannot be exactly determined. Seroprevalence surveys done by the Centers for Disease Control and Prevention (CDC) during 1988–1989 at 20 clinics around the United States showed a median seroprevalence of HIV infection of 3.4% (range 0–46%) among patients with active tuberculosis.[26] Rates of HIV infection were noted to be much higher in East Coast cities such as New York, Boston, and Miami than in other regions. Using a different approach to estimating the impact of HIV on tuberculosis in the United States, the CDC evaluated hospitalizations by young adults during the 1985–1990 period and determined that 21% of persons hospitalized with tuberculosis were co-infected with HIV.[27] In a national survey of death certificates of patients who died from tuberculosis in 1993, approximately 24% were known to be co-infected with HIV.[28]

More recent data appear to show a decrease in the absolute number of HIV-related tuberculosis cases in the United States and in the percentage of cases of tuberculosis that occur in HIV-infected people. In 1993 HIV status was known for only 7447 (30%) of all persons with active tuberculosis in the United States; and of these, 3678 were HIV-positive.[25] By 1998 there were 8229 persons with tuberculosis whose serostatus was known, and the number of HIV-infected persons had decreased to 1824. As noted above, these data are not complete due to the voluntary nature of HIV testing. A more complete data set evaluated the impact of HIV on tuberculosis in Atlanta[29]: From 1991 to 1997 HIV serostatus was determined for 85% of the 1378 patients with tuberculosis, and HIV infection as a cofactor decreased from a peak of 45% of tuberculosis cases in 1994 to a low of 25% of cases in 1997. Similarly, in San Francisco the case rate of tuberculosis in HIV-positive persons declined from 492 per 100,000 in 1991 to 66 per 100,000 in 1997.[30]

The incidence of tuberculosis among HIV-infected persons has been reported by several groups and varies widely by region. A prospective study conducted at six centers in the United States found that among 1130 HIV-infected persons without AIDS the incidence of tuberculosis was 0.7 [95% confidence interval (CI) 0.5 to 1.0] cases/100 person-years,[31] a finding similar to that of a Baltimore retrospective cohort study of persons with counts less than 300 CD4 cells/mm^3, which found an incidence of 0.4 (95% CI 0.1 to 0.9)/100 person-years.[32] A national study conducted using death certificate information found that of 24,230 HIV-infected patients who died in 1992 there were 4.1% who were reported to also have had tuberculosis.[33]

▲ CLINICAL SYNDROME

Effect of HIV Infection on the Presentation of Tuberculosis

Tuberculosis is frequently the first manifestation of HIV infection, so all patients with tuberculosis should be tested for HIV. The CD4+ T-lymphocyte count in patients with HIV and tuberculosis has varied widely; in a series from San Francisco,[34] for example, the median CD4+ T-lymphocyte count was 326/mm^3, whereas a series from New York showed a median CD4+ T-lymphocyte count of 72/mm^3.[35] This may reflect two different populations, with reactivated tuberculosis predominating in persons with high CD4+ T-lymphocyte cell counts and primary tuberculosis occurring mainly in persons with advanced HIV infection.

Pulmonary tuberculosis is the major manifestation of tuberculosis in both HIV-positive and HIV-negative populations. Extrapulmonary disease, however, is more common in HIV-infected patients and is directly correlated with the CD4+ T-lymphocyte count. In a study of 97 patients with HIV and tuberculosis, 70% of patients with 100 CD4 cells/mm^3 or less had extrapulmonary disease, compared with only 28% of patients with more than 300 cells/mm^3.[36] Common sites of extrapulmonary disease in the series included blood (positive in 22/75 patients cultured), bone marrow, and lymph nodes. Other organs reported to be infected with tuberculosis were liver, spleen, and kidney. Tuberculous meningitis occurs much more commonly in patients with AIDS. In a series of 455 HIV-infected Spanish patients with tuberculosis, 45 (10%) had tuberculous meningitis.[37] In this series the clinical manifestations of meningeal involvement were similar in patients with and without HIV infection and included fever (89%), headache (60%), and altered level of consciousness (43%).

Whether patients have pulmonary disease, extrapulmonary disease, or both, almost all patients have systemic manifestations of tuberculosis. Most patients are febrile, and almost half report night sweats, cough, or weight loss.[38] These protean manifestations should alert the clinician to the possibility of tuberculosis, although they are nonspecific and may be secondary to other complications of HIV infection.

Effect of Tuberculosis on the Course of HIV Infection

In addition to the impact of HIV infection on the natural history and clinical manifestations of tuberculosis, the occurrence of tuberculosis affects the clinical course of HIV infection.[39] Patients with active tuberculosis have been found to have a dramatic increase in HIV RNA levels, which decrease with successful therapy of the tuberculosis.[40] The clinical impact of tuberculosis and the progression of HIV disease can be measured as increased numbers of opportunistic infections and as an increase in mortality.

Whalen and colleagues reported a cohort study of 106 HIV-infected patients with active tuberculosis and 106 HIV-infected controls matched for CD4 cells.[41] Patients with active tuberculosis developed opportunistic infections at a relative risk of 1.42 (95% CI 0.94–2.11) compared to patients without tuberculosis. In this study, 45 patients in the tuberculosis group died—6 as a result of tuberculosis—compared to 30 deaths among the control patients. Tuberculosis was found to be an independent predictor of death resulting from HIV infection, even when the six deaths directly caused by tuberculosis were removed.

▲ DIAGNOSIS

Skin Testing

Tuberculin skin testing with PPD remains the only method for detecting latent tuberculosis and can be used as an adjunct for the diagnosis of active disease. The only strength for which diagnostic cutoff points have been developed is the 5 tuberculin unit (5-TU) dose, which is the only dose that should be used when diagnosing tuberculosis. Other tests that use tuberculin, such as the tine test and the multitest CMI (Connaught Laboratories), are not standardized; and although they may be used for screening, they should not be relied on as a diagnostic test for infection with *M. tuberculosis*. PPD skin tests should be applied using the standard Mantoux technique, with the induration measured between 48 and 72 hours. Tests read later than 72 hours that are still positive are valid, but tests read after 72 hours that are negative should be repeated.

The definition of a positive PPD test depends on the underlying risk factors for tuberculosis infection and the ability of the host to respond to the antigenic stimulant.[42] As shown in Table 33–1, a 5 mm or more induration is considered positive for all HIV-infected persons. A patient whose HIV status is unknown and who has had close contact with someone who has active tuberculosis is also considered positive with a 5 mm induration. Injection drug users not known to be HIV-infected are considered positive with a 10 mm induration.

Tuberculin skin testing is a crude diagnostic tool, with both false-positive and false-negative results. PPD skin testing is based on a delayed-type hypersensitivity (DTH) response, which is a function of cell-mediated immunity. DTH responses are frequently reduced in patients with advanced HIV infection, which leads to an increase in false-negative skin tests.[43] Several methods have been proposed to improve the accuracy of PPD tests in HIV-positive persons. One approach has been to provide a second, or "booster," PPD dose 1 to 3 weeks after a negative initial test. This approach is based on the ability to detect latent tuberculosis in elderly persons using such a strategy.[44] In a Community Programs for Clinical Research on AIDS (CPCRA) study of 709 HIV-infected persons in the United States who were initially tuberculin-negative, only 18 (2.7%) responded to a second (booster) test.[45] A study by Hecker and colleagues found a booster response in 17 (29%) of 58 persons studied in Uganda.[46] The low yield with the booster test in the United States does not suggest it for routine use, but it may be worthwhile in individual circumstances. A second suggestion has been to lower the cutoff point for a positive PPD in HIV-infected persons to 2 mm to reduce the number of misclassified persons.[47] Other studies have found that, in fact, few HIV-positive persons have PPD reactions between 2 and 5 mm,[45,48] and the current standard remains 5 mm for a positive test in HIV-infected persons.

Another approach that has been suggested to reduce the number of persons misclassified because of the results of PPD testing has been to include an anergy panel to identify persons who are anergic and unable to react to PPD or any DTH test, or persons not anergic, who presumably would be PPD-positive if infected with latent tuberculosis. In 1991 the CDC suggested that anergy testing be done on a routine basis for HIV-infected persons using two antigens (e.g., mumps skin test antigen and tetanus toxoid) in addition to PPD.[43] More recently, however, data have shown the results of anergy testing to be unstable and unreliable in HIV-infected persons.[49,50] Of particular importance when emphasizing the problems of anergy testing is the report from the Pulmonary Complications of HIV Infection group, which followed 491 HIV-infected persons.[50] This group identified 46 persons who were initially PPD-positive and then were later PPD-negative. At the time of a negative PPD reaction, 18 (39%) had a positive mumps skin test. A positive mumps, or anergy, test and a negative PPD would have usually been interpreted as "proof" that the patient was not infected with *M. tuberculosis* when in fact these were examples of a false-negative PPD in a nonanergic patient. The CDC has evaluated the accumulated data and revised their guidelines for anergy testing.[51] Although it is acknowledged that anergy testing may have a role as a prognostic factor in HIV infection[52,53] and may be of value in limited situations, anergy testing is no longer recommended for routine use in tuberculosis screening programs of HIV-infected persons.

▲ **Table 33–1.** DEFINITION OF A POSITIVE PPD TEST

Induration	Risk Factors for Tuberculosis
≥5 mm	HIV infection Close contact with an active case Chest radiograph suggestive of tuberculosis Patients with organ transplants or otherwise immunocompromised
≥10 mm	Injection drug use Residence in high congregate setting (e.g., prison, jail, nursing home, shelter) Recent arrival from a high-prevalence country Renal failure, diabetes, malignancy, or other condition that increases the risk of active tuberculosis Local determination of high-prevalence group
≥15 mm	No known risk factors for tuberculosis

Radiographic Examination

Pulmonary disease is the most common manifestation of tuberculosis. Whether alone or in conjunction with extrapulmonary disease, the lungs are involved in 68% to 100%

of HIV-infected persons with tuberculosis.[15,35,36,38,54] In all patients who are HIV-infected, a chest radiograph should be obtained at the time of the first evaluation regardless of PPD status. In addition, a chest radiograph should be obtained in all persons suspected of having active tuberculosis and in all those with a newly positive PPD.

The pulmonary manifestations of tuberculosis differ somewhat in HIV-positive and HIV-negative patients. In a large series of 422 patients with tuberculosis in Zimbabwe, HIV-infected patients were less likely to have upper lobe infiltrates (43% vs. 67%) and more likely to have pleural, lymph node, miliary, or pericardial abnormalities (38% vs. 20%).[55] In another series from Africa, cavitary lesions appeared to be less common in HIV-infected persons (23% vs. 40%).[56] Series of cases from the United States have also reported chest films demonstrating a higher prevalence of adenopathy, diffuse infiltrates, and pleural effusions than would be expected in HIV-negative patients with tuberculosis.[35,36] These "atypical" pulmonary manifestations of tuberculosis are more common in patients with less than 200 CD4 cells/mm^3, and may represent primary infection.

In persons suspected of having extrapulmonary disease, additional radiographic tests may be indicated. In particular, computed tomography (CT) scans of the chest and abdomen are useful for detecting tuberculous lymphadenopathy. CT scans are also useful for detecting tuberculomas in the brain and liver as well as genitourinary tract disease.

Bacteriologic Examination

Isolation of *M. tuberculosis* is required to make a definitive diagnosis of tuberculosis, but tuberculosis may be treated and reported based on clinical evidence alone. Sputum is the most common source for detecting *M. tuberculosis*. It should be obtained for three consecutive days, preferably morning specimens. For persons unable to cough, sputum induction using inhalation of saline is helpful. For samples of sputum being examined for tuberculosis, the laboratory should be advised to process any sample, even if it does not meet the specifications for the presence of polymorphonuclear leukocytes, which are usually required for cultures for routine bacteria.

A smear positive for acid-fast bacilli (AFB) occurs in about 60% of persons with HIV infection who have a positive culture for *M. tuberculosis*,[57] the same yield as HIV-negative individuals. A positive AFB smear is not proof of tuberculosis because *Mycobacterium avium* and *Mycobacterium kansasii* also commonly result in positive smears.

Technology has recently been developed to detect the presence of *M. tuberculosis* directly in sputum. These direct amplification probes have the advantage of identifying the presence of *M. tuberculosis* within hours. Both of the tests currently under widespread use, the Gen-Probe MTD (Gen-Probe, San Diego, CA, USA) and the Amplicor *M. tuberculosis test* (Roche Diagnostic Systems, Branchburg, NJ, USA), have excellent sensitivity and specificity for AFB-positive specimens, and an enhanced version of the MTD test has been approved for use in AFB smear-negative specimens.[58–60] These tests have been validated only for sputum samples and not for detecting extrapulmonary disease. The accuracy of these tests for diagnosing tuberculosis in HIV-positive patients may or may not differ from the data published because only small numbers of HIV-positive patients have been included in studies to date.

Regardless of the result of the smear or the direct probes, all samples should be processed for mycobacterial culture. Liquid culture techniques should be used to reduce the time of detection. Whereas the initial BACTEC broth depended on a radiometric system,[61] nonradiometric rapid broth systems have become available.[62,63] These various systems detect the growth of mycobacteria within 1 to 2 weeks, compared with 3 to 6 weeks for traditional solid media. Liquid cultures that are positive for mycobacteria should be probed using a direct DNA probe to ascertain if the organism is *M. tuberculosis* or some other mycobacterium.[64]

Although any HIV-infected person with a positive culture for *M. tuberculosis* must be aggressively followed and evaluated for treatment, it has become apparent that some patients diagnosed with "tuberculosis" are in fact diagnosed falsely owing to laboratory error.[65] This should be particularly considered in the setting of low clinical suspicion and a single positive culture. These false-positives have been due to multiple factors, including contamination of equipment such as bronchoscopes, laboratory cross-contamination, and reporting errors. In published series the median rate of false-positive cultures for *M. tuberculosis* was 3.1%.[65] If contamination is suspected, restriction fragment length polymorphism (RFLP) analysis has proved helpful for clinical decision-making for HIV-infected persons.[66]

All isolates of *M. tuberculosis* should be tested for drug susceptibility. Laboratories using broth systems usually are able to report susceptibility results within 3 to 4 weeks from the time the sample is obtained compared to 8 to 12 weeks from laboratories using conventional solid media.

Mycobacteremia occurs in patients with disseminated tuberculosis as well as disease that appears clinically confined to the lungs. In one study of 27 consecutive HIV-infected persons with tuberculosis, 7 (26%) had positive blood cultures, including 5 (83%) of 6 persons with extrapulmonary disease and 4 (8%) of 53 persons with pulmonary disease.[67] Other studies have reported bacteremia rates up to 42% in persons with both HIV and tuberculosis[54]; because of this, blood cultures for mycobacteria should be obtained whenever tuberculosis is suspected in HIV-infected patients. Blood cultures for mycobacteria has been shown to be useful in developing nations, where more invasive tests may be unavailable.[68,69]

Approach to Diagnosing Active Tuberculosis

Patients suspected of having tuberculosis should be evaluated rapidly for their personal medical care and their potential threat to public health. Figure 33–1 represents a diagnostic approach. A reaction of 5 mm or more to a PPD skin test means that it is likely the patient is infected with *M. tuberculosis*, although it does not necessarily imply that there is active disease. In a person with a past negative test, a newly positive PPD test is a matter of particular concern because it may indicate that the person has a

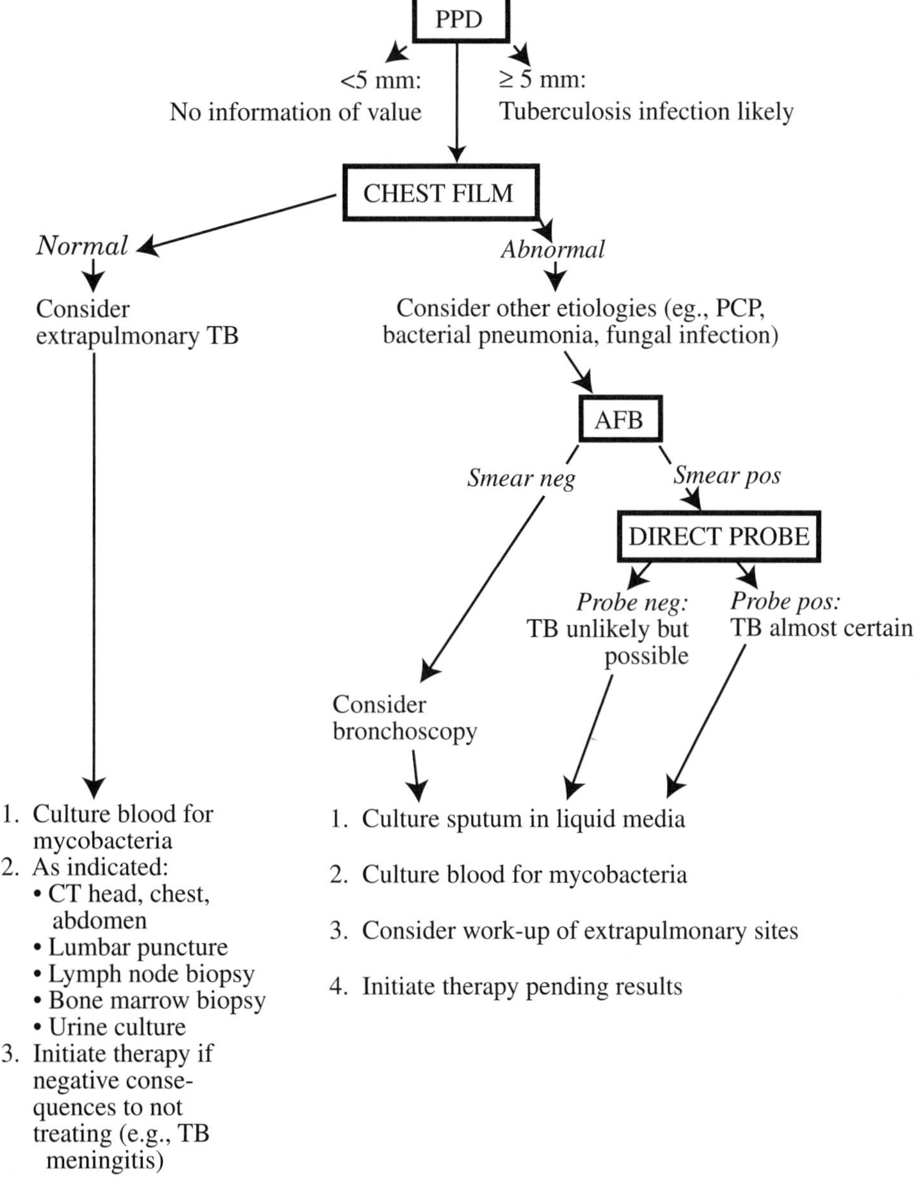

Figure 33–1. Diagnostic approaches for suspected tuberculosis (TB).

primary infection. A negative PPD test is of no diagnostic value and should not dissuade further workup.

A chest film should be obtained from all patients. As discussed above, any abnormality should be considered as consistent with tuberculosis. Other etiologies for pulmonary infiltrates should be considered, including *Pneumocystis carinii* pneumonia, bacterial and fungal infections, and malignancies.[70] Sputum for AFB testing should be obtained from any patient with an abnormal chest film in whom tuberculosis is suspected. In asymptomatic persons with normal chest films, routine collection of sputum for AFB testing has a low yield and should not be done routinely.[71] Patients with a negative AFB smear should be considered for bronchoscopy, with or without biopsy.[72]

Patients with AFB-positive sputum may benefit from a direct application test. A positive test makes tuberculosis almost certain, but the specimen should always be cultured for definitive proof and susceptibility testing. Ten percent of individuals who are AFB-positive with a negative direct amplification test have positive *M. tuberculosis* cultures; therefore one must consider the underlying likelihood of tuberculosis before deciding on whether to continue isolation of the patient and whether to treat for tuberculosis. An injection drug user in New York City with an abnormal chest film is, for example, more likely to have for tuberculosis and should probably be kept in isolation and on treatment than the homosexual man with a normal chest film living in Portland, Oregon. An American Thoracic Society workshop considered the implications of various therapeutic and public health actions based on direct amplification results, and it published a set of recommendations for using these tests.[58] In addition, the CDC has suggested an algorithm for using these tests in persons with smear-negative disease.[60]

▲ **Table 33–2.** MANIFESTATIONS OF DISEASE DUE TO *M. TUBERCULOSIS* AND *M. AVIUM* COMPLEX IN PATIENTS WITH HIV INFECTION

Manifestation	Presence of Tuberculosis	Disseminated MAC
Preexisting complications of HIV	Possible	Usual
CD4 count	Any	<50
Pulmonary involvement	Common	Rare
Chest film	Abnormal	Normal
Anemia	Mild	Severe
Mycobacteremia	10–40%	80–90%

MAC, *Mycobacterium avium* complex.

Other than *M. tuberculosis*, the other common organism most likely to occur as a positive AFB smear in persons with HIV is *M. avium* complex, but the diseases caused by these two mycobacteria are usually easily distinguished (Table 33–2). Patients with disseminated *M. avium* usually present with less than 50 CD4 cells/mm^3, a normal chest film, anemia, and liver function abnormalities,[73] whereas tuberculosis occurs at any CD4+ T-lymphocyte count and usually is associated with pulmonary disease.

Regardless of sputum smear results, sputum and blood specimens should be sent for culture. In patients in whom extrapulmonary disease is suspected, other diagnostic tests and cultures are be indicated based on the likely site of the infection.

In persons with a high likelihood of disease, therapy should usually be initiated pending results of the cultures. Presumptive therapy may benefit the patient in terms of controlling the tuberculosis and reducing HIV replication.[40] In addition, early therapy of pulmonary tuberculosis reduces the potential spread of organisms. Presumptive therapy of extrapulmonary tuberculosis must be based on the likelihood of disease and the consequences of not treating it. For example, tuberculous meningitis had a 21% mortality rate in one series of AIDS patients[37] and so treatment should be instituted rapidly. For both pulmonary and extrapulmonary disease, treatment may be viewed as a diagnostic tool, with the response to therapy serving as proof of tuberculosis if cultures are unavailable.[74]

▲ TREATMENT

Recommended Regimens

The recommended initial therapy for tuberculosis includes four primary drugs: isoniazid, rifampin, pyrazinamide, and ethambutol[75–77] (Table 33–3). Isoniazid, rifampin, and pyrazinamide are critical to this regimen for reducing the total duration of therapy. There are few areas in the United States where resistance is so uncommon that a 3-day initial regimen would be recommended. Ethambutol may be dropped from the regimen as soon as the organism is shown to be susceptible to the other three drugs. Because of the propensity of HIV-infected persons to develop

▲ **Table 33–3.** TREATMENT REGIMENS FOR TUBERCULOSIS

Preferred Regimen
Initial 2 months
Isoniazid[a]
Rifampin[b]
Pyrazinamide
Ethambutol[c]
Final 4 months
Isoniazid
Rifampin
Alternative Regimen for Patients Intolerant to Pyrazinamide
For 9–12 months
Isoniazid
Rifampin
Ethambutol

[a]A 50-mg dose of pyridoxine should be given daily to all HIV-infected patients receiving isoniazid.
[b]Rifabutin may be substituted for rifampin if protease inhibitors or nonnucleoside reverse transcriptase inhibitors are being used.
[c]Ethambutol should be included in areas where there is 4% or more isoniazid drug resistance until drug susceptibility results are available.

peripheral neuropathy, 50 mg of pyridoxine should be given to all persons receiving isoniazid. For patients with pan-susceptible disease, 2 months of isoniazid, rifampin, and pyrazinamide followed by 4 months more of isoniazid and rifampin is considered adequate for HIV-negative patients. Most HIV-positive patients clear their sputum rapidly,[78] and a 6-month regimen is considered adequate.[77] In a study in Zaire, HIV-infected patients treated for 12 months had a lower relapse rate than patients treated for 6 months (1.9% vs. 9.0%).[79] It is unclear whether this difference was due to the initial therapy or to reinfection in patients living in a high-incidence region of the world. In a U.S. study, there was no difference in outcome between 6 months versus 9 months of treatment for tuberculosis in HIV-infected persons.[80] For patients not given pyrazinamide, a 9- to 12-month regimen of isoniazid and rifampin is mandatory.[75]

Rifapentine is a long-acting rifamycin recently approved for treatment of tuberculosis in the United States. In a study of the treatment of tuberculosis conducted by the Tuberculosis Trials Consortium (TBTC), rifapentine given once weekly with isoniazid in the continuation phase of therapy (final 4 months) was as effective as twice-weekly rifampin and isoniazid.[81] In HIV-positive patients treated with rifapentine, however, the regimen was found to be ineffective, with a high risk of relapse due to rifampin-resistant organisms.[82] Therefore rifapentine should not be used to treat HIV-infected persons with tuberculosis.

The major difficulty of successfully treating tuberculosis is patient adherence to the drug regimen.[83] Taking drugs inappropriately has become one of the main reasons for increased levels of drug-resistant tuberculosis in the United States.[84] Directly observed treatment (DOT) is now recommended for consideration for all patients being treated for tuberculosis.[75] In a study in Tarrant County, Texas, DOT was demonstrated to reduce relapse and to decrease rates of both primary and acquired drug resistance.[85] DOT programs have been proven cost-effective.[86]

The dosages for the individual drugs are given in Table 33–4. Most patients are given daily treatment for a minimum of 2 weeks and either twice- or thrice-weekly therapy

▲ **Table 33–4.** DOSAGE RECOMMENDATIONS FOR INITIAL TREATMENT OF TUBERCULOSIS IN CHILDREN AND ADULTS

Drug	Daily Dose		Twice-weekly Dose		Thrice-weekly Dose	
	Children	Adults	Children	Adults	Children	Adults
Isoniazid (mg/kg)	10–20 (max 300 mg)	5 (max 300 mg)	20–40 (max 900 mg)	15 (max 900 mg)	20–40 (max 900 mg)	15 (max 900 mg)
Rifampin (mg/kg)	10–20 (max 600 mg)	10 (max 600 mg)	10–20 (max 600 mg)	10 (max 600 mg)	10–20 (max 600 mg)	10 (max 600 mg)
Pyrazinamide (mg/kg)	15–30 (max 2 g)	15–30 (max 2 g)	50–70 (max 4 g)	50–70 (max 4 g)	50–70 (max 3 g)	50–70 (max 3 g)
Ethambutol (mg/kg)[a]	15–25	15–25	50	50	25–30	25–30
Streptomycin (mg/kg)	20–40 (max 1.0 g)	15 (max 1.0 g)	25–30 (max 1.5 g)	25–30 (max 1.5 g)	25–30 (max 1.5 g)	25–30 (max 1.5 g)

Children are defined as those 12 years of age.

[a]Ethambutol is generally not recommended for children whose visual acuity cannot be monitored (<8 years of age). However, ethambutol should be considered for all children with organisms resistant to other drugs when susceptibility to ethambutol has been demonstrated or susceptibility is likely.

From American Thoracic Society. Treatment of tuberculosis and tuberculosis infection in adults and children. Am J Respir Crit Care Med 149:1359, 1994.)

by DOT for the remainder of the regimen. Patients not receiving DOT should receive daily therapy throughout the course of their treatment, preferably using a fixed combination of isoniazid plus rifampin (Rifamate, Aventis) or isoniazid plus rifampin plus pyrazinamide (Rifater, Aventis). By not allowing single-drug therapy, these fixed-dose regimens prevent the development of drug resistance.[87]

Adverse Effects and Drug Interactions

The major side effects and drug interactions of the primary tuberculosis drugs are listed in Table 33–5. Rifampin is a potent inducer of the microsomal P_{450} system and induces metabolism of many drugs handled by this system, including the protease inhibitors and nonnucleoside reverse transcriptase inhibitors (NNRTIs).[88–90] Because of resultant subtherapeutic levels, rifampin should not be used with any of the protease inhibitors or NNRTIs. Although recent CDC guidelines suggest the possible use of rifampin with efavirenz or ritonavir,[90] most experts substitute rifabutin when using any of the protease inhibitors or NNRTIs.

▲ **Table 33–5.** PRIMARY ANTITUBERCULOUS DRUGS

Drug	Major Adverse Effects	Major Drug Interactions
Isoniazid	Liver function abnormalities Peripheral neuropathy Fever	↑ Phenytoin
Rifampin[a]	Liver function abnormalities Rash Acute renal failure Fever	↓ Protease inhibitors ↓ Nonnucleoside reverse transcriptase inihibtors ↓ Methodone ↓ Coumadin derivatives ↓ Fluconazole, ketoconazole ↓ Oral contraceptives ↓ Digoxin ↓ Cyclosporin
Pyrazinamide	Liver function abnormalities Uric acid elevations Polyarthralgia Photosensitivity	
Ethambutol	Optic neuritis (more common at >15 mg/kg/day)	
Streptomycin	Ototoxicity Nephropathy	Increase in nephrotoxicity with vancomycin and pentamidine

[a]Should not be used with protease inhibitors or nonnucleoside reverse transcriptase inhibitors owing to a decrease in the level of these drugs.

When treating HIV-infected individuals with active tuberculosis, it is important to provide optimal treatment for both infections. If the patient is not in need of antiretroviral therapy or is only on nucleoside agents, the tuberculosis treatment should include rifampin. If the patient is receiving indinavir, saquinavir, ritonavir, nelfinavir, amprenavir, lopinavir, efavirenz, or nevirapine, rifabutin should be used in place of rifampin in the treatment regimen.[77] Delavirdine cannot be used with either rifampin or rifabutin. Rifabutin is a less potent inducer of the cytochrome P_{450} enzyme and is compatible (with dose modifications) with the agents listed above.[89,90] Table 33–6 lists the appropriate doses of rifabutin when used with currently available agents. Rifabutin can be used at full dose (300 mg daily or twice weekly) if the patient is receiving only nucleoside agents. It should be noted that HIV-infected patients may have highly complex pharmacokinetics due to host factors and drug–drug interactions. The recommended dose changes are based on limited data, and patients with evidence of rifabutin toxicity (e.g., such as uveitis, liver abnormalities, neutropenia) may need to have the dose of rifabutin lowered or the drug stopped completely.

Rifabutin is extremely active against *M. tuberculosis* in vitro and has proven to be clinically effective for treating active tuberculosis.[91] There are limited data on the efficacy of rifabutin to treat tuberculosis when combined with protease inhibitors or NNRTIs. One series reported 25 patients with active tuberculosis treated with a rifabutin-containing regimen while also receiving indinavir or nelfinavir.[92] All 25 patients were cured of their tuberculosis with no relapses occurring at a median of 13 months of follow-up after therapy. Moreover, patients had a positive response to their antiretroviral regimen while on rifabutin, showing increased CD4 cells and a decreased HIV load.

▲ **Table 33–6.** RIFABUTIN DOSE WITH ANTIRETROVIRAL THERAPY

Antiretroviral Drug Regimen	TB Treatment Phase	Action
Indinavir, nelfinavir, amprenavir[a]	Daily	↓ Rifabutin to 150 mg qd
Indinavir, nelfinavir, amprenavir	Intermittent	Use 300 mg twice weekly
Saquinavir[b]	Any phase	Use 300 mg daily or twice weekly
Ritonavir (any dose)	Any phase	↓ Rifabutin to 150 mg twice weekly
Delavirdine	Any phase	Do not use rifabutin
Efavirenz (EFV)	Any phase	↑ Rifabutin to 600 mg qd or twice weekly
Nevirapine (NEV)	Any phase	Use 300 mg daily or twice weekly
Lopinavir/ritonavir	Any phase	↓ Rifabutin to 150 mg twice weekly
PI (except RTV) + NNRTI (EFV or NEV)	Any phase	Use 300 mg daily or twice weekly
Evidence of rifabutin toxicity[c]	Intermittent	↓ Rifabutin to 150 mg twice weekly

NNRTI, nonnucleoside reverse transcriptase inhibitors; PI, protease inhibitor; RTV, ritonavir.

[a]Unclear if doses of PIs should be changed when used with rifabutin (RBT): can consider ↑ indinavir to 1000 mg q8h, ↑ nelfinavir to 1000 mg tid or 1250 mg bid.

[b]Saquinavir, as single PI, may not be optimal with RBT.

[c]Uveitis, vomiting after doses, myalgias, skin pigmentation, and neutropenia.

Response in HIV-Infected Persons

Patients with HIV infection respond well to standard antituberculosis regimens.[34,35,93–97] Time to sputum conversion, clinical and radiographic improvement, and overall rates of cure appear to be similar in HIV-positive and HIV-negative patients. Mortality has consistently been reported as higher than expected in HIV-positive patients, with most of the deaths secondary to the underlying HIV disease. In one series of 89 patients with HIV and tuberculosis, 40 patients died during a mean follow-up of 22 months[94]; only three of these deaths, however, were attributed to tuberculosis. Reports have noted median survival as short as 16 to 22 months following diagnosis of tuberculosis,[34,35,97,98] and mortality may be related to tuberculosis-induced increased replication of HIV.[40,41]

Adverse reactions to antituberculosis drugs in HIV-infected persons were initially reported to be higher than expected, with 18% of 132 patients in one series altering therapy as a result of reactions.[93] However, studies directly comparing HIV-positive and HIV-negative patients treated for tuberculosis in the same setting have reported no difference in the rate of adverse events.[34,97]

Drug absorption has been reported to be a problem in HIV-positive patients. In a study of 26 patients with HIV infection and active tuberculosis, 2-hour serum levels were below the predicted minimum for at least one drug for 21 (81%) of the patients.[99] Rifampin and ethambutol were consistently low, although patients on fluconazole had normal rifampin levels. In a study of HIV-infected persons without tuberculosis and HIV-negative controls, the HIV-infected persons were found to have 24% to 32% lower serum levels of pyrazinamide and rifampin.[100] Another study of HIV-positive patients being treated for tuberculosis found no difference in serum levels compared with HIV-negative controls.[101] Because most persons respond appropriately to antituberculosis therapy, routine serum monitoring is not indicated; it should, however, be considered for patients who fail to improve despite adherence to medication.[89]

Drug Resistance

Drug-resistant tuberculosis occurs through the improper use of antituberculous drugs. Common factors leading to acquired resistance include an initially inadequate regimen, failure to recognize nonadherence, and addition of a single drug to a failing regimen.[84] The likelihood of primary drug resistance is based in part on the place where the tuberculosis was contracted because rates of resistance vary widely throughout the world. A survey of drug-resistant tuberculosis reported rates of resistance to isoniazid as high as 10% in Africa and 17% in Asia, while remaining at less than 10% in Europe.[102] Rates of resistance to rifampin remain low in most locations. A 1991 nationwide survey of tuberculosis in the United States found that 8.2% of new cases were resistant to isoniazid and 3.5% to rifampin.[103] Multidrug-resistant (MDR) tuberculosis, defined as resistance to both isoniazid and rifampin, occurred in 3.5% of all cases, with the highest rates occurring in persons living in New York and New Jersey and in those with recurrent disease. Due to nationwide improvements in treatment of active cases, increased use of directly observed therapy, and better use of infection control measures, the rate of drug-resistant tuberculosis has decreased in the United States. In 1999 isoniazid resistance was reported for 7.2% and MDR for 1.1% of new cases of tuberculosis in the United States.[25]

In 1991 the CDC reported outbreaks of MDR tuberculosis among HIV-infected persons in hospitals in New York and Florida.[104] Most of these initial, and subsequent, outbreaks were due to improper infection control techniques: The consequence was primary spread of tuberculosis to immunocompromised HIV-infected patients.[18,24,38,105–108] The problem of drug-resistant and MDR tuberculosis has been centered in New York City, with 19% of patients treated there in April 1991 reported to have MDR tuberculosis.[109] In that survey, patients with HIV infection were more than six times more likely to have MDR tuberculosis than persons without documented HIV infection. A more recent CPCRA survey evaluated drug-resistant tuberculosis in eight metropolitan regions in the United States:[110] In the New York City area, 37% of HIV-positive patients had drug-resistant isolates compared to 18% of HIV-negative individuals; in areas other than New York, resistance rates were approximately 15% in both groups. The problem of MDR tuberculosis remained centered in New York in that survey.

Treatment of patients with drug-resistant tuberculosis is complex and must be guided by susceptibility results. It is imperative that patients receive at least two drugs to which the organism is susceptible.[111] For patients with monoresistance to isoniazid, a 6- to 9-month regimen of rifampin (or rifabutin), ethambutol, and pyrazinamide is usually effective.

For patients resistant to rifampin, an 18-month regimen of isoniazid and ethambutol is effective, or one could use a 9-month regimen of isoniazid, streptomycin, and pyrazinamide.[77] For patients resistant to both isoniazid and rifampin, a regimen of four active drugs should be employed guided by susceptibility patterns. The doses and major adverse effects of the second-line antituberculous drugs are listed in Table 33–7. The quinolone drugs have been widely used to treat tuberculosis and should be considered in resistant cases.[112] An aminoglycoside should always be given to patients with MDR disease. Rifabutin is active in approximately 25% of isolates with rifampin resistance.[113]

The clinical outcome in patients with drug-resistant tuberculosis depends on the pattern of resistance and the immune state of the patient. In HIV-negative patients with MDR isolates, response rates have been reported (by the group at the National Jewish Center for Immunology and Respiratory Medicine) to be as low as 56%.[114] During the early outbreaks of MDR tuberculosis among HIV-infected patients, mortality was high, with a median survival time of only 2.1 months in one report.[38] In a series of MDR tuberculosis patients from New York City from 1983 to 1993, HIV-infected patients had a median survival of 6.8 months, but it was longer for those who had early initiation of appropriate treatment.[115] Many of the deaths were due to the underlying advanced HIV disease. In a more recent multicenter series of MDR tuberculosis, 25% of patients had died at 12 months and 35% at 18 months.[116] Treatment outcomes in patients with resistance that is not of the MDR type have been markedly better.[97]

Paradoxical Reactions

Transient worsening of signs and symptoms of tuberculosis soon after initiation of antituberculosis therapy is referred to as a "paradoxical reaction."[77] Such reactions have been noted to occur much more commonly in HIV-infected patients who are beginning antiretroviral therapy while being treated for tuberculosis. In one series from Florida, paradoxical reactions were noted in 1 of 55 (2%) HIV-negative patients being treated for tuberculosis compared with 12 of 33 (36%) HIV-infected patients.[117] The paradoxical reactions were more closely associated in time with the initiation of antiretroviral therapy than the initiation of tuberculosis treatment. Patients have most frequently had worsening fever and lymphadenitis.[117–119] In addition, many patients experience worsening of their chest radiograph abnormalities.[120]

Although the exact mechanism responsible for the transient worsening is not known, it is hypothesized that it is due to an improved immune response to the mycobacterium, as patients frequently have a decrease in HIV load, an increase in CD4 cells, and a return of the tuberculin skin test response at the time of the paradoxical reaction.[66,77,117] It is important to evaluate for other causes of fever and deterioration, such as intercurrent infections, inadequate tuberculosis treatment, or nonadherence to drugs. Most often patients improve with continuation of the initial regimen, although some require a short course of steroids (2 to 3 weeks).

▲ **Table 33–7.** SECONDARY ANTITUBERCULOSIS DRUGS

Drug	Usual Daily Dose	Major Adverse Effects
Levofloxacin	500 mg PO qd	GI upset CNS abnormalities
Ciprofloxacin	500–750 mg PO bid	GI upset CNS abnormalities
Capreomycin	15 mg/kg IM qd (1 g max)	Ototoxicity Nephrotoxicity
Kanamycin	15 mg/kg IM qd (1 g max)	Ototoxicity Nephrotoxicity
Amikacin	15 mg/kg IM qd (1 g max)	Ototoxicity Nephrotoxicity
Rifabutin[a]	300 mg PO qd	Liver function abnormalities Neutropenia
Clofazimine	100–200/mg PO qd	Skin discoloration GI upset
Ethionamide	15 mg/kg PO qd (1 g max)	Liver function abnormalities Neurologic disorders
Cycloserine	15 mg/kg PO qd (1 g max)	Psychiatric abnormalities Convulsions Neuropathy

CNS, central nervous system; GI, gastrointestinal.
[a]Dose must be adjusted when combined with certain other HIV therapies; see Table 33–6.

Approach to Therapy

Most patients suspected of having active tuberculosis should be started on therapy while cultures are pending. If drug resistance is not suspected, the initial regimen should be isoniazid, rifampin, pyrazinamide, ethambutol, and pyridoxine (Fig. 33–2). Rifabutin should be substituted for rifampin if a protease inhibitor or NNRTI is being used. If drug resistance is suspected because of prior treatment, at least two new drugs should be added. If primary resistance is suspected based on epidemiologic data, a minimum of five drugs should be used. DOT is mandatory for patients suspected of having resistant organisms, and it is highly recommended for all patients. Susceptibility results should be used to determine the final regimen: Patients with pan-susceptible organisms should complete standard therapy, and an individual regimen should be developed for patients with resistant organisms. Patients with extrapulmonary disease usually receive the same regimens as those with pulmonary diseases. Patients with bone and joint tuberculosis and meningiomas may require longer treatment.

Patients must be educated about their medications and the possible adverse effects, and they are instructed to report any abnormalities as soon as they are noted. This is particularly important for symptoms associated with hepatitis because isoniazid-associated deaths have been reported and are estimated to occur in approximately 23 of 100,000 people receiving this drug.[121] Patients should have a formal evaluation for clinical response and adverse events at monthly intervals. Monthly liver function tests may be indicated while patients are on isoniazid, rifampin, or pyrazinamide if baseline results are abnormal or if symptoms develop. If toxicity occurs, the offending drug should be removed and the regimen altered, which may necessitate modifying the overall length of treatment.

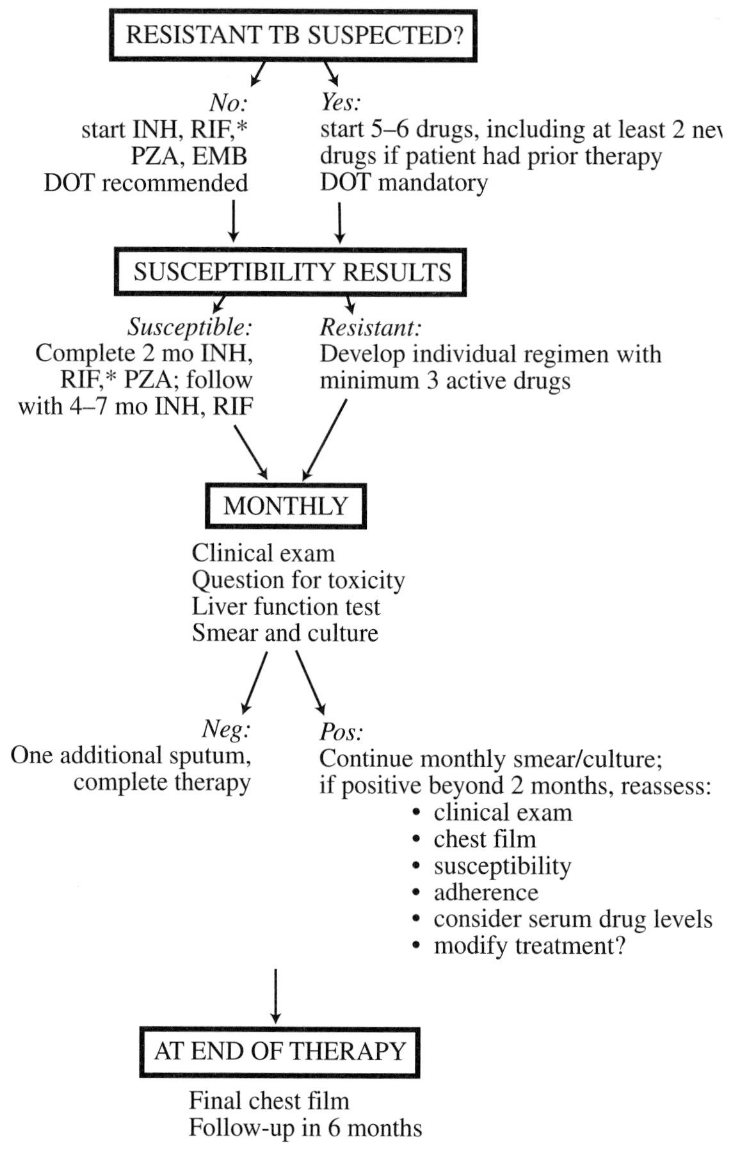

Figure 33–2. Treatment of active tuberculosis.

Patients who experience worsening of symptoms after therapy is initiated should be considered to be having a possible paradoxical reaction. Patients who have an increase in fever or a worsening lymphadenopathy or chest radiograph should be evaluated for possible concurrent illnesses or drug toxicities. In addition, adherence to their medications must be ensured and consideration given to the possibility that the tuberculosis therapy is failing because of resistant organisms. Usually patients can be successfully treated through a paradoxical reaction with no change in therapy. For severe paradoxical reactions, a 2- to 3-week course of steroid therapy may be beneficial.

Sputum should be obtained monthly for smears and culture. Patients who remain positive longer than 2 months should be closely evaluated for their clinical response and for adherence to the treatment regimen. Repeating the chest radiograph and susceptibility testing of the organism should be done at 2 months if the response to therapy is deemed inadequate. Serum drug levels should be considered for patients not responding adequately.

Patients who complete therapy should have a repeat chest film as a new baseline. Relapse is uncommon, and there is no need for lifelong isoniazid. A follow-up visit at 6 months is recommended for evaluation, and visits beyond that time should be individualized but should include additional visits for those who were slow to respond or had drug-resistant isolates.

▲ PREVENTION

Treatment of Latent Tuberculosis Infection (Preventive Therapy)

It is estimated that there are more than 80,000 persons co-infected with HIV and *M. tuberculosis* in North America and more than 5 million in the world.[2] Without

▲ **Table 33-8.** EFFICACY OF ISONIAZID PROPHYLAXIS IN
▲ HIV-INFECTED PERSONS

Reference	TB rate per 100 person-years	
	INH	No INH
13	1.70	10.0
124	1.08	3.41
14	0–8.9	16.2
125	0.50	10.4
126	0	9.7

intervention, these individuals develop active tuberculosis at a rate of 5% to 10% per year.[12–15] To provide treatment of latent tuberculosis infection (chemoprophylaxis), it is important to identify these co-infected individuals by applying a PPD skin test at the time of initial evaluation and yearly thereafter for PPD-negative individuals. It is particularly important to identify and treat HIV-infected persons exposed to a recent case of tuberculosis, as these individuals are at highest risk of developing active disease.[121]

For the past 30 years isoniazid has been accepted as the standard means of preventing reactivation tuberculosis.[123] Controlled and noncontrolled studies of HIV-infected patients have demonstrated the efficacy of isoniazid in reducing active tuberculosis in PPD-positive patients (Table 33–8).[13,14,124–127] In a controlled study of isoniazid versus no isoniazid for HIV-positive, PPD-positive patients, Pape et al. reported a reduction of active tuberculosis from 10.0/100 person-years to 1.7/100 person-years;[13] in a placebo-controlled trial of 6 months of isoniazid, Whalen et al. showed a reduction from 3.41 cases/100 person-years to 1.08 cases/100 person-years.[124] The other three studies noted in Table 33–8 report observational data rates of tuberculosis occurring in HIV-positive, PPD-positive patients who did or did not take isoniazid. In all three reports, the rate of tuberculosis was significantly reduced by taking isoniazid.

The most common adverse effect of isoniazid when used for prophylaxis is chemical and clinical hepatitis. In a study of 1000 HIV-infected patients receiving isoniazid preventive therapy during the era prior to HIV, 1.7% developed symptomatic hepatitis and an additional 4.7% had asymptomatic hepatitis.[128] HIV-infected persons have not experienced unusual reactions to isoniazid.

The current recommendation is that HIV-positive, PPD-positive patients receive daily isoniazid for 9 months[77,129,130] (Table 33–9). For persons who are unable to take their own medication, isoniazid may be given by DOT as 900 mg twice weekly, although the efficacy of this regimen has not been proven.[131] A 2-month regimen of daily rifampin and pyrazinamide was compared to 1 year of isoniazid for prevention of tuberculosis in HIV-positive, PPD-positive persons; the 2-month regimen was found to be equivalent to 12 months of isoniazid[132] and is an acceptable regimen for preventing tuberculosis in patients exposed to susceptible or isoniazid-resistant organisms. This regimen must be given daily to achieve maximum benefit.[130] Rifampin given as single-drug therapy for 4 months has some supportive data for efficacy, and it can be given to persons exposed to isoniazid-resistant tuberculosis or those started on rifampin

▲ **Table 33-9.** CHEMOPROPHYLAXIS OF TUBERCULOSIS FOR
▲ HIV-INFECTED PATIENTS

Drugs	Dosage
Standard regimen	
Isoniazid	300 mg PO qd × 9 months
Rifampin[a] +	600 mg PO qd } × 2 months
Pyrazinamide	20 mg/kg qd
Alternatives	
Isoniazid	900 mg PO twice weekly (DOT) × 9 months
Rifampin[a]	600 mg PO qd × 4 months
Alternatives for exposure to MDR-TB	
Levofloxacin +	500 mg qd }
Ethambutol	15 mg/kg qd
Ciprofloxacin +	750 mg PO bid } × 12 months
Ethambutol	15 mg/kg qd
Pyrazinamide +	20 mg/kg qd } × 12 months
Ethambutol	15 mg/kg qd

DOT, directly observed therapy.
[a]Rifabutin maybe substituted for rifampin; see Table 33–6 for correct dosing of rifabutin.

and pyrazinamide but unable to take pyrazinamide.[130] As noted above, rifampin cannot be used with the current protease inhibitors or NNRTIs, and rifabutin may be considered as a substitute. For persons exposed to MDR tuberculosis, preventive therapy should be based on individual susceptibility patterns. Ethambutol combined with either pyrazinamide or a fluoroquinolone such as levofloxacin or ciprofloxacin for 12 months should be used in situations where the susceptibility pattern is unknown.[133]

Many HIV-infected patients with latent tuberculosis cannot be identified because of anergy. Based on data showing that certain high-risk anergic patients develop active tuberculosis at rates of 3.4 to 12.4/100 person-years,[14,15,124,125] the CDC suggested in 1991 that consideration be given to preventive therapy for HIV-infected persons who are anergic and belong to *groups in which the prevalence of tuberculosis infection is 10% or higher*.[43] This strategy was tested in a CPCRA study of 517 high-risk, HIV-infected, anergic patients who were randomized to receive 6 months of isoniazid or a matched placebo.[134] Because only 0.9 cases of active tuberculosis per 100 person-years were reported in the placebo group, isoniazid could not be demonstrated to be beneficial. Whalen et al. were also unable to show a benefit for isoniazid prophylaxis for anergic patients in Uganda.[124] Based on these studies and data showing anergy testing to be highly variable and unstable,[48–50] the CDC now suggests that anergy testing not be done routinely and that only those PPD-negative patients exposed to an active case of tuberculosis should receive chemoprophylaxis.[51,77]

Approach to Treatment of Latent Tuberculosis Infection (Preventive Therapy)

All HIV-infected patients should receive 5 tuberculin units (TU) of PPD and undergo chest radiography at the time of their initial presentation (Fig. 33–3). Any person with a chest film or clinical symptoms suggestive of active tuberculosis should be evaluated (Fig. 33–1). Persons with a negative PPD test (<5 mm induration) should receive

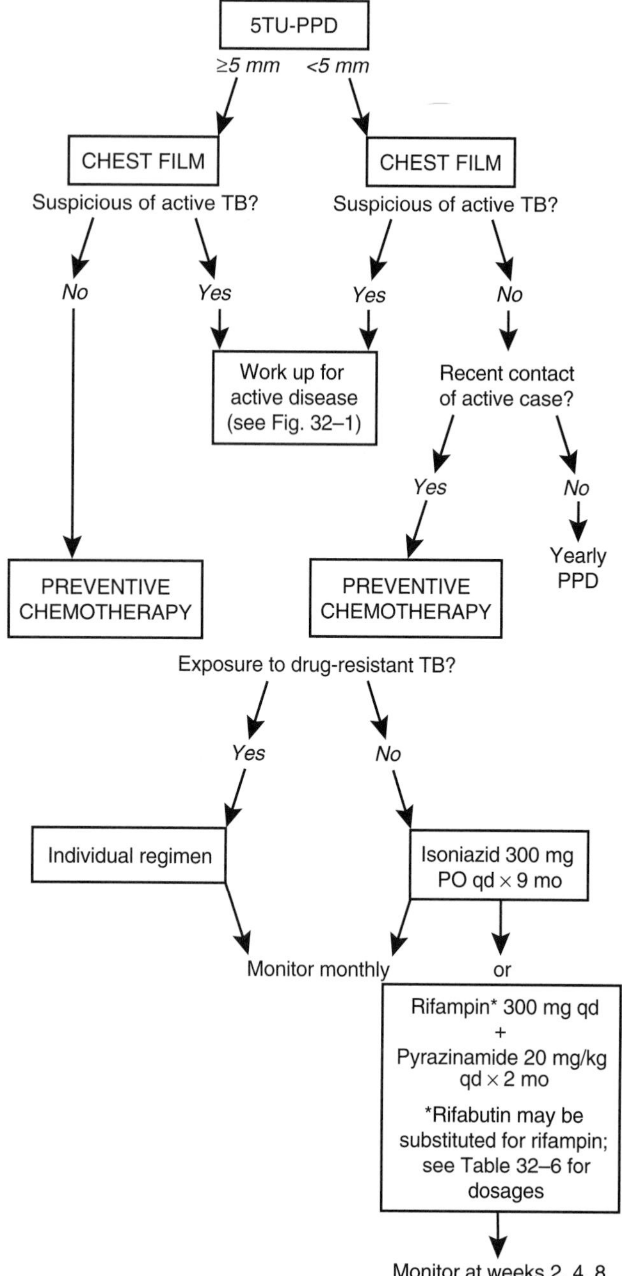

Figure 33–3. Approach to the prevention of tuberculosis in HIV-infected persons.

treatment for latent tuberculosis infection (chemoprophylaxis) only if recently exposed to an active case of tuberculosis. Persons with a negative PPD test should be reevaluated yearly if they are at risk for acquiring disease or more frequently if exposed to active tuberculosis. It is also reasonable to reevaluate a person's PPD reaction if, in response to antiretroviral therapy, there has been a rise in CD4+ T-lymphocyte count to more than 200/mm^3.

Persons with a positive PPD test, negative chest film, and no evidence suggestive of active tuberculosis should receive a chemoprophylaxis regimen of 300 mg isoniazid daily for 9 months or a 2-month regimen of rifampin (or rifabutin) and pyrazinamide.[129,130,134a] The rifabutin dose may have to be adjusted, depending on other HIV therapies (Table 33–6). Patients exposed to drug-resistant organisms must be given one of the alternative regimens listed in Table 33–9. Patients on isoniazid chemoprophylaxis should be evaluated monthly to monitor toxicity and to encourage adherence to their regimen. Patients on rifampin (or rifabutin) and pyrazinamide should be evaluated at weeks 2, 4, 6, and 8 with liver function tests at baseline and weeks 2, 4 and 6. Such frequent monitoring is recommended to enhance compliance for this short regimen and to assess toxicity for a regimen that has not undergone extensive field testing. CDC has reported 23 cases of severe or fatal lung injury associated with rifampin and pyrizinamide therapy for latent tuberculosis infection. None of these cases occurred in patients with HIV infection. However, the American Thoracic Society and CDC now recommend that this regimen be used with caution, especially in patients taking other medications associated with liver injury, or those with alcoholism. This regimen is not recommended for patients with underlying liver disease or those with a history of INH-associated liver disease. CDC also recommends that no more than a 2 week drug supply should be dispersed to enhance compliance with toxicity monitoring. Patients on isoniazid should be subjected to baseline liver function tests (at least a serum bilirubin and serum aminotransferase), which should be repeated at regular intervals if abnormal at baseline or if clinical symptoms suggest hepatitis. Asymptomatic aminotransferase increases are expected and usually do not require that treatment be stopped. Treatment should be stopped and not resumed if the serum aminotransferase level is substantially above baseline.

Prevention of Primary Infection

Spread of both susceptible and drug-resistant isolates of *M. tuberculosis* among HIV-infected persons has been reported in a variety of settings, including hospitals, prisons, shelters, and group homes.[18,20–24,38,104–108,135–137] The common theme in these outbreaks was the rapid spread of organisms from patients with active tuberculosis to immunocompromised HIV-infected persons who subsequently developed primary tuberculosis. These outbreaks were due to the lack of adequate infection control procedures, usually stemming from lack of recognition of the active case. HIV-infected patients appear as likely to spread tuberculosis as HIV-negative patients,[138] and both smear-negative and smear-positive patients are capable of transmitting the mycobacterium to others.[139]

The increased public awareness and improved funding of programs for tuberculosis treatment and control have resulted in a marked nationwide decrease in the number of new cases of tuberculosis.[25] In New York City, new cases of tuberculosis in HIV-infected persons decreased 24%, from 2386 cases in 1991–1992 to 1810 cases in 1993–1994.[140] As of 1999, New York City reported a further reduction to a total of 1540 cases of tuberculosis, both HIV-infected and all others.[25] This decrease in the number of new cases is thought to represent principally the impact of primary prevention.

Basic principles of infection control have been found to be extremely effective at preventing spread of tuberculosis among patients and from patients to health care workers.[141] The basic tenet of tuberculosis control is early recognition, isolation, and treatment of patients with active tuberculosis.[142] Patients with abnormal chest films must be identified immediately and a decision made about the need for isolation. Some facilities with high rates of tuberculosis have developed a policy of isolation for all persons with abnormal chest films pending results of sputum cultures. The implementation of this policy at Grady Memorial Hospital in Atlanta resulted in PPD conversion rates among health care workers decreasing from 8% to 1% per year.[143] This decrease in conversion rates among health care workers would be expected to benefit the patients as well by lowering the rate of tuberculosis transmission in the facility. When a patient is suspected to have tuberculosis, some institutions maintain isolation until three adequate sputum specimens have been shown to be smear-negative or one bronchoalveolar lavage is smear-negative. However, if a patient is truly suspected to have tuberculosis, it is probably preferable to maintain isolation until cultures have been assessed for at least 2 weeks, as smear-negative patients with tuberculosis can and do transmit disease. Patients who are smear-positive should remain in isolation until they show signs of response (e.g., decreased fever and cough, improved roentgenograms, negative smear).

Health care workers have been documented to have acquired tuberculosis from HIV-infected patients.[104,108] The rapid identification and placement of the patient in a proper isolation room is the most critical element in controlling spread of infection.[141] Isolation rooms should be under negative pressure, with at least six air exchanges per hour. Upper-room ultraviolet germicidal irradiation may be used as an adjunct to ventilation and may be useful in large areas such as waiting rooms or emergency departments, where negative ventilation is not feasible. Patients should be kept in isolation until there is a clear response to therapy, as evidenced by alleviation of clinical symptoms and a negative AFB smear. Patients suspected of having drug-resistant disease should be kept in isolation pending documentation of their drug susceptibility pattern. Particulate respiratory air masks have been the focus of controversy in the safety of health care workers.[144,145] Although these protective devices should be worn by all health care workers involved with patients suspected of having tuberculosis, for controlling the spread of the organism they are secondary in importance to identifying and isolating the patients.

A CDC survey of occupations of persons reported with active tuberculosis showed rates of tuberculosis cases among health care workers (6.7/100,000) to be similar to those in the general population.[146] The risk of acquiring tuberculosis from working with HIV-infected individuals was evaluated in a study of 1014 health care workers involved in AIDS care and research.[147] The PPD conversion rate was found to be 1.8/100 person-years, essentially the same range as reported for other health care workers in general medical care. HIV-infected persons who are health care workers should be warned about the risk of acquiring tuberculosis in the workplace,[142] but mandatory exclusion of HIV-infected caregivers from taking care of patients with tuberculosis is not justified.[148]

REFERENCES

1. World Health Organization. Groups at Risk: WHO Report on the Tuberculosis Epidemic. Geneva, World Health Organization, 1996.
2. Raviglione MC, Sinder DE, Kochi A. Global epidemiology of tuberculosis: morbidity and mortality of a worldwide epidemic. JAMA 273:220, 1995.
3. DeCock KM, Binkin NJ, Zuber NJ, et al. Research issues involving HIV-associated tuberculosis in resource-poor countries. JAMA 276:1502, 1996.
4. Dye C, Scheele S, Dolin P, et al. Global burden of tuberculosis: estimated incidence, prevalence, and mortality by country. JAMA 282:677, 1999.
5. Kirk O, Gatel JM, Mocroft A, et al. Infections with *Mycobacterium tuberculosis* and *Mycobacterium avium* among HIV-infected patients after the introduction of highly active antiretroviral therapy. Am J Respir Crit Care Med 162:865, 2000.
6. Odhiambo JA, Borgdorff MW, Kiambih FM, et al. Tuberculosis and the HIV epidemic: increasing annual risk of tuberculosis infection in Kenya, 1986–1996. Am J Public Health 89:1078, 1999.
7. Rieder HL, Cauthen GM, Comstock GW, et al. Epidemiology of tuberculosis in the United States. Epidemiol Rev 11:79, 1989.
8. Canwell MF, Snider DE, Cauthen GM, et al. Epidemiology of tuberculosis in the United States, 1985 through 1992. JAMA 272:535, 1994.
9. Brudney K, Dobkin J. Resurgent tuberculosis in New York City: human immunodeficiency virus, homelessness, and the decline of tuberculosis control programs. Am Rev Respir Dis 144:745, 1991.
10. Girardi E, Raviglione MC, Antonucci G, et al. Impact of the HIV epidemic on the spread of other diseases: the case of tuberculosis. AIDS 14(suppl 3):S47, 2000.
11. Murray JF. The white plague: down and out, or up and coming? Am Rev Respir Dis 140:1788, 1989.
12. Selwyn PA, Hartel D, Lewis VA, et al. A prospective study of the risk of tuberculosis among intravenous drug users with human immunodeficiency virus infection. N Engl J Med 320:545, 1989.
13. Pape JW, Jean SS, Ho JL, et al. Effect of isoniazid on the incidence of active tuberculosis and progression of HIV infection. Lancet 342:268, 1993.
14. Guelar A, Gattell JM, Verdejo J, et al. A prospective study of the risk of tuberculosis among HIV-infected patients. AIDS 7:1345, 1993.
15. Antonucci G, Girardi E, Raviglione MC, et al. Risk factors for tuberculosis in HIV-infected persons: a prospective cohort study. JAMA 274:143, 1995.
16. Small PM, Hopewell PC, Singh SP, et al. The epidemiology of tuberculosis in San Francisco: a population-based study using conventional and molecular methods. N Engl J Med 330:1703, 1994.
17. Alland D, Kalkut GE, Moss AR, et al. Transmission of tuberculosis in New York City: an analysis by DNA fingerprinting and conventional epidemiologic methods. N Engl J Med 330:1710, 1994.
18. Edlin BR, Tokars JI, Grieco MH, et al: An outbreak of multidrug-resistant tuberculosis among hospitalized patients with the acquired immunodeficiency syndrome. N Engl J Med 326:1514, 1992.
19. Daley CL, Small PM, Schecter GF, et al. An outbreak of tuberculosis with accelerated progression among persons infected with the human immunodeficiency virus. N Engl J Med 326:231, 1992.
20. Centers for Disease Control and Prevention. Drug-susceptible tuberculosis outbreak in a state correctional facility housing HIV-infected inmates: South Carolina, 1999–2000. MMWR Morbid Mortal Wkly Rep 49:46, 2000.
21. Moss AR, Hahn JA, Tulsky JP, et al. Tuberculosis in the homeless: a prospective study. Am J Respir Crit Care Med 162:460, 2000.
22. Yaganehdoost A, Graviss EA, Ross MW, et al. Complex transmission dynamics of clonally related virulent *Mycobacterium tuberculosis* associated with barhopping by predominantly human immunodeficiency virus-positive gay men. J Infect Dis 180:1245, 1999.
23. Centers for Disease Control and Prevention. HIV-related tuberculosis in a transgender network: Baltimore, Maryland, and New York City area, 1998–2000. MMWR Morbid Mortal Wkly Rep 49:15, 2000.

24. Small PM, Shafer RW, Hopewell PC, et al. Exogenous reinfection with multidrug-resistant *Mycobacterium tuberculosis* in patients with advanced HIV infection. N Engl J Med 328:1137, 1993.
25. Centers for Disease Control and Prevention. Reported tuberculosis in the United States, 1999. Atlanta, CDC, August 2000.
26. Onorato IM, McCray E. Prevalence of human immunodeficiency virus infection among patients attending tuberculosis clinics in the United States. J Infect Dis 165:87, 1992.
27. Rosenblum LS, Castro KG, Dooley S, et al. Effect of HIV infection and tuberculosis on hospitalizations and cost of care for young adults in the United States, 1985 to 1990. Ann Intern Med 121:786, 1994.
28. Selik RM, Karon JM, Ward JW. Effect of the human immunodeficiency virus epidemic on mortality from opportunistic infections in the United States in 1993. J Infect Dis 176:632, 1997.
29. Sotir MJ, Parrott P, Metchock B, et al. Tuberculosis in the inner city: impact of a continuing epidemic in the 1990s. Clin Infect Dis 29:1138, 1999.
30. Jasmer RM, Hahn JA, Small PM, et al. A molecular epidemiologic analysis of tuberculosis trends in San Francisco, 1991–1997. Ann Intern Med 130:971, 1999.
31. Markowitz N, Hansen NI, Hopewell PC. Incidence of tuberculosis in the United States among HIV-infected persons. Ann Intern Med 126:123, 1997.
32. Moore RD, Chaisson RE. Natural history of opportunistic disease in an HIV-infected urban clinical cohort. Ann Intern Med 124:636, 1996.
33. Selik RM, Chu SY, Ward JW. Trends in infectious diseases and cancers among persons dying of HIV infection in the United States from 1987 to 1992. Ann Intern Med 123:933, 1995.
34. Theuer CP, Hopewell PC, Elias D. Human immunodeficiency virus infection in tuberculosis patients. J Infect Dis 162:8, 1990.
35. Alpert PL, Munsiff SS, Gourevitch MN, et al. A prospective study of tuberculosis and human immunodeficiency virus infection: clinical manifestations and factors associated with survival. Clin Infect Dis 24:661, 1997.
36. Jones BE, Young SM, Antoniskis D, et al. Relationship of the manifestations of tuberculosis to CD4 cell counts in patients with human immunodeficiency virus infection. Am Rev Respir Dis 148:1292, 1993.
37. Berenguer J, Moreno S, Laguna F, et al. Tuberculous meningitis in patients infected with the human immunodeficiency virus. N Engl J Med 326:668, 1992.
38. Fischl MA, Daikos GL, Uttamchandani RB, et al. Clinical presentation and outcome of patients wit HIV infection and tuberculosis caused by multiple-drug-resistant bacilli. Ann Intern Med 117:184, 1992.
39. Del Amo J, Malin AS, Pozniak A, et al. Does tuberculosis accelerate the progression of HIV disease? Evidence from basic science and epidemiology. AIDS 13:1151, 1999.
40. Goleeti D, Weissman D, Jackson RW, et al. Effect of *Mycobacterium tuberculosis* on HIV replication: role of immune activation. J Immunol 157:1271, 1996.
41. Whalen C, Horsburgh CR, Hom D, et al. Accelerated course of human immunodeficiency virus infection after tuberculosis. Am J Respir Crit Care Med 151:129, 1995.
42. American Thoracic Society. Diagnostic standards and classification of tuberculosis in adults and children. Am J Respir Crit Care Med 161:1376, 2000.
43. Centers for Disease Control and Prevention. Purified protein derivative tuberculin anergy and HIV infection: guidelines for anergy testing and management of anergic persons at risk of tuberculosis. MMWR Morbid Mortal Wkly Rep 40(RR-5):27, 1991.
44. Gordin FM, Perez-Stable EJ, Flaherty D, et al. Evaluation of a third sequential tuberculin skin test in a chronic care population. Am Rev Respir Dis 137:153, 1986.
45. Webster CT, Gordin FM, Matts JP, et al. Two-stage tuberculin skin testing in individuals with human immunodeficiency virus infection. Am J Respir Crit Care Med 151:805, 1995.
46. Hecker MT, Johnson JL, Whalen CC, et al. Two-step tuberculin skin testing in HIV-infected persons in Uganda. Am J Respir Crit Care Med 155:81, 1997.
47. Graham NH, Nelson KE, Solomon L, et al. Prevalence of tuberculin positivity and skin test anergy in HIV-1-seropositive and seronegative intravenous drug users. JAMA 267:369, 1992.
48. Gourevitch MN, Hartel D, Schoenbaum EE, et al. Lack of association of induration size with HIV infection among drug users reacting to tuberculin. Am J Respir Crit Care Med 154:1029, 1996.
49. Caiaffa WT, Graham NM, Galai N, et al. Instability of delayed-type hypersensitivity skin test anergy in human immunodeficiency virus infection. Arch Intern Med 155:2111, 1995.
50. Chin DP, Osmond D, Page-Shafer K, et al. Reliability of anergy skin testing in persons with HIV infection. Am J Respir Crit Care Med 153:1982, 1996.
51. Centers for Disease Control and Prevention. Anergy skin testing and preventive therapy for HIV-infected persons, revised recommendations. MMWR Morbid Mortal Wkly Rep 46(RR-15):1, 1997.
52. Birx DL, Brundage J, Larson K, et al. The prognostic utility of delayed-type hypersensitivity skin testing in the evaluation of HIV-infected patients. J Acquir Immune Defic Syndr 6:1248, 1993.
53. Gordin FM, Hartigan PM, Klimas NG, et al. Delayed-type hypersensitivity skin tests are an independent predictor of human immunodeficiency virus disease progression. J Infect Dis 169:893, 1994.
54. Barnes PF, Bloch AB, Davidson PT, et al. Tuberculosis in patients with human immunodeficiency virus infection. N Engl J Med 324:1644, 1991.
55. Pozniak AL, MacLeod GA, Ndlovu D, et al. Clinical and chest radiographic features of tuberculosis associated with human immunodeficiency virus in Zimbabwe. Am J Respir Crit Care Med 152:1558, 1995.
56. Mlika-Cabanne N, Brauner M, Mugusi F, et al. Radiographic abnormalities in tuberculosis and risk of coexisting human immunodeficiency virus infection. Am J Respir Crit Care Med 152:786, 1995.
57. Smith RL, Yew K, Berkowitz KA, et al. Factors affecting the yield of acid-fast sputum smears in patients with HIV and tuberculosis. Chest 106:684, 1994.
58. American Thoracic Society Workshop. Rapid diagnostic tests for tuberculosis: what is the appropriate use? Am J Respir Crit Care Med 155:1804, 1997.
59. Catanzaro A, Perry S, Clarridge JE, et al. The role of clinical suspicion in evaluating a new diagnostic test for active tuberculosis: results of a multicenter prospective trial. JAMA 283:639, 2000.
60. Centers for Disease Control and Prevention. Update: nucleic acid amplification tests for tuberculosis. MMWR Morbid Mortal Wkly Rep 49:593, 2000.
61. Kirihara JM, Hillier SL, Coyle MB. Improved detection times for *Mycobacterium avium* complex and *Mycobacterium tuberculosis* with the BACTEC radiometric system. J Clin Microbiol 22:841, 1985.
62. Zuhre Badak F, Kiski DL, Setterquist S, et al. Comparison of mycobacterial growth indicator tube with BACTEC 460 for detection and recovery of mycobacteria from clinical specimens. J Clin Microbiol 34:2236, 1996.
63. Zanetti S, Ardito F, Sechi L, et al. Evaluation of a nonradiometric system (BACTEC 9000 MB) for detection of mycobacteria in human clinical samples. J Clin Microbiol 35:2072, 1997.
64. Peterson EM, Lu R, Floyd C, et al. Direct identification of *Mycobacterium tuberculosis*, *Mycobacterium avium*, and *Mycobacterium intracellulare* from amplified primary cultures in BACTEC media using DNA probes. J Clin Microbiol 27:1543, 1989.
65. Burman WJ, Reves RR. Review of false-positive cultures for *Mycobacterium tuberculosis* and recommendations for avoiding unnecessary treatment. Clin Infect Dis 31:1390, 2000.
66. Havlir DV, Barnes PF. Tuberculosis in patients with human immunodeficiency virus infection. N Engl J Med 340:367, 1999.
67. Shafer RW, Goldberg R, Sierra M, et al. Frequency of *Mycobacterium tuberculosis* bacteremia in patients with tuberculosis in an area endemic for AIDS. Am Rev Respir Dis 140:1611, 1989.
68. McDonald LC, Archibald LK, Rheanpumikankit S, et al. Unrecognised *Mycobacterium tuberculosis* bacteraemia among hospital inpatients in less developed countries. Lancet 354:1159, 1999.
69. Archibald LK, McDonald LC, Rheanpumikankit S, et al. Fever and human immunodeficiency virus infection as sentinels for emerging mycobacterial and fungal bloodstream infections in hospitalized patients 15 years old, Bangkok. J Infect Dis 180:87, 1999.
70. Hirschitick RE, Glassroth J, Jordan MC, et al. Bacterial pneumonia in persons infected with the human immunodeficiency virus. N Engl J Med 333:845, 1995.
71. Kvale PA, Hansen NI, Markowitz N, et al. Routine analysis of induced sputum is not an effective strategy for screening persons infected with human immunodeficiency virus for *Mycobacterium tuberculosis* or *Pneumocystis carinii*. Clin Infect Dis 19:410, 1994.

72. Salzman SH, Schindel ML, Aranda CP, et al. The role of bronchoscopy in the diagnosis of pulmonary tuberculosis in patients at risk for HIV infection. Chest 102:143, 1992.
73. Gordin FM, Cohn DL, Sullam PM, et al. Early manifestations of disseminated *Mycobacterium avium* complex disease: a prospective evaluation. J Infect Dis 176:126, 1997.
74. Schluger NW, Rom WN. Current approaches to the diagnosis of active pulmonary tuberculosis. Am J Respir Crit Care Med 149:264, 1994.
75. American Thoracic Society. Treatment of tuberculosis and tuberculosis infection in adults and children. Am J Respir Crit Care Med 149:1359, 1994.
76. Horsburgh CR Jr, Feldman S, Ridzon R. Practice guidelines for the treatment of tuberculosis. Clin Infect Dis 31:633, 2000.
77. Centers for Disease Control and Prevention. Prevention and treatment of tuberculosis among patients infected with human immunodeficiency virus: principles of therapy and revised recommendations. MMWR Morbid Mortal Wkly Rep 47(RR-20):1, 1998.
78. Brindle RJ, Nunn PP, Githui W, et al. Quantitative bacillary response to treatment in HIV-associated pulmonary tuberculosis. Am Rev Respir Dis 147:958, 1993.
79. Perriens JH, St Louis ME, Mukadi YB, et al. Pulmonary tuberculosis in HIV-infected patients in Zaire. N Engl J Med 332:779, 1995.
80. El-Sadr WM, Perlman DC, Matts JP, et al. Evaluation of an intensive intermittent-induction regimen and duration of short-course treatment for human immunodeficiency virus-related pulmonary tuberculosis. Clin Infect Dis 26:1148, 1998.
81. Vernon A. Abstracts 2000 International Conference of the American Thoracic Society: TBTC study 22 (rifapentine trial): preliminary results in HIV-negative patients. Am J Respir Crit Care Med 161:A252, 2000.
82. Vernon A, Burman W, Benator D, et al. Acquired rifamycin monoresistance in patients with HIV-related tuberculosis treated with once-weekly rifapentine and isoniazid. Lancet 353:1843, 1999.
83. Sumartojo E. When tuberculosis treatment fails. Am Rev Respir Dis 147:1311, 1993.
84. Mahmoudi A, Iseman MD. Pitfalls in the care of patients with tuberculosis. JAMA 270:65, 1993.
85. Weis SE, Slocum PC, Blaise FX, et al. The effect of directly observed therapy on the rates of drug resistance and relapse in tuberculosis. N Engl J Med 330:1179, 1994.
86. Moore RD, Chaulk CP, Griffiths R, et al. Cost-effectiveness of directly observed versus self-administered therapy for tuberculosis. Am J Respir Crit Care Med 154:1013, 1996.
87. Moulding T, Dutt AK, Reichman LB. Fixed-dose combinations of antituberculous medications to prevent drug resistance. Ann Intern Med 122:951, 1995.
88. Centers for Disease Control and Prevention. Clinical update: impact of HIV protease inhibitors on the treatment of HIV-infected tuberculosis patients with rifampin. MMWR Morbid Mortal Wkly Rep 45:921, 1996.
89. Burman WJ, Gallicano K, Peloquin C. Therapeutic implications of drug interactions in the treatment of human immunodeficiency virus-related tuberculosis. Clin Infect Dis 28:419, 1999.
90. Centers for Disease Control and Prevention. Updated guidelines for the use of rifabutin or rifampin for the treatment and prevention of tuberculosis among HIV-infected patients taking protease inhibitors or nonnucleoside reverse transcriptase inhibitors. MMWR Morbid Mortal Wkly Rep 49:185, 2000.
91. McGregor MM, Olliaro P, Wolmarans L, et al. Efficacy and safety of rifabutin in the treatment of patients with newly diagnosed pulmonary tuberculosis. Am J Respir Crit Care Med 154:1462, 1996.
92. Narita M, Stambaugh JJ, Hollender ES, et al. Use of rifabutin with protease inhibitors for human immunodeficiency virus-infected patients with tuberculosis. Clin Infect Dis 30:779, 2000.
93. Small PM, Schecter GF, Goodman PC, et al. Treatment of tuberculosis in patients with advanced human immunodeficiency virus infection. N Engl J Med 324:289, 1991.
94. Jones BE, Otaya M, Antoniskis D, et al. A prospective evaluation of antituberculosis therapy in patients with human immunodeficiency virus infection. Am J Respir Crit Care Med 150:1499, 1994.
95. Schluger NW. Issues in the treatment of active tuberculosis in human immunodeficiency virus-infected patients. Clin Infect Dis 28:130, 1999.
96. Murray J, Sonnenberg P, Shearer SC, et al. Human immunodeficiency virus and the outcome of treatment for new and recurrent pulmonary tuberculosis in African patients. Am J Respir Crit Care Med 159:733, 1999.
97. Chaisson RE, Clermont HC, Holt EA, et al. Six-month supervised intermittent tuberculosis therapy in Haitain patients with and without HIV infection. Am J Respir Crit Care Med 154:1034, 1996.
98. Whalen C, Okwera A, Johnson J, et al. Predictors of survival in human immunodeficiency virus-infected patients with pulmonary tuberculosis. Am J Respir Crit Care Med 153:1977, 1996.
99. Peloquin CA, Nitta AT, Burman WJ, et al. Low antituberculosis drug concentrations in patients with AIDS. Ann Pharmacother 30:919, 1996.
100. Sahai J, Gallicano K, Swick L, et al. Reduced plasma concentrations of antituberculosis drugs in patients with HIV infection. Ann Intern Med 127:289, 1997.
101. Choudhri SH, Hawken M, Gathua S, et al. Pharmacokinetics of antimycobacterial drugs in patients with tuberculosis, AIDS, and diarrhea. Clin Infect Dis 25:104, 1997.
102. Cohn DL, Bustreo F, Raviglione MC. Drug-resistant tuberculosis: review of the worldwide situation and the WHO/IUATLD global surveillance project. Clin Infect Dis 24(suppl 1):S121, 1997.
103. Bloch AB, Cauthen GM, Onorato IM, et al. Nationwide survey of drug-resistant tuberculosis in the United States. JAMA 271:665, 1994.
104. Centers for Disease Control. Nosocomial transmission of multidrug-resistant tuberculosis among HIV-infected persons: Florida and New York, 1988–1991. MMWR Morbid Mortal Wkly Rep 40:585, 1991.
105. Centers for Disease Control. Transmission of multidrug-resistant tuberculosis among immunocompromised persons, correctional system: New York, 1991. JAMA 268:855, 1992.
106. Cleveland JL, Kent J, Gooch BF, et al. Multidrug-resistant *Mycobacterium tuberculosis* in an HIV dental clinic. Infect Control Hosp Epidemiol 16:7, 1995.
107. Frieden TR, Sherman LF, Maw KL, et al. A multi-institutional outbreak of highly drug-resistant tuberculosis. JAMA 276:1229, 1996.
108. Kenyon TA, Ridzon R, Luskin-Hawk R, et al. A nosocomial outbreak of multidrug-resistant tuberculosis. Ann Intern Med 127:32, 1997.
109. Frieden TR, Sterling T, Pablos-Mendez A, et al. The emergence of drug-resistant tuberculosis in New York City. N Engl J Med 328:521, 1993.
110. Gordin FM, Nelson ET, Matts JP, et al. The impact of human immunodeficiency virus infection of drug-resistant tuberculosis. Am J Respir Crit Care Med 154:1478, 1996.
111. Iseman MD. Treatment of multidrug-resistant tuberculosis. N Engl J Med 329:784, 1993.
112. Hong Kong Chest Service/British Medical Research Council. A controlled study of rifabutin and an uncontrolled study of ofloxacin in the retreatment of patients with pulmonary tuberculosis resistant to isoniazid, streptomycin and rifampicin. Tuber Lung Dis 73:59, 1992.
113. Heifets LB, Lindholm-Levy PJ, Iseman MD. Rifabutine: minimal inhibitory and bactericidal concentrations for *Mycobacterium tuberculosis*. Am Rev Respir Dis 137:719, 1988.
114. Goble M, Iseman MD, Madsen LA, et al. Treatment of 171 patients with pulmonary tuberculosis resistant to isoniazid and rifampin. N Engl J Med 328:527, 1993.
115. Park MM, Davis AL, Schluger NW, et al. Outcome of MDR-TB patients, 1983–1993; prolonged survival with appropriate therapy. Am J Respir Crit Care Med 153:317, 1996.
116. Telzak EE, Chrigwin KD, Nelson ET, et al. Predictors for multidrug-resistant tuberculosis among HIV-infected patients and response to specific drug regimens: Terry Beirn Community Programs for Clinical Research on AIDS (CPCRA) and the AIDS Clinical Trials Group (ACTG), National Institutes of Health. Int J Tuberc Lung Dis 3:337, 1999.
117. Narita M, Ashkin D, Hollender ES, et al. Paradoxical worsening of tuberculosis following antiretroviral therapy in patients with AIDS. Am J Respir Crit Care Med 158:157, 1998.
118. Hill AR, Mateo F, Hudak A. Transient exacerbation of tuberculous lymphadenitis during chemotherapy in patients with AIDS. Clin Infect Dis 19:774, 1994.
119. Chien JW, Johnson JL. Paradoxical reactions in HIV and pulmonary TB. Chest 114:933, 1998.
120. Fishman JE, Saraf-Lavi E, Narita M, et al. Pulmonary tuberculosis in AIDS patients: transient chest radiographic worsening after initiation of antiretroviral therapy. AJR Am J Roentgenol 174:43, 2000.

121. Snider DE, Caras GJ. Isoniazid-associated hepatitis deaths: a review of available information. Am Rev Respir Dis 145:494, 1992.
122. Centers for Disease Control and Prevention. Missed opportunities for prevention of tuberculosis among persons with HIV infection—selected locations, United States, 1996–1997. MMWR Morbid Mortal Wkly Rep 49:685, 2000.
123. Snider DE, Caras GJ, Koplan JP. Preventive therapy with isoniazid: cost-effectiveness of different durations of therapy. JAMA 255:1579, 1986.
124. Whalen CC, Johnson JL, Okwera A, et al. A trial of three regimens to prevent tuberculosis in Ugandan adults infected with the human immunodeficiency virus. N Engl J Med 337:801, 1997.
125. Moreno S, Baraia-Etxaburu J, Bouza E, et al. Risk for developing tuberculosis among anergic patients infected with HIV. Ann Intern Med 119:194, 1993.
126. Selwyn PA, Sckell BM, Alcabes P, et al. High risk of active tuberculosis in HIV-infected drug users with cutaneous anergy. JAMA 268:504, 1992.
127. Bucher HC, Griffith LE, Guyatt GH, et al. Isoniazid prophylaxis for tuberculosis in HIV infection: a meta-analysis of randomized controlled trials. AIDS 13:501, 1999.
128. Byrd RB, Horn BR, Solomon DA, et al. Toxic effects of isoniazid in tuberculosis chemoprophylaxis. JAMA 241:1239, 1979.
129. USHPS/IDSA Prevention of Opportunistic Infections Working Group. 2001 USPHS/IDSA guidelines for the prevention of opportunistic infections in persons infected with human immunodeficiency virus. http://www.hivatis.org.
130. American Thoracic Society/Centers for Disease Control and Prevention. Targeted tuberculin testing and treatment of latent tuberculosis infection. Am J Respir Crit Care Med 161:S221, 2000.
131. Nazar-Stewart V, Nolan CM. Results of a directly observed intermittent isoniazid preventive therapy program in a shelter for homeless men. Am Rev Respir Dis 148:57, 1992.
132. Gordin F, Chaisson R, Matts J, et al. Rifampin and pyrazinamide vs isoniazid for prevention of tuberculosis in HIV-infected persons an international randomized trial. JAMA 283:1445, 2000.
133. Centers for Disease Control and Prevention. Management of persons exposed to multidrug-resistant tuberculosis. MMWR Morbid Mortal Wkly Rep 41(RR-11):59, 1992.
134. Gordin FM, Matts JP, Miller C, et al. A controlled trial of isoniazid in persons with anergy and human immunodeficiency virus infection who are at high risk for tuberculosis. N Engl J Med 337:315, 1997.
134a. CDC. Update: Fatal and severe liver injuries associated with Rifampin and Pyrazinamide for latent tuberculosis infection and retrovirus in American Thoracic Society of CDC Recommendation–United States 2001. MMWR Morbid Mortal Wkly Rep 50:335, 2001.
135. Dooley SW, Villarino ME, Lawrence M, et al. Nosocomial transmission of tuberculosis in a hospital unit for HIV-infected patients. JAMA 267:2632, 1992.
136. Ritacco V, DiLonardo M, Reniero A, et al. Nosocomial spread of human immunodeficiency virus-related multidrug-resistant tuberculosis in Buenos Aires. J Infect Dis 176:637, 1997.
137. Zolopa AR, Hahn JA, Gorter R, et al. HIV and tuberculosis infection in San Francisco's homeless adults. JAMA 272:455, 1994.
138. Espinal MA, Perez EN, Baez J, et al. Infectiousness of *Mycobacterium tuberculosis* in HIV-1-infected patients with tuberculosis: a prospective study. Lancet 355:275, 2000.
139. Behr MA, Warren SA, Salamon H, et al. Transmission of *Mycobacterium tuberculosis* from patients smear-negative for acid-fast bacilli. Lancet 353:444, 1999.
140. Frieden TR, Fujiwara PI, Washko RM, et al. Tuberculosis in New York City: turning the tide. N Engl J Med 333:229, 1995.
141. McGowan JE. Nosocomial tuberculosis: new progress in control and prevention. Clin Infect Dis 21:489, 1995.
142. Centers for Disease Control. Guidelines for preventing the transmission of *Mycobacterium tuberculosis* in health-care facilities, 1994. MMWR Morbid Mortal Wkly Rep 43(RR-13):1, 1994.
143. Blumberg HM, Watkins DL, Berschling JD, et al. Preventing the nosocomial transmission of tuberculosis. Ann Intern Med 122:658, 1995.
144. Nettleman MD, Frederickson M, Good NL, et al. Tuberculosis control strategies: the cost of particulate respirators. Ann Intern Med 121:37, 1994.
145. Adal KA, Anglim AM, Palumbo CL, et al. The use of high-efficiency particulate air-filter respirators to protect hospital workers from tuberculosis. N Engl J Med 331:169, 1994.
146. McKenna MT, Hutton M, Cauthen G, et al. The association between occupation and tuberculosis. Am J Respir Crit Care Med 154:587, 1996.
147. Zahnow K, Hillman D, Matts J, et al. Tuberculosis skin test conversion rates among health care workers providing HIV care. In: Abstracts of the 35th Interscience Conference on Antimicrobial Agents and Chemotherapy. Washington, DC, American Society for Microbiology, 1995, p 220.
148. Bayer R, Dublier NN, Landesman S, et al. The dual epidemics of tuberculosis and AIDS: ethical and policy issues in screening and treatment. Am J Public Health 83:649, 1993.

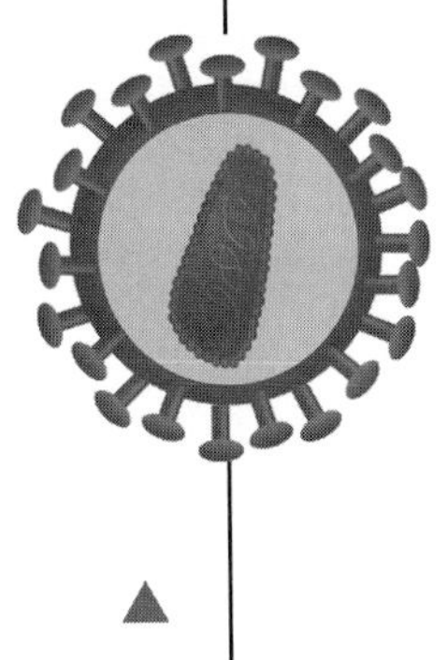

CHAPTER 34

Mycobacterium avium Complex and Other Atypical Mycobacterial Infections

Constance A. Benson, MD

Mycobacterium avium complex (MAC) disease in patients with acquired immunodeficiency syndrome (AIDS) and advanced immunosuppression, in the absence of potent antiretroviral therapy, is generally associated with disseminated multiorgan infection. Early symptoms may be minimal and may precede detectable mycobacteremia by several weeks.[1,2] Although mycobacteremia may be intermittent, transient, or absent, untreated disease in most patients with advanced immunosuppression progresses to result in clinically apparent symptoms, sustained bacteremia, and widespread infiltration of reticuloendothelial and organ tissue.[1–7] Those with established blood and widespread tissue infection report symptoms that include fever, drenching sweats, weight loss, wasting, fatigue, diarrhea, and abdominal pain.[1,3–6] Focal lymphadenitis and fever, or other localized tissue infections caused by *M. avium*, unaccompanied by bacteremia or disseminated tissue or organ involvement, has been described in patients with advanced immunosuppression who experience a substantial increase in the CD4+ T-lymphocyte count (100 cells/μl or higher) after initiation of potent combination antiretroviral therapy.[8–10] Similarly, an inflammatory response that mimics active *M. avium* disease may occur in those with previously established but quiescent or treated *M. avium* tissue infection who have rapid and substantial increases in CD4+ T-lymphocyte counts after starting potent antiretroviral therapy.[8–10] Signs and symptoms may be clinically indistinguishable from those of an infection but are often unaccompanied by detectable mycobacterial replication or growth in culture or tissue samples. In patients not receiving, or who have not immunologically responded to, potent combination antiretroviral therapies, localized disease had been uncommonly reported. The localized syndromes described in human immunodeficiency virus (HIV)-infected individuals include a diarrheal malabsorption syndrome resembling Whipple's disease, cervical or mesenteric lymphadenitis pneumonitis, pericarditis, osteomyelitis, skin or soft tissue abscesses, an enlarging genital ulcer, or central nervous system infection[4,11–16] (C. Benson, personal observations).

The most frequently observed laboratory abnormalities in those with disseminated *M. avium* disease are anemia, elevated liver alkaline phosphatase, and decreased serum albumin.[3–6,17] Neutropenia or thrombocytopenia (or both) may accompany bone marrow infiltration. Hepatomegaly, splenomegaly, or central (paratracheal, retroperitoneal, or para-aortic) lymphadenopathy may be detected on physical examination or by radiographic or other imaging studies.[3,4,18] With the exception of focal lymphadenitis, peripheral lymphadenopathy is uncommon. Other focal symptoms, signs, or laboratory abnormalities may occur in the context of the localized disease syndromes previously described.

PATHOGEN

The *M. avium* complex is comprised of two predominant species, *M. avium* and *M. intracellulare*, and several unspeciated mycobacteria.[3,19] MAC organisms are considered nonphotochromogenic, although production of yellow pigment by older colonies grown under select conditions has been reported.[20] Growth on solid media is generally slow, but growth can be detected radiometrically in liquid media within 7 to 10 days depending on inoculum size and laboratory conditions.[21] The colonial morphotype on solid media is determined by the glycopeptidolipid content of the cell wall, the characteristic that distinguishes serovars. Of the more than 28 identified serovars, types 1 to 6, 8 to 11, and 21 are *M. avium*, and types 7, 12 to 20, and 25 are *M. intracellulare*.[20,22] Types 1, 4, and 8 of *M. avium* are most frequently associated with disease in persons with AIDS in the United States and developed countries.[20,22]

Previous studies have shown that more than 95% of isolates of MAC recovered from patients with AIDS and disseminated MAC disease are *M. avium*.[23–27] In contrast, 40% of MAC isolates from non-HIV-infected individuals are *M. intracellulare*.[26] Characteristics of individual serovars and unique host genetic or immune factors may determine differences in the prevailing organisms causing disease in different hosts or geographic regions.[28]

Up to 25% of persons with AIDS and disseminated *M. avium* disease may be infected with two or more genetically distinct strains of *M. avium*.[29–31] The clinical significance of this finding is unknown, although in one study different strains recovered before and during treatment demonstrated disparate susceptibility to antimicrobial agents.[29–31]

▲ EPIDEMIOLOGY

Mycobacterium avium complex organisms can be recovered from a number of environmental reservoirs, including water, soil, domestic and farm animals, birds, foods, and some tobacco products.[27,32,33] Early studies evaluating delayed-type hypersensitivity responses to skin testing with purified protein derivative. Battey indicated a high prevalence of responses among persons residing in the southeastern part of the United States.[34] Studies using a more specific mycobacterial antigen, sensitin, derived from *M. avium* suggest that 7% to 12% of adults in the United States, Kenya, Trinidad, and Finland have been previously exposed to or infected with *M. avium*.[35] Although environmental reservoirs of *M. avium* also exist in developing countries or regions, MAC disease is uncommon among patients with AIDS in these areas.[35,36] Hypotheses suggested to explain this observation are that the high prevalence of latent or active *M. tuberculosis* infection in developing countries confers partial immunity to atypical mycobacterial infection or that biologic characteristics among local environmental serovars of MAC diminish their virulence.[4,36,37]

The environmental source of infection for individuals who develop active disease, with rare exception, is indeterminate. Von Reyn et al. described two small clusters of HIV-infected individuals with disseminated MAC disease from whom MAC isolates were recovered and found to be genetically identical to isolates recovered from potable water supplies in the same hospitals in which these patients had previously been hospitalized.[38] Household water supplies have also been shown to be "contaminated" with environmental strains of *M. avium*.[39] Von Reyn and colleagues further reported an association between ingestion of raw fish, prior bronchoscopy, or treatment with granulocyte colony-stimulating factor and an increased risk of developing disseminated MAC disease.[40] Similarly, Horsburgh et al. demonstrated an association between ingestion of hard cheese and an increased risk of developing MAC bacteremia.[41] In the latter two studies an association was also noted between daily showering or occupational exposure to water and a decreased risk of developing MAC bacteremia.[40,41] These findings notwithstanding, no environmental exposure or behavior has been consistently associated with the subsequent development of MAC disease in susceptible persons; therefore behaviors aimed at avoidance of exposure cannot be expected to result in a decreased risk of developing disease for susceptible individuals.[42–44]

Prior to the advent of effective chemoprophylaxis and potent combination antiretroviral therapy, the incidence of disseminated MAC disease in persons with AIDS ranged from approximately 20% to 40%.[5,6,45,46] There has been a dramatic decline in the incidence of opportunistic infections overall and specifically in *M. avium* disease during the modern era of potent combination antiretroviral therapy. The clinical event rate in one study comparing two drugs for prophylaxis of *Pneumocystis carinii* pneumonia in subjects intolerant of trimethoprim-sulfamethoxazole declined from 64 per 100 patient-years during the first year of follow-up to 34 per 100 patient-years during the second year; the proportion of study subjects who used protease inhibitor therapies increased from none at the beginning of the first year to 72% at the end of the second year of the study.[47] In the Centers for Disease Control and Prevention (CDC)-sponsored HIV Outpatient Study (HOPS), the overall proportion of persons followed with AIDS who had CD4+ T-lymphocyte counts of less than 100 cells/μl and who developed an opportunistic infection in 1995 was 26.9%, compared with 18.1% in 1996; the rate declined from 4.8% during the fourth quarter of 1996 to 3.0% during the second quarter of 1997 coincident with the increased use of protease inhibitor therapy.[48] Similar rates of decrease of opportunistic infections were reported by investigators following implementation of protease inhibitor therapies in Europe.[49,50] Additional studies have indicated that rates of *M. avium* disease in similar populations have declined in concert with the rates of other opportunistic infections.[51–53] For patients who enrolled in ACTG 320, a clinical trial comparing treatment with zidovudine/lamivudine with zidovudine/lamivudine/indinavir, the overall rate of occurrence of MAC disease for those with a baseline CD4+ T-lymphocyte count of less than 50 cells/μl was 2.0 cases per 100 patient-years.[51] Similarly, in two randomized clinical trials evaluating azithromycin or placebo for prophylaxis of MAC disease in patients on potent combination antiretroviral therapy who had an increase in their CD4+ T-lymphocyte counts from less than 50 cells/μl to more than 100 cells/μl at entry, the overall rate of MAC disease was fewer than two cases per 100 patient-years of follow-up.[52,53] These rates are considerably lower than those reported for previous years in the absence of potent antiretroviral therapy and chemoprophylaxis.

The increased susceptibility of HIV-infected persons with advanced immunosuppression to disseminated *M. avium* disease has not been fully explained. CD4+ and CD8+ T-lymphocytes, macrophages, natural killer (NK) cells, $\gamma\delta$ T cells, and the host of cytokines produced by these cells in response to mycobacterial antigen stimulation represent the primary immune response to infection with

MAC organisms.[54–65] Among the cytokines most central to the host immune response to MAC appear to be interleukin-12 (IL-12), interferon-γ (IFNγ), tumor necrosis factor-α (TNFα), IL-6, and IL-10.[54–65] Animal studies show that TNFα is essential for the development of protective immunity to MAC and contributes to the reduction of intracellular growth of MAC.[66,67] IL-12 stimulates IFNγ production, and both play key roles in the immune defense against MAC disease. In mice lacking these cytokines after targeted gene deletions and in humans with genetic defects of IL-12 or IFNγ production or expression, increased susceptibility to MAC infection and severe forms of disseminated MAC disease ensue.[65,68–73] IL-6 promotes *M. avium* growth, and IL-10 appears to inhibit production of TNFα and IL-12; IL-10 also down-regulates expression of co-stimulatory molecules on *M. avium*-infected monocytes, resulting in inhibition of IFNγ production.[65,74–77] Whereas in vitro macrophage function and response to IFNγ and the induction and expression of TNFα appear to be similar in HIV-infected individuals and uninfected controls, both HIV-infected and HIV-uninfected individuals with established MAC disease have been reported to have increased expression of IL-6, decreased production of or single cell cytokine expression of IFNγ and IL-12, and increased production of IL-10 by peripheral blood mononuclear cells.[62–65,78,79] These data suggest that, in addition to CD4+ T-lymphocyte depletion and loss of CD4+ T-cells, perturbations of these cytokines are involved in the increased propensity of HIV-infected individuals to develop disseminated MAC disease. Functionally as well, untreated HIV-infected patients have significantly reduced lymphoproliferative responses to *M. avium.*[64]

The most important risk factor for or predictor of the development of disseminated *M. avium* disease is advanced immunosuppression, as indicated by a CD4+ T-lymphocyte count of less than 50 cells/μl.[43–53] This remains true in patients treated with potent antiretroviral therapy.[49–53] High plasma HIV-1 RNA levels (>100,000 copies/ml) and a prior opportunistic infection, particularly cytomegalovirus disease, also contribute to the hazard of developing *M. avium* disease.[45,46,80–83]

Data regarding the relative risk of developing a specific opportunistic infection in those receiving potent combination antiretroviral therapies are limited, but trends clearly indicate substantial declines attributed not only to increases in CD4+ T-lymphocyte counts in response to therapy but also to more effective control of HIV-1 replication. For example, in the DACS 071 study, a retrospective analysis of the risk of developing opportunistic infections in patients who participated in the virology substudies of the ACTG 116B/117, 175, and 241 trials, the risk of developing disseminated *M. avium* disease was reduced threefold at 24 months for those who experienced even a modest decline in the plasma HIV-1 RNA level of 0.5 $\log_{10}$ copies/ml 8 weeks following initiation of combination antiretroviral therapies that included nucleoside or nonnucleoside reverse transcriptase inhibitors (or both).[82] In an evaluation of the relation between viral load and the occurrence of MAC disease (among other opportunistic infections), investigators from the Multicenter AIDS Cohort Study (MACS) showed that the relative hazard of developing *M. avium* disease for those with a baseline HIV-1 RNA level of 30,000 to 60,000 copies/ml was 1.29; it increased to 9.85 for those with a baseline HIV-1 RNA level of 60,000 to 90,000 copies/ml and to 14.97 for those with a baseline HIV-1 RNA of more than 90,000 copies/ml.[83] HIV-1 RNA level and CD4+ T-lymphocyte count were independent predictors of risk. In the ACTG 320 trial, significant predictors of a shorter time to development of MAC disease were a 1 $\log_{10}$ copies/ml increment in baseline HIV-1 RNA with at least a 0.5 $\log_{10}$ copies/ml decrease in HIV-1 RNA at week 8 of therapy, as well as a less than 10 cell increase in CD4+ T-lymphocyte count in response to antiretroviral therapy by week 8.[51]

Physiologic factors that contribute to the risk of developing *M. avium* bacteremia and disease in immunosuppressed individuals include colonization of the respiratory or gastrointestinal tract. Acid-fast bacilli (AFB) smears and cultures of stool or sputum may demonstrate the presence of *M. avium* prior to detection of mycobacteremia in up to 25% to 33% of HIV-infected individuals who subsequently develop disseminated *M. avium* disease.[84,85] Colonization of the gastrointestinal or respiratory tract, when detected, appears to have a positive predictive value approaching 60% in a profoundly immunocompromised patient population; however, the utility of screening cultures of these sites to detect colonization is limited because most of the patients are not colonized. Furthermore, when colonization can be demonstrated, it may be transient and not followed by the development of disseminated disease.[84,85]

Most prospective studies have not suggested differences in the incidence of *M. avium* disease according to gender, racial or ethnic group, age, or geographic distribution.[5,42,45,46,80,86] However, data collected among homosexual or bisexual men in the MACS indicated that those living in Baltimore (6.9%) or Los Angeles (5.6%) had a higher incidence of MAC disease than those in Chicago (2.6%) or Pittsburgh (0%).[80] In another study evaluating the geographic and seasonal variation in *M. avium* bacteremia among patients with AIDS receiving placebo in a randomized clinical trial of *M. avium* prophylaxis, those with the highest risk were patients in south central regions of the United States, whereas those with the lowest risk resided in northern states and Canada.[87] There also appeared to be a trend toward decreased numbers of cases in northern states during summer months compared to other seasons.

▲ TRANSMISSION

The mode of transmission for *M. avium* infection is thought to be inhalation, aspiration, or ingestion via respiratory or gastrointestinal tract portals of entry. Support for this contention includes laboratory studies demonstrating that *M. avium* can be experimentally aerosolized from environmental sources, and that organisms recovered from environmental aerosols are genetically similar to clinical isolates.[88,89] Data that support the gastrointestinal route as the predominant portal of entry for HIV-infected patients include the not-infrequent finding of extensive infiltration of the gastrointestinal tract and intra-abdominal organs in those with disseminated disease and the finding that disseminated disease rapidly follows intraoral or intrarectal challenge of the beige mouse or immunosuppressed murine or rat models with *M. avium*.[84,85,90–93] Household or close contact of those with *M. avium* disease are not at increased risk of developing disease, and isolates recovered from individuals, in general, do not appear to be genetically related, indicating that person-to-person transmission is unlikely.[29,41] However, at least one study has demonstrated multiple clusters of two or three patients infected with four genetically unique strains of *M. avium*; the investigators concluded that their data suggested a common environmental source rather than person-to-person spread.[31]

▲ DIAGNOSIS

Disseminated *M. avium* disease is diagnosed when a compatible clinical syndrome is present coupled with the recovery of *M. avium* from cultures of blood, bone marrow, or other normally sterile tissue or body fluids. The disease may be asymptomatic or only mildly symptomatic early; in this setting low-level mycobacteremia may produce intermittently positive blood cultures, and a small proportion of patients may have extensive infiltration of bone marrow or other reticuloendothelial organs in the absence of mycobacteremia.[1,3,94,95]

Isolation of *Mycobacterium*

Use of an Isolator (Wampole Laboratories, Cranbury, NJ, USA) or similar blood culture system and subsequent inoculation of blood into Bactec 12B liquid medium or direct inoculation of specimens into Bactec 13A bottles (Bactec; Becton-Dickinson, Sparks, MD, USA) followed by radiometric detection of growth are the most frequently employed methods for isolating *M. avium* from blood.[96] Inoculation onto solid media (e.g., Middlebrook 7H10/11 or Lowenstein-Jensen media) is most useful when quantification of mycobacteria is necessary, but adequate growth requires longer incubation. Species-specific DNA probes, high-performance liquid chromatography, or biochemical tests can be used to identify such organisms as *M. avium*, *M. intracellulare*, or other mycobacteria. Polymerase chain reaction assays for the detection of MAC species in clinical samples have not reached a level of sensitivity requisite for diagnostic clinical use.[96–98] Depending on the size of the inoculum, the average time required to cultivate and identify *M. avium* using liquid media, radiometric detection of growth, and DNA probe identification generally ranges from 7 to 14 days.[21,99,100]

Other ancillary studies that may be useful for diagnosing disseminated MAC disease for HIV-infected patients at risk include AFB smears or stool cultures, biopsies of clinically suspect tissues or organs, radiographic imaging of the abdomen or mediastinum to detect lymphadenopathy, or other studies aimed at recovery of organisms from focal infection sites. The yield of these procedures is generally dependent on the presence of symptoms, signs, or laboratory abnormalities related to the involved sites. The finding of MAC in sputum or stool in HIV-infected individuals may represent colonization rather than disease. Treatment should not be initiated based on these findings alone unless there is other evidence to indicate the presence of active disease.

Susceptibility Testing

Testing *M. avium* for susceptibility to antimicrobial agents can be accomplished using conventional agar proportion, agar dilution, broth dilution, or radiometric broth macrodilution techniques. Each may produce differing results depending on the assay and laboratory conditions used. The most widely recommended method for use in clinical laboratories in the United States is radiometric broth macrodilution utilizing Bactec technology.[101] The technical performance of assays using this method has been described in detail elsewhere.[96,101]

The use of susceptibility test results to guide selection of initial regimens for treatment of *M. avium* disease remains controversial. In early published studies characterizing treatment of pulmonary disease in nonimmunocompromised patients, the use of four to six drugs to which the isolate was susceptible was reportedly associated with improved clinical outcome.[102] In clinical trials of patients with AIDS, a relation between pretreatment susceptibility test results and the microbiologic and clinical responses has been demonstrated primarily for clarithromycin, azithromycin, and, less compellingly, rifabutin.[103–105] Relapses caused by clarithromycin- or azithromycin-resistant isolates have been reported when these agents are used as monotherapy during prophylaxis or treatment of *M. avium* disease, although relapse also occurs in those receiving multiple drug therapy, presumably as a result of poor adherence, poor absorption, the use of ineffective companion drugs, or drug–drug interactions. Thus far evidence indicates that *M. avium* resistance to clarithromycin is due to single-step mutations in the V domain of the 23S rRNA gene; these mutations confer cross-resistance to azithromycin and probably other macrolides.[106,107]

Breakpoints for the interpretation of susceptibility test results have been proposed for clarithromycin, azithromycin, and rifabutin based on data from prospective clinical trials.[96,101] Minimum inhibitory concentrations (MICs) of 32 μg/ml or more for clarithromycin or 256 μg/ml or more for azithromycin are the suggested thresholds for determining resistance based on the Bactec method for radiometric susceptibility testing.[96,101] It has been further suggested by some that the criteria for resistance should be based on the peak concentration achieved in serum after administration of therapeutic doses of drugs; however, clarithromycin, azithromycin, and rifabutin readily penetrate cells and tissue, often to levels far exceeding the MIC of most susceptible *M. avium* organisms. *M. avium* survives and replicates within macrophages, where these levels may be highest. This point should be considered when establishing resistance breakpoints or determining the clinical significance of susceptibility test results or serum or plasma concentrations of antimycobacterial drugs.

▲ **Table 34–1.** ANTIMYCOBACTERIAL DRUGS SUGGESTED FOR TREATMENT OF DISSEMINATED *MYCOBACTERIUM AVIUM* DISEASE
▲ IN PATIENTS WITH AIDS

Drug	Adult Dose	Common Adverse Reactions	Common Drug Interactions
Initial Therapy Agents			
Clarithromycin	500 mg bid[a]	Nausea, vomiting, abdominal pain, diarrhea, dysgeusia, rash, elevated liver transaminases, hearing loss, mania(?)	↑ Rifabutin levels; contraindicated with astemizole, terfenadine
Azithromycin	500–600 mg/d[a]	Diarrhea, nausea, vomiting, abdominal pain, rash, elevated liver transaminases	
Ethambutol	15 mg/kg/d	Nausea, vomiting, abdominal pain, diarrhea, hepatitis, optic neuritis, peripheral neuropathy (rare)	
Rifabutin	300–600 mg/d[b]	Nausea, vomiting, abdominal pain, diarrhea, rash, uveitis, brown-orange discoloration of body fluids, neutropenia, arthralgia, myositis, elevated liver transaminases	↑ Clarithromycin, ↓ protease inhibitor (PI) levels (indinavir, saquinavir, nelfinavir) amprenavir); PIs increase rifabutin levels, dose
Secondary Agents			
Ciprofloxacin	500–750 mg bid	Nausea, vomiting, abdominal pain, diarrhea, rash, insomnia, tremors, mental status changes	Aluminum-containing antacids inhibit absorption
Amikacin	10–15 mg/kg/d	Ototoxicity (cochlear and vestibular), nephrotoxicity	

[a]Clarithromycin, 500 mg bid, is the dose approved by the U.S. Food and Drug Administration (FDA) for prophylaxis and treatment of *Mycobacterium avium* complex (MAC) disease. Azithromycin 1200 mg once per week is approved for prophylaxis of MAC disease.
[b]Rifabutin, 300 mg/day, is the dose approved by the FDA for prophylaxis of MAC disease; dose increases to 450–600 mg/day are suggested when used with efavirenz.
Data from refs. 2, 20, 127–145.

▲ TREATMENT OF *M. AVIUM* DISEASE

Initial Therapy

Available antimicrobial agents with demonstrated activity in human clinical trials, alone or in combination regimens, for the treatment of *M. avium* disease include clarithromycin, azithromycin, rifabutin, ethambutol, and possibly ciprofloxacin and amikacin.[1,4,103,108–120] These agents, their commonly recommended adult doses, and their most common side effects are summarized in Table 34–1.[3,4,108,121–126]

Initial treatment of *M. avium* disease consists of a combination of at least two antimycobacterial drugs to prevent or delay the emergence of resistance.[44,126] Clarithromycin or azithromycin is the preferred first agent, although data regarding the efficacy of azithromycin are more limited than for clarithromycin.[44,126] Ethambutol is the recommended second drug. A third or fourth drug selected from among rifabutin, ciprofloxacin, or parenteral amikacin may be added for those with more severe or extensive symptoms or disease.[3,4,114,108,121] Alleviation of fever and a decline in the quantity of mycobacteria in blood or tissue can be expected within 2 to 4 weeks after initiation of appropriate therapy; for those with widespread tissue involvement or high levels of mycobacteremia, a longer duration of treatment may be required before a clinical response is observed. Susceptibility testing is not generally recommended as a guide to initial therapy because of the lack of standardization of methods and limited correlation of results with clinical and microbiologic outcome.[101,103–105,108,126] Experts recommend testing the susceptibility of MAC isolates to clarithromycin or azithromycin for patients who fail to respond to the initial therapy, who relapse after an initial response, or who develop MAC disease while receiving a macrolide for prophylaxis, although most patients who fail clarithromycin or azithromycin prophylaxis have isolates susceptible to these drugs at the time MAC disease is detected.[146,147]

Maintenance Therapy (Secondary Prophylaxis)

Revised U.S. Public Health Service/Infectious Disease Society of America (USPHS/IDSA) guidelines recommend that therapy for disseminated MAC disease in patients with AIDS be continued for life unless sustained immune recovery occurs with potent antiretroviral therapy.[44,126,127] The availability of potent combination antiretroviral therapy has altered the outcome of MAC disease in many individuals such that the disease can be effectively "cured" in select patients.[148,149] Studies presented to date are summarized in Table 34–2. In one small observational study, four patients

▲ **Table 34–2.** DISCONTINUATION OF SECONDARY PROPHYLAXIS
▲ FOR DISSEMINATED MAC

Study	No.	CD4 Criteria	Viral[a] Load Criteria	Follow-up (months)	Relapses While CD4 >100/mm^3
Aberg[148]	4	>100	<10,000	8–13	0
Shafran[150]	33	Variable	Variable	17 (median)	0[b]
Zeller[149]	26	Variable	Variable	7–58	2

[a]Copies per milliliter.
[b]Patient relapsed after stopping HAART.

who responded to potent antiretroviral therapy with sustained increases in CD4+ T-lymphocyte counts to more than 100 cells/μl and suppression of plasma HIV-1 RNA levels to less than 10,000 copies/ml had antimycobacterial therapy stopped after 1 year of treatment with a macrolide-containing regimen and after demonstrating the absence of active disease by negative blood and bone marrow cultures. None had relapsed during the 8 to 13 months of observation following discontinuation of antimycobacterial therapy.[148] Evaluation of small numbers of patients in several more largely observational studies indicate that patients with established MAC disease who have completed a 12 month or longer course of MAC treatment remain asymptomatic and have an increase in the CD4+ T-lymphocyte count to levels higher than 100 cells/μl for 6 months or longer on potent antiretroviral therapy are at low risk for recurrence of MAC disease. Hence the revised USPHS/IDSA guidelines now indicate that discontinuation of chronic maintenance therapy can be safely considered in patients who meet these criteria.[44,127,148–150] A prospective clinical trial evaluating the safety of discontinuing antimycobacterial treatment in this setting has been completed and supports the safety of this approach (C.A. Benson, personal communication).

Review of Clinical Trials

The early data from human clinical trials upon which the USPHS Task Force recommendations and USPHS/IDSA guidelines for treatment of disseminated *M. avium* disease are based are captured in a series of what are now largely historical studies. The more recent of these, conducted during the "modern era" of antimycobacterial or antiretroviral therapy (or both), are briefly discussed in the following text.[103,109,111–115,117,151–154] An algorithm characterizing current treatment recommendations can be found in Figure 34–1.

Perhaps the most clinically important study of treatment for *M. avium* disease in individuals with AIDS is that conducted by the Canadian HIV Trials Network; this study established the efficacy of a clarithromycin-containing regimen compared with more conventional antimycobacterial therapy. In this study, 187 patients with AIDS and symptomatic MAC bacteremia were randomized to receive a combination of rifampin/ethambutol/clofazimine/ciprofloxacin or clarithromycin (1 g twice daily)/ethambutol/rifabutin (600 mg/day).[112] Of the two treatments, the clarithromycin regimen more effectively in cleared MAC bacteremia (69% vs. 30%; $P < 0.001$) and was associated with improved survival (8.7 vs. 5.2 months; $P < 0.001$).[112] In this study the rifabutin dose was reduced to 300 mg/day after approximately half of the patients assigned to the clarithromycin/ethambutol/rifabutin arm developed uveitis, which was attributed to a previously unrecognized drug interaction between clarithromycin and rifabutin.[155,156] A dose-response relation with rifabutin was suggested by the finding that the 600 mg/day dose was associated with a higher proportion of patients who cleared their mycobacteremia but who developed uveitis than was the 300 mg/day dose.

A series of randomized clinical trials of similar design have compared combinations of two- or three-drug

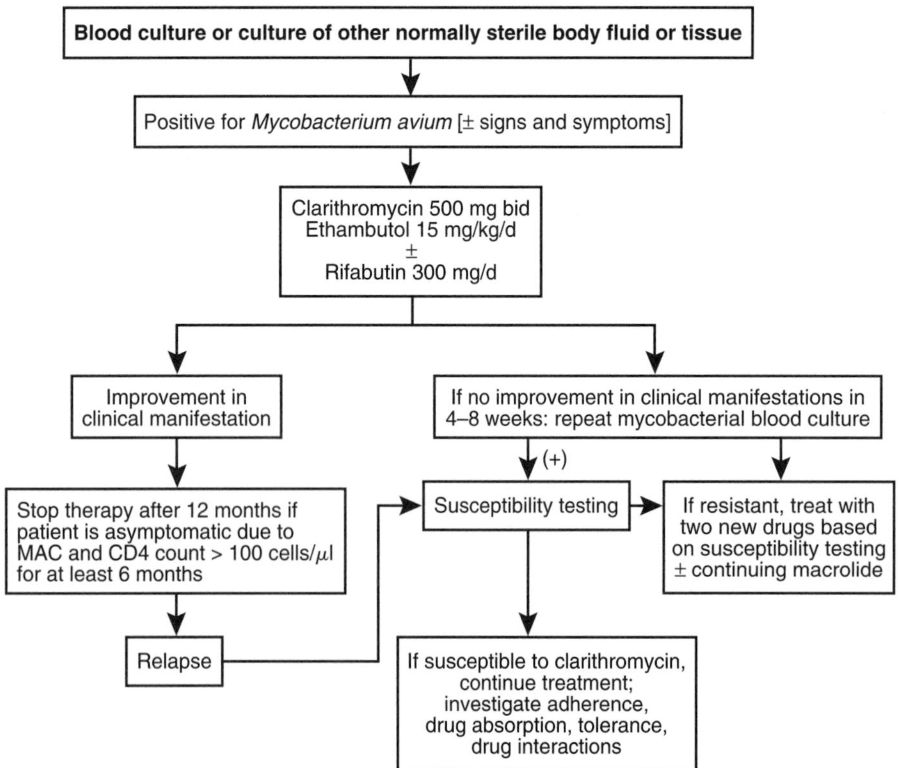

Figure 34–1. Algorithm for treatment of disseminated *Mycobacterium avium* complex disease in patients with AIDS.

clarithromycin-containing regimens for treatment of MAC disease. In the first of these trials, Chaisson et al. evaluated 89 patients with AIDS and *M. avium* bacteremia who were randomized to receive either clarithromycin/ethambutol or clarithromycin/ethambutol/clofazimine.[117] The randomization of patients failed to circumvent significantly disparate baseline quantitative colony counts between the two arms [152 colony-forming units (CFU)/ml vs. 1907 CFU/ml, respectively], although they were otherwise demographically and clinically comparable. The proportion of patients who cleared *M. avium* bacteremia reported improved symptoms, and relapses were similar.[117] However, patients randomized to the three-drug arm had a higher rate of treatment-limiting side effects and a higher mortality rate. In a Cox proportional hazards analysis of factors associated with decreased survival, the baseline quantitative colony counts of *M. avium* in blood ($P = 0.043$) and treatment with clofazimine ($P = 0.045$) were independent predictors of decreased survival.

Dube and coinvestigators evaluated 95 patients with AIDS and MAC bacteremia who were randomized to receive either clarithromycin/clofazimine or clarithromycin/clofazimine/ethambutol.[115] The primary endpoint of this study was the time to relapse; although early clinical and microbiologic outcome was the same for the two treatment arms, 68% of patients receiving two drugs had relapsed by 36 weeks of therapy compared with only 12% of those receiving the three-drug regimen ($P = 0.004$).[115] All patients who relapsed had clarithromycin-resistant isolates recovered from blood. Ethambutol appeared to contribute to a reduced likelihood of relapse and emergence of clarithromycin-resistant *M. avium* in this study.

In a third study, 144 HIV-infected patients were randomized to receive clarithromycin/ethambutol/rifabutin (450 mg/day) or clarithromycin/clofazimine; 22 patients randomized to the two-drug arm relapsed compared with only 6 receiving three drugs ($P < 0.001$).[113] Of the 22 patients in the two-drug arm who relapsed, clarithromycin-resistant isolates were recovered from 21, whereas resistant isolates were found in only 2 of 6 in the three-drug arm.[113] Both groups had similar clinical responses with similar reductions in symptoms after 2 and 6 months of treatment, respectively.

Gordin and colleagues compared the combination of clarithromycin/ethambutol with clarithromycin/ethambutol/rifabutin (300 mg/day) in 198 patients with AIDS and MAC bacteremia.[114] At week 16 a total of 63% and 61% of patients in the three-drug arm or the two-drug arm, respectively, had a bacteriologic response to therapy ($P = 0.81$), and no differences were reported in clinical improvement or median survival. Median survivals were 439 and 398 days for the three- and two-drug arms, respectively. Moreover, no overall differences were noted with regard to the development of clarithromycin resistance; however, when only those with a bacteriologic response were included in the analysis, a more 2% receiving all three drugs had a clarithromycin-resistant MAC isolate recovered during therapy, while 14% of those receiving only clarithromycin/ethambutol developed clarithromycin resistance ($P = 0.055$).[114]

A fifth study evaluated 203 patients randomized to receive clarithromycin plus ethambutol, rifabutin, or both.[157] The primary endpoint was a complete microbiologic response defined as two consecutive negative MAC blood cultures at least 1 week apart by week 12 of treatment. The proportion of patients with a complete microbiologic response at week 12 did not differ significantly among the three regimens. The proportions of patients with a complete microbiologic response at any time during follow-up were 55%, 46%, and 70%, respectively. The proportion who experienced a relapse on clarithromycin/rifabutin (24%) was significantly higher than that for the three-drug regimen (6%) ($P = 0.027$) and marginally significantly higher than for clarithromycin/ethambutol (7%) ($P = 0.057$). The rate of emergence of clarithromycin resistance was greater on clarithromycin/rifabutin than in the other two arms. There was an overall significant difference in time to death ($P = 0.020$, log-rank test), with improved survival for those randomized to the three-drug arm compared to either of the two-drug arms.[157]

Finally, in a factorial study design attempting to address the potency of higher doses of clarithromycin for treatment of *M. avium* disease, Cohn et al. randomized patients with AIDS and *M. avium* bacteremia to receive one of two doses of clarithromycin, 500 or 1000 mg twice daily, combined with ethambutol, and they secondarily randomized patients to receive either rifabutin or clofazimine.[116] The study was terminated early because of excess mortality observed in the higher-dose clarithromycin arm coupled with the data from previously reported clinical trials indicating the lack of benefit of clofazimine and its association with increased mortality. As with the previous studies demonstrating the association of higher doses of clarithromycin with increased early mortality in patients being treated for *M. avium* disease, the cause was not apparent and the association was unrelated to adverse events, baseline clinical characteristics, or laboratory abnormalities.[103,116]

Although comparative data are limited, in general clarithromycin and azithromycin may be used interchangeably.[158,159] In the largest published comparative study to date, 246 patients with disseminated MAC disease were randomized to receive azithromycin 250 mg once daily, azithromycin 600 mg once daily, or clarithromycin 500 mg twice daily, each in combination with ethambutol.[159] The azithromycin 250 mg arm was halted after an interim analysis showed a lower rate of clearance of MAC bacteremia. At 24 weeks of therapy, the proportion of patients who experienced two consecutive negative MAC blood cultures was similar for both the azithromycin 600 mg qd ($n = 68$) and clarithromycin ($n = 57$) arms (46% and 56%, respectively; $P = 0.24$). The likelihood of relapse, the recovery of resistant isolates following relapse, and mortality were also similar for both treatment arms.[159]

For patients who fail to respond to the initial treatment or who relapse after an initial response, many experts recommend testing *M. avium* isolates for susceptibility to clarithromycin, azithromycin, and rifabutin and then using these data to craft a new multidrug regimen consisting of at least two new drugs not previously used and to which the isolate is susceptible. It is unclear whether continuing clarithromycin or azithromycin in the face of resistance provides additional benefit. Preliminary results were reported from one small study in which eight patients who relapsed with a clarithromycin-resistant MAC isolate while receiving a combination of clarithromycin and clofazimine were treated with "salvage" regimens that consisted of continuing a macrolide coupled with ethambutol and one or more additional drugs; five of eight patients had a 1 $\log_{10}$ copies/ml or more decline in mycobacterial colony counts per milliliter of blood, and two of the eight became culture-negative.[160] Because the number of drugs with activity against *M. avium* in this setting is limited, salvage regimens, if constructed in this manner, will likely consist of two or more of the following: ethambutol, rifabutin, ciprofloxacin, or amikacin with or without continuing a macrolide. Liposomal amikacin, an investigational agent, could also be considered.[161] Based on its lack of efficacy in randomized trials and its association with increased mortality, clofazimine should generally not be used. Other second-line agents, such as ethionamide or thiacetazone, have been anecdotally combined with these drugs as "salvage" therapy, but their role in this setting is unknown. None of these approaches has been evaluated in controlled clinical trials in this patient population.

Adjunctive Immunomodulator Therapy for Disseminated MAC Disease in Patients with AIDS

Adjunctive treatment of *M. avium* complex disease with immunomodulators remains controversial. Interferon-γ (IFNγ), tumor necrosis factor-α (TNFα, granulocyte/macrophage colony-stimulating factor (GM-CSF), and interleukin-12 (IL-12), alone or in combination with other cytokines, appear to inhibit intracellular replication or enhance in vitro intracellular killing of *M. avium*.[3,55–79] The use of these agents or immunomodulators that influence their production may be an attractive adjuvant treatment for those who fail more conventional antimycobacterial therapy. Some pilot human clinical trials suggest that this approach may have merit.

In a small clinical trial, HIV-infected patients with *M. avium* bacteremia were randomized to receive azithromycin alone or azithromycin plus GM-CSF for 4 weeks; preliminary results indicated that GM-CSF use was associated with enhanced monocyte activation and intracellular *M. avium* killing.[162] Holland and colleagues described their experience using IFNγ as an adjunct along with antimycobacterial drugs in seven HIV-seronegative patients with disseminated *M. avium* or other nontuberculous mycobacterial infections refractory to standard therapy; the result was a reduction in clinical symptoms and number of mycobacteria in blood within 8 weeks.[163] In an anecdotal report, Wormser et al. reported that five patients with AIDS and disseminated *M. avium* disease unresponsive to conventional antimycobacterial therapy had weight gain, reduced fever, and improvement of a number of laboratory abnormalities after the addition of dexamethasone (2 mg/day) to their antimycobacterial treatment.[164] Finally, preliminary data are available from a retrospective analysis comparing 52 patients with disseminated *M. avium* disease who received standard antimycobacterial therapy plus prednisone 0.5 mg/kg/day with 41 patients who received only antimycobacterial therapy. The data demonstrated lower mortality, higher CD4+ T-lymphocyte counts, and greater weight gain over a 1-year observation period in those receiving adjunctive prednisone therapy.[165] The interpretation of these data may be limited, however, because other underlying disease factors and the type of and response to antiretroviral therapy were not controlled; moreover patients were not treated with standard antiretroviral or antimycobacterial therapies according to a protocol. A study of IL-12 in patients with AIDS and advanced immunosuppression has been recently completed, but no data are yet available regarding the utility of this approach.

Although these preliminary findings are promising, the substantial improvement in immunologic function resulting from treatment with potent combination antiretroviral therapy may reduce the incidence of "refractory" *M. avium* disease, making this investigational approach unnecessary.

Primary Prophylaxis for Disseminated MAC Disease in Patients with AIDS

The USPHS/IDSA guidelines for preventing of opportunistic infections recommend chemoprophylaxis for disseminated MAC disease for all HIV-infected adults and adolescents who have a CD4+ T-lymphocyte count of less than 50 cells/μl (and for infants and children with similar age-adjusted CD4+ T-lymphocyte counts).[44,127] The first-line agents recommended for prophylaxis include clarithromycin 500 mg twice daily or azithromycin 1200 mg once a week. These agents also reduce the risk of respiratory bacterial infections and probably *Pneumocystis carinii* pneumonia.[44,127,147,166,167] Rifabutin 300 mg/day is recommended as a second-line alternative. Although the combination of azithromycin and rifabutin was found to be more effective than either single drug in one clinical trial, the higher rate of adverse effects and cost preclude its general use.[44,127,147] Because the combination of clarithromycin/rifabutin was shown to be no more effective than clarithromycin alone, it too is not recommended.[44,146] The clinical trials that formed the basis for these recommendations are reiterated in the following paragraphs. An algorithm summarizing current prophylaxis guidelines can be seen in Figure 34–2.

In the first of these studies, HIV-infected individuals with CD4+ T-lymphocyte counts of less than 100 cells/μl were randomized to receive clarithromycin 500 mg twice daily or placebo for prevention of *M. avium* disease; the incidence of *M. avium* bacteremia (5.6% for those randomized to clarithromycin) was reduced by 69% compared to that seen with placebo (15.5%).[166] The reduction in incidence was accompanied by an increase in the duration of survival (> 700 days) for patients receiving clarithromycin versus those receiving placebo (573 days; $P < 0.01$). Of 19 isolates recovered from patients who developed *M. avium* bacteremia while on clarithromycin prophylaxis, 11 were resistant to clarithromycin; isolates from these patients had minimum inhibitory concentrations (MICs) of 512 μg/ml or more.[166] Despite the seemingly high rate of clarithromycin resistance among breakthrough isolates in this study, only 2% of patients receiving clarithromycin prophylaxis developed *M. avium* disease caused by a clarithromycin-resistant organism.

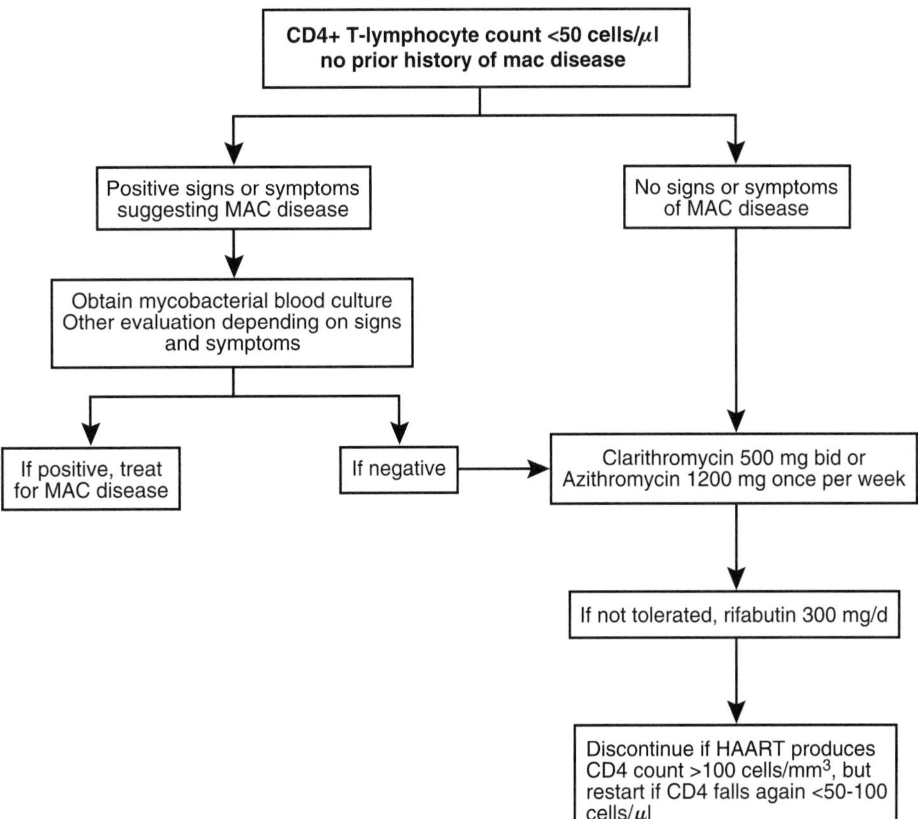

Figure 34–2. Algorithm for primary chemoprophylaxis of *Mycobacterium avium* complex disease in patients with AIDS.

In a smaller but similarly designed clinical trial, 181 HIV-infected individuals were randomized to receive either azithromycin 1200 mg once a week or placebo.[168] Of the 85 patients who received azithromycin 7 (8.2%) developed MAC disease compared to 20 (23.3%) of the 86 who received placebo ($P = 0.002$). Gastrointestinal adverse events predominated and were treatment-limiting in 8% of those randomized to azithromycin compared with 2% of those randomized to placebo ($P = 0.09$). Survival and emergence of azithromycin resistance did not differ between the two arms, although the study was not powered to detect a survival difference.

Data from these and two other studies established the superiority of clarithromycin, azithromycin, and rifabutin over placebo for prevention of MAC disease in HIV-infected patients with advanced immunosuppression.[86,166,168,169] Two additional clinical trials compared azithromycin or clarithromycin with rifabutin or combinations of azithromycin/rifabutin or clarithromycin/rifabutin.[146,147] The first evaluated azithromycin 1200 mg once a week, rifabutin 300 mg/day, or their combination in 669 HIV-infected individuals with CD4+ T-lymphocyte counts of less than 100 cells/μl at entry.[147] Of the 199 patients who received azithromycin plus rifabutin, 5 (2.5%) developed *M. avium* disease compared with 18 of 204 (8.8%) randomized to azithromycin and 25 of 207 (12.1%) randomized to rifabutin.[97] The combination of azithromycin and rifabutin was more effective than either single agent for reducing the occurrence of *M. avium* disease ($P < 0.001$ and 0.01, respectively, for the rifabutin and azithromycin comparisons); and azithromycin was more effective than rifabutin ($P = 0.006$). No survival differences were observed among the three treatment arms. Treatment-limiting adverse effects were more common among those receiving the two-drug combination than others with either single agent. Azithromycin- or clarithromycin-resistant *M. avium* isolates were recovered from 2 of 18 patients (11%) randomized to azithromycin and none of those randomized to the other two arms. There were no differences among the treatment arms with regard to recovery of rifabutin-resistant isolates. Rates of *P. carinii* pneumonia and respiratory bacterial infections were reduced for patients who received an azithromycin-containing regimen compared with those who received rifabutin alone.

In the second study, clarithromycin 500 mg twice daily was compared with rifabutin 300 mg/day and their combination in 1178 HIV-infected persons with CD4+ T-lymphocyte counts of 100 cells/μl or less at entry.[146] Of the 398 patients randomized to receive clarithromycin, 36 (9%) developed *M. avium* disease versus 59 of 391 (15%) randomized to rifabutin and 26 of 389 (7%) receiving the combination.[146] Clarithromycin and the combination were more effective than rifabutin ($P < 0.001$) in reducing the occurrence of *M. avium* disease, but the two clarithromycin-containing arms were equally effective. As with the previously described study, the combination of clarithromycin/rifabutin was associated with a higher rate of treatment-limiting adverse effects; gastrointestinal side effects and uveitis predominated. No differences in survival among the three treatment arms were observed. Of the *M. avium* isolates recovered from patients who failed prophylaxis, 29% from those randomized to clarithromycin and 25% from those randomized to the combination were resistant to clarithromycin and azithromycin; there were no differences among the treatment arms with regard to recovery of isolates resistant to rifabutin. Overall, approximately 2% of patients randomized to a clarithromycin-containing regimen broke through with a clarithromycin-resistant isolate.

The results of placebo-controlled trials have clearly shown that chemoprophylaxis is associated with improved survival compared to observation and serial monitoring of blood cultures followed by initiation of antimycobacterial therapy for those receiving placebo. However, the availability of more potent antiretroviral therapies that suppress HIV replication, improve immune function, and increase CD4+ T-lymphocyte counts to levels above those associated with increased risk has resulted in a marked decline in the incidence of *M. avium* disease, has altered the clinical manifestations of disease, and has improved the response to antimycobacterial therapy and mortality associated with *M. avium* disease.[47–51] Two randomized clinical trials have demonstrated the safety of discontinuing MAC prophylaxis for patients who have had a sustained increase in their CD4+ T-lymphocyte counts from a nadir of less than 50 cells/μl to more than 100 cells/μl while receiving potent combination antiretroviral therapies.[52,53] Currier et al. studied 643 HIV-1-infected patients who met this entry criterion and who were randomized to receive azithromycin 1200 mg once weekly or placebo.[53] During a median of 16 months of follow-up, only two cases of MAC disease occurred in the placebo group and none in the azithromycin group. The calculated incidence rate in the placebo group was only 0.5 event per 100 person-years [95% confidence interval (CI), 0.06 to 1.83 per 100 person-years]. There was no statistically significant difference in incidence for placebo versus azithromycin. In a similarly designed study conducted by El Sadr and colleagues, no cases of MAC disease occurred among 512 patients followed for a median of 12 months.[52] Based on these data, USPHS/IDSA guidelines recommend that primary prophylaxis be discontinued for patients who have responded to highly active antiretroviral therapy (HAART) with an increase in CD4+ T-lymphocyte count to levels higher than 100 cells/μl for at least 3 months.[127] For those who experience a subsequent decline in CD4+ T-lymphocyte count to less than 100 cells/μl, MAC prophylaxis should be restarted.[127]

Drug Interactions Among Agents Used for Treatment or Prophylaxis of MAC Disease

For those who require prophylaxis or treatment for MAC disease, the potential for significant drug interactions with agents used for prophylaxis or treatment remains problematic. The most clinically important are those occurring with drugs metabolized by the cytochrome P_{450} enzyme system in the liver or intestinal tract. Clarithromycin, a potent inhibitor of the 3A4 isoenzyme of the cytochrome P_{450} system, is associated with a bidirectional interaction with rifabutin, a moderately potent inducer of CYP 3A4. Competitive inhibition of CYP 3A4 by clarithromycin is associated with a 77% increase in rifabutin and 25-desacetyl rifabutin plasma concentrations when the two drugs are co-administered.[129,158,170] Increased rifabutin levels have been associated with the development of uveitis and other adverse effects of rifabutin.[128,155] Co-administration of rifabutin and clarithromycin also results in a 50% reduction in the clarithromycin area under the concentration curve (AUC), although there is wide individual variation.[129,158] Reduced serum or plasma concentrations may have little if any clinical impact for these drugs, which are highly concentrated in macrophages where they exert activity against replicating intracellular mycobacteria; treatment trials utilizing these agents in combination suggest that the clinical impact is small.[146,157] A similar magnitude of increase in rifabutin levels when co-administered with fluconazole appeared to enhance the efficacy of rifabutin in preventing *M. avium* disease in one study.[129,130] A comparable interaction between azithromycin and rifabutin has not been described.

Drug interactions between the protease inhibitor and nonnucleoside reverse transcriptase inhibitor (NNRTI) antiretroviral drugs and rifabutin or clarithromycin make management of antimycobacterial therapy and prophylaxis for MAC disease complex for those who require co-administration of these agents. Ritonavir is both a potent inhibitor and an inducer of CYP 3A4.[131] Indinavir, nelfinavir, and amprenavir are reversible and less potent inhibitors of CYP 3A4 than ritonavir and probably produce comparable levels of inhibition.[131] Saquinavir appears to be the least potent inhibitor. Ritonavir inhibits the metabolism of clarithromycin to its 14-hydroxy metabolite; the result is an increase in the clarithromycin AUC of about 77%, a decrease in the 14-hydroxy metabolite of about 99%, and an overall increase of 35% to 40% in clarithromycin exposure.[132,133] Clarithromycin increases the ritonavir AUC by only about 12%. The interaction between indinavir and clarithromycin appears to be similar, producing a comparable increase in clarithromycin exposure. No dose adjustment for clarithromycin or, conversely, for ritonavir or indinavir when either is co-administered with clarithromycin, is currently recommended for patients with normal renal function. Data fully evaluating interactions between nelfinavir, saquinavir, amprenavir, or other protease inhibitors and clarithromycin are not available. Efavirenz may induce the metabolism of clarithromycin in a manner similar to that of the protease inhibitors (i.e., resulting in a decrease in serum concentration of the parent drug but an increase in the serum concentration of the 14-hydroxy active metabolite.)[127,134] Although no studies have evaluated the clinical significance of this interaction, careful monitoring is advised when these agents are used together.

The resultant interaction when ritonavir and rifabutin are co-administered is substantial. Ritonavir 500 mg every 12 hours given with rifabutin 150 mg daily produces a fourfold increase in the AUC of rifabutin, a 35-fold increase in the AUC of the major metabolite, and an overall seven-fold increase in rifabutin exposure; rifabutin in this dose does not alter the AUC of ritonavir.[135,136] When used in combination with ritonavir, the dose of rifabutin should be reduced to 150 mg every other day. The interaction between rifabutin and indinavir, amprenavir, or nelfinavir is less great. Conventional doses of indinavir given concomitantly with rifabutin 300 mg/day result in an increase in the rifabutin AUC by about 204% and a decrease in the indinavir AUC by about 32%.[137] A similar magnitude of interaction has been demonstrated between nelfinavir or amprenavir and rifabutin; a dose reduction of rifabutin to 150 mg/day is recommended for patients co-administered either indinavir or nelfinavir with rifabutin.[138,139] When saquinavir (hard gel capsule formulation) in doses of 600 mg three times daily is combined with of rifabutin 300 mg/day, the AUC of saquinavir is reduced by approximately 40%; coupled with the poor oral bioavailability of this formulation of saquinavir, the data indicate that these drugs should not be used together.[140,141] The magnitude of the interaction between rifabutin and the soft gel capsule formulation of saquinavir is unclear; these two drugs also should probably not be combined. There are sparse data characterizing the interactions of clarithromycin or rifabutin with lopinavir/ritonavir or other ritonavir-enhanced protease inhibitor combinations. Thus rifabutin in particular should be used with caution when given to patients treated with ritonavir-enhanced protease inhibitor regimens. The doses should be adjusted to at least the same levels as recommended when the protease inhibitor is used alone, and patients should be carefully monitored for rifabutin-associated toxicity.[127]

The NNRTIs are also metabolized by the CYP 3A4 isoenzyme, although as a class the drug interactions associated with them are not the same for all drugs in the class. Nevirapine and efavirenz induce CYP 3A4, whereas delavirdine inhibits this isoenzyme.[131,142,144] Pharmacokinetic interactions between all of these agents and clarithromycin have not been fully evaluated, although preliminary data for efavirenz indicate that it reduces the clarithromycin AUC by approximately 39%.[145] Rifabutin induces the metabolism of the NNRTIs. A fivefold increase in delavirdine clearance has been reported when delavirdine and rifabutin are co-administered, although interindividual variability is substantial; delavirdine inhibits rifabutin metabolism, resulting in an increased rifabutin AUC.[143] Efavirenz and rifabutin appear to induce each other's metabolism, although to what degree is unclear; data from interaction studies with rifampin suggest that rifampin reduces the efavirenz AUC by about 34%, although again there appears to be substantial interindividual variability.[142,144] A rifabutin dose adjustment to 450 to 600 mg/day has been suggested when it is used with efavirenz.[127,134] No dose adjustment is recommended when rifabutin and nevirapine are used in combination. When the NNRTIs are used in combination with protease inhibitors, it is unknown which level of interaction is likely to predominate among the multiple drugs. Careful monitoring of adverse effects and antiviral activity is necessary; and in many instances avoidance of rifabutin use is advisable where feasible.

▲ *MYCOBACTERIUM KANSASII* INFECTION

The most common clinical manifestations of disease caused by *M. kansasii* among individuals with HIV infection include fever, pulmonary symptoms, and pulmonary infiltrates.[171–179] In series of reported cases of *M. kansasii* disease in HIV-infected patients, the proportion of those with cavitary lung disease ranges from 0% to 53%; most of those without cavitary disease had interstitial or alveolar infiltrates on chest radiographs.[171–179] Although pulmonary disease predominates, extrapulmonary or disseminated disease occurs in a substantial proportion as well, ranging from 10% to 39%.[171–179] Although early reports suggested that the gastrointestinal tract was a common area of extrapulmonary involvement, more recent observations fail to confirm this as a frequent finding, with isolation from blood or bone marrow being the more common manifestation of disseminated disease. For patients who are symptomatic, fever, cough with or without sputum production, dyspnea, abdominal pain, and weight loss are reportedly the most common clinical symptoms.[171–179]

Most patients with HIV infection who develop disease caused by *M. kansasii* have CD4+ T-lymphocyte counts of less than 100 cells/μl. As with other opportunistic infections during the era of potent combination antiretroviral therapy for HIV infection, the incidence of disease caused by *M. kansasii* has declined, although there were insufficient data available at any time during the epidemic to evaluate the overall incidence of this opportunistic infection. Several reports have suggested a higher prevalence of disease caused by *M. kansasii* among individuals living in the central Midwestern portions of the United States and among injection drug users; the largest numbers of cases among patients with HIV infection in the United States have been reported from Kansas City and Chicago.[171–179]

As with other mycobacterial infections in this patient population, the diagnosis depends on the presence of a compatible clinical syndrome coupled with isolation of *M. kansasii* from respiratory secretions, blood, or other body fluids or tissue. As with *M. avium,* inoculation of specimens into Bactec 12B liquid medium or direct inoculation of specimens into Bactec 13A bottles, followed by radiometric detection of growth, is the preferred method for isolating of *M. kansasii.* Middlebrook 7H10/11 or Lowenstein-Jensen solid media can also be used. Species-specific DNA probes, high-performance liquid chromatography, or biochemical tests can also be used to identify organisms such as *M. kansasii.*

The cornerstones of combination therapy for *M. kansasii* infection are rifampin and ethambutol. Most isolates are relatively resistant to isoniazid; the latter is usually included in suggested treatment regimens, however, although its contribution is unclear. The organism is variably susceptible to other second-line antimycobacterial drugs, including clarithromycin.[178,179] In vitro susceptibility testing is generally recommended as a guide to therapy, although randomized clinical trials establishing a predictive relation between in vitro susceptibility test results and clinical and microbiologic responses have not been reported. The recommended duration of treatment is 12 to 18 months for immunocompetent individuals. There are no prospective data to determine the most appropriate duration of treatment for those co-infected with HIV. As with treatment for *M. avium,* many experts continue therapy for 12 to 18 months and then discontinue it for those who have responded to potent combination antiretroviral therapy.

▲ **Table 34–3.** OTHER ATYPICAL MYCOBACTERIAL INFECTIONS IN HIV-INFECTED INDIVIDUALS: ASSOCIATED CLINICAL SYNDROMES
▲ AND SUGGESTED TREATMENT REGIMENS

Mycobacterium Species	Clinical Syndrome	Suggested Treatment Regimen(s)
M. genovense	Disseminated multiorgan infection similar to *M. avium* (molecular techniques are required for species identification)	Clarithromycin, ethambutol, and rifamycins (amikacin and ciprofloxacin have been included in some reports with variable response)
M. scrofulaceum	Cervical lymphadenitis; disseminated disease (rare)	Surgical excision may be the treatment of choice; clarithromycin, azithromycin, rifabutin, with or without streptomycin, cycloserine, and sulfonamides appear to have activity
M. xenopi	Pulmonary nodules or diffuse reticulonodular infiltrates	Clarithromycin, ethambutol, rifabutin, streptomycin or amikacin
M. haemophilum	Cutaneous lesions; disseminated disease (the organism grows optimally at 32°C and requires iron-containing media for optimal growth)	Isoniazid, rifampin, and ethambutol are most commonly recommended; clarithromycin, minocycline, doxycycline, ciprofloxacin, and amikacin have in vitro activity
M. bovis	Disseminated multiorgan disease (may be seen following bacille Calmette Guérin vaccination); cavitary pulmonary disease mimicking pulmonary tuberculosis	Isoniazid, rifampin, ethambutol, streptomycin
M. chelonei	Skin, soft tissue, bone, and joint infections with the potential for sinus tract formation	Amikacin, doxycycline, erythromycin, imipenem, tobramycin all have variable in vitro activity; combinations of these may be effective in vivo
M. fortuitum	Cutaneous lesions; soft tissue; bone; disseminated multiorgan disease; isolated central nervous system (CNS) disease	Clarithromycin, amikacin, cefoxitin, sulfonamides, doxycycline, fluoroquinolones
M. marinum	Cutaneous lesions; soft tissue; bone; usually associated with water exposure	Rifampin, ethambutol, minocycline; or clarithromycin
M. malmoense	Cavitary pulmonary disease with fever, night sweats, weight loss; CNS ring-enhancing lesions with fever, headache, neurologic symptoms	Clarithromycin or azithromycin, rifabutin, ethambutol, and ciprofloxacin have been used; resistance to isoniazid, rifampin, ethambutol demonstrated in vitro
M. celatum	Disseminated multiorgan disease with cavitary pulmonary lesions (in one case)	Clarithromycin, amikacin, ciprofloxacin

From Brown BA, Wallace RJ Jr. Infections due to nontuberculous mycobacteria. In: Mandell G, Bennett JE, Dolin R (eds) Principles and Practice of Infectious Diseases, 5th ed. Philadelphia, Churchill Livingstone, 2000, p 2630; and Arasteh KN, Cordes C, Ewers M, et al. HIV-related nontuberculous mycobacterial infection: incidence, survival analysis, and associated risk factors. Eur J Med Res 5:424, 2000.

▲ OTHER ATYPICAL MYCOBACTERIAL INFECTIONS IN HIV-INFECTED PATIENTS

A number of other atypical mycobacteria infrequently cause disease in HIV-infected individuals. The organisms, the most commonly recognized associated clinical syndromes, and suggested treatment regimens are summarized in Table 34–3.[180–188]

REFERENCES

1. Kemper CA, Havlir D, Bartok AE, et al. Transient bacteremia due to Mycobacterium avium complex in patients with AIDS. J Infect Dis 170:488, 1994.
2. Gordin FM, Cohn DL, Sullam PM, et al. Early manifestations of disseminated Mycobacterium avium complex disease: a prospective evaluation. J Infect Dis 176:126, 1997.
3. Inderlied CB, Kemper CA, Bermudez LEM. The Mycobacterium avium complex. Clin Microbiol Rev 6:266, 1993.
4. Benson CA, Ellner JJ. Mycobacterium avium complex infection and AIDS: advances in theory and practice. Clin Infect Dis 17:7, 1993.
5. Havlik JA Jr, Horsburgh CR Jr, Metchock B, et al. Disseminated Mycobacterium avium complex infection: clinical identification and epidemiologic trends. J Infect Dis 165:577, 1992.
6. Benson CA. Disease due to the Mycobacterium avium complex in patients with AIDS: epidemiology and clinical syndrome. Clin Infect Dis 18:S-218, 1994.
7. Torriani FJ, McCutchan JA, Bozzette SA, et al. Autopsy findings in AIDS patients with Mycobacterium avium complex bacteremia. J Infect Dis 170:1601, 1994.
8. Phillips P, Kwiatkowski MB, Copland M, et al. Mycobacterial lymphadenitis associated with the initiation of combination antiretroviral therapy. J Acquir Immune Defic Syndr Hum Retrovirol 20:122, 1999.
9. Race E, Adelson-Mitty J, Kriegel GR, et al. Focal mycobacterial lymphadenitis following initiation of protease-inhibitor therapy in patients with advanced HIV-1 disease. Lancet 351:252, 1998.
10. Cabie A, Abel S, Brebion A, et al. Mycobacterial lymphadenitis after initiation of highly active antiretroviral therapy. Eur J Clin Microbiol Infect Dis 17:812, 1998.
11. Packer SJ, Cesario T, Williams JH Jr. Mycobacterium avium complex infection presenting as endobronchial lesions in immunosuppressed patients. Ann Intern Med 109:389, 1988.
12. Barbaro DJ, Orcutt VL, Coldiron BM. Mycobacterium avium-Mycobacterium intracellulare infection limited to the skin and lymph nodes in patients with AIDS. Rev Infect Dis 11:635, 1989.
13. Kerns E, Benson C, Spear J, et al. Pericardial disease in patients with HIV infection. In: Program and Abstracts of the 31st Interscience Conference on Antimicrobial Agents and Chemotherapy. Washington, DC, American Society for Microbiology, 1991, p 191, abstract 551.
14. Hellyer TJ, Brown IN, Taylor MB, et al. Gastrointestinal involvement in Mycobacterium avium-intracellulare infection of patients with HIV. J Infect 26:55, 1993.
15. Owen RL, Roth RI, St. Hilaire RJ, et al. Pseudo Whipple's disease intestinal infection with Mycobacterium avium intracellulare (M. avium) in acquired immune deficiency syndrome (AIDS). Gastroenterology 84:1267, 1983.

16. Jacob CN, Henein SS, Heurich AE, et al. Nontuberculous mycobacterial infection of the central nervous system in patients with AIDS. South Med J 86:638, 1993.
17. Gascon P, Sathe SS, Rameshwar P. Impaired erythropoiesis in the acquired immunodeficiency syndrome with disseminated Mycobacterium avium complex. Am J Med 94:41, 1993.
18. Marinelli DL, Albelda SM, Williams TM, et al. Nontuberculous mycobacterial infection in AIDS: clinical, pathologic, and radiographic features. Radiology 160:77, 1986.
19. Wolinsky E. Nontuberculous mycobacteria and associated diseases. Am Rev Respir Dis 119:107, 1979.
20. Havlir DV, Ellner JJ. Mycobacterium avium complex. In: Mandell G, Bennett JE, Dolin R (eds) Principles and Practice of Infectious Diseases, 4th ed. New York, Churchill Livingstone, 1994, p 2250.
21. Anagyros P, Astill DSJ, Lim ISL. Comparison of improved BACTEC and Lowenstein-Jensen media for culture of mycobacteria from clinical specimens. J Clin Microbiol 28:1288, 1990.
22. Saito H, Tomioka H, Sato H, et al. Identification of various serovar of Mycobacterium avium complex by using DNA probes specific for Mycobacterium avium and Mycobacterium intracellulare. J Clin Microbiol 28:1694, 1990.
23. Horsburgh CR Jr, Cohn DL, Roberts RB, et al. Mycobacterium avium-M. intracellulare isolates from patients with or without acquired immunodeficiency syndrome. Antimicrob Agents Chemother 30:955, 1986.
24. Tsang AY, Denner JC, Brennan PJ, et al. Clinical and epidemiological importance of typing Mycobacterium avium complex isolates. J Clin Microbiol 30:479, 1992.
25. Yakrus MA, Good RC. Geographic distribution, frequency, and specimen source of Mycobacterium avium complex serotypes isolated from patients with acquired immunodeficiency syndrome. J Clin Microbiol 28:926, 1990.
26. Guthertz LS, Damsker B, Bottone EJ, et al. Mycobacterium avium and Mycobacterium intracellulare infections in patients with and without AIDS. J Infect Dis 160:1037, 1989.
27. Horsburgh CR Jr, Selik RM. The epidemiology of disseminated nontuberculous mycobacterial infection in the acquired immunodeficiency syndrome (AIDS). Am Rev Respir Dis 139:4, 1989.
28. Reddy VM, Parikh K, Luna-Herrera J, et al. Comparison of virulence of Mycobacterium avium complex (MAC) strains isolated from AIDS and non-AIDS patients. Microb Pathog 16:121, 1994.
29. Arbeit RD, Slutsky A, Barber TW, et al. Genetic diversity among strains of Mycobacterium avium causing monoclonal and polyclonal bacteremia in patients with AIDS. J Infect Dis 167:1384, 1993.
30. Slutsky AM, Arbeit RD, Barber TW, et al. Polyclonal infections due to Mycobacterium avium complex in patients with AIDS detected by pulsed-field gel electrophoresis of sequential clinical isolates. J Clin Microbiol 32:1773, 1994.
31. Mazurek GH, Chin DP, Hartman S, et al. Genetic similarity among Mycobacterium avium isolates from blood, stool, and sputum of persons with AIDS. J Infect Dis 176:976, 1997.
32. Iseman MD, Corpe RF, O'Brien RJ, et al. Disease due to Mycobacterium avium-intracellulare. Chest 87:139S, 1985.
33. Eaton T, Falkinham JO III, von Reyn CF. Recovery of Mycobacterium avium from cigarettes. J Clin Microbiol 33:2757, 1995.
34. Edwards LB, Palmer CE. Epidemiology studies of tuberculin sensitivity. I. Preliminary results with purified protein derivatives prepared from atypical acid fast organisms. Am J Hyg 68:213, 1958.
35. Gilks CF, Brindle RJ, Mwachari C, et al. Disseminated Mycobacterium avium infection among HIV-infected patients in Kenya. J Acquir Immune Defic Syndr 8:195, 1995.
36. Morrissey AB, Aisu TO, Falkinham JO III, et al. Absence of Mycobacterium avium complex disease in patients with AIDS in Uganda. J Acquir Immune Defic Syndr 5:477, 1992.
37. Von Reyn CF, Barber TW, Arbeit RD, et al. Evidence of previous infection with Mycobacterium avium-Mycobacterium intracellulare complex among healthy subjects: an international study of dominant mycobacterial skin test reactions. J Infect Dis 168:1553, 1993.
38. Von Reyn CF, Maslow JN, Barber TW, et al. Persistent colonization of potable water as a source of Mycobacterium avium infection in AIDS. Lancet 343:1137, 1994.
39. Montecalvo M, Forester G, Tsang A, et al. Colonization of potable water with Mycobacterium avium complex in homes of HIV-infected persons. Lancet 343:1639, 1994.
40. Von Reyn CF, Arbeit RD, Tosteson ANA, et al. The international epidemiology of disseminated Mycobacterium avium complex infection in AIDS. AIDS 10:1025, 1996.
41. Horsburgh CR Jr, Chin DP, Yajko DM, et al. Environmental risk factors for acquisition of Mycobacterium avium complex in persons with human immunodeficiency virus infection. J Infect Dis 170:362, 1994.
42. Ostroff SM, Spiegel RA, Feinberg J, et al. Preventing disseminated Mycobacterium avium complex disease in patients infected with human immunodeficiency virus. Clin Infect Dis 21(suppl 1):S72, 1995.
43. USPHS/IDSA Prevention of Opportunistic Infections Working Group. 1997 USPHS/IDSA guidelines for the prevention of opportunistic infections in persons infected with human immunodeficiency virus. MMWR Morb Mortal Wkly Rep 46(RR-12), 1997.
44. USPHS/IDSA Prevention of Opportunistic Infections Working Group. 1999 USPHS/IDSA guidelines for the prevention of opportunistic infections in persons infected with human immunodeficiency virus. MMWR Morb Mortal Wkly Rep 48(RR-10), 1999.
45. Nightingale SD, Byrd LT, Southern PM, et al. Incidence of Mycobacterium avium-intracellulare complex bacteremia in human immunodeficiency virus-positive patients. J Infect Dis 165:1082, 1992.
46. Chaisson RE, Moore RD, Richman DD, et al. Incidence and natural history of Mycobacterium avium complex infections in patients with advanced human immunodeficiency virus disease treated with zidovudine. Am Rev Respir Dis 146:285, 1992.
47. Murphy R, El-Sadr W, Cheung T, et al. Impact of protease inhibitor containing regimens on the risk of developing opportunistic infections and mortality in the CPCRA 034/ACTG 277 Study. In: Abstracts of the 5th Conference on Retroviruses and Opportunistic Infections, Chicago. Alexandria, VA, Foundation for Retrovirology and Human Health, 1998, p 113, abstract 181.
48. Palella F, Delaney K, Moorman A, et al. Declining morbidity and mortality among patients with advanced human immunodeficiency virus infection. N Engl J Med 338:853, 1998.
49. Ledergerber B, Egger M, Erard V, et al. AIDS-related opportunistic illnesses occurring after initiation of potent antiretroviral therapy: the Swiss HIV Cohort Study. JAMA 282:2220, 1999.
50. Mocroft A, Katlama C, Johnson AM, et al. AIDS across Europe, 1994–1998: the Eurosida study. Lancet 356:291, 2000.
51. Currier JS, Williams PL, Grimes JM, et al. Incidence rates and risk factors for opportunistic infections in a phase III trial comparing indinavir + ZDV + 3TC to ZDV + 3TC. In: Abstracts of the 5th Conference on Retroviruses and Opportunistic Infections, Chicago. Alexandria, VA, Foundation for Retrovirology and Human Health, 1998, p 127, abstract 257.
52. El-Sadr WM, Burman WJ, Grant LB, et al. Discontinuation of prophylaxis against Mycobacterium avium complex disease in HIV-infected patients who have a response to antiretroviral therapy. N Engl J Med 342:1085, 2000.
53. Currier JS, Williams PL, Koletar SL, et al. Discontinuation of Mycobacterium avium complex prophylaxis in patients with antiretroviral therapy-induced increases in CD4+ T-lymphocyte count: a randomized, double-blind, placebo-controlled trial. Ann Intern Med 133:493, 2000.
54. Benson CA. Mycobacterium avium-intracellulare complex disease. In: Schlossberg D (ed). Tuberculosis and Nontuberculosis Mycobacterial Infections, 4th ed. WB Saunders, Philadelphia, 1999, pp 351–371.
55. Bermudez LE. Immunobiology of Mycobacterium avium infection. Eur J Clin Microbiol Infect Dis 13:1000, 1994.
56. Bermudez LE, Young LS. Natural killer cell dependent mycobacteriostatic and mycobactericidal activity in human macrophages. J Immunol 146:265, 1991.
57. Barnes PF, Grisso CL, Abrams JS, et al. Gamma-delta T lymphocytes in human tuberculosis. J Infect Dis 165:506, 1992.
58. Katz P, Yeager H, Whalen G, et al. Natural killer cell-mediated lysis of Mycobacterium avium complex infected macrophages. J Clin Immunol 10:71, 1990.
59. Blanchard DK, McMillen S, Hoffman SL, Djeu JY. Mycobacterial induction of activated killer cells: possible role of tyrosine kinase activity in interleukin-2 receptor-α expression. Infect Immun 60:2843, 1992.
60. Blanchard DK, Michelini-Norris MB, Pearson CA, et al. Mycobacterium avium-intracellulare induces interleukin-6 from human monocytes and large granular lymphocytes. Blood 77:2218, 1991.

61. Toba H, Crawford JT, Ellner JJ. Pathogenicity of Mycobacterium avium for human monocytes: absence of macrophage-activating factor activity of gamma interferon. Infect Immun 57:239, 1989.
62. MacArthur RD, Lederman MM, Benson CA, et al. Effects of Mycobacterium avium complex-infection treatment on cytokine expression in human immunodeficiency virus-infected persons: results of AIDS Clinical Trials Group Protocol 853. J Infect Dis 181:1486, 2000.
63. Tsukaguchi K, Yoneda T, Okamura H, et al. Defective T cell function for inhibition of growth of Mycobacterium avium-intracellulare complex (MAC) in patients with MAC disease: restoration by cytokines. J Infect Dis 182:1664, 2000.
64. Havlir DV, Schrier RD, Torriani FJ, et al. Effect of potent antiretroviral therapy on immune responses to Mycobacterium avium in human immunodeficiency virus-infected subjects. J Infect Dis 182:1658, 2000.
65. Vankayalapati R, Wizel B, Samten B, et al. Cytokine profiles in immunocompetent persons infected with Mycobacterium avium complex. J Infect Dis 183:478, 2001.
66. Ehlers S, Benini J, Kutsch S, et al. Fata granuloma necrosis without exacerbated mycobacterial growth in tumor necrosis factor receptor p55 gene-deficient mice intravenously infected with Mycobacterium avium. Infect Immun 67:3571, 1999.
67. Bermudez LE, Stevens P, Kolonoski P, et al. Treatment of experimental disseminated Mycobacterium avium complex infection in mice with recombinant IL-2 and tumor necrosis factor. J Immunol 143:2996, 1989.
68. Silva RA, Pais TF, Appelberg R. Evaluation of IL-12 immunotherapy and vaccine design in experimental Mycobacterium avium infections. J Immunol 161:5578, 1998.
69. Doherty TM, Sher A. IL-12 promotes drug-induced clearance of Mycobacterium avium infection in mice. J Immunol 160:5428, 1998.
70. Frutch DM, Holland SM. Defective monocyte costimulation for IFN-gamma production in familial disseminated Mycobacterium avium complex infection: abnormal IL-12 regulation. J Immunol 157:411, 1996.
71. Altare F, Durandy A, Lammas D, et al. Impairment of mycobacterial immunity in human interleukin-12 receptor deficiency. Science 280:1432, 1998.
72. Newport MJ, Huxley CM, Huston S, et al. A mutation in the interferon-gamma receptor gene and susceptibility to mycobacterial infection. N Engl J Med 335:1941, 1996.
73. Holland SM, Eisenstein EM, Kuhns DB, et al. Treatment of refractory disseminated nontuberculous mycobacterial infection with interferon gamma. N Engl J Med 330:1348, 1994.
74. Bermudez LE, Wu M, Petrofsky M, Young LS. Interleukin-6 antagonizes tumor necrosis factor-mediated mycobacteriostatic and mycobactericidal activities in macrophages. Infect Immun 60:4245, 1992.
75. Balcewicz-Sablinska MK, Gan H, Remold HG. Interleukin 10 produced by macrophages inoculated with Mycobacterium avium attenuates mycobacteria-induced apoptosis by reduction of tumor necrosis factor-alpha activity. J Infect Dis 180:1230, 1999.
76. Gong J, Zhang M, Modlin RL, et al. Interleukin-10 downregulates Mycobacterium tuberculosis-induced Th1 responses and CTLA-4 expression. Infect Immun 64:913, 1996.
77. Rojas RE, Balaji KN, Subramanian A, Boom WH. Regulation of human $CD4^+$ $\alpha\beta$ T-cell-receptor-positive (TCR^+) and gamma delta TCR^+ T-cell responses to Mycobacterium tuberculosis by interleukin-10 and transforming growth factor beta. Infect Immun 67:6461, 1999.
78. Johnson JL, Shiratsuchi H, Toba H, Ellner JJ. Preservation of monocyte effector functions against Mycobacterium avium-M. intracellulare in patients with AIDS. Infect Immun 59:3639, 1991.
79. Johnson JL, Shiratsuchi H, Toossi Z, Ellner JJ. Altered IL-1 expression and compartmentalization in monocytes from patients with AIDS stimulated with Mycobacterium avium complex. J Clin Immunol 17:387, 1997.
80. Hoover DR, Graham NMH, Bacellar B, et al. An epidemiologic analysis of Mycobacterium avium complex disease in homosexual men infected with human immunodeficiency virus type 1. Clin Infect Dis 20:1250, 1995.
81. Finkelstein DM, Williams PL, Molenberghs G, et al. Patterns of opportunistic infections in patients with HIV infection. J Acquir Immune Defic Syndr Hum Retrovirol 12:38, 1996.
82. Williams PL, Currier JS, Swindells S. Joint effects of HIV-1 RNA levels and CD4 lymphocyte cells on the risk of specific opportunistic infections. AIDS 13:1035, 1999.
83. Lyles RH, Chu C, Mellors JW, et al. Prognostic value of plasma HIV RNA in the natural history of Pneumocystis carinii pneumonia, cytomegalovirus and Mycobacterium avium complex. AIDS 13:341, 1999.
84. Havlik JA Jr, Metchock B, Thompson SE III, et al. A prospective evaluation of Mycobacterium avium complex colonization of the respiratory and gastrointestinal tracts of persons with human immunodeficiency virus infection. J Infect Dis 168:1045, 1994.
85. Chin DP, Hopewell PC, Yajko DM, et al. Mycobacterium avium complex in the respiratory or gastrointestinal tract and the risk of M. avium complex bacteremia in patients with human immunodeficiency virus infection. J Infect Dis 169:289, 1994.
86. Nightingale SD, Cameron DW, Gordin FM, et al. Two controlled trials of rifabutin prophylaxis against Mycobacterium avium complex infection in AIDS. N Engl J Med 329:828, 1993.
87. Horsburgh C Jr, Schoenfelder JR, Gordin FM, et al. Geographic and seasonal variation in Mycobacterium avium bacteremia among North American patients with AIDS. Am J Med Sci 313:341, 1997.
88. Fry KL, Meissner PS, Falkinham JO. Epidemiology of infection by nontuberculous mycobacteria. VI. Identification and use of epidemiologic markers for studies of Mycobacterium avium, M. intracellulare, and M. scrofulaceum. Am Rev Respir Dis 134:39, 1986.
89. Parker BC, Ford MA, Gruft H, et al. Epidemiology of infection by nontuberculous mycobacteria. IV. Preferential aerosolization of Mycobacterium intracellulare from natural waters. Am Rev Respir Dis 128:652, 1983.
90. Gray JR, Rabeneck L. Atypical mycobacterial infection of the gastrointestinal tract in AIDS patients. Am J Gastroenterol 84:1521, 1989.
91. Bermudez LE, Petrofsky M, Kolonoski P, et al. An animal model of Mycobacterium avium complex disseminated infection after colonization of the intestinal tract. J Infect Dis 165:75, 1992.
92. Brown ST, Edwards FF, Bernard EM, et al. Progressive disseminated infection with Mycobacterium avium complex after intravenous and oral challenge in cyclosporine-treated rats. J Infect Dis 164:922, 1991.
93. Orme IM, Furney SK, Roberts AD. Dissemination of enteric Mycobacterium avium infections in mice rendered immunodeficient by thymectomy and CD4 depletion or by prior infection with murine AIDS retrovirus. Infect Immun 60:4747, 1992.
94. Torriani F, Behling C, McCutchan JA, et al. Disseminated Mycobacterium avium complex: correlation between blood cultures and tissue burden. J Infect Dis 173:942, 1996.
95. Hafner R, Inderlied CB, Peterson DM, et al. Correlation of quantitative bone marrow and blood cultures in AIDS patients with disseminated Mycobacterium avium complex infection. J Infect Dis 180:438, 1999.
96. Inderlied CB. Microbiology and minimum inhibitory concentration testing for Mycobacterium avium prophylaxis. Am J Med 102:2, 1997.
97. Thierry D, Vincent V, Clement F, et al. Isolation of specific DNA fragments of Mycobacterium avium and their possible use in diagnosis. J Clin Microbiol 31:1048, 1993.
98. Van der Giessen JWB, Eger A, Haagsma J, et al. Rapid detection and identification of Mycobacterium avium by amplification of 16s rRNA sequences. J Clin Microbiol 31:2509, 1993.
99. Shanson DC, Dryden MS. Comparison of methods for isolating Mycobacterium avium-intracellulare from blood of patients with AIDS. J Clin Pathol 41:687, 1988.
100. Evans KD, Nakasome AS, Sutherland PA, et al. Identification of Mycobacterium tuberculosis and Mycobacterium avium-M. intracellulare directly from primary BACTEC7 cultures by using acridinium-ester labelled DNA probes. J Clin Microbiol 30:2427, 1992.
101. Heifets L, Lindholm-Levy P, Libonati J, et al. Radiometric broth macrodilution method for determination of minimal inhibitory concentrations (MIC) with Mycobacterium avium complex isolates: proposed guidelines. Denver, CO, National Jewish Center for Immunology and Respiratory Medicine, 1993.
102. Horsburgh C, Mason U, Heifets L, et al. Response to therapy of pulmonary Mycobacterium avium intracellulare infection correlates with results of in vitro susceptibility testing. Am Rev Respir Dis 135:418, 1987.
103. Chaisson RE, Benson CA, Dube MP, et al. Clarithromycin therapy for bacteremic Mycobacterium avium complex disease in patients with AIDS. Ann Intern Med 121:905, 1994.
104. Heifets L, Mor N, Vanderkolk J. Mycobacterium avium strains resistant to clarithromycin and azithromycin. Antimicrob Agents Chemother 37:2364, 1993.

105. Shafran SD, Talbot JA, Chomyc S, et al. Does in vitro susceptibility to rifabutin and ethambutol predict the response to treatment of Mycobacterium avium complex bacteremia with rifabutin, ethambutol, and clarithromycin? Canandian HIV Trials Network Protocol 010 Study Group. Clin Infect Dis 27:1401, 1998.
106. Meier A, Heifets L, Wallace RJ Jr, et al. Molecular mechanisms of clarithromycin resistance in Mycobacterium avium: observation of multiple 23S rDNA mutations in a clonal population. J Infect Dis 174:354, 1996.
107. Nash KA, Inderlied CB. Genetic basis of macrolide resistance in Mycobacterium avium isolated from patients with disseminated disease. Antimicrob Agents Chemother 39:2625, 1995.
108. Benson CA. Treatment of disseminated disease due to the Mycobacterium avium complex in patients with AIDS. Clin Infect Dis 18(suppl):S237, 1994.
109. Young LS, Wiviott L, Wu M, et al. Azithromycin for treatment of Mycobacterium avium-intracellulare complex infection in patients with AIDS. Lancet 388:1107, 1991.
110. Jacobson MA, Yajko D, Northfelt D, et al. Randomized, placebo controlled trial of rifampin, ethambutol and ciprofloxacin for AIDS patients with disseminated Mycobacterium avium complex infection. J Infect Dis 168:112, 1993.
111. Kemper CA, Meng RC, Nussbaum J, et al. Treatment of Mycobacterium avium complex bacteremia in AIDS with a four-drug oral regimen. Ann Intern Med 116:466, 1992.
112. Shafran SD, Singer J, Zarowney DP, et al. A comparison of two regimens for the treatment of Mycobacterium avium complex bacteremia in AIDS: rifabutin, ethambutol, and clarithromycin versus rifampin, ethambutol, clofazimine, and ciprofloxacin. N Engl J Med 335:377, 1996.
113. May T, Brel F, Beuscart C, et al. Comparison of combination therapy regimens for treatment of human immunodeficiency virus-infected patients with disseminated bacteremia due to Mycobacterium avium. Clin Infect Dis 25:621, 1997.
114. Gordin FM, Sullam PM, Shafran SD, et al. A randomized, placebo-controlled study of rifabutin added to a regimen of clarithromycin and ethambutol for treatment of disseminated infection with Mycobacterium avium complex. Clin Infect Dis 28:1080, 1999.
115. Dube MP, Sattler F, Torriani F, et al. A randomized evaluation of ethambutol for prevention of relapse and drug resistance during treatment of Mycobacterium avium complex bacteremia with clarithromycin-based combination therapy. J Infect Dis 176:1225, 1997.
116. Cohn DL, Fisher EJ, Peng GT, et al. A prospective randomized trial of four three-drug regimens in the treatment of disseminated Mycobacterium avium complex disease in AIDS patients: excess mortality associated with high-dose clarithromycin. Clin Infect Dis 29:125, 1999.
117. Chaisson RE, Keiser P, Pierce M, et al. Clarithromycin and ethambutol with or without clofazimine for the treatment of bacteremic Mycobacterium avium complex disease in patients with HIV infection. AIDS 11:311, 1997.
118. Wallace R Jr, Brown B, Griffith D, et al. Initial clarithromycin monotherapy for Mycobacterium avium-intracellulare complex lung disease. Am J Respir Crit Care Med 149:1335, 1994.
119. Wallace RJ Jr, Brown BA, Griffith DE, et al. Clarithromycin regimens for pulmonary Mycobacterium avium complex: the first 50 patients. Am J Respir Crit Care Med 153:1766, 1996.
120. Griffith DE, Brown BA, Girard WM, et al. Azithromycin activity against Mycobacterium avium complex lung disease in HIV negative patients. Clin Infect Dis 23:983, 1996.
121. Korvick JA, Benson CA. Advances in the treatment and prophylaxis of Mycobacterium avium complex in individuals infected with human immunodeficiency virus. In: Korvick JA, Benson CA (eds) Mycobacterium avium Complex Infection: Progress in Research and Treatment. New York, Marcel Dekker, 1996, p 241.
122. Clarithromycin (Biaxin) package insert/product monograph. Abbott Park, IL, Abbott Laboratories, 1995.
123. Azithromycin (Zithromax) package insert/product monograph. New York, Pfizer, 1996.
124. Rifabutin (Mycobutin) package insert/product monograph. Kalamazoo, MI, Pharmacia & Upjohn, 1995.
125. Benson CA, Sha BE. Management of disseminated Mycobacterium avium complex disease in HIV-infected women. In: Cotton D, Watts HD (eds) The Medical Management of AIDS in Women. New York, Wiley-Liss, 1997, p 269.
126. Masur H, Public Health Service Task Force on Prophylaxis and Therapy for Mycobacterium avium Complex. Recommendations on prophylaxis and therapy for disseminated Mycobacterium avium complex disease in patients infected with the human immunodeficiency virus. N Engl J Med 329:898, 1993.
127. U.S. Public Health Service/Infectious Disease Society of America Guidelines for Prevention of Opportunistic Infections in Persons with AIDS. www.hivatis.org.
128. Fuller JD, Stanfield LED, Craven DE. Rifabutin prophylaxis and uveitis [letter]. N Engl J Med 330:1315, 1994.
129. Trapnell CB, Narang PK, Li R, et al. Increased plasma rifabutin levels with concomitant fluconazole therapy in HIV-infected patients. Ann Intern Med 124:573, 1996.
130. Narang PK, Trapnell CB, Schoenfelder JR, et al. Fluconazole and enhanced effect of rifabutin prophylaxis [letter]. N Engl J Med 330:1316, 1994.
131. Piscitelli SC, Flexner C, Minor JR, et al. Drug interactions in patients infected with human immunodeficiency virus. Clin Infect Dis 23:685, 1996.
132. Norvir (Ritonavir) package insert/product monograph. Abbott Park, IL, Abbott Laboratories, 1996.
133. Ouellet D, Hsu A, Granneman GR, et al. Assessment of the pharmacokinetic interaction between ritonavir and clarithromycin [abstract PI-58]. Clin Pharmacol Ther 59:143, 1996.
134. Centers for Disease Control and Prevention. Notice to readers: updated guidelines for the use of rifabutin or rifampin for the treatment and prevention of tuberculosis among HIV-infected patients taking protease inhibitors or nonnucleoside reverse transcriptase inhibitors. MMWR Morb Mortal Wkly 49:183, 2000.
135. Cato A, Cavanaugh JH, Shi H, et al. Assessment of multiple doses of ritonavir on the pharmacokinetics of rifabutin. In: Abstracts of the XIth International Conference on AIDS, Vancouver, 1996, p 89, abstract Mo.B.1199.
136. Sun E, Heath-Chiozzi M, Cameron DW, et al. Concurrent ritonavir and rifabutin increases the risk of rifabutin associated adverse effects. In: Abstracts of the XIth International Conference on AIDS, Vancouver, 1996, p 18, abstract Mo.B.171.
137. Hamzeh F, Benson C, Gerber J, et al. Steady-state pharmacokinetic interaction of modified-dose indinavir and rifabutin. In: Abstracts of the 7th Conference on Retroviruses and Opportunistic Infections, San Francisco. Alexandria, VA, Foundation for Retrovirology and Human Health, 2000, p 92, abstract 90.
138. Crixivan (Indinavir) package insert/product monograph. West Point, PA, Merck, 1996.
139. Viracept (Nelfinavir) package insert/product monograph. La Jolla, CA, Agouron, 1998.
140. Invirase (saquinavir) package insert/product monograph. Nutley, NJ, Hoffman-LaRoche, 1996.
141. Sahai J, Stewart F, Swick L, et al. Rifabutin (RBT) reduces saquinavir (SAQ) plasma levels in HIV-infected patients. In: Program and Abstracts of the 36th Interscience Conference on Antimicrobial Agents and Chemotherapy, New Orleans. Washington, DC, American Society for Microbiology, 1996, p 6, abstract A27.
142. Viramune (nevirapine) package insert/product monograph. Columbus, OH, Roxane, 1997.
143. Borin MT, Cox SR, Driver MR, et al. Effect of rifabutin on delavirdine pharmacokinetics in HIV^+ patients. In: Program and Abstracts of the 34th Interscience Conference on Antimicrobial Agents and Chemotherapy. Washington, DC, American Society for Microbiology, 1994, p 81, abstract A48.
144. Benson CA. Critical drug interactions with agents used for prophylaxis and treatment of Mycobacterium avium complex infections. Am J Med 102:32, 1997.
145. Efavirenz (Sustiva) data on file. Wilmington, DE, DuPont Merck, 1998.
146. Benson CA, Williams PL, Cohn DL, et al. Clarithromycin or rifabutin alone or in combination for primary prophylaxis of Mycobacterium avium complex disease in patients with AIDS: a randomized, double-blind, placebo-controlled trial. J Infect Dis 181:1289, 2000.
147. Havlir DV, Dube MP, Sattler FR, et al. Prophylaxis against disseminated Mycobacterium avium complex with weekly azithromycin, daily rifabutin, or both. N Engl J Med 335:392, 1996.
148. Aberg JA, Yajko DM, Jacobson MA. Eradication of AIDS-related disseminated Mycobacterium avium complex infection after 12 months

of antimycobacterial therapy combined with highly active antiretroviral therapy J Infect Dis 178:1446, 1998.

149. Zeller V, Jovan M, Truffaaut, et al. Discontinuing maintenance treatment for Pneumocystis pneumonia, toxoplasmic encephalitis, and disseminated Mycobacterium avium complex infection. Presented at the 1st IAS Conference on HIV Pathogenesis and Treatment, Buenos Aires, 2001, p 302, abstract 739.
150. Shafran SD, Gill MJ, Lalonde RG, et al. Successful discontinuation of MAC therapy following effective HAART. In: Abstracts of the 8th Conference on Retroviruses and Opportunistic Infections, Chicago. Alexandria, VA, Foundation for Retrovirology and Human Health, 2001, p 208, abstract 547.
151. Chiu J, Nussbaum J, Bozzette S, et al. Treatment of disseminated Mycobacterium avium complex infection in AIDS with amikacin, ethambutol, rifampin, and ciprofloxacin. Ann Intern Med 113:358, 1990.
152. Kemper CA, Havlir D, Haghighat D, et al. The individual microbiologic effect of three antimycobacterial agents, clofazimine, ethambutol and rifampin, on Mycobacterium avium complex bacteremia in patients with AIDS. J Infect Dis 170:157, 1994.
153. Parenti D, Ellner J, Hafner R, et al. A phase II/III trial of rifampin (RIF), ciprofloxacin (CIPRO), clofazimine (CLOF), ethambutol (ETH), amikacin (AK) in the treatment of disseminated Mycobacterium avium (MAC) infection in HIV-infected individuals. In: Abstracts of the 2nd National Conference on Human Retroviruses and Related Diseases. Washington, DC, American Society for Microbiology, 1995, p 56, abstract 6.
154. Dautzenberg B, Truffot C, Legris S, et al. Activity of clarithromycin against Mycobacterium avium infection in patients with acquired immune deficiency syndrome: a controlled clinical trial. Am Rev Respir Dis 144:564, 1991.
155. Shafran SD, Deschenes J, Miller M, et al. Uveitis and pseudojaundice during a regimen of clarithromycin, rifabutin, and ethambutol [letter]. N Engl J Med 330:438, 1994.
156. Hafner R, Bethel J, Power M, et al. Tolerance and pharmacokinetic interactions of rifabutin and clarithromycin in human immunodeficiency virus-infected volunteers. Antimicrob Agents Chemother 42:631, 1998.
157. Benson CA, Williams PL, Currier JS, et al. ACTG 223: an open, prospective, randomized study comparing efficacy and safety of clarithromycin (C) plus ethambutol (E), rifabutin (R) or both for treatment (Rx) of MAC disease in patients with AIDS. In: Abstracts of the 6th Conference on Retroviruses and Opportunistic Infections, Chicago. Alexandria, VA, Foundation for Retrovirology and Human Health, 1999, abstract 249.
158. Ward TT, Rimland D, Kauffman C, et al. Randomized, open label trial of azithromycin plus ethambutol versus clarithromycin plus ethambutol therapy for Mycobacterium avium complex bacteremia in patients with human immunodeficiency virus infection. Clin Infect Dis 27:1278, 1998.
159. Dunne M, Fessel J, Kumar P, et al. A randomized, double-blind trial comparing azithromycin and clarithromycin in the treatment of disseminated Mycobacterium avium infection in patients with human immunodeficiency virus. Clin Infect Dis 31:1245, 2000.
160. Dube MP, Torriani F, See D, et al. Successful short-term suppression of clarithromycin-resistant Mycobacterium avium complex bacteremia in AIDS: California Collaborative Treatment Group. Clin Infect Dis 28:136, 1999.
161. Nelson M, Richardson S, Gazzard BS. Liposomal amikacin for the treatment of non-tuberculous mycobacteria in HIV disease. In: Conference Record, 12th World AIDS Conference, Geneva, 1998, abstract 22170.
162. Kemper CA, Bermudez L, Deresinski S. Immunomodulatory treatment of Mycobacterium avium complex bacteremia in patients with AIDS by use of recombinant granulocyte macrophage colony-stimulating factor. J Infect Dis 177:914, 1998.
163. Holland SM, Eisenstein DM, Kuhns DB, et al. Treatment of refractory disseminated nontuberculous mycobacterial infection with interferon gamma: a preliminary report. N Engl J Med 330:1348, 1994.
164. Wormser GP, Horowitz H, Dworkin B. Low-dose dexamethasone as adjuvant therapy for disseminated Mycobacterium avium complex infections in AIDS patients. Antimicrob Agents Chemother 38:2215, 1994.
165. Graves M, Salvato P, Thompson C. MAIC and the effect of prednisone on disease progression in AIDS patients. In: Abstracts of the XIth International Conference on AIDS, Vancouver, 1996, p 119, abstract Mo.B.1371.
166. Pierce M, Crampton S, Henry D, et al. A randomized trial of clarithromycin as prophylaxis against disseminated Mycobacterium avium complex infection in patients with advanced acquired immunodeficiency syndrome. N Engl J Med 335:392, 1996.
167. Currier J, Williams P, Feinberg J, et al. Impact of prophylaxis for Mycobacterium avium complex on bacterial infections in patients with advanced human immunodeficiency virus disease. Clin Infect Dis 32:1615, 2001.
168. Oldfield EC, Dickinson G, Chung R, et al. Once weekly azithromycin for the prevention of Mycobacterium avium complex (MAC complex) infection in AIDS patients. Clin Infect Dis 26:611, 1998.
169. Moore RD, Chaisson RE. Survival analysis of two controlled trials of rifabutin prophylaxis against Mycobacterium avium complex in AIDS. AIDS 9:1337, 1995.
170. Wallace RJ Jr, Brown BA, Griffith DE, et al. Reduced serum levels of clarithromycin in patients treated with multidrug regimens including rifampin or rifabutin for Mycobacterium avium-M. intracellulare infection. J Infect Dis 171:747, 1995.
171. Bamberger DM, Driks MR, Gupta MR, et al. Mycobacterium kansasii among patients infected with human immunodeficiency virus in Kansas City. Clin Infect Dis 18:395, 1994.
172. Levine B, Chaisson RE. Mycobacterium kansasii: a cause of treatable pulmonary disease associated with advanced human immunodeficiency virus (HIV) infection. Ann Intern Med 114:861, 1991.
173. Valainis GT, Cardona LM, Greer DL. The spectrum of Mycobacterium kansasii disease associated with HIV-1 infected patients. J Acquir Immune Defic Syndr 4:516, 1991.
174. Sherer R, Sable R, Sonnenberg M, et al. Disseminated infection with Mycobacterium kansasii in the acquired immunodeficiency syndrome. Ann Intern Med 105:710, 1986.
175. Carpenter JL, Parks JM. Mycobacterium kansasii infections in patients positive for human immunodeficiency virus. Rev Infect Dis 13:789, 1991.
176. Pintado V, Fortun J, Casado JL, Gomez-Mampaso E. Mycobacterium kansasii pericarditis as a presentation of AIDS. Infection 29:48, 2001.
177. Pintado V, Gomez-Mampaso E, Martin-Davila P, et al. Mycobacterium kansasii infection in patients infected with the human immunodeficiency virus. Eur J Clin Microbiol Infect Dis 18:582, 1999.
178. Graybill JR, Bocanegra R. Treatment alternatives for Mycobacterium kansasii. J Antimicrobial Chemother 47:417, 2001.
179. Burman WJ, Stone BL, Brown BA, et al. AIDS-related Mycobacterium kansasii infection with initial resistance to clarithromycin. Diagn Microbiol Infect Dis 31:369, 1998.
180. Straus WL, Ostroff SM, Jernigan DB, et al. Clinical and epidemiologic characteristics of Mycobacterium haemophilum, an emerging pathogen in immunocompromised patients. Ann Intern Med 120:118, 1994.
181. El-Helou P, Rachlis A, Fong I, et al. Mycobacterium xenopi infection in patients with human immunodeficiency virus infection. Clin Infect Dis 25:206, 1997.
182. Hirschel B, Chang HR, Mach N, et al. Fatal infection with a novel unidentified mycobacterium in a man with the acquired immunodeficiency syndrome. N Engl J Med 323:109, 1990.
183. Bessesen MT, Shlay J, Stone-Venohr B, et al. Disseminated Mycobacterium genovense infection: clinical and microbiological features and response to therapy. AIDS 7:1357, 1993.
184. Albrecht H, Rusch-Gerdes S, Stellbrink H-J, et al. Treatment of disseminated Mycobacterium genovense infection. AIDS 9:659, 1995.
185. Fakih M, Chapalamadugu S, Ricart A, et al. Mycobacterium malmoense bacteremia in two AIDS patients. J Clin Microbiol 34:731, 1996.
186. Tortoli E, Piersimoni C, Bacosi D, et al. Isolation of the newly described species Mycobacterium celatum from AIDS patients. J Clin Microbiol 33:137, 1995.
187. Brown BA, Wallace RJ Jr. Infections due to nontuberculous mycobacteria. In: Mandell G, Bennett JE, Dolin R (eds) Principles and Practice of Infectious Diseases, 5th ed. Philadelphia, Churchill Livingstone, 2000, p 2630.
188. Arasteh KN, Cordes C, Ewers M, et al. HIV-related nontuberculous mycobacterial infection: incidence, survival analysis, and associated risk factors. Eur J Med Res 5:424, 2000.

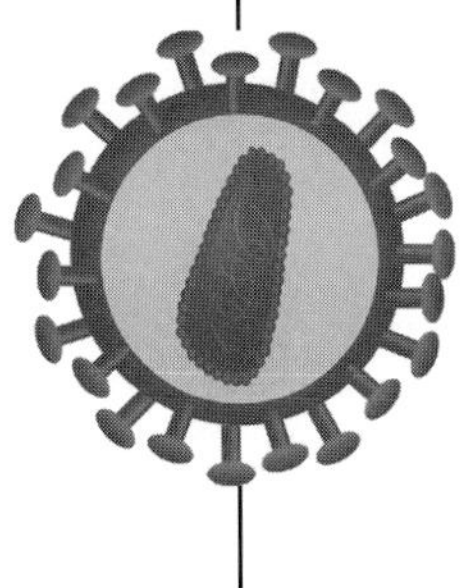

CHAPTER 35

Bartonellosis

Jane E. Koehler, MD

▲ CLINICAL PRESENTATION

The spectrum of disease caused by *Bartonella* species includes cat scratch disease (*B. henselae)*, bacillary angiomatosis *(B. henselae, B. quintana*), bacillary peliosis (*B. henselae*), endocarditis (*B. henselae, B. quintana, B. elizabethae*), bacteremia (*B. henselae, B. quintana, B. vinsonii* subsp. *arupensis*), trench fever (*B. quintana*), meningitis/neuroretinitis (*B. henselae, B. grahamii, B. vinsonii* subsp. *arupensis*), Oroya fever (*B. bacilliformis*), and verruga peruana (*B. bacilliformis*).[1,2] *Bartonella* infections occur in both immunocompromised and immunocompetent patients, but some of the disease manifestations are related to the degree of immunocompromise. Cat scratch disease, a granulomatous lymphadenitis, usually occurs in immunocompetent individuals or in patients early in the course of human immunodeficiency virus (HIV) infection. In contrast, bacillary angiomatosis and bacillary peliosis occur almost exclusively in severely immunocompromised individuals, especially in patients with late stage HIV infection (the median CD4 cell count in a series of patients with bacillary angiomatosis and peliosis was 22/mm^3).

Bacillary angiomatosis lesions are caused by infection with *B. henselae* or *B. quintana*.[4,5] These lesions often are not recognized for several reasons: They can be impossible to distinguish clinically from Kaposi sarcoma lesions,[6] and can have diverse presentations.[7] Bacillary angiomatosis has been described most frequently in skin (as angiomatous papules, pedunculated lesions, or subcutaneous masses). These vascular proliferative lesions also occur in bone, the gastrointestinal and respiratory tracts, lymph nodes, and the central nervous system. A closely related angiomatous lesion of the liver and spleen, known as parenchymal bacillary peliosis,[8] is caused by *B. henselae*.[5]

Some manifestations of *Bartonella* infection, including endocarditis, bacteremia, and meningitis, occur in patients regardless of the degree of immunocompromise. In immunocompetent individuals, cat scratch disease and other manifestations of *Bartonella* infection are usually self-limited, and there are no prospective or compelling data that antibiotic treatment affects the course of *Bartonella* infection in people with a normal immune system. In contrast, *Bartonella* infections in HIV-infected patients are more severe and can even be fatal[9]; therefore all immunocompromised patients with *Bartonella* infection should be treated with appropriate antimicrobial therapy.

▲ TAXONOMY

Infections with *Bartonella* were first identified in the United States because of the acquired immunodeficiency syndrome (AIDS) epidemic. In 1983 Stoler et al. identified an HIV-infected patient with subcutaneous lesions.[10] They subsequently identified numerous bacilli in the lesions by electron microscopy and treated the patient with erythromycin. The lesions resolved, and little additional information became known about the causative organism until 1990, when bacterial DNA was extracted from biopsied bacillary angiomatosis tissue from HIV-infected patients. This molecular analysis led to identification of the organism as being closely related to the agent of trench fever, *Rochalimaea quintana*.[11] The new species also was isolated from the blood of HIV-infected patients[12] and subsequently was named *R. henselae*.[13,14] This species was thought to be the sole agent of bacillary angiomatosis until the bacilli were isolated directly from cutaneous bacillary angiomatosis lesions, and *R. quintana* also was found to cause bacillary angiomatosis in immunocompromised patients.[4]

Brenner et al. found that members of the *Rochalimaea* genus were closely related to the sole species of the genus *Bartonella, B. bacilliformis*; and in 1993 all *Rochalimaea* species (*R. henselae, R. quintana, R. elizabethae, R. vinsonii*) were merged into the *Bartonella* genus.[15] Another genus, *Grahamella,* was subsequently merged with *Bartonella,* adding three more species to the genus, all of which infect small mammals: *B. taylorii, B. grahamii, B. doshiae.*[16] An additional four species were isolated from small mammals, including *B. clarridgeiae, B. tribocorum, B. alsatica,* and *B. koehlerae.*[2] There are currently 12 extant species of *Bartonella,* five of which have been associated with human infection: *B. bacilliformis, B. elizabethae, B. henselae, B. vinsonii* subsp. *arupensis, B. quintana.* Only *B. henselae* and *B. quintana* have been associated with disease in HIV-infected patients.

▲ BIOLOGY AND EPIDEMIOLOGY

Before the bacillary angiomatosis bacillus was identified, epidemiologic studies revealed that development of bacillary angiomatosis was statistically significantly associated with cat contact, cat scratches, and cat bites.[17] Further investigation of household cats belonging to four patients who developed bacillary angiomatosis revealed that all seven cats of these patients were bacteremic with *B. henselae,* the same species that caused the bacillary angiomatosis in these patients.[18] Surveys of the cats in the greater San Francisco Bay area demonstrated that 41% of the 61 pet and pound cats were bacteremic with *B. henselae,* although no illness could be demonstrated in any of the infected cats.[18]

Because of this high prevalence of *B. henselae* bacteremia, and the demonstration that viable *B. henselae* could be cultured from cat fleas infesting bacteremic cats, the cat flea was suspected to be a vector of *B. henselae.* Further evidence implicating the cat flea as an arthropod vector of *B. henselae* was provided by the correlation between the increased prevalence of flea infestation and increased *B. henselae* seroprevalence in cats tested in different regions of the United States.[19] Definitive demonstration of transmission of *B. henselae* from cat to cat was provided when fleas were combed from cats bacteremic with *B. henselae* and placed on specific-pathogen-free cats in an arthropod-free university facility. The recipient cats developed high-level *B. henselae* bacteremia within 2 weeks of experimental infestation and seroconverted several weeks later.[20]

Based on the initial epidemiology study in 1993,[17] it was evident that although most of the patients had developed bacillary angiomatosis after traumatic cat contact, nearly one-third of the patients had no cat contact prior to developing bacillary angiomatosis. After the second species, *B. quintana,* was found to cause bacillary angiomatosis, it was suspected that these patients without cat contact might have developed bacillary angiomatosis infection caused by *B. quintana.* By determining the infecting species for 49 patients with bacillary angiomatosis and comparing exposures of these patients with their 96 matched controls, it was demonstrated that patients infected with *B. henselae* had a statistically significant association with cat contact, including having received cat bites, cat scratches, and cat flea bites.[5] The patients with bacillary angiomatosis caused by *B. quintana,* however, had a statistically significant exposure to the body louse and were of lower socioeconomic status than their matched controls.[5] This contemporary association between the body louse and *B. quintana* corroborates historical data demonstrating that the spread of *B. quintana* among the soldiers occurred via body lice, causing an epidemic of trench fever that affected tens of thousands of troops in World War I.[21]

Each *Bartonella* species is believed to have one or more mammalian reservoir(s): the domestic cat for *B. henselae, B. koehlerae,* and *B. clarridgeiae*; the human for *B. quintana* and *B. bacilliformis*; rabbits for *B. alsatica;* and moles, voles, rats, and mice for *B. vinsonii, B. taylorii, B. doshiae, B. grahamii, B. elizabethae,* and *B. tribocorum.* Arthropod vectors of *Bartonella* species have not been studied as extensively as the reservoirs, but in addition to the cat flea vector (*Ctenocephalides felis*) of *B. henselae*[20] another flea, *Xenopsylla cheopis,* transmitted *Bartonella* spp. to voles.[22] The sandfly *Lutzomyia verrucarum* is the natural arthropod vector known to transmit *B. bacilliformis* among humans in the Peruvian Andes.[23] Little information is currently known about arthropod vectors of other *Bartonella* species.

▲ MICROBIOLOGY

Bartonella species are small, slowly growing, fastidious gram-negative rods. Two species have flagella and are motile: *B. bacilliformis* and *B. clarridgeiae.*[24] The *Bartonella* bacilli are relatively inert biochemically and are not able to oxidize glucose. *Bartonella* species are able to utilize glutamate and succinate as carbon sources, and hemin or serum supplementation of growth media permits optimal growth on artificial media.[25] The colony morphology of primary isolates differs for *B. henselae* (rough, with pitting of the agar) and *B. quintana* (smooth, without pitting of the agar).[5]

▲ DIAGNOSIS

Direct Detection

Bartonella species can be detected in biopsied bacillary angiomatosis tissue using the hematoxylin and eosin (H&E) stain and, optimally, the Warthin-Starry silver stain (Tables 35–1 and 35–2). For cutaneous bacillary angiomatosis lesions, a 5 mm punch biopsy specimen usually provides adequate tissue for diagnosis (for small papules or subcutaneous nodules). The vascular proliferative changes identified by H&E staining are usually highly characteristic.[26] Newly formed, capillary-size blood vessels can be identified and are

▲ **Table 35–1.** MANIFESTATIONS OF *BARTONELLA* INFECTION IN HIV-INFECTED PATIENTS

Manifestation	Diagnostic Approach
Skin	Biopsy with W-S staining
May resemble Kaposi sarcoma	
Angiomatous nodule	
Friable vascular lesion	
Red papule	
Pedunculated lesion	
Deep subcutaneous mass	
Bone	
Extremely painful osteolysis	Biopsy with W-S staining
Lytic lesions on radiograph (technetium-positive)	
Lymph nodes	
Enlargement	Biopsy with W-S staining
Heart	
Valve vegetation	Echo, blood culture (lysis-centrifugation method or EDTA tube)
Valve insufficiency	
Blood	
Thrombosis, fever	Blood culture (echo to rule out endocarditis)
Liver/spleen	
Hypodense lesions—CT	Biopsy with W-S staining (monitor for bleeding)
Hepatosplenomegaly—CT	
Elevated LFTs (alkaline phosphatase)	
Pancytopenia	
Thrombocytopenia	
Other	
Brain, gastrointestinal, pulmonary, others	Biopsy with W-S staining

CT, computed tomography; echo, echocardiography; LFT, liver function tests; W-S, Warthin-Starry stain.
From Koehler JE. *Bartonella*-associated infections in HIV-infected patients. AIDS Clin Care 7:97, 1995. Copyright 1995, Massachusetts Medical Society, with permission.

lined with protruberant endothelial cells. Adjacent to these regions of vascular proliferation are clusters of granular, amphophilic material that represent microcolonies of *Bartonella* bacteria; distinct bacilli are revealed in these granular deposits when the Warthin-Starry silver stain is used. In situ immunohistochemical staining also has been useful for direct visualization of *Bartonella* bacilli in biopsied tissue from bacillary angiomatosis and bacillary peliosis lesions.[27]

▲ **Table 35–2.** *BARTONELLA* LABORATORY DIAGNOSIS

Method	Comments
Histopathology	Check for (H&E staining) Lobular, vascular proliferation Neutrophils and debris Basophilic granular material Protruberant endothelial cells Check for darkly staining bacilli (Warthin-Starry stain)
Blood culture	Lysis-centrifugation or EDTA tubes, onto fresh chocolate and rabbit blood agars Incubate in 5% CO_2 at 35°C for 21 days Accessible to many laboratories
Culture of tissue biopsy	Experimental Co-cultivation of endothelial cells with homogenate
Serology	Centers for Disease Control and Prevention indirect immunofluorescence antibody test

From Koehler JE: *Bartonella*-associated infections in HIV-infected patients. AIDS Clin Care 7:97, 1995. Copyright 1995, Massachusetts Medical Society, with permission.

Culture

The extremely fastidious nature of *Bartonella* bacilli has made isolation difficult or impossible in the clinical microbiology laboratory setting of most hospitals. Isolation is best achieved using enriched agar: optimally, heart infusion agar with 5% defibrinated rabbit blood for *B. henselae*[12] and chocolate agar (including IsovitaleX and hemoglobin) for *B. quintana*.[4] There are distinct differences in the preference of *B. quintana* and *B. henselae* for these two agar compositions.[5] Both agar types should be inoculated with homogenized biopsied bacillary angiomatosis tissue or blood to optimize recovery of either species. Cultures should be incubated for up to 4 weeks in a 5% CO_2-enriched, moist environment; *Bartonella* colonies usually are not identifiable until 8 days after inoculation.[5] Co-cultivation of biopsied tissue with endothelial cell monolayers is usually a more sensitive technique for isolating *Bartonella* species.[4]

Isolation from blood is optimally achieved using EDTA blood tubes or (EDTA-ethylenediamine-tetraacetic acid) the lysis-centrifugation system (Wampole, Cranbury, NJ, USA).[12] This is a primary isolation system that involves immediate centrifugation of the tube filled with 10 ml of blood, followed by plating the pellet onto fresh agar. Many blood culture systems do not detect *Bartonella*; detection of *Bartonella* in these culture systems requires blind passage of blood culture bottle contents onto agar, centrifuging onto endothelial shell vials,[28] or staining with acridine orange.[29]

Serology

A serologic test was developed by the Centers for Disease Control and Prevention (CDC) using co-cultivation of *Bartonella* species with Vero cells. This indirect immunofluorescence antibody (IFA) test has good sensitivity and specificity for detecting *Bartonella* infection in immunocompetent individuals with cat scratch disease, although it does not distinguish between *B. henselae* and *B. quintana* infection.[30] This test also appears to be useful for detecting *Bartonella* infection in immunocompromised patients with bacillary angiomatosis.[31]

In Vitro Susceptibility Testing

As for many fastidious bacteria, antibiotic susceptibility testing for *Bartonella* species is not standardized. In addition, there is little correlation between the in vitro susceptibilities of *Bartonella* isolates and the in vivo treatment experience for a number of antibiotics. This is especially true for cell wall active antibiotics such as penicillin and first-generation cephalosporins. For the Fuller-type strain of

B. quintana, early studies found excellent in vitro susceptibility for penicillin, with a 50% minimum inhibitory concentration (MIC_{50}) of 0.024 and a 90% MIC (MIC_{90}) of 0.035 μg/ml[32]; yet there are many reports of treatment failures and even dramatic progression of bacillary angiomatosis disease in patients receiving penicillin.[7,33] The role for routine antimicrobial susceptibility testing of *Bartonella* isolates is therefore not clear and is currently not of practical value.

In one study, 28 antibiotics were tested with 14 *Bartonella* isolates using an agar dilution method.[34] As previously demonstrated in vitro, the *Bartonella* strains usually were susceptible to penicillins (MIC_{90} ranging from 0.015 to 0.060 μg/ml). In addition to nine strains of *B. quintana,* the other species of *Bartonella* tested (one strain of *B. vinsonii,* one strain of *B. elizabethae,* three strains of *B. henselae*) were susceptible to erythromycin, doxycycline, and rifampin. These isolates also were susceptible to azithromycin and clarithromycin. Indeed, all *Bartonella* isolates tested to date have shown in vitro susceptibility to erythromycin and tetracycline, with the exception of one isolate reported by Colson et al. that had an MIC higher than 256 μg/ml to erythromycin and clarithromycin but with retesting was susceptible with an MIC of 0.06 μg/ml.[35] Treatment with ciprofloxacin and rifampin was continued in this patient; a subsequent relapse isolate also was susceptible to both erythromycin and clarithromycin with an MIC of 0.06 μg/ml. The significance of this transiently elevated MIC to macrolides is unclear.

Susceptibility of 10 *B. henselae* isolates to erythromycin, azithromycin, rifampin, doxycycline, ciprofloxacin, and vancomycin were evaluated using the E-test in another study.[36] Good correlation was found between the agar dilution method and E-test susceptibilities for erythromycin, azi-thromycin, doxycycline, and rifampin. Because the E-test is much easier to perform than the agar dilution method, susceptibility testing using the E-test may be the most practical method for determining susceptibilities for *Bartonella* isolates.

▲ THERAPY

Approach to Therapy: In Vivo Treatment Experience

Treatment of *Bartonella* infections in HIV-infected patients has not been studied systematically or in any trials, but dozens of anecdotal cases have been reported in the literature. The initially described patient with bacillary angiomatosis was treated successfully with erythromycin,[10] and the first prospectively identified case at San Francisco General Hospital, a patient with *B. quintana* osteomyelitis, was cured following treatment with 4 months of erythromycin therapy.[33] We have a cumulative experience of treating more than 50 patients with biopsy-proved bacillary angiomatosis, bacillary peliosis hepatis, and *Bartonella* bacteremia. Our experience and that of others treating bacillary angiomatosis patients, as reported in the literature, demonstrate that erythromycin and doxycycline have excellent in vivo activity for treatment of bacillary angiomatosis. Additionally, tetracycline, rifampin, and newer macrolides (clarithromycin and azithromycin) seem to have in vivo efficacy against *Bartonella* infections in HIV-infected patients (summarized by Koehler and Tappero[7] and Maurin and Raoult[37]).

Anecdotal reports describe a treatment response of *Bartonella* infection to ciprofloxacin, but we have observed progression of bacillary angiomatosis during treatment with ciprofloxacin.[38] We also have isolated *Bartonella* species from patients being treated with gentamicin, trimethoprim-sulfamethoxazole, and first-generation cephalosporins; hence we do not recommend treatment with these antibiotics.[5]

Several other studies have provided evidence that macrolides and tetracyclines may be efficacious in the treatment of *Bartonella* infection. A placebo-controlled, prospective study of azithromycin treatment of immunocompetent patients with cat scratch disease was reported by Bass et al.[39] At 30 days after initiation of treatment, there was an 80% decrease in sonographically documented lymph node volume in the azithromycin-treated group compared with controls. Studies of cats experimentally infected with *B. henselae* also have substantiated the favorable clinical treatment experience with a macrolide or a tetracycline, as well as the lack of response of *Bartonella* infections to ciprofloxacin therapy.[40] In one study 25 cats were infected with *B. henselae* and then treated with one of four antibiotics: tetracycline, amoxicillin, erythromycin, or enrofloxacin (a fluoroquinolone). Blood specimens were obtained for culture during antibiotic treatment, and the numbers of *B. henselae* bacilli in the blood were quantitated; only tetracycline or erythromycin administration decreased the number of bacteria at any time during the period after infection, although there was no significant difference among the antibiotics with regard to apparent resolution of bacteremia in these cats.

Specific Drugs with Dose and Administration

The drug of choice for treatment of HIV-infected patients with bacillary angiomatosis, bacillary peliosis, or *Bartonella* bacteremia is erythromycin or doxycycline (Fig. 35–1). Erythromycin and doxycycline appear to have equivalent activity when treating bacillary angiomatosis; additionally, there does not appear to be a difference in treatment response whether bacillary angiomatosis is caused by *B. henselae* or *B. quintana*. Dosing for erythromycin should be 500 mg q6h PO or IV and for doxycycline 100 mg q12h PO or IV. Because of our more extensive experience with erythromycin than with other antibiotics, we usually initiate therapy for bacillary angiomatosis with erythromycin. However, doxycycline therapy is preferred over erythromycin in several settings: when *Bartonella* infection involves the central nervous system, when severe gastrointestinal symptoms are present, or when the twice-daily dosing for doxycycline is likely to increase compliance.

Intravenous therapy is recommended for patients with severe disease, especially in those with gastrointestinal involvement, nausea, and vomiting and in whom drug absorption may be impaired. Intravenous therapy also should be administered to patients with osteomyelitis and endocarditis. In extremely ill patients, treatment with combination therapy may be warranted; Rifampin has demonstrated in vivo activity and can be added to doxycycline or erythromycin. Treat-

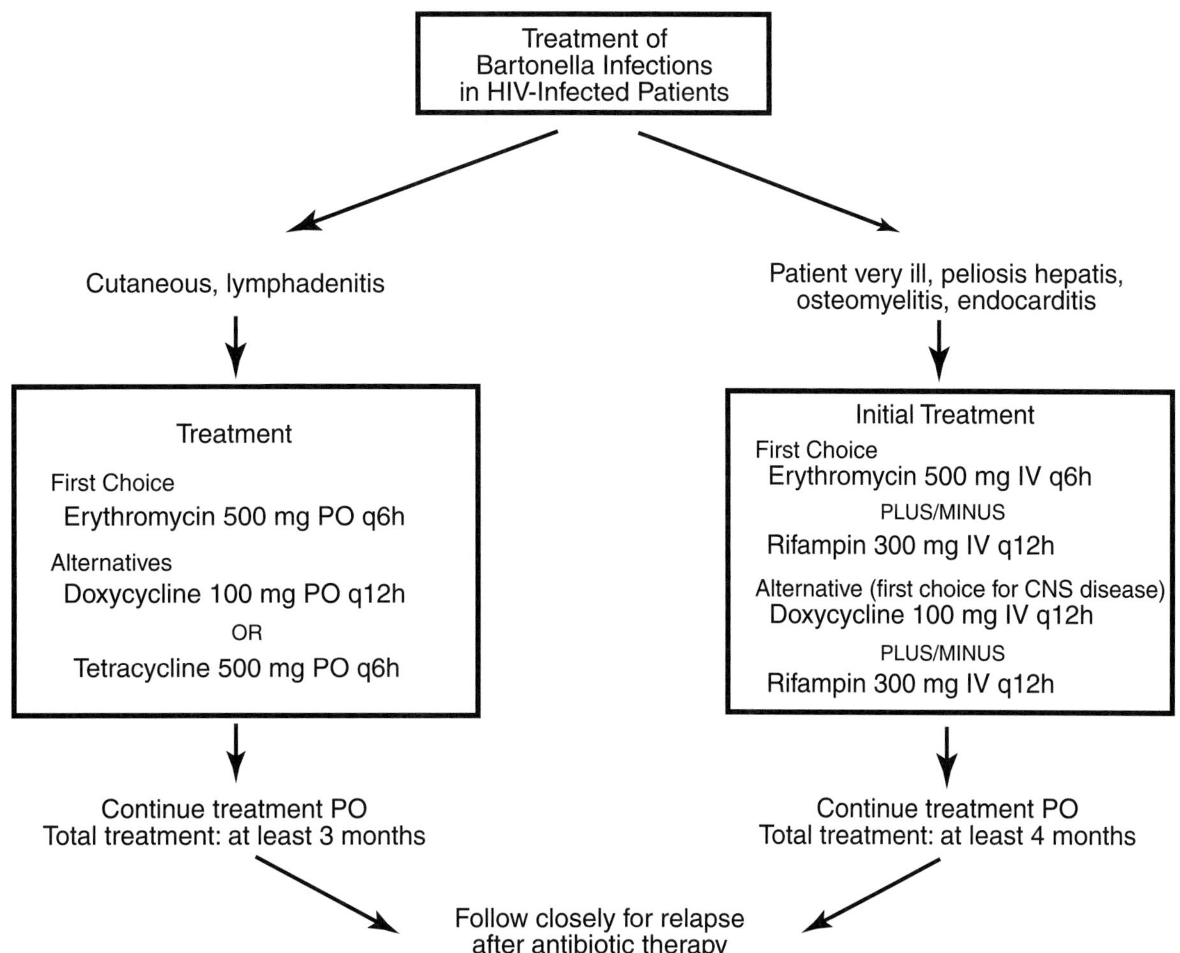

Figure 35–1. Algorithm for treatment of *Bartonella* infections in HIV-infected individuals. Note that therapy or prophylaxis regimens for *Mycobacterium avium* complex that include a macrolide may treat or prevent *Bartonella* infections. (From Koehler JE. Bartonella-associated infections in HIV-infected patients. AIDS Clin Care 7:97, 1995. Copyright 1995, Massachusetts Medical Society, with permission.)

ment with rifampin alone should be avoided because of the high rate at which many bacteria develop spontaneous rifampin resistance. For patients whose infection fails to respond after 10 days of treatment, therapy should be changed to the other first-line drug and rifampin added. It may also be beneficial to administer antibiotics intravenously to patients not responding after 10 days of oral therapy.

Toxicities/Complications and Their Management

Immunocompromised patients may develop a Jarisch-Herxheimer-like reaction after the first several doses of antibiotics for *Bartonella* infection.[4] Physicians should anticipate this possibility because it may be mistaken for an adverse drug reaction, resulting in an unnecessary change of antibiotic therapy. Patients should be informed, and those with severe respiratory or cardiovascular compromise should be monitored carefully after institution of antibiotic therapy.

Adverse reactions most frequently reported during erythromycin treatment include gastrointestinal symptoms (abdominal cramps, nausea, vomiting, diarrhea) with the oral or the intravenous route and thrombophlebitis with the intravenous route. Serious interactions can occur with concomitantly administered erythromycin and cisapride, cyclosporin, tacrolimus, theophylline (theophylline toxicity), warfarin (increased anticoagulation), digoxin (digoxin toxicity), and astemizole or terfenadine (torsades de pointes).[41]

Doxycycline-associated erosive esophagitis also has been well described and most frequently occurs when a dose is taken with only a small amount of liquid just before retiring.[42] Patients should take the evening doxycycline dose several hours before bedtime with a large amount of liquid. Doxycycline can cause gastrointestinal symptoms, dental discoloration in children, and photosensitivity reactions. Interactions of tetracyclines with oral anticoagulants may increase anticoagulation and if given with oral contraceptive hormones may result in decreased efficacy resulting in pregnancy.[43]

Recommendations for Optimal Approach to Therapy

Most patients with apparently focal bacillary angiomatosis actually have systemic disease. We found that half of the patients with bacillary angiomatosis were bacteremic with a *Bartonella* species.[5] Because of this and the propensity for relapse of *Bartonella* infections treated for a short duration, we recommend that all HIV-infected patients with *Bartonella* infection receive at least 3 to 4 months of antibiotic treatment (3 months for uncomplicated cutaneous bacillary angiomatosis and 4 months for osteomyelitis, bacillary peliosis, or CNS involvement) (Fig. 35–1). Before beginning therapy, patients with cutaneous bacillary angiomatosis should be carefully evaluated for the presence of disease at another site that might require a longer duration of therapy (e.g., endocarditis or osteomyelitis). Careful cardiac examination should be performed for any signs of endocarditis, and any patient with bacillary angiomatosis and a cardiac murmur should undergo echocardiography. If bony or deep soft tissue tenderness is identified on physical examination the patient should undergo a bone scan.

Although the largest number of HIV-infected patients have been successfully treated with erythromycin or doxycycline, other antibiotics should be considered in patients unable to tolerate either of these drugs. Experience with alternative antibiotics is limited, but they include tetracycline (which was efficacious in an HIV-infected patient with bacillary angiomatosis[4]) and the newer macrolides. Azithromycin may be a useful alternative in patients unable to comply with two- or four-times-daily dosing with doxycycline or erythromycin. An azithromycin dose of 500 mg q24h PO was used for 28 to 90 days to treat 5 of the 10 immunocompetent patients with *B. quintana* bacteremia reported by Spach et al.[44] Another report described treatment of an immunocompromised patient with bacillary angiomatosis using azithromycin 1 g q24h PO.[45] There are a few reports of treating immunocompetent patients with clarithromycin (250 mg q12h PO),[46,47] and either of these macrolides seems to be a reasonable alternative if erythromycin cannot be used.

Resolution of infection can be documented by abdominal computed tomography (CT) scanning (peliosis hepatis) or technetium 99m bone scans (osteomyelitis). Most patients describe alleviation of fever, anorexia, and pain within 1 to 2 weeks. Cutaneous lesions usually resolve after 1 to 2 months of antibiotic treatment, although hyperpigmentation may persist at the site of bacillary angiomatosis lesions indefinitely. Hepatic lesions may require 2 to 3 months to resolve.

▲ PREVENTION

Environmental and Behavioral Factors

The principal reservoir and vectors for *B. henselae* have been identified, and some recommendations can be made to decrease the potential for human infection with this *Bartonella* species. The domestic cat is the major reservoir[18] and the most common vector of *B. henselae* for humans via scratches and bites.[48,49] The arthropod vector for *B. henselae*, the cat flea, readily transmits this species among cats.[20] Although transmission of *B. henselae* to humans has never been demonstrated, control of flea infestation decreases the potential for human exposure to *B. henselae* by reducing contamination of cat claws due to scratching and by decreasing feline infection. HIV-infected patients need not give up their pet cats but should wash cat wounds immediately with soap and water, avoid rough play with cats, and make their medical caregiver aware that they have a pet cat. If an immunocompromised individual wishes to acquire a pet cat, it preferably should be a mature cat (more than 1 year old); older cats are less likely to be bacteremic and less likely to scratch.[50] Testing cats for *B. henselae* infection or treating of bacteremic cats is not recommended.[50] It is not evident whether the bacterium can be eradicated from the cat, and giving the cat antibiotics incurs additional risk of scratches and bites for the owner.

Bartonella quintana is transmitted by the body louse from human to human, and patients of low socioeconomic status are at highest risk for lice infestation.[5,44] The only current recommendation for preventing bacillary angiomatosis due to *B. quintana* is to avoid louse infestation, and caregivers should consider *Bartonella* infection in the differential diagnosis of homeless HIV-infected individuals with fever or vascular cutaneous lesions.

Approach to Prevention-Specific Drugs

Primary prophylactic regimens for *Bartonella* infections have not been studied systematically, and there is no current recommendation for primary prophylaxis. However, our case-control study of 49 patients with bacillary angiomatosis found that the macrolide class of antibiotics (e.g., erythromycin, clarithromycin) was the only class that was protective.[5] Trimethoprim-sulfamethoxazole, ciprofloxacin, dapsone, penicillin, and cephalosporin antibiotic classes were not protective against developing *Bartonella* infection. It is likely that regimens that include a macrolide or rifabutin for prophylaxis or treatment of *Mycobacterium avium* complex infection simultaneously provide prophylaxis or treatment of *Bartonella* infection.

After cessation of treatment for documented *Bartonella* infection, patients should be monitored carefully for relapse. *Bartonella* infection may recur at the same site or at a new site months later.[4] For patients who develop relapse of *Bartonella* infection, lifelong secondary prophylaxis with a macrolide or doxycycline should be instituted after retreatment.[51]

Acknowledgments: Dr. Koehler was supported by funds from the NIH R01 AI43703 and the California University-wide AIDS Research Program.

REFERENCES

1. Koehler JE. Bartonella: an emerging human pathogen. In: Scheld WM, Armstrong D, Hughes JM (eds) Emerging Infections I. Washington, DC, American Society for Microbiology Press, 1998, p 147.
2. Cunningham ET Jr, Koehler JE. Ocular bartonellosis. Am J Ophthalmol 130:340, 2000.
3. Mohle-Boetani JC, Koehler JE, Berger TG, et al. Bacillary angiomatosis and bacillary peliosis in patients infected with human immunodeficiency virus: clinical characteristics in a case-control study. Clin Infect Dis 22:794, 1996.
4. Koehler JE, Quinn FD, Berger TG, et al. Isolation of *Rochalimaea* species from cutaneous and osseous lesions of bacillary angiomatosis. N Engl J Med 327:1625, 1992.

5. Koehler JE, Sanchez MA, Garrido CS, et al. Molecular epidemiology of *Bartonella* infections in patients with bacillary angiomatosis-peliosis. N Engl J Med 337:1876, 1997.
6. Berger TG, Tappero JW. Kaymen A, LeBoit PE. Bacillary (epithelioid) angiomatosis and concurrent Kaposi's sarcoma in acquired immunodeficiency syndrome. Arch Dermatol 125:1543, 1989.
7. Koehler JE, Tappero JW. Bacillary angiomatosis and bacillary peliosis in patients infected with human immunodeficiency virus. Clin Infect Dis 17:612, 1993.
8. Perkocha LA, Geaghan SM, Yen TSB, et al. Clinical and pathological features of bacillary peliosis hepatis in association with human immunodeficiency virus infection. N Engl J Med 323:1581, 1990.
9. Cockerell CJ, Whitlow MA, Webster GF, Friedman-Kien AE. Epithelioid angiomatosis: a distinct vascular disorder in patients with the acquired immunodeficiency syndrome or AIDS-related complex. Lancet 2:654, 1987.
10. Stoler MH, Bonfiglio TA, Steigbigel RT, Pereira M. An atypical subcutaneous infection associated with acquired immune deficiency syndrome. Am J Clin Pathol 80:714, 1983.
11. Relman DA, Loutit JS, Schmidt TM, et al. The agent of bacillary angiomatosis: an approach to the identification of uncultured pathogens. N Engl J Med 323:1573, 1990.
12. Slater LN, Welch DF, Hensel D, Coody DW. A newly recognized fastidious gram-negative pathogen as a cause of fever and bacteremia. N Engl J Med 323:1587, 1990.
13. Regnery RL, Anderson BE, Clarridge JE, et al. Characterization of a novel *Rochalimaea* species, *R. henselae* sp. nov., isolated from blood of a febrile, human immunodeficiency virus-positive patient. J Clin Microbiol 30:265, 1992.
14. Welch DF, Pickett DA, Slater LN, et al. *Rochalimaea henselae* sp. nov., a cause of septicemia, bacillary angiomatosis, and parenchymal bacillary peliosis. J Clin Microbiol 30:275, 1992.
15. Brenner DJ, O'Connor SP, Winkler HH, Steigerwalt AG. Proposals to unify the genera *Bartonella* and *Rochalimaea*, with descriptions of *Bartonella quintana* comb. nov., *Bartonella vinsonii* comb. nov., *Bartonella henselae* comb. nov., and *Bartonella elizabethae* comb. nov., and to remove the family *Bartonellaceae* from the order *Rickettsiales*. Int J Syst Bacteriol 43:777, 1993.
16. Birtles RJ, Harrison TG, Saunders NA, Molyneux DH. Proposals to unify the genera *Grahamella* and *Bartonella*, with descriptions of *Bartonella talpae* comb. nov., *Bartonella peromysci* comb. nov., and three new species, *Bartonella grahamii* sp. nov., *Bartonella taylorii* sp. nov., and *Bartonella doshiae* sp. nov. Int J Syst Bacteriol 45:1, 1995.
17. Tappero JW, Mohle-Boetani J, Koehler JE, et al. The epidemiology of bacillary angiomatosis and bacillary peliosis. JAMA 269:770, 1993.
18. Koehler JE, Glaser CA, Tappero JW. *Rochalimaea henselae* infection: a new zoonosis with the domestic cat as reservoir. JAMA 271:531, 1994.
19. Jameson P, Greene C, Regnery R, et al. Prevalence of *Bartonella henselae* antibodies in pet cats throughout regions of North America. J Infect Dis 172:1145, 1995.
20. Chomel BB, Kasten RW, Floyd-Hawkins K, et al. Experimental transmission of *Bartonella henselae* by the cat flea. J Clin Microbiol 34:1952, 1996.
21. Strong RP. Trench Fever: Report of Commission, Medical Research Committee, American Red Cross. Oxford, Oxford University Press, 1918.
22. Von Krampitz HE. Weitere Untersuchungen an Grahamella Brumpt 1911. Tropenmed Parasitol 13:34, 1962.
23. Weinman D, Kreier JP. *Bartonella* and *Grahamella*. In: Kreier JP (ed) *Parasitic Protozoa,* vol 4. San Diego, Academic Press, 1977, p 197.
24. Lawson PA, Collins MD. Description of *Bartonella clarridgeiae* sp. nov. isolated from the cat of a patient with *Bartonella henselae* septicemia. Med Microbiol Lett 5:64, 1996.
25. Myers WF, Osterman JV, Wisseman CL Jr. Nutritional studies of *Rickettsia quintana*: nature of the hematin requirement. J Bacteriol 109:89, 1972.
26. LeBoit PE, Berger TG, Egbert BM, et al. Bacillary angiomatosis: the histopathology and differential diagnosis of a pseudoneoplastic infection in patients with human immunodeficiency virus disease. Am J Surg Pathol 13:909, 1989.
27. Reed JA, Brigati DJ, Flynn SD, et al. Immunocytochemical identification of *Rochalimaea henselae* in bacillary (epithelioid) angiomatosis, parenchymal bacillary peliosis, and persistent fever with bacteremia. Am J Surg Pathol 16:650, 1992.
28. La Scola B, Raoult D. Culture of *Bartonella quintana* and *Bartonella henselae* from human samples: a 5-year experience (1993–1998). J Clin Microbiol 37:1899, 1999.
29. Dougherty MJ, Spach DH, Larson AM, et al. Evaluation of an extended blood culture protocol to isolate fastidious organisms from patients with AIDS. J Clin Microbiol 34:2444, 1996.
30. Dalton MJ, Robinson LE, Cooper J, et al. Use of *Bartonella antigens* for serologic diagnosis of cat-scratch disease at a national referral center. Arch Intern Med 155:1670, 1995.
31. Tappero J, Regnery R, Koehler J. Detection of serologic response to Rochalimaea henselae in patients with bacillary angiomatosis (BA) by immunofluorescent antibody (IFA) testing. Presented at the 32nd Interscience Conference on Antimicrobial Agents and Chemotherapy, American Society for Microbiology, 1992.
32. Myers WF, Grossman DM, Wisseman CLJ. Antibiotic susceptibility patterns in *Rochalimaea quintana*, the agent of trench fever. Antimicrob Agents Chemother 25:690, 1984.
33. Koehler JE, LeBoit PE, Egbert BM, Berger TG. Cutaneous vascular lesions and disseminated cat-scratch disease in patients with the acquired immunodeficiency syndrome (AIDS) and AIDS-related complex. Ann Intern Med 109:449, 1988.
34. Maurin M, Gasquet S, Ducco C, Raoult D. MICs of 28 antibiotic compounds for 14 *Bartonella* (formerly *Rochalimaea*) isolates. Antimicrob Agents Chemother 39:2387, 1995.
35. Colson P, Lebrun L, Drancourt M, et al. Multiple recurrent bacillary angiomatosis due to *Bartonella quintana* in an HIV-infected patient [letter]. Eur J Clin Microbiol Infect Dis 15:178, 1996.
36. Wolfson C, Branley J, Gottlieb T. The E test for antimicrobial susceptibility testing of *Bartonella henselae*. J Antimicrob Chemother 38:963, 1996.
37. Maurin M, Raoult D. Antimicrobial susceptibility of *Rochalimaea quintana, Rochalimaea vinsonii*, and the newly recognized *Rochalimaea henselae*. J Antimicrob Chemother 32:587, 1993.
38. Tappero JW, Koehler JE. Cat scratch disease and bacillary angiomatosis [letter]. JAMA 266:1938, 1991.
39. Bass JW, Freitas BC, Freitas AD, et al. Prospective randomized double blind placebo-controlled evaluation of azithromycin for treatment of cat-scratch disease. Pediatr Infect Dis J 17:447, 1998.
40. Regnery RL, Rooney JA, Johnson AM, et al. Experimentally induced *Bartonella henselae* infections followed by challenge exposure and antimicrobial therapy in cats. Am J Vet Res 57:1714, 1996.
41. Steigbigel NH. Macrolides and clindamycin. In: Mandell GL, Bennett JE, Dolin R (eds) Principles and Practice of Infectious Diseases. New York, Churchill Livingstone, 2000, p 366.
42. Kikendall JW, Friedman AC, Oyewole MA, et al. Pill-induced esophageal injury: case reports and review of the medical literature. Dig Dis Sci 28:174, 1983.
43. Standiford HC. Tetracyclines and chloramphenicol. In: Mandell GL, Bennett JE, Dolin R (eds) Principles and Practice of Infectious Diseases. New York, Churchill Livingstone, 2000, p 336.
44. Spach DH, Kanter AS, Dougherty MJ, et al. *Bartonella* (*Rochalimaea*) *quintana* bacteremia in inner-city patients with chronic alcoholism. N Engl J Med 332:424, 1995.
45. Guerra LG, Neira CJ, Boman D, et al. Rapid response of AIDS-related bacillary angiomatosis to azithromycin. Clin Infect Dis 17:264, 1993.
46. Bakker RC, van Heukelem H, van de Sandt MM, Bergmans AM. [Visceral granulomas and pericardial effusion caused by a *Bartonella henselae* infection.] Ned Tijdschr Geneeskd 141:388, 1997.
47. Heizmann WR, Schalasta G, Moling O, Pegoretti S. [Cat scratch disease: Bartonella henselae antibodies and DNA detection in regional lymphadenopathy.] Dtsch Med Wochenschr 121:622, 1996.
48. Carithers HA. Cat-scratch disease: an overview based on a study of 1,200 patients. Am J Dis Child 139:1124, 1985.
49. Margileth AM. Cat scratch disease: a therapeutic dilemma. Vet Clin North Am 17:91, 1987.
50. Regnery RL, Childs JE, Koehler JE. Infections associated with *Bartonella* species in persons infected with human immunodeficiency virus. Clin Infect Dis 21 (suppl 1):S94, 1995.
51. Centers for Disease Control and Prevention. 1999 USPHS/IDSA guideline for the prevention of opportunistic infections in persons infected with human immunodeficiency virus. MMWR Morbid Mortal Wkly Rep 48 (RR-10):1, 1999.

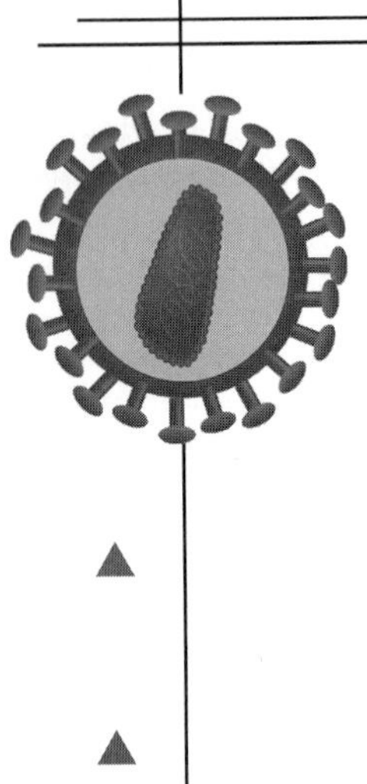

CHAPTER 36

Cryptococcosis

Judith A. Aberg, MD
William G. Powderly, MD

Disseminated cryptococcosis has been the most common life-threatening fungal infection in patients with acquired immunodeficiency syndrome (AIDS), affecting up to 8% of patients with advanced human immunodeficiency virus (HIV) infection.[1–3] The most common manifestation is meningoencephalitis, although disseminated disease is well described, and localized infection of many organs can occur. Carefully conducted clinical trials have helped define effective therapy for this infection, although many issues in management remain unresolved. This chapter reviews the microbiology, pathogenesis, epidemiology, clinical syndromes, and treatment of cryptococcosis in patients with AIDS.

▲ MICROBIOLOGY

There are more than 20 known species of *Cryptococcus,*[4] but *Cryptococcus neoformans* is essentially the only human pathogen, although there have been isolated case reports of infection with *Cryptococcus albidus* and *Cryptococcus laurenti. C. neoformans* is an encapsulated, round to oval yeast that reproduces by narrow-based budding. It has a surrounding polysaccharide capsule ranging from 1 μm to more than 30 μm when cultivated in the laboratory.[5] In its natural environment, it is smaller and poorly encapsulated. Mycelia are produced bearing basidiospores ranging from 1 to 8 μm in its perfect state *(Filobasidiella neoformans). F. neoformans* has never been isolated from patients or in nature.[6] During the exponential growth phase of *Cryptococcus,* the generation or doubling time ranges from 2.5 to 6.0 hours.

There are two pathogenic varieties, *C. neoformans* var. *neoformans* and *C. neoformans* var. *gattii,* which can be distinguished on the basis of capsular serotypes.[5,7] These two varieties differ in geographic distribution; but their growth requirements for temperature, phenol oxidase production, and capsule formation are similar. They can also be distinguished by growth characteristics on canavanine-glycine-bromthymol blue agar. The serotypes of *C. neoformans* are designated A, B, C, and D based on antigenic determinants on the polysaccharide capsule.[8] Serotypes A and D (*C. neoformans* var. *neoformans*) are the most common cause of infection and are most often seen in immunocompromised hosts. Serotypes B and C (*C. neoformans* var. *gattii*) are endemic in Australia and southern California, are usually isolated from normal hosts, and have a predilection for invading the central nervous system (CNS).[9,10] Although the incidence of cryptococcosis in AIDS patients appears to vary geographically, even in areas where var. *gattii* is endemic, most of the isolates from patients with AIDS are var. *neoformans.*[11,12] The genotypic features of *C. neoformans* were actively pursued during the 1990s, now with more than 20 genes cloned and sequenced.[13–27] Electrophoretic karyotyping has identified 12 genes in *C. neoformans* var. *neoformans* compared to 13 genes in *C. neoformans* var. *gattii.*[14]

▲ PATHOGENESIS AND HOST DEFENSE MECHANISMS

It is postulated that initial infection occurs via inhalation of the basidiospores or unencapsulated forms, leading to subsequent colonization of the airways and subsequent respiratory infection.[8,28] *C. neoformans* has been isolated from the nasopharynx of approximately 50% of AIDS patients with cryptococcosis, whereas *C. neoformans* has not been isolated from AIDS patients without cryptococcosis.[29] The initial immune response correlates best with polymorphonuclear leukocyte activity more than macrophage activity. However, the role of pulmonary macrophages is paramount in the host's control of the yeast inoculum,[30] and complement-mediated phagocytosis appears to be the primary initial defense against cryptococcal invasion.[5] Other host–yeast interactions, such as the role of CD4+ and CD8+ T cells, as well as the role of cytokines, also appear to be important.[30–33] It is clear that the absence of an intact cell-mediated response results in ineffective ingestion and killing of the organism, leading to dissemination and increased cryptococcal burden. In murine models both CD4+ and CD8+ T cells are required to inhibit cryptococcosis. Natural killer (NK) cells also appear to have a limited role.[30,34] Specifically, interleukin-2 (IL-2)-activated T and NK cells can inhibit *C. neoformans*[35] The role of humoral immunity in the control of cryptococcal infections is controversial. In vitro studies of antibodies to the soluble capsular polysaccharide of *C. neoformans* have revealed enhanced phagocytosis, increased fungicidal activity of leukocytes, and increased fungistatic activity of NK cells.[36–39] Animal models of both polyclonal and monoclonal antibody immunization have had varying results.[40–43]

Factors associated with the virulence of *C. neoformans* include its polysaccharide capsule, production of melanin, the mating type, and growth at 37°C (thermotolerance).[44–46] The polysaccharide capsule, composed mainly of glucuronoxylomannan, was the first *C. neoformans* virulence factor associated with disease.[47] There is also some evidence of an interaction between *C. neoformans* and HIV-1 in vitro. Soluble *C. neoformans* capsular polysaccharide is able to enhance HIV infection in cultured cells, subsequent production of HIV-1, and in vitro production of syncytia.[48] Additionally, a study of dual immunocytochemical staining for HIV-1 and cryptococcal antigen in brain tissue of AIDS patients showing anatomic co-localization of both pathogens suggests a possible synergistic effect of virus and yeast in vivo.[49]

Cryptococcus neoformans is distinguished from other yeasts by its ability to assimilate urea and its possession of membrane-bound phenol oxidase enzymes, which are able to convert phenolic compounds into melanin. *Cryptococcus neoformans* strains that produce melanin are more virulent in mouse models than strains that do not produce melanin.[38,39] In addition, murine cells with melanin appear more resistant to phagocytosis.[45] It is postulated that the propensity of *C. neoformans* to invade the CNS may be due to its ability to synthesize melanin from catecholamines, which are present in large concentrations there.[49]

▲ EPIDEMIOLOGY

In the developed world prior to the use of more effective antiretroviral therapy, approximately 5% to 10% of patients with AIDS developed cryptococcal meningitis. In 1991 the annual prevalence of cryptococcosis among HIV-infected patients in New York was estimated to be 6.1% to 8.5%.[50] There is considerable geographic variation in the prevalence of cryptococcal infection. In the United States it is more common in residents east of the Mississippi River.[51] The incidence of cryptococcosis among AIDS patients is higher in Africa and Southeast Asia than the United States, whereas it appears less often in Europe.[9] The male/female ratio among AIDS patients is essentially 1:1. Cryptococcosis in children with AIDS is less common, with a prevalence rate of approximately 1.4%.[52] The clinical and laboratory characteristics of cryptococcosis in children is comparable to those seen in adults.

More than three-fourths of the cases associated with AIDS develop when the CD4 count falls below 50 cells/μl.[51] Cryptococcosis is the initial AIDS-defining illness in 50% to 60% of patients and thus tends to be seen more commonly in patients in whom HIV infection has not yet been diagnosed. Risk factors that have been suggested for the development of cryptococcosis include black race, injection drug use, cigarette smoking, and several environmental exposures (presumed areas where pigeon droppings accumulate). No differences in demographic variables, HIV risk factors, or stage of AIDS was found in a recent case-controlled study. It is of note that the investigators were unable to detect an increased risk of the development of cryptococcal meningitis in patients who had received short and episodic courses of steroids.[53]

The annual incidence of invasive *C. neoformans* in the United States has declined in HIV-infected patients during the years since 1990. Between 1987 and 1992, cryptococcosis decreased from sixth to ninth place in rank order for infections associated with death in HIV-infected persons.[3] This epidemiologic trend preceded the use of highly active antiretroviral therapy and has been temporally associated with the increased use of fluconazole since its licensure in 1990.[54] It is of note that in a large prospective, population-based surveillance study patients who had received fluconazole were significantly less likely to develop cryptococcosis, and decreases in the incidence of cryptococcosis from 1992 to 1994 were attributed to the increased use of azoles.[55]

A 56.5% decrease in the incidence of cryptococcal meningitis was reported between 1996 and 1997 at San Francisco General Hospital, correlating with a 30% increased use of potent antiretroviral therapy that included a protease inhibitor.[56] However, the decrease in incidence of crytococcosis was even more dramatic when one compared the 1995 incidence with 1996 prior to the introduction of protease inhibitors. This suggests that patients may have been receiving benefit from the use of nucleosides alone as well as the use of azoles. Furthermore, the incidence of cryptococcal meningitis had increased 30% between 1997 and 1998 and has remained constant, occurring primarily in individuals not taking potent antiretroviral therapy.[57]

▲ CLINICAL FEATURES AND DIAGNOSIS

Central Nervous System Disease

The most common manifestation of cryptococcosis is meningoencephalitis. The time span between the appearance of symptoms and diagnosis ranges from days to months.[58] The clinical presentation may be nonspecific (Fig.

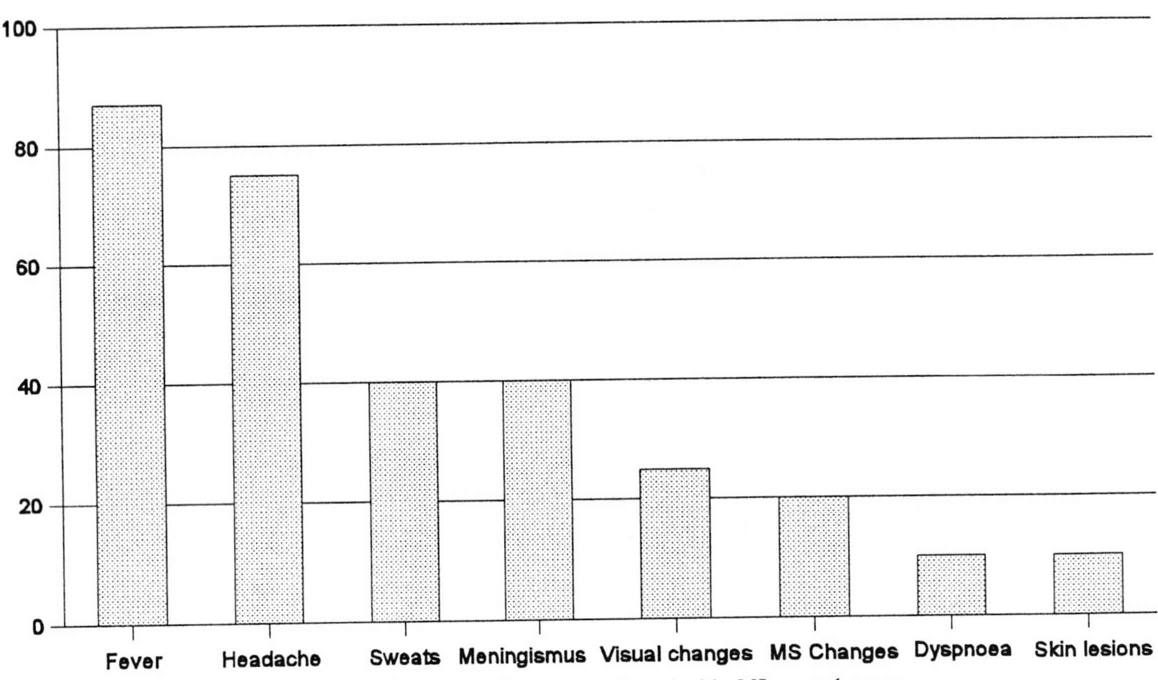

Figure 36–1. Symptoms of cryptococcal meningitis. MS, mental status.

36–1), although infection typically presents as a subacute process.[59] Symptoms may range from headache, nausea, irritability, and decline in cognitive function to frank obtundation. Physical findings may include fever and abnormal neurologic examination, with cranial nerve palsies, hyperreflexia, and papilledema. Complications of CNS infection include hydrocephalus, motor or sensory deficits, cerebellar dysfunction, seizures, and dementia. Prompt inclusion of *C. neoformans* in the differential diagnosis of acute and chronic meningitis for susceptible hosts should allow for prompt brain imaging study followed by lumbar puncture once a mass lesion has been ruled out. Although focal lesions caused by intracerebral granulomas (cryptococcomas) may be seen on computed tomography or magnetic resonance imaging, they are uncommon in patients with AIDS.[60] Acute cryptococcal meningitis in patients with AIDS is often complicated by cerebral edema. Assessment should include measuring the opening pressure by manometry in all patients. The opening pressure is usually higher than 25 cm H_2O in 60% of patients.[61] Abnormal findings in the composition of cerebrospinal fluid (CSF) include a lymphocytic pleocytosis, elevated protein, and low glucose.[59] However, as many as 20% of patients have no clear abnormality in the CSF profile despite positive cultures for *C. neoformans.* Therefore finding a normal CSF should not exclude the possibility of cryptococcal infection. Detection of CSF cryptococcal antigen by rapid diagnostic testing should prompt initiation of therapy.

Pulmonary Cryptococcosis

Although the lung is most likely the entry portal, isolated pulmonary cryptococcosis is diagnosed less frequently than meningitis in AIDS patients.[62,63] However, pulmonary involvement in the presence of disseminated disease is common. More than 10% of patients with disseminated disease may have acute respiratory failure.[64] It is unclear if disseminated disease always represents progression of pulmonary disease because many patients have no evidence of pulmonary involvement at the time of diagnosis of disseminated disease. Given the relatively nonspecific clinical signs and symptoms, variable radiographic signs, and increased frequency of other pulmonary opportunistic infections, it is likely that cryptococcal pneumonia is underdiagnosed and not recognized until dissemination. In a retrospective study aimed at determining the etiology of pulmonary symptoms in HIV-positive patients with cryptococcal meningitis, 14 of 18 patients (78%) reported respiratory symptoms within 4 months prior to the diagnosis of cryptococcal meningitis.[65] Other reviews suggest that 63% to 90% of HIV-infected patients with pulmonary cryptococcosis have concomitant extrapulmonary disease.[62,66] However, pulmonary disease may not always be cryptococcal in origin; approximately 15% of HIV-infected patients with proven cryptococcal disease have a second pulmonary pathogen, such as *Pneumocystis carinii, Mycobacterium tuberculosis,* or nontuberculous mycobacteria.[62,67]

In a retrospective chart review of 210 patients with cryptococcal disease,[64] independent variables predictive of acute respiratory failure included black race, lactacte dehydrogenase level of ≥ 500 IU/L, the presence of interstitial infiltrates, and the presence of cutaneous lesions. Mortality was 100% for the 19 patients in whom the respiratory failure could be attributed solely to cryptococcosis.

Patients with pulmonary cryptococcosis may present with cough, fever, malaise, shortness of breath, pleuritic pain, and an abnormal chest radiograph. Chest radiographs typically reveal focal or diffuse infiltrates similar to other opportunistic pathogens, particularly *Pneumocystis carinii* pneumonia (PCP). Other chest radiographic findings not as commonly seen include solitary subpleural nodules, mass-like infiltrates with consolidation, hilar and mediastinal adenopathy, and pleural effusions. Rarely, cavitation and empyema have been reported.[68]

Patients with apparently isolated cryptococcal pneumonia should be evaluated for cryptococcal meningitis with a lumbar puncture even in the absence of neurologic signs or symptoms. In addition, antifungal therapy should be initiated because early treatment of localized pulmonary cryptococcosis can be effective and can prevent dissemination.[69]

Other Organ Involvement

Cryptococcosis in HIV-positive patients is typically disseminated; and up to three-fourths of patients with meningitis have positive blood cultures. A small percentage of patients with cryptococcosis present initially with extrapulmonary, nonmeningeal disease, although many are subsequently found to have meningitis. Infections of the skin, joints, eye, adrenal glands, gastrointestinal tract, liver, pancreas, peritoneum, heart, prostate, and urinary tract have been described.[70–77] The prostate can serve as a reservoir of infection and is a potential source of reinfection after completion of therapy.[78] Cutaneous cryptococcosis is usually a sign of dissemination but may precede evidence of disease elsewhere by several weeks.[70,79] The lesions vary greatly and mimic many other dermatologic entities. The most typical have an appearance resembling molluscum contagiosum,[80] but cryptococcal skin disease may present as pustules, vesicles, plaques, abscesses, cellulitis, purpura, draining sinus, or subcutaneous swelling.[81]

Atypical Presentations

Unlike infections with *Mycobacterium avium* complex and cytomegalovirus, there have been few reported cases of unusual manifestations of cryptococcal disease associated with highly active antiretroviral therapy (HAART). One report[82] suggested that three patients had partial immune reconstitution unmasking latent cryptococcal therapy but it is unclear if these cases truly represented immune reconstitution. Two of the patients developed cryptococcal meningitis shortly after starting HAART; both patients had nadir CD4+ T-lymphocyte counts less than 50 cells/μl and CD4+ T-lymphocyte counts less than 150 cells/μl after "therapy" at the time they were diagnosed with cryptococcal meningitis. The CSF analyses were typical of those seen with cryptococcal meningitis. A third patient with a recent history of cryptococcal meningitis on itraconazole developed aseptic meningitis with leukocytosis 10 days after starting HAART. This patient's therapy was not altered, and the meningeal symptoms resolved spontaneously. There have also been two reports of cryptococcal lymphadenitis in patients receiving potent antiretroviral therapy.[83,84]

Diagnostic Evaluation

The diagnosis is confirmed by isolating *Cryptococcus* from a sterile body site or by histopathology; the diagnosis can also be inferred by detecting cryptococcal capsular antigen in serum or CSF. The India ink stain, which outlines the polysaccharide capsule, is positive on direct examination of the CSF in approximately 80% of patients. Encapsulated yeasts seen after alcian blue, mucicarmine, or Gomori methenamine silver staining are diagnostic of *Cryptococcus*. Other stains, such as Fontana-Masson and periodic acid-Schiff, reveal yeast cells but are not specific for *Cryptococcus*.

Cryptococcal antigen in the CSF is produced locally in the subarachnoid space by the invading yeast and does not represent active or passive diffusion from the serum into the CNS. Soluble circulating serum cryptococcal antigen (sCRAG) has been found only in patients with substantial infection. Several commercial latex agglutination tests (LAT) kits and one enzyme-linked immunoassay (EIA) test for detection of cryptococcal antigen in serum and CSF are widely available. The detection of CRAG in serum and CSF by latex agglutination is rapid and has a sensitivity and specificity of more than 95%.[85,86] Comparative performance of four LATs and one EIA commercially available test revealed high concordance of all tests for CSF specimens, with sensitivities of 93% to 100% and specificities of 93% to 98%.[86] Pronase-containing latex tests reduce the number of false-positive sCRAGs.[86] False-positives can also occur secondary to infection with *Trichosporon beigelii,* which cross-reacts with the antigen.[87] In addition, false-positives have occurred secondary to residual disinfectant on laboratory test slides.[88] False-negatives may occur with low cryptococcal antigen concentrations. Although serum cryptococcal antigens are positive in 95% to 99% of cryptococcal meningitis cases, a positive result does not indicate that CNS invasion is present. Conversely, a negative sCRAG suggests that the patient is unlikely to have CNS disease; the test may be useful for screening symptomatic patients. The utility of sCRAG in asymptomatic HIV patients as a screening tool has not been adequately studied.[89] Although routine screening for cryptococcal antigen in asymptomatic patients is not recommended, if a positive titer (>1:8) is noted in an asymptomatic patient, therapy may be appropriate[89] because of the risk of its progressing to disseminated disease.

There is little value in serial measurements of CSF and sCRAG for routine management of cryptococcal meningitis.[90,91] CSF cryptococcal antigen titers should decrease after effective therapy. However, there is no evidence to support following the serum antigen serially, which shows no correlation with the outcome of antifungal therapy.[92] Management decisions should be based on an individual clinical assessment, not relying on cryptococcal antigen titers alone.

▲ TREATMENT

The reported acute mortality with treatment in patients with AIDS is 10% to 25%.[59,93–95] Prior to AIDS the standard therapy for cryptococcal meningitis had been to use the combination of amphotericin B and flucytosine, with a trend toward using lower doses of amphotericin B and a shorter duration of treatment.[96,97] A study of HIV-negative patients conducted by the National Institute of Allergy and Infectious Diseases (NIAID)-sponsored Mycosis Study Group (MSG)[96] compared 4 weeks of combination therapy with a 6-week course. That study was designed to randomize patients at the end of a uniform 4-week course of combination therapy. Only 91 of 181 patients initially treated were randomized. Of these 91 patients, cure or improvement was seen in 75% of those receiving 4 weeks of therapy compared with 85% of those in the 6-week cohort. There was no difference in toxicity between the two regimens. It is important to note that 31 of 80 nonrandomized patients died, giving a 17% overall acute mortality rate with this treatment for cryptococcal meningitis. The conclusions from this study were that 4 weeks of combination therapy was acceptable for patients who did not have risk factors that correlated with a high frequency of relapse.

Although there were few HIV-positive patients in the trial, one important risk factor that was predictive of relapse was immunosuppression. Thus more prolonged courses of amphotericin B and flucytosine were used initially in the AIDS epidemic. However, early reports of the experience with the amphotericin B/flucytosine regimens in patients with AIDS were not favorable. Indeed, data suggested that flucytosine was too toxic in AIDS patients and was not beneficial.[59]

The poor outcomes and increased incidence of cryptococcal meningitis in AIDS led to a search for more effective primary treatment. This became particularly relevant with the availability of the orally active antifungal triazoles fluconazole and itraconazole (Table 36–1). Initial experience with these agents was encouraging[98–101] and led to a number of controlled comparative trials (Table 36–2).

A small randomized, controlled study compared fluconazole 400 mg/day to amphotericin B plus flucytosine in AIDS patients.[102] Patients were initially given amphotericin B 0.7 mg/kg/day for 7 days; the frequency was then changed to three times a week for 9 weeks. Of 14 patients randomized to fluconazole, 8 failed, in contrast to no failures among those given combination therapy. Of the 16 fluconazole patients, 4 died; there were no deaths among six patients in the combination group. The trial was terminated early because of the higher failure and mortality rates seen in the fluconazole group. Another small study compared itraconazole 200 mg bid with amphotericin B 0.3 mg/kg/day plus flucytosine 150 mg/kg/day.[103] A 41%

▲ **Table 36–1.** DRUGS USED TO TREAT CRYPTOCOCCAL INFECTION

Agent	Usual Dose(s)	Side Effects	Drug Interactions	Comments
Amphotericin B	Amphotericin B (deoxycholate) 0.7–1.0 mg/kg/d Liposomal amphotericin B 3–6 mg/kg/d Amphotericin B lipid complex 5 mg/kg/d	Immediate hypersensitivity reactions, fever, hypotension, nausea and vomiting during administration, hypokalemia, nephropathy	Nephrotoxic drugs (e.g., aminoglycosides, pentamidine, foscarnet, cidofovir)	
Flucytosine	25 mg/kg q6h	Gastrointestinal, bone marrow suppression	Nephrotoxic drugs	Dosage must be reduced in patients with renal dysfunction
Fluconazole	400 mg/d (acute therapy); 200 mg/d (suppressive therapy)	Nausea, rash, hepatitis	Rifabutin (increased rifabutin levels); rifampin (decreased fluconazole levels)	
Itraconazole	200–400 mg bid PO	Nausea, abdominal pain, rash, headache, edema, hypokalemia	Rifamycin, ritonavir, phenobarbital, phenytoin all decrease itraconazole levels. Effect of nevirapine is unknown. The drug should not be used concomitantly with terfenadine or astemizole. Antacids, H_2-blockers decrease itraconazole absorption. Itraconazole itself acts as a moderate inhibitor of the cytochrome P_{450} system and can increase levels of indinavir, cyclosporin, digoxin, and phenytoin	Absorption of itraconazole is dependent on food and gastric acid and may be erratic. The newer solution is better absorbed

▲ **Table 36–2.** RANDOMIZED TRIALS OF TREATMENT OF CRYPTOCOCCAL MENINGITIS IN AIDS

Trial	Agents (Dose)	No. of Patients	Mycologic Response[a] (%)	Comments
Primary Infection				
Larsen[102]	Amphotericin B (0.7 mg/kg/d) and flucytosine (5-FC) (150 mg/kg/d) *vs.*	7	100	Study stopped because of increased mortality in fluconazole group
	Fluconazole 200 mg qd	14	43	
De Gans[103]	Amphotericin B (0.3 mg/kg/d) and 5-FC (150 mg/kg/d) *vs.*	11	100	Amphotericin B regimen superior
	Itraconazole 200 mg twice daily	14	50	
Saag[104]	Amphotericin (0.4 mg/kg/d)[b]	63	40	No significant difference between regimens
	Fluconazole 200–400 g/d[c]	131	34	
Moskovitz[105]	Fluconazole 400 mg daily *vs.*	40	41	Study confined to patients with "good prognostic features"
	Itraconazole 200 mg twice daily	33	38	
Van der Horst[106]	*Part A*[d]			
	Amphotericin B (0.7 mg/kg/d) *vs.*	179	51	Difference between arms in part A were not significant (NS) (P = 0.06)
	Amphotericin B (0.7 mg/kg/d) plus 5-FC (100 mg/kg/d)	202	60	
	Part B[e]			Differences in second part were NS, but the null hypothesis that fluconazole was superior could not be rejected
	Fluconazole 400 mg/d *vs.*	151	72	
	Itraconazole 400 mg/d	155	60	
Hamill[107]	Amphotericin B deoxycholate (0.7 mg/kg/d *vs.*	87	54	All patients received 2 weeks of amphotericin followed by fluconazole for a total of 10 weeks. Differences in responses between groups were NS. More nephrotoxicity in amphotericin deoxycholate arm
	Liposomal amphotericin B (3 mg/kg/d) *vs.*	86	63	
	Liposomal amphotericin B (6 mg/kg/d)	94	54	
Suppressive Therapy				
Bozzette[108]	Fluconazole 200 mg/d *vs.*	34	3	Fluconazole superior
	Placebo	27	37	
Powderly[109]	Fluconazole 200 mg PO qd *vs.*	119	2	Fluconazole superior (P <0.001)
	Amphotericin B 1 mg/kg IV q wk	88	18	
Saag[110]	Fluconazole 200 mg/d *vs.*	52	4	Fluconazole superior (P = 0.003)
	Itraconazole 200 mg/d	57	23	

[a]Response is defined as mycologic clearance (CSF cultures negative) by the end of treatment (6–10 weeks depending on study; 2 weeks for Part A of van der Horst study and for Hamill study) for the acute trials and as relapse rate for the suppressive trials.
[b]Median dose. Investigators were allowed to use any dose from 0.3 to 0.6 mg/kg/day. 5-FC was used in 14% of patients.
[c]Patients were treated with 200 mg initially; dose could be increased to 400 mg at the investigator, discretion.
[d]Part A was followed for the first 2 weeks of treatment.
[e]Part B was followed during weeks 3–10 of treatment.

failure rate was reported in the itraconazole group compared to no failures in the combination group for primary treatment. More relapses were seen in the group initially treated with itraconazole.

In contrast to these apparently superior results with amphotericin B, a randomized, prospective trial conducted by the NIAID[104] comparing fluconazole to amphotericin B for treatment of acute cryptococcal meningitis in AIDS failed to show any significant differences in outcomes between the two regimens. The median dose of amphotericin B in this study was 0.4 mg/kg; flucytosine, the use of which was at the discretion of the investigators, was rarely employed. Fewer than 50% of patients in either group were successfully treated, as judged by clearance of cryptococci from their CSF cultures. However, there were hints of differences between the two regimens. Although there was no significant difference in the overall mortality between the two groups, the mortality was higher during the first 2 weeks of therapy with fluconazole. As with some other trials, the dose of amphotericin B may have been too low.

Initial therapy with azoles alone does not appear to be the most effective approach to treatment. A study comparing itraconazole 200 mg bid PO and fluconazole 400 mg daily PO as primary treatment of cryptococcal meningitis in patients with AIDS showed no statistical significance in CSF sterilization between the two groups.[105] However, the study was terminated early partly because the clinical response rate was only approximately 40%. Thus no prospective randomized trial of triazoles given as initial therapy to unselected patients has shown a response rate higher than 50%.

In light of these data, the NIAID's MSG and AIDS Clinical Trials Group (ACTG) investigated a strategy of induction amphotericin B (for 2 weeks) followed by azole treatment. Patients with cryptococcal meningitis were randomized to receive 2 weeks of amphotericin B (0.7 mg/kg/day) with either flucytosine (25 mg/kg every 6 hours) or matching placebo. The ACTG 159/MSG 017 study addressed two questions: Does adding flucytosine to amphotericin B as induction therapy for cryptococcal meningitis improve the 2- or 10-week survival compared to induction with amphotericin B alone? Is itraconazole as effective as fluconazole in suppressing relapse of cryptococcal meningitis during the maintenance phase of treatment? At the end of 2 weeks patients who were stable or improved were again randomized to receive either fluconazole 400 mg/day or itraconazole 200 mg bid. The acute mortality with this regimen was 6%, which compares favorably with anything previously reported for cryptococcal meningitis in AIDS patients.[106] The addition of flucytosine to amphotericin B did not significantly improve the mortality rate or the clinical course. However, flucytosine was well tolerated, and there was a trend to a better CSF sterilization rate with its use (60% of patients assigned to amphotericin B plus flucytosine were culture-negative at 2 weeks, compared with 51% of patients who received amphotericin B alone). Furthermore, the use of flucytosine as initial therapy has been associated with a decreased risk of later relapse of cryptococcal meningitis. In the second (azole) phase of the MSG/ACTG trial, there was no significant difference in clinical symptoms, response rate, or mortality among patients randomized to either fluconazole or itraconazole, although trends favored fluconazole. An open-label Italian study of this strategic approach (high-dose amphotericin B followed by triazoles) was also associated with favorable outcomes.[111] Of 31 patients treated in this fashion, 29 (94%) responded to therapy, and there were no deaths resulting from cryptococcosis. Thus it is reasonable to recommend this approach as a standard one for the treatment of acute cryptococcal meningitis in AIDS (Fig. 36–2). The Infectious Diseases Society of America (IDSA) recently released practice guidelines endorsing this strategy. In patients unable to tolerate flucytosine, amphotericin B alone is an acceptable alternative.[112]

Outcome from acute cryptococcal infection is worse in patients who have abnormal mental status before treatment is initiated.[104] In addition, patients who have positive blood cultures for *C. neoformans,* high titers of cryptococcal antigen in their CSF, or a low CSF white blood cell count have generally fared worse with therapy. At this point it is not clear whether a different strategy (e.g., a more prolonged induction period with amphotericin B) is warranted for such patients.

Although the data to date suggest that azole therapy alone is not optimal initial treatment, there is still considerable interest in the possibility of a completely oral regimen. The experience with higher doses of fluconazole does not suggest that this would be sufficiently active. However, the initial experience with the combination of fluconazole (400 mg/day) with flucytosine (150 mg/kg/day) as primary treatment resulted in promising response rates in selected patients.[113] After 10 weeks of therapy, 75% of CSF cultures were negative within a median time of 23 days, which was less than previously reported times with either drug alone. Almost 30% of patients had dose-limiting adverse effects from flucytosine mandating its discontinuation. Additional studies suggest that the combination of flucytosine and high doses of fluconazole (800 to 2000 mg/day) are associated with initial response rates of more than 70%, comparable to those seen in trials of amphotericin B plus flucytosine.[114] A small number of patients have also been treated successfully with the combination of itraconazole

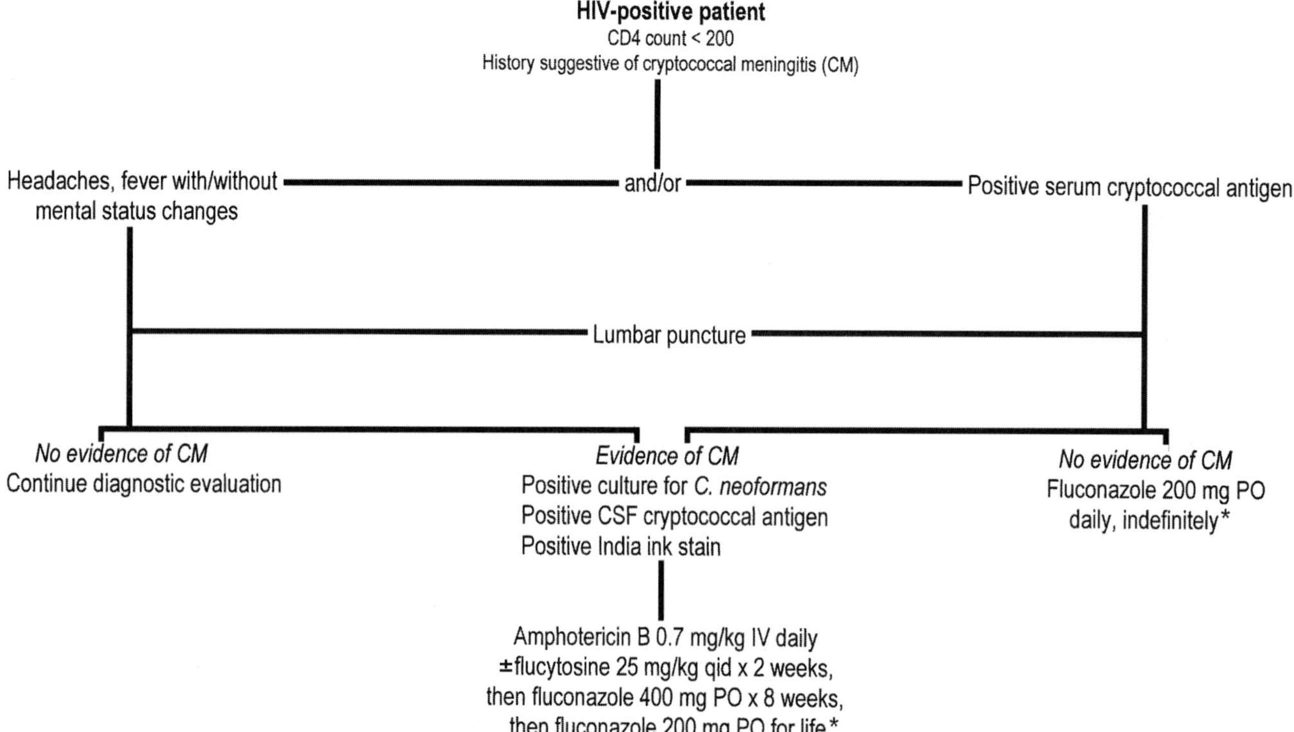

Figure 36–2. Algorithm for the diagnosis and treatment of cryptococcal meningitis. *Recent evidence suggests fluconazole secondary prophylaxis may be discontinued if the patients CD, count rises above 100–200 cells/μl and is sustained at this level for greater than 6 months (see text).

and flucytosine.[115] These data clearly suggest that this combination merits more extensive investigation, and that it may emerge as a useful alternative to parenteral amphotericin B-based regimens.

Another area of active investigation is the use of alternative formulations of amphotericin B. The use of amphotericin mixed with Intralipid has attracted some attention. In a randomized comparison of amphotericin B deoxycholate and amphotericin B/Intralipid for the treatment of AIDS-associated cryptococcal meningitis, an increased incidence of anemia and nephrotoxicity was noted in the group taking the Intralipid preparation.[116] The Intralipid preparation did reduce the incidence of infusion-related adverse reactions and was associated with a trend toward an improved mycologic cure; but given that there was no benefit in the renal toxicity or clinical outcome, its use cannot be recommended. A randomized study comparing the amphotericin B–lipid complex with amphotericin B deoxycholate in 55 HIV-positive patients with cryptococcal meningitis noted less hematologic and nephrotoxicity in the lipid complex arm.[117] There was a trend favoring "standard" amphotericin B in terms of the mycologic outcome. Small randomized studies[118,119] of liposomal amphotericin B compared with conventional amphotericin B noted an earlier CSF sterilization rate in patients randomized to the liposomal preparation. A larger randomized comparision of amphotericin B with liposomal amphotericin B[107] found similar clinical effects but less toxicity with the liposomal product. However, given that dose-limiting toxicity is rare with 2 weeks of amphotericin B deoxycholate, the role of the much more expensive liposomal preparation is still uncertain.

One aspect of managing acute cryptococcal meningitis in AIDS patients that has become more apparent in recent years is that clinical deterioration may be due to mechanical events associated with increased intracranial pressure, and that this aspect may not respond rapidly to antifungal therapy.[120,121] Baseline pressures appear to be predictive of outcome. In the recent MSG/ACTG trial,[61] among 381 patients enrolled, pretreatment opening pressures were reported for 221. The mean opening pressure at baseline for survivors was 27.9 ± 10.0 cm H_2O; for those who died, the median pressure was 29.4 ± 17.0 cm H_2O. Among the 21 patients who died during the initial 2 weeks of therapy, 12 had had a baseline CSF pressure measured; 6 of these patients had a pressure of 35 cm H_2O or higher. Two of the other patients who died had opening pressures of more than 55 cm H_2O immediately prior to death. There were statistically significant differences in survival between patients whose CSF pressure was less than 19 cm H_2O and those with pressures of 25 or 35 cm H_2O or more, with survival among these with the highest pressures being significantly less than those in patients whose pressures were normal.[61]

Ten patients with HIV-associated cryptococcal meningitis complicated by elevated intracranial pressure (range 26 to 60 cm H_2O) were prospectively followed.[122] High-volume lumbar puncture defined as removal of 20 to 30 ml CSF was performed one or two times daily. All patients returned to their baseline level of consciousness following normalization of their CSF pressure, and all 10 remain alive (range 7 to 24 months). Eight patients eventually required placement of lumbar peritoneal shunts, only one of which has subsequently been removed.

These data do not prove a causal relation between the pressure and outcome, nor do they prove that lowering pressure improves the prognosis. Nevertheless, they suggest that all patients with cryptococcal meningitis should have their opening pressure measured when a lumbar puncture is performed, and strong consideration should be given to reducing such pressure (by repeated lumbar punctures, a lumbar drain, or a shunt) if the opening pressure is high (>25 cm H_2O).

Patients with AIDS and cryptococcal meningitis require lifelong maintenance therapy. This was demonstrated in a placebo-controlled, double-blind, randomized trial evaluating the effectiveness of fluconazole for maintenance therapy after successful primary treatment with amphotericin B alone or in combination with flucytosine in patients with AIDS.[108] The risk of recurrence in the placebo group was significantly higher than that in the fluconazole group. It is of note that 22% of the placebo group in that trial were found to have clinically silent, recurrent cryptococcal infection in the urinary tract after prostatic massage. Other trials have confirmed that fluconazole 200 mg/day is the most effective maintenance therapy for cryptococcal meningitis. A trial comparing fluconazole 200 mg/day and amphotericin B 1 mg/kg/week for suppressive therapy of cryptococcal meningitis in AIDS patients[109] showed that the amphotericin B group had significantly more relapses, increased drug-related adverse events, and more bacterial infections, including bacteremia. A more recent comparison of fluconazole 200 mg/day versus itraconazole 200 mg/day was terminated by its Data Safety Monitoring Board after preliminary results revealed a CSF culture relapse rate of 4% in AIDS patients receiving fluconazole compared to 23% relapse in the itraconazole group.[110]

Until 2001, the U.S. Public Health Service (USPHS) and IDSA guidelines had recommended maintenance therapy with fluconazole for life.[112,123] Recently the USPHS guidelines have changed secondary prophylaxis recommendations for most opportunistic pathogens to reflect data revealing that it is safe to discontinue secondary prophylaxis in patients who have had a sustained immunologic response on HAART. It seems reasonable to assume that it would be safe to discontinue secondary prophylaxis in patients with a history of disseminated fungal disease who have had sustained immunologic responses. There have been four case series of safely discontinuing secondary prophylaxis in patients with cryptococcal meningitis. In one study,[124] six patients with disseminated cryptococcal disease including one patient with a history of a brain abscess discontinued antifungal prophylaxis after 1 year of prophylaxis and a sustained CD4+ T-lymphocyte count of more than 150 cells/μl (range 178 to 525 cells/μl) on HAART. One patient had positive CSF CRAG and sCRAG tests at the time of enrollment. In a second observational study, 16 of 33 patients voluntarily discontinued maintenance therapy when their mean CD4 and T-lymphocyte counts were 113 cells/μl: mean follow-up was 15.2 months.[124a] In another study,[125] six patients including three with an sCRAGs titer of more than 1:8 discontinued antifungal prophylaxis after a median 11 months of HAART with a CD4+ T-lymphocyte count higher than 100 cells/μl. None of the patients in these three studies has had a recurrence of cryptococcosis. Another recent study has been published.[125a]

Thus, the USPHS guidelines for 2001 recommend discontinuation of secondary prophylaxis if patients have successfully completed a course of initial therapy for cryptococcosis, remain asymptomatic with respect to signs and symptoms of their cryptococcosis, and have a sustained increase (i.e., ≥6 months) in their CD4 and T-lymphoctye counts to >100–200 cells/μl following HAART. Some experts would perform a lumbar puncture to determine if the CSF were culture negative before stopping therapy even if patients were asymptomatic, but many experts do not believe this is necessary. Maintenance therapy should be restarted if the CD4 and T-lymphocyte count falls to <100–200 cells/μl.

Most relapses that do occur appear to be associated with the same strain of *C. neoformans* that caused the initial infection.[126–128] In general, these strains have not been associated with changes in antifungal susceptibility (especially to fluconazole, the usual suppressive treatment). This suggests that relapse generally is due to recurrence rather than a new infection (although new infection can occur[129]) and that the major problem in such cases appears to be compliance with antifungal therapy. A small number of cases associated with the acquisition of fluconazole resistance have been reported,[130–134] as have isolated cases of cryptococcal meningitis caused by amphotericin B-resistant strains.[135] In one study, 28 isolates from 25 patients were tested for fluconazole susceptibility, and they correlated with clinical outcomes. Therapeutic failure was observed in five patients who were infected with isolates for which the fluconazole minimum inhibitory concentrations (MICs) were 16 μg/ml or more.[136] Of these five patients, four died from active cryptococcal disease. Of the 20 patients with fluconazole-susceptible isolates, only two patients died, both unrelated to cryptococcal disease. These findings suggest that fluconazole susceptibility may be useful for predicting the clinical response. In addition, a previous study suggested that fluconazole susceptibility may be useful for determining if fluconazole can be used as primary therapy.[137]

Although not currently a major issue, close attention must be given to monitoring whether azole-resistant cryptococcal disease becomes a future problem. Management of these resistant cases is largely anecdotal. In one case of amphotericin B-resistant disease,[135] the patient ultimately responded well to the combination of fluconazole and flucytosine. It is possible that this combination (especially with higher azole dosages) would be effective in cases associated with azole resistance; however, the most prudent course would be to treat with amphotericin B and flucytosine and to give maintenance therapy with intermittent amphotericin B.

▲ PREVENTION

Several studies have suggested that fluconazole can prevent many cases of cryptococcal meningitis in patients with AIDS.[51] Indeed, the declining incidence of this infection has been attributed to widespread use of fluconazole. A randomized trial comparing fluconazole 200 mg/day with clotrimazole troches for prevention of fungal infections in AIDS patients demonstrated a 2-year invasive fungal infection rate of 2.8% in the fluconazole group compared to 9.1% in the clotrimazole group, with a sevenfold reduction in the risk of cryptococcosis[138] (Table 36–3). These prospective trial data are supported by a case-controlled analysis of the effect of exposure to fluconazole on the risk of developing cryptococcal meningitis in AIDS patients.[141] A higher percentage (36%) of patients without cryptococcal meningitis had received fluconazole sometime during the preceding 6 months compared to 11% of patients with cryptococcal meningitis. Other studies have indicated that fluconazole doses lower than 200 mg/day may be effective in preventing cryptococcosis. A double-blind, randomized study comparing weekly fluconazole with daily fluconazole for the prevention of fungal infections reported equivalent effects in preventing cryptococcal disease, although the weekly regimen was less effective in suppressing oral candidiasis.[139] A study of fluconazole 200 mg three times weekly given to 231 HIV-infected individuals noted the occurrence of cryptococcal meningitis in one patient (0.4%).[142] There is also evidence that itraconazole is effective in preventing cryptococcosis. The MSG conducted a prospective, randomized trial of itraconazole 200 mg/day compared with placebo in HIV-infected patients with CD4 counts less than 150 cells/mm^3 who resided in areas endemic for histoplasmosis.[140] Cryptococcal infection occurred

▲ **Table 36–3.** RANDOMIZED COMPARATIVE TRIALS OF PREVENTION OF CRYPTOCOCCAL INFECTION IN HIV-POSITIVE PATIENTS

Trial	Agents Used	Target Populations	No. of Patients	Rates of Cryptococcal Infection (%)	Comments
Powderly[138]	Fluconazole, 200 mg qd *vs.*	CD4+ T-lymphocyte count < 200/mm^3	217	0.9	Fluconazole superior as prophylaxis (*P* < 0.001), but no survival benefit noted
	Clotrimazole troches 5 times daily		211	7.1	
Havlir[139]	Fluconazole 200 mg daily *vs.*	CD4+ T-lymphocyte count < 100/mm^3	316	0.3	Difference between two regimens not significant
	Fluconazole 400 mg once weekly		317	1.6	
McKinsey[104]	Itraconazole *vs.*	CD4+ T-lymphocyte count < 150/mm^3	149	0.7	Itraconazole significantly delayed cryptococcosis (*P* < 0.001); no survival benefit
	Placebo		146	5.4	

in one patient assigned to itraconazole compared with eight cases of cryptococcosis in patients receiving placebo. As with the fluconazole studies, no survival benefit was noted. Thus despite clear evidence of a protective effect, the overall utility of routine use of fluconazole as primary prophylaxis in advanced HIV disease is unclear. There is considerable concern that prolonged usage of fluconazole may result in acquired resistance to fluconazole, especially in *Candida* species.[143,144] At this point, the recommended guidelines from the USPHS and IDSA for prophylaxis in patients with HIV infection do not endorse routine use of primary antifungal prophylaxis.[123]

▲ FUTURE ISSUES

Several cytokines show some potential as adjunctive therapy for infection based on a number of in vitro and animal studies. Interferon-γ activates macrophages for fungicidal activity against *C. neoformans.*[30,33] In murine models of intraperitoneal and CNS infection with *C. neoformans,* recombinant interferon-γ improved survival, especially when combined with amphotericin B.[145,146] A randomized, double-blind, placebo-controlled, dose-range, Phase II study of the safety and antifungal activity of subcutaneous recombinant interferon-γ 1b (rIFN-γ1b) in conjunction with standard therapy in patients with acute cryptococcal meningitis is currently in progress. Results from a pilot study presented in late 2001 did not show striking clinical benefit.[146a]

Tumor necrosis factor-α (TNFα) can enhance the complement-dependent phagocytosis of *C. neoformans* by murine macrophages in vitro.[147] In addition, monoclonal antibodies against TNFα enhanced mortality in response to experimental disseminated cryptococcosis.[147] IL-2 has been demonstrated to activate T cells for cytokine production of macrophages, adherence to *C. neoformans,* and inhibition of growth.[148] IL-12 alone and in combination with fluconazole significantly reduced the development of systemic cryptococcal infection in a murine infection model.[149]

Basal fungistatic anticryptococcal activity of peripheral blood monocytes for AIDS patients is significantly reduced compared that in HIV-seronegative controls. Treatment of monocytes with granulocyte/macrophage colony-stimulating factor (GM-CSF) from AIDS patients resulted in increased fungistatic activity, and the combination of GM-CSF with fluconazole resulted in increased fungicidal activity. The effects of GM-CSF treatment in monocytes included enhanced phagocytic activity, increased superoxide anion generation, and up-regulation of CD11b/CD18 expression.[150]

Monoclonal antibodies have also been investigated for their therapeutic potential. Monoclonal antibodies to *C. neoformans* glucuronoxylomannan have been demonstrated to enhance fluconazole and amphotericin B in a murine model.[151,152] In addition, a series of patients receiving serum antibody adjuvant therapy with amphotericin B for *C. neoformans* infection suggests the possibility of clinical benefit.[153] Antibody-based therapy for cryptococcal disease is currently under investigation.[154] The MSG is currently conducting a Phase I evaluation of the safety and pharmacodynamic activity of the murine-derived anti-cryptococcal antibody 18B7 in HIV-infected subjects who have responded to therapy for cryptococcal meningitis.

Although chemoprophylaxis is relatively successful in patients with AIDS, as noted above, it is not routinely recommended. An alternative strategy for prevention is to consider vaccination early during the HIV infection in the hope of eliciting a protective response. Current investigational strategies include passive antibody administration (which is likely not to be practical) and immunization with glucuronoxylomannan–tetanus toxoid conjugate.[155–157]

REFERENCES

1. Dismukes WE. Cryptococcal meningitis in patients with AIDS. J Infect Dis 157:624, 1988.
2. Powderly WG. Cryptococcal meningitis and AIDS. Clin Infect Dis 17:837, 1993.
3. Selik RM, Chu SY, Ward JW. Trends in infectious diseases and cancers among persons dying of HIV infection in the United States from 1987 to 1992. Ann Intern Med 123:933, 1995.
4. Kwon-Chung KJ, Bennett JE. Cryptococcosis. In: Medical Mycology. Philadelphia, Lea & Febiger, 1992, p 397.
5. Kwon-Chung KJ, Kozel TR, Edman JC, et al. Recent advances in biology and immunology of Cryptococcus neoformans. J Med Vet Mycol 30:133, 1992.
6. Madrenys N, De Vroey C, Raes-Wuytack C, et al. Identification of the perfect state of Cryptococcus neoformans from 195 clinical isolates including 84 from AIDS patients. Mycopathologia 123:65, 1993.
7. Cherniak R, Reiss E, Slodki ME, et al. Structure and antigenic activity of the capsular polysaccharide of Cryptococcus neoformans serotype. Ann Mol Immunol 17:10, 1980.
8. Levitz SM. The ecology of Cryptococcus neoformans and the epidemiology of cryptococcosis. Rev Infect Dis 13:1163, 1991.
9. Ellis DH, Pfeiffer TJ. Ecology, life cycle, and infectious propagule of Cryptococcus neoformans. Lancet 336:923, 1990.
10. Speed B, Dunt D. Clinical and host differences between infections with the two varieties of Cryptococcus neoformans. Clin Infect Dis 21:28, 1995.
11. Rinaldi MG, Drutz DJ, Howell A, et al. Serotypes of Cryptococcus neoformans in patients with AIDS. J Infect Dis 153:642, 1986.
12. Shimizu RY, Howard DH, Clancy MN. The variety of Cryptococcus neoformans in patients with AIDS. J Infect Dis 154:1042, 1986.
13. Restrepo BI, Barbour AG. Cloning of 18S and 25S rDNAs from the pathologic fungus Cryptococcus neoformans. J Bacteriol 171:5596, 1989.
14. Wickes BL, Moore TDE, Kwon-Chung KJ. Comparison of the electrophoretic karyotypes and chromosomal location of ten genes in the two varieties of Cryptococcus neoformans. Microbiology 140:543, 1994.
15. Perfect JR, Toffaletti DL, Rude TH. The gene encoding phosphoribosylaminomidazole carboxylase (*ADE2*) is essential for growth of Cryptococcus neoformans in cerebrospinal fluid. Infect Immun 61:4446, 1993.
16. Parker AR, Moore TDE, Edman JC, et al. Cloning sequence analysis and expression of the gene encoding imidazole glycerol phosphate dehydratase in Cryptococcus neoformans. Gene 145:135, 1994.
17. Chang YC, Kwon-Chung KJ. Complementation of a capsule-deficient mutation of Cryptococcus neoformans restores its virulence. Mol Cell Biol 14:4912, 1994.
18. Williamson PR. Biochemical and molecular characterization of the diphenol oxidase of Cryptococcus neoformans: identification as a laccase. J Bacteriol 176:656, 1994.
19. Perfect JR, Rude TH, Wong B, et al. Identification of a Cryptococcus neoformans gene that directs expression of the cryptic Saccharomyces cerevisiae mannitol dehydrogenase gene. J Bacteriol 178:5257, 1996.
20. Lodge JK, Johnson RL, Weinberg RA, et al. Comparison of myristoyl-CoA:protein N-myristoyltransferases from three pathogenic fungi: Cryptococcus neoformans, Histoplasma capsulatum, and Candida albicans. J Biol Chem 269:2996, 1994.

21. Cox GM, Rude TH, Dykstra CC, et al. Actin gene from Cryptococcus neoformans: structure and phylogenetic analysis. J Med Vet Mycol 33:261, 1995.
22. Cruz MC, Bartlett MS, Edlind TD. In vitro susceptibility of the opportunistic fungus Cryptococcus neoformans to anthelmintic benzimidazoles. Antimicrob Agents Chemother 38:378, 1994.
23. Perfect JR, Rude TH, Penning LM, et al. Cloning the Cryptococcus neoformans TRP1 gene by complementation in Saccharomyces cerevisiae. Gene 122:213, 1992.
24. Moore TDE, Edman JC. The a mating type locus of Cryptococcus neoformans contains a peptide pheromone gene. Mol Cell Biol 13:1962, 1993.
25. Livi LL, Edman U, Schneider GP, et al. Cloning, expression and characterization of thymidylate synthase from Crptococcus neoformans. Gene 150:221, 1994.
26. Tolkacheva T, McNamara P, Piekarz E, et al. Cloning of a Cryptococcus neoformans gene, GPA1, encoding a G-protein a subunit homolog. Infect Immun 62:2849, 1994.
27. Jacobson ES, Ayers DJ, Harrell AC. Genetic and phenotypic characterization of capsule mutants of Cryptococcus neoformans. J Bacteriol 150:1292, 1982.
28. Bulmer GS. Twenty-five years with Cryptococcus neoformans. Mycopathologia 109:111, 1990.
29. Sukroongreung S, Eampokalap B, Tansuphaswadikul S, et al. Recovery of Cryptococcus neoformans from the nasopharynx of AIDS patients. Mycopathologia 143:131, 1999.
30. Perfect JR, Granger DL, Durack DT. Effects of antifungal agents and gamma interferon on macrophage cytotoxicity for fungi and tumor cells. J Infect Dis 156:316, 1987.
31. Huffnagle GB, Yates JL, Lipscomb MF. Immunity to a pulmonary Cryptococcus neoformans infection requires both CD4+ and CD8+ T-cells. J Exp Med 173:793, 1991.
32. Flesch IE, Schwamberger G, Kaufman SH. Fungicidal activity of IFN-gamma activated macrophages: extracellular killing of Cryptococcus neoformans. J Immunol 142:3219, 1989.
33. Roseff SA, Levitz SM. Effect of endothelial cells on phagocyte-mediated anticryptococcal activity. Infect Immun 61:3818, 1993.
34. Salkowski CA, Balish E. Role of natural killer cells in resistance to systemic cryptococcosis. J Leukoc Biol 50:151, 1991.
35. Levitz SM, Dupont MP. Phenotypic and functional characterization of human leukocytes activated by interleukin-2 to directly inhibit growth of Cryptococcus neoformans in vitro. J Clin Invest 91:1490, 1993.
36. Miller MF, Mitchell T, Storkus WJ, et al. Human natural killer cells do not inhibit growth of Cryptococcus neoformans in the absence of antibody. Infect Immun 58:639, 1990.
37. Mukherjee S, Lee SC, Casadevall A. Antibodies to Cryptococcus neoformans glucuronoxylomannan enhance antifungal activity of murine macrophages. Infect Immun 63:573, 1995.
38. Kwon-Chung KJ, Rhodes JC. Encapsulation and melanin formation as indicators of virulence in Cryptococcus neoformans. Infect Immun 51:218, 1986.
39. Rhodes JC, Polacheck I, Kwon-Chung KJ. Phenoloxidase activity and virulence in isogenic strains of Cryptococcus neoformans. Infect Immun 36:1175, 1982.
40. Casadevall A. Antibody immunity and invasive fungal infections. Infect Immun 63:4211, 1995.
41. Gadebusch HH. Passive immunization against Cryptococcus neoformans. Proc Soc Exp Biol Med 98:611, 1958.
42. Mukherjee J, Lee S, Scharff MD, et al. Monoclonal antibodies to Cryptococcus neoformans capsular polysaccharide modify the course of intravenous infection in mice. Infect Immun 62:1079, 1994.
43. Mukherjee J, Scharff MD, Casadevall A. Protective murine monoclonal antibodies to Cryptococcus neoformans. Infect Immun 60:4534, 1992.
44. Murphy JW, Mosley RL, Cherniak R, et al. Serological, electrophoretic, and biological properties of Cryptococcus neoformans antigens. Infect Immun 56:424, 1988.
45. Wang Y, Aisen P, Casadevall A. Cryptococcus neoformans melanin and virulence: mechanism of action. Infect Immun 63:3131, 1995.
46. Kwon-Chung KJ, Edman JC, Wickes BL. Genetic association of mating types and virulence in Cryptococcus neoformans. Infect Immun 60:602, 1992.
47. Evans EE, Kessel JF. The antigenic composition of Cryptococcus neoformans: serologic studies with the capsular polysaccharide. J Immunol 67:109, 1951.
48. Pettoello-Mantovani M, Casadevall A, Kollmann TR, et al. Enhancement of HIV-1 infection by the capsular polysaccharide of Cryptococcus neoformans. Lancet 339:21, 1992.
49. Lee SC, Casadevall A. Polysaccharide antigen in brain tissue of AIDS patients with cryptococcal meningitis. Clin Infect Dis 23:194, 1996.
50. Currie BP, Casadevall A. Estimation of the prevalence of cryptococcal infection among patients infected with the human immunodeficiency virus in New York City. Clin Infect Dis 19:1029, 1994.
51. Pinner RW, Hajjeh RA, Powderly WG. Prospects for preventing cryptococcosis in persons infected with human immunodeficiency virus. Clin Infect Dis 21(suppl 1):S103, 1995.
52. Abadi J, Nachman S, Kressle AB, Pirofski L. Cryptococcosis in children with AIDS. Clin Infect Dis 28:309, 1999.
53. Oursler KAK, Moore RD, Chaisson R. Risk factors for cryptococcal meningitis in HIV-infected patients. AIDS Res Hum Retroviruses 15:625, 1999.
54. McNeil JI, Kan VL. Decline in the incidence of cryptococcosis among HIV-infected patients. J Acquir Immune Defic Syndr Hum Retrovirol 9:206, 1995.
55. Hajjeh RA, Conn LA, Stephens DS, et al. Cryptococcosis: population-based multistate active surveillance and risk factor in human immunodeficiency virus-infected persons. J Infect Dis 179:449, 1999.
56. Holtzer CD, Jacobson MA, Hadley WK, et al. Decline in the rate of specific opportunistic infections at San Francisco General Hospital, 1994–1997. AIDS 12:1931, 1998.
57. Koo JJ, Aberg JA. Increase in the rate of AIDS-related opportunistic infections at San Francisco General Hospital in the era of potent antiretroviral therapy [abstract]. Presented at the XIII International AIDS Conference, Durban, South Africa, July 2000.
58. Rozenbaum R, Goncalves AJR. Clinical epidemiological study of 171 cases of cryptococcosis. Clin Infect Dis 18:369, 1994.
59. Chuck SL, Sande MA. Infections with Cryptococcus neoformans in the acquired immunodeficiency syndrome. N Engl J Med 321:794, 1989.
60. Dismukes WE. Management of cryptococcosis. Clin Infect Dis 17(suppl):S507, 1993.
61. Graybill JR, Sobel J, Saag M, et al. Diagnosis and management of Increased Intracranial pressure in patients with AIDS and cryptococcal meningitis. Clin Infect Dis 30:47, 2000.
62. Cameron ML, Bartlett JA, Gallis HA, et al. Manifestations of pulmonary cryptococcosis in patients with acquired immunodeficiency syndrome. Rev Infect Dis 13:64, 1991.
63. Clark RA, Greer DL, Valainis GT, et al. Cryptococcus neoformans pulmonary infection in HIV-1-infected patients. J Acquir Immune Defic Syndr Hum Retrovirol 3:480, 1990.
64. Visnegarwala F, Graviss EA, Lacke CE, et al. Acute respiratory failure associated with cryptococcosis in patients with AIDS: analysis of predictive factors. Clin Infect Dis 27:1231, 1998.
65. Driver JA, Saunders CA, Heinze-Lacey B, et al. Cryptococcal pneumonia in AIDS: is cryptococcal meningitis preceded by clinically recognizable pneumonia? J Acquir Immune Defic Syndr Hum Retrovirol 9:168, 1995.
66. Clark RA, Greer DL, Atkinson W, et al. Spectrum of Cryptococcus neoformans infection in 68 patients infected with human immunodeficiency virus. Rev Infect Dis 12:768, 1990.
67. Mulanovich VE, Dismukes WE, Markowitz N. Cryptococcal empyemia: case report and review. Clin Infect Dis 20:1396, 1995.
68. Darras-Joly C, Chevret S, Wolff M, et al. Cryptococcus neoformans infection in France: epidemiologic features of and early prognostic parameters for 76 patients who were infected with human immunodeficiency virus. Clin Infect Dis 23:369, 1996.
69. Meyohas MC, Roux P, Bollens D, et al. Pulmonary cryptococcosis: localized and disseminated infections in 27 patients with AIDS. Clin Infect Dis 21:628, 1995.
70. Murakawa GJ, Kerschmann R, Berger T. Cutaneous Cryptococcus infection and AIDS: report of 12 cases and review of the literature. Arch Dermatol 132:545, 1996.
71. Lewis W, Lipsick J, Cammarosano C. Cryptococcal myocarditis in acquired immune deficiency syndrome. Am J Cardiol 55:1240, 1985.
72. Lafont A, Wolff M, Marche C, et al. Overwhelming myocarditis due to Cryptococcus neoformans in an AIDS patient. Lancet 2:1145, 1987.
73. Ricciardi DD, Sepkowitz DV, Berkowitz LB, et al. Cryptococcal arthritis in a patient with acquired immune deficiency syndrome: case report and review of the literature. J Rheumatol 13:455, 1986.

74. Morinelli EN, Dugel PU, Riffenburgh R, et al. Infectious multifocal choroiditis in patients with acquired immune deficiency syndrome. Ophthalmology 100:1014, 1993.
75. Bonacini M, Nussbaum J, Ahluwalia C. Gastrointestinal, hepatic, and pancreatic involvement with Cryptococcus neoformans in AIDS. J Clin Gastroenterol 12:295, 1990.
76. Finazzi R, Guffanti M, Cernuschi M, et al. Unusual presentation of cryptococcosis in a patient with AIDS. Clin Infect Dis 22:709, 1996.
77. Ndimbie OK, Dekker A, Martinez AJ, et al. Prostatic sequestration of Cryptococcus neoformans in immunocompromised persons treated for cryptococcal meningoencephalitis. Histol Histopathol 9:643, 1994.
78. Larsen RA, Bozzette S, McCutchan JA, et al. Persistent Cryptococcus neoformans of the prostate after successful treatment of meningitis. Ann Intern Med 111:125, 1989.
79. Penneys NS. Skin Manifestations of AIDS. Philadelphia, JB Lippincott, 1990.
80. Concus AP, Helfand RF, Imber MJ, et al. Cutaneous cryptococcosis mimicking molluscum contagiosum in a patient with AIDS. J Infect Dis 158:897, 1988.
81. Manfredi R, Mazzoni A, Nanetti A, et al. Morphologic features and clinical significance of skin involvement in patients with AIDS-related cryptococcosis. Acta Derm Venereol 76:72, 1996.
82. Woods ML, MacGinley R, Eisen DP, Allworth AM. HIV combination therapy: partial immune reconstitution unmasking latent cryptococcal infection. AIDS 12:1491, 1998.
83. Blanche P, Gombert B, Ginsburg C, et al. HIV combination therapy: immune restitution causing cryptococcal lymphadenitis dramatically improved by anti-inflammatory therapy. Scand J Infect Dis. 30:615, 1998.
84. Lanzafame M, Trevenzoli M, Carretta G, et al. Mediastinal lymphadenitis due to cryptococcal infection in HIV-positive patients on highly active antiretroviral therapy. Chest 116:848, 1999.
85. Currie BP, Freundlich LF, Soto MA, et al. False-negative cerebrospinal fluid cryptococcal latex agglutination tests for patients with culture-positive cryptococcal meningitis. J Clin Microbiol 31:2519, 1993.
86. Tanner DC, Weinstein MP, Fedoview B, et al. Comparison of commercial kits for detection of cryptococcal antigen. J Clin Microbiol 32:1680, 1993.
87. McManus EJ, Jones JM. Detection of a Trichosporon beigelii antigen cross reactive with Cryptococcus neoformans capsular polysaccharide in serum from a patient with disseminated Trichosporon infection. J Clin Microbiol 21:681, 1985.
88. Blevins LB, Fenn J, Segal H, et al. False-positive cryptococcal antigen latex agglutination caused by disinfectants and soaps. J Clin Microbiol 33:1674, 1995.
89. Feldmeser M, Harris C, Reichberg S, et al. Serum cryptococcal antigen in patients with AIDS. Clin Infect Dis 23:827, 1996.
90. Powderly WG, Cloud GA, Dismukes WE, et al. Measurement of cryptococcal antigen in serum and cerebrospinal fluid: value in the management of AIDS-associated cryptococcal meningitis. Clin Infect Dis 18:789, 1994.
91. Powderly WG, Tuazon C, Cloud GA, et al. Serum and CSF cryptococcal antigen in management of cryptococcal meningitis in AIDS. In: Abstracts of the 4th National Conference on Human Retroviruses and Related Infections, Washington, DC. Alexandria, VA, Westover Management Group, 1997, abstract 6.
92. Aberg JA, Watson J, Segal M, Chang LW. Clinical utility of monitoring serum cryptococcal antigen (sCRAG) in patients with AIDS-related cryptococcal disease. HIV Clin Trials 1:1, 2000.
93. Zuger A, Louie E, Holzman RS, et al. Cryptococcal disease in patients with the acquired immunodeficiency syndrome: diagnostic features and outcome of treatment. Ann Intern Med 104:234, 1986.
94. Kovacs JA, Kovacs AA, Polis M, et al. Cryptococcosis in the acquired immunodeficiency syndrome. Ann Intern Med 103:533, 1985.
95. Eng RH, Bishburg E, Smith S, et al. Cryptococcal infections in the acquired immune deficiency syndrome. Am J Med 81:19, 1986.
96. Bennett JE, Dismukes WE, Duma RJ, et al. A comparison of amphotericin B alone and combined with flucytosine in the treatment of cryptococcal meningitis. N Engl J Med 301:126, 1979.
97. Dismukes WE, Cloud G, Gallis H, et al. Treatment of cryptococcal meningitis with combination of amphotericin B and flucytosine for four as compared with six weeks. N Engl J Med 317:334, 1987.
98. Dupont B, Hilmarsdottir I, Datry A, et al. Cryptococcal meningitis in AIDS patients: a pilot study of fluconazole therapy in 52 patients. In: vanden Bossche H, Mackenzie DWR, Cauwenbergh G, et al (eds) Mycosis in AIDS Patients. New York, Plenum Press, 1990, p 287.
99. Denning DW, Tucker RM, Hanson LH, et al. Itraconazole therapy for cryptococcal meningitis and cryptococcosis. Arch Intern Med 149:2301, 1989.
100. Denning DW, Tucker RM, Hostetler JS, et al. Oral itraconazole therapy of cryptococcal meningitis and cryptococcosis in patients with AIDS. In: vanden Bossche H, Mackenzie DWR, Cauwenbergh G, et al (eds) Mycosis in AIDS Patients. New York, Plenum Press, 1990, p 305.
101. Robinson PA, Knirsch AK, Joseph JA. Fluconazole for life-threatening fungal infections in patients who cannot be treated with conventional antifungal therapy. Rev Infect Dis 12(suppl 3):S349, 1990.
102. Larsen RA, Leal M, Chan L. Fluconazole compared with amphotericin B plus flucytosine for cryptococcal meningitis in AIDS. Ann Intern Med 113:183, 1990.
103. De Gans J, Portegies P, Tiessens G, et al. Itraconazole compared with amphotericin B plus flucytosine in AIDS patients with cryptococcal meningitis. AIDS 6:185, 1992.
104. Saag MS, Powderly WG, Cloud GA, et al. Comparison of amphotericin B with fluconazole in the treatment of acute AIDS-associated cryptococcal meningitis. N Engl J Med 326:83, 1992.
105. Moskovitz BL, Wiesinger B, Cryptococcal Meningitis Research Group. Randomized comparative trial of itraconazole and fluconazole for treatment of AIDS-related cryptococcal meningitis. In: Abstracts of the 1st National Conference on Human Retroviruses. Washington, DC, American Society for Microbiology, 1994, p 61.
106. Van der Horst CM, Saag MS, Cloud GA, et al: Treatment of cryptococcal meningitis associated with the acquired immunodeficiency syndrome. N Engl J Med 337:15, 1997.
107. Hamill RJ, Sobel J, el-Sadr W, et al. Randomized double blind trial of AmBisome (liposomal amphotericin B) and amphotericin B in acute cryptococcal meningitis in AIDS patients. In: Program and Abstracts of the 39th ICAAC; September, 1999. San Francisco, American. Society of Microbiology, abstract 1161.
108. Bozzette SA, Larsen R, Chiu J, et al. A controlled trial of maintenance therapy with fluconazole after treatment of cryptococcal meningitis in the acquired immunodeficiency syndrome. N Engl J Med 324:580, 1991.
109. Powderly WG, Saag MS, Cloud GA, et al. A controlled trial of fluconazole or amphotericin B to prevent relapse of cryptococcal meningitis in patients with the acquired immunodeficiency syndrome. N Engl J Med 326:793, 1992.
110. Saag MS,Cloud GA, Graybill R, NIAID Mycoses Study Group. A comparison of fluconazole versus itraconazole as maintenance therapy for AIDS-associated cryptococcal meningitis. Clin Infect Dis 28:291, 1999.
111. De Lalla F, Pellizzer G, Vaglia A, et al. Amphotericin B as primary therapy for cryptococcosis in AIDS patients: reliability of relatively high doses administered over a relatively short period. Clin Infect Dis 20:263, 1995.
112. Saag MS, Graybill RJ, Larsen, RA, MSG Cryptococcal Subproject. Practice guidelines for the management of cryptococcal disease. Clin Infect Dis 30:710, 2000.
113. Larsen RA, Bozzette SA, Jones BE, et al. Fluconazole combined with flucytosine for the treatment of cryptococcal meningitis in patients with AIDS. Clin Infect Dis 19:741, 1994.
114. Milefchik E, Leal M, Haubrich R, et al. A Phase II dose escalation trial of high dose fluconazole with and without flucytosine for AIDS associated cryptococcal meningitis. In: Abstracts of the 4th Conference on Retroviruses and Opportunistic Infections, Washington, DC. Alexandria, VA, Westover Management Group, 1997, abstract 5.
115. Viviani MA, Tortorano AM, Langer M, et al. Experience with itraconazole in cryptococcosis and aspergillosis. J Infect 18:151, 1989.
116. Joly V, Aubry P, Ndayiragide A, et al. Randomized comparison of amphotericin B deoxycholate dissolved in dextrose or Intralipid for the treatment of AIDS-associated cryptococcal meningitis. Clin Infect Dis 23:556, 1996.
117. Sharkey PK, Graybill JR, Johnson ES, et al. Amphotericin B lipid complex compared with amphotericin B in the treatment of cryptococcal meningitis in patients with AIDS. Clin Infect Dis 22:315, 1996.
118. Coker RJ, Viviani M, Gazzarxd BG, et al. Treatment of cryptococcosis with liposomal amphotericin B (AmBisome) in 23 patients with AIDS. AIDS 7:829, 1993.

119. Leenders ACAP, Reiss P, Portegeis P, et al. Liposomal amphotericin B (AmBisome) compared with amphotericin B both followed by oral fluconazole in the treatment of AIDS-associated cryptococcal meningitis. AIDS 11:1463, 1997.
120. Denning DW, Armstrong RW, Lewis BH, et al. Elevated cerebrospinal fluid pressures in patients with cryptococcal meningitis and acquired immunodeficiency syndrome. Am J Med 91:267, 1991.
121. Malessa R, Krams M, Hengge U. Elevation of intracranial pressure in acute AIDS-related cryptococcal meningitis. Clin Investigator 72:1020, 1994.
122. Fessler RD, Sobel J, Guyot L, et al. Management of elevated intracranial pressure in patients with cryptococcal meningitis. J Acquir Immune Defic Syndr Hum Retrovirol 17:137, 1998.
123. USPHS/IDSA Prevention of Opportunistic Infections Working Group. 2001 USPHS/IDSA guidelines for the prevention of opportunistic infections in persons infected with human immunodeficiency virus. http://www.hivatis.org.
124. Aberg JA, Price RW, Heeren DM, et al. Discontinuation of antifungal therapy for cryptococcosis following immunologic response to antiretroviral therapy [abstract]. Presented at the 7th Conference on Retroviruses and Opportunistic Infections, San Francisco, January 2000, abstract L10e.
124a. Mussini C, Cossarizza A, Pezzotti P, et al. Discontinuation or continuation of maintenance therapy for cryptococcal meningitis in patients with AIDS Treated with HAART. In: Progress and Abstracts of the 8th Conference on Retroviruses and Opportunistic Infections, Chicago, February 2001, abstract 546.
125. Martinez E, Garcia-Viejo MA, Marcos MA. Discontinuation of secondary prophylaxis for cryptococcal meningitis in HIV-infected patients responding to highly active antiretroviral therapy. AIDS 14:2615, 2000.
125a. Masur H, Kaplan JE, Holmes KK. Guidelines for preventing opportunistic infections among HIV infected persons–2002. Recommendations of the U.S. Public Health Service and the Infectious Disease Society of America. Ann Intern Med 2002; 137: in press.
126. Spitzer ED, Spitzer SG, Freundlich LF, et al. Persistence of initial infection in recurrent Cryptococcus neoformans meningitis. Lancet 341:595, 1993.
127. Casadevall X, Spitzer ED, Webb D, et al. Susceptibilities of serial Cryptococcus neoformans isolates from patients with recurrent cryptococcal meningitis to amphotericin B and fluconazole. Antimicrob Agents Chemother 37:1383, 1993.
128. Brandt ME, Pfaller MA, Hajjeh R, et al. Molecular subtypes and antifungal susceptibilities of serial Cryptococcus neoformans isolates in human immunodeficiency virus infected patients. J Infect Dis 174:812, 1996.
129. Haynes KA, Sullivan DJ, Coleman DC, et al. Involvement of multiple Cryptococcus neoformans strains in a single episode of cryptococcosis and reinfection with novel strains in recurrent infection demonstrated by random amplification of polymorphic DNA and DNA fingerprinting. J Clin Microbiol 33:99, 1995.
130. Paugam A, Dupouy-Camet J, Blanche P, et al. Increased fluconazole resistance of Cryptococcus neoformans isolated from a patient with AIDS and recurrent meningitis. Clin Infect Dis 19:975, 1994.
131. Birley HD, Johnson EM, McDonald P, et al. Azole drug resistance as a cause of clinical relapse in AIDS patients with cryptococcal meningitis. Int J STD AIDS 6:353, 1995.
132. Armengou A, Porcar C, Mascaro J, et al. Possible development of resistance to fluconazole during suppressive therapy for AIDS-associated cryptococcal meningitis. Clin Infect Dis 23:1337, 1996.
133. Berg J, Clancy CJ, Nguyen MH. The hidden danger of primary fluconazole prophylaxis for patients with AIDS. Clin Infect Dis 26:186, 1998.
134. Smith NH, Graviss EA, Hashmey R, et al. Multi-drug-resistant cryptococcal meningitis in an AIDS patient. In: Abstracts of the 35th Annual Meeting of the Infectious Diseases Society of America. Alexandria, VA, Infectious Diseases Society of America, 1997, abstract 529.
135. Powderly WG, Keath EJ, Sokol-Anderson M, et al. Amphotericin-B resistant Cryptococcus neoformans in a patient with AIDS. Infect Dis Clin Pract 1:314, 1992.
136. Aller AI, Martin-Mazuelos E, Lozano F, et al. Correlation of fluconazole MICs with clinical outcome in cryptococcal infection. Antimicrob Agents Chemother 44:1544, 2000.
137. Witt MD, Lewis RJ, Larsen RA, et al. Identification of patients with acute AIDS-associated cryptococcal meningitis who can be effectively treated with fluconazole: the role of antifungal susceptibility testing. Clin Infect Dis 22:322, 1996.
138. Powderly WG, Finkelstein D, Feinberg J, et al. A randomized trial comparing fluconazole with clotrimazole troches for the prevention of fungal infections in patients with advanced human immunodeficiency virus infection. N Engl J Med 332:700, 1995.
139. Havlir DV, Dube MP, McCutchan JA, et al. Prophylaxis with weekly versus daily fluconazole for fungal infections in patients with AIDS. Clin Infect Dis 27:1369, 1998.
140. McKinsey DS, Wheat LJ, Cloud GA, et al. Itraconazole prophylaxis for fungal infections in patients with advanced human immunodeficiency virus infection: randomized, placebo-controlled, double-blind study: National Institute of Allergy and Infectious Diseases Mycoses Study Group. Clin Infect Dis 28:1049, 1999.
141. Quagliarello VJ, Viscoli C, Visconti RI. Primary prevention of cryptococcal meningitis by fluconazole in HIV-infected patients. Lancet 345:548, 1995.
142. Singh N, Barnish MJ, Berman S, et al. Low-dose fluconazole as primary prophylaxis for cryptococcal infection in AIDS patients with CD4+ T lymphocyte counts of < or = 100/mm^3: demonstration of efficacy in a positive, multicenter trial. Clin Infect Dis 23:1282, 1996.
143. Maenza JR, Keruly JC, Moore RD, et al. Risk factors for fluconazole-resistant candidiasis in human immunodeficiency virus-infected patients. J Infect Dis 173:219, 1996.
144. Fichtenbaum CJ, Powderly WG. Azole-resistant candidiasis. Clin Infect Dis 26:556, 1998.
145. Joly V, Saint-Julien L, Carbon C, et al. In vivo activity of interferon-gamma in combination with amphotericin B in the treatment of experimental cryptococcosis. J Infect Dis 170:1331, 1994.
146. Lutz JE, Clemons KV, Stevens DA. Enhancement of antifungal chemotherapy by interferon-gamma in experimental systemic cryptococcosis. J Antimicrob Chemother 46:437, 2000.
146a. Pappas PG, Bustamante B, Ticona R, et al. Adjunctive interferon gamma for treatment of cryptococcal meningitis. A randomized double blind pilot study. In: Abstracts of the 41st Interference Conference on Antimicrobial Agents and Chemotherapy, Chicago, 2001, abstract 1272.
147. Collins HL, Bancroft GJ. Cytokine enhancement of complement-dependent phagocytosis by macrophages: synergy of tumor necrosis factor-α and granulocyte-macrophage colony-stimulating factor for phagocytosis of Cryptococcus neoformans. Eur J Immunol 22:1447, 1992.
148. Levitz SM. Activation of human peripheral blood mononuclear cells by interleukin-2 and granulocye-macrophage colony-stimulating factor to inhibit Cryptococcus neoformans. Infect Immun 59:3393, 1991.
149. Clemons KV, Brummer E, Stevens DA. Cytokine treatment of central nervous system infection: efficacy of interleukin-12 alone and synergy with conventional antifungal therapy in experimental cryptococcosis. Antimicrob Agents Chemother 38:460, 1994.
150. Tascini C, Vecchiarelli A, Preziosi R, et al. Granulocyte-macrophage colony-stimulating factor and fluconazole enhance anti-cryptococcal activity of monocytes from AIDS patients. AIDS 13:49, 1999.
151. Mukherjee J, Feldmesser M, Scharff MD, et al. Monoclonal antibodies to Cryptococcus neoformans glucuronoxylomannan enhance fluconazole efficacy. Antimicrob Agents Chemother 39:1398, 1995.
152. Mukherjee J, Zuckier LS, Scharff MD, et al. Therapeutic efficacy of monoclonal antibodies to Cryptococcus neoformans glucuronoxylomannan alone and in combination with amphotericin B. Antimicrob Agents Chemother 38:580, 1994.
153. Gordon MA, Casadevall A. Serum therapy for cryptococcal meningitis. Clin Infect Dis 21:1477, 1995.
154. Casadevall A, Scharff MD. Return to the past: the case for antibody-based therapies in infectious diseases. Clin Infect Dis 21:150, 1995.
155. Zebedee SL, Koduri RK, Mukherjee J, et al. Mouse-human immunoglobulin G1 chimeric antibodies with activities against Cryptococcus neoformans. Antimicrob Agents Chemother 38:1507, 1994.
156. Devi SJN, Schneerson R, Egan W, et al. Cryptococcus neoformans serotype A glucuronoxylomannan protein conjugate vaccine: synthesis, characterization and immunogenicity. Infect Immun 59:370, 1991.
157. Mukherjee J, Casadevall A, Scharff MD. Molecular characterization of the humoral responses to Cryptococcus neoformans infection and glucuronoxylomannan-tetanus toxoid conjugate immunization. J Exp Med 177:1105, 1993.

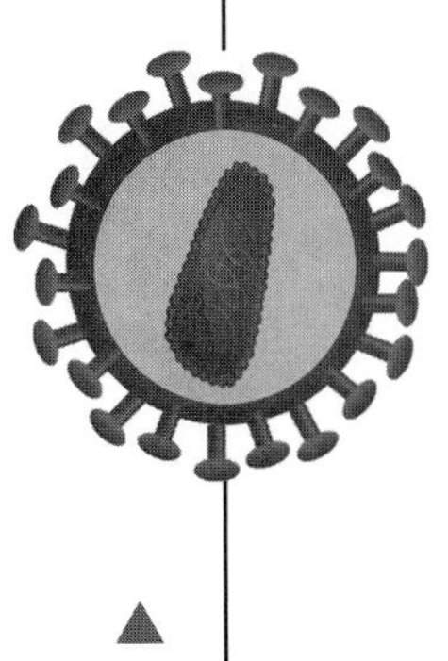

CHAPTER 37

Histoplasmosis

Joe Wheat, MD

▲ PATHOGEN

Clinical Findings

Disseminated disease occurs in 95% of cases of histoplasmosis in patients with acquired immunodeficiency syndrome (AIDS), but localized pulmonary disease may be seen in those with high CD4+ T-lymphocyte counts, typically above 300/μl. About 90% of cases of disseminated histoplasmosis have occurred in patients with CD4+ T-lymphocyte counts below 200/μl, and the median CD4+ T-lymphocyte count was below 30/μl in two studies.[1,2] Patients usually present with fever, fatigue, and weight loss; one-half exhibit respiratory symptoms (cough and dyspnea). Common physical findings include hepatosplenomegaly and lymphadenopathy. The course may be rapidly fatal, but a subacute presentation over 1 to 3 months is characteristic.

Patients infrequently (< 10%) present with shock, respiratory insufficiency, and hepatic and renal failure. This sepsis presentation represents a late manifestation of histoplasmosis, usually occurring in patients who delayed seeking care until they were severely ill. Nearly half of patients who present with a sepsis-like illness die within a week of diagnosis.[3,4]

Central nervous system histoplasmosis occurs in 10% to 20% of cases. Patients may present with lymphocytic meningitis, focal brain lesions, or diffuse encephalitis.[3,5,6] Patients complain of fever and headache and often demonstrate mental status changes. Seizures or focal neurologic deficits may occur in patients with brain involvement.[3,5] The cerebrospinal fluid (CSF) shows lymphocytic pleocytosis, protein elevation, and hypoglycorrhachia in those with meningitis. Single or multiple enhancing brain lesions may be seen by computed tomography (CT) scans or magnetic resonance imaging (MRI) in patients with cerebral involvement. The prognosis is worse in patients with neurologic findings than in those without these complications.[3]

Gastrointestinal manifestations including diarrhea, abdominal pain, intestinal obstruction or perforation, bleeding, or peritonitis complicate about 10% of cases.[7-9] A spectrum of lesions, including plaques, ulcerations, pseudopolyps, small (3 to 8 mm) nodules, thickened intestinal folds, luminal masses, and strictures, may occur anywhere along the gastrointestinal tract but are more common in the small intestines and right colon.[10-14] Misdiagnosis (e.g., cancer or inflammatory bowel disease) is common.[7,11,14] Omental and mesenteric nodules causing peritonitis and ascites have been reported.[8] Perforation also has occurred resulting from transmural necrosis of the small intestine. Biopsies of intestinal lesions show necrotizing granulomas containing yeast forms of *Histoplasma capsulatum.*

Dermatologic findings, seen in 10% of cases, include erythematous or hyperpigmented papules, pustules, folliculitis, plaques with ulcerations, nodules, eczematous changes, erythema multiforme, and rosacea-like rashes.[15-19] *H. capsulatum* organisms may be seen in biopsies of skin lesions, providing a rapid diagnosis. Rare manifestations include adrenal insufficiency,[20] pericarditis, pleuritis,[21] pancreatitis,[3] prostatitis,[22] and retinitis.[23,24]

Taxonomy

Histoplasma capsulatum var. *capsulatum* is an ascomycete whose teleomorphic state is *Ajellomyces capsulatus.*[25] It is classified in the family Arthrodermataceae, order Onygenales of the Ascomycotina. Other varieties include *H. capsulatum* var. *duboisii* and *farciminosum*.

Biology

Histoplasma capsulatum grows as a mold in the soil and is found primarily in microfoci containing large amounts of rotted guano where starlings have roosted or bats have inhabited. The mold is comprised of hyphae bearing large tuberculate macroconidia (8 to 14 μm in diameter), which are characteristic of *H. capsulatum,* and smaller microconidia (2 to 5 μm), which are the infectious form of the organism (Fig. 37–1). It causes infection when conidia are inhaled. At temperatures above 35°C *H. capsulatum* grows as a yeast measuring 2 to 3 $\times$ 3 to 4 μm in diameter. The yeast form is typically found in infected tissues (Fig. 37–1). Old foci of infection may reactivate in immunosuppressed individuals with quiescent histoplasmosis. Person-to-person transmission does not occur, except possibly in rare cases of direct inoculation in persons with genital lesions caused by histoplasmosis.

Cellular immunity plays the key role in defense against *H. capsulatum.* With development of specific T cell-mediated immunity, cytokines including interferon-γ and interleukin-12 (IL-12) arm macrophages to kill the fungus and halt progression of the disease.[26] If cell-mediated immunity is impaired, an appropriate immune response to the infection cannot occur, leading to a progressive disseminated infection. Macrophages from human immunodeficiency virus (HIV)-infected patients demonstrate impaired fungicidal activity against *H. capsulatum.*[27]

Epidemiology

Histoplasmosis occurs in 2% to 5% of patients with AIDS from endemic areas and up to 25% from selected cities in the United States (Kansas City, Indianapolis, Nashville, Memphis).[3,21] Cases in patients in the endemic region usually are caused by exogenous exposure but less commonly result from reactivation of an old infection.

Histoplasmosis occurs in fewer than 1% of patients from nonendemic areas, where reactivation of latent infection is

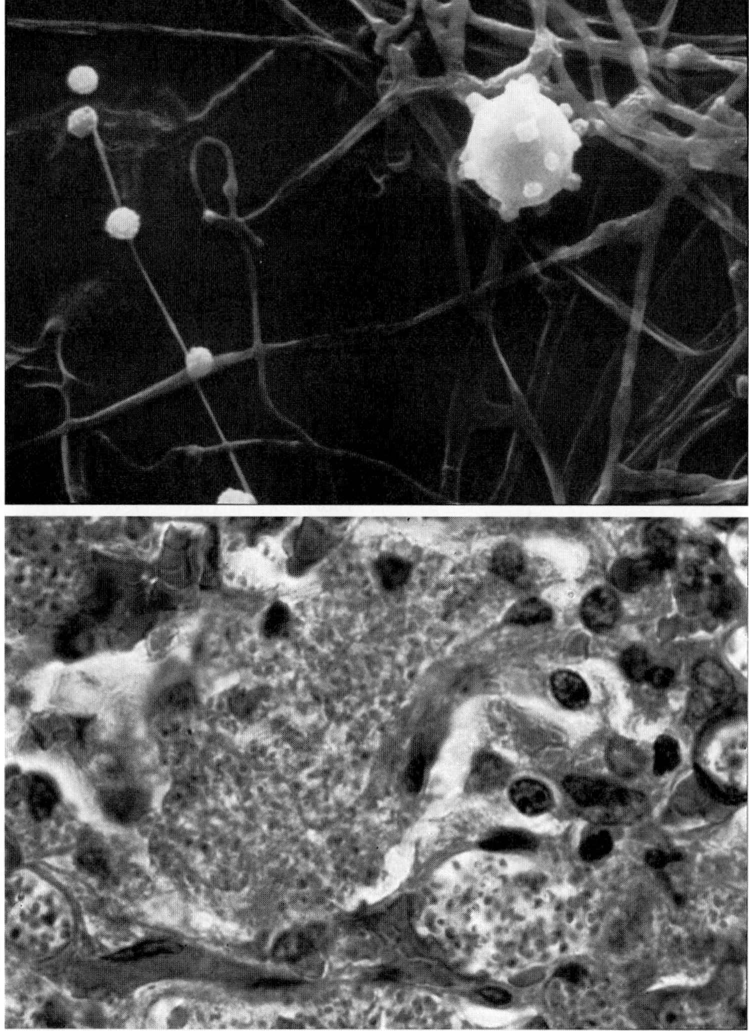

Figure 37–1. *Top,* Electron micrographs showing mold phase from a culture with large tuberculated macroconidia and smaller microconidia. *Bottom,* Hematoxylin and eosin stain showing intracellular yeasts in tissue.

more likely than exogenous infection.[28] Identification of a mitochondrial DNA pattern characteristic of Latin American strains in Puerto Rican immigrants supports this hypothesis.[28] Disseminated histoplasmosis was identified at autopsy in 8% of patients with AIDS from Brazil and 44% from Venezuela.[29] Cutaneous involvement appears to be more common in South American cases. Cases also have been reported in Europe, Africa, and Southeast Asia. Infection with *H. capsulatum* var. *duboisii* has been reported in patients with AIDS who have lived in Africa.[30,31]

Microbiology

Growth on mycologic media at 25° to 30°C is slow, requiring incubation for up to 4 weeks. Mold colonies vary from white to buff brown. Definitive identification requires conversion of the mold to the yeast, demonstration of specific reactivity with anti-*H. capsulatum* antiserum (exoantigen tests), or reactivity with DNA probes specific for *Histoplasma* mRNA.[32]

▲ DIAGNOSIS

Direct Detection

Staining of tissue sections using a variety of staining techniques (Giemsa, Gram, hematoxylin and eosin, Wright) reveals yeast cells measuring about 3 μm in diameter, with occasional buds (Fig. 37–1). Wright stains of blood smears may permit rapid diagnosis in up to one-half of patients (Table 37–1). Yeasts may be identified more easily using special fungal stains such as Gomori methenamine silver (GMS). The highest yield is from bone marrow, positive in 50% to 75% of patients.[3,33,34] *H. capsulatum* may be seen in peripheral blood smears in patients with more se-vere manifestations.[33–36] Care must be taken when interpreting fungal stains, however, as other organisms (especially *Candida glabrata* and *Pneumocystis carinii* and staining artifacts may be misidentified as *H. capsulatum.*

Antigen Detection

Detection of antigen in body fluids permits rapid diagnosis of disseminated histoplasmosis.[37–39] Guidelines for diagnosis using a battery of serologic and mycologic tests are reviewed in Figure 37–2. Antigen is detected in the urine of 95% and the serum of 85% of patients with disseminated histoplasmosis.[38] Antigen may be detected in bronchoalveolar lavage fluid[40] and cerebrospinal fluid[41,42] of patients with pulmonary or meningeal involvement. Tests for antigen may be falsely negative in patients with mild clinical manifestations or localized sites of dissemination such as gastrointestinal or skin ulcers, and they may be falsely positive in those with other systemic mycoses caused by organisms that contain cross-reactive antigens (*Blastomyces dermatitidis, Penicillium marneffei, Paracoccidioides braziliensis*).[43] Testing is available at the Histoplasmosis Reference Laboratory; no other laboratories perform this test. Information about shipping of specimens can be obtained as follows: 1-800-HISTODG; fax 317-630-8605; e-mail histodgn@iupui.edu; internet www.iupui.edu/~histodgn.

Cultures

Histoplasma capsulatum can be isolated from blood, bone marrow, respiratory secretions, or localized lesions in more than 85% of cases.[3,34–36,38] Centrifugation-lysis methods are superior to other blood culture methods. Cultures from respiratory specimens are positive in 50% to 75% of cases. However, isolation of *H. capsulatum* may take 2 to 4 weeks, delaying diagnosis and initiation of therapy. Fungal cultures should be held for 4 weeks because of the slow growth rate. Blood cultures should be performed in all cases. Biopsies of bone marrow, liver, or other tissues may provide a diagnosis if fungal stains and tests for antigen are negative.

Serologic Tests

High levels of antibodies develop within 4 to 6 weeks and peak over the next few months. Serologic tests are

▲ **Table 37–1.** DIAGNOSTIC APPROACH

Test	Sensitivity (%)	Recommend	Comment
Skin test	<5	No	Not of use for diagnosis of histoplasmosis and may boost antibodies
Serology			
Immunodiffusion	50	Yes	M band may persist for years
Complement fixation	60	Yes	Titers ≥ 1:32 more indicative of active infection
Antigen testing			Rapid diagnosis, within one work day
Urine	95	Yes	False-negative in mild cases
Serum	80	Yes	Useful for monitoring therapy in conjunction with test on urine
Alveolar lavage	70	Yes	More sensitive than fungal stain
CSF	50	Yes	Borderline levels (1–2 units) may be seen in patients without meningitis
Cultures	85	Yes	Blood and bone marrow most sensitive, but cultures from other sites of infection also recommended
Fungal stains	50	Yes	Rapid diagnosis but requires experienced pathologist and sensitivity lower than antigen detection

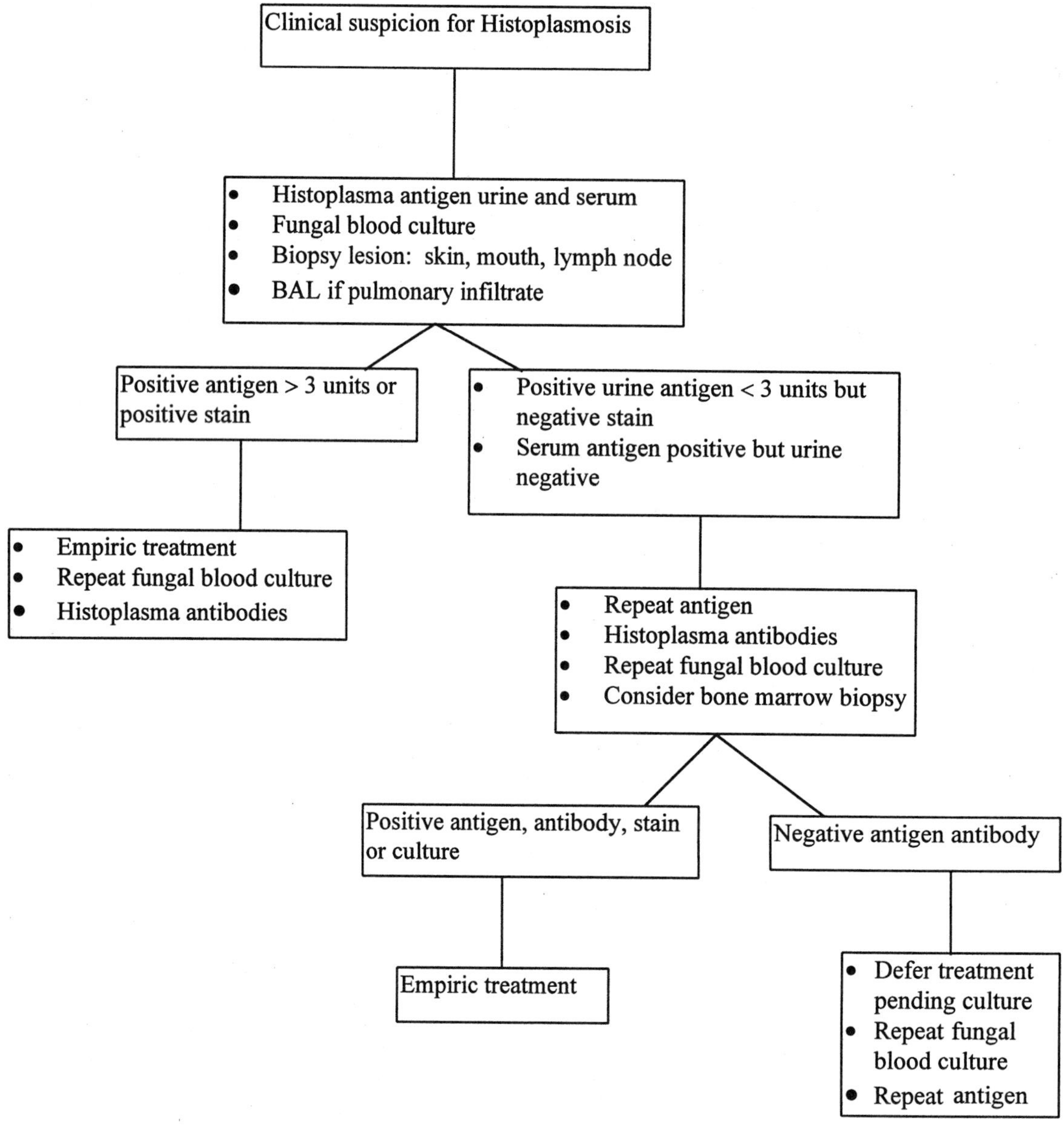

Figure 37–2. Algorithm for evaluating suspected histoplasmosis.

positive in more than two-thirds of cases in patients with AIDS.[3,38] The immunodiffusion and complement fixation tests should be performed to achieve maximum sensitivity and are recommended for all patients suspected of having histoplasmosis. Complement fixation test results are expressed as titers, and positive results in serum range from 1:8 to 1:512 or more. Titers of 1:32 or more are more diagnostic of active infection; but titers of 1:8 and 1:16 should not be disregarded, as they occur in up to 20% of cases. Titers of 1:8 and 1:16 and M-precipitin bands by immunodiffusion also may represent past infection and must be interpreted cautiously to avoid misdiagnosis of histoplasmosis in patients with other infectious, inflammatory, or malignant diseases. When testing CSF, it should begin with undiluted fluid; detection of reactivity at any titer is considered positive. Whereas the immunodiffusion test is simple to perform and can be done at most hospital laboratories, the complement fixation test should be performed only at laboratories that are experienced with this technology using standardized reagents. Testing is available at the Histoplasmosis Reference Laboratory. Serologic tests may provide the sole basis for diagnosis.

Skin Tests

Histoplasmin skin tests are not useful for diagnosing histoplasmosis and should not be performed. Furthermore, skin testing reagents for histoplasmosis are no longer produced. Skin tests would be expected to be negative in patients with AIDS who have disseminated histoplasmosis because of the defect in cell-mediated immunity associated with advanced HIV infection. In a study of HIV-positive volunteers from endemic areas who had CD4+ T-lymphocyte counts below 150/μl, only 2.4% had positive histoplasmin skin tests.[44] The expected skin test positivity in healthy individuals who reside in endemic areas is 50% to 80%. Skin tests boost antibody levels, confounding the use of serologic tests for diagnosing histoplasmosis. Skin testing is inappropriate for diagnosis but may be useful when assessing immune function and risk for histoplasmosis. A positive skin test might indicate intact immunity and resistance to infection with *H. capsulatum,* a hypothesis yet to be tested. Other methods to test for cellular immunity include the lymphoproliferative response and induced interferon-γ production upon incubation with *Histoplasma* antigens, tests that are available only in research laboratories.

▲ TREATMENT

Approach to Therapy

Disseminated histoplasmosis is a progressive, fatal infection in patients with AIDS. Treatment guidelines are summarized in Figure 37–3 and take into account the severity of the illness and other factors that may affect selection of antifungal agents. Patients who recover following treatment relapse within 3 to 18 months if suppressive therapy is not used.[3] Thus treatment includes an induction phase to produce a clinical remission and a suppressive maintenance phase to prevent relapse.

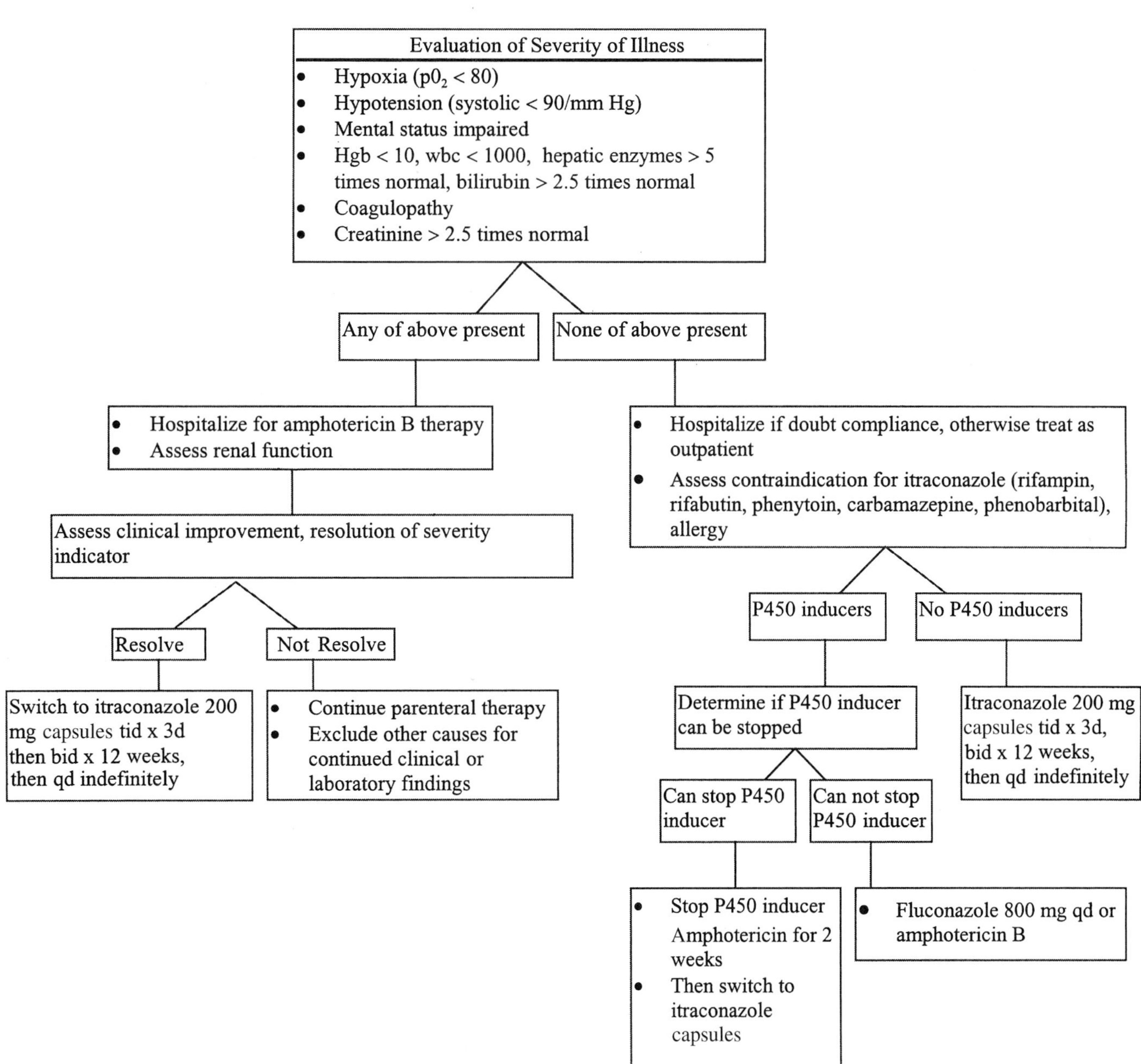

Figure 37–3. Selection of antifungal therapy for histoplasmosis.

Liposomal amphotericin B (AmBisome) is more effective than the standard deoxycholate formulation of amphotericin B in patients with moderately severe or severe clinical manifestations of disseminated histoplamosis, inducing a more rapid, more complete response, lowering mortality, and reducing toxicity.[45] The role of the intravenous formulation of itraconazole for treatment of hospitalized cases remains to be determined, but it would be an alternative in patients who cannot take any of the amphotericin B formulations because of toxicity or allergy. Hospitalization is indicated for persons with marked laboratory abnormalities, neurologic impairment, hypoxia, hypotension, or serious concurrent infections, or who are difficult to treat and monitor at home. Oral therapy with itraconazole is effective in persons with mild illness who are not ill enough to require hospitalization. Posaconazole and voriconazole also are active against *H. capsulatum* and may prove to be alternatives to the standard agents, but they have not been studied in humans. The echinocandidin caspofungin has minimal in vitro or in vivo activity against histoplasmosis and should not be used for this indication.

Histoplasma antigen levels fall with therapy[1,3,46] and increase with relapse.[47] An antigen increase of more than two units suggests recurrence and supports further laboratory evaluation and consideration of resuming of induction therapy. Use of the antigen test to diagnose relapse requires measurement of antigen levels at 4- to 6-month intervals.[48]

Specific Drugs

Liposomal Amphotericin B

A prospective, double-blind study in patients with AIDS and disseminated histoplasmosis showed liposomal amphotericin B *(AmBisome)* to be more effective than the standard deoxycholate formulation.[45] With a 2:1 randomization to liposomal amphotericin B 3 mg/kg/day (n = 51) versus the deoxycholate formulation (n = 22) for 2 weeks followed by itraconazole, a clinical response by week 2 occurred in 88% of the liposomal group versus 64% of the standard treatment group (P = 0.014) (Table 37–2). Patients receiving the liposomal preparation also defervesced more rapidly (P = 0.09) and exhibited improved survival (P = 0.04). There were three deaths due to histoplasmosis in the standard treatment group versus a single death in the liposomal amphotericin B group, the latter caused by staphylococcal bacteremia rather than histoplasmosis. These findings support use of the liposomal preparation for moderately severe or severe cases. The other lipid preparations have not been studied in histoplasmosis and should not be presumed to be as effective as liposomal amphotericin B.

Amphotericin B

Amphotericin B is highly effective in patients who are not severely ill. Of 56 AIDS patients with non-life-threatening manifestations, 55 (98%) experienced a clinical remission[4] (Table 37–2). Clinical improvement occurred within 1 week in more than 80% of patients.[3,50] The mortality is high, however, in patients with severe manifestations, including shock or respiratory failure. Of 17 patients presenting with the sepsis syndrome at the Indiana University Hospitals, 8 (47%) died despite amphotericin B treatment. Often impaired renal function worsened during treatment and precluded aggressive therapy with daily doses of 50 mg of amphotericin B. Amphotericin B also was less effective in patients with meningitis; of 13 patients, 8 died (62%) during treatment.[3]

Itraconazole

Itraconazole capsules 200 mg three times daily for 3 days, then twice daily for 12 weeks, was effective therapy for patients with mild or moderate clinical manifestations of histoplasmosis, inducing remission in 85% of cases.[2] Fever resolved within 1 week in most patients. Treatment failures occurred in those with more severe clinical manifestations and in one patient with undetectable itraconazole blood concentrations. Itraconazole does not penetrate the CSF and has not been evaluated for treatment of *Histoplasma* meningitis. Blood concentrations should be monitored, and concentrations of at least 1 μg/ml by bioassay [about 300 ng/ml by high performance liquid chromatography (hplc)] are therapeutic for treatment of histoplasmosis.

Itraconazole requires an acidic pH for solubilization and should be given with food or Cola.[51] If patients must receive H_2-blockers or omeprazole, a new oral solution formulation of itraconazole overcomes problems associated with reduced gastric acidity. P_{450} inducers (rifampin, rifabutin, phenytoin, phenobarbital) reduce itraconazole blood concentrations and should be avoided (Table 37–3). The solution formulation of itraconazole may circumvent the problem

▲ **Table 37–2.** OUTCOME OF INDUCTION THERAPY FOR HISTOPLASMOSIS

Treatment	No.	Dose	Response (%)	Study
Amphotericin[a]	73	~50 mg/d	88	Wheat[3]
Severe disease	17		53	Wheat[4]
Moderate	56		98	Wheat[4]
Amphotericin B[b]	22	0.7 mg/kg/d × 14 days	64	Johnson[45]
Liposomal amphotericin B[b]	51	3 mg/kg/d × 14 days	88	Johnson[45]
Itraconazole[b]	59	400 mg/d	88	Wheat[2]
Fluconazole[b]	49	800 mg/d	74	Wheat[49]
Ketoconazole[a]	11	200–400 mg/d	9	Wheat[3]

[a]Data obtained by retrospective chart review of cases at Indiana University Medical Center hospitals.

[b]Results from prospective controlled clinical trials conducted by investigators of the AIDS Clinical Trials Group, Mycoses Study Group, or both.

▲ **Table 37–3.** IMPORTANT TRIAZOLE–P_{450} DRUG INTERACTIONS

P_{450} Inducers that Reduce Itraconazole Concentration
Rifampin (Rifadin)[52]
Rifabutin (Mycobutin)
Isoniazid
Carbamazepine (Tegretol)[52]
Phenobarbital
Phenytoin (Dilantin)[52]
Itraconazole and Fluconazole Delays Increased Levels of
Terfenadine (Seldane)[53,54a]
Astemizole (Hismanal)
Cisapride (Propulsid)
Midazolam (Versed)[55]
Triazolam (Halcion)
Simvastatin (Zocor)
Lovastatin (Mevacor)
Phenytoin (Dilantin)[56]
Cyclosporin (Sandimmune)[57,58]
Tacrolimus (Prograf)
Oral hypoglycemics
Coumadin[59]
Digitalis[60]
Calcium channel blockers
Quinidine
Protease inhibitors: ritonavir, indinavir, saquinavir, nelfinavir

[a]Concurrent administration of medications in italics should be strictly avoided because of profound reduction of itraconazole blood levels with rifampin and rifabutin and the potential for life-threatening adverse events with terfenadine, astemizole, cisapride, triazolam, and midazolam.

with absorption and interactions with medications that reduce gastric acidity but still interact with P_{450} inducers.

Itraconazole inhibits hepatic P_{450} enzymes and thus slows the metabolism and increases the blood concentrations of many other drugs. Concurrent treatment with the following medications can cause serious toxicities and should be avoided: terfenadine (Seldane), astemizole (Hismanal), cisapride (Propulsid), triazolam (Halcion), lovastatin (Mevacor), and simvastatin (Zocor). Itraconazole also increases the concentrations of phenytoin, warfarin (Coumadin), oral hypoglycemics, digitalis, calcium-channel blockers, midazolam (Versed), cyclosporin, tacrolimus (Prograf), and antiretroviral protease inhibitors and may potentiate their toxicities. Concurrent therapy with itraconazole and these agents should be monitored to prevent complications.

Itraconazole has been well tolerated, requiring discontinuation in fewer than 10% of patients.[1,2] The most common side effects are gastrointestinal and include nausea (10%), vomiting (5%), diarrhea (3%), and abdominal pain (1%). Rash occurs in 5% to 10% of cases and can be severe. Patients who have experienced rashes caused by itraconazole have been successfully treated with itraconazole following desensitization.[61] Hypertension, edema, and hypokalemia may occur, particularly in patients receiving high doses (600 mg/day).[62–64] Ventricular fibrillation caused by itraconazole-induced hypokalemia has been reported.[65] Liver enzyme elevation occurs in 4% of patients, but clinically significant hepatitis is rare.[66]

Fluconazole

Fluconazole, at a dose of 800 mg/day, induced remission in 74% of AIDS patients with mild to moderately severe manifestations of disseminated histoplasmosis (Table 37–2), but one-third relapsed during maintenance treatment with 400 mg/day.[49] The poorer response to fluconazole than to itraconazole is caused by its reduced in vitro activity for *H. capsulatum* and is further aggravated by the development of resistance during therapy.[67] Fluconazole achieves high levels in CSF and may play a role in the treatment of meningitis.

Ketoconazole

Ketoconazole is not an acceptable treatment for histoplasmosis in patients with AIDS. Fewer than 10% of patients with AIDS responded to ketoconazole induction therapy, (Table 37–2).[3,68] Reasons for ketoconazole's ineffectiveness may be poor absorption[69] or noncompliance caused by gastrointestinal side effects.

Others

The newer triazoles, such as Schering 59562, may offer advantages over itraconazole and should be studied for treatment of histoplasmosis.

Maintenance Treatment

Suppressive maintenance treatment is indicated to prevent relapse. Relapse occurred in 35%[68] to 80%[3] of patients who did not receive maintenance therapy. Amphotericin B (50 to 100 mg weekly or biweekly)[3,70] and itraconazole (200 to 400 mg daily)[1] are more than 90% effective as maintenance therapy (Table 37–4). Fluconazole is less effective. Relapse occurred in 12% of patients receiving 100 to 400 mg of fluconazole for maintenance after completing induction therapy with amphotericin B in a retrospective trial[73] and in 31% of those in a prospective trial receiving fluconazole 400 mg/day after successful induction therapy with 800 mg/day.[49]

Itraconazole 200 mg once or twice daily to maintain blood concentrations of at least 1 μg/ml (by bioassay) is the maintenance treatment of choice. Guidelines for use of serum concentrations of itraconazole and antigen levels in serum and urine to follow patients during maintenance therapy are summarized in Figure 37–4. Reasons for treatment failure may include poor compliance with therapy, use of other medications that interfere with the absorption or accelerate the metabolism of itraconazole, or malabsorption. Failure of fluconazole maintenance

▲ **Table 37–4.** OUTCOME OF MAINTENANCE THERAPY FOR HISTOPLASMOSIS

Treatment	No.	Response (%)	Study
Amphotericin 50 mg/wk	21	81	McKinsey[71]
Itraconazole			
400 mg	42	92	Wheat[1]
200 mg	46	89	Hecht[72]
Fluconazole			
100–400 mg	72	88	Norris[73]
400 mg	36	64	Wheat[49]
Ketoconazole 200–400 mg	20	50	Wheat[3]

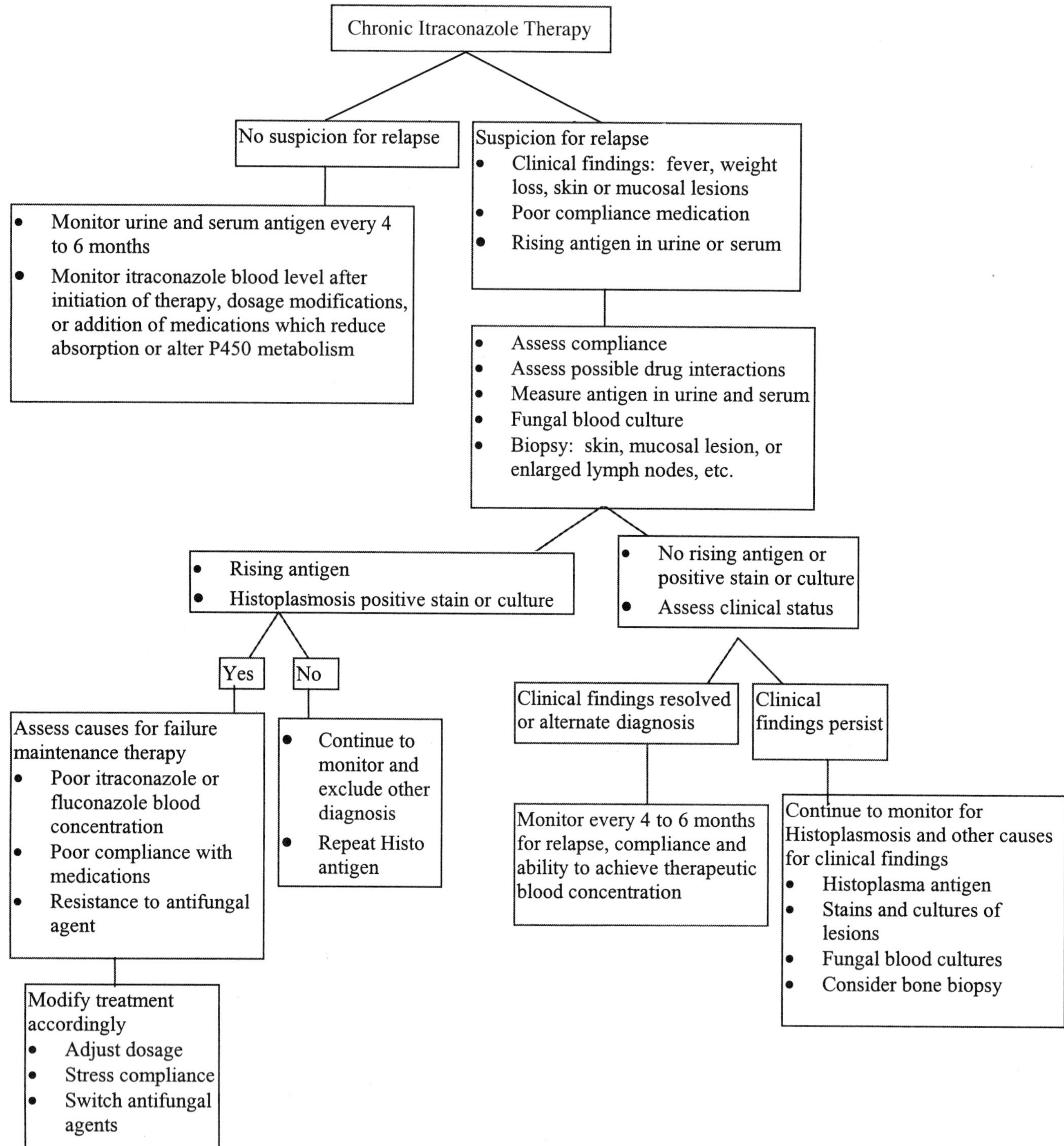

Figure 37–4. Follow-up of patients receiving therapy for histoplasmosis.

therapy may be caused by development of resistance during therapy.[67]

A study is in progress to determine if chronic maintenance therapy can be safely stopped in patients who are in remission, with *Histoplasma* antigen concentrations in urine and serum at less than 4 units, who have completed at least 1 year of treatment, and who have experienced improvement in their CD4+ T-lymphocyte count to more than 150 cells/mm^3 following potent antiretroviral therapy. To date, of more than 30 patients enrolled in that study, none has relapsed.

Recommendations for Treatment

Liposomal amphotericin B (AmBisome) 3 mg/kg/day is the treatment of choice for patients with moderately severe or

▲ **Table 37–5.** GUIDELINES FOR TREATMENT

Severity	Drug	Dose	Duration
Induction			
Mild	Itraconazole[a]	400 mg/d	3 Months
Moderate or severe	Liposomal amphotericin B then itraconazole	3 mg/kg/d	0.5–2.0 Weeks
		400 mg/d	10 Weeks
Maintenance			
	Itraconazole[a]	200 mg/d	Life
		or	
		400 mg/d[2]	Life

[a]Fluconazole is an alternative if itraconazole is contraindicated, using 800 mg/day for induction and 600–800 mg/day for maintenance. Itraconazole 200 mg twice daily should be continued if the bioassay concentration is below 4 μg/ml on 200 mg twice daily.

severe clinical manifestations of histoplasmosis who require hospitalization, (Table 37–5; Fig. 37–3). If the deoxycholate formulation of amphotericin B is used, the dose should be 50 mg/day or 1 mg/kg in individuals weighing less than 50 kg, and it should be given for 3 to 14 days followed by treatment with itraconazole.

Itraconazole 200 mg three times daily for 3 days, then twice daily for 3 months, is recommended for patients with mild or moderate manifestations of histoplasmosis. The capsule formulation should be given with food or Cola, and the solution should be given on an empty stomach for the best absorption. Rifampin and rifabutin must be strictly avoided, and treatment with other agents that induce hepatic P_{450} enzymes should be strongly discouraged. The oral solution formulation should be used in patients who require treatment with H_2-blockers or omeprazole, have thrush refractory to treatment with the capsules, or have low blood concentrations while receiving the capsules. Blood concentrations should be measured during the second week of therapy about 2 hours after a dose. Fluconazole 800 mg/day might be used in patients who require treatment with rifampin or rifabutin, have undetectable itraconazole blood concentrations, or have meningitis. Patients receiving fluconazole for histoplasmosis should be followed closely for relapse.[67] Voriconazole or posaconazole also may play a role in patients unable to take itraconazole.

▲ PREVENTION

Fluconazole did not prevent histoplasmosis in a trial of persons with CD4+ T-lymphocyte counts below 200/μl, although the sample size and incidence of histoplasmosis were inadequate to assess its efficacy fully for this purpose.[74] In that study, histoplasmosis occurred in 1.4% of persons receiving fluconazole versus 2.4% of those receiving clotrimazole, (Table 37–6). A trial comparing itraconazole 200 mg/day versus placebo in persons with CD4+ T-lymphocyte counts below 150/μl showed more than a twofold reduction of histoplasmosis in the itraconazole group (2.7% vs. 6.8%).[75] Itraconazole also prevented cryptococcosis (eight cases in the control group versus one in the itraconazole group). It is note that three of the four patients who developed histoplasmosis and the single patient who developed cryptococcal meningitis in the itraconazole group had stopped prophylaxis several months earlier. All of the histoplasmosis and cryptococcosis cases occurred in patients with CD4+ T-lymphocyte counts below 100/mm^3. Itraconazole failed to prevent recurrent oral candidiasis or esophagitis, which occurred in about 15% of patients in both groups and appeared to select for resistance to both itraconazole and fluconazole.[76] Prophylaxis had no impact on survival, however, probably because of the excellent outcome in patients who are followed closely in clinical trials. Prophylaxis warrants consideration in areas with high combined rates of histoplasmosis and cryptococcosis (about 10% per year in patients with CD4+ T-lymphocyte counts below 100/μl).

▲ **Table 37–6.** TRIALS OF PROPHYLAXIS FOR HISTOPLASMOSIS

Study	Regimen	Breakthrough rate[a]
Powderly[74]	Fluconazole 200 mg/d	3/217 (1.4%)
	Clotrimazole 50 mg/d	5/211 (2.4%)
McKinsey[75]	Itraconazole 200 mg/d	4/149 (2.7%)[b]
	Placebo	10/146 (6.8%)

[a]Number/total (percent) who developed histoplasmosis.
[b]Of the four who developed histoplasmosis on the itraconazole arm of the study, three had stopped the itraconazole more than a month before the illness.

REFERENCES

1. Wheat J, Hafner R, Wulfson M, et al. Prevention of relapse of histoplasmosis with itraconazole in patients with the acquired immunodeficiency syndrome. Ann Intern Med 118:610, 1993.
2. Wheat J, Hafner R, Korzun AH, et al. Itraconazole treatment of disseminated histoplasmosis in patients with the acquired immunodeficiency syndrome. Am J Med 98:336, 1995.
3. Wheat LJ, Connolly-Stringfield PA, Baker RL, et al. Disseminated histoplasmosis in the acquired immune deficiency syndrome: clinical findings, diagnosis and treatment, and review of the literature. Medicine 69:361, 1990.
4. Wheat L. Histoplasmosis in the acquired immunodeficiency syndrome. Curr Top Med Mycol 7:7, 1996.
5. Wheat LJ, Batteiger BE, Sathapatayavongs B. Histoplasma capsulatum infections of the central nervous system: a clinical review. Medicine 69:244, 1990.
6. Anaissie E, Fainstein V, Samo T, et al. Central nervous system histoplasmosis: an unappreciated complication of the acquired immunodeficiency syndrome. Am J Med 84:215, 1988.
7. Clarkston WK, Bonacini M, Peterson I. Colitis due to Histoplasma capsulatum in the acquired immune deficiency syndrome. Am J Gastroenterol 86:913, 1991.
8. Alterman DD, Cho KC. Histoplasmosis involving the omentum in an AIDS patient: CT demonstration. J Comput Assist Tomogr 12:664, 1988.

9. Lamps LW, Molina CP, West AB, et al. The pathologic spectrum of gastrointestinal and hepatic histoplasmosis. Am J Clin Pathol 113:64, 2000.
10. Eisig S, Boguslaw B, Cooperband B, Phelan J. Oral manifestations of disseminated histoplasmosis in acquired immunodeficiency syndrome: report of two cases and review of the literature. J Oral Maxillofac Surg 49:310, 1991.
11. Forsmark CE, Wilcox CM, Darragh TM, Cello JP. Disseminated histoplasmosis in AIDS: an unusual case of esophageal involvement and gastrointestinal bleeding. Gastrointest Endosc 36:604, 1990.
12. Machado AA, Coelho ICB, Roselino AMF, et al. Histoplasmosis in individuals with acquired immunodeficiency syndrome (AIDS): report of six cases with cutaneous-mucosal involvement. Mycopathologic 115:13, 1991.
13. Heinic GS, Greenspan D, MacPhail LA, et al. Oral Histoplasma capsulatum infection in association with HIV infection: a case report. J Oral Pathol Med 21:85, 1992.
14. Graham BS, McKinsey DS, Driks MR, Smith DL. Colonic histoplasmosis in acquired immunodeficiency syndrome: report of two cases. Dis Colon Rectum 34:185, 1991.
15. Eidbo J, Sanchez RL, Tschen JA, Ellner KM. Cutaneous manifestations of histoplasmosis in the acquired immune deficiency syndrome. Am J Surg Pathol 17:110, 1993.
16. Cohen PR, Bank DE, Silvers DN, Grossman ME. Cutaneous lesions of disseminated histoplasmosis in human immunodeficiency virus-infected patients. J Am Acad Dermatol 23:422, 1990.
17. Barton EN, Roberts L, Ince WE et al. Cutaneous histoplasmosis in the acquired immune deficiency syndrome: a report of three cases from Trinidad. Trop Geogr Med 40:153, 1988.
18. Wasserteil V, Jimenez-Acosta FJ, Kerdel FA. Disseminated histoplasmosis presenting as a rosacea-like eruption in a patient with the acquired immunodeficiency syndrome. Int J Dermatol 29:649, 1990.
19. Ferrandiz C, Ribera M. Eosinophilic pustular folliculitis in patients with acquired immunodeficiency syndrome. Int J Dermatol 31:193, 1992.
20. Radin DR. Disseminated histoplasmosis: abdominal CT findings in 16 patients. AJR Am J Roentgenol 157:955, 1991.
21. Marshall BC, Cox JK Jr, Carroll KC, Morrison RE. Case report: histoplasmosis as a cause of pleural effusion in the acquired immunodeficiency syndrome. Am J Med Sci 300:98, 1990.
22. Zighelboim J, Goldfarb RA, Mody D, et al. Prostatic abscess due to Histoplasma capsulatum in a patient with the acquired immunodeficiency syndrome. J Urol 147:167, 1992.
23. Macher A, Rodrigues MM, Kaplan W, et al. Disseminated bilateral chorioretinitis due to Histoplasma capsulatum in a patient with the acquired immunodeficiency syndrome. Ophthalmology 92:1159, 1985.
24. Specht CS, Mitchell KT, Bauman AE, Gupta M. Ocular histoplasmosis with retinitis in a patient with acquired immune deficiency syndrome. Ophthalmology 98:1356, 1991.
25. Bowman BH, Taylor JW, White TJ. Molecular evolution of the fungi: human pathogens. Mol Biol Evol 9:893, 1992.
26. Zhou P, Sieve MC, Bennett J, et al. IL-12 prevents mortality in mice infected with Histoplasma capsulatum through induction of IFN-gamma. J Immunol 155:785, 1995.
27. Chaturvedi S, Frame P, Newman SL. Macrophages from human immunodeficiency virus-positive persons are defective in host defense against Histoplasma capsulatum. J Infect Dis 171:320, 1995.
28. Keath EJ, Kobayashi GS, Medoff G. Typing of Histoplasma capsulatum by restriction fragment length polymorphisms in a nuclear gene. J Clin Microbiol 30:2104, 1992.
29. Murillo J, Castro KG. HIV infection and AIDS in Latin America. Infect Dis Clin North Am 8:1, 1994.
30. Arendt V, Coremans-Pelseneer J, Gottlob R, et al. African histoplasmosis in a Belgian AIDS patient. Mycoses 34:59, 1991.
31. Carme B, Itoua Ngaporo A, Ngolet A, et al. Disseminated African histoplasmosis in a Congolese patient with AIDS. J Med Vet Mycol 30:245, 1992.
32. Stockman L, Clark KA, Hunt JM, Roberts GD. Evalutation of commericially available acridinium ester-labeled chemiluminescent DNA probes for culture identification of Blastomyces dermatitidis, Coccidioides immitis, Cryptococcus neoformans, and Histoplasma capsulatum. J Clin Microbiol 31:845, 1993.
33. Kurtin PJ, McKinsey DS, Gupta MR, Driks M. Histoplasmosis in patients with acquired immunodeficiency syndrome: hematologic and bone marrow manifestations. Am J Clin Pathol 93:367, 1990.
34. Zarabi CM, Thomas R, Adesokan A. Diagnosis of systemic histoplasmosis in patients with AIDS. South Med J 85:1171, 1992.
35. Nightingale SD, Parks JM, Pounders SM, et al. Disseminated histoplasmosis in patients with AIDS. South Med J 83:624, 1990.
36. Neubauer MA, Bodensteiner DC. Disseminated histoplasmosis in patients with AIDS. South Med J 85:1166, 1992.
37. Wheat LJ, Kohler RB, Tewari RP. Diagnosis of disseminated histoplasmosis by detection of Histoplasma capsulatum antigen in serum and urine specimens. N Engl J Med 314:83, 1986.
38. Williams B, Fojtasek M, Connolly-Stringfield P, Wheat J. Diagnosis of histoplasmosis by antigen detection during an outbreak in Indianapolis, Ind. Arch Pathol Lab Med 118:1205, 1994.
39. Zimmerman SE, French MLV, Kleiman MB, Wheat LJ. Evaluation of an enzyme-linked immunosorbent assay that uses ferrous metal beads for determination of antihistoplasmal immunoglobulins G and M. J Clin Microbiol 28:59, 1990.
40. Wheat LJ, Connolly-Stringfield PA, Williams B, et al. Diagnosis of histoplasmosis in patients with the acquired immunodeficiency syndrome by detection of Histoplasma capsulatum polysaccharide antigen in bronchoalveolar lavage fluid. Am Rev Respir Dis 145:1421, 1992.
41. Wheat LJ, Kohler RB, Tewari RP, et al. Significance of Histoplasma antigen in the cerebrospinal fluid of patients with meningitis. Arch Intern Med 149:302, 1989.
42. Wheat LJ. Diagnosis and management of fungal infections in AIDS. Curr Opin Infect Dis 6:617, 1993.
43. Wheat J, Wheat H, Connolly P, et al. Cross-reactivity in Histoplasma capsulatum variety capsulatum antigen assays of urine samples from patients with endemic mycoses. Clin Infect Dis 24:1169, 1997.
44. McKinsey DS, Spiegel RA, Hutwagner L, et al. Prospective study of histoplasmosis in patients infected with human immunodeficiency virus: incidence, risk factors, and pathophysiology. Clin Infect Dis 24:1195, 1997.
45. Johnson PC, Wheat LJ, Cloud GA, et al. Safety and efficacy of liposomal amphotericin B compared with conventional amphotericin B for induction therapy of histoplasmosis in patients with AIDS. Ann Intern Med 137:105, 2002.
46. Wheat LJ, Connolly-Stringfield P, Blair R, et al. Effect of successful treatment with amphotericin B on Histoplasma capsulatum variety *capsulatum* polysaccharide antigen levels in patients with AIDS and histoplasmosis. Am J Med 92:153, 1992.
47. Wheat LJ, Connolly-Stringfield P, Blair R, et al. Histoplasmosis relapse in patients with AIDS: detection using Histoplasma capsulatum variety *capsulatum* antigen levels. Ann Intern Med 115:936, 1991.
48. Buckley HR, Richardson MD, Evans EGV, Wheat LJ. Immunodiagnosis of invasive fungal infection. J Med Vet Mycol 30(suppl 1):249, 1992.
49. Wheat J, MaWhinney S, Hafner R, et al. Treatment of histoplasmosis with fluconazole in patients with acquired immunodeficiency syndrome. Am J Med 103:223, 1997.
50. Sathapatayavongs B, Batteiger BE, Wheat LJ, et al. Clinical and laboratory features of disseminated histoplasmosis during two large urban outbreaks. Medicine 62:263, 1983.
51. Chin TWF, Loeb M, Fong IW. Effects of an acidic beverage (Coca-Cola) on absorption of ketoconazole. Antimicrob Agents Chemother 39:1671, 1995.
52. Tucker RM, Denning DW, Hanson LH, et al. Interaction of azoles with rifampin, phenytoin, and carbamazepine: in vitro and clinical observations. Clin Infect Dis 14:165, 1992.
53. Honig PK, Wortham DC, Hull R, et al. Itraconazole affects single-dose terfenadine pharmacokinetics and cardiac repolarization pharmacodynamics. J Clin Pharmacol 33:1201, 1993.
54. Honig PK, Wortham DC, Zamani K, et al. The effect of fluconazole on the steady-state pharmacokinetics and electrocardiographic pharmacodynamics of terfenadine in humans. Clin Pharmacol Ther 53:630, 1993.
55. Olkkola KT, Backman JT, Neuvonen PJ. Midazolam should be avoided in patients receiving the systemic antimycotics ketoconazole or itraconazole. Clin Pharmacol Ther 55:481, 1994.
56. Blum RA, Wilton JH, Hilligoss DM, et al. Effect of fluconazole on the disposition of phenytoin. Clin Pharmacol Ther 49:420, 1991.
57. Kramer MR, Marshall SE, Denning DW, et al. Cyclosporine and itraconazole interaction in heart and lung transplant recipients. Ann Intern Med 113:327, 1990.
58. Sorenson AL, Lovdahl M, Hewitt JM, et al. Effects of ketoconazole on cyclosporine metabolism in renal allograft recipients. Transplant Proc 26:2822, 1994.

59. Crussell-Porter LL, Rindone JP, Ford MA, Jaskar DW. Low-dose fluconazole therapy potentiates the hypoprothrombinemic response of warfarin sodium. Arch Intern Med 153:102, 1993.
60. Sachs MK, Blanchard LM, Green PJ. Interaction of itraconazole and digoxin. Clin Infect Dis 16:400, 1993.
61. Bittleman DB, Stapleton J, Casale TB. Report of successful desensitization to itraconazole. J Allergy Clin Immunol 94:270, 1994.
62. Tucker RM, Haq Y, Denning DW, Stevens DA. Adverse events associated with itraconazole in 189 patients on chronic therapy. J Antimicrob Chemother 26:561, 1990.
63. Rosen T. Debilitating edema associated with itraconazole therapy. Arch Dermatol 130:260, 1994.
64. Sharkey PK, Rinaldi MG, Dunn JF, et al. High-dose itraconazole in the treatment of severe mycoses. Antimicrob Agents Chemother 35:707, 1991.
65. Nelson MR, Smith D, Erskine D, Gazzard BG. Ventricular fibrillation secondary to itraconazole induced hypokalaemia. J Infect 26:348, 1993.
66. Lavrijsen APM, Balmus KJ, Nugteren-Huying WM, et al. Hepatic injury associated with itraconazole. Lancet 340:251, 1992.
67. Wheat J, Marichal P, Vanden Bossche H, et al. Hypothesis on the mechanism of resistance to fluconazole in Histoplasma capsulatum. Antimicrob Agents Chemother 41:410, 1997.
68. Sarosi GA, Johnson PC. Disseminated histoplasmosis in patients infected with human immunodeficiency virus. Clin Infect Dis 14(suppl 1):S60, 1992.
69. Lake-Bakaar G, Tom W, Lake-Bakaar D, et al. Gastropathy and ketoconazole malabsorption in the acquired immunodeficiency syndrome (AIDS). Ann Intern Med 15:471, 1988.
70. McKinsey DS, Gupta MR, Driks M, et al. Histoplasmosis in patients with AIDS: efficacy of maintenance amphotericin B therapy. Am J Med 92:225, 1992.
71. McKinsey DS, Gupta MR, Riddler SA, et al. Long-term amphotericin B therapy for disseminated histoplasmosis in patients with the acquired immune deficiency syndrome. Ann Intern Med 111:655, 1989.
72. Hecht FM, Wheat J, Korzun AH, et al. Itraconazole maintenance treatment for histoplasmosis in AIDS: a prospective, multicenter trial. J Acquir Immune Defic Syndr Hum Retrovirol 16:100, 1997.
73. Norris S, Wheat J, McKinsey D, et al. Prevention of relapse of histoplasmosis with fluconazole in patients with the acquired immunodeficiency syndrome. Am J Med 96:504, 1994.
74. Powderly WG, Finkelstein DM, Feinberg J, et al. A randomized trial comparing fluconazole with clotrimazole troches for the prevention of fungal infections in patients with advanced human immunodeficiency virus infection. N Engl J Med 332:700, 1995.
75. McKinsey DS, Wheat LJ, Cloud GA, et al. Itraconazole prophylaxis for fungal infections in patients with advanced human immunodeficiency virus infection: randomized, placebo-controlled, double-blind study. Clin Infect Dis 28:1049, 1999.
76. Goldman M, Cloud GA, Smedema M, et al. Does long-term itraconazole prophylaxis result in in vitro azole resistance in mucosal Candida albicans isolates from persons with advanced human immunodeficiency virus infection? Antimicrob Agents Chemother 44:1585, 2000.

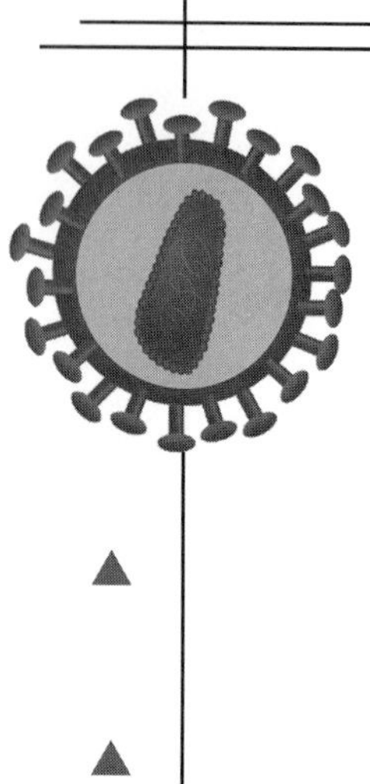

CHAPTER 38

Coccidioidomycosis

Neil M. Ampel, MD

Coccidioidomycosis is an infection caused by the dimorphic fungus *Coccidioides immitis*. The endemic region for this mycosis is confined to the Western hemisphere from California to Argentina. Areas of endemicity tend to coincide with distinct geographic and climatic conditions, principally consisting of alkaline soil in arid, warm regions with relatively mild winters and hot summers. In the United States the endemic region extends from the San Joaquin Valley of California, from which the common name for coccidioidomycosis, valley fever, is derived, to western Texas.[1,2] The areas of highest endemicity are the southern San Joaquin Valley and the region encompassing Phoenix and Tucson in south-central Arizona.[1–3]

In the soil *C. immitis* exists as a mold in which alternating hyphal cells degenerate. The intervening live cells, called arthroconidia, may dislodge and become airborne, particularly in dry, windy conditions. If inhaled by a susceptible host, the arthroconidia can reach the alveolus and begin infection. Once infection occurs, *C. immitis* undergoes a unique transformation among the pathogenic fungi. The outer wall rounds up and internal septations form to yield the spherule stage. These septations give rise to internal endospores. Spherules may rupture and release packets of endospores, propagating the infection within the host.

Among immunocompetent individuals, infection with *C. immitis* is completely asymptomatic in two-thirds of all cases. The other third usually have nonspecific pulmonary symptoms. Approximately 5% of all patients develop chronic disease, either persistent pulmonary illness or infection disseminated beyond the thoracic cavity.[2,4] Patients who develop chronic disease may have been asymptomatic or had symptoms at the time of the initial infection.

Clinical and in vitro studies have all indicated that cell-mediated immunity is important in host defense against coccidioidomycosis.[5–7] In particular, patients who have mild, self-limited disease usually manifest delayed-type hypersensitivity upon skin testing with coccidioidal antigens and have minimal serum antibody responses. On the other hand, patients with chronic, active disease, particularly those with disseminated infection, usually lack coccidioidal delayed-type hypersensitivity and have high serum anti-coccidioidal antibody titers.[5] Because of this, it is not surprising that coccidioidomycosis is recognized as an opportunistic infection among patients with human immunodeficiency virus (HIV) infection, particularly among those living in the coccidioidal endemic area.[8,9]

▲ EPIDEMIOLOGY

During the early part of the HIV epidemic, coccidioidomycosis was not recognized as an opportunistic process in persons infected with HIV. One reason was that the initial epicenters of the HIV epidemic in North America, including the Los Angeles basin, were not in areas endemic for coccidioidomycosis, and reports of cases were sporadic.[10–15] Another reason was that symptomatic coccidioidomycosis often occurs in individuals with no underlying immunodeficiency. The first series of cases of coccidioidomycosis occurring among HIV-infected persons was reported by Bronnimann and colleagues in 1987.[16] In that report, 7 of 27 patients with acquired immunodeficiency syndrome (AIDS) living in southern Arizona developed symptomatic coccidioidomycosis. Six of the seven had diffuse, nodular pulmonary infiltrates, and five had detectable anti-coccidioidal antibodies in their sera; all died within 14 months of the diagnosis of coccidioidomycosis. Since that report, two large case series[17,18] and one prospective study[8] have been reported, expanding our understanding of the clinical expression and epidemiology of coccidioidomycosis during HIV infection.

The impact of coccidioidomycosis on patients infected with HIV infection is not geographically uniform. In Arizona 8.2% of all patients reported to the Centers for Disease Control and Prevention (CDS) as having AIDS had concomitant coccidioidomycosis, compared to only 0.3% nationwide.[9] The impact of coccidioidomycosis on HIV-infected persons living in Arizona is substantial. In 1993 ten percent of all hospitalizations among HIV-infected persons included a discharge diagnosis of coccidioidomycosis. Conversely, 44% of all hospitalizations for coccidioidomycosis during the same year were among HIV-infected patients.[3]

In the CDC study[9] only 0.5% of all patients with AIDS in California were reported to have concomitant coccidioidomycosis. However, the impact of HIV infection on the development of active coccidioidomycosis appears to be significantly greater in the coccidioidal endemic areas within the state. Using data from the California State Health Department, Rutherford found that 3.5% of patients living in Kern County, a known coccidioidal endemic area, were reported to have coccidioidomycosis as their AIDS-defining diagnosis compared to only 0.3% for the entire state.[19]

These data indicate that coccidioidomycosis has become a major opportunistic infection in coccidioidal endemic areas, illustrated by the results of a prospective study from Arizona.[8] In that study, 170 HIV-infected persons who were without active coccidioidomycosis on entry were followed over time. After 41 months 13 of these subjects had developed active coccidioidomycosis, yielding an estimated cumulative incidence of nearly 25%. Only two risk factors, a CD4+ T-lymphocyte count less than 250/μl and the clinical diagnosis of AIDS, were associated with the development of active coccidioidomycosis. Length of stay in the endemic area, history of a prior diagnosis of coccidioidomycosis, and a positive coccidioidal skin test were not associated with a risk of developing active coccidioidomycosis, suggesting that most clinical disease was due to primary infection. Moreover, 11 of the 13 subjects who developed active coccidioidomycosis had either focal or diffuse pulmonary involvement.

For the cases that occur outside the endemic area, reactivation remains the principal way in which patients develop active coccidioidomycosis. Whether there are immunologic and epidemiologic differences between those who develop active coccidioidomycosis in the coccidioidal endemic area compared to those who develop it outside this area is not known. In addition, the only data currently available on coccidioidomycosis and HIV infection are from the United States. Whether coccidioidomycosis will become a major opportunistic infection among HIV-infected persons living in other coccidioidal endemic regions, such as in northern Mexico and Argentina, is not known.

The incidence of most infectious opportunistic infections has declined since the advent of highly active antiretroviral therapy (HAART),[20] and it is reasonable to presume that a decline in the incidence of coccidioidomycosis among those with HIV infection has also occurred. In a retrospective analysis of cases of coccidioidomycosis in southern Arizona from 1994 through 1997,[21] a period that spans the initiation of the use of HAART, the number of cases of coccidioidomycosis among those with HIV infection declined from 77 in 1995 to 15 in 1997. Although no subsequent studies have been performed, the number of cases of coccidioidomycosis among those with HIV infection seen in clinics in the endemic area appears to be lower than that observed prior to the HAART era.

▲ CLINICAL MANIFESTATIONS

The clinical spectrum of coccidioidomycosis among HIV-infected persons has been documented in several case series reports.[8,17,18] Diffuse pneumonia is the most common presentation. This is a devastating form of coccidioidomycosis, with 70% mortality within 1 month.[16–18,22] It presents most often in patients with peripheral blood CD4+ T-lymphocyte counts of less than 50/μl, is frequently associated with fungemia, and undoubtedly represents an acute, severe form of disseminated disease. The presentation is nonspecific, with complaints of fever, night sweats, weight loss, and dyspnea. The chest radiograph reveals diffuse pulmonary nodules with increased interstitial markings, described as "reticulonodular." In some patients this nodularity is striking (Fig. 38–1a), whereas in others the radiographic appearance is more subtle and suggestive of *Pneumocystis carinii* pneumonia (Fig. 38–1b). Concurrent pneumocystosis occurs in up to 30% of patients with diffuse, reticulonodular coccidioidomycosis.[17,23] Even with prompt antifungal therapy, this form of coccidioidomycosis is often rapidly fatal.[17,18]

The second most frequent presentation is focal pneumonia.[17,18] This presentation is more likely to occur in more immunocompetent patients with higher peripheral blood CD4+ T-lymphocyte counts. Patients usually complain of cough, either nonproductive or productive of only scanty sputum, associated with pleuritic chest pain and fever. Bacterial pneumonia is usually the first diagnosis considered. However, the symptoms persist despite antibiotic therapy. The chest radiograph initially reveals a focal alveolar infiltrate (Fig. 38–2). Over time, usually weeks, this infiltrate becomes nodular. The prognosis of focal pulmonary coccidioidomycosis in the HIV-infected patients is better than among those with diffuse pulmonary disease. In one study[17] the median survival of those with focal pulmonary disease was 5 months compared to 1 month in those with diffuse pulmonary disease. Currently, the survival of HIV-infected patients with focal pulmonary coccidioidomycosis who receive appropriate antifungal and antiretroviral therapy is probably not different from patients at a similar stage of HIV illness without coccidioidomycosis.

The most frequent manifestation of disseminated coccidioidomycosis in the HIV-infected patient is meningitis. Coccidioidal meningitis in patients without HIV infection usually presents with headache and decreased mental status, which occurs over weeks to months, usually with no other symptoms of active coccidioidomycosis.[24] The presentation

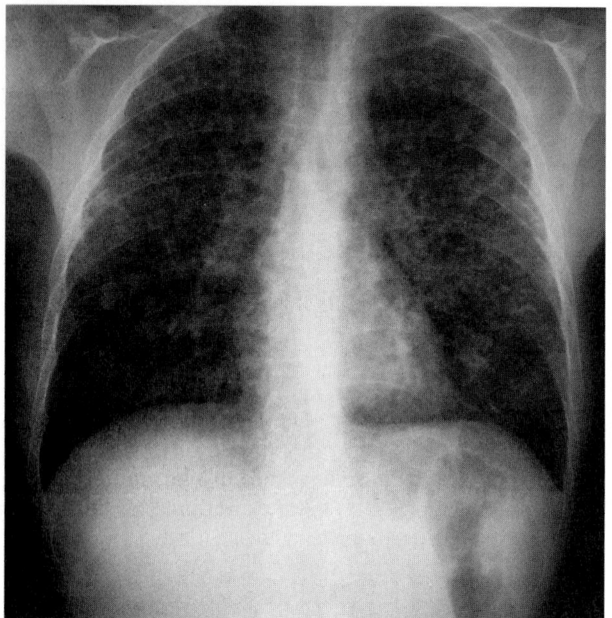

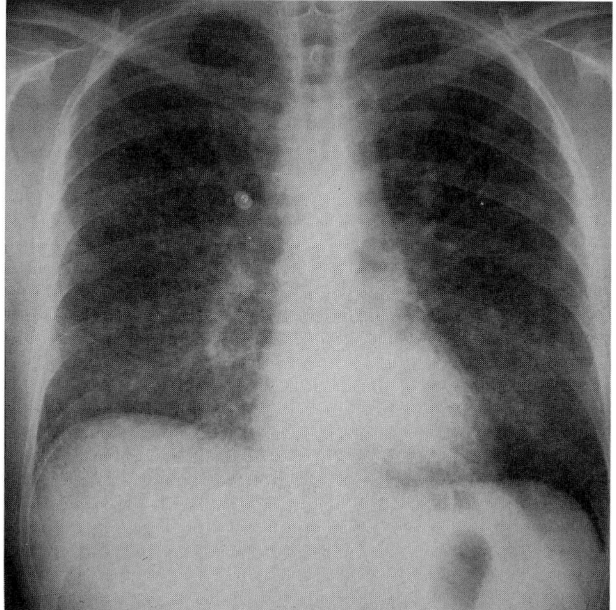

Figure 38–1. Two HIV-infected patients with diffuse reticulonodular coccidioidomycosis. *A*, Chest radiograph from one patient shows diffuse nodularity. *B*, Chest radiograph from another patient reveals a finer, more reticular appearance.

is similar in the HIV-infected patient except that concurrent pulmonary involvement, particularly reticulonodular pneumonia, is more likely to be present.[18] The cerebrospinal fluid (CSF) profile of HIV-infected patients is the same as in other groups of patients. There is a lymphocytic pleocytosis with hypoglycorrhachia. The finding of eosinophils in the CSF is further suggestive.

Other manifestations of disseminated coccidioidomycosis in the HIV-infected patient include cutaneous disease, lymph node involvement, and bone and joint disease. These generally present in a manner similar to that seen in patients without HIV infection, with the exception that bone and joint disease tends to be uncommon in HIV-infected patients. Another form of disseminated coccidioidomycosis is hepatosplenic involvement, manifesting as fever, inanition, elevated coccidioidal serologic titers, and an enlarged liver and spleen. This presentation is similar to that seen with disseminated histoplasmosis in the HIV-infected patient.[25]

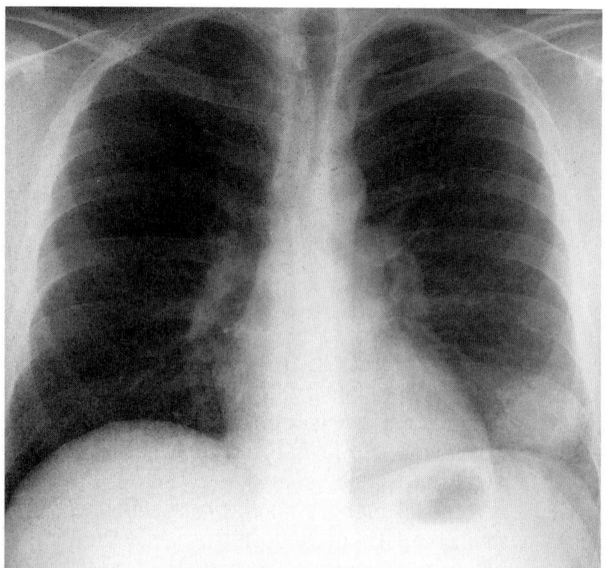

Figure 38–2. Focal, primary coccidioidomycosis in a patient with HIV infection. Chest radiograph reveals a rounded infiltrate in the left lower lobe.

A unique presentation of coccidioidomycosis in the HIV-infected person is a positive serum antibody reaction without clinical manifestations of illness.[8,17] In one study, 5 of 13 individuals with positive coccidioidal serologic tests as their only manifestation of coccidioidomycosis subsequently developed active disease 4 to 35 months after the positive serology was first noted. In four instances patients developed pulmonary coccidioidomycosis, and in the fifth case hepatosplenic coccidioidomycosis occurred. Prior use of antifungal therapy did not significantly reduce the risk of developing active coccidioidomycosis, but the doses and duration of therapy varied considerably. The median peripheral blood CD4+ T-lymphocyte count at the time of development of the positive serologic test was 89/μl, whereas it was 10/μl at the time of development of active disease. Most of the positive tests were of the complement-fixing type, with titers ranging from 1:2 to 1:128.[26] These data suggest that a positive coccidioidal antibody test in an HIV-infected person represents true infection with a significant risk for the development of clinically active disease.

▲ DIAGNOSIS

The first principle when establishing the diagnosis of coccidioidomycosis in the HIV-infected patient is to consider it. Whether within or outside the endemic area, the diagnosis

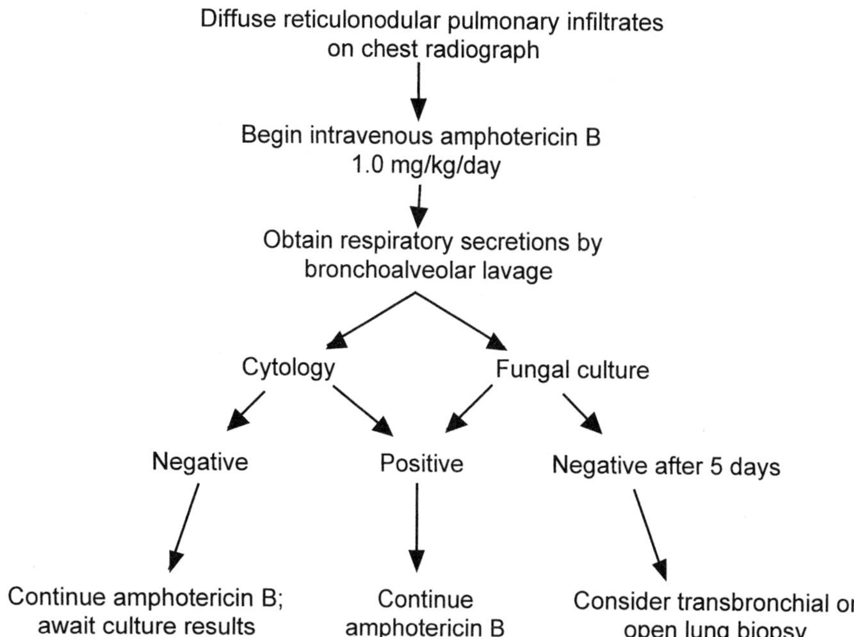

Figure 38-3. Algorithm for the diagnosis and management of diffuse, reticulonodular pulmonary coccidioidomycosis in the HIV-infected patient.

should be entertained in any HIV-infected patient who presents with a diffuse pneumonia, a focal pneumonia not responsive to antibacterial agents, or a lymphocytic meningitis.

There are two general approaches to diagnosing coccidioidomycosis in the HIV-infected patient (Figs. 38–3 and 38–4). The first is to obtain a clinical specimen and directly examine it for the presence of *C. immitis*. With pulmonary involvement, either expectorated sputum or a respiratory sample obtained by bronchoscopy is useful. Direct examination of tissue from biopsy of involved tissue is often required to diagnose cutaneous, lymphoid, or hepatosplenic coccidioidomycosis or the rare case of bone and joint coccidioidomycosis. With meningitis CSF samples rarely reveal the presence of the fungus, and the diagnosis is usually established indirectly by serology.

Once a clinical specimen is in hand, there are several tests available to detect *C. immitis*. The KOH test is commonly used on sputum and respiratory samples. This test is simple to perform, but it has a low yield. The Papanicolaou or Gomori-methenamine stains, particularly when used on a pellet obtained by bronchoalveolar lavage (BAL), have the advantage of allowing identification of spherules of *C. immitis* as well as *Pneumocystis carinii*. However, the yield

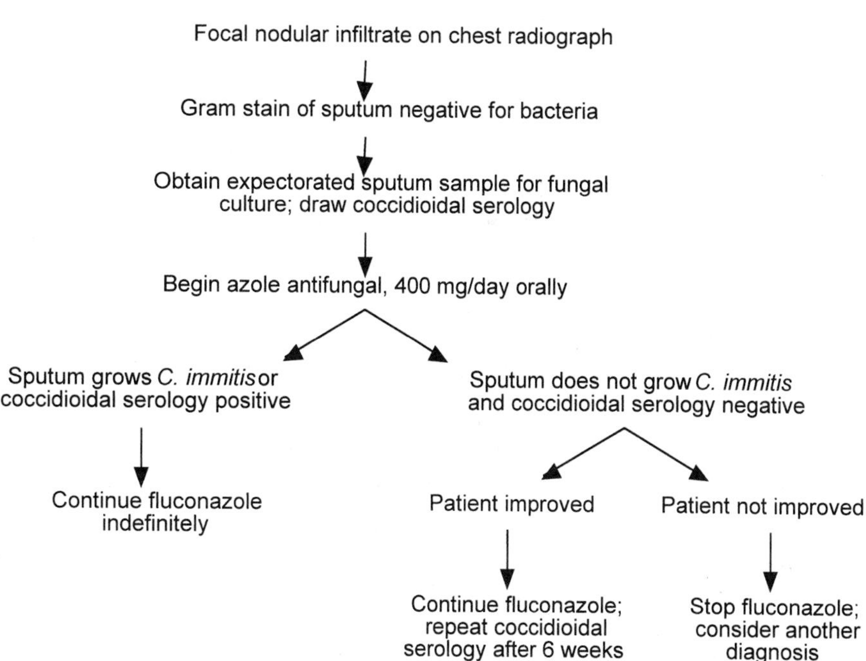

Figure 38-4. Algorithm for the diagnosis and management of focal pulmonary coccidioidomycosis in the HIV-infected patient.

of such cytologic stains for coccidioidomycosis may be as low as 40% in patients with HIV infection.[27] For biopsy specimens, examination of fixed samples stained by hematoxylin-eosin usually reveal the presence of spherules. The Gomori-methenamine stain, by staining spherules and endospores black, may make the organisms more easily identifiable, but it is more time-consuming.

Many clinicians are under the misapprehension that *C. immitis* is fastidious and difficult to cultivate. The fungus usually displays visible colonies in culture in as few as 3 to 7 days on a variety of culture media.[4] However, cultures to detect *C. immitis* should only be performed by laboratories with extensive experience owing to the highly infectious nature of the organism and the resultant risk to laboratory personnel. Culture of respiratory samples and biopsy specimens has a high yield. In one study, culture of respiratory samples revealed the presence of *C. immitis* in 69% of cases. Cultures of lung biopsy specimens were positive in 80%.[18] Therefore any clinical specimen suggestive of containing *C. immitis* should be cultured.

Sequences unique to *C. immitis* have been identified on the gene encoding 18S ribosomal RNA,[28] making genomic identification of the fungus within clinical specimens a possibility. Although genomic identification is now used to confirm the identification of *C. immitis* once it is visibly growing,[29] no assays are currently available for direct identification in clinical specimens. In addition, no test is clinically available to detect antigenemia or antigenuria in patients with coccidioidomycosis.

Without direct evidence of *C. immitis*, detection of anti-coccidioidal antibodies in the serum and CSF has been frequently used to establish the diagnosis of coccidioidomycosis. Understanding coccidioidal serology is complicated by the antiquated nomenclature and changing methodology.[30] Two types of antibody are recognized. Antibodies of the immunoglobulin M (IgM) type, first detected using the tube precipitins (TP) method, occur early in the course of disease or during acute reactivation. Serum titers of anti-coccidioidal IgM antibodies do not predict outcome, and they are rarely positive in the CSF in those with coccidioidal meningitis. In contrast, IgG antibodies, first detected by complement fixation (CF), arise later during the course of disease and are useful for diagnosing meningitis; and serum and CSF titers are helpful for following the course of disease.

In addition to the TP and CF methods, latex agglutination (LA), immunodiffusion (ID), and an enzyme immunoassay (EIA) are also available for detecting anti-coccidioidal antibodies. The LA test is useful only for detecting IgM antibodies and has a high false-positive rate. Any positive result should be confirmed by another method.[30] The ID technique, which detects both TP (IDTP) and CF (IDCF) antibodies, is extremely sensitive and specific.[30,31] The commercially available Premier EIA (Meridian Diagnostics, Cincinnati, OH, USA) detects both IgM and IgG antibodies and appears to be as sensitive and specific as ID,[31–33] although false-positives has been reported.[31] None of these antibody detection systems has been formally studied using samples from HIV-infected patients.

In individuals with HIV infection and coccidioidomycosis, tests for anti-coccidioidal antibodies in the serum are positive at the time of diagnosis in 68% to 100% of patients.[17,18,34] IgG-type antibodies are more likely to be positive than the IgM types.[17] Although some HIV-infected patients never develop positive serologic tests for coccidioidomycosis despite active infection,[34] serology remains an important diagnostic tool for most patients.

▲ TREATMENT

Currently, there are two classes of systemic antifungal agents available for the treatment of coccidioidomycosis in the HIV-infected patient (Table 38–1; Figs. 38–3 and 38–4). The first, amphotericin B, is a polyene antibiotic first introduced in 1955 as a deoxycholate dispersion (Fungizone). Although useful in the treatment of coccidioidomycosis, this form of amphotericin B has numerous drawbacks, including the need for intravenous administration and the appearance of multiple toxicities.[35] Moreover, intravenous amphotericin B is not useful for treating coccidioidal meningitis. For this form of disease, intrathecal administration is required.[36] When using intravenous amphotericin B in the deoxycholate formulation for the treatment of coccidioidomycosis, an initial daily dosage of 1.0 to 1.5 mg/kg should be prescribed. In recent years, several new formulations of amphotericin B have become available for clinical use, including a lipid dispersion (ABLC, ABEL-

▲ TABLE 38–1. RECOMMENDATIONS REGARDING TREATMENT OF ▲ COCCIDIOIDOMYCOSIS IN ADULT PATIENTS INFECTED WITH HIV

Type of Disease	Recommended Therapy	Alternative Therapy
Diffuse pneumonia	IV amphotericin B, 1.0–1.5 mg/kg/d[a]	Fluconazole or itraconazole, at least 400 mg/day[b]
Focal pneumonia	Oral fluconazole or itraconazole, at least 400 mg/day[b]	Amphotericin B 1.0–1.5 mg/kg/d IV followed by oral fluconazole or itraconazole, at least 400 mg/day[b]
Meningitis	Oral fluconazole or itraconazole, beginning at 800 mg/day	Intrathecal amphotericin B[c]
Other forms of dissemination	Oral fluconazole or itraconazole, at least 400 mg/day[b]	Amphotericin B 1.0–1.5 mg/kg/d IV followed by oral fluconazole or itraconazole, at least 400 mg/day[b]
Positive serology only	Oral fluconazole or itraconazole, at least 400 mg/day[b]	Observation

Normal renal and hepatic function is assumed. For all instances of coccidioidomycosis during HIV infection, lifelong therapy is recommended.

[a]Assumes use of the deoxycholate preparation (Fungizone).

[b]Fluconazole preferred because of better absorption, with fewer drug interactions.

[c]Should be administered by someone with prior experience.

CET), a cholesteryl colloidal dispersion (ABCD, Amphotec), and a true liposomal preparation (AmBisome). Despite their reduced toxicity, the efficacy data in animal models and human studies are incomplete.[37–39] Further data are needed[40] before the use of these newer formulations can be recommended for initial treatment of coccidioidomycosis. Currently, their use should be reserved for patients who develop toxicity due to the deoxycholate formulation.[41]

The second group of agents available are the orally absorbable azole antifungals, which include ketoconazole, fluconazole, and itraconazole. Ketoconazole for the treatment of coccidioidomycosis has largely been supplanted by the newer triazoles fluconazole and itraconazole. Although used extensively for the treatment of coccidioidomycosis, neither of these agents is currently approved by the U.S. Food and Drug Administration (FDA) for this purpose.[42] In a variety of studies, both drugs have been found to be useful for treating most forms of coccidioidomycosis in persons without HIV infection.[43–47] However, relapse after therapy is discontinued has been frequent for both drugs.[43,47] Fluconazole and itraconazole differ in terms of their absorption, protein binding, and metabolism.[48] Whereas fluconazole is well absorbed from the gastrointestinal tract and is not affected by food or gastric acid,[49] itraconazole requires the presence of acid for maximum absorption, often a problem in HIV-infected persons.[50]

In study directly comparing fluconazole to itraconazole for the management of coccidioidomycosis, 198 subjects with various forms of chronic coccidioidomycosis were evaluated; 7 had concomitant HIV infection.[51] Among all the subjects, there were no statistically significant differences between those who received fluconazole and those who received itraconazole after 8 months of therapy. In addition, although specific details of the response among those subjects with HIV infection were not provided, HIV infection was not found to be a risk factor for therapy failure. Finally, serum levels of itraconazole did not predict response. Given these data, either fluconazole or itraconazole appears to be an appropriate choice for treating coccidioidomycosis, including among those with HIV infection. Whichever azole antifungal is chosen for therapy, the initial daily dosage for the adult should be at least 400 mg[43,47] to ensure an optimal response. Data suggest that azole antifungals are associated with congenital anomalies.[52] Caution is therefore advised when treating pregnant females with azole antifungals as therapy for coccidioidomycosis; if these agents are used in any female with childbearing potential, they must be combined with effective contraception.

Azole antifungals, particularly ketoconazole and itraconazole, are potent inhibitors of the cytochrome P_{450} (CYP) 3A4 enzyme system.[53] Therefore they may interact with the metabolism of a variety of other drugs. Well recognized interactions of these agents include increased plasma levels of warfarin, phenytoin, digoxin, and cyclosporin. Itraconazole in particular may cause marked increases in the levels of the antihistamines terfenadine and astemazole, resulting in life-threatening cardiac arrhythmias.[48] Fluconazole has been shown to increase the plasma levels of rifabutin, an effect associated with an increase risk of uveitis,[54] and it may retard zidovudine metabolism.[55] There are few data on interaction of azole antifungals with HIV-1 protease inhibitors, but the potential exists. Although azole antifungals and HIV-1 protease inhibitors competitively inhibit CYP 3A4, HIV-1 protease inhibitors are also substrates for CYP 3A4.[53] Based on this it would be expected that azole antifungals, particularly ketoconazole and itraconazole, would increase plasma levels of HIV-1 protease inhibitors. In fact, this appears to be the case.[56] No adverse effects of this interaction have been reported to date.

In the absence of clinical trials, the therapeutic approach to coccidioidomycosis in the patient with HIV infection must be empiric. Determinations about therapy should revolve around the extent of clinical illness, the degree of immunodeficiency, and the site of infection. Unlike the situation in patients without immunodeficiency, therapy should be considered for all forms of coccidioidomycosis in the HIV-infected patient. Currently, there are no standardized methods for antifungal susceptibility testing of *C. immitis,* and there are no data about antifungal resistance detected by any in vitro technique or about clinical outcome.

Most HIV-infected patients who present with focal pulmonary coccidioidomycosis are clinically stable and do not require hospitalization. Given this scenario, therapy with an oral azole antifungal at an initial dosage of 400 mg/day is a reasonable approach. Response can be measured by the alleviation of clinical symptoms, resolution of the pulmonary process on the chest radiograph, and a diminution of serum anti-coccidioidal antibody titers over time. Serum titers may be negative at the time of diagnosis, rise to a peak as the patient responds to therapy over the next weeks to months, and then fall. Hence a rising serologic titer should not be the only factor when determining whether a patient has initially responded to therapy. Among those who respond to therapy, the initial alveolar infiltrate on the chest radiograph develops sharp, rounded borders and in many cases becomes a nodule. It is important that the initial coccidioidal pneumonia be documented because the nodule could later be confused with a pulmonary malignancy.

Diffuse, reticulonodular pneumonia is associated with extremely high mortality[17,18] and requires aggressive treatment. Intravenous amphotericin B is recommended as the initial therapy. Given the significant mortality associated with this form of coccidioidomycosis in HIV-infected patients, a pertinent question is whether amphotericin B should be combined with another antifungal agent. There is no evidence that the addition of flucytosine to amphotericin B is useful for treating coccidioidomycosis. Because azole antifungals inhibit the synthesis of fungal ergosterol whereas amphotericin B acts by binding to ergosterol, the combination of amphotericin B with azole antifungals is potentially antagonistic. However, in vitro, animal, and human data have provided no consistent evidence of such antagonism.[57] Moreover, amphotericin B and azole antifungals have been frequently combined by clinicians treating coccidioidomycosis, particularly meningitis. Hence, in patients failing to respond to amphotericin B, the addition of an azole antifungal can be considered with the caveat that are no data on whether this combination leads to an improved outcome. In patients who respond to the initial amphotericin B therapy, the frequency of infusions can be slowly tapered from daily therapy to two or three times each week. In all cases, once the patient is clinically stable on amphotericin B, therapy can be gradually changed to an oral azole antifungal.

The management of coccidioidal meningitis has changed dramatically since the Mycoses Study Group reported that treatment with oral fluconazole results in a nearly 80% response rate.[46] In that study of 50 patients, 9 had concomitant HIV infection. Of these nine, three did not respond to fluconazole, with two dying and one requiring intrathecal amphotericin B. Although the two deaths were not directly related to coccidioidomycosis, both patients had evidence of continued active coccidioidal infection at the time of death. Of the six patients who responded, all required fluconazole 800 mg/day. Four of these subjects maintained their improvement over at least 15 months; one developed hydrocephalus; and one required reinstitution of intrathecal amphotericin B.

Given these findings, treatment of coccidioidal meningitis in HIV-infected patients should begin with fluconazole at a daily dose of 800 mg. Itraconazole has also been found to have activity in coccidioidal meningitis in patients without HIV infection,[44] but no data exist on its use in the HIV-infected patient. Failure of azole antifungal therapy should lead to the use of intrathecal amphotericin B, just as it would in the patient without HIV infection. Concomitant pulmonary coccidioidomycosis, especially diffuse pulmonary involvement, is a frequent occurrence in patients with HIV infection and coccidioidal meningitis.[18] Therefore combined intravenous amphotericin B and oral or intravenous fluconazole therapy is a reasonable choice for initial antifungal therapy in such patients. As discussed above, clinical antagonism with this combination has not been reported. The goal of combination therapy in this situation is not to provide antifungal synergism but, rather, to treat both manifestations of coccidioidomycosis optimally. Once the patient has clinically responded, oral azole antifungal therapy alone can be prescribed. Therapy should be lifelong,[58] and daily azole antifungal doses of at least 400 mg should be maintained.

Other forms of extrathoracic disseminated coccidioidomycosis in HIV-infected patients appear to respond to antifungal therapy in a manner similar to those without HIV infection. In such cases, if the patient is severely ill and requires hospitalization, initial therapy with amphotericin B is warranted. For those who are clinically stable and are being managed as outpatients, oral azole antifungal therapy is a reasonable choice.

There are two therapeutic options for patients who present with positive coccidioidal serologic tests without evidence of active clinical disease. The first is to follow such patients over time, repeating the serologic tests every 3 to 4 months. If overt clinical disease develops or if the serologic titer progressively increases, antifungal therapy is warranted. The second approach is to begin antifungal therapy with an oral azole antifungal at a daily dose of 400 mg immediately. The patient should still be followed every 3 to 4 months for the development of clinical illness and for assessment of the anti-coccidioidal antibody response. With appropriate therapy the serologic titers should diminish over time.

Any HIV-infected patient with coccidioidomycosis should be followed approximately every 4 months to ensure control of disease. The most important test is the serum anti-coccidioidal antibody titer. With appropriate therapy, that titer should progressively diminish over time. In most patients who clinically respond, the serum antibody titer becomes undetectable. However, in some patients it nadirs at a low but detectable level. This is acceptable if the patient is clinically well. Increasing titers, particularly of twofold or higher dilutions, should raise the question of treatment failure and result in a careful clinical and radiologic assessment for recrudescent disease. In patients who appear to be failing azole antifungal therapy, increasing the daily dose may regain control of the infection. In other patients, amphotericin B is required.

Currently, lifelong high-dose therapy of coccidioidomycosis is recommended for the HIV-infected patient. However, the effect of immune reconstitution associated with HAART has not been well studied in coccidioidomycosis. Undoubtedly, there are some patients, particularly those who are undergoing aggressive antiretroviral therapy and who have elevated CD4+ T-lymphocyte counts, who may not require such therapy. Preliminary data suggest that there is specific immune response to coccidioidal antigens at peripheral blood CD4+ T-lymphocyte counts above 200/μl.[59] Given this, one approach among patients with peripheral blood CD4+ T-lymphocyte counts over 200/μl who are on effective antiretroviral therapy is to taper the daily dose of antifungals slowly and follow the patient's clinical course and the serum antibody titer closely. For example, in a patient with focal pulmonary infection, after 6 to 12 months of fluconazole or itraconazole therapy at 400 mg/day, the dose could be reduced to 200 mg/day. Given the high risk of relapse that occurs with coccidioidomycosis, even among patients without HIV infection,[43,47] subsequent reduction in azole antifungal therapy in the HIV-infected patient should be done cautiously. For patients with coccidioidal meningitis, the daily azole antifungal dosage should be at least 400 mg, and discontination of therapy is not advised.[58]

▲ PREVENTION

There are few data on whether azole antifungal therapy prevents the development of active coccidioidomycosis for HIV-infected patients living in the coccidioidal endemic area. In one retrospective study[21] the use of azole antifungals was associated with a diminished risk of subsequent coccidioidomycosis among HIV-infected persons living in the coccidioidal endemic region who had concomitant oropharyngeal or esophageal candidiasis but not among other groups of HIV-infected patients. Given the cost, risk of drug interactions, and risk of developing fungal resistance, particularly of *Candida albicans*,[60] azole antifungals to prevent the development of symptomatic coccidioidomycosis cannot be generally recommended. For HIV-infected patients living in the coccidioidal endemic area, monitoring anti-coccidioidal antibody serum tests at intervals of every 4 to 6 months is reasonable. The development of a new positive test suggests possible new infection and requires either close follow-up or initiation of antifungal therapy. Outside the endemic area, serial testing for anti-coccidioidal antibodies is unlikely to be useful. Delayed-type hypersensitivity to coccidioidal antigens does not predict the development of active coccidioidomycosis,[8] and skin testing for coccidioidomycosis is not recommended, either within or outside the coccidioidal endemic area.

Many persons infected with HIV are concerned about visiting areas in the coccidioidal endemic region for fear of contracting coccidioidomycosis. Although it would be prudent for such persons to avoid behaviors associated with an increased risk of acquiring coccidioidomycosis, such as working closely with the desert soil or incurring extensive exposure to outdoor dust, there are no compelling data that such patients should absolutely avoid visiting this region. Patients who are immunodeficient due to HIV infection are at risk for infection with a variety of agents that reside in the environment in many parts of the world. Therefore, HIV-infected persons should be aware of local environmental pathogens, be aware of ways to minimize their risk of acquiring them, and make decisions about visiting local areas based on these risks and their own needs and desires about such visits.

REFERENCES

1. Pappagianis D. Epidemiology of coccidioidomycosis. In: McGinnis M (ed) Current Topics in Medical Mycology, vol 2. New York, Springer-Verlag, 1988, pp 199–238.
2. Galgiani JN. Coccidioidomycosis. West J Med 159:153, 1993.
3. CDC. Coccidioidomycosis—Arizona, 1990–1995. MMWR Morbid Mortal Wkly Rep 45:1069, 1996.
4. Stevens DA. Coccidioidomycosis. N Engl J Med 332:1077, 1995.
5. Drutz DJ, Catanzaro A. Coccidioidomycosis: state of the art; parts I and II. Am Rev Respir Dis 117:559, 727, 1978.
6. Ampel NM, Bejarano GC, Salas SD, Galgiani JN. In vitro assessment of cellular immunity in human coccidioidomycosis: relationship between dermal hypersensitivity, lymphocyte transformation, and lymphokine production by peripheral blood mononuclear cells from healthy adults. J Infect Dis 165:710, 1992.
7. Corry DB, Ampel NM, Christian L, et al. Cytokine production by peripheral blood mononuclear cells in human coccidioidomycosis. J Infect Dis 174:440, 1996.
8. Ampel NM, Dols CL, Galgiani JN. Coccidioidomycosis during human immunodeficiency virus infection: results of a prospective study in a coccidioidal endemic area. Am J Med 94:235, 1993.
9. Jones JL, Fleming PL, Ciesielski CA, et al. Coccidioidomycosis among persons with AIDS in the United States. J Infect Dis 171:961, 1995.
10. Abrams DI, Robia M, Blumenfeld W, et al. Disseminated coccidioidomycosis in AIDS [letter]. N Engl J Med 310:986, 1984.
11. Kovacs A, Forthal DN, Kovacs JA, Overturf GD. Disseminated coccidioidomycosis in a patient with acquired immune deficiency syndrome. West J Med 140:447, 1984.
12. Roberts CJ. Coccidioidomycosis in acquired immune deficiency syndrome: depressed humoral as well as cellular immunity. Am J Med 76:734, 1984.
13. Macher AM, De Vinatea ML, Koch Y, et al. Case for diagnosis: AIDS. Milit Med 151:M57, 1986.
14. Wolf JE, Little JR, Pappagianis D, Kobayashi GS. Disseminated coccidioidomycosis in a patient with the acquired immune deficiency syndrome. Diagn Microbiol Infect Dis 5:331, 1986.
15. Jarvik JG, Hesselink JR, Wiley C, et al. Coccidioidomycotic brain abscess in an HIV-infected man. West J Med 149:83, 1988.
16. Bronnimann DA, Adam RD, Galgiani JN, et al. Coccidioidomycosis in the acquired immunodeficiency syndrome. Ann Intern Med 106:372, 1987.
17. Fish DG, Ampel NM, Galgiani JN, et al. Coccidioidomycosis during human immunodeficiency virus infection: a review of 77 patients. Medicine 69:384, 1990.
18. Singh VR, Smith DK, Lawrence J, et al. Coccidioidomycosis in patients infected with human immunodeficiency virus: review of 91 cases at a single institution. Clin Infect Dis 23:563, 1996.
19. Rutherford GW. Epidemiology of AIDS-related coccidioidomycosis in California. In: XI International Conference on AIDS, Vancouver, 1996, abstract Mo.C.1407.
20. Palella FJ Jr, Delaney KM, Moorman AC, et al. Declining morbidity and mortality among patients with advanced human immunodeficiency virus infection: HIV Outpatient Study Investigators. N Engl J Med 338:853, 1998.
21. Woods CW, McRill C, Plikaytis BD, et al. Coccidioidomycosis in human immunodeficiency virus-infected persons in Arizona, 1994–1997: incidence, risk factors, and prevention. J Infect Dis 181:1428, 2000.
22. Ampel NM, Ryan KJ, Carry PJ, et al. Fungemia due to Coccidioides immitis: an analysis of 16 episodes in 15 patients and a review of the literature. Medicine 65:312, 1986.
23. Mahaffey KW, Hippenmeyer CL, Mandel R, Ampel NM. Unrecognized coccidioidomycosis complicating Pneumocystis carinii pneumonia in patients infected with the human immunodeficiency virus and treated with corticosteroids: a report of two cases. Arch Intern Med 153:1496, 1993.
24. Bouza E, Dreyer JS, Hewitt WL, Meyer RD. Coccidioidal meningitis. Medicine 60:139, 1981.
25. Wheat LJ, Connolly-Stringfield PA, Baker RL, et al. Disseminated histoplasmosis in the acquired immune deficiency syndrome: clinical findings, diagnosis and treatment, and review of the literature. Medicine 69:361, 1990.
26. Arguinchona HL, Ampel NM, Dols CL, et al. Persistent coccidioidal seropositivity without clinical evidence of active coccidioidomycosis in patients infected with human immunodeficiency virus. Clin Infect Dis 20:1281, 1995.
27. DiTomasso JP, Ampel NM, Sobonya RE, Bloom JW. Bronchoscopic diagnosis of pulmonary coccidioidomycosis: comparison of cytology, culture, and transbronchial biopsy. Diagn Microbiol Infect Dis 18:83, 1994.
28. Bowman BH, Taylor JW, White TJ. Molecular evolution of the fungi: human pathogens. Mol Biol Evol 9:893, 1992.
29. Stockman L, Clark KA, Hunt JM, Roberts GD. Evaluation of commercially available acridinium ester-labeled chemiluminescent DNA probes for culture identification of Blastomyces dermatitidis, Coccidioides immitis, Cryptococcus neoformans, and Histoplasma capsulatum. J Clin Microbiol 31:845, 1993.
30. Pappagianis D. Serology of coccidioidomycosis. Clin Microbiol Rev 3:247, 1990.
31. Kaufman L, Sekhon AS, Moledina N, et al. Comparative evaluation of commercial Premier EIA and microimmunodiffusion and complement fixation tests for Coccidioides immitis antibodies. J Clin Microbiol 33:618, 1995.
32. Martins TB, Jaskowski TD, Mouritsen CL, Hill HR. Comparison of commercially available enzyme immunoassay with traditional serological tests for detection of antibodies to Coccidioides immitis. J Clin Microbiol 33:940, 1995.
33. Zartarian M, Peterson EM, de la Maza LM. Detection of antibodies to Coccidioides immitis by enzyme immunoassay. Am J Clin Pathol 107:148, 1997.
34. Antoniskis D, Larsen RA, Akil B, et al. Seronegative disseminated coccidioidomycosis in patients with HIV infection. AIDS 4:691, 1990.
35. Gallis HA, Drew RH, Pickard WW. Amphotericin B: 30 years of clinical experience. Rev Infect Dis 12:308, 1990.
36. Labadie EL, Hamilton RH. Survival improvement in coccidioidal meningitis by high-dose intrathecal amphotericin B. Arch Intern Med 146:2013, 1986.
37. Sharkey PK, Lipke R, Renteria A, et al. Amphotericin B lipid complex (ABLC) in treatment (Rx) of coccidioidomycosis (C). In: 31st Interscience Conference on Antimicrobial Agents and Chemotherapy. Chicago, American Society for Microbiology, 1991, abstract 742.
38. Hotstetler JS, Caldwell JW, Johnson RH, et al. Coccidioidal infections treated with amphotericin B colloid dispersion (Amphocil or ABCD). In: 32nd Interscience Conference on Antimicrobial Agents and Chemotherapy. Anaheim, CA, American Society for Microbiology, 1992, abstract 628.
39. Albert MM, Adams K, Luther MJ, et al. Efficacy of AmBisome in murine coccidioidomycosis. J Med Vet Mycol 32:467, 1994.
40. Graybill JR. Lipid formulations for amphotericin B: does the emperor need new clothes. Ann Intern Med 124:921, 1996.
41. Koehler AP, Cheng AF, Chu KC, et al. Successful treatment of disseminated coccidioidomycosis with amphotericin B lipid complex. J Infect 36:113, 1998.

42. Mirels LF, Stevens DA. Update on the treatment of coccidioidomycosis. West J Med 166:58, 1997.
43. Graybill JR, Stevens DA, Galgiani JN, et al. Itraconazole treatment of coccidioidomycosis. Am J Med 89:282, 1990.
44. Tucker RM, Denning DW, Dupont B, Stevens DA. Itraconazole therapy for chronic coccidioidal meningitis. Ann Intern Med 112:108, 1990.
45. Tucker RM, Galgiani JN, Denning DW, et al. Treatment of coccidioidal meningitis with fluconazole. Rev Infect Dis 12:S380, 1990.
46. Galgiani JN, Catanzaro A, Cloud GA, et al. Fluconazole therapy for coccidioidal meningitis: the NIAID-Mycoses Study Group. Ann Intern Med 119:28, 1993.
47. Catanzaro A, Galgiani JN, Levine BE, et al. Fluconazole in the treatment of chronic pulmonary and nonmeningeal disseminated coccidioidomycosis. Am J Med 98:249, 1995.
48. Como JA, Dismukes WE. Oral azole drugs as systemic antifungal therapy. N Engl J Med 330:263, 1994.
49. Blum RA, D'Andrea DT, Florentino BM, et al. Increased gastric pH and the bioavailability of fluconazole and ketoconazole. Ann Intern Med 114:755, 1991.
50. Lake-Bakaar G, Tom W, Lake-Bakaar D, et al. Gastropathy and ketoconazole malabsorption in the acquired immunodeficiency syndrome (AIDS). Ann Intern Med 109:471, 1988.
51. Galgiani JN, Catanzaro A, Cloud GA, et al. Comparison of oral fluconazole and itraconazole for progressive, nonmeningeal coccidioidomycosis: a randomized, double-blind trial. Ann Intern Med 133:676, 2000.
52. Pursley TJ, Blomquist IK, Abraham J, et al. Fluconazole-induced congenital anomalies in three infants. Clin Infect Dis 22:336, 1996.
53. Dresser GK, Spence JD, Bailey DG. Pharmacokinetic-pharmacodynamic consequences and clinical relevance of cytochrome P450 3A4 inhibition. Clin Pharmacokinet 38:41, 2000.
54. Trapnell CB, Narang PK, Li R, Lavelle JP. Increased plasma rifabutin levels with concomitant fluconazole therapy in HIV-infected patients. Ann Intern Med 124:573, 1996.
55. Sahai J, Gallicano K, Pakuts AL, Cameron DW. Effect of fluconazole on zidovudine pharmacokinetics in patients infected with human immunodeficiency virus. J Infect Dis 169:103, 1994.
56. Koks CH, van Heeswijk RP, Veldkamp AI, et al. Itraconazole as an alternative for ritonavir liquid formulation when combined with saquinavir [letter]. AIDS 14:89, 2000.
57. Sugar AM. Use of amphotericin B with azole antifungal drugs: what are we doing? Antimicrobiol Agent Chemother 39:1907, 1995.
58. Dewsnupp DH, Galgiani JN, Graybill JR, et al. Is it ever safe to stop azole therapy for Coccidioides immitis meningitis? Ann Intern Med 124:305, 1996.
59. Ampel NM, Kramer LA, Kerekes KM, et al. Human immune response to the coccidioidal antigen preparation T27K by flow cytometry of whole blood. In: 38th Annual Meeting of the Infectious Diseases Society of America, New Orleans, 2000.
60. Maenza JR, Keruly JC, Moore RD, et al. Risk factors for fluconazole-resistant candidiasis in human immunodeficiency virus-infected patients. J Infect Dis 173:219, 1996.

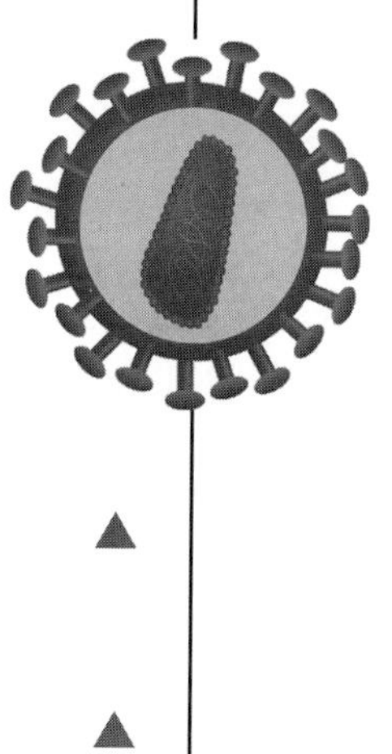

CHAPTER 39
Candidiasis

Carl J. Fichtenbaum, MD

PATHOGEN

Oropharyngeal candidiasis (OPC) was among the initial manifestations recognized in association with human immunodeficiency virus (HIV) infection.[1,2] Mucocutaneous candidiasis typically affects most persons with advanced untreated HIV infection. Its importance is often obscured by the occurrence of other severe opportunistic infections seen with acquired immunodeficiency syndrome (AIDS). OPC may be a sentinel event for the detection or progression of HIV disease, presenting months or years before more severe opportunistic disease.[3–5] Despite the frequency of mucosal disease, disseminated or invasive infections with *Candida* and related yeasts are surprisingly uncommon.

Although usually associated with slight morbidity, OPC can be clinically significant. Severe OPC can interfere with the administration of medications and adequate nutritional intake and may spread to the esophagus.[6] Symptoms may include burning pain, altered taste sensation, and difficulty swallowing liquids and solids. Many patients are asymptomatic. Pseudomembranous candidiasis, or thrush (white plaques on the buccal mucosa, gums, or tongue), is the most common presentation for OPC. Less commonly persons have acute atrophic candidiasis (erythematous) or chronic hyperplastic candidiasis (leukoplakia) involving the tongue.

Esophageal candidiasis is usually accompanied by the presence of OPC. Typically, dysphagia and odynophagia are described. Esophageal involvement is asymptomatic in as many as 40% of patients with OPC.[6] Esophageal disease occasionally presents in the absence of clinically detectable oropharyngeal disease.

Vulvovaginal candidiasis is an important concern for women with HIV infection. Vulvar candidiasis manifests as a morbilliform rash involving the intertriginous areas with satellite lesions on the thighs. Vaginal disease generally presents as a creamy-white abnormal vaginal discharge. Common symptoms include pruritus, vulvar or vaginal pain, dysuria, and dyspareunia. The vagina may appear erythematous, and white plaques are often seen.

Invasive candidiasis typically occurs in persons with more advanced disease and other risk factors (e.g., indwelling venous catheters).[7,8] Bloodstream infections, meningitis, intra-abdominal infections, and osteomyelitis have been described. The clinical manifestations of invasive candidiasis are similar to those of HIV-seronegative persons. The pathogenesis typically involves disruption of a mucosal or skin surface barrier that cannot be attributed to HIV infection alone, perhaps explaining the relative paucity of invasive disease.

Taxonomy and Biology

Yeasts are fungi that grow as single cells and reproduce by budding. They are distinguished on the basis of the presence or absence of capsules, the size and shape of the yeast cells, the mechanism of daughter formation, the formation of true or pseudohyphae, and the presence of sexual spores, along with physiologic data. *Candida albicans* is the predominant causative agent of all forms of mucocutaneous candidiasis. Less frequently, *C. glabrata, C. parapsilosis, C. tropicalis, C. krusei,* and several other species cause disease. More recently, *C. dubliniesis* has been identified as a separate species from its phenotypically similar relative *C. albicans*.[9–11]

Candida species are normal inhabitants of the human gastrointestinal tract and may be recovered from the mouths of up to one-third of normal individuals and two-thirds of those with advanced HIV disease.[12,13] Colonization with a more inherently resistant organism is more common in advanced HIV infection (CD4+ T-lymphocyte counts of <50 cells/μl).[13] Most of the disease is caused by organisms that are part of the normal flora of an individual, although rare cases of person-to-person transmission have been documented.[14]

Microbiology

The individual *Candida* strains affecting persons with HIV infection are typically not different from those in other immunosuppressed hosts.[15] *Candida dubliniesis* is more commonly identified in HIV-infected persons, though its clinical significance is, at this point, indistinguishable from that of *C. albicans*.[9–11] There are no detectable differences in the virulence of strains isolated from HIV-infected or HIV-uninfected persons. Recurrent disease can result from the same species or strains of *Candida* or because of a change in either.[15–18] The emergence of different strains or species is more likely in persons exposed to antifungal therapy with low CD4+ T-lymphocyte counts.[19]

Epidemiology

Mucocutaneous candidiasis occurs in three forms in persons with HIV infection: oropharyngeal, esophageal, and vulvovaginal disease. Oropharyngeal and vulvovaginal disease are the most common forms. Historically, up to 90% of persons with advanced untreated HIV infection developed OPC, with 60% having at least one episode per year with frequent recurrences (50% to 60%).[12,18,20–28] Esophageal candidiasis occurred less frequently (10% to 20%) but was the leading cause of esophageal disease.[29–31] Vaginal candidiasis has been noted in 27% to 60% of women, similar to the rates of oropharyngeal disease.[32–34] However, the incidence appears to be similar in HIV-infected and HIV-uninfected women.[35,36] It is noteable that 75% of all women of childbearing age develop vaginal candidiasis, and 40% have a second occurrence. Few women (<5%) experience frequent recurrences (defined as four or more infections during a 12-month period).

Two factors have affected the epidemiology of mucocutaneous candidiasis. The first was the widespread use of antifungal agents, particularly the azoles. Continuous use of azoles led to a decline in the prevalence of mucosal candidiasis while leading to the emergence of refractory infections. More importantly, the introduction of highly active antiretroviral therapy (HAART) resulted in a significant decline in the incidence of a number of opportunistic illnesses [e.g., *Pneumocystis carinii* pneumonia and cytomegalovirus (CMV)].[37–39] In turn, the incidence of mucocutaneous forms of candidiasis declined precipitously. For example, Cauda et al. reported a significant difference in the incidence of recurrent OPC in patients treated with protease inhibitors compared with those not treated with protease inhibitors (7% vs. 36%).[40] Similarly, Martins et al. reported a decline in the incidence of OPC from 30% to 4% over a 1-year period in persons on HAART.[41]

A number of factors are important in the development of mucocutaneous candidiasis. The level of immunosuppression is paramount.[23] Other host factors important to the defense against *Candida* infections include blood group secretor status, salivary flow rates, epithelial barrier, antimicrobial constituents of saliva, the presence of normal bacterial flora, and local immunity.[24,42] Several studies suggest impairment of a number of anti-*Candida* host defense mechanisms in persons with HIV infection.[23,25,26] High levels of HIV-1 RNA in the plasma have been associated with increased rates of mucocutaneous candidiasis and colonization with *Candida*.[43,44] It is noteable that the relationship between the level of immunosuppression and vaginal candidiasis may not be as strong. In one cross-sectional study of 833 HIV-infected and 427 HIV-uninfected women the annual incidence of vaginal candidiasis was similar in the two groups (9%).[35]

There are few studies describing the incidence and prevalence of nonesophageal invasive candidiasis in HIV-infected persons. The incidence is probably less than 1%.[7,8] Most studies are restricted to case series or anecdotal reports.

▲ DIAGNOSIS

Clinical Appearance

The diagnosis of OPC is usually made by its characteristic clinical appearance (Fig. 39–1). Recovery of an organism is not required to diagnose candidiasis. Oropharyngeal cultures often demonstrate *Candida* species but alone are not diagnostic because colonization is common.[20] The diagnosis of OPC can be confirmed by examining a 10% KOH slide preparation of a scraping of an active lesion, which demonstrates characteristic pseudohyphae and budding yeast. A KOH preparation is not mandatory for diagnosing OPC. A presumptive diagnosis of OPC can be made by visual detection of characteristic lesions, with resolution of those lesions in response to antifungal therapy. Culture is usually not necessary on the first episode of OPC unless the lesions fail to clear with appropriate antifungal therapy. In patients with poorly responsive OPC, a culture should be prepared to look for inherently drug resistant yeasts or those that respond poorly to certain azoles (e.g., *C. kruseii* or *C. glabrata*). Clinicians should note that many microbiology laboratories report yeast cultures as either *C. albicans* or C. non-*albicans* species based on the germ tube test; a request must be made if further characterization is desired. Distinction between *C. albicans* and *C. dubliniesis* can be difficult and is not routinely done in most clinical microbiology laboratories.[9] Biopsies of oral lesions are rarely helpful or indicated.

A presumptive diagnosis of *Candida* esophagitis is appropriate in a patient with dysphagia or odynophagia (or both) who has OPC (Fig. 39–2). Upper endoscopy can be used to confirm esophageal involvement; a barium swallow test may be used, but it is less sensitive and specific than endoscopy.

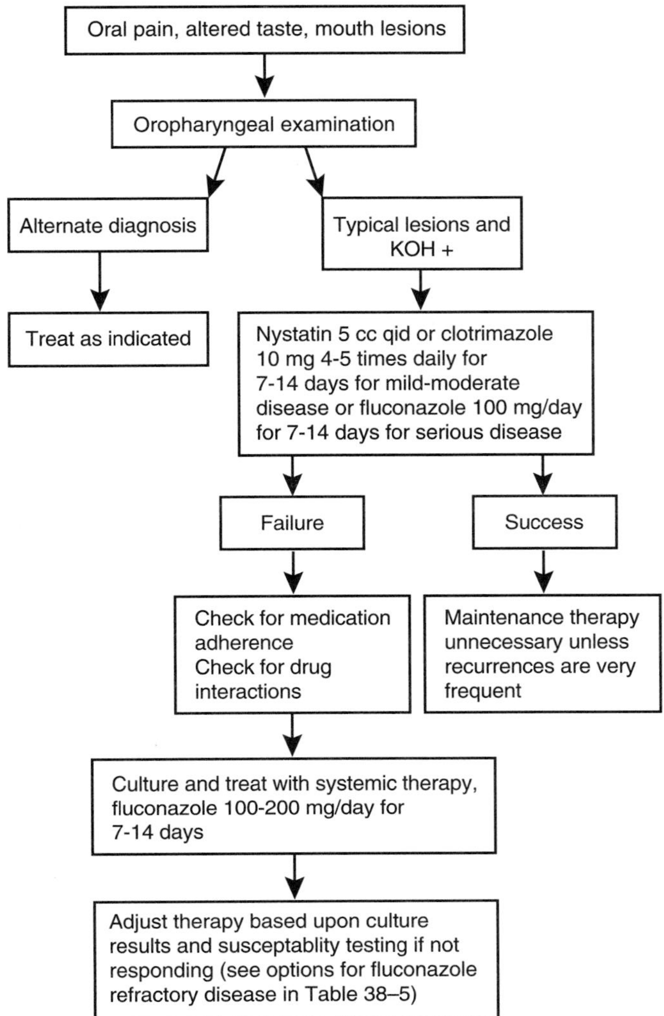

Figure 39–1. Diagnosis and treatment of oral candidiasis.

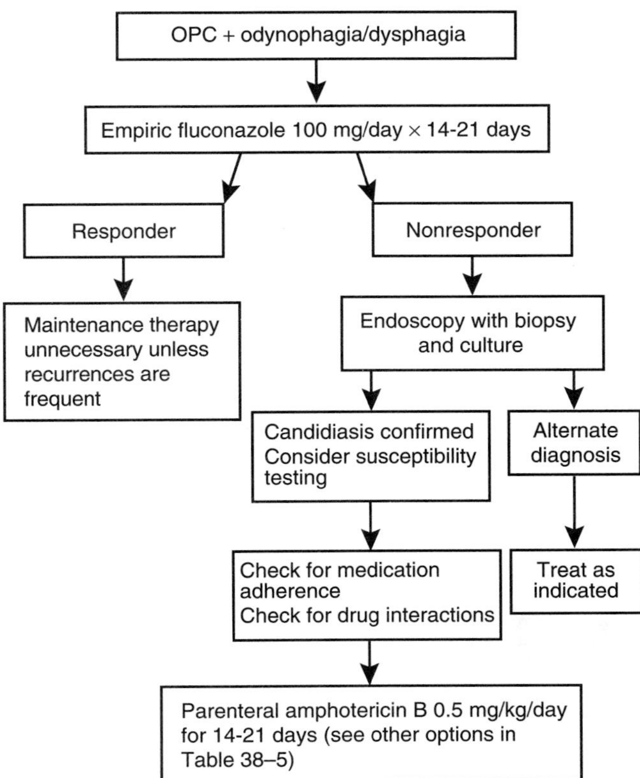

Figure 39–2. Diagnosis and treatment of esophageal candidiasis.

These studies are not uniformly required unless a patient fails to improve with appropriate systemic antifungal therapy.[31] If a patient with OPC does not resolve the esophageal symptoms despite resolution of the oral lesions, endoscopy is indicated to exclude other causes of esophagitis (e.g., CMV, herpes simplex virus, aphthous ulcers). The diagnosis of *Candida* esophagitis is confirmed by the presence of yeast forms on histologic examination of esophageal lesions. Specimens culture for should be obtained from patients who require endoscopy to look for drug-resistant yeast.

Candida vaginitis is diagnosed based on the presence of a characteristic clinical appearance and observation of yeast forms on a microscopic examination (Fig. 39–3). A KOH preparation should always be done on vaginal lesions to confirm the diagnosis of candidiasis because there are a number of other conditions that appear similar (e.g., trichomoniasis). Routine cultures are rarely helpful in the absence of KOH-positive lesions because yeasts are normal inhabitants of the vaginal mucosa. A culture should be prepared if a patient fails to respond to standard antifungal therapy. Vulvar disease is typically diagnosed by its characteristic appearance.

Invasive disease is typically diagnosed by demonstrating the presence of *Candida* on microscopic examination along with the recovery of *Candida* from a sterile site (e.g., bone biopsy, cerebrospinal fluid). Bloodstream infections are usually diagnosed when more than one set of aerobic cultures are positive for *Candida* (Fig. 39–4). In the presence of appropriate clinical symptoms (fever, sepsis) without an alternative explanation, a single positive blood culture for *Candida* should be considered significant. The diagnosis of invasive candidiasis from other nonsterile sites can be challenging. It is not always possible to obtain appropriate specimens, and one must often resort to the use of clinical judgment to make a presumptive diagnosis of invasive disease.

Drug Resistance and Susceptibility Testing

Antifungal susceptibility testing is gradually becoming standardized. The National Committee on Clinical Laboratory Standards (NCCLS) has definitions for in vitro susceptibilities for selected agents using standard methodologies (Table 39–1).[45] The most common methods for in vitro testing are the macrotube and microtiter broth dilution assays. In vitro susceptibilities should not be used routinely to guide the choice of antifungal agents because there is not a clear correlation between clinical response and susceptibility testing.

Despite the technical limitations, a number of studies have documented that in vitro resistance to antifungal

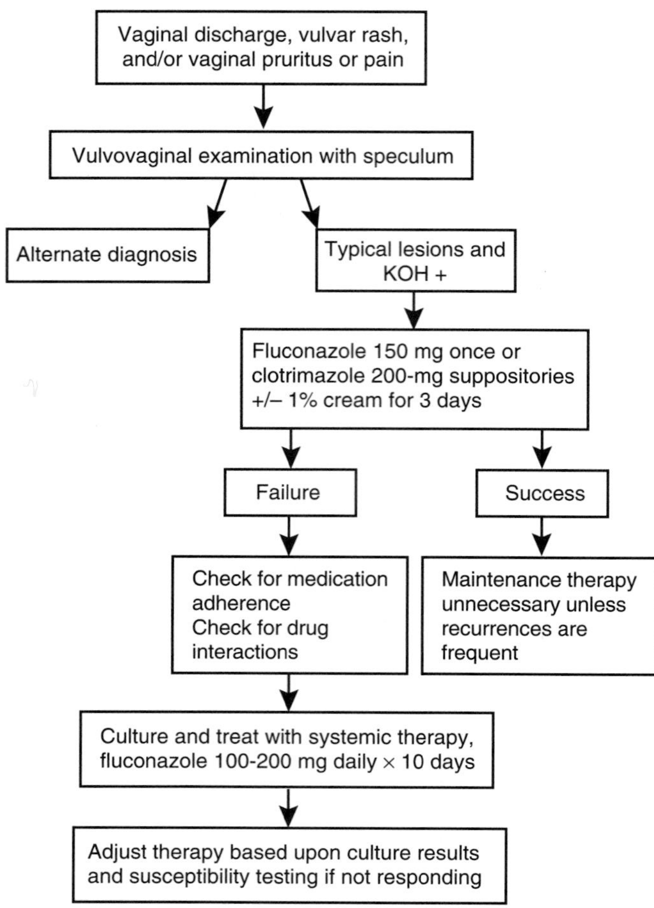

Figure 39–3. Diagnosis and treatment of vaginal candidiasis.

medications is common.[13,19,46–57] The incidence of resistance varies widely in these studies. Overall, the rates of fluconazole resistance vary from 5% to 56%.[13,19,46–50] The rates of ketoconazole and itraconazole resistance have been less frequently reported but vary from 0% to 25%.[51–55,58] Amphotericin B resistance is extremely uncommon but has been reported.[58] Much of the variance in the rates of in vitro resistance can be explained by several factors: differences in the level of host immunosuppression; prior exposure to antifungal agents; the design of the study (longitudinal versus cross-sectional); the prevalence of non-*albicans Candida* species; and differences in the in vitro methods used.[19,55,58]

There are several mechanisms that explain in vitro resistance to antifungal drugs, including target alteration, reduced cell permeability, and active efflux of the drug out of the cell.[59–62] Some yeasts have single drug resistance, whereas others are multidrug-resistant. Azole resistance has been demonstrated in yeasts containing alterations in the enzymes that were the target of their action or were involved in ergosterol biosynthesis. The cytochrome P_{450}-dependent 14α-sterol demethylase (P_{450}) and)^{5,6} -sterol desaturase are two enzymes that, when altered, result in azole resistance.[59,60] The relative incidence of these various mechanisms of resistance is unknown. Furthermore, it is not clear whether certain mechanisms

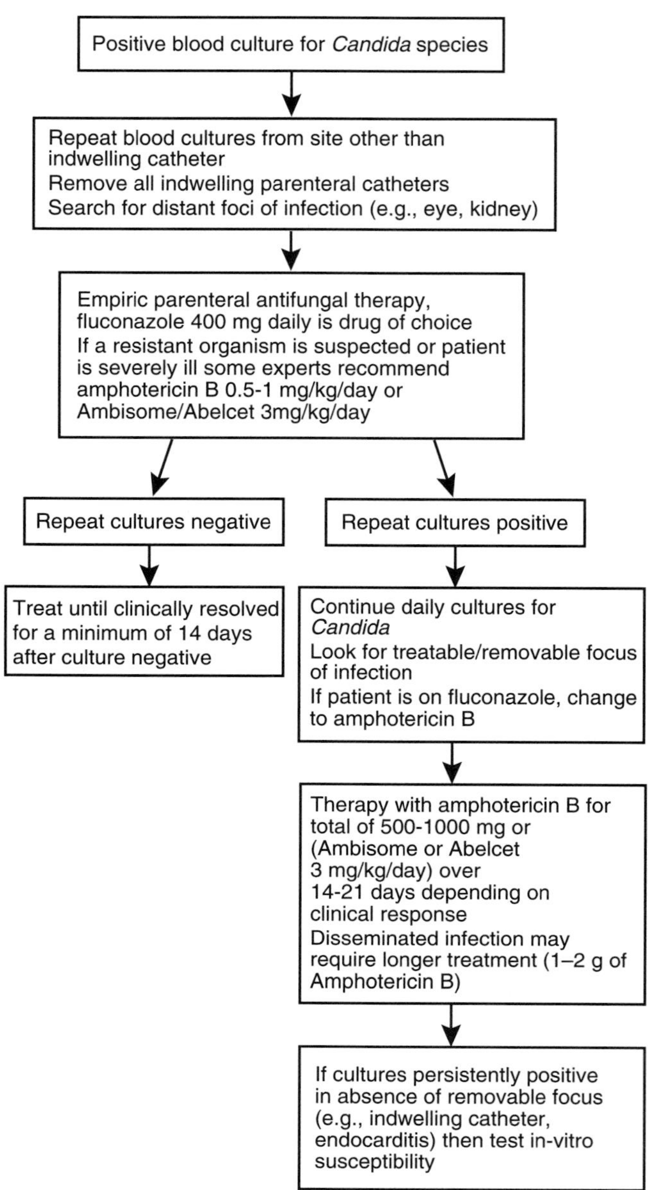

Figure 39–4. Diagnosis and treatment of candidemia.

of resistance may be overcome by higher dosing of the drug.

▲ THERAPY

Numerous agents are effective against candidiasis (Table 39–2). Important factors that determine clinical response in addition to the choice of antifungal agent include the extent and severity of disease, patient adherence to the regimen, and the pharmacodynamic/pharmacokinetic properties of the drug. Treatment of OPC and vaginal candidiasis is relatively simple, with most types responding to therapy. Overall, there have been few clinical differences in randomized studies comparing topical with systemic therapy. Mild OPC or vulvovaginal disease can often be treated success-

Table 39–1. DEFINITION OF IN VITRO RESISTANCE FOR *CANDIDA* SPECIES

	Range of MICs (μg/ml)		
Antifungal Agent	Susceptible	Susceptible-Dose Dependent	Resistant
Itraconazole	≤0.125	0.25–0.50	≥1.0
Fluconazole	≤8.0	16–32	>64.0
Amphotericin B	≤1.0	—	≥2.0

MIC, minimum inhibitory concentration.
Adapted from NCCLS standard definitions for antifungal susceptibilities using microbroth or macrotube dilution methodology. From Rex JH, Pfaller MA, Galgiani JN, et al. Development of interpretive breakpoints for antifungal susceptibility testing: conceptual framework and analysis of in vitro-in vivo correlation data for fluconazole, itraconazole, and Candida infections. Clin Infect Dis 24:235, 1997, with permission.

fully with topical therapy. Moderate and severe episodes typically require systemic therapy. Esophagitis and other invasive disease always require systemic therapy.

Antifungal Agents

There are various classes of antifungal agents: (1) the polyenes (nystatin and amphotericin B), which work by binding to ergosterol in the fungal cell membrane, inducing osmotic instability and loss of membrane integrity; (2) the azoles, including the imidazoles (clotrimazole) and triazoles (ketoconazole, itraconazole, fluconazole, voriconazole, ravuconazole, posaconazole), which inhibit fungal cytochrome P_{450}-dependent enzymes, resulting in impaired ergosterol biosynthesis and depletion of ergosterol from the fungal cell membrane; (3) pyrimidine synthesis inhibitors, including 5-fluorocytosine, which inhibits DNA and RNA synthesis in fungal organisms; and (4) newer agents such as the candins (caspofungin, formerly MK-0991 and V-Echinocandin, formerly LY303366), which are cyclic lipopeptides that inhibit β 1,3-glucan synthase, an enzyme involved in fungal wall cell biosynthesis.

Nystatin is used in a topical preparation. The oral form is not absorbed and has minimal side effects other than dysgeusia. Clotrimazole is available as a spray, solution, and troche for oral usage. Clotrimazole has few side effects and is poorly absorbed from the gastrointestinal tract. Flucytosine is available as a tablet and has a number of associated side effects, including nausea, vomiting, diarrhea, gastrointestinal bleeding, renal insufficiency, hepatitis, thrombocytopenia, anemia, and leukopenia.

Flucytosine is rarely used alone because of the rapid emergence of resistant organisms on therapy. It is sometimes used in combination with fluconazole for refractory candidiasis and has been used adjunctively for difficult-to-treat invasive candidiasis. Flucytosine levels should be maintained between 50 and 100 μg/ml.

Amphotericin B is available in parenteral forms (Amphotericin B, liposomal Amphotericin B, Abelcet, and ABCD). Adverse effects from the parenteral preparation include fever, chills, electrolyte disturbances, and renal insufficiency. The oral formulation is no longer commercially available. Many pharmacies can mix the parenteral form into an oral preparation, though it is not standardized. For example, our pharmacy mixes the powder in sterile water (50 mg/5 ml) and dilutes this mixture in sugar-free Jell-O (200 mg amphotericin B/480 ml). The usual dose of the oral preparation is usually 100 to 500 mg four times daily to treat fluconazolerefractory infections. There are few adverse effects from the oral preparation with the exception of poor taste. Parenteral amphotericin B comes as deoxycholate, liposome, and lipid complex preparations. The latter two (AmBisome and Abelcet) are liposomal preparations typically used in doses of 3 to 5 mg/kg/day for *Candida* infections.

Ketoconazole is rarely used as an oral formulation in the United States. It is available as a tablet or cream. Oral absorption is enhanced when the gastric pH is less than 4.0. Achlorhydria has been documented in HIV-infected patients and, when present, may interfere with ketoconazole absorption.[63] Because of the more frequent incidence of adverse effects, less predictable absorption, and higher frequency of drug–drug interactions (all relative to other available azoles), oral ketoconazole is rarely used.

Itraconazole is a triazole compound available in a cyclodextrin suspension, capsule, or intravenous preparation. The cyclodextrin suspension has enhanced bioavailability compared to the capsule formulation. Absorption is improved when taken after a full meal.

Fluconazole was the first triazole compound released in the United States. It is more completely absorbed than itraconazole or ketoconazole because its absorption is not dependent on gastric acidity or food intake. It is available in suspension, tablet, and parenteral forms.

Voriconazole is a triazole that was recently approved. It comes in tablet and parenteral forms. It does not appear to have any advantages over currently available triazoles for the treatment of most *Candida* infections although it appears to have enhanced activity against Aspergillus and several other molds. In general, the side effects of ketoconazole, itraconazole, fluconazole, posaconazole, and voriconazole are similar. The more commonly reported side effects are headache, dyspepsia, diarrhea, nausea, vomiting, hepatitis, and skin rash.[64] Voriconazole can cause reversible mild abnormal vision.[65] Prolonged administration of azoles may require surveillance of liver enzymes to monitor for hepatotoxicity. There are a number of significant drug interactions with each of these medications (Table 39–3).

Caspofungin acetate is a newly released candin that is available in parenteral form for the treatment of refractory *Aspergillus* infections. It is effective for oral and esophageal candidiasis including fluconazole-refractory disease.[65a,65b,66] In a randomized double blind study of caspofungin vs. amphotericin B for the treatment of Candidal esophagitis involving 128 patients, 80% of whom were HIV infected, caspofungin was at least as effective as amphotericin B (endoscopic use rates were 74% for caspofungin 50 mg, 89% for caspofungin 70%, and 63% for amphotericin B 0.5 mg/kg). Therapy was discontinued due to toxicity in 24% of patients treated with amphotericin B compared to 4% and 7% for patients treated with the two caspofungin doses.[65a] There are several other candins under investigation, though none is currently available in an oral formulation. Adverse events such as fever, nausea, vomiting, flushing, and infused-vein complications are typically mild.[66]

Table 39–2. THERAPEUTIC OPTIONS FOR MUCOSAL CANDIDIASIS

Medication	Dosage	Important Toxicities
Oropharyngeal Candidiasis		
Clotrimazole troches	10 mg 4–5 times/d × 7–14 days	Altered taste, GI upset
Nystatin suspension	100,000 units/cc 5 cc qid × 7–14 days	GI upset
Ketoconazole	200 mg/d × 7–14 days	GI upset, hepatitis, endocrine effects
Itraconazole	100 mg/d × 7–14 days	GI upset, hepatitis
Fluconazole	100 mg/d × 7–14 days	GI upset, hepatitis
Esophageal Candidiasis		
Fluconazole[a]	100 mg/d × 14–21 days	GI upset, hepatitis
Ketoconazole	400 mg/d × 14–21 days	GI upset, hepatitis, endocrine effects
Itraconazole	200 mg/d × 14–21 days	GI upset, hepatitis
Parenteral amphotericin B	0.5 mg/kg/d × 14–21 days	Renal failure, electrolyte losses, fever, chills, sweats
Liposomal amphotericin B products[b]	3 mg/kg/d × 14–21 days	Fever, chills, sweats, electrolyte losses, renal insufficiency uncommon
Voriconazole	200 mg bid × 14–21 days	GI upset, hepatitis, visual impairment
Caspofungin	50–70 mg/d × 14–21 days	Fever, nausea, vomiting, infusion-associated phlebitis
Vulvovaginal Candidiasis[c]		
Fluconazole	150 mg once	Minimal GI upset
Butoconazole		
2% Cream	5 g at bedtime × 3 days	Local irritation
2% Cream	5 g once	Local irritation
Clotrimazole		
Suppositories[d]	100 mg × 7 days	Local irritation
Suppositories[d]	200 mg × 3 days	Local irritation
1% Cream	5 g bid × 3 days	Local irritation
1% Cream	5 g/d × 7 days	Local irritation
Miconazole		
Suppositories[d]	100 mg/d × 7 days	Local irritation
2% Cream	5 g/d × 7 days	Local irritation
4% Cream	5 g at bedtime × 3 days	Local irritation
Nystatin tablets[d]	100,000 unit tablet × 14 days	Local irritation
Tioconazole 6.5% cream	4.6 g single dose	Local irritation
Terconazole		
0.4% Cream	5 g/d × 7 days	Local irritation
0.8% Cream	5 g/d × 3 days	Local irritation
Suppository 80 mg[d]	1 each day × 3 days	Local irritation

GI, gastrointestinal
[a]Drug of choice.
[b]Includes amphotericin B lipid complex (ABLC), liposomal amphotericin B.
[c]Nonprescription alternatives available for most topical drugs with treatment for 3 to 7 days.
[d]Presence of vulvar disease requires additional use of cream directly on rash for 3 to 7 days.

Many antifungal treatment studies for mucocutaneous candidiasis suffer from one or more weaknesses, such as small numbers of patients, heterogeneous populations, short follow-up, and a nonblinded design. In particular, no study has stratified patients by CD4+ T-lymphocyte count. This is important because persons with low CD4+ T-lymphocyte counts appear to respond more slowly to treatment; they have lower rates of fungal eradication and higher relapse rates than persons with less advanced disease. Another important weakness is that there are no reported treatment trials for vulvovaginal candidiasis in women with HIV infection. Recommendations for the treatment of vulvovaginal disease are made based on data from the nonHIV-infected population.

A number of controlled trials of currently approved medications for the treatment of oral and esophageal candidiasis are listed in Table 39–4. Response rates range from 34% to 100% in studies of treatment for oral and esophageal disease.[27,67–69,72–76] In clinical experience, the response rates to standard antifungal treatments are on the order of 75% to 95%. There are few significant differences in response rates between topical and systemic therapies or among the various systemic therapies for OPC. Thus it is reasonable to conclude that clotrimazole, ketoconazole, fluconazole, itraconazole, and voriconazole are probably equivalent for acute treatment of most cases of OPC. Mild cases of OPC should probably be treated with clotrimazole or nystatin initially for 7 to 14 days. Nonresponsive cases or patients with more severe disease should use fluconazole 100 mg/day or itraconazole 200/day for 7 to 14 days. The treatment of esophageal candidiasis has not been as well studied as that of OPC. Response rates to systemic therapies are generally quite good. Fluconazole (21 days duration) is the drug of choice for this entity. Susceptibility testing in routine cases of OPC or esophageal candidiasis need not be performed. It should be reserved for patients who fail systemic therapy with fluconazole or amphotericin B.

The cure rates for vulvovaginal candidiasis range from 72% to 98% in most trials of persons without HIV infection.[77–81] Historically, treatment for vulvovaginal candidiasis typically consisted of topical therapy for 7 days. How-

▲ **Table 39–3.** IMPORTANT DRUG INTERACTIONS WITH SELECTED ANTIFUNGAL MEDICATIONS

Interacting Drug	Antifungal	Effect and Manifestations
Anticoagulants, oral	F, K, V	Anticoagulant levels (prolonged prothrombin time, bleeding)
Antihistamines: H_1-blockers (excluding loratadine)	I, F, K	Antihistamine levels (ventricular arrhythmias)
Carbamazepine	I	Itraconazole levels (decreased efficacy)
Cisapride	I, F, K	Cisapride levels (ventricular arrhythmias)
Contraceptives, oral	I, F, K	Efficacy of oral contraceptives (pregnancy)
Cyclosporin/tacrolimus	I, F, K, V	CSA/tacrolimus level (CSA/tacrolimus toxicity)
Didanosine	I, K	Complex interaction with levels of involved drugs
Digoxin	I	Digoxin levels (digitalis toxicity)
HMG-CoA inhibitors	I, F, K	HMG-CoA inhibitor levels (rhabdomyolysis)
Oral hypoglycemics	F, K	Oral hypoglycemic effect (hypoglycemia)
Isoniazid	I, F, K	I, F, K levels (decreased efficacy)
H_2-blockers/proton pump	I, K, V	I, K levels (decreased efficacy); V levels with omeprazole
Phenytoin	I, F, K, V	Complex (I, K, V levels; V, F, phenytoin levels)
Rifabutin	F, V	F levels (uveitis); V levels (decreased efficacy)
Rifampin	I, F, K, V	I, F, K levels (decreased efficacy)
Theophylline	I, F, K	Theophylline levels (toxicity)

F, fluconazole; I, itraconazole; K, ketoconazole; V, voriconazole; HMG-CoA, 3-hydroxy-3-methylglutaryl coenzyme A; CSA, cyclosporin A.
Voriconazole is the newest triazole, and not all drug interactions have been evaluated/reported.

ever, shorter courses (3 days) and single-dose therapy is often effective. Sobel et al. compared a one-time dose of 150 mg of fluconazole with 7 days of topical therapy with clotrimazole (100 mg vaginal suppositories).[81] The clinical cure rate by day 35 was equivalent in the two groups (75%). Mycologic eradication rates at day 35 were 63% for the fluconazole group and 57% for the clotrimazole group. Clinical experience in women with HIV infection is generally positive with either topical or systemic therapy, but relapse rates are quite high.[34] Single-dose therapy with fluconazole is simple and effective. In patients who fail, it is reasonable to treat with clotrimazole suppositories with or without cream for 3 to 7 days before using longer courses of systemic fluconazole.

The recommendation for treating nonesophageal forms of invasive candidiasis is similar to that for HIV-seronegative persons. It is beyond the scope of this chapter to review all the alternative approaches to the use systemic antifungals for invasive candidiasis. In general, though, bloodstream infections may be treated with fluconazole 400 mg/day or amphotericin B 0.5 to 1.0 mg/kg/day for 2 to 4 weeks (Fig. 39–4). Indwelling vascular devices typically should be removed if possible. Amphotericin B has been the mainstay of treatment for most deep-seated *Candida* infections, though azoles are increasingly being used. Typically, the duration of treatment is 4 to 6 weeks. Lipid complex formulations of amphotericin B are also increasingly being used to avoid the toxicity of amphotericin B deoxycholate, though there appears to be no advantage in efficacy. The typical starting dose for liposomal preparations is 3 mg/kg/day. The use of these agents should be reserved for subjects intolerant of amphotericin B deoxycholate or with preexisting renal insufficiency.

There are no prospective trials using real-time in vitro susceptibility testing to guide the choice of antifungal therapy. This is likely explained by the facts that most *Candida* infections respond to empiric therapy, and in vitro testing is not yet as reliable as antibiotic susceptibility testing against bacteria. There are patients with fungal organisms that are "resistant" by in vitro testing that respond to therapy. Less commonly, some patients fail to respond to therapy despite having a relatively "sensitive" organism isolated. Most clinicians prescribe empiric therapy and reserve susceptibility testing for nonresponders to systemic therapy with fluconazole or amphotericin B. Thus although there are now standard definitions for what constitutes in vitro resistance, there is still much work to be done in this area before it can be used as a guide to therapy.

Refractory Candidiasis

Reports of refractory OPC and esophageal disease began emerging in 1990.[13,46–48,82–96] Refractory vaginal candidiasis has remained relatively uncommon.[97] Refractory disease is defined as the failure to respond to antifungal treatment with appropriate doses for a standard duration of time (e.g., 14 days).[13,98] Fluconazole-refractory disease emerged as the focus because there was significant morbidity, treatment often required the use of parenteral agents, and fluconazole was the most commonly prescribed antifungal agent. The annual incidence of fluconazole-refractory OPC has been reported to be 4% to 5% in patients with advanced HIV infection during the pre-HAART era.[13,34] Like most other opportunistic infections, fluconazole-refractory OPC is less common with the widespread use of HAART. Amphotericin B-refractory disease is exceedingly uncommon.[99–102] It is of note that clinical failures may also result from inadequate drug absorption or drug interactions that decrease the levels of some antifungal medications.[63,103,104]

Refractory candidiasis tends to occur in persons with advanced HIV disease (CD4+ T-lymphocyte counts of <50 cells/μl) who have been exposed to antifungal therapy on a continuous, chronic basis.[13] Maenza and colleagues reported a longer median duration of exposure to antifungal therapy (419 vs. 118 days, $P<0.001$) and of systemic azole therapy (272 vs. 14 days, $P<0.001$) in persons who had fluconazole-refractory OPC compared to matched controls.[86] Other factors that may predict the development of refractory candidiasis include use of prophylactic trimethoprim-

▲ **Table 39–4.** CLINICAL TRIALS FOR TREATMENT OF HIV-ASSOCIATED ORAL AND ESOPHAGEAL CANDIDIASIS

Medication	Clinical Response	Mycologic Response	Relapse Rate	Study
Oral Candidiasis				
Fluconazole				
100 mg/d × 14 d	100% (*n* = 16)	75%	60% at day 42	Koletar[67]
100 mg/d × 14 d	98% (*n* = 152)	65%	34% at day 42	Pons[27]
50 mg/d × 28 d	100% (*n* = 17)	87%	46% at day 30	DeWit[68]
200 mg/d × 14 d[a]	42% (*n* = 38)	NA	62%	Barchiesi[69]
100 mg/d × 14 d	83% (*n* = 94)	51%	37% at day 30	Vazquez[70]
100 mg/d × 14 d	83% (*n* = 160)	68%	38%	Nieto[71]
Clotrimazole				
10 mg 5×/d × 14 d	94% (*n* = 136)	48%	40% at day 42	Pons[27]
10 mg 5×/d × 14 d	65% (*n* = 17)	20%	14% at day 42	Koletar[67]
Ketoconazole				
200 mg/d × 28 d	75% (*n* = 16)	69%	11% at day 30	DeWit[68]
200 mg bid × 28 d	93% (*n* = 40)	73%	>80% at day 90	Smith[28]
200 mg/d × 14 d	60% (*n* = 52)	62%	80% at day 60	de Repentigny[72]
400 mg/d × 12 d[a]	34% (*n* = 39)	NA	22%	Barchiesi[69]
Itraconazole				
200 mg/d × 14 d	71% (*n* = 46)	63%	80% at day 60	de Repentigny[72]
200 mg/d × 28 d	93% (*n* = 46)	72%	>80% at day 90	Smith[28]
Posaconazole				
50 mg/d × 14 d	74% (*n* = 98)	36%	41% at day 30	Vazquez[70]
100 mg/d × 14 d	80% (*n* = 102)	37%	38% at day 30	Vazquez[70]
200 mg/d × 14 d	74% (*n* = 91)	35%	35% at day 30	Vazquez[70]
400 mg/d × 14 d	83% (*n* = 100)	40%	36% at day 30	Vazquez[70]
200 mg/d × 14 d	82% (*n* = 169)	68%	31%	Nieto[71]
Esophageal Candidiasis				
Fluconazole				
100 mg/d × 21 d[b]	85% (*n* = 72)	NA	NA	Laine[73]
200 mg/d × 2–6 wks	90% (*n* = 141)	NA	NA	Dupont[65]
Itraconazole				
200 mg/d × 28 d	100% (*n* = 12)	NA	58% at day 60	de Repentigny[72]
Ketoconazole				
200 mg/d × 21 d[b]	65% (*n* = 71)	NA	NA	Laine[73]
200 mg/d × 28 d	91% (*n* = 19)	NA	82% at day 60	de Repentigny[72]
Voriconazole				
200 mg bid × 2–6 wks	95% (*n* = 115)	NA	NA	Dupont[65]
Caspofungin				
50 mg/d × 14 d	74%	80%	NA	Villanueva[65a]
70 mg/d × 14 d	81%	96%	NA	

NA, not available.
[a]Median duration of therapy (range 6–46 days).
[b]Treatment given for 14 days after patient was asymptomatic minimum 21 days up to 8 weeks.

sulfamethoxazole and a history of prior opportunistic illnesses such as *Mycobacterium avium* complex disease.[13] Similarly, chronic exposure to itraconazole results in higher rates of in vitro resistance, although these isolates typically remain susceptible to fluconazole.[105]

Refractory candidiasis is often difficult to treat and may become increasingly less responsive to therapy over time. The most important step is to determine what medications and dosages have been tried and whether adherence with therapy was adequate. Removal of any interacting medications or increasing the dose of the antifungal agent is curative in some persons. In general, persons with OPC unresponsive to clotrimazole, nystatin, ketoconazole, or itraconazole tablets respond to fluconazole. Persons with OPC unresponsive to fluconazole 200 mg daily given for 2 weeks are less likely to respond to higher doses but sometimes do.

There are a number of options for fluconazole-refractory disease (Table 39–5). Few controlled studies of these approaches and no comparative studies have been reported. Parenteral amphotericin B remains the drug of choice for persons with severe disease or esophageal involvement. For mild to moderate fluconazole-refractory OPC, itraconazole cyclodextrin or amphotericin B oral suspension are reasonable choices.[106–112] Overall, the response rates for itraconazole cyclodextrin are somewhere between 50% and 60% and are slightly lower for oral amphotericin B solution (oral solution of amphotericin B is not currently commercially available). Anecdotal success and in vitro susceptibility to fluconazole-resistant isolates has been reported with voriconazole and with caspofungin.[113,114] Treatment with protease inhibitors has been noted to result in clinical improvement in difficult-to-treat cases.[115] Protease inhibitors have also been shown to inhibit *Candida* secretory aspartic proteases demonstrating direct antifungal activity for *Candida*, though the clinical significance of this finding remains unclear.[116–118] Optimization of antiretroviral therapy (potent therapy with or without protease inhibitors) in persons with refractory disease is essential. The duration of treatment for refractory disease is based on the response,

▲ **Table 39–5.** THERAPEUTIC OPTIONS FOR FLUCONAZOLE-REFRACTORY MUCOSAL CANDIDIASIS

Medication	Dosage
Topical Therapy	
Clotrimazole troches	100–500 mg 4–5 times daily
Gentian violet	Apply to oropharynx once (may repeat weekly as needed)
Amphotericin B oral solution[a]	100 mg/ml, 5 ml PO qid
Systemic Therapy	
Fluconazole tablets	400–800 mg PO qd or bid
± Flucytosine	100–150 mg/kg/d PO qid
Itraconazole tablets	200–400 mg PO qd or bid
Itraconazole solution[a]	40 mg/ml, 2.5–5.0 ml PO bid
Parenteral amphotericin B	0.5–1.0 mg/kg/d IV qd
Lipid formulations of amphotericin B	3 mg/kg/d IV qd
Caspofungin[b]	50–70 mg IV qd
Non-FDA-Approved Therapy (Compassionate Use)	
Voriconazole[c]	200 mg bid
Adjunctive Therapy	
Potent antiretroviral therapy	RT inhibitors + protease Inhibitors
GM-CSF[b]	300 μg SC 3–5 times weekly

Granulocyte/macrophage colony-stimulating factor; RT, reverse transcriptase.
Duration of treatment should be a minimum of 21–28 days.
[a]Controlled study supports use of this treatment for fluconazole-refractory candidiasis.
[b]Not FDA-approved for the treatment of *Candida* infections.
[c]Investigational.

but typically a 14-day regimen is required for OPC or vaginal disease and 21 to 28 days for esophageal disease. Relapse rates are high in persons with refractory disease, and maintenance suppressive therapy is universally required.[112]

▲ NEW ANTIFUNGAL MEDICATIONS

There are a number of new antifungals in varying phases of clinical development including triazoles, echinocandins, sordarins, chitin synthase inhibitors, and topoisomerase inhibitors. Several new agents in the former two categories are nearing approval in the United States. In vitro activity of three new azoles—posaconazole, ravuconazole, voriconazole—appears to be quite good for *Candida* species. The latter agent was recently approved.[113,119–121] Dupont et al. presented data on a blinded, randomized study of voriconazole 200 mg twice daily versus fluconazole 200 mg daily for the treatment of esophageal candidiasis.[65] There was no difference in the number of persons with endoscopically proven cure after 2 to 6 weeks of therapy: 94.8% of the voriconazole group (n = 115) versus 90.1% of the fluconazole group (n = 141). Posaconazole 100 mg suspension/day compared favorably to fluconazole 100 mg suspension/day for treating OPC in persons with HIV infection.[70] The clinical cure rate was 92% (n = 169) for posaconazole versus 93% (n = 160) for fluconazole. Similarly, posaconazole compared favorably to fluconazole in a dose-ranging study for the treatment of oral candidiasis associated with HIV infection.[71] Caspofungin (recently released as Cancidas), V-Echinocandin, and FK-463 are members of the candins, a novel class of antifungals. These agents also show promise in the treatment of *Candida* infections but are limited to parenteral administration at present.[122–124] Caspofungin may be useful in subjects with mucosal or invasive candidiasis who fail or are intolerant of standard and liposomal preparations of amphotericin B. Data on the efficacy with caspofungin for the treatment of various forms of candidiasis in persons with HIV infection are limited. Several of these newer agents can be obtained on a compassionate-use basis, particularly for treating azole- and polyene-refractory mucosal candidiasis.

▲ PREVENTION

The most important method for preventing mucocutaneous candidiasis is reversal of the immunodeficiency associated with HIV infection. Potent antiretroviral therapy is likely the single best intervention to reduce the incidence of mucocutaneous candidiasis. Several studies have demonstrated a decline in the rate of colonization and clinical disease with the use of potent antiretroviral therapy.[40,41,43,44] This decline has been correlated with reduced HIV-1 RNA levels in plasma.[41,43,44] Other possible interventions include smoking cessation, good oral hygiene, avoidance of unnecessary antibiotics and steroids, and specific antifungal medications.

Although recurrent mucocutaneous candidiasis is frequent in persons with untreated advanced HIV infection, the indications for prophylactic antifungal therapy remain uncertain. A randomized study comparing clotrimazole to fluconazole demonstrated that fluconazole can prevent invasive fungal infections such as cryptococcosis and esophageal candidiasis,[125] but there was no survival advantage in the study. Weekly fluconazole prophylaxis has also been studied for the prevention of OPC and vulvovaginal disease.[34,126,127] Schuman et al. reported decreases in the incidence of both OPC [relative risk (RR) 0.50; 95% confidence interval (CI) 0.33 to 0.71] and vulvovaginal disease (RR 0.56; 95% CI 0.41 to 0.77) in a study of 323 women with moderately advanced HIV infection who took weekly doses of fluconazole 200 mg (median follow-up 29 months).[34] Thus although one can reduce the risk of mucocutaneous candidiasis, there is no survival advantage. Furthermore, several studies have demonstrated that continuous, long-term exposure to antifungal agents such as fluconazole can lead to the emergence of resistance and refractory infections.[13] Consequently, the United States Public Health Service—Infectious Disease Society guidelines and most experts do not recommend universal primary antifungal prophylaxis.

The use of secondary prophylaxis should be individualized. Some experts recommend prophylaxis in persons with a prior episode of esophageal candidiasis.[128,129] In general, persons with occasional disease or infrequent recurrences of OPC (fewer than three episodes per year) can be treated for each episode. An alternative approach is to provide the patient with a supply of antifungal medications that can be initiated at the earliest sign of recurrence. This alternative may be useful for adherent, well educated patients with frequent or disabling episodes (or both). Persons with frequent recurrences or complications that result in nutritional impairment or severe esophageal disease may be a group that can benefit from secondary prophylaxis, particularly as the CD4+ T-lymphocyte count declines. Some experts recommend prophylaxis in persons with advanced HIV disease when prescribing antibiotics or corticosteroids, such as in a patient with *Pneumocystis carinii* pneumonia. If one decides to use prophylaxis, the most published experience is with daily, thrice-weekly, or weekly fluconazole. Ketoconazole and itraconazole are probably also useful but have not been evaluated in controlled trials. Topical therapy is useful in some patients. In summary, continuous use of antifungal agents should be reserved for persons with frequent or severe recurrences of mucosal candidiasis to avoid the emergence of drug resistance, avoid drug interactions, simplify already complex drug regimens, avoid drug toxicity, and lower the cost of treatment.

REFERENCES

1. Gottlieb MS, Schroff R, Schanker HM. Pneumocystis carinii pneumonia and mucosal candidiasis in previously healthy homosexual men: evidence of a new acquired cellular immunodeficiency. N Engl J Med 305:1425, 1981.
2. Masur H, Michelis MA, Greene JB, et al. An outbreak of community-acquired Pneumocystis carinii pneumonia: initial manifestation of cellular immune dysfunction. N Engl J Med 305:1431, 1981.
3. Klein RS, Harris CA, Small CB, et al. Oral candidiasis in high-risk patients as the initial manifestation of the acquired immunodeficiency syndrome. N Engl J Med 311:354, 1984.
4. Dodd CL, Greenspan D, Katz MH, et al. Oral candidiasis in HIV infection: pseudomembranous and erythematous candidiasis show similar rates of progression to AIDS. AIDS 5:1339, 1991.
5. Katz MH, Greenspan D, Westenhouse J, et al. Progression to AIDS in HIV-infected homosexual and bisexual men with hairy leukoplakia and oral candidiasis. AIDS 6:95, 1992.
6. Tavitian A, Raufman JP, Rosenthal LE. Oral candidiasis as a marker for esophageal candidiasis in the acquired immunodeficiency syndrome. Ann Intern Med 104:54, 1986.
7. Launay O, Lortholary O, Bouges-Michel C, et al. Candidemia: a nosocomial complication in adults with late-stage AIDS. Clin Infect Dis 26:1134, 1998.
8. Tumbarello M, Tacconelli E, de Gaetano Donati K, et al. Candidemia in HIV-Infected subjects. Eur J Clin Microbiol Infect Dis 18:478, 1999.
9. Tintelnot K, Haase G, Seibold M, et al. Evaluation of phenotypic markers for selection and identification of Candida dubliniensis. J Clin Microbiol 38:1599, 2000.
10. Scholing S, Kortinga HC, Froschb M, Muhlschlegel F. The role of Candida dubliniensis in oral candidiasis in human immunodeficiency virus-infected individuals. Crit Rev Microbiol 26:59, 2000.
11. Jabra-rizk MA, Falkler WA, Merz WG, et al. Retrospective identification and characterization of Candida dubliniensis isolates among Candida albicans clinical laboratory isolates from human immunodeficiency virus (HIV)-infected and non-HIV-infected individuals. J Clin Microbiol 38:2423, 2000.
12. Odds FC. Candida and Candidosis. London, Baillière Tindall, 1988, p 117.
13. Fichtenbaum CJ, Koletar S, Yiannoutsos C, et al. Refractory mucosal candidiasis in advanced human immunodeficiency virus infection. Clin Infect Dis 30:749, 2000.
14. Barchiesi F, Hollis RJ, Del Poeta M, et al. Transmission of fluconazole-resistant Candida albicans between patients with AIDS and oropharyngeal candidiasis documented by pulsed-field gel electrophoresis. Clin Infect Dis 21:561, 1995.
15. Powderly WG, Robinson K, Keath EJ. Molecular typing of Candida albicans isolated from oral lesions of HIV-infected individuals. AIDS 6:81, 1992.
16. Powderly WG. Mucosal candidiasis caused by non-albicans species of Candida in HIV-positive patients. AIDS 6:604, 1992.
17. Bruatto M, Vidotto V, Marinuzzi G, et al. Candida albicans biotypes in human immunodeficiency virus type 1-infected patients with oral candidiasis before and after antifungal therapy. J Clin Microbiol 29:726, 1991.
18. Scmid J, Odds FC, Wiselka MJ, et al. Genetic similarity and maintenance of Candida albicans strains from a group of AIDS patients, demonstrated by DNA fingerprinting. J Clin Microbiol 30:935, 1992.
19. Korting HC, Ollert M, Georgii A, et al. In vitro susceptibilities and biotypes of Candida albicans isolates from the oral cavities of patients infected with human immunodeficiency virus. J Clin Microbiol 26:2626, 1988.
20. Feigal DW, Katz MH, Greenspan D, et al. The prevalence of oral lesions in HIV-infected homosexual and bisexual men: three San Francisco epidemiological cohorts. AIDS 5:519, 1991.
21. Pindborg JJ. Oral candidiasis in HIV infection. In: Robertson PB, Greenspan JS (eds) Perspectives on Oral Manifestations of AIDS. Littleton, MA, PSG Publishing, 1988, p 23.
22. Holmstrup P, Samaranayake LP. Acute and AIDS-related oral candidosis. In: Samaranayake LP, MacFarlane TW (eds) Oral Candidosis. London, Wright, 1990, p 133.
23. McCarthy GM, Mackie ID, Koval J, et al. Factors associated with increased frequency of HIV-related oral candidiasis. J Oral Pathol Med 20:332, 1991.
24. Epstein JB, Truelove EL, Izutzu KT. Oral candidiasis: pathogenesis and host defense. Rev Infect Dis 6:96, 1984.
25. McCarthy GM. Host factors associated with HIV-related oral candidiasis. Oral Surg Oral Med Oral Pathol 73:181, 1992.
26. Yeh CK, Fox PC, Ship JA, et al. Oral defense mechanisms are impaired early in HIV-1 infected patients. J Acquir Immune Defic Syndr 1:361, 1988.
27. Pons VG, Greenspan D, Koletar S, Multicenter Study Group. Comparative study of fluconazole and clotrimazole troches for the treatment of oral thrush in AIDS. J Acquir Immune Defic Syndr 6:1311, 1993.
28. Smith DE, Midgley J, Allan M, et al. Itraconazole versus ketoconazole in the treatment of oral and esophageal candidosis in patients infected with HIV. AIDS 5:1367, 1991.
29. Selik RM, Starcher ET, Curran JW. Opportunistic diseases reported in AIDS patients: frequencies, associations, and trends. AIDS 1:175, 1987.
30. Moore RD, Chaisson RE. Natural history of opportunistic disease in an HIV-infected urban clinical cohort. Ann Intern Med 124:633, 1996.
31. Wilcox CM, Alexander LN, Clark WS, et al. Fluconazole compared with endoscopy for human immunodeficiency virus-infected patients with esophageal symptoms. Gastroenterology 110:2803, 1996.
32. Duerr A, Sierra M, Clarke L, et al. Vaginal candidiasis among HIV-infected women. In: Proceedings of the IXth International Conference on AIDS, Berlin, 1993, vol I, abstract PO-B01-0880:282.
33. Sha B, Benson C, Pottage J, et al. HIV infection in women: a six year longitudinal, observational study. In: Proceedings of the IXth International Conference on AIDS, Berlin, 1993, vol I, abstract PO-B01-0891:283.
34. Schuman P, Capps L, Peng G, et al. Weekly fluconazole for the prevention of mucosal candidiasis in women with HIV infection. Ann Intern Med 126:689, 1997.
35. White MH. Is vulvovaginal candidiasis an AIDS-related illness? Clin Infect Dis 22(suppl 2):S124, 1996.
36. Schuman P, Sobel JD, Ohmit SE, et al. Mucosal candidal colonization and candidiasis in women with or at risk for human immunodeficiency virus infection. Clin Infect Dis 27:1161, 1998.
37. Mouton Y, Alfandari S, Valette M, et al. Impact of protease inhibitors on AIDS defining events and hospitalization in 10 French AIDS reference centers. AIDS 11:F101, 1997.
38. Palella FJ, Delaney KM, Moorman AC, et al. Declining morbidity and mortality among patients with advanced human immunodeficiency virus infection: HIV Outpatient Study investigators. N Engl J Med 338:853, 1998.
39. Hammer SM, Squires KE, Hughes MO, et al. A controlled trial of two nucleosides plus indinavir in persons with human immunodeficiency infection and CD4 cell counts of 200 per cubic millimeters or less. N Engl J Med 337:725, 1997.
40. Cauda R, Tacconelli E, Tumbarello M, et al. Role of protease inhibitors in preventing recurrent oral candidosis in patients with HIV infection: a prospective case-control study. J Acquir Immune Defic Syndr 21:20, 1999.
41. Martins MD, Lozano-Chiu M, Rex JH. Declining rates of oropharyngeal candidiasis and carriage of Candida albicans associated with

trends toward reduced rates of carriage of fluconazole-resistant C. albicans in human immunodeficiency virus-infected patients. Clin Infect Dis 27:1291, 1998.

42. Steele C, Leigh J, Swoboda R, Fidel PL. Growth inhibition of Candida by human oral epithelial cells. J Infect Dis 182:1479, 2000.
43. Gottfredsson M, Cox GM, Indridason OS, et al. Association of plasma levels of human immunodeficiency virus type 1 RNA and oropharngeal Candida colonization. J Infect Dis 180:534, 1999.
44. Dios P, Ocampo A, Otero I, et al. Changes in oropharyngeal colonization and infection by Candida albicans in human immunodeficiency virus-infected patients. J Infect Dis 183:355, 2001.
45. Rex JH, Pfaller MA, Galgiani JN, et al. Development of interpretive breakpoints for antifungal susceptibility testing: conceptual framework and analysis of in vitro-in vivo correlation data for fluconazole, itraconazole, and Candida infections. Clin Infect Dis 24:235, 1997.
46. Heinic GS, Stevens DA, Greenspan D, et al. Fluconazole-resistant Candida in AIDS patients. Oral Surg Oral Med Oral Pathol 76:711, 1993.
47. Quereda C, Polanco AM, Giner C, et al. Correlation between in vitro resistance to fluconazole and clinical outcome of oropharyngeal candidiasis in HIV-infected patients. Eur J Clin Microbiol Infect Dis 15:30, 1996.
48. Maenza JR, Merz WG, Romagnoli MJ, et al. Infection due to fluconazole-resistant Candida in AIDS patients: prevalence and microbiology. Clin Infect Dis 24:28, 1997.
49. Pfaller MA, Rhine-Chalberg J, Redding SW, et al. Variations in fluconazole susceptibility and electrophoretic karyotype among oral isolates of Candida albicans from patients with AIDS and oral candidiasis. J Clin Microbiol 32:59, 1994.
50. Laguna F, Rodriquez-Tudela JL, Martinez-Suarez JV, et al. Patterns of fluconazole susceptibility in isolates from human immunodeficiency virus-infected patients with oropharyngeal candidiasis due to Candida albicans. Clin Infect Dis 24:124, 1997.
51. Barchieshi F, Colombo AL, McGough DA, et al. In vitro activity of itraconazole against fluconazole-susceptible and -resistant Candida albicans isolates from oral cavities of patients infected with human immunodeficiency virus. Antimicrob Agents Chemother 38:1530, 1994.
52. He X, Tiballi RN, Zarins LT, et al. Azole resistance in oropharyngeal Candida albicans strains isolated from patients infected with human immunodeficiency virus. Antimicrob Agents Chemother 38:2495, 1994.
53. Fan-Havard P, Capano D, Smith SM, et al. Development of resistance in Candida isolates from patients receiving prolonged antifungal therapy. Antimicrob Agents Chemother 35:2302, 1991.
54. St Germain G, Dion C, Espinel-Ingroff A, et al. Ketoconazole and itraconazole susceptibility of Candida albicans isolated from patients infected with HIV. J Antimicrob Chemother 36:109, 1995.
55. Cameron ML, Schell WA, Bruch S, et al. Correlation of in vitro fluconazole resistance of Candida isolates in relation to therapy and symptoms of individuals seropositive for human immunodeficiency virus type 1. Antimicrob Agents Chemother 37:2449, 1993.
56. Chavenet P, Lopez J, Grappin M, et al. Cross-sectional study of the susceptibility of Candida isolates to antifungal drugs and in vitro-in vivo correlation in HIV-infected patients. AIDS 8:945, 1994.
57. Sangeorozan JA, Bradley SF, Xiaogang H, et al. Epidemiology of oral candidiasis in HIV-infected patients: colonization, infection, treatment and emergence of fluconazole resistance. Am J Med 97:339, 1994.
58. Ruhnke M, Eigler A, Tennagen I, et al. Emergence of fluconazole-resistant strains of Candida albicans in patients with recurrent oropharyngeal candidosis and human immunodeficiency virus infection. J Clin Microbiol 32:2092, 1994.
59. Hitchcock CA. Resistance of Candida albicans to antifungal agents. Biochem Soc Trans 132:1039, 1993.
60. Vanden Bossche H, Marichal P, Odds F. Molecular mechanisms of drug resistance in fungi. Trends Microbiol 2:393, 1994.
61. Ryley JF, Wilson RG, Barrett-Boe KJ. Azole resistance in Candida albicans. J Med Vet Mycol 22:53, 1984.
62. Crombie T, Falconer DJ, Hitchcock CA. Fluconazole resistance due to energy-dependent efflux in Candida glabrata. Antimicrob Agents Chemother 39:1696, 1996.
63. Lake-Bakaar G, Tom W, Lake-Bakaar D, et al. Gastropathy and ketoconazole malabsorption in the acquired immunodeficiency syndrome (AIDS). Ann Intern Med 109:471, 1988.
64. Munoz P, Moreno S, Berenguer J, et al. Fluconazole-related hepatotoxicity in patients with acquired immunodeficiency syndrome. Arch Intern Med 151:1020, 1991.
65. Dupont B, Ally R, Burke J, et al. A double-blind, randomized, multicenter trial of voriconzole (vori) vs. fluconazole (flu) for the treatment of esophageal candidiasis (EC) in immunocompromised adults. In: Proceedings of the 40th Interscience Conference on Antimicrobial Agents and Chemotherapy, Toronto, 2000, abstract 706.

65a. Villanueva A, Arathoon EG, Gotazzo E, et al. A randomized double blind study of Caspofungin versus Amphotericin for the treatment of candidal esophagitis. Clin Infect Dis 33:1529, 2001.

65b. Keating GM, Jarvis B. Caspofungin. Drugs 61:1121, 2001.

66. Maertens J, Raad I, Sable CA, et al. Multicenter, noncomparative study to evaluate the safety and efficacy of caspofungin (CAS) in adults with invasive aspergillosis (IA) and refractory (R) or intolerant (I) to amphotericin B (AMB), AMB lipid formulations (Lipid AMB), or azoles. In: Proceedings of the 40th Interscience Conference on Antimicrobial Agents and Chemotherapy, Toronto, 2000, abstract 706.
67. Koletar SL, Russell JA, Fass RJ, et al. Comparison of oral fluconazole and clotrimazole troches as treatment for oral candidiasis in patients infected with human immunodeficiency virus. Antimicrob Agents Chemother 34:2267, 1990.
68. De Wit S, Goosens H, Weerts D, et al. Comparison of fluconazole and ketoconazole for oropharyngeal candidiasis in AIDS. Lancet 1:746, 1989.
69. Barchiesi F, Giacometti A, Arzeni D, et al. Fluconazole and ketoconazole in the treatment of oral and esophageal candidiasis in AIDS patients. J Chemother 4:381, 1992.
70. Vazquez JA, Northland R, Miller S, et al. Posaconazole compared to fluconazole for oral candidiasis in HIV-positive patients. In: Proceedings of the 40th Interscience Conference on Antimicrobial Agents and Chemotherapy, Toronto, 2000, abstract 1107.
71. Nieto L, Northland R, Pittisuttithum P, et al. Posaconazole equivalent to fluconazole in the treatment of oropharyngeal candidiasis. In: Proceedings of the 40th Interscience Conference on Antimicrobial Agents and Chemotherapy, Toronto, 2000, abstract 1108.
72. De Repentigny L, Ratelle J. Comparison of itraconazole and ketoconazole in HIV-positive patients with oropharyngeal or esophageal candidiasis. Chemotherapy 42:374, 1996.
73. Laine L, Dretler RH, Conteas CN, et al. Fluconazole compared with ketoconazole for the treatment of Candida esophagitis in AIDS. Ann Intern Med 117:655, 1992.
74. Lim SG, Lee CA, Hales M, et al. Fluconazole for oropharyngeal candidiasis in anti-HIV positive hemophiliacs. Aliment Pharmacol Ther 5:199, 1991.
75. De Wit S, Urbain D, Rahir F, et al. Efficacy of oral fluconazole in the treatment of AIDS associated esophageal candidiasis. Eur J Clin Microbiol Infect Dis 10:503, 1991.
76. Chave JP, Francioli P, Hirschel B, et al. Single-dose therapy for esophageal candidiasis with fluconazole. AIDS 4:1034, 1990.
77. Kutzer E, Oittner R, Leodolter S, et al. A comparison of fluconazole and ketoconazole in the oral treatment of vaginal candidiasis: report of a double-blind multicentre trial. Eur J Obstet Gynecol Reprod Biol 29:305, 1988.
78. Van Huesden AM, Merkus HM, Corbeij RS, et al. Single-dose oral fluconazole versus single-dose topical miconazole for the treatment of acute vulvovaginal candidiosis. Acta Obstet Gynecol Scand 69:417, 1990.
79. Woolley PD, Higgins SP. Comparison of clotrimazole, fluconazole and itraconazole in vaginal candidiasis. Br J Clin Pract 49:65, 1995.
80. Anonymous. A comparison of single-dose oral fluconazole with 3-day intravaginal clotrimazole in the treatment of vaginal candidiasis: report of an international multicentre trial. Br J Obstet Gynaecol 96:226, 1989.
81. Sobel JD, Brooker D, Stein GE, et al. Single oral dose fluconazole compared with conventional clotrimazole topical therapy of Candida vaginitis. Am J Obstet Gynecol 172:1263, 1995.
82. Baily GG, Perry FM, Denning DW, et al. Fluconazole-resistant candidosis in an HIV cohort. AIDS 8:787, 1994.
83. Boken DJ, Swindells S, Rinaldi MG. Fluconazole-resistant Candida albicans. Clin Infect Dis 17:1018, 1993.
84. Newman SL, Flanigan TP, Fisher A, et al. Clinically significant mucosal candidiasis resistant to fluconazole treatment in patients with AIDS. Clin Infect Dis 19:684, 1994.
85. White A, Goetz MB. Azole-resistant Candida albicans: report of two cases of resistance to fluconazole and review. Clin Infect Dis 19:687, 1994.
86. Maenza JR, Keruly JC, Moore RD, et al. Risk factors for fluconazole-resistant candidiasis in human immunodeficiency virus-infected patients. Clin Infect Dis 173:219, 1996.

87. Fox R, Neal KR, Leen CLS, et al. Fluconazole resistant Candida in AIDS. J Infect 22:202, 1991.
88. Kitchen VS, Savage M, Harris JRW. Candida albicans resistance in AIDS. J Infect 22:204, 1991.
89. Smith D, Boag F, Midgley J, et al. Fluconazole resistant Candida in AIDS. J Infect 23:345, 1992.
90. Willocks L, Leen CLS, Brettle RP, et al. Fluconazole resistance in AIDS patients. J Antimicrob Chemother 28:937, 1991.
91. Arilla MC, Carbonero JL, Schneider J, et al. Vulvovaginal candidiasis refractory to treatment with fluconazole. Eur J Obstet Gynaecol 44:77, 1992.
92. Sanguineti A, Carmichael JK, Campbell K. Fluconazole-resistant Candida albicans after long-term suppressive therapy. Arch Intern Med 153:1122, 1993.
93. Redding S, Smith J, Farinacci G, et al. Resistance of Candida albicans to fluconazole during treatment of oropharyngeal candidiasis in a patient with AIDS: documentation by in vitro susceptibility testing and DNA subtype analysis. Clin Infect Dis 18:240, 1994.
94. Troillet N, Durussel C, Bille J, et al. Correlation between in vitro susceptibility of Candida albicans and fluconazole-resistant oropharyngeal candidiasis in HIV-infected patients. Eur J Clin Microbiol Infect Dis 12:911, 1993.
95. Cartledge JD, Midgley J, Gazzard BG. Relative growth measurement of Candida species in a single concentration of fluconazole predicts the clinical response to fluconazole in HIV infected patients with oral candidosis. J Antimicrob Chemother 37:275, 1996.
96. Horn CA, Washburn RG, Givner LB, et al. Azole-resistant oropharyngeal and esophageal candidiasis in patients with AIDS. AIDS 9:533, 1995.
97. Arilla MC, Carbonero JL, Schneider J, et al. Vulvovaginal candidiasis refractory to treatment with fluconazole. Eur J Obstet Gynecol Reprod Biol 44:77, 1992.
98. Fichtenbaum CJ, Powderly WG. Refractory and resistant mucosal candidiasis in the acquired immunodeficiency syndrome. Clin Infect Dis 26:556, 1998.
99. Berman S, Ho M. Highly resistant esophageal candidiasis in patients with AIDS. In: Proceedings of the IXth International Conference on AIDS, Berlin, 1993, vol I, abstract PO-B09-1405:369.
100. Dick JD, Merz WG, Saral R. Incidence of polyene-resistant yeasts recovered from clinical specimens. Antimicrob Agents Chemother 18:158, 1980.
101. Kwon-Chung KJ, Bennett JE. Principles of antifungal therapy. In: Medical Mycology. Philadelphia, Lea & Febiger, 1992, p 81.
102. Powderly WG, Kobayashi GS, Herzig GP, et al. Amphotericin resistant yeast infection in severely immunocompromised patients. Am J Med 84:826, 1988.
103. Blum RA, D'Andrea DT, Florentino BM, et al. Increased gastric pH and the bioavailability of fluconazole and ketoconazole. Ann Intern Med 114:755, 1991.
104. Kaltenbach G, Leveque D, Peter JD, et al. Pharmacokinetic interaction between itraconazole and rifampin in Yucatan miniature pigs. Antimicrob Agents Chemother 40:2043, 1996.
105. Goldman M, Cloud GA, Smedema M, et al. Does long-term itraconazole prophylaxis result in in vitro azole resistance in mucosal Candida albicans isolates from persons with advanced human immunodeficiency virus infection? Antimicrob Agents Chemother 44:1585, 2000.
106. Dewsnup DH, Stevens DA. Efficacy of oral amphotericin B in AIDS patients with thrush clinically resistant to fluconazole. J Med Vet Mycol 32:389, 1994.
107. Nguyen MT, Weiss PG, Labarre RC, et al. Oral amphotericin B in the treatment or oral candidiasis due to azole-resistant Candida species. In: Abstracts of the Annual Meeting of the Infectious Diseases Society of America, Orlando, 1994, abstract 287.
108. Fichtenbaum CJ, Zackin R, Rajicic N, et al. Amphotericin B oral suspension for fluconazole-resistant oral candidiasis in HIV-infected patients. AIDS 14:845, 2000.
109. Cartledge JD, Midgley J, Youle M, et al. Itraconazole cyclodextrin solution: effective treatment for HIV-related candidosis unresponsive to other azole therapy. J Antimicrob Chemother 33:1071, 1994.
110. Phillips P, Zemcov J, Mahmood W, et al. Itraconazole cyclodextrin solution for fluconazole-refractory oropharyngeal candidiasis in AIDS: correlation of clinical response with in-vitro susceptibility. AIDS 10:1369, 1996.
111. Saag MS, Fessel WJ, Kaufman CA, et al. Treatment of fluconazole refractory oropharyngeal candidiasis with itraconazole oral solution in HIV-positive patients. AIDS Res Hum Retroviruses 15:1413, 1999.
112. Moskovitz B, Wu J, Baruch A, et al. Long term safety and efficacy of itraconazole oral solution for the treatment of fluconazole refractory oropharyngeal candidiasis in HIV positive patients. In: Proceedings of the 4th Conference on Retroviruses and Opportunistic Infections, Washington, DC, January 1997, abstract 325.
113. Ruhnke M, Schmidt-Westhausen A, Trautmann M. In vitro activities of voriconazole (UK-109,496) against fluconazole-susceptible and resistant Candida albicans isolates from oral cavities of patients with human immunodeficiency virus infection. Antimicrob Agents Chemother 41:575, 1997.
114. Hegener P, Troke PF, Fatkenheuer G, et al. Treatment of fluconazole-resistant candidiasis with voriconazole in patients with AIDS. AIDS 12:2227, 1998.
115. Zingman BS. Resolution of refractory AIDS-related mucosal candidiasis after initiation of didanosine plus saquinavir. N Engl J Med 334:1674, 1996.
116. Borg-von Zepelin M, Meyer I, Thomssen R, et al. HIV-protease inhibitors reduce cell adherence of Candida albicans strains by inhibition of yeast secreted aspartic proteases. J Invest Dermatol 113:747, 1999.
117. Naglik JR, Newport G, White TC, et al. In vivo analysis of secreted aspartyl proteinase expression in human oral candidiasis. Infect Immun 67:2482, 1999.
118. Korting HC, Schaller M, Eder G, et al. Effects of the human immunodeficiency virus (HIV) proteinase inhibitors saquinavir and indinavir on in vitro activities of secreted aspartyl proteinases of Candida albicans isolates from HIV-infected patients. Antimicrob Agents Chemother 43:2038, 1999.
119. Pfaller MA, Messer SA, Hollis RJ, et al. In vitro susceptibilities of Candida bloodstream isolates to the new triazole antifungal agents BMS-207147, Sch 56592, and voriconazole. Antimicrob Agents Chemother 42:3242, 1998.
120. Chavez M, Bernal S, Valverde A, et al. In-vitro activity of voriconazole (UK-109,496), LY303366 and other antifungal agents against oral Candida spp: isolates from HIV-infected patients. J Antimicrob Chemother 44:697, 1999.
121. Cacciapuoti A, Loebenberg D, Corcoran E, et al. In vitro and in vivo activities of SCH 56592 (posaconazole), a new triazole antifungal agent, against Aspergillus and Candida. Antimicrob Agents Chemother 44:2017, 2000.
122. Pettengell K, Ross D, Kluyts T, et al. A multicenter study of the echinocandin antifungal FK463 for the treatment of esophageal candidiasis in HIV positive patients. In: Proceedings of the 40th Interscience Conference on Antimicrobial Agents and Chemotherapy, Toronto, 2000, abstract 1104.
123. Brown GL, White RJ, Turik M. Phase II, randomized, open label study of two intravenous dosing regimens of V-Echinocandin in the treatment of esophageal candidiasis. In: Proceedings of the 40th Interscience Conference on Antimicrobial Agents and Chemotherapy, Toronto, 2000, abstract 1106.
124. Hicks PS, Dorso KL, Gerckens LS, et al. Comparative in vitro susceptibility of clinical trial isolates to the echinocandin antifungal caspofungin (Cancidas™, MK-0991). In: Proceedings of the 40th Interscience Conference on Antimicrobial Agents and Chemotherapy, Toronto, 2000, abstract 193.
125. Powderly WG, Finkelstein DM, Feinberg J, et al. A randomized trial comparing fluconazole with clotrimazole troches for the prevention of fungal infections in patients with advanced human immunodeficiency virus infection. N Engl J Med 332:700, 1995.
126. Leen CLS, Dunbar EM, Ellis ME, et al. Once-weekly fluconazole to prevent recurrence of oropharyngeal candidiasis in patients with AIDS and AIDS-related complex: a double-blind placebo-controlled study. J Infect 21:55, 1990.
127. Marriott DJE, Jones PD, Hoy JF, et al. Fluconazole once a week as secondary prophylaxis against oropharyngeal candidiasis in HIV-infected patients. Med J Aust 158:312, 1993.
128. Esposito R, Castagna A, Foppa CU. Maintenance therapy of oropharyngeal candidiasis in HIV-infected patients with fluconazole. AIDS 4:1033, 1990.
129. Agresti MB, de Bernardis F, Mondello F, et al. Clinical and mycological evaluation of fluconazole in the secondary prophylaxis of esophageal candidiasis in AIDS patients. Eur J Epidemiol 10:17, 1994.

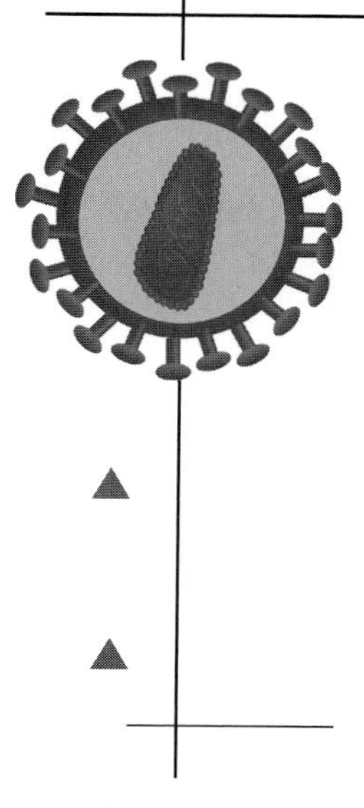

CHAPTER 40

Mycoses Caused by Moulds

John R. Graybill, MD
Thomas F. Patterson, MD

Infections caused by moulds are uncommon but important causes of invasive mycoses in patients with advanced acquired immunodeficiency syndrome (AIDS). The most common fungal infections are due to *Candida* species and *Cryptococcus neoformans*. Less commonly seen are the endemic dimorphic mycoses, such as those due to *Histoplasma capsulatum* and *Coccidioides immitis*. The least commonly encountered mycoses are the miscellaneous infections caused by organisms grouped as primary mycelial fungi, or moulds.[1,2] Since the development of highly active antiretroviral therapy (HAART), infections with moulds have decreased. Most often patients have advanced human immunodeficiency virus (HIV) infection with CD4+ T-lymphocyte counts usually less than 200/mm^3 (often less than 50/mm^3) with uncontrolled HIV viral replication. Other risk factors, such as neutropenia, injection drug use, malignancy, the use of corticosteroids or intravenous catheters, and other chronic medical illness, are frequently present.[3,4] The clinical presentation of these fungi ranges from sinusitis and soft pulmonary infection to localized deep tissue abscess and widely disseminated disease (Table 40–1). The possibility of a fungal infection must be considered early to allow prompt diagnosis and institution of antifungal therapy and surgical intervention as needed. Long-term suppressive therapy for these mycoses is often required because relapse is frequent. With immunologic reconstitution during HAART, some physicians have elected to stop suppressive or prophylactic therapy for certain nonfungal infections and for *Candida*. This practice is not yet widely done for moulds.

▲ PATHOGENS AND EPIDEMIOLOGY

The mycologic classification of moulds includes dimorphic pathogens (organisms that exist in nature as moulds but are seen as yeasts or yeast-like organisms in tissue), agents of hyalohyphomycosis (lightly pigmented moulds) or phaeohyphomycosis (darkly pigmented moulds), and Zygomycetes (fungi with wide, rarely septated hyphae). This chapter includes infections caused by dimorphic pathogens other than *C. immitis* and *H. capsulatum* (*Paracoccidioides brasiliensis*, *Blastomyces dermatitidis*, *Penicillium marnefeii*, *Sporothrix schenckii*); agents of hyalohyphomycosis (*Aspergillus*, *Fusarium*, *Pseudallescheria*, *Trichosporon*, other less commonly encountered hyaline moulds); Zygomycetes (*Rhizopus* species, other members of the order Mucorales); and agents of phaeohyphomycosis (*Alterneria*, *Bipolaris*, *Exophiala*, other dematiaceous moulds).

Infection by moulds most commonly occurs by inhaling conidia (*B. dermatitidis*, *P. brasiliensis*, probably *P. marneffei*, *Aspergillus* species, Zygomycetes). However, intravenous injection of conidia through injection drug use (Zygomycetes, *Aspergillus* species) or direct percutaneous inoculation (*S. schenckii*, agents of phaeohyphomycosis) also occur. After infection, progression or resolution depends on the specific fungal pathogen and the immunocompetence of the patient. *Aspergillus*, Zygomycetes, and even rare fungal agents of human disease such as *Schizophyllum commune* (mushroom) have caused infection in the maxillary sinuses of patients with AIDS.[5–7]

These mycoses generally occur during late stages of AIDS, causing widely disseminated infection. Other risk

▲ **Table 40–1.** CLINICAL MANIFESTATIONS OF SELECTED MOULD INFECTIONS IN PATIENTS WITH AIDS

Organism	Clinical Manifestations
Agents of Hyalohyphomycosis	
Aspergillus spp.	Pulmonary, sinusitis, cutaneous, focal abscess, disseminated disease
Pseudallescheria spp.	Pneumonia, sinusitis, endocarditis, disseminated disease, meningitis
Fusarium spp.	Fungemia, endocarditis, disseminated infection
Chrysosporium spp.	Osteomyelitis
Trichosporon spp.	Catheter-related fungemia
Geotrichum spp.	Esophageal ulcer
Penicillium decumbens	Disseminated infection
Agents of Phaeohyphomycosis	
Alterneria spp.	Nasal soft tissue infection, sinusitis
Exophiala spp.	Esophagitis, soft tissue infection
Hormonema spp.	Liver abscess
Cladophialophora bantiana	Brain abscess, pulmonary
Phialophora spp.	Disseminated infection
Bipolaris spp.	Endophthalmitis
Scedosporium prolificans	Disseminated infection
Agents of Zygomycosis	
Rhizopus arrhizus	Orbit, soft tissue, sinus
Absidia corymbifera	Renal abscesses, pharyngeal, pulmonary
Cunninghamella bertholletiae	Soft tissue abscess
Mucor spp.	Sinus

Data from Cunliffe NA, Denning DW. Uncommon invasive mycoses in AIDS. AIDS 9:411, 1995; and Minamoto GY, Rosenberg AS. Fungal infections in patients with the acquired immunodeficiency syndrome. Med Clin North Am 81:381, 1997.

factors, such as neutropenia, use of corticosteroids, cytomegalovirus infection, and chemotherapy, compound the risk of becoming infected with many moulds, such as *Aspergillus*.

▲ DIAGNOSIS AND THERAPY

Diagnosis for all of these infections depends on direct demonstration of the pathogen by histopathology or culture (Table 40–2). Serologic testing for antibody may be useful for some mycoses (paracoccidioidomycosis, blastomycosis, coccidioidomycosis), but such tests may be negative in the severely immunocompromised patient and, if negative, may not be helpful. Except for histoplasmosis, antigen tests for these organisms are not generally available for clinical use. A culture from any site is usually sufficient to establish a diagnosis of infection because most of these organisms do not usually cause colonization. A major exception is *Aspergillus,* which may colonize the respiratory tract and not be associated with active infection.[8] Other moulds occasionally colonize the respiratory tract or sinuses without causing invasive disease. The diagnosis of invasive infection should be considered in patients with a compatible clinical syndrome.

Treatment of the invasive moulds has evolved considerably in recent years. Until recently amphotericin B has been the unchallenged standard therapy for most of these organisms. More recently, drugs such as lipid formulations of amphotericin B, the newer triazoles (e.g., posaconazole and voriconazole), and the echinocandins (e.g., caspofungin and micafungin) have shown significant efficacy; and in some situations they may be or become the drugs of choice.[9–11] The large number of patients infected with the various fungal pathogens has enabled multicenter studies to define treatment regimens for many mycoses. However, the number of patients infected with a specific species of mould remains small, so treatment regimens and approaches to therapy remain largely anecdotal. However, as the patients infected with these organisms has continued to increase, the Infectious Disease Society of America published guidelines for managing fungal infections (though mostly in non-HIV-infected patients).[12–14] An approach to therapy is summarized in Figure 40–1. Most important is a high index of suspicion for the diagnosis, particularly in patients with risk factors for invasive infections. Positive

▲ **Table 40–2.** DIAGNOSIS OF MOULD INFECTIONS IN PATIENTS WITH AIDS

Organism	Tissue Characteristics	Serology/Others
Agents of hyalohyphomycosis		
Aspergillus spp.	Septated, acute-angle branching	Antibody not useful; antigen investigational
Other agents	Indistinguishable from *Aspergillus* spp.	Serology not available for *Fusarium* spp.; *Fusarium* may grow from blood cultures
Agents of phaeohyphomycosis	Irregular hyphae, confirm melanin with specific Masson-Fontana stain	Serology not available
Agents of zygomycosis	Wide, rarely septated hyphae	Serology not available; may not grow from homogenized tissues

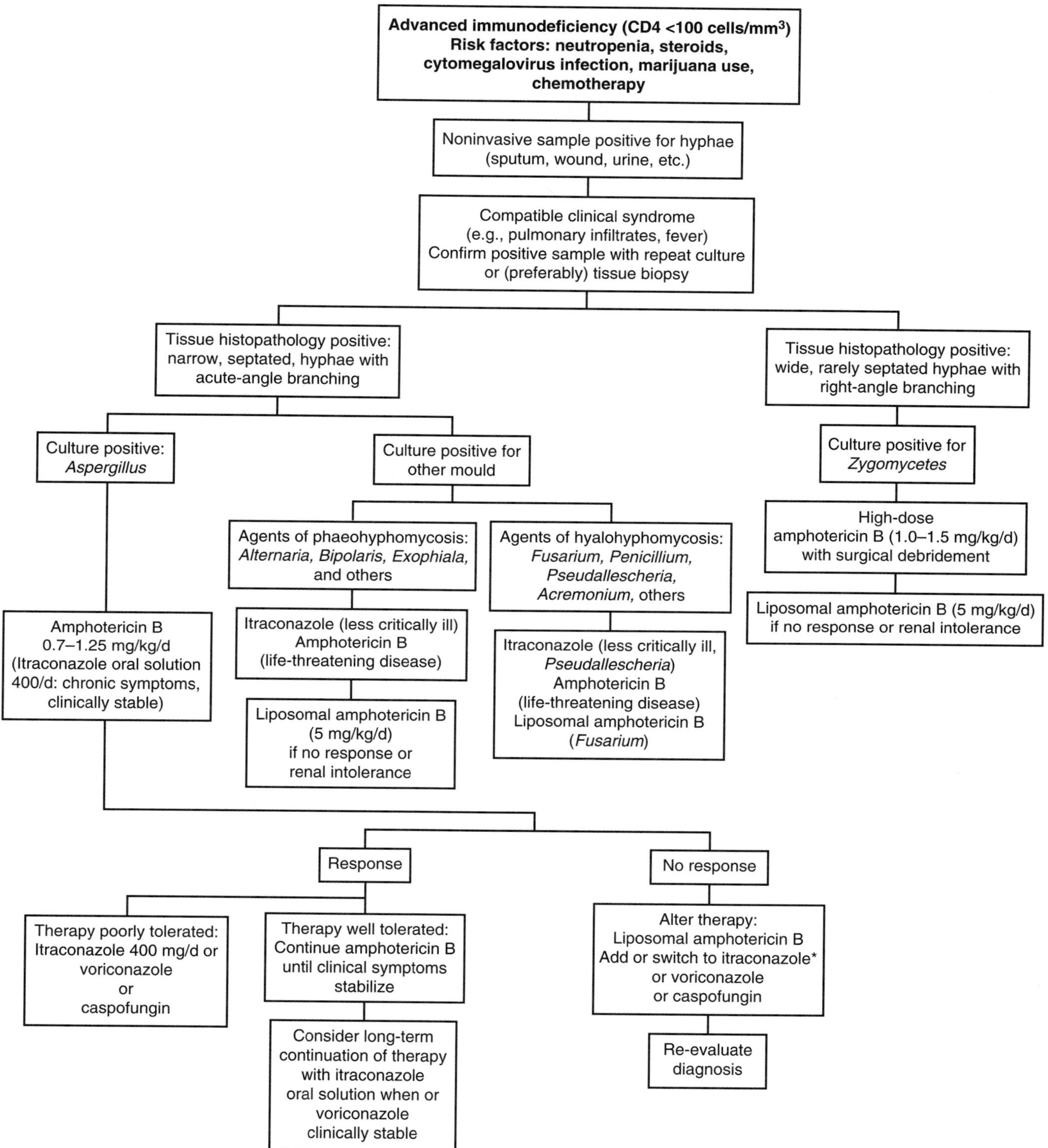

Figure 40–1. Algorithm of management of invasive mould infections in patients with AIDS. *Potential for antagonism of amphotericin B and itraconazole remains controversial.

cultures from noninvasive samples (e.g., sputum, wounds, urine) may indicate infection, particularly if they are repeatedly positive. Bronchoalveolar lavage and, when appropriate, tissue biopsies should be undertaken to confirm the presence of hyphae. Culture specimens should be obtained to confirm the specific mould, as treatment options may vary.

Antifungal therapy with high-dose amphotericin B (0.7 to 1.5 mg/kg/day) should be initiated promptly in most patients with life-threatening disease. Exceptions are patients known to be infected with an amphotericin B-resistant pathogen such as *Aspergillus terreus* or *Pseudallescheria boydii*.[15,16] Adjunctive surgical resection of isolated lesions (as may occur with *Aspergillus* when lesions are juxtaposed to the pulmonary artery) or débridement of infection caused by the Zygomycetes may improve outcome. The newer azoles, particularly itraconazole, and the newer azoles undergoing development, such as voriconazole and posaconazole,[17] have activity against many of these pathogens (except for the Zygomycetes, and even for these organisms activity with posaconazole has been suggested). Itraconazole solution increases the bioavailability of oral itraconazole and is now used parenterally as well. The use of itraconazole orally especially in capsule form, has been largely limited to patients with less severe infection.[18] In patients intolerant of high-dose amphotericin B and with progressive infection or nephrotoxicity, liposomal forms of amphotericin may improve the efficacy of therapy.[19,20] An entirely new class of antifungal agents is available in the echinocandins. These agents act rapidly and noncompetively to target the cell walls of *Candida* and *Aspergillus*. The spectrum is not yet well defined beyond *Candida* and *Aspergillus* species. Echinocardins are not excreted renally and have no nephrotoxicity.[21,22]

An initial course of amphotericin B should be administered in critically ill patients, usually for a minimum of 2 weeks or until stabilization of the disease and resolution of the underlying risk factors such as neutropenia. Following "induction" therapy with amphotericin B, high-dose azole therapy (usually with itraconazole or voriconazole for moulds) is possible for some patients.[23]

Following initial "induction" and "consolidation" therapy, long-term suppressive therapy with an oral azole is warranted for most mould infections. Long-term survival with many of these infections is uncommon unless the HIV-induced immunosuppression is corrected.

▲ "DIMORPHIC" MYCOSES (*SPOROTHRIX, PENICILLIUM, BLASTOMYCES*)

Pathogen

The dimorphic mycoses are caused by fungi that are pathogenic to normal and immune hosts. These organisms tend to occur in certain limited geographic areas or have specific epidemiologic niches (Table 40–3). The mycoses caused by these organisms include those due to endemic fungi, histoplasmosis, coccidioidomycosis, paracoccidioidomycosis, blastomycosis, penicilliosis (caused by the fungus *Penicillium marneffei*), and sporotrichosis. Among the agents of dimorphicmycoses, *Sporothrix schenckii* does not occur in a specific geographic zone but does occur in the specific setting of exposure to contaminated vegetative material such as moss and rosebush thorns. All are dimorphic; that is, they have an infectious mycelial form in nature and a yeast or yeast-like parasitic form in humans. Histoplasmosis and coccidioidomycosis are discussed in Chapters 37 and 38, respectively.

The infectious particle is the conidium, or spore. All of the dimorphic pathogens may infect by inhalation, although *Sporothrix* infection often is due to percutaneous inoculation.[24] Within a short time after infection occurs, the conidia are ingested by macrophages or monocytes within hours to days the fungus converts to the parasitic form. Infection is ultimately controlled by cell-mediated immune responses. However, in patients with HIV infection, T-helper cell (T_H2) responses are depressed or ablated. The fungus may grow and spread locally or hematogenously without much restriction. In patients with AIDS the endemic mycoses are more frequently disseminated compared to their presentation in non-HIV-infected hosts. The clinical manifestations of these diseases in HIV-infected patients are summarized in Table 40–3.

Some infections caused by dimorphic pathogens remain uncommon in patients with AIDS. For example, paracoccidioidomycosis is the major endemic mycosis in South America, but infection in patients with AIDS is rare.[25] When the disease does occur in AIDS patients, its presentation is distinct from that seen in normal hosts. In immunocompetent subjects paracoccidioidomycosis is associated with chronic progressive pulmonary granulomatous disease and dense fibrosis progressing over years. In patients with AIDS there is much more rapid progression, and the disease closely resembles disseminated histoplasmosis, with mucocutaneous skin lesions, miliary pulmonary infiltrates, and adrenal insufficiency being significant components. Meningitis may also occur, but fibrosis is not a major component of this form of disease. Blastomycosis is also uncommon in AIDS patients, occurring mainly as a late complication in those with advanced AIDS.[26,27] In immunocompetent hosts blastomycosis is associated with pulmonary fibrosis or skin infection; in patients with AIDS, however, there is widely disseminated infection, including meningitis.[28,29]

In contrast, penicilliosis caused by the dimorphic fungus *P. marneffei* has become the major endemic fungus of Southeast Asia, appearing particularly in southern China and northern Thailand.[30,31] Penicilliosis may occur in

▲ **Table 40–3.** CHARACTERISTICS OF DIMORPHIC MYCOSES IN PATIENTS WITH AIDS

Mycosis	Geographic Location	Frequency/Form
Histoplasmosis	US/Latin America	30% HIV local/disseminated infection, reticuloendothelial system
Coccidioidomycosis	Southwest US/Latin America	Locally common/primary and reactivation
Blastomycosis	US/scattered worldwide	Rare/pulmonary, disseminated
Paracoccidioidomycosis	South America	Rare/disseminated
Penicilliosis	Southeast Asia	Local 20% HIV/disseminated, pulmonary and skin
Sporotrichosis	Scattered worldwide	Uncommon/cutaneous, disseminated disease

immunocompetent patients but more commonly is seen as an opportunistic infection of AIDS. Multisystem involvement with pulmonary, skin, and visceral lesions is similar in AIDS and non-AIDS patients. Penicilliosis is a febrile wasting disease associated with symptoms that mimic other granulomatous diseases such as tuberculosis or histoplasmosis. There are commonly seen cutaneous lesions with umbilicated centers. These lesions resemble molluscum contagiosum. Like *Histoplasma*, *P. marneffei* may be recovered in blood cultures; however, in contrast to *H. capsulatum*, the yeasts of *Penicillium* divide by fission rather than by budding, so a central zone of clearing between the yeasts may be observed.

Sporotrichosis is most commonly associated with lymphocutaneous disease in immunocompetent patients.[32] However, infection may also result from inhalation of conidia, so pulmonary infection and disseminated disease may occur. Widespread disease involving joints and the lungs and other tissues is more common in HIV-infected patients. Meningitis, which is usually rare in sporotrichosis, has been reported in a few patients with HIV infection.[24,33] Untreated, these pathogens may spontaneously resolve in immunocompetent patients; but in patients with immunodeficiency such as AIDS, these mycoses are commonly progressive and lethal.

Diagnosis

The fungi causing all of these dimorphic mycoses exist in nature in their mycelial forms. This is presumably related to nutritional requirements and, for *B. dermatitidis* and *P. marneffei*, may be related to animal vectors of disease (beavers and bamboo rats, respectively). *Paracoccidioides brasiliensis* is found in certain moist tropical forest areas, but its natural habitat or vector within those zones is unclear. It has been associated with agricultural occupations (including farming) and gold mining. *Sporothrix schenckii* is also associated with outdoor activities, particularly trauma from garden exposures and sphagnum moss. Although sporotrichosis is found as far north as Canada, a number of small hyperendemic zones have been seen in tropical countries, where this infection is more common than in temperate climates.[34]

It is assumed that nutritional requirements also in large part dictate the endemic zones of these fungi. The endemic zone for blastomycosis in North America and the zone for paracoccidioidomycosis in South America largely overlap the endemic zones for histoplasmosis. However, relatively few cases of blastomycosis or paracoccidioidomycosis are associated with AIDS, whereas histoplasmosis is a major pathogen in AIDS patients. The clear rural associations of infection with *B. dermatitidis* or *P. braziliensis* are offered as a contrast to histoplasmosis, which is seen in both urban and rural settings and is associated with construction. Late reactivation of disease appears to be less common with paracoccidioidomycosis than histoplasmosis. Another factor that may play a role in "suppressing" paracoccidioidomycosis is the frequent use of trimethoprim-sulfamethoxazole (TMP-SMX) for preventing pneumocystosis. TMP-SMX is active against *P. brasiliensis* as well, so a secondary benefit of preventing *P. brasiliensis* is theoretically possible.[19]

These dimorphic pathogens are identified by culture or presumptively by identifying distinct tissue forms on tissue samples. *B. dermatitidis*, *S. schenckii*, and *P. marneffei* grow readily as mycelia on usual fungal media such as Sabouraud dextrose agar. *P. marneffei* produces a distinctive red pigment that diffuses out into the medium and facilitates identification. Mycelial cultures may take up to a month to grow at room temperature. *P. brasiliensis* grows slowly in the mycelial phase and requires a temperature range of 18° to 22°C and McVeigh Morton agar to grow optimally.[35]

Although a mycologist may distinguish these dimorphic pathogens in mycelial form, the clinician encounters them more often in biopsy specimens. Infection can be diagnosed by identifying the distinctive tissue forms of the organisms. Normally the fungi are seen associated with granulomas (*P. brasiliensis*, *P. marneffei*) or mixed granuloma and pyogenic reactions (*B. dermatiditis*, *S. schenckii*). In patients with AIDS, however, there may be a much less intact granulomatous reaction.

Cultures may be prepared from sputum, cutaneous lesions, lymph nodes, or urine. Blood can be cultured by the isolator technique or using the BacTech system. Culture may require up to a month for growth to be detected, and it is sometimes falsely negative because of failure of the organism to convert from the parasitic form to the mycelial form in vitro. It is much more rapid and feasible to identify the organism in tissue using the Gomori methenamine silver stain or periodic acid-Schiff, each of which stains the cell walls. The presence of these organisms on tissue biopsy, wet mount, or culture is indicative of infection and may be associated with pulmonary or disseminated disease.

Serologic testing is less useful than with histoplasmosis (which can be diagnosed with antigen testing) or coccidioidomycosis (for which positive antibody results correlate with the disease). Antibody tests are available for paracoccidioidomycosis and blastomycosis.[29,35] Although the antibodies measured can be useful for diagnosis and their titers tend to rise with worsening disease, they are not protective. There is some cross reaction (especially for *B. dermatitidis*) with *H. capsulatum* and *C. immitis*. There is a serologic test for sporotrichosis, but it is not widely used. A serologic test has been developed for *P. marneffei* disease but is still not used routinely.[36] Antibody testing may be less useful in patients with HIV infection, particularly during the late stages when antibodies are poorly produced. Fungal antibody tests are routinely available through clinical or reference laboratories. Antigen testing is clinically available only for histoplasmosis (Histoplasmosis Reference Laboratory, Indianapolis, IN, USA).

Susceptibility testing of the endemic mycoses remains nonstandardized. In general, modification of the standard yeast susceptibility testing method of the National Committee for Clinical Laboratory Standards is used, but incubation is carried out for longer periods. As a practical tool, susceptibility testing has been correlated with clinical response for *P. marneffei,* and for *H. capsulatum* for which amphotericin B and itraconazole are more potent in vitro than fluconazole, with corresponding clinical results.[37]

Therapy

Treatment approaches for the endemic mycoses are relatively well established, although there have been no prospective, comparative trials for any of these infections in patients with AIDS (Fig. 40–1). Experience with these infections in non-HIV-infected patients and results of clinical trials of HIV-infected patients with histoplasmosis and coccidioidomycosis allow some general guidelines.[14,38] First, if the patient is severely ill, amphotericin B remains the standard therapy. Amphotericin B is usually infused intravenously over 2 to 4 hours at 0.7 to 1.0 mg/kg daily or up to twice the dose on alternate days. After a time defined by the onset of clear clinical improvement, usually a minimum of 2 weeks, the patient may be switched to an azole. An exception may be sporotrichosis, in which a patient may be refractory to amphotericin B but respond to itraconazole.[39] If a patient is only moderately ill, therapy may be begun with an azole.

The most potent antifungal azole now widely available for these mycoses is itraconazole,[35,40–42] which is administered as capsules at oral doses from 50 mg/day (*P. brasiliensis*) through 200 to 400 mg/day (for the others). Because the drug is cleared slowly by the liver and clearance is dose-dependent, a loading dose of up to 800 mg/day may be given for the first 2 to 3 days. Itraconazole solution may produce serum concentrations that are double those seen with capsules, so a lower dose may be sufficient. Because absorption of itraconazole is somewhat erratic, an intravenous form has been developed using the same vehicle. The loading dose is 200 mg twice daily for the first day, then 200 mg once daily for adults.[43,44] Before commencing itraconazole, it is important to ascertain that the patient is not receiving concurrent agents that alter the metabolism of itraconazole. Specific cautions to itraconazole use include concurrent medications such as rifampin, rifabutin, phenytoin, and others that induce hepatic degrading cytochrome P_{450} enzymes.[45] Specific cautions also stem from itraconazole delaying excretion of concurrently administered drugs, including terfenadine, astemizole, loperamide, and lovastatin. Tacrolimus and cyclosporin must be monitored closely because their concentrations may rise. Similar events may occur with the protease inhibitors, which are metabolized through the cytochrome P_{450} enzyme system. Nevirapine may accelerate itraconazole clearance. Reverse transcriptase inhibitors are not problematic.

For paracoccidioidomycosis and blastomycosis, the most extensive reports of treatment efficacy were accumulated from data before itraconazole had gained widespread use, and our recommendation for itraconazole is based on experience with non-HIV-infected patients. The response rate to itraconazole in non-HIV-infected patients with sporotrichosis is close to 100% for lymphocutaneous disease and more than 70% for patients with disseminated disease.[41,46] However, only 71% of patients with lymphocutaneous disease and 31% of patients with disseminated disease responded to fluconazole.[14,40] The outcome for blastomycosis and sporotrichosis in AIDS patients is generally much worse with disseminated disease than with local pulmonary disease (blastomycosis and paracoccidioidomycosis) or cutaneous disease (sporotrichosis). Meningitis caused by *S. schenckii* is rare and does not respond well to treatment.[24,27] Blastomycosis in AIDS patients is strongly associated with central nervous system involvement (46% of 24 patients), with the mortality 90% in this group.[26]

The patient is stabilized on "consolidation" therapy (400 mg/day capsular form), after which the dose may be lowered eventually to 200 mg/day for chronic suppression and prevention of relapse. All of these infections are associated with relapse if treatment is interrupted. With effective antiretroviral therapy, it is possible that immune recovery will prevent relapse if treatment is interrupted. At what level of CD4 count or what duration of therapy this may be done has not been determined.

Alternative agents for treating the endemic mycoses include fluconazole, which has more attractive kinetics and fewer drug interactions. Fluconazole is less efficacious than itraconazole for penicilliosis, sporotrichosis, blastomycosis, histoplasmosis, and paracoccidioidomycosis.[37,47,48] The newer azoles, including posaconazole and voriconazole, also have activity against these organisms. Posaconazole, an investigational new triazole, appears to be a particularly attractive alternative for these agents based on its extremely potent in vitro and animal model activity against a wide variety of filamentous mycoses. Limited clinical experience with coccidioidomycosis, including disseminated disease in HIV-infected and non-HIV-infected patients, suggests that the clinical response to posaconazole may be more rapid and complete than with any other antifungal agent. A small (unpublished) study of 20 patients treated for up to 6 months (non-HIV-infected) supported rapid, complete response of the infection.[49] Given the potential for posaconazole in coccidioidomycosis, the most challenging of the endemic mycoses, it is likely (but speculative) that posaconazole will be highly effective treatment for the other dimorphic mycoses.

Prevention

There are no proven ways to eliminate the risk of infection with these dimorphic pathogens.

▲ AGENTS OF HYALOHYPHOMYCOSIS (*ASPERGILLUS*, *FUSARIUM*, *PSEUDALLESCHERIA*)

Agents of hyalohyphomycosis are a diverse group of lightly pigmented (hyaline) moulds. The most important of these organisms is *Aspergillus*, but other moulds, such as *Fusarium* species, *Pseudallescheria boydii*, and *Chrysosporium* species, have also been reported occasionally in patients with advanced AIDS[50] (Table 40–1). Since the advent of HAART, these infections have become rare in HIV patients but are ever more common in patients with leukemia/lymphoma.[51] Nevertheless, they remain potential pathogens in patients with advanced AIDS and uncontrolled viral replication. They appear similar to each other and to *Aspergillus* in tissue, so cultures are needed to confirm the specific agent causing the disease. The risk factors for these infections include advanced immunodeficiency, with CD4+ T-lymphocyte counts usually less than 50/mm^3, and other alterations in host defenses, such as neutropenia, malignancy, indwelling catheters, and co-morbid conditions such as diabetes mellitis.[3]

Aspergillus

Invasive aspergillosis was not defined as an opportunistic infection of AIDS because of the relative obscurity of that infection in the original cases of AIDS. Although the frequency of these infections increased for some years, they have once again become uncommon. The clinical presentation of invasive aspergillosis with AIDS includes pulmonary disease, sinusitis, cutaneous infection, localized abscesses including vertebral infection, brain abscess, and renal disease as well as widely disseminated infection.[51,52] Colonization with *Aspergillus* has been reported to occur in approximately 5% of AIDS patients in some series, although the rate of proven invasive disease was less than 1%.[8] The course of aspergillosis is frequently unremitting, although aggressive antifungal therapy may suppress clinical symptoms and prolong survival.[53] The course may not be fulminant as frequently occurs in other immunosuppressed patients, such as profoundly neutropenic patients and those undergoing bone marrow transplantation. In patients with more chronic symptoms, a high index of suspicion is needed to establish the diagnosis.[54]

The most common species associated with infection in most medical centers is *Aspergillus fumigatus*, though other species may be found. The usual route of infection is through inhalation of conidia, which are ubiquitous and found in air, dust, ventilation systems, plants, soil, and environmental surfaces. Cutaneous infection may also occur in association with indwelling intravenous catheters or injection drug use.[55]

The major host defenses against *Aspergillus* species are neutrophils (which inhibit conidia) and macrophages (which kill conidia).[56] Thus HIV-infected patients with impaired neutrophils, such as those undergoing cytotoxic chemotherapy, therapy for opportunistic infections that cause neutropenia, or therapy for malignancy, are at greatest risk for infection. Patients with impaired macrophage function, as occurs with the use of corticosteroids, are also at increased risk. However, some patients with HIV infection do not have other identifiable risks, so HIV infection may independently increase the risk of *Aspergillus* infection.[56,57]

Diagnosis

The diagnosis of invasive aspergillosis is suggested by repeated isolation of the organism from noninvasive samples such as sputum, particularly in a high risk patient with compatible clinical symptoms.[58] The diagnosis is established by demonstrating hyphae in tissue samples (Fig. 40–2). The presence of hyphae consistent with *Aspergillus* on bronchoalveolar lavage samples in an HIV-infected patient with a compatible clinical syndrome is often sufficient to allow institution of empiric therapy. Evaluation of bronchoalveolar lavage and, in selected patients, a tissue biopsy are important for confirming that invasion rather than colonization is present and to determine if other opportunistic pathogens are present. A culture is necessary because other agents of hyalohyphomycosis may appear indistinguishable on a tissue biopsy. Susceptibility testing is not standardized and is not generally useful, although *Aspergillus* strains resistant to itraconazole have been reported.[59]

Nonculture methods can also be used to help establish a diagnosis of invasive aspergillosis. Chest radiographs are usually abnormal in patients with invasive infection, but patients with ulcerative tracheobronchitis may not show pulmonary infiltrates. Radiographically invasive pulmonary aspergillosis appears most commonly as diffuse infiltrates (25%), focal infiltrates (22%), cavitary lesions (36%), bronchial aspergillosis with atelectasis (14%), and other nonspecific findings (3%).[60] Computed tomography of the chest may show an early halo or air-crescent sign, indicating the presence of infection, although these findings may be less specific in nonneutropenic patients.[61] Their presence has led some clinicians to institute therapy early, which may improve outcomes or at least delay progression.

Antigen detection of galactomannan has undergone continuing investigation, particularly in patients with leukemia and lymphoma.[62,63] Maertens et al. have summarized encouraging studies in which predisposed patients are monitored twice weekly for antigenemia and, if positive, are subjected to other confirmatory tests and treated for presumptive disease.[64] The polymerase chain reaction (PCR) may be less specific than testing for the presence of galactomannan for diagnosis.[65] There is uncertainty over whether these methods, even if used routinely in patients at high risk for fulminating disease (leukemia, bone marrow transplant), can detect the patient who has progressive but less aggressive disease, as is more typical for the patient with AIDS. Furthermore, a large-scale screening program would be extremely costly for the few patients who might be identified.

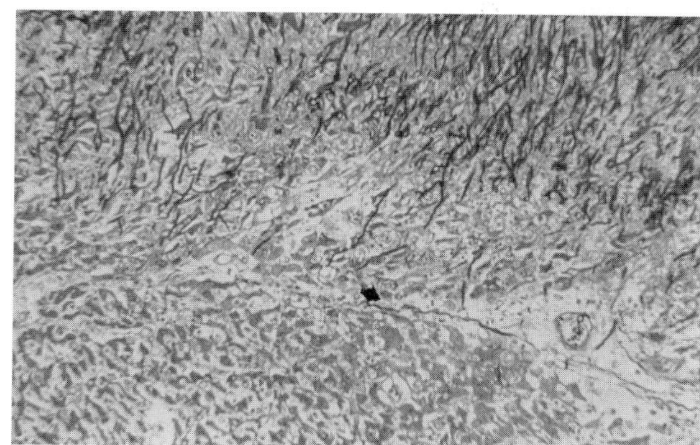

Figure 40–2. Histopathologic appearance of *Aspergillus* species hyphae (silver stain).

Therapy and Prevention

Initial therapy for invasive aspergillosis should be with high-dose amphotericin B (0.7 to 1.5 mg/kg/day) in most patients, although response rates are poor. This likely reflects the critically ill status of patients selected for therapy. Liposomal amphotericin B preparations may be effective and are often used if patients are at high risk for nephrotoxicity or show indications of renal toxicity. Doses of 5 to 10 mg/kg/day have been used for both AmBisome and Abelcet.

Itraconazole has also been used, usually following an initial course of amphotericin B.[23] Response rates to itraconazole capsules at initial doses of 600 mg/day for 3 days followed by 400 mg/day produced partial responses or stabilization of symptoms in 7 of the 11 AIDS patients (63%) treated.[66] However, progression of underlying disease eventually occurred in all patients.

During the past few years new agents have appeared that may be quite effective. Caspofungin is the first of a new class of antifungal drugs, the echinocandins. This drug acts rapidly to stop growth of the fungal cell wall and appears to be fungicidal for growing tips of *Aspergillus* hyphae. At present caspofungin is licensed for salvage therapy of acute invasive aspergillosis, and the experience (with an overall response rate of approximately 45%) has been limited in patients with AIDS.[67] The main disadvantage of this class of drug is the need for intravenous administration. Advantages include few drug interactions, no need to adjust the dose in the presence of renal failure, and minimal to no hepatic or renal toxicity. Aspergillosis is the only mycelial infection in which this class of drugs has thus far been evaluated.

Other agents offering great promise include voriconazole and posaconazole.[10,17,68,69] They have been found as effective (40% to 50%) as caspofungin in salvage studies of invasive aspergillosis. Results of comparative trials indicate that voriconazole offers a significant advantage over Amphotericin B for primary therapy of invasive aspergillosis as well. (Division of Antiviral Drug Advisory Committee, September 2001) Voriconazole is likely to become the drug of choice for invasive aspergillosis. Advantages of these compounds include oral and (for voriconazole) parenteral administration; limitations include the well known range of drug interactions for broad-spectrum triazoles. Voriconazole also has associated transient visual toxicity, which manifests as "brightness" in visual perception.

Unfortunately, limited data are published on either of these new triazoles or caspofungin at this stage of their development. Although these drugs provide some basis for hope, thus far the response rates to antifungal agents in invasive aspergillosis for the highest risk patients remain dismal. If there is no response to antiretrovirals, death occurs a median of 2 to 4 months after diagnosis. Even if control of infection is achieved, which is seen in a limited number of patients for more than 12 months, recrudescence is common. Clinicians often use combination therapy in desperate situations (i.e., combinations of amphotericin B with azole therapy, caspofungin, or both). Whether such combination therapy is advantageous is unknown.

In patients with localized disease, surgical resection of pulmonary nodules or visceral abscesses may improve outcome. Patients with cutaneous and catheter-related infection also respond to local intervention combined with aggressive antifungal therapy. Patients with endobronchial lesions are also effectively treated with itraconazole therapy.[70,71]

Infection with *Aspergillus* species is not readily prevented because patients are constantly exposed to conidia. Prophylaxis with antifungal agents is not indicated because of the rarity of this infection. However, the judicious use of steroids and the reversal of neutropenia may decrease the number of patients at risk for infection.[56]

Other Agents (*Fusarium*, *Pseudallescheria*, *Chrysosporium*)

An increasing number of other agents of hyalohyphomycosis have been reported to cause invasive mycoses in patients with AIDS. These organisms include a collection of hyaline moulds such as *Fusarium* species, *Pseudallescheria boydii*, *Chrysosporium* species, *Geotrichum*, *Trichosporon beigelii*, and *Penicillium* species[72–78] (Table 40–1).

The risk factors for infection are similar to those for *Aspergillus*, and the clinical presentations of these infections may all be similar to that of invasive aspergillosis. The clinical presentations include sinusitis, pulmonary infection, localized abscesses, cutaneous infection, and (fusarium) fungemia that may be associated with disseminated infection.

In tissue, all of these organisms appear as branched, septated hyphae that are indistinguishable from those of *Aspergillus* or other molds (Fig. 40–3). Specific diagnosis requires culture of the organism from tissue. Standard treatment for most of these organisms has been amphotericin B, although some of these organisms are clinically and mycologically resistant to amphotericin B, including *Fusarium* and *Pseudallescheria*.[76,77,79] Posaconazole and voriconazole have both been used with success in the treatment of *Pseudallescheria* and *Fusarium* infections and are likely to become drugs of choice, although only limited data are available at present.[80–83] Voriconazole may be quite effective against *Scedosporium apiospermium* (63% of 27 patients responding) but appears less effective against

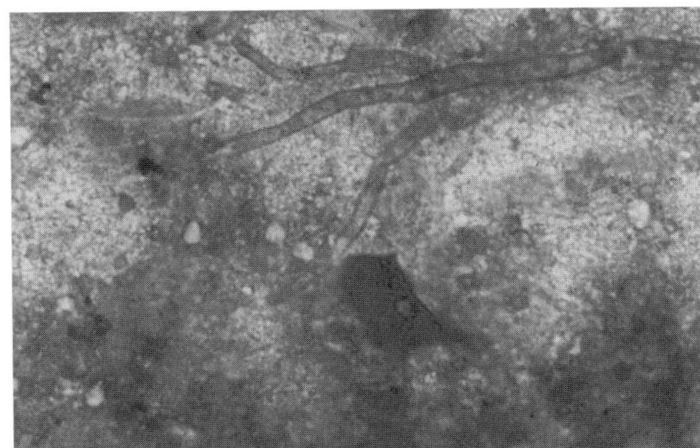

Figure 40–3. Histopathologic appearance of an agent of hyalohyphomycosis in tissue (periodic acid-Schiff stain).

Scedosporium prolificans (two of seven patients responding).[84] Antifungal agents to prevent these mycoses are not indicated because they remain rare. Early consideration for the diagnosis and prompt initiation of therapy may improve prognosis. Lifelong suppressive antifungal therapy may be needed though improved antiretroviral therapy raises the possibility of limited duration of treatment.

▲ AGENTS OF PHAEOHYPHOMYCOSIS (*CLADOPHIALOPHORA*, *ALTERNERIA*, *EXOPHIALA*)

Pathogens

Agents of phaeohyphomycosis comprise a group of opportunistic molds that are dematiaceous, or darkly pigmented (Table 40–1). These emerging pathogens remain rare in patients with AIDS. There are many genera of fungi in this group, but they infrequently cause infections in patients with HIV.[93] These opportunistic fungi do not cause infections specifically in HIV-infected patients but do cause disease in certain epidemiologic settings.

As with other moulds, infection usually occurs by inhalation of conidia. It usual starts in the sinuses or the lungs. Alternatively, infection may follow percutaneous inoculation.[89,92] Fungemia may also occur.[94]

The pathogenicity of these organisms is quite variable. In immunocompetent patients or those with minimal host defense abnormalities, phaeohyphomycosis may proceed with the development of sinusitis or pneumonia over months to years, and there may be direct invasion of the brain from the sinuses.[95] There may also be a significant component of hypersensitivity, with eosinophils and Charcot-Leyden crystals in sinus aspirates. Subcutaneous lesions may gradually enlarge over months. Colonies of the dematiaceous fungi are dark-colored. Many of these fungi, such as *Cladophialophora* species, are neurotropic and may cause brain abscesses.[96] These fungi may infect the individual at any stage of AIDS, but they are commonly associated with a more rapid course in those with late AIDS.

The organisms are found in decaying vegetation and are abundant in nature but of sufficiently low virulence that only scattered infections occur. They thrive best in an acidic, glucose-rich environment and are readily killed by polymorphonuclear leukocytes. Thus neutropenia and uncontrolled diabetes are risk factors for infection. Traumatic inoculation while gardening is a major mode of infection.

Diagnosis and Therapy

Agents of phaeohyphomycosis are characterized by production of black melanin pigment, which may be seen histopathologically and in gross lesions. The mycelia are quite variable, and identification is made by examining conidia in culture. As with endemic mycoses, the diagnosis is made by culture or biopsy. Unlike the endemic mycoses, in which the morphology of the parasitic form is distinctive, these mycoses may present with "mycelia sterilia," a mould culture that does not sporulate and thus does not allow identification. Masson-Fontana staining of tissue specimens is useful for staining the melanin in the hyphae, and it allows a specific diagnosis of an agent of phaeohyphomycosis (Fig. 40–4). Culture specimens are best obtained from normally sterile sites (e.g., biopsy of a subcutaneous lesion or sinus aspirate). These organisms may be found colonizing the respiratory tract from sputum samples, so a tissue biopsy may be needed to establish a diagnosis of invasive infection.

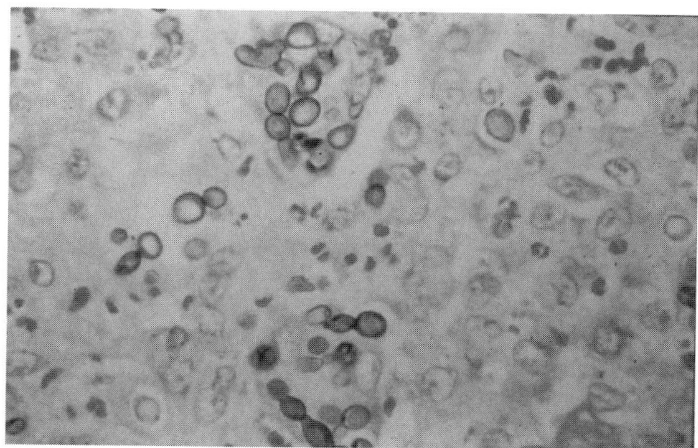

Figure 40–4. Histopathologic appearance of an agent of phaeohyphomycosis in tissue (Masson-Fontana stain).

Therapy is commonly initiated with amphotericin B. However, in vitro activity of the azoles has been demonstrated against many of the agents of phaeohyphomycosis, so itraconazole is a possible alternative for patients with less serious infection and for long-term suppressive therapy. Itraconazole is more active in vitro than ketoconazole or fluconazole, although few clinical reports have evaluated fluconazole in these infections. Because these mycoses are uncommon and there are no comparative trials of antifungals, animal studies have been used to evaluate the efficacy of antifungals against some of these pathogens.[97]

Itraconazole should be used at initial loading doses of 600 to 800 mg/day for 3 days and then continued at 400 mg/day.[98,99] For patients with central nervous system (CNS) involvement, continuing a dose of 600 mg/day has controlled progression of the disease. Several new antifungal triazoles, including voriconazole and posaconazole[100] have been effective in vitro or in animal models of these infections.[100,101] Voriconazole has been clinically effective in a few patients. The new echinocandins also have potent activity in vitro against some agents of phaeohyphomycosis, but there is no clinical experience with them.[102] There are no known ways to prevent these unusual mycoses.

▲ ZYGOMYCOSIS

Pathogens and Diagnosis (*Rhizopus* Species, *Absidia*, *Mucor*, *Rhizomucor*, *Cunninghamella*)

Zygomycetes such as *Rhizopus* species, *Absidia*, *Mucor*, *Rhizomucor*, and *Cunninghamella* commonly cause rhinocerebral disease or pneumonia in patients with diabetes

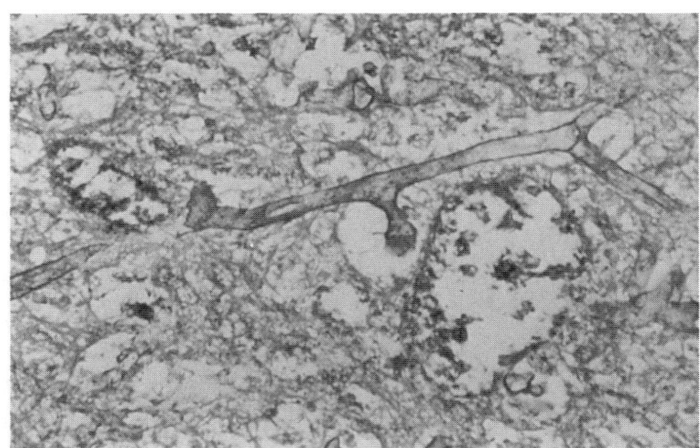

Figure 40–5. Histopathologic appearance of an agent of zygomycosis in tissue (silver stain).

or neutropenia[103] (Table 40–1). These organisms have been reported uncommonly in patients with AIDS but may cause localized deep tissue abscesses in organs including the kidney, liver, spleen, and stomach.[104] Some of these infections progress rather slowly in patients with AIDS and respond well to surgery and to antifungal therapy with amphotericin B.[105] Disseminated infection, including infections in the CNS, may also occur; it tends to be aggressive and has a poor outcome, with mortality rates of 80% or more.[6,106,107]

Risk factors for infection include injection drug use, neutropenia, the use of corticosteroids, and diabetes. In most cases the route of infection is presumed to be through contamination of injected drugs, although inhalation of conidia is also possible.

Zygomycosis is diagnosed by demonstrating wide, rarely septated hyphae with right-angle branching in tissue (Fig. 40–5). Hematoxylin-eosin stains Zygomycetes' mycelia densely, usually much more than those of *Aspergillus*. However, the individual species must be identified in vitro in cultures, where distinctive microscopic and macroscopic features, such as the presence or absence of rhizoids (rootlike structures) or characteristics of sporangia, allow a specific diagnosis. Zygomycetes grow rapidly on culture media, usually within a day, using routine fungal media. However, when tissue is homogenized before culture, the mycelium may be broken up sufficiently that it does not grow in culture. Serologic testing is not useful for these organisms.

Therapy and Prevention

Zygomycoses are not considered responsive to azole antifungals, although in vitro and in animal studies posaconazole shows good activity against Zygomycetes. In our experience, two patients with lung transplants and zygomycosis responded to posaconazole therapy (J.R. Graybill, unpublished observations). Specific organisms (e.g., some strains of *Absidia*) are susceptible in vitro to itraconazole, although clinical experience is limited. Zygomycosis is treated with surgical débridement and amphotericin B in the traditional formulation or as lipid formulations.[3,19,108] The experience in HIV-infected patients is so limited that chronic management of survivors is unclear.

This infection is rare in HIV patients, and the results of treatment are mixed, with a usually poor outcome if the CNS is involved but a better outcome if the disease is localized to the skin or other organs. In some cases surgical resection is appropriate and necessary to control the infection. Specific measures to prevent these rare mycoses are not possible.

REFERENCES

1. Cunliffe NA, Denning DW. Uncommon invasive mycoses in AIDS. AIDS 9:411, 1995.
2. Perfect JR, Schell WA. The new fungal opportunists are coming. Clin Infect Dis 22(suppl 2):S112, 1996.
3. Minamoto GY, Rosenberg AS. Fungal infections in patients with the acquired immunodeficiency syndrome. Med Clin North Am 81:381, 1997.
4. Ampel N. Emerging issues and fungal pathogens in patients with the acquired immunodeficiency syndrome. Emerg Infect Dis 2:109, 1997.
5. Teh W, Matti BS, Marisiddaiah H, Minamoto GY. Aspergillus sinusitis in patients with AIDS: report of three cases and review. Clin Infect Dis 21:529, 1995.
6. Blatt SP, Lucey DR, DeHoff D, Zellmer RB. Rhinocerebral zygomycosis in a patient with AIDS. J Infect Dis 17:948, 1993.
7. Rosenthal J, Katz R, DuBois DB, et al. Chronic maxillary sinusitis associated with the mushroom Schizophyllum commune in a patient with AIDS. Clin Infect Dis 14:46, 1992.
8. Pursell KJ, Telzak EE, Armstrong D. Aspergillus species colonization and invasive disease in patients with AIDS. Clin Infect Dis 14:141, 1992.
9. Hiemenz JW, Walsh TJ. Lipid formulations of amphotericin B: recent progress and future directions. Clin Infect Dis 22(suppl 2):S133, 1996.
10. Schlamm H, Corey L, Brown J, Perfect J. Voriconazole for salvage treatment of invasive aspergillosis. Presented at the 38th Annual Meeting of the Infectious Disease Society of America, 2000, p 93, abstract 304.
11. Perfect J, Lutsar I, Gonzalez-Ruiz. Voriconazole (VORI) for treatment of resistant and rare fungal pathogens. Presented at the 38th Annual Meeting of the Infectious Disease Society of America, 2000, p 93, abstract 303.
12. Stevens DA, Kan VL, Judson MA, et al. Practice guidelines for diseases caused by Aspergillus. Clin Infect Dis 30:696, 2000.
13. Galgiani JN, Ampel NM, Catanzaro A, et al. Practice guidelines for the treatment of coccidioidomycosis. Clin Infect Dis 30:658, 2000.
14. Kauffman CA, Hajjeh R, Chapman SW, Mycoses SG. Practice guidelines for the management of patients with sporotrichosis. Clin Infect Dis 30:684, 2000.
15. Dannaoui E, Borel E, Persat F, et al. Amphotericin B resistance of Aspergillus terreus in a murine model of disseminated aspergillosis. J Med Microbiol 49:601, 2000.
16. Walsh TJ, Peter J, McGough DA, et al. Activities of amphotericin B and antifungal azoles alone and in combination against Pseudallescheria boydii. Antimicrob Agents Chemother 39:1361, 1995.
17. Denning DW, Del Favero A, Gluckman E, et al. The efficacy and tolerability of UK109,496 (Voriconazole) in the treatment of invasive aspergillosis. Presented at the 13th Congress of the International Society for Human and Animal Mycology, 1997, p 217, abstract P552.
18. Willems L, van der Geest R, de Beule K. Itraconazole oral solution and intravenous formulations: a review of pharmacokinetics and pharmacodynamics. J Clin Pharm Ther 26:159, 2001.
19. Walsh TJ, Hiemenz JW, Seibel NL, et al. Amphotericin B lipid complex for invasive fungal infections: analysis of safety and efficacy in 556 cases. Clin Infect Dis 26:1383, 1998.
20. Fisher EW, Toma A, Fisher PH. Rhinocerebral mucormycois: therapy with amphotericin B lipid complex. Arch Intern Med 156:337, 1996.
21. Hector RF. Compounds active against cell walls of medically important fungi. Clin Microbiol Rev 6:1, 1993.
22. Ernst EJ, Klepser ME, Pfaller M. Postantifungal effects of echinocandin, azole, and polyene antifungal agents against Candida albicans

and Cryptococcus neoformans. Antimicrob Agents Chemother 44:1108, 2000.
23. Patterson TF, Kirkpatrick WR, White M, et al. Invasive aspergillosis: disease spectrum, treatment practices, and outcomes. Medicine 79:250, 2000.
24. Donabedian RM, O'Donnell E, Olszewski C, et al. Disseminated cutaneous and meningeal sporotrichosis in an AIDS patient. Diagn Microbiol Infect Dis 18:111, 1994.
25. Goldani LZ, Sugar AM. Paracoccidioidomycosis and AIDS: an overview. Clin Infect Dis 21:1275, 1995.
26. Witzig RS, Hoadley DJ, Greer DL, et al. Blastomycosis and human immunodeficiency virus: three new cases and review. South Med J 87:715, 1994.
27. Pappas PG, Pottage JC, Powderly WG, et al. Blastomycosis in patients with acquired immunodeficiency syndrome. Ann Intern Med 116:847, 1992.
28. Tan G, Kaufman L, Peterson EM, De la Maza LM. Disseminated atypical blastomycosis in two patients with AIDS. Clin Infect Dis 16:107, 1993.
29. Bradsher RW. Blastomycosis. Clin Infect Dis 14(suppl 1):S82, 1992.
30. Wong SSY, Siau H, Yuen KY. Penicilliosis marneffei: West meets East. J Med Microbiol 48:973, 1999.
31. Supparatpinyo K, Khamwan C, Baosoung V, et al. Disseminated Penicillium marneffei infection in Southeast Asia. Lancet 344:110, 1994.
32. Kauffman CA. Old and new therapies for sporotrichosis. Clin Infect Dis 21:981, 1995.
33. Penn CC, Goldstein E, Bartholomew WR. Sporothrix schenckii meningitis in a patient with AIDS. Clin Infect Dis 15:568, 1992.
34. Pappas PG, Tellez I, Deep AE, et al. Sporotrichosis in Peru: description of an area of hyperendemicity. Clin Infect Dis 30:65, 2000.
35. Brummer E, Castaneda E, Restrepo A. Paracoccidioidomycosis: an update. Clin Microbiol Rev 6:89, 1993.
36. Yuen K, Wong SS, Tsang DN, Chau P. Serodiagnosis of Penicillium marneffei infection. Lancet 344:444, 1994.
37. Supparatpinyo K, Nelson KE, Merz WG, et al. Response to antifungal therapy by human immunodeficiency virus-infected patients with disseminated Penicillium marneffei infections and in vitro susceptibilities of isolates from clinical specimens. Antimicrob Agents Chemother 37:2407, 1993.
38. Chapman SW, Bradsher RW Jr, Campbell GD Jr, et al. Practice guidelines for the management of patients with blastomycosis. Clin Infect Dis 30:679, 2000.
39. Bolao F, Podzamczer D, Ventin M, Gudiol F. Efficacy of acute phase and maintenance therapy with itraconazole in an AIDS patient with sporotrichosis. Eur J Clin Microbiol Infect Dis 13:609, 1994.
40. Kauffman CA, Pappas PG, McKinsey DS, et al. Treatment of lymphocutaneous and visceral sporotrichosis with fluconazole. Clin Infect Dis 22:46, 1996.
41. Winn RE, Anderson JG, Piper J, et al. Systemic sporotrichosis treated with itraconazole. Clin Infect Dis 17:210, 1993.
42. Oscherwitz SL, Rinaldi MG. Correspondence: disseminated sporotrichosis in a patient infected with human immunodeficiency virus. Clin Infect Dis 15:568, 1992.
43. Caillot D, Bassaris H, Seifert WF, et al. Efficacy, safety, and pharmacokinetics of intravenous (IV) followed by oral itraconazole (ITR) in patients (pts) with invasive pulmonary aspergillosis (IPA). Presented at the 39th Interscience Conference on Antimicrobial Agents and Chemotherapy, 1999, p 574, abstract 1643.
44. Boogaerts MA, Maertens J, Van Der Geest R, et al. Pharmacokinetics and safety of a 7-day administration of intravenous itraconazole followed by a 14-day administration of itraconazole oral solution in patients with hematologic malignancy. Antimicrob Agents Chemother 45:981, 2001.
45. Como JA, Dismukes WE. Oral azole drugs as systemic antifungal therapy. N Engl J Med 330:263, 1994.
46. Sharkey-Mathis PK, Kauffman CA, Graybill JR, et al. Treatment of sporotrichosis with itraconazole. Am J Med 95:279, 1993.
47. Pappas PG, Bradsher RW, Chapman SW, et al. Treatment of blastomycosis with fluconazole: a pilot study. Clin Infect Dis 20:267, 1995.
48. Kauffman CA. Sporotrichosis. Clin Infect Dis 29:231, 1999.
49. Graybill JR, Stevens DA, Galgiani JN, et al. Itraconazole treatment of coccidiodomycosis. Am J Med 89:292, 1990.
50. Schell WA. New aspects of emerging fungal pathogens: a multifaceted challenge. Clin Lab Med 15:365, 1995.
51. Denning D. Invasive aspergillosis. Clin Infect Dis 26:781, 1998.
52. Mylonakis E, Paliou M, Sax PE, et al. Central nervous system aspergillosis in patients with human immunodeficiency virus infection: report of 6 cases and review. Medicine (Baltimore) 79:269, 2000.
53. Lortholary O, Meyohas M-C, DuPont B, et al. Invasive aspergillosis in patients with acquired immunodeficiency syndrome: report of 33 cases. Am J Med 95:177, 1993.
54. Mylonakis E, Rich JD, Flanigan T. Muscle abscess due to Aspergillus fumigatus in a patients with AIDS. Clin Infect Dis 23:1323, 1996.
55. Smith WF, Wallace MR. Cutaneous aspergillosis. Cutis 59:138, 1997.
56. Khoo SH, Denning DW. Invasive aspergillosis in patients with AIDS. Clin Infect Dis 19(suppl 1):S41, 1994.
57. Minamoto GY, Barlam TF, Vander Els NJ. Invasive aspergillosis in patients with AIDS. Clin Infect Dis 14:66, 1992.
58. Horvath JA, Dummer S. The use of respiratory-tract cultures in the diagnosis of invasive pulmonary aspergillosis. Am J Med 100:171, 1996.
59. Denning DW, Venkateswarlu K, Oakley KL, et al. Itraconazole resistance in Aspergillus fumigatus. Antimicrob Agents Chemother 41:1364, 1997.
60. Miller WTJ, Sais GT, Frank I. Pulmonary aspergillosis in patients with AIDS: clinical and radiographic correlations. Chest 105:32, 1994.
61. Caillot D, Casanovas O, Bernard A. Improved management of invasive pulmonary aspergillosis in neutropenic patients using early thoracic computed tomographic scan and surgery. J Clin Oncol 15:139, 1997.
62. Fortun J, Martin-Davila P, Alvarez ME, et al. Aspergillus antigenemia sandwich-enzyme immunoassay test as a serodiagnostic method for invasive aspergillosis in liver transplant recipients. Transplantation 71:145, 2001.
63. Chumpitazi BFF, Pinel C, Lebeau B, et al. Aspergillus fumigatus antigen detection in sera from patients at risk for invasive aspergillosis. J Clin Microbiol 38:438, 2000.
64. Maertens J, Verhaegen J, Lagrou K, et al. Screening for circulating galactomannan as a noninvasive diagnostic tool for invasive aspergillosis in prolonged neutropenic patients and stem cell transplantation recipients: a prospective validation. Blood 97:1604, 2001.
65. Becker MJ, de Marie S, Willemse D, et al. Quantitative galactomannan detection is superior to PCR in diagnosing and monitoring invasive pulmonary aspergillosis in an experimental rat model. J Clin Microbiol 38:1434, 2000.
66. Denning DW, Lee JY, Hostetler JS, et al. NIAID Mycoses Study Group multicenter trial of oral itraconazole therapy for invasive aspergillosis. Am J Med 97:135, 1994.
67. Maertens J, Raad I, Sable CA, et al. Multicenter, noncomparative study to evaluate the safety and efficacy of caspofungin (CAS) in adults with invasive aspergillosis (IA) refractory (R) or intolerant (I) to standard therapy (ST). Presented at the 40th Interscience Conference on Antimicrobial Agents and Chemotherapy, 2000, p 371, abstract 1103.
68. Kirkpatrick WR, McAtee RK, Fothergill AW, et al. Efficacy of SCH56592 in a rabbit model of invasive aspergillosis. Antimicrob Agents Chemother 44:780, 1999.
69. Graybill JR, Bocanegra R, Luther M, Loebenberg D. SCH56592 treatment of murine invasive aspergillosis. J Antimicrob Chemother 42:539, 1998.
70. Kemper CA, Hostetler JS, Follansbee SE, et al. Ulcerative and plaque-like tracheobronchitis due to infection with Aspergillus in patients with AIDS. Clin Infect Dis 17:344, 1993.
71. Dal Conte I, Riva G, Obert R. Tracheobronchial aspergillosis in a patient with AIDS treated with aerosolized amphoteriicn B combined with itraconazole. Mycoses 39:371, 1996.
72. Barchiesi F, Morbiducci V, Ancarani D, et al. Trichosporon beigelii fungemia in an AIDS patient. AIDS 7:139, 1993.
73. Leaf HL, Simberkoff MS. Invasive trichosporonosis in a patient with acquired immunodeficiency syndrome. J Infect Dis 160:356, 1989.
74. Alvarez S. Systemic infection caused by Penicillium decumbens in a patient with acquired immunodeficiency syndrome. J Infect Dis 162:283, 1990.
75. Raffanti SP, Fyfe B, Carreiro S, et al. Native valve endocarditis due to Pseudallescheria boydii in a patient with AIDS. Rev Infect Dis 12:993, 1990.
76. Eljaschewitsch J, Sandfort J, Tintelnot K. Port-a-cath related Fusarium oxysporum infection in an HIV-infected patient: treatment with liposomal amphotericin B. Mycoses 39:115, 1996.

77. Glasgow BJ, Engstrom RE Jr, Holland GN, et al. Bilateral endogenous Fusarium endophthalmitis associated with acquired immunodeficiency syndrome. Arch Ophthalmol 114:873, 1996.
78. Torssander J, Carlsson B, von Krogh G. Trichosporon beigelii: increased occurrence in homosexual men. Mykosen 28:355, 1985.
79. Meyer RD, Gaultier CR, Yamashita JT, et al. Fungal sinusitis in patients with AIDS: report of 4 cases and review of the literature. Medicine (Baltimore) 73:69, 1994.
80. Muñoz P, Marín M, Tornero P, et al. Successful outcome of Scedosporium apiospermum disseminated infection treated with voriconazole in a patient receiving corticosteroid therapy. Clin Infect Dis 31:1499, 2000.
81. Nesky MA, McDougal EC, Peacock JE Jr. Pseudallescheria boydii brain abscess successfully treated with voriconazole and surgical drainage: case report and literature review of central nervous system pseudallescheriasis. Clin Infect Dis 31:673, 2000.
82. Lozano-Chiu M, Arikan S, Paetznick VL, et al. Treatment of murine fusariosis with SCH 56592. Antimicrob Agents Chemother 43:589, 1999.
83. Hachem R, Raad II, Afif CM. An open, non-comparative multicenter study to evaluate efficacy and safety of posaconazole (SCH56592) in the treatment of invasive fungal infections (IFI) refractory (R) to or intolerant to (I) standard therapy (ST). Presented at the 40th Interscience Conference on Antimicrobial Agents and Chemotherapy, 2000, p 372, abstract 1109.
84. Torre-Cisneros J, Gonzalez-Ruiz A, Hodges MR, Lutsar I. Voriconazole (VORI) for the treatment of S. apiospermium and S. prolificans. Presented at the 38th Annual Meeting of the Infectious Disease Society of America, 2001, p 93, abstract 305.
85. Walsh TJ, Gonzalez C, Roilides E, et al. Fungemia in children infected with the human immunodeficiency virus: new epidemiologic patterns, emerging pathogens, and improved outcome with antifungal therapy. Clin Infect Dis 20:900, 1995.
86. De Hoog GS, Queiroz-Tellez F, Haase G. Black fungi: clinical and pathogenic approaches. Med Mycol 38(suppl 1):243, 2000.
87. Dugan JM, Wolff MD, Kauffman CA. Phialophora verrucosa infection in an AIDS patient. Mycoses 38:215, 1995.
88. Dhar J, Carey PB. Scopulariopsis brevicaulis skin lesions from an AIDS patient. AIDS 7:1283, 1993.
89. Sudduth EJ, Crumbley AJ, Farrar WE. Phaeohyphomycosis due to Exophiala species: clinical spectrum of disease in humans. Clin Infect Dis 15:639, 1992.
90. Nenoff P, Horn LC, Schwenke H. Disseminated mycosis due to Scedosprium prolificans in an AIDS patient with Burkitt lymphoma. Mycoses 39:461, 1996.
91. Brenner SA, Morgan J, Rickert PD. Cladophialophora bantiana isolated from an AIDS patient with pulmonary infiltrates. J Med Vet Mycol 34:427, 1996.
92. Shugar MA, Montgomery WW, Hyslop NE. Alternaria sinusitis. Ann Otol Rhinol Laryngol 90:251, 1981.
93. Rossman SN, Cernoch PL, David JR. Dematiaceous fungi are an increasing cause of human disease. Clin Infect Dis 22:73, 1996.
94. Nachman S, Alpan O, Malowitz R, Spitzer ED. Catheter-associated fungemia due to Wangiella (Exophiala) dermatitidis. J Clin Microbiol 34:1011, 1996.
95. Mukherji SK, Castillo M. Cerebral phaeohyphomycosis caused by Xylohypha bantiana: MR findings. AJR Am J Roentgenol 164:1304, 1995.
96. Rock JP, Camins MB, Chandler WF. Cerebral phaeohyphomycosis caused by Ramichloridium obovoideum (Ramichloridium mackenziei): case report—comments. Neurosurgery 45:375, 1999.
97. Dixon DM, Polak A. In vitro and in vivo drug studies with three agents of central nervous system phaeohyphomycosis. Chemotherapy 33:129, 1987.
98. Sharkey PK, Rinaldi MG, Dunn JF, et al. High dose itraconazole in the treatment of severe mycoses. Antimicrob Agents Chemother 35:707, 1991.
99. Sharkey PK, Graybill JR, Rinaldi MG, et al. Itraconazole treatment of phaeohyphomycosis. J Am Acad Dermatol 23:577, 1990.
100. Al-Abdely HM, Najvar L, Bocanegra R, et al. SCH 56592, amphotericin B, or itraconazole therapy of experimental murine cerebral phaeohyphomycosis due to Ramichloridium obovoideum ("Ramichloridium mackenziei"). Antimicrob Agents Chemother 44:1159, 2000.
101. Espinel-Ingroff A. In vitro fungicidal activities of voriconazole, itraconazole, and amphotericin B against opportunistic moniliaceous and dematiaceous fungi. J Clin Microbiol 39:954, 2001.
102. Del Poeta M, Schell WA, Perfect J. In vitro antifungal activity of pneumocandin L-743, 872 against a variety of clinically significant molds. Antimicrob Agents Chemother 41:1835, 1997.
103. Kontoyiannis DP, Wessel VC, Bodey GP, Rolston KVI. Zygomycosis in the 1990s in a tertiary-care cancer center. Clin Infect Dis 30:851, 2000.
104. Sanchez MR, Ponge-Wilson I, Moy JA. Zygomycosis and HIV infection. J Am Acad Dermatol 30:904, 1994.
105. Levy E, Bia MJ. Isolated renal mucormycosis: case report and review. J Am Soc Nephrol 5:2014, 1995.
106. Nagy-Agren SE, Chu P, Smith GJ. Zygomycosis (mucor-mycosis) and HIV infection: report of three cases and review. J Acquir Immune-Defic Syndr 10:441, 1995.
107. Micozzi MS, Wetli CV. Intravenous amphetamine abuse, primary cerebral mucormycosis, and aquired immunodeficiency. J Forensic Sci 30:504, 1985.
108. Lister J. Amphotericin B lipid complex (Abelcet®) in the treatment of invasive mycoses: the North American experience. Eur J Haematol 56(suppl 57):18, 1996.

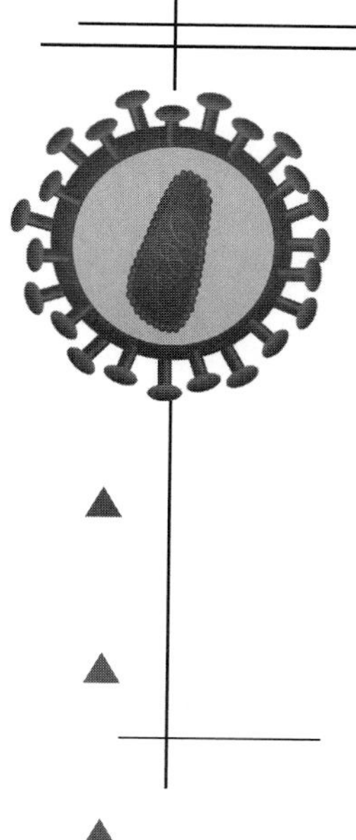

CHAPTER 41

Herpes Simplex Virus Infections

John C. Pottage, Jr., MD
Harold A. Kessler, MD

▲ PATHOGEN

Herpes simplex virus type 1 (HSV-1) and type 2 (HSV-2) are common pathogens in human immunodeficiency virus (HIV)-infected patients. Seroprevalence surveys of adults in the United States indicate that 50% to 70% of individuals are infected with HSV-1 and 15% to 33% with HSV-2.[1–3] There are increased seroprevalence rates for both HSV-1 and HSV-2 associated with HIV infection,[3] and during the era prior to the widespread use of highly active antiretroviral therapy (HAART) 4.4% of acquired immunodeficiency syndrome (AIDS)-defining illnesses in HIV-infected patients were due to severe HSV-1 or HSV-2 infection.[4] Several studies have shown that there is an increased incidence of HSV-related genital ulcer disease in HIV-infected women compared to HIV-infected men.[5–8] It has been noted that the overall incidence of clinically evident HSV infection in HIV-infected patients has declined, associated with the increased use of HAART.[9]

Herpes simplex virus has a double-stranded DNA enclosed in an icosahedral capsid that is surrounded by a lipid envelope. The most characteristic biologic property of these viruses is the ability to induce latency and periodically cause reactivation of infections.[10,11] The incubation period is 2 to 12 days. Spread is person to person via contact with infected body secretions. Primary infection occurs following initial introduction of the virus through the skin or mucous membranes. Following local replication, the virus travels along the sensory nerves and establishes latency in the dorsal nerve root ganglia. Reactivation disease occurs when the virus travels back along the sensory nerves and replicates in the mucocutaneous region that was initially infected. Although reactivation disease is generally of shorter duration and consists of milder symptoms than primary infection, it should be noted that both primary and reactivation infections are often clinically asymptomatic.[10,11]

The most common clinical manifestation of HSV is the development of vesicular and ulcerative lesions in the orolabial and/or genital regions. HSV-1 is associated with approximately 70% of orolabial infections and HSV-2 with approximately 70% of genital infections. Symptoms are more severe and prolonged in HIV-infected patients with advanced disease than in immunocompetent patients.[10–14] Symptoms begin with painful, erythematous papules that quickly become vesicles and soon ulcerate. These ulcerations then crust and heal. In the untreated healthy host, the time course from the development of papules to healing is approximately 14 to 28 days for primary disease. The course of reactivation disease is considerably shorter. Painful, tender regional lymphadenopathy often accompanies these lesions, particularly in patients with primary infection.[10,11]

In HIV-infected patients, most morbidity is associated with HSV infections in the genital and perirectal region.[12–14] Most serious infections occur in patients with less than 200 CD4 cells/mm^3. Untreated, the time course of HSV is often prolonged. Ulcerative lesions are often present for more than 1 to 3 months. In patients with advanced HIV infection, recurrences become more frequent, severe, and prolonged if left untreated. Multiple ulcerations can become confluent and involve extensive areas of the perineum. Heaped-up verrucous lesions caused by HSV-2, resembling condyloma acuminata, have been reported.[15] Asymptomatic shedding of HSV-2 is more prolonged in both HIV-infected men and women compared to HIV-uninfected patients.[16,17]

Proctitis caused by HSV has been described primarily in HIV-infected male patients.[18–20] They usually present with fever, pruritus, rectal pain, and tenesmus. A rectal discharge may be present. Additionally, difficulty urinating, impotence, and the presence of sacral paresthesia may be present. External lesions and inguinal lymphadenopathy frequently accompany this syndrome. Sigmoidoscopy shows large ulcerations. HSV-2 is responsible for most cases of proctitis. Concomitant infection with *Neisseria gonorrhoeae* has also been noted.[18–20]

As with genital and perirectal disease, orolabial HSV infections are more severe and prolonged in HIV-infected patients.[14,21] Lesions can occur on any mucosal surface, most commonly the lips, palate, or gingiva. Most cases are reactivated disease and most commonly consist of one or two ulcerations. Co-infection with other pathogens such as cytomegalovirus (CMV) or *Histoplasma* has been reported.[22]

Mucocutaneous forms of HSV infection located in other parts of the body, such as herpetic whitlow or paronychia, have been reported in association with HIV infection.[23–25] As is the case for disease in the genital and orolabial regions, cutaneous disease can be more severe and prolonged than that seen in the immunocompetent host.

Following mucocutaneous disease, the next most common clinical manifestation of HSV infection in HIV-infected patients is HSV esophagitis.[26–29] This AIDS-defining complication is seen usually in patients with less than 50 CD4 cells/mm^3. The symptoms are clinically indistinguishable from esophagitis caused by *Candida* species. Odynophagia or burning retrosternal pain is common. Orolabial ulcerations are present in approximately 38% to 80% of patients with HSV esophagitis.[26,29] Endoscopically, most herpetic lesions are seen in the distal third of the esophagus.[26] Rare complications include esophageal strictures and perforation.[30,31]

Visceral or disseminated HSV infection in HIV-infected patients is uncommon. Case reports of hepatitis, pneumonia, or encephalitis have been noted. Most cases of HSV encephalitis are caused by HSV-1 and are frequently associated with evidence of CMV encephalitis.[32] In immunocompetent patients herpes simplex encephalitis usually occurs in the temporal lobe, whereas in HIV-infected patients encephalitis has involved diverse areas of the brain outside the limbic system as well as the brain stem.[32] Myelitis caused by HSV has also been reported.[32]

▲ DIAGNOSIS

Mucocutaneous vesicular ulcerative disease in patients with HIV infection can have multiple causes, including disseminated CMV, varicella-zoster virus (VZV), or disseminated cryptococcal infection; histoplasmosis; squamous cell carcinoma; and pustular dermatosis. Therefore it is important to establish a firm microbiologic diagnosis, particularly if a typical-appearing lesion does not respond to acyclovir (Fig. 41–1). The laboratory diagnosis of HSV includes culture, cytopathologic techniques, HSV antigen detection by immunologic methods, nucleic acid detection by polymerase chain reaction (PCR), and serology. Traditionally, a viral culture has been the cornerstone of the laboratory diagnosis of HSV. Specimens are most likely to yield virus if they are taken from vesicles within the first 1 to 2 days after formation.[10,33] It should be noted that patients with chronic mucocutaneous HSV disease often have prolonged periods of shedding.[12,14,16,17] Following inoculation into tissue culture, a cytopathic effect with ballooning degeneration and multinucleated giant cells occurs within 1 to 2 days. Typing for HSV-1 or HSV-2 can be done using type-specific monoclonal antibodies, although this is not important for therapy.[10,11,33] Viral isolation is especially important if acyclovir resistance is suspected because viral susceptibility testing can be performed.[34]

Cytopathologic examination of scrapings of ulcerations can be quickly performed. The Tzanck smear shows typical multinucleated giant cells characteristic of herpesvirus infection but does not differentiate HSV from VZV.[10,11,33] Additionally, it is not as sensitive as a culture, with a positivity rate of approximately 40% to 50%. More sensitive approaches include antigen detection methods with monoclonal antibodies and DNA detection with the use of PCR techniques.[35]

Polymerase chain reaction detection of HSV DNA in cerebrospinal fluid is widely used to establish a diagnosis of HSV encephalitis. In addition to diagnosis, quantification of PCR and persistence of PCR reactivity after treatment may help determine the prognosis of infection and the risk of relapse.[36,37]

Sensitive type-specific serologic tests have been developed,[38] but detecting antibodies to HSV-1 or HSV-2 has no role in the diagnosis of active vesicular ulcerative disease. It does provide specific information as to whether the patient has been previously infected with the virus.

In vitro antiviral susceptibility testing of HSV has not been standardized, and the results can be variable. Routine use of susceptibility testing is not indicated for the management of uncomplicated episodes of HSV disease and should be reserved for episodes that appear to be unresponsive to acyclovir therapy (Fig. 41–1). Because standard plaque reduction assays can be time-consuming, several techniques have been developed for more rapid screening for acyclovir resistance. These methods have been reviewed elsewhere.[34,39]

▲ TREATMENT

Mucocutaneous Disease

Initial therapy for mucocutaneous HSV infections in HIV-infected patients is similar to that for patients who are not immunocompromised. Therapy is divided into that for primary infection and that for recurrent infection. Recurrent disease is treated either in an episodic fashion or as continuous suppressive therapy. Treatment leads to amelioration of the signs and symptoms of HSV disease and decreases the time to healing and shedding of the virus.

The treatment for primary infection is oral or intravenous acyclovir (Table 41–1). Therapy is given for a 10- to 14-day course or until the lesions have become crusted over. Alternative agents are famciclovir or valacyclovir. It should be noted that no studies involving famciclovir or

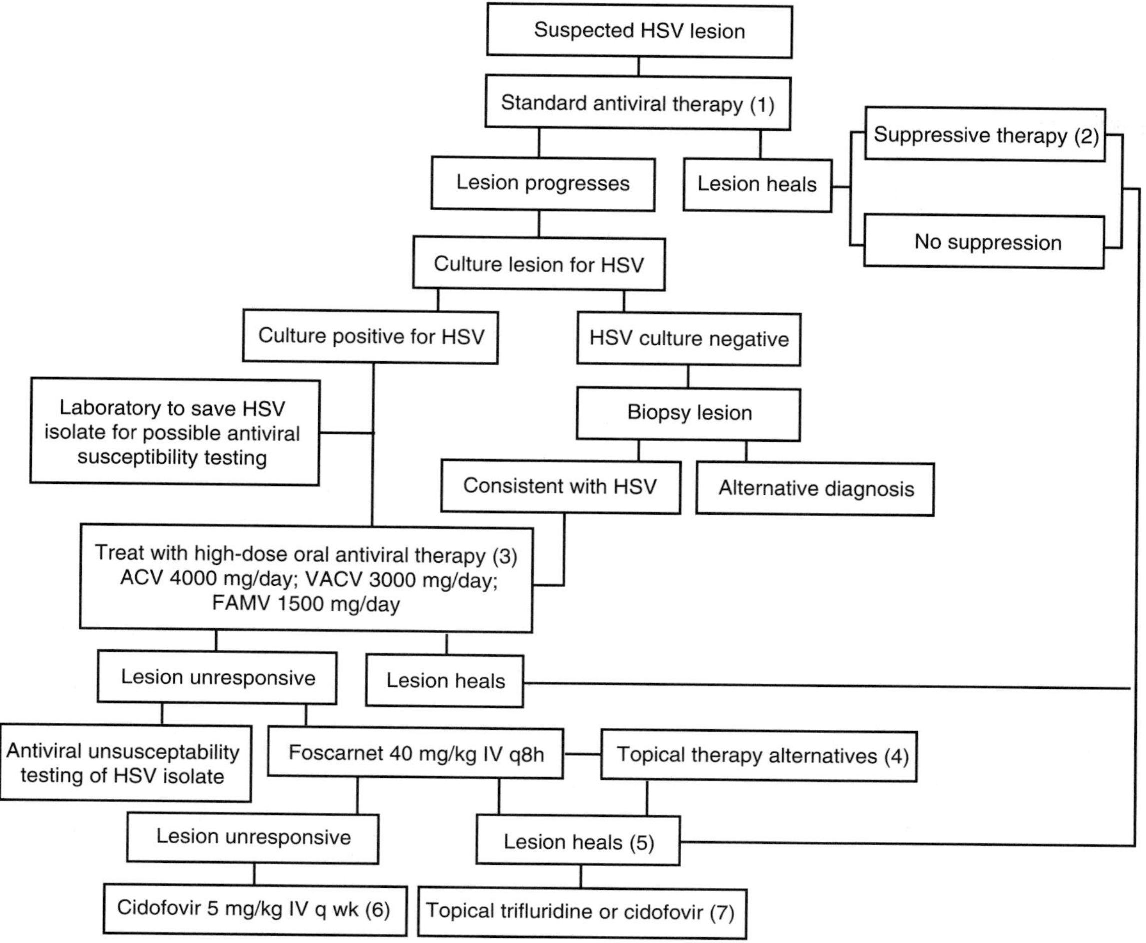

Figure 41–1. Algorithm for the management of herpes simplex disease in patients with HIV infection. (1) See text for discussion of currently recommended therapies. (2) See text for discussion of management of recurrent HSV disease. (3) See text for discussion of the management of acyclovir-unresponsive HSV disease (ACV, acyclovir; FAMV, famciclovir; VACV, valacyclovir). (4) See text for discussion of trifluridine ophthalmic solution, foscarnet cream, and cidofovir gel. (5) See text for discussion of the long-term management of acyclovir-resistant HSV disease. (6) Parenteral cidofovir not currently approved for the treatment of acyclovir-resistant HSV disease; dose based on therapy for CMV infection. (7) Cidofovir gel; Food and Drug Administration approval not being pursued by the manufacturer (Gilead Sciences).

valacyclovir for the treatment of primary mucocutaneous HSV infection in HIV patients have been reported. In patients with severe disease or who are unable to tolerate or absorb oral medications, intravenous acyclovir (5 mg/kg every 8 hours) should be used. The treatment course is 7 to 10 days or until the lesions have crusted over. Patients can be switched to oral acyclovir to complete the course of therapy when they are clinically improved and able to tolerate oral medications.[40–43]

Recurrent disease treatment is individualized to the patient's needs. Episodic therapy is usually patient-initiated. The treatment of choice in this instance is also acyclovir. Alternate agents include famciclovir 500 mg PO twice daily or valacyclovir 500 mg PO twice daily.[41,44,45] A comparative study in HIV-infected patients with mucocutaneous HSV infection of famciclovir (500 mg PO twice daily) and acyclovir (400 mg PO five times a day) showed that there was no difference between these agents in decreasing the time to complete healing and reducing new lesion formation.[46] It should be noted that the dosage of famciclovir that was used in this trial was higher than the dosage used to treat non-HIV-infected patients, which is 125 mg PO twice daily. Studies in HIV-infected patients treated with this lower dosage have not been reported; and whether this lower dose would be equally efficacious in HIV-infected patients, particularly those with less immunosuppression, is unclear. In general, recurrent infection is treated for 5 to 7 days. In patients with advanced HIV infection, improvement may take up to 14 days.

Continuous suppressive therapy should be considered for patients who have frequent symptomatic recurrent infections (Table 41–2). Frequent recurrences are usually defined as three or more outbreaks during a 6-month period. Acyclovir given at a dose of 400 mg PO twice daily is the treatment of choice for suppressive therapy.[40–42] Alternative agents include famciclovir 250 mg PO twice daily and valacyclovir 500 mg PO twice daily or 1000 mg PO once daily.[25,47] Optimization of HAART may decrease the need

▲ **Table 41–1.** TREATMENT FOR HERPES SIMPLEX VIRUS DISEASE IN PATIENTS WITH HIV INFECTION

Drug	Dose: Initial Disease	Dose: Recurrent Disease	Toxicity	Interactions
Acyclovir	5 mg/kg IV q8h × 10–14 days[a] *or* 200–400 mg PO 5×/day × 10–14 days	200–400 mg PO 5×/day × 5–10 days[b]	Phlebitis with IV formulation. Reversible nephrotoxicity (rare with these doses of drug). Neurotoxicity (rare with these doses of drug in the absence of decreased renal function)	If given with nephrotoxic drugs reduce dose with decreasing CrCl Cimetidine and probenecid increase acyclovir levels
Valacyclovir	1000 mg PO bid × 10–14 days[c]	500 mg PO bid × 5–10 days	Same as for oral acyclovir. Thrombotic microangiopathy (rare)[d]	Same as for acyclovir
Famciclovir	500 mg PO bid × 10–14 days[e]	500 mg PO bid × 5–10 days	No serious adverse events	If given with nephrotoxic drugs reduce dose with decreasing CrCl

CrCl, creatinine clearance.
[a]Decision on intravenous versus oral therapy based on clinical severity; switch to oral therapy as soon as a good clinical response is achieved.
[b]Intravenous therapy may initially be necessary for patients with severe oral or esophageal disease.
[c]Limited clinical data in HIV-infected patients; not approved for immunocompromised hosts.
[d]Reported in small number of patients with advanced HIV disease on prolonged high dose (8 g/day) therapy for cytomegalovirus (CMV) retinitis prophylaxis.
[e]Limited clinical data; not approved for treatment of initial disease.

of continuous suppressive therapy and should form an important component of this therapeutic strategy.

Although there has not been an increase in acyclovir resistance in immunocompetent patients treated with prolonged courses of acyclovir (>6 years of therapy), there have been increasing reports of acyclovir resistance in patients with advanced HIV infection.[34,48,49] Treatment of HIV-infected patients with recurrent HSV disease with episodic therapy rather than continuous suppression has been advocated as a way to decrease exposure to acyclovir. Whether this reduces the likelihood of acyclovir-resistant disease has not been established.

Acyclovir-Unresponsive Disease

Although the overall incidence of acyclovir resistance remains low, there have been reports of HIV-infected patients with severe debilitating chronic mucocutaneous disease caused by acyclovir-resistant HSV.[24,34,50,51] Additionally, patients with esophagitis and visceral disease caused by acyclovir-resistant HSV have been described.[34,52,53] Typically, these patients have advanced HIV disease with less than 50 CD4 cells/mm^3. The patients with mucocutaneous disease have large, progressive, deeply ulcerated lesions that frequently develop satellite lesions. Symptoms can be present for months. Additionally, viral shedding is prolonged.[34,50,51]

Acyclovir resistance should be suspected in HIV-infected patients with mucocutaneous HSV infections that do not respond to acyclovir therapy within 14 days (Fig. 41–1). At this time, repeat cultures should be performed and the HSV isolate saved for antiviral susceptibility testing. Not all patients with HSV infection unresponsive to oral acyclovir have acyclovir resistance. Therefore patients should first be treated with higher doses of acyclovir (800 mg PO every 4 hours five times per day). Alternatively, famciclovir or valacyclovir, which have enhanced oral bioavailability, may be tried (Fig. 41–1; Table 41–1). Continuous-infusion acyclovir (1.5 to 2.0 mg/kg/hr) has also been reported to be beneficial for treatment of acyclovir-resistant HSV.[54,55] If these regimens fail, antiviral susceptibility testing can be performed and alternative therapy considered. Treatment of acyclovir-resistant HSV is with foscarnet[34,41,51,56–58] given intravenously at a dose of 40 mg/kg three times daily (Table 41–3). Treatment is continued until the lesions have crusted over and reepithelialized, which usually takes at least 2 to 3 weeks. It is interesting that following resolution of lesions caused by acyclovir-resistant HSV, recurrent in-

▲ **Table 41–2.** CHRONIC SUPPRESSIVE TREATMENT FOR RECURRENT HERPES SIMPLEX VIRUS DISEASE IN PATIENTS WITH HIV INFECTION

Drug	Dose	Toxicity	Interactions
Acyclovir	200 mg PO bid *or* 400 mg PO bid	Reversible nephrotoxicity (rare with these doses). Neurotoxicity (rare with these does in the absence of decreased renal function)	If given with nephrotoxic drugs, reduce dose with decreasing CrCl. Cimetidine and probenecid increase acyclovir levels
Valacyclovir	1000 mg PO q day[a]	Same as for oral acyclovir. Thrombotic microangiopathy (rare)[b]	Same as for acyclovir
Famciclovir	250 mg PO bid[c]	No serious adverse events	If given with nephrotoxic drugs, reduce dose with decreasing CrCl

CrCl, creatine clearance.
[a]Limited clinical data; not approved for immunocompromised hosts.
[b]Reported in small number of patients with advanced HIV disease on prolonged high dose (8 g/day) therapy for CMV retinitis prophylaxis.
[c]Limited clinical data; not approved for immunocompromised hosts.

▲ **Table 41–3.** TREATMENT FOR ACYCLOVIR-RESISTANT HSV DISEASE IN PATIENTS WITH HIV INFECTION

Drug	Dose	Toxicity	Interactions
Systemic Therapy			
Foscarnet	40 mg/kg IV q8h × 10–14 days; may require longer duration depending on rate of reepithelialization	Nephrotoxicity, electrolyte distrubances (particularly related to calcium), nausea/irritability, genital ulceration	Increased risk of nephrotoxicity if administered with other nephrotoxic drugs
Cidofovir[a]	5 mg/kg IV q wk × 2–4 weeks; may require longer duration depending on rate of reepithelialization	Nephrotoxicity (must be co-administered with probenecid); neutropenia, uveitis, alopecia, hypotony; probenecid toxic effects include rash, fever, nausea, fatigue	Increased risk of nephrotoxicity if administered with other nephrotoxic drugs; probenecid increases levels of most drugs excreted by proximal tubules[b]
Topical Therapy			
Trifluridine	Ophthalmic solution applied to lesion tid until healed[c]	Minor local irritation including itching and stinging (uncommon)	None
Foscarnet cream 1%[d]	Apply to lesion 5×/day until healed	Skin ulceration, local irritation, fever	None
Cidofovir gel 1%[e]	Apply to lesion q day × 5 days; may be repeated 10 days after first application is completed	Minor local irritation including pain, burning, pruritus	None

[a]Not currently approved for this indication.

[b]Zidovudine dose should be reduced by 50% or withheld on the day of infusion only. Rifampin, ketoprofen, chlorpropamide, dapsone, methotrexate, trimethoprim-sulfamethoxasole, zalcitibine, and NSAID should be on the day of dosing only.

[c]After gentle gauze débridement of the lesion with hydrogen peroxide, a thin layer of trifluridine is applied to the lesion with overlapping of the edges, and a sterile Teflon gauze covering with polymyxin-bacitracin ointment applied is used to cover the lesion. Not currently approved for this indication.

[d]Currently not available in the United States (Astra Pharmaceutical Products).

[e]FDA approval not being pursued by manufacturer (Gilead Sciences).

fections often are caused by HSV isolates sensitive to acyclovir. This indicates that latent infection may be maintained by a virus population different from that found in the acute, cutaneous lesions.[57]

Intravenous cidofovir has been used to treat a small number of patients with acyclovir-resistant HSV disease.[59–63] Most of these patients were bone marrow transplant patients, and roughly half of the patients had foscarnet-resistant isolates in addition to acyclovir resistance. Although there was evidence of response, toxicities from cidofovir and concomitant probenecid were problematic.[59–62] Further studies are needed to define the role of intravenous cidofovir in the treatment of HIV-infected patients with acyclovir-resistant HSV disease, and its use should be reserved for patients with disease unresponsive to acyclovir and foscarnet.

Acyclovir-resistant HSV mucocutaneous disease has also been successfully treated topically. Antiviral agents that have been used in this fashion include trifluridine, cidofovir, and foscarnet.[53–69]

Trifluridine ophthalmic solution is applied to the HSV lesions in a thin layer and covered with a nonabsorbable gauze to which polymyxin B/bacitracin ointment has been applied. Lesions are cleansed with hydrogen peroxide and gentle gauze débridement between applications. This treatment is given every 8 hours until the lesions have reepithelialized. In a pilot study, approximately 30% of the patients had complete healing in a median time of 7 weeks, and 30% of the patients failed therapy. There was essentially no toxicity. However, application of the solution is unwieldy.[64]

Compared to a placebo, topical gel cidofovir at 0.3% to 1.0% applied once daily for 5 days was associated with decreased pain and viral shedding, and it accelerated healing of lesions. Thirty percent of the patients had complete healing within a median time of 21 days. Site reactions to the topical gel cidofovir (consisting of pain, burning, or pruritus) occurred in 23% of the patients and were not considered serious. Little systemic absorption of cidofovir occurred and then only in patients with the largest lesions.[67]

A pilot study using 1% foscarnet cream for treatment of acyclovir-resistant HSV in HIV patients has been reported.[69] Patients were treated five times daily for approximately 1 month. Of these 20 patients, 8 showed complete healing. There also was a decline in viral shedding and pain. Four patients developed application site reactions. Plasma foscarnet levels were not detected.[69]

In summary, treatment of acyclovir-resistant HSV disease should be individualized. Patients with extensive disease must be treated with intravenous foscarnet. The role of intravenous cidofovir is presently unknown. Patients with more limited disease may be treated with topical agents. Clearly, more experience must be gained regarding topical therapy. Additionally, improvement of the underlying immunodeficiency with potent HAART regimens may also improve the outcome of therapy in these patients.

In addition to acyclovir-resistant herpes simplex, isolates of HSV with foscarnet resistance have been described in HIV-infected patients.[67,70] As do patients with acyclovir-resistant HSV, these patients also have advanced HIV disease, and they have had extensive exposure to foscarnet.

The mechanism is a mutation in the DNA polymerase gene.[67] These isolates may be sensitive to acyclovir, which can be used as therapy.[67] It is of note that isolates with both foscarnet and acyclovir resistance have also been described. Treatment with cidofovir may be effective in this situation.[60,67]

Visceral Disease

The treatment of HSV esophagitis or proctitis is intravenous acyclovir (5 mg/kg every 8 hours), oral acyclovir (400 mg every 4 hours five times daily), or oral valacyclovir (500 mg every 12 hours) for a 10- to 14-day course.[19,20,26,28,40,41] Concurrent use of potent HAART regimens has been associated with a reduction in recurrent symptoms and improved survival in patients with HIV-associated HSV esophagitis.[71] Visceral or central nervous system (CNS) disease is generally treated with intravenous acyclovir (10 mg/kg every 8 hours) for 14 to 21 days.[30-32]

▲ PHARMACOLOGY OF ANTIVIRAL AGENTS USED TO TREAT HSV

Acyclovir

Acyclovir is an acyclic nucleoside analogue of guanosine with potent antiviral activity against HSV-1 and HSV-2. The drug is monophosphorylated by a herpesvirus-specific thymidine kinase (TK) to acyclovir monophosphate. Host cellular kinases then convert acyclovir monophosphate to acyclovir triphosphate, which inhibits viral DNA polymerase and incorporates into viral DNA, resulting in chain termination of the growing DNA chain.[40,41] Acyclovir resistance can occur through one of three mechanisms: (1) TK deficiency; (2) altered acyclovir affinity for TK; or (3) altered acyclovir affinity for DNA polymerase. Most (>90%) resistant isolates are characterized by TK deficiency.[34]

Acyclovir may be administered intravenously, orally, and topically. It is widely distributed in the body but only penetrates the cerebrospinal fluid at approximately 50% of the plasma level. Acyclovir has a half-life of approximately 2.5 hours and is excreted through the kidneys. Dosage adjustment is needed for patients with renal failure. Acyclovir has an oral bioavailability of approximately 15% to 30%. Topically applied acyclovir has no systemic absorption and has limited clinical utility.[40,42,72]

Acyclovir is an extremely well tolerated drug.[73] Phlebitis and pain occasionally follow intravenous infusion. High doses of acyclovir (30 mg/kg/day) may lead to reversible renal failure as a result of crystallization of the drug in renal tubules. Patients must be well hydrated when high doses of intravenous acyclovir are administered, and the drug should be infused over at least 1 hour. Neurologic symptoms consisting of mental status changes and seizures have been reported to occur rarely and are associated with elevated acyclovir levels.[74] These symptoms resolve with discontinuation of acyclovir. Oral acyclovir has been associated with gastrointestinal disturbances, including nausea and vomiting. An erythematous maculopapular rash has uncommonly been reported to occur. A short-lived stinging or burning sensation is the only toxicity related to the topical administration of acyclovir.[40,42,72,73]

Valacyclovir

Valacyclovir is the L-valyl ester prodrug of acyclovir. Following oral administration, valacyclovir is converted to acyclovir and L-valine in the intestine and liver. The bioavailability of acyclovir following oral ingestion of a 1000 mg dose of valacyclovir is approximately 50%. The conversion of valacyclovir to acyclovir is more than 99%. Once converted to acyclovir, its pharmacology is that of acyclovir.[75,76]

The toxicity of valacyclovir is of special note in HIV-infected patients. A thrombotic microangiopathy syndrome similar to thrombotic thrombocytopenic purpura/hemolytic-uremic syndrome has been reported to occur in HIV-infected patients with advanced disease treated with valacyclovir at higher dosages (8 g/day) than those used for the treatment of HSV infection[77]; this information is still included as a warning in the current package insert.[78] However, there was a recent case report of the association of this syndrome in a patient with advanced HIV infection (CD4 count 98 cells/mm^3) who had been receiving valacyclovir at a dose of 500 mg PO twice daily for suppressive HSV therapy for 1 year.[79] It therefore seems prudent to avoid the use of valacyclovir in doses exceeding 3000 mg/day for more than a 7- to 14-day course in patients with advanced HIV disease (CD4+ T-lymphocyte counts <100 cells/mm^3). Other toxicities involving the gastrointestinal system, CNS, and kidneys are the same as those seen with acyclovir.[76,77]

At the present time, valacyclovir is indicated for episodic treatment of reactivated HSV infection and suppressive treatment of frequent reactivation HSV infection. The usual dose for treatment of episodic disease is 500 mg PO every 12 hours in patients with normal renal function. In patients with a creatinine clearance of less than 30 ml/min, the dose should be reduced to 500 mg PO every 24 hours.[77] For suppressive therapy the usual dose is 500 or 1000 mg PO once daily.[77,80]

Famciclovir

Famciclovir is the prodrug of penciclovir, an antiviral agent with excellent in vitro activity against HSV-1 and HSV-2. Following oral ingestion of famciclovir, the drug is metabolized by deacetylation and oxidation to penciclovir by the intestine and liver. Similarly to acyclovir, penciclovir is initially monophosphorylated by the HSV TK and then triphosphorylated by a host cellular kinase. Penciclovir triphosphate inhibits HSV DNA polymerase. Viral resistance is similar to that of acyclovir. Famciclovir is not effective in the treatment of TK-deficient mutants.[81-83]

Famciclovir is administered only orally and has penciclovir bioavailability of approximately 77% following a 500 mg dose (of famciclovir). Famciclovir is eliminated by the kidneys. Dose modifications must be made in patients with renal failure.[82,83] Famciclovir is well tolerated. The most common adverse events associated with it are headaches and gastrointestinal symptoms, primarily nausea and diarrhea.[83]

At the present time, famciclovir is approved for episodic treatment of reactivation HSV disease and suppressive therapy of frequent reactivation HSV disease. The usual dosage for episodic therapy is 500 mg PO twice daily for HIV-infected patients, and for suppressive therapy the usual dose is 250 mg PO twice daily. In patients with a creatinine clearance of 20 to 40 ml/min famciclovir should be given as 125 mg PO every 24 hours, and in patients with a creatinine clearance of less than 20 ml/min the dose should be 125 mg PO every 48 hours.[82,83]

Foscarnet

Foscarnet is a pyrophosphate analogue that interferes with pyrophosphate binding sites on DNA polymerase. Unlike acyclovir and penciclovir, foscarnet does not require phosphorylation for its antiviral activity.[42,84] Viral isolates resistant to acyclovir and penciclovir are sensitive to foscarnet. Foscarnet resistance caused by altered DNA polymerase has been described in HIV-infected patients. These patients can be treated successfully with acyclovir.[70]

Foscarnet is available only as an intravenous formulation; a topical cream formulation is investigational.[69] The drug penetrates the CNS. It is not metabolized and is excreted by the kidneys. Dosage adjustments are necessary for patients with decreased creatinine clearance. The normal dosage of foscarnet for treatment of HSV disease is 40 mg/kg every 8 hours.[42,84,85]

The most serious toxicity associated with foscarnet is nephrotoxicity, which occurs to some degree in virtually all patients treated with foscarnet. Renal failure is generally reversible following discontinuation of foscarnet. Foscarnet chelates divalent metal ions and so may be associated with hypocalcemia, hypophosphatemia, and hypomagnesemia. CNS toxicity (consisting mainly of seizures) has been associated with elevated levels of foscarnet. Elevated liver enzymes, anemia, leukopenia, and thrombocytopenia have been associated with foscarnet usage.[84,85]

Cidofovir

Cidofovir is a monophosphate nucleotide analogue of cytosine that undergoes intracellular phosphorylation to its diphosphate form by cellular kinases and blocks HSV DNA polymerase.[86] Cidofovir is active against acyclovir-resistant HSV. An HSV-2 isolate has been described that has diminished susceptibility for cidofovir as the result of a mutation in the HSV DNA polymerase.[87]

Currently, cidofovir is available only as an intravenous formulation; a topical gel formulation is not available at present, although individual pharmacies can prepare a gel if desired.[68] Cidofovir is given intravenously in doses of 3 to 5 mg/kg. Eighty percent of the drug is excreted unchanged in the urine. The plasma half-life is 2.4 to 3.2 hours, but the intracellular half life is 50 to 60 hours, which is the rationale for once-weekly dosing.[86,88] Probenecid blocks the tubular secretion of cidofovir and results in increased serum levels.

The major toxicity of cidofovir is renal tubular toxicity. Proteinuria frequently occurs with high dosages of cidofovir (>3.0 mg/kg). Probenecid, which offers some protection against the renal toxicity, must be administered before and after cidofovir dosing. Saline infusions have been used to decrease nephrotoxicity. Probenecid, a sulfa-derived compound, has been associated with toxicity that includes nausea, vomiting, headaches, fevers, and flushing.[54,86]

Presently, cidofovir is approved only for treatment of CMV disease. The role of cidofovir, intravenously or topically, in the treatment of HSV disease is reserved for treatment of acyclovir- and foscarnet resistant HSV disease.

▲ PREVENTION

Primary prophylaxis with acyclovir to prevent acquisition of HSV is not recommended for HIV-infected patients.[4,89] Efforts to prevent initial exposure to HSV with latex condoms are important. Sexual contact should be avoided when lesions are present in either partner.[89]

The first step in long-term suppression of HSV disease is optimization of a potent HAART regimen. Following that step, suppression of reactivation HSV disease can be performed successfully with chronic acyclovir. However, in view of the ease of treating patients episodically and the possible risk for the development of acyclovir resistance, it is recommended that suppressive therapy be reserved for only those patients with disabling and frequent recurrences. The use of valacyclovir or famciclovir for chronic suppressive therapy in the HIV-infected patient should probably be avoided until more long-term data (>1 year) are available. Recurrent disease with acyclovir-resistant HSV can be treated episodically with foscarnet. Isolates from recurrent episodes of acyclovir-resistant HSV disease that have been treated with foscarnet may be susceptible to acyclovir, but the role for chronic suppressive therapy with acyclovir in these patients is unknown.[56]

REFERENCES

1. Gibson JJ, Hornung CA, Alexander GR, et al. A cross-sectional study of herpes simplex virus 1 and 2 in college students: occurrence and determinants of infection. J Infect Dis 162:306, 1990.
2. Johnson RE, Nahmias AJ, Magder LS, et al. A seroepidemiologic survey of the prevalence of herpes simplex virus type 2 in the United States. N Engl J Med 321:7, 1989.
3. Siegel D, Golden E, Washington AE, et al. Prevalence and correlates of herpes simplex infections: the population based AIDS in multiethnic neighborhoods study. JAMA 268:1702, 1992.
4. Stewart JA, Reef SE, Pellett PE, et al. Herpes virus infection in persons infected with human immunodeficiency virus. Clin Infect Dis 21(suppl 1):S114, 1995.
5. LaGuardia KD, White MH, Saigo PE, et al. Genital ulcer disease in women infected with human immunodeficiency virus. Am J Obstet Gynecol 172:553, 1995.
6. Anderson J, Clark RA, Watts DH, et al. Idiopathic genital ulcers in women infected with human immunodeficiency virus. J Acquir Immun Defic Syndr Hum Retrovirol 13:343, 1996.
7. Cu-Uvin S, Flanigan TP, Rich JD, et al. Human immunodeficiency virus infection and acquired immunodeficiency syndrome among North American women. Am J Med 105:316, 1996.

8. Sobel JD. Gynecologic infections in human immunodeficiency virus-infected women. Clin Infect Dis 31:1225, 2000.
9. Patton LL, McKaig R, Strauss R, et al. Changing prevalence of oral manifestations of human immuno-deficiency virus in the era of protease inhibitor therapy. Oral Surg Oral Med Oral Pathol Oral Radiol Endod 89:299, 2000.
10. Corey L, Adams HG, Brown ZA, et al. Genital herpes simplex virus infections: clinical manifestations, course and complications. Ann Intern Med 98:958, 1983.
11. Corey L, Spear PG. Infections with herpes simplex viruses. N Engl J Med 314:686, 749, 1986.
12. Siegal FP, Lopez C, Hammer GS, et al. Severe acquired immunodeficiency in male homosexuals, manifested by chronic perianal ulcerative herpes simplex lesions. N Engl J Med 305:1439, 1981.
13. Quinnan GV Jr, Masur H, Rook AH, et al. Herpes virus infections in the acquired immunodeficiency syndrome. JAMA 252:72, 1984.
14. Safrin S, Ashley R, Houlihan C, et al. Clinical and serologic features of herpes simplex virus infection in patients with AIDS. AIDS 5:1107, 1990.
15. Tony P, Mutasim DF. Herpes simplex virus infection masquerading as condyloma acuminata in a patient with HIV disease. Br J Dermatol 134:797, 1996.
16. Augenbaum M, Feldman J, Chirgwin K, et al. Increased genital shedding of herpes simplex 2 in HIV-seropositive women. Ann Intern Med 123:845, 1995.
17. Schacker T, Zeh J, Hui-lin H, et al. Frequency of symptomatic and asymptomatic herpes simplex virus 2 reactivations among human immunodeficiency virus-infected men. J Infect Dis 170:1616, 1998.
18. Goodell SE, Quinn TC, Mkrtichian E, et al. Herpes simplex virus proctitis in homosexual men. N Engl J Med 308:858, 1983.
19. Rompalo AM, Mertz GJ, Davis LG, et al. Oral acyclovir for treatment of first episode herpes simplex virus proctitis. JAMA 259:2879, 1988.
20. Rompalo AM. Diagnosis and treatment of sexually acquired proctitis and proctocolitis: an update. Clin Infect Dis 28(suppl 1):S84, 1999.
21. Itin PH, Lautenschlager S, Fluckiger R. Oral manifestations in HIV infected patients: diagnosis and management. J Am Acad Dermatol 29:749, 1993.
22. Regezi JA, Eversole LR, Barker BF, et al. Herpes simplex and cytomegalovirus coinfected oral ulcers in HIV-positive patients. Oral Surg Oral Med Oral Pathol 81:55, 1996.
23. Gill MJ, Arlette J, Bucham K. Herpes simplex virus infection of the hand: a profile of 79 cases. Am J Med 84:89, 1988.
24. Norris SA, Kessler HA, Fife KH. Severe progressive herpetic whitlow caused by an acyclovir-resistant virus in a patient with AIDS. J Infect Dis 157:209, 1988.
25. Giani G, Quirino T, Sacrini F, et al. Destructive mucocutaneous phagedenic herpes simplex virus infection in an HIV-infected patient who had a partial response to interferon and ultraviolet rays. Clin Infect Dis 22:381, 1996.
26. Genereau T, Lorthollary O, Bonchaud O, et al. Herpes simplex esophagitis in patients with AIDS: report of 34 cases. Clin Infect Dis 22:926, 1996.
27. Bonacini M, Young T, Laine L. The cause of esophageal symptoms in human immunodeficiency virus infection: a prospective study of 110 patients. Arch Intern Med 151:1567, 1991.
28. Wilcox CM, Schwartz DA, Clark WS. Esophageal ulceration in human immunodeficiency virus infection: causes, response to therapy, and long term outcome. Ann Intern Med 123:143, 1995.
29. Wilcox CM, Straub RF, Clark WS. Prospective evaluation of oropharyngeal findings in human immunodeficiency virus-infected patients with esophageal ulceration. Am J Gastroenterol 90:1938, 1995.
30. Wilcox CM. Esophageal strictures complicating ulcerative esophagitis in patients with AIDS. Am J Gastroenterol 94:339, 1999.
31. Dieckhaus KD, Hill DR. Boerhaave's syndrome due to herpes simplex virus type 1 esophagitis in a patient with AIDS. Clin Infect Dis 26:1244,1998.
32. Chretien F, Belech L, Hilton DA, et al. Herpes simplex virus type 1 encephalitis in acquired immunodeficiency syndrome. Neuropathol Appl Neurobiol 22:394, 1996.
33. Corey L, Holmes KK. Genital herpes simplex virus infections: current concepts in diagnosis, therapy, and prevention. Ann Intern Med 98:972, 1983.
34. Pottage JC Jr, Kessler HA. Herpes simplex virus resistance to acyclovir: clinical relevance. Infect Agents Dis 4:115, 1995.
35. Do Nascimento MC, Sumita LM, de Souza VA, Pannuti CS. Detection and direct typing of herpes simplex virus in perianal ulcers of patients with AIDS by PCR. J Clin Microbiol 36:848, 1998.
36. Cinque P, Vago L, Marenzi R, et al. Herpes simplex virus infections of the central nervous system in human immunodeficiency virus-infected patients: clinical management by polymerase chain reaction assay of cerebrospinal fluid. Clin Infect Dis 27:303, 1998.
37. Domingues RB, Lakeman FD, Mayo MS, Whitley RJ. Application of competitive PCR to cerebrospinal fluid samples from patients with herpes simplex encephalitis. J Clin Microbiol 36:2229, 1998.
38. Koutsky LA, Stevens CE, Holmes KK, et al. Under diagnosis of genital herpes by current clinical and viral-isolation procedures. N Engl J Med 326:1533, 1992.
39. De la Iglesia P, Melon S, Lopez B, et al. Rapid screening tests for determining in vitro susceptibility of herpes simplex virus clinical isolates. J Clin Microbiol 36:2389, 1998.
40. Whitley RJ, Gnann JW Jr. Acyclovir: a decade later. N Engl J Med 327:782, 1992.
41. Klepser ME, Klepser TB. Drug treatment of HIV-related opportunistic infections. Drugs 53:40, 1997.
42. Pottage JC Jr. Antifungal and antiviral therapy. In: Parrillo JE, Bone RC (eds) Critical Care Medicine: Principles of Diagnosis and Management. St. Louis, Mosby Year Book, 1995, p 969.
43. Wood MJ. Antivirals in the context of HIV disease. J Antimicrob Chemother 37(suppl B):97, 1996.
44. Sacks SL, Aoki FY, Diaz-Mitoma F, et al. Patient initiated, twice daily oral famciclovir for early recurrent genital herpes: a randomized double blind multicenter trial. JAMA 276:44, 1996.
45. Smiley ML, International Valaciclovir HSV Study Group. Valaciclovir and acyclovir for the treatment of recurrent genital herpes simplex virus infections. In: Abstracts of the 37th Interscience Conference on Antimicrobial Agents and Chemotherapy, Toronto. Washington, DC, American Society for Microbiology, 1997, abstract 1210.
46. Romanowski B, Aoki FY, Martel AY, et al. Efficacy and safety of famciclovir for treating mucocutaneous herpes simplex infection in HIV-infected individuals. AIDS 14:1211, 2000.
47. Mertz GJ, Loveless MO, Levin MJ, et al. Oral famciclovir for suppression of recurrent genital herpes simplex virus infection in women: a multicenter, double blind placebo controlled study. Arch Intern Med 157:343, 1997.
48. Reyes M, Graber J, Reeves WC. Acyclovir-resistant HSV: initial results from a National Surveillance System. In: Abstracts of the 35th Annual Meeting of the Infectious Diseases Society of America, San Francisco. Alexandria, VA, Infectious Diseases Society of America, 1997, abstract 55.
49. Fife KH, Crumpacker CS, Mertz GJ, et al. Acyclovir study: recurrence and resistance of herpes simplex virus following cessation of greater than or equal to 6 years of chronic suppression with acyclovir. Infect Dis 169:1338, 1994.
50. Erlich KS, Mills J, Chatis P, et al. Acyclovir-resistant herpes simplex virus infections in patients with the acquired immunodeficiency syndrome. N Engl J Med 320:293, 1989.
51. Chatis PA, Miller CH, Schrager LE, et al. Successful treatment with foscarnet of an acyclovir-resistant mucocutaneous infection with herpes simplex virus in a patient with acquired immunodeficiency syndrome. N Engl J Med 320:297, 1989.
52. Sacks SL, Wanklin RJ, Reece DJ, et al. Progressive esophagitis from acyclovir-resistant herpes simplex. Ann Intern Med 111:893, 1989.
53. Gateley A, Gander RM, Johnson PC, et al. Herpes simplex virus type 2 meningoencephalitis resistant to acyclovir in a patient with AIDS. J Infect Dis 161:711, 1990.
54. Engel JP, Englund JA, Fletcher CV, et al. Treatment of resistant herpes simplex virus with continuous infusion acyclovir. JAMA 263:1662, 1990.
55. Fletcher CV, Englund JA, Bean B, et al. Continuous infusion of high-dose acyclovir for serious herpes virus infections. Antimicrob Agents Chemother 33:1375, 1989.
56. Safrin S, Assauleem T, Follansbee S, et al. Foscarnet therapy for acyclovir-resistant mucocutaneous herpes simplex virus infection in 26 AIDS patients: preliminary data. J Infect Dis 161:1078, 1990.
57. Safrin S, Crumpacker C, Chatis P, et al. A controlled trial comparing foscarnet with vidarabine for acyclovir resistant mucocutaneous herpes simplex in the acquired immunodeficiency syndrome. N Engl J Med 325:551, 1991.

58. Hardy WD. Foscarnet treatment of acyclovir-resistant herpes simplex virus infection in patients with the acquired immunodeficiency syndrome: preliminary results of a controlled randomized, regimen-comparative trial. Am J Med 92(suppl 2A):305, 1992.
59. Lalezari JP, Drew WL, Glutzer E, et al. Treatment with intravenous (s)-1-(3-hydroxy-2-phosphonylmethoxypropyl)cytosine of acyclovir-resistant mucocutaneous infection with herpes simplex virus in a patient with AIDS. J Infect Dis 170:550, 1994.
60. Chen Y, Scieux C, Garrait V, et al. Resistant herpes simplex virus type 1 infection: an emerging concern after allogeneic stem cell transplantation. Clin Infect Dis 31:927, 2000.
61. LoPresti AE, Levine JF, Munk GB, et al. Successful treatment of an acyclovir- and foscarnet-resistant herpes simplex virus type 1 lesion with intravenous cidofovir. Clin Infect Dis 26:512, 1998.
62. Martinez CM, Luks-Golger DB. Cidofovir use in acyclovir-resistant herpes infection. Ann Pharmacother 31:1519, 1997.
63. Birch CJ, Tyssen DP, Tacheddjian G, et al. Clinical effects and in vitro studies of trifluorothymidine combined with interferon for treatment of drug resistant and sensitive herpes simplex virus infections. J Infect Dis 166:108, 1992.
64. Kessler HA, Hurwitz C, Farthing C, et al. Pilot study of topical trifluridine for the treatment of acyclovir-resistant mucocutaneous herpes simplex disease in patients with AIDS (ACTG 172). J Acquir Immun Defic Syndr 12:147, 1996.
65. Amiu AR, Robinson MR, Smith DD, et al. Trifluorothymidine 0.5% ointment in the treatment of acyclovir resistant mucocutaneous herpes simplex in AIDS [letter]. AIDS 10:1051, 1996.
66. Snoeck R, Andrei G, DeClercq E, et al. A new topical treatment for resistant herpes simplex infections [letter]. N Engl J Med 327:968, 1993.
67. Snoeck R, Andei G, Gerard M, et al. Successful treatment of progressive mucocutaneous infection due to acyclovir and foscarnet resistant herpes simplex virus with (S)-1-(3-hydroxy-2-phosphonylmethoxypropyl)cytosine (HPMPC). Clin Infect Dis 18:570, 1994.
68. Lalezari J, Schacker T, Feinberg J, et al. A randomized, double blind, placebo-controlled study of cidofovir gel for the treatment of acyclovir-unresponsive mucocutaneous herpes simplex virus infections in patients with AIDS. J Infect Dis 17:862, 1997.
69. Javaly K, Wohlfeiler M, Kalayjian R, et al. Treatment of mucocutaneous herpes simplex virus infections unresponsive to acyclovir with topical foscarnet cream in AIDS patients: a phase I/II study. J Acquir Immune Defic Syndr 21:301, 1999.
70. Safrin S, Kemmerly S, Plotkin B, et al. Foscarnet-resistant herpes simplex virus infection in patients with AIDS. J Infect Dis 169:193, 1994.
71. Bini EJ, Micale PL, Weinshel EH. Natural history of HIV-associated esophageal disease in the era of protease inhibitor therapy. Dig Dis Sci 45:1301, 2000.
72. Laskin OL. Acyclovir: pharmacology and clinical experience. Arch Intern Med 144:1241, 1984.
73. Tilson HH, Engl CR, Andrews EB. Safety of acyclovir: a summary of the first ten years experience. J Med Virol 41(suppl 1):67, 1993.
74. Haefeli WE, Schoenberger RAZ, Weiss P, et al. Acyclovir-induced neurotoxicity: concentration-side effect relationship in acyclovir overdose. Am J Med 94:212, 1993.
75. Weller S, Blum MR, Doucette M, et al. Pharmacokinetics of acyclovir prodrug valaciclovir after escalating single and multiple-dose administration to normal volunteers. Clin Pharmacol Ther 54:595, 1993.
76. Jacobson MA, Gallant J, Wang LH, et al. Phase 1 trial of valaciclovir, the L-valyl ester of acyclovir, in patients with advanced human immunodeficiency virus disease. Antimicrob Agents Chemother 38:1534, 1994.
77. Valtrex (valacyclovir hydrochloride) caplets: product information. Research Triangle Park, NC, Glaxo Wellcome, 1996.
78. Valtrex (valcyclovir hydrochloride). In: Physicians Desk Reference, 55th ed. Montvale, NJ, Medical Economics Library, 2001.
79. Rivaud E, Massiani MA, Vincent F, et al. Valacyclovir hydrochloride therapy and thrombotic thrombocytopenic purpura in an HIV-infected patient. Arch Intern Med 160:1707, 2000.
80. Ormrod D, Scott LJ, Perry CM. Valacyclovir: a review of its long term utility in the management of genital herpes simplex virus and cytomegalovirus infections. Drugs 59:839, 2000.
81. Earnshaw DL, Bacon TH, Darlison SJ, et al. Mode of antiviral action of penciclovir in MRC-5 cells infected with herpes simplex virus type 1 (HSV-1), HSV-2, and varicella-zoster virus. Antimicrob Agents Chemother 36:2747, 1992.
82. Pue M, Benet LZ. Pharmacokinetics of famciclovir in man. Antiviral Chem Chemother 4(suppl 1):47, 1993.
83. Saltzman R, Jurewicz R, Boon R. Safety of famciclovir in patients with herpes zoster and genital herpes. Antimicrob Agents Chemother 38:2454, 1994.
84. Oberg B. Antiviral effects of phosphonoformate (PFA, foscarnet sodium). Pharmacol Ther 40:213, 1989.
85. Jacobson MA. Review of the toxicities of foscarnet. J Acquir Immune Defic Syndr 5(suppl 2):511, 1992.
86. Lea AP, Bryson HM. Cidofovir. Drugs 52:225, 1996.
87. Mendel DB, Tai CY, Barkhimer DB, et al. Characterization of an in vitro selected herpes simplex virus type 2 (HSV-2) strain with decreased susceptibility to cidofovir. In: Abstracts of the 4th Conference on Retroviruses and Opportunistic Infections. Alexandria, VA, Westover Management Group, 1997, abstract 681.
88. Cundy KC, Petty BG, Flaherty J, et al. Clinical pharmacokinetics of cidofovir in human immunodeficiency virus-infected patients. Antimicrob Agents Chemother 39:1247, 1995.
89. Centers for Disease Control and Prevention. USPHS/IDSA guidelines for the prevention of opportunistic infections in persons infected with human immunodeficiency virus. Clin Infect Dis 30(suppl 1):S1, 2000.

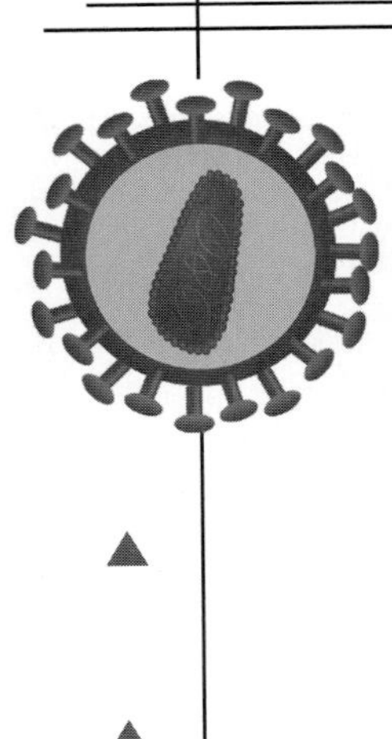

CHAPTER 42

Varicella-Zoster Virus Infections

John W. Gnann, Jr., MD

Diseases caused by all human herpesviruses, including varicella-zoster virus (VZV), occur with increased frequency in patients with human immunodeficiency virus (HIV) infection.[1] Among HIV-seropositive children, primary VZV infection (varicella) is associated with a higher rate of complications than is seen among immunocompetent children.[2] An association between recurrent VZV disease (herpes zoster) and acquired immunodeficiency syndrome (AIDS) has been noted since the onset of the pandemic.[3–8] As with herpes simplex virus (HSV) infections and tuberculosis, herpes zoster can occur in HIV-infected individuals with relatively high CD4+ T-lymphocyte counts and may be the initial opportunistic infection.[5,9–11] In most HIV-seropositive patients, herpes zoster presents as a self-limited cutaneous eruption in a dermatomal distribution. A variety of complications have been described that are associated with increased morbidity and occasional mortality. A unique feature of herpes zoster in patients with HIV infection is a propensity for multiple recurrences.

▲ VARICELLA-ZOSTER VIRUS INFECTIONS

VZV causes two clinically distinct diseases. Varicella (or chickenpox) is a common, extremely contagious acute illness that occurs in epidemics among school-age children and is characterized by a generalized vesicular rash. Like all herpesviruses, VZV establishes latency following primary infection. Reactivation of latent VZV results in herpes zoster (or shingles), a localized cutaneous eruption that is most common among the elderly. Complications of both varicella and herpes zoster are more frequent in immunocompromised patients.

Biology of Varicella-Zoster Virus

The VZV shares structural characteristics with other members of the family Herpesviridae. The intact virion is approximately 180 to 200 nm in diameter and is composed of an icosohedral nucleocapsid, an amorphous tegument, and a lipid-containing envelope with external glycoprotein spikes.[12,13] The VZV genome consists of a linear double-stranded DNA molecule containing about 125,000 basepairs (bp) and is organized with unique long (UL) (104.5 kb) and unique short (US) (5.2 kb) regions flanked by inverted repeat sequences.[14,15] VZV encodes approximately 33 polypeptides, including five glycoproteins. VZV can be propagated in vitro in a restricted variety of cell culture monolayers, mostly of human or simian origin. In human embryonic lung fibroblasts, cytopathic effects begin as a focal process with subsequent cell-to-cell spread. Approximately 8 to 10 hours after infection, virus-specific immunofluorescence can be detected in cells adjacent to the initial focus of infection. VZV is highly cell-associated with limited release of infectious virions into the culture media.

Pathogenesis of VZV Infections

Varicella

Humans are the only known reservoir for VZV. Primary infection occurs when a susceptible individual is exposed to airborne virus via the respiratory route. Patients with chickenpox are contagious for about 2 days prior to rash onset and 4 to 5 days thereafter. Varicella is most often acquired following exposure to another person with active chickenpox, but infection can also result from close exposure to a patient with herpes zoster. Varicella is highly infectious, and attack rates of 60% to 90% have been observed among household contacts.[16] VZV in airborne droplets enters the susceptible host via mucosal surfaces of the conjunctivae, oropharynx, or upper respiratory tract, then undergoes an initial round of replication in cervical lymph nodes.[17] When local immune responses are overcome, primary viremia occurs with widespread dissemination of VZV to the reticuloendothelial system. Following additional cycles of replication, a second viremic phase occurs about 1 week after the initial viremia and is accompanied by the onset of clinical symptoms.[18] VZV localizes to endothelial cells of cutaneous capillaries and then extends to epithelial cells of the epidermis where replication results in formation of the characteristic vesicles. In the normal host, viremia and new vesicle formation continue for 3 to 5 days until humoral and cellular immune responses appear.[19]

There is no convincing evidence that varicella acts as a cofactor to accelerate the progression of HIV disease. Although VZV can transactivate long terminal repeat (LTR) sequences of HIV in vitro,[20] clinical studies have not demonstrated an impact of varicella on CD4+ T-lymphocyte counts.[21,22] This is important because use of a live varicella vaccine in HIV-infected children could not be considered if VZV functioned as a cofactor.

Herpes Zoster

As VZV replicates in the skin during acute varicella, some virions are transported via sensory nerves to the corresponding dorsal root ganglia where latent infection is established.[23,24] VZV periodically reactivates and undergoes limited gene expression, but replication is suppressed by immunity before any clinical symptoms result.[25] The specific immune responses that limit reactivation of VZV in the sensory ganglia are not well defined. The most important factor that predisposes to the development of herpes zoster is a decline or suppression of VZV-specific cellular immunity, which occurs naturally with aging or can be induced by immunosuppressive illness or therapy.[26] Following reactivation and replication in the ganglion, VZV moves via axonal transport along the sensory nerve to the skin where the virus again replicates in epithelial cells, producing the characteristic dermatomal vesicular rash of herpes zoster. In contrast to the varied lesion stages seen in varicella, most zoster lesions are in the same stage of development.

Investigators initially described herpes zoster as an early sentinel marker of HIV seropositivity.[5,10,11,27,28] Although herpes zoster can occur in patients with any CD4+ lymphocyte count, the incidence is higher among individuals with advanced HIV disease.[28–32] In a survey of 175 cases reported from an American cohort, the incidence of herpes zoster was substantially higher in patients with CD4+ lymphocyte counts of less than 100 cells per cubic millimeter (4.1% annually) than in patients with counts of more than 500 cells per cubic millimeter (2.2% annually).[33] Some conflicting data exist, but prednisone therapy probably does not significantly increase the risk of herpes zoster in HIV-infected patients.[34]

Herpes zoster was originally considered a marker for rapid progression of HIV disease.[5,10,27,35] However, larger studies controlled for age and for CD4+ T-lymphocyte counts have clearly demonstrated that the development of herpes zoster is not significantly associated with the rate of disease progression to AIDS.[29,32,36–39]

As has previously been observed with infections caused by cytomegalovirus (CMV) and mycobacteria, immune reconstitution following initiation of highly active antiretroviral therapy (HAART) may be associated with an increased frequency of VZV reactivation.[40–42] Between 4 and 16 weeks after beginning combination antiretroviral therapy (containing a protease inhibitor or nonnucleoside reverse transcriptase inhibitor), the risk of herpes zoster increases two- to fourfold from baseline. In one study, 24 (8%) of 316 patients beginning combination antiretroviral therapy developed herpes zoster after a mean of 5 weeks.[42] During the 6 months following the start of combination antiretroviral therapy, the incidence of herpes zoster exceeds 90 episodes per 1000 person-years.[40,42] The percentage of CD8+ lymphocytes at baseline and the magnitude of their increase at 1 month after initiation of drug therapy is strongly associated with an increased risk of herpes zoster.[40,42] The immunologic mechanisms that account for this observation are not fully understood. The clinical presentation and natural history of herpes zoster in the setting of immune reconstitution does not seem to differ from that seen in other HIV-infected patients.[40,42]

Epidemiology of VZV Infections

Varicella

In the United States, varicella epidemics occur annually during the late winter and early spring, with numbers of cases peaking in March.[43] During the prevaccine era about 3.8 million cases of varicella occurred each year in the United States, which is approximately equal to the annual birth cohort.[43] About 50% to 60% of varicella cases occurred in children between the ages of 5 and 9 years, and 90% of cases were in children under 15 years of age. Serologic surveys demonstrated that more than 95% of the U.S. population had been infected by VZV by age 20. Introduction of the varicella vaccine in the United States in 1995 has resulted in striking changes in the epidemiology of chickenpox. By monitoring vaccine and disease activity at three sentinel sites, the Centers for Disease Control and Prevention (CDC) showed that vaccine coverage among preschool-age children increased from 40% in 1997 to 70% in 1999.[44] Between 1995 and 1999 the varicella incidence declined 80% in the surveillance areas, accompanied by an attenuation of disease seasonality. The greatest decline in incidence was seen in children aged 1 to 4 years.[44]

Herpes Zoster

The annual incidence of herpes zoster in the United States is 1.5 to 3.0 cases per 1000 population. An incidence of 2.0 cases per 1000 persons would project to about 500,000 cases of herpes zoster annually in the United States.

Increasing age is clearly the most important risk factor for the development of herpes zoster. There is a significant increase in the age-specific incidence of herpes zoster beginning at around age 55; individuals over 75 years of age have a herpes zoster incidence of about 10 cases per 1000 person-years.[45,46] These figures predict that an immunocompetent individual living to be 70 years of age has a 10% to 20% risk of developing herpes zoster at some point during his or her lifetime. Shingles occurs with equal frequency in men and women, and there is no seasonal association.

The other well defined risk factor for herpes zoster is altered cell-mediated immunity, as seen in patients with lymphoproliferative malignancies, organ transplant recipients, and AIDS patients. Results from several prospective studies have confirmed the incidence rates for herpes zoster in HIV-infected individuals to be about 30 to 50 cases per 1000 person-years.[28,29,31–33,47,48] In a surveillance study conducted in San Francisco, the incidence of herpes zoster among HIV-seropositive men was 29.4 cases per 1000 person-years compared with 2.0 cases per 1000 person-years among a control group of HIV-seronegative gay men.[29] HIV infection was associated with an increased relative risk (RR) of herpes zoster in all age groups [RR 16.9; 95% confidence interval (CI) 8.7 to 32.6].[29] The cumulative proportion of men developing herpes zoster increased linearly; by 12 years after the diagnosis of HIV infection, 30% of the patients had developed herpes zoster. Among patients with herpes zoster, 22% experienced more than one episode of shingles.[29] In a similar prospective study conducted in The Netherlands, the incidence of herpes zoster among HIV-seropositive patients was 51.5 cases per 1000 person-years, with a 41% cumulative incidence over 10 years; in the HIV-seronegative control population, the zoster incidence was 3.31 cases per 1000 person-years, with a 10-year cumulative incidence of 3%.[32] Prospective studies in Uganda yielded similar results.[48] These observations confirm that the incidence of herpes zoster is about 15-fold higher among HIV-infected individuals than among age-matched seronegative controls. As a corollary, the possibility of HIV infection should be considered in otherwise healthy patients less than 55 years of age who present with herpes zoster. In African populations where the prevalence of HIV infection is high, more than 90% of patients presenting with a new diagnosis of herpes zoster were found to be HIV-infected.[9,10,49]

Clinical Presentation

Varicella

Varicella is usually a benign disease in healthy children, although symptoms are frequently more severe in adolescents and adults.[50,51] Symptoms develop after an incubation period of about 15 days. The appearance of the rash is sometimes preceded by a brief (1 to 2 days) prodrome of fever, malaise, headache, and anorexia. Cutaneous lesions begin as pink macules that quickly become papular and evolve into fragile vesicles 1 to 4 mm in diameter surrounded by a zone of erythema. The lesions first appear on the head, progress to the trunk, and finally to the extremities. The rash of varicella is characterized by rapid evolution of lesions during 8 to 12 hours and by successive crops of new lesions. Consequently, lesions at all stages of development are present simultaneously. New vesicle formation continues for 2 to 4 days, accompanied by pruritus, fever, headache, malaise, and anorexia. The rash peaks at about the fifth day with a lesion count of about 250 to 500 (lower in children under 5 years of age and higher in adults). With the influx of inflammatory cells, vesicles pustulate and then crust. The scabs detach after 1 to 3 weeks, and the lesions usually heal without scarring.

Varicella does not appear to be unusually severe in most HIV-seropositive children.[52,53] However, the natural history of varicella in this population is difficult to ascertain from the literature, as most published reports are based on retrospective studies of hospitalized patients or referral populations that likely overestimate the frequency of complications.[2,54–56] The clinical presentation of varicella is similar to that seen in immunocompetent children, although some investigators have reported a longer duration of new lesion formation and higher median lesion counts.[2,54,55,57] In a prospective, case-controlled study of 30 HIV-infected children with chickenpox, 29 of the cases were scored as mild or moderate in severity, even among the children who received no treatment with acyclovir.[21] The only serious complication was one severe case of varicella pneumonia.[21] The manifestations of varicella were judged to be less severe in HIV-infected children than in children with acute leukemia.[21]

A variety of varicella complications in HIV-infected children have been reported, although reliable incidence figures are not available. An inverse correlation between CD4+ lymphocyte counts and complication rates has been suggested[54] but not substantiated in other studies.[2,58] Cutaneous complications of varicella may include hemorrhagic skin lesions or bacterial superinfections.[2] Visceral dissemination of VZV may manifest by disseminated intravascular coagulopathy, pneumonitis, hepatitis, or encephalitis.[2,54,55,59,60] Deaths attributable to chickenpox in children with HIV infection are rare and are usually due to pneumonitis.[2,54]

Following an episode of varicella, HIV-infected children are at high risk for persistent or recurrent VZV infections.[21,52] In a few reported cases the cutaneous lesions of primary varicella failed to heal and remained VZV culture-positive; this was usually associated with a very low CD4+ T-lymphocyte count.[59] More often, children develop recurrent cutaneous VZV infections months to years after the primary infection.[54,58,61,62] In a population of 480 HIV-infected children, 117 episodes of VZV infection were identified in 73 patients.[59] Of the 73 children, 38 (53%) had recurrent VZV infections; the mean interval from the first to second episode was 17 months. Among 22 children with primary varicella who were followed for 24 months, 10 (45%) had recurrent VZV disease. CD4+ T-lymphocyte counts were no different between children who experienced recurrences and those who did not. Five of the recurrences were classic herpes zoster, and the other five were described as "recurrent varicella" with a widespread cutaneous rash.[59] In most cases "recurrent varicella" probably results from VZV reactivation and is actually generalized cutaneous zoster (as has been previously described in other immunocompromised populations), although true reacquisition due to failed immune responses occur occasionally. Seroconversion following varicella was documented by enzyme-linked immunosorbent assay (ELISA) testing of acute and convalescent sera in six of eight HIV-infected children.[58]

About 95% of HIV-infected adults have antibody against VZV as a result of childhood varicella, and antibody levels are well preserved even in patients with advanced AIDS.[63,64] However, when chickenpox does occur in HIV-infected adults, the disease may produce significant morbidity, including VZV pneumonia.[55,65] In a series of five HIV-seropositive adults with varicella, three had uncomplicated courses, one had possible central nervous system (CNS) involvement, and one had possible CNS infection plus hepatitis and thrombocytopenia.[63] All five patients improved with acyclovir therapy. Four developed VZV antibody, and one had herpes zoster 2 years after varicella.[63] Recurrent varicella-like eruptions, as described above in children, have also been reported in adults.[55,66]

Herpes Zoster

Herpes zoster presents as a painful cutaneous eruption in a dermatomal distribution. The inflammatory changes that occur as latent VZV reactivates in the sensory ganglion produce discomfort in the corresponding dermatome. The patient may report sensations ranging from mild itching or tingling to severe pain that precedes the development of the skin lesions by 1 to 5 days (or rarely weeks). The cutaneous eruption, appearing in the skin segment innervated by a single sensory ganglion, is unilateral and does not cross the midline (Fig. 42–1A). Overlap of lesions into adjacent dermatomes occurs in 20% of cases. The most common sites for herpes zoster are the thoracic dermatomes (50% of cases), followed by cranial nerve (15%), cervical (15%), lumbar (15%), and sacral (5%) dermatomes.[67] During the acute phase of herpes zoster, most patients experience dermatomal pruritus and pain, which can be quite severe. Patients may also complain of headache, photophobia, and malaise; but significant fever is rare. Skin changes begin with an erythematous maculopapular rash followed by the appearance of clear vesicles (Figs. 42–1B). New vesicle formation typically continues for 3 to 5 days followed by lesion pustulation and scabbing. Bacterial superinfection of the cutaneous lesions occurs in 10% to 15% of cases.[11,31] Skin lesions heal within 2 to 4 weeks, often leaving skin scarring and permanent pigmentation changes. In rare cases, patients develop dermatomal neuralgic pain but do not progress to the cutaneous eruption phase, a condition termed zoster sine herpete.[68] In the normal host, the most frequent complication of herpes zoster is chronic pain, traditionally termed postherpetic neuralgia (PHN). The incidence and the duration of PHN are markedly increased in elderly individuals.[45]

Patients with deficiencies of cell-mediated immunity, including AIDS, have a high incidence of herpes zoster and an increased likelihood of complications.[69] Most cases of herpes zoster in HIV-seropositive patients are clinically similar to shingles seen in the immunocompetent host, although distinctive features such as frequent recurrences and atypical lesions are well described. Herpes zoster involving multiple nonadjacent dermatomes has occasionally been observed in HIV-infected patients.[11,70,71] A high frequency of herpes zoster involving the first division of the trigeminal nerve (herpes zoster ophthalmicus, or HZO) among HIV-infected patients was reported from both the United States[4,72–74] and Africa.[75,76] However, prospective studies have shown that about 15% of herpes zoster cases in HIV-seropositive patients involve cranial dermatomes, which is similar to the frequency seen in immunocompetent patients.[31,70] Because of the prominent symptoms and cosmetic issues associated with facial herpes zoster, patients with HZO may be more likely to seek care. For example, studies conducted in Ethiopia and Miami showed that 81 of 85 (95%) and 29 of 112 (26%) patients, respectively, presenting with HZO were found to be HIV-seropositive.[74,76] HZO warrants aggressive therapy to prevent ocular complications such as conjunctivitis, keratitis (both acute and chronic), iritis, and uveitis.[77–79]

Patients infected with HIV have a much higher frequency of recurrent shingles than is seen in immunocompetent persons or in other populations of immunocompromised patients. About 20% to 30% of HIV-infected patients

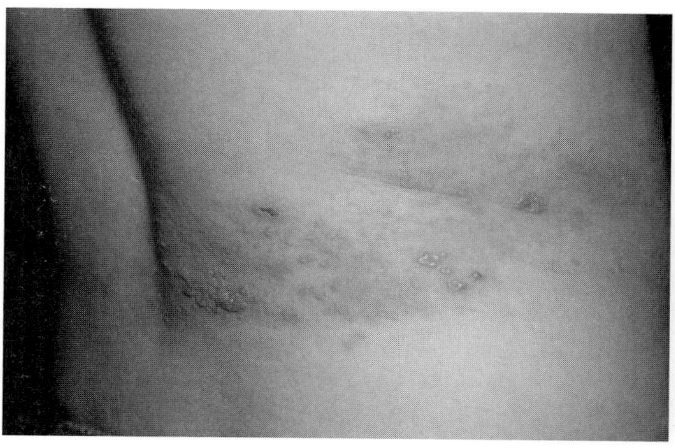

A

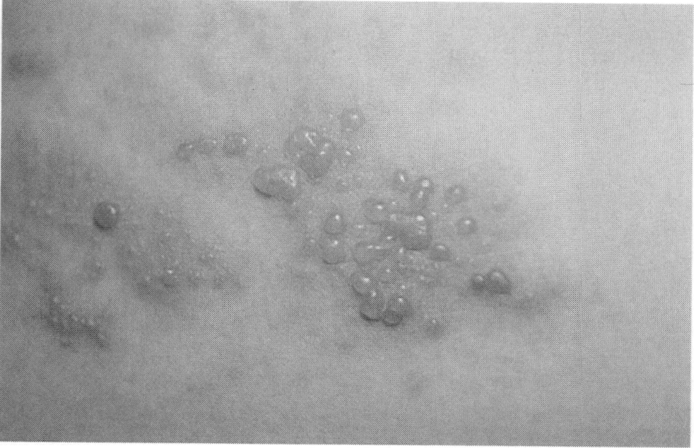

B

Figure 42–1. Typical cutaneous eruption of herpes zoster. *A*, Shingles involving the right T_{10} dermatome. *B*, Vesicles characteristic of early VZV infection.

develop one or more subsequent episodes of herpes zoster, which may involve the same or different dermatomes.[10,29,31] The probability of a recurrence of zoster within 1 year of the index episode is about 12%.[38,80]

Whereas herpes zoster is uncommon in healthy children, shingles is frequently diagnosed in HIV-infected children.[21,81] In a prospective study, 8 of 30 HIV-infected children with documented varicella subsequently developed herpes zoster.[21] The average interval between varicella and zoster was about 24 months,[21,81] although intervals as short as 2 months have been reported.[82] A low CD4+ T-lymphocyte count at the onset of varicella has been reported to correlate strongly with an increased risk of subsequent herpes zoster.[21] Investigators at the National Cancer Institute reported a series of 11 HIV-seropositive children with frequently recurring herpes zoster, averaging five episodes per child over 25 months. Of the 58 discrete episodes documented, 29 were characterized as localized herpes zoster, 9 cases involved multiple dermatomes, and 20 cases had cutaneous dissemination; there were no cases of visceral dissemination and no deaths.[81]

VZV can cause atypical skin lesions in HIV-seropositive patients that are not characteristic of either classic varicella or herpes zoster.[83] Aberrant presentations include disseminated varicella-like lesions,[55,84] disseminated verrucous or hyperkeratotic lesions,[61,85–91] disseminated ecthymatous lesions,[92,93] and disseminated pinpoint papules.[94] The most common atypical manifestation in HIV-seropositive patients is multiple hyperkeratotic lesions, measuring 3 to 20 mm in diameter, that follow no dermatomal distribution and may be chronic, persisting for months or years (Fig. 42–2A). A second dermatologic variant is ecthymatous VZV lesions, presenting with multiple large (10 to 30 mm) punched-out ulcerations with a central black eschar and a peripheral rim of vesicles (Fig. 42–2B). The atypical appearance of these lesions may be linked to abnormal expression of VZV glycoproteins.[95] Making the correct diagnosis requires a high index of suspicion, with confirmation provided by viral culture or lesion biopsy. Importantly, a significant number of these atypical verrucous or ecthymatous lesions are caused by acyclovir-resistant strains of VZV.[62,85,96–98] VZV isolates obtained from these atypical lesions should routinely be submitted for antiviral susceptibility testing.

Most herpes zoster-related complications occur in patients with CD4+ lymphocyte counts of less than 200 cells per cubic millimeter.[31,70] A review of 23 cases of VZV dissemination in patients with HIV infection documented that most of these patients experienced zoster involving several contiguous dermatomes, extensive local skin necrosis, and cutaneous dissemination of lesions.[99,100] Visceral dissemination of VZV to lung or liver has rarely, if ever, been documented as a complication of herpes zoster in AIDS patients.[81,99,101]

The occurrence of PHN does not appear to differ markedly between HIV-infected and seronegative patients with herpes zoster. About 10% to 15% of HIV-seropositive patients report PHN as a complication following herpes zoster.[31] The primary predictors for chronic pain are older age and severity of pain at presentation.[102]

The primary target organ for herpes zoster dissemination in patients with HIV infection is the CNS.[103] CNS involvement may occur simultaneously with the cutaneous eruption, follow the acute episode of herpes zoster by weeks or months, or occur in patients with no documented history of cutaneous herpes zoster.[104,105] A variety of neurologic syndromes attributed to VZV infection have been described in HIV-infected patients, including multifocal leukoencephalitis,[106,107] ventriculitis,[108] myelitis and myeloradiculitis,[71,109–113] cranial nerve palsies and focal brain stem lesions,[114–117] and aseptic meningitis.[31] A chronic, progressive form of VZV encephalitis attributed to small vessel vasculopathy has been diagnosed in several AIDS patients.[60,118–120] Virtually all of these diagnoses of VZV neurologic diseases were in AIDS patients with markedly depleted CD4+ lymphocytes. Approximately 30% to 40% of these patients had no recognized recent history of cutaneous VZV infection. In cases in which antecedent herpes zoster had been diagnosed, the skin lesions often preceded the neurologic symptoms by months.

Acute retinal necrosis (ARN) caused by VZV has previously been described in immunocompetent patients. More aggressive variants of this disease have been recognized in

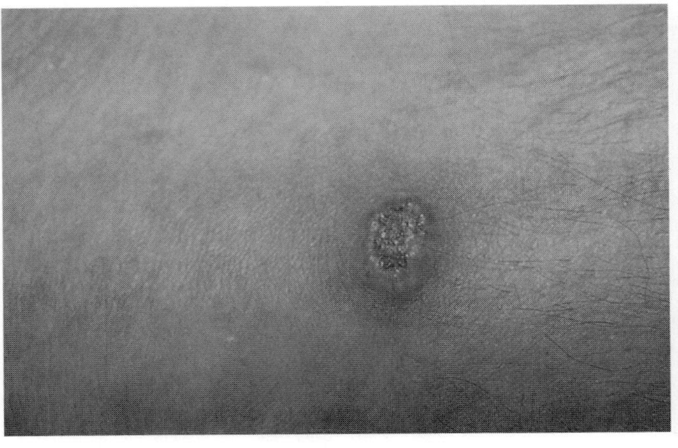

A

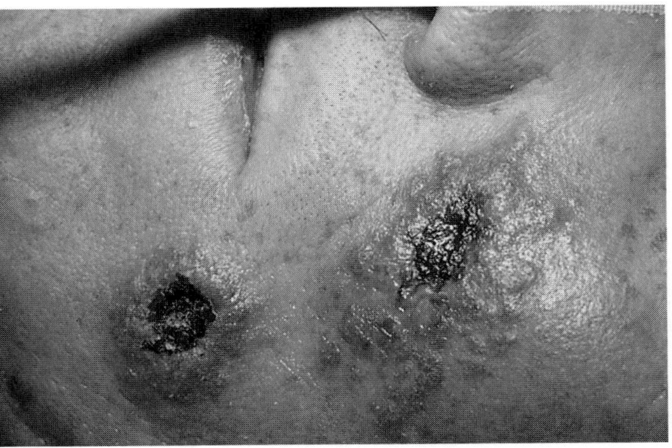

B

Figure 42–2. Atypical cutaneous lesions caused by acyclovir-resistant VZV. *A*, Hyperkeratotic nodule on the forearm. *B*, Facial echthymatous ulcerations with rim of vesicles.

patients with AIDS and were termed varicella-zoster virus retinitis (VZVR), progressive outer retinal necrosis (PORN), and rapidly progressive herpetic retinal necrosis (RPHRN).[121-125] The RPHRN syndrome is seen almost exclusively in AIDS patients with CD4+ lymphocyte counts of less than 100 cells per cubic millimeter.[124,126,127] This form of VZV retinitis may occur concurrently with active herpes zoster or, more frequently, develops weeks or months after the acute episode of herpes zoster has resolved.[121,128] RPHRN can occur after HZO or after herpes zoster involving a remote dermatome. The retinitis begins with multifocal necrotizing lesions involving the peripheral retina. Most patients present with unilateral involvement, but progression to bilateral disease occurs frequently.[124,125,129] The funduscopic examination reveals granular, yellowish, nonhemorrhagic lesions that rapidly extend and coalesce, often resulting in retinal detachment. There is a relative lack of intraocular inflammatory changes. RPHRN rapidly progresses to confluent full-thickness retinal necrosis (which differs from the slow progression seen with CMV retinitis) and results in blindness in 75% to 85% of involved eyes.[74,122,124,126] The etiologic role of VZV in most cases of RPHRN has been established by demonstrating of virus by culture or the polymerase chain reaction (PCR) from choroid, vitreous fluid, and retinal biopsies[123,130,131] HSV occasionally causes an identical syndrome.[124,132]

▲ DIAGNOSIS OF VZV INFECTIONS

The appearance of varicella is quite distinctive, and a clinical diagnosis is usually accurate and reliable (Fig. 42–3). The presentation of a child with mild constitutional symptoms, a diffuse vesicular rash, and no history of chickenpox is strongly suggestive of the diagnosis, especially during an epidemic. Herpes zoster, with its characteristic vesicular rash, is also readily diagnosed on the basis of clinical appearance, although the diagnosis may be initially obscure in patients who present with dermatomal neuralgic pain prior to the development of skin lesions. The skin disease most commonly confused with herpes zoster is zosteriform HSV infection, which appears in a dermatome-like distribution (most commonly in the sacral area) and may closely mimic the appearance of shingles.[133]

Serologic techniques can be used to determine susceptibility to VZV infection and to document rising antibody titers in patients with acute varicella. Serum immunoglobulin G (IgG) becomes detectable several days after the onset of varicella, and titers peak at 2 to 3 weeks, so routine serologic tests provide only a retrospective diagnosis. Acute infection can be confirmed by VZV-specific serum IgM titers,[134] but antigen detection techniques are usually faster and more reliable. Patients with herpes zoster are VZV-seropositive at the time of disease onset, but most show a significant rise in antibody titer during the convalescence phase.[135] Elevated antibody titers in CSF can be measured to support the diagnosis of VZV CNS infection.[136] A variety of methods have been used to detect VZV antibodies, but most laboratories have now adopted an ELISA or a latex agglutination (LA) assay for VZV serodiagnosis. The ELISA is capable of detecting IgG or IgM responses, is a reliable indicator of immune status following natural infection, and is readily automated.[137,138] However, the ELISA may not be sufficiently sensitive to measure vaccine-induced immunity.[139] The LA assay is rapid, simple, inexpensive, and highly sensitive but cannot be automated or used to detect IgM.[140] The fluorescent antibody to membrane antigen (FAMA) test is also highly sensitive but not widely available.

Unlike HSV or CMV, VZV is not shed asymptomatically. Consequently, demonstration of VZV virions, antigens, or nucleic acids in tissues (other than sensory ganglia) or body fluids is diagnostic of active infection. VZV can be identified in infected tissues by histopathology or electron microscopy, but visualization of multinucleated giant cells with inclusion bodies or herpesvirus virions does not distinguish between VZV and HSV. Immunohistochemical staining of viral antigens can provide a more specific diagnosis.[141] Direct fluorescent antigen (DFA) staining using

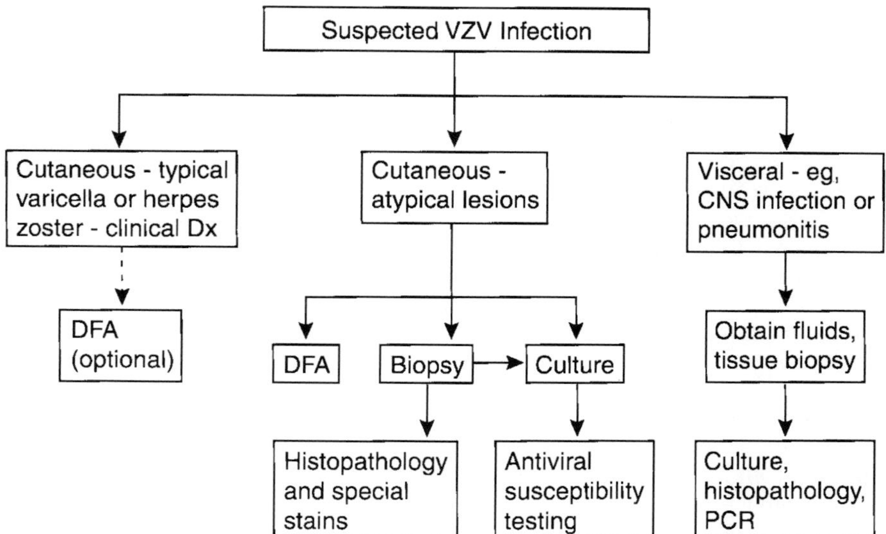

Figure 42–3. Diagnostic approach to VZV infections in HIV-seropositive patients. DFA, direct fluorescent antigen (test).

fluorescein-conjugated monoclonal antibodies to detect VZV glycoproteins in infected epithelial cells is especially helpful for making a rapid diagnosis when the clinical presentation is atypical (Fig. 42–4). This simple, rapid technique is more sensitive than virus culture, especially in later stages of VZV infection when virus isolation becomes more difficult.[135,142] In a population of 92 HIV-infected adults with suspected herpes zoster, DFA and viral culture were positive in 85 of 92 (92%) and 60 of 92 (65%) patients, respectively.[135] To perform the DFA assay, epithelial cells are scraped from the base of a vesicle or ulcer with a scalpel blade, smeared on a glass slide, fixed with cold acetone, stained with fluorescein-conjugated monoclonal antibodies, and then examined using a fluorescence microscope.[143–145] By using virus-specific monoclonal antibodies, HSV can be readily distinguished from VZV, making DFA staining a much more powerful technique than a simple Tzanck preparation.

The use of the PCR to detect VZV nucleic acids in clinical specimens is emerging as an important diagnostic tool.[105,146,147] The PCR overcomes the difficulties inherent in culturing labile VZV and has been used successfully to detect viral DNA in cerebrospinal fluid (CSF) from patients with VZV encephalitis[107,148–150] and in ocular fluids and tissues from VZV retinitis cases.[123,131,151]

Viral culture currently remains the benchmark method for diagnosing active VZV infection. VZV can be cultured by inoculating vesicular fluid onto monolayers of human fetal diploid kidney or lung cells. Unlike HSV, VZV is extremely labile, and every effort should be made to minimize the time spent for specimen transport and storage. Ideally, fluid should be aspirated from clear vesicles using a tuberculin syringe containing 0.2 ml of medium, inoculated directly into tissue culture at the bedside (or taken immediately to the laboratory), and then incubated at 36°C in 5% CO_2 atmosphere.[69] If no vesicles or pustules are available for aspiration, the clinician should carefully remove overlying debris or crusts from the freshest lesions available, swab the underlying ulcers, and place the swab directly into viral transport medium for rapid delivery on ice to the laboratory. Characteristic cytopathic effects are usually seen in tissue culture in 3 to 7 days, although cultures should be held for 14 days before they are declared negative. The culture process can be accelerated by using centrifugation cultures in shell vials.[152] Identification of the isolate can be confirmed by staining the monolayer with VZV-specific monoclonal antibodies.[153] In general, viral culture for VZV is highly specific but slow, insensitive, and expensive.

Diseases caused by strains of VZV resistant to acyclovir have been reported in a substantial number of HIV-seropositive patients.[96] Resistance, which never occurs in immunocompetent patients, is usually seen in severely immunocompromised patients with extensive previous exposure to acyclovir or similar drugs. In vitro studies of acyclovir-resistant isolates have documented a variety of mutations in the thymidine kinase gene that result in production of an enzyme that is truncated and nonfunctional or has altered substrate specificity.[97,154] Patients with VZV infections who fail to respond to conventional antiviral therapy or who present with chronic atypical lesions should have specimens submitted to a reference laboratory for VZV culture and drug-susceptibility testing. The plaque reduction assay, which measures inhibition of viral plaque formation in the presence of the antiviral drug, is the classic method for susceptibility testing.[155] Because clinical isolates of VZV are strongly cell-associated, the assay must be performed using infected cell suspensions, which makes the plaque reduction assay technically demanding for VZV. An alternative approach is to measure the effect of antiviral compounds on in vitro viral DNA synthesis. DNA-DNA hybridization test kits are commercially available (Hybriwix Probe Systems; Diagnostic Hybrids, Athens, OH, USA) for VZV susceptibility testing. The assay measures VZV DNA production by hybridizing ^{125}I-labeled single-stranded DNA probes with viral DNA and measuring the reduction of radioactivity counts at various drug concentrations. Compared with the plaque-reduction assay, DNA-DNA hybridization is more rapid but requires specialized reagents and equipment. A third method for susceptibility testing utilizes enzyme-linked immunoassays performed on fixed, infected cell monolayers to evaluate drug activity against VZV.[156] For each of these methods, VZV resistance is defined as a three- to fourfold increase in the effective drug concentration required to inhibit 50% of the replication of the clinical isolate (IC_{50}) compared to a VZV control isolate.[96,155,157] Isolates that are resistant to acyclovir are usually also resistant to drugs with similar mechanisms of action, including penciclovir and ganciclovir. VZV resistance to foscarnet, a drug that utilizes a different mechanism of action, is rare.[158,159]

Diagnosing VZV infection of the CNS can be difficult, especially in cases where there is no concomitant cutaneous disease. Examination of the CSF usually reveals a moderate lymphocytic pleocytosis, normal to moderately elevated protein, and normal glucose. The PCR for VZV DNA in CSF should be positive in more than 75% of cases.[105] In one series of 34 HIV-infected patients with VZV neurologic complications, the mean CSF white blood cell count was 126/mm^3, the mean protein concentration was 230 mg/dl, and the PCR was positive for VZV in all cases.[103] In patients with chronic VZV encephalitis, magnetic resonance imaging (MRI) may show a characteristic picture of multifocal lesions located in deep white matter and at the gray–white matter junction.[105,107,120]

▲ THERAPY OF VZV INFECTIONS

Treatment of Varicella

Chickenpox is associated with low rates of morbidity and mortality among immunocompetent children, and supportive care is usually sufficient. Astringent soaks and antipyretics (e.g., acetaminophen) provide symptomatic relief. Aspirin (possibly associated with Reye syndrome) and nonsteroidal antiinflammatory drugs (possibly associated with necrotizing fasciitis) should be avoided. Trimming fingernails closely helps prevent bacterial superinfections caused by scratching the lesions. If bacterial cellulitis develops, antibiotics may be required. Oral acyclovir has been evaluated for treatment of uncomplicated varicella in immunocompetent children,

▲ **Table 42–1.** ANTIVIRAL DRUGS FOR VZV INFECTIONS IN AIDS PATIENTS

Drug	Indication	Dose[a]	Major Toxicities
Acyclovir	Varicella or herpes zoster	20 mg/kg (or 800 mg) PO 5 times daily until healed (≥7 d)	None; minor nausea or headache
	Disseminated or visceral VZV infection	10 mg/kg IV q8h × ≥7 d	Nephrotoxicity (rare), CNS disturbances (rare)
Famciclovir	Herpes zoster	500 mg PO q8h until healed (≥7 d)	None; minor nausea or headache
Valacyclovir	Herpes zoster	1.0 g q8h until healed (≥7 d)	? Associated with TTP/HUS; minor nausea or headache
Foscarnet	Acyclovir-resistant VZV infections	60–90 mg/kg IV q12h until healed (≥10 d)	Nephrotoxicity (common), electrolyte disturbances (common), seizures, arrhythmias, anemia, genital ulcers

HUS, hemolytic-uremic syndrome; TTP, thrombotic thrombocytopenic purpura.
[a]Doses given are for adults with normal renal function.

adolescents, and adults.[160–162] In these studies, initiation of acyclovir therapy within 24 hours of rash onset reduced the time to cessation of new lesion formation, the number of lesions, and constitutional symptoms, including fever. The dose of oral acyclovir for chickenpox is 20 mg/kg (up to a maximum of 800 mg) five times daily (Table 42–1). Unlike acyclovir, valacyclovir and famciclovir are not available as suspensions and have not been evaluated extensively for treatment of varicella, although the properties of these drugs suggest that they should be at least as effective as acyclovir. No controlled prospective studies of antiviral therapy for chickenpox in HIV-infected children have been reported, so recommendations must be derived from anecdotal experience or from data derived in other populations (Fig. 42–4). Most clinicians prescribe oral antiviral therapy, reserving intravenous acyclovir for patients with unusually severe or complicated infections.[21,59,63]

Treatment of Herpes Zoster

Three oral antiviral drugs are currently approved in the United States for treating herpes zoster (Table 42–1). In the normal host, acyclovir, valacyclovir, and famciclovir have all been demonstrated to reduce the duration of viral shedding, accelerate cessation of new lesion formation, accelerate the events of cutaneous healing, and limit the duration of pain when therapy is initiated within 72 hours of the onset of herpes zoster.[163–166] Because of their superior pharmacokinetic properties, valacyclovir and famciclovir are currently considered the preferred drugs for herpes zoster.[167] Appropriate supportive care can help make patients with herpes zoster more comfortable. Skin lesions should be kept clean and dry to reduce the risk of bacterial superinfection. Astringent soaks (e.g., Domeboro solution) may be soothing. Most patients with acute herpes zoster have significant pain and require therapy with opioid analgesics.

Prospectively acquired data to guide clinicians when selecting antiviral therapy for herpes zoster in HIV-seropositive patients are currently limited (Fig. 42–5). Nearly 300 HIV-infected patients with herpes zoster were enrolled in controlled studies comparing orally administered acyclovir (800 mg five times daily) with sorivudine (40 mg once daily).[80,168] Times to cessation of new vesicle formation, total crusting, and resolution of zoster-associated pain were 3 to 4 days, 7 to 8 days, and about 60 days, respectively.[80] Although sorivudine was shown to be the superior treatment, development of that compound was halted because of concerns about interactions with 5-fluorouracil. However, these studies clearly confirmed the efficacy and safety of oral antiviral therapy for herpes zoster in patients with HIV infection. Famciclovir was judged to be effective and safe for herpes zoster in AIDS patients when evaluated in a small, open-label clinical trial.[169] Valacyclovir has not been systematically evaluated as a treatment for herpes zoster in HIV-infected patients, although anecdotal clinical experience suggests therapeutic benefit. Long-term administration of antiherpesvirus drugs to prevent recurrences of herpes zoster is not routinely recommended.

The value of anti-VZV therapy in patients presenting with herpes zoster of more than 72 hours duration has not been determined. Patients who have signs of ongoing VZV replication (evidenced by new vesicle formation) can likely benefit from antiviral therapy. Patients who have HZO should also be treated to reduce the risk of serious ocular complications, even when presenting beyond 72 hours.[170,171] Antiviral therapy is unlikely to be useful for patients whose lesions are crusted or scabbed. Because of the documented risk of relapsing infection, VZV disease in HIV-seropositive patients should be treated until all lesions are completely resolved, which is often longer than the standard 7 to 10 day course. What impact anti-VZV therapy may have on the risk of subsequent complications such as CNS infection or retinitis is unknown. Adjunctive therapy of herpes zoster with corticosteroids has not been evaluated in HIV-infected patients and is not currently recommended.[172,173] The effect of therapy on zoster sine herpete[68] is also not established, although some clinicians advocate a trial of antiviral therapy in an attempt to ameliorate symptoms.

Most clinicians select intravenous acyclovir as the drug of choice to treat severe or complicated herpes zoster in HIV-infected patients, although this approach has not been studied in a prospective fashion. The literature contains case reports documenting successful therapy of neurologic complications, including myelitis, with intravenous acyclovir.[174–176] Some investigators have recommended intravenous acyclovir for initial therapy of HZO in HIV-infected patients, although oral therapy appears adequate in most cases.[177]

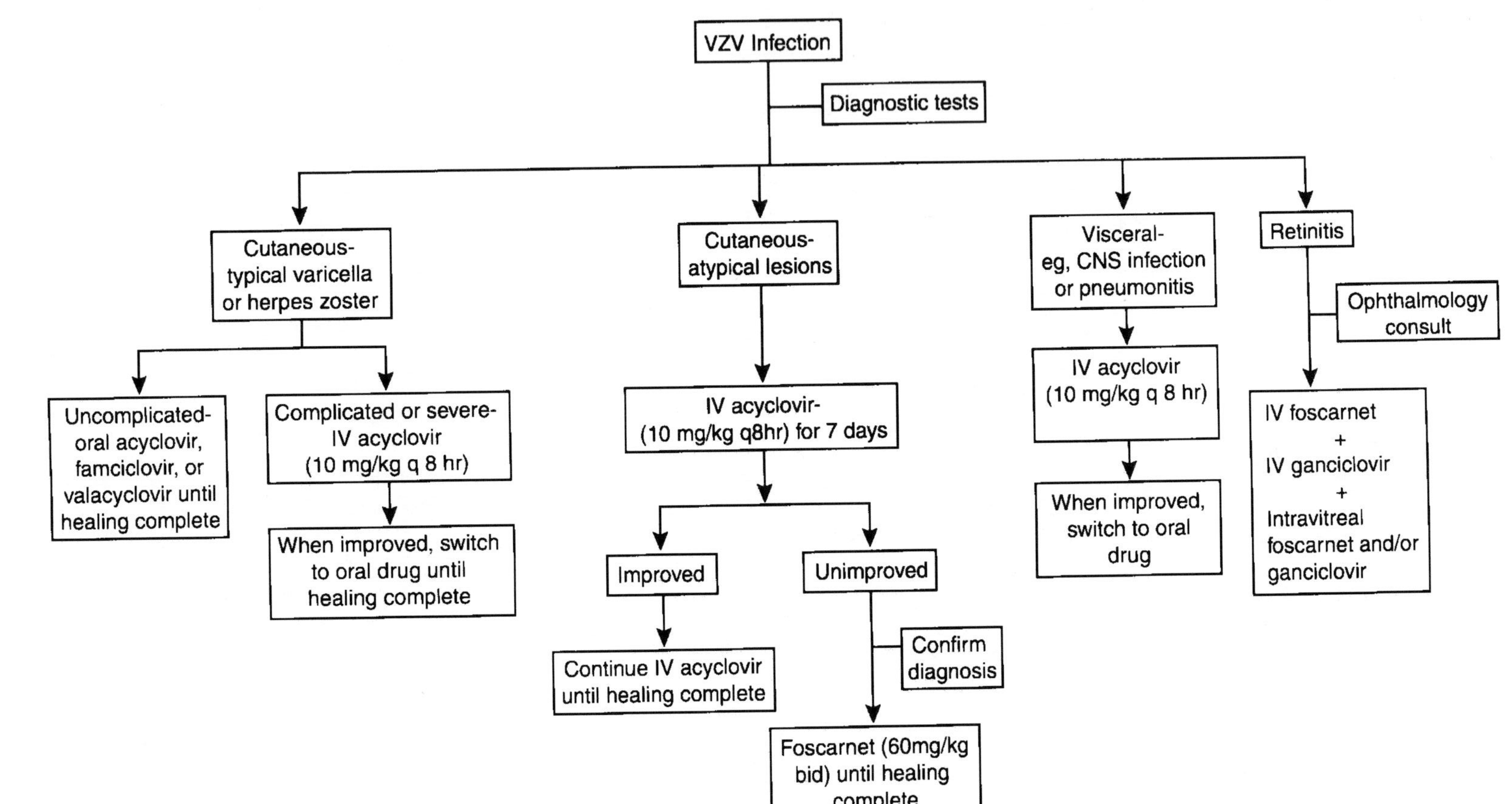

Figure 42–4. Approach to therapy of VZV infections in HIV-seropositive patients.

Optimal antiviral therapy for VZV-induced, rapidly progressive herpetic retinal necrosis remains undefined. Responses to intravenous acyclovir or ganciclovir have been inconsistent and disappointing.[178] Several case reports have documented preservation of vision in patients treated with a combination of intravenous ganciclovir plus foscarnet, with or without intravitreal ganciclovir.[179,180] The optimal duration of induction therapy and options for long-term maintenance therapy have not been established.

Management of Acyclovir-Resistant VZV Infections

The first acyclovir-resistant isolate of VZV was recovered from an HIV-infected child in 1988.[62] Additional case reports have provided a better picture of the characteristic features of disease caused by acyclovir-resistant VZV.[85,96,98,157,181,182] Virtually all cases have been described in AIDS patients with very low CD4+ T-lymphocyte counts, and most patients had been treated previously with acyclovir. Most isolates resistant to acyclovir are also resistant to valacyclovir, famciclovir, penciclovir, and ganciclovir, all of which depend on viral thymidine kinase for activation. A strong association exists between acyclovir-resistant VZV and the presence of atypical skin lesions.[62,85,96,97] One report described four HIV-seropositive adults undergoing chronic suppressive acyclovir therapy who developed disseminated hyperkeratotic papules that failed to respond to acyclovir.[96] In vitro susceptibility testing confirmed that the VZV isolates were acyclovir-resistant, with a mean IC_{50} for acyclovir of 20 μg/ml, compared with 0.75 μg/ml for reference strain VZV_{Oka}.[96] Patients with chronic or atypical VZV-positive lesions merit a thorough evaluation for the possibility of acyclovir-resistant virus. In addition, the possibility of acyclovir resistance should be strongly considered in patients who develop VZV disease while undergoing suppressive ganciclovir therapy for CMV infection.

The drug of choice for treatment of acyclovir-resistant VZV disease is foscarnet, a viral DNA polymerase inhibitor that is not dependent on thymidine kinase for activation.[183–185] In a series of 13 patients with AIDS and acyclovir-resistant VZV infection treated with intravenous foscarnet, 10 patients (77%) had complete lesion healing after a mean of 17.8 days of therapy.[185] Of the 10 responding patients, 5 subsequently had a herpes zoster recurrence after a median of 110 days. Most cases of disease caused by acyclovir-resistant VZV have been limited to cutaneous involvement, although a few instances of visceral infection caused by acyclovir-resistant VZV have been reported, including cases of retinal necrosis[186] and meningoradiculitis.[187]

Fortunately, VZV isolates resistant to acyclovir-type drugs and to foscarnet have been encountered infrequently.[158,188] The molecular biology of these dually resistant isolates has not been fully explored, but a mutation in the viral DNA polymerase could account for both acyclovir and foscarnet resistance.[159] Cidofovir would likely retain activity against these isolates and could be tried in patients with disease caused by dually resistant VZV, although there are no data available to validate this approach.

Although the mechanisms that lead to the development of acyclovir resistance are incompletely understood, clinical data indicate that many cases are associated with inadequate dosing of acyclovir for either acute therapy or long-term suppression, possibly allowing selection of thymidine kinase-deficient mutants. Clinicians using acyclovir or related drugs for treatment of varicella or herpes zoster in AIDS patients should utilize the full therapeutic dose (which is higher than the dose required to treat HSV infections) and continue therapy until VZV lesions have completely resolved.[90,96]

Drugs for Treatment of VZV Infections

Acyclovir

Acyclovir is a selective inhibitor of the replication of HSV-1, HSV-2, and VZV.[189,190] The drug is converted by virus-encoded thymidine kinase to its monophosphate derivative, a reaction that does not occur to any significant extent in uninfected cells.[191] Subsequent diphosphorylation and triphosphorylation steps are catalyzed by cellular enzymes, producing high acyclovir triphosphate concentrations in HSV- or VZV-infected cells. Acyclovir triphosphate inhibits viral DNA synthesis by competing with deoxyguanosine triphosphate as a substrate for viral DNA polymerase.[192] When acyclovir triphosphate is incorporated into the viral DNA chain, it functions as an obligate chain terminator because it lacks the 3′-hydroxyl group required for further chain elongation. Viral DNA polymerase is tightly associated with the terminated DNA chain and is functionally inactivated.[193] Because viral DNA polymerase has much greater affinity for acyclovir triphosphate than does cellular DNA polymerase, there is little incorporation of acyclovir into cellular DNA.[194] In vitro, acyclovir exhibits good activity against HSV-1, HSV-2, and VZV, with median IC_{50} values of approximately 0.04, 0.10, and 0.50 g/ml, respectively.[155,195,196] Thus the concentration of acyclovir required to inhibit replication in vitro is 5- to 10-fold higher for VZV than for HSV.

Acyclovir is available in topical, oral, and intravenous formulations. The topical preparation consists of 5% acyclovir in a polyethylene glycol ointment base; it should not be used to treat VZV infections. Oral acyclovir preparations include a 200 mg capsule, 400 and 800 mg tablets, and a suspension (200 mg/5 ml). Following oral administration, acyclovir is slowly and incompletely absorbed; its oral bioavailability is approximately 15% to 30%.[197] After oral administration of multiple doses of 200 or 800 mg of acyclovir, mean plasma peak concentrations at steady state are about 0.6 and 1.6 g/ml, respectively.[198] Steady-state peak plasma acyclovir concentrations after intravenous doses of 5 or 10 mg/kg body weight every 8 hours are about 10 and 20 g/ml, respectively.[199] Acyclovir penetrates well into most tissues, including the CNS. Acyclovir is minimally metabolized, and about 85% is excreted unchanged in the urine via glomerular filtration and renal tubular secretion. The terminal half-life of acyclovir in plasma is 2 to 3 hours in adults with normal renal function.

The dose of oral acyclovir for chickenpox is 20 mg/kg (up to a maximum of 800 mg) four times daily (Table 42–1). Adults with herpes zoster can be treated with oral acyclovir at a dose of 800 mg five times daily. For patients with severe renal insufficiency (creatinine clearance <10 ml/min), the dose of oral acyclovir should be reduced to 800 mg every 12 hours. Patients with unusually severe or disseminated VZV infection should be treated with intravenous acyclovir at a dose of 10 mg/kg (or 500 mg/m^2) every 8 hours. In patients whose creatinine clearance is 25 to 50 ml/min or 10 to 25 ml/min, the dosing interval for intravenous acyclovir should be extended to 12 or 24 hours, respectively. If the creatinine clearance is less than 10 ml/min, the intravenous acyclovir dose should be reduced by 50% and given every 24 hours.[200] Acyclovir is readily removed by hemodialysis but not by peritoneal dialysis.

Acyclovir is extremely well tolerated and has few significant adverse effects. With intravenous acyclovir therapy, inflammation and phlebitis occasionally follow localized drug extravasation.[201] Renal dysfunction resulting from accumulation of acyclovir crystals in the kidney has been observed after administration of large doses of acyclovir by rapid intravenous infusion, but it is uncommon and usually reversible.[202,203] The risk of nephrotoxicity can be minimized by administering acyclovir by slow infusion (over 1 hour) and ensuring adequate hydration. A few reports have linked intravenous administration of acyclovir with CNS disturbances, including agitation, hallucinations, disorientation, tremors, and myoclonus.[204–206] Neurotoxicity has most often been recognized in elderly patients with underlying CNS abnormalities and renal insufficiency.[207,208] Neurotoxicity and nephrotoxicity are rarely associated with oral acyclovir therapy. The safety of oral acyclovir for long-term administration has been established in patients receiving the drug for many years for suppression of recurrent genital herpes.[209] Although the drug is not approved for use during pregnancy, acyclovir has been used to treat VZV infections in pregnant women without evidence of maternal or fetal toxicity.[210]

Significant interactions between acyclovir and other drugs are extremely uncommon. Probenecid decreases the renal clearance of acyclovir and can prolong the plasma excretion half-life. Additive acyclovir-induced nephrotoxicity in patients receiving concomitant cyclosporin A therapy has been suggested but does not appear to be clinically important.[211] Lethargy has been reported in a few patients receiving both acyclovir and zidovudine, but a causative role for acyclovir has not been established.[212]

Valacyclovir

Valacyclovir is an orally administered prodrug of acyclovir designed to overcome the problem of poor oral bioavailability of the parent compound. Valacyclovir, the L-valine ester of acyclovir, is well absorbed from the gastrointestinal tract via a stereospecific transporter; it undergoes essentially complete first-pass conversion to acyclovir via enzymatic hydrolysis.[213] With this prodrug formulation, the bioavailability of acyclovir is increased by about three- to fivefold. After a 1 g oral dose of valacyclovir, the peak plasma concentration of acyclovir is in the range of 5 to 6 μg/ml, and the plasma valacyclovir level is less than 0.3 μg/ml. Valacyclovir administered at a dose of 2.0 g orally 4 times daily produces a plasma acyclovir area under the curve (AUC) level approximately the same as that produced by acyclovir given intravenously at a dose of 10 mg/kg every 8 hours.[214] The pharmacokinetic profile of valacyclovir is similar in patients with AIDS and normal volunteers.[215] Following enzymatic conversion to acyclovir, the mechanism of action, spectrum of activity, and pharmacokinetic properties are the same as those described above for the parent compound. The dose of valacyclovir for herpes zoster in adults with normal renal function is 1 g orally 3 times daily (Table 42–1).

In large-scale clinical trials of therapy for herpes zoster in the normal host, valacyclovir was well tolerated, with an adverse event profile similar to that of oral acyclovir.[165] High-dose valacyclovir (2 g four times daily) was evaluated as prophylaxis for CMV infection in AIDS patients.[216] In that clinical trial, a subset of patients developed a microangiopathic disorder (hemolytic anemia, thrombocytopenia, fever, renal dysfunction, altered mental status singly or in combination) resembling thrombotic thrombocytopenic purpura or the hemolytic-uremic syndrome.[217] Although there was a statistically significant association between the development of this syndrome and ingestion of high-dose valacyclovir, a causal association with valacyclovir has not been proven. Importantly, thrombotic microangiopathy has not been reported in patients taking valacyclovir at conventional doses (up to 3 g/day).

Famciclovir

Just as valacyclovir is a prodrug of acyclovir, famciclovir is a prodrug of the antiviral compound penciclovir. Because penciclovir is poorly absorbed, famciclovir (the diacetyl ester of 6-deoxypenciclovir) has been developed as the oral formulation.[218] The bioavailability of penciclovir after oral administration of famciclovir is about 77%.[219] Penciclovir is an acyclic guanine derivative similar to acyclovir in structure, mechanism of action, and spectrum of activity. There are some qualitative differences in the mechanism of action between penciclovir and acyclovir in terms of rates of phosphorylation, stability, intracellular concentration of the triphosphate derivative, and affinity for viral DNA polymerase.[220] Penciclovir triphosphate achieves high intracellular concentrations and has an extended intracellular half-life of about 9 hours in VZV-infected cells. However, compared with acyclovir triphosphate, penciclovir triphosphate has a much lower affinity for viral DNA polymerase.[220] Unlike acyclovir triphosphate, penciclovir triphosphate is not an obligate DNA chain terminator. The in vitro activity of penciclovir against HSV-1, HSV-2, and VZV is similar to that of acyclovir, with average IC_{50} values of 0.4, 1.5, and 4.0 μg/ml, respectively, in MRC-5 cells.[218,221] Following a single oral dose of 500 mg of famciclovir, a peak plasma concentration of penciclovir of about 3.5 μg/ml is achieved at 1 hour.[222] Penciclovir is not metabolized but is eliminated unchanged in urine, with an elimination half-life of about 2 hours after intravenous administration.[222,223]

The recommended dose for famciclovir for treatment of herpes zoster in adults is 500 mg every 8 hours (Table 42–1).[166,169] When the patient's creatinine clearance is 40 to 59 ml/min or 20 to 39 ml/min, the famciclovir dosing interval should be extended to 12 or 24 hours, respectively; when the creatinine clearance is less than 20 ml/min, the famciclovir dose for herpes zoster is 250 mg every 48 hours. The adverse effects most frequently reported by patients participating in clinical trials of famciclovir were headache and nausea, although they did not differ significantly between famciclovir and placebo recipients.[166,224] Co-administration of cimetidine or theophylline increases the penciclovir AUC about 20%. Co-administration of famciclovir and digoxin results in a 19% increase in the peak digoxin concentration but no change in the AUC. None of these drug interactions is considered clinically significant.[225]

Foscarnet

Although foscarnet is used primarily to treat CMV infections, the drug also plays an important role in therapy for infections caused by acyclovir-resistant HSV and VZV.[184,188] Foscarnet (phosphonoformic acid) is a pyrophosphate analogue that functions as an inhibitor of viral DNA polymerase by blocking the pyrophosphate-binding site.[226] Unlike the acyclovir-like drugs discussed above, foscarnet is not a nucleoside analogue, does not require intracellular activation by thymidine kinase, and is not incorporated into the viral DNA chain.[227,228] Therefore thymidine kinase-deficient HSV and VZV isolates that are resistant to acyclovir and related drugs remain susceptible to foscarnet. In addition to HSV and VZV, foscarnet has in vitro activity against CMV, Epstein-Barr virus (EBV), human herpesvirus-6 (HHV-6), hepatitis B virus (HBV), and HIV.[228]

Foscarnet has poor oral bioavailability and is given only by the intravenous route.[229] Peak plasma concentrations after steady-state dosing at 60 or 90 mg/kg every 8 hours are about 150 and 208 μg/ml, respectively.[229–231] Foscarnet is not metabolized, and about 80% of an administered dose is excreted unchanged in the urine by glomerular filtration and tubular secretion.[228] About 20% of the foscarnet dose is retained in bone, presumably due to the drug's structural similarity to inorganic phosphate.[231,232] This results in a complex pattern of drug disposition in which the initial elimination half-life is about 3.5 hours followed by a prolonged terminal half-life as drug is released from bone.[229,230] CSF levels demonstrate wide interpatient variability but average about 66% of plasma levels at steady state.[233,234] Foscarnet is cleared by hemodialysis.[235]

The appropriate dose of foscarnet for treatment of acyclovir-resistant VZV infections has not been assessed systematically. In one study, four of five patients responded to a foscarnet dose of 40 mg/kg every 8 hours (Table 42–1).[184] Other investigators used a higher dose of foscarnet (100 mg/kg every 12 hours) and achieved lesion healing in 10 of 13 patients.[185] Clinicians should carefully follow guidelines published in the package insert for adjusting foscarnet doses in patients with renal insufficiency. Serum creatinine levels should be checked at least three times weekly in patients on foscarnet and the dosage adjusted accordingly.

The most important adverse effect associated with foscarnet therapy is nephrotoxicity.[236–239] Dose-limiting renal toxicity occurs in at least 15% to 20% of patients treated with foscarnet for CMV retinitis.[236,239] Loading the patient with intravenous saline prior to foscarnet dosing can help reduce the risk of nephrotoxicity.[238] In most cases the renal dysfunction reverses when foscarnet therapy is discontinued. Foscarnet can induce a variety of electrolyte and metabolic abnormalities, most notably hypocalcemia.[240,241] Hypercalcemia, hypomagnesemia, hypokalemia, and hypo- and hyperphosphatemia have also been reported. The immediate decline in ionized serum calcium that can occur with foscarnet infusion may be caused by formation of a complex between foscarnet and free calcium.[240] Further depletion of total serum calcium seen with long-term drug administration may be due to renal calcium wasting, abnormal bone metabolism, concurrent hypomagnesemia, or some combination of these factors.[240,241] Foscarnet-induced electrolyte disturbances can predispose the patient to cardiac arrhythmias, tetany, altered mental status, or seizures.[239] To avoid serious adverse effects that can result from bolus infusion, foscarnet must be administered with an infusion pump over a duration of at least 1 hour. Foscarnet is much less myelosuppressive than ganciclovir, but anemia is reported in 20% to 50% of AIDS patients receiving foscarnet.[228] Patients, especially uncircumcised males, may develop genital ulcerations as a result of local toxicity from high foscarnet concentrations in urine.[242,243] The safety of foscarnet during pregnancy has not been established.

Specific drug interactions with foscarnet have not been described, although there is significant potential for additive toxicity.[225] Concurrent therapy with foscarnet and intravenous pentamidine can result in severe, potentially fatal hypocalcemia. Similarly, use of other nephrotoxic drugs such as amphotericin B or aminoglycosides in patients receiving foscarnet can compound the risk of serious nephrotoxicity.[239]

Other Drugs

Vidarabine has in vitro activity against acyclovir-resistant strains of VZV but has not proven to be clinically effective.[62,157] A topical preparation of *trifluridine*, a thymidine analogue, has been used successfully to treat cutaneous lesions caused by acyclovir-resistant VZV.[244] *Cidofovir*, an intravenous acyclic phosphonate nucleotide analogue developed primarily for CMV therapy, also has good activity against VZV and may be the best option in patients with acyclovir-resistant VZV infections who cannot tolerate foscarnet and for those rare patients with VZV isolates resistant to both acyclovir and foscarnet.[245,246]

▲ PREVENTION OF VZV INFECTIONS

Serologic Testing

The presence of serum VZV-specific IgG indicates that an individual has previously been infected or vaccinated and is not at risk for primary varicella. As discussed above, the more sensitive latex agglutination assay (rather than ELISA) must be used to detect serum IgG reliably after varicella vaccination. The magnitude of the anti-VZV antibody titer does not predict risk for developing herpes zoster. Serologic surveys have shown that about 95% of HIV-infected adults have VZV antibodies.[63,64] Children or adults with no clinical history of chickenpox, herpes zoster, or varicella vaccination can be tested to determine susceptibility.

Varicella Vaccine

A live, attenuated varicella vaccine containing VZV_{Oka} strain has been available for use in the United States since 1995. The varicella vaccine is safe and effective among healthy children. The vaccine provides 70% to 90% protection against infection and 95% protection against severe disease for at least 7 to 10 years.[247,248] Investigations of the role of varicella vaccine in HIV-seropositive persons are ongoing. In a study of 41 HIV-infected children with relatively well preserved immunity (CDC stage N1 or A1), varicella vaccine was well tolerated and did not affect the HIV viral load.[249] Two months after the second dose of vaccine, 60% of recipients had detectable serum anti-VZV antibody, and 83% had a positive response in a lymphocyte proliferation assay against VZV antigen.[249] On the basis of these data and in view of the potential morbidity caused by chickenpox, advisory groups now recommend that HIV-seropositive children who are asymptomatic or mildly symptomatic (CDC stage N1 or A1) should receive varicella vaccine.[250,251] Little information is available regarding the safety and efficacy of varicella vaccination in HIV-seropositive adults. HIV-seronegative/VZV-seronegative household contacts of HIV-seropositive/VZV-seronegative individuals should be vaccinated.[252]

Postexposure Prophylaxis

Persons infected with HIV who are VZV-seronegative should receive prophylactic treatment after close exposure to an individual with active VZV disease. The goal is to prevent or modify symptomatic chickenpox. Three options can be considered: passive immunoprophylaxis with immune globulin; chemoprophylaxis with an antiviral drug (e.g., acyclovir); or postexposure vaccination.

Passive Immunoprophylaxis

Advisory committees have recommended administration of varicella-zoster immune globulin (VZIG) to VZV-seronegative/HIV-seropositive children or adults who have a recognized close exposure to VZV (to a patient with either chickenpox or herpes zoster).[251,252] In many cases VZIG administration does not prevent infection in the susceptible host but delays the onset of varicella and reduces the severity of the resulting illness.[22,59] Placebo-controlled trials in other (non-AIDS) immunocompromised children have demonstrated that VZIG ameliorates the severity of chickenpox and reduces the risk of disseminated infection by about 75%.[253,254] For maximal efficacy, VZIG must be given as soon as possible after exposure ($\leq$96 hours). VZIG is administered by deep intramuscular injection at a dose of 125 units/10 kg (to a maximum of 625 units). Intravenous immunoglobulin (IVIG) also contains substantial amounts of VZV-specific IgG and can be used if VZIG is not immediately available. Unfortunately, if the VZV exposure is unrecognized (which is often the case), the opportunity for VZIG administration is missed. The efficacy of VZIG prophylaxis in HIV-seropositive children or adults has not been evaluated prospectively.

Chemoprophylaxis

Prophylactic administration of acyclovir following VZV exposure has been studied to a limited extent in susceptible immunocompetent children but not in children with HIV infection. In studies of healthy children conducted in Japan, varicella developed in 16% of the children prophylactically treated with acyclovir and in 100% of the children in the control group.[255] About 80% of children prophylactically treated with acyclovir subsequently seroconverted, indicating VZV infection without significant disease.[256] However, additional data are required before this approach can be routinely recommended in either immunocompetent or immunocompromised populations. A suggested (but unvalidated) regimen is acyclovir 200 mg orally four or five times daily for 21 days beginning 5 days after exposure.[252]

Postexposure Vaccination

Small clinical trials in immunocompetent populations have shown that postexposure immunization of susceptible children and adults can prevent varicella.[257,258] Administration of varicella vaccine to a VZV-seronegative individual within 3 to 4 days of VZV exposure provides a protective (or partially protective) immune response. Up to one-half of patients receiving a postexposure vaccination may still develop some signs or symptoms of chickenpox, but the disease manifestations are usually mild. This approach may be appropriate for HIV-infected patients who are asymptomatic and not significantly immunosuppressed but has not been evaluated prospectively. In appropriate populations, postexposure VZV vaccination may prove to be more effective and less expensive than preemptive antiviral therapy.

REFERENCES

1. Stewart JA, Reef SE, Pellett PE, et al. Herpesvirus infections in persons infected with human immunodeficiency virus. Clin Infect Dis 21(suppl 1):S114, 1995.
2. Leibovitz E, Cooper D, Giurgiutiu D, et al. Varicella zoster virus infection in Romanian children infected with the human immunodeficiency virus. Pediatrics 92:838, 1993.
3. Masur H, Michelis MA, Greene JB, et al. An outbreak of community-acquired *Pneumonocystis carinii* pneumonia: initial manifestation of cellular immune dysfunction. N Engl J Med 305:1431, 1981.
4. Cole EL, Meister DM, Calabrese LH, et al. Herpes zoster ophthalmicus and acquired immune deficiency syndrome. Arch Ophthalmol 102:1027, 1984.
5. Friedman-Kien AE, Lafleur FL, Gendler E, et al. Herpes zoster: a possible early clinical sign for development of acquired immunodeficiency syndrome in high-risk individuals. J Am Acad Dermatol 14:1023, 1986.
6. Verroust F, Lemay D, Laurian Y. High frequency of herpes zoster in young hemophiliacs [letter]. N Engl J Med 316:166, 1987.
7. Payne CMER, Farthing C, Byron N, et al. Shingles in seven homosexuals. Lancet 1:103, 1984.
8. Quinnan GV, Masur H, Rook AH, et al. Herpesvirus infections in the acquired immune deficiency syndrome. JAMA 252:72, 1984.
9. Van de Perre P, Bakkers E, Batungwanayo J, et al. Herpes zoster in African patients: an early manifestation of HIV infection. Scand J Infect Dis 20:277, 1988.

10. Colebunders R, Mann JM, Francis H, et al. Herpes zoster in African patients: a clinical predictor of human immunodeficiency virus infection. J Infect Dis 157:314, 1988.
11. Tyndall MW, Nasio J, Agoki E, et al. Herpes zoster as the initial presentation of human immunodeficiency virus type 1 infection in Kenya. Clin Infect Dis 21:1035, 1995.
12. Davison AJ. The fourteenth Fleming lecture: varicella-zoster virus. J Gen Virol 72:475, 1991.
13. Grose C. Glycoproteins encoded by varicella-zoster virus: biosynthesis, phosphorylation and intracellular trafficking. Annu Rev Microbiol 44:59, 1990.
14. Ostrove JM. Molecular biology of varciella-zoster virus. Adv Virus Res 38:45, 1990.
15. Davison AJ, Scott JE. The complete DNA sequence of varicella-zoster virus. J Gen Virol 67:1759, 1986.
16. Gordon JE. Chickenpox: an epidemiologic review. Am J Med Sci 244:362, 1962.
17. Grose C. Variation on a theme by Fenner: the pathogenesis of chickenpox. Pediatrics 68:735, 1981.
18. Sawyer MH, Wu YN, Chamberlin CJ, et al. Detection of varciella-zoster virus DNA in the oropharynx and blood of patients with varicella. J Infect Dis 166:885, 1992.
19. Arvin AM, Kinney-Thomas E, Shriver K, et al. Immunity to varicella-zoster viral glycoproteins gpI (gp 90/58) and gpIII (gp 118) and to a nonglycosylated protein, p170. J Immunol 137:1346, 1986.
20. Gendelman H, Phelps W, Feigenbaum L. Trans-activation of the human immunodeficiency virus long terminal repeat sequence by DNA viruses. Proc Natl Acad Sci USA 83:9759, 1986.
21. Gershon AA, Mervish N, LaRussa P, et al. Varicella-zoster virus infection in children with underlying human immunodeficiency virus infection. J Infect Dis 176:1496, 1997.
22. Aronson JE, McSherry G, Hoyt L, et al. Varicella does not appear to be a cofactor for human immunodeficiency virus infection in children. Pediatr Infect Dis J 11:1004, 1992.
23. Gilden DH, Mahalingam R, Dueland AN, et al. Herpes zoster: pathogenesis and latency. Prog Med Virol 39:19, 1992.
24. Meier JL, Straus SE. Comparative biology of latent varicella-zoster virus and herpes simplex virus infections. J Infect Dis 166:S13, 1992.
25. Croen KD, Straus SE. Varicella-zoster latency. Annu Rev Microbiol 45:265, 1991.
26. Burke BL, Steele RW, Beard OW, et al. Immune response to varicella-zoster in the aged. Arch Intern Med 142:291, 1982.
27. Melbye M, Grossman RJ, Goedert JJ, et al. Risk of AIDS after herpes zoster. Lancet 1:728, 1987.
28. Rogues A-M, Dupon M, Ladner J, et al. Herpes zoster and human immunodeficiency virus infection: a cohort study of 101 co-infected patients. J Infect Dis 168:245, 1993.
29. Buchbinder SP, Katz MH, Hessol NA, et al. Herpes zoster and human immunodeficiency virus infection. J Infect Dis 166:1153, 1992.
30. Holmberg S, Buchbinder SP, Conley LJ, et al. The spectrum of medical conditions and symptoms before acquired immunodeficiency syndrome in homosexual and bisexual men. Am J Epidemiol 141:395, 1995.
31. Glesby MJ, Moore RD, Chaisson RE. Clinical spectrum of herpes zoster in adults infected with human immunodeficiency virus. Clin Infect Dis 21:370, 1995.
32. Veenstra J, Krol A, Van Praag RME, et al. Herpes zoster, immunological deterioration, and disease progression. AIDS 9:1153, 1995.
33. Engels EA, Rosenberg PS, Biggar RJ. Zoster incidence in human immunodeficiency virus-infected hemophiliacs and homosexual men, 1984–1997. District of Columbia Gay Cohort Study; Multicenter Hemophilia Cohort Study. J Infect Dis 180:1784, 1999.
34. Keiser P, Jodcus J, Horton H, et al. Prednisone therapy is not associated with increased risk of herpetic infections in patients infected with human immunodeficiency virus. Clin Infect Dis 23:201, 1996.
35. Van Griensven GJP, de Vroome EMM, de Wolf F, et al. Risk factors for progression of human immunodeficiency virus (HIV) infection among seroconverted and seropositive homosexual men. Am J Epidemiol 132:203, 1990.
36. Alliegro MB, Dorrucci M, Pezzotti P, et al. Herpes zoster and progression to AIDS in a cohort of individuals who seroconverted to human immunodeficiency virus. Clin Infect Dis 23:990, 1996.
37. Moss AR, Bacchetti P, Osmond D, et al. Seropositivity for HIV and the development of AIDS or AIDS related conditions: three-year follow-up of the San Francisco General Hospital Cohort. BMJ 296:745, 1988.
38. Glesby MJ, Moore RD, Chaisson RE, et al. Herpes zoster in patients with advanced human immonodeficiency virus infection treated with zidovudine. J Infect Dis 168:1264, 1993.
39. McNulty A, Li Y, Radtke U, et al. Herpes zoster and the stage and prognosis of HIV-1 infection. Genitourin Med 73:467, 1997.
40. Martinez E, Gatell J, Moran Y, et al. High incidence of herpes zoster in patients with AIDS soon after therapy with protease inhibitors. Clin Infect Dis 27:1510, 1998.
41. Aldeen T, Hay P, Davidson F, et al. Herpes zoster infection in HIV-seropositive patients associated with highly active antiretroviral therapy. AIDS 12:1719, 1998.
42. Domingo P, Torres OH, Ris J, et al. Herpes zoster as an immune reconstitution disease after initiation of combination antiretroviral therapy in patients with human immunodeficiency virus type-1 infection. Am J Med 110:605, 2001.
43. Preblud SR, Orensetin WA, Bart KJ. Varicella: clinical manifestations, epidemiology and health impact in children. Pediatr Infect Dis J 3:505, 1984.
44. Seward J, Watson B, Peterson C, et al. Decline in varicella incidence and hospitalizations in sentinel surveillance areas in the United States, 1995–2000. Presented at the Fourth International Conference on Varicella, Herpes Zoster, and Post-Herpetic Neuralgia, LaJolla, CA, 2001, abstract 11.
45. Ragozzino MW, Melton LJI, Kurland LT, et al. Population-based study of herpes zoster and its sequelae. Medicine (Baltimore) 61:310, 1982.
46. Donahue JG, Choo PW, Manson JE, et al. The incidence of herpes zoster. Arch Intern Med 155:1605, 1995.
47. Moore PS, Gao SJ, Dominguez G, et al. Primary characterization of a herpesvirus agent associated with Kaposi's sarcoma. J Virol 70:549, 1996.
48. Morgan D, Mahe C, Malamba S, et al. Herpes zoster and HIV-1 infection in a rural Ugandan cohort. AIDS 15:223, 2001.
49. Naburi AE, Leppard B. Herpes zoster and HIV infection in Tanzania. Int J STD AIDS 11:254, 2000.
50. Ross AH. Modification of chickenpox in family contacts by administration of gamma globulin. N Engl J Med 267:369, 1962.
51. Straus SE, Ostrove JM, Inchauspe G, et al. Varicella-zoster virus infections. Ann Intern Med 108:221, 1988.
52. Derryck A, LaRussa P, Steinberg S, et al. Varicella and zoster in children with human immunodeficiency virus infection. Pediatr Infect Dis J 17:931, 1998.
53. Rongkavilit C, Mitchell CD, Nachman S. Varicella zoster infection in HIV-infected children. Paediatr Drugs 2:291, 2000.
54. Jura E, Chadwick EG, Josephs SH, et al. Varicella-zoster virus infections in children infected with human immunodeficiency virus. Pediatr Infect Dis J 8:586, 1989.
55. Perronne C, Lazanas M, Leport C, et al. Varicella in patients infected with the human immunodeficiency virus. Arch Dermatol 126:1033, 1990.
56. Srugo I, Israele V, Wittek AE, et al. Clinical manifestations of varicella-zoster infections in human immunodeficiency virus-infected children. Am J Dis Child 147:742, 1993.
57. Zampogna JC, Flowers FP. Persistent verrucous varicella as the initial manifestation of HIV infection. J Am Acad Dermatol 44:391, 2001.
58. Kelley R, Mancao M, Sawyer M, et al. Varicella in children with perinatally acquired human immunodeficiency virus infection. J Pediatr 124:271, 1994.
59. Von Seidlein L, Gilette SG, Bryson Y, et al. Frequent recurrence and persistence of varicella-zoster virus infections in children infected with human immunodeficiency virus type 1. J Pediatr 128:52, 1996.
60. Silliman CC, Tedder D, Ogle JW, et al. Unsuspected varicella-zoster virus encephalitis in a child with acquired immunodeficiency sydrome. J Pediatr 123:418, 1993.
61. Janier M, Hillion B, Baccard M, et al. Chronic varicella zoster infection in acquired immunodeficiency syndrome. J Am Acad Dermatol 18:584, 1988.
62. Pahwa S, Biron K, Lim W, et al. Continuous varicella-zoster infection associated with acyclovir resistance in a child with AIDS. JAMA 260:2879, 1988.
63. Wallace MR, Hooper DG, Pyne JM, et al. Varicella immunity and clinical disease in HIV-infected adults. South Med J 87:74, 1994.

64. Clark R, Wilson S, Williams T. Varicella immunity in women infected with the human immunodeficiency virus [letter]. Clin Infect Dis 19:1165, 1994.
65. Fraisse P, Faller M, Rey D, et al. Recurrent varicella pneumonia complicating an endogenous reactivation of chickenpox in an HIV-infected adult patient. Eur Respir J 11:776, 1998.
66. Baran J, Khatib R. Recrudescence of initial cutaneous lesions after crusting of chickenpox in an adult with advanced AIDS suggests prolonged local viral persistence. Clin Infect Dis 24:741, 1997.
67. Hope-Simpson RE. The nature of herpes zoster: a long-term study and a new hypothesis. Proc R Soc Med 58:9, 1965.
68. Gilden DH, Dueland AN, Devlin ME, et al: Varicella-zoster virus reactivation without rash. J Infect Dis 166(suppl 1):S30, 1992.
69. Balfour HH. Varicella-zoster virus infections in immunocompromised hosts. Am J Med 85:68, 1988.
70. Veenstra J, van Praag RM, Krol A, et al. Complications of varicella zoster virus reactivation in HIV-infected homosexual men. AIDS 10:393, 1996.
71. Edelstein H. Multidermatomal herpes zoster in an AIDS patient. Clin Infect Dis 19:975, 1994.
72. Jabs DA, Green WR, Fox R, et al. Ocular manifestations of acquired immune deficiency syndrome. Ophthalmology 96:1092, 1989.
73. Sandor E, Croxson TS, Millman A, et al. Herpes zoster ophthalmicus in patients at high risk for AIDS [letter]. N Engl J Med 310:1118, 1984.
74. Sellitti TP, Huang AJW, Schiffman J, et al. Association of herpes zoster ophthalmicus with acquired immunodeficiency syndrome and acute retinal necrosis. Am J Ophthalmol 116:297, 1993.
75. Kestelyn P, Stevens AM, Bakkers E, et al. Severe herpes zoster ophthalmicus in young African adults: a marker for HTLV-III seropositivity. Br J Ophthalmol 71:806, 1987.
76. Bayu S, Alemayehu W. Clinical profile of herpes zoster ophthalmicus in Ethiopians. Clin Infect Dis 24:1256, 1997.
77. Engstrom RE, Holland GN. Chronic herpes zoster virus keratitis associated with the acquired immunodeficiency syndrome. Am J Ophthalmol 105:556, 1988.
78. Litoff D, Catalano RA. Herpes zoster optic neuritis in human immunodeficiency virus infection. Arch Ophthalmol 108:782, 1990.
79. Chern KC, Conrad D, Holland GN, et al. Chronic varicella-zoster virus epithelial keratitis in patients with acquired immunodeficiency syndrome. Arch Ophthalmol 116:1011, 1998.
80. Gnann JW, Crumpacker CS, Lalezari JP, et al. Sorivudine versus acyclovir for treatment of dermatomal herpes zoster in human immunodeficiency virus-infected patients: results from a randomized, controlled clinical trial. Antimicrob Agents Chemother 42:1139, 1998.
81. Freifeld AG, Marchigiani D, Lewis L, et al. Frequently recurrent zoster in children with AIDS. Presented at the 35th ICAAC, San Francisco, 1995, abstract H90.
82. Patterson LER, Butler KM, Edwards MS. Clinical herpes zoster shortly following primary varicella in two HIV-infected children. Clin Pediatr 28:354, 1989.
83. Cohen JI, Brunell PA, Straus SE, et al. Recent advances in varicella-zoster virus infection. Ann Intern Med 130:922, 1999.
84. Lokke-Jensen B, Weismann K, Mathiesen L, et al. Atypical varicella-zoster infection in AIDS. Acta Derm Venereol 73:123, 1993.
85. LeBoit PE, Limova M, Yen TSB, et al. Chronic verrucous varicella-zoster virus infection in patients with the acquired immunodeficiency syndrome (AIDS): histologic and molecular biologic findings. Am J Dermatopathol 14:1, 1992.
86. Tronnier M, Plettenberg A, Meigel WN, et al. Recurrent verrucous herpes zoster in an HIV patient: demonstration of the virus by immunofluorescence and electron microscopy. Eur J Dermatol 4:604, 1994.
87. Vaughan-Jones SA, McGibbon DH, Bradbeer CS. Chronic verrucous varicella-zoster infection in a patient with AIDS. Clin Exp Dermatol 19:327, 1994.
88. Disler RS, Dover JS. Chronic localized herpes zoster in the acquired immunodeficiency syndrome. Arch Dermatol 126:1105, 1990.
89. Grossman MC, Grossman ME. Chronic hyperkeratotic herpes zoster and human immunodeficiency virus infection. J Am Acad Dermatol 28:306, 1993.
90. Hoppenjans WB, Bibler MR, Orme RL, et al. Prolonged cutaneous herpes zoster in acquired immunodeficiency syndrome. Arch Dermatol 126:1048, 1990.
91. Kimya-Asadi A, Tausk FA, Nousari HC. Verrucous varicella zoster virus lesions associated with acquired immunodeficiency syndrome. Int J Dermatol 39:77, 2000.
92. Gilson IH, Barnett JH, Conant MA, et al. Disseminated ecthymatous herpes varicella zoster virus infection in patients with acquired immunodeficiency syndrome. J Am Acad Dermatol 20:637, 1989.
93. Alessi E, Cusini M, Zerboni R. Unusual varicella zoster virus infection in patients with the acquired immunodeficiency syndrome. Arch Dermatol 124:1011, 1988.
94. Castanet J, Rodots S, Lacour JP, et al. Chronic varicella presenting as disseminated pinpoint-sized papules in a man infected with the human immunodeficiency virus. Dermatology 192:84, 1996.
95. Nikkels AF, Rentier B, Piérard GE. Chronic varicella-zoster virus skin lesions in patients with human immunodeficiency virus are related to decreased expression of gE and gB. J Infect Dis 176:261, 1997.
96. Jacobson MA, Berger TG, Fikrig S, et al. Acyclovir-resistant varicella zoster virus infection after chronic oral acyclovir therapy in patients with the acquired immunodeficiency syndrome (AIDS). Ann Intern Med 112:187, 1990.
97. Boivin G, Edelman CK, Pedneault L, et al. Phenotypic and genotypic characterization of acyclovir-resistant varicella zoster viruses isolated from persons with AIDS. J Infect Dis 170:68, 1994.
98. Lyall EGH, Ogilvie MM, Smith NM, et al. Acyclovir resistant varicella zoster and HIV infection. Arch Dis Child 70:133, 1994.
99. Cohen PR, Beltrani VP, Grossman ME. Disseminated herpes zoster in patients with human immunodeficiency virus infection. Am J Med 84:1076, 1988.
100. Cohen PR, Grossman ME. Clinical features of human immunodeficiency virus-associated disseminated herpes zoster virus infection—a review of the literature. Clin Exp Dermatol 14:273, 1989.
101. Williamson BC. Disseminated herpes zoster in a human immunodeficiency virus-positive homosexual man without complications. Cutis 40:485, 1987.
102. Harrison RA, Soong S, Weiss HL, et al. A mixed model for factors predictive of pain in AIDS patients with herpes zoster. J Pain Symptom Manage 17:410, 1999.
103. De La Blanchardiere A, Rozenberg F, Caumes E, et al. Neurological complications of varicella-zoster virus infection in adults with human immunodeficiency virus infection. Scand J Infect Dis 32:263, 2000.
104. Gray F, Bélec L, Lescs MC, et al. Varicella-zoster virus infection of the central nervous system in the acquired immune deficiency syndrome. Brain 117:987, 1994.
105. Iten A, Chatelard P, Vuadens P, et al. Impact of cerebrospinal fluid PCR on the management of HIV-infected patients with varicella-zoster virus infection of the central nervous system. J Neurovirol 5:172, 1999.
106. Gray F, Mohr M, Rozenberg F, et al. Varicella-zoster virus encephalitis in acquired immunodeficiency syndrome: a report of four cases. Neuropathol Appl Neurobiol 18:502, 1992.
107. Brown M, Scarborough M, Brink N, et al. Varicella zoster virus-associated neurological disease in HIV-infected patients. Int J STD AIDS 12:79, 2001.
108. Chrétien F, Gray F, Lescs MC, et al. Acute varicella-zoster virus ventriculitis and meningomyeloradiculitis in acquired immunodeficiency syndrome. Acta Neuropathol (Berl) 86:659, 1993.
109. Snoeck R, Andrei G, Gérard M, et al. Successful treatment of progressive mucocutaneous infection due to acyclovir- and foscarnet-resistant herpes simplex virus with (S)-1-(3-hydroxy-2-phosphonylmethoxypropyl)cytosine (HPMPC). Clin Infect Dis 18:570, 1994.
110. Janssen RS, Saykin AJ, Kaplan JE, et al. Neurological complications of human immunodeficiency virus infection in patients with lymphadenopathy syndrome. Ann Neurol 23:49, 1988.
111. Gómez-Tortosa E, Gadea I, Gegúndez MI, et al. Development of myelopathy before herpes zoster rash in patients with AIDS. Clin Infect Dis 18:810, 1994.
112. Manian FA, Kindred M, Fulling KH. Chronic varicella-zoster virus myelitis without cutaneous eruption in a patient with AIDS: report of a fatal case. Clin Infect Dis 21:986, 1995.
113. Kenyon LC, Dulaney E, Montone KT, et al. Varicella-zoster ventriculo-encephalitis and spinal cord infarction in a patient with AIDS. Acta Neuropathol (Berl) 92:202, 1996.
114. Bélec L, Gherardi R, Georges AJ, et al. Peripheral facial paralysis and HIV infection: report of four African cases and review of the literature. J Neurol 236:411, 1989.

115. Mishell JH, Applebaum EL. Ramsay-Hunt syndrome in a patient with HIV infection. Otolaryngol Head Neck Surg 102:177, 1990.
116. Moulignier A, Pialoux G, Dega H, et al. Brain stem encephalitis due to varicella-zoster virus in a patient with AIDS. Clin Infect Dis 20:1378, 1995.
117. Rosenblum MK. Bulbar encephalitis complicating trigeminal zoster in the acquired immune deficiency syndrome. Hum Pathol 20:292, 1989.
118. Gilden DH, Murray RS, Wellish M, et al. Chronic progressive varicella-zoster virus encephalitis in an AIDS patients. Neurology 1988:1150, 1988.
119. Ryder JW, Croen K, Kleinschmidt-Demasters BK, et al. Progressive encephalitis three months after resolution of cutaneous zoster in a patient with AIDS. Ann Neurol 19:182, 1986.
120. Gilden DH, Kleinschmidt-DeMaster BK, LaGuardia JJ, et al. Neurologic complications of the reactivation of varicella-zoster virus. N Engl J Med 342:635, 2000.
121. Forster DJ, Dugel PU, Frangieh GT, et al. Rapidly progressive outer retinal necrosis in the acquired immunodeficiency syndrome. Am J Ophthalmol 110:341, 1990.
122. Margolis TP, Lowder CY, Holland GN, et al. Varicella-zoster virus retinitis in patients with the acquired immunodeficiency sydrome. Am J Ophthalmol 112:119, 1991.
123. Engstrom RE, Holland GN, Maryolis TP, et al. The progressive outer retinal necrosis syndrome: a variant of necrotizing herpetic retinopathy in patients with AIDS. Ophthalmology 101:1488, 1994.
124. Ormerod LD, Larkin JA, Margo CA, et al. Rapidly progressive herpetic retinal necrosis: a blinding disease characteristic of advanced AIDS. Clin Infect Dis 26:34, 1998.
125. Moorthy RS, Weinberg DV, Teich SA, et al. Management of varicella zoster virus retinitis in AIDS. Br J Ophthalmol 81:189, 1997.
126. Batisse D, Eliaszewicz M, Zazoan L, et al. Acute retinal necrosis in the course of AIDS: study of 26 cases. AIDS 10:55, 1996.
127. Miller RF, Brink NS, Cartledge J, et al. Necrotising herpetic retinopathy in patients with advance HIV disease. Genitourin Med 73:462, 1997.
128. Hellinger WC, Bolling JP, Smith TF, et al. Varicella-zoster virus retinitis in a patient with AIDS-related complex: case report and brief review of the acute retinal necrosis syndrome. Clin Infect Dis 16:208, 1993.
129. Chambers RB, Derick RJ, Davidorf FH, et al. Varicella-zoster retinitis in human immunodeficiency virus infection. Arch Ophthalmol 107:960, 1989.
130. Garweg J, Böhnke M. Varicella-zoster virus is strongly associated with atypical necrotizing herpetic retinopathies. Clin Infect Dis 24:603, 1997.
131. Short GA, Margolis TP, Kuppermann BD, et al. A polymerase chain reaction-based assay for diagnosing varicella-zoster virus retinitis in patients with acquired immunodeficiency syndrome. Am J Ophthalmol 123:157, 1997.
132. Kashiwase M, Sata T, Yamauchi Y, et al. Progressive outer retinal necrosis caused by herpes simplex virus type 1 in a patient with acquired immunodeficiency syndrome. Ophthalmology 107:790, 2000.
133. Kalman CM, Laskin OL. Herpes zoster and zosteriform herpes simplex virus infections in immunocompetent adults. Am J Med 81:775, 1986.
134. Brunell PA, Gershon AA, Uduman SA, et al. Varicella-zoster immunoglobulins during varicella, latency, and zoster. J Infect Dis 132:49, 1975.
135. Dahl H, Marcoccia J, Linde A. Antigen detection: the method of choice in comparison with virus isolation and serology for laboratory diagnosis of herpes zoster in human immunodeficiency virus-infected patient. J Clin Microbiol 35:345, 1997.
136. Forsberg P, Kam-Hansen S, Fryden A. Production of specific antibodies by cerebrospinal fluid lymphocytes in patients with herpes zoster, mumps, meningitis and herpes simplex virus encephalitis. Scand J Immunol 24:261, 1986.
137. Shanley J, Myer M, Edmond B, et al. Enzyme-linked immunosorbent assay for detection of antibody to varicella-zoster virus. J Clin Microbiol 15:208, 1982.
138. Wasmuth EW, Miller WJ. Sensitive enzyme-linked immunosorbent assay for antibody to varicella-zoster virus using purified VZV glycoprotein antigen. J Med Virol 32:189, 1990.
139. American Academy of Pediatrics. Committee on Infectious Diseases. varicella vaccine update. Pediatrics 105:136, 2000.
140. Steinberg SP, Gerson AA. Measurement of antibodies to varicella-zoster virus by using a latex agglutination test. J Clin Microbiol 29:1527, 1991.
141. Schmidt NJ, Gallo D, Devin V, et al. Direct immunofluorescence staining for detection of herpes simplex and varicella-zoster virus antigens in vesicular lesions and certain tissue specimens. J Clin Microbiol 12:651, 1980.
142. Perez JL, Garcia A, Niubo J, et al. Comparison of techniques and evaluation of three commercial monoclonal antibodies for laboratory diagnosis of varicella-zoster virus in mucocutaneous specimens. J Clin Microbiol 32:1610, 1994.
143. Gleaves CA, Lee CF, Bustamante CI, et al. Use of murine monoclonal antibodies for laboratory diagnosis of varicella-zoster infections. J Clin Microbiol 26:1623, 1988.
144. Rawlinson WD, Dwyer DE, Gibbons VL, et al. Rapid diagnosis of varicella-zoster virus infection with a monoclonal antibody based direct immunofluorescence technique. J Virol Methods 23:13, 1989.
145. Nahass GT, Goldstein BA, Zhu WY, et al. Comparision of Tzanck smear, viral culture, and DNA diagnostic methods in detection of herpes simplex and varicella-zoster infection. JAMA 268:2541, 1992.
146. Dlugosch D, Eis-Hubinger AM, Kleim JP, et al. Diagnosis of acute and latent varicella-zoster virus infections using the polymerase chain reaction. J Med Virol 35:136, 1992.
147. Kido S, Ozake T, Asada H, et al. Detection of varicella-zoster virus (VZV) DNA in clinical samples from patients with VZV by the polymerase chain reaction. J Clin Microbiol 29:76, 1991.
148. Burke DG, Kalayjian RC, Vann VR, et al. Polymerase chain reaction and clinical significance of varicella-zoster virus in cerebrospinal fluid from human immunodeficiency virus-infected patients. J Infect Dis 176:1080, 1997.
149. Cinque P, Bossolasco S, Vago L, et al. Varicella-zoster virus (VZV) DNA in cerebrospinal fluid of patients infected with human immunodeficiency virus: VZV disease of the central nervous system or subclinical reactivation of VZV infection? Clin Infect Dis 25:634, 1997.
150. Shoji J, Honda Y, Murai I, et al. Detection of varicella-zoster virus DNA by polymerase chain reaction in cerebrospinal fluid of patients with herpes zoster meningitis. J Neurol 239:69, 1992.
151. Danise A, Cinque P, Vergani S, et al. Use of polymerase chain reaction assays of aqueous humor in the differential diagnosis of retinitis in patients infected with human immunodeficiency virus. Clin Infect Dis 24:1100, 1997.
152. Schirm J, Meulenberg J, Pastoor GM, et al. Rapid detection of varicella-zoster virus in clinical specimens using monoclonal antibodies on shell vials and smears. J Med Virol 28:1, 1989.
153. Weigle KA, Grose C. Common expression of varicella-zoster viral glycoprotein antigens in vitro and in chickenpox and zoster vesicles. J Infect Dis 148:630, 1983.
154. Talarico CL, Phelps WC, Biron KK. Analysis of the thymidine kinase genes from acyclovir-resistant mutants of varicella-zoster virus isolated from patients with AIDS. J Virol 67:1024, 1993.
155. Biron KK, Elion GB. In vitro susceptibility of varicella-zoster virus to acyclovir. Antimicrob Agents Chemother 18:443, 1980.
156. Berkowitz FE, Levin MJ. Use of an enzyme-linked immunosorbent assay performed directly on fixed infected cell monolayers for evaluating drugs against varicella-zoster virus. Antimicrob Agents Chemother 28:207, 1985.
157. Linnemann CC, Biron KK, Hoppenjans WG, et al. Emergence of acyclovir-resistant varicella zoster virus in an AIDS patient on prolonged acyclovir therapy. AIDS 4:577, 1990.
158. Fillet A-M, Visse B, Caumes E, et al. Foscarnet-resistant multidermatomal zoster in a patient with AIDS. Clin Infect Dis 21:1348, 1995.
159. Visse B, Dumont B, Huraux JM, et al. Single amino acid change in DNA polymerase is associated with foscarnet resistance in a varicella-zoster virus strain recovered from a patient with AIDS. J Infect Dis 178(suppl 1):S55, 1998.
160. Dunkle LM, Arvin AM, Whitley RJ, et al. A controlled trial of acyclovir for chickenpox in normal children. N Engl J Med 325:1539, 1991.
161. Balfour HH, Rotbart HA, Feldman S, et al. Acyclovir treatment of varicella in otherwise healthy adolescents. Pedatrics 120:627, 1992.
162. Wallace MR, Bowler WA, Murray NB. Treatment of adult varicella with oral acyclovir. Ann Intern Med 117:358, 1992.
163. Huff JC, Bean B, Balfour HH, et al. Therapy of herpes zoster with oral acyclovir. Am J Med 85(suppl 2A):84, 1988.
164. Wood MJ, Kay R, Dworkin RH, et al. Oral acyclovir therapy accelerates pain resolution in patients with herpes zoster: a meta-analysis of placebo-controlled trials. Clin Infect Dis 22:341, 1996.

165. Beutner KR, Friedman DJ, Forszpaniak C, et al. Valaciclovir compared with acyclovir for improved therapy for herpes zoster in immunocompetent adults. Antimicrob Agents Chemother 39:1546, 1995.
166. Tyring S, Barbarash RA, Nahlik JE, et al. Famciclovir for the treatment of acute herpes zoster: effects on acute disease and post-herpetic neuralgia: a randomized, double-blind, placebo-controlled trial. Ann Intern Med 123:89, 1995.
167. Tyring SK, Beutner KR, Tucker BA, et al. Antiviral therapy for herpes zoster: randomized, controlled clinical trial of valacyclovir and famciclovir therapy in immunocompetent patients 50 years and older. Arch Fam Med 9:863, 2000.
168. Bodsworth NJ, Boag F, Burdge D, et al. Evaluation of sorivudine (BV-araU) versus acyclovir in the treatment of acute localized herpes zoster in human immunodeficiency virus-infected adults. J Infect Dis 176:103, 1997.
169. Sullivan M, Skiest D, Signs D, et al. Famciclovir in the management of acute herpes zoster (HZ) in the HIV-positive patients. Presented at the Fourth Conference on Retroviruses and Opportunistic Infections, Washington, DC, 1997, abstract 704.
170. Holland GN. Acquired immune deficiency syndrome and ophthalmology: the first decade. Am J Ophthalmol 114:86, 1992.
171. Cobo LM. Corneal complications of herpes zoster ophthalmicus. Cornea 7:50, 1988.
172. Wood MJ, Johnson RW, McKendrick MW, et al. A randomized trial of acyclovir for 7 days or 21 days with and without prednisolone for treatment of acute herpes zoster. N Engl J Med 330:896, 1994.
173. Whitley RJ, Weiss H, Gnann JW, et al. Acyclovir with and without prednisone for the treatment of herpes zoster: a randomized, placebo-controlled trial; the National Institute of Allergy and Infectious Diseases Collaborative Antiviral Study Group. Ann Intern Med 125:376, 1996.
174. Poscher ME. Successful treatment of varicella-zoster virus meningoencephalitis in patients with AIDS: report of 4 cases and review. AIDS 8:1115, 1994.
175. De Silva SM, Mark AS, Gilden DH, et al. Zoster myelitis: improvement with antiviral therapy in two cases. Neurology 47:929, 1996.
176. Lionnet F, Pulik M, Genet P, et al. Myelitis due to varicella-zoster virus in 2 patients with AIDS: successful treatment with acyclovir. Clin Infect Dis 22:138, 1996.
177. Seiff SR, Margolis T, Graham SH, et al. Use of intravenous acyclovir for treatment of herpes zoster ophthalmicus in patients at risk for AIDS. Ann Ophthalmol 20:480, 1988.
178. Johnston WH, Holland GN, Engstrom RE, et al. Recurrence of presumed varicella-zoster virus retinopathy in patients with acquired immune deficiency syndrome. Am J Ophthalmol 116:42, 1993.
179. Galindez OA, Sabates NR, Whitacre MW, et al. Rapidly progressive outer retinal necrosis caused by varicella zoster virus in a patient infected with human immunodeficiency virus. Clin Infect Dis 22:149, 1996.
180. Perez-Blazquez E, Traspas R, Mendez MI, et al. Intravitreal ganciclovir treatment in progressive outer retinal necrosis. Am J Ophthalmol 124:418, 1997.
181. Bernhard P, Obel N. Chronic ulcerating acyclovir-resistant varicella zoster lesions in an AIDS patient. Scand J Infect Dis 27:623, 1995.
182. Smith KJ, Kahlter DC, Davis C, et al. Acyclovir-resistant varicella zoster responsive to foscarnet. Arch Dermatol 127:1069, 1991.
183. Balfour HH, Benson C, Braun J, et al. Management of acyclovir-resistant herpes simplex and varicella-zoster virus infections. J Acquir Immune Defic Syndr 7:254, 1994.
184. Safrin S, Berger TG, Gilson I, et al. Foscarnet therapy in five patients with AIDS and acyclovir-resistant varicella-zoster virus infection. Ann Intern Med 115:19, 1991.
185. Breton G, Fillet AM, Katlama C, et al. Acyclovir-resistant herpes zoster in human immunodeficiency virus-infected patients: results of foscarnet therapy. Clin Infect Dis 27:1525, 1998.
186. Wunderli W, Miner R, Wintsch J, et al. Outer retinal necrosis due to a strain of varicella-zoster virus resistant to acyclovir, ganciclovir, and sorivudine. Clin Infect Dis 22:864, 1996.
187. Snoeck R, Gérard M, Sadzot-Delvaux C, et al. Meningoradiculitis due to acyclovir-resistant varicella-zoster virus in a patient with AIDS [letter]. J Infect Dis 168:1330, 1993.
188. Safrin S, Crumpacker C, Chatis P, et al. A controlled trial comparing foscarnet with vidarabine for acyclovir resistant mucocutaneous herpes simplex in the acquired immunodeficiency syndrome. N Engl J Med 325:551, 1991.
189. Elion GB, Furman PA, Fyfe JA, et al. Selectivity of action of an antiherpetic agent, 9-(2-hydroxyethoxymethyl) guanine. Proc Natl Acad Sci USA 74:5716, 1977.
190. Schaeffer HJ, Beauchamp L, Miranda PD, et al. 9-(2-Hydroxyethoxymethyl)guanine activity against viruses of the herpes group. Nature 272:583, 1978.
191. Fyfe JA, Keller PM, Furman PA, et al. Thymidine kinase from herpes simplex virus phosphorylates the new antiviral compound, 9-(2-hydroxyethoxymethyl)guanine. J Biol Chem 253:8721, 1978.
192. Derse D, Chang Y-C, Furman PA, et al. Inhibition of purified human and herpes simplex virus-induced DNA polymerase by 9-(2-hydroxyethoxymethyl) guanine (acyclovir) triphosphate: effects on primer-template function. J Biol Chem 256:11447, 1981.
193. Furman PA, St Clair MH, Spector T. Acyclovir triphosphate is a suicide inactivator of the herpes simplex virus DNA polymerase. J Biol Chem 259:9575, 1984.
194. Furman PA, St Clair MH, Fyfe JA, et al. Inhibition of herpes simplex virus-induced DNA polymerase activity and viral DNA replication by 9-(2-hydroxyethoxy methyl)guanine and its triphosphate. J Virol 32:72, 1979.
195. Collins P, Bauer DJ: The activity in vitro against herpes virus of 9-(2-hydroxyethoxymethyl)guanine (acycloguanosine), a new antiviral agent. J Antimicrob Chemother 5:431, 1979.
196. Crumpacker CS, Schnipper LE, Zaia JA, et al. Growth inhibition by acycloguanosine of herpes viruses isolated from human infections. Antimicrob Agents Chemother 15:642, 1979.
197. DeMiranda P, Blum MR. Pharmacokinetics of acyclovir after intravenous and oral administration. J Antimicrob Chemother 12:29, 1983.
198. Laskin OL. Acyclovir: pharmacology and clinical experience. Arch Intern Med 144:1241, 1984.
199. Whitley RJ, Blum MR, Barton N, et al. Pharmacokinetics of acyclovir in humans following intravenous administration: a model for the development of parenteral antivirals. Am J Med 73:165, 1982.
200. Brigden D, Whiteman P: The clinical pharmacology of acyclovir and its prodrugs. Scand J Infect Dis Suppl 47:33, 1985.
201. Keeney RE, Kirk LE, Brigden D. Acyclovir tolerance in humans. Am J Med 73(suppl 1A):176, 1982.
202. Sawyer MH, Webb DE, Barlow JE, et al. Acyclovir-induced renal failure: clinical cause and histology. Am J Med 84:1067, 1988.
203. Speigal DM, Lau K. Acute renal failure and coma secondary to acyclovir therapy. JAMA 255:1882, 1986.
204. Wade JC, Meyers JD. Neurologic symptoms associated with parenteral acyclovir treatment after marrow transplantation. Ann Intern Med 98:921, 1983.
205. Cohen SMZ, Minkove JA, Zebley JW, et al. Severe but reversible neurotoxicity from acyclovir. Ann Intern Med 100:920, 1984.
206. Feldman S, Rodman J, Gregory B. Excessive serum concentrations of acyclovir and neurotoxicity. J Infect Dis 157:385, 1988.
207. Haefeli WE, Schoenenberger RA, Weiss P, et al. Acyclovir-induced neurotoxicity: concentration side effect relationship in acyclovir overdose. Am J Med 94:212, 1993.
208. Bean B, Aeppli D. Adverse effects of high-dose intravenous acyclovir in ambulatory patients with acute zoster. J Infect Dis 151:362, 1985.
209. Goldberg LH, Kaufman R, Kurtz TO, et al. Long-term suppression of recurrent genital herpes with acyclovir: a 5-year benchmark. Arch Dermatol 129:582, 1993.
210. Reiff-Eldridge R, Heffner CR, Ephross SA, et al. Monitoring pregnancy outcomes after prenatal drug exposure through prospective pregnancy registries: a pharmaceutical company commitment. Am J Obstet Gynecol 182:159, 2000.
211. Shepp DH, Dandliker PS, Meyers JD. Treatment of varicella-zoster infection in severely immunocompromised patients: a randomized comparison of acyclovir and vidarabine. N Engl J Med 314:208, 1986.
212. Cooper DA, Pehrson PO, Pederson C, et al. The efficacy and safety of zidovudine alone or as a cofactor with acyclovir for the treatment of patients with AIDS-related complex: a double-blind, randomized trial. AIDS 7:197, 1993.
213. Burnette TC, de Miranda P. Purification and characterization of an enzyme from rat liver that hydrolyzes 256U87, the L-valyl ester prodrug of acyclovir (Zovirax) [abstract]. Antiviral Res 20(suppl 1):115, 1993.
214. Weller S, Blum MR, Doucette M, et al. Pharmacokinetics of the acyclovir pro-drug valaciclovir after escalating single- and multiple-dose administration to normal volunteers. Clin Pharmacol Ther 54:595, 1993.

215. Jacobson MA, Gallant J, Wang LH, et al. Phase I trial of valaciclovir, the L-valyl ester of acyclovir, in patients with advanced human immunodeficiency virus disease. Antimicrob Agents Chemother 38:1534, 1994.
216. Feinberg JE, Hurwitz S, Cooper D, et al. A randomized, double-blind trial of valaciclovir prophylaxis for cytomegalovirus disease in patients with advanced human immunodeficiency virus infection. J Infect Dis 177:48, 1998.
217. Bell WR, Chulay JD, Feinberg JE. Manifestations resembling thrombotic microangiopathy in patients with advanced human immunodeficiency virus (HIV) disease in a cytomegalovirus prophylaxis trial (ACTG 204). Medicine (Baltimore) 76:369, 1997.
218. Vere Hodge RA: Famciclovir and penciclovir. the mode of action of famciclovir including its conversion to penciclovir. Antivir Chem Chemother 42:67, 1993.
219. Pue MA, Benet LZ. Pharmacokinetics of famciclovir. Antivir Chem Chemother 4(suppl 1):47, 1993.
220. Earnshaw DL, Bacon TH, Darlison SJ, et al. Mode of antiviral action of penciclovir in MRC-5 cells infected with herpes simplex virus type 1, HSV-2, and varicella-zoster virus. Antimicrob Agents Chemother 36:2747, 1992.
221. Weinberg A, Bate BJ, Masters HB, et al. In vitro activities of penciclovir and acyclovir against herpes simplex virus types 1 and 2. Antimicrob Agents Chemother 36:2037, 1992.
222. Pue MA, Pratt SK, Fairless AJ, et al. Linear pharmacokinetics of penciclovir following administration of single oral doses of famciclovir 125, 250, 500, and 750 mg to healthy volunteers. J Antimicrob Chemother 33:119, 1994.
223. Fowles SE, Pierce DM, Prince WT. The tolerance to and pharmacokinetics of penciclovir (BRL 39123A), a novel antiherpes agent, administered by intravenous infusion to healthy subjects. Eur J Clin Pharmacol 43:513, 1992.
224. Schacker T, Hu HL, Koelle DM, et al. Famciclovir for the suppression of symptomatic and asymptomatic herpes simplex virus reactivation in HIV-infected persons. Ann Intern Med 128:21, 1998.
225. Taburet AM, Singlas E. Drug interactions with antiviral drugs. Clin Pharmacokinet 30:385, 1996.
226. Helgstrand E, Erikkson B, Johansson NG, et al. Trisodium phosphonoformate, a new antiviral compound. Science 201:819, 1978.
227. Crumpacker CS. Mechanism of action of foscarnet against viral polymerases. Am J Med 92(suppl 2A):3S, 1992.
228. Chrisp P, Clissold SP. Foscarnet: a review of its antiviral activity, pharmacokinetic properties and therapeutic use in immunocompromised patients with cytomegalovirus retinitis. Drugs 41:104, 1991.
229. Aweeka F, Gambertoglio J, Mills J, et al. Pharmacokinetics of intermittently administered intravenous foscarnet in the treatment of acquired immunodeficiency syndrome patients with serious cytomegalovirus retinitis. Antimicrob Agents Chemother 33:742, 1989.
230. Wagstaff AJ, Bryson HM. Foscarnet: a reappraisal of its antiviral activity, pharmacokinetic properties and therapeutic use in immunocompromised patients with viral infections. Drugs 48:199, 1994.
231. Jacobson MA, Polsky B, Causey D, et al. Pharmacodynamic relationship of pharmacokinetic parameters of maintenance doses of foscarnet and clinical outcome of cytomegalovirus retinitis. Antimicrob Agents Chemother 38:1190, 1994.
232. Sjovall J, Karlsson A, Ogenstad S, et al. Pharmacokinetics and absorption of foscarnet after intravenous and oral administration to patients with human immunodeficiency virus. Clin Pharmacol Ther 44:65, 1988.
233. Sjovall J, Bergdahl S, Movin G, et al. Pharmacokinetics of foscarnet and distribution to cerebrospinal fluid after intravenous infusion in patients with human immunodeficiency virus infection. Antimicrob Agents Chemother 33:1023, 1989.
234. Hengge UR, Brockmeyer NH, Malessa R, et al. Foscarnet penetrates the blood-brain barrier: rationale for therapy of cytomegalovirus encephalitis. Antimicrob Agents Chemother 37:1010, 1993.
235. MacGregor RR, Graziani AL, Weiss R, et al. Successful foscarnet therapy for cytomegalovirus retinitis in an AIDS patient undergoing hemodialysis: rationale for empiric dosing and plasma level monitoring. J Infect Dis 164:785, 1991.
236. Studies of Ocular Complications of AIDS (SOCA) Research Group. Morbidity and toxic effects associated with ganciclovir or foscarnet therapy in a randomized cytomegalovirus retinitis trial. Arch Intern Med 155:65, 1995.
237. Cacoub P, Deray G, Baumelou A, et al. Acute renal failure induced by foscarnet: four cases. Clin Nephrol 29:315, 1988.
238. Deray G, Martinez F, Katlama C, et al. Foscarnet nephrotoxicity: mechanism, incidence and prevention. Am J Nephrol 9:316, 1989.
239. Jacobson MA. Review of the toxicities of foscarnet. J Acquir Immune Defic Syndr 5(suppl 1):S11, 1992.
240. Jacobson MA, Gambertoglio JG, Aweeka FT, et al. Foscarnet-induced hypocalcemia and effects of foscarnet on calcium metabolism. J Clin Endocrinol Metab 72:1130, 1991.
241. Guillaume MP, Karmali R, Gergmann P, et al. Unusual prolonged hypocalcemia due to foscarnet in a patient with AIDS. Clin Infect Dis 25:932, 1997.
242. Fergueux S, Salmon D, Picard C, et al. Penile ulceration with foscarnet. Lancet 335:547, 1990.
243. Gross AS, Dretler RH. Foscarnet-induced penile ulcer in uncircumcised patients with AIDS. Clin Infect Dis 17:1076, 1993.
244. Ives DV, Stanat SC, Biron KK. Successful treatment of acyclovir-resistant zoster with topical triflurothymidine. Presented at the 2nd National Conference on Human Retroviruses, Washington, DC, 1995, abstract 292.
245. Lalezari JP, Drew WL, Glutzer E, et al. Treatment with intravenous (S)-1-[3-hydroxy-2-(phosphonylmethoxy)propyl]-cytosine of acyclovir-resistant mucocutaneous infection with herpes simplex virus in a patient with AIDS. J Infect Dis 170:570, 1994.
246. Cundy KC, Petty BG, Flaherty J, et al. Clinical pharmacokinetics of cidofovir in human immunodeficiency virus-infected patients. Antimicrob Agents Chemother 39:1247, 1995.
247. Vazquez M, LaRussa PS, Gershon AA, et al. The effectiveness of the varicella vaccine in clinical practice. N Engl J Med 344:955, 2001.
248. White CJ. Varicella-zoster virus vaccine. Clin Infect Dis 24:753, 1997.
249. Levin MJ, Gershon AA, Weinberg A, et al. Immunization of HIV-infected children with varicella vaccine. J Pediatr 139:305, 2001.
250. American Academy of Pediatrics Committee on Infectious Diseases. Varicella vaccine update. Pediatrics 105:136, 2000.
251. Centers for Disease Control and Prevention. Prevention of varicella: update recommendations of the Advisory Committee on Immunization Practices (ACIP). MMWR Morb Mortal Wkly Rep 48:1, 1999.
252. Kaplan JE, Masur H, Holmes KK, et al. 1999 USPHS/IDSA guidelines for the prevention of opportunistic infections in persons infected with human immunodeficiency virus. Clin Infect Dis 30(suppl 1):S29, 2000.
253. Orenstein WA, Heymann DL, Ellis RJ, et al. Prophylaxis of varicella in high-risk children: dose response effect of zoster immunoglobulin. J Pediatr 98:368, 1981.
254. Zaia JA, Levin MJ, Preblud SR, et al. Evaluation of varicella-zoster immune globulin: protection of immunosuppressed children after household exposure to varicella. J Infect Dis 147:737, 1983.
255. Asano Y, Yoshikawa T, Suga S, et al. Postexposure prophylaxis of varicella in family contacts by oral acyclovir. Pediatrics 92:219, 1993.
256. Suga S, Yoshikawa T, Ozaki T, et al. Effect of oral acyclovir against primary and secondary viraemia in incubation period of varicella. Arch Dis Child 69:639, 1993.
257. Salzman MB, Garcia C. Postexposure varicella vaccination in siblings of children with active varicella. Pediatr Infect Dis J 17:256, 1998.
258. Watson B, Seward J, Yang A, et al. Postexposure effectiveness of varicella vaccine. Pediatrics 105:84, 2000.

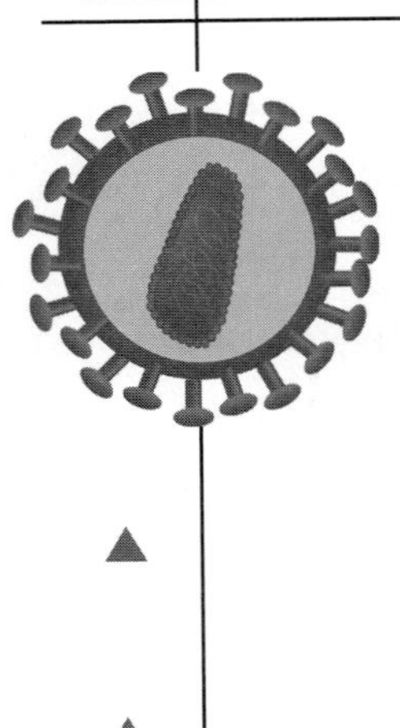

CHAPTER 43

Cytomegalovirus Disease

Michael A. Polis, MD, MPH

End-organ disease due to cytomegalovirus (CMV) occurs late in the course of human immunodeficiency virus (HIV) infection. The increased use of highly active antiretroviral therapy (HAART) including protease inhibitors and nonnucleoside reverse transcriptase inhibitors (NNRTIs) for the treatment of HIV infection has led to improved immunocompetence and a decrease in the incidence of opportunistic infections, including CMV, in persons with HIV infection. Immune reconstitution due to HAART is the most important therapeutic intervention for long-term management of CMV disease in persons with HIV infection.

Large databases of HIV-infected persons, such as the Centers for Disease Control and Prevention (CDC) Adult Spectrum of Disease Project, have shown that the incidence of CMV disease in the United States decreased by approximately 80% between 1992 and 1998.[1] CMV-associated diseases are still seen in persons who do not have access to HAART and present with advanced HIV infection and in those who do not respond to antiretroviral therapy. The most common end-organ presentation is retinitis, occurring in approximately 80% to 90% of persons with CMV disease. Colitis or esophagitis occur in about 10% of HIV-infected persons with CMV disease. Pneumonitis, adrenalitis, and neurologic disease occur much less frequently.[2,3]

PATHOGEN

Taxonomy

Human CMV is a large, linear, double-stranded DNA virus of the Betaherpesvirinae subfamily of the Herpesviridae. The subclassification is based on its slow growth in vitro and its strict species specificity.[4] CMV looks like a typical herpesvirus by electron microscopy: The DNA is contained within a capsid of 162 hexagonal capsomeres surrounded by the tegument, which in turn is surrounded by a lipid envelope.

Biology

In vivo CMV-infected cells are found in tissues of epithelial and endothelial origin, whereas in vitro CMV replication is fully permissive only in human fibroblasts.[4] In nonimmunosuppressed persons, disease due to CMV is most commonly associated with heterophile-negative infectious mononucleosis. As with other herpesviruses, primary infection is usually followed by persistent infection with the potential for latent virus to reactivate. In immunocompromised hosts, reactivation can be associated with dissemination of the virus and severe end-organ disease. The specific sites of reactivation vary dramatically according to the specific underlying immunosuppressive disease. Similarly, the diagnostic and prognostic significance of isolating CMV and the approach to prevention and therapy differ markedly in these various immunosuppressive diseases. Clinicians must recognize the clinical implications of these differences.

Epidemiology

In HIV-infected persons, as with most other opportunistic infections associated with HIV infection, CMV disease appears to be due to reactivation of the latent virus in a previously infected host. Although more than 90% of persons with HIV

All material in this chapter is in the public domain, with the exception of any borrowed figures or tables.

infection have antibodies to CMV, indicating prior infection, the clinical manifestations of CMV disease do not generally present until the CD4+ T-lymphocyte count drops below 100 cells per microliter.[5,6] In one study from Australia, which assessed 31 persons with HIV infection and CMV retinitis who had CD4+ lymphocyte determinations performed within the 2 months before or 1 month after the diagnosis of CMV retinitis, the mean and median CD4+ T-lymphocyte counts were 29 and 17 cells per microliter, respectively.[7] In a multicenter observational cohort of 1002 HIV-infected persons with fewer than 250 CD4+ T-lymphocytes per microliter receiving zidovudine, disease due to CMV developed in 109 persons.[2] Kaplan-Meier estimates of the proportion of persons who developed CMV disease was 21.4% at 2 years for persons entering the study with fewer than 100 CD4+ T-lymphocytes per microliter and 10.3% for persons with initial counts higher than 100 cells per microliter. Of the 109 persons developing CMV disease, 93 (85.3%) were diagnosed with retinitis, 10 (9.2%) with esophagitis, 3 with both retinitis and esophagitis, 8 (7.3%) with colitis, and 1 each with gastritis, hepatitis, and encephalitis. A smaller study of 135 persons with fewer than 250 CD4+ T-lymphocytes per microliter found the Kaplan-Meier estimate for the development of CMV retinitis to be 42% within 27 months for the group with fewer than 50 CD4+ T-lymphocytes per microliter.[8] Of the 26 persons developing CMV retinitis, 24 had CD+ T-lymphocyte counts of less than 50 cells per microliter before developing CMV retinitis; the other 2 persons had counts of 60 and 160 cells per microliter 7 and 11 months before the diagnosis, respectively. The mean time from the first CD4+ T-lymphocyte count of less than 50 cells per microliter until the diagnosis of CMV retinitis was 13.1 months. Since 1990, when cases of *Pneumocystis carinii* pneumonia (PCP) reported to the CDC began to decrease owing to the widespread use of prophylaxis to prevent PCP, cases of acquired immunodeficiency syndrome (AIDS)-defining CMV retinitis increased. (Total cases of CMV retinitis, however, did not decrease.) A prospectively followed cohort of 844 men were followed before the development of an AIDS-related opportunistic infection. Among those who received PCP prophylaxis, CMV disease was the initial AIDS-related opportunistic infection in 9.4% of men compared to 3.1% of men who did not receive PCP prophylaxis. The lifetime occurrences of CMV disease were 44.9% and 24.8% in those groups, respectively.[9] The CDC's Adult Spectrum of Disease Project found that persons who received HAART presented with CMV disease at slightly higher CD4+ T-lymphocyte counts than persons not receiving HAART, but the small difference was not likely to be clinically significant.[1]

Disease due to primary infection with CMV is rarely recognized in persons with HIV infection. More than 90% of persons with AIDS in the United States have evidence of prior infection with CMV.[10] Reactivation of the latent infection may result in systemic signs and symptoms such as fevers, myalgias, leukopenia, and weight loss in addition to symptoms attributable to end-organ disease. The diagnosis of CMV in organs such as the colon and lung requires the identification of characteristic histopathologic findings of the pathognomonic "owl's eye" intranuclear and smaller intracytoplasmic inclusion bodies on tissue specimens.

Viremia with CMV is common in asymptomatic persons with low CD4+ T-lymphocyte counts (i.e., < 50 to 100 cells per microliter). In addition, in the absence of clinical disease, rare cells containing CMV inclusion bodies may be seen on histopathologic specimens even when other pathogens are causing organ dysfunction. In these cases, there are many examples where patients recovered with treatment for the other pathogen but no treatment for CMV. Thus for most syndromes CMV disease should be diagnosed only when many typical CMV inclusion-containing cells are seen with an associated inflammatory response in the appropriate clinical setting. Because of the difficulty obtaining appropriate tissue specimens, the diagnosis of retinitis due to CMV is not determined by histopathologic findings but by the characteristic appearance of a hard or fluffy exudate often associated with hemorrhage and perivascular sheathing in the retina.

Commonly, but not invariably, CMV retinitis is associated with CMV viruria and CMV viremia.[11] In one study from the National Institutes of Health, 9 of 26 (35%) HIV-infected, CMV-viremic persons with fewer than 200 CD4+ T-lymphocytes per microliter developed disease due to CMV within 6 months compared with 6 of 74 (8%) persons without CMV viremia ($P = 0.003$).[12] Similarly, 13 of 47 (28%) persons who were CMV viruric with fewer than 200 CD4+ T-lymphocytes per microliter developed CMV within 6 months compared with only 2 of 43 (5%) persons without CMV viruria ($P = 0.008$). However, though CMV blood and cultures were useful for identifying persons with a high likelihood of developing end-organ disease due to CMV, their positive predictive values were poor and were not useful clinically. Positive CMV cultures are more a reflection of the patients' underlying immunologic status and are strongly correlated with declining CD4+ T-lymphocyte counts. A similar, prospective study of 28 persons with AIDS and CMV viremia found that 50% of these persons developed end-organ disease due to CMV in 16.6 months.[13] There is little role for the use of virologic cultures or antibody testing in the diagnosis of CMV disease in persons with HIV infection except perhaps for diagnosing neurologic disease.

Data on the use of a qualitative CMV-specific polymerase chain reaction (PCR) on whole blood suggests that this test may be both more sensitive and specific for the development of CMV disease. In a prospective cohort of 97 HIV-infected persons with fewer than 50 CD4+ T-lymphocytes per microliter followed every 3 months with CMV PCR, 16 of 27 persons (59%) who were CMV-positive by PCR at baseline developed CMV disease within 12 months compared with only 3 of 70 persons (4%) who were initially CMV-negative.[14] In a cohort of 94 HIV-infected individuals without CMV disease at baseline, a qualitative plasma CMV PCR was more sensitive and specific (89% and 75%, respectively) than either urine CMV cultures (85% and 29%, respectively) or leukocyte cultures (38% and 74%, respectively) for the identification of persons developing CMV disease within 12 months.[15] Quantitative CMV PCR was able to increase the specificity of the assay at some cost to the sensitivity.

In an analysis of 619 persons with AIDS who participated in a study of the efficacy of oral ganciclovir for the prevention of CMV disease, CMV DNA was quantitated by PCR.[16] A positive baseline plasma CMV DNA PCR was associated with a 2.5-fold risk of death, and each log increase in CMV DNA load was associated with a 3.1-fold increased risk for CMV disease and a 2.2-fold increase in mortality ($P < 0.001$ for both).[16] Commercial PCR assays for CMV are currently available, but these study data have not translated into widespread clinical use in HIV-infected persons. The identification of persons at high risk for the development of CMV disease may allow the development of preemptive therapeutic strategies to prevent end-organ disease due to CMV; but because of the overwhelming impact of HAART in the management of persons with advanced HIV infection, such strategies are of marginal use, at present, in persons with HIV infection.

▲ NATURAL HISTORY AND DIAGNOSIS

Retinitis

Retinitis due to CMV results from the hematogenous dissemination of CMV after reactivation of a latent CMV infection.[5] Progression of the infection within the retina is generally to contiguous cells. Lesions near the macula or optic nerve (zone 1) commonly produce complaints of decreased visual acuity or defects in the visual field. Retinal lesions at least 1500 μm from the edge of the optic nerve and at least 3000 μm from the center of the fovea (zones 2 and 3) or anterior to the equator of the eye may be asymptomatic or present with the complaint of "floaters" or loss of peripheral vision. CMV retinitis is not associated with pain or photophobia.

Visual loss due to CMV retinitis occurs in several ways. Direct infection of the retinal cells by CMV causes retinal necrosis, which may result in a visual field defect or scotoma, depending on where in the retina the lesion occurs. This permanent, irreversible loss of vision is not amenable to therapy and depends on the location and extent of the retinal necrosis. Normal central vision may be preserved if the macula is not involved. Second, retinal involvement of the area near the macula may produce edema in the macula and loss of central visual acuity. The macular edema and loss of visual acuity are potentially reversible if recognized and treated promptly before the retinal cells are infected. Third, after infection with CMV and subsequent retinal necrosis, the retina is left as a thin, atrophic tissue that is susceptible to breaks and detachment.[17] Retinal detachment occurs commonly in persons with CMV retinitis and presents with the sudden onset of floaters, flashing lights, loss of visual field, and decreased visual acuity. Retinal detachments can be repaired; but owing to the nature of the atrophic retinal tissue they frequently recur. One series of 145 patients with CMV retinitis found a cumulative probability of retinal detachment of 50% one year after diagnosis of CMV retinitis.[18] More recent data suggest that the incidence of retinal detachments is approximately 18% at 6 months and 36% at 12 months: and it is markedly reduced in persons receiving HAART.[19] Data from randomized controlled trials using standard treatment with ganciclovir, foscarnet, or cidofovir showed that the median time to relapse after successful initial therapy of CMV retinitis, in the absence of HAART, ranges from 50 to 120 days.[11, 20–22]

Because of the difficulty of obtaining retinal tissue for histopathologic examination, CMV retinitis is diagnosed based on the appearance of the characteristic perivascular fluffy yellow-white retinal infiltrate that is often associated with retinal hemorrhage. The portion of the vessels near the lesion may appear to be sheathed. Occasionally, the lesions present with a granular, rather than fluffy, appearance.[5] Progression of retinitis is in a characteristic "brushfire" pattern, with a granular, white leading edge advancing before an atrophic, gliotic scar. Progression is irregular and occurs in fits and starts. In a study performed before the availability of HAART using serial, masked retinal photographs, the median progression rate at which disease approached the fovea in 17 untreated patients was found to be 24.0 μm/day compared with a median progression rate of 11.5 μm/day in 14 patients treated with ganciclovir.[23] Patients with AIDS and CMV retinitis, who are not being treated with HAART and have not reconstituted their immune system, usually have minimal inflammation of the vitreous. CMV retinitis usually presents unilaterally but, untreated, becomes bilateral in most cases. The presence of positive blood cultures for CMV is neither necessary nor sufficient to make the diagnosis of CMV retinitis. In one study, although all 24 patients had positive urine cultures for CMV at the time of diagnosis of CMV retinitis, only 15 of 24 (63%) had positive blood cultures.[11] The presence of serum antibodies to CMV is of no utility for establishing a diagnosis of CMV retinitis inasmuch as patients with other causes of retinitis usually have immunoglobulin G (IgG) antibodies to CMV. Retinitis in a CMV-seronegative individual would make a diagnosis of CMV retinitis highly improbable.

Other ocular lesions that occur in HIV-infected persons are in the differential diagnosis of CMV retinitis.[24] Cotton-wool spots are microinfarctions of the retinal nerve fiber layer that occur commonly in persons with HIV infection and may present similar to an early CMV retinitis.[25] These small, white lesions do not affect vision and spontaneously regress over several weeks. In the setting of an HIV-infected person with fewer than 100 CD4+ T-lymphocytes per microliter, it is critical to ensure that lesions that appear to be cotton-wool spots regress and do not progress as would be expected with CMV retinitis. Acute retinal necrosis, caused by herpes zoster, presents with either peripheral retinal vascular occlusion overlying a white, necrotic retina or, when more central vessels are involved, ischemia due to central vascular occlusion.[26] Intraocular lymphomas may present with small retinochoroidal infiltrates, optic nerve head swelling, and vascular sheathing. Toxoplasmic chorioretinitis may be unifocal or multifocal but is usually associated with a moderate to severe inflammatory reaction in the vitreous, which helps differentiate it from CMV retinitis.[27] *Pneumocystis carinii* chorioretinitis appears as multifocal, white-yellow raised choroidal lesions with minimal inflammation.[28] Other, rare causes of ocular disease in persons with HIV infection include syphilis, *Mycobacterium tuberculosis*, *Cryptococcus*, and *Candida infections,* and histoplasmosis.[29]

Gastrointestinal Disease

CMV Esophagitis

Esophagitis due to CMV is a common cause of odynophagia in persons with AIDS.[29] *Candida* more characteristically causes dysplasia. CMV esophagitis is much less common than *Candida* esophagitis, which occurs in approximately 10% of persons with AIDS who develop CMV disease.[2] The definitive diagnosis of CMV esophagitis is established by biopsy evidence of CMV with an inflammatory response in the appropriate clinical setting. The presence of extensive large, shallow ulcers of the distal esophagus is the hallmark of the disease. Pathologically, the large intranuclear inclusion bodies characteristic of CMV can be seen in the endothelial cells at the edge of the ulcer and are required to confirm the diagnosis.[30] Immunohistochemical stains may add to the sensitivity of routine hematoxylin and eosin staining for CMV. Culturing CMV from a biopsy or brushing of the esophagus is not sufficient to establish the diagnosis of CMV esophagitis because many persons with low CD4+ T-lymphocyte counts are viremic and have positive cultures for CMV in the absence of clinical disease.[12]

Other entities in the differential diagnosis of CMV esophagitis include esophagitis due to herpes simplex, reflux or peptic ulcer disease, histoplasmosis, Kaposi sarcoma, lymphoma, HIV infection, *M. tuberculosis* infection, and rarely *Mycobacterium avium-intracellulare* complex infection, cryptosporidial infection, and *Pneumocystis carinii* pneumonia.[31] Because of the relative prevalence of *Candida* esophagitis in this population, many clinicians treat esophageal symptoms empirically, especially in the presence of oral thrush. Empiric therapy usually consists of fluconazole for presumptive *Candida* esophagitis, endoscoping only those persons who fail to respond.[32] Persons with CMV or *Candida* esophagitis typically present with CD4+ T-lymphocyte counts of less than 50 cells per microliter, whereas persons with esophageal candidiasis, but not CMV, can present with counts between 50 and 400 cells per microliter.[7,11]

CMV Colitis

Colitis due to CMV occurs in fewer than 10% of persons with AIDS in whom disease due to CMV is diagnosed.[2] Fever, weight loss, anorexia, abdominal pain, debilitating diarrhea, and malaise are frequently present. Extensive hemorrhage and perforation can be life-threatening complications.[33] The symptoms are nonspecific and may be similar those due to other gastrointestinal pathogens, such as *Cryptosporidium*, *Microsporidium*, *Cyclospora cayetanensis*, *Mycobacterium avium* complex, *Giardia lamblia*, *Entamoeba histolytica*, *Salmonella*, and *Shigella* or the gastrointestinal involvement seen with lymphoma or Kaposi sarcoma. The radiographic manifestations of CMV colitis are nonspecific and may mimic the findings of other inflammatory bowel conditions, including ulcerative colitis.[34] Colonoscopic or rectal biopsy with histopathologic identification of characteristic intranuclear and intracytoplasmic inclusions is required for diagnosis. Identification of CMV by culture or even on histopathologic specimens may not be sufficient to implicate CMV; frequently multiple pathogens may coexist and must be considered in persons with advanced HIV infection.[35]

Pneumonitis

Although CMV can be cultured routinely from throat washings, pulmonary secretions, bronchoalveolar lavage specimens, and autopsy lung tissue, CMV is seldom implicated antemortem as an isolated pathogen causing pneumonitis in persons with HIV infection.[36] Foci of CMV inclusion bodies and pneumonitis are often found at autopsy. In one study from San Francisco, although CMV was cultured from bronchial alveolar lavage fluid or transbronchial biopsy specimens in 54 of 111 patients diagnosed with their first episode of *P. carinii* pneumonia, the presence of CMV had no impact on the long-term survival, acute death rate, or length of hospital stay.[37] Of 17 persons with biopsy-diagnosed CMV pneumonitis, no clinical, radiographic, or histologic findings distinguished persons with CMV as the sole pathogen from those with other, concomitant pathogens.[38]

Pneumonitis due to CMV generally presents as an interstitial pneumonitis in an individual with advanced HIV infection. Shortness of breath, dyspnea on exertion, a nonproductive cough, and hypoxemia are characteristic. CMV pneumonitis should be diagnosed only in the setting of pulmonary infiltrates by identifying multiple CMV inclusion bodies in lung tissue of appropriate clinical specimens in the absence of other pathogens that are more commonly associated with pneumonitis in this population, such as *P. carinii*, *M. tuberculosis*, *Histoplasma capsulatum*, *Coccidioides immitis*, *Cryptococcus neoformans*, or bacterial pathogens such as *Streptococcus pneumoniae* or *Haemophilus influenzae*. Treatment should be considered for persons with histologic evidence of CMV infection who do not respond to treatment of other pathogens.

Neurologic Disease

Cytomegalovirus has been found to be associated with various neurologic infections in persons with HIV infection, particularly ventriculoencephalitis[39–45] and ascending polyradiculopathy.[46–49] Ventriculoencephalitis usually occurs in advanced HIV infection in persons with a prior CMV disease diagnosis. Patients typically present with lethargy, confusion, and fever; but the clinical presentation may overlap that of HIV encephalitis. The cerebrospinal fluid (CSF) generally shows a pleocytosis that may be polymorphonuclear, low to normal glucose levels, and normal to elevated protein levels. The single clinical presentation of CMV end-organ disease where CMV culture is helpful for diagnosing the disease is neurologic disease. PCR techniques are superior to culture for detection of CMV.[44,45] Periventricular enhancement of computed tomography (CT) or magnetic resource imaging (MRI) scales are suggestive of CMV ventriculoencephalitis rather than HIV-related neurologic disease.

Polyradiculopathy caused by CMV is characterized by urinary retention and progressive bilateral leg weakness.[46–49] The clinical symptoms generally progress over several weeks to include loss of bowel and bladder control and flaccid paraplegia. A spastic myelopathy has been reported, and sacral paresthesia may occur. The CSF often shows a pleocytosis that is usually polymorphonuclear, hypoglycorrhachia, and elevated protein levels. PCR techniques are superior to culture for detection of CMV.

Although CMV is found in the central nervous system (CNS) in up to 25% of persons in autopsy studies,[39,40,50] the incidence of CMV neurologic disease antemortem appears to be low.

Other CMV-Associated Diseases

CMV Adrenalitis

Involvement of the adrenal glands with CMV is frequently reported in autopsy studies of persons with HIV infection, with the involvement documented in as many as 64 of 83 (77%)[51] and 42 of 71 (59%)[50] persons in two autopsy studies. Patients rarely manifest adrenal insufficiency by laboratory or clinical parameters. Adrenalitis due to CMV is uncommonly diagnosed premortem, but hypoadrenalism is occasionally documented in persons with CMV disease by the cosyntropin stimulation test.[52]

CMV Hepatitis and Biliary Disease

Although CMV involvement of the liver and biliary tract is often seen in autopsy specimens, clinical hepatitis due to CMV is rare in persons with HIV infection.[2] Biliary tract or hepatic involvement by CMV may present with right upper quadrant pain and elevated alkaline phosphatase, but infections with *Cryptosporidium* and *M. avium-intracellulare* complex are more common with this presentation. In one series of 66 consecutive persons with AIDS and first-episode gastrointestinal CMV disease, 22 patients presented with esophagitis, 28 with colitis, 9 with sclerosing cholangitis, and only 2 with acute hepatitis.[53]

▲ THERAPY

Specific therapies for CMV disease are summarized in Table 43–1. Drug susceptibilities and pharmacokinetic values are summarized in Table 43–2.

Specific Treatments

The U.S. Food and Drug Administration (FDA) has approved seven approaches to CMV therapy for patients with HIV (Table 43–3).

Ganciclovir

Initial Therapy with Intravenous Ganciclovir

The first major advance in the treatment for CMV disease was the development of ganciclovir, an agent highly specific for human herpesviruses. Ganciclovir is a nucleoside analogue whose activity depends on inhibition of herpesvirus DNA polymerases. It requires phosphorylation in CMV-infected cells, and most strains of CMV resistant to ganciclovir are unable to phosphorylate ganciclovir. The CMV UL97 open reading frame codes for a protein kinase capable of phosphorylating ganciclovir in CMV-infected cells.[54,55] Ganciclovir is virustatic against CMV. Thus when treatment for disease is stopped, viral spread and progression of disease characteristically begin again.[6] Prior to the introduction of HAART, lifelong daily therapy was required, most often intravenously through an indwelling catheter. An oral formulation of ganciclovir is available but is poorly absorbed and is not as clinically effective as the intravenous formulation.[56,57]

When given intravenously by a 1-hour infusion, the standard 5 mg/kg dose of ganciclovir reaches a maximum concentration in the plasma at the end of infusion of approximately 6 μg/ml (24 μM).[57] Trough levels 11 hours after infusion are approximately 1 μg/ml (4 μM). The initial distribution half-life ($t_{1/2}$) is about 0.76 hour, and the terminal elimination $t_{1/2}$ is 3.60 hours.[57] Orally, ganciclovir is less than 10% bioavailable. Most studies report that for human CMV isolates the 50% inhibition (ID_{50}) of viral plaque formation is attained by concentrations of ganciclovir between 0.4 and 11.0 μM.[6,58]

Ganciclovir was licensed by the FDA in 1988. The recommended dosing of ganciclovir for the treatment of CMV retinitis in persons with AIDS is 5 mg/kg IV twice daily for a 14- to 21-day induction period followed by a 5 mg/kg daily indefinite maintenance phase. The terms "induction" and "maintenance" may be misnomers inasmuch as progression of CMV retinitis is regularly seen during the maintenance phase with ganciclovir and foscarnet (Table 43–1). Patients with progression during the maintenance phase are routinely retreated with the twice-daily regimen. Ganciclovir at 1000 mg PO thrice daily is approved for maintenance therapy of CMV retinitis but should not be used in persons whose central visual acuity is threatened if progression of disease should occur. Valganciclovir was licensed by the FDA in 2001 and is likely to supplant oral ganciclovir as the oral anti-CMV agent of choice.

In a compilation of clinical data, treatment with ganciclovir resulted in the improvement or stabilization of CMV retinitis in 80% to 90% of patients.[59] The median time to clinical progression in these uncontrolled studies appeared to be as long as 145 days from the diagnosis of CMV retinitis while continuing some maintenance therapy with ganciclovir. One large, uncontrolled series reported the outcomes of 105 immunocompromised (primarily AIDS) patients who were treated with ganciclovir for CMV retinitis. Analysis of a subset of these patients selected for their ability to tolerate a prolonged course of therapy and who had high-dose maintenance therapy (25 to 35 mg/kg per week) after induction therapy showed that the mean time to progression of retinitis was 18 weeks. This result, however, is based on subset analysis; these patients were selected for their ability to tolerate a prolonged course of relatively high-dose ganciclovir without the development of neutropenia. The results of other trials indicate that with standard doses of both agents there is no difference in the

Table 43–1. THERAPIES FOR AIDS-ASSOCIATED CMV RETINITIS

Parameter	Ganciclovir IV	Foscarnet IV	Combined GCV IV/FOS IV	Valganciclovir PO	GCV Implant	Intravitreal Cidofovir IV	Fomivirsen
Median time to first retinitis progression	47–104 d	53–93 d	129 d	160 d	216–226 d	64–120 d	71 d
Induction regimen	5 mg/kg q12h for 14–21 d	90 mg/kg q12h for 14–21 d	FOS 90 mg/kg IV q12h and GCV 5 mg/kg IV qd, both for 14–21 d	900 mg PO bid for 14–21 days	Intraocular implantation via pars plana of GCV (4.5 mg) implant; requires concomitant oral therapy	5 mg/kg q wk for 2 weeks with probenecid and IV fluids before and after therapy	Intravitreal injection of 0.05 ml (330 μg) q 2 wk for 2 doses
Maintenance	5 mg/kg qd	90–120 mg/kg qd	FOS 90–120 mg/kg and GCV 5 mg/kg IV both qd	900 mg PO qd	Requires replacement q 5–8 mo	5 mg/kg q 2 wk	0.05 ml q 4 wk
Adverse effects	Neutropenia, thrombocytopenia, catheter sepsis	Nephrotoxicity, electrolyte abnormalities, catheter sepsis, genital ulceration	Same as GCV and FOS	Same as GCV	Surgical complications, transient blurred vision, infection, hemorrhage	Nephrotoxicity, uveitis, hypotony	Abnormal or blurred vision, eye pain, ocular inflammation
Comments	Higher doses may be used for refractory disease Dosage should be adjusted for creatinine clearance < 70 ml/min	Dosage should be adjusted based on recent creatinine clearance Requires hydration with 0.9% saline to reduce nephrotoxicity	Dosages of either may be increased based on prior drug experience	Few data have been reported regarding the efficacy of VAL as initial therapy for CMV retinitis	Oral ganciclovir has been recommended to prevent systemic CMV disease; VAL is a better choice	Requires dose reduction to 3 mg/kg for increase in serum creatinine by 0.3–0.4 mg/dl	Limited to persons with refractory disease
Main toxicities, side effects	Requires IV therapy Bone marrow toxicity	Requires IV therapy Renal toxicity	Requires frequent infusions; toxicities of both agents	Bone marrow toxicity	Surgical risks No coverage for systemic disease	Requires IV therapy Renal toxicity	Requires intravitreal therapy

FOS, foscarnet; GCV, ganciclovir; VAL, valganciclovir.

▲ **Table 43–2.** REPORTED ANTI-CMV DRUG SUSCEPTIBILITY AND PHARMACOKINETIC VALUES

Drug	ED_{50} (μg/ml)	Plasma Concentration (μg/ml)		Intravitreal Concentration (μg/ml)		Half-life (hr)		
		C_{max}	C_{min}	C_{max}	C_{min}	Plasma	Intracellular	Intravitreal
Ganciclovir	1.50	—	—	—	—	—	16.5[a]	13.3
5 mg/kg	—	8.2	0.05	0.6–1.8	0.2	—	—	—
1000 mg PO tid	—	1.2	0.23					
200 μg, Intravitreal	—	—	—	17.9	NA	—	—	—
4.5 mg intraocular device	—	—	—	0.69–7.40	0.69–7.40	—	—	—
Valganciclovir[b]	1.50	—	—	—	—	—	—	—
900 mg PO bid	—	5.6	NA	—	—	4.1	—	—
Foscarnet	120.00	—	—	—	—	—	—	—
90 mg/kg IV q12h	—	181	16	—	57	3.4	—	32
2400 μg intravitreal	—	—	—	269	NA	—	—	—
Cidofovir	0.63	—	—	—	—	—	—	—
5 mg/kg q2wk[c]	—	25	NA	—	—	3.2	65[b]	—

C_{max}, maximum concentration; C_{min}, minimum concentration; ED_{50}, drug concentration that inhibits by 50% the in vitro replication of clinical CMV isolates obtained from patients who have not been treated with the drug; NA, not available.
[a]Ganciclovir triphosphate.
[b]Ganciclovir levels measured.
[c]Co-administered with probenecid 4 g PO over 8 hours.

rate of progression of CMV retinitis in AIDS patients treated with either ganciclovir or foscarnet.[11,20,21] Clinical examination tends to overestimate the time to progression compared with data based on rigorous photographic endpoints.[56,59–61]

The results of a randomized, controlled trial comparing ganciclovir with delayed therapy using strictly graded retinal photographs demonstrated that progression of retinitis while on ganciclovir occurred within a median of 50.5 days, compared with the progression on delayed therapy, which occurred within a median of 15 days.[20] Similarly, the results of the Studies of the Ocular Complications of AIDS (SOCA) trial demonstrated that the median time to progression of CMV retinitis while on ganciclovir was 56 days.[21]

In an open study of ganciclovir for the treatment of CMV esophagitis, among 10 evaluable patients treated with an induction regimen of 2.5 mg/kg IV q8 h or 5 mg/kg IV q12 h for 10 days, 5 persons had a good response, 3 had a partial response, and 2 had no response to therapy.[29] In general, in the absence of HAART, there is a high rate of relapse of CMV esophagitis in persons who receive intermittent therapy. The decision about whether to use daily, lifelong treatment or intermittent, high-dose therapy for esophagitis due to CMV must be individualized. Maintenance therapy should be considered, particularly after a relapse (Fig. 43–1).

▲ **Table 43–3.** ANTI-CMV AGENTS

Drug	Year of FDA Approval
Ganciclovir IV	1989
Foscarnet IV	1991
Ganciclovir capsules	1994
Ganciclovir implant	1996
Cidofovir IV	1996
Fomivirsen injectable	1998
Valganciclovir	2001

Ganciclovir has been evaluated in a multicenter, double-blind, placebo-controlled trial for the treatment of CMV colitis in persons with AIDS.[62] Although the trial lasted only 14 days and was too short to demonstrate colonic healing and resolution of diarrhea, colonoscopy scores reflecting inflammation and positive cultures for CMV from the colon and urine significantly decreased in patients on the ganciclovir arm. Most experienced clinicians recommend that treatment for CMV colitis should be given for 3 to 6 weeks. Unlike CMV retinitis, because the cells lining the gastrointestinal tract regenerate rapidly, therapy can often wait for the development of moderate to severe symptoms to justify the use of a systemic therapy with not inconsiderable toxicities. As with esophagitis, maintenance therapy is not necessarily required but should be strongly considered after a relapse. In a randomized, controlled trial of 48 patients with biopsy-proven gastrointestinal CMV disease comparing intravenous ganciclovir (n = 22) with intravenous foscarnet (n = 26), 73% of subjects had a good or complete clinical response to a 2- to 4-week trial of either drug, with more than 83% of the subjects demonstrating an endoscopic response.[63]

The utility of ganciclovir therapy in the treatment of CMV in other organ systems is not proven by randomized controlled trials. Although the combination of ganciclovir with high-dose intravenous immunoglobulin has been suggested to be more effective than ganciclovir alone in the treatment of CMV pneumonitis in bone marrow transplant recipients using historical controls,[64,65] the addition of intravenous immunoglobulin has not shown any benefit over ganciclovir alone in persons with AIDS.[66] The response of pneumonitis to intravenous ganciclovir has been reported to be better than 60%.[38] Response is probably better when patients are treated before the disease is severe. The role for maintenance

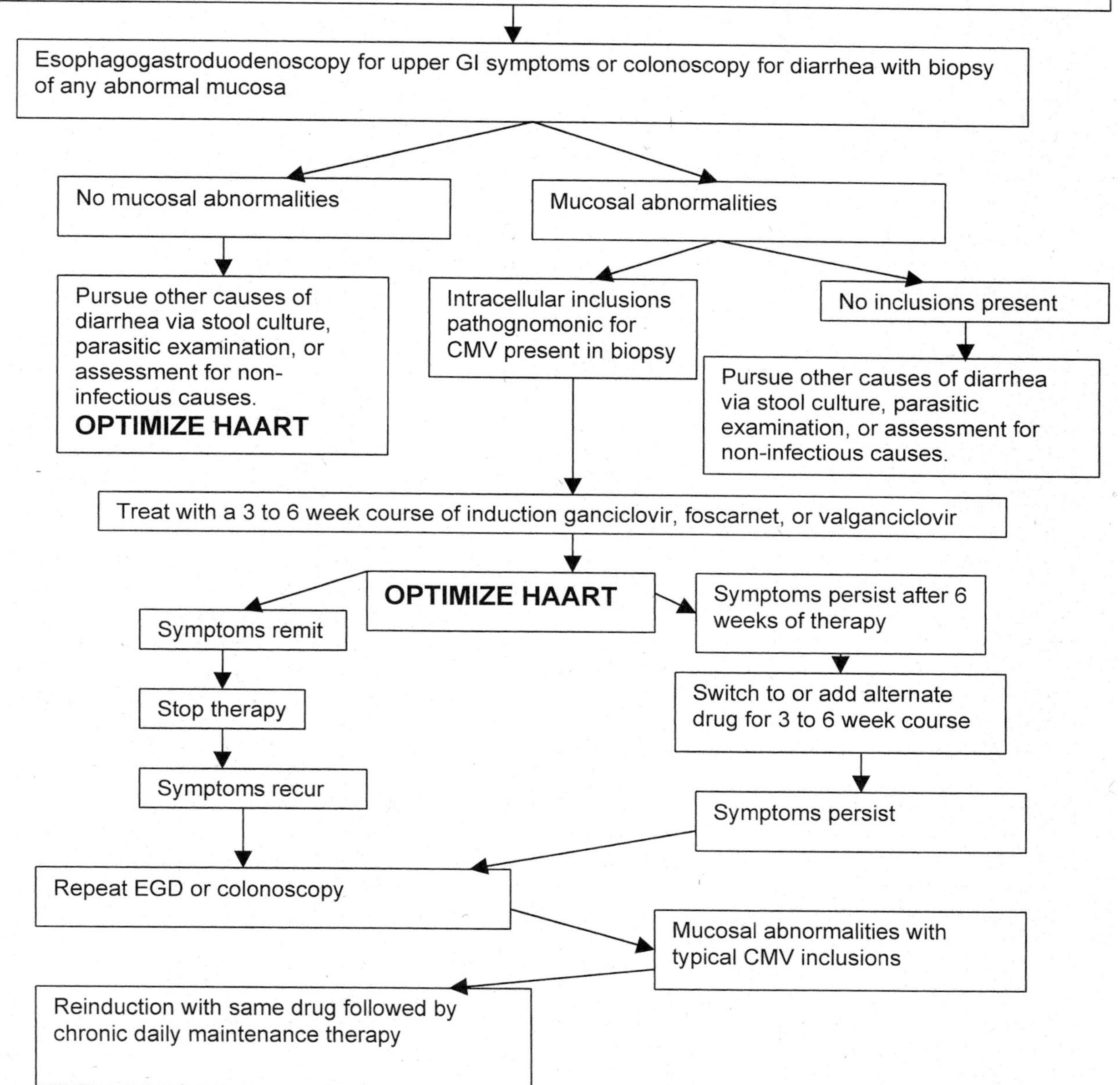

Figure 43–1. Algorithm for diagnosing and treating CMV gastrointestinal (GI) disease. EGD, esophagogastroduodenoscopy.

therapy for CMV pneumonitis has not been established (Figure 43–2). Many clinicians recommend such maintenance, however, so long as the CD4+ T-lymphocyte count remains below 100 to 150 cells per microliter. For neurologic disease, initiating therapy promptly is critical for an optimal clinical response. Most clinicians treat CMV neurologic disease with ganciclovir. Some data suggest that combination therapy with ganciclovir and foscarnet is best for stabilizing or improving the response[67] (Figs. 43–3, 43–4).

Cytomegalovirus viremia may be associated with subclinical involvement of other organ systems. Viremia in the absence of attributable clinical disease is not recommended. Treatment of CMV viremia when no other pathogen has

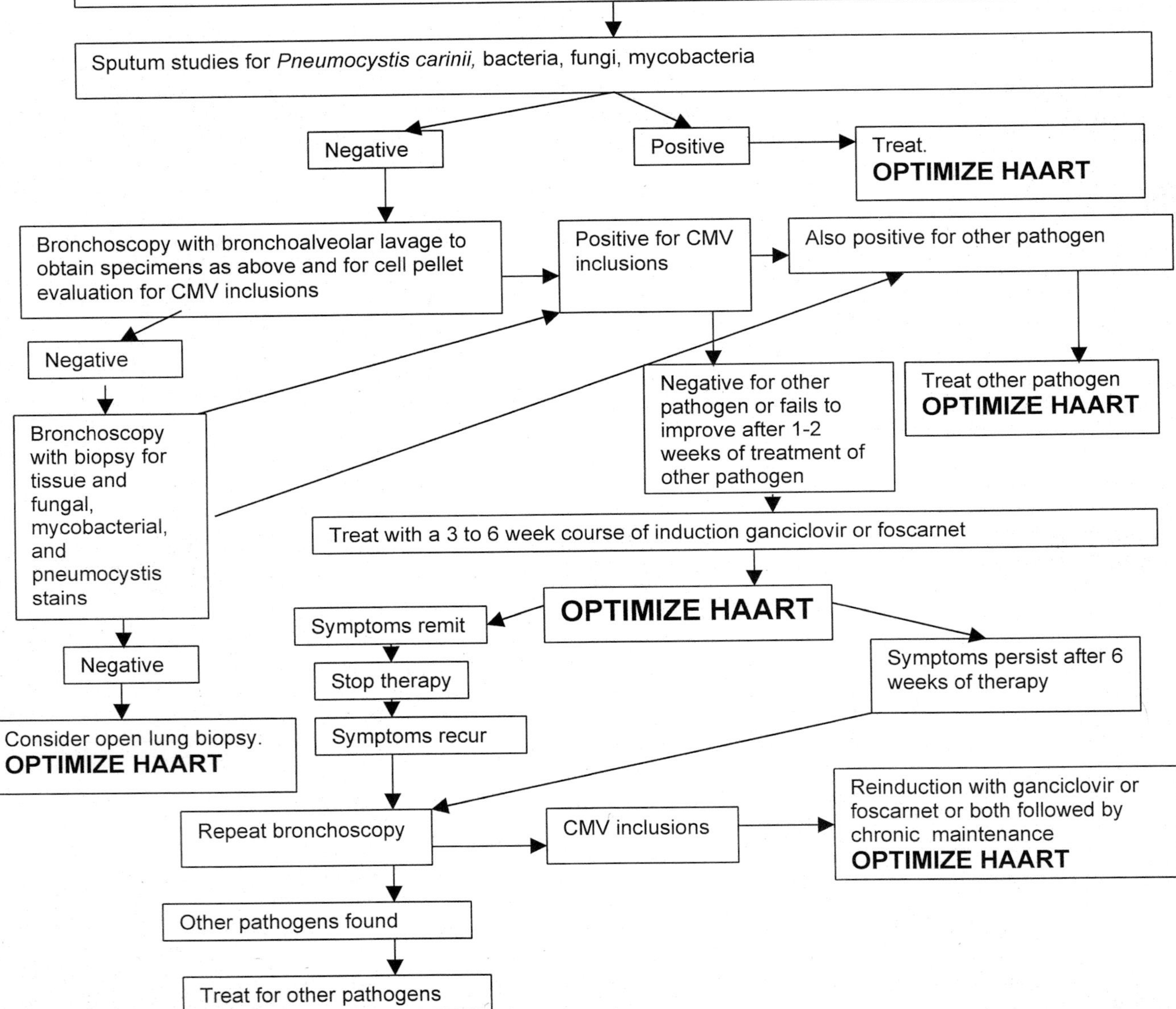

Figure 43–2. Algorithm for diagnosing and treating CMV pulmonary disease.

been identified after thorough investigation is rarely warranted in patients with fever or wasting.

Neutropenia and thrombocytopenia are the major dose-limiting toxicities of ganciclovir therapy (Table 43–1). Because ganciclovir and zidovudine are both myelosuppressive, it is difficult to administer these agents concurrently.[68] In one study, only 18% of 29 persons with CMV disease were able to tolerate full doses of ganciclovir with 600 mg of zidovudine daily.[69] In the randomized trial comparing initial therapy with ganciclovir versus foscarnet for the treatment of CMV retinitis, 14 of 127 (11%) patients required switching from ganciclovir to foscarnet: 9 of 14 for progression of retinitis but only 1 of 14 for drug toxicity.[21] Limited in vitro data suggest that the antiretroviral activity of both zidovudine and didanosine may be antagonized by ganciclovir.[69]

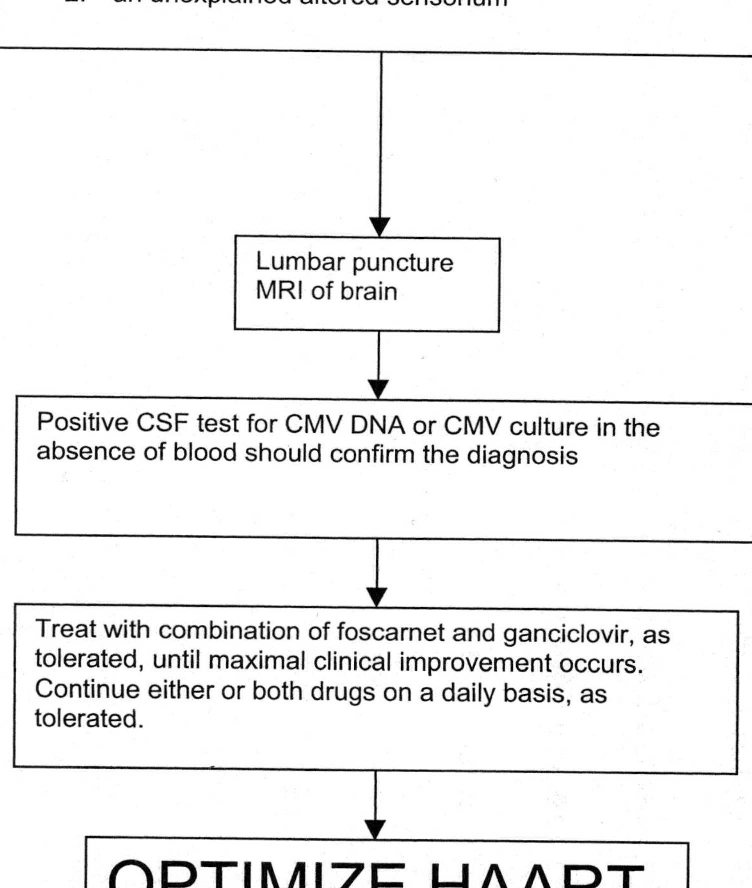

Figure 43-3. Algorithm for diagnosing and treating CMV encephalitis.

Intravitreal Ganciclovir

Intravitreal injections of ganciclovir have been used for the treatment of CMV retinitis in persons unable or unwilling to tolerate systemic therapy with ganciclovir or foscarnet.[70-72] The concentration of ganciclovir in intravitreal fluid immediately after injection has been as high as 65 μM.[71] Concentrations higher than the ID_{50} for most strains of CMV can be maintained for 60 hours after a single 400 μg injection.[72] Two injections of 400 μg of ganciclovir per week are given for 2 to 3 weeks during an induction period, followed by weekly maintenance injections. Alternatively, a single 2 mg injection may be given weekly. This alternative therapy effectively prevents the progression of CMV retinitis without the systemic toxicity of ganciclovir and without significant toxicity to the retina. Rarely, retinal detachment, intraocular infection, intravitreal hemorrhage, or damage to the lens occurs.

Ganciclovir Intraocular Device

Local administration of ganciclovir can be accomplished using a ganciclovir intraocular device, licensed by the FDA for the treatment of CMV retinitis in 1996. This implant device releases ganciclovir into the vitreous cavity at a rate of approximately 1.40 μg/hr for a period of 6 to 9 months. It is surgically implanted in the affected eye during a simple surgical procedure that does not require an overnight hospital stay. Recovery time is generally of the order of several days, but persons tend to have decreased visual acuity in the implanted eye for 4 weeks.[73] In a randomized, controlled clinical trial patients with peripheral CMV retinitis received either immediate implantation of the device or were closely monitored; the median time to progression of retinitis was 15 days in eyes in the delayed treatment group ($n = 16$) compared with 226 days in the immediate treatment group ($n = 14$) ($P < 0.00001$).[73] In eight persons in whom vitreous levels of ganciclovir were obtained, the mean vitreous drug

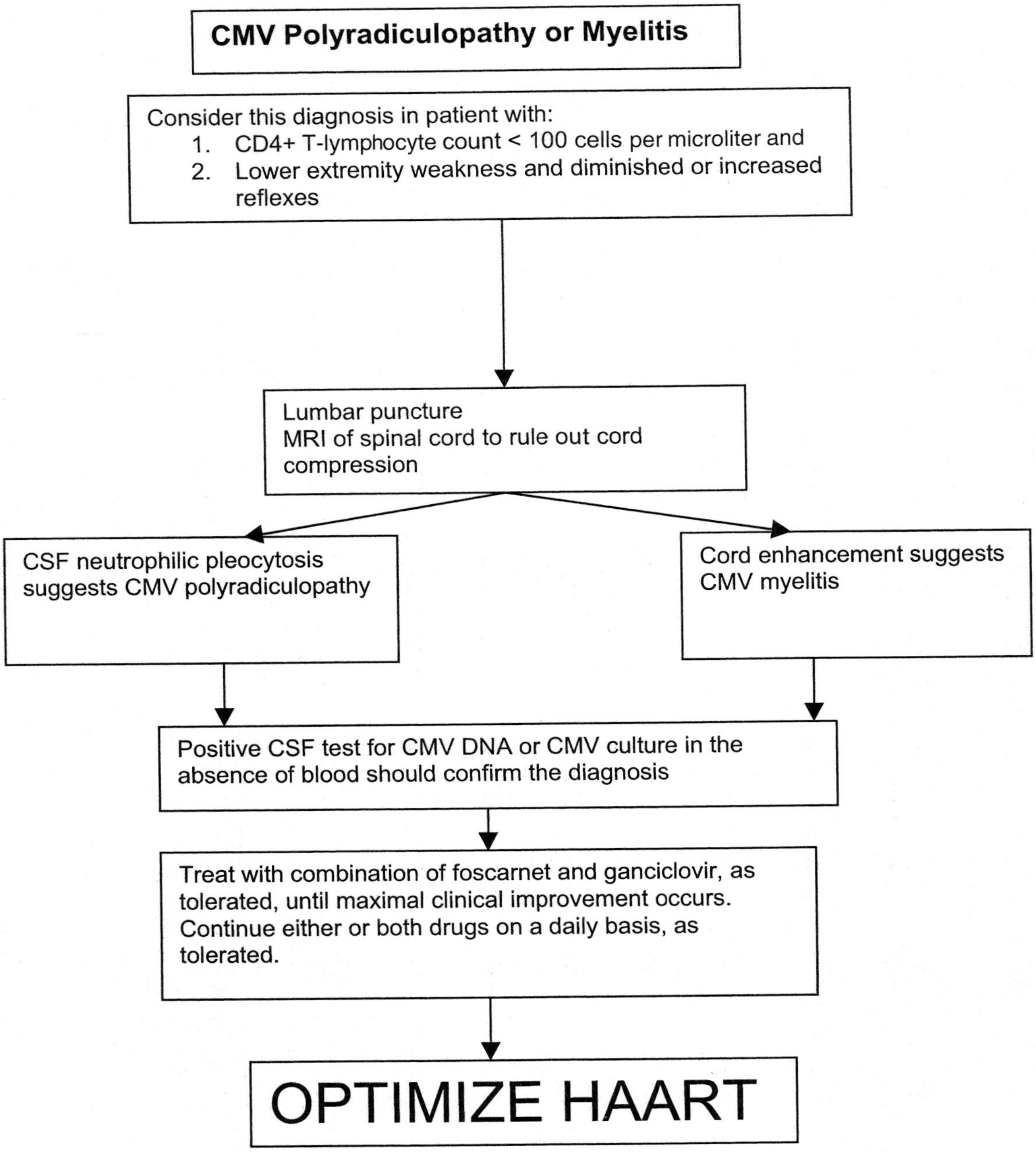

Figure 43–4. Algorithm for diagnosing and treating CMV polyradiculopathy or myelitis.

level was 4.1 μg/ml, roughly four times the concentration in the eye obtained with intravenous ganciclovir. The major complications of the trial included the risk of CMV retinitis development in the fellow eye (estimated at 50% at 6 months) and the development of visceral CMV disease in 31% of patients. Seven late retinal detachments occurred in this study, but because retinal detachment occurs in those with treated and untreated CMV retinitis[17–19] it appears that an increased rate of early, surgically associated retinal detachment may be balanced by a decreased rate of late retinal detachments due to better control of the CMV retinitis.

A randomized, controlled clinical trial compared the use of intravenous ganciclovir with that of two ganciclovir implant devices releasing ganciclovir at different rates.[74] The median time to progression of retinitis was 191 days (71 eyes) and 221 days (75 eyes) with the two implants, compared with 71 days (76 eyes) with intravenous ganciclovir ($P < 0.001$). Extraocular CMV disease occurred more commonly in persons with the implant devices than in those receiving intravenous ganciclovir (10.3% vs. 0%; $P = 0.04$). Vitreous hemorrhage, which was generally transient, occurred in 7.8% of eyes. Endophthalmitis was reported in three eyes. Retinal detachments were reported in 11.9% of eyes receiving implants compared with 5.1% of the eyes of persons receiving intravenous ganciclovir. There was no indication of a significant difference in mortality between the groups on this study.[74]

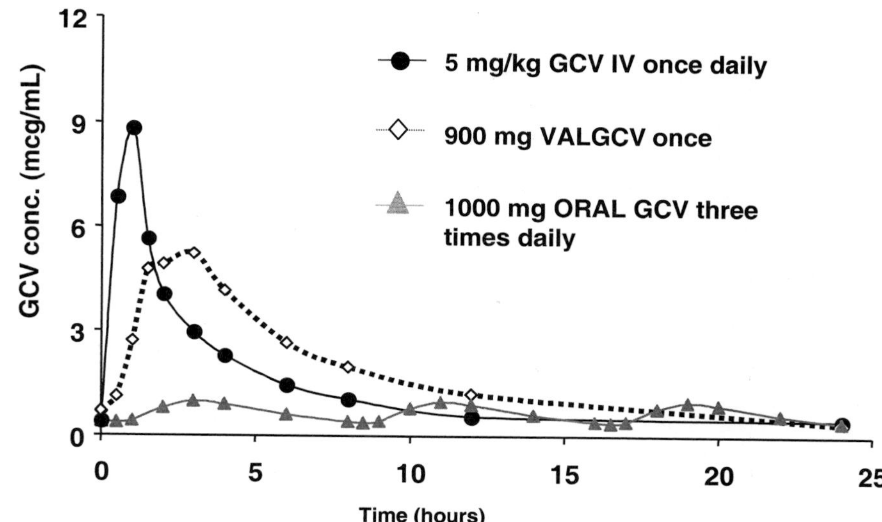

Figure 43–5. Ganciclovir plasma concentration-time profiles in HIV+/CMV+ patients.

To evaluate the efficacy of oral ganciclovir in combination with the ganciclovir implant to control the development of extraocular and fellow-eye CMV disease, a multicenter, three-arm randomized clinical trial comparing the use of the implant alone versus the implant with co-administration of oral ganciclovir (1500 mg PO thrice daily) versus standard intravenous ganciclovir was conducted.[75] In 377 patients with AIDS and CMV retinitis restricted to one eye, after 6 months of treatment the development of extraocular CMV disease or CMV retinitis in the fellow eye was 37.8%, 22.4%, and 17.9% in the three groups, respectively, a statistically significant finding comparing either the combination or the intravenous ganciclovir groups with the implant-alone group. It is of note that the rate of development of Kaposi sarcoma was similarly decreased, occurring in 11.3 %, 2.7%, and 1.5% of the three groups, respectively. This is the first time that use of an antiviral agent in a randomized clinical trial decreased the incidence of Kaposi sarcoma. With the availability of valganciclovir in 2001 and the higher plasma levels of ganciclovir achieved with valganciclovir compared with oral ganciclovir, it is likely that the use of oral ganciclovir may be of historical interest only.

Complications seen with use of the ganciclovir implant are associated with the insertion procedure and include retinal detachment and, rarely, intraocular hemorrhage or infection. The incidence of surgical complications may decrease with increased familiarity with the procedure. Persons may have multiple devices implanted to control CMV retinitis once the ganciclovir is spent. It is controversial whether to perform scheduled surgical replacement of these devices at 5 to 8 months after implantation or to replace them once the CMV disease progresses. The implant device is especially useful in individuals who are unable or incapable of administering daily intravenous therapy. It may also have a role in individuals who require temporary therapy for CMV retinitis while waiting for a response after initiating HAART, although oral valganciclovir is probably preferable. Finally, because of the increased intraocular levels of ganciclovir achieved with the implant device compared to systemic administration of ganciclovir, it may be useful in persons who do not respond to systemic ganciclovir. In those circumstances it may be prudent to treat with intravitreal ganciclovir initially to determine if higher levels of ganciclovir would be useful or if high-level resistance to ganciclovir is present.

Oral Valganciclovir

Valganciclovir was approved for both induction and maintenance therapy of CMV retinitis in 2001.[76] Few clinical data have been published for valganciclovir. Induction therapy for CMV retinitis is 900 mg PO bid for 2 to 3 weeks followed by indefinite maintenance therapy of 900 mg PO daily. The oral administration of 900 mg of valganciclovir results in serum ganciclovir levels approximating those obtained with 5 mg/kg IV (Fig. 43–5).[77] The results of a randomized, open-label controlled study of 160 patients with AIDS and newly diagnosed CMV retinitis randomized to receive either valganciclovir or intravenous ganciclovir at the standard doses were recently reported[78] and are available on the FDA website.[79] After 4 weeks of either oral valganciclovir or Intravenous ganciclovir, all patients in the study received valganciclovir maintenance therapy at a dose of 900 mg daily. Among each group of 80 subjects, 7 had progression of their CMV retinitis at 4 weeks determined by a masked review of retinal photographs. Two persons in the intravenous ganciclovir arm and one person in the valganciclovir arm died. Interestingly, detection of CMV by PCR at week 4 was similar in the two arms (Table 43–4).

Table 43–4. DETECTION OF CMV IN URINE, BLOOD, OR SEMEN OF PATIENTS WITH CMV RETINITIS

Test	Incidence of CMV	
	IV GCV	Val-GCV
Baseline		
PCR (Plasma)	51% (39/76)	40% (31/77)
Culture (Any)	65% (46/71)	46% (33/71)
Week 4		
PCR (Plasma)	3% (2/70)	4% (3/71)
Culture (Any)	6% (4/64)	7% (4/58)

GCV, ganciclovir; PCR, polymerase chain reaction; Val-GCV, valganciclovir.

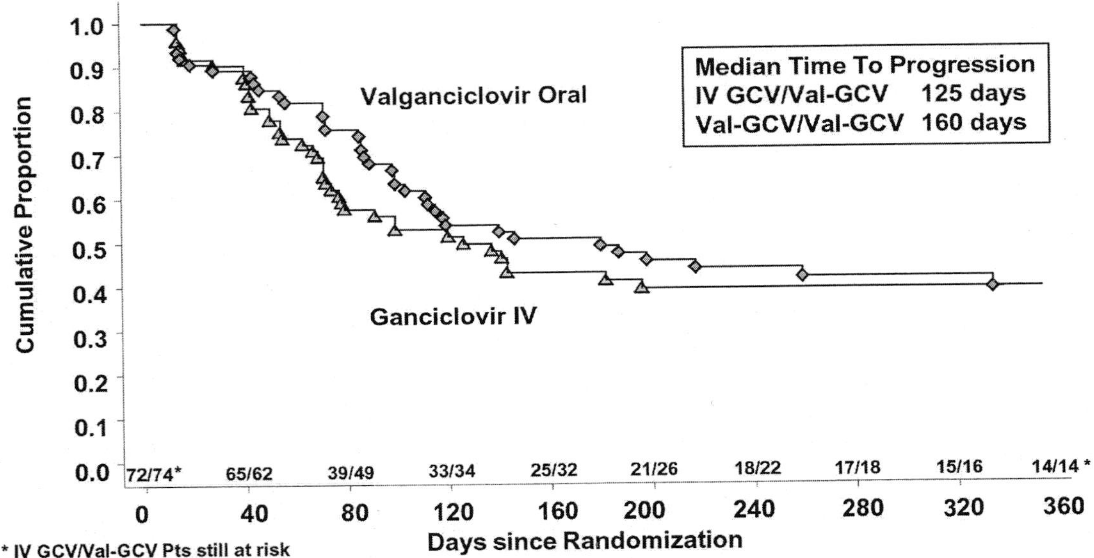

Figure 43–6. CMV retinitis maintenance therapy: IV ganciclovir versus oral valganciclovir. Time to progression determined by retinal photography.

The median time to progression of retinitis in the valganciclovir-alone arm was 160 days, compared with 125 days in the intravenous ganciclovir to valganciclovir arm, which is much longer than the median times observed in similar randomized trials conducted before the introduction of HAART (Fig. 43–6). The incidence of adverse events in the two study arms was similar (Table 43–5). It is likely that valganciclovir, owing to its better bioavailability, will entirely supplant the use of oral ganciclovir and potentially a major portion of the use of intravenous ganciclovir.

Foscarnet

Intravenous Administration

Foscarnet, or trisodium phosphonoformate hexahydrate, was approved by the FDA in 1991. The recommended regimen for CMV retinitis in persons with AIDS is 90 mg/kg IV q12 h for an induction period of 2 to 3 weeks followed by an indefinite 90 mg/kg IV daily for maintenance (Table 43–1). As with ganciclovir, the terms "induction" and "maintenance," though commonly used, may be misnomers; the half-lives of both ganciclovir and foscarnet are both relatively short, and therapeutic drug levels against CMV of each may not be maintained during most of the day during the "maintenance" phase of therapy. This probably accounts for the routine progression of CMV retinitis while on the "maintenance" phase of therapy with either agent. Patients experiencing progression of CMV retinitis during the maintenance phase are routinely retreated with "induction" doses of foscarnet.

Table 43–5. IV GANCICLOVIR VS. ORAL VALGANCICLOVIR: ADVERSE EVENTS

Adverse Event	IV GCV (n = 79)	Val-GCV (n = 79)
Diarrhea	8 (10%)	13 (16%)
Nausea	11 (14%)	6 (8%)
Vomiting	8 (10%)	6 (8%)
Catheter-related	9 (11%)	2 (3%)
Neutropenia	5 (6%)	5 (6%)
< 500 cells/dl	10 (13%)	12 (15%)
< 500–750 cells/dl	0	1 (1%)
Platelets < 50,000/dl	0	1 (1%)

Foscarnet is an antiviral agent with activity against CMV and other human herpesviruses and HIV. Foscarnet inhibits DNA polymerases and prevents chain elongation by blocking nucleoside-binding sites of all herpesviruses. Specifically, foscarnet prevents cleavage of pyrophosphate from adenine triphosphate and, unlike ganciclovir, does not require phosphorylation in virally infected cells.[6] In addition to having inhibitory activity against the DNA polymerases of herpes simplex 1 and 2 and CMV, foscarnet has activity against the reverse transcriptase of HIV.[80–82]

Oral preparations of foscarnet have been absorbed poorly and have resulted in plasma concentrations that are inadequate to inhibit herpesvirus or HIV replication.[83] In humans, pharmacokinetic studies have been performed using both intermittent and continuous foscarnet infusions. Administration of foscarnet 60 mg/kg (or less depending on creatinine clearance) every 8 hours to eight patients with AIDS and CMV retinitis resulted in a mean plasma $t_{1/2}$ of 4.5 hours and steady-state peak plasma concentrations ranging between 272 and 876 μM, well above the drug concentrations that inhibit in vitro viral replication by 50% (ID_{50}) of susceptible viruses. Trough concentrations of 57 to 225 μM were sometimes lower than susceptible virus ID_{50} values. Plasma clearance was directly related to renal function; two patients with impaired creatinine clearance had delayed clearance and higher plasma concentrations of foscarnet.[84]

Continuous infusion of foscarnet (0.14 to 0.19 mg/kg/min for 8 to 21 days) in 13 patients with HIV infection and generalized lymphadenopathy or AIDS resulted in a mean plasma $t_{1/2}$ of 6.8 hours.[85] At steady state, 79% to 92% of the dose was excreted unchanged in the urine. After 8 days, small amounts of foscarnet could still be measured in the urine of all patients; and in one patient trace amounts were measurable 2.3 years after infusion. Persistent urinary levels are probably due to slow release from bone. CSF levels of foscarnet measured in five subjects found a mean CSF/plasma concentration ratio of 43%. Four of the subjects, however, had elevated CSF protein, suggesting a preexisting meningeal barrier defect.[85]

Foscarnet also inhibits the reverse transcriptase of HIV and, correspondingly, the replication of HIV.[82,86] Like ganciclovir, foscarnet is only virustatic; and prior to the availability of HAART lifelong treatment of disease was generally required. The major toxicities of foscarnet are its effects on renal function and serum electrolytes. The need for concurrent or preadministration of a saline solution to minimize renal dysfunction requires a longer infusion period than with ganciclovir.[87] Therefore foscarnet should be infused over at least 1 hour with an infusion pump. This is especially true when other nephrotoxic agents are also being administered. Frequent monitoring of serum creatinine, creatinine clearance, and serum electrolytes is required.

Uncontrolled trials initially demonstrated the efficacy of foscarnet in the treatment of CMV retinitis in AIDS patients.[88–90] In a randomized, controlled trial of foscarnet, 24 AIDS patients with CMV retinitis who were not in immediate danger of losing central visual acuity were entered onto a trial with a 1:1 assignment to either an immediate or delayed treatment group.[11] Among those patients, 13 received immediate induction therapy with foscarnet (60 mg IV q8 h for 21 days followed by 90 mg IV daily as maintenance therapy), and 11 patients were assigned to delayed therapy. The endpoint of the trial was defined as the time when any evaluable lesion progressed 750 μm (one-half the diameter of the optic disc) over a 750 μm front or when any new retinal lesion due to CMV appeared. The mean time to progression of retinitis was 13.3 weeks (median 7.5 weeks) in the foscarnet group versus 3.2 weeks (median 3.0 weeks) in the delayed therapy group from endpoints determined from retinal photographs obtained weekly and read at a masked reading center. Patients in the delayed therapy arm received foscarnet when retinitis progressed. This trial design became the model by which other trials of therapeutic agents for CMV retinitis were tested. Persons receiving immediate therapy with foscarnet frequently had conversion of CMV blood and urine cultures from positive to negative, whereas conversion of cultures in those not receiving therapy was a rare event. Although foscarnet only delayed the progression of retinitis in most patients on maintenance therapy, progression could generally be halted by another induction course of foscarnet or by increasing the maintenance dose.

In the SOCA study comparing foscarnet and ganciclovir directly, no difference in the time to progression of CMV retinitis was found between the two arms, with a median time to progression of 59 days in the foscarnet arm and 56 days in the ganciclovir arm.

Clinical trials have demonstrated the clinical utility of foscarnet against gastrointestinal infections due to CMV.[53,63,91] In one study in patients with AIDS, 18 episodes of esophagitis and 27 episodes of colitis were treated with foscarnet, 20 mg/kg over 10 to 30 minutes followed by a continuous infusion of 200 mg/kg over 24 hours for a total of 3 weeks of therapy.[91] Symptoms and mucosal ulcerations resolved in 15 of 16 episodes of esophagitis in which therapy was completed, for a response rate of 94%. Three patients had a relapse of CMV esophagitis at 1, 4, and 7 months after therapy; two of these cases were successfully retreated with foscarnet and remained in remission 9 months later. Of the remaining 12 patients, 8 died a mean 5.8 months later without recurrence of esophagitis, suggesting that maintenance therapy may not be necessary for sustained remission of CMV esophagitis.

Of 18 initial episodes of CMV colitis in which foscarnet therapy was completed, 11 had a complete response, 6 had a partial response, and 1 had no response. In the six with partial responses, other pathogens were also present. Therefore, 11 of 12 initial episodes of colitis due to CMV alone responded to foscarnet for a response rate of 92%. Two patients with relapses responded to either foscarnet or ganciclovir. The one case that did not respond to foscarnet also failed to respond to ganciclovir.[91] Similar rates of response were found with intermittent infusions of foscarnet.[53]

In comparison, 42 immunocompromised (primarily AIDS) patients treated with ganciclovir for upper (esophagitis and gastritis) and lower (enteritis and colitis) CMV gastrointestinal disease had a response rate of 83%. Some of these patients received maintenance or repeat therapy as a result of disease relapses.[59] In a randomized, controlled trial of 48 patients with biopsy-proven gastrointestinal CMV disease comparing intravenous ganciclovir and foscarnet, equivalent clinical and endoscopic responses to a 2- to 4-week trial of either was seen.[63]

The utility of foscarnet therapy in the treatment of CMV pneumonitis, CNS disease, viremia, or other infections due to CMV is largely anecdotal. Data suggest efficacy rates similar to those for ganciclovir.[64]

Foscarnet is not commonly associated with neutropenia and can usually be administered along with zidovudine (Table 43–1).[11,21] Elevations in serum creatinine are perhaps the most common laboratory abnormality encountered and occur more frequently when other nephrotoxic agents are administered at the same time. These elevations are almost always reversible with reduction or discontinuation of therapy. In one study[87] elevations in serum creatinine of more than 25% over baseline occurred in 66% of 56 episodes of CMV infection treated with foscarnet. Acute renal failure requiring temporary hemodialysis occurred in one instance. In this same report, a series of 27 patients were prehydrated with 2.5 L of normal saline per day before and during the administration of foscarnet. Only one patient in this group developed an elevated serum creatinine level. Autopsy of one patient revealed acute tubular necrosis, suggesting it as one mechanism of foscarnet-associated renal toxicity. The major toxicities of foscarnet in the randomized immediate versus delayed treatment study included abnormalities in serum electrolytes, neutropenia ($>$500 cells/μl), increased red blood cell transfusion requirements, nausea that required discontinuation of therapy in two instances, and seizures.[11] The seizures occurred in the setting of preexisting toxoplasmic encephalitis in one patient and cryptococcal disease in the other. In the third instance the patient had a known idiopathic seizure disorder and suffered a seizure after initiation of foscarnet therapy. The occurrence of seizures in this study suggests that foscarnet may lower the seizure threshold in those who are already predisposed.[11,21] Seizures have also been reported in several patients with elevated serum levels of foscarnet due to administration of inappropriately large doses. In a randomized trial comparing initial therapy of foscarnet with ganciclovir for the treatment of CMV retinitis, 39 of 107 (36%) patients required switching from foscarnet to ganciclovir, 22 of 39 for drug-related toxicity, and 9 of 39 for progression of retinitis,[21] demonstrating that foscarnet is generally less well tolerated than ganciclovir.

In regard to abnormalities in serum electrolytes, one study reported low serum ionized calcium in six patients immediately after foscarnet infusion, although total serum calcium remained normal.[92] The combination of foscarnet with intravenous pentamidine was associated with severe hypocalcemia in four patients with AIDS and *P. carinii* pneumonia. After discontinuing one of the drugs, the serum calcium level returned to normal in three patients, but the fourth patient died with severe hypocalcemia.[93] Other less commonly occurring adverse experiences associated with foscarnet therapy include genital and oral ulcerations, generalized cutaneous rash, and nephrogenic diabetes insipidus.

Intravitreal Administration

Intravitreal injections of foscarnet have also been used to treat CMV retinitis in persons unable or unwilling to tolerate systemic foscarnet.[94] The regimen of two injections, 2400 μg of foscarnet per injection given for 2 to 3 weeks during an induction period followed by weekly maintenance injections, is similar to that of ganciclovir. This alternative therapy appears to be as effective and safe as intravitreal ganciclovir for preventing the progression of CMV infection, but there are few published long-term data available.

Cidofovir

Initial Studies

Cidofovir, a nucleotide analogue with activity against all herpesviruses, was licensed for the treatment of CMV retinitis in 1996. Though the terminal $t_{1/2}$ of cidofovir is approximately 2.6 hours, a fraction of the drug appears to be excreted in a slow elimination phase, suggesting that phosphorylated metabolites of cidofovir may have long intracellular half-lives.[95] Early data suggested that clinically tolerated effective doses of cidofovir could be administered as infrequently as every 2 weeks.[96,97] Nephrotoxicity was found to be a relatively common toxicity of cidofovir therapy, and it was necessary to administer saline hydration and large doses of probenecid around the time of infusion of cidofovir to block the uptake of cidofovir by the proximal renal tubular cells.[96,97]

Two randomized, clinical trials have been conducted comparing intravenous cidofovir with deferred therapy in persons with advanced HIV infection and peripheral CMV retinitis (Table 43–1).[22,98] In the first trial, using a previously established trial design,[11,20] persons were randomized to receive immediate therapy (n = 25) with cidofovir 5 mg/kg IV weekly for 2 weeks for induction therapy, then every 2 weeks for maintenance (with probenecid on the day of infusion, 2 g PO 3 hours prior to infusion and 1 g 2 and 8 hours after infusion), or deferred treatment (n = 23) until progression of retinitis. Progression of retinitis was documented by masked reading of retinal photographs. The median time to progression of CMV retinitis was 120 days in the immediate treatment group compared with 22 days in the deferred treatment group ($P < 0.001$). Asymptomatic neutropenia and proteinuria occurred in 15% and 12% of patients, respectively. Cidofovir was discontinued in 10 of 41 patients (24%) because of treatment-limiting nephrotoxicity. Mild to moderate constitutional symptoms or nausea occurred in 23 of 41 patients (56%), but they were treatment-limiting in only 3 (7%).

Using similar eligibility criteria, the second trial randomized patients to: (1) deferred treatment (n = 26); (2) high-dose treatment using the same dose of cidofovir as in the first trial (n = 12); and (3) low-dose treatment with cidofovir 5 mg/kg weekly for 2 weeks then 3 mg/kg every 2 weeks for maintenance.[98] Probenecid was given on the day of cidofovir administration using the same regimen as the first trial. The median time to progression was 21 days in the deferred treatment group and 64 days in the low-dose treatment group; progression had not yet recurred in the high-dose treatment group at the time of data closure. Patients receiving cidofovir in this trial also developed a significant incidence of proteinuria and reactions to probenecid; the data suggested that the use of probenecid, hydration, and careful monitoring of patients receiving cidofovir may have minimized but not prevented nephrotoxicity.[98] Four patients on this trial were noted to have ocular hypotony, defined as an intraocular pressure of less than 5 mm Hg and a decrease by at least 50% from baseline.

Another report has raised a concern about the development of iritis in association with the administration of cidofovir.[99] Iritis, defined as an increase in anterior chamber cells accompanied by photophobia, redness, pain, or blurred vision, occurred in 11 of 43 persons (26%) receiving cidofovir in three medical centers. Most patients with iritis were successfully managed with topical corticosteroids and cycloplegics and were able to continue to receive cidofovir. The development of iritis in association with cidofovir was potentially confounded by the use of protease inhibitors in 10 of the 11 persons with iritis, suggesting that the inflammatory response may be a therapeutic response to the institution of HAART rather than drug toxicity due to cidofovir.[99] It is of note that 4 of the 11 patients with iritis also developed hypotony (low intraocular pressure). The hypotony was associated with clinically significant events including choroidal or retinal detachments, a macular fold, or a reduction in visual acuity in five of the six eyes (two persons had bilateral hypotony).

The data from the two randomized clinical trials suggest that cidofovir is at least as effective as ganciclovir or foscarnet for controlling CMV retinitis, but it has not been compared directly to these agents in controlled clinical trials, and the results of analysis of the time-to-progression curves were somewhat different in the different studies.[11,20,22,98] The incidence of treatment-limiting toxicities of cidofovir (or probenecid) may be greater than those of ganciclovir or foscarnet, but the convenience of an every-2-week therapy compared with daily intravenous therapy and the need to maintain a chronic indwelling catheter for ganciclovir or foscarnet is a major advantage for the use of cidofovir (Table 43–1). Close monitoring of renal function and ocular pressure is required when administering cidofovir.

Few clinical data on the efficacy of cidofovir for extraocular CMV disease are available. Intravenous cidofovir appears to be ineffective in suppressing CMV viremia.[22,97,98] Treatment of extraocular CMV diseases with cidofovir should not be routinely attempted.

Intravitreal Administration

Similar to ganciclovir and foscarnet, cidofovir has been administered effectively by the intravitreal route.[100] Cidofovir, 20 μg intravitreally (with probenecid, as with intravenous administration of cidofovir) was administered to 32 eyes of 22 patients at 5- to 6-week intervals for a mean follow-up period of 15.3 weeks (range 5 to 44 weeks). Only 2 of 32 eyes developed progression of CMV retinitis during the study period. Mild iritis developed after 14 of 101 injections (14%) that had been preceded by the administration of probenecid but responded within 2 weeks to topical steroids and cycloplegics. Two cases of hypotony (6%) requiring treatment discontinuation and associated with significant visual loss, one irreversible, occurred. The incidence of visual loss from hypotony precludes the routine intravitreal use of cidofovir.

Intravitreal Fomivirsen

Fomivirsen is an oligonucleotide antisense compound that can only be administered intravitreally. It is indicated in persons with CMV retinitis intolerant of or resistant to other therapies.[101] Fomivirsen is given by intravitreal injections of 0.05 ml (330 μg) every 2 weeks for two doses, then every 4 weeks. Contraindications include hypersensitivity to fomivirsen or receipt of intravenous or intravitreal administration of cidofovir within the previous 2 to 4 weeks. Side effects include abnormal or blurred vision, eye pain, ocular inflammation, and increased intraocular pressure. In persons with unilateral, peripheral CMV retinitis, treatment with fomivirsen 165 μg weekly for 3 weeks and then every other week resulted in a median time-to-disease progression of 71 days compared to 14 days for persons in whom therapy was delayed until the CMV retinitis progressed. In persons with sight-threatening, refractory CMV retinitis, treatment with fomivirsen 330 μg weekly for 2 to 3 weeks and then every 2 to 4 weeks resulted in a median time-to-disease progression of 90 days, significantly delaying disease progression.[102]

Drug Resistance

With the increased use of ganciclovir and the use of it for longer periods of time due to the improved survival of persons with AIDS, ganciclovir-resistant CMV has been reported with increasing frequency.[103] In one study of 72 CMV-viruric AIDS patients treated with ganciclovir for CMV disease and followed prospectively for the development of ganciclovir-resistant CMV, no resistant strains of CMV were found in 31 randomly chosen patients before therapy or 7 culture-positive patients treated for less than 3 months.[104] After 3 months of therapy, only 20% of persons remained culture-positive; 5 of 13 (38%) randomly chosen positives, or 8% overall, were found to have ganciclovir-resistant strains with an IC_{50} higher than 12 μM. However, there appears to be a decreasing sensitivity of strains of CMV to ganciclovir in persons receiving the drug for extended periods, suggesting that the progressive shortening of the time between relapses of CMV retinitis may be due in part to decreasing sensitivity of the virus.[105] In a cohort of persons with CMV retinitis followed at a single site, CMV developed resistance to ganciclovir at a rate of approximately 11% at 6 months and 28% at 9 months of continuous therapy with ganciclovir.[106] Low-level ganciclovir resistance (IC_{50} 8 to 30 μM) is mediated by mutations in the UL97 viral phosphotransferase gene, whereas high-level ganciclovir resistance ($IC_{50} > 30$ μM) is mediated predominantly by combined UL97 and UL54 viral DNA polymerase gene mutations.[107]

Treatment with foscarnet has been successful for ganciclovir-resistant CMV retinitis.[108] The development of foscarnet-resistant strains of CMV are directly related to duration of therapy, and they appear at a rate of approximately 26% after 6 months and 37% after 9 months of continuous therapy.[109] Unlike ganciclovir, foscarnet does not require viral phosphotransferase to be activated, so low-level ganciclovir-resistant isolates are usually sensitive to foscarnet.[110] Resistance to foscarnet is mediated largely by mutations in the CMV polymerase gene but at a site distinct from those that mediate high-level resistance to ganciclovir and cidofovir.[111] Most isolates of CMV resistant to ganciclovir and cidofovir are likely to be sensitive to foscarnet.

Resistance mutations in the CMV polymerase gene causing resistance to ganciclovir overlap those of cidofovir, suggesting that persons with CMV with high-level resistance to ganciclovir may also be resistant to cidofovir. Strains of CMV with low-level resistance to ganciclovir (due to CMV protein kinase mutations) are likely to be susceptible to cidofovir.[107] Foscarnet may be used for strains of CMV resistant to ganciclovir and cidofovir.[111]

Salvage Therapy for Cytomegalovirus Retinitis

Despite continued therapy with prolonged maintenance doses of therapeutic agents, most persons with CMV retinitis develop progression of their disease. Simple progressions can be treated with reinduction doses of any of the agents, though successive progressions of retinitis occur at progressively shorter intervals. In a CMV retinitis retreatment trial, there appeared to be no benefit when switching from ganciclovir to foscarnet or from foscarnet to ganciclovir in individuals who developed early progression of their CMV retinitis.[112] Higher doses of ganciclovir have been safely administered, though often in conjunction with colony-stimulating factors to prevent neutropenia. Doses up to 10 mg/kg IV twice daily can be given and may overcome low-level resistance due to protein kinase mutations but are not likely to overcome high-level resistance due to polymerase mutations.[107,111] Higher doses of foscarnet and cidofovir are difficult to administer owing to the potential for nephrotoxicity of these agents.

In persons intolerant to intravenous therapy, the ganciclovir implant may be useful for treating progressive disease. It should be used with caution, however, in individuals who have received intravenous ganciclovir for an extended period and may be resistant to ganciclovir. In these individuals, it may be prudent to administer a test dose of intravitreal ganciclovir and monitor the response prior to subjecting patients to the surgical procedure of inserting the implant.

Laboratory data have suggested that the co-administration of ganciclovir and foscarnet have synergistic activity against CMV,[113] prompting initiation of a clinical trial of this combination for persons whose CMV retinitis progressed through continued monotherapy with either ganciclovir or foscarnet.[112] In this controlled clinical trial, patients with progressive CMV retinitis were randomized to receive high-dose ganciclovir (n = 94), high-dose foscarnet (n = 89), or a combination regimen of standard doses of ganciclovir and foscarnet (n = 96). Persons receiving the combination regimen had a longer time to progression (median 4.3 months) compared with persons receiving ganciclovir (2.0 months) or foscarnet (1.3 months) ($P < 0.001$). Though persons did not have any significant laboratory toxicities associated with the combination therapy compared with either monotherapy, there was a significant adverse effect on quality of life in persons receiving combination therapy due to the requirement for two intravenous infusions daily.[112]

▲ CONTRIBUTION TO MORTALITY OF CMV IN PERSONS WITH AIDS

Before 1988 the survival of individuals diagnosed with CMV retinitis in conjunction with HIV infection ranged from 1 to 6 months.[60,113–115] With the increasing familiarity with the diagnosis of this CMV disease and the availability of ganciclovir after 1988 to treat it, survival after diagnosis of CMV retinitis increased to 5 to 13 months.[21,115,116] Two of these studies have suggested a survival benefit in patients treated with ganciclovir compared with untreated patients or patients not responding to ganciclovir. Holland et al. reported that patients treated with ganciclovir survived a median of 7 months compared with untreated patients, who survived a median of only 2 months.[115] Jabs et al. reported that patients who responded to treatment with ganciclovir had a median survival of 10.0 months, compared with a median survival of only 2.3 months among patients who did not have a complete response.[117] A retrospective study evaluating the effect of foscarnet on survival found no difference in the median survival time from the diagnosis of CMV retinitis between patients treated with ganciclovir (8 months, n = 56) and those treated with foscarnet (9 months, n = 21).[116] In a randomized clinical trial of initial therapy with ganciclovir compared with foscarnet for the treatment of CMV retinitis, persons randomized to the foscarnet arm of the trial (n = 107) had a significantly increased survival (12.6 months) compared with those randomized to the ganciclovir arm (8.5 months, n = 127).[21] This increase in survival was not confounded by the differential use of specific antiretroviral agents. A long-term follow-up of the randomized foscarnet trial independently corroborated the extended survival of foscarnet-treated persons with a median survival of that cohort of 13.5 months.[118] Much of this survival difference will change based on the use of more HAART for HIV infection. At present, the use of HAART has enabled persons with CMV retinitis and AIDS to discontinue therapy for CMV retinitis; the median survival in persons with CMV retinitis who have responded to HAART has not been determined.

▲ NEW ANTI-CMV AGENTS

The current therapies for CMV infection all suffer from significant toxicities and limited efficacy.[119] A number of novel, potentially effective compounds are in preclinical and clinical evaluation. Unfortunately, none of these agents is sufficiently advanced in its development to suggest that it may be available within the next 2 years.[120] An orally bioavailable benzimidazole riboside 1263W94 has potent, selective activity in vitro against CMV by inhibiting CMV DNA synthesis via a mechanism that does not require phosphorylation and does not involve DNA polymerase. Clinical CMV isolates resistant to ganciclovir appear to be susceptible to 1263W94.[121] Methylenecyclopropane analogues of nucleosides have now been tested against clinical isolates of human CMV and have demonstrated activity comparable to that of ganciclovir, suggesting the need for further evaluation of these and similar compounds.[122]

▲ PREVENTION

Primary Disease

In the first prospective, double-blind study to be completed for prophylaxis of CMV disease, 725 HIV-infected persons with advanced disease were randomized to receive either oral ganciclovir (1 g PO three times daily) or placebo.[123] At 18 months, CMV disease, retinitis, and colitis occurred, respectively, in 39%, 39%, and 4% of persons receiving placebo but in only 20%, 18%, and 2%, respectively, of patients treated with ganciclovir. A second study failed to show that oral ganciclovir was beneficial, but this study was limited by lack of routine ophthalmologic examinations and perhaps a lower rate of ascertainment of endpoints.[124] There is no role for acyclovir in the therapy or prevention of CMV disease in persons with HIV infection.

The 2001 U.S. Public Health Service/Infections Disease Society of America (USPHS/IDSA) guidelines for the pre-

Table 43–6. FOLLOW-UP OF PATIENTS WITH CMV RETINITIS WHO DISCONTINUED MAINTENANCE THERAPY DUE TO IMMUNE RECONSTITUTION

Study	No. of Patients	CD4+ T-Lymphocyte Count (cells/μl): Required for Inclusion in Study	CD4+ T-Lymphocyte Count (cells/μl): Median Count at Study Entry	Median Duration of HAART at Study Entry (months)	Median Duration of Follow-up (months)	Relapses (no.)
Tural[126]	7	> 150	233	NR	9	0
MacDonald[127]	22	> 50	161	NR	16	3
Whitcup[128]	14	> 150	315	NR	18	0
Jabs[129]	15	> 100	297	17.0	8	0
Jouan[130]	48	> 75	239	18.0	11	2
Berenguer[131]	36	> 100	287	17.5	21	1

HAART, highly active antiretroviral therapy; NR, not reported.

vention of opportunistic infections in persons infected with HIV recommended that prophylaxis with oral ganciclovir be considered an option for HIV-infected patients who are CMV-seropositive with fewer than 50 CD4+ T-lymphocytes per microliter, but that it should not be considered the standard of care.[125] Despite some indications that primary prophylaxis could prevent disease, this intervention was not recommended because: (1) long-term vision does not differ in patients who receive prophylaxis compared to those whose disease is treated when it occurs; (2) the regimen is expensive; (3) the regimen requires taking 12 large tablets per day, which is difficult for adherence; (4) chronic therapy would be likely to induce resistance; and (5) chronic therapy would be associated with toxicities such as cytopenia. The availability of valganciclovir offers a drug that would be easier to take (i.e., fewer pills per day). However, the impact of chronic therapy for primary prophylaxis on long-term vision as well as cost, adherence, toxicity, and resistance remain issues that are likely to deter health care providers and patients from undertaking primary prophylaxis with this agent. If patients at especially high risk could be identified among those with very low CD4+ T-lymphocyte counts (e.g., by quantitative PCR) then primary prophylaxis (or preemptive therapy) might be more attractive.

The most important intervention to prevent CMV disease is maintenance of the individual's CD4+ T-lymphocyte count above 100 cells per microliter, most often with the use of HAART.

Secondary Disease (Maintenance Therapy)

As already noted, once CMV retinitis occurs, it is likely to recur promptly in patients with persistently low CD4+ T-lymphocyte counts unless maintenance therapy is administered. CMV disease of other organs is also likely to recur, although the limited data available suggest that recurrence is not as frequent as with retinitis. The maintenance regimens recommended are listed in Table 43–1.

Some individuals with advanced HIV infection and CMV retinitis who have had immune reconstitution in response to potent antiretroviral therapy manifested by sustained increases in their CD4+ T-lymphocyte counts to more than 100 to 150 cells per microliter have discontinued their maintenance CMV therapy and have not had progression of disease for up to 12 months (Table 43–6).[126–134] Follow-up of these case series (presented in abstract form) have suggested that the progression CMV retinitis can be delayed or prevented for more than 3 years with judicious use of potent antiretroviral therapy.[135] The USPHS/IDSA guidelines recommended that discontinuation of maintenance therapy for CMV retinitis should be considered in patients with sustained increases in CD4+ T-lymphocyte counts to these levels.[125] Decisions to discontinue therapy should be made in consultation with an ophthalmologist and should evaluate factors such as the magnitude and duration of the CD4+ T-lymphocyte count increase, the anatomic location and extent of the retinitis, vision in the contralateral eye, and the availability of regular ophthalmologic evaluation. Relapses have generally occurred when the CD4+ T-lymphocyte counts have dropped below 50 cells per microliter.[136] Relapses have occurred in persons with CD4+ T-lymphocyte counts higher than 100 cells per microliter as well, but to date such relapses have been highly unusual.[137]

IMMUNE RECOVERY UVEITIS

The ability to discontinue specific anti-CMV therapy is not without its problems. The immune reconstitution associated with the use of HAART has also been associated with the development of an immune recovery-associated uveitis.[138,139] This entity is characterized by posterior segment inflammation, including vitreitis, papillitis, and optic disk and macular edema. Clinically important complications of immune-recovery uveitis included cataract and epiretinal membrane formation and loss of visual acuity. This entity is common in persons with CMV retinitis who have substantial increases in their CD4+ T-lymphocyte counts. One study diagnosed this problem in 19 of 30 patients (63%) responding to HAART with an annual incidence of 83 per 100 person-years.[138] A second study found evidence of intraocular inflammation in 22 of 23 eyes, with CMV retinitis in 16 patients who discontinued CMV therapy after responding to HAART.[139]

A third study found immune recovery uveitis much less frequently; only 6 persons among 33 responding to HAART were found to have immune recovery uveitis, for an incidence of 11 per 100 person-years.[140] This lower rate may be related to a less dramatic response to HAART in this population and the retrospective nature of the study.[140]

▲ SCREENING FOR DISEASE DUE TO CMV

There is no consensus regarding the screening of persons for CMV disease. The diseases rarely occur in persons with more than 100 CD4+ T-lymphocytes per microliter,[2,7,8] so screening these persons seems not to be cost or time-effective. Screening blood and urine cultures for CMV has poor specificity and poor sensitivity for detecting persons who will subsequently develop CMV disease.[12,13] The early diagnosis of CMV colitis or esophagitis before the onset of moderate to severe symptoms is unlikely to benefit most patients because, due to the toxicities of the agents available for treatment, most patients tolerate mild disease before beginning therapy. Additionally, because the cells that line the colon and esophagus reproduce rapidly, later treatment with ganciclovir or foscarnet usually produces no permanent morbidity.

The early diagnosis of CMV retinitis is more important. Because retinal cells do not regenerate, delay in diagnosis can lead to spread of the disease and permanent loss of vision. Early diagnosis is critical to the management of CMV retinitis. Many experts recommend a baseline dilated ophthalmologic examination by the time the CD4+ T-lymphocyte count falls below 100 cells per microliter. Because most persons with CMV retinitis present with some symptoms (either vision changes or "floaters") it is most important to query patients about any subtle visual changes, discuss with susceptible persons the early signs of CMV disease, and bring them to the attention of their health care provider. Some experienced clinicians recommend to their patients that they test their own visual fields using standard grids, and others have dilated ophthalmologic examinations performed on their patients with low CD4+ T-lymphocyte counts every 2 to 3 months. Whether these routines are better than close questioning about visual symptoms is unknown.

REFERENCES

1. Kaplan JE, Hanson DL, Dworkin MS, et al. Epidemiology of human immunodeficiency virus-associated opportunistic infections in the United States in the era of highly active antiretroviral therapy. Clin Infect Dis 30:S5–S14, 2000.
2. Gallant JE, Moore RD, Richman DD, et al. Zidovudine Epidemiology Study Group: incidence and natural history of cytomegalovirus disease in patients with advanced human immunodeficiency virus disease treated with zidovudine. J Infect Dis 166:1223–1227, 1992.
3. Whitley RJ, Jacobson MA, Friedberg DN, et al. Guidelines for the treatment of cytomegalovirus diseases in patients with AIDS in the era of potent antiretroviral therapy: recommendations of an international panel. Arch Intern Med 158:957–969, 1998.
4. Griffiths PD, Emery VC. Cytomegalovirus. In: Richman DD, Whitley RJ, Hayden FG (eds) Clinical Virology. New York, Churchill Livingstone, 1997, p 445–470.
5. Bloom JN, Palestine AG. The diagnosis of cytomegalovirus retinitis. Ann Intern Med 109:963–969, 1988.
6. Drew WL. Cytomegalovirus infection in patients with AIDS. Clin Infect Dis 14:608–615, 1992.
7. Crowe SM, Carlin JB, Stewart KI, et al. Predictive value of CD4 lymphocyte numbers for the development of opportunistic infections and malignancies in HIV-infected persons. J Acquir Immune Defic Syndr 4:770–776, 1991.
8. Pertel P, Hirschtick R, Phair J, et al. Risk of developing cytomegalovirus retinitis in persons infected with the human immunodeficiency virus. J Acquir Immune Defic Syndr 5:1069–1074, 1992.
9. Hoover DR, Saah AJ, Bacellar H, et al. Clinical manifestations of AIDS in the era of Pneumocystis prophylaxis. N Engl J Med 329:1922–1926, 1993.
10. Jacobson MA, Mills J. Serious cytomegalovirus disease in the acquired immunodeficiency syndrome (AIDS): clinical findings, diagnosis, and treatment. Ann Intern Med 108:585–594, 1988.
11. Palestine AG, Polis MA, De Smet MD, et al. A randomized, controlled trial of foscarnet in the treatment of cytomegalovirus retinitis in patients with AIDS. Ann Intern Med 115:665–673, 1991.
12. Zurlo JJ, O'Neill D, Polis MA, et al. Lack of clinical utility of cytomegalovirus blood and urine cultures in patients with HIV infection. Ann Intern Med 118:12–17, 1993.
13. Salmon D, Lacassin F, Harzic M, et al. Predictive value of cytomegalovirus viraemia for the occurrence of CMV organ involvement in AIDS. J Med Virol 32:160–163, 1990.
14. Bowen EF, Sabin CA, Wilson P, et al. Cytomegalovirus (CMV) viraemia detected by polymerase chain reaction identifies a group of HIV-positive patients at high risk of CMV disease. AIDS 11:889–893, 1997.
15. Shinkai M, Bozzette SA, Powderly W, et al. Utility of urine and leukocyte cultures and plasma DNA polymerase chain reaction for identification of AIDS patients at risk for developing human cytomegalovirus disease. J Infect Dis 175:302–308, 1997.
16. Spector SA, Wong R, Hsia K, et al. Plasma cytomegalovirus (CMV) DNA load predicts CMV disease and survival in AIDS patients. J Clin Invest 101:497–502, 1998.
17. Freeman WR, Henderly DE, Wan WL, et al. Prevalence, pathophysiology, and treatment of rhegmatogenous retinal detachment in treated cytomegalovirus retinitis. Am J Ophthalmol 103:527–536, 1987.
18. Jabs DA, Enger C, Haller J, deBustros S. Retinal detachments in patients with cytomegalovirus retinitis. Arch Ophthalmol 109:794–799, 1991.
19. Kempen JH, Jabs DA, Dunn JP, et al. Retinal detachment risk in cytomegalovirus retinitis related to the acquired immunodeficiency syndrome. Arch Ophthalmol 119:33–40, 2001.
20. Spector SA, Weingeist T, Pollard RB, et al. A randomized, controlled study of intravenous ganciclovir therapy for with cytomegalovirus peripheral retinitis in patients with AIDS. J Infect Dis 168:557–563, 1993.
21. Studies of the Ocular Complications of AIDS Research Group, AIDS Clinical Trials Group. Mortality in patients with the acquired immunodeficiency syndrome treated with either foscarnet or ganciclovir for cytomegalovirus retinitis. N Engl J Med 326:213–220, 1992.
22. Lalezari JP, Stagg RJ, Kuppermann BD, et al. Intravenous cidofovir for peripheral CMV retinitis in patients with AIDS. Ann Intern Med 126:257–263, 1997.
23. Holland G, Shuler JD. Progression rates of cytomegalovirus retinopathy in ganciclovir-treated and untreated patients. Arch Ophthalmol 110:1435–1442, 1992.
24. De Smet MD. Differential diagnosis of retinitis and choroiditis in patients with acquired immunodeficiency syndrome. Am J Med 92(suppl 2A):17S–21S, 1992.
25. O'Donnell JJ, Jacobson MA. Cotton-wool spots and cytomegalovirus in AIDS. Int Ophthalmol Clin 29:105–107, 1987.
26. Engstrom RE, Holland GN, Margolis TP, et al. The progressive outer retinal necrosis syndrome: a variant of necrotizing herpetic retinopathy in patients with AIDS. Ophthalmology 101:1488–1502, 1994.
27. Holland GN, Engstrom RE, Glasgow BJ, et al. Ocular toxoplasmosis in patients with the acquired immunodeficiency syndrome. Am J Ophthalmol 106:653–657, 1988.
28. Dugel PU, Rao NA, Forester DJ. *Pneumocystis carinii* choroiditis after long-term aerosolized pentamidine therapy. Am J Ophthalmol 110:113–117, 1990.
29. Wilcox CM, Diehl DL, Cello JP, et al. Cytomegalovirus esophagitis in patients with AIDS: a clinical, endoscopic, and pathologic correlation. Ann Intern Med 113:589–593, 1990.
30. Dieterich DT, Wilcox CM. Diagnosis and treatment of esophageal diseases associated with HIV infection. Am J Gastroenterol 91:2265–2269, 1996.

31. Wilcox CM. Esophageal disease in the acquired immunodeficiency syndrome: etiology, diagnosis, and management. Am J Med 92:412–421, 1992.
32. Porro GB, Parente F, Cernuschi M. The diagnosis of esophageal candidiasis in patients with acquired immune deficiency syndrome: is endoscopy always necessary? Am J Gastroenterol 84:143–146, 1989.
33. Dieterich DT, Rahmin M. Cytomegalovirus colitis in AIDS: presentation in 44 patients and a review of the literature. J Acquir Immune Defic Syndr 4(suppl 1):S29–S35, 1991.
34. Frager DH, Frager JD, Wolf EL, et al. Cytomegalovirus colitis in acquired immune deficiency syndrome: radiologic spectrum. Gastrointest Radiol 11:241–246, 1986.
35. Smith PD, Lane HC, Gill VJ, et al. Intestinal infections in patients with the acquired immunodeficiency syndrome (AIDS). Ann Intern Med 108:328–333, 1988.
36. Wallace JM, Hannah J. Cytomegalovirus pneumonitis in patients with AIDS: findings in an autopsy series. Chest 82:198–203, 1987.
37. Jacobson MA, Mills J, Rush J, et al. Morbidity and mortality of patients with AIDS and first-episode *Pneumocystis carinii* pneumonia unaffected by concomitant pulmonary cytomegalovirus infection. Am Rev Respir Dis 144:6–9, 1991.
38. Rodriguez-Barradas MC, Stool E, Musher DM, et al. Diagnosing and treating cytomegalovirus pneumonia in patients with AIDS. Clin Infect Dis 23:76–81, 1996.
39. Petito CK, Cho ES, Lemann W, et al. Neuropathology of acquired immunodeficiency syndrome (AIDS): an autopsy review. J Neuropathol Exp Neurol 45:635–646, 1986.
40. Morgello S, Cho ES, Nielsen S, et al. Cytomegalovirus encephalitis in patients with acquired immunodeficiency syndrome: an autopsy study of 30 cases and a review of the literature. Hum Pathol 18:289–297, 1987.
41. Kalayjian RC, Cohen ML, Bonomo RA, Flanigan TP. Cytomegalovirus ventriculoencephalitis in AIDS: a syndrome with distinct clinical and pathological features. Medicine (Baltimore) 72:67–77, 1993.
42. Holland NR, Power C, Mathews VP, et al. Cytomegalovirus encephalitis in acquired immunodeficiency syndrome (AIDS). Neurology 44:507–514, 1994.
43. Arribas JR, Storch GA, Clifford DB, Tselis AC. Cytomegalovirus encephalitis. Ann Intern Med 125:577–587, 1996.
44. Arribas JR, Clifford DB, Fichtenbaum CJ, et al. Level of cytomegalovirus (CMV) DNA in cerebrospinal fluid of subjects with AIDS and CMV infection of the central nervous system. J Infect Dis 172:527–531, 1995.
45. Wolf DG, Spector SA. Diagnosis of human cytomegalovirus central nervous system disease in AIDS patients by DNA amplification from cerebrospinal fluid. J Infect Dis 166:1412–1415, 1992.
46. Behar R, Wiley C, McCutchan JA. Cytomegalovirus polyradiculopathy in acquired immune deficiency syndrome. Neurology 37:557–561, 1987.
47. McCutchan JA. Cytomegalovirus infections of the nervous system in patients with AIDS. Clin Infect Dis 20:747–754, 1995.
48. Olney RK. Acute lumbosacral polyradiculopathy in acquired immunodeficiency syndrome: experience in 23 patients. Ann Neurol 35:53–58, 1994.
49. Miller RF, Fox JD, Thomas P, et al. Acute lumbosacral polyradiculopathy due to cytomegalovirus in advanced HIV disease: CSF findings in 17 patients. J Neurol Neurosurg Psychiatry 61:456–460, 1996.
50. McKenzie R, Travis WD, Dolan SA, et al. The causes of death in patients with human immunodeficiency virus infection: a clinical and pathologic study with emphasis on the role of pulmonary diseases. Medicine (Baltimore) 70:326–343, 1991.
51. Bricaire F, Marche C, Zoubi D, et al. Adrenocortical lesions and AIDS [letter]. Lancet 1:881, 1988.
52. Greene LW, Cole W, Greene LB, et al. Adrenal insufficiency as a complication of the acquired immunodeficiency syndrome. Ann Intern Med 101:497–498, 1984.
53. Blanshard C. Treatment of HIV-related cytomegalovirus disease of the gastrointestinal tract with foscarnet. J Acquir Immun Defic Syndr 5(suppl 1):S25–S28, 1992.
54. Littler E, Stuart AD, Chee MS. Human cytomegalovirus UL97 open reading frame encodes a protein that phosphorylates the antiviral nucleoside analogue ganciclovir. Nature 358:160–162, 1992.
55. Sullivan V, Talarico CL, Stanat SC, et al. A protein kinase homologue controls phosphorylation of ganciclovir in human cytomegalovirus-infected cells. Nature 358:162–164, 1992.
56. Drew WL, Ives D, Lalezari JP, et al. Oral ganciclovir as maintenance treatment for cytomegalovirus retinitis in patients with AIDS. N Engl J Med 333:615–620, 1995.
57. Sommadossi JP, Bevan R, Ling T, et al. Clinical pharmacokinetics of ganciclovir in patients with normal and impaired renal function. Rev Infect Dis 10(suppl 3):S507–S514, 1988.
58. Faulds D, Heel RC. Ganciclovir: a review of its antiviral activity, pharmacokinetic properties and therapeutic efficacy in cytomegalovirus infections. Drugs 4:597–638, 1990.
59. Buhles WC, Mastre BJ, Tinker AJ, et al. Ganciclovir treatment of life- or sight-threatening cytomegalovirus infection: experience in 314 immunocompromised patients. Rev Infect Dis 10(suppl 3):S495–S504, 1988.
60. Palestine AG, Rodrigues MM, Macher AM, et al. Ophthalmic involvement in acquired immunodeficiency syndrome. Ophthalmology 91:1092–1099, 1984.
61. Jacobson MA, O'Donnell JJ, Mills J. Foscarnet treatment of cytomegalovirus retinitis in patients with the acquired immunodeficiency syndrome. Antimicrob Agents Chemother 33:736–741, 1989.
62. Dieterich DT, Kotler DP, Busch DF, et al. Ganciclovir treatment of cytomegalovirus colitis in AIDS: a randomized, double-blind, placebo-controlled multicenter study. J Infect Dis 167:278–282, 1993.
63. Blanshard C, Benhamou Y, Dohin E, et al. Treatment of AIDS-associated gastrointestinal cytomegalovirus infection with foscarnet and ganciclovir: a randomized comparison. J Infect Dis 172:622–628, 1995.
64. Emanuel D, Cunningham I, Jules-Elysee K, et al. Cytomegalovirus pneumonia after bone-marrow transplantation successfully treated with the combination of ganciclovir and high-dose intravenous immune globulin. Ann Intern Med 109:777–782, 1988.
65. Reed EC, Bowden RA, Dandliker PS, et al. Treatment of cytomegalovirus pneumonia with ganciclovir and intravenous cytomegalovirus immunoglobulin in patients with bone marrow transplants. Ann Intern Med 109:783–788, 1988.
66. Jacobson MA, O'Donnell JJ, Rousell R, et al. Failure of adjunctive cytomegalovirus intravenous immune globulin to improve efficacy of ganciclovir in patients with acquired immunodeficiency syndrome and cytomegalovirus retinitis: a phase I study. Antimicrob Agents Chemother 34:176–178, 1990.
67. Anduze-Faris BM, Fillet AM, Gozlan J, et al. Induction and maintenance therapy of cytomegalovirus central nervous system infection in HIV-infected patients. AIDS 14:517–524, 1999.
68. Hochster H, Dieterich D, Bozzette S, et al. Toxicity of combined ganciclovir and zidovudine for cytomegalovirus disease associated with AIDS. Ann Intern Med 113:111–117, 1990.
69. Medina DJ, Hsiung GD, Mellors JW. Ganciclovir antagonizes the anti-human immunodeficiency virus activity of zidovudine and didanosine in vitro. Antimicrob Agents Chemother 36:1127–1130, 1992.
70. Cantrill HL, Henry K, Melroe NH, et al. Treatment of cytomegalovirus retinitis with intravitreal ganciclovir: long-term results. Ophthalmology 69:367–374, 1989.
71. Henry K, Cantrill H, Fletcher C, et al. Use of intravitreal ganciclovir (dihydroxy propoxymethyl guanine) for cytomegalovirus retinitis in a patient with AIDS. Am J Ophthalmol 103:17–23, 1987.
72. Schulman J, Peyman GA, Horton MR, et al. Intraocular 9-([2-hydroxy-1-(hydroxymethyl) ethoxy] methyl) guanine levels after intravitreal and subconjunctival administration. Ophthalmic Surg 17:429–432, 1986.
73. Martin DF, Parks DJ, Mellow SD, et al. Treatment of cytomegalovirus retinitis with an intraocular sustained-release ganciclovir implant. Arch Ophthalmol 112:1531–1539, 1994.
74. Musch DC, Martin DF, Gordon JF, et al. Treatment of cytomegalovirus retinitis with a sustained-release ganciclovir implant. N Engl J Med 337:83–90, 1997.
75. Martin D, Kuppermann B, Wolitz R, et al. Oral ganciclovir for patients with cytomegalovirus retinitis treated with a ganciclovir implant. N Engl J Med 340:1063–1070, 1999.
76. Anonymous. Valganciclovir, a more potent oral therapy for CMV retinitis in AIDS, approved by FDA. Clin Infect Dis 32:ii, 2001.
77. Brown F, Banken L, Saywell K, et al. Pharmacokinetics of valganciclovir and ganciclovir following multiple oral dosages of valganciclovir in HIV- and CMV-seropositive volunteers. Clin Pharmacokinet 37:167–176, 1999.
78. Martin DF, Sierra-Madero J, Walmsley S, et al. A controlled trial of valganciclovir as induction therapy for cytomegalovirus retinitis. N Engl J Med 346:1119–1126, 2002.

79. Food and Drug Administration. Antiviral Drugs Advisory Committee Meetings: valganciclovir. http : //www.fda.gov/cder/audiences/acspage/antiviral meetings1.htm, February 27, 2001.
80. Ostrander M, Cheng Y-C. Properties of herpes simplex virus type 1 and type 2 DNA polymerase. Biochim Biophys Acta 609:232–245, 1980.
81. Eriksson B, Öberg B, Wahren B. Pyrophosphate analogues as inhibitors of DNA polymerases of cytomegalovirus, herpes simplex virus and cellular origin, Biochim Biophys Acta 696:115–123, 1982.
82. Sandstrom EG, Byington RE, Kaplan JC, Hirsch MS. Inhibition of human T-cell lymphotrophic virus type III in vitro by phosphonoformate. Lancet 1:1480–1482, 1985.
83. Sjövall J, Karlsson A, Ogenstad S, et al. Pharmacokinetics and absorption of foscarnet after intravenous and oral administration to patients with human immunodeficiency virus. Clin Pharmacol Ther 44:65–73, 1988.
84. Aweeka F, Gambertoglio J, Mills J, Jacobson MA. Pharmacokinetics of intermittently administered intravenous foscarnet in the treatment of acquired immunodeficiency syndrome patients with serious cytomegalovirus retinitis. Antimicrob Agents Chemother 33:742–745, 1989.
85. Sjövall J, Bergdahl S, Movin G, et al. Pharmacokinetics of foscarnet and distribution to cerebrospinal fluid after intravenous infusion in patients with human immunodeficiency virus infection. Antimicrob Agents Chemother 33:1023–1031, 1989.
86. Oberg B. Antiviral effects of phosphonoformate (PFA, foscarnet sodium). Pharmacol Ther 19:387–415, 1989.
87. Deray G, Martinez F, Katlama C, et al. Foscarnet nephrotoxicity: mechanism, incidence, and prevention. Am J Nephrol 9:316–321, 1989.
88. Walmsley SL, Chew E, Read SE, et al. Treatment of cytomegalovirus retinitis with trisodium phosphonoformate hexahydrate (foscarnet). J Infect Dis 157:569–572, 1988.
89. Lehoang P, Girard B, Robinet M, et al. Foscarnet in the treatment of cytomegalovirus retinitis in acquired immune deficiency syndrome. Ophthalmology 96:865–874, 1989.
90. Fanning MM, Read SE, Benson M, et al. Foscarnet therapy of cytomegalovirus retinitis in AIDS. J Acquir Immune Defic Syndr 3:472–479, 1990.
91. Nelson MR, Connolly GM, Hawkins DA, Gazzard BG. Foscarnet in the treatment of cytomegalovirus infection of the esophagus and colon in patients with the acquired immune deficiency syndrome. Am J Gastroenterol 86:876–881, 1991.
92. Jacobson MA, Gambertoglio JG, Aweeka FT, et al. Foscarnet-induced hypocalcemia and effects of foscarnet on calcium metabolism. J Clin Endocrinol Metab 72:1130–1135, 1991.
93. Youle MS, Clarbour J, Gazzard B, Chanas A. Severe hypocalcaemia in AIDS patients treated with foscarnet and pentamidine. Lancet 1:1455–1456, 1988.
94. Díaz-Llopis M, Chipont E, Sanchez S, et al. Intravitreal foscarnet for cytomegalovirus retinitis in a patient with acquired immunodeficiency syndrome. Am J Ophthalmol 114:742–747, 1992.
95. Cundy KC, Petty BG, Flaherty J, et al. Clinical pharmacokinetics of cidofovir in human immunodeficiency virus-infected patients. Antimicrob Agents Chemother 115:686–688, 1995.
96. Lalezari JP, Drew Wl, Glutzer E, et al. (S)-1-[3-Hydroxy-2-(phosphonylmethoxy)propyl]cytosine (cidofovir): results of a phase I/II study of a novel antiviral nucleotide analogue. J Infect Dis 171:788–796, 1995.
97. Polis MA, Spooner KM, Baird BF, et al. Anticytomegaloviral activity and safety of cidofovir in patients with human immunodeficiency virus infection and cytomegalovirus viruria. Antimicrob Agents Chemother 39:882–886, 1995.
98. Studies of the Ocular Complications of AIDS Research Group in collaboration with the AIDS Clinical Trials Group: parenteral cidofovir for cytomegalovirus retinitis in patients with AIDS: the HPMPC peripheral cytomegalovirus retinitis trial. Ann Intern Med 126:264–274, 1997.
99. Davis JL, Taskintuna I, Freeman WR, et al. Iritis and hypotony after treatment with intravenous cidofovir for cytomegalovirus retinitis. Arch Ophthalmol 115:733–737, 1997.
100. Rahhal FM, Arevalo JF, Chavez de la Paz E, et al. Treatment of cytomegalovirus retinitis with intravitreous cidofovir in patients with AIDS: a preliminary report. Ann Intern Med 125:98–103, 1996.
101. DeSmet MD, Meenken CJ, van den Horn GJ. Fomivirsen: a phosphorothioate oligonucleotide for the treatment of CMV retinitis. Ocul Immunol Inflamm 7:189–198, 1999.
102. Perry CM, Balfour JAB. Formivirsen. Drugs 57:375–380, 1999.
103. Erice A, Chou S, Biron KK, et al. Progressive disease due to ganciclovir-resistant cytomegalovirus in immunocompromised patients. N Engl J Med 320:289–293, 1989.
104. Drew WL, Miner RC, Busch DF, et al. Prevalence of resistance in patients receiving ganciclovir for serious cytomegalovirus infection. J Infect Dis 163:716–719, 1991.
105. Studies of the Ocular Complications of AIDS (SOCA) in collaboration with the AIDS Clinical Trials Group: cytomegalovirus (CMV) culture results, drug resistance, and clinical outcome in patients with AIDS and CMV retinitis treated with foscarnet or ganciclovir. J Infect Dis 176:50–58, 1997.
106. Jabs DA, Enger C, Dunn JP, et al. Cytomegalovirus retinitis and viral resistance: ganciclovir resistance. J Infect Dis 177:770–773, 1998.
107. Smith IL, Cherrington JM, Jiles RE, et al. High-level resistance of cytomegalovirus to ganciclovir is associated with alterations in both the UL97 and DNA polymerase genes. J Infect Dis 176:69–77, 1997.
108. Jacobson MA, Drew WL, Feinberg J, et al. Foscarnet therapy for ganciclovir-resistant cytomegalovirus retinitis in patients with AIDS. J Infect Dis 163:1348–1351, 1991.
109. Jabs DA, Enger C, Forman M, et al. Incidence of foscarnet resistance and cidofovir resistance in patients treated for cytomegalovirus retinitis. Antimicrob Agents Chemother 42:2240–2244, 1998.
110. Erice A, Gil-Roda C, Perez JL, et al. Antiviral susceptibilities and analysis of UL97 and DNA polymerase sequences of clinical cytomegalovirus isolates from immunocompromised patients. J Infect Dis 175:1087–1092, 1997.
111. Baldanti F, Underwood MR, Stanat SC, et al. Single amino acid changes in the DNA polymerase confer foscarnet resistance and slow-growth phenotype, while mutations in the UL97-encoded phosphotransferase confer ganciclovir resistance in three double-resistant human cytomegalovirus strains recovered from patients with AIDS. J Virol 70:1390–1395, 1996.
112. Studies of Ocular Complications of AIDS Research Group, AIDS Clinical Trials Group. Combination foscarnet and ganciclovir therapy vs. monotherapy for the treatment of relapsed cytomegalovirus retinitis in patients with AIDS: the Cytomegalovirus Retreatment Trial. Arch Ophthalmol 114:23–33, 1996.
113. Henderly DE, Freeman WR, Causey DM, Rao NA. Cytomegalovirus retinitis and response to therapy with ganciclovir. Ophthalmology 94:425–434, 1987.
114. Jacobson MA, O'Donnell JJ, Porteous D, et al. Retinal and gastrointestinal disease due to cytomegalovirus in patients with the acquired immune deficiency syndrome: prevalence, natural history, and response to ganciclovir therapy. Q J Med 254:473–486, 1988.
115. Holland GN, Sison RF, Jatulis DE, et al. Survival of patients with the acquired immune deficiency syndrome after development of cytomegalovirus retinopathy. Ophthalmology 97:204–211, 1990.
116. Harb GE, Bacchetti P, Jacobson MA. Survival of patients with AIDS and cytomegalovirus disease treated with ganciclovir or foscarnet. AIDS 5:959–965, 1991.
117. Jabs DA, Enger C, Bartlett JG. Cytomegalovirus retinitis and acquired immunodeficiency syndrome. Ophthalmology 107:75–80, 1989.
118. Polis MA, De Smet MD, Baird BF, et al. Increased survival of a cohort of patients with acquired immunodeficiency syndrome and cytomegalovirus retinitis who received sodium phosphonoformate (foscarnet). Am J Med 94:185–190, 1993.
119. Griffiths PD. Cytomegalovirus therapy: current constraints and future opportunities. Curr Opin Infect Dis 14:765–768, 2001.
120. Martinez A, Castro A, Gil C, et al. Recent strategies in the development of new human cytomegalovirus inhibitors. Med Res Rev 21:227–244, 2001.
121. McSharry JJ, McADonough A, Oson B, et al. Inhibition of ganciclovir-susceptible and -resistant human cytomegalovirus clinical isolates by the benximidazole l-riboside 1263W94. Clin Diagn Lab Immunol 8:1279–1281, 2001.
122. Rybak RJ, Harline CB, Qiu YL, et al. In vitro activities of methylenecyclopropane analogues of nucleosides and their phosphoralaninate prodrugs against cytomegalovirus and other herpescirus infections. Antimicrob Agents Chemother 44:1506–1511, 2000.
123. Spector SA, McKinley GF, Lalezari JP, et al. Oral ganciclovir for the prevention of cytomegalovirus disease in persons with AIDS. N Engl J Med 334:1491–1497, 1996.
124. Brosgart CL, Torres RA, Thompson MA, et al. A randomized, placebo-controlled trial of the safety an efficacy of oral ganciclovir

for prophylaxis of CMV disease in HIV-infected individuals with severe immunosuppression. AIDS 12:269, 1998.

125. 2001 USPHS/IDSA guidelines for the prevention of opportunistic infections in persons infected with human immunodeficiency virus. http://www.hivatis.org/trtgdlns.html#Opportunistic.
126. Tural C, Romeu J, Sicrera G, et al. Long-lasting remission of cytomegalovirus retinitis without maintenance therapy in human immunodeficiency virus-infected patients. J Infect Dis 105:1259–1264, 1998.
127. MacDonald JC, Torriani FJ, Morse LS, et al. Lack of reactivation of cytomegalovirus (CMV) retinitis after stopping CMV maintenance therapy in AIDS patients with sustained elevations in CD4 T cells in response to highly active antiretroviral therapy. J Infect Dis 177:1182–1187, 1998.
128. Whitcup SM, Fortin E, Lindblad AS, et al. Discontinuation of anti-cytomegalovirus therapy in persons with HIV infection and cytomegalovirus retinitis. JAMA 282:1633–1637, 1999.
129. Jabs DA, Bolton SG, Dunn JP, et al. Discontinuing anticytomegalovirus therapy in patients with immune reconstitution after combination antiretroviral therapy. Am J Ophthalmol 126:817–822, 1998.
130. Jouan M, Saves H, Tubiana R, et al. Discontinuation of maintenance therapy for cytomegalovirus retinitis in HIV infected patients receiving highly active antiretroviral therapy: Restimop study team. AIDS 15:23–31, 2001.
131. Berenguer J, Gonzalez J, Pulido F, et al. Discontinuation of secondary prophylaxis in patients with cytomegalovirus retinitis who have responded to highly active antiretroviral therapy. Clin Infect Dis 34: electronically released, 2002.
132. Whitcup SM, Fortin E, Nussenblatt RB, et al. Therapeutic effect of combination antiretroviral therapy on cytomegalovirus retinitis. JAMA 277:1519–1520, 1997.
133. Vrabec TR, Baldassano VF, Whitcup SM. Discontinuation of maintenance therapy in patients with quiescent cytomegalovirus retinitis and elevated CD4+ counts. Ophthalmology 105:1259–1264, 1998.
134. Macdonald JC, Karavellas M, Torriani FJ, et al. Highly active antiretroviral therapy-related immune recovery in AIDS patients with cytomegalovirus retinitis. Ophthalmology 107:877–883, 2000.
135. Monastra R, Rock D, Robinson M, et al. Continued 5-year increase in CD4+ lymphocyte counts in response to potent antiretroviral therapy in a cohort of advanced HIV-infected subjects discontinuing therapy for cytomegalovirus retinitis. Presented at the 1st IAS Conference on HIV Pathogenesis and Treatment. Buenos Aires, July 2001, abstract 652.
136. Torriani FJ, Freeman WR, MacDonald JC, et al. CMV retinitis recurs after stopping treatment in virological and immunological failures of potent antiretroviral therapy. AIDS 14:173–180, 2000.
137. Johnson SC, Benson CA, Johnson DW, et al. Recurrences of cytomegalovirus retinitis in a human immunodeficiency virus-infected patient, despite potent antiretroviral therapy and apparent immune reconstitution. Clin Infect Dis 32:815–819, 2001.
138. Karavellas MP, Plummer DJ, Macdonald JC, et al. Incidence of immune recovery vitritis in cytomegalovirus retinitis patients following institution of successful highly active antiretroviral therapy. J Infect Dis 179:697–700, 1999.
139. Robinson MR, Reed G, Csaky KG, et al. Immune-recovery uveitis in patients with cytomegalovirus retinitis taking highly active antiretroviral therapy. Am J Ophthalmol 120:49–56, 2000.
140. Nguyen QD, Kempen JH, Bolton SG, et al. Immune recovery uveitis in patients with AIDS and cytomegalovirus retinitis after highly active antiretroviral therapy. Am J Ophthalmol 129:634–639, 2000.

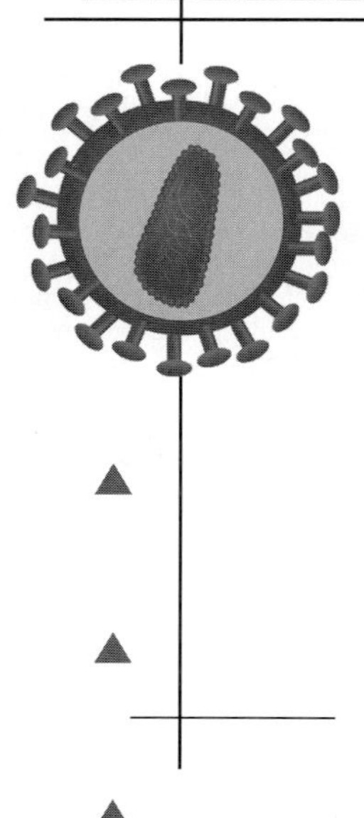

CHAPTER 44

Human Herpesvirus-6 and Herpesvirus-7 Infections

David W. Kimberlin, MD
John W. Gnann, Jr., MD

In 1986 a novel virus was isolated from six patients with lymphoproliferative syndromes, two of whom were also infected with the human immunodeficiency virus (HIV).[1] Molecular and structural characterization of the new virus revealed an icosahedral core structure of 162 capsomeres, indicating that it was a herpesvirus. Because of the initial belief that the new virus selectively infected freshly isolated human B cells, the virus was given the name human B-lymphotropic virus.[1] Subsequent investigation revealed a broader cell tropism, with notable T cell lymphotropism.[2] For this reason, current nomenclature refers to this virus as human herpesvirus-6 (HHV-6).

Four years after the discovery of HHV-6, Frenkel and colleagues isolated another novel virus from the CD4+ T-lymphocytes of a healthy adult.[3] Designated human herpesvirus-7 (HHV-7), this new virus is closely related to HHV-6,[4] exhibiting partial antigenic cross-reactivity with HHV-6.[5,6] In 1994 DNA from the eighth member of the human herpesvirus family was isolated from Kaposi's sarcoma lesions of HIV-infected individuals. Human herpesvirus-8, or Kaposi's sarcoma-associated herpesvirus, is discussed in Chapter 45.

Thus in less than a decade the number of known human herpesviruses increased from five to eight. New technologic advances (peripheral blood mononuclear cell [PBMC] culture, representational difference analysis) and the emergence of the acquired immunodeficiency syndrome (AIDS) epidemic converged to create the circumstances necessary for this remarkable pace of discovery. Two of the three new herpesviruses were initially isolated from AIDS patients, and all three may prove to cause disease in severely immunocompromised persons. This chapter reviews the current knowledge of HHV-6 and HHV-7 biology and the possible impact of these viruses in HIV-infected persons. Although much work is needed to elucidate fully the clinical implications of co-infection with HHV-6 or HHV-7 in HIV-infected persons, preliminary data suggest that an enhanced appreciation of these new herpesviruses may expand the understanding of HIV infection and disease progression. Moreover, such lines of investigation may ultimately provide information on which therapeutic strategies for disease intervention can be based.

▲ HUMAN HERPESVIRUS-6

Since its discovery in AIDS patients, HHV-6 has been implicated as a possible pathogen in HIV-infected persons or a cofactor in HIV disease progression. As researchers investigated and characterized HHV-6 in HIV-infected adults, Yamanishi and colleagues pursued its association with disease in immunocompetent children, discovering in 1988 that HHV-6 caused the common childhood disease exanthem subitum (roseola).[7] As with all herpesviruses, HHV-6 establishes latency following primary infection during childhood, and reactivation from latency can result in active viral replication in both immunocompromised and immunocompetent persons.

Virology

Classification

Human herpesvirus-6 is a member of the Herpesviridae family. Genomic analysis places HHV-6 among the β-herpesviruses, along with human cytomegalovirus (CMV) and HHV-7. Similarities with respect to amino acid sequences, gene organization, and putative protein functions suggest that

HHV-6 is closely related to both CMV and HHV-7.[3,8,9] On the basis of DNA restriction analysis, in vitro tropism studies, and antigenic relations defined by reactivities of monoclonal antibodies, HHV-6 can be separated into two variants: variant A (HHV-6A) and variant B (HHV-6B).[10] Characteristic HHV-6A isolates include GS (the original isolate) and U 1102 (iso lated from a Ugandan AIDS patient).[1,11] The prototypic HHV-6B isolate is Z 29, isolated from a Zairian AIDS patient.[12] The intravariant nucleotide sequence homology ranges from 97% to 100% and the intervariant homology from 94% to 96%.[13,14]

Although the first isolate of HHV-6 (GS) was a variant A strain, only HHV-6B strains have been definitively proven to cause disease (exanthem subitum during childhood, as described later). At the current time it is unclear if HHV-6A causes any disease. Variant A strains of HHV-6 are mainly isolated from AIDS patients or persons with lymphoproliferative disorders, whereas HHV-6B strains are primarily recovered from patients with exanthem subitum.

Viral Composition

Virion Structure

An enveloped virus, HHV-6 has an icosahedral nucleocapsid consisting of 162 capsomeres.[15] The capsid diameter measures 95 to 105 nm, with the diameter of the nucleoid being 60 to 80 nm. The nucleocapsid is surrounded by a dense, prominent tegument 25 to 40 nm thick.[15] Extracellular enveloped virions range from 160 to 200 nm, comparable to that of herpes simplex virus.

Genomic Structure and Genetic Content

Contained within the nucleocapsid of HHV-6 is a linear, double-stranded DNA molecule of 160 to 170 kb. The genome consists of a 143-kb unique sequence (U) flanked by direct repeats, DRL (left) and DRR (right), of approximately 10 to 13 kb.[16] The variation in length is due to the heterogeneous (het) region at the left end of both DR elements.[17,18] The mean G + C content is 43%.[8,16,17] The complete nucleotide sequences of HHV-6A (U 1102) and more recently of HHV-6B (Z29) have been reported.[16,19] The genomes contain 102 and 119 distinct open reading frames likely to encode proteins, respectively, with genes arranged co-linearly with those in the genome of CMV. The overall nucleotide sequence identity between HHV-6A and HHV-6B is 90%.[19] Complete nucleotide results have also been reported recently for HHV-6B (HST).[20]

Protein Properties

More than 30 polypeptides encoded by HHV-6 have been identified in virions and infected cells.[21,22] The molecular weight of these proteins ranges from 30,000 to 200,000, and the proteins include six or seven glycoproteins.

In Vitro Biologic Properties

HHV-6 exhibits predominantly CD4+ T-lymphocyte tropism.[2,23,27] It can be isolated from CD4+ CD8− and CD3+ CD4+ mature T lymphocytes but not from CD4− CD8+, CD4− CD8−, or CD3− T cells.[23] Additionally, HHV-6 can be propagated in CD4+ CD8+, CD4+ CD8−, and CD3+ CD4+ cells with mature phenotypes and rarely in CD4− CD8+ human cord blood mononuclear cells (CBMCs).[23] The HHV-6 receptor has recently been identified as the CD46 molecule.[24] The HIV-1 receptors and co-receptors CD4, CXCR4, and CCR5 are not receptors for HHV-6.[25,26] At the organ level, co-infection with HHV-6 and HHV-7 results in increased quantities of HHV-6 viral genome.[28] Likewise, reactivation of HHV-6 by infection with HHV-7 has been achieved in vitro.[29]

Efficient HHV-6 replication in primary cell culture requires both prior mitogen activation of primary T cells, as provided by phytohemagglutinin (PHA),[1,12] and full progression of the cell cycle, as demonstrated by the requirement for interleukin-2 (IL-2).[30] Mitogenic anti-CD3 monoclonal antibodies can also enhance HHV-6 replication.[31]

The HHV-6A and HHV-6B strains have both been adapted by serial passage to replicate in continuous cell lines. Established human cell lines that support HHV-6A replication include those of T cell (including the T-lymphoblastoid cell line HSB-2), B cell, megakaryocyte, and glial cell lineages, as well as transformed cervical epithelial cells.[18] HHV-6B strains replicate well in the Molt-3 T cell line and the T cell lymphoma line MT-4.[30,32]

The cytopathic effect (CPE) of HHV-6 is first visible in culture 3 to 5 days following infection. The CPE is characterized by refractile enlargement of some of the lymphocytes and occasional multinucleated cells. Lytic degeneration of the infected cells occurs following the development of CPE.

Epidemiology

Geographic Distribution

Seroprevalence studies of HHV-6 infection have demonstrated remarkable reproducibility from widely separated regions of the globe. With rare exceptions,[33] the prevalence of antibodies to HHV-6 is high among populations throughout the world.

Incidence and Prevalence of Infection

Epidemiologic studies in normal children have shown that most primary HHV-6 infections occur within the first year of life.[34,35] HHV-6 immunoglobulin G (IgG) can be detected in more than 90% of neonates,[36,37] reflecting both the high seroprevalence of HHV-6 among adults[37,38] and the active transport of HHV-6 IgG across the placenta.[35] The prevalence of HHV-6 IgG drops significantly by 4 to 6 months of life as maternal antibodies decline, then increases through the third year of life and remains high into adulthood.[34,35,37] The highest geometric mean titers of HHV-6 antibody occur during the first 3 years of life, indicating a predominant clustering of primary infections in infants and toddlers.[35,38] More than 90% of normal children become infected with HHV-6 by 12 months of life,[37] and virtually 100% acquire infection by 3 years of age.[38]

Transmission

Although the mode(s) of transmission of HHV-6 has yet to be proven definitively, most children probably acquire infection through contact with the secretions of adult caretakers shedding the virus in saliva.[39–42] Reports of culture isolation of HHV-6 from the saliva of healthy adults[40,42] and adult patients infected with HIV[42] document salivary shedding in more than 85% of persons. Viral shedding in saliva is intermittent,[43] and the serum antibody titer to HHV-6 does not correlate with the ability to isolate HHV-6 from saliva samples.[42] HHV-6 DNA can be detected by polymerase chain reaction (PCR) in saliva or PBMCs of more than 90% of healthy individuals.[44,45] Using in situ hybridization and immunohistochemical staining, HHV-6 DNA and HHV-6 protein expression have been demonstrated in tissue from submandibular glands,[39] parotid glands,[39] salivary glands,[41] and bronchial glands.[41] Although breast milk is unlikely to be an important source of early HHV-6 infection,[46] several reports suggest that HHV-6 may infect an infant congenitally or perinatally.[47–50] Definitive proof of such transmission, however, remains elusive.

Pathogenesis

Viral Replication and Latency

Analysis of pathologic specimens reveals that HHV-6 can infect a wide variety of cell and tissue types. During acute infection, infection of lymphocytes, macrophages, histiocytes, endothelial cells, and epithelial cells occurs, with CD4+ T-lymphocytes being the predominant target cell type in the blood. The cell target of HHV-6 in the oropharynx during primary infection remains under investigation. HHV-6 has been shown to establish latency in mononuclear cells.[51]

Immune Responses to HHV-6 Infection

Humoral Immune Response

The protective effect of antibody is suggested by the epidemiology of HHV-6 infection. As noted above, passively acquired maternal antibody wanes over the first 6 months of infancy; and during the next 6 months of life the number of children acquiring HHV-6 for the first time approaches 90%.[37] This finding suggests that maternal antibody provides protection against primary HHV-6 infection. Additionally, during primary HHV-6 infection the clearance of viremia coincides with the appearance of HHV-6B-specific neutralizing antibody,[52] again suggesting the importance of the humoral arm of the immune response to HHV-6.

Following primary HHV-6 infection, IgM-neutralizing antibodies appear within 5 to 7 days. Maximum IgM titers appear at 2 to 3 weeks, and the titers then decline and reach undetectable levels after 2 months.[53] Host IgG responses following primary HHV-6 infection develop 7 to 10 days following the febrile period.[54] Serologic evidence of previous infection manifested by HHV-6 IgG is maintained indefinitely.

Cellular Immune Response

The T cell immune responses against HHV-6 infection are readily identified in healthy adult populations, and HHV-6-specific T cell clones have been isolated.[55,56] Moreover, the importance of the cellular component of the host immune response in maintaining latency is suggested by the increased frequency of HHV-6 reactivation in solid organ transplant recipients.[57] Complete understanding of the role of cellular immunity in primary HHV-6 infection and in viral reactivation from latency awaits further investigation.

Clinical Relevance of HHV-6

The only disease for which HHV-6B has been shown definitively to be the causative agent is exanthem subitum (roseola), a common disease of childhood.[7,54] In addition, HHV-6B is a major cause of emergency room visits and hospitalizations for infants and young children.[48] HHV-6 produces a spectrum of neurologic diseases as well, including encephalitis and febrile seizures.[58–60]

Clinical Relevance in Relation to HIV Infection

In Vitro Data

Because HHV-6 was initially isolated from two HIV-positive patients and exhibits CD4+ cell tropism, it was hypothesized that HHV-6 may act as a cofactor in the acceleration of HIV infection to AIDS in patients co-infected with the two viruses. Initial evaluation of possible interactions between HHV-6 and HIV led to the discovery that the viruses can simultaneously infect the same CD4+ T-lymphocytes under experimental conditions.[2,61] Studies evaluating the impact of HHV-6 co-infection on active HIV viral replication in vitro have yielded contradictory results, with some investigations documenting enhanced HIV replication,[61–63] whereas others reported inhibition of HIV replication.[12,64–67] HHV-6 infection in the presence of HIV *tat* results in significantly higher HIV long terminal repeat (LTR) activation than that observed by *tat* or HHV-6 alone, indicating that HHV-6 and *tat* interact synergistically.[68,69] Effects of co-infection on HHV-6 replication are less impressive: HHV-6 replication is unaffected[65,66] or slightly inhibited[64] in cells co-infected with HIV. However, expression of HIV-1 *tat* inhibits HHV-6 replication more dramatically, as shown by a 3.6- to 15.4-fold reduction in yield of infectious virus.[68]

HHV-6 induces expression of CD4 receptor molecules on the cell membranes of infected lymphocytes and natural killer cells, rendering them susceptible to co-infection with HIV.[27,70,71] In vitro studies demonstrate that such co-infection leads to accelerated cellular apoptosis.[61,71] Induction of CD4 molecules on the surface of T cell clones is not dependent on viral DNA replication, suggesting that such up-regulation may be mediated by early gene expression or virion protein(s).[72] HHV-6 has been shown to down-regulate the HIV-1 co-receptor CXCR4,[26] possibly offsetting the potential biologic impact on HIV of HHV-6-mediated CD4 receptor up-regulation.

Perhaps most interestingly, numerous investigators have demonstrated that HHV-6 can *trans*-activate the LTR promoter of HIV.[61,62,68,73–83] Such transcriptional activation occurs in an NF-κB- or Spl-binding-site-dependent manner.[62,74,76,81,83] Co-expression of HIV-1 *tat* transactivating protein produces enhanced transcriptional activation.[62,68] Transactivation of the HIV LTR is accomplished by both HHV-6A and HHV-6B, although HHV-6B induction requires T cells to be stimulated, whereas induction by HHV-6A can occur in either stimulated or resting T cells.[74]

Loci of HHV-6A that are capable of HIV-1 LTR transactivation are depicted in Figure 44–1.[18] These loci contain homologues of the CMV UL36-38 and CMV US22 gene families,[74–79] a portion of the putative DNA polymerase accessory protein,[82] putative IE genes,[75] and sequences of unknown function.[74,81]

In Vivo Data

The consequence of HHV-6 on HIV infection in vivo has been inadequately evaluated. Of the few published clinical reports that have evaluated the potential interaction between these two viruses from epidemiologic and pathologic perspectives, conflicting results have emerged. In a study of the prevalence of HHV-6 seropositivity in a cohort of HIV-1-infected patients, the frequency of HHV-6 seropositivity was significantly lower in patients who had a slower decline in CD4 cells, compared to patients with rapidly declining CD4+ T-lymphocyte counts and to the general population.[84] This finding suggests a role for HHV-6 co-infection in the progression of HIV-1 disease. HHV-6 DNA has been detected primarily in HIV-infected patients with high CD4+ T-lymphocyte counts in some studies[62,85,86] and primarily in patients with low CD4+ T-lymphocyte counts in others.[87] A small longitudinal study of HIV-infected patients has demonstrated that HHV-6 reactivation was followed by a temporary decrease in CD4+ T-lymphocyte counts and by a progressive, dramatic loss of CD4 cells during the following 18 months.[88]

HHV-6 DNA is present in the peripheral lymph nodes and spleens of recent HIV-1 seroconverters at a frequency and distribution similar to that of control tissues from individuals not infected with HIV.[89] In patients with advanced HIV disease, however, HHV-6 can disseminate widely to visceral organs, including the lungs of patients who died of pneumonitis.[90–92] AIDS patients have significantly higher HHV-6 viral loads in these visceral organs than do patients who are not infected with HIV.[92] Furthermore, HIV-infected patients whose organs are co-infected with HHV-6 have higher concentrations of HIV proviral DNA in those organs, compared with HIV-infected persons who are not co-infected with HHV-6.[28,93]

HHV-6 DNA has been detected by PCR in the colonic mucosa of HIV-seropositive patients with diarrhea undergoing intestinal biopsy.[94] A study involving serologic evaluation of Romanian children with nonprogressive HIV disease found that current or recent HHV-6 infection appeared to be associated with the development of pneumonitis,[95] although other reports have not correlated HHV-6 with respiratory disorders in HIV-infected patients.[96] HHV-6 has been correlated with pneumonitis in other immunocompetent and immunocompromised pediatric populations, however.[97] Several reports have documented the presence of HHV-6

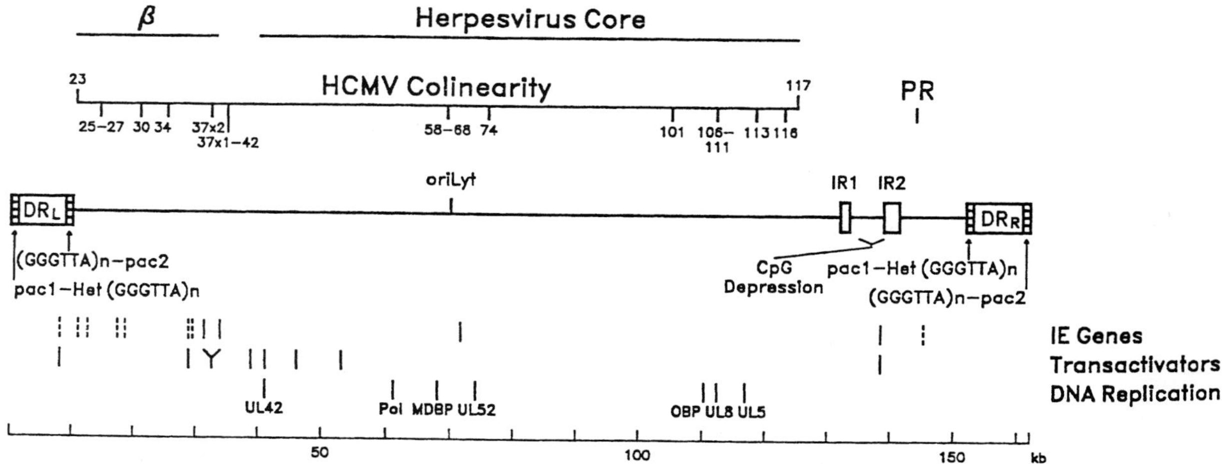

Figure 44–1. Human herpesvirus-6 (HHV-6) genomic and genetic architecture. Note a 162-kb HHV-6 genome with a 141-kb segment of DNA bracketed by 10-kb DR elements, both copies of DR being flanked by arrays of (GGGTTA)$_n$, with the arrays at the left end of DR being more heterogeneous [het(GGGTTA)$_n$]. The portion of the genome co-linear with human cytomegalovirus (HCMV) from HCMV UL23 to HCMV UL117 is indicated, with HCMV UL genes that have no obvious HHV-6 homologue shown below the line. Numerous genes present in HHV-6 but not in HCMV are interspersed in this region but are not shown. Regions containing genes thus far found only in the β-herpesviruses HHV-6 and HCMV (β) and those conserved across the herpesvirus family (herpesvirus core) are shown. Locations are shown for the parvovirus replication protein homologue (PR), oriLyt, the CpG depressed region, the CACATA repeat motif (IR1), the putative immediate early enhancer (IR2), proven and putative immediate early genes identified as described in the text (HCMV US22 homologues are indicated by broken lines), segments of DNA that can transactivate HIV long terminal repeat in transient expression assays (HIV LTR), and the homologues of the seven viral genes necessary for HSV-1 lytic origin-dependent DNA replication: polymerase accessory factor (UL42); DNA polymerase (Pol); major DNA-binding protein (MDBP); helicase-primase components (UL52, UL8, UL5); origin binding protein (OBP). (From Pellett PE, Black JB. Human herpesvirus 6. In: Fields BN, Knipe DM, Howley PM, et al. [eds]. Fields Virology. Philadelphia, Lippincott-Raven, 1996, p 2587, with permission.)

antigens and DNA in retinal lesions from patients with AIDS-associated retinitis, with CMV or HIV-1 usually being present concomitantly.[98–102] In vitro studies have proven that HIV-1 and HHV-6 are capable of simultaneously infecting corneal epithelial cells.[103] Several studies have suggested that HHV-6 can be detected infrequently from cerebrospinal fluid of HIV-infected persons, although its pathogenicity in such settings has been called into question and may relate to co-pathogens such as CMV.[104–106]

Although the studies cited above suggest that HHV-6 plays a role as cofactor in HIV disease progression, other reports have found no correlation between HHV-6 infection and the course of the HIV infection.[107–112] Investigations in animal models have also failed to demonstrate a clinical consequence of simultaneous infection with HHV-6 and HIV.[113]

With limited exceptions,[49,95] each of the in vivo studies to date involved only adult patients. Because HHV-6 establishes latency following primary infection during childhood, an inherent difficulty with clinical evaluations of the possible interaction(s) between HHV-6 and HIV-1 is distinguishing causality. That is, it is difficult to determine if HHV-6 reactivation results in progression of HIV-1 disease, or if progression of HIV-1 disease (with its corresponding decline in immunoregulatory function) results in reactivation of HHV-6. In an effort to assess the impact of primary HHV-6 acquisition on HIV viral dynamics and disease course, Thai and Japanese investigators evaluated 227 infants born to HIV-infected women. The cumulative infection rates of HHV-6 at 6 and 12 months of age were significantly lower in HIV-infected children (11% and 33%, respectively) than in uninfected children (28% and 78%, respectively; $P < 0.001$).[49] Similar findings have been observed by one of the authors of this chapter (D.K.) in an analysis of specimens obtained from patients enrolled in the National Institutes of Health (NIH)-sponsored Women and Infants Transmission Study (WITS). HIV-infected infants without HHV-6 co-infection had lower rates of HIV disease progression at 12 months of life than did co-infected patients (42% vs. 100%; $P < 0.05$), suggesting an association of HHV-6 infection and progression of HIV disease in children with vertically acquired HIV infection.[49]

Diagnosis

Diagnosis of HHV-6 infection is accomplished both serologically and virologically. As with other herpesvirus infections for which latency is established, documentation of primary infection is less difficult than establishing viral reactivation. In general, a four-fold or greater rise in anti-HHV-6 antibody titer between acute and convalescent serum samples suggests that active viral replication has occurred. Detection of HHV-6 IgM in infants and young children is a reliable marker of primary infection, although extrapolation to adults is problematic because IgM can be detected during HHV-6 reactivation.[114] In organ transplant recipients, reactivation of HHV-6 can produce IgM neutralizing antibody responses that persist for 2 to 3 months and then become undetectable 5 to 6 months after transplantation.[53] Furthermore, avidity of IgG antibodies to HHV-6, as determined by elution with urea, can distinguish between primary and recurrent infection: with primary infection low-avidity antibody is detected that matures to high avidity within 5 months, whereas with recurrent infection high-avidity antibody is present from the time of viral reactivation from latency.[115]

Detection of HHV-6 by viral culture provides indisputable evidence of active HHV-6 infection. Likewise, detection of HHV-6 DNA in cell-free plasma specimens suggests the presence of active HHV-6 replication in vivo,[116,117] as does detection by reverse transcriptase (RT)-PCR assay.[118]

Prevention and Treatment

Given the ubiquity of HHV-6 during early childhood and the lack of an effective vaccine, prevention of primary HHV-6 infection is not feasible. However, prevention of HHV-6 reactivation from latency with antiviral therapy may be possible. Data suggesting such a possibility come from investigations in organ transplant recipients. In one report HHV-6 DNA was repeatedly assayed by PCR in peripheral blood leukocytes from 37 allogeneic bone marrow transplant patients.[119] Nine of these patients received high-dose acyclovir prophylactically against CMV infection. HHV-6 DNA was detected in 3 (33%) of the patients so treated compared with 23 of 28 (82%) of the group without acyclovir prophylaxis ($P = 0.01$). The proportion of HHV-6-positive samples within the first 3 months after bone marrow transplantation was significantly lower among the patients who received acyclovir (5/51 vs. 52/158; $P < 0.01$). In none of the nine patients in the acyclovir group was HHV-6 DNA detected when the samples were diluted at 1:10, compared with 11 of 28 patients in the group who did not receive high-dose acyclovir ($P = 0.01$).[119] Whether similar beneficial effects of acyclovir prophylaxis of HHV-6 reactivation can be demonstrated in HIV-infected patients remains to be determined.

Antiviral susceptibility patterns of HHV-6 closely resemble those of CMV. Several investigators have analyzed the in vitro sensitivity of HHV-6 to antiviral agents currently used to treat herpesvirus infections.[120–125] HHV-6 multiplication is readily inhibited by foscarnet, cidofovir, and ganciclovir at levels that are easily achievable in the plasma of humans. Although acyclovir also has an inhibitory effect against HHV-6, it is much less active than the other antiviral agents listed above. Despite these in vitro findings, there have been no controlled prospective clinical evaluations of antiviral therapy for HHV-6 infections, and only anecdotal reports exist in the literature.[126]

▲ HUMAN HERPESVIRUS-7

In 1990 Frenkel and colleagues discovered another new herpesvirus (HHV-7) in cultures of CD4+ T-lymphocytes.[3] As with HHV-6, growth of HHV-7 in vitro requires co-cultivation of activated CD4+ T cells with fresh PBMCs or cord blood mononuclear cells (CBMCs). Such activation can be achieved utilizing the polyclonal T cell mitogen PHA in addition to IL-2. Although the potential for in vivo interaction between HHV-7 and HIV exists, a paucity of data precludes even preliminary speculation in this regard. Therefore, this review of HHV-7 is relatively brief, focusing on basic knowledge from which possible interactions with HIV may be postulated.

Biologic Properties

As with HHV-6, HHV-7 exhibits CD4+ T-lymphocyte tropism,[3,9] with the CD4 cell surface molecule being a critical component of the HHV-7 receptor.[127] Specifically, selective, progressive down-regulation of the surface membrane expression of CD4 was observed in human CD4+ T cells during the course of HHV-7 infection. Addition of murine monoclonal antibodies directed against CD4 or the recombinant soluble form of human CD4 resulted in dose-dependent inhibition of HHV-7 infection in primary CD4+ T-lymphocytes. In the same study, a marked reciprocal interference was observed between HHV-7 and HIV, with prior exposure of CD4+ T cells to HHV-7 dramatically interfering with infection by both primary and in vitro-passaged HIV-1 isolates. Similarly, persistent infection with HIV-1 or treatment with the soluble form of gp 120 rendered CD4+ T cells resistant to HHV-7 infection.[127]

The HIV-1 co-receptors CXCR4 and CCR5 are not receptors for HHV-7.[26,128] Two studies found that HHV-7 down-regulates CXCR4 by a mechanism independent of CD4,[26,129] whereas one study failed to confirm this observation.[128] If true, such down-regulation would provide further in vitro evidence suggesting interference of HIV replication by HHV-7. HHV-7 can provide a transactivating function, mediating reactivation of HHV-6 from latency[130]; and co-infection with HHV-6 and HHV-7 within an organ results in increased quantities of HHV-7 viral genome.[28]

Epidemiology

Primary HHV-7 infection usually occurs during childhood, although the age of infection appears to be somewhat later than the very early age documented for HHV-6. In one study, the mean age at which HHV-7 seroconversion occurred was 17 months versus a mean age of 11 months for HHV-6.[131] Most adults have serologic evidence of prior HHV-7 infection.[132]

Transmission

Data suggest that the salivary glands may be the site of HHV-7 replication and transmission. Among blood donors in Germany, HHV-7 DNA was detected by PCR in 95.5% of saliva specimens and 66.1% of blood buffy coat specimens.[133] HHV-7 DNA was detected by PCR in 75% of the salivary glands of Italian patients with parotid tumors and in 55% of salivary samples from healthy adults.[134] In the same Italian study, HHV-7 DNA was detected with similar frequency in saliva from donors with the common cold or recurrent aphthous ulcerations, but saliva specimens from HIV-infected patients harbored HHV-7 with higher frequency (81%) and increased viral load.[134] Among healthy adults in Japan, HHV-7 DNA was detected by PCR in 89.7% of saliva samples, and the viral load detected in saliva remained constant over time.[43] In addition to persistent replication in salivary gland tissue, HHV-7 establishes latency in peripheral blood T cells.[135]

Clinical Relevance of HHV-7

As yet HHV-7 has not been definitively shown to cause a specific disease. The strongest data for the association of HHV-7 with clinical disease implicate it as a cause of first or second episodes of exanthem subitum.[131,136] HHV-7 may also be associated with febrile seizures and other neurologic manifestations as well as with minor upper respiratory tract infections.[58,60,136–138]

With limited exceptions, knowledge of specific viral interactions between HHV-7 and HIV in vivo is almost completely lacking. HHV-7 is detected more frequently and in greater amounts in the saliva of HIV-infected persons, as described above.[134] Lymph node tissue from HIV-infected persons also is more likely to demonstrate immunohistochemical evidence of HHV-7 infection than that of HIV-negative patients.[139]

Treatment

In vitro analysis suggests that foscarnet and cidofovir are most active against HHV-7, with ganciclovir and penciclovir having less activity and acyclovir showing no activity.[122,140] A study of ganciclovir therapy in renal transplant recipients failed to demonstrate any effect of treatment on the incidence of HHV-7 viremia, suggesting that HHV-7 is resistant to ganciclovir in vivo.[141]

▲ CONCLUSIONS

Investigations of the recently discovered herpesviruses HHV-6 and HHV-7 have yielded intriguing suggestions of in vivo interactions with HIV. Systematic evaluation of such potential interactions has not yet been carried out in a definitive manner. It is likely that such research will enhance our understanding of the natural history of HIV infection and could provide the avenues for improved therapeutic strategies. The potential for HHV-6 and HHV-7 to cause significant opportunistic infections in HIV-infected persons also requires additional investigation.

REFERENCES

1. Salahuddin SZ, Ablashi DV, Markham PD, et al. Isolation of a new virus, HBLV, in patients with lymphoproliferative disorders. Science 234:596, 1986.
2. Lusso P, Markham PD, Tschachler E, et al. In vitro cellular tropism of human B-lymphotropic virus (human herpesvirus-6). J Exp Med 167:1659, 1988.
3. Frenkel N, Schirmer EC, Wyatt LS, et al. Isolation of a new herpesvirus from human CD4+ T cells. Proc Natl Acad Sci USA 87:748, 1990.

4. Mukai T, Isegawa Y, Yamanishi K. Identification of the major capsid protein gene of human herpesvirus 7. Virus Res 37:55, 1995.
5. Wyatt LS, Rodriguez WJ, Balachandran N, et al. Human herpesvirus 7: antigenic properties and prevalence in children and adults. J Virol 65:6260, 1991.
6. Frenkel N, Wyatt LS. HHV-6 and HHV-7 as exogenous agents in human lymphocytes. Dev Biol Stand 76:259, 1992.
7. Yamanishi K, Okuno T, Shiraki K, et al. Identification of human herpesvirus-6 as a causal agent for exanthem subitum. Lancet 1:1065, 1988.
8. Lawrence GL, Chee M, Craxton MA, et al. Human herpesvirus 6 is closely related to human cytomegalovirus. J Virol 64:287, 1990.
9. Berneman ZN, Ablashi DV, Li G, et al. Human herpesvirus 7 is a T-lymphotropic virus and is related to, but significantly different from, human herpesvirus 6 and human cytomegalovirus. Proc Natl Acad Sci USA 89:10552, 1992.
10. Ablashi D, Agut H, Berneman Z, et al. Human herpesvirus-6 strain groups: a nomenclature. Arch Virol 129:363, 1993.
11. Downing RG, Sewankambo N, Serwadda D, et al. Isolation of human lymphotropic herpesvirus from Uganda. Lancet 2:390, 1987.
12. Lopez C, Pellett P, Stewart J, et al. Characteristics of human herpesvirus-6. J Infect Dis 157:1271, 1988.
13. Aubin J-T, Collandre H, Candotti D, et al. Several groups among human herpesvirus-6 strains can be distinguished by Southern blotting and polymerase chain reaction. J Clin Microbiol 29:367, 1991.
14. Aubin J-T, Agut H, Collandre H, et al. Antigenic and genetic differentiation of two putative types of human herpesvirus-6. J Virol Methods 41:223, 1993.
15. Biberfeld P, Kramarsky B, Salahuddin SZ, et al. Ultrastructural characterization of a new human B lymphotropic DNA virus (human herpesvirus 6) isolated from patients with lymphoproliferative disease. J Natl Cancer Inst 79:933, 1987.
16. Gompels UA, Nicholas J, Lawrence G, et al. The DNA sequence of human herpesvirus-6: structure, coding content, and genome evolution. Virology 209:29, 1995.
17. Lindquester GJ, Pellett PE. Properties of the human herpesvirus 6 strain Z 29 genome: G-C content, length, and presence of variable-length directly repeated terminal sequence elements. Virology 182:102, 1991.
18. Pellett PE, Black JB. Human herpesvirus 6. In: Fields BN, Knipe DM, Howley PM, et al (eds) Fields' Virology. Philadelphia, Lippincott-Raven, 1996, p 2587.
19. Dominguez G, Dambaugh TR, Stamey FR, et al. Human herpesvirus 6B genome sequence: coding content and comparison with human herpesvirus 6A. J Virol 73:8040, 1999.
20. Isegawa Y, Mukai T, Nakano K, et al. Comparison of the complete DNA sequences of human herpesvirus 6 variants A and B. J Virol 73:8053, 1999.
21. Balachandran N, Amelse RE, Zhou WW, et al. Identification of proteins specific for human herpesvirus 6-infected human T cells. J Virol 63:2835, 1989.
22. Shiraki K, Okuno T, Yamanishi K, et al. Virion and nonstructural polypeptides of human herpesvirus-6. Virus Res 13:173, 1989.
23. Takahashi K, Sonoda S, Higashi K, et al. Predominant CD4 T-lymphocyte tropism of human herpesvirus 6-related virus. J Virol 63:3161, 1989.
24. Santoro F, Kennedy PE, Locatelli G, et al. CD46 is a cellular receptor for human herpesvirus 6. Cell 99:817, 1999.
25. Lusso P, Gallo RC, DeRocco SE, et al. CD4 is not the membrane receptor for HHV-6. Lancet 1:730, 1989.
26. Yasukawa M, Hasegawa A, Sakai I, et al. Down-regulation of CXCR4 by human herpesvirus 6 (HHV-6) and HHV-7. J Immunol 162:5417, 1999.
27. Lusso P, Malnati MS, Garzino-Demo A, et al. Infection of natural killer cells by human herpesvirus 6. Nature 362:458, 1993.
28. Emery VC, Atkins MC, Bowen EF, et al. Interactions between beta-herpesviruses and human immunodeficiency virus in vivo: evidence for increased human immunodeficiency viral load in the presence of human herpesvirus 6. J Med Virol 57:278, 1999.
29. Tanaka-Taya K, Kondo T, Nakagawa N, et al. Reactivation of human herpesvirus 6 by infection of human herpesvirus 7. J Med Virol 60:284, 2000.
30. Black JB, Sanderlin KC, Goldsmith CS, et al. Growth properties of human herpesvirus-6 strain Z29. J Virol Methods 26:133, 1989.
31. Kikuta H, Lu H, Tomizawa K, et al. Enhancement of human herpesvirus 6 replication in adult human lymphocytes by monoclonal antibody to CD3. J Infect Dis 161:1085, 1990.
32. Ablashi DV, Balachandran N, Josephs SF, et al. Genomic polymorphism, growth properties, and immunologic variations in human herpesvirus-6 isolates. Virology 184:545, 1991.
33. Yadav M, Umamaheswari S, Ablashi DV. Low prevalence of antibody to human herpesvirus-6 (HHV-6) in Kadazans. Southeast Asian J Trop Med Public Health 21:259, 1990.
34. Farr TJ, Harnett GB, Pietroboni GR, et al. The distribution of antibodies to HHV-6 compared with other herpesviruses in young children. Epidemiol Infect 105:603, 1990.
35. Yoshikawa T, Suga S, Asano Y, et al. Distribution of antibodies to a causative agent of exanthem subitum (human herpesvirus-6) in healthy individuals. Pediatrics 84:675, 1989.
36. Knowles WA, Gardner SD. High prevalence of antibody to human herpesvirus-6 and seroconversion associated with rash in two infants. Lancet 2:912, 1988.
37. Leach CT, Sumaya CV, Brown NA. Human herpesvirus-6: clinical implications of a recently discovered, ubiquitous agent. J Pediatr 121:173, 1992.
38. Brown NA, Sumaya CV, Liu C-R, et al. Fall in human herpesvirus 6 seropositivity with age. Lancet 2:396, 1988.
39. Fox JD, Briggs M, Ward PA, et al. Human herpesvirus 6 in salivary glands. Lancet 336:590, 1990.
40. Harnett GB, Farr TJ, Pietroboni GR, et al. Frequent shedding of human herpesvirus 6 in saliva. J Med Virol 30:128, 1990.
41. Krueger GRF, Wassermann K, DeClerck LS, et al. Latent herpesvirus-6 in salivary and bronchial glands. Lancet 336:1255, 1990.
42. Levy JA, Greenspan D, Ferro F, et al. Frequent isolation of HHV-6 from saliva and high seroprevalence of the virus in the population. Lancet 335:1047, 1990.
43. Fujiwara N, Namba H, Ohuchi R, et al. Monitoring of human herpesvirus-6 and -7 genomes in saliva samples of healthy adults by competitive quantitative PCR. J Med Virol 61:208, 2000.
44. Cone RW, Huang ML, Ashley R, et al. Human herpesvirus 6 DNA in peripheral blood cells and saliva from immunocompetent individuals. J Clin Microbiol 31:1262, 1993.
45. Aberle SW, Mandl CW, Kunz C, Popow-Kraupp T. Presence of human herpesvirus 6 variants A and B in saliva and peripheral blood mononuclear cells of healthy adults. J Clin Microbiol 34:3223, 1996.
46. Takahashi K, Sonoda S, Kawakami K, et al. Human herpesvirus 6 and exanthem subitum. Lancet 1:1463, 1988.
47. Dunne WM Jr, Demmler GJ. Serological evidence for congenital transmission of human herpesvirus 6. Lancet 340:121, 1992.
48. Hall CB, Long CE, Schnabel KC, et al. Human herpesvirus-6 infection in children: a prospective study of complications and reactivation. N Engl J Med 331:432, 1994.
49. Kositanont U, Wasi C, Wanprapar N, et al. Primary infection of human herpesvirus 6 in children with vertical infection of human immunodeficiency virus type 1. J Infect Dis 180:50, 1999.
50. Dahl H, Fjaertoft G, Norsted T, et al. Reactivation of human herpesvirus 6 during pregnancy. J Infect Dis 180:2035, 1999.
51. Yoshikawa T, Suzuki K, Ihira M, et al. Human herpesvirus 6 latently infects mononuclear cells but not liver tissue. J Clin Pathol 52:65, 1999.
52. Asano Y, Yoshikawa T, Suga S, et al. Viremia and neutralizing antibody response in infants with exanthem subitum. J Pediatr 114:535, 1989.
53. Suga S, Yoshikawa T, Asano Y, et al. IgM neutralizing antibody responses to human herpesvirus-6 in patients with exanthem subitum or organ transplantation. Microbiol Immunol 36:495, 1992.
54. Ueda K, Kusuhara K, Hirose M, et al. Exanthem subitum and antibody to human herpesvirus-6. J Infect Dis 159:750, 1989.
55. Yakushijin Y, Yasukawa M, Kobayashi Y. T-cell immune response to human herpesvirus-6 in healthy adults. Microbiol Immunol 35:655, 1991.
56. Yasukawa M, Yakushijin Y, Furukawa M, et al. Specificity analysis of human $CD4^+$ T-cell clones directed against human herpesvirus 6 (HHV-6), HHV-7, and human cytomegalovirus. J Virol 67:6259, 1993.
57. Singh N, Carrigan DR. Human herpesvirus-6 in transplantation: an emerging pathogen. Ann Intern Med 124:1065, 1996.
58. Kimberlin DW, Whitley RJ. Human herpesvirus-6: neurologic implications of a newly-described viral pathogen. J Neurovirol 4:474, 1998.

59. Chan PK, Ng HK, Hui M, et al. Presence of human herpesviruses 6, 7, and 8 DNA sequences in normal brain tissue. J Med Virol 59:491, 1999.
60. Yoshikawa T, Ihira M, Suzuki K, et al. Invasion by human herpesvirus 6 and human herpesvirus 7 of the central nervous system in patients with neurological signs and symptoms. Arch Dis Child 83:170, 2000.
61. Lusso P, Ensoli B, Markham PD, et al. Productive dual infection of human CD4$^+$ T lymphocytes by HIV-1 and HHV-6. Nature 337:370, 1989.
62. Knox KK, Carrigan DR. Active HHV-6 infection in the lymph nodes of HIV-infected patients: in vitro evidence that HHV-6 can break HIV latency. J Acquir Immune Defic Syndr 11:370, 1996.
63. Ensoli B, Lusso P, Schachter F, et al. Human herpes virus-6 increases HIV-1 expression in co-infected T cells via nuclear factors binding to the HIV-1 enhancer. EMBO J 8:3019, 1989.
64. Levy JA, Landay A, Lennette ET. Human herpesvirus 6 inhibits human immunodeficiency virus type 1 replication in cell culture. J Clin Microbiol 28:2362, 1990.
65. Pietroboni GR, Harnett GB, Farr TJ, et al. Human herpes virus type 6 (HHV-6) and its in vitro effect on human immunodeficiency virus (HIV). J Clin Pathol 41:1310, 1988.
66. Asada H, Klaus-Kovtun V, Golding H, et al. Human herpesvirus 6 infects dendritic cells and suppresses human immunodeficiency virus type 1 replication in coinfected cultures. J Virol 73:4019, 1999.
67. Bonura F, Perna AM, Vitale F, et al. Inhibition of human immunodeficiency virus 1 (HIV-1) by variant B of human herpesvirus 6 (HHV-6). New Microbiol 22:161, 1999.
68. Di Luca D, Secchiero P, Bovenzi P, et al. Reciprocal in vitro interactions between human herpesvirus-6 and HIV-1 Tat. AIDS 5:1095, 1991.
69. Garzino-Demo A, Chen M, Lusso P, et al. Enhancement of TAT-induced transactivation of the HIV-1 LTR by two genomic fragments of HHV-6. J Med Virol 50:20–24, 1996.
70. Lusso P, De Maria A, Malnati M, et al. Induction of CD4 and susceptibility to HIV-1 infection in human CD8$^+$ T lymphocytes by human herpesvirus 6. Nature 349:533, 1991.
71. Schonnebeck M, Krueger GR, Braun M, et al. Human herpesvirus-6 infection may predispose cells to superinfection by other viruses. In Vivo 5:255, 1991.
72. Lusso P, Malnati M, De Maria A, et al. Productive infection of CD4$^+$ and CD8$^+$ mature human T cell populations and clones by human herpesvirus 6: transcriptional downregulation of CD3. J Immunol 147:685, 1991.
73. Horvat RT, Wood C, Balachandran N. Transactivation of human immunodeficiency virus promoter by human herpesvirus 6. J Virol 63:970, 1989.
74. Horvat RT, Wood C, Josephs SF, et al. Transactivation of the human immunodeficiency virus promoter by human herpesvirus 6 (HHV-6) strains GS and Z-29 in primary human T lymphocytes and identification of transactivating HHV-6(GS) gene fragments. J Virol 65:2895, 1991.
75. Martin ME, Nicholas J, Thomson BJ, et al. Identification of a transactivating function mapping to the putative immediate-early locus of human herpesvirus 6. J Virol 65:5381, 1991.
76. Geng YQ, Chandran B, Josephs SF, et al. Identification and characterization of a human herpesvirus 6 gene segment that trans activates the human immunodeficiency virus type 1 promoter. J Virol 66:1564, 1992.
77. Kashanchi F, Thompson J, Sadaie MR, et al. Transcriptional activation of minimal HIV-l promoter by ORF-1 protein expressed from the SalI-L fragment of human herpesvirus 6. Virology 201:95, 1994.
78. Nicholas J, Martin ME. Nucleotide sequence analysis of a 38.5-kilobase-pair region of the genome of human herpesvirus 6 encoding human cytomegalovirus immediate-early gene homologs and transactivating functions. J Virol 68:597, 1994.
79. Thompson J, Choudhury S, Kashanchi F, et al. A transforming fragment within the direct repeat region of human herpesvirus type 6 that transactivates HIV-1. Oncogene 9:1167, 1994.
80. Thomson BJ, Weindler FW, Gray D, et al. Human herpesvirus 6 (HHV-6) is a helper virus for adeno-associated virus type 2 (AAV-2) and the AAV-2 rep gene homologue in HHV-6 can mediate AAV-2 DNA replication and regulate gene expression. Virology 204:304, 1994.
81. Wang J, Jones C, Norcross M, et al. Identification and characterization of a human herpesvirus 6 gene segment capable of transactivating the human immunodeficiency virus type 1 long terminal repeat in an Sp1 binding site-dependent manner. J Virol 68:1706, 1994.
82. Zhou Y, Chang CK, Qian G, et al. trans-Activation of the HIV promoter by a cDNA and its genomic clones of human herpesvirus-6. Virology 199:311, 1994.
83. McCarthy M, Auger D, He J, Wood C. Cytomegalovirus and human herpesvirus-6 trans-activate the HIV-1 long terminal repeat via multiple response regions in human fetal astrocytes. J Neurovirol 4:495, 1998.
84. Chen H, Pesce AM, Carbonari M, et al. Absence of antibodies to human herpesvirus-6 in patients with slowly-progressive human immunodeficiency virus type 1 infection. Eur J Epidemiol 8:217, 1992.
85. Fairfax MR, Schacker T, Cone RW, et al. Human herpesvirus 6 DNA in blood cells of human immunodeficiency virus-infected men: correlation of high levels with high CD4 cell counts. J Infect Dis 169:1342, 1994.
86. Fabio G, Knight SN, Kidd IM, et al. Prospective study of human herpesvirus 6, human herpesvirus 7, and cytomegalovirus infections in human immunodeficiency virus-positive patients. J Clin Microbiol 35:2657, 1997.
87. Blázquez VM, Madueño JA, Jurado R, et al. Human herpesvirus-6 and the course of human immunodeficiency virus infection. J Acquir Immune Defic Syndr 9:389, 1995.
88. Iuliano R, Trovato R, Lico S, et al. Human herpesvirus-6 reactivation in a longitudinal study of two HIV-l infected patients. J Med Virol 51:259, 1997.
89. Madea B, Roewert HJ, Krueger GR, et al. Search for early lesions following human immunodeficiency virus type 1 infection: a study of six individuals who died a violent death after seroconversion. Arch Pathol Lab Med 114:379, 1990.
90. Corbellino M, Lusso P, Gallo RC, et al. Disseminated human herpesvirus 6 infection in AIDS. Lancet 342:1242, 1993.
91. Knox KK, Carrigan DR. Disseminated active HHV-6 infections in patients with AIDS. Lancet 343:577, 1994.
92. Clark DA, Ait-Khaled M, Wheeler AC, et al. Quantification of human herpesvirus 6 in immunocompetent persons and post-mortem tissues from AIDS patients by PCR. J Gen Virol 77:2271, 1996.
93. Knox KK, Carrigan DR. Active HHV-6 infection in the lymph nodes of HIV-infected patients: in vitro evidence that HHV-6 can break HIV latency. J Acquir Immune Defic Syndr 11:370, 1996.
94. Gautheret A, Monfort L, Poirel L, et al. Human cytomegalovirus, human herpesvirus-6 and human herpesvirus-7 DNA in colonic mucosa from HIV-seropositive patients with diarrhea. In: Abstracts of the XIth International Conference on AIDS, Vancouver, 1996, abstract 1224.
95. Nigro G, Luzi G, Krzysztofiak A, et al. Detection of IgM antibodies to human herpesvirus 6 in Romanian children with nonprogressive human immunodeficiency virus disease. Pediatr Infect Dis J 14:891, 1995.
96. Portolani M, Fabio G, Pecorari M, et al. Search for human herpesvirus 6 and human cytomegalovirus in bronchoalveolar lavage from patients with human immunodeficiency virus-1 and respiratory disorders. J Med Virol 48:179, 1996.
97. Hammerling JA, Lambrecht RS, Kehl KS, Carrigan DR. Prevalence of human herpesvirus 6 in lung tissue from children with pneumonitis. J Clin Pathol 49:802, 1996.
98. Reux I, Fillet AM, Agut H, et al. In situ detection of human herpesvirus 6 in retinitis associated with acquired immunodeficiency syndrome. Am J Ophthalmol 114:375, 1992.
99. Qavi HB, Green MT, SeGall GK, et al. Transcriptional activity of HIV-l and HHV-6 in retinal lesions from AIDS patients. Invest Ophthalmol Vis Sci 33:2759, 1992.
100. Qavi HB, Green MT, Pearson G, et al. Possible role of HHV-6 in the development of AIDS retinitis. In Vivo 8:527, 1994.
101. Qavi HB, Green MT, Lewis DE, et al. HIV-1 and HHV-6 antigens and transcripts in retinas of patients with AIDS in the absence of human cytomegalovirus. Invest Ophthalmol Vis Sci 36:2040, 1995.
102. Fillet AM, Reux I, Joberty C, et al. Detection of human herpes virus 6 in AIDS-associated retinitis by means of in situ hybridization, polymerase chain reaction and immunohistochemistry. J Med Virol 49:289, 1996.
103. Qavi HB, Xu B, Green MT, et al. Morphological and ultrastructural changes induced in corneal epithelial cells by HIV-l and HHV-6 in vitro. Curr Eye Res 15:597, 1996.

104. Quereda C, Corral I, Laguna F, et al. Diagnostic utility of a multiplex herpesvirus PCR assay performed with cerebrospinal fluid from human immunodeficiency virus-infected patients with neurological disorders. J Clin Microbiol 38:3061, 2000.
105. Bossolasco S, Marenzi R, Dahl H, et al. Human herpesvirus 6 in cerebrospinal fluid of patients infected with HIV: frequency and clinical significance. J Neurol Neurosurg Psychiatry 67:789, 1999.
106. Cinque P, Vago L, Dahl H, et al. Polymerase chain reaction on cerebrospinal fluid for diagnosis of virus-associated opportunistic diseases of the central nervous system in HIV-infected patients. AIDS 10:951, 1996.
107. Brown NA, Kovacs A, Lui CR, et al. Prevalence of antibody to human herpesvirus 6 among blood donors infected with HIV. Lancet 2:1146, 1988.
108. Essers S, Schwinn A, ter Meulen J, et al. Seroepidemiological correlations of antibodies to human herpesviruses and human immunodeficiency virus type 1 in African patients. Eur J Epidemiol 7:658, 1991.
109. Fox J, Briggs M, Tedder RS. Antibody to human herpesvirus 6 in HIV-1 positive and negative homosexual men. Lancet 2:396, 1988.
110. Spira TJ, Bozeman LH, Sanderlin KC, et al. Lack of correlation between human herpesvirus-6 infection and the course of human immunodeficiency virus infection. J Infect Dis 161:567, 1990.
111. Gautheret A, Aubin JT, Fauveau V, et al. Rate of detection of human herpesvirus-6 at different stages of HIV infection. Eur J Clin Microbiol Infect Dis 14:820, 1995.
112. Dorrucci M, Rezza G, Andreoni M, et al. Serum IgG antibodies to human herpesvirus-6 (HHV-6) do not predict the progression of HIV disease to AIDS. Eur J Epidemiol 15:317, 1999.
113. Gobbi A, Stoddart CA, Locatelli G, et al. Coinfection of SCID-hu Thy/Liv mice with human herpesvirus 6 and human immunodeficiency virus type 1. J Virol 74:8726, 2000.
114. Fox JD, Ward P, Briggs M, et al. Production of IgM antibody to HHV6 in reactivation and primary infection. Epidemiol Infect 104:289, 1990.
115. Ward RN, Gray JJ, Joslin ME, et al. Avidity of IgG antibodies to human herpesvirus-6 distinguishes primary from recurrent infection in organ transplant recipients and excludes cross-reactivity with other herpesviruses. J Med Virol 39:44, 1993.
116. Huang L-M, Kuo P-F, Lee C-Y, et al. Detection of human herpesvirus-6 DNA by polymerase chain reaction in serum or plasma. J Med Virol 38:7, 1992.
117. Secchiero P, Carrigan DR, Asano Y, et al. Detection of human herpesvirus 6 in plasma of children with primary infection and immunosuppressed patients by polymerase chain reaction. J Infect Dis 171:273, 1995.
118. Norton RA, Caserta MT, Hall CB, et al. Detection of human herpesvirus 6 by reverse transcription-PCR. J Clin Microbial 37:3672, 1999.
119. Wang F-Z, Dahl H, Linde A, et al. Lymphotropic herpesviruses in allogeneic bone marrow transplantation. Blood 88:3615, 1996.
120. Agut H, Collandre H, Aubin J-T, et al. In vitro sensitivity of human herpesvirus-6 to antiviral drugs. Res Virol 140:219, 1989.
121. Russler SK, Tapper MA, Garrigan DR. Susceptibility of human herpesvirus 6 to acyclovir and ganciclovir. Lancet 2:382, 1989.
122. Yoshida M, Yamada M, Chatterjee S, et al. A method for detection of HHV-6 antigens and its use for evaluating antiviral drugs. J Virol Methods 58:137, 1996.
123. Yoshida M, Yamada M, Tsukazaki T, et al. Comparison of antiviral compounds against human herpesvirus 6 and 7. Antiviral Res 40:73, 1998.
124. Burns WH, Sandford GR. Susceptibility of human herpesvirus 6 to antivirals in vitro. J Infect Dis 162:634, 1990.
125. Manichanh C, Grenot P, Gautheret-Dejean A, et al. Susceptibility of human herpesvirus 6 to antiviral compounds by flow cytometry analysis. Cytometry 40:135, 2000.
126. Bethge W, Beck R, Jahn G, et al. Successful treatment of human herpesvirus-6 encephalitis after bone marrow transplantation. Bone Marrow Transplant 24:1245, 1999.
127. Lusso P, Secchiero P, Crowley RW, et al. CD4 is a critical component of the receptor for human herpesvirus 7: interference with human immunodeficiency virus. Proc Natl Acad Sci USA 91:3872, 1994.
128. Zhang Y, Hatse S, De Clercq E, Schols D. CXC-chemokine receptor 4 is not a coreceptor for human herpesvirus 7 entry into CD4(+) T cells. J Virol 74:2011, 2000.
129. Secchiero P, Zella D, Barabitskaja O, et al. Progressive and persistent downregulation of surface CXCR4 in CD4(+) T cells infected with human herpesvirus 7. Blood 92:4521, 1998.
130. Katsafanas GC, Schirmer EC, Wyatt LS, et al. In vitro activation of human herpesvirus 6 and 7 from latency. Proc Natl Acad Sci USA 93:9788, 1996.
131. Torigoe S, Kumamoto T, Koide W, et al. Clinical manifestations associated with human herpesvirus 7 infection. Arch Dis Child 72:518, 1995.
132. Secchiero P, Berneman ZN, Gallo RC, et al. Biological and molecular characteristics of human herpesvirus 7: in vitro growth optimization and development of a syncytia inhibition test. Virology 202:506, 1994.
133. Wilborn F, Schmidt CA, Lorenz F, et al. Human herpesvirus type 7 in blood donors: detection by the polymerase chain reaction. J Med Virol 47:65, 1995.
134. Di Luca D, Mirandola P, Ravaioli T, et al. Human herpesviruses 6 and 7 in salivary glands and shedding in saliva of healthy and human immunodeficiency virus positive individuals. J Med Virol 45:462, 1995.
135. Black JB, Pellett PE. Human herpesvirus 7. Rev Med Virol 9:245, 1999.
136. Tanaka K, Kondo T, Torigoe S, et al. Human herpesvirus 7: another causal agent for roseola (exanthem subitum). J Pediatr 125:1, 1994.
137. Caserta M, Hall CB, Schnabel K, et al. Human herpesvirus-7 (HHV-7) infection in U.S. children [abstract 996]. Pediatr Res 39:168A, 1996.
138. Van den Berg JS, van Zeijl JH, Rotteveel JJ, et al. Neuroinvasion by human herpesvirus type 7 in a case of exanthem subitum with severe neurologic manifestations. Neurology 52:1077, 1999.
139. Kempf W, Muller B, Maurer R, et al. Increased expression of human herpesvirus 7 in lymphoid organs of AIDS patients. J Clin Virol 16:193, 2000.
140. Zhang Y, Schols D, De Clercq E. Selective activity of various antiviral compounds against HHV-7 infection. Antiviral Res 43:23, 1999.
141. Brennan DC, Storch GA, Singer GG, et al. The prevalence of human herpesvirus-7 in renal transplant recipients is unaffected by oral or intravenous ganciclovir. J Infect Dis 181:1557, 2000.

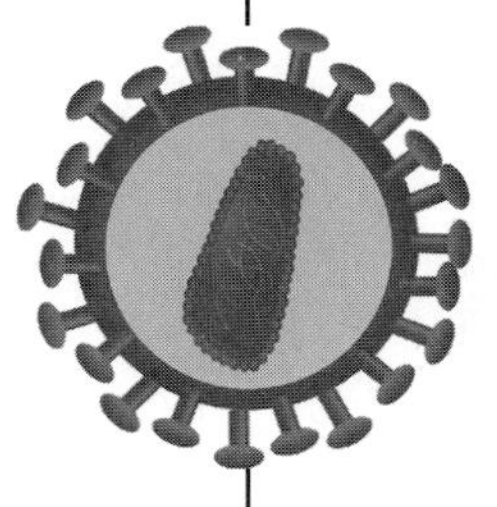

CHAPTER 45

Epstein-Barr Virus and Kaposi's Sarcoma-Associated Herpesvirus

Eric C. Johannsen, MD

Epstein-Barr virus (EBV), the agent of infectious mononucleosis in young adults, is associated with the human immunodeficiency virus (HIV)-related syndromes of oral hairy leukoplakia and non-Hodgkin's lymphoma including primary central nervous system (CNS) lymphoma and Burkitt's-like anaplastic lymphomas. In other populations it has been implicated in the pathogenesis of post-transplant lymphoproliferative disease, nasopharyngeal carcinoma, and some forms of Hodgkin's disease. An infectious etiology was long suspected for Kaposi's sarcoma (KS) based on epidemiologic evidence. The identification of a herpesvirus, closely related to EBV, in KS biopsies has markedly advanced our understanding of this disease. Information on this virus, called human herpesvirus-8 or KS-associated herpesvirus (KSHV), has accumulated rapidly, and the complete sequence of the virus was reported just 2 years after its discovery. KSHV has been subsequently linked to other forms of neoplasia: primary effusion lymphoma and the multicentric form of Castleman's disease. EBV and KSHV, like all herpesviruses, can switch a latent form of infection in which most of the viral genes are not expressed and the genome is maintained in the nucleus by cellular machinery. It is well established that EBV genes expressed during latent infection drive B lymphocytes to proliferate and are almost certainly responsible for EBV's association with malignancy. The pathophysiology of KSHV-related diseases is less completely understood, but expression of viral genes during latency appears to play a prominent role. The natural history and pathophysiology of these two viruses and implications for therapy are reviewed herein.

▲ TAXONOMY

Based on genomic organization and biologic characteristics, EBV and KSHV belong to the Gammaherpesvirinae subfamily of herpesviruses (Fig. 45–1). All herpesvirus virions consist of a linear, double-stranded DNA genome within an icosahedral nucleocapsid, an amorphous tegument, and a lipid bilayer envelope.[1] The genomes range in size from about 170 kb (KSHV) to about 184 kb (EBV) and encode almost 100 proteins each. The two strains of EBV (types I and II) show an overall divergence of less than 4% and are indistinguishable on clinical grounds or by commercially available serologic tests.[2] Infection with type I EBV is far more prevalent in most populations, although type II infection among HIV-infected patients is increased relative to the general population, as is co-infection with types I and II. Five major subtypes of KSHV have been designated A to E.[3,4] Unlike EBV, KSHV subtypes demonstrate distinct geographic distribution: A and C predominate in Europe with C extending to Asia and the Americas as well; B is predominantly in Africa; and D and E are restricted to Oceania or Amerindian populations.[4,5] It is not currently known if the biologic properties of these subtypes differ significantly.

▲ EPSTEIN-BARR VIRUS

Natural History

Infection with EBV is transmitted by contact with the oral secretions of seropositive individuals. Primary infection in children is generally asymptomatic, whereas many adults

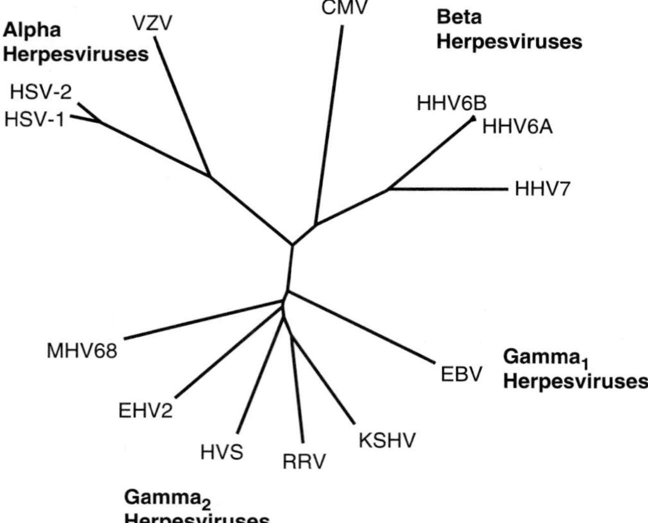

Figure 45–1. Phylogenetic tree of Kaposi's sarcoma-assoicated herpesvirus (KSHV) and Epstein-Barr virus (EBV) based on a comparison of amino acid sequences of the viral DNA polymerase. The α and β subfamily groupings are labeled. KSHV is more closely related to many nonhuman γ-herpesviruses, which form the rhadinovirus (or γ_2-herpesvirus) genus, than to EBV, which is a member of the genus lymphocryptovirus (or γ_1-herpesvirus). Comparison of the phylogenetic tree of host organisms (not shown) to the rhadinovirus tree reveals a similar branching pattern. This suggests that a common primate ancestor was infected with an ancestral rhadinovirus that co-speciated with its host. The divergence of γ_1- and γ_2-herpesviruses is even more ancient. EHV2, equine herpesvirus 2; HVS, herpesvirus siamiri; MHV68, murine herpesvirus 68. RRV rhesus rhadinovirus.

and adolescents experience the typical symptoms of infectious mononucleosis: fever, lymphadenopathy, pharyngitis. The virus replicates in the oropharynx and spreads to B lymphocytes by binding to the receptor for the d region of the third component of complement (C3d receptor, also known as CR2 or CD21). EBV induces a growth transformation of infected B lymphocytes, and these proliferating B cells incite a brisk cytotoxic T cell response. It is these reactive T cells that account for the atypical lymphocytosis, or "mononucleosis," of acute infection and are ultimately responsible for containing the infection.

After resolution of primary infection, EBV, like all herpesviruses, establishes a persistent latent infection in the host and is able to reactivate periodically. Latent infection, which occurs in B lymphocytes, is characterized by cessation of most viral gene expression and maintenance of the viral genome as a circular episome by cellular machinery. In vitro, lymphocytes latently infected with EBV are transformed into lymphoblastoid cell lines and can be propagated indefinitely. In vivo, EBV transformation of B lymphocytes is controlled by specific cytotoxic T lymphocytes but can result in lymphoproliferative disease in immunosuppressed individuals. Approximately 1 in 10^6 lymphocytes is latently infected with EBV and serves as the reservoir for reactivation. Virions released from lymphocytes undergo lytic replication in the oral epithelium and are shed in the saliva of seropositive individuals.

Epidemiology

Seroepidemiologic studies show that more than 95% adults are infected with EBV. In developing countries primary infection occurs during infancy or early childhood; but in affluent populations of industrial countries as many as one-third of infections occur during adolescence or early adulthood. With the exception of vertical transmission of HIV, EBV infection precedes HIV infection. Studies in children who acquired HIV infection by vertical transmission reveal that EBV seroconversion, at least in this HIV-positive population, did not have an appreciable affect on clinically important parameters such as CD4 count or viral load.[6,7] Moreover, primary infection appears to be largely asymptomatic, although one study noted an increased incidence of hepatosplenomegaly. By contrast, many studies have shown a significant increase in the frequency of oral shedding of EBV by HIV-positive persons.[6,8,9] As previously stated, type II EBV infection, rare outside Africa and New Guinea, is present in about half of the HIV-positive population, and at least half of these individuals are co-infected with both types I and II. In nonendemic areas, acquisition of type II EBV infection appears to be closely linked to sexual behavior.[10,11]

Pathogenesis/Molecular Biology

Multiple factors probably account for the relation between HIV and EBV infections. First, acquired immunodeficiency syndrome (AIDS) patients have 10 to 20 times as many circulating EBV-infected B cells. T lymphocytes from these patients have been shown to suppress EBV-positive B cells less effectively than do T cells from normal controls.[12] Increased salivary shedding of EBV in the HIV population indicates that control of lytic infection is also impaired. Host factors also appear to be important as evidenced by the observation that HIV-positive persons with the 3′A allele of the stromal cell-derived growth factor 1 (SDF-1) chemokine have a twofold increased risk of non-Hodgkin's lymphoma (NHL) in the heterozygous state and a fourfold increase when the host is homozygous.[13,14] The chemokine receptor 5 variant CCR5Δ32 and the chemokine receptor 2 variant CCR2-64I, which are protective against progression to AIDS, were investigated in one study. They found that the CCR5Δ32 allele conferred a threefold lower risk of developing NHL, but carrying CCR2-64I had no effect on NHL risk.[13]

Epstein-Barr virus-associated disease is distinctive because it is largely caused by latent infection not by reactivation of lytic infection. Oral hairy leukoplakia, caused by extensive EBV replication in oral epithelium, represents a notable exception. The term latent infection refers to the fact that viral particles are not produced, but this should not be taken to mean that EBV infection of B lymphocytes is passive. In fact, EBV can express as many as two membrane proteins (LMP1 and LMP2), six nuclear proteins (EBV nuclear antigens or EBNAs), and two untranslated RNAs (EBERs) during latency (Table 45–1).[1] It is these viral proteins that transform B lymphocytes into lymphoblastoid cell lines and are almost certainly responsible for EBV's association with malignancy. *LMP1,* the major viral oncogene, induces a growth-promoting signal that mimics a

▲ **Table 45–1.** PATTERNS OF LATENT EBV GENE EXPRESSION

	Latent Gene Expression Pattern						
Type	LMP-1	LMP-2	EBNA-1	EBNA-2 EBNA-LP	EBNA-3s	EBERs	**Occurrence**
I	—	—	+	—	—	+	Burkitt's lymphoma
II	+	+	+	—	—	+	NPC, Hodgkin's disease; peripheral T cell lymphoma
III	+	+	+	+	+	+	Infectious mononucleosis; LCL; XLPD; PTLD
N.A.	—	+	+	—	—	+	Healthy carrier

For historical reasons, the nomenclature of latent EBV gene expression derives from patterns of gene expression seen in EBV-related tumors.
EBER, EBV-encoded RNA; EBNA, EBV nuclear antigen; EBV, Epstein-Barr virus; LCL, lymphoblastoid cell line; LMP, latent membrane protein; NPC, nasopharyngeal carcinoma; PTLD, posttransplant lymphoproliferative disease; XLPD, X-linked lymphoproliferative disease.
From Kieff E, Rickison AB. Epstein-Barr virus and its replication. In: Knipe D, Howley P (eds) Fields Virology, 4th ed. Philadelphia, Lippincott, Williams & Wilkins, 2001; and Cohen JI. Epstein-Barr virus infection. N Engl J Med 343:481, 2000.

constitutively active form of the B cell surface molecule CD40.[16-18] The nuclear protein EBNA-1 ensures that the viral episome is maintained by cell machinery.[19] A second nuclear protein, EBNA-2, is a powerful activator of transcription that targets downstream elements of the Notch signaling pathway to induce expression of both viral and cellular genes, including *c-myc*.[20–22] The function of the remaining four nuclear proteins is less completely understood, but they may modulate the effects of EBNA-2.

The expression of all 10 latent EBV genes, referred to as type III latency, induces a potent immune response and is seen in the peripheral blood of normal hosts only during infectious mononucleosis. After resolution of primary infection, more restricted latent gene expression is observed. Continued EBNA-1 expression ensures maintenance of the viral genome; and because EBNA-1 can inhibit its own processing for presentation on class I major histocompatibility complex (MHC) molecules, it does not incite a significant immune response.[23] The EBERs and LMP2 also continue to be expressed; and though they appear not to have a direct role in lymphocyte transformation, they may be important for the biology of EBV in vivo.[24,25] For example, LMP2 has been shown to interact with signaling proteins downstream of the B cell receptor to prevent B cell activation. Because this signal frequently induces lytic replication, the purpose of LMP2 may be to preserve EBV in a latent state of infection.[26,27] Reversion to type III latency likely occurs at some low frequency, as normal individuals maintain lifelong strong cytotoxic T cell responses against type III latency antigens. In fact, one study suggested that type III latency is frequently observed in tonsillar B cells of normal hosts.[28] In immunocompromised hosts, the balance between immune clearance and B cell proliferation is disturbed. The lymphoproliferative syndromes seen in these hosts probably represent the in vivo equivalent of lymphoblastoid cell line transformation.

Primary Infection

For obscure reasons, primary EBV infection is accompanied approximately 90% of the time by antibodies that react with antigens found on sheep, horse, and beef erythrocytes. Detection of these so-called heterophile antibodies forms the basis for commercial assays such as the Monospot test.[29] Heterophile antibodies can be found in 5% to 10% of the healthy adult population; and in the setting of immune dysregulation by HIV the rate may be even higher. In children (the only HIV-positive population likely to be EBV-naive) primary EBV infection is heterophile-negative in about one-half of cases. When diagnostic uncertainty exists, specific antibodies to EBV proteins can be measured.

Immunoglobulin M (IgM) antibodies to viral capsid antigen (VCA) are present in 90% of acute infections and absent in the general population, so their presence is essentially diagnostic of primary infection.[29,30] By contrast, a fourfold rise in VCA IgG titers can be demonstrated in only 10% to 20% of cases because titers are generally already high upon initial presentation. Measurement of other antibodies is probably of limited clinical utility. One possible exception is that seroconversion to anti-EBNA antibodies occurs relatively late and can be used to confirm recent EBV infection in a patient previously documented to be anti-VCA-positive and anti-EBNA-negative.[31] Although virus can be cultured from the saliva, this assay is of little clinical use because it is slow, unable to distinguish acute infection from the viral shedding seen in healthy adults, and not generally available. Because primary EBV infection can be closely mimicked by the symptoms seen in HIV primary infection, measurement of an HIV viral load should always be considered in any person presenting with symptoms suggestive of infectious mononucleosis.[32]

Oral Hairy Leukoplakia

Oral hairy leukoplakia (OHL) presents as a corrugated, or "hairy," white lesion on the lateral surface of the tongue that is not removed by gentle scraping. It is a nonmalignant lesion caused by unchecked lytic replication of EBV.[33,34] OHL is seen in about 20% of persons with asymptomatic HIV infection and becomes more common with advanced disease.[35] Development of OHL is associated with more rapid progression to AIDS and death after controlling for the CD4 count.[36,37] It is also seen in other immunosuppressed persons, including bone marrow and solid organ transplant recipients.[38,39] Rarely, OHL is seen in the

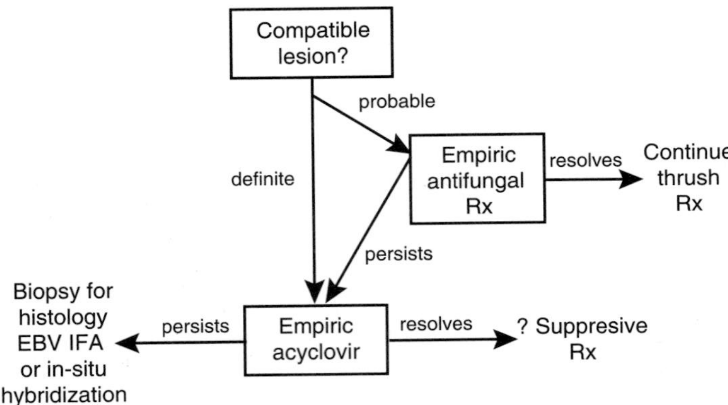

Figure 45–2. Diagnostic approach to oral hairy leukoplakia. Treatment should be considered for bothersome or symptomatic lesions. IFA, immunofluorescence assay.

absence of immunosuppression, but its presence demands that HIV be excluded.[40] The diagnosis of OHL (Fig. 45–2) is generally based on the typical appearance of the lesions in the appropriate clinical setting. The differential includes oral candidiasis, which can be distinguished by the ease of its removal from the tongue, an empiric trial of antifungal therapy, or both. Biopsy for histology and in situ hybridization or immunofluorescence staining for EBV is rarely necessary but can confirm the diagnosis. Polymerase chain reaction (PCR) detection of EBV in "oral scrapings" is neither sensitive nor specific for OHL.[41]

Persons with OHL are frequently asymptomatic, and lesions were reported to resolve spontaneously in 37% of a cohort followed for 1 year.[42] Treatment of symptomatic OHL is limited by the lack of large placebo-controlled trials in biopsy-proven cases. In an early study, Resnick et al. treated 6 of 13 OHL patients with acyclovir (3.2 g/day for 20 days) and observed regression in 5.[43] All five cases recurred with cessation of therapy, and no spontaneous regression was seen in the seven patients who refused therapy. Other authors have reported similar results.[44–46] Desciclovir (750 mg/day), an analogue of acyclovir, produced a similar complete response followed by relapse in eight patients treated by Greenspan et al.[47] Foscarnet and ganciclovir, which also inhibit EBV replication, have been associated with resolution of OHL in the context of treatment of cytomegalovirus (CMV)-related disease.[48,49] Less impressive results were seen in a study of acyclovir for CMV prophylaxis in which 19 of 32 (59%) who had OHL on entry improved on acyclovir versus 13 of 30 (43%) in the placebo group.[50] Moreover, there appeared to be no prophylactic benefit: The incidence of new OHL in the placebo group was 16% compared to 14% in the acyclovir group (118 patients in each group).

Zidovudine has also been shown to have activity against EBV in vitro, and alleviation of OHL during zidovudine therapy has been reported,[51,52] although other studies have shown little benefit of zidovudine.[42] Resolution with potent combination antiretroviral regimens is anticipated, and one observational study documented a decreasing prevalence of OHL.[53]

Topical therapy of OHL has also met with some success. Treatment with podophyllum resin 25% in one study resulted in remissions lasting 2 to 28 weeks.[54] A second observer-blinded study demonstrated marked improvement (relative to the untreated side) within 2 days of a single application.[55] Side effects were minimal, including slight burning or pain and transient dysgeusia.

Non-Hodgkin's Lymphoma

Unlike the rate of opportunistic infections, the incidence of non-Hodgkin's lymphoma in the HIV-positive population has not decreased with the advent of effective antiretroviral therapy.[56] In addition to primary effusion lymphoma (discussed under Kaposi's Sarcoma-Associated Herpesvirus), HIV infection carries a substantially increased risk of two forms of EBV-related B cell lymphomas. The first, Burkitt's-like lymphomas, generally occur early in the course of HIV infection and are EBV-positive 30% to 40% of the time.[57,58] Presentation at multiple extranodal sites and aggressive growth are the norm. The tumors contain the typical *c-myc* translocations of Burkitt's lymphomas.[59] As with classic Burkitt's lymphoma, the precise role of EBV in pathogenesis is not clear. When present, EBV episomes are monoclonal, implying that EBV infection preceded tumor expansion.[60] However, latent EBV gene expression in these tumors is restricted to EBNA-1 and the EBERs, which do not have well established oncogenic properties.

The second EBV-related B cell lymphoma seen with HIV infection is diffuse large-cell lymphoma (DLCL), which bears a striking resemblance to posttransplant lymphoproliferative disease (PTLD). As with PTLD, it occurs in the setting of profound immunosuppression; those with the lowest CD4 counts for the longest time are at greatest risk. Presentation as a primary CNS lymphoma is frequent, and essentially all CNS lymphomas are EBV-positive, whereas about two-thirds of DLCLs outside the CNS are EBV-positive.[57] The frequency of type I versus type II EBV in these tumors roughly parallels their prevalence in the HIV-positive population.[61–63] The pattern of EBV latent gene expression in DLCL and PTLD resemble that of lymphoblastoid cell lines.[64–66] Both diseases probably represent EBV-driven B cell proliferation that has escaped immune control.

The diagnosis of EBV-related non-Hodgkin's lymphoma generally rests on the histology and in situ hybridization for EBV gene products of appropriate biopsy material. A consistent correlation between serum EBV viral load and risk of PTLD is observed among solid organ and bone marrow transplant recipients.[67–71] Limited data suggest that this correlation extends to DLCL in HIV-positive patients.[72] Not surprisingly, many persons without DLCL have detectable amounts of EBV DNA in their serum. Moreover, EBV serum viral load can correlate poorly with clinical response during treatment.[73] Further studies are required before a role for serum EBV PCR can be entertained in HIV-infected patients.

The approach to CNS mass lesions in AIDS patients is discussed in Chapter 52 (see Fig. 52–2). The magnetic resonance imaging (MRI) and computed tomography (CT) appearance of primary CNS lymphoma are not sufficiently specific to exclude infectious etiologies. Single-photon emission CT (SPECT) or positron emission tomography (PET) scanning may be helpful, although the specificity is still likely to be insufficient by itself to establish a definitive diagnosis in difficult cases.[74,75] Unlike the results seen for serum, PCR for EBV DNA in the cerebrospinal fluid (CSF) has high sensitivity and specificity (>90%).[76–78] It has been suggested that the combination of PET scanning and EBV PCR may avoid the need for most biopsies.[74] However, as primary CNS lymphoma is seen only in those who are profoundly immunosuppressed, this diagnosis should be confirmed by biopsy in patients with CD4 counts higher than 100 mm^3.

The prognosis of AIDS-related DLCL has been poor, but treatment strategies are rapidly evolving. The mainstay PTLD treatment—reduction of immunosuppression—can be accomplished with antiretroviral therapy, but immune reconstitution may not be sufficiently rapid to obviate the need for cytotoxic therapy. Treatment of primary CNS lymphoma remains problematic, with reported median survival rates of less than 2 months.[79] Radiation therapy can increase median survival to about 4 months and dramatically improve quality of life. The role of systemic chemotherapy for primary CNS disease is under investigation. Treatment of non-Hodgkin's lymphoma outside the CNS begins with a complete staging workup that includes a complete blood count (CBC); lactate dehydrogenase (LDH) assay; CT of the abdomen, pelvis, and chest; bone marrow biopsy; and lumbar puncture (to exclude concurrent leptomeningeal disease). Systemic chemotherapy is required, even in cases that appear to be localized. The results of various regimens have been reviewed (see Chapter 49).[56]

Modulation of the host immune response is an intriguing direction for future therapy. The use of donor cytotoxic T cells has been investigated for the treatment of PTLD in bone marrow transplant patients. In one study the lymphoma resolution was observed in 90% of patients receiving donor lymphocytes; about one-third relapsed, however, and many experienced graft-versus-host disease (GVHD).[80] EBV-specific cytotoxic T cells have been used for prophylaxis[81,82] and treatment[83] of PTLD and appear to be less frequently associated with GVHD. Immunomodulatory therapy has also produced promising results: interferon-α produced complete regression in 8 of 14 PTLD patients.[84] Use of neutralizing monoclonal antibodies to interleutein-6 (IL-6), a cytokine known to play a critical autocrine role in EBV-mediated lymphoproliferation, has been shown to decrease tumor incidence and prolong survival in a mouse model.[85,86] Other monoclonal antibodies have been used to target tumor cells for immune clearance. Antibodies against CD21 (the EBV receptor) and CD24 (found on the surface of all B cells) produced complete remission in 61% of patients.[87] The recent U.S. Food and Drug Administration (FDA) approval of rituximab, a monoclonal antibody against CD20 (found on all B cells except plasma cells), for the treatment of low-grade B cell lymphomas was followed by a series of case reports of its efficacy for PTLD.[88–91] At present there are no reports of rituximab use in patients with HIV-associated lymphoma.

Perhaps the most controversial aspect of treating EBV-associated lymphoma is the role of antiviral therapy. Despite strong evidence that latent EBV infection is central to the pathogenesis of these malignancies, interest in antiviral therapy persists. Several justifications for this interest have been advanced. First, PTLD in pediatric patients frequently occurs in the setting of primary EBV infection. The use of acyclovir (or similar agents) in this setting may limit the extent of spread of the virus to the B cell compartment. It has also been argued that lytic gene expression, reported in some tumors,[92] may allow antiviral agents to act against some fraction of EBV-positive tumor cells. Several investigators report successful treatment of EBV-associated lymphomas with regimens that include acyclovir, foscarnet, or ganciclovir, though no well controlled trials exist to support or refute this practice.[93–96] A retrospective study by Fong et al. suggested that acyclovir may find a role in the prevention of EBV-associated lymphoma.[97] They found that patients receiving high doses, low or intermittent doses, or no acyclovir developed non-Hodgkin's lymphoma at rates of 7%, 16%, and 25%, respectively. The distribution of CNS lymphoma (3%, 9%, 5%, respectively) did not correlate with acyclovir exposure, and the proportion of non-CNS lymphomas that were EBV-positive was not determined. An earlier study found no decrease in non-Hodgkin's lymphoma associated with acyclovir exposure.[98] Such a prophylactic effect, if confirmed by a prospective trial, would be surprising in light of earlier data that acyclovir treatment has no effect on the number of circulating EBV-positive B cells.[99]

One antiviral drug that has shown activity against EBV during latent infection is hydroxyurea. In vitro this drug can eliminate EBV genomes from tissue culture cell lines. Slobod et al. reported a limited response to hydroxyurea in two patients with primary CNS lymphoma.[100]

See Chapter 51 for a further discussion of the diagnosis and therapy of non-Hodgkin's lymphoma in patients with AIDS.

Other EBV-Associated Diseases

Lymphoid interstitial pneumonitis is characterized by diffuse interstitial pulmonary infiltrates. It occurs primarily in children infected with HIV but is also seen in adults. EBV proteins and DNA have been detected in biopsy specimens from affected children.[101]

Epstein-Barr virus genomes have also been found in leiomyosarcoma biopsy specimens from children with AIDS.[102] These authors were able to demonstrate that the tumors expressed the EBV receptor (CD21) and did not find any evidence that EBV was associated with smooth muscle tumors of HIV-negative patients.

Two other EBV-associated diseases deserve mention. Nasopharyngeal carcinoma (NPC), a disease endemic in southern China and among the Inuit, is strongly associated with EBV infection.[2] There does not appear to be an appreciably increased incidence of NPC in the HIV-positive population. Hodgkin's disease, particularly the mixed-cellularity and lymphocyte-depleted forms, has also been linked to EBV infection. There is probably a modestly increased risk for HIV-positive persons in whom the disease tends to follow a more aggressive course.[103]

▲ KAPOSI'S SARCOMA-ASSOCIATED HERPESVIRUS

Natural History/Epidemiology

Although advances in the molecular biology of KSHV have outpaced our understanding of its natural history, epidemiologic studies were critical for establishing an infectious etiology for KS. A transmissible agent had long been suspected, and intensive investigation had even uncovered ultrastructural evidence for a herpesvirus in KS tissue,[104] but repeated efforts failed to isolate a pathogen. This changed in 1994 when Chang and colleagues, using a novel technique called representational difference analysis, succeeded in isolating two DNA sequences from KS tumors that ultimately proved to be from KSHV.[105] They later stated that epidemiologic evidence was a critical determinant of their decision to continue to search for a "Kaposi sarcoma agent."[106] Particularly compelling was surveillance data from the Centers for Disease Control and Prevention (CDC), which established that men who have sex with men (MSM) were 20 times more likely to have KS than similarly immunodeficient hemophiliac men.[107,108] Remarkably, much of what we know about the natural history of KSHV today could be deduced from studying the epidemiology of KS. Infection with the KS agent is relatively uncommon in the general population; it is transmitted by sexual or parasexual practices common among homosexual men but inefficiently transmitted by blood or blood products.

The identification of a specific pathogen enabled investigators to prove that the same virus was associated with all forms of KS: classic, endemic, AIDS- and transplant-related.[105,109] KSHV was subsequently linked to a rare form of HIV-associated lymphoma called primary effusion lymphoma and the multicentric form of Castleman's disease.[110–112] The diversity of assays used to measure KSHV antibodies has complicated estimates of KSHV seroprevalence. For example, assays that measure antibodies to latent KSHV antigens yield prevalence rates consistently lower than assays that measure antibodies to lytic antigens. Nevertheless, it can be safely stated that KSHV infection is not ubiquitous and displays distinct geographic variation. The KSHV seropositivity in the general population of the United States and western Europe is in the range of 1% to 5%.[113–115] This increases to 10% to 20% in certain regions of Mediterranean countries where classic KS is found[115–118] and may be as high as 30% to 80% in parts of sub-Saharan Africa.[118–124] In Western countries the KSHV seroprevalence among HIV-negative homosexual men is approximately 11% to 20% and rises to 30% to 54% in HIV-positive gay men; but among other HIV risk groups it is comparable to that seen in the general population.[114,125–127] One retrospective study found that a cohort of HIV-positive homosexual men seroconverted to KSHV 33 months (median) prior to the development of KS.[113]

The precise mode of transmission of KSHV is unclear. In endemic countries acquisition during childhood appears to be common, indicating that the mode of transmission may be different from that in the MSM population. The marked geographic variation in seroprevalence indicates that transmission is inefficient relative to herpesviruses such as EBV. The observed clustering in families suggests transmission between siblings or from mother to child. However, transmission by breastfeeding is unlikely because seroconversion appears to occur predominantly after the age of 2 years.[128] Studies of MSM cohorts have suggested that HIV positivity, increasing number of sexual partners, a history of a partner with KS, orogenital sex, and even use of inhaled amyl nitrate capsules were independent risk factors for KSHV seroconversion.[126,129–133] In heterosexual populations, birth in Africa appears to be the strongest risk factor.[130] Some studies have observed elevated rates of KSHV positivity at sexually transmitted disease clinics or among female workers, though other studies did not find evidence for heterosexual transmission.[114,115,130,134,135] KSHV DNA was found in the semen of HIV-infected persons but not in samples from healthy donors.[136] Viral loads appear to be about two logs higher in saliva than in semen or blood, and infectious virions have been recovered from saliva specimens.[137,138] These findings raise the possibility that the orogenital insertive sex poses a greater risk of KSHV acquisition than orogenital receptive sex.

A few potential cases of primary KSHV infection have been reported in the literature. Using banked serum samples, Oksenhendler et al. retrospectively documented seroconversion in a 43-year-old HIV-positive man 5 weeks prior to presentation with fever, arthralgia, cervical mass, and splenomegaly.[139] Interestingly, although pathologic examination of the cervical nodes revealed foci of KS, the patient never developed clinically evident KS despite 9 years of follow-up. Luppi et al. reported seroconversion to KSHV in two cadaveric renal transplant recipients from the same KSHV-positive donor.[140] The first patient, a 61-year-old man with idiopathic end-stage renal disease, presented with KS involving cervical lymph nodes, tracheobronchial tract, and gastrointestinal tract 4 months after transplant. The second patient, a 44-year-old man with membranoproliferative glomerulonephritis, also became symptomatic about 4 months after transplant with fever, splenomegaly, and pancytopenia. Finally, a 1-month-old female infant with DiGeorge syndrome, diagnosed with GVHD due to engrafted maternal cells, was found to have multiorgan dissemination of KSHV by PCR and in situ hybridization at autopsy.[141]

Pathogenesis/Molecular Biology

Whether KS represents a true malignancy or semimalignant angioproliferation is still a contested issue. The histology of these lesions is complex, involving spindle cells, endothelial cells, extravasated erythrocytes, and a variable inflammatory infiltrate. The spindle cells are believed to be the neoplastic component of KS lesions. However, examinations of spindle cells for clonality have produced conflicting results. The finding of polyclonal spindle cells by some investigators suggests that KS is an angioproliferation, whereas reports of spindle cell monoclonality are more consistent with a true malignancy.[142-145] One potentially unifying explanation for these discrepant observations is that KS begins as a polyclonal proliferation with a propensity to evolve into a true malignancy. In support of this theory is that late (nodular) KS has more frequently been monoclonal.

Despite uncertainty about the exact nature of KS, evidence continues to accumulate that KSHV plays a central role in its pathogenesis. Within the limits of current assays, KSHV seroconversion precedes the development of KS.[113,135] KSHV genomes are present in the spindle cells of KS lesions, in primary effusion lymphoma (PEL) cells, and in plasmablasts found in the mantle zone of the multicentric form of Castleman's disease.[110,112,146-148] One of the assays used to determine clonality, terminal repeat analysis, also reveals that KSHV infection of PEL and most KS spindle cells occur prior to neoplastic expansion.[145] There is good reason to believe that the presence of KSHV early in the evolution of these tumors reflects a causal relation. The sequencing of the KSHV genome[149] provided a large number of candidate genes to explain KSHV's relation to neoplastic transformation (Table 45–2). Some, such as v-*cyclin* or v-*FLIP*, were related to cells involved in cellular growth or antiapoptosis. Others, namely *K1, K9 (VIRF-1), K12,* and *vIL-8R,* have demonstrated transforming properties in standard assays. Whether any of these mediate KSHV's association with neoplasia remains to be determined. Similar genes in the EBV genome such as the *bcl2* homologue proved to have no role in transformation.

Several lines of evidence suggest that KSHV infection of KS spindle cells represents a latent viral infection. First is the inability to detect mRNA coding for conserved structural (i.e., lytic) proteins in spindle cells.[156,157] By contrast, mRNA for latency-associated nuclear antigen (LANA) is readily detected.[158] Expression of v-*FLIP,* v-*cyclin,* and *K12* (kaposin), genes associated with latent infection in PEL cell lines, has also been demonstrated.[156,157,159-161] The demonstration that KSHV genomes in KS lesions are present as viral episomes suggests that the role of KSHV in KS may indeed be analogous to that played by EBV-associated tumors.[159] Therefore many of the most promising genes from Table 45–2 are not expressed in KS spindle cells, although it is possible that a few cells entering the lytic phase allow these genes to play a paracrine role in tumorigenesis.

There are only limited analogies between the pathogenesis of latent KSHV infection and latent EBV infection. The divergence between these two viruses is vastly greater in the latent genes than the divergence between lytic, particularly structural, genes. Only one KSHV latent gene, *LANA,* has a clearly established EBV functional homologue. LANA has been demonstrated to be a sequence-specific DNA binding protein that recognizes a GC-rich sequence found in the terminal repeat region of the genome. It appears to function in a manner analogous to EBNA-1 in maintenance of the viral genome.[162,163] LANA is also reported to have other functions not shared by EBNA-1.[164-166] Further study is required to determine the importance and specific role of the other KSHV genes expressed in latency.

▲ **Table 45–2.** KSHV GENES THAT MAY PROMOTE NEOPLASIA

Reading Frame	Gene Product	Putative Function	Expression Pattern
K1	Membrane protein	Transforms rodent fibroblasts	Lytic
K2	vIL-6	B lymphocyte growth factor	Lytic
K4 K4.1 K6	vMIP-2 vMIP-3 vMIP-1	Cytokine analogues (of macrophage inhibitory protein)—may induce angiogenesis via cytokine receptors	Lytic
ORF16	vBcl-2	Inhibitor of apoptosis	Lytic
K9	vIRF-1	Inhibits interferon signaling; can transform rodent fibroblasts	Lytic
K10.5	LANA2, vIRF3	May inhibit *p53*-induced apoptosis	Latent
K12	Kaposin	Membrane protein; can transform rodent fibroblasts	?Latent
K13	vFLIP	Inhibits apoptosis	Latent
ORF72	v-cyclin	Stimulates cell division via cyclin-dependent kinases (CDKs) and makes CDKs resistant to inhibition	Latent
ORF73	LANA	Genome maintenance	Latent
ORF74	vIL-8R	Constitutively active cytokine receptor; transforms rodent . cells	Lytic

LANA, latency-associated nuclear antigen; ORF, open reading frame. The prefix "v" refers to a viral homologue of a cell gene.

Data are from Sun R, Lin SF, Staskus K, et al. Kinetics of Kaposi's sarcoma-associated herpesvirus gene expression. J Virol 73:2232, 1999; Callahan J, Pai S, Cotter M, et al. Distinct patterns of viral antigen expression in Epstein-Barr virus and Kaposi's sarcoma-associated herpesvirus coinfected body-cavity-based lymphoma cell lines: potential switches in latent gene expression due to coinfection. Virology 262:18, 1999; Jenner RG, Alba MM, Boshoff C, et al. Kaposi's sarcoma-associated herpesvirus latent and lytic gene expression as revealed by DNA arrays. J Virol 75:891, 2001; Schulz TF. Kaposi's sarcoma-associated herpesvirus (human herpesvirus-8). J Gen Virol 79:1573, 1998; Schulz TF. Kaposi's sarcoma-associated herpesvirus (human herpesvirus 8): epidemiology and pathogenesis. J Antimicrob Chemother 45(suppl T3):15, 2000; and Katano H, Sata T. Human herpesvirus 8: virology, epidemiology and related diseases. Jpn J Infect Dis 53:137, 2000.

Kaposi's Sarcoma

Kaposi's sarcoma was initially described in 1872 as a rare, indolent tumor occurring in elderly men of Mediterranean descent (classic KS). Subsequently, the disease was found to be endemic in portions of eastern Africa. Endemic KS was more aggressive, often presented in children with lymphadenopathy instead of skin lesions, and was frequently fatal. KS was later seen in organ transplant recipients; and its occurrence at an unexpectedly high rate among MSM heralded the HIV epidemic. Although the distribution of cases of classic KS is probably attributable to KSHV seroprevalence in these regions, the environmental or genetic cofactors that interact to produce the more aggressive endemic form of KS are unknown. Even immunodeficiency is not the straightforward risk factor it appears to be. AIDS patients in Gambia rarely present with KS, despite the high seroprevalence of KSHV in this region. Interestingly, HIV-2 infection is much more common in this region than HIV-1 infection, yet most reported cases of AIDS-associated KS are in patients infected with HIV-1.[118]

A detailed description of the treatment of KS is presented in Chapter 50. As with EBV-associated disease, the role of antiviral therapy is unclear. In vitro studies have established that foscarnet, ganciclovir, and cidofovir can inhibit KSHV replication, whereas acyclovir does not.[167–170] Several studies have reported a reduced rate of KS lesion appearance in patients taking ganciclovir or foscarnet but not in those taking acyclovir.[98,171–174] Surprisingly, two small studies found foscarnet administration to be associated with KS lesion regression.[175,176] Another study demonstrated that patients who were receiving intravenous foscarnet or ganciclovir still had detectable levels of KSHV in peripheral blood mononuclear cells.[177] Larger studies are required to define a role for antiviral agents in the treatment of KSHV disease.

Primary Effusion Lymphoma

Primary effusion lymphoma (PEL), formerly called body cavity-based lymphoma, represents a rare HIV-associated disease that presents as a malignant effusion in the pleural, pericardial, or peritoneal space. PEL cells are consistently KSHV-positive and frequently co-infected with EBV.[110] PEL is of monoclonal origin, and KSHV infection appears to occur early in tumorigenesis.[145] Cell lines have been established, and phorbal esters can induce lytic replication and produce infectious virions. This system has been used extensively to determine which KSHV genes are expressed during viral latency.

Multicentric Castleman's Disease

Angiofollicular lymphoid hyperplasia, or Castleman's disease, consists of two distinct clinical entities with similar histology.[178] The localized form presents as a solitary mass, and excision is generally curative. By contrast, the multicentric form (MCD) presents with diffuse lymphadenopathy and constitutional symptoms and is an aggressive, usually fatal disorder. Biopsies of MCD have shown KSHV to be present in mantle zone large immunoblastic B cells of these lesions.[160] Those diagnosed with MCD are at increased risk of subsequent development of lymphoma or KS. HIV infection is associated with MCD, and 75% of HIV-positive MCD patients subsequently develop KS.[179] In contrast to other KSHV-associated neoplasia, MCD is clearly a polyclonal disorder.[180] It has been associated with high levels of IL-6, which are thought to play an important paracrine role in stimulating growth.[181–184] The increased rate of lytic KSHV infection in MCD may permit the lytic *vIL-6* gene and/or other lytic genes to participate in the pathogenesis of MCD.[185,186] There are no data in the literature regarding the use of antiviral agents for the treatment of MCD. Because lytic infection is more prominent in MCD lesions, it appears to be an important avenue for future study.

REFERENCES

1. Kieff E, Rickison AB. Epstein-Barr virus and its replication. In: Knipe D, Howley P (eds) Fields Virology, 4th ed. Philadelphia, Lippincott, Williams & Wilkins, 2001.
2. Rickinson AB, Kieff E. Epstein-Barr virus. In: Knipe DM, Howley PM (eds) Fields Virology, 4th ed. Philadelphia, Lippincott, Williams & Wilkins, 2001.
3. Zong JC, Ciufo DM, Alcendor DJ, et al. High-level variability in the ORF-K1 membrane protein gene at the left end of the Kaposi's sarcoma-associated herpesvirus genome defines four major virus subtypes and multiple variants or clades in different human populations. J Virol 73:4156, 1999.
4. Biggar RJ, Whitby D, Marshall V, et al. Human herpesvirus 8 in Brazilian Amerindians: a hyperendemic population with a new subtype. J Infect Dis 181:1562, 2000.
5. Hayward GS. KSHV strains: the origins and global spread of the virus. Semin Cancer Biol 9:187, 1999.
6. Jenson H, McIntosh K, Pitt J, et al. Natural history of primary Epstein-Barr virus infection in children of mothers infected with human immunodeficiency virus type 1. J Infect Dis 179:1395, 1999.
7. Pedneault L, Lapointe N, Alfieri C, et al. Natural history of Epstein-Barr virus infection in a prospective pediatric cohort born to human immunodeficiency virus-infected mothers. J Infect Dis 177:1087, 1998.
8. Luxton JC, Williams I, Weller I, et al. Epstein-Barr virus infection of HIV-seropositive individuals is transiently suppressed by high-dose acyclovir treatment. AIDS 7:1337, 1993.
9. Ferbas J, Rahman MA, Kingsley LA, et al. Frequent oropharyngeal shedding of Epstein-Barr virus in homosexual men during early HIV infection. AIDS 6:1273, 1992.
10. Yao QY, Croom-Carter DS, Tierney RJ, et al. Epidemiology of infection with Epstein-Barr virus types 1 and 2: lessons from the study of a T-cell-immunocompromised hemophilic cohort. J Virol 72:4352, 1998.
11. Van Baarle D, Hovenkamp E, Dukers NH, et al. High prevalence of Epstein-Barr virus type 2 among homosexual men is caused by sexual transmission. J Infect Dis 181:2045, 2000.
12. Birx DL, Redfield RR, Tosato G. Defective regulation of Epstein-Barr virus infection in patients with acquired immunodeficiency syndrome (AIDS) or AIDS-related disorders. N Engl J Med 314:874, 1986.
13. Rabkin CS, Yang Q, Goedert JJ, et al. Chemokine and chemokine receptor gene variants and risk of non-Hodgkin's lymphoma in human immunodeficiency virus-1-infected individuals. Blood 93:1838, 1999.
14. Dean M, Jacobson LP, McFarlane G, et al. Reduced risk of AIDS lymphoma in individuals heterozygous for the CCR5-delta32 mutation. Cancer Res 59:3561, 1999.
15. Cohen JI. Epstein-Barr virus infection. N Engl J Med 343:481, 2000.
16. Mosialos G, Birkenbach M, Yalamanchili R, et al. The Epstein-Barr virus transforming protein LMP1 engages signaling proteins for the tumor necrosis factor receptor family. Cell 80:389, 1995.

17. Izumi KM, Kieff ED. The Epstein-Barr virus oncogene product latent membrane protein 1 engages the tumor necrosis factor receptor-associated death domain protein to mediate B lymphocyte growth transformation and activate NF-kappaB. Proc Natl Acad Sci USA 94:12592, 1997.
18. Izumi KM, Kaye KM, Kieff ED. The Epstein-Barr virus LMP1 amino acid sequence that engages tumor necrosis factor receptor associated factors is critical for primary B lymphocyte growth transformation. Proc Natl Acad Sci USA 94:1447, 1997.
19. Yates J, Warren N, Reisman D, et al. A cis-acting element from the Epstein-Barr viral genome that permits stable replication of recombinant plasmids in latently infected cells. Proc Natl Acad Sci USA 81:3806, 1984.
20. Henkel T, Ling PD, Hayward SD, et al. Mediation of Epstein-Barr virus EBNA2 transactivation by recombination signal-binding protein J kappa. Science 265:92, 1994.
21. Grossman SR, Johannsen E, Tong X, et al. The Epstein-Barr virus nuclear antigen 2 transactivator is directed to response elements by the J kappa recombination signal binding protein. Proc Natl Acad Sci USA 91:7568, 1994.
22. Kaiser C, Laux G, Eick D, et al. The proto-oncogene c-myc is a direct target gene of Epstein-Barr virus nuclear antigen 2. J Virol 73:4481, 1999.
23. Levitskaya J, Sharipo A, Leonchiks A, et al. Inhibition of ubiquitin/proteasome-dependent protein degradation by the Gly-Ala repeat domain of the Epstein-Barr virus nuclear antigen 1. Proc Natl Acad Sci USA 94:12616, 1997.
24. Swaminathan S, Tomkinson B, Kieff E. Recombinant Epstein-Barr virus with small RNA (EBER) genes deleted transforms lymphocytes and replicates in vitro. Proc Natl Acad Sci USA 88:1546, 1991.
25. Longnecker R, Miller CL, Miao XQ, et al. The last seven transmembrane and carboxy-terminal cytoplasmic domains of Epstein-Barr virus latent membrane protein 2 (LMP2) are dispensable for lymphocyte infection and growth transformation in vitro. J Virol 67:2006, 1993.
26. Miller CL, Lee JH, Kieff E, et al. Epstein-Barr virus protein LMP2A regulates reactivation from latency by negatively regulating tyrosine kinases involved in sIg-mediated signal transduction. Infect Agents Dis 3:128, 1994.
27. Longnecker R. Epstein-Barr virus latency: LMP2, a regulator or means for Epstein-Barr virus persistence? Adv Cancer Res 79:175, 2000.
28. Babcock JG, Hochberg D, Thorley-Lawson AD. The expression pattern of Epstein-Barr virus latent genes in vivo is dependent upon the differentiation stage of the infected B cell. Immunity 13:497, 2000.
29. Evans AS, Niederman JC, Cenabre LC, et al. A prospective evaluation of heterophile and Epstein-Barr virus-specific IgM antibody tests in clinical and subclinical infectious mononucleosis: specificity and sensitivity of the tests and persistence of antibody. J Infect Dis 132:546, 1975.
30. Henle W, Henle G, Niederman JC, et al. Antibodies to early antigens induced by Epstein-Barr virus in infectious mononucleosis. J Infect Dis 124:58, 1971.
31. Henie G, Henle W, Horwitz CA. Antibodies to Epstein-Barr virus-associated nuclear antigen in infectious mononucleosis. J Infect Dis 130:231, 1974.
32. Schacker T, Collier AC, Hughes J, et al. Clinical and epidemiologic features of primary HIV infection. Ann Intern Med 125:257, 1996.
33. Greenspan JS, Greenspan D, Lennette ET, et al. Replication of Epstein-Barr virus within the epithelial cells of oral "hairy" leukoplakia, an AIDS-associated lesion. N Engl J Med 313:1564, 1985.
34. Triantos D, Porter SR, Scully C, et al. Oral hairy leukoplakia: clinicopathologic features, pathogenesis, diagnosis, and clinical significance. Clin Infect Dis 25:1392, 1997.
35. Feigal DW, Katz MH, Greenspan D, et al. The prevalence of oral lesions in HIV-infected homosexual and bisexual men: three San Francisco epidemiological cohorts. AIDS 5:519, 1991.
36. Greenspan D, Greenspan JS, Hearst NG, et al. Relation of oral hairy leukoplakia to infection with the human immunodeficiency virus and the risk of developing AIDS. J Infect Dis 155:475, 1987.
37. Katz MH, Greenspan D, Westenhouse J, et al. Progression to AIDS in HIV-infected homosexual and bisexual men with hairy leukoplakia and oral candidiasis. AIDS 6:95, 1992.
38. Epstein JB, Sherlock CH, Greenspan JS. Hairy leukoplakia-like lesions following bone-marrow transplantation. AIDS 5:101, 1991.
39. Greenspan D, Greenspan JS, de Souza Y, et al. Oral hairy leukoplakia in an HIV-negative renal transplant recipient. J Oral Pathol Med 18:32, 1989.
40. Wurapa AK, Luque AE, Menegus MA. Oral hairy leukoplakia: a manifestation of primary infection with Epstein-Barr virus? Scand J Infect Dis 31:505, 1999.
41. Scully C, Porter SR, Di Alberti L, et al. Detection of Epstein-Barr virus in oral scrapes in HIV infection, in hairy leukoplakia, and in healthy non-HIV-infected people. J Oral Pathol Med 27:480, 1998.
42. Katz MH, Greenspan D, Heinic GS, et al. Resolution of hairy leukoplakia: an observational trial of zidovudine versus no treatment. J Infect Dis 164:1240, 1991.
43. Resnick L, Herbst JS, Ablashi DV, et al. Regression of oral hairy leukoplakia after orally administered acyclovir therapy. JAMA 259:384, 1988.
44. Glick M, Pliskin ME. Regression of oral hairy leukoplakia after oral administration of acyclovir. Gen Dent 38:374, 1990.
45. Laskaris G, Laskaris M, Theodoridou M. Oral hairy leukoplakia in a child with AIDS. Oral Surg Oral Med Oral Pathol Oral Radiol Endod 79:570, 1995.
46. Naher H, Helfrich S, Hartmann M, et al. [EBV replication and therapy of oral hairy leukoplakia using acyclovir.] Hautarzt 41:680, 1990.
47. Greenspan D, De Souza YG, Conant MA, et al. Efficacy of desciclovir in the treatment of Epstein-Barr virus infection in oral hairy leukoplakia. J Acquir Immune Defic Syndr 3:571, 1990.
48. Newman C, Polk BF. Resolution of oral hairy leukoplakia during therapy with 9-(1,3-dihydroxy-2-propoxymethyl)guanine (DHPG). Ann Intern Med 107:348, 1987.
49. Albrecht H, Stellbrink HJ, Brewster D, et al. Resolution of oral hairy leukoplakia during treatment with foscarnet. AIDS 8:1014, 1994.
50. Youle MS, Gazzard BG, Johnson MA, et al. Effects of high-dose oral acyclovir on herpesvirus disease and survival in patients with advanced HIV disease: a double-blind, placebo-controlled study. European-Australian Acyclovir Study Group. AIDS 8:641, 1994.
51. Kessler HA, Benson CA, Urbanski P. Regression of oral hairy leukoplakia during zidovudine therapy. Arch Intern Med 148:2496, 1988.
52. Phelan JA, Klein RS. Resolution of oral hairy leukoplakia during treatment with azidothymidine. Oral Surg Oral Med Oral Pathol 65:717, 1988.
53. Patton LL, McKaig R, Strauss R, et al. Changing prevalence of oral manifestations of human immuno-deficiency virus in the era of protease inhibitor therapy. Oral Surg Oral Med Oral Pathol Oral Radiol Endod 89:299, 2000.
54. Lozada-Nur F, Costa C. Retrospective findings of the clinical benefits of podophyllum resin 25% sol on hairy leukoplakia: clinical results in nine patients. Oral Surg Oral Med Oral Pathol 73:555, 1992.
55. Gowdey G, Lee RK, Carpenter WM. Treatment of HIV-related hairy leukoplakia with podophyllum resin 25% solution. Oral Surg Oral Med Oral Pathol Oral Radiol Endod 79:64, 1995.
56. Levine AM. Acquired immunodeficiency syndrome-related lymphoma: clinical aspects. Semin Oncol 27:442, 2000.
57. Hamilton-Dutoit SJ, Raphael M, Audouin J, et al. In situ demonstration of Epstein-Barr virus small RNAs (EBER 1) in acquired immunodeficiency syndrome-related lymphomas: correlation with tumor morphology and primary site. Blood 82:619, 1993.
58. Subar M, Neri A, Inghirami G, et al. Frequent c-myc oncogene activation and infrequent presence of Epstein-Barr virus genome in AIDS-associated lymphoma. Blood 72:667, 1988.
59. Chaganti RS, Jhanwar SC, Koziner B, et al. Specific translocations characterize Burkitt's-like lymphoma of homosexual men with the acquired immunodeficiency syndrome. Blood 61:1265, 1983.
60. Neri A, Barriga F, Inghirami G, et al. Epstein-Barr virus infection precedes clonal expansion in Burkitt's and acquired immunodeficiency syndrome-associated lymphoma. Blood 77:1092, 1991.
61. Boyle MJ, Sewell WA, Sculley TB, et al. Subtypes of Epstein-Barr virus in human immunodeficiency virus-associated non-Hodgkin lymphoma. Blood 78:3004, 1991.
62. Gunthel CJ, Ng V, McGrath M, et al. Association of Epstein-Barr virus types 1 and 2 with acquired immunodeficiency syndrome-related primary central nervous system lymphomas. Blood 83:618, 1994.
63. Van Baarle D, Hovenkamp E, Kersten MJ, et al. Direct Epstein-Barr virus (EBV) typing on peripheral blood mononuclear cells: no association between EBV type 2 infection or superinfection and the devel-

opment of acquired immunodeficiency syndrome-related non-Hodgkin's lymphoma. Blood 93:3949, 1999.

64. Hamilton-Dutoit SJ, Rea D, Raphael M, et al. Epstein-Barr virus-latent gene expression and tumor cell phenotype in acquired immunodeficiency syndrome-related non-Hodgkin's lymphoma. correlation of lymphoma phenotype with three distinct patterns of viral latency. Am J Pathol 143:1072, 1993.
65. Rea D, Delecluse HJ, Hamilton-Dutoit SJ, et al. Epstein-Barr virus latent and replicative gene expression in post-transplant lymphoproliferative disorders and AIDS-related non-Hodgkin's lymphomas: French Study Group of Pathology for HIV-associated Tumors. Ann Oncol 5:113, 1994.
66. Brink AA, Dukers DF, van den Brule AJ, et al. Presence of Epstein-Barr virus latency type III at the single cell level in post-transplantation lymphoproliferative disorders and AIDS related lymphomas. J Clin Pathol 50:911, 1997.
67. Savoie A, Perpete C, Carpentier L, et al. Direct correlation between the load of Epstein-Barr virus-infected lymphocytes in the peripheral blood of pediatric transplant patients and risk of lymphoproliferative disease. Blood 83:2715, 1994.
68. Rooney CM, Loftin SK, Holladay MS, et al. Early identification of Epstein-Barr virus-associated post-transplantation lymphoproliferative disease. Br J Haematol 89:98, 1995.
69. Rowe DT, Qu L, Reyes J, et al. Use of quantitative competitive PCR to measure Epstein-Barr virus genome load in the peripheral blood of pediatric transplant patients with lymphoproliferative disorders. J Clin Microbiol 35:1612, 1997.
70. Lucas KG, Burton RL, Zimmerman SE, et al. Semiquantitative Epstein-Barr virus (EBV) polymerase chain reaction for the determination of patients at risk for EBV-induced lymphoproliferative disease after stem cell transplantation. Blood 91:3654, 1998.
71. Green M, Bueno J, Rowe D, et al. Predictive negative value of persistent low Epstein-Barr virus viral load after intestinal transplantation in children. Transplantation 70:593, 2000.
72. Laroche C, Drouet EB, Brousset P, et al. Measurement by the polymerase chain reaction of the Epstein-Barr virus load in infectious mononucleosis and AIDS-related non-Hodgkin's lymphomas. J Med Virol 46:66, 1995.
73. Yang J, Tao Q, Flinn IW, et al. Characterization of Epstein-Barr virus-infected B cells in patients with posttransplantation lymphoproliferative disease: disappearance after rituximab therapy does not predict clinical response. Blood 96:4055, 2000.
74. Antinori A, De Rossi G, Ammassari A, et al. Value of combined approach with thallium-201 single-photon emission computed tomography and Epstein-Barr virus DNA polymerase chain reaction in CSF for the diagnosis of AIDS-related primary CNS lymphoma. J Clin Oncol 17:554, 1999.
75. Hoffman JM, Waskin HA, Schifter T, et al. FDG-PET in differentiating lymphoma from nonmalignant central nervous system lesions in patients with AIDS. J Nucl Med 34:567, 1993.
76. Cinque P, Brytting M, Vago L, et al. Epstein-Barr virus DNA in cerebrospinal fluid from patients with AIDS-related primary lymphoma of the central nervous system. Lancet 342:398, 1993.
77. Cingolani A, Gastaldi R, Fassone L, et al. Epstein-Barr virus infection is predictive of CNS involvement in systemic AIDS-related non-Hodgkin's lymphomas. J Clin Oncol 18:3325, 2000.
78. Broccolo F, Iuliano R, Careddu AM, et al. Detection of lymphotropic herpesvirus DNA by polymerase chain reaction in cerebrospinal fluid of AIDS patients with neurological disease. Acta Virol 44:137, 2000.
79. Bower M, Fife K, Sullivan A, et al. Treatment outcome in presumed and confirmed AIDS-related primary cerebral lymphoma. Eur J Cancer 35:601, 1999.
80. O'Reilly RJ, Small TN, Papadopoulos E, et al. Biology and adoptive cell therapy of Epstein-Barr virus-associated lymphoproliferative disorders in recipients of marrow allografts. Immunol Rev 157:195, 1997.
81. Rooney CM, Smith CA, Ng CY, et al. Use of gene-modified virus-specific T lymphocytes to control Epstein-Barr-virus-related lymphoproliferation. Lancet 345:9, 1995.
82. Heslop HE, Rooney CM. Adoptive cellular immunotherapy for EBV lymphoproliferative disease. Immunol Rev 157:217, 1997.
83. Rooney CM, Smith CA, Ng CY, et al. Infusion of cytotoxic T cells for the prevention and treatment of Epstein-Barr virus-induced lymphoma in allogeneic transplant recipients. Blood 92:1549, 1998.
84. Davis CL, Wood BL, Sabath DE, et al. Interferon-alpha treatment of posttransplant lymphoproliferative disorder in recipients of solid organ transplants. Transplantation 66:1770, 1998.
85. Mauray S, Fuzzati-Armentero MT, Trouillet P, et al. Epstein-Barr virus-dependent lymphoproliferative disease: critical role of IL-6. Eur J Immunol 30:2065, 2000.
86. Tosato G, Tanner J, Jones KD, et al. Identification of interleukin-6 as an autocrine growth factor for Epstein-Barr virus-immortalized B cells. J Virol 64:3033, 1990.
87. Benkerrou M, Jais JP, Leblond V, et al. Anti-B-cell monoclonal antibody treatment of severe posttransplant B-lymphoproliferative disorder: prognostic factors and long-term outcome. Blood 92:3137, 1998.
88. Cook RC, Connors JM, Gascoyne RD, et al. Treatment of post-transplant lymphoproliferative disease with rituximab monoclonal antibody after lung transplantation. Lancet 354:1698, 1999.
89. Niedermeyer J, Hoffmeyer F, Hertenstein B, et al. Treatment of lymphoproliferative disease with rituximab. Lancet 355:499, 2000.
90. Zompi S, Tulliez M, Conti F, et al. Rituximab (anti-CD20 monoclonal antibody) for the treatment of patients with clonal lymphoproliferative disorders after orthotopic liver transplantation: a report of three cases. J Hepatol 32:521, 2000.
91. Oertel SH, Anagnostopoulos I, Bechstein WO, et al. Treatment of posttransplant lymphoproliferative disorder with the anti-CD20 monoclonal antibody rituximab alone in an adult after liver transplantation: a new drug in therapy of patients with posttransplant lymphoproliferative disorder after solid organ transplantation? Transplantation 69:430, 2000.
92. Pallesen G, Hamilton-Dutoit SJ, Rowe M, et al. Expression of Epstein-Barr virus replicative proteins in AIDS-related non-Hodgkin's lymphoma cells. J Pathol 165:289, 1991.
93. Raez L, Cabral L, Cai JP, et al. Treatment of AIDS-related primary central nervous system lymphoma with zidovudine, ganciclovir, and interleukin 2. AIDS Res Hum Retroviruses 15:713, 1999.
94. Brockmeyer NH, Pohl G, Mertins L. Combination of chemotherapy and antiviral therapy for Epstein-Barr virus-associated non-Hodgkin's lymphoma of high grade malignancy in cases of HIV infection. Eur J Med Res 2:133, 1997.
95. Oertel SH, Ruhnke MS, Anagnostopoulos I, et al. Treatment of Epstein-Barr virus-induced posttransplantation lymphoproliferative disorder with foscarnet alone in an adult after simultaneous heart and renal transplantation. Transplantation 67:765, 1999.
96. Schmidt W, Anagnostopoulos I, Scherubl H. Virostatic therapy for advanced lymphoproliferation associated with the Epstein-Barr virus in an HIV-infected patient. N Engl J Med 342:440, 2000.
97. Fong IW, Ho J, Toy C, et al. Value of long-term administration of acyclovir and similar agents for protecting against AIDS-related lymphoma: case-control and historical cohort studies. Clin Infect Dis 30:757, 2000.
98. Ioannidis JP, Collier AC, Cooper DA, et al. Clinical efficacy of high-dose acyclovir in patients with human immunodeficiency virus infection: a meta-analysis of randomized individual patient data. J Infect Dis 178:349, 1998.
99. Yao QY, Ogan P, Rowe M, et al. Epstein-Barr virus-infected B cells persist in the circulation of acyclovir-treated virus carriers. Int J Cancer 43:67, 1989.
100. Slobod KS, Taylor GH, Sandlund JT, et al. Epstein-Barr virus-targeted therapy for AIDS-related primary lymphoma of the central nervous system. Lancet 356:1493, 2000.
101. Andiman WA, Eastman R, Martin K, et al. Opportunistic lymphoproliferations associated with Epstein-Barr viral DNA in infants and children with AIDS. Lancet 2:1390, 1985.
102. McClain KL, Leach CT, Jenson HB, et al. Association of Epstein-Barr virus with leiomyosarcomas in children with AIDS. N Engl J Med 332:12, 1995.
103. Spina M, Vaccher E, Nasti G, et al. Human immunodeficiency virus-associated Hodgkin's disease. Semin Oncol 27:480, 2000.
104. Giraldo G, Beth E, Buonaguro FM. Kaposi's sarcoma: a natural model of interrelationships between viruses, immunologic responses, genetics, and oncogenesis. Antibiot Chemother 32:1, 1983.
105. Chang Y, Cesarman E, Pessin MS, et al. Identification of herpesvirus-like DNA sequences in AIDS-associated Kaposi's sarcoma. Science 266:1865, 1994.
106. Moore PS, Chang Y. Kaposi's sarcoma (KS), KS-associated herpesvirus, and the criteria for causality in the age of molecular biology. Am J Epidemiol 147:217, 1998.

107. Beral V, Peterman TA, Berkelman RL, et al. Kaposi's sarcoma among persons with AIDS: a sexually transmitted infection? Lancet 335:123, 1990.
108. Albrecht H, Helm EB, Plettenberg A, et al. Kaposi's sarcoma in HIV infected women in Germany: more evidence for sexual transmission: a report of 10 cases and review of the literature. Genitourin Med 70:394, 1994.
109. Moore PS, Chang Y. Detection of herpesvirus-like DNA sequences in Kaposi's sarcoma in patients with and without HIV infection. N Engl J Med 332:1181, 1995.
110. Cesarman E, Chang Y, Moore PS, et al. Kaposi's sarcoma-associated herpesvirus-like DNA sequences in AIDS-related body-cavity-based lymphomas. N Engl J Med 332:1186, 1995.
111. Nador RG, Cesarman E, Chadburn A, et al. Primary effusion lymphoma: a distinct clinicopathologic entity associated with the Kaposi's sarcoma-associated herpesvirus. Blood 88:645, 1996.
112. Soulier J, Grollet L, Oksenhendler E, et al. Kaposi's sarcoma-associated herpesvirus-like DNA sequences in multicentric Castleman's disease. Blood 86:1276, 1995.
113. Gao SJ, Kingsley L, Hoover DR, et al. Seroconversion to antibodies against Kaposi's sarcoma-associated herpesvirus-related latent nuclear antigens before the development of Kaposi's sarcoma. N Engl J Med 335:233, 1996.
114. Kedes DH, Operskalski E, Busch M, et al. The seroepidemiology of human herpesvirus 8 (Kaposi's sarcoma-associated herpesvirus): distribution of infection in KS risk groups and evidence for sexual transmission. Nat Med 2:918, 1996.
115. Simpson GR, Schulz TF, Whitby D, et al. Prevalence of Kaposi's sarcoma associated herpesvirus infection measured by antibodies to recombinant capsid protein and latent immunofluorescence antigen. Lancet 348:1133, 1996.
116. Whitby D, Luppi M, Barozzi P, et al. Human herpesvirus 8 seroprevalence in blood donors and lymphoma patients from different regions of Italy. J Natl Cancer Inst 90:395, 1998.
117. Calabro ML, Sheldon J, Favero A, et al. Seroprevalence of Kaposi's sarcoma-associated herpesvirus/human herpesvirus 8 in several regions of Italy. J Hum Virol 1:207, 1998.
118. Ariyoshi K, Schim van der Loeff M, Cook P, et al. Kaposi's sarcoma in the Gambia, West Africa is less frequent in human immunodeficiency virus type 2 than in human immunodeficiency virus type 1 infection despite a high prevalence of human herpesvirus 8. J Hum Virol 1:193, 1998.
119. Mayama S, Cuevas LE, Sheldon J, et al. Prevalence and transmission of Kaposi's sarcoma-associated herpesvirus (human herpesvirus 8) in Ugandan children and adolescents. Int J Cancer 77:817, 1998.
120. Bestetti G, Renon G, Mauclere P, et al. High seroprevalence of human herpesvirus-8 in pregnant women and prostitutes from Cameroon. AIDS 12:541, 1998.
121. Bourboulia D, Whitby D, Boshoff C, et al. Serologic evidence for mother-to-child transmission of Kaposi sarcoma-associated herpesvirus infection. JAMA 280:31, 1998.
122. Sitas F, Carrara H, Beral V, et al. Antibodies against human herpesvirus 8 in black South African patients with cancer. N Engl J Med 340:1863, 1999.
123. Gessain A, Mauclere P, van Beveren M, et al. Human herpesvirus 8 primary infection occurs during childhood in Cameroon, Central Africa. Int J Cancer 81:189, 1999.
124. Chatlynne LG, Ablashi DV. Seroepidemiology of Kaposi's sarcoma-associated herpesvirus (KSHV). Semin Cancer Biol 9:175, 1999.
125. Schulz TF. KSHV (HHV8) infection. J Infect 41:125, 2000.
126. Pauk J, Huang ML, Brodie SJ, et al. Mucosal shedding of human herpesvirus 8 in men. N Engl J Med 343:1369, 2000.
127. Perna AM, Bonura F, Vitale F, et al. Antibodies to human herpes virus type 8 (HHV8) in general population and in individuals at risk for sexually transmitted diseases in western Sicily. Int J Epidemiol 29:175, 2000.
128. Lyall EG, Patton GS, Sheldon J, et al. Evidence for horizontal and not vertical transmission of human herpesvirus 8 in children born to human immunodeficiency virus-infected mothers. Pediatr Infect Dis J 18:795, 1999.
129. Dukers NH, Renwick N, Prins M, et al. Risk factors for human herpesvirus 8 seropositivity and seroconversion in a cohort of homosexual men. Am J Epidemiol 151:213, 2000.
130. Smith NA, Sabin CA, Gopal R, et al. Serologic evidence of human herpesvirus 8 transmission by homosexual but not heterosexual sex. J Infect Dis 180:600, 1999.
131. Martin JN, Ganem DE, Osmond DH, et al. Sexual transmission and the natural history of human herpesvirus 8 infection. N Engl J Med 338:948, 1998.
132. Goudsmit J, Renwick N, Dukers NH, et al. Human herpesvirus 8 infections in the Amsterdam cohort studies (1984–1997): analysis of seroconversions to ORF65 and ORF73. Proc Natl Acad Sci USA 97:4838, 2000.
133. Blackbourn DJ, Osmond D, Levy JA, et al. Increased human herpesvirus 8 seroprevalence in young homosexual men who have multiple sex contacts with different partners. J Infect Dis 179:237, 1999.
134. Sosa C, Klaskala W, Chandran B, et al. Human herpesvirus 8 as a potential sexually transmitted agent in Honduras. J Infect Dis 178:547, 1998.
135. Lennette ET, Blackbourn DJ, Levy JA. Antibodies to human herpesvirus type 8 in the general population and in Kaposi's sarcoma patients. Lancet 348:858, 1996.
136. Howard MR, Whitby D, Bahadur G, et al. Detection of human herpesvirus 8 DNA in semen from HIV-infected individuals but not healthy semen donors. AIDS 11:F15, 1997.
137. LaDuca JR, Love JL, Abbott LZ, et al. Detection of human herpesvirus 8 DNA sequences in tissues and bodily fluids. J Infect Dis 178:1610, 1998.
138. Vieira J, Huang ML, Koelle DM, et al. Transmissible Kaposi's sarcoma-associated herpesvirus (human herpesvirus 8) in saliva of men with a history of Kaposi's sarcoma. J Virol 71:7083, 1997.
139. Oksenhendler E, Cazals-Hatem D, Schulz TF, et al. Transient angiolymphoid hyperplasia and Kaposi's sarcoma after primary infection with human herpesvirus 8 in a patient with human immunodeficiency virus infection. N Engl J Med 338:1585, 1998.
140. Luppi M, Barozzi P, Schulz TF, et al. Bone marrow failure associated with human herpesvirus 8 infection after transplantation. N Engl J Med 343:1378, 2000.
141. Sanchez-Velasco P, Ocejo-Vinyals JG, Flores R, et al. Simultaneous multiorgan presence of human herpesvirus 8 and restricted lymphotropism of Epstein-Barr virus DNA sequences in a human immunodeficiency virus-negative immunodeficient infant. J Infect Dis 183:338, 2001.
142. Delabesse E, Oksenhendler E, Lebbe C, et al. Molecular analysis of clonality in Kaposi's sarcoma. J Clin Pathol 50:664, 1997.
143. Rabkin CS, Janz S, Lash A, et al. Monoclonal origin of multicentric Kaposi's sarcoma lesions. N Engl J Med 336:988, 1997.
144. Gill PS, Tsai YC, Rao AP, et al. Evidence for multiclonality in multicentric Kaposi's sarcoma. Proc Natl Acad Sci USA 95:8257, 1998.
145. Judde JG, Lacoste V, Briere J, et al. Monoclonality or oligoclonality of human herpesvirus 8 terminal repeat sequences in Kaposi's sarcoma and other diseases. J Natl Cancer Inst 92:729, 2000.
146. Li JJ, Huang YQ, Cockerell CJ, et al. Localization of human herpes-like virus type 8 in vascular endothelial cells and perivascular spindle-shaped cells of Kaposi's sarcoma lesions by in situ hybridization. Am J Pathol 148:1741, 1996.
147. Kennedy MM, Cooper K, Howells DD, et al. Identification of HHV8 in early Kaposi's sarcoma: implications for Kaposi's sarcoma pathogenesis. Mol Pathol 51:14, 1998.
148. Boshoff C, Schulz TF, Kennedy MM, et al. Kaposi's sarcoma-associated herpesvirus infects endothelial and spindle cells. Nat Med 1:1274, 1995.
149. Russo JJ, Bohenzky RA, Chien MC, et al. Nucleotide sequence of the Kaposi sarcoma-associated herpesvirus (HHV8). Proc Natl Acad Sci USA 93:14862, 1996.
150. Sun R, Lin SF, Staskus K, et al. Kinetics of Kaposi's sarcoma-associated herpesvirus gene expression. J Virol 73:2232, 1999.
151. Callahan J, Pai S, Cotter M, et al. Distinct patterns of viral antigen expression in Epstein-Barr virus and Kaposi's sarcoma-associated herpesvirus coinfected body-cavity-based lymphoma cell lines: potential switches in latent gene expression due to coinfection. Virology 262:18, 1999.
152. Jenner RG, Alba MM, Boshoff C, et al. Kaposi's sarcoma-associated herpesvirus latent and lytic gene expression as revealed by DNA arrays. J Virol 75:891, 2001.
153. Schulz TF. Kaposi's sarcoma-associated herpesvirus (human herpesvirus-8). J Gen Virol 79:1573, 1998.

154. Schulz TF. Kaposi's sarcoma-associated herpesvirus (human herpesvirus 8): epidemiology and pathogenesis. J Antimicrob Chemother 45(suppl T3):15, 2000.
155. Katano H, Sata T. Human herpesvirus 8: virology, epidemiology and related diseases. Jpn J Infect Dis 53:137, 2000.
156. Staskus KA, Zhong W, Gebhard K, et al. Kaposi's sarcoma-associated herpesvirus gene expression in endothelial (spindle) tumor cells. J Virol 71:715, 1997.
157. Blasig C, Zietz C, Haar B, et al. Monocytes in Kaposi's sarcoma lesions are productively infected by human herpesvirus 8. J Virol 71:7963, 1997.
158. Katano H, Sato Y, Kurata T, et al. High expression of HHV-8-encoded ORF73 protein in spindle-shaped cells of Kaposi's sarcoma. Am J Pathol 155:47, 1999.
159. Decker LL, Shankar P, Khan G, et al. The Kaposi sarcoma-associated herpesvirus (KSHV) is present as an intact latent genome in KS tissue but replicates in the peripheral blood mononuclear cells of KS patients. J Exp Med 184:283, 1996.
160. Dupin N, Fisher C, Kellam P, et al. Distribution of human herpesvirus-8 latently infected cells in Kaposi's sarcoma, multicentric Castleman's disease, and primary effusion lymphoma. Proc Natl Acad Sci USA 96:4546, 1999.
161. Kellam P, Bourboulia D, Dupin N, et al. Characterization of monoclonal antibodies raised against the latent nuclear antigen of human herpesvirus 8. J Virol 73:5149, 1999.
162. Ballestas ME, Chatis PA, Kaye KM. Efficient persistence of extrachromosomal KSHV DNA mediated by latency-associated nuclear antigen. Science 284:641, 1999.
163. Cotter MA, Robertson ES. The latency-associated nuclear antigen tethers the Kaposi's sarcoma-associated herpesvirus genome to host chromosomes in body cavity-based lymphoma cells. Virology 264:254, 1999.
164. Friborg J, Kong W, Hottiger MO, et al. p53 Inhibition by the LANA protein of KSHV protects against cell death. Nature 402:889, 1999.
165. Lim C, Sohn H, Gwack Y, et al. Latency-associated nuclear antigen of Kaposi's sarcoma-associated herpesvirus (human herpesvirus-8) binds ATF4/CREB2 and inhibits its transcriptional activation activity. J Gen Virol 81 (Pt 11):2645, 2000.
166. Renne R, Barry C, Dittmer D, et al. Modulation of cellular and viral gene expression by the latency-associated nuclear antigen of Kaposi's sarcoma-associated herpesvirus. J Virol 75:458, 2001.
167. Kedes DH, Ganem D. Sensitivity of Kaposi's sarcoma-associated herpesvirus replication to antiviral drugs: implications for potential therapy. J Clin Invest 99:2082, 1997.
168. Medveczky MM, Horvath E, Lund T, et al. In vitro antiviral drug sensitivity of the Kaposi's sarcoma-associated herpesvirus. AIDS 11:1327, 1997.
169. Neyts J, De Clercq E. Antiviral drug susceptibility of human herpesvirus 8. Antimicrob Agents Chemother 41:2754, 1997.
170. Cannon JS, Hamzeh F, Moore S, et al. Human herpesvirus 8-encoded thymidine kinase and phosphotransferase homologues confer sensitivity to ganciclovir. J Virol 73:4786, 1999.
171. Jones JL, Hanson DL, Chu SY, et al. AIDS-associated Kaposi's sarcoma. Science 267:1078, 1995.
172. Glesby MJ, Hoover DR, Weng S, et al. Use of antiherpes drugs and the risk of Kaposi's sarcoma: data from the Multicenter AIDS Cohort Study. J Infect Dis 173:1477, 1996.
173. Mocroft A, Youle M, Gazzard B, et al. Anti-herpesvirus treatment and risk of Kaposi's sarcoma in HIV infection. Royal Free/Chelsea and Westminster Hospitals Collaborative Group. AIDS 10:1101, 1996.
174. Martin DF, Kuppermann BD, Wolitz RA, et al. Oral ganciclovir for patients with cytomegalovirus retinitis treated with a ganciclovir implant. Roche Ganciclovir Study Group. N Engl J Med 340:1063, 1999.
175. Morfeldt L, Torssander J. Long-term remission of Kaposi's sarcoma following foscarnet treatment in HIV-infected patients. Scand J Infect Dis 26:749, 1994.
176. Robles R, Lugo D, Gee L, et al. Effect of antiviral drugs used to treat cytomegalovirus end-organ disease on subsequent course of previously diagnosed Kaposi's sarcoma in patients with AIDS. J Acquir Immune Defic Syndr Hum Retrovirol 20:34, 1999.
177. Humphrey RW, O'Brien TR, Newcomb FM, et al. Kaposi's sarcoma (KS)-associated herpesvirus-like DNA sequences in peripheral blood mononuclear cells: association with KS and persistence in patients receiving anti-herpesvirus drugs. Blood 88:297, 1996.
178. Herrada J, Cabanillas F, Rice L, et al. The clinical behavior of localized and multicentric Castleman disease. Ann Intern Med 128:657, 1998.
179. O'Leary JJ, Kennedy MM, McGee JO. Kaposi's sarcoma associated herpesvirus (KSHV/HHV 8): epidemiology, molecular biology and tissue distribution. Mol Pathol 50:4, 1997.
180. Soulier J, Grollet L, Oksenhendler E, et al. Molecular analysis of clonality in Castleman's disease. Blood 86:1131, 1995.
181. Cannon JS, Nicholas J, Orenstein JM, et al. Heterogeneity of viral IL-6 expression in HHV-8-associated diseases. J Infect Dis 180:824, 1999.
182. Oksenhendler E, Carcelain G, Aoki Y, et al. High levels of human herpesvirus 8 viral load, human interleukin-6, interleukin-10, and C reactive protein correlate with exacerbation of multicentric Castleman disease in HIV-infected patients. Blood 96:2069, 2000.
183. Kim JE, Kim CJ, Park IA, et al. Clinicopathologic study of Castleman's disease in Korea. J Korean Med Sci 15:393, 2000.
184. Mori Y, Nishimoto N, Ohno M, et al. Human herpesvirus 8-encoded interleukin-6 homologue (viral IL-6) induces endogenous human IL-6 secretion. J Med Virol 61:332, 2000.
185. Parravinci C, Corbellino M, Paulli M, et al. Expression of a virus-derived cytokine, KSHV vIL-6, in HIV-seronegative Castleman's disease. Am J Pathol 151:1517, 1997.
186. Katano H, Sato Y, Kurata T, et al. Expression and localization of human herpesvirus 8-encoded proteins in primary effusion lymphoma, Kaposi's sarcoma, and multicentric Castleman's disease. Virology 269:335, 2000.

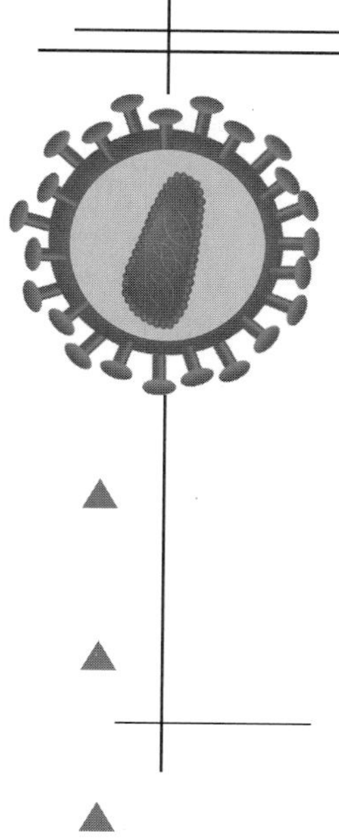

CHAPTER 46

Hepatitis Viruses

Mark Sulkowski, MD
David L. Thomas, MD, MPH

Human immunodeficiency virus (HIV)-infected persons have an increased incidence of viral hepatitis and an accelerated course of chronic liver disease. Accordingly, the U.S. Public Health Service (USPHS) and Infectious Diseases Society of America (IDSA) consider management of viral hepatitis in their report on opportunistic infections in persons with HIV.[1] In this chapter the viral hepatitis agents that pose the greatest threat to HIV-infected patients are considered. For each virus, we discuss the agent, epidemiology/natural history, diagnosis, treatment, and prevention. Emphasis is placed on clinical issues of greatest importance to the HIV-infected patient. Readers are also referred to Chapter 65, where the subject of liver disease in the HIV-infected patient is discussed.

▲ HEPATITIS A VIRUS

Hepatitis A virus (HAV) is a nonenveloped, positive-stranded, RNA-containing virus classified as a hepatovirus in the Picornaviridae family[2,3] (Table 46–1). The 7.5-kb HAV genome encodes at least four capsid proteins (VP1 to VP4) and nonstructural peptides, including an RNA-dependent RNA polymerase and a protease.[4] Although more than 100 strains and four distinct HAV genotypes have been recognized, there is only one HAV serotype.[5,6] Thus antibody elicited by vaccination or infection with any HAV strain protects against infection worldwide. HAV is relatively resistant to acidity and heat, and contaminated materials may harbor infective organisms for months.[7] In contrast to the lipid-enveloped hepatitis B and C viruses, HAV is stable in bile and remains infectious when excreted in feces.

Epidemiology and Natural History

Hepatitis A virus is principally transmitted by ingestion of food or beverage contaminated with HAV-containing feces. HAV is infrequently parenterally transmitted, such as when HAV-containing blood products are transfused and when injection drug users share needles with someone during their brief period of viremia. HAV may also be transmitted by certain sexual practices among men having intercourse with other men.

The prevalence of HAV infection is high in places where sanitary conditions are low. More than 90% of adults in developing countries have had HAV infection, as have more than 60% of adults over the age of 60 in the United States. HAV outbreaks and high prevalence rates have been reported among injection drug users and men who have sex with men.[8,9] Thus the incidence of HAV infection is probably higher overall among HIV-infected persons, reflecting increased transmission in crowded urban areas and these shared transmission routes.

Replication of HAV occurs within a week of inoculation and peaks 2 to 3 weeks after exposure, just before the onset of symptoms.[10] During replication, HAV may be recovered from stool or serum, although concentrations in stool are 1000 times higher than in serum.[11] When sensitive tests such as the polymerase chain reaction (PCR) are used, HAV RNA can be detected in stool and serum weeks before and, in some cases, months after the onset of symptoms.[10,12] However, in healthy adults, infectivity is substantially reduced 1 to 2 weeks after symptoms begin.

After an incubation of 2 to 4 weeks, jaundice occurs in about two-thirds of adults with HAV infection, although the frequency varies substantially in various outbreak reports.

▲ **Table 46–1.** VIRAL HEPATITIS AGENTS

Characteristic	HAV	HBV	HCV	HDV	HEV
Virology	RNA	DNA	RNA	RNA	RNA
Usual source	Feces	Blood/blood-contaminated fluids	Blood/blood-contaminated fluids	Blood/blood-contaminated fluids	Feces
Transmission	Fecal-oral	Percutaneous, permucosal	Percutaneous, permucosal	Percutaneous, permucosal	Fecal-oral
Chronic infections	No	Yes	Yes	Yes	No
Medical prevention[a]	IG; immunization	HBIG; immunization	None	Immunization (for HBV)	Non approved (2001)

IG, immunoglobulin; HBIG, hepatitis B immunoglobulin.
[a]See text for details of pre- and postexposure prevention. All infections can be avoided by reducing exposure.

In some persons cholestasis may be profound and prolonged (*prolonged cholestasis*), and in others hepatitis recurs months after apparent initial recovery (*relapsing hepatitis*). However, HAV infection does not become chronic like HBV or HCV infections.

A coexisting HIV infection does not appear to modify the natural history of HAV infection. However, marked increases in HIV viral load have been reported in HIV-infected persons with acute hepatitis A.[13] In addition, HAV infection can be mistaken for antiretroviral toxicity, or other HIV-related liver conditions (see Chapter 65).

Diagnosis

Infection with HAV elicits immunoglobin M(IgM) antibodies (IgM anti-HAV) that can be detected at the onset of symptoms (jaundice), peaking 4 to 6 weeks after exposure, and persisting for 3 to 12 months[14] (Table 46–2). Thus IgM anti-HAV indicates current or recent HAV infection. Within a week of IgM anti-HAV, IgG antibodies (IgG anti-HAV) are formed that have neutralizing activity and may persist for life.[6] Therefore serum IgG anti-HAV without IgM anti-HAV represents past HAV infection and protection against infection. Anti-HAV elicited by vaccination may not be detected by commercially available assays.

Treatment

No medical treatment is indicated for persons with hepatitis A. HAV infection should be reported to the local health department and secondary cases prevented by providing intramuscular immune globulin within 1 week to persons exposed to the index case in the approximately 10-day period before jaundice.[15]

Prevention

Before exposure, HAV infection can be prevented by vaccination or immune globulin administration.[15] HAV vaccination is indicated for persons at increased risk including many HIV-infected persons, such as men who have sex with men or injection drug users, persons with chronic hepatitis, and travelers to HAV endemic areas. Although postvaccination anti-HAV titers are somewhat lower than in persons without HIV infection, HAV vaccine is safe and well tolerated in HIV-infected persons.[16,17] Because of the high prevalence of HAV infection in this population, prevaccination screening for antibody to hepatitis A (anti-HAV IgG) is generally cost-effective and should be performed.[18]

▲ **Table 46–2.** DIAGNOSIS OF VIRAL HEPATITIS

Type of Hepatitis	Acute Infection	Chronic Infection	Supplemental Tests	Comments
HAV	IgM anti-HAV	N/A	HAV RNA[a]	IgG anti-HAV indicates prior infection and protective immunity
HBV	HBsAg and IgM anti-HBc	HBsAg	HBeAg, HBV DNA	Chronic infection is defined as persistence of HBsAg >6 months
HCV	Anti-HCV HCV RNA	Anti-HCV[b]	HCV RNA, RIBA	HCV RNA may be detectable as early as 2 weeks after exposure
HDV	HBsAg and anti-HDV	HBsAg	HDV RNA[a]	
HEV	IgM anti-HEV	N/A	HEV RNA[a]	

HBeAg, hepatitis B early antigen; HBsAg, hepatitis B surface antigen; IgM, immunoglobulin M; N/A, not applicable; RIBA, recombinant immunoblot assay.
[a]Not commercially available.
[b]Can be negative with advanced immunosuppression, such as HIV with a CD4 count of less than 200/mm^3 and hemodialysis.

▲ HEPATITIS B VIRUS

The hepatitis B virus (HBV) is an enveloped, incompletely double-stranded DNA virus of the family Hepadnaviridae.[19,20] The 3200-base HBV genome encodes three circulating particles, including the complete 42-nm virion, smaller 22-nm diameter spheres, and rod-like particles 22 × 200 nm.[21] The primary protein of the HBV envelope is the hepatitis B surface antigen (HBsAg), which contains a group-specific determinant (a) shared by all HBsAg preparations and two pairs of subtype determinants (d,y and w,r).[22] The HBV core gene encodes the hepatitis B core antigen (HBcAg), which does not circulate freely in serum, and the hepatitis B e antigen (HBeAg), which when present in serum correlates with high concentrations of HBV virions and infectivity.[23,24]

Circular HBV DNA is closed, then reverse-transcribed to RNA transcripts that contain the necessary enzyme activities and code for viral progeny.[20] During replication nonlethal mutations can accumulate, such as one in the precore region that interrupts translation of the HBeAg, resulting in e antigen-negative chronic hepatitis B.[25] Another mutation in the surface envelope gene inhibits expression of the "a" subtype determinant, resulting in a variant that may not be neutralized by antibodies induced by the recombinant HBV vaccines.[26] In persons taking lamivudine, mutations also can accumulate in the catalytic center of the reverse transcriptase domain, the YMDD motif, as discussed under Treatment.[27]

Epidemiology and Natural History

HBV can be transmitted by sexual intercourse, percutaneous exposure, or from mother to infant. In the United States HBV is most often transmitted by sexual intercourse (both heterosexual and between men) followed by injection drug use.[28] In Asia and sub-Saharan Africa, HBV is principally transmitted from mother to infant or during early childhood.

An estimated 300 million persons have chronic HBV infection worldwide compared with just over 1 million in the United States.[29,30] Because the routes of transmission are similar, there is evidence of prior or ongoing HBV infection in many HIV-infected persons.[31,32]

The outcome of HBV infection varies according to the age of acquisition and the immune status of the host. HBV infection persists in 50% to 90% of persons infected at birth or early childhood. In contrast, among adults, fewer than 5% of HBV infections become chronic.[33] Recovery from HBV infection is characterized by clearance of HBsAg and HBeAg from blood in association with formation of antibodies to both antigens.[33] The highest incidence of viral recovery is during the first year after infection, but spontaneous clearance of HBsAg and HBeAg can occur indefinitely. It is now appreciated that HBV DNA can be detected in some persons with serologic evidence of recovery, indicating there is ongoing replication that is contained by a vigorous immune response.[34,35] This incomplete clearance probably explains relapses that have been reported in immunosuppressed persons such as those with acquired immunodeficiency syndrome (AIDS).[36]

Among those in whom HBsAg is persistently detected, some never develop substantial liver enzyme elevation or significant histologic disease and are referred to as chronic carriers.[37–39] Typically, chronic carrier sera contains HBsAg, HBV DNA, and antibody to HBeAg but not HBeAg. Others with persistent HBsAg develop significant liver disease (chronic active hepatitis) that can progress to cirrhosis or hepatocellular cancer.[38,40] Persons at risk for cirrhosis usually have HBsAg and HBeAg in their sera, although hepatocellular cancer and even cirrhosis can occur in those who have cleared HBeAg. Among HIV-uninfected carriers who have HBsAg and antibodies to HBeAg, the aspartate aminotransferase level may be the best noninvasive measure of HBV disease activity; the stage of disease in HBeAg-positive persons is typically assessed by liver biopsy.[41] Nonetheless, at least one published guideline for the treatment of chronic hepatitis B is chiefly predicated on the results of liver enzyme and HBV serologic testing, rather than liver histology.[41a] Few data are available to guide management of HBV infection in HIV-infected persons. It is reasonable to perform a liver biopsy to stage disease on HBeAg-positive HIV-infected persons, unless survival is limited (e.g., uncontrolled, advanced HIV infection), biopsy is contraindicated (e.g., bleeding cannot be safely controlled), or HBV treatment is not anticipated.

The natural history of hepatitis B is modified by HIV infection which has been associated with higher rates of HBV persistence (HBsAg and HBeAg detection) and relapse (reemergence of HBsAg, HBeAg or both).[36,42] Among those with persistent HBV infection the severity of liver disease has been reported to be both increased and decreased, differences that may be related to the duration of HIV/HBV co-infection, immune status, and alcohol use.[43–46] Antiretroviral-related immune restoration has been associated with spontaneous recovery from chronic HBV infection.[47] Effects of HBV infection on HIV natural history are less apparent but may include a higher incidence of liver enzyme elevations associated with antiretroviral therapy.[48]

Diagnosis

Ongoing HBV infection is diagnosed by detecting viral antigens (HBsAg or HBeAg) or HBV DNA in blood (Table 46–2). When infection is acute, IgM antibodies to the core protein are also detected, generally together with HBV antigens and DNA.[49] When infection has been ongoing for more than 12 months, IgG (but not IgM) antibodies to the core protein are detectable along with viral antigens and DNA.[33] The presence of HBeAg is important as an indicator of a high degree of infectivity and potential disease.[24,50]

When there is recovery from acute hepatitis B, HBeAg and HBsAg are no longer detectable in blood, although low levels of HBV DNA may be detected with sensitive assays, as already mentioned (Fig. 46–1).[34,35,51,52] With recovery, antibodies to HBV antigens are detectable, including antibody to the surface, e, and core antigens.[33,51] Because recombinant and serum-derived HBV vaccines include HBsAg antigen determinants, prior vaccination and immunity are reflected by the presence of anti-HBs in serum.[53]

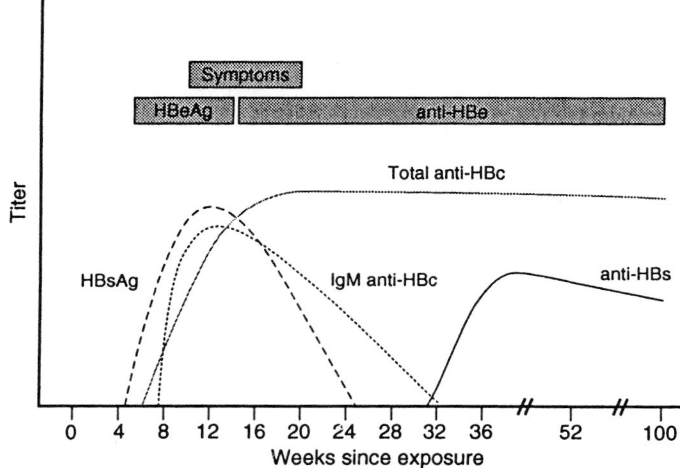

Figure 46–1. Typical serologic course of acute hepatitis B virus (HBV) infection with recovery. HBeAg, hepatitis B early antigen; HBsAg, hepatitis B surface antigen; HBc, hepatitis B core [antigen]. (From Centers for Disease Control and Prevention, Atlanta.)

Antibodies can be detected to HBV core in some persons without HBsAg, HBeAg, or antibodies to these antigens.[54,55] Isolated HBV core antibody serology occurs frequently in injection drug users (who are generally HCV-infected) and among both HIV-infected and HIV-uninfected persons.[32,56,57] The probability that isolated antibody to HBV core represents HBV infection (versus a false-positive reaction) is related to the prevalence of HBV infection and the anti-core antibody titer. For example, in low-prevalence settings, such as among volunteer blood donors, persons with low titers of antibody to HBV core without other HBV markers uncommonly have anamnestic responses to HBV vaccination, (detection of antibody to surface antigen) after a single dose suggesting that these may be false-positive anticore reactions.[58] However, patients with isolated hepatitis B core antibodies who are at high risk for HBV infection and those with high titer core antibodies are more likely to have evidence of prior HBV infection, indicated by anamnestic responses to vaccine or detection of HBV DNA by PCR.[56,59] In fact, in one study of HBsAg-negative patients with liver disease, HBV DNA was detected in 33% of HCV-positive and 14% of HCV-negative patients.[59] Two-thirds of the HBV DNA-positive, HBsAg-negative patients in this study had antibody to hepatitis B core, and 33% had cirrhosis. Although the severity of liver disease in HBsAg-negative persons requires further evaluation, it is reasonable to assume that many persons with isolated HBV core serology have or have had HBV infection.

Treatment

Two medications are approved by the U.S. Food and Drug Administration (FDA) for treatment of chronic hepatitis B in the United States: interferon-α (5 million units SC daily or 10 million units SC thrice weekly for 4 months) or lamivudine (100 mg PO daily, duration of therapy not specified) (Table 46–3). In a meta-analysis of placebo-controlled studies, interferon-α treatment was associated with a 33% chance of HBeAg clearance compared to 12% for untreated controls.[60] There are few studies of the success of interferon-α treatment of patients with HIV/HBV co-infection.

Lamivudine is an oral nucleoside analogue that inhibits both HIV and HBV reverse transcriptase activity. In a 1-year, placebo-controlled trial of Asian patients with hepatitis B, oral lamivudine therapy (100 mg/day) was associated with HBeAg conversion and HBV DNA suppression (16%), improved hepatic necroinflammatory activity (56%), and few serious adverse events.[61] Lamivudine use also has been associated with HBV DNA suppression and improved liver enzymes among HIV/HBV co-infected persons.[62] In one study of persons with pretreatment HBV levels above 5 pg/ml who were treated with lamivudine 300 to 600 mg/day, more than 90% achieved HBV levels less than 5 pg/ml.[63] In the CAESAR study, HIV-infected patients taking zidovudine were randomized to receive placebo, lamivudine, or lamivudine plus loviride. In a retrospective evaluation of HBsAg-positive patients, HBV DNA levels were suppressed more often in patients taking lamivudine than in the controls.[62] Long-term studies are still needed to evaluate the efficacy of lamivudine in decreasing hepatic fibrosis and liver failure in HIV/HBV co-infected patients.

Mutations (YMDD) may accumulate in the catalytic site of the HBV reverse transcriptase.[61] YMDD mutations occur in 10% to 20% of persons and correlate with resurgent infection (elevated liver enzymes and HBV DNA levels).[61] Similar rates of accumulation have been reported in HIV-infected patients.[63,64] These findings suggest that the use of more than one antiviral agent may be better, and lamivudine-resistant variants may be susceptible in vitro to other reverse transcriptase inhibitors such as adefovir and tenofovir.[65,65a] However, the clinical effect of combined nucleoside analogue therapy has not been demonstrated in HIV/HBV co-infected persons.

Once lamivudine treatment is stopped, hepatitis B can recur. In some HIV/HBV-infected patients, the resurgence of hepatitis B has been severe after lamivudine withdrawal.[66,67] However, because lamivudine withdrawal usually is followed by another antiretroviral regimen, it may be difficult to dissect the role of resurgent hepatitis B or the effect of the new medications, either causing hepatic toxicity directly or through immune reconstitution (see Chapter 65). Although there is a paucity of supporting data, some authorities recommend that HBsAg-positive patients receive

▲ **Table 46–3.** TREATMENT OF CHRONIC VIRAL HEPATITIS

Type of Hepatitis	Drug	Dose	Duration	Comments
HBV	Interferon α-2b (IFNα2b)	5 MIU qd 10 MIU tiw	4 months	Consider PEG-IFNα (no data)
	Lamivudine	150 mg bid	12 months or indefinite	Lamivudine 100 mg/day is the FDA-approved dose for the treatment of HBV. However, in the setting of HIV co-infection 150 mg bid is preferred
	Adefovir	10 mg qd?	?	Investigational (not FDA-approved). In vitro and in vivo activity against lamivudine-resistant mutants
HDV (with HBV)	IFNα	5 MIU daily?	6 months or indefinite	Higher IFNα dose and longer duration may be better. Preliminary studies have failed to demonstrate activity of lamivudine
HCV	IFNα2a or 2b or IFNαcon-1	3 MIU tiw (9 μg tiw for IFNαcon-1)	12 months	
	IFNα2b plus ribavirin	3 MIU tiw plus ribavirin (1000mg–1200mg/d)	12 months	
	PEG-IFNα2a (Hoffmann La-Roche)	180 μg weekly	12 months	Dosage of 90 μg/week used in studies of maintenance therapy
	PEG-IFNα2b (Schering-Plough)	1.0 μg/kg weekly	12 months	Dosage of 0.5 μg/kg/week used in studies of maintenance therapy
	PEG-IFNα2b or 2a plus ribavirin	1.5 μg/kg weekly plus 1000–1200 mg/day	12 months	Combination with PEG-IFNα2a not yet approved in U.S.; data suggests higher SVR in genotype 1 than with standard combination

MIU, million international units; PEG, polyethylene glycol; SVR, sustained virologic response; tiw, three times a week.

lamivudine therapy indefinitely. In HIV/HBV coinfected patients, additional antiretroviral agents should be used with lamivudine to prevent development of HIV nucleoside resistant mutations.

Prevention

Vaccination and observance of universal precautions are the chief methods for preventing HBV infection before exposures occur.[68–70] HBV vaccination is indicated for all children and adults who are at increased risk of HBV infection, including virtually all HIV-infected persons, persons with multiple sexual partners, men who have sex with men, and injection drug users. The vaccine used in most developed nations is a recombinant surface antigen expressed in yeast.[71] When used as licensed (three doses administered intradeltoid), more than 95% of adults develop antibody responses that are considered protective.[71] Within 6 months after the third dose of vaccination, antibody titers decline, and many adults serorevert.[71] However, those in whom antibody to HBsAg was initially detected but then became undetectable (< 10 IU/L) are not considered to be at risk of complications of HBV infection, even though some have developed antibodies to hepatitis B core, indicating that infection occurred. Postvaccination antibody testing is recommended 1–2 months after the third vaccine dose for persons with an increased risk of exposure.[72,73]

In HIV-infected persons HBV vaccination appears to be safe, as measured by the increase in HIV viral load or subsequent progression of HIV infection.[74,75] HBV vaccine immunogenicity is reduced in HIV-infected persons, especially those with low CD4 lymphocyte counts.[75] Improved HBV vaccine responses have been described in HIV-infected patients who were given three additional vaccine injections.[76] In addition, higher doses of vaccination have been used to improve the serologic responses among hemodialysis patients. Neither of these measures is currently routinely recommended to prevent hepatitis B in persons with HIV infection.

Infection with HBV can also be prevented during the first week after exposure (Table 46–4). Persons exposed to HBV-contaminated blood or body fluids who are susceptible to HBV (i.e., do not have anti-HBs or prior documented seroconversion) should receive HBV vaccination and hepatitis B immune globulin (HBIG).[72,73]

▲ **Table 46–4.** RECOMMENDED POSTEXPOSURE PROPHYLAXIS FOR HEPATITIS B VIRUS

Exposed Person's Status	Treatment According to Source HBsAg Status		
	Positive	Negative	Not known
Unvaccinated	HBIG × 1, vaccinate	Vaccinate	Vaccinate
Previously vaccinated			
Known responder	None	None	None
Known nonresponder	HBIG × 2 or HBIG and vaccinate	None	
Response unknown	Test for anti-HBs If adequate, none If inadequate, HBIG and vaccine booster	None	If known high-risk source, treat as if source were HBsAg-positive

Based on Centers for Disease Control and Prevention recommendations.
HBIG, HBV immune globulin 0.06 ml/kg IM. HBsAg, hepatitis B surface antigen. Vaccinate means three doses of HBV vaccine (0, 1, and 6 months). Anti-HBs is the antibody to HBV surface antigen. Responder means demonstration of anti-HB. Booster means one dose of vaccine.

▲ HEPATITIS C VIRUS

The hepatitis C virus (HCV) is a spherical, enveloped RNA virus, classified within the *Hepacivirus* genus of the Flaviviridae family. The positive-sense, single-stranded, approximately 9.6-kb RNA genome contains a single large (about 3000-amino-acid) open reading frame flanked by 3′ and 5′ untranslated regions.[77] The open reading frame encodes for at least 10 proteins including four structural proteins (core protein, envelope proteins E1 and E2, NS2A) and six nonstructural proteins (*cis*-active Zn^{2+}-dependent proteinase, serine proteinase, NTPase, RNA helicase, NS3 proteinase cofactor, RNA-dependent RNA polymerase).

Replication of HCV chiefly occurs in the cytoplasm of hepatocytes, although some studies have suggested that replication may occur in some other cell types, such as B cells, T cells, and monocytes. In chronically infected humans, mathematic models of HCV kinetics suggest that up to 1.0×10^{12} virons are produced daily with a half-life of about 2.5 hours.[78] This high level of virion turnover coupled with the lack of proofreading by the RNA polymerase results in the rapid accumulation of mutations, estimated at a rate of 0.90×10^{-3} 1.92×10^{-3} base substitutions per year.[79,80] Consequently, within each infected person, HCV exists as a quasispecies, a group of closely related variants that typically share 91% to 99% sequence identity. HCV sequences from different individuals may have less than 60% RNA identity, and six major genotypes have been identified.[81] HCV strains are further classified into subtypes that typically share 75% to 85% nucleotide sequence identity.[82–84] Although the natural history of HCV genotypes does not seem to vary, there are dramatic intergenotypic differences in responsiveness to interferon-based therapies.

Epidemiology and Natural History

Epidemiology

Hepatitis C virus is transmitted chiefly by percutaneous exposure to blood. Although transfusion of contaminated blood and blood products was once a major source of HCV transmission, HCV transmission by administration of clotting factors diminished during the mid-1980s because of viral inactivation procedure and use of recombinant products. In addition, during the early 1990s when blood donations were routinely screened for HCV antibody, the incidence of post-transfusion HCV infection dropped to less than 1:100,000 per unit transfused in the United States.[85,86] After 1999 the risk of transfusion transmission of HCV declined even further because of routine screening of donations for HCV RNA. Injection drug use is the leading route of HCV transmission in the United States. Indeed, worldwide, 50% to 90% of injection drug users are HCV-infected as a consequence of sharing contaminated needles and drug-use equipment.[87–90]

The HCV can also be transmitted between sexual partners and from mother to infant.[91] A higher than expected HCV prevalence is frequently found in persons reporting high risk sexual practices (e.g., multiple sexual partners), and 15% to 20% of persons with acute hepatitis C have an anti-HCV-positive partner or admit having had multiple sexual partners during the 6 months before illness onset, in the absence of other risk factors for infection.[88] In addition, in one study women attending a clinic for sexually transmitted diseases (STDs) were threefold more likely to have HCV infection if their sexual partner was HCV-infected.[92] On the other hand, in at least five studies the prevalence of HCV infection was less than 2% among long-term sexual partners of HCV-infected individuals.[93–97] Furthermore, a higher than expected prevalence of HCV infection has been found in only a few studies of men who have sex with men. In addition, although HIV co-infection has been associated with increased HCV transmission between sexual partners, the prevalence of HCV in a sexual partner is at least fivefold less than for HIV.[97,98] Thus although there is evidence that HCV may be transmitted sexually, intercourse appears to be a relatively inefficient mode of transmission.

The HCV infection occurs in approximately 2% to 5% of infants born to HCV-positive mothers.[91] However, the incidence of mother–infant transmission increases approximately threefold if the mother is co-infected with HIV.[99,100] In addition, in one study an increased rate of HIV transmission was found among infants born to mothers who were co-infected with HIV and HCV.[101]

Because of shared routes of transmission, HCV and HIV co-infection is common. In the United States there are thought to be 100,000 to 240,000 persons co-infected with HCV and HIV, representing 15% to 30% of the estimated

800,000 individuals with HIV infection. Similar data have been reported from Europe; 33% of more than 3000 patients with HIV infection followed in the EuroSIDA cohort study had evidence of HCV infection.[102] However, the prevalence of HCV/HIV co-infection varies depending on the route of HIV infection. HCV is approximately 10-fold more likely than HIV to be transmitted by an accidental needlestick exposure and is acquired more readily than HIV by injection drug users.[89,94,103] Thus 50% to 90% of persons who acquire HIV from injecting drugs are also HCV-infected. Similarly, more than 50% of hemophiliacs who were exposed to unscreened, non-heat-treated blood products had HCV/HIV co-infection.[104] HCV infection is less common (<10%) in men who acquired HIV infection from same-sex intercourse.[92,105]

Natural History

After acute infection, approximately 15% of individuals clear virus from the blood and presumably have fully recovered from infection.[106,107] The remaining 70% to 85% of acutely infected persons have viremia that persists for life. In some chronically infected persons, alanine aminotransferase (ALT) levels are persistently elevated or normal. However, in most persons they fluctuate and are poor predictors of liver disease.[108] Some persistently infected persons develop hepatic fibrosis that progresses to cirrhosis, liver failure, or hepatocellular carcinoma.[109] The probability of cirrhosis after 20 years of infection is estimated to be 5% to 25%, depending on the population studied.[109–111] After cirrhosis has developed, the rates of progression to liver failure and hepatocellular carcinoma are estimated to be approximately 2% to 4% and 1% to 7% per year, respectively.[112]

Unfortunately, disease progression for an individual patient cannot be predicted by currently available laboratory tests. The magnitude or the pattern of ALT elevation does not correlate well with disease outcome.[113] Unlike the HIV RNA level, which is highly correlated with HIV disease progression, the HCV RNA level is not closely associated with the outcome of hepatitis C.[114–116] The best tool for evaluating the stage of infection is liver biopsy, but even liver histology is an imperfect indicator of the ultimate disease course.[117]

HIV Infection Impact on Hepatitis C Progression

Infection with HIV has been reported to exacerbate several steps in the natural history of hepatitis C. In one study, HIV-infected persons were less likely to have cleared viremia than those without HIV.[116] HIV infection has also been associated with a higher HCV RNA viral load and a more rapid progression of HCV-related liver disease.[118–126] Eyster and colleagues reported that HCV RNA levels were higher in hemophiliacs who became HIV-infected than in those who remained HIV-negative, and liver failure occurred exclusively in HIV/HCV co-infected patients.[122,123] Similarly, Darby and coworkers studied mortality from liver disease and hepatocellular carcinoma among 4865 men with hemophilia who were exposed to HCV-contaminated blood products. At all ages the cumulative risk of liver-related death was 1.4% (range 0.7% to 3.0%) for HIV-uninfected men and 6.5% (range 4.5% to 9.5%) for HIV-infected men.[124] Lesens and colleagues found that the risk of progressive liver disease was sevenfold higher in hemophiliacs with HCV/HIV co-infection than in those with HCV infection alone.[125] Among HCV-infected persons who chiefly acquired HCV from injection drug use, Pol and coworkers found that HIV co-infection was an independent risk factor for the development of cirrhosis.[126] Thomas and colleagues did not detect more end-stage liver disease in HIV-infected members of a study of 1667 HCV-infected current and former intravenous drug users (IDUs).[116] However, in that study there were many competing causes of mortality in the HIV-positive group.

In addition to increasing the proportion of HCV-infected persons who develop cirrhosis, HIV co-infection appears to decrease the time to cirrhosis. For example, in the study by Darby et al. liver failure occurred frequently within 10 years of the first exposure to HCV, suggesting that HIV infection abbreviates the typical 15 to 20-year natural history of hepatitis C.[124]

As survival among HIV-infected patients increases owing to the use of potent antiretroviral therapies and the prophylaxis of traditional opportunistic pathogens, hepatitis C-related morbidity and mortality should increase among HIV-infected patients. Indeed, HCV-related liver disease has been reported to be a major cause of hospital admissions and deaths among HIV-infected persons.[127,128]

HCV Infection Impact on HIV Disease Progression

There are conflicting reports about the effect of HCV infection on the natural history of HIV disease. In a prospective study of 416 HIV seroconverters the 51.4% who were HCV co-infected had an HIV progression rate similar to those without HCV infection.[129] However, the reported follow-up averaged only 3 years. Among 1742 patients, Sulkowski and coworkers found that HCV infection was not independently associated with progression to AIDS or death after adjusting for exposure to highly active antiretroviral therapy (HAART) and HIV suppression.[130] Conversely, Sabin and coworkers found that HIV/HCV co-infected hemophiliacs with HCV genotype 1 infection experienced a more rapid progression to AIDS and death than did those infected with other genotypes.[131] Piroth et al. reported that HCV co-infection was associated with more rapid clinical and immunologic progression among HIV-infected patients with CD cell counts higher than 600 cells/mm^3.[132] Similarly, Lesens and coworkers found that co-infected individuals progressed rapidly to AIDS after the development of clinically significant liver disease.[125] Among 3111 patients receiving potent antiretroviral therapy, Greub and colleagues reported that HCV-infected persons had a modestly increased risk of progression to a new AIDS-defining event or death, even among the subgroup with continuous suppression of HIV replication. Interestingly, Greub and coworkers also found that the magnitude of the CD4 cell increase following effective anti-HIV therapy was significantly less than that observed in HCV-uninfected persons, suggesting that HCV co-infection may blunt immune recovery following HAART.[133]

HCV Co-infection and HAART-Associated Hepatotoxicity

Antiretroviral drugs, such as zidovudine and HIV-1 protease inhibitors, have been associated with hepatotoxicity, which may interrupt HIV therapy and cause significant morbidity and mortality.[134–137] Some but not all studies suggest that drug-induced hepatotoxicity may be more common among patients with HIV/HCV co-infection, particularly with the use of HIV-1 protease inhibitors and antituberculosis drugs.[137,138] The mechanism of enhanced drug-induced hepatotoxicity among co-infected patients is unknown but may be the result of underlying HCV-related liver disease or immune reconstitution with enhanced cytolytic anti-HCV immune activity.[139–141] Although co-infected patients may be at increased risk for the development of hepatotoxicity, 88% of a large cohort of HCV co-infected patients prospectively studied did not experience significant hepatotoxicity following HAART, and no irreversible outcomes were observed among the patients experiencing toxicity.[137] Thus the available evidence suggests that antiretroviral therapies can be safely administered to HIV-infected patients with chronic hepatitis C; however, serum liver enzymes should be closely monitored in these patients.[1] Although there are currently no established guidelines for the management of antiretroviral-associated hepatotoxicity, some studies have suggested that it is not necessary to discontinue antiretroviral therapy unless patients are symptomatic or develop significant elevations in liver enzymes ($>5 \times$ upper limit of normal).[48]

Diagnosis

All HIV-infected persons should be screened for HCV infection because of the high prevalence of HCV infection in this group.[1] HCV screening should be done with enzyme immunoassays (EIA) licensed for the detection of antibody to HCV in blood.[142] Patients with positive anti-HCV results by EIA should have confirmatory testing performed using either supplemental antibody testing (RIBA) or reverse transcriptase-polymerase chain reaction (RT-PCR) for HCV RNA. The latter test is preferred by these authors to confirm HCV infection in HIV-infected persons. The detection of HCV RNA in a person with a positive anti-HCV result indicates current infection. However, because some persons with chronic HCV infection experience intermittent viremia, a single undetectable HCV RNA result must be interpreted cautiously.[106] Anti-HCV titers may decline to undetectable levels in persons with advanced immunodeficiency (CD4+ T-lymphocyte count $<100/mm^3$). Likewise, in patients with acute HCV infection, anti-HCV EIA may remain undetectable for weeks.[142,143] Thus HCV RNA should be assessed in the blood when HCV infection is suspected in persons with negative anti-HCV results. The clinical significance of quantitative HCV RNA level (i.e., viral load) in HIV-infected patients is not known and should not be interpreted based on the well described relation of HIV viral load and HIV disease progression.[115]

Management

All HIV-infected individuals with chronic HCV infection should be counseled to prevent liver damage and HCV transmission and should be evaluated for chronic liver disease and consideration of anti-HCV treatment. Because alcohol ingestion, particularly in quantities of more than 50 g (4 drinks) per day, accelerates the progression of liver disease and significantly increases the risk of cirrhosis, all HIV/HCV-infected patients should be advised to abstain from alcohol use.[91,144–146] Counseling regarding household and sexual practices to prevent HIV transmission also should be effective to prevent HCV transmission.

The HIV-infected patients with chronic HCV infection who are susceptible to HAV or HBV infections should be vaccinated because most of these patients have risk factors for acquiring HAV and HBV infection.[15] In addition, HCV-infected patients with chronic liver disease who become infected with HAV are at increased risk for fulminant hepatitis.[147]

The HIV/HCV co-infected patients should be evaluated for the presence of chronic liver disease. Assessments of disease severity should include a history and physical examination to look for signs and symptoms of chronic liver disease, measurement of blood albumin, prothrombin time, direct bilirubin assay, and platelet count to determine hepatic function; evaluation of liver histology by biopsy is appropriate in many patients. Measurements of the serum ALT level and HCV RNA level are important to establish that the infection is ongoing, but these tests provide only limited information regarding HCV disease severity.[108,114] The liver biopsy provides important information about HCV-related disease activity and fibrosis stage and may exclude alternative causes of liver disease. Most studies indicate that liver biopsy can be safely performed in HIV-infected individuals.[148]

Treatment

As of mid-2002 there were no published guidelines for treating HCV infection in HIV-infected persons. Nonetheless, principles for the treatment of HIV-uninfected persons are useful. Treatment is currently recommended for patients with chronic hepatitis C who are at the greatest risk for progression to cirrhosis, as characterized by persistently elevated ALT levels, detectable HCV RNA, and histologic findings of portal or bridging fibrosis or at least moderate degrees of inflammation or necrosis.[149] Because HIV-infected patients have a greater progression of liver disease and, during the era of HAART, have substantially prolonged survival, the impetus to treat HCV infection should be at least as strong as in HCV-infected adults without HIV.

Two distinct benefits have been attributed to HCV treatment. First, it is possible to eradicate the infection, referred to as a sustained virologic response (undetectable HCV RNA at the end of treatment and 6 months later). Marcellin and colleagues reported that 96% of patients with no detectable HCV RNA 6 months after therapy maintained their virologic response and experienced sustained histologic improvement during long-term follow-up.[150] Similarly, Lau and coworkers reported that five patients with 6-month post-treatment virologic responses also had favorable clinical and histologic outcomes 6 to 13 years after therapy, with no detectable HCV RNA in the serum and liver tissue.[151] Soriano and coworkers have reported that a sustained virologic response can be achieved in persons with HIV/HCV co-infection.[152,153]

A second potential benefit of HCV treatment is a reduction in the risk of liver failure and liver cancer.[154–156] Although there are relatively few data linking HCV treatment to long-term outcomes, it is important to note that this benefit does not appear to be restricted to patients with sustained virologic response. These preliminary data form the basis for treating patients at the greatest risk for end-stage liver disease (e.g., those with advanced hepatic fibrosis) to prevent hepatic decompensation without regard to virologic response. If substantiated, this approach could be especially pertinent to HIV/HCV co-infected patients who generally have more liver disease, lower sustained virologic response, and limited access to orthotopic liver transplantation compared to HCV-infected adults without HIV.[157]

These medical regimens have been approved by the FDA for the treatment of chronic HCV infection: monotherapy with interferon-α2b, interferon-α2a, interferon-αcon-1, or polyethylene glycol (PEG)ylated interferon-α2b and combination therapy with interferon-α2b plus ribavirin. Few studies have been reported that examined the use of interferon-α for treatment of chronic HCV infection in HIV-infected patients (Table 46–5). Boyer and coworkers reported a sustained biochemical response in only 1 of 12 HIV-infected patients receiving interferon-α.[167] Similarly, Marriott and colleagues found that only 3 of 14 HIV-infected patients treated with interferon-α for 1 year achieved a sustained virologic response.[168] On the other hand, in the largest published study, Soriano and the Spanish Hepatitis Study Group treated 90 co-infected patients (CD4+ T-lymphocyte counts >200 cells/mm^3) with interferon-α for 12 months. In an intention-to-treat analysis, 18 (20%) of 90 HIV-infected patients achieved a sustained virologic response to therapy determined 12 months after the end of therapy; as expected, the sustained response was associated with pretreatment CD4+ T-lymphocyte counts of more than 500 cells/mm^3. Although 10 patients in this study had a more than 50% reduction in CD4+ T-lymphocyte count, it was reversible in 3 patients and medication was generally well tolerated.[152,153] Thus based on limited data, interferon-α therapy appears to be reasonably well tolerated and may be effective for the treatment of HCV infection in HIV-infected patients.

Among HIV-uninfected patients, randomized, placebo-controlled clinical trails have clearly demonstrated that interferon-α plus ribavirin combination therapy is more effective than interferon alone for the treatment of chronic HCV infection.[169,170] Studies are currently underway in the United States and Europe, but there are few published data addressing the safety and efficacy of interferon-α2b and ribavirin therapy in HIV-infected persons. Several retrospective treatment series have suggested that interferon-α2b plus ribavirin is reasonably well tolerated and may lead to the eradication of HCV infection in some HIV-infected patients.[165,171–173] Among HIV-uninfected persons, pretreatment factors associated with sustained virologic response to combination therapy include infection with HCV genotype 2 or 3, low HCV RNA level (<3.5 million copies/ml), little or no portal fibrosis on liver biopsy, female gender, and age less than 40 years.[174] Such factors have not been adequately defined in the treatment of HIV/HCV co-infected persons.

Table 46–5. SELECTED CLINICAL TRIALS OF INTERFERON-α AND INTERFERON-α PLUS RIBAVIRIN FOR TREATING CHRONIC HCV IN HIV-INFECTED PERSONS

Study	Year	No.	Treatment Regimen	Response (%)	Comments
Boyer[158]	1992	12	IFNα1, 2, or 3 MIU × 4–6 months	33.0	ALT response reported
Marriott[159]	1993	14	IFNα2a 9 MIU daily then taper × 12 months	21.0	HCV RNA undetectable in 3 patients
Mauss[160]	1995	9	IFNα2b	33.0	
Soriano[161]	1996	90	IFNα2b 5 MIU tiw × 3 months then 3 MIU × 9 months	20.0	HCV RNA response data shown as intention-to-treat
Mauss[162]	1998	17	IFNα	29.0	HCV eradication associated with higher CD4+ T-lymphocyte count
Causse[163]	2000	64	IFNα2a 3 MIU tiw × 6 months	12.5	Retrospective cohort; ALT response reported
Prestileo[164]	2000	41	IFNα3 MIU tiw then dose increase	2.4	All patients had prior IDU; 10 patients had drug relapse
Zylberberg[165]	2000	21	IFNα3 MIU tiw + RBV 1000–1200 mg/day	14.3	Retrospective cohort; all patients had previously failed to respond to IFN
Landau[166]	2000	20	IFNα2b 3 MIU tiw + RBV 500–600 mg/day	50.0	End-of-treatment HCV RNA response reported

ALT, alanine aminotransferase; IDU, intravenous drug use; IFN, interferon.

More recently, the addition of the inert PEG moiety to the interferon-α molecule has allowed once-weekly subcutaneous injection, which provides continuous exposure to the active interferon molecule. In HIV-uninfected persons, randomized clinical trials have demonstrated that both PEGylated interferon-α2a (branched 40-kDa PEG; Pegasys, Hoffmann La-Roche, Nutley NJ, USA) and PEGylated interferon-α2b (linear, 12-kDa PEG, PegIntron, Schering-Plough, Kenilworth, NJ, USA) are more effective than standard interferon-α monotherapy with a similar adverse effect profile.[175–177] PEGylated interferon-α has also been studied in combination with ribavirin. Among 1730 HIV-uninfected patients with chronic HCV infection, Manns and colleagues demonstrated higher sustained virologic response rates among HCV genotype 1 infected persons receiving PEGylated interferon-α2b once weekly plus ribavirin (42%) than those receiving standard interferon-α2b thrice weekly plus ribavirin (33%).[178] Thus based on the ease of administration (once-weekly injection) and the superior efficacy of PEG-interferon-α plus ribavirin in patients infected with HCV genotype 1, it is anticipated combination therapy with PEG-interferon-α will largely replace the use of standard interferon-α in combination with ribavirin for the treatment of chronic HCV infection. Studies of PEGylated interferon-α with and without ribavirin are currently underway, but no data have been reported regarding its safety and effectiveness for the treatment of HIV/HCV co-infected persons.

Interferon-α therapy is associated with many adverse effects,[179] most of which are relatively minor, treatable with adjunctive therapies, and in most cases reversible with discontinuation of therapy. With the first several doses of interferon-α most (60% to 90%) patients experience influenza-like symptoms (e.g., fever, malaise, tachycardia, chills, headache, arthalgia, myalgia). However, these symptoms usually subside after the first several injections, and their intensity may be ameliorated by acetaminophen or nonsteroidal antiinflammatory drugs (NSAIDs). Fatigue, malaise, anorexia, weight loss, skin rash, and reversible alopecia can occur months into therapy.

Additionally, neuropsychiatric side effects (irritability, insomnia, mood and cognitive changes) are observed in 25% to 60% of patients but generally can be managed effectively with pharmacologic agents. Rarely, depression is severe, and suicides have been reported in persons taking interferon-α. Interferon-associated thyroid dysfunction occurs in about 4% of patients and may take the form of thyroiditis, hypothyroidism, or hyperthyroidism.[180] With careful monitoring of thyroid function (thyroid-stimulating hormone) during therapy, this condition is rarely symptomatic; however, the thyroid dysfunction may be irreversible, and long-term thyroid replacement therapy may be required. Interferon may also cause neutropenia, mild anemia, and thrombocytopenia, adverse events that are often minor and may respond to dose reduction or the administration of filgrastim (granulocyte colony-stimulating factor).

Ribavirin also causes side effects. During the first 4 weeks of therapy approximately 80% of patients develop a dose-related hemolytic anemia. With interferon-α2b and ribavirin combination therapy, the hemoglobin level usually decreases by 2 to 3 g/dl, sometimes associated with fatigue, shortness of breath, and headache. In rare circumstances anemia occurs more rapidly and has caused angina and myocardial infarction. Thus ribavirin should be used cautiously in persons with preexisting cardiac disease, and older patients or those with significant cardiac risk factors should undergo pretreatment cardiac testing. Ribavirin-associated anemia is reversible with dose reduction or discontinuation (or both). In addition, preliminary evidence suggests that epoetin alfa can effectively increase the hemoglobin level in some patients experiencing ribavirin-associated anemia.[181] Ribavirin-induced anemia may be a greater problem in HIV co-infected patients owing to the high prevalence of anemia and limited myeloid reserves that may exist as a result of co-morbid diseases or concurrent drug toxicity.[182] Ribavirin may also be associated with rash, pruritus, nasal congestion, cough, and gout. Importantly, ribavirin causes birth defects and must not be administered to pregnant women or men intending to conceive. All men and women receiving ribavirin therapy must be counseled to use two forms of effective contraception during therapy and for a period of 6 months after discontinuation because of the long half-life of ribavirin.

An additional concern regarding the use of ribavirin in HIV-infected persons is the potential for drug–drug interactions between ribavirin, a guanosine nucleoside analogue, and anti-HIV nucleoside analogues. In vitro, ribavirin appears to inhibit the anti-HIV activity of pyrimidine 2′,3′-dideoxynucleosides (including zidovudine, zalcitabine, and stavudine) through inhibition of their intracellular phosphorylation.[183–185] Conversely, ribavirin may increase the intracellular conversion of didanosine to its active metabolite, which appears to enhance its anti-HIV activity in vitro but may also increase its in vivo toxicity in vivo, including mitochondrial effects.[185–187] Although in vivo studies of potential drug–drug interactions have not been completed, several small case series reported to date have failed to detect clinically significant interaction between ribavirin and nucleoside analogues.[171,173]

Despite the uncertainties and limitations of currently available HCV treatment strategies, HCV treatment may be beneficial for some HCV/HIV co-infected persons. However, many HIV-infected patients have co-morbid conditions, such as major depressive illness, cytopenias, and active illicit drug or alcohol use, which may prevent or complicate interferon-α plus ribavirin therapy. HCV treatment in co-infected patients should be coordinated by health care providers with experience treating both HIV and HCV disease (Table 46–6).

Prevention

Infection with HCV currently cannot be prevented by vaccination or administration of immune globulin. HCV infection can be avoided by adhering to counseling typically provided to HIV-infected persons to prevent HIV transmission. In particular, patients should be counseled to stop using injection drugs, and those who continue to inject drugs should be counseled to use safer injection practices to reduce harm.[1,166]

▲ **Table 46–6.** TREATMENT ALGORITHM FOR HEPATITIS C

Before Starting Therapy

Review HIV disease status including CD4 count, HIV RNA level, use of antiretroviral therapy and active opportunistic diseases.
Examine co-morbid conditions such as depression, drug and alcohol use, and cardiopulmonary disease.
Consider a liver biopsy to confirm the diagnosis of hepatitis C virus (HCV), assess the grade and stage of disease, and rule out other diagnoses. In situations where a liver biopsy is contraindicated or the patient declines, therapy can be given without a pretreatment liver biopsy.
Measure serum HCV RNA by polymerase chain reaction (PCR) to document that viremia is present.
Test for HCV genotype to help determine the probability of virologic response.
Measure blood counts and aminotransferases to establish a baseline for these values.
Counsel the patient about the relative risks and benefits of treatment. Side effects should be thoroughly discussed.

During Therapy

Measure blood counts and aminotransferases at weeks 2 and 4 and at 4- to 8-week intervals thereafter. Consider concurrent administration of filgrastim in the management of interferon-associated neutropenia.
Measure HIV RNA, absolute CD4+ T lymphocyte count, and percentage CD4 at 12-week intervals.
Adjust the dose of ribavirin downward (200 mg at a time) if significant anemia occurs (hemoglobin less than 10 g/dl or hematocrit <30%); stop ribavirin if severe anemia occurs (hemoglobin <8.5 g/dl or hematocrit <26%). Consider concurrent administration of epoetin alfa (40,000 IU by subcutaneous injection weekly) for management of treatment-related anemia.
Evaluate for neuropsychiatric complications monthly (depression screen). Consider use of antidepressants (e.g., SSRIs) and/or consultation with a mental health provider.
Measure thyroid-stimulating hormone levels every 3–6 months during therapy.
Measure HCV RNA by PCR at 24 weeks. If HCV RNA is still present, stop therapy. If HCV RNA is negative, continue therapy for at least another 24 weeks.
Reinforce the need to practice strict birth control during therapy and for 6 months thereafter.
At the end of therapy, test HCV RNA by PCR to assess whether there is an end-of-treatment response.

After Therapy

Measure aminotransferases every 2 months for 6 months.
Six months after stopping therapy, test for HCV RNA by PCR. If HCV RNA is still negative, the chance for a long-term virologic response is high; relapses have rarely been reported after this point.

SSRIs, selective serotonin receptor inhibitors.
Adapted from National Institute of Diabetes and Digestive and Kidney Disease (NIDDK). Chronic Hepatitis C: Current Disease Management. http//www.niddk.nih.gov.

REFERENCES

1. Centers for Disease Control and Prevention. 2002 USPHS/IDSA guidelines for the prevention of opportunistic infections in persons infected with human immunodeficiency virus: disease-specific recommendations; USPHS/IDSA Prevention of Opportunistic Infections Working Group; US Public Health Services/Infectious Diseases Society of America. MMWR Morbid Mortal Wkly Rep 51:1, 2002 and www.nivatis.org.
2. Feinstone SM, Kapikian AZ, Purcell RH. Hepatitis A: detection by immune electron microscopy of a viruslike antigen associated with acute illness. Science 182:1026, 1973.
3. Siegl G, Frosner GG, Gauss-Muller V, et al. The physicochemical properties of infectious hepatitis A virons. J Gen Virol 57:331, 1981.
4. Baroudy BM, Ticehurst JR, Miele TA, et al. Sequence analysis of hepatitis A virus cDNA coding for capsid proteins and RNA polymerase. Proc Natl Acad Sci USA 82:2143, 1985.
5. Lemon SM. Type A viral hepatitis: new developments in an old disease. N Engl J Med 313:1059, 1985.
6. Lemon SM, Binn LN. Serum neutralizing antibody response to hepatitis A virus. J Infect Dis 148:1033, 1983.
7. Sobsey MD, Shields PA, Hauchman FS, et al. Survival and persistence of hepatitis A virus in environmental samples. In: Zuckerman AJ (ed). Viral Hepatitis and Liver Disease. New York, Alan R. Liss, 1988, pp 121–124.
8. Villano SA, Nelson KE, Vlahov D, et al. Hepatitis A among homosexual men and injection drug users: more evidence for vaccination. Clin Infect Dis 25:726, 1997.
9. Corey L, Holmes KK. Sexual transmission of hepatitis A in homosexual men: incidence and mechanism. N Engl J Med 302:435, 1980.
10. Koff RS. Hepatitis A. Lancet 351:1643, 1998.
11. Coulepis AG, Locarnini SA, Lehmann NI, Gust ID. Detection of hepatitis A virus in the feces of patients with naturally acquired infections. J Infect Dis 141:151, 1980.
12. Fujiwara K, Yokosuka O, Ehata T, et al. Frequent detection of hepatitis a viral RNA in serum during the early convalescent phase of acute hepatitis A. Hepatology 26:1634, 1997.
13. Ridolfo AL, Rusconi S, Antinori S, et al. Persisting HIV-1 replication triggered by acute hepatitis A virus infection. Antivir Ther 5:15, 2000.
14. Decker RH, Overby LR, Ling CM, et al. Serologic studies of transmission of hepatitis A in humans. J Infect Dis 139:74, 1979.
15. Centers for Disease Control and Prevention. Prevention of hepatitis A through active or passive immunization: recommendations of the Advisory Committee on Immunization Practices (ACIP). MMWR Morbid Mortal Wkly Rep 48(RR-12):1, 1999.
16. Hess G, Clemens R, Bienzle U, et al. Immunogenicity and safety of an inactivated hepatitis A vaccine in anti-HIV positive and negative homosexual men. J Med Virol 46:40, 1995.
17. Santagostino E, Gringeri A, Rocino A, et al. Patterns of immunogenicity of an inactivated hepatitis A vaccine in anti-HIV positive and negative hemophilic patients. Thromb Haemost 72:508, 1994.
18. Das A. An economic analysis of different strategies of immunization against hepatitis A virus in developed countries. Hepatology 29:548, 1999.
19. Tiolles P, Pourcel C, Dejean A. The hepatitis B virus. Nature 317:489, 1985.
20. Lee WM. Hepatitis B virus infection. N Engl J Med 337:1733, 1997.
21. Bayer ME, Blumberg BS, Werner B. Particles associated with Austrialia antigen in the sera of patients with leukemia, Down's syndrome and hepatitis. Nature 218:1057, 1968.
22. Molnar-Kimber KL, Jarocki-Witek V, Dheer SK, et al. Distinctive properties of the hepatitis B virus envelope proteins. J Virol 62:407, 1988.
23. Miller RH. Proteolytic self-cleavage of hepatitis B virus core protein may generate serum e antigen. Science 236:722, 1987.
24. Alter HJ, Seeff LB, Kaplan PM, et al. Type B hepatitis: the infectivity of blood positive for e antigen and DNA polymerase after accidental needlestick exposure. N Engl J Med 295:909, 1976.
25. Carman WF, Jacyna MR, Hadziyannis S, et al. Mutation preventing formation of hepatitis B e antigen in patients with chronic hepatitis B infection. Lancet 2:588, 1989.
26. Carman WF, Zanetti AR, Karayiannis P, et al. Vaccine induced escape mutant of hepatitis B virus. Lancet 326:325, 1990.

27. Benhamou Y, Bochet M, Thibault V, et al. Long-term incidence of hepatitis B virus resistance to lamivudine in human immunodeficiency virus-infected patients. Hepatology 30:1302, 1999.
28. Alter MJ, Hadler SC, Margolis HS, et al. The changing epidemiology of hepatitis B in the United States: need for alternative vaccination strategies. JAMA 263:1218, 1990.
29. Centers for Disease Control and Prevention. Hepatitis B vaccination of adolescents—California, Louisiana, and Oregon, 1992–1994. MMWR Morbid Mortal Wkly Rep 43:605, 1994.
30. Coleman PJ, McQuillan GM, Moyer LA, et al. Incidence of hepatitis B virus infection in the United States, 1976–1994: estimates from the national health and nutrition examination surveys. J Infect Dis 178:954, 1998.
31. Thomas DL, Cannon RO, Shapiro CN, et al. Hepatitis C, hepatitis B, and human immunodeficiency virus infections among non-intravenous drug-using patients attending clinics for sexually transmitted diseases. J Infect Dis 169:990, 1994.
32. Levine OS, Vlahov D, Koehler J, et al. Seroepidemiology of hepatitis B virus in a population of injecting drug users: association with drug injection patterns. Am J Epidemiol 142:331, 1995.
33. Seeff LB, Beebe GW, Hoofnagle JH, et al. A serologic follow-up of the 1942 epidemic of post-vaccination hepatitis in the United States Army. N Engl J Med 316:965, 1987.
34. Rehermann B, Ferrari C, Pasquinelli C, Chisari FV. The hepatitis B virus persists for decades after patients' recovery from acute viral hepatitis despite active maintenance of a cytotoxic T-lymphocyte response. Nat Med 2:1104, 1996.
35. Yotsuyanagi H, Yasuda K, Iino S, et al. Persistent viremia after recovery from self-limited acute hepatitis B. Hepatology 27:1377, 1998.
36. Vento S, Di Perri G, Garofano T, et al. Reactivation of hepatitis B in AIDS [letter]. Lancet 2:108, 1989.
37. Fattovich G, Brollo L, Alberti A, et al. Long-term follow-up of anti-HBe-positive chronic active hepatitis B. Hepatology 8:1651, 1988.
38. Weissberg JI, Andres LL, Smith CI, et al. Survival in chronic hepatitis B: an analysis of 379 patients. Ann Intern Med 101:613, 1984.
39. De Franchis R, Meucci G, Vecchi M, et al. The natural history of asymptomatic hepatitis B surface antigen carriers. Ann Intern Med 118:191, 1993.
40. Beasley RP, Hwang LY, Lin CC, Chien CS. Hepatocellular carcinoma and hepatitis B virus: a prospective study of 22707 men in Taiwan. Lancet 2:1129, 1981.
41. Ter Borg F, ten Kate FJW, Cuypers HTM, et al. Relation between laboratory test results and histological hepatitis activity in individuals positive for hepatitis B surface antigen and antibodies to hepatitis B e antigen. Lancet 351:1914, 1998.
41a. Lok ASF, McMahon BJ. Chronic hepatitis B—AASLD Practice Guidelines. Hepatology 34:1225, 2001.
42. Bodsworth N, Donovan B, Nightingale BN. The effect of concurrent human immunodeficiency virus infection on chronic hepatitis B: a study of 150 homosexual men. J Infect Dis 160:577, 1989.
43. Rustgi VK, Hoofnagle JH, Gerin JL, et al. Hepatitis B virus infection in the acquired immunodeficiency syndrome. Ann Intern Med 101:795, 1984.
44. Perrillo RP, Regenstein FG, Roodman ST. Chronic hepatitis B in asymptomatic homosexual men with antibody to the human immunodeficiency virus. Ann Intern Med 105:382, 1986.
45. Scharschmidt BF, Held MJ, Hollander HH, et al. Hepatitis B in patients with HIV infection: relationship to AIDS and patient survival. Ann Intern Med 117:837, 1992.
46. Gilson RJ, Hawkins AE, Beecham MR, et al. Interactions between HIV and hepatitis B virus in homosexual men: effects on the natural history of infection. AIDS 11:597, 1997.
47. Piroth L, Grappin M, Buisson M, et al. Hepatitis B virus seroconversion in HIV-HBV coinfected patients treated with highly active antiretroviral therapy [letter]. J Acquir Immune Defic Syndr 23:356, 2000.
48. Den Brinker M, Wit FW, Wertheim-van Dillen PM, et al. Hepatitis B and C virus co-infection and the risk for hepatotoxicity of highly active antiretroviral therapy in HIV-1 infection. AIDS 14:2895, 2000.
49. Chau KH, Hargie MP, Decker RH, et al. Serodiagnosis of recent hepatitis B infection by IgM class anti-HBc. Hepatology 3:142, 1983.
50. Hadziyannis SJ, Lieberman HM, Karvountzis GG, Shafritz DA. Analysis of liver disease, nuclear HBcAg, viral replication, and hepatitis B virus DNA in liver and serum of HBeAg vs. anti-HBe positive carriers of hepatitis B virus. Hepatology 3:656, 1983.
51. Hoofnagle JH, Dusheiko GM, Seeff LB, et al. Seroconversion from hepatitis B e antigen to antibody in chronic type B hepatitis. Ann Intern Med 94:744, 1981.
52. Krugman S, Overby LR, Mushahwar IK, et al. Viral hepatitis, type B: studies on natural history and prevention re-examined. N Engl J Med 300:101, 1979.
53. Scolnick EM, McLean AA, West DJ, et al. Clinical evaluation in healthy adults of a hepatitis B vaccine made by recombinant DNA. JAMA 251:2812, 1984.
54. Draelos M, Morgan T, Schifman RB, Sampliner RE. Significance of isolated antibody to hepatitis B core antigen determined by immune response to hepatitis B vaccination. JAMA 258:1193, 1987.
55. Lok AS, Lai CL, Wu PC. Prevalence of isolated antibody to hepatitis B core antigen in an area endemic for hepatitis B virus infection: implications in hepatitis B vaccination programs. Hepatology 8:766, 1988.
56. Davaro RE, Cheeseman SH, Keroack MA, Ellison RT III. The significance of isolated antibody to hepatitis B core antigen seropositivity in patients infected with human immunodeficiency virus. Clin Infect Dis 23:189, 1996.
57. Jilg W, Sieger E, Zachoval R, Schätzl H. Individuals with antibodies against hepatitis B core antigen as the only serological marker for hepatitis B infection: high percentage of carriers of hepatitis B and C virus. J Hepatol 23:14, 1995.
58. Aoki SK, Finegold D, Kuramoto IK, et al. Significance of antibody to hepatitis B core antigen in blood donors as determined by their serologic response to hepatitis B vaccine. Transfusion 33:362, 1993.
59. Cacciola I, Pollicino T, Squadrito G, et al. Occult hepatitis B virus infection in patients with chronic hepatitis C liver disease. N Engl J Med 341:22, 1999.
60. Wong DK, Cheung AM, O'Rourke K, et al. Effect of alfa-interferon treatment in patients with hepatitis B e antigen-positive chronic hepatitis B. Ann Intern Med 119:312, 1993.
61. Lai CL, Chien RN, Leung NWY, et al. A one-year trial of lamivudine for chronic hepatitis B. N Engl J Med 339:61, 1998.
62. Dore GJ, Cooper DA, Barrett C, et al. Dual efficacy of lamivudine treatment in human immunodeficiency virus/hepatitis B virus-coinfected persons in a randomized, controlled study (CAESAR): the CAESAR coordinating committee. J Infect Dis 180:607, 1999.
63. Benhamou Y, Katlama C, Lunel F, et al. Effects of lamivudine on replication of hepatitis B virus in HIV-infected men. Ann Intern Med 125:705, 1996.
64. Pillay D, Cane PA, Ratcliffe D, et al. Evolution of lamivudine-resistant hepatitis B virus and HIV-1 in co-infected individuals: an analysis of the CAESAR study: CAESAR coordinating committee. AIDS 14:1111, 2000.
65. Ono-Nita SK, Kato N, Shiratori Y, et al. Susceptibility of lamivudine-resistant hepatitis B virus to other reverse transcriptase inhibitors. J Clin Invest 103:1635, 1999.
65a. Benhamon Y, Bochet M, Thibault V, et al. Safety and efficacy of adefovir dipivoxil in patients co-infected with HIV–1 and lamivudine-resistant hepatitis B virus: an open–label pilot study. Lancet 358:718, 2001.
66. Bessesen M, Ives D, Condreay L, et al. Chronic active hepatitis B exacerbations in human immunodeficiency virus-infected patients following development of resistance to or withdrawal of lamivudine. Clin Infect Dis 28:1032, 1999.
67. Neau D, Schvoerer E, Robert D, et al. Hepatitis B exacerbation with a precore mutant virus following withdrawal of lamivudine in a human immunodeficiency virus-infected patient. J Infect 41:192, 2000.
68. Szmuness W, Stevens CE, Harley EJ, et al. Hepatitis B vaccine: demonstration of efficacy in a controlled clinical trial in a high-risk population in the United States. N Engl J Med 303:833, 1980.
69. Hadler SC, Francis DP, Maynard JE, et al. Long-term immunogenicity and efficacy of hepatitis B vaccine in homosexual men. N Engl J Med 315:209, 1986.
70. Chang MH, Chen CJ, Lai MS, et al. Universal hepatitis B vaccination in Taiwan and the incidence of hepatocellular carcinoma in children: Taiwan Childhood Hepatoma Study Group. N Engl J Med 336:1855, 1997.
71. Lemon SM, Thomas DL. Drug therapy: vaccines to prevent viral hepatitis. N Engl J Med 336:196, 1997.
72. Centers for Disease Control and Prevention. Immunization of health care workers: recommendations of the Advisory Committee on Im-

munization Practices and the Hospital Infection Control Practices Advisory Committee. MMWR Morbid Mortal Wkly Rep 46(RR18):22, 1997.

73. Centers for Disease Control and Prevention. The hepatitis B virus: a comprehensive strategy for eliminating transmission in the United States through universal childhood vaccination. MMWR Morbid Mortal Wkly Rep 40:1, 1991.
74. Cheeseman SH, Davaro RE, Ellison RT. Hepatitis B vaccination and plasma HIV-1 RNA. N Engl J Med 334:1272, 1996.
75. Collier AC, Corey L, Murphy VL, Handsfield HH. Antibody to human immunodeficiency virus and suboptimal response to hepatitis B vaccination. Ann Intern Med 109:101, 1988.
76. Rey D, Krantz V, Partisani M, et al. Increasing the number of hepatitis B vaccine injections augments anti-HBs response rate in HIV-infected patients: effects on HIV-1 viral load. Vaccine 18:1161, 2000.
77. Choo QL, Richman KH, Han JH, et al. Genetic organization and diversity of the hepatitis C virus. Proc Natl Acad Sci USA 88:2451, 1991.
78. Neumann AU, Lam NP, Dahari H, et al. Hepatitis C viral dynamics in vivo and the antiviral efficacy of interferon-alpha therapy. Science 282:103, 1998.
79. Ogata N, Alter HJ, Miller RH, Purcell RH. Nucleotide sequence and mutation rate of the H strain of hepatitis C virus. Proc Natl Acad Sci USA 88:3392, 1991.
80. Abe K, Inchauspe G, Fujisawa K. Genomic characterization and mutation rate of hepatitis C virus isolated from a patient who contracted hepatitis during an epidemic of non-A, non-B hepatitis in Japan. J Gen Virol 73:2725, 1992.
81. Stuyver L, Rossau R, Wyseur A, et al. Typing of hepatitis C virus isolates and characterization of new subtypes using a line probe assay. J Gen Virol 74:1093, 1993.
82. Simmonds P, Holmes EC, Cha T-A, et al. Classification of hepatitis C virus into six major genotypes and a series of subtypes by phylogenetic analysis of the NS-5 region. J Gen Virol 74:2391, 1993.
83. Zein NN, Rakela J, Krawitt EL, et al. Hepatitis C virus genotypes in the United States: epidemiology, pathogenicity, and response to interferon therapy. Ann Intern Med 125:634, 1996.
84. Lau JYN, Davis GL, Prescott LE, et al. Distribution of hepatitis C virus genotypes determined by line probe assay inpatients with chronic hepatitis C seen at tertiary referral centers in the United States. Ann Intern Med 124:868, 1996.
85. Donahue JG, Munoz A, Ness PM, et al. The declining risk of post-transfusion hepatitis C virus infection. N Engl J Med 327:369, 1992.
86. Schreiber GB, Busch MP, Kleinman SH, Korelitz JJ. The risk of transfusion-transmitted viral infections: the Retrovirus Epidemiology Donor Study. N Engl J Med 334:1685, 1996.
87. Thomas DL, Vlahov D, Solomon L, et al. Correlates of hepatitis C virus infections among injection drug users in Baltimore. Medicine 74:212, 1995.
88. Alter MJ, Hadler SC, Judson FN, et al. Risk factors for acute non-A, non-B hepatitis in the United States and association with hepatitis C virus infection. JAMA 264:2231, 1990.
89. Villano SA, Vlahov D, Nelson KE, et al. Incidence and risk factors for hepatitis C among injection drug users in Baltimore, Maryland. J Clin Microbiol 35:3274, 1997.
90. Van Ameijden EJ, van den Hoek JA, Mientjes GH, Coutinho RA. A longitudinal study on the incidence and transmission patterns of HIV, HBV and HCV infection among drug users in Amsterdam. Eur J Epidemiol 9:255, 1993.
91. Centers for Disease Control and Prevention. Recommendations for prevention and control of hepatitis C virus (HCV) infection and HCV-related chronic disease. MMWR Morbid Mortal Wkly Rep 47(RR-19):1, 1998.
92. Thomas DL, Zenilman JM, Alter HJ, et al. Sexual transmission of hepatitis C virus among patients attending sexually transmitted diseases clinics in Baltimore: an analysis of 309 sex partnerships. J Infect Dis 171:768, 1995.
93. Conry-Cantilena C, Vanraden MT, Gibble J, et al. Routes of infection, viremia, and liver disease in blood donors found to have hepatitis C virus infection. N Engl J Med 334:1691, 1996.
94. Everhart JE, Di Bisceglie AM, Murray LM, et al. Risk for non-A, non-B (type C) hepatitis through sexual or household contact with chronic carriers. Ann Intern Med 112:544, 1990.
95. Gordon SC, Patel AH, Kulesza GW, et al. Lack of evidence for the heterosexual transmission of hepatitis C. Am J Gastroenterol 87:1849, 1992.
96. Brettler DB, Mannucci PM, Gringeri A, et al. The low risk of hepatitis C virus transmission among sexual partners of hepatitis C-infected hemophilic males: an international, multicenter study. Blood 80:540, 1992.
97. Osmond DH, Padian NS, Sheppard HW, et al. Risk factors for hepatitis C virus seropositivity in heterosexual couples. JAMA 269:361, 1993.
98. Eyster ME, Alter HJ, Aledort LM, et al. Heterosexual co-transmission of hepatitis C virus (HCV) and human immunodeficiency virus (HIV). Ann Intern Med 115:764, 1991.
99. Thomas DL, Villano SA, Riester KA, et al. Perinatal transmission of hepatitis C virus from human immunodeficiency virus type 1-infected mothers. J Infect Dis 177:1480, 1998.
100. Zanetti AR, Tanzi E, Paccagnini S, et al. Mother-to-infant transmission of hepatitis C virus. Lancet 345:289, 1995.
101. Hershow RC, Riester KA, Lew J, et al. Increased vertical transmission of human immunodeficiency virus from hepatitis C virus-coinfected mothers. J Infect Dis 176:414, 1997.
102. Stubbe L, Soriano V, Antunes F, et al. Hepatitis C in the EuroSIDA cohort of European HIV-infected patients: prevalence and prognostic value. Presented at the 12th World AIDS Conference, Geneva, July 1998, abstract 22261.
103. Kiyosawa K, Sodeyama T, Tanaka E, et al. Hepatitis C in hospital employees with needlestick injuries. Ann Intern Med 115:367, 1991.
104. Makris M, Preston FE, Triger DR, et al. Hepatitis C antibody and chronic liver disease in haemophilia. Lancet 335:1117, 1990.
105. Donahue JG, Nelson KE, Munoz A, et al. Antibody to hepatitis C virus among cardiac surgery patients, homosexual men, and intravenous drug users in Baltimore, Maryland. Am J Epidemiol 134:1206, 1991.
106. Villano SA, Vlahov D, Nelson KE, et al. Persistence of viremia and the importance of long-term follow-up after acute hepatitis C infection. Hepatology 29:908, 1999.
107. Alter MJ, Margolis HS, Krawczynski K, et al. The natural history of community acquired hepatitis C in the United States. N Engl J Med 327:1899, 1992.
108. Inglesby TV, Rai R, Astemborski J, et al. A prospective, community-based evaluation of liver enzymes in individuals with hepatitis C after drug use. Hepatology 29:590, 1999.
109. Tong MJ, El-Farra NS, Reikes AR, Co RL. Clinical outcomes after transfusion-associated hepatitis C. N Engl J Med 332:1463, 1995.
110. Seeff LB, Buskell-Bales ZB, Wright EC, et al. Long-term mortality after transfusion-associated non-A, non-B hepatitis. N Engl J Med 327:1906, 1992.
111. Kenny-Walsh E. Clinical outcomes after hepatitis C infection from contaminated anti-D immune globulin: Irish Hepatology Research Group. N Engl J Med 340:1228, 1999.
112. Fattovich G, Giustina G, Degos F, et al. Morbidity and mortality in compensated cirrhosis C: a follow-up study of 384 patients. Gastroenterology 112:463, 1997.
113. Mathurin P, Moussalli J, Cadranel JF, et al. Slow progression rate of fibrosis in hepatitis C virus patients with persistently normal alanine transaminase activity. Hepatology 27:868, 1998.
114. Fanning L, Kenny E, Sheehan M, et al. Viral load and clinicopathological features of chronic hepatitis C (1b) in a homogeneous patient population. Hepatology 29:904, 1999.
115. Mellors JW, Rinaldo CRJ, Gupta P, et al. Prognosis in HIV-1 infection predicted by the quantity of virus in plasma. Science 272:1167, 1996.
116. Thomas DL, Astemborski J, Rai RM, et al. The natural history of hepatitis C virus infection: host, viral, and environmental factors. JAMA 284:450, 2000.
117. Perrillo RP. The role of liver biopsy in hepatitis C. Hepatology 26:57S, 1997.
118. Thomas DL, Astemborski J, Vlahov D, et al. Determinants of the quantity of hepatitis C virus RNA. J Infect Dis 181:844, 2000.
119. Thomas DL, Shih JW, Alter HJ, et al. Effect of human immunodeficiency virus on hepatitis C virus infection among injecting drug users. J Infect Dis 174:690, 1996.
120. Telfer P, Sabin C, Devereux H, et al. The progression of HCV-associated liver disease in a cohort of hemophiliac patients. Br J Haematol 87:555, 1994.

121. Sherman KE, O'Brien J, Gutierrez AG, et al. Quantitative evaluation of hepatitis C virus RNA in patients with concurrent human immunodeficiency virus infections. J Clin Microbiol 31:2679, 1993.
122. Eyster ME, Fried MW, Di Bisceglie AM, Goedert JJ. Increasing hepatitis C virus RNA levels in hemophiliacs: relationship to human immunodeficiency virus infection and liver disease. Blood 84:1020, 1994.
123. Eyster ME, Diamondstone LS, Lien JM, et al. Natural history of hepatitis C virus infection in multitransfused hemophiliacs: effect of coinfection with human immunodeficiency virus: the Multicenter Hemophilia Cohort Study. J Acquir Immune Defic Syndr 6:602, 1993.
124. Darby SC, Ewart DW, Giangrande PL, et al. Mortality from liver cancer and liver disease in haemophilic men and boys in UK given blood products contaminated with hepatitis C. Lancet 350:1425, 1997.
125. Lesens O, Deschenes M, Steben M, et al. Hepatitis C virus is related to progressive liver disease in human immunodeficiency virus-positive hemophiliacs and should be treated as an opportunistic infection. J Infect Dis 179:1254, 1999.
126. Pol S, Lamorthe B, Thi NT, et al. Retrospective analysis of the impact of HIV infection and alcohol use on chronic hepatitis C in a large cohort of drug users. J Hepatol 28:945, 1998.
127. Soriano V, Garcia-Samaniego J, Valencia E, et al. Impact of chronic liver disease due to hepatitis viruses as cause of hospital admission and death in HIV-infected drug users. Eur J Epidemiol 15:1, 1999.
128. Bica I, McGovern B, Dhar R, et al. Increasing mortality due to end-stage liver disease in patients with human immunodeficiency virus infection. Clin Infect Dis 32:492, 2001.
129. Dorrucci M, Pezzotti P, Phillips AN, et al. Coinfection of hepatitis C virus with human immunodeficiency virus and progression to AIDS. J Infect Dis 172:1503, 1995.
130. Sulkowski MS, Moore RD, Mehta SH, et al. Hepatis C and progression of HIV disease. JAMA 288:241, 2002.
131. Sabin CA, Telfer P, Phillips AN, et al. The association between hepatitis C virus genotype and human immunodeficiency virus disease progression in a cohort of hemophilic men. J Infect Dis 175:164, 1997.
132. Piroth L, Duong M, Quantin C, et al. Does hepatitis C virus co-infection accelerate clinical and immunological evolution of HIV-infected patients? AIDS 12:381, 1998.
133. Greub G, Ledergerber B, Battegay M, et al. Clinical progression, survival, and immune recovery during antiretroviral therapy in patients with HIV-1 and hepatitis C virus coinfection: the Swiss HIV Cohort Study. Lancet 356:1800, 2000.
134. Brau N, Leaf HL, Wieczorek RL, Margolis DM. Severe hepatitis in three AIDS patients treated with indinavir. Lancet 349:924, 1997.
135. Arribas JR, Ibanez C, Ruiz-Antoran B, et al. Acute hepatitis in HIV-infected patients during ritonavir treatment. AIDS 12:1722, 1998.
136. Rodriguez-Rosado R, Garcia-Samaniego J, Soriano V. Hepatotoxicity after introduction of highly active antiretroviral therapy. AIDS 12:1256, 1998.
137. Sulkowski MS, Thomas DL, Chaisson RE, Moore RD. Hepatotoxicity associated with antiretroviral therapy in adults infected with human immunodeficiency virus and the role of hepatitis C or B virus infection. JAMA 283:74, 2000.
138. Ungo JR, Jones D, Ashkin D, et al. Antituberculosis drug-induced hepatotoxicity: the role of hepatitis C virus and the human immunodeficiency virus. Am J Respir Crit Care Med 157:1871, 1998.
139. Vento S, Garofano T, Renzini C, et al. Enhancement of hepatitis C virus replication and liver damage in HIV-coinfected patients on antiretroviral combination therapy. AIDS 12:116, 1998.
140. John M, Flexman J, French MAH. Hepatitis C virus-associated hepatitis following treatment of HIV-infected patients with HIV protease inhibitors: an immune restoration disease? AIDS 12:2289, 1998.
141. Zylberberg H, Pialoux G, Carnot F, et al. Rapidly evolving hepatitis C virus-related cirrhosis in a human immunodeficiency virus-infected patient receiving triple antiretroviral therapy. Clin Infect Dis 27:1255, 1998.
142. Thio CL, Nolt KR, Astemborski J, et al. Screening for hepatitis C virus in human immunodeficiency virus-infected individuals. J Clin Microbiol 38:575, 2000.
143. Chamot E, Hirschel B, Wintsch J, et al. Loss of antibodies against hepatitis C virus in HIV-seropositive intravenous drug users. AIDS 4:1275, 1990.
144. Frieden TR, Ozick L, McCord C, et al. Chronic liver disease in central Harlem: the role of alcohol and viral hepatitis. Hepatology 29:883, 1999.
145. Wiley TE, McCarthy M, Breidi L, Layden TJ. Impact of alcohol on the histological and clinical progression of hepatitis C infection. Hepatology 28:805, 1998.
146. Poynard T, Bedossa P, Opolon P. Natural history of liver fibrosis progression in patients with chronic hepatitis C. Lancet 349:825, 1997.
147. Vento S, Garofano T, Renzini C, et al. Fulminant hepatitis associated with hepatitis A virus superinfection in patients with chronic hepatitis C. N Engl J Med 338:286, 1998.
148. Poles MA, Dieterich DT, Schwarz ED, et al. Liver biopsy findings in 501 patients infected with human immunodeficiency virus (HIV). J Acquir Immune Defic Syndr Hum Retrovirol 11:170, 1996.
149. National Institutes of Health consensus development conference panel statement: management of hepatitis C. Hepatology 26:2S, 1997.
150. Marcellin P, Boyer N, Gervais A, et al. Long-term histologic improvement and loss of detectable intrahepatic HCV RNA in patients with chronic hepatitis C and sustained response to interferon-α therapy. Ann Intern Med 127:875, 1997.
151. Lau DTY, Kleiner DE, Ghany MG, et al. 10-Year follow-up after interferon-alpha therapy for chronic hepatitis C. Hepatology 28:1121, 1998.
152. Soriano V, García-Samaniego J, Bravo R, et al. Interferon α for the treatment of chronic hepatitis C in patients infected with human immunodeficiency virus. Clin Infect Dis 23:585, 1996.
153. Soriano V, Bravo R, García-Samaniego J, et al. Relapses of chronic hepatitis C in HIV-infected patients who responded to interferon therapy. AIDS 11:400, 1997.
154. Effect of interferon-alpha on progression of cirrhosis to hepatocellular carcinoma: a retrospective cohort study: International Interferon-alpha Hepatocellular Carcinoma Study Group. Lancet 351:1535, 1998.
155. Nishiguchi S, Kuroki T, Nakatani S, et al. Randomised trial of effects of interferon-α on incidence of hepatocellular carcinoma in chronic active hepatitis C with cirrhosis. Lancet 346:1051, 1995.
156. Nishiguchi S, Shiomi S, Nakatani S, et al. Prevention of hepatocellular carcinoma in patients with chronic active hepatitis C and cirrhosis. Lancet 357:196, 2001.
157. Sulkowski MS, Mast EE, Seeff LB, Thomas DL. Hepatitis C virus infection as an opportunistic disease in persons infected with human immunodeficiency virus. Clin Infect Dis 30(suppl 1):S77, 2000.
158. Boyer N, Marcellin P, Degott C, et al. Recombinant interferon-alpha for chronic hepatitis C in patients positive for antibody to human immunodeficiency virus. J Infect Dis 165:723, 1992.
159. Marriott E, Navas S, Del Romero J, et al. Treatment with recombinant alpha-interferon of chronic hepatitis C in anti-HIV-positive patients. J Med Virol 40:107, 1993.
160. Mauss S, Heintges T, Adams O, et al. Treatment of chronic hepatitis C with interferon-alpha in patients infected with the human immunodeficiency virus. Hepatogastroenterology 42:528, 1995.
161. Soriano V, García-Samaniego J, Bravo R, et al. Interferon α for the treatment of chronic hepatitis C in patients infected with human immunodeficiency virus. Clin Infect Dis 23:585, 1996.
162. Mauss S, Klinker H, Ulmer A, et al. Response to treatment of chronic hepatitis C with interferon α in patients infected with HIV-1 is associated with higher CD4+ cell count. Infection 26:20, 1998.
163. Causse X, Payen JL, Izopet J, et al. Does HIV-infection influence the response of chronic hepatitis C to interferon treatment? A French multicenter prospective study: French Multicenter Study Group. J Hepatol 32:1003, 2000.
164. Prestileo T, Mazzola G, Di Lorenzo F, et al. Response-adjusted alpha-interferon therapy for chronic hepatitis C in HIV-infected patients. Int J Antimicrob Agents 16:373, 2000.
165. Zylberberg H, Benhamou Y, Lagneaux JL, et al. Safety and efficacy of interferon-ribavirin combination therapy in HCV-HIV coinfected subjects: an early report. Gut 47:694, 2000.
166. Landau A, Batisse D, Van Huyen JP, et al. Efficacy and safety of combination therapy with interferon-alpha2b and ribavirin for chronic hepatitis C in HIV-infected patients. AIDS 14:839, 2000.
167. Boyer N, Marcellin P, Degott C, et al. Recombinant Interferon-alpha for chronic hepatitis C in patients positive for antibody to human immunodeficiency virus. J Infect Dis 165:723, 1992.
168. Marriott E, Navas S, Del Romero J, et al. Treatment with recombinant alpha-interferon of chronic hepatitis C in anti-HIV-positive patients. J Med Virol 40:107, 1993.

169. Poynard T, Marcellin P, Lee SS, et al. Randomised trial of interferon α2b plus ribavirin for 48 weeks or for 24 weeks versus interferon α2b plus placebo for 48 weeks for treatment of chronic infection with hepatitis C virus. Lancet 352:1426, 1998.
170. McHutchison JG, Gordon SC, Schiff ER, et al. Interferon alfa-2b alone or in combination with ribavirin as initial treatment for chronic hepatitis C. N Engl J Med 339:1485, 1998.
171. Landau A, Batisse D, Piketty C, et al. Lack of interference between ribavirin and nucleosidic analogues in HIV/HCV co-infected individuals undergoing concomitant antiretroviral and anti-HCV combination therapy. AIDS 14:1857, 2000.
172. Landau A, Batisse D, Piketty C, Kazatchkine MD. Effect of interferon and ribavirin on HIV viral load. AIDS 14:96, 2000.
173. Zylberberg H, Benhamou Y, Lagneaux JL, et al. Safety and efficacy of interferon-ribavirin combination therapy in HCV-HIV coinfected subjects: an early report. Gut 47:694, 2000.
174. Poynard T, McHutchison J, Goodman Z, et al. Is an "a la carte" combination interferon alfa-2b plus ribavirin regimen possible for the first line treatment in patients with chronic hepatitis C? The ALGOVIRC project group. Hepatology 31:211, 2000.
175. Zeuzem S, Feinman SV, Rasenack J, et al. PEGinterferon alfa-2a in patients with chronic hepatitis C. N Engl J Med 343:1666, 2000.
176. Heathcote EJ, Shiffman ML, Cooksley WG, et al. PEGinterferon alfa-2a in patients with chronic hepatitis C and cirrhosis. N Engl J Med 343:1673, 2000.
177. Trepo C, Lindsay K, Niederau C, et al. PEGylated interferon alfa-2b monotherapy is superior to interferon alfa-2b for the treatment of chronic hepatitis C [abstract GS2/08]. J Hepatol 32(suppl 2):29, 2000.
178. Manns MP, McHutchison JG, Gordon S, et al. PEGinterferon alfa-2b plus ribavirin compared with interferon alfa-2b plus ribavirin for the treatment of chronic hepatitis C: a randomized trial. Lancet 358:958, 2001.
179. Dusheiko G. Side effects of alpha interferon in chronic hepatitis C. Hepatology 26:112S, 1997.
180. Deutsch M, Dourakis S, Manesis EK, et al. Thyroid abnormalities in chronic viral hepatitis and their relationship to interferon alfa therapy. Hepatology 26:206, 1997.
181. Dieterich DT, Wasserman R, Brau N, et al. Once-weekly recombinant human erythropoetin (epoetin alfa) facilitates optimal ribavirin (RBV) dosing in hepatitis C virus (HCV)-infected patients receiving interferon-α-2b combination therapy [abstract 104956]. Gastroenterology 120:A-64, 2001.
182. Moore RD. Human immunodeficiency virus infection, anemia, and survival. Clin Infect Dis 29:44, 1999.
183. Vogt MW, Hartshorn KL, Furman PA, et al. Ribavirin antagonizes the effect of azidothymidine on HIV replication. Science 235:1376, 1987.
184. Hoggard PG, Kewn S, Barry MG, et al. Effects of drugs on 2′,3′-dideoxy-2′,3′-didehydrothymidine phosphorylation in vitro. Antimicrob Agents Chemother 41:1231, 1997.
185. Baba M, Pauwels R, Balzarini J, et al. Ribavirin antagonizes inhibitory effects of pyrimidine 2′,3′-dideoxynucleosides but enhances inhibitory effects of purine 2′,3′-dideoxynucleosides on replication of human immunodeficiency virus in vitro. Antimicrob Agents Chemother 31:1613, 1987.
186. Lafeuillade A, Hittinger G, Chadapaud S. Increased mitochondrial toxicity with ribavirin in HIV/HCV coinfection. Lancet 357:280, 2001.
187. Japour AJ, Lertora JJ, Meehan PM, et al. A phase-I study of the safety, pharmacokinetics, and antiviral activity of combination didanosine and ribavirin in patients with HIV-1 disease: AIDS Clinical Trials Group 231 Protocol Team. J Acquir Immune Defic Syndr Hum Retrovirol 13:235, 1996.

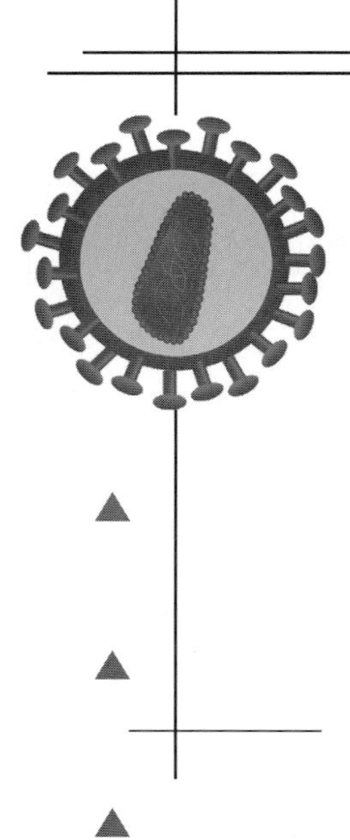

CHAPTER 47

Sexually Transmitted Human Papillomavirus Infection

William Bonnez, MD

Human papillomaviruses (HPVs) represent a large group of viruses that infect mostly the squamous epithelia of the body. They cause latent, asymptomatic infections as well as neoplasms that range from benign warts to malignant squamous cell carcinoma, particularly of the cervix. A subgroup of HPVs has a predilection for the anogenital tract (Table 47–1). Because these genital HPVs are mostly sexually transmitted, they are likely to be encountered in the human immunodeficiency virus (HIV)-infected population. Although the host factors that control HPV infections are poorly understood, immunosuppression and immunodeficiencies tend to be associated with HPV diseases that are more florid and more difficult to eradicate or control than in the immunocompetent host. Consequently, sexually transmitted HPV diseases in the HIV-infected patient create management problems for the practitioner. This chapter describes the resources and approaches that are available.

PATHOGEN

The HPVs are circular, double-stranded DNA, nonenveloped viruses that belong to the *Papillomavirus* genus of the Papillomaviridae family. The nucleic acid is enclosed in a 55 nm diameter icosahedral capsid composed of 72 pentamers. One strand of the DNA encodes all the open reading frames (ORFs). The genome can be divided into three parts. The first is a noncoding region, or upstream regulatory region (URR), that contains the origin of replication as well as a promoter sequence and binding sites for various viral and cellular regulatory proteins. Downstream of the URR are a group of "early" ORFs (E1, E2, E4, E5, E6, E7) that encode for nonstructural proteins. E1 is involved in viral replication, as is E2, which also regulates viral expression. E4 produces an abundant cytoplasmic protein that associates with the intermediate filament network but whose role is obscure. E5 is believed to contribute to malignant transformation, a role that has been well established for E6 and E7 of high-risk oncogenic HPVs. The E6 protein binds to p53, a major tumor suppressor protein, and induces its degradation. Similarly, the E7 protein binds and inactivates other tumor suppressor molecules, the retinoblastoma protein (pRB) and pRB-associated proteins. Both p53 and pRB exert essential control on cellular replication and apoptosis. E6 and E7 also interact with many other cellular proteins. The late ORFs are the third component of the genome and are made up of two ORFs, L1 and L2, encoding for structural proteins: the major and minor capsid proteins, respectively. In malignant lesions, HPV DNA is typically found to be integrated into the host genome. This integration always disrupts the E2 ORFs but never the E6 and E7 ORFs, which become unregulated. There is minimal evidence that HIV interacts directly with HPV.[1–4]

Because of the difficulty of growing HPVs experimentally, the classification of HPVs has been based on genotypes rather than serotypes. HPV types are distinct if they share less than 90% of the DNA sequence homology for the L1 ORF with one another. More than 220 HPV types have been identified so far, and 91 types have been characterized (Current taxonomic information is kept on the Internet at http://hpv-web.lanl.gov.) Each type tends to be associated with particular tissue specificity, pathology, and oncogenic risk (Table 47–1).

Thus three main groups of HPV diseases can be delineated. The first consists of cutaneous warts, which include the common warts found on hands and soles, deep plantar

▲ **Table 47–1.** GENITAL HPV TYPES AND THEIR DISEASE ASSOCIATION*

Disease	HPV Types[a]	
	Frequent Association	Less-frequent Association
Condylomata acuminata	6, 11	30,[b] 42, 43, 44, 45,[b] 51,[b] 54, 55, 70[b]
Intraepithelial neoplasias		
Unspecified		30,[b] 34, 39,[b] 40, 53, 57, 59,[b] 61, 62, 64, 66,[b] 67, 68,[b] 69, 71
Low grade	6, 11	16,[b] 18,[b] 31,[b] 33,[b] 35,[b] 42, 43, 44, 45,[b] 51,[b] 52,[b] 74,[c] 86, 87
High grade	16,[b] 18[b]	6, 11, 31,[b] 33,[b] 35,[b] 39,[b] 42, 44, 45,[b] 51,[b] 52,[b] 56,[b] 58,[b] 66[b]
Bowen's disease	16[b]	31,[b] 34
Bowenoid papulosis	16[b]	34, 39,[b] 42, 45,[b] 67[b]
Cervical (and other genital) carcinomas	16,[b] 18[b]	31,[b] 33,[b] 35,[b] 39,[b] 45,[b] 51,[b] 52,[b] 56,[b] 58,[b] 59,[b] 66,[b] 68,[b] 70[b]
Recurrent respiratory papillomatosis	6, 11	
Conjunctival papillomas and carcinomas	6, 11, 16[b]	

The author is grateful to Dr. Ethel-Michele de Villiers (HPV Reference Center, Heidelberg, Germany) and Dr. Gérard Orth (Institut Pasteur, Paris, France) for sharing information.

[a]The distinction between "frequent" and "less frequent" is arbitrary in many instances. Large descriptive statistics of HPV type distribution by disease are not available for most HPV types. Moreover, many HPV types have been sought or identified only once.

[b]Types with high malignant potential or isolated in only one or a few lesions that were malignant.

[c]Type first recovered from immunosuppressed or HIV-infected patients.

warts, and flat warts. HIV infection increases the prevalence of these lesions; they are not discussed further here.

The second group corresponds to epidermodysplasia verruciformis, a rare condition that develops in adults and is governed by genetic factors. It manifests as flat wart-like lesions, plaques, or pityriasis versicolor-like lesions that have a high risk of evolving into malignant squamous cell carcinomas. No association with HIV infection has been described for this condition.

The third group includes the genital or mucosal HPV diseases. They involve the external genitalia and anus and, in females, the vagina and cervix as well. Their manifestations can be subclinical or full-blown, the latter being the only state relevant to treatment. The diseases range from the typically benign warts (or condylomas) to preinvasive and invasive cancers (mostly squamous cell carcinomas). The preinvasive cancers are called intraepithelial neoplasias (also improperly named dysplasias).

Although condylomas or warts can be present on the vagina, cervix, or anal canal, anogenital (venereal) warts usually refer to exophytic lesions of the external anogenital area; they are also called condylomata acuminata (singular: condyloma acuminatum). Condylomata acuminata on occasion are extremely large (giant condylomas). They may then adopt a locally invasive behavior and be called condylomatous carcinomas or Buschke-Löwenstein tumors.

The intraepithelial neoplasias are a group of conditions defined by the proliferation in the anogenital stratified epithelium of basaloid (basal-appearing) cells with an excess of mitotic figures (dysplasia). Three grades are recognized, from the less severe to the more severe, based on the proportion of the epithelium involved in this process. Thus the process involves up to the lower third of the epithelium in grade 1 (I), more than one-third but less than two-thirds in grade 2 (II), and more than two-thirds in grade 3 (III). In carcinoma in situ (CIS), a form of intraepithelial neoplasia grade 3, the full thickness of the epithelium is involved. Breakage of the basement membrane by this cellular proliferation represents invasion and the ultimate stage of evolution of an intraepithelial neoplasia: squamous cell carcinoma. Originally devised for the cervix (Fig. 47–1), this simple histologic classification scheme is also used for other locations, giving rise to various acronyms: CIN for cervical intraepithelial neoplasia, VAIN for the vagina, VIN for the vulva, PIN for the penis, and AIN for the anus. Other conditions developing on the external genitalia are simply clinical variants of intraepithelial neoplasias. They include bowenoid papulosis (pigmented papules with a condylomatous cytoarchitecture); Bowen's disease (CIS presenting as a flat, red to brown plaque with well demarcated borders and a scaly surface); and erythroplasia of Queyrat (Bowen's disease of the glans penis). Condylomas and intraepithelial neoplasias of the cervix typically arise in the transformation zone, the virtual space between the location of the squamocolumnar–epithelial junction at birth and the current location of this junction, which with age recedes toward the endocervix. Similarly, in the anus it is in the area of squamous metaplasia, at the junction of the squamous and glandular epithelium, that one finds AIN and carcinomas.

If only based on the fact that they are in part caused by the same HPV types, these diseases are related. Another relation, histopathologic, has been particularly well documented for the cervix, where a lesion may progress from condyloma or CIN grade 1 to CIN grades 2 and 3 and cancer. This progression is not necessarily predictable, however; it may not even occur, some of its stages may be missed, and up to grade 3 it may revert. Importantly, the risk of progression or regression is related to the HPV type causing the process, molecular variants within HPV types, HPV viral load, and persistence. Figure 47–1 illustrates the relation between HPV type and disease grade in greater detail in the case of uterine cervix involvement.

Two minor groups of diseases are related to the genital HPV diseases because they are caused by the same HPV types and are mostly sexually transmitted: recurrent respiratory papillomatosis and oral condylomas. Although risk factors for the acquisition of recurrent respiratory papillomatosis include receptive oral sex in adults and vaginal delivery in children, for unclear reasons the disease seems to be rare in HIV-infected individuals. Oral HPV diseases include condylomas resulting from sexual transmission. Only histology helps distinguish them from other oral warts associated with cutaneous HPV types that are not sexually

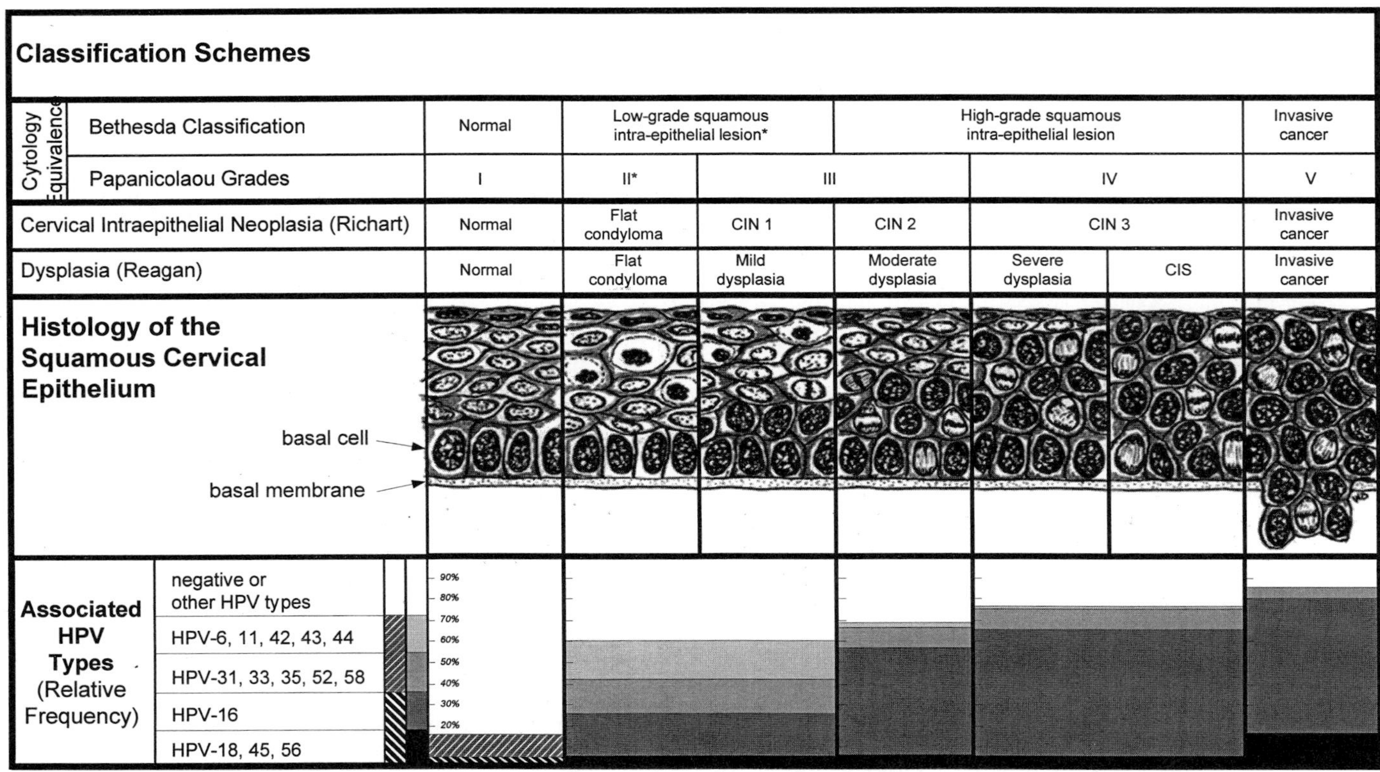

Figure 47–1. Nomenclature, histologic features, and distribution of associated HPV types in HPV-related cervical lesions. The dysplasia and cervical intraepithelial neoplasia classifications are primarily histologic categories that are also used for cytology, whereas the Bethesda classification is designed mainly for cytology (see text for details). *This category also includes benign cell changes, reactive changes, atypical squamous cells of undetermined significance (ASCUS), and atypical glandular cells of unknown significance (AGUS).

transmitted. Heck's disease (focal epithelial hyperplasia), an uncommon florid oral papillomatosis predominantly caused by HPV type 13, has been described in HIV patients associated with HPV-32.[5,6]

Anogenital HPV infections are particularly common in the general population, but the prevalence varies with the method of diagnosis and, as would be expected for agents that are mostly sexually transmitted, the age of the population. For example, in one study, using a polymerase chain reaction (PCR) assay, 49% of women between the ages of 20 and 25 years had HPV in their cervix in contrast to 34% of women 26 to 50 years of age.[7] Based on cytology, the rates fall to about 1% to 5% depending on age and diagnostic criteria.[8] It is estimated that approximately 1% of the population has condyloma acuminatum.[8] These numbers exemplify the large size of the virus reservoir in the population at large. Sexual transmission is by far the major mode of dissemination; and although direct evidence is lacking, it is probably more efficient if the infection causes full-blown disease rather than latency or subclinical disease.

Three types of anogenital HPV diseases are clearly overrepresented in the HIV-seropositive population compared to the seronegative population: condyloma acuminatum, AIN (in men and in women to a lesser extent), and CIN (Table 47–2).[9–19] A large population survey has shown that in patients who have AIDS the relative risks of in situ or invasive squamous cell carcinomas are increased in several anatomic locations: cervix, vulva/vagina, anus (both genders), penis, and (men only) tonsils and conjunctiva.[18]

These findings are consistent with the observation that HIV infection is associated with anogenital infections involving high risk rather than low risk HPV genotypes and with more persistent, high HPV viral loads.[11,16,25–32] Other factors, such as smoking and young age, independently contribute to the risk of anogenital HPV infection and disease.[15,19,33]

The nature of the link between HIV and HPV infections seems to be behavioral and immunologic, but the details are not well defined. Because both infections are sexually transmitted, it is obvious that they share some of the same behavioral risk factors. However, if oral sex seems to be a risk factor for adult-onset recurrent respiratory papillomatosis in the general population, it not clear why this entity is not more common in HIV-infected patients.[34] HIV infection depresses the immune defenses that control HPV infections. Accordingly, the more severe the HIV infection (as measured by the progression to AIDS, CD4 cell count, or HIV viral load) the higher is the risk of finding high risk HPV DNA in the anogenital tract, condylomata acuminata, or preinvasive squamous cell carcinoma in the cervix and anus of men and women.[15,19,22,25,31,35–37] It is also not surprising that because of the HIV-induced immunosuppression HPV diseases in these patients tend to be more severe and intractable, and they recur more frequently.[38–45]

▲ **Table 47–2.** SELECTED EPIDEMIOLOGIC DATA ON THE RELATION BETWEEN HPV DISEASE AND HIV

Population and Pathology	No. of Individuals with Pathology/total (%)		Odds Ratio[a]
	HIV+	HIV−	
Homosexual men[20]			
With history of anal warts	28/48 (58%)	13/44 (30%)	3.3*
With history of penile warts	4/49 (8%)	7/46 (15%)	0.5
Presence of anal warts	12/49 (24%)	6/45 (13%)	2.1
Presence of anal HPV DNA[b]	13/49 (26%)	3/47 (6%)	5.3*
Homosexual men with anogenital warts[14]			
With abnormal anal cytology	159/346 (46%)	26/261 (10%)	7.7*
With anal HSIL	8/346 (2.3%)	0/261 (0%)	+*
STD clinic population, Haiti[21]			
Anogenital warts	43/374 (11.4%)	28/548 (5.1%)	2.4*
Women with anogenital warts[22]	22/253 (8.7%)	8/660 (1.2%)	7.8*
Women[23]			
With LSIL	33/135 (94.3%)	8/101 (7.9%)	3.5*
With HSIL	15/135 (11.1%)	1/101 (0.9%)	12.5*
Women, IVDA[24]			
With presence of cervical HPV DNA[c]	30/53 (57%)	7/55 (13%)	8.9*
With presence of anal HPV DNA[c]	40/52 (77%)	28/50 (56%)	2.6*

HSIL, high-grade SIL; IVDA, intravenous drug abuser; LSIL, low-grade SIL; SIL, squamous intraepithelial lesion; STD, sexually transmitted disease.
[a]An asterisk indicates $P < 0.05$.
[b]By a combination of dot blot and Southern blot.
[c]By PCR assay.

This simple biologic explanation is not sufficient, however; otherwise the risk of invasive cervical cancer should rise as patients progress to acquired immunodeficiency syndrome (AIDS). On the basis of that expectation, in 1993 the Centers for Disease Control and Prevention (CDC) had included cervical cancer as an AIDS-defining illness.[46] The failure for the expectation to materialize clearly has been a surprise. It has since been reasoned that because cervical cancer takes about a decade to develop in the general population, the limited survival of HIV patients did not permit a sufficient number of cervical cancers to occur for the trend to be detected. This interpretation is losing strength because ever-larger surveys still do not detect even a trend.[18,47] It has also been proposed that intensified screening programs in combination with improved antiretroviral treatments might have curbed the progression of CIN to invasive cancer. However, the introduction of highly active antiretroviral therapy had no effect on the incidence of invasive cervical carcinoma in an Italian cohort study.[47a] In Africa where cervical cancer screening programs and antiretroviral therapy are rarely available, the increase in the incidence of cervical cancers in the HIV population has been much more limited, when present, than in the developed world.[48–51] We do not know if, when noted, this increase correlates with the degree of immunosuppression or some important covariates of HIV infection.[51] The issue remains to be clarified, but this does not change the need for attentive screening for HPV-related anogenital cancers in the HIV population.

▲ DIAGNOSIS

All available treatment modalities are directed at eradicating HPV disease rather than HPV infection. Therefore, disease diagnosis is more relevant than proving HPV infection. To detect HPV disease, the clinician depends on clinical methods, cytology, colposcopy, and histology. It is clear that the diagnosis of HPV infection and the typing of its agents are likely to play an important role in the future. Because HPVs cannot yet be grown and propagated in vitro, the diagnosis of HPV infection depends on the detection of HPV DNA. Serology is useful in epidemiology but has no place in clinical practice.

Clinical Diagnosis

Diagnosis of anogenital HPV diseases in HIV-infected patients requires a history and physical examination. The history should focus on symptoms of the anogenital area (itching, discomfort, pain, bleeding, change of appearance) and inquiries about changes that affect sexual intercourse, urination, and defecation. Anorectal symptoms are particularly common in patients with AIN grade 3 and minimally invasive anal cancer and should not be ignored.[52] If a diagnosis has already been established, one should assess its psychological impact and note the treatment received for the present condition and possible previous occurrences. To ensure future treatment compliance, it is wise to inquire about the patient's experience with prior treatment. It is also important to document how the diagnosis was made (e.g., clinically, cytologically, biopsy), because it may be open to revision. A sexual history should identify age at first intercourse, number of past and present sexual partners, sexual practices, and use of barrier methods of contraception and sexually transmitted disease (STD) prevention. The history and treatment of other STDs should be also recorded as well as the histories of warts, intraepithelial neoplasias, or cancers in the sexual partners.

The physical examination of the male patient is typically carried out with the subject leaning back against the end of the examining table and standing in front of the seated clinician. For the anal examination the patient turns back, legs apart, the torso bent and applied against the table. A tilting, proctologic examination table is helpful, if available. Alternatively, the patient can be examined in lateral decubitus and genuflected. For the female, the entire examination is conducted with the patient in the lithotomy position, legs placed in stirrups. Good lighting is essential. The examiner should wear gloves; the use of aprons, gown, mask, and eye-protective equipment should be tailored to the circumstances of the examination and to the additional procedures performed. Physical examination of the external genitalia can be augmented by the application for 1 to 5 minutes of gauzes soaked in 3% to 5% acetic acid (white vinegar). This is most helpful for detecting small or maculopapular HPV lesions because they tend to be acetowhite, particularly on the nonkeratinized ("mucosal") epithelia. However, acetowhitening is not a specific test when used alone and treatment should only be directed at papular lesions consistent with warts. The use of a magnifying glass or, better, a colposcope assists the diagnosis further. An anoscopic examination should be done if there are anal symptoms, a history of anal-receptive intercourse, or perianal warts (see Therapy).[53] Anoscopic diagnosis requires some familiarity, and proper evaluation should be left to experts. The diagnosis can be aided with a colposcope and prior application of 1% acetic acid. Because lesions rarely extend beyond the pectinate line, a sigmoid examination is not routinely indicated.[54,55] In women, a speculum examination of the vagina and cervix should be done to at least rule out gross abnormalities and obtain a Papanicolaou (Pap) smear, if indicated (see Prevention). Application of acetic acid and use of a colposcope aid the diagnosis considerably, but such skills are usually beyond those of the primary care practitioner. An examination of the oral cavity should be considered to exclude associated oral warts. Whenever the proper diagnosis is in doubt, especially if intraepithelial neoplasia or cancer is in the differential diagnosis, a biopsy should be considered. This particularly applies to pigmented lesions and anal, vaginal, or cervical lesions. The use of anatomic diagrams to document the lesions is strongly recommended because they facilitate subsequent evaluations.

Cytology and Colposcopy

Cervical cytology in the form of the Pap smear is an important tool for detecting and managing HPV diseases of the cervix. Several methods and instruments have been designed to collect the cervical cells.[56] Ideally, one uses a wooden Ayre spatula. The longer lip is placed in the cervical os, and the spatula is rotated 360 degrees. A Dacron swab or, better, an endocervical brush is then introduced in the os and rotated 180 degrees. The material collected on the spatula and on the brush are then respectively smeared and rolled on the same side of a glass slide bearing the patient's identification. The slide is immediately exposed to a fixative, either with a spray or by immersion in a transport jar filled with alcohol. A Cervex brush ("broom") substitutes advantageously for the Ayre spatula and brush when the cells are collected for liquid-based cytology (ThinPrep; AutoCyte). This newer technology allows better preparation of the sample, increases the sensitivity for the detection of SIL, but is more costly and time-consuming than traditional cytology.[57,58] Figure 47–1 illustrates the correspondence between the various histologic and cytologic classification schemes for HPV cervical lesions. The Bethesda classification, established in 1988, and revised in 1992, and 2001, calls for establishing the adequacy of the sample, categorizing the cytology, and recommending management and follow-up (www.bethesda2001.cancer.gov).[59,60] Squamous cell abnormalities fall into four categories: (1) atypical squamous cells (a) of undetermined significance (ASC-US), or (b) but HSIL cannot be excluded (ASC-H) (both subcategories used to be grouped as ASCUS); (2) low-grade squamous intraepithelial lesion; (3) high-grade intraepithelial lesion; (4) squamous cell carcinoma. The sensitivity and specificity of the Pap smear for detecting CIN in HIV-seropositive women were found in one study to be 81% and 87%, respectively.[61] For detecting cervical carcinoma in the general population, the same numbers are 80.0% and 99.4%.[62] These are optimal figures.[58] The Pap smear is not a diagnostic test, but because it is inexpensive and can be repeated frequently it remains an excellent, so far essential screening tool.

Colposcopy plays a role in the evaluation of an abnormal Pap smear. In that context, it has two connected purposes: the visual identification of lesions and the selection of biopsy sites for histologic confirmation. The colposcope is simply a binocular microscope with a long focal length (300 to 350 mm) and its own light source that permits detailed inspection of the cervix exposed with a vaginal speculum. With its complete implementation, the colposcopic examination includes application of 5% acetic acid and possibly an iodine (Lugol) solution (Schiller test). Lesion identification is based on one of several scoring systems that rely on elements such as color, shape of the margins, and vessel appearance. If abnormalities are present, colposcopy should be supplemented by biopsies for a more reliable histologic diagnosis.

Cytologic screening has been extended to the anal canal. The technique requires introduction of a Dacron swab moistened with saline or water, or a cervical cytobrush, into the anal canal more than 2 cm from the anal margin.[63] The swab is rotated as it is withdrawn and then rolled over a glass slide bearing the patient's identification. The slide is promptly fixed and processed as for a Pap smear. The sensitivity and specificity of anal cytology for the diagnosis of AIN (excluding ASCUS) in HIV-seropositive homosexual men are 46% and 81%, respectively.[64] Therefore, as for the cervix, anal cytology should be viewed more as a screening tool than a diagnostic tool. Anal cytology screening for SIL in HIV-positive and HIV-negative homosexual and bisexual men appears to be cost-effective when theoretical models are analyzed.[65,66] Nevertheless, it cannot be widely recommended at this time for several reasons.[67] There is a lack of clinically validated screening strategies adapted to the various populations at risk. We also do not know the natural evolution of high-grade anal SIL. In addition, the medical and surgical treatment options are limited, and their impact on the prevention of anal cancer is unknown. Another difficulty is the need to train physicians in the proper collection of anal cytology samples and how to evaluate, biopsy, and treat a cytology-positive patient with anoscopy under magnified optics ("high resolution anoscopy").

Histology

Histologic diagnosis is used to confirm the diagnosis of HPV disease. The histologic material may be an operative sample or a biopsy specimen obtained by scalpel, scissors, punch, forceps, or electrosurgical or laser excision. Buffered formalin is the fixative of choice if subsequent in situ hybridization techniques are contemplated. Although diagnostic criteria are well recognized, particularly for the cervix, sampling variations, the size and condition of the sample, and intra- and interobserver variabilities can still affect the accuracy of the diagnosis. One study has shown that the interobserver reproducibility of cervical histology is no better than that of cervical cytology and is only moderate with both techniques.[68]

Nucleic Acid Detection Assays

Nucleic acid detection assays permit the diagnosis of HPV infection and typing of the virus. The material submitted for analysis can be cells collected from scraping, cervical lavage, or tissue. The Hybrid Capture II assay (Digene Diagnostics) is the only test approved by the U.S. Food and Drug Administration (FDA) that is available to the practitioner. This proprietary assay is based on liquid phase hybridization. Cells or DNA extracted from the tissue sample are denatured in an alkaline solution. Two pools of RNA probes are added in parallel. Probes in pool A hybridize low risk HPV types (6, 11, 42, 43, 44), whereas in pool B they hybridize high risk HPV types (16, 18, 31, 33, 35, 39, 45, 51, 52, 56, 58, 59, 68). The hybrid DNA-RNA is immobilized by an antibody coating the wells of a microtiter plate and is recognized by an antibody conjugated to alkaline phosphatase that generates a chemoluminescent signal. The assay is rapid, resilient to cross-contamination, and quantitative. Investigators have also developed various assays based on the PCR for HPV DNA detection and typing. The Hybrid Capture II assay and PCR have comparable sensitivities, but PCR is more type-specific.[69,70]

Although the relation between HPV type and the risk of progression of CIN is well established in the HIV-negative and HIV-positive populations,[16,71–73] there are still several obstacles to the use of typing information when making management decisions. For example, one lacks information on the reliability of these assays in standard clinical practice. Another concern is that HPV infections of the cervix are about 10 times more common than CIN or cervical carcinoma. Furthermore, the presence of high risk HPV does not lead to cancer in many patients. Consequently, at present, HPV DNA typing is not recommended in routine practice. However, the results of several large studies have helped define its place in cervical cancer screening.[70,74,75] Guidelines on the place of HPV testing in the management of cervical squamous lesions are expected to be released in March of 2002. Specific recommendations do not exist for the HIV population. The place, if any, of HPV typing for the anus is unknown.

▲ THERAPY

This section focuses on condyloma acuminatum, a condition whose treatment and management are amenable to direct intervention by the primary care practitioner. Intraepithelial neoplasias and cancer, which mostly concern the cervix and anus, typically necessitate specialized care; only those aspects that are relevant for the primary care practitioner are discussed here.

Approach to Therapy

Condyloma Acuminatum

A wide variety of options are available for the treatment of condyloma acuminatum; unfortunately, none is satisfactory. Treatments are often ineffective, painful, and costly. Therefore it is important to discuss with the patient the goals and limitations of treatment.

Goals of Therapy

The psychological effect of condyloma acuminatum in the general population tends to be overlooked, yet it is an important reason for seeking treatment.[76] In fact, about half of the patients report a significant psychosexual impact either before or after treatment.[77–80] It is not known if the HIV-seropositive population is similarly affected, or if the social stigma of an additional STD is a reason for seeking treatment.

In the general population three-fourths of patients are asymptomatic, and treatment is initiated for cosmetic reasons.[81] There are no data on the frequency and nature of symptoms in HIV-seropositive patients, but symptoms such as itching and less frequently burning, pain, discomfort, discharge, bleeding, and dyspareunia may be indications for treatment. In pregnant women, warts may partially obstruct the birth canal or compromise hemostasis and repair of lacerations and incisions after delivery.

Treatment should be directed at the disease, not the infection, although the latter may be more extensive than the former.[82,83] Current treatments are considered ineffective for eliminating HPV infection. For example, laser vaporization of the entire mucosal surface of the lower genital tract of women with histologic evidence of HPV infection failed to eradicate the infection in most patients, and it was associated with severe morbidity.[84] Similar disappointing results have been obtained in men.[85]

No information is available on the prevalence of condyloma acuminatum and other anogenital HPV diseases in the sexual partners of HIV-seropositive patients with condyloma acuminatum. However, several studies in the general population have indicated that 40% to 70% of sexual partners of patients with anogenital HPV disease have lesions, which are macroscopic in half the cases.[86,87] Treating the male partner of women with CIN or subclinical genital

HPV infection has failed to have an impact on the patient's condition.[84,88] Whether the reverse situation—treating the female partner—helps the male patient is unknown. At present, the CDC does not advocate tracing and treating sexual partners for HPV disease.[89] The sexual partners of HIV-seropositive patients are more likely to be evaluated for HPV disease when traced for HIV infection or other STDs.

There is an association between condyloma acuminatum and the presence of cervical or anal intraepithelial neoplasias and cancer in HIV patients.[90] As yet there is no other evidence to indicate that treatment of condyloma acuminatum, even intra-anal, has an effect on these conditions. Vulvar and penile cancers are too rare for studies to be able to gauge an effect from treating condyloma acuminatum. Thus so long as one can be reassured that it is condyloma acuminatum, not intraepithelial neoplasia or cancer, cancer prevention should not be a reason for treating condyloma acuminatum.

Risks of Therapy

Frequent but usually transient adverse effects can be expected for the various treatment modalities of condyloma acuminatum. Permanent complications are rarer and include scarring and loss of tissue. Little is known of the psychosexual impact of the various therapies. Because recurrences or incomplete responses to treatment are common, some patients are exposed to several therapeutic attempts that increase the cumulative risk of durable side effects. Costs, which can be particularly high with certain forms of treatment, are another concern.

Therapeutic abstention is definitely an option to consider, provided one is confident that the patient has only condylomata acuminata, not intraepithelial neoplasia or cancer, and that regular follow-up is possible. Although HIV-seropositive patients may have more recalcitrant and longer-standing disease than their HIV-seronegative counterparts, this is not uniformly the case.[38,43] The natural history of condyloma acuminatum is poorly known, especially among those who are HIV-seropositive. In the nonimmunocompromised host, the experience with the placebo recipients in controlled clinical trials suggests that one can expect a 5% to 20% rate of spontaneous resolution of condyloma acuminatum within 3 to 4 months.[91–96]

Other Anogenital HPV Diseases

The three general principles that apply to the management of intra-anal warts and anogenital intraepithelial neoplasias are simple. First is the need to make a tissue diagnosis. Biopsies are essential, but sampling errors are a problem. For example, cervical punch biopsies of the cervix may underdiagnose HPV disease in HIV-seropositive women.[97]

The second principle is to apply the proper treatment, which should be left to experts. The third, extremely important principle is to follow the patient on a regular basis. In at least half of the HIV-seropositive patients treated for CIN, disease recurs, with a risk that increases with the falling CD4 cell count.[39,44,98] Screening is part of the management for cervical HPV diseases.

Effect of HIV Antiviral Treatment on HPV Disease

The effect of antiretroviral treatment [highly active antiretroviral treatment (HAART) in particular] on the natural history of anogenital, HPV diseases cannot be firmly ascertained at present because the data are conflicting and suffer from methodologic limitations. In a cohort of 107 HIV-positive women who had had at least two study visits, Luque et al. noted that the prevalence of abnormal Pap smears was higher (relative risk 2.1), in women who were not on antiretroviral therapy than in those who were, and that these Pap smears were more likely to remain abnormal (relative risk 2.2).[99] In a study of 49 women with cervical cytologic abnormalities, Heard et al. observed that the initiation of HAART was associated with regression of the abnormalities in 3 of 13 (23%) women with HSIL and in 9 of 21 (43%) with LSIL,[100] but the prevalence of HPV infection did not change. In a retrospective study of 56 women with CIN, Robinson et al. noted that HAART was associated with lower rates of recurrence, persistence, and progression.[101] Luque et al. also found that HAART was associated with a lower incidence of Pap smear abnormalities in a prospective survey of 178 women.[102] In a multicenter study, Minkoff et al. reported that after initiation of HAART women were 1.4 times more likely to have cervical lesion regression, and 1.5 less likely to have progression.[102a] In contrast, Del Mistro et al. did not see an impact of HAART on the evolution of cervical SIL or CIN in a cohort of 229 patients.[103] HAART did not change the risk of developing cervical SIL over a median duration of 15 months in a cohort study of 168 women, 74 of whom received HAART.[103a] Using anal cytology, anal biopsies, and CD4 cell count, Palefsky et al. followed 98 HIV-positive men over two 6-month periods, before and after the initiation of HAART.[104] They did not see an effect of HAART on the evolution of anal lesions. Jones et al. also failed to detect changes that might be associated with HAART in the incidence trends of invasive cervical cancer in nine U.S. cities from January 1994 through June 1997.[105] Dorrucci et al. made similar observations in Italy.[47a] No data are available about the effect of antiretroviral treatment about anogenital warts. However, HAART has been associated with a three fold increase in the incidence of oral warts.[105a]

Available Treatment Modalities

Treatment modalities for condyloma acuminatum are many, a reflection of the limitations of them all. To choose among them is complicated by the relative paucity of well conducted comparative trials. Even some commonly used treatments have never been submitted to a double-blind, placebo-controlled, randomized trial. The most commonly used or best studied treatment modalities are emphasized in this section. The available information presented has been derived from studies done largely, if not exclusively, in immunocompetent patients. For the most part, one can only extrapolate this knowledge to the HIV-positive population, remembering that a successful treatment response may be less frequent, recurrences more common, disease more extensive, and side effects different. Table 47–3 sum-

Table 47–3. DRUGS COMMONLY USED TO TREAT CONDYLOMA ACUMINATUM

Drug	Formulations	Presentation	Typical Dosing Regimen	Common Potential Toxicities	Comments
Podophyllin	Podophyllum (USP)[a] Podocon-25 Podofin	— Bottle 15 ml Bottle 15 ml	q wk, ≤6 applications with a cotton-tipped applicator	Itching, pain, inflammation, chemical burns, ulcerations, scarring, contact dermatitis; systemic penetration and toxicities are possible if large doses are delivered	Applied by the practitioner Application on healthy skin is to be avoided; may use protective ointment (e.g., zinc oxide-based paste) Do not treat more than 10 cm^2 of skin area or overapply the drug Do not leave medication on for more than 24 hours. Best to wash off by the end of the day Not to be used in pregnant women; discouraged for nursing women
Podofilox (podophyllotoxin)	Condylox 0.5% solution[a] or gel[a]	Bottle 3.5 ml with cotton-tipped applicators or 3.5 g gel tube	Therapeutic: bid applications, ×3 consecutive days/wk, ≤4 cycles Suppressive: qd applications, ×3 consecutive days/wk, ≤8 cycles	Same as with podophyllin No contact dermatitis	Self-applied, after demonstration of technique and lesions to be treated Application on healthy skin is to be avoided; may use protective ointment when using the solution (e.g., zinc oxide-based paste) Do not treat more than 10 cm^2 of skin area or apply more than 0.5 ml of the drug Effectiveness and safety beyond 8 weeks has not been determined for suppressive use Not to be used in pregnant women; discouraged for nursing women
Bi- and trichloracetic acids	Bichloracetic Acid 80% Tri-Chlor 80%	Bottle 10 ml Bottle 15 ml	q wk, ≤6 applications with a cotton-tipped applicator or wooden stick	Itching pain, inflammation, chemical burns, ulcerations, scarring	Applied by the practitioner Application on healthy skin is to be avoided; may use protective ointment (e.g., zinc oxide-based paste) or buffer the excess acid with talcum powder or bicarbonate soda Can be used in pregnant and nursing women
5-Fluorouracil	Efudex 5% cream Fluroplex 1% cream and solution	Tube 25 g Tube 30 g or Bottle 30 ml	Many regimens have been recommended from bid to qowk (see the literature[106–117] Applied externally with the fingers (finger cots may be used) or internally with a vaginal applicator	Itching, pain, inflammation, chemical burns, ulcerations, mucosal denudation, scarring, contact dermatitis	Self-applied; fingers should be washed afterward Use is discouraged in pregnant women

Table continued on following page

Table 47–3. DRUGS COMMONLY USED TO TREAT CONDYLOMA ACUMINATUM *Continued*

Drug	Formulations	Presentation	Typical Dosing Regimen	Common Potential Toxicities	Comments
Interferon (IFN) injection				Fever, chills, malaise, headache, myalgia, fatigue	Intralesional injection is the most effective. IFN is injected at the base of the lesion Systemic injection SC or IM Systemic reactions are usually mild with the intralesional injections. They may be blunted by taking acetaminophen or an nonsteroidal antiinflammatory agent prior to the injection Monitoring the complete blood count and liver enzymes is recommended when systemic reactions are anticipated
IFNα_{n3}	Alferon N[a]	5 MIU/vial	250,000 IU/wart (total ≤2.5 MIU) biw, ≤8wk[118]		
IFNα2b	Intron A[a]	10 MIU/vial	1 MIU/wart (≤5 warts), tiw, ×3wk[119–125]		
IFNα2a	Roferon-A	Various formulations	See the literature[b126–128]		
IFNβ1a	Avonex	6.6 MIU/vial	See the literature[129,130]		
IFNγ1b	Actimmune	3.0 MIU/vial	See the literature[131,132]		
IFNβ1b	Betaseron	9.6 MIU/vial	See the literature[122]		
Imiquimod	Aldara 5% cream[a]	Box of 12 single-use 250 mg packets	qod applications, ×3/week, ≤16 wk	Itching, burning, erythema, erosion, excoriation, edema	Self-applied; fingers should be washed afterward Anogenital area should be washed 6–10 hours after cream application No data available about use in nursing or pregnant women Cream weakens condoms and diaphragms; sex should be avoided the day the cream is applied

bid, twice daily; biw, twice weekly; MIU, million international units; qd, once daily; qod, every other day; qwk, once weekly; qowk, every other week; tiw, thrice weekly.

[a]These products have been approved by the FDA for the treatment of condyloma acuminatum.

[b]References are given only for studies using intralesional injections. Studies of other routes of administration are reported elsewhere.[133,134]

marizes practical information on the drugs commonly used to treat condyloma acuminatum.

Laser therapy, electrosurgery, and cryotherapy are the three most common approaches offered for the treatment of CIN or AIN. Cold-blade surgery is sometimes required. Choosing among these therapies is guided by personal experience, reported case series, availability of equipment, and some technical considerations. A limited but growing experience with some of these approaches in the HIV-seropositive population has been reported.

Podophyllin/Podofilox

Podophyllin is a natural product extracted from the rhizome of the American mandrake (May apple, *Podophyllum peltatum*), a plant indigenous to eastern North America. In the rest of the world, podophyllin is also prepared from the more potent Indian species, *P. emodi. Juniperus* species can also be used. The two major groups of compounds found in podophyllin resin are flavonols and lignans. The antiwart activity is limited to the lignans and principally to podophyllotoxin, which represents about 10% of the preparation.[135] Podofilox is now the generic name of podophyllotoxin. Like colchicine, it binds tubulin and inhibits microtubule polymerization.[136] This causes disruption of the mitotic spindle and mitosis, and there is disruption of the other cellular functions dependent on the integrity of microtubules. In addition, podofilox may directly damage HPV DNA.[137]

Table 47–3 describes how podophyllin and podofilox are used and prescribed for treatment of condyloma acuminatum. Being a purified, standardized product, podofilox has a more predictable effect than podophyllin. It is also more active and less toxic on a weight basis, permitting the drug to be applied by the patient.[138,139] The toxicity of podophyllin is well documented. In addition to the local side effects listed in Table 47–3,[140,141] the medication can be readily absorbed through the skin and cause systemic side effects including death.[142] Gastrointestinal manifestations (nausea and vomiting) usually precede neurologic signs, which include motor and sensory neuropathy that can be irreversible, seizure, and coma. Leukopenia, leukocytosis, and pancytopenia have been reported. Other affected organs include the lungs (tachypnea, respiratory failure) and the kidneys (hematuria, renal failure). The mutagenic[143] and abortifacient[144] properties of podophyllin are contraindications for its use during pregnancy. Skin biopsies obtained after application of podophyllin should be interpreted with great caution. The drug causes skin necrosis in the lower third of the epidermis, and the presence of large keratinocytes with disrupted chromatin (podophyllin cells) or mitoses can be misinterpreted for intraepithelial neoplasia.[145,146] Podophyllin has been associated with contact dermatitis caused by the benzoin vehicle or guaiacum wood contaminants. Toxicity due to podofilox is less well known than that of podophyllin but appears to be similar.[142]

Since the 1940s there have been many reports on the use and efficacy of podophyllin and, later, podofilox for the treatment of anogenital warts. The efficacy can be best ascertained from the many randomized comparative trials.[147–166] Reported rates of a complete response to podophyllin vary widely, from 22% to 100%, but mostly range from 35% to 50%. They are inferior to those of the other standard forms of treatment (excisional surgery, electrodesiccation, cryotherapy, podofilox). Recurrences are common (typically 40% to 70%), so the net complete response rates are even lower, ranging from 25% to 45% (the longer the follow-up, the higher the recurrences rate). Overall, podofilox is more effective than podophyllin, but the complete response rates associated with its use range from 20% to 100%, typically 60% to 70%; and recurrences are common (30% to 50%), bringing the net complete response rate to a common range of 30% to 50%.

Prophylactic application of podofilox after the lesions disappear does prevent recurrences.[167] Podofilox 0.5% self-applied once a day for 3 consecutive days a week for 8 weeks after condylomata acuminata had been eradicated with either podofilox or cryotherapy resulted in only 2 of 21 patients (19%) having recurrences. In contrast, 12 of 24 patients (50%) treated with only the vehicle recurred. The durability of this effect is unknown. Information on the use of podophyllin or podofilox in HIV-seropositive patients is limited. Beck et al. treated 31 patients with anal condylomas using 5% podophyllin and found a 26% recurrence rate at a mean 12 months later.[168] Orkin and Smith observed worse results in their study: 17 of their 21 patients (81%) treated with podophyllin failed.[169] Podofilox has also been associated with a poor outcome. After a single cycle of podofilox 0.5% solution applied twice a day for 3 consecutive days, 8 of 18 HIV-seronegative patients (45.5%) were free of condylomata acuminata after 6 months of follow-up compared to only 1 of 15 HIV-seropositive patients ($P = 0.02$).[42]

Bichloracetic Acid and Trichloroacetic Acid

Bichloracetic and trichloroacetic (TCA) acids have long been used, predominantly by gynecologists, but also by proctologists. They induce acid hydrolysis, which is responsible for their keratolytic action. They may bind to the cellular proteins, acting as a cauterizing, fixative agent.[170] They also readily destroy HPV DNA. Only 1 of 14 condyloma acuminata patients (7%) treated in vitro by TCA yielded HPV DNA by PCR.[134] Table 47–3 lists dosages and administration of bichloracetic and trichloroacetic acids and their side effects. Discomfort, ulcerations, and scabbing are some of the adverse reactions that occur in about two-thirds of the patients. They are more common than with cryotherapy.[171,172] Widely used, these agents have been submitted to limited evaluation, and only TCA has been compared to other standard therapies.[171–173] TCA appears to be equivalent to cryotherapy in terms of the complete response rate (about 65% to 80%) and recurrence rate, with about half of the patients remaining free of disease.[171] Acids are safe for the treatment of pregnant women.

5-Fluorouracil and Nucleoside Derivatives

5-Fluorouracil (5-FU) is a pyrimidine antagonist. A structural analogue of thymidine, it interferes with the synthesis of DNA and to a lesser extent of RNA by blocking the methylation of deoxyuridylic acid into thymidylic acid.

Dividing cells are particularly sensitive to its action, and the compound has been widely used topically by dermatologists to treat diverse conditions.

Various topical regimens with 5-FU have been applied for the treatment and prophylaxis of condyloma acuminatum, vaginal warts, and intraepithelial neoplasias of the vagina and cervix.[106–117] 5-FU has been applied twice daily to weekly for durations ranging from a few days to 10 weeks. The frequency and nature of the side effects depend on the regimens used and the sites treated. Pain, itching, burning, and hyperpigmentation are the most common local adverse reactions, affecting approximately half of the patients. More serious reactions have also been noted, such as contact and allergic dermatitis and chronic vaginal ulcerations,[174–177] which has discouraged many practitioners from using this drug. Twice-weekly applications are much better tolerated than daily applications, without an apparent difference in efficacy.[115] Reportedly, fair-skinned individuals are particularly prone to local side effects.[178] Rarer but significant complications should be mentioned: leukopenia, thrombocytopenia, toxic granulations, and eosinophilia as well as the development of vaginal adenosis and vaginal clear cell carcinoma.[179] Administration of 5-FU has not been associated with congenital malformations, but the safety of this drug during pregnancy is not established.[180]

Intrameatal warts seem to be particularly responsive to 5-FU treatment, usually administered daily for 3 to 14 days.[108,109,181] Krebs observed that 16 of 20 patients (80%) with vaginal warts had a long-term (median 16 months) complete response after treatment with bedtime application of 1.5 g of 5% 5-FU cream once a week for 10 weeks.[114] Similarly, intravaginal or vulvar 5-FU prophylaxis against recurrences after treatment of vaginal and vulvar warts, respectively, appeared to be effective in non-HIV patients.[113,182] In the HIV population, a placebo-controlled trial evaluated the efficacy of 1% 5-FU gel in 60 women with intravaginal warts, all of whom were receiving zidovudine 250 mg three times a day.[183] The 5-FU preparation was self-administered for 4 weeks: every other day 3 times a week at bedtime by deep intravaginal application of 4 ml. Sixteen weeks after treatment initiation the complete response rates were 83.4% in the 5-FU group and 13.3% in the placebo group. Side effects included mild erythema, vaginal erosion, and edema. No patients dropped out of the study.

Anecdotal case series suggest that 5-FU might be useful for treatment of anogenital intraepithelial neoplasias in the general population, a claim that remains to be evaluated properly.[184] In addition, 5% 5-FU cream, applied daily, has been used successfully in combination with 5% imiquimod cream three times a week for treatment of AIN grade 3 lesions in an HIV-positive man.[185] Better evidence supports the use of 5-FU as secondary prophylaxis of CIN in HIV patients.[186] In a recent trial (ACTG 200), 101 HIV-positive women who had undergone ablative or excisional treatment for CIN were randomized to receive either topical vaginal 5% 5-FU cream (2 g) self-administered twice a week or nothing. Of the 50 (28%) women in the 5-FU group, 14 developed CIN recurrences compared to 24 of 51 (47%) in the observation group ($P < 0.05$). Moreover, in the 5-FU group recurrences tended to appear later and were more likely to be CIN grade 1 than CIN grade 2 or 3.

Cidofovir (Vistide), or (*S*)-1-(3-hydroxy-2-phosphonylmethoxypropyl)cytosine, is an acyclic nucleotide analogue that is available for treating of cytomegalovirus (CMV) retinitis. Intralesional injection of the compound has been found effective in a small number of patients, HIV infected or not, with condyloma acuminatum, recurrent respiratory papillomatosis, VIN, and upper digestive HPV tumors.[187–191] A topical gel formulation of 1% cidofovir gel (Forvade) has been evaluated in a Phase II trial for treating condyloma acuminatum in immunocompetent patients.[192] It was administered daily for 5 days every other week for up to six cycles. One-third of the patients were randomized to receive placebo. At the end of the treatment period (12 weeks), 9 of 19 (47%) patients treated with cidofovir had a complete response compared to none of 11 patients in the placebo group ($P = 0.01$). Various strengths (0.3%, 1%, 3%) of cidofovir gel applied daily for 5 or 10 days every other week for up to three cycles were evaluated in an open Phase I/II study conducted in HIV-positive patients with anogenital warts.[190] Overall, 7 of 46 (15%) patients had a complete response. All treatment regimens appeared equipotent. Cidofovir 1% gel was also administered three times every other day on biopsy-proven CIN grade 3 lesions in 15 immunocompetent women.[193] One month later the cervix was excised, and 7 of 15 (47%) of the specimens showed complete histologic resolution; four of them also demonstrated disappearance of HPV DNA. Topical cidofovir 1% has been associated with complete eradication of recurrent VIN grade 3 lesions in an HIV-negative woman.[191] A 1% cream preparation was used to obtain the resolution of recalcitrant oral papillomatosis in an AIDS patient.[193a] Cidofovir gel or cream is currently not available commercially but can be made up by a pharmacist upon request. Cidofovir is a potential carcinogen, and caution should be exercised with its use.

Cryotherapy

Cryotherapy is one of the most common forms of treatment for anogenital HPV diseases and other dermatologic conditions. Solid carbon dioxide (carbonic ice; boiling temperature −78.5°C), nitrous oxide (−89.5°C), and especially liquid nitrogen (−196°C) are the principal cryogenic agents. Cold can be applied with cryogenic pencils or cotton swabs, but the most common modes of delivery are sprays for external lesions and cryoprobes of various sizes for internal lesions. Cryoprobes carry the potential risk of virus transmission, which is avoided with sprays.[194] Cryotherapy techniques are varied and empiric.[195–197] A common approach is to spray or cool the wart for 20 to 30 seconds until a 1- to 2-mm ice halo forms around the lesion. Some practitioners allow the lesion to thaw completely and then freeze it again.

Cold injury causes necrosis of the tissue but little HPV DNA destruction.[137,198] The patient experiences a brief stinging sensation followed by numbness. Upon thawing, about half of the patients report discomfort: itching, burning, or pain.[199,200] Uterine cramping follows cervical cryotherapy. Aggressive treatment may cause blisters and pronounced edema and should be avoided. One-fourth of the patients treated for condyloma acuminatum have skin discoloration at the treatment site 6 months later.[199]

The efficacy of cryotherapy for the treatment of condyloma acuminatum has been demonstrated in several open studies.[152,171,172,201–209] Unfortunately, although it is a common approach, there have been few randomized comparative trials. This makes it difficult to define confidently the role of cryotherapy. Typically, 65% to 85% of patients have a complete response with a 20% to 40% recurrence rate. When recurrences are taken into account, the complete response rate with cryotherapy is about 60%, which makes it a better choke than podophyllin and podofilox, equivalent to TCA, but slightly inferior to electrosurgery. Cryotherapy is particularly well suited for the care of meatal warts and the pregnant patient.

Along with electrosurgery and laser surgery, cryotherapy is used to treat internal HPV diseases (condylomas and intraepithelial neoplasias). These three techniques appear to have similar efficacies.[201,210] Compared to laser therapy, cryotherapy of the cervix is more painful and associated with longer symptomatic bleeding and vaginal discharge.[212] The cervix can be treated with cryotherapy during pregnancy.[213]

Cold-Blade Surgery

Surgical excision is one of the simplest radical approaches to the treatment of condyloma acuminatum. Thomson and Grace described the current technique developed for the treatment of anal warts.[214] The skin is disinfected and the base of the lesion is infiltrated with an anesthetic such as lidocaine. The resultant swelling aids in demarcating the margins of the lesion. Epinephrine (1:100,000) may be added to the anesthetic to give better hemostatic control. The lesion is excised with curved (iridectomy) scissors, and bleeding is controlled by pressure with a gauze and application of 30% TCA or another hemostatic agent. The procedure is remarkably well tolerated. After the brief stinging pain of the anesthesia, little is felt by the patient, who later may experience mild local discomfort or itching. Frank pain is rare.[148] Slight bleeding of the wound is often noted but is self-limited. Hypopigmentation, the most common long-term complication, occurs a small number of patients, and hypertrophic scarring is rare.[215] A variation of cold-blade surgery is the use of micro-resectors for internal lesions.[216]

Net complete response rates vary from 46% to 92% with cold-blade surgery.[148,214,221–222] Typically, the procedure is reserved for patients with few lesions, and this potential selection bias may contribute to the excellent efficacy of this technique. Cold-blade surgery is often used in combination with other therapies such as podophyllin, fulguration (electrosurgery), or both, with no evidence that outcomes are improved. In HIV-seropositive patients, cold-blade surgery has been combined with fulguration for the treatment of anal condylomas. Results of these open, retrospective case series have been mixed. Beck et al. found a recurrence rate of only 4% in 27 patients followed for a mean of 1 year.[168] Miles et al. treated 24 patients; of the 15 available for follow-up 1 month later, 7 required additional treatment.[223] The addition of systemic interferon-γ does not lower the recurrences rate.[224] Wound healing after anorectal surgery for condylomata acuminata is usually not a problem in the HIV-seropositive patient, although it may be significantly delayed in the more severely immunocompromised patients (CD4 count < 50 cells/μl) or those with anal cancer.[225,226]

Cold-blade surgery applied to the treatment of cervical HPV diseases is known as conization.[227] It consists of excising a large cone of the cervix that includes the endocervix (the exocervix forms the base of the cone). Conization is now being largely replaced by less aggressive treatment options: electrosurgery, laser surgery, cryotherapy. Even for the rare indications of conization such as endocervical CIN or microinvasion, adapted laser and electrosurgical techniques (laser or loop electrosurgical excision cone biopsy) have replaced the traditional scalpel excision. As with all surgical procedures that generate biologic fluids potentially infected with HIV, the operator should wear gloves, apron or gown, mask, and eye protection.

Electrosurgery

Electrosurgical techniques are diverse and not necessarily interchangeable.[228] Depending on the number of electrodes used contact (or not) with the lesion, and the type, intensity, frequency, and wave shape of the current delivered, one recognizes, in an unfortunately often muddled nomenclature, electrofulguration (electrodesiccation), electrocoagulation, electrosection, and electrocautery. Although electrosurgery is often used by surgeons and dermatologists to treat HPV diseases, it has undergone little rigorous evaluation.

Vuori et al. reported that 58 of 100 patients with condyloma acuminatum treated with electrocoagulation had a complete response.[229] One important randomized study compared cryotherapy, 20% podophyllin, and electrodesiccation.[152] All three treatments were administered weekly until a complete response was evident or for up to 6 weeks. Electrosurgery was the best treatment, with 83 of 88 patients (94%) having a complete response; cryotherapy, was next best, with 68 complete responses in 86 patients (79%), followed by podophyllin, with 26 complete responses in 63 patients (41%) (all differences were statistically significant). A 3- to 5-month follow-up indicated that only about one-fifth of the patients treated with electrosurgery or cryotherapy had a recurrnce, compared to two-fifths of those treated with podophyllin. The intralesional administration of interferon-α as adjuvant to electrosurgery may reduce the rate of recurrence. In one study patients treated with electrocautery were randomized to receive 5 million units of interferon-α-2b (IFNα2b) in each lesion site (up to a total dose of 25 million units) for 2 to 3 days, or nothing.[119] Altogether, 31% of the 22 interferon-treated patients had recurrences compared to 45% of the 11 non-interferon-treated patients ($P = 0.03$). In another study, patients with anal condylomas treated by surgical excision and electrosurgery were randomized to receive the addition of 500,000 units of IFNαn3 or saline in each quadrant of the anal canal.[230] After a mean follow-up of 16 weeks, 3 of 25 interferon recipients (12%) had recurrences compared to 7 of 18 saline recipients (39%) ($P = 0.07$). Interestingly, half of the patients in this study were HIV-seropositive. They exhibited the same favorable response to interferon as the seronegative patients. Thirty-eight HIV-seropositive patients with anogenital warts were treated with electrocautery and IFNβ (3 million units/day IM for 10 days) and then were randomized to receive IFNβ as maintenance three times a week for 1 month or 3 months.[231] No significant differences in the recurrence rates were observed for the two groups.

Electrosurgical procedures on the external genitalia are painful, but effective topical anesthesia could be obtained with EMLA cream (lidocaine and prilocaine) in 90% of men and 40% of women.[232] Another complication is scarring.[152]

Over the past decade electrosurgical techniques have emerged as among the most popular approaches for the management of CIN.[233] These techniques, which come in several varieties, are known as large loop excision of the transitional zone (LLETZ) or the loop electrosurgical excision procedure (LEEP).[234,235] They provide a diagnostic specimen and a therapeutic procedure in one intervention. Under the proper indications, about 95% of treatment-naive patients remain free of disease regardless of CIN grade. Local anesthesia is typically required, but these procedures are well tolerated, with minimal subsequent pain, bleeding, and vaginal discharge. Fertility does not seem to be affected.[236] Electrosurgical procedures should be avoided on a pregnant cervix. Chang et al. have used high resolution anoscopy followed by excisional biopsy and electrosurgery to treat anal HSIL.[236a] All eight HIV seronegative men had a complete resolution sustained for a mean 2.5 years. In contrast, only 6 of 29 HIV seropositive men had a persistent complete response for a mean of 2 years.

Electrosurgery, like laser surgery, emits a plume of smoke that must be evacuated because, as discussed in the next section, it poses a potential infectious risk to the operator and assistants.[237,238]

Laser Surgery

Lasers are optical devices that generate a powerful beam of monochromatic and highly collimated light (the electromagnetic waves have the same wavelength, travel in parallel planes, and are in phase). Various types of medical lasers are available. The pulse dye, argon, and KTP lasers have been used for the treatment of HPV disease, but the one that is best adapted to anogenital surgery is the CO_2 laser.[239-245] Its infrared wavelength (10,600 nm) is well absorbed by water, which converts the energy to heat. That heat is responsible for vaporizing the lesion. A focused, narrow, high-energy beam is used for cutting and excision. A defocusing device allows a broader spot, convenient for tissue destruction and ablation. The lower energy density of the beam causes less tissue vaporization but more thermal conductive damage ("brushing" technique), resulting in coagulation of the cellular proteins; it can also be used for hemostasis. A pulsed output provides greater control for the operator. The laser light can be delivered through a handheld device, which is convenient for external lesions, or more commonly through the colposcope by a set of mirrors and lenses.

Laser surgery is applicable to the full range of anogenital HPV diseases.[178,240-245] Typically, laser procedures are conducted under topical anesthesia (EMLA cream or injectable anesthetics), but general anesthesia is required in some patients because of pain or the extent of the lesions. In addition to pain in the external genitalia, bleeding, discharge, tissue swelling, dysuria, meatal stenosis, and scarring occur in up to one-fourth of patients.[178,215,246-249] For vaginal and cervical procedures, symptomatic bleeding and vaginal discharge are minimal, usually lasting less than a week.[212] Pregnancy is not a contraindication to laser surgery.

Laser surgery and electrocoagulation generate smoke that contains HPV DNA; it can be found in the surgeon's upper respiratory tract and on the walls of the surgical suite.[237,238,250,251] It represents a true infectious risk because laser surgeons appear to be at increased risk of developing hand and nasopharyngeal warts.[252] In addition to the protections already customary for surgeons working with HIV-infected individuals (gloves, gown, mask, and goggles), a smoke evacuation system should be used.

Although the general principles of laser surgery are well defined, the technique is difficult to evaluate from the literature because individual techniques and skills vary appreciably. A review of laser surgery for the treatment of condyloma acuminatum in retrospective case series and randomized comparative trials in the general population indicates that the more rigorous the evaluation the poorer is the efficacy.[82,127,128,215,224,246-249,252-266] Although laser surgery provides an immediate complete response in 90% to 100% of patients, in the better designed studies 50% to 65% of the patients experience a relapse. Systemic interferon therapy has been given as an adjuvant to laser surgery to prevent wart recurrence. The results have been inconsistent, with either doubling of the net complete response rate[127,263] or no effect.[128,224,265]

There are few strict comparative studies of laser surgery versus electrosurgery or cryotherapy for treating CIN. The available data suggest that all these techniques yield similar results.[201-212,233,267-269] The main limitations of laser surgery are cost and the availability of a skilled practitioner.

Photodynamic laser therapy relies on the laser light to activate selectively the cytotoxicity of a photosensitizing compound applied topically (5-aminolevulinic acid, 5-ALA) or systemically [e.g., *meso*-tetra(*m*-hydroxyphenyl) porphyrin (*m*-THPP) or 5-ALA]. Photodynamic laser therapy is a technique in development whose application for the treatment of condyloma acuiminatum and CIN has so far been limited.[270,271]

Interferon and Cytokine Inducers

Interferons comprise a group of cytokines recognized for their immunomodulatory, antitumor, and antiviral properties. There are three classes of these proteins: α, β, γ. IFNα and IFNβ share the same cellular receptor and some physicochemical properties.[133] IFNγ is distinct. IFN has been used since 1972 to treat HPV diseases, but the demonstration in 1982 that bovine interferon could eradicate bovine papillomavirus infection in vitro gave a great impetus to further basic and clinical investigations.

Interferons are produced in cell cultures (e.g., IFNβ and IFNαn1) or by recombinant technology (e.g., IFNα2a, IFNα2b, IFNα2c), as full, truncated, consensus, or hybrid gene products. Because they have been used extensively to treat various diseases, their clinical adverse effects are well recognized. These effects are in part dose-related and are typically reversible upon cessation of the drug. The most common symptoms include fever, chills, malaise, headache, myalgia, and fatigue, which occur several hours after administration but rarely persist beyond 24 hours. Acetaminophen or nonsteroidal antiinflammatory agents, if taken at the time of drug administration, can blunt these side effects. Side effects wane with repeated administration of the drug. More serious side effects include lethargy, confusion, anxiety, depression, weight loss, anorexia, nausea, vomiting, alopecia, insomnia, and peripheral neuropathies. Biologic alterations may be noted, particularly neutropenia, thrombocytopenia, a rise in serum transaminases, and occasionally anemia and hypertriglyceridemia. Antibodies may form, possibly compromising efficacy. Interferons are contraindicated during pregnancy.

Interferons are some of the best studied treatments for HPV disease. These investigations have examined various diseases, various interferon classes, different dosages and schedules of administration, and different routes of administration.

For the treatment of condyloma acuminatum, the topical route has been generally disappointing.[272–275] The excellent results of Syed et al. with a natural IFNα cream or gel are unusual in this respect.[161,162,276] The application of an IFNβ gel after excisional or ablative therapy for genital warts might be effective for preventing recurrence.[277] Topical IFN preparations are not available in the United States. The best and more consistent results have been obtained with intralesional interferon.[119–134] The limitations of this approach include fastidiousness, a limit on the number of lesions that can be treated at one session, and the pain associated with the injection. Other side effects are usually minimal. The most important obstacle raised against intralesional interferon in HIV-infected patients is the report by Douglas et al.[278] They administered, in up to three warts per patient, 1 million IU of IFNα2a three times a week for 4 weeks. At 16 weeks' follow-up, none of 8 HIV-seropositive patients had a complete response compared to 11 of 21 HIV-seronegative patients (52%) ($P = 0.01$).

Systemic administration of interferon for the treatment of condyloma acuminatum has been largely ineffective when evaluated in randomized, rigorous studies. There is little reason to believe that it would be more effective in HIV-seropositive patients.[133] As mentioned in previous sections, interferons have been used in combination with other treatment modalities. They also have been extensively evaluated when used with cryotherapy or podophyllin, and their effect has been disappointing.[199,200,279] Interferons have also been used for the treatment of CIN. The experience remains largely unconvincing of their efficacy and role in the management of this condition.[280–283] No data are available at present on the use of the new long-acting, PEGylated IFNα2a and IFNα2b.

Imiquimod [1-(2-methylpropyl)-1*H*-imidazo[4,5-*c*]quinolin-4-amine] is an imidazoquinolineamine derivative with immunomodulating properties. In particular, it is an inducer of IFNα and other cytokines.[284] The drug has demonstrated excellent activity as a topical preparation for the treatment of condyloma acuminatum. It has been approved for that indication by the FDA as a 5% cream (Aldara). In one double-blind, randomized study 108 patients were treated with a 5% cream or vehicle, every other day three times a week for up to 8 weeks.[285] At the end of therapy no patients in the vehicle group had a complete response compared to 37% in the imiquimod group ($P < 0.001$). Only 3 of 16 patients (19%) had recurrences within 10 weeks of follow-up. In another study patients were randomized to self-apply 5% imiquimod, 1% imiquimod, or placebo cream[94] with the same frequency but for up to 16 weeks. The complete response rates were 50% (54/109), 21% (21/102), and 11% (11/100), respectively. The differences between the 5% imiquimod group and either of the two other groups were statistically significant ($P < 0.001$). The response was much better in females than in males irrespective of treatment. The recurrence rates in the three groups were 13%, 0%, and 10%, respectively. A similar randomized, double-blind trial was conducted to evaluate daily rather than thrice-weekly imiquimod self-administration.[286] At the end of the 16-week treatment period the complete response rates were 52% (49/94) in the 5% imiquimod group, 14% (13/90) in the 1% imiquimod group, and 4% (3/95) in the placebo cream group ($P < 0.0001$). As in the previous trial, women responded better than men; for instance, in the 5% imiquimod group there was a complete response rate of 64% (27/42) in women compared to 42% (22/52) in men. A fourth randomized trial was done in men to evaluate self-application of 5% imiquimod cream three times a week, once daily, twice daily, or three times a day.[287] Complete response rates at 16 weeks were similar in all four groups (ranging from 24% to 35%) without evidence of a dose-response effect. As in the previous trials, the magnitude of the side effects was directly related to the dose and were most severe with more frequent application than with daily application. A dose-range study was also done to determine the optimal dosing for the treatment of foreskin-associated warts in uncircumcised men.[288] Imiquimod cream 5%, every other day three times a week was best, yielding a 62% complete response rate. A 2% imiquimod cream, in development for the European market and applied once daily (men) or twice daily (women) for 3 consecutive days per week for up to 4 weeks (men) or 6 weeks (women), has been evaluated for the self-treatment of genital warts.[95,96] Excellent complete response rates were reported at the end of the treatment period: 70% (21/30) for the men in the imiquimod group compared to 10% (3/30) in the placebo group, and 73% (22/30) for the women with imiquimod compared to 3% (1/30) with placebo ($P < 0.0001$ in either comparison).

Imiquimod has been evaluated in HIV-infected patients for the treatment of condyloma acuminatum. A randomized, placebo-controlled study enrolled 97 men and 3 women with CD4 cell counts higher than 99 cells/μl.[289] Patients were self-treated with 5% imiquimod cream every other day, three times a week for up to 16 weeks. Two-thirds ($n = 65$) were randomized to imiquimod and one-third ($n = 35$) to placebo. Tolerance was similar to that in immunocompetent hosts, but the complete response rate was poor: 11% in the imiquimod group and 6% in the placebo group ($P = 0.49$). However, 38% of patients receiving imiquimod had at least 50% or more wart clearance, compared to 14% of the placebo recipients ($P = 0.01$). Although imiquimod has been strongly advocated as an adjunct to other modalities for the treatment of condyloma acuminatum in HIV patients, this regimen has not been rigorously evaluated.[290] There is an anecdotal observation in an HIV-positive man to support the use of topical imiquimod in combination with 5-FU for the treatment of anal squamous cell carcinoma.[185]

Side effects of imiquimod are local and include itching and burning sensations, as well as erythema, erosion, and swelling. All are well tolerated by the patients, especially at the FDA-approved dosing of three times a week.

Other Modalities

Retinoids (e.g., tretinoin, isotretinoin, etretinate) are synthetic derivatives of retinol, a vitamin A analogue.[291] They increase desquamation and inhibit the proliferation of keratinocytes, including cells infected by HPV.[292] This and the observation that vitamin A and other vitamins may play a role in the etiology of CIN led to the evaluation of these compounds for the treatment and prophylaxis of anogenital HPV diseases.[293,294] Isotretinoin given to eight subjects, 1 mg/kg PO for 6 weeks, had no effect on their condylomata acuminata.[295] Similarly, 0.05% tretinoin cream was found ineffective for the topical treatment of anogenital warts.[296] Retinoids were found to be more successful for the treatment of CIN. Meyskens et al. randomized 301 women with CIN grade 2 or 3 to receive cervical caps with sponges containing 1 ml of 0.372% tretinoin cream or vehicle. The treatment was applied daily for 4 days the first month and daily for 2 days at months 3 and 6. Tretinoin was effective at reducing the grade of CIN grade 2 (43% for tretinoin compared to 27% for the vehicle; $P = 0.04$) but not of CIN grade 3.[297] Vaginal discharge was the most severe side effect. Only anecdotal evidence supports the use of retinoids in HIV-seropositive men or women with intraepithelial neoplasia.[298,299] A Phase III study comparing oral isotretinoin with observation only for the treatment of CIN grade 1 in HIV-seropositive women (ACTG 293) has now completed enrollment.

Cimetidine is a histamine receptor antagonist for which several claims of efficacy for the treatment of cutaneous warts have dissipated with the negative results of randomized, double-blind studies.[300] It is thus unlikely that the case report of cimetidine successfully treating condyloma acuminatum in the presence of HIV infection can be confirmed.[301]

▲ **Table 47–4.** SUGGESTED APPROACHES TO THE
▲ TREATMENT OF SEXUALLY TRANSMITTED HPV DISEASES

Type of Wart or Lesion	Treatment Options	
	First line	Second line
Condylomata acuminata	Podofilox[a] Imiquimod[a] Cryotherapy Trichloroacetic acid Scissor excision (if few and small lesions) Podophyllin	Electrosurgery Laser surgery *Third line:* interferon
Oral warts	Cryotherapy Electrosurgery	Cold-blade excision
Urethral meatus warts	Cryotherapy Podofilox[a] 5-Fluorouracil	Podophyllin Electrocautery
Anal warts	Cold-blade surgery Trichloroacetic acid Cryotherapy	Electrosurgery Laser surgery
Vaginal warts	Cryotherapy (liquid nitrogen spray, not a cryoprobe) Trichloroacetic acid 5-Fluorouracil (secondary prophylaxis)	Laser surgery
Cervical warts	Electrosurgery (LEEP) Cryotherapy Laser surgery	
Intraepithelial neoplasia		
External genitalia	Laser surgery Cryotherapy (penis)	Cold-blade surgery
Anal	Cryotherapy Trichloroacetic acid Podophyllin Cold-blade surgery	Electrosurgery
Vaginal	Laser surgery	5-Fluorouracil (secondary prophylaxis)
Cervical	Electrosurgery (LEEP) Cryotherapy Laser surgery	

LEEP, loop electrosurgical excision procedure.
[a]These treatments are applied be the patient for home-based therapy.

Recommendations for Optimal Approach to Therapy

Condyloma Acuminatum

Table 47–4 summarizes the suggested treatment approaches to condyloma acuminatum in the HIV-infected patient. These recommendations are tentative and are largely derived from the experience already reviewed with immunocompetent patients. Various treatment guidelines have been issued[89,134,302,303] that should give the reader a sense of the uncertainties attached to any treatment recommendations.

In addition to efficacy and tolerance, cost is a factor to consider when choosing a treatment. Several cost-effectiveness analyses have been reported, and their assumptions are sufficiently arguable and their conclusions sufficiently conflicting that their general usefulness is limited. However, they may help practitioners determine the most cost-effective options in their own practice. Often convenience and availability are the deciding factors, but the treatment methods are not necessarily interchangeable. If the patient is pregnant, cryotherapy or TCA is the treatment of choice. If few lesions are present, one should consider scissor excision. Large, numerous lesions may be best treated by laser surgery.

In HIV-infected patients with condyloma acuminatum, it is important to ensure proper follow-up, particularly if a patient has failed several treatments, so preinvasive malignancies can be detected. Such monitoring should be integrated into the management of the HIV infection. One must also realize that, at least in immunocompetent patients, refractoriness to previous treatments is not a strong

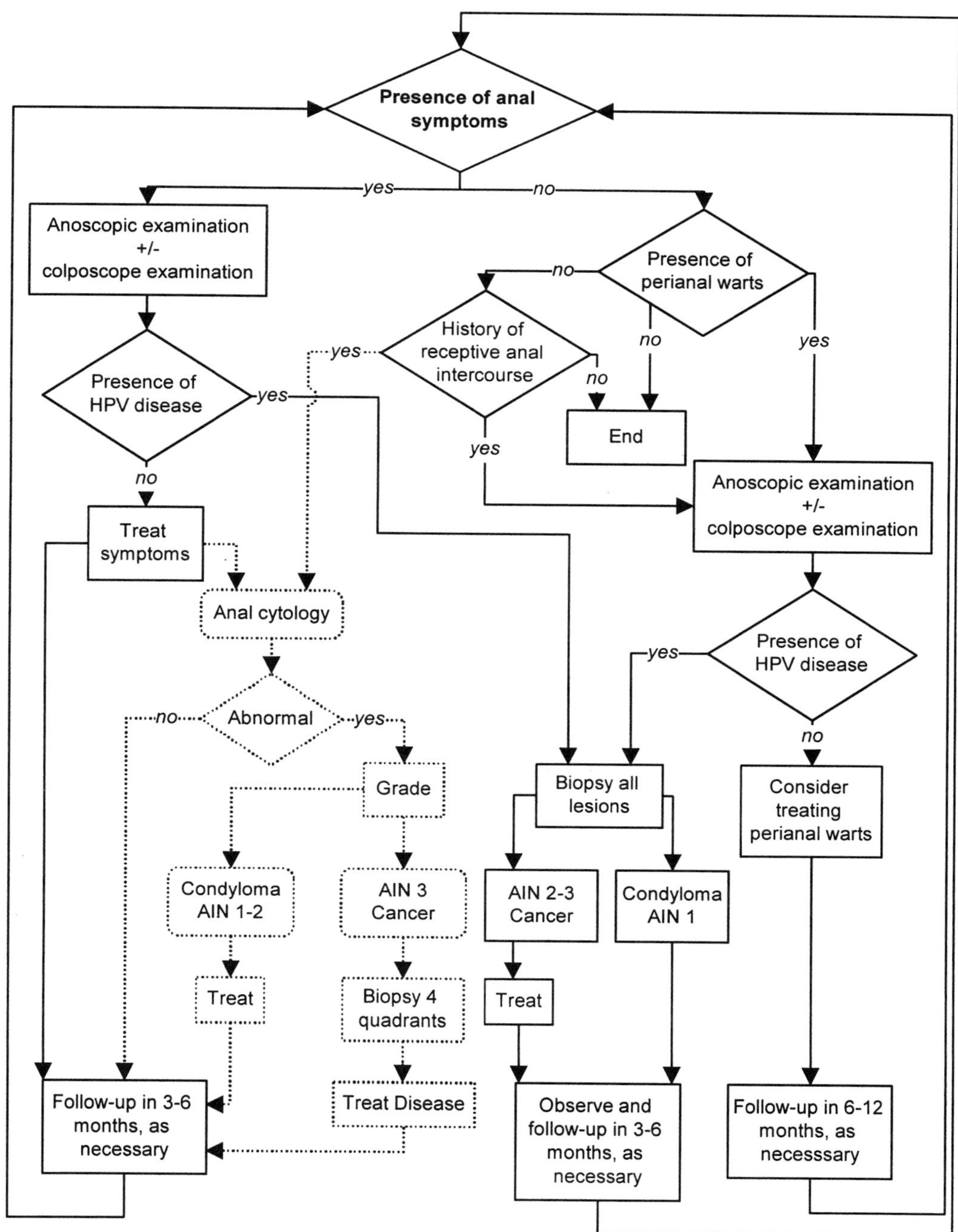

Figure 47–2. Suggested management of anal HPV diseases. The dashed pathways refer to the potential place of anal cytology, a tool that remains to be validated.

predictor of resistance to future, even identical treatments.[199,200]

Other HPV Diseases

As a general principle, the management of intraepithelial neoplasias is best left in the hands of the expert. First, the diagnosis is established, and then the patient is advised, with referral as necessary. Figure 47–2 offers a suggested approach for the management of anal HPV diseases. Note that anal cytology is not yet a validated procedure, and it is incorporated into the algorithm simply to indicate how it might be used.[65,304]

Figures 47–3 and 47–4 provide a suggested general guide for the management of cervical HPV diseases. The largely empirical nature of these schemes leaves room for variations.[305] Cryotherapy and LEEP are less expensive and less technically demanding than laser surgery.[233,306] Other considerations apply as well. Cervical LEEP is contraindicated during pregnancy. Cryotherapy may not be optimal if the lesion extends toward the endocervix, is large, or cannot be covered by the cryoprobe. Laser

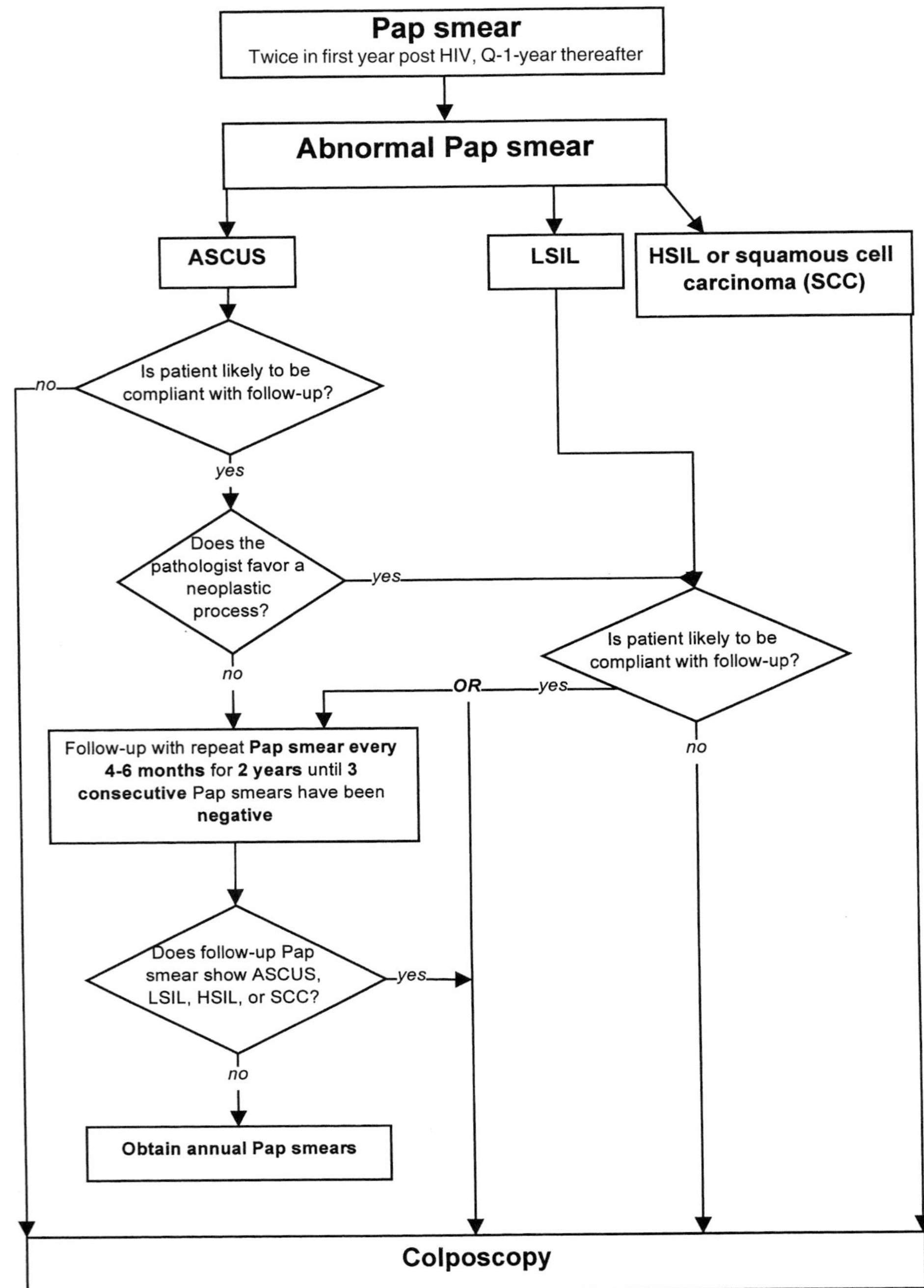

Figure 47–3. Management of the abnormal Papanicolaou smear in the HIV-seropositive woman according to the 2002 U.S. Public Health Service/Infectious Diseases Society of America guidelines. HSIL, high-grade squamous intraepithelial lesion; LSIL, low-grade squamous intraepithelial lesion; SCC, squamous cell carcinoma.

surgery may have an advantage if the lesions are particularly large or extend to the vaginal fornices. LEEP is not only conservative to the cervix but has the unique advantage of providing a tissue sample that allows diagnostic verification. This has been the justification for the concept of "see and treat."[306,307] The idea is to treat the patient at the time of diagnostic colposcopy, dispense with the punch biopsies, reduce costs, and avoid losing the patient to follow-up. In the general population, this approach seems appropriate for the lesions that are unequivocally CINs as seen by cytology and colposcopy.[308] The role of the see-and-treat approach remains to be defined in the HIV-infected population.

Patient Advice and Support

The psychosexual impact of genital warts is well recognized in the general population but not in the HIV-infected subsect.[76] The patient may be referred to resources available to the HIV-infected population for advice and support as well

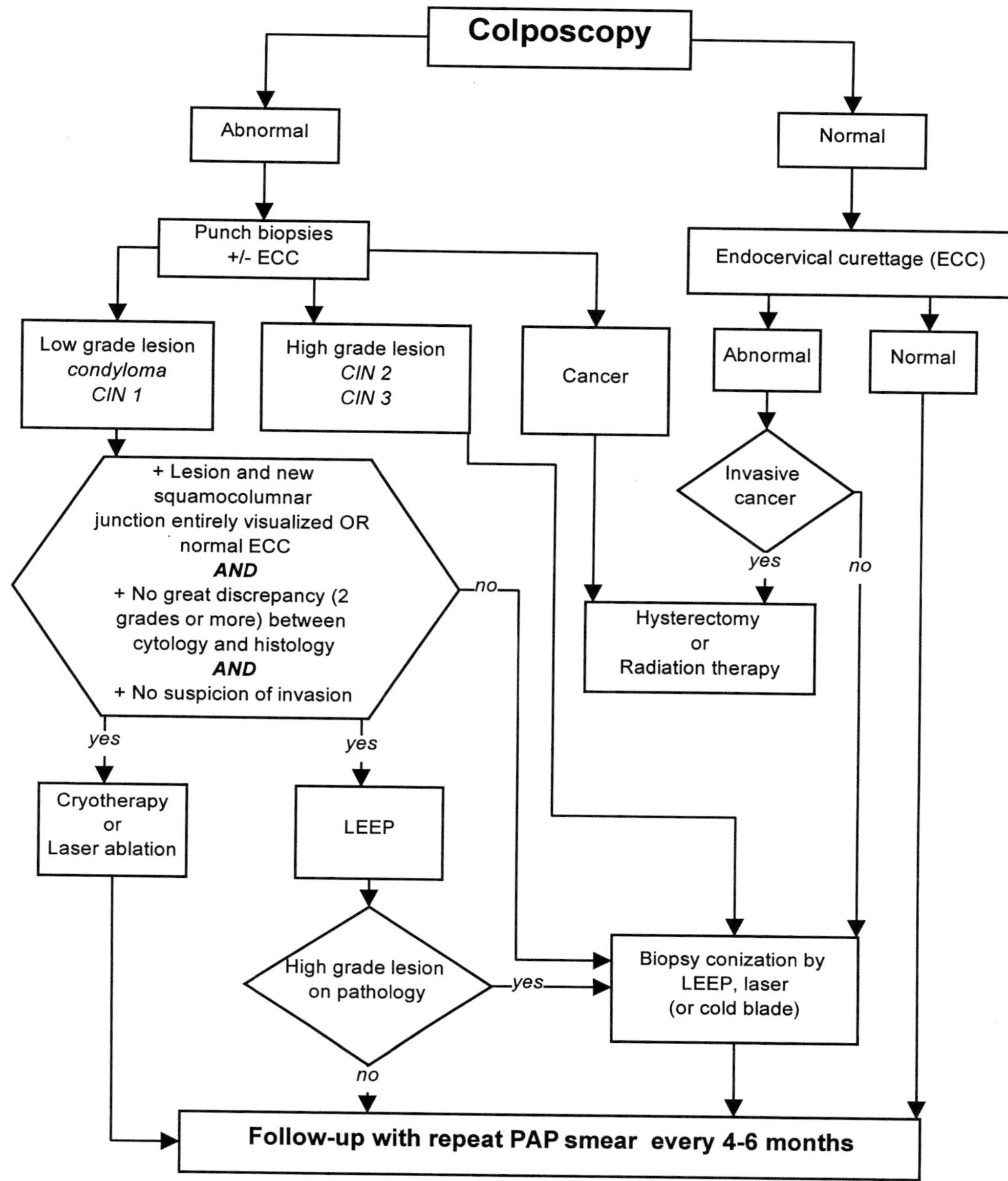

Figure 47–4. Suggested approach to cervical HPV diseases based on colposcopic evaluation. ECC, endocervical curettage.

as to resources devoted to HPV diseases. One such resource is the Centers for Disease Control and Prevention (CDC) (http://www.cdc.gov/nchstp/dstd/dstd.html) whose hotline is accessible at 1-800-227-8922 (Monday through Friday, 8:00 a.m. to 11:00 p.m.). Another is the American Social Health Association (ASHA) (http://www.ashastd.org) hotline at 1-877-478-5878 (Monday through Friday, 2:00 p.m. to 7:00 p.m.).

▲ PREVENTION

Approach to Prevention

The measures taken by health practitioners to prevent nosocomial transmission of HIV to other patients are adequate for HPVs. Disposable material should not be reused; instruments are sterilized and surfaces decontaminated with a 1:10 household bleach (5.25% sodium hypochlorite) solution. As mentioned earlier, special precautions must be taken by the operator during electrosurgery and laser surgery.

The best method of prevention is screening. At this point screening with the Pap smear can only be recommended for HPV cervical disease. Table 47–5 and Figure 47–3 detail current U.S. Public Health Service/Infectious Diseases of America (USPHS/IDSA) guidelines for the prevention of cervical and anal intraepithelial neoplasia and cancer in HIV-seropositive patients.[310,311] There is considerable debate about the best screening and management strategies for HIV-positive patients. For example, biannual Pap smears have been recommended for HIV-positive women with normal cytology.[305,312] Nevertheless, the guide-

Table 47–5. 1997 USPHS/IDSA GUIDELINES FOR THE PREVENTION OF HPV-ASSOCIATED CERVICAL AND ANAL INTRAEPITHELIAL NEOPLASIAS AND CANCERS IN HIV-INFECTED PATIENTS

HPV-Associated Genital Epithelial Cancers in HIV-Infected Women
After a complete history of previous cervical disease has been obtained, HIV-infected women should have a pelvic examination and a Papanicolaou (Pap) smear. The Pap smear should be obtained twice during the first year after diagnosis of HIV infection and if the results are normal annually thereafter.
If the results of the Pap smear are abnormal, care should be provided according to the Interim Guidelines for Management of Abnormal Cytology reported by a National Cancer Institute Consensus Panel[309] and briefly summarized in Figure 47–3.
The risks for recurrence of squamous intraepithelial lesions and cervical cancer after conventional therapy are increased among HIV-infected women. The prevention of illness associated with recurrence depends on careful follow-up of patients after treatment. Patients should be monitored with frequent cytologic screening and, when indicated, with colposcopic examination for recurrent lesions.
HPV-Associated AIN and Anal Cancer in HIV-Infected Men Who Have Sex with Men
Although the risks for AIN and anal cancer are increased among HIV-infected men who have sex with men, the role of anal cytologic screening and treatment of AIN in preventing anal cancer in these men is not well defined. Therefore, no recommendations can be made for periodic anal cytologic screening for the detection and treatment of AIN.

AIN, anal intraepithelial neoplasia.

Adapted from Centers for Disease Control and Prevention. 1997 USPHS/IDSA guidelines for the prevention of opportunistic infections in persons infected with human immunodeficiency virus, MMWR Most Mortal Wkly Rep 46(RR-12):1, 1997.

lines outlined in Table 47–5 have been validated by an extensive cost-effectiveness analysis.[313]

Prophylaxis

The use of condoms and other barrier methods is recommended to prevent HIV and other sexually transmitted infections.[310,311] This advice is germane to HPV infections because cervical or vaginal lesions may bleed, and vaginal HIV RNA levels rise after treatment for CIN.[314] The effectiveness of condoms for preventing the transmission of HPV infections and diseases is not firmly established. The evidence suggests that condoms may reduce the amount of HPV transferred, thus lessening the chance of genital warts, CIN, and cervical cancer developing.[315–319] Spermicidal agents may have a weak protective effect.[320] Povidone-iodine reduces the infectivity of papillomavirus in vitro; and sodium dodecyl sulfate (SDS), a common additive, inactivates both HIV and HPV.[317,321] However, the clinical efficacy of these compounds remains to be demonstrated. Smoking should be discouraged because it may cause HPV infection to progress to condyloma acuminatum.[33]

There are no available primary chemoprophylaxis methods for HPV infections or diseases. Efforts are ongoing to evaluate whether the progression of established CIN can be halted or reverted. Retinoids have been used for this purpose (see Therapy). 5-FU is effective for the secondary prophylaxis of CIN in HIV-infected women (see Therapy).[186] In the general population, podofilox can prevent the recurrence of condyloma acuminatum, but it is only a short-term solution.[167]

Vaccines

No vaccines are available for the treatment or prophylaxis of HPV infections and diseases. However, an intensive effort to develop such vaccines is underway.[322,323] Promising results have been obtained with human papillomavirus prophylactic vaccines based on virus-like particles.[324,325]

▲ CONCLUSIONS

Sexually transmitted HPV diseases are a substantial problem in the HIV-infected population because they are frequent and can progress to various anogenital cancers. Longer survival may mean a greater chance for some lesions to progress to cancer. Unfortunately, our means of detecting, treating, and preventing these diseases are presently deficient. Although these diseases are caused by a viral infection, none of the treatments so far available is truly antiviral. A drug development effort must be fostered. Management and screening strategies have been developed in the general population largely by an empirical approach, but their multiplicity is an invitation to conduct more scientific prospective evaluations to identify the best approaches in both the general population and HIV-infected patients. Finally, HPV vaccines hold good promise, but their development is likely to take many years.

REFERENCES

1. Vernon SD, Hart CE, Reeves WC, Icenogle JP. The HIV-1 tat protein enhances E2-dependent human papillomavirus 16 transcription. Virus Res 27:133, 1993.
2. Buonaguro FM, Tornesello ML, Buonaguro L, et al. Role of HIV as cofactor in HPV oncogenesis: in vitro evidence of virus interactions. Antibiot Chemother 46:102, 1994.
3. Toy EP, Rodriguez-Rodriguez L, McCance D, et al. Induction of cell-cycle arrest in cervical cancer cells by the human immunodeficiency virus type 1 viral protein R. Obstet Gynecol 95:141, 2000.
4. Dolei A, Curreli S, Marongiu P, et al. Human immunodeficiency virus infection in vitro activates naturally integrated human papillomavirus type 18 and induces synthesis of the L1 capsid protein. J Gen Virol 80:2937, 1999.
5. Vilmer C, Cavelier-Balloy B, Pinquier L, et al. Focal epithelial hyperplasia and multifocal human papillomavirus infection in an HIV-seropositive man. J Am Acad Dermatol 30:497, 1994.
6. Viraben R, Aquilina CA, Brousset P, Bazex J. Focal epithelial hyperplasia (Heck disease) associated with AIDS. Dermatology 193:261, 1996.
7. Ley C, Bauer HM, Reingold A, et al. Determinants of genital human papillomavirus infection in young women. J Natl Cancer Inst 83:997, 1991.
8. Koutsky L. Epidemiology of genital human papillomavirus infection. Am J Med 102:3, 1997.
9. Northfelt DW, Swift PS, Palefsky JM. Anal neoplasia: pathogenesis, diagnosis, and management. Hematol Oncol Clin North Am 10:1177, 1996.
10. Robinson WR, Morris CB. Cervical neoplasia: pathogenesis, diagnosis, and management. Hematol Oncol Clin North Am 10:1163, 1996.

11. Sun X-W, Kuhn L, Ellerbrock TV, et al. Human papillomavirus infection in women infected with the human immunodeficiency virus. N Engl J Med 337:1343, 1997.
12. Palefsky JM, Holly EA, Ralston ML, et al. High incidence of anal high-grade squamous intra-epithelial lesions among HIV-positive and HIV-negative homosexual and bisexual men. AIDS 12:495, 1998.
13. Aynaud O, Piron D, Barrasso R, Poveda JD. Comparison of clinical, histological, and virological symptoms of HPV in HIV-1 infected men and immunocompetent subjects. Sex Transm Infect 74:32, 1998.
14. Palefsky JM, Holly EA, Ralston ML, et al. Anal squamous intraepithelial lesions in HIV-positive and HIV-negative homosexual and bisexual men: prevalence and risk factors. J Acquir Immun Defic Syndr Hum Retrovirol 17:320, 1998.
15. Palefsky JM, Minkoff H, Kalish LA, et al. Cervicovaginal human papillomavirus infection in human immunodeficiency virus-1 (HIV)-positive and high-risk HIV-negative women. J Natl Cancer Inst 91:226, 1999.
16. Ellerbrock TV, Chiasson MA, Bush TJ, et al. Incidence of cervical squamous intraepithelial lesions in HIV-infected women. JAMA 283:1031, 2000.
17. Moscicki AB, Ellenberg JH, Vermund SH, et al. Prevalence of and risks for cervical human papillomavirus infection and squamous intraepithelial lesions in adolescent girls: impact of infection with human immunodeficiency virus. Arch Pediatr Adolesc Med 154:127, 2000.
18. Frisch M, Biggar RJ, Goedert JJ. Human papillomavirus-associated cancers in patients with human immunodeficiency virus infection and acquired immunodeficiency syndrome. J Natl Cancer Inst 92:1500, 2000.
19. Palefsky JM, Holly EA, Ralston ML, et al. Prevalence and risk factors for anal human papillomavirus infection in human immunodeficiency virus (HIV)-positive and high risk HIV-negative women. J Infect Dis 183:383, 2001.
20. Kiviat N, Rompalo A, Bowden R, et al. Anal human papillomavirus infection among human immunodeficiency virus-seropositive and -seronegative men. J Infect Dis 162:358, 1990.
21. Mellon LR, Gélin-Charlot C, Grand'Pierre R, et al. Prevalence of STDs among HIV^+ and HIV^- patients in an STD clinic in Haiti. Abstr Int Conf AIDS 10:459C, 1994.
22. Chirgwin KD, Feldman J, Augenbraun M, et al. Incidence of venereal warts in human immunodeficiency virus-infected and uninfected women. J Infect Dis 172:235, 1995.
23. Rezza G, Giuliani M, Branca M, et al. Determinants of squamous intraepithelial lesions (SIL) on Pap smear: the role of HPV infection and of HIV-1-induced immunosuppression. DIANAIDS Collaborative Study Group. Eur J Epidemiol 13:937, 1997.
24. Williams AB, Darragh TM, Vranizan K, et al. Anal and cervical human papillomavirus infection and risk of anal and cervical epithelial abnormalities in human immunodeficiency virus-infected women. Obstet Gynecol 83:205, 1994.
25. Klein RS, Ho GYF, Vermund SH, et al. Risk factors for squamous intraepithelial lesions on Pap smear in women at risk for human immunodeficiency virus infection. J Infect Dis 170:1404, 1994.
26. Critchlow CW, Surawicz CM, Holmes KK, et al. Prospective study of high grade anal squamous intraepithelial neoplasia in a cohort of homosexual men: influence of HIV infection, immunosuppression and human papillomavirus infection. AIDS 9:1255, 1995.
27. Hillemanns P, Ellerbrock TV, McPhillips S, et al. Prevalence of anal human papillomavirus infection and anal cytologic abnormalities in HIV-seropositive women. AIDS 10:1641, 1996.
28. Langley CL, Benga-De E, Critchlow CW, et al. HIV-1, HIV-2, human papillomavirus infection and cervical neoplasia in high-risk African women. AIDS 10:413, 1996.
29. St Louis ME, Icenogle JP, Manzila T, et al. Genital types of papillomavirus in children of women with HIV-1 infection in Kinshasa, Zaire. Int J Cancer 54:181, 1993.
30. Ahdieh L, Muñoz A, Vlahov D, et al. Cervical neoplasia and repeated positivity of human papillomavirus infection in human immunodeficiency virus-seropositive and -seronegative women. Am J Epidemiol 151:1148, 2000.
31. Friedman HB, Saah AJ, Sherman ME, et al. Human papillomavirus, anal squamous intraepithelial lesions, and human immunodeficiency virus in a cohort of gay men. J Infect Dis 178:45, 1998.
32. Heard I, Tassie JM, Schmitz V, et al. Increased risk of cervical disease among human immunodeficiency virus-infected women with severe immunosuppression and high human papillomavirus load. Obstet Gynecol 96:403, 2000.
33. Feldman JG, Chirgwin K, Dehovitz JA, Minkoff H. The association of smoking and risk of condyloma acuminatum in women. Obstet Gynecol 89:346, 1997.
34. Derkay CS. Recurrent respiratory papillomatosis. Laryngoscope 111:57, 2001.
35. Ho GY, Burk RD, Fleming I, Klein RS. Risk of genital human papillomavirus infection in women with human immunodeficiency virus-induced immunosuppression. Int J Cancer 56:788, 1994.
36. Luque AE, Demeter LM, Reichman RC. Association of human papillomavirus infection and disease with magnitude of human immunodeficiency virus type 1 (HIV-1) RNA plasma level among women with HIV-1 infection. J Infect Dis 179:1405, 1999.
37. Lie AK, Isaksen CV, Skarsvag S, Haugen OA. Human papillomavirus (HPV) in high-grade cervical intraepithelial neoplasia (CIN) detected by morphology and polymerase chain reaction (PCR): a cytohistologic correlation of 277 cases treated by laser conization. Cytopathology 10:112, 1999.
38. McMillan A, Bishop PE. Clinical course of anogenital warts in men infected with human immunodeficiency virus. Genitourin Med 65:225, 1989.
39. Wright TC Jr, Koulos J, Schnoll F, et al. Cervical intraepithelial neoplasia in women infected with the human immunodeficiency virus: outcome after loop electrosurgical excision. Gynecol Oncol 55:253, 1994.
40. Palefsky JM. Anal human papillomavirus infection and anal cancer in HIV-positive individuals: an emerging problem. AIDS 8:283, 1994.
41. Heard I, Bergeron C, Jeannel D, et al. Papanicolaou smears in human immunodeficiency virus-seropositive women during follow-up. Obstet Gynecol 86:749, 1995.
42. Kilewo CD, Urassa WK, Pallangyo K, et al. Response to podophyllotoxin treatment of genital warts in relation to HIV-1 infection among patients in Dar es Salaam, Tanzania. Int J STD AIDS 6:114, 1995.
43. Von Krogh G, Wikström A, Syrjänen K, Syrjänen S. Anal and penile condylomas in HIV-negative and HIV-positive men: clinical, histological and virological characteristics correlated to therapeutic outcome. Acta Derm Venereol (Stockh) 75:470, 1995.
44. Fruchter RG, Maiman M, Sedlis A, et al. Multiple recurrences of cervical intraepithelial neoplasia in women with the human immunodeficiency virus. Obstet Gynecol 87:338, 1996.
45. Cappiello G, Garbuglia AR, Salvi R, et al. HIV infection increases the risk of squamous intra-epithelial lesions in women with HPV infection: an analysis of HPV genotypes. Int J Cancer 72:982, 1997.
46. Anonymous. 1993 Revised classification system for HIV infection and expanded surveillance case definition for AIDS among adolescents and adults. MMWR Morbid Mortal Wkly Rep 41(RR-17):1, 1992.
47. Frisch M, Biggar RJ, Engels EA, et al. Association of cancer with AIDS-related immunosuppression in adults. JAMA 285:1736, 2001.
47a. Dorrucci M, Suligoi B, Serraino D, et al. Incidence of invasive cervical cancer in a cohort of HIV-seropositive women before and after the introduction of highly active antiretroviral therapy. J Acquir Immun Defic Syndr Hum Retrovirol 26:377, 2001.
48. Beral V, Newton R. Overview of the epidemiology of immunodeficiency-associated cancers. J Natl Cancer Inst Monogr 23:1, 1998.
49. La Ruche G, Ramon R, Mensah-Ado I, et al. Squamous intraepithelial lesions of the cervix, invasive cervical carcinoma, and immunosuppression induced by human immunodeficiency virus in Africa: Dyscer-CI Group. Cancer 82:2401, 1998.
50. Newton R, Ziegler J, Beral V. A case-control study of human immunodeficiency virus infection and cancer in adults and children residing in Kampala, Uganda. Int J Cancer 92:622, 2001.
51. Sitas F, Pacella-Norman R, Carrara H, et al. The spectrum of HIV-1 related cancers in South Africa. Int J Cancer 88:489, 2000.
52. Forti RL, Medwell SJ, Aboulafia DM, et al. Clinical presentation of minimally invasive and in situ squamous cell carcinoma of the anus in homosexual men. Clin Infect Dis 21:603, 1995.
53. Schlappner OLA, Schaffer EA. Anorectal condylomata acuminata: a missed part of the condyloma spectrum. Can Med Assoc J 118:172, 1978.

54. McMillan A. Sigmoidoscopy: a necessary procedure in the routine investigation of homosexual men? Genitourin Med 63:44, 1987.
55. Parker BJ, Cossart YE, Thompson CH, et al. The clinical management and laboratory assessment of anal warts. Med J Aust 147:59, 1987.
56. Martin-Hirsch P, Lilford R, Jarvis G, Kitchener HC. Efficacy of cervical-smear collection devices: a systematic review and meta-analysis. Lancet 354:1763, 1999.
57. Bishop JW, Marshall CJ, Bentz JS. New technologies in gynecology oncology. J Reprod Med 45:701, 2000.
58. Nanda K, McCrory DC, Myers ER, et al. Accuracy of the Papanicolaou test in screening for and follow-up of cervical cytologic abnormalities: a systematic review. Ann Intern Med 132:810, 2000.
59. Anonymous. The revised Bethesda system for reporting cervical/vaginal cytologic diagnoses: report of the 1991 Bethesda workshop. Acta Cytol 36:273, 1992.
60. Kurman RJ, Henson DE, Herbst AL, et al. Interim guidelines for management of abnormal cervical cytology. JAMA 271:1866, 1994.
61. Wright TC Jr, Ellerbrock TV, Chiasson MA, et al. Cervical intraepithelial neoplasia in women infected with human immunodeficiency virus: prevalence, risk factors, and validity of Papanicolaou smears: New York Cervical Disease Study. Obstet Gynecol 84:591, 1994.
62. Soost HJ, Lange HJ, Lehmacher W, Ruffing-Kullmann B. The validation of cervical cytology: sensitivity, specificity, and predictive values. Acta Cytol 35:8, 1991.
63. Northfelt DW. Anal neoplasia in persons with HIV infection. AIDS Clin Care 8:63, 1996.
64. Palefsky JM, Holly EA, Hogeboom CJ, et al. Anal cytology as a screening tool for anal squamous intraepithelial lesions. J Acquir Immun Defic Syndr Hum Retrovir 14:415, 1997.
65. Goldie SJ, Kuntz KM, Weinstein MC, et al. The clinical effectiveness and cost-effectiveness of screening for anal squamous intraepithelial lesions in homosexual and bisexual HIV-positive men. JAMA 281:1822, 1999.
66. Fairley CK, Chen S, Tabrizi S, et al. Influence of quartile of menstrual cycle on pellet volume of specimens from tampons and isolation of human papillomavirus. J Infect Dis 166:1199, 1992.
67. Palefsky JM. Anal squamous intraepithelial lesions in human immunodeficiency virus-positive men and women. Semin Oncol 27:471, 2000.
68. Stoler MH, Schiffman M. Atypical squamous cells of undetermined significance: low-grade squamous intraepithelial lesion triage study (ALTS) group: interobserver reproducibility of cervical cytologic and histologic interpretations; realistic estimates from the ASCUS-LSIL Triage Study. JAMA 285:1500, 2001.
69. Peyton CL, Schiffman M, Lorincz AT, et al. Comparison of PCR- and hybrid capture-based human papillomavirus detection systems using multiple cervical specimen collection strategies. J Clin Microbiol 36:3248, 1998.
70. Anonymous. Human papillomavirus testing for triage of women with cytologic evidence of low-grade squamous intraepithelial lesions: baseline data from a randomized trial: the Atypical Squamous Cells of Undetermined Significance/Low-Grade Squamous Intraepithelial Lesions Triage Study (ALTS) group. J Natl Cancer Inst 92:397, 2000.
71. Lorincz AT, Reid R, Jenson AB, et al. Human papillomavirus infection of the cervix: relative risk associations of 15 common anogenital types. Obstet Gynecol 79:328, 1992.
72. Petry KU, Bohmer G, Iftner T, et al. Human papillomavirus testing in primary screening for cervical cancer of human immunodeficiency virus-infected women, 1990–1998. Gynecol Oncol 75:427, 1999.
73. Womack SD, Chirenje ZM, Gaffikin L, et al. HPV-based cervical cancer screening in a population at high risk for HIV infection. Int J Cancer 85:206, 2000.
74. Manos MM, Kinney WK, Hurley LB, et al. Identifying women with cervical neoplasia: using human papillomavirus DNA testing for equivocal Papanicolaou results. JAMA 281:1605, 1999.
75. Solomon D, Schiffman M, Tarone R, ALTS Group. Comparison of three management strategies for patients with atypical squamous cells of undetermined significance: baseline results from a randomized trial. J Natl Cancer Inst 93:293, 2001.
76. Maw RD, Reitano M, Roy M. An international survey of patients with genital warts: perceptions regarding treatment and impact on lifestyle. Int J STD AIDS 9:571, 1998.
77. Persson G, Gösta Dahlöf L, Krantz I. Physical and psychological effects of anogenital warts on female patients. Sex Transm Dis 20:10, 1993.
78. Voog E, Löwhagen G-B. Follow-up of men with genital papilloma virus infection: psychosexual aspects. Acta Derm Venereol (Stockh) 72:185, 1992.
79. Filiberti A, Tamburini M, Stefanon B, et al. Psychological aspects of genital human papillomavirus infection: a preliminary report. J Psychosom Obstet Gynaecol 14:145, 1993.
80. Sheppard S, White M, Walzman M. Genital warts: just a nuisance? Genitourin Med 71:194, 1995.
81. Chuang T-Y, Perry HO, Kurland LT, Ilstrup DM. Condyloma acuminatum in Rochester, Minn, 1950–1978. I. Epidemiology and clinical features. Arch Dermatol 120:469, 1984.
82. Ferenczy A, Mitao M, Nagai N, et al. Latent papillomavirus and recurring genital warts. N Engl J Med 313:784, 1985.
83. Ward KA, Winter PC, Walsh M, et al. Detection of human papillomavirus by the polymerase chain reaction in histologically normal penile skin adjacent to penile warts. Sex Transm Dis 21:83, 1994.
84. Riva JM, Sedlacek TV, Cunnane MF, Mangan CE. Extended carbon dioxide laser vaporization in the treatment of subclinical papillomavirus infection of the lower genital tract. Obstet Gynecol 73:25, 1989.
85. Carpiniello VL, Zderic SA, Malloy TR, Sedlacek T. Carbon dioxide laser therapy of subclinical condyloma found by magnified penile surface scanning. Urology 29:608, 1987.
86. Höckenström T, Jonassen F, Knutsson F, et al. High prevalence of cervical dysplasia in female consorts of men with genital warts. Acta Derm Venereol (Stockh) 67:511, 1987.
87. Barrasso R. HPV-related genital lesions in men. In: Muñoz N, Bosch FX, Shah KV, Meheus A (eds) The Epidemiology of Cervical Cancer and Human Papillomavirus. IARC Scientific Publications No. 119. Lyon, International Agency for Research on Cancer, 1992, pp 85–92.
88. Krebs H-B, Helmkamp BF. Does the treatment of genital condylomata in men decrease the treatment failure rate of cervical dysplasia in the female sexual partner? Obstet Gynecol 76:660, 1990.
89. Anonymous. 1998 Guidelines for the treatment of sexually transmitted diseases. MMWR Morbid Mortal Wkly Rep 47(RR-1):1, 1998.
90. Anonymous. Human papillomaviruses. IARC Monogr Eval Carcinog Risks Hum 94:1, 1995.
91. Schonfeld A, Nitke S, Schattner A, et al. Intramuscular human interferon-β injections in treatment of condylomata acuminata. Lancet 1:1038, 1984.
92. Reichman RC, Oakes D, Bonnez W, et al. Treatment of condyloma acuminatum with three different alpha interferon preparations administered parenterally: a double-blind, placebo-controlled trial. J Infect Dis 162:1270, 1990.
93. Condylomata International Collaborative Study Group. Recurrent condylomata acuminata treated with recombinant interferon alfa-2a: a multicenter double-blind placebo-controlled clinical trial. JAMA 265:2684, 1991.
94. Edwards L, Ferenczy A, Eron L, et al. Self-administered topical 5-percent imiquimod cream for external anogenital warts. Arch Dermatol 134:25, 1998.
95. Syed TA, Ahmadpour OA, Ahmad SA, Ahmad SH. Management of female genital warts with an analog of imiquimod 2% in cream: a randomized, double-blind, placebo-controlled study. J Dermatol 25:429, 1998.
96. Syed TA, Hadi SM, Qureshi ZA, et al. Treatment of external genital warts in men with imiquimod 2% in cream: a placebo-controlled, double-blind study. Infect 41:148, 2000.
97. Del Priore G, Gilmore PR, Maag T, et al. Colposcopic biopsies versus loop electrosurgical excision procedure cone histology in human immunodeficiency virus-positive women. J Reprod Med 41:653, 1996.
98. Cuthill S, Maiman M, Fruchter RG, et al. Complications after treatment of cervical intraepithelial neoplasia in women infected with the human immunodeficiency virus. J Reprod Med 40:823, 1995.
99. Luque AE, Li H, Demeter LM, Reichman RC. Effect of antiretroviral therapy (ARVT) on human papillomavirus (HPV) infection and disease among HIV-infected women [abstract]. Presented at the 8th Conference Retrovirus Opportunistic Infections, Chicago, February 2001, p 724.

100. Heard I, Schmitz V, Costagliola D, et al. Early regression of cervical lesions in HIV-seropositive women receiving highly active antiretroviral therapy. AIDS 12:1459, 1998.
101. Robinson WR, Hamilton CA, Michaels SH, Kissinger P. Effect of excisional therapy and highly active antiretroviral therapy on cervical intraepithelial neoplasia in women infected with human immunodeficiency virus. Am J Obstet Gynecol 184:538, 2001.
102. Luque AE, Li H, Demeter LM, Reichman RC. Effect of highly active antiretroviral therapy (HAART) on human papillomavirus (HPV) infection and disease among HIV-infected women. In: Abstracts 40th Interscience Conference on Antimicrobials and Chemotherapy, 2000, p 66.
102a. Minkoff H, Ahdieh L, Massad LS, et al. The effect of highly active antiretroviral therapy on cervical cytologic changes associated with oncogenic HPV among HIV-infected women. AIDS 15:2157, 2001.
103. Del Mistro A, Franzetti M, Cattelan A, et al. Clinical and virological features of HPV-associated genital lesions in HIV-infected women. In: Abstracts of the 3rd National AIDS Malignancy Conference, May 1999, p 11.
103a. Lillo F, Ferrari D, Veglia F, et al. Human papillomavirus infection and associated cervical disease in human immunodefiency virus-infected women: effect of highly active antiretroviral therapy. J Infect Dis 184:547, 2001.
104. Palefsky JM, Holly EA, Ralston ML, et al. Effect of highly active antiretroviral therapy on the natural history of anal squamous intraepithelial lesions and human papillomavirus infection. J Acquir Immun Defic Syndr Hum Retrovirol 28:422, 2001.
105. Jones JL, Hanson DL, Dworkin MS, et al. Effect of antiretroviral therapy on recent trends in selected cancers among HIV-infected persons. J Acquir Immune Defic Syndr 21:S11, 1999.
105a. Greenspan D, Canchola AJ, MacPhail LA, et al. Effect of highly active antiretroviral therapy on frequency of oral warts. Lancet 357:1411, 2001.
106. Nel WS, Fourie ED. Immunotherapy and 5% topical 5-fluoro-uracil ointment in the treatment of condylomata acuminata. S Afr Med J 47:45, 1973.
107. Haye KR. Treatment of condyloma acuminata with 5 per cent: 5-fluorouracil (5-FU) cream. Br J Vener Dis 50:466, 1974.
108. Dretler SP, Klein LA. The eradication of intraurethral condyloma acuminata with 5 per cent 5-fluorouracil cream. J Urol 113:195, 1975.
109. Von Krogh G. 5-Fluoro-uracil cream in the successful treatment of therapeutically refractory condylomata acuminata of the urinary meatus. Acta Derm Venereol (Stockh) 56:297, 1976.
110. Wallin J. 5-Fluorouracil in the treatment of penile and urethral condylomata acuminata. Br J Vener Dis 53:240, 1977.
111. Von Krogh G. The beneficial effect of 1% 5-fluorouracil in 70% ethanol on therapeutically refractory condylomas in the preputial cavity. Sex Transm Dis 5:137, 1978.
112. Pareek S. Treatment of condyloma acuminatum with 5% 5-fluorouracil. Br J Vener Dis 55:65, 1979.
113. Krebs H-B. Prophylactic topical 5-fluorouracil following treatment of human papillomavirus-associated lesions of the vulva and vagina. Obstet Gynecol 68:837, 1986.
114. Krebs H-B. Treatment of vaginal condylomata acuminata by weekly topical application of 5-fluorouracil. Obstet Gynecol 70:68, 1987.
115. Krebs H-B. Treatment of extensive vulvar condylomata acuminata with topical 5-fluorouracil. South Med J 83:761, 1990.
116. Pride G. Treatment of large lower genital tract condylomata acuminata with topical 5-fluorouracil. J Reprod Med 35:384, 1990.
117. Bergman A, Nalick R. Genital human papillomavirus infection in men: diagnosis and treatment with a laser and 5-fluorouracil. J Reprod Med 36:363, 1991.
118. Friedman-Kien A, Eron LJ, Conant M, et al. Natural interferon alfa for treatment of condylomata acuminata. JAMA 259:533, 1988.
119. Tiedemann K-H, Ernst T-M. Kombinationstherapie von rezidivierenden Condylomata acuminata mit Elektrokaustik und Alpha-2-Interferon. Akt Dermatol 14:200, 1988.
120. Vance JC, Bart BJ, Hansen RC, et al. Intralesional recombinant alpha-2 interferon for the treatment of patients with condyloma acuminatum or verruca plantaris. Arch Dermatol 122:272, 1986.
121. Eron LJ, Judson F, Tucker S, et al. Interferon therapy for condylomata acuminata. N Engl J Med 315:1059, 1986.
122. Reichman RC, Oakes D, Bonnez W, et al. Treatment of condyloma acuminatum with three different interferons administered intralesionally: a double-blind, placebo-controlled trial. Ann Intern Med 108:675, 1988.
123. Welander CE, Homesley HD, Smiles KA, Peets EA. Intralesional interferon alfa-2b for the treatment of genital warts. Am J Obstet Gynecol 162:348, 1990.
124. Douglas JM Jr, Eron LJ, Judson FN, et al. A randomized trial of combination therapy with intralesional interferon α_{2b} and podophyllin versus podophyllin alone for the therapy of anogenital warts. J Infect Dis 162:52, 1990.
125. Bart BJ, Vance JC, Krywonis N, et al. Treatment of condylomata acuminata: comparing intralesional alpha-2b interferon combined with liquid nitrogen to liquid nitrogen alone. J Invest Dermatol 90:545, 1988.
126. Handley JM, Horner T, Maw RD, et al. Subcutaneous interferon alpha 2a combined with cryotherapy vs cryotherapy alone in the treatment of primary anogenital warts: a randomised observer blind placebo controlled study. Genitourin Med 67:297, 1991.
127. Reid R, Greenberg MD, Pizzuti DJ, et al. Superficial laser vulvectomy. V. Surgical debulking is enhanced by adjuvant systemic interferon. Am J Obstet Gynecol 166:815, 1992.
128. Condylomata International Collaborative Study Group. Randomized placebo-controlled double-blind combined therapy with laser surgery and systemic interferon-alpha 2a in the treatment of anogenital condylomata acuminatum. J Infect Dis 167:824, 1993.
129. Bornstein J, Pascal B, Zarfati D, et al. Recombinant human interferon-beta for condylomata acuminata: a randomized, double-blind, placebo-controlled study of intralesional therapy. Int J STD AIDS 8:614, 1997.
130. Dinsmore W, Jordan J, O'Mahony C, et al. Recombinant human interferon-beta in the treatment of condylomata acuminata. Int J STD AIDS 8:622, 1997.
131. Trizna Z, Evans T, Bruce S, et al. A randomized phase II study comparing four different interferon therapies in patients with recalcitrant condylomata acuminata. Sex Transm Dis 25:361, 1998.
132. Gaspari AA, Zalka A. Interferon gamma immunotherapy for generalized verrucosis in the setting of chronic immunodeficiency. J Am Acad Dermatol 38(Pt 1):286, 1998.
133. Rockley PF, Tyring SK. Interferons alpha, beta and gamma therapy of anogenital human papillomavirus infections. Pharmacol Ther 65:265, 1995.
134. Beutner KR, Wiley DJ, Douglas JM, et al. Genital warts and their treatment. Clin Infect Dis 28(suppl 1):S37, 1998.
135. Sullivan M, Hearin JT. Treatment of condylomata acuminata with podophyllotoxin. South Med J 41:336, 1948.
136. Wilson L, Bamburg JR, Mizel SB, et al. Interaction of drugs with microtubule proteins. Fed Proc 33:158, 1974.
137. Zhu W-Y, Blauvelt A, Goldstein BA, et al. Detection with the polymerase chain reaction of human papillomavirus DNA in condylomata acuminata treated in vitro with liquid nitrogen, trichloracetic acid, and podophyllin. J Am Acad Dermatol 26:710, 1992.
138. Von Krogh G. Topical treatment of penile condylomata acuminata with podophyllin, podophyllotoxin and colchicine. Acta Derm Venereol (Stockh) 58:163, 1978.
139. White C, Sparks RA. Podophyllotoxin: is it user friendly? Genitourin Med 67:174, 1991.
140. Fisher AA. Severe systemic and local reactions to topical podophyllum resin. Cutis 28:233,236,242,248,266, 1981.
141. Finkle TH, Frishwasser EJ. Treatment of penile condylomata acuminata with podophylin: observations on the prevention of balanitis. J Invest Dermatol 8:199, 1947.
142. Beutner KR. Podophyllotoxin in the treatment of genital human papillomavirus infection: a review. Semin Dermatol 6:10, 1987.
143. Ferguson LR, Pearson A. Chromosomal changes in Chinese hamster AA8 cells caused by podophyllin, a common treatment for genital warts. Mutat Res 266:231, 1992.
144. Chamberlain MJ, Reynolds AL, Yeoman WB. Toxic effect of podophyllum application in pregnancy. BMJ 3:391, 1972.
145. Sullivan M, King LS. Effects of resin of podophyllum on normal skin, condylomata acuminata and verruca vulgares. Arch Dermatol Syphilol 56:30, 1947.
146. Wade TR, Ackerman AB. The effects of resin of podophyllin on condyloma acuminatum. Am J Dermatopathol 6:109, 1984.

147. Lassus A, Haukka K, Forsström S. Podophyllotoxin for treatment of genital warts in males: a comparison with conventional podophyllin therapy. Eur J Sex Transm Dis 2:31, 1984.
148. Jensen SL. Comparison of podophyllin application with simple surgical excision in clearance and recurrence of perianal condylomata acuminata. Lancet 2:1146, 1985.
149. Petersen CS, Worm A-M, Kroon S, Tikjob G. Podophyllotoxin 5% and podophyllin 20% in the treatment of ano-genital warts: a comparative double-blind study. Eur J Sex Transm Dis 2:155, 1985.
150. Edwards A, Atma-Ram A, Thin RN. Podophyllotoxin 0.5% *v* podophyllin 20% to treat penile warts. Genitourin Med 64:263, 1988.
151. Beutner KR, Friedman-Kien AE, Artman NN, et al. Patient-applied podofilox for treatment of genital warts. Lancet 1:831, 1989.
152. Stone KM, Becker TM, Hadgu A, Kraus SJ. Treatment of external genital warts: a randomised clinical trial comparing podophyllin, cryotherapy, and electrodesiccation. Genitourin Med 66:16, 1990.
153. Kirby P, Dunne A, King DH, Corey L. Double-blind randomized clinical trial of self-administered podofilox solution versus vehicle in the treatment of genital warts. Am J Med 88:465, 1990.
154. Mazurkiewicz W, Jablonska S. Clinical efficacy of Condyline (0.5% podophyllotoxin) solution and cream versus podophyllin in the treatment of external condylomata acuminata. J Dermatol Treat 1:123, 1990.
155. Greenberg MD, Rutledge LH, Reid R, et al. A double-blind, randomized trial of 0.5% podofilox and placebo for the treatment of genital warts in women. Obstet Gynecol 77:735, 1991.
156. Condylomata International Collaborative Study Group. A comparison of interferon alfa-2a and podophyllin in the treatment of primary condylomata acuminata. Genitourin Med 67:394, 1991.
157. Von Krogh G, Hellberg D. Self-treatment using a 0.5% podophyllotoxin cream of external genital condylomata acuminata in women: a placebo-controlled, double-blind study. Sex Transm Dis 19:170, 1992.
158. Syed TA, Lundin S. Topical treatment of penile condylomata acuminata with podophyllotoxin 0.3% solution, 0.3% cream and 0.15% cream: a comparative open study. Dermatology 187:30, 1993.
159. Von Krogh G. Self-treatment using 0.25%–0.50% podophyllotoxin-ethanol solutions against penile condylomata acuminata: a placebo-controlled comparative study. Genitourin Med 70:105, 1994.
160. Syed TA, Lundin S, Ahmad SA. Topical 0.3% and 0.5% podophyllotoxin cream for self-treatment of condylomata acuminata in women: a placebo-controlled, double-blind study. Dermatology 189:142, 1994.
161. Syed TA, Cheema KM, Khayyami M, et al. Human leukocyte interferon-alpha versus podophyllotoxin in cream for the treatment of genital warts in males: a placebo-controlled, double-blind, comparative study. Dermatology 191:129, 1995.
162. Syed TA, Khayyami M, Kriz D, et al. Management of genital warts in women with human leukocyte interferon-alpha vs. podophyllotoxin in cream: a placebo-controlled, double-blind, comparative study. J Mol Med 73:255, 1995.
163. Hellberg D, Svarrer T, Nilsson S, Valentin J. Self-treatment of female external genital warts with 0.5% podophyllotoxin cream (Condyline) vs weekly applications of 20% podophyllin solution. Int J STD AIDS 6:257, 1995.
164. Strand A, Brinkeborn RM, Siboulet A. Topical treatment of genital warts in men, an open study of podophyllotoxin cream compared with solution. Genitourin Med 71:387, 1995.
165. Claesson U, Lassus A, Happonen H, et al. Topical treatment of venereal warts: a comparative open study of podophyllotoxin cream versus solution. Int J STD AIDS 7:429, 1996.
166. White DJ, Billingham C, Chapman S, et al. Podophyllin 0.5% or 2.0% *v* podophyllotoxin 0.5% for the self-treatment of penile warts: a double-blind randomised study. Genitourin Med 73:184, 1997.
167. Bonnez W, Elswick RK Jr, Bailey-Farchione A, et al. Efficacy and safety of 0.5% podofilox solution in the treatment and suppression of anogenital warts. Am J Med 96:420, 1994.
168. Beck DE, Jaso RG, Zajac RA. Surgical management of anal condylomata in the HIV-positive patient. Dis Colon Rectum 33:180, 1990.
169. Orkin BA, Smith LE. Perineal manifestations of HIV infection. Dis Colon Rectum 35:310, 1992.
170. Weiner M, Semah D, Schewach-Millet M, Cesarini J-P. Preclinical and clinical evaluation of topical acid products for skin tumors. Clin Pharmacol Ther 33:77, 1983.
171. Godley MJ, Bradbeer CS, Gellan M, Thin RNT. Cryotherapy compared with trichloracetic acid in treating genital warts. Genitourin Med 63:390, 1987.
172. Abdullah AN, Walzman M, Wade A. Treatment of external genital warts comparing cryotherapy (liquid nitrogen) and trichloracetic acid. Sex Transm Dis 20:344, 1993.
173. Gabriel G, Thin RNT. Treatment of anogenital warts: comparison to trichloracetic acid and podophyllin versus podophyllin alone. Br J Vener Dis 59:124, 1983.
174. Shelley WB, Shelley ED. Scrotal dermatitis caused by 5-fluorouracil (Efudex). J Am Acad Dermatol 19:929, 1988.
175. Goette DK, Odom RB. Allergic contact dermatitis to topical fluorouracil. Arch Dermatol 113:1058, 1977.
176. Mansell PWA, Litwin MS, Ichinose H, Krementz ET. Delayed hypersensitivity to 5-fluorouracil following topical chemotherapy of cutaneous cancers. Cancer Res 35:1288, 1975.
177. Krebs H-B, Helmkamp BF. Chronic ulcerations following topical therapy with 5-fluorouracil for vaginal human papillomavirus-associated lesions. Obstet Gynecol 78:205, 1991.
178. Reid R. The management of genital condylomas, intraepithelial neoplasia, and vulvodynia. Obstet Gynecol Clin North Am 23:917, 1996.
179. Goodman A, Zukerberg LR, Nikrui N, Scully RE. Vaginal adenosis and clear cell carcinoma after 5-fluorouracil treatment for condylomas. Cancer 68:1628, 1991.
180. Odom LD, Plouffe L Jr, Butler WJ. 5-Fluorouracil exposure during the period of conception: report on two cases. Obstet Gynecol 163:76, 1990.
181. De Benedictis JT, Marmar JL, Praiss DE. Intraurethral condylomata acuminata: management and a review of the literature. J Urol 118:767, 1977.
182. Reid R, Greenberg MD, Lörincz AT, et al. Superficial laser vulvectomy. IV. Extended laser vaporization and adjunctive 5-fluorouracil therapy of human papillomavirus-associated vulvar disease. Obstet Gynecol 76:439, 1990.
183. Syed TA, Quresh ZA, Ahmad SA, Shahida M. Management of intravaginal warts in HIV-infected women with a dual combination therapy: 5-fluorouracil (1%) in injectable hydrophyllic gel and zidovudine 250 mg [abstract]. Presented at the National HIV Prevention Conference, August-September, 1999, 105.
184. Sillman FH, Sedlis A, Boyce JG. A review of lower genital intraepithelial neoplasia and the use of topical 5-fluorouracil. Obstet Gynecol Surv 40:190, 1985.
185. Pehoushek J, Smith KJ. Imiquimod and 5% fluorouracil therapy for anal and perianal squamous cell carcinoma in situ in an HIV-1-positive man. Arch Dermatol 137:14, 2001.
186. Maiman M, Watts DH, Andersen J, et al. Vaginal 5-fluorouracil for high-grade cervical dysplasia in human immunodeficiency virus infection: a randomized trial. Obstet Gynecol 94:954, 1999.
187. Van Cutsem E, Snoeck R, van Ranst M, et al. Successful treatment of a squamous papilloma of the hypopharynx-esophagus by local injections of (*S*)-1-(3-hydroxy-2-phosphonyl-methoxypropyl) cytosine. J Med Virol 45:230, 1995.
188. Snoeck R, van Ranst M, Andrei G, et al. Treatment of anogenital papillomavirus infections with an acyclic nucleoside phosphonate analogue. N Engl J Med 333:943, 1995.
189. Snoeck R, Wellens W, Desloovere C, et al. Treatment of severe recurrent laryngeal papillomatosis by local injections of (*S*-1-(3-hydroxy-2-phosphonylmethoxypropyl)cytosine (Cidofovir). Antiviral Res 30:A25, 1996.
190. Douglas J, Corey L, Tyring S, et al. A phase I/II study of cidofovir topical gel for refractory condyloma acuminatum in patients with HIV infection. In: Abstracts 4th Conference on Retroviral Opportunistic Infections, 1997, p 677.
191. Koonsaeng S, Verschraegen C, Freedman R, et al. Successful treatment of recurrent vulvar intraepithelial neoplasia resistant to interferon and isotretinoin with cidofovir. J Med Virol 64:195, 2001.
192. Snoeck R, Bossens M, Parent D, et al. Phase II double-blind, placebo-controlled study of the safety and efficacy of cidofovir topical gel for the treatment of patients with human papillomavirus infection. Clin Infect Dis 33:597, 2001.

193. Snoeck R, Noel JC, Muller C, et al. Cidofovir, a new approach for the treatment of cervix intraepithelial neoplasia grade III (CIN III). J Med Virol 60:205, 2000.
193a. Calista D. Resolution of recalcitrant human papillomavirus gingival infection with topical cidofovir. Oral Surg Oral Med Oral Pathol Oral Radiol Endod 90:713, 2000.
194. Jones SK, Darville JM. Transmission of virus particles by cryotherapy and multi-use caustic pencils: a problem to dermatologists? Br J Dermatol 121:481, 1989.
195. Kuflik EG, Lubritz RR, Torre D. Cryotherapy. Dermatol Clin 2:319, 1984.
196. Dachow-Siwiec E. Technique of cryotherapy. Clin Dermatol 3:185, 1985.
197. Hatch KD. Cryotherapy. Baillieres Clin Obstet Gynaecol 9:133, 1995.
198. Grimmett RH. Liquid nitrogen therapy. Arch Dermatol 83:563, 1961.
199. Bonnez W, Oakes D, Bailey-Farchione A, et al. A randomized, double-blind, placebo-controlled trial of systemically administered alpha-, beta-, or gamma-interferon in combination with cryotherapy for the treatment of condyloma acuminatum. J Infect Dis 171:1081, 1995.
200. Bonnez W, Oakes D, Bailey-Farchione A, et al. A randomized, double-blind trial of parenteral low dose versus high dose interferon-β in combination with cryotherapy for treatment of condyloma acuminatum. Antiviral Res 35:41, 1997.
201. Ghosh AK. Cryosurgery of genital warts in cases in which podophyllin treatment failed or was contraindicated. Br J Vener Dis 53:49, 1977.
202. Balsdon MJ. Cryosurgery of genital warts. Br J Vener Dis 54:352, 1978.
203. Simmons PD, Langlet F, Thin RNT. Cryotherapy versus electrocautery in the treatment of genital warts. Br J Vener Dis 57:273, 1981.
204. Dodi G, Infantino A, Moretti R, et al. Cryotherapy of anorectal warts and condylomata. Cryosurgery 19:287, 1982.
205. Bergman A, Bhatia NN, Broen EM. Cryotherapy for treatment of genital condylomata during pregnancy. J Reprod Med 29:432, 1984.
206. Bashi SA. Cryotherapy versus podophyllin in the treatment of genital warts. Int J Dermatol 24:535, 1985.
207. Sand PK, Shen W, Bowen LW, Ostergard DR. Cryotherapy for the treatment of proximal urethral condyloma acuminatum. J Urol 137:874, 1987.
208. Matsunaga J, Bergman A, Bhatia NN. Genital condylomata acuminata in pregnancy: effectiveness, safety and pregancy outcome following cryotherapy. Br J Obstet Gynaecol 94:168, 1987.
209. Damstra RJ, van Vloten WA. Cryotherapy in the treatment of condylomata acuminata: a controlled study of 64 patients. J Dermatol Surg Oncol 17:273, 1991.
210. Cox JT. Management of cervical intraepithelial neoplasia. Lancet 353:857, 1999.
211. Martin-Hirsch PL, Paraskevaidis E, Kitchener H. Surgery for cervical intraepithelial neoplasia. Cochrane Database of Systematic Reviews [computer file] CD001318, 2000.
212. Wetchler SJ. Treatment of cervical intraepithelial neoplasia with the CO_2 laser: laser versus cryotherapy: a review of effectiveness and cost. Obstet Gynecol Surv 39:469, 1984.
213. Bergman A, Matsunaga J, Bhatia NN. Cervical cryotherapy for condylomata acuminata during pregnancy. Obstet Gynecol 69:47, 1987.
214. Thomson JPS, Grace RH. The treatment of perianal and anal condylomata acuminata. J R Soc Med 71:180, 1978.
215. Duus BR, Philipsen T, Christensen JD, et al. Refractory condylomata acuminata: a controlled clinical trial of carbon dioxide laser versus conventional surgical treatment. Genitourin Med 61:59, 1985.
216. Myer CM III, Willging JP, McMurray S, Cotton RT. Use of a laryngeal micro resector system. Laryngoscope 109(Pt 1):1165, 1999.
217. Gollock JM, Slatford K, Hunter JM. Scissor excision of anogenital warts. Br J Vener Dis 58:400, 1982.
218. Khawaja HT. Treatment of condyloma acuminatum. Lancet 1:208, 1986.
219. Khawaja HT. Podophyllin versus scissor excision in the treatment of perianal condylomata acuminata: a prospective study. Br J Surg 76:1067, 1989.
220. Simmons PD, Thompson JPS. Scissor excision of penile warts: case report. Genitourin Med 62:277, 1986.
221. McMillan A, Scott GR. Outpatient treatment of perianal warts by scissor excision. Genitourin Med 63:114, 1987.
222. Bonnez W, Oakes D, Choi A, et al. Therapeutic efficacy and complications of excisional biopsy of condyloma acuminatum. Sex Transm Dis 23:273, 1996.
223. Miles AJG, Mellor CH, Gazzard B, et al. Surgical management of anorectal disease in HIV-positive homosexuals. Br J Surg 77:869, 1990.
224. Zouboulis CC, Büttner P, Orfanos CE. Systemic interferon gamma as adjuvant therapy for refractory anogenital warts: a randomized clinical trial and meta-analysis of the available data. Arch Dermatol 128:1413, 1992.
225. Burke EC, Orloff SL, Freise CE, et al. Wound healing after anorectal surgery in human immunodeficiency virus-infected patients. Arch Surg 126:1267, 1991.
226. Lord RVN. Anorectal surgery in patients infected with human immunodeficiency virus: factors associated with delayed wound healing. Ann Surg 226:92, 1997.
227. Jones HW III. Cone biopsy in the management of cervical intraepithelial neoplasia. Clin Obstet Gynecol 26:968, 1983.
228. Odell RC. Electrosurgery: principles and safety issues. Clin Obstet Gynecol 38:610, 1995.
229. Vuori J, Alfthan O, Pyrhönen S, et al. Treatment of condyloma acuminata in male patients. Eur Urol 3:213, 1977.
230. Fleshner PR, Freilich MI. Adjuvant interferon for anal condyloma: a prospective, randomized trial. Dis Colon Rectum 37:1255, 1994.
231. Orani AM, Fossati M, Bolis D, et al. Efficacy and safety evaluation on combination therapy with systemic interferon beta and electrocautery in the anogenital warts treatment of HIV-seropositive patients. Abstr Int Conf AIDS 9:PO-B08-1326, 1993.
232. Hallén A, Ljunghall K, Wallin J. Topical anesthesia with local anesthetic (lidocaine and prilocaine, EMLA) cream for cautery of genital warts. Genitourin Med 63:316, 1987.
233. Wright TC, Richart RM, Ferenczy A. Electrosurgery for HPV-Related Diseases of the Lower Genital Tract. New York, Arthur Vision, 1991.
234. Wright TC Jr, Gagnon S, Richart RM, Ferenczy A. Treatment of cervical intraepithelial neoplasia using the loop electrosurgical excision procedure. Obstet Gynecol 79:173, 1992.
235. Prendiville W. Large loop excision of the transformation zone. Clin Obstet Gynecol 38:622, 1995.
236. Bigrigg A, Haffenden DK, Sheehan AL, et al. Efficacy and safety of large-loop excision of the transformation zone. Lancet 343:32, 1994.
236a. Chang GJ, Berry JM, Jay N, et al. Surgical treatment of high-grade anal squamous intraepithelial lesions—a prospective study. Dis Colon Rect (in press) (communicated by JM Palefsky).
237. Sawchuk WS, Weber PJ, Lowy DR, Dzubow LM. Infectious papillomavirus in the vapor of warts treated with carbon dioxide laser or electrocoagulation: detection and protection. J Am Acad Dermatol 21:41, 1989.
238. Bergbrant I-M, Samuelsson L, Olofsson S, et al. Polymerase chain reaction for monitoring human papillomavirus contamination of medical personnel during treatment of genital warts with CO_2 laser and electrocoagulation. Acta Derm Venereol (Stockh) 74:393, 1994.
239. Herd RM, Dover JS, Arndt KA. Basic laser principles. Dermatol Clin 15:355, 1997.
240. Dover JS, Arndt KA, Dinehart SM, et al. Guidelines/Outcomes Committee: guidelines of care for laser surgery. J Am Acad Dermatol 41:484, 1999.
241. Hruza GJ. Laser treatment of warts and other epidermal and dermal lesions. Dermatol Clin 15:487, 1997.
242. Dorsey JH. Laser surgery for cervical intraepithelial neoplasia. Obstet Gynecol Clin North Am 18:475, 1991.
243. Reid R. Laser surgery of the vulva. Obstet Gynecol Clin North Am 18:491, 1991.
244. Ferenczy A. Laser treatment of genital human papillomavirus infections in the male patient. Obstet Gynecol Clin North Am 18:525, 1991.
245. Bhatta KM. Lasers in urology. Lasers Surg Med 16:312, 1995.
246. Bellina JH. The use of the carbon dioxide laser in the management of condyloma acuminatum with eight-year follow-up. Am J Obstet Gynecol 147:375, 1983.

247. Calkins JW, Masterson BJ, Magrina JF, Capen CV. Management of condylomata acuminata with the carbon dioxide laser. Obstet Gynecol 59:105, 1982.
248. Krogh J, Beuke H-P, Miskowiak J, et al. Long-term results of carbon dioxide laser treatment of meatal condylomata acuminata. Br J Urol 65:621, 1990.
249. Bar-Am A, Shilon M, Peyser MR, et al. Treatment of male genital condylomatous lesions by carbon dioxide laser after failure of previous nonlaser methods. J Am Acad Dermatol 24:87, 1991.
250. Garden JM, O'Banion MK, Shelnitz LS, et al. Papillomavirus in the vapor of carbon dioxide laser-treated verrucae. JAMA 259:1199, 1988.
251. Kashima HK, Kessis T, Mounts P, Shah K. Polymerase chain reaction identification of human papillomavirus DNA in CO_2 laser plume from recurrent respiratory papillomatosis. Otolaryngol Head Neck Surg 104:191, 1991.
252. Gloster HM Jr, Roenigk RK. Risk of acquiring human papillomavirus from the plume produced by the carbon dioxide laser in the treatment of warts. J Am Acad Dermatol 32:436, 1995.
253. Baggish MS. Carbon dioxide laser treatment for condylomata acuminata venereal infections. Obstet Gynecol 55:711, 1980.
254. Ferenczy A. Using the laser to treat vulvar condylomata acuminata and intraepidermal neoplasia. Can Med Assoc J 128:135, 1983.
255. Kryger-Baggesen N, Larsen JF, Pedersen PH. CO_2-laser treatment of condylomata acuminata. Acta Obstet Gynecol Scand 63:341, 1984.
256. Ferenczy A. Treating genital condyloma during pregnancy with the carbon dioxide laser. Am J Obstet Gynecol 148:9, 1984.
257. Reid R. Superficial laser vulvectomy. I. The efficacy of extended superficial ablation for refractory and very extensive condylomas. Am J Obstet Gynecol 151:1047, 1985.
258. Baggish MS. Improved laser techniques for the elimination of genital and extragenital warts. Am J Obstet Gynecol 153:545, 1985.
259. Krebs H-B, Wheelock JB. The CO_2 laser for recurrent and therapy-resistant condylomata acuminata. J Reprod Med 30:489, 1985.
260. Graversen PH, Baggi P, Rosenkilde P. Laser treatment of recurrent urethral condylomata acuminata in men. Scand J Urol Nephrol 24:163, 1990.
261. Larsen J, Petersen CS. The patient with refractory genital warts in the STD-clinic. Dan Med Bull 37:194,1990.
262. Geraci A, Thomas G, Lavigne J, Levy M. Relative efficacy of laser versus radio-frequency ablation of anogenital condylomata. Abstr Int Conf AIDS 6:2020, 1990.
263. Hohenleutner U, Landthaler M, Braun-Falco O. Postoperative adjuvante Therapie mit Interferon-alfa-2b nach Laserchirurgie von Condylomata acuminata. Hautarzt 41:545, 1990.
264. Petersen CS, Bjerring P, Larsen J, et al. Systemic interferon alpha-2b increases the cure rate in laser treated patients with multiple persistent genital warts: a placebo-controlled study. Genitourin Med 67:99, 1991.
265. Nieminen P, Aho M, Lehtinen M, et al. Treatment of genital HPV infection with carbon dioxide laser and systemic interferon alpha-2b. Sex Transm Dis 21:65, 1994.
266. Klutke JJ, Bergman A. Interferon as an adjuvant treatment for genital condyloma acuminatum. Int J Gynaecol Obstet 49:171, 1995.
267. Morris M, Tortolero-Luna G, Malpica A, et al. Cervical intraepithelial neoplasia and cervical cancer. Obstet Gynecol Clin North Am 23:347, 1996.
268. Townsend DE, Richart RM. Cryotherapy and carbon dioxide laser management of cervical intraepithelial neoplasia: a controlled comparison. Obstet Gynecol 61:75, 1983.
269. Mathevet P, Dargent D, Roy M, Beau G. A randomized prospective study comparing three techniques of conization: cold-knife, laser, and LEEP. Gynecol Oncol 54:175, 1994.
270. Bissonnette R, Lui H. Current status of photodynamic therapy in dermatology. Dermatol Clin 15:507, 1997.
271. Abdel-Hady ES, Martin-Hirsch P, Duggan-Keen M, et al. Immunological and viral factors associated with the response of vulval intraepithelial neoplasia to photodynamic therapy. Cancer Res 61:192, 2001.
272. Vesterinen E, Meyer B, Cantell K, Purola E. Topical treatment of flat vaginal condyloma with human leukocyte interferon. Obstet Gynecol 64:535, 1984.
273. Vesterinen E, Meyer B, Purola E, Cantell K. Treatment of vaginal flat condyloma with interferon cream. Lancet 1:157, 1984.
274. Keay S, Teng N, Eisenberg M, et al. Topical interferon for treating condyloma acuminata in women. J Infect Dis 158:934, 1988.
275. Frega A, Stentella P, Direnzi F, et al. Assessment of self application of four topical agents on genital warts in women. J Eur Acad Dermatol Venereol 8:112, 1997.
276. Syed TA, Ahmadpour OA. Human leukocyte derived interferon-alpha in a hydrophilic gel for the treatment of intravaginal warts in women: a placebo-controlled, double-blind study. Int J STD AIDS 9:769, 1998.
277. Gross G, Rogozinski T, Schofer H, et al. Recombinant interferon beta gel as an adjuvant in the treatment of recurrent genital warts: results of a placebo-controlled double-blind study in 120 patients. Dermatology 196:330, 1998.
278. Douglas JM, Rogers M, Judson FN. The effect of asymptomatic infection with HTLV-III on the response of anogenital warts in intralesional treatment with recombinant α_2 interferon. J Infect Dis 154:331, 1986.
279. Armstrong DK, Maw RD, Dinsmore WW, et al. A randomised, double-blind, parallel group study to compare subcutaneous interferon alpha-2a plus podophyllin with placebo plus podophyllin in the treatment of primary condylomata acuminata. Genitourin Med 70:389, 1994.
280. Yliskoski M, Cantell K, Syrjänen K, Syrjänen S. Topical treatment with human leukocyte interferon of HPV 16 infections associated with cervical and vaginal intraepithelial neoplasia. Gynecol Oncol 36:353, 1990.
281. Bornstein J, Ben-David Y, Atad J, et al. Treatment of cervical intraepithelial neoplasia and invasive squamous cell carcinoma by interferon. Obstet Gynecol Surv 48:251, 1993.
282. Rotola A, Costa S, Di Luca D, et al. Beta-interferon treatment of cervical intraepithelial neoplasia: a multicenter clinical trial. Intervirology 38:325, 1995.
283. Gonzalez-Sanchez JL, Martinez-Chequer JC, Barahona-Bustillos E, Andrade-Manzano AF. Randomized placebo-controlled evaluation of intramuscular interferon beta treatment of recurrent human papillomavirus. Obstet Gynecol 97:621, 2001.
284. Sauder DN. Immunomodulatory and pharmacologic properties of imiquimod. J Am Acad Dermatol 43:S6, 2000.
285. Spruance S, Douglas J, Hougham A, et al. Multicenter trial of 5% imiquimod (IQ) cream for the treatment of genital and perianal warts. In: Abstracts 33rd Interscience Conference on Antimicrobial Chemotherapy, 1993, p 1432.
286. Beutner KR, Tyring SK, Trofatter KF Jr, et al. Imiquimod, a patient-applied immune-response modifier for treatment of external genital warts. Antimicrob Agents Chemother 42:789, 1998.
287. Fife KH, Ferenczy A, Douglas JM Jr, et al. Treatment of external genital warts in men using 5% imiquimod cream applied three times a week, once daily, twice daily, or three times a day. Sex Transm Dis 28:226, 2001.
288. Gollnick H, Barasso R, Jappe U, et al. Safety and efficacy of imiquimod 5% cream in the treatment of penile genital warts in uncircumcised men when applied three times weekly or once per day. Int J STD AIDS 12:22, 2001.
289. Gilson RJ, Shupack JL, Friedman-Kien AE, et al. A randomized, controlled, safety study using imiquimod for the topical treatment of anogenital warts in HIV-infected patients: Imiquimod Study Group. AIDS 13:2397, 1999.
290. Conant MA. Immunomodulatory therapy in the management of viral infections in patients with HIV infection. J Am Acad Dermatol 43(Pt 2):S27, 2000.
291. Orfanos CE, Ehlert R, Gollnick H. The retinoids: a review of their clinical pharmacology and therapeutic use. Drugs 34:459, 1987.
292. Eckert RL, Agarwal C, Hembree JR, et al. Human cervical cancer: retinoids, interferon and human papillomavirus. Adv Exp Med Biol 375:31, 1995.
293. Schneider A, Shah K. The role of vitamins in the etiology of cervical neoplasia: an epidemiological review. Arch Gynecol Obstet 246:1, 1989.
294. Mitchell MF, Hittelman WK, Lotan R, et al. Chemoprevention trials and surrogate end point biomarkers in the cervix. Cancer 76(suppl):1956, 1995.
295. Olsen EA, Kelly FF, Vollner RT, et al. Comparative study of systemic interferon alfa-n1 and isotretinoin in the treatment of resistant condylomata acuminata. J Am Acad Dermatol 20:1023, 1989.

296. Handley J, Dinsmore W. Topical tretinoin in the treatment of anogenital warts. Sex Transm Dis 19:181, 1992.
297. Meyskens FL Jr, Surwit E, Moon TE, et al. Enhancement of regression of cervical intraepithelial neoplasia II (moderate dysplasia) with topically applied all-trans-retinoic acid: a randomized trial. J Natl Cancer Inst 86:539, 1994.
298. Ampel NM, Stout ML, Garewal HS. Persistent ulcer associated with human papillomavirus type 33 in a patient with AIDS: successful treatment with isotretinoin. Rev Infect Dis 12:1004, 1990.
299. Del Priore G, Herron MM. Retinoids for vulvar dysplasia in the HIV-infected patient. Int J Gynaecol Obstet 55:77, 1996.
300. Rogers CJ, Gibney MD, Siegfried EC, et al. Cimetidine therapy for recalcitrant warts in adults: is it any better than placebo? J Am Acad Dermatol 41:123, 1999.
301. Wargon O. Cimetidine for mucosal warts in an HIV positive adult. Aust J Dermatol 37:149, 1996.
302. Beutner KR, Reitano MV, Richwald GA, Wiley DJ. External genital warts: report of the American Medical Association Consensus Conference. Clin Infect Dis 27:796, 1998.
303. Von Krogh G, Lacey CJ, Gross G, et al. European course on HPV associated pathology: guidelines for primary care physicians for the diagnosis and management of anogenital warts. Sex Transm Infect 76:162, 2000.
304. Volberding P. Looking behind: time for anal cancer screening. Am J Med 108:674, 2000.
305. Maiman M. Management of cervical neoplasia in human immunodeficiency virus-infected women. J Natl Cancer Inst Monogr 23:43, 1998.
306. Montz FJ. Management of high-grade cervical intraepithelial neoplasia and low-grade squamous intraepithelial lesion and potential complications. Clin Obstet Gynecol 43:394, 2000.
307. Murdoch JB. The case for early intervention ("see and treat") in patients with dyskaryosis on routine cervical screening. Int J STD AIDS 6:415, 1995.
308. Ferenczy A, Choukroun D, Arseneau J. Loop electrosurgical excision procedure for squamous intraepithelial lesions of the cervix: advantages and potential pitfalls. Obstet Gynecol 87:332, 1996.
309. Abramson AL, Shikowitz MJ, Mullooly VM, et al. Variable light-dose effect on photodynamic therapy for laryngeal papillomas. Arch Otolaryngol Head Neck Surg 120:852, 1994.
310. Kaplan JE, Masur H, Holmes KK. Prevention of opportunistic infections in persons infected with human immunodeficiency virus. Clin Infect Dis 25(suppl 3):S299, 1997.
311. Centers for Disease Control and Prevention. 1997 USPHS/IDSA guidelines for the prevention of opportunistic infections in persons infected with human immunodeficiency virus. MMWR Morb Mortal Wkly Rep 46(RR-12):1, 1997.
312. Marlink R, Kao H, Hsieh E. Clinical care issues for women living with HIV and AIDS in the United States. AIDS Res Hum Retroviruses 17:1, 2001.
313. Goldie SJ, Weinstein MC, Kuntz KM, Freedberg KA. The costs, clinical benefits, and cost-effectiveness of screening for cervical cancer in HIV-infected women. Ann Intern Med 130:97, 1999.
314. Wright TC, Hart C, Ellerbrock TV, Lennox J. Treatment of CIN increases vaginal HIV RNA level. In: Abstracts of the 4th Conference on Retroviral Opportunistic Infections, 1997, p 338.
315. Evans BA, Kell PD, Bond RA, MacRae KD. Heterosexual relationships and condom-use in the spread of sexually transmitted diseases to women. Genitourin Med 71:291, 1995.
316. Silverman BG, Gross TP. Use and effectiveness of condoms during anal intercourse: a review. Sex Transm Dis 24:11, 1997.
317. Division of STD Prevention. Prevention of Genital HPV Infection and Sequelae: Report of an External Consultants' Meeting. Atlanta, Centers for Disease Control and Prevention (CDC), 1999.
318. Wen LM, Estcourt CS, Simpson JM, Mindel A. Risk factors for the acquisition of genital warts: are condoms protective? Sex Transm Infect 75:312, 1999.
319. Halperin DT. Heterosexual anal intercourse: prevalence, cultural factors, and HIV infection and other health risks. Part I. AIDS Patient Care STDs 13:717, 1999.
320. Hildesheim A, Brinton LA, Mallin K, et al. Barrier and spermicidal contraceptive methods and risk of invasive cervical cancer. Epidemiology 1:266, 1990.
321. Sokal DC, Hermonat PL. Inactivation of papillomavirus by low concentrations of povidone-iodine. Sex Transm Dis 22:22, 1995.
322. Breitburd F, Coursaget P. Human papillomavirus vaccines. Semin Cancer Biol 9:431, 1999.
323. Da Silva DM, Eiben GL, Fausch SC, et al. Cervical cancer vaccines: emerging concepts and developments. J Cell Physiol 186:169, 2001.
324. Harro CD, Pang Y-YS, Roden RBS, et al. Safety and immunogenicity trial in adult volunteers of a human papillomavirus 16 L1 virus-like particle vaccine. J Natl Cancer Inst 93:284, 2001.
325. Evans TG, Bonnez W, Rose RC, et al. A phase 1 study of a recombinant viruslike particle vaccine against human papillomavirus type 11 in healthy adult volunteers. J Infect Dis 183:1485, 2001.

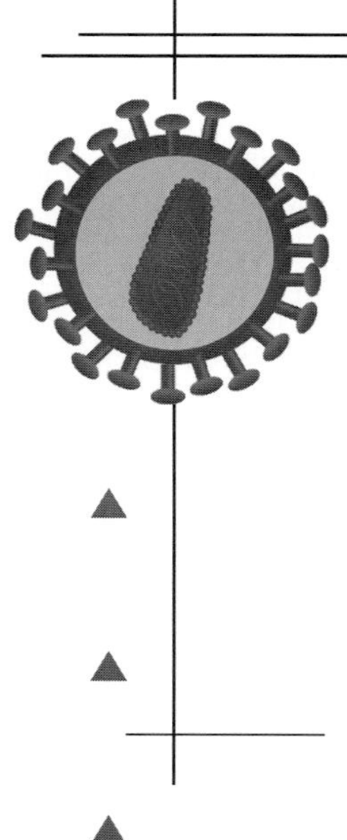

CHAPTER 48

JC Virus Neurologic Infection

Colin D. Hall, MB, ChB

Progressive multifocal leukoencephalopathy (PML) was initially described by Astrom and colleagues in 1958[1] as a complication of chronic leukemia and Hodgkin's disease. It has since been recognized in association with an increasing number of conditions associated with human immunodeficiency. It became more prevalent with the aggressive use of therapeutic immunosuppressive agents during the 1960s and 1970s but was still regarded as a rare disease until the acquired immunodeficiency syndrome (AIDS) epidemic, with its resulting large pool of immunocompromised patients. PML is an AIDS-defining illness and one of the common opportunistic infections of the brain in this population, found in up to 8% of patients at autopsy.[2–5] In 10% to 55% of cases it has been reported as the presenting manifestation of human immunodeficiency virus (HIV) infection.[6–8] PML is rare in those with pediatric AIDS, but it does occur.[9,10]

In 1971 Padgett and colleagues isolated the viral agent etiologically responsible for PML from the brain of an infected patient, and named it JC virus (JCV), from the initials of the patient.[11] JCV is a polyomavirus. It is similar to the other human polyomavirus, BK, and to simian immunodeficiency virus 40 (SV40). JCV is ubiquitous in humans and is usually acquired by the time of adolescence; more than 70% of the adult population generate a humoral response.[12,13] The precise mode of transmission is not established, although it is suspected to be via the respiratory tract.[1]

There are no known symptoms associated with the initial infection with JCV, and the only known clinical manifestations of PML are the results of nervous system involvement. It has an insidious onset with progressive neurologic dysfunction, generally without fever or headache. It is primarily a disease of white matter but sometimes involves gray matter structures and may therefore result in a wide spectrum of neurologic symptoms and signs. The most common initial clinical findings reported in AIDS patients with PML include painless progressive monoparetic or hemiparetic limb weakness or sensory loss, gait difficulty, and visual disturbance. Subtle or overt alteration of mental status may accompany other manifestations; occasionally the initial presentation is encephalopathy without focal findings. The course is generally rapidly progressive over weeks, with the development of more diffuse lesions, including brain stem disease with cranial nerve involvement and eventually coma with vegetative signs.

▲ DIAGNOSIS

The diagnosis of PML is based primarily on clinical findings and a compatible magnetic resonance imaging (MRI) picture (Figs. 48–1 and 48–2). The diagnosis is confirmed by establishing the presence of JCV and ruling out other opportunistic infections.

The clinical presentation depends on the location of the active infection. Because it may involve any area of the brain, brain stem, or cerebellum, PML must be considered in any patient presenting with central nervous system disease.

Abnormalities seen on computed tomography (CT) scans are typically hypodense white matter lesions without mass effect. Only rarely do these lesions enhance with contrast. MRI is more sensitive than CT and typically reveals more involvement.[14–16] Lesions on MRI are primarily but not exclusively of white matter and appear as single or multiple

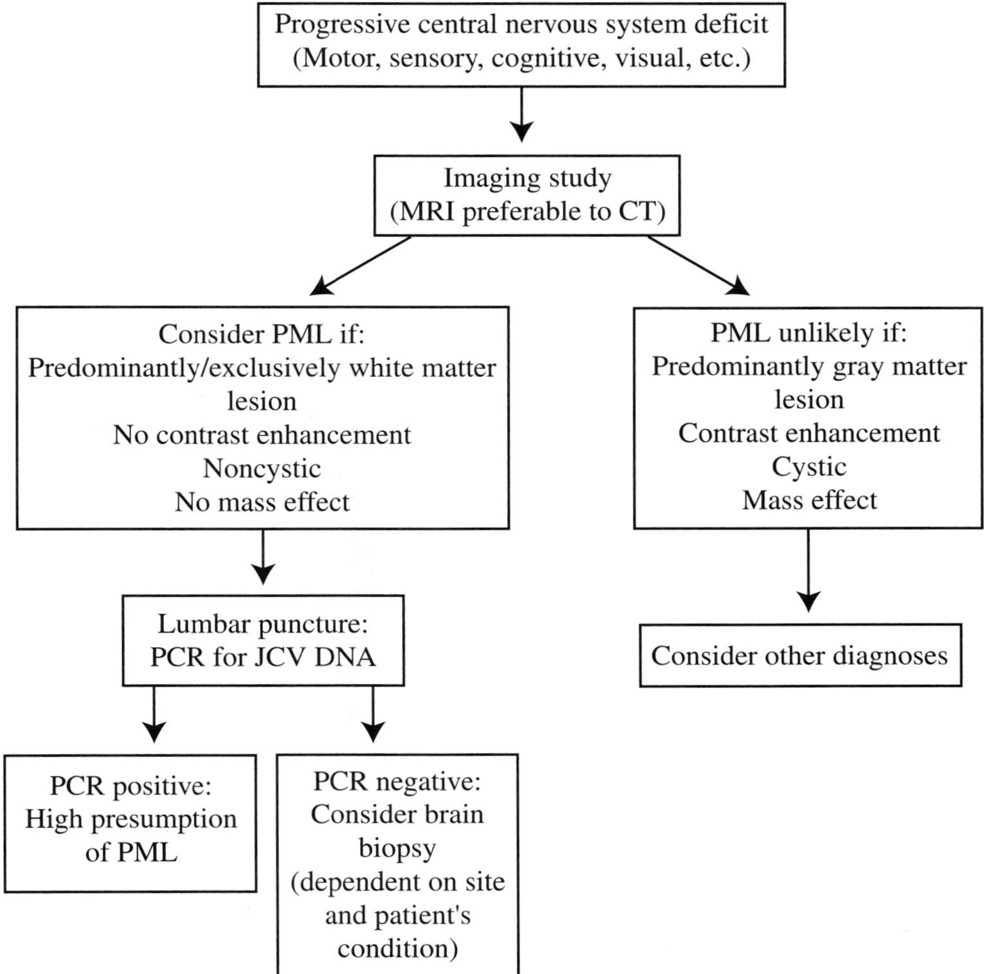

Figure 48–1. Diagnostic algorithm for progressive multifocal leukoencephalopathy (PML).

large or small bright areas on T2-weighted images, again generally without contrast enhancement or mass effect (Fig. 48–2). T1-weighted images are invariably of low density. However, it is not always possible to exclude other lesions, including lymphoma and HIV encephalitis, by MRI. Furthermore, although MRI is of paramount importance as a diagnostic tool, there is no evidence that the number or size of the lesions found has any prognostic significance.[17] Magnetic resonance spectroscopy is currently under evaluation as an additional diagnostic tool.[18] Typically, spectroscopy shows an elevated choline/creatine ratio, but this is not a specific finding.

Routine testing for antibodies to JCV is not of value for establishing the diagnosis of PML. Immunoglobulin G (IgG) antibody identification by hemagglutination inhibition is positive in most healthy adults worldwide. The titer does not rise with active disease, and there is generally a lack of IgM antibody in either serum or cerebrospinal fluid (CSF), indicating that PML results from reactivation of a latent infection.[13]

Routine CSF analysis is generally not helpful. Although some elevation of cell count, protein, and immunoglobulin may be found,[2] it is not clear that it occurs more often than in HIV-infected patients without PML.[19]

Until the past few years, the definitive diagnosis has depended on the pathologic examination, although the advent of CSF JCV polymerase chain reaction (PCR) analysis has now minimized the need for brain biopsy. The typical appearance on biopsy is multiple areas of demyelination at the corticomedullary junction, extending in severe cases into large areas of white matter (Fig. 48–3). With advanced disease gray matter may also be involved. The oligodendrocytes have large, deeply staining nuclei, many with inclusions and large numbers of virions (Fig. 48–4). Reactive astrocytosis is generally present, and there may be giant astrocytes similar to those found in glioblastoma multiforme.[20] Neurons are not infected. HIV-infected patients have a higher incidence of large, confluent lesions with prominent necrosis and a higher incidence of marked perivascular inflammatory infiltrates than do patients with other causes of immunocompromise.[21]

Stereotactic brain biopsy causes less morbidity than open biopsy and is generally the preferred procedure,[22,23] but it does not always provide adequate tissue for a defini-

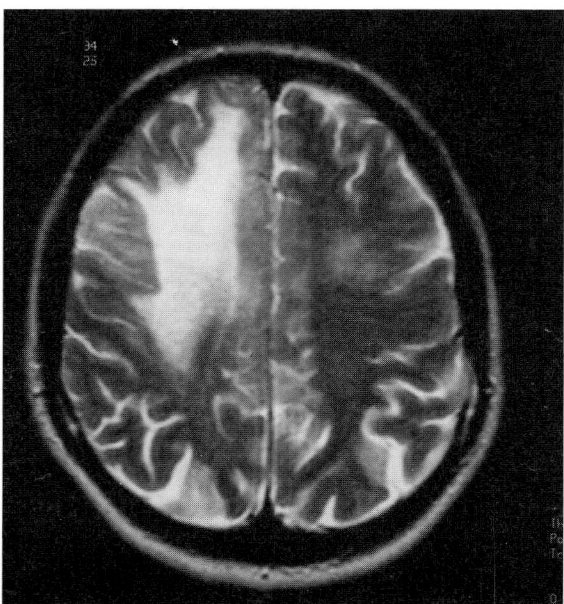

Figure 48–2. T2-weighted MRI scan of the brain in a patient with PML. There is a large lesion in the right anterior hemisphere, with smaller lesions in the left frontal lobe and both occipital lobes.

tive microscopic diagnosis. The use of in situ hybridization techniques[24] and immunocytochemistry increases the diagnostic potential of stereotactic biopsy, and these are useful adjunctive diagnostic tools.[25,26] Utilizing the PCR, JCV DNA has been identified in the brains of HIV-infected patients with and without PML and in uninfected control brains. This presumably reflects indolent infection of brain tissue and suggests that the PCR of brain biopsy tissue is too sensitive for a specific diagnosis of active disease.[27–29]

Since the early 1990s there has been great interest in the possibility that analysis of easily accessible body fluids can provide a reliable method for diagnosis, sparing the patient the need for brain biopsy. It is clear that the kidney may act as a viral reservoir in healthy populations; and in several series 20% to 80% of urine samples from healthy adults with no specific immune deficiency have yielded isolates of JCV.[30,31] PCR in urine is thus unsuitable for diagnosing the disease. The same is true for peripheral blood evaluation. Fifteen percent of samples from healthy subjects without immunocompromise yield positive JCV PCR results.[32] Tornatore et al. detected JCV DNA in lymphocytes in 89% of patients with PML and in 38% of asymptomatic HIV-positive patients[33]; Dubois et al. found JCV DNA in lymphocytes in more than 40% of HIV-infected patients without PML.[34]

Much greater specificity has been achieved through the evaluation of CSF. Weber et al. identified JCV DNA in CSF from each of three HIV-infected patients with PML but in none of 30 HIV-infected patients without PML.[35] Later the same group reported CSF analysis from 28 patients with PML and 82 HIV-infected patients without PML. JCV DNA was detected in 82% of the PML patients and none of the controls.[36] De Luca and colleagues evaluated CSF from 19 patients with clinical PML and 83 patients with advanced HIV disease but no evidence of PML. Nested PCR had 74% sensitivity and 100% specificity, with no positive results in the patients without PML.[37] McGuire et al., using conditions optimized to detect one viral copy in 50 μg CSF, reported 92% sensitivity and 92% specificity.[38] Thus it is now accepted, even for clinical trials, that a firm diagnosis of PML can be reached based on typical clinical and radiologic appearances plus a positive JCV DNA analysis in CSF. Brain biopsy confirmation would then be required only if the CSF evaluation was negative, if the clinical picture was

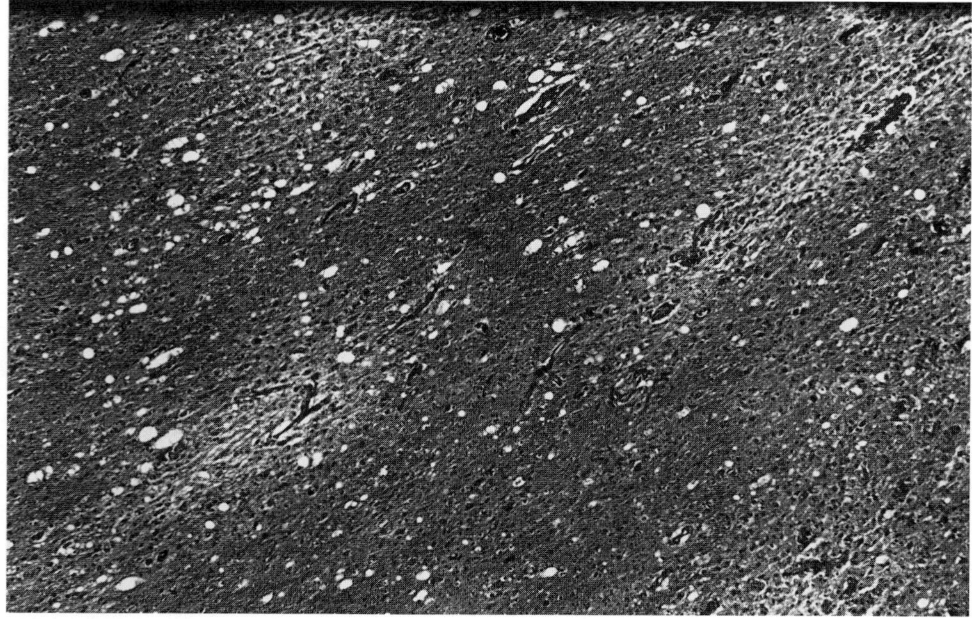

Figure 48–3. Multiple foci of demyelination unaccompained by significant inflammatory infiltrate. (×45)

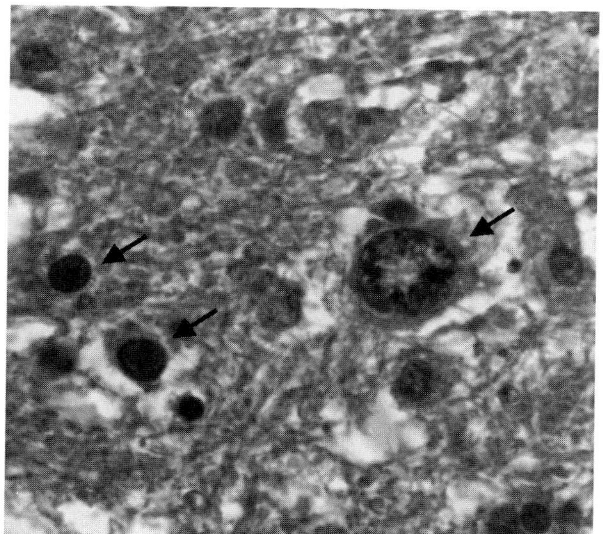

Figure 48–4. Hyperchromatic, enlarged nuclei of infected oligodendrocytes (small arrows) and atypical bizarre astrocyte (large arrow). (×150)

atypical, or if there was concern about a concomitant condition, such as lymphoma. Current treatment trials are being based on this algorithm. It is generally accepted that more than 90% of patients with PML have positive JCV PCR in the CSF, and this does not occur in normal subjects or HIV-infected patients without PML. However a number of studies have demonstrated that all CSF samples are not positive; so in cases with a high clinical suspicion and an initially negative PCR, repeat CSF evaluation may be helpful. A further complication when interpreting the CSF results is the observation in a number of trials that treatment with highly active antiretroviral therapy (HAART) may be associated with disappearance of JCV from the CSF.[39,40] The JCV viral load in the CSF also appears to be of prognostic value: the higher the number of copies, the worse the prognosis.[41,42] PCR for JCV is available commercially through the laboratories listed in Table 48–1.

▲ **Table 48–1.** LABORATORIES OFFERING JC VIRUS POLYMERASE CHAIN REACTION

Molecular Microbiology Mayo Medical Laboratories Mayo Clinic 200 First Street S.W. Rochester, MN 55905 (Tel. 1-800-533-1710)
Diagnostic Virology Laboratory University of Colorado Health Sciences Center 4200 East 9th Avenue Room MS1632 Denver, CO 80220 (Tel. 303-372-8182)
Virolab, Inc. 1204 10th Street Berkeley, CA 94710 (Tel. 510-524-6201)

It is recognized among clinicians that occasional cases appear clinically and radiographically to be typical of PML but do not have JCV PCR positivity in the CSF or in areas of demyelinating brain tissue. It is not clear whether these cases are due to JCV mutation that is not labeled by current probes or to a different, as yet unidentified virus.

▲ THERAPY

Other than the maintenance of immune function, there are no measures for prophylaxis or prevention of PML. With the emerging exception of optimizing HAART for HIV therapy, no drugs have proven to be of value against JCV.

The prognosis for HIV-infected patients who develop PML is grave. Wiley and colleagues theorized that the prognosis may be worse in HIV infection because JCV, in addition to its direct toxicity, may increase ingress to the brain of HIV-infected macrophages.[43] Median survival from the time of diagnosis has generally been 2.6 to 4.0 months.[21,39,44] However, approximately 10% of HIV-infected patients have a more protracted course, with stabilization over months or years and occasionally with apparent reduction or resolution of lesions.[45,46] This has made it difficult to assess treatment efficacy.

Completed Studies

The infrequency of the disease before the AIDS epidemic precluded the development of adequately controlled studies, and therapeutic measures were based on anecdotal case reports using agents with theoretical potential efficacy. A number of such agents have been tried, some suggesting benefit in single cases or small series.

Immunocompromise is a common factor in the development of PML. In the AIDS population, antiretroviral agents, by improving immune function, might be expected to have the potential to reverse or retard the progression of disease. There is strong evidence to support this from uncontrolled case reports and incidence studies of populations before and after the era of HAART. In 1988 Fiala et al. first reported improvement in an AIDS patient with suspected PML following the administration of zidovudine (AZT).[47] In 1990 Conway et al. reported a case of biopsy-proven PML in an AIDS patient with marked improvement following AZT administration.[48] Britton and colleagues reported that 7 of 26 patients stabilized or showed improvement on antiretroviral therapy alone.[49] Not all investigators reported positive results during the pre-HAART era.[50] The ACTG 243 study, primarily designed to evaluate cytosine arabinoside (ara-C), encouraged the use of moderately high-dose AZT (900 mg/day) in combination with another antiretroviral, generally didanosine (ddI) or zalcitabine (ddC), in each of its three arms. There was no control arm against which to compare the effects of antiretroviral therapy, but the mean survival in the three arms, approximately 3 months, suggests there was no significant improvement over historical survival figures.[39] Based on retrospective and prospective cohort studies and individual case reports, there is good evidence that treatment with HAART has resulted in improved survival of patients with PML.[51–55] However, even in the studies showing the best responses, most patients continue to decline and succumb to the disease.

Other nucleoside analogues, which interfere with DNA synthesis, have proven efficacy against some viral infections. However, these agents may have different antiviral effects against different viruses within the same family.[13] Adenine arabinoside[56,57] and iododeoxyuridine[58] have been unsuccessful in altering the clinical course of PML. Isolated reports and small case studies suggested encouraging results with ara-C, which has fairly powerful antiviral effects in cell culture studies.[59] These reports suggested that some patients benefited from intravenous treatment, some from intrathecal treatment, and some from a combination; and they included both HIV-infected patients and those with other reasons for immunocompromise.[49,60–65]

Not all investigators have reported positive effects from ara-C.[66–68] To address the question, the Neurologic AIDS Research Consortium, in conjunction with the AIDS Clinical Trials Group, designed a three-arm study (ACTG 243) to compare the efficacy of high-dose antiretroviral therapy alone versus antiretroviral therapy plus either intravenous or intrathecal ara-C (Table 48–2). The study was terminated in June 1993 after interim analysis demonstrated no benefit in either the intravenous or the intrathecal arm; and ara-C, which is associated with major bone marrow toxicity, can no longer be recommended as therapy when delivered by intravenous or intraventricular injection.[39]

An interesting development in the ara-C story is being pursued by Levy and colleagues at Northwestern University. They have shown in animal studies that infusion of the drug into the ventricular system results in extremely low penetration of the brain parenchyma. They have also shown that continuous perfusion in nanomolar dosage by a catheter inserted into the brain substance rather than the ventricle leads to highly satisfactory drug levels in the brain extracellular space, with apparent safety, at least in the animal model. Levy is currently conducting a small, highly intensive Phase I open-label study in humans to test the safety of this method of administration. If it is found to be successful, future retesting of the compound using this means of delivery may be indicated. Other than the Levy study there is no possibility for current treatment using this approach.[69]

On the theory that PML is the result of activated JCV-infected B lymphocytes gaining access to the brain, and because heparin sulfate in animal models prevents activated lymphocytes from crossing the blood-brain barrier,[70] Major et al. conducted an uncontrolled trial of low-dose heparin sulfate in HIV-infected patients with PML and reported initially encouraging results.[13] Subjects treated with 5000 units of subcutaneous heparin twice a day appeared to form fewer new lesions than a control group, but the numbers were too small for statistical significance (S. Houff, personal communication).

Interferon-α

Based on its beneficial effect on the treatment of other papillomaviruses, including human papillomavirus-associated genital warts and laryngeal papillomatosis,[71,72] and on its effect on SV40 suppression in vitro,[73] interferon-α has been postulated as therapy for PML. There are reports of the efficacy of interferon-α in non-AIDS PML.[74,75] The two reports in AIDS patients have not been encouraging. In an uncontrolled, open-label multicenter study, Berger et al. treated 15 patients with biopsy-confirmed PML with up to 18 million units of interferon-α per day by subcutaneous injection.[76] Although two patients appeared to stabilize during treatment, there was reason to believe both had the protracted form of the disease described in 10% of AIDS patients, rather than a response to the medication. Counihan et al. treated four AIDS patients with pathologically confirmed PML with 5 million to 10 million units of subcutaneous interferon-α per day for 4 to 12 weeks and noted no clinical response.[77] McArthur presented a retrospective analysis of the Johns Hopkins University experience with interferon-α in HIV infection.[78] Forty patients were treated with 3 million units per day. Although there was an initial impression that survival was improved, multivariate analysis demonstrated that the difference was entirely explained by the concomitant use of HAART.[79]

Cidofovir

Cidofovir is a nucleoside analogue that is highly active in vitro against mouse and primate polyomaviruses, including SV40.[80] It also has a demonstrable in vivo antiviral effect against papillomavirus-induced condylomas.[81] It has therapeutic effect in an animal model of cytomegalovirus (CMV) encephalitis[82] and in CMV retinitis in humans,[83,84] suggesting that it crosses the blood-brain barrier. Although it has not been shown to have efficacy against JCV in vitro and indeed showed cellular toxicity,[85] it was thought there was enough reason to evaluate its effects in PML.

▲ **Table 48–2.** TRIALS OF PML THERAPY

Study	Study Design	Result	Comment
Hall[39] (ACTG 243)	Open label, three arms ARVs alone (AZT + ddI/ddC) ARVs + IV Ara-C ARVs + IT Ara-C	No efficacy	Only prospective, biopsy-confirmed study of PML to date
Marra[86] (ACTG 363)	Open label, cidofovir + HAART	No clear benefit	24 Patients; 11 died from PML
Dupont[94]	Open label, topotecon	No clear benefit	11 Patients; 7 died from PML

AraC, cytosine arabinoside; ARVs, antiretrovirals; AZT, zidovudine; ddC, dideoxycytidine; ddI, didanosine; HAART, highly active antiretroviral therapy; IT, intrathecal; PML, progressive multifocal leukoencephalopathy.

There have been a number of reports on the use of cidofovir with in patients PML and AIDS. The ACTG 363 trial studied 24 subjects in an open-label study to evaluate the safety of cidofovir.[86] All were receiving HAART. Of the 24 subjects, 12 died, 11 from progressive PML. Only 13 patients were able to continue to week 8 of the study. Two of them showed more than 25% improvement. This is not convincingly better than in historical controls. Two European studies showed slightly more promise. De Luca et al., in a multicenter observational study, reviewed 26 patients treated with HAART alone and 14 with HAART and cidofovir.[87] Altogether, 24% of the HAART-alone group and 57% of the HAART plus cidofovir group had improved after 2 months, and 87% of the cidofovir-treated patients attained undetectable JC virus DNA in the cerebrospinal fluid (CSF) compared to 42% of those given HAART alone. The 1-year cumulative probability of survival was 0.67 with cidofovir and 0.31 without (log-rank test, $P = 0.01$). Gasnault reviewed the French Hospital Database on HIV in patients with both proven and presumptive PML.[88] Altogether, 22 patients were treated with HAART alone and 24 with HAART and cidofovir. At 4 to 12 months after PML diagnosis the cidofovir-treated group had a significantly better survival rate. There was no difference in the neurologic deficit or in JC virus DNA clearance from the CSF. There have also been case reports of patients with PML on HAART who improved when cidofovir was added.[89]

The treatment has been similar across studies. For example, in the ACTG 363 trial cidofovir was given as 5 mg/kg IV over 1 hour.[86] Three doses of probenecid were given orally with each administration: 1.5 g 3 hours prior to infusion and then 750 mg 2 hours after infusion and again 8 hours after infusion. The infusion was weekly for the first two doses, then every other week for a total of 13 doses.

The concomitant antiretroviral agents used in these studies have not been consistent, and both the degree of disability and the time between diagnosis and treatment have varied. Thus although there is some encouragement, and there may be enough evidence to pursue a more rigorous study, the positive results must be evaluated with reserve, particularly in light of the ara-C experience.

Topoisomerase Inhibitors

The JC virus has tissue tropism for oligodendrocytes and to a lesser extent for astrocytes but not for neurons. The primary determinant of this neurotropism is believed to be the glial-restricted expression of the viral early protein.[90,91] One step in this early DNA replication depends on recruitment of the cellular enzyme topoisomerase 1. The enzyme binds to one of the DNA strands. Causing a nick in the strand allows the helix to swivel, releasing topologic strain. The topoisomerase inhibitor camptothecin and its analogues have been shown to block SV40 and JCV replication in vitro,[92] and camptothecin and topotecan inhibit JCV DNA replication in glioma cells.[93] Controlled clinical studies have been designed using the camptothecin analogues topotecan and 9-aminocamptothecin. Topotecan has less protein binding than camptothecan and reaches CSF levels that are 30% those in blood. Dupont et al. have reported on the results of treatment of 11 patients[94]; 8 showed no clinical response, and 7 died of PML, although one showed improvement on MRI. The other three subjects did appear to show clinical improvement; two are surviving after 140 weeks, and one died from PML after 84 weeks. Hematologic toxicity was common. In a smaller treatment trial of topotecan, Houff found a high degree of toxicity with no clear benefit (S. Houff, personal communication).

Interleukin-2

Przepiorka et al. reported on a patient with low-grade lymphoma without HIV infection who developed PML and responded to treatment with continuous infusion of interleukin-2 (IL-2) at 0.5 MU/m^2/day.[95] The improvement had persisted for over a year after therapy was terminated. There was complete resolution of symptoms, and a general improvement in immune parameters. The investigators suggested that the improvement was due to up-regulation of cytokines by IL-2. Although this observation deserves further study, it represents only one patient, without HIV infection; hence at this stage IL-2 cannot be recommended as routine therapy.

Drugs in Development

There are no drugs currently in development.

▲ RECOMMENDATIONS

Progressive multifocal leukoencephalopathy remains one of the most devastating opportunistic infections associated with AIDS. It is important to rule out treatable infections of the brain, including toxoplasmosis, lymphoma, CMV infection, syphilis, cryptococcosis, and other fungal infections. This is generally possible by evaluating the clinical presentation in combination with CSF analysis and neuroradiologic evaluation. Confirmatory diagnosis of PML by brain biopsy is now rarely required, even in the setting of clinical trials. In the face of a negative PCR, the decision to proceed to brain biopsy must be made individually, taking into account the patient's clinical condition, the likelihood of missing a treatable condition, and the site of the lesion(s) versus the danger of biopsy.

At this time the first approach to treatment should be to maximize the patient's ability to resist progression using HAART. There is no information on whether there is an advantage for any particular HAART regimen.

For patients who fail to respond to HAART alone, the treating physician should consider the addition of cidofovir, although its benefit is far from proven. At least 4 weeks of HAART therapy appears to be required before a beneficial effect becomes apparent; but the prognosis is poor enough that if there is continued rapid neurologic decline even during the first month of HAART it may be reasonable to initiate cidofovir emergently. The fact that up to 10% of patients have a more protracted course allows us to offer some hope to patients and their families, but at the same time they should be warned that in most cases the average survival duration from diagnosis continues to be only a few months.

REFERENCES

1. Astrom KE, Mancell EL, Richardson EP. Progressive multifocal leukoencephalopathy: a hitherto unrecognized complication of chronic lymphatic leukemia and Hodgkin's disease. Brain 81:93, 1958.
2. Berger JR, Kaszovitz B, Post JD, et al. Progressive multifocal leukoencephalopathy associated with human immunodeficiency virus infection. Ann Intern Med 107:78, 1987.
3. Petito CK, Cho ES, Lemann W, et al. Neuropathology of acquired immunodeficiency syndrome (AIDS): an autopsy review. J Neuropathol Exp Neurol 45:635, 1986.
4. Krupp LB, Lipton RB, Swerdlow ML, et al. Progressive multifocal leukoencephalopathy: clinical and radiographic features. Ann Neurol 17:344, 1985.
5. Lang W, Miklossy J, Deruaz JP, et al. Neuropathology of acquired immunodeficiency syndrome (AIDS): a report of 135 consecutive cases from Switzerland. Acta Neuropathol (Berl) 77:379, 1989.
6. Levy RM, Bredesen DE, Rosenblum ML. Neurological manifestations of the acquired immune deficiency syndrome (AIDS): experience at UCSF and review of the literature. J Neurosurg 62:475, 1985.
7. Hansman ML, Whiteman MD, Donovan Post MJ, et al. Progressive multifocal leukoencephalopathy in 47 HIV-seropositive patients: neuroimaging with clinical and pathological correlation. Radiology 187:233, 1993.
8. Li A, Cook D. Symptomatology and clinical course in AIDS patients with progressive multifocal leukoencephalopathy (PML). In: Abstracts of the XIth International Conference on AIDS, Vancouver, 1996, p 105, abstract We.B.3282.
9. Berger JR, Scott G, Albrecht, J, et al. Progressive multifocal leukoencephalopathy in HIV-1 infected children. AIDS 6:837, 1992.
10. Vandersteenhoven JJ, Dbaino G, Boyko OB, et al. Progressive multifocal leukoencephalopathy in pediatric acquired immunodeficiency syndrome. Pediatr Infect Dis J 11:232, 1992.
11. Padgett BL, Walker DL, ZuRhein GM, et al. Cultivation of papova-like virus from human brain with progressive multifocal leukoencephalopathy. Lancet 1:1257, 1971.
12. Walker DL, Padgett BL. The epidemiology of human polyoma viruses. In: Sever JL, Madden DL (eds) Polyomaviruses and Human Neurological Diseases. New York, Alan R. Liss, 1983, p 99.
13. Major EO, Amemiya K, Tornatore CS, et al. Pathogenesis and molecular biology of progressive multifocal leukoencephalopathy, the JC virus-induced demyelinating disease of the human brain. Clin Microbiol Rev 5:49, 1992.
14. Trotot PM, Vazeux R, Yamashita HK, et al. MRI pattern of progressive multifocal leukoencephalopathy in AIDS: pathological correlations. J Neuroradiol 17:233, 1990.
15. Mark AS, Atlas SW. Progressive multifocal leukoencephalopathy in patients with AIDS: appearance on MR images. Radiology 173:517, 1989.
16. Whiteman ML, Post MJ, Berger JR, et al. Progressive multifocal leukoencephalopathy in 47 HIV seropositive patients: neuroimaging with clinical and pathological correlation. Radiology 187:233, 1993.
17. Post M, Yiannoutsos C, Dimpson D, et al. Progressive multifocal leukoencephalopathy in AIDS: are there any MR findings useful to patient management and predictive of patient survival. Am J Neuroradiol 20:1896, 1999.
18. Chang L, Miller B, McBride D, et al. Brain lesions in patients with AIDS: H-1 MR spectroscopy. Radiology 197:525, 1995.
19. Hall CD, Snyder CR, Messenheimer JA, et al. Cerebrospinal fluid in human immunodeficiency virus infection. Ann Clin Lab Sci 22:139, 1992.
20. Walker DL. Progressive multifocal leukoencephalopathy. In: Vinken PJ, Brun GW (eds) Handbook of Clinical Neurology, vol 3. Amsterdam, Elsevier Science, 1985, p 503.
21. Kuchelmeister K, Gullotta F, Bergmann M, et al. Die progressive multifokale Leukoenzephalopathie (PML) bei AIDS: morphologische und topographische Besonderheiten. Verh Dtsch Ges Pathol 75:189, 1991.
22. Chappell ET, Gutherie BL, Orenstein J. The role of stereotactic biopsy in the management of HIV-related focal brain lesions. Neurosurgery 30:825, 1992.
23. MacArthyr RD, Nandi P, McMillen L, et al. CT guided brain biopsy findings in HIV infected persons: a retrospective review of 44 cases at an urban medical center. In: Abstracts of the XIth International Conference on AIDS, Vancouver, 1996, p 106, abstract We.B.3286.
24. Greenlee J, Kenney PM. Immunoenzymatic labelling of JC papovavirus T antigen in brains of patients with progressive multifocal leukoencephalopathy. Acta Neuropathol (Berl) 71:150, 1986.
25. Hulette CM, Downey BT, Burger PC. Progressive multifocal leukoencephalopathy: diagnosis by in situ hybridization with a bioactinylated JC virus DNA probe using an automated histomatic code-on slide stainer. Am J Surg Pathol 15:791, 1991.
26. Aksamit A. Nonradioactive in situ hybridization in progressive multifocal leukoencephalopathy. Mayo Clin Proc 68:899, 1993.
27. Quinlivan EB, Norris M, Bouldin TW, et al. Subclinical central nervous system infection with JC virus in patients with AIDS. J Infect Dis 16:80, 1992.
28. Elsner C, Dorries K. Evidence of human polyomavirus BK and JC infection in normal brain tissue. Virology 191:72, 1992.
29. White FA, Ishaq M, Stoner GL, et al. JC virus DNA is present in many human brain samples from patients without progressive multifocal leukoencephalopathy. J Virol 66:5726, 1992.
30. Agostini HT, Ryschkewitsch CF, Stoner GL. Genotype profile of human polyomavirus JC excreted in urine of immunocompetent individuals. J Clin Microbiol 34:159, 1996.
31. Martin JD, Padgett BL, Walker DL. Characterization of tissue culture-induced heterogenicity in DNA from independent isolates of JC virus. J Gen Virol 64:2271, 1983.
32. Clifford DB, Major EO. The biology of JC virus and progressive multifocal leukoencephalopathy. J Neurovirol 7:279, 2001.
33. Tornatore C, Berger JR, Houff SA, et al. Detection of JC virus DNA in peripheral lymphocytes from patients with and without progressive multifocal leukoencephalopathy. Ann Neurol 32:454, 1992.
34. Dubois VL, Lafon ME, Ragnaud JM, et al. JC virus mRNA in the peripheral blood of JC-positive HIV-infected patients. In: Abstracts of the XIth International Conference on AIDS, Vancouver, 1996, p 262, abstract Th.A.4054.
35. Weber T, Turner RW, Frey SE, et al. Progressive multifocal leukoencephalopathy diagnosed by amplification of JC virus-specific DNA from cerebrospinal fluid. AIDS 8:49, 1994.
36. Weber T, Turner RW, Frey S, et al. Specific diagnosis of progressive multifocal leukoencephalopathy by polymerase chain reaction. J Infect Dis 169:1138, 1994.
37. De Luca A, Cingolani A, Linzanlone A, et al. Improved detection of JC virus DNA in cerebrospinal fluid for diagnosis of AIDS-related progressive multifocal leukoencephalopathy. J Clin Microbiol 34:1343, 1996.
38. McGuire D, Barhite S, Hollander H, et al. JC virus DNA in cerebrospinal fluid of human immunodeficiency virus-infected patients: predictive value for progressive multifocal leukoencephalopathy. Ann Neurol 37:395, 1995.
39. Hall C, Dafni U, Simpson D, et al. Failure of cytarabine in progressive multifocal leukoencephalopathy associated with human immunodeficiency virus infection. N Engl J Med 338:1345, 1998.
40. Giudici B, Vaz B, Bossolasco S, et al. Highly active antiretroviral therapy and progressive multifocal leukencephalopathy: effects on cerebrospinal fluid markers of JC virus replication and immune response. Clin Infect Dis 30:95, 2000.
41. Yiannoutsos C, Major E, Curfman B, et al. Relation of JC virus DNA in the cerebrospinal fluid to survival in acquired immunodeficiency syndrome patients with biopsy proven progressive multifocal leukoencephalopathy. Ann Neurol 45:817, 1999.
42. Gasnault J, Taoufik Y, Goujard C, et al. Prolonged survival without neurological improvement in patients with AIDS-related progressive multifocal leukoencephalopathy on potent combined antiretroviral therapy. J Neurovirol 5:421, 1999.
43. Wiley CA, Grafe M, Kennedy C, et al. Human immunodeficiency virus (HIV) and JC virus in acquired immune deficiency syndrome (AIDS) patients with progressive multifocal leukoencephalopathy. Acta Neuropathol (Berl) 76:338, 1988.
44. Karahalios D, Breit R, Dal Canto MC, et al. Progressive multifocal leukoencephalopathy in patients with HIV infection: lack of impact of early diagnosis by stereotactic brain biopsy. J Acquir Immune Defic Syndr 5:1030, 1992.
45. Berger J, Muke L. Prolonged survival and partial recovery in AIDS-associated progressive multifocal leukoencephalopathy. Neurology 38:1060, 1988.
46. Berger JR, Pall L, Whiteman M. Progressive multifocal leukoencephalopathy in HIV infection. Neurology 46:A286, 1996.
47. Fiala M, Cone LA, Cohen N, et al. Responses of neurologic complications of AIDS to 3′-azido-3′-dithymidine and 9-(1,3-dihydroxy-2-propoxymethyl) guanine. 1. Clinical features. Rev Infect Dis 10:250, 1988.
48. Conway B, Halliday WC, Brunham RC. Human immunodeficiency virus-associated progressive multifocal leukoencephalopathy: apparent response to 3′-azido-3′-deoxythymidine. Rev Infect Dis 12:479, 1990.

49. Britton CB, Romagnoli M, Sisti M, et al. Analysis of outcome and response to intrathecal ara-C in 26 patients. In: Abstracts of the Conference on Neuroscience of HIV Infection: Basic and Clinical Frontiers, Amsterdam, July 1992, p 40.
50. Garrote FJ, Molina JA, Lacambra C, et al. The inefficacy of zidovudine (AZT) in progressive multifocal leukoencephalopathy (PML) associated with the acquired immunodeficiency syndrome (AIDS). Rev Clin Esp 187:404, 1990.
51. Tassie JM, Gasnault J, Benata M, et al. Survival improvement of AIDS-related progressive multifocal leukoencephalopathy in the era of protease inhibitors. AIDS 13:1881, 1999.
52. Bethany E, Aromin C, Flaningan TP, et al. Prolonged remission of AIDS-associated progressive multifocal leukoencephalopathy with combined antiretroviral therapy. In: Abstracts of the XIth International Conference on AIDS, Vancouver, 1996, p 222, abstract Th.B.183.
53. Tashima K, Farrar D, Elliot NC, et al. Resolution of AIDS-related opportunistic infections with addition of protease inhibitor treatment. In: Abstracts of the 4th Conference on Retroviruses and Opportunistic Infections, Washington, DC. Alexandria, VA, Westover Management Group, 1997, p 129, abstract 355.
54. Clifford D, Neurologic AIDS Research Consortium. Natural history of progressive multifocal leukoencephalopathy in AIDS modified by antiretroviral therapy. J Neurovirol 4:346, 1998.
55. De Luca A, Giancola ML, Ammassari A, et al. The effects of potent antiretroviral therapy and JC virus load in cerebrospinal fluid on clinical outcome of patients with AIDS-associated progressive multifocal leukoencephalopathy. J Infect Dis 182:1077, 2000.
56. Rand KH, Johnson KP, Rubenstein LJ, et al. Adenine arabinoside in the treatment of progressive multifocal leukoencephalopathy: use of virus containing cells in the urine to assess response to therapy. Ann Neurol 1:458, 1977.
57. Wolinsky JS, Johnson KP, Rand K, et al. Progressive multifocal leukoencephalopathy: clinical pathological correlates and failure of a drug trial in two patients. Trans Am Neurol Assoc 101:81, 1976.
58. Taray D, Holden EM, Segarra JM, et al. 5-Iodo-2-deoxyuridine (IUDR) (NSC-396621) given intraventricularly in the treatment of progressive multifocal leukoencephalopathy. J Infect Dis 162:838, 1973.
59. Zaky DA, Betts RF, Douglas RG, et al. Varicella-zoster virus and subcutaneous cytarabine: correlation of in vitro sensitivities to blood levels. Antimicrob Agents Chemother 7:229, 1975.
60. Bauer WR, Turel AP, Johnson KP. Progressive multifocal leukoencephalopathy and cytarabine. JAMA 226:174, 1973.
61. Marriott PJ, O'Brien MD, Mackenzie IC, et al. Progressive multifocal leukoencephalopathy: remission with cytarabine. J Neurol Neurosurg Psychiatry 38:205, 1975.
62. O'Riordan T, Daly PA, Hutchinson M, et al. Progressive multifocal leukoencephalopathy: remission with cytarabine. J Infect 20:51, 1990.
63. Portegies P, Algra AR, Hollak CE, et al. Response to cytarabine in progressive multifocal leukoencephalopathy in AIDS. Lancet 337:680, 1991.
64. Nicoli F, Chave B, Peragut JC, et al. Efficacy of cytarabine in progressive multifocal leukoencephalopathy in AIDS. Lancet 339:306, 1992.
65. Lidman C, Lindqvist L, Mathiesen T, et al. Progressive multifocal leukoencephalopathy in AIDS. AIDS 5:1039, 1990.
66. Antoniri A, De Luca A, Ammassari A, et al. Failure of cytarabine and increased JC virus-DNA burden in the cerebrospinal fluid of patients with AIDS-related progressive multifocal leukoencephalopathy. AIDS 8:7, 1994.
67. Van Horn GF, Bastien FO, Moake JL. Progressive multifocal leukoencephalopathy: failure of response to corticosteroids, transfer factor and cytarabine. Neurology 28:794, 1978.
68. Urtizberea JA, Flament-Saillour M, Clair B, et al. Cytarabine for progressive multifocal leukoencephaly (PML) in AIDS patients. Int Conf AIDS 9:421, 1993.
69. Levy RM, Major R, Ali MJ, et al. Convection-enhanced intraparenchymal delivery (CEID) of cytosine arabinoside (AraC) for the treatment of HIV-related progressive multifocal leukoencephalopathy. J Neurovirol 7:386, 2001.
70. Houff SA, Major EO, Katz D, et al. Involvement of JC virus-infected mononuclear cells from the bone marrow and spleen in the pathogenesis of progressive multifocal leukoencephalopathy. N Engl J Med 318:301, 1988.
71. Howley PM, Schlegel R. The human papilloma viruses: an overview. Am J Med 85:155, 1988.
72. Finter NB, Chapman S, Dowd P, et al. The use of interferon alpha in virus infections. Drugs 42:749, 1991.
73. Yamamoto K, Yamaguchi N, Kinichrio O. Mechanism of interferon-induced inhibition of early simian virus 40 (SV40) function. Virology 68:58, 1975.
74. Colosimo C, Lebon P, Martelli M, et al. Alpha interferon therapy in a case of probable progressive multifocal leukoencephalopathy. Acta Neurol Belg 1:24, 1992.
75. Steiger MJ, Tarnesby G, Gable S, et al. Successful outcome of progressive multifocal leukoencephalopathy with cytarabine and interferon. Ann Neurol 33:407, 1993.
76. Berger JR, Pall L, McArthur J, et al. A pilot study of recombinant alpha 2a interferon in the treatment of AIDS-related progressive multifocal leukoencephalopathy. Neurology 42(suppl 3):257, 1992.
77. Counihan TJ, Venna N, Craven D, et al. Alpha interferon in AIDS-related progressive multifocal leukoencephalopathy. J Neuro-AIDS 1:79, 1996.
78. Huang SS, Skolasky RL, Dal Pan GJ, et al. Survival prolongation in HIV-associated progressive multifocal leukoencephalopathy treated with alpha-interferon: an observational study. J Neurovirol 4:324, 1998.
79. Geshwind MD, Skolasky RI, Royal WS, McArthur JC. The relative contributions of HAART and alpha-interferon for therapy of progressive multifocal leukoencephalopathy in AIDS. J Neurovirol 7:353, 2001.
80. Andrei G, Snoeck R, Vandeputte M, et al. Activity of various compounds against murine and human polyomaviruses. Antimicrob Agents Chemother 41:587, 1997.
81. Snoeck R, Van Ranst M, Andrei G, et al. Treatment of anogenital papillomavirus infection with an acyclic nucleoside phosphate analogue. N Engl J Med 333:943, 1995.
82. Neyts J, Sobis H, Snoeck R, et al. Efficacy of (S)-1-(3-hydroxy-2-phosphonylmethoxypropyl)-cytosine and 9-(1,3-dihydroxyl-2-propoxymethyl)-guanine in the treatment of intracerebral murine cytomegalovirus infections in immunocompetent and immunodeficient mice. Eur J Clin Microbiol Infect Dis 12:269, 1993.
83. Polis M, Spooner K, Baird B, et al. Anticytomegaloviral activity and safety of cidofovir in patients with human immunodeficiency virus infection and cytomegalovirus viruria. Antimicrob Agents Chemother 39:882, 1995.
84. Lalezari J, Kemper C, Stagg R, et al. A randomized, controlled study of the safety and efficacy of intravenous cidofovir (CDV, HPMPC) for the treatment of relapsing cytomegalovirus retinitis in patients with AIDS. In: Abstracts of the XIth International Conference on AIDS, Vancouver, 1996, p 26, abstract Th.B.304.
85. Ho J, Major EO. The efficacy of nucleoside analogs against JC virus multiplication in a persistently infected human fetal brain cell line. J Neurovirol 4:451, 1998.
86. Marra C, Rajicic N, Barker D, et al. Prospective pilot study of cidofovir for HIV-associated progressive multifocal leukoencephalopathy. In: 8th Conference on Retroviruses and Opportunistic Infections, Chicago February 2001, abstract 597.
87. De Luca A, Giancola ML, Ammassari A, et al. Cidofovir added to HAART improves virological and clinical outcome in AIDS-associated progressive multifocal leukoencephalopathy. AIDS 14:F117, 2000.
88. Gasnault J, Kousignian P, Kahraman M, et al. Cidofovir in AIDS-associated progressive multifocal leukoencephalopathy: a monocenter observational study with clinical and JC virus load monitoring. J Neurovirol 7:386, 2001.
89. Portilla H, Boix V, Roman F, et al. Progressive multifocal leukoencephalopathy treated with cidofovir in HIV-infected patients receiving highly active anti-retroviral therapy. J Infect 41:182, 2000.
90. Small JA, Scangos GA, Cork L, et al. The early region of human papovavirus JC induces dysmyelination in transgenic mice. Cell 46:13, 1986.
91. Raj GV, Khalili K. Transcription regulation: lessons from the human neurotropic polyoma virus, JCV. Virology 213:283, 1995.
92. Tsao YP, Russo A, Nyamuswa G, et al. Interaction between replication forks and topoisomerase I-DNA cleavable complexes: studies in a cell-free SV40 DNA replication system. Cancer Res 53:5908, 1993.
93. Kerr DA, Chang CF, Gordon J, et al. Inhibition of human neurotropic virus (JCV) DNA replication in glial cells by camptothecin. Virology 196:612, 1993.
94. Dupont D, Fish D, McGuire D, et al. Continuous infusion of topotecan in AIDS-associated progressive multifocal leukoencephalopathy. In: 8th Conference on Retroviruses and Opportunistic Infections, Chicago, February 2001, abstract 597.
95. Przepiorka D, Jaeckle KA, Birdwell RR, et al. Successful treatment of progressive multifocal leukoencephalopathy with low-dose interleukin-2. Bone Marrow Transplant 20:983, 1997.

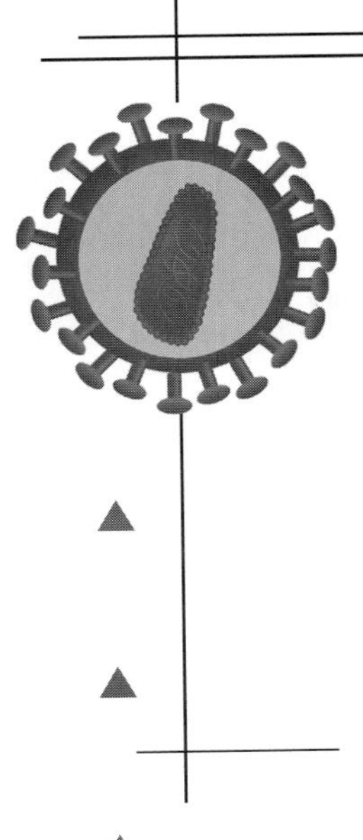

CHAPTER 49
Sexually Transmitted Diseases

Edward W. Hook, III, MD
Jane R. Schwebke, MD

When considering sexually transmitted disease (STD) management for patients with concomitant human immunodeficiency virus (HIV) infection, a common question is whether the therapy recommended for persons without HIV will work as well and, if not, if there is a relation between the person's HIV disease stage and the therapeutic response. Although the bulk of this chapter addresses these questions, a second, increasingly important issue relates to the context in which the STD is encountered and mandates unique counseling interventions. In some patients STDs or problems encountered during the management of these infections may be an indicator of the presence of HIV infection. In addition, patients presenting with uncomplicated STDs create the opportunity for HIV counseling and testing. Thus the presence of the STD may be a sentinel event, leading to the diagnosis of HIV infection. In patients already infected with HIV, STDs are important indicators of continuing unprotected sexual activity and signal the need for further patient counseling or intervention for STD control.

CONTEXTUAL CONSIDERATIONS OF STD DIAGNOSIS IN HIV PATIENTS

Clinics for STD diagnosis and treatment are important sites for identifying HIV-infected patients and a major focus of public health HIV counseling and testing efforts. In 1994 more than 26% of all HIV infections identified by publicly funded HIV counseling and testing occurred in STD clinics.[1] In a variety of other settings, the clinical presentation of at-risk patients to hospitals and clinics may lead clinicians to undertake HIV testing. For instance, a clinical diagnosis of neurosyphilis in a young patient,[2,3] a particularly severe presentation of an anogenital herpes infection,[4] or the presentation of pelvic inflammatory disease (PID) with tuboovarian abscess should serve as sentinel events that signal clinicians to perform HIV counseling and testing.[5–7] Each of these presentations has been associated with substantially increased HIV seroprevalence. HIV-infected persons identified in this way have most often been asymptomatic with the exception of their STD-related symptoms. Initial management of this group of patients is generally no different than for other persons with similar STD presentations. Once treated for the STD, the patients are then usually referred to other specialized clinics for HIV-related care. In a few STD clinics HIV care has been integrated into routine patient management.

A growing body of literature indicates that even following a diagnosis of HIV otherwise asymptomatic HIV-infected patients may continue to have unprotected sexual intercourse and, in this context, may acquire new STDs.[8–10] These STDs in turn, increase the likelihood of HIV transmission to HIV-uninfected sex partners. For example, HIV-infected men with gonococcal or nongonococcal urethritis have eightfold increased HIV concentrations in their ejaculate compared to HIV-infected men without urethritis.[11,12] In addition, increased HIV shedding in men with urethritis persists for far longer periods (up to 2 weeks) than causative agents can be recovered.[11] Similarly, in women inflammatory genital tract infections are associated with increased CD4+ T-lymphocyte concentrations in genital secretions, a finding also associated with increased local concentrations of HIV virus and thus increased HIV transmission.[13] These observations help explain observed reductions in HIV transmission accomplished through aggressive

STD control efforts and support the World Health Organization recommendations that STD control is a critical component of efforts to reduce HIV transmission.[12,14,15] A new STD diagnosis in a person with known HIV infection represents a failure of safer sex counseling and provides an important opportunity for intervention to reduce risks for continuing HIV/STD transmission. Regular testing (screening) for treatable STDs is now recommended for all HIV-infected persons by the Centers for Disease Control and Prevention (CDC) and the Institute of Medicine.[16,17]

In the United States, several studies have demonstrated the increased risk of STD acquisition among established patients with HIV. In the first such study of its type, Zenilman et al.[8] found that more than 10% of 615 HIV-seropositive Baltimore STD clinic patients who received STD posttest counseling went on to return with newly acquired, treatable infections. Although the STD incidence was lower than for patients without HIV infection, in HIV-seropositive patients the relatively high incidence of STDs such as gonorrhea, nongonococcal urethritis, trichomoniasis, and syphilis during the 6- to 24-month period after being informed of HIV infection (median interval to the diagnosis of a new STD was 4.8 months), suggests continuing unprotected sexual exposure to others and therefore continuing risk for HIV transmission as well.[8] These observations were subsequently confirmed by Otten et al.,[9] who found that 6.5% of Miami STD clinic patients who received posttest counseling following HIV diagnosis returned to the clinic within 6 months with a new case of gonorrhea. Although, as in Baltimore, this figure represents a lower STD incidence than for patients from the same clinics who were HIV-seronegative, it is striking that more than 10% of known HIV-seropositive patients per year were acquiring new STDs.

Such observations are not limited to STD clinic patients. Among 118 women attending a St. Louis HIV clinic for continuing care, newly acquired STDs were noted in 32% over 19 months of follow-up, and 10 women (8%) became pregnant.[10] Studies of a large cohort of men who have sex with men (MSM) living in San Francisco document greater numbers of recent sex partners in HIV-infected MSM than in those who are seronegative. Increasing self-reports of unprotected rectal intercourse among HIV-infected MSM (from 37% in 1993–1994 to 50% in 1996–1997) and frequent (> 50%) sex with partners of unknown or discordant HIV infection status[18,19] provide two important messages for health care providers taking care of HIV-infected patients: (1) continued risk reduction and safer sex counseling should be included as a standard component of ongoing care for HIV infection to help prevent spread of infection to others; and (2) regular screening for newly acquired STDs is an important element for providing continuing care for patients with HIV infection.

▲ BACTERIAL STDs

The clinical manifestations of STDs reflect host–pathogen interactions and are influenced by changes in the immune status of infected persons. Therefore the presentation of STDs among HIV-infected patients may vary when compared to those without HIV. Similarly, because antimicrobial therapy augments host responses to infection, therapeutic responses may also differ in HIV-infected persons. Current treatment recommendations for STDs in patients with HIV are presented in Table 49–1.

Syphilis

Syphilis has been and continues to be a common co-infection with HIV.[20–22] Early in the HIV epidemic strong associations were noted between genital ulcer disease and the risk for HIV infection.[12,23] In the United States these associations were particularly strong for persons with serologic evidence of syphilis infection.[23] Numerous case reports and small series also suggested that in persons with HIV infectious syphilis might be a more aggressive illness, the incidence of clinical neurosyphilis might be increased, serologic response to infection might be modified, and the recommended therapy for syphilis (benzathine penicillin) might be less effective than in persons without HIV. Many of these initial observations were made at a time when the incidence of syphilis, which had been relatively stable in the United States, was increasing at a rate of 10% to 15% per year.[24]

Although there may be shifts in the clinical spectrum of disease manifestations and serologic response to infection, they are changes in degree rather than more dramatic, quantum changes in syphilis presentation among persons co-infected with HIV.[25–27] For example, although HIV-infected patients are somewhat more likely to present with secondary manifestations of syphilis (generally with lower CD4+ T-lymphocyte concentrations),[25] there are no specific manifestations of syphilis unique to HIV-infected persons. Any patient with syphilis should be considered to be at risk for HIV infection, not just those with particularly striking clinical manifestations of disease.

Similarly, although there have been reports of delayed development of reactive serologic tests for syphilis [i.e., Venereal Disease Research Laboratory (VDRL)[28] or rapid plasma reagin (RPR) tests], in most HIV-infected patients with syphilis serologic tests are reliable for both diagnosis and follow-up subsequent to treatment.[25–28] Some studies have found that after correction for stage of infection and history of prior syphilis HIV-infected persons with syphilis tend to have higher RPR or VDRL titers, but the overlap between the groups does not permit differences in the serologic test for syphilis titers to be used for differentiating HIV-infected patients with syphilis from HIV-seronegative patients with syphilis.[25]

Likewise, early concerns regarding neurologic invasion by *Treponema pallidum,* the contribution of central nervous system (CNS) invasion to the risk of treatment failure, and the role of lumbar puncture have been topics of much discussion regarding HIV-infected individuals. More recent studies, however, suggest that lumbar puncture may not help to predict outcomes of therapy for patients with early syphilis. In contrast, the relatively high prevalence of asymptomatic neurosyphilis in HIV-infected patients with latent syphilis[15,29] may warrant continued emphasis on this procedure for patients diagnosed with HIV who are found

▲ **Table 49–1.** THERAPY FOR SELECTED STDs IN PATIENTS WITH HIV INFECTION

Disease	Drug	Regimen	Comments
Syphilis			
Primary or secondary	Benzathine penicillin G *or*	2.4 MU IM × 1 dose	Some experts prefer three weekly injections of benzathine penicillin rather than one; and some prefer LP as part of the evaluation.
	Doxycycline	100 mg PO bid × 14 d	
Early latent	Benzathine penicillin G *or*	2.4 MU IM × 1 dose	Consider LP to rule out neurosyphilis.
	Doxycycline	100 mg PO bid × 14 d	
Latent, late latent, *or* unknown	Benzathine penicillin G *or*	2.4 MU IM q wk × 3	LP indicated.
	Doxycycline	100 mg PO bid × 28 d	
Tertiary	Benzathine penicillin G	2.4 MU IM q wk × 3	LP indicated.
Neurosyphilis	Aqueous penicillin G *or*	18–24 MU IV qd × 10–14 d	
	Procaine penicillin	2.4 MU IM qd × 10–14 d with probenicid 500 mg PO qd × 14 d	
Chlamydia trachomatis infection (cervicitis, urethritis)	Azithromycin *or*	1 g PO × 1 dose	Test of cure not necessary unless symptoms persist.
	Doxycycline *or*	100 mg PO bid × 7 d	
	Ofloxacin *or*	300 mg PO bid × 7 d	
	Erythromycin *or*	500 mg PO qid × 7 d	
	Erythromycin ethylsuccinate	400 mg PO qid × 7 d	
Granuloma Inguinale	Doxycycline *or*	100 mg PO bid for ≥ 3 wk	Until lesions heal, strongly consider adding an aminoglycoside (e.g., gentamicin).
	TMP-SMX *or*	1 DS tab PO bid x ≥ 3 wk	
	Erythromycin *or*	500 mg PO qd × ≥ 3 wk	
	Ciprofloxacin	750 mg PO bid × ≥ 3 wk	
Herpes Simplex Virus Infection			
Primary genital	Acyclovir *or*	400 mg PO tid × 7–10 d	
	Valacyclovir *or*	1.0 g PO bid × 7–10 d	
	Famciclovir	250 mg PO tid × 7–10 d	
		500 mg PO bid × 7–10 d	
Recurrent genital	Acyclovir *or*	400 mg PO tid? 5 d	
		200 mg PO 5/day × 5 d	
		800 mg PO bid × 5 d	
	Valacyclovir *or*	500 mg PO bid × 5 d	
	Famciclovir	125 mg PO bid × 5 d	
Suppression genital	Acyclovir *or*	400 mg PO bid	
	Valacyclovir *or*	500–1000 mg qd	
	Famciclovir	250 mg PO bid	
Acyclovir-resistant	Foscarnet *or*	40 mg/kg IV q8h	Until clinical resolution.
	Cidofovir	1% gel qd × ≥ 5 d	

to have latent syphilis of unknown duration (i.e., a reactive serologic test for syphilis and no history of treatment).

Finally, based on case reports and small series, many questions have been raised regarding the adequacy of currently recommended therapy for early syphilis in patients with HIV infection[2,3] (Table 49–1). These reports described dramatic presentations of treatment failure with clinical neurosyphilis at a time when syphilis in general and neurosyphilis in particular were relatively rare diseases. Major questions related to syphilis therapy for HIV-infected patients include the following: Was treatment failure for HIV-infected patients with early syphilis more common than in patients without HIV infection? Did lumbar puncture in patients with early syphilis play a role in predicting which individuals were at risk for treatment failure? What was the role of lumbar puncture for screening HIV-infected patients with reactive serologic tests for syphilis to assess the risk for progressive neurosyphilis?

Many of these questions were addressed in a large, prospectively conducted, randomized controlled trial comparing currently recommended therapy for early (primary, secondary, early latent) syphilis using benzathine penicillin G, 2.4 million units IM, to the same recommended therapy given with supplementary, high-dose oral therapy using amoxicillin 6.0 g daily plus probenicid 500 mg tid for 10 days.[27] The latter therapeutic regimen was chosen on the basis of reports indicating that cerebrospinal fluid (CSF) penicillin concentrations achieved by this combination reached treponemicidal levels. In the larger study 541 patients, including 101 HIV-infected individuals, were enrolled and followed. Although serologic treatment failures (failure of serologic tests for syphilis to decline two or more dilutions at 12 months following therapy) were higher than had been anticipated in both HIV-infected and HIV-seronegative patients (21% and 16%, respectively), the difference was not statistically significant. Furthermore, although addition of the enhanced treatment regimen was relatively well tolerated, it did not significantly improve the response to therapy. Equally important was the observation that in this group of more than 500 patients only a single clinically defined treatment failure was observed. Based on these observations, the authors concluded that current recommendations for treating early syphilis with single intramuscular injections of 2.4 million units of benzathine penicillin were adequate for most patients irrespective of the presence or absence of HIV infection.

The apparent contradiction between the results of this carefully conducted study and the observations of many

▲ **Table 49–1.** THERAPY FOR SELECTED STDs IN PATIENTS WITH HIV INFECTION *Continued*

Disease	Drug	Regimen	Comments
Mucocutaneous (nongenital)	Acyclovir *or*	400 mg PO tid × 5–10 d	Until lesions resolve. If severe, acyclovir 5–10 mg/kg q8h. If encephalitis, 10 mg/kg q8h is needed.
	Famcyclovir *or*	250 mg PO tid × 5–10 d	
	Valacyclovir	1.0 g PO bid × 5–10 d	
Chancroid	Azithromycin *or*	1 g PO × 1 dose	
	Ceftriaxone *or*	250 mg IM × 1 dose	
	Ciprofloxacin *or*	500 mg PO bid × 3 d	
	Erythromycin base	500 mg PO qid × 7 d	
Bacterial Vaginosis	Metronidazole *or*	500 mg PO bid × 7 d	
	Metronidazole gel 0.75% *or*	One application (0.5 g) intravaginally qd or bid × 5 d	
	Clindamycin cream 2% *or*	One application (5 g) intravaginally hs × 7 d	
	Clindamycin	300 mg PO bid × 7 d	Some experts do not recommend this.
Gonorrhea			
Cervix, urethra, rectum	Cefixime *or*	400 mg PO × 1 dose	
	Ceftriaxone *or*	125 mg IM × 1 dose	
	Ciprofloxacin *or*	500 mg PO × 1 dose	
	Ofloxacin *plus*	400 mg PO × 1 dose	
	Azithromycin *or*	1 g PO × 1 dose	
	Doxycycline	100 mg PO bid × 7 d	Co-treatment for *C. trachomatis* is recommended.
Pharynx	Ceftriaxone *or*	125 mg IM × 1 dose	
	Ciprofloxacin *or*	500 mg PO × 1 dose	
	Ofloxacin *plus*	400 mg PO × 1 dose	
	Azithromycin *or*	1 gm PO × 1 dose	Co-treatment for *C. trachomatis*.
	Doxycycline	100 mg PO bid × 7 d	
Lymphogranuloma Venereum	Doxycycline *or*	100 mg PO bid × 21 d	
	Erythromycin	500 mg PO qid × 21 d	
Nongonococcal Urethritis	Azithromycin *or*	1 gm PO × 1 dose	
	Doxycycline *or*	100 mg PO bid × 7 d	
	Ofloxacin	300 mg PO bid × 7 d	
	Erythromycin ethylsuccinate *or*	800 mg PO qid × 7 d	
	Erythromycin base	500 mg PO qid × 7 d	
Persistent Urethritis	Metronidazole *or*	2 gm PO × 1 dose	
	Erythromycin base *or*	500 mg PO qid × 7 d	
	Erythromycin ethylsuccinate	800 mg PO qid × 7 d	

LP, lumbar puncture; MU, million units; STDs, sexually transmitted diseases; TMP-SMX, trimethoprim-sulfamethoxazole.

clinicians who sensed that they were seeing more individuals failing syphilis therapy, and that those individuals often had coexisting HIV infection, may be partially explained by a report by Malone and coworkers.[30] In their study of 56 HIV-infected patients with syphilis followed for an average of 28 months, treatment failures occurred in 18% (10 patients). Interestingly, however, 6 of the 10 treatment failures occurred 12 to 24 months after therapy, substantially beyond the period of observation used in most syphilis treatment studies, including the randomized controlled trial cited above. Synthesis of these data, a number of other reports in the literature, and clinical observations suggests that although treatment failure is somewhat more common in HIV-infected patients than non-HIV-infected patients clinically apparent treatment failures in either group are relatively rare. In addition, intervals of a year or more may occur between receipt of therapy and evidence of treatment failure. Thus there is no basis for recommending that more intensive treatment be given to HIV-infected patients diagnosed with syphilis. More careful, prolonged follow-up of therapy is recommended for HIV-infected patients with syphilis.[15]

Another important question addressed in the large study mentioned above is whether invasion of the CNS by *T. pallidum,* which occurs in more than 20% of all patients with early syphilis, is a harbinger of subsequent treatment failure.[27,31] This question arose related in part to a study by Lukehart et al.,[31] who isolated *T. pallidum* from CSF in 12 of 40 patients (30%) with early syphilis. They found that in 3 HIV-seropositive patients undergoing follow-up lumbar puncture viable *T. pallidum* was still present in CSF following therapy with 2.4 million units of benzathine penicillin G. In the randomized prospective treatment trial[27] referenced above, however, although *T. pallidum* was found at the time of enrollment in 24% of the 131 patients who underwent lumbar puncture and in 7 of 35 who were tested following therapy, none had clinically evident neurosyphilis. Moreover, the rate of *T. pallidum* detection did not vary according to the HIV status or treatment outcome as measured serologically. These data suggest that aggressive efforts to perform lumbar punctures as prognostic tests for early syphilis patients with HIV infection are not currently warranted.

Gonococcal and Chlamydial Infections

There are no formal studies of therapy for gonorrhea and chlamydial infections in HIV-infected patients. These infections are relatively common in persons with HIV infections, and they increase the risk for HIV transmission and acquisition.[11,12,32,33] There are no data to suggest that treatment failures are more common in this group. Thus currently recommended therapy for uncomplicated *Neisseria gonorrhoeae* and *Chlamydia trachomatis* infections remain appropriate therapy for HIV-infected persons[15] (Table 49–1).

Bacterial Vaginosis

There are increasing data to suggest that abnormal vaginal flora, such as that typical of bacterial vaginosis (BV), facilitates the acquisition of STDs including HIV.[34–36] Studies have evaluated associations between HIV infection and BV using three complementary measures: clinical diagnosis of BV; Gram stain demonstration of BV-associated changes in vaginal flora (reduced lactobacilli and increased concentrations of anaerobic and facultative anaerobic bacteria); or cultures for hydrogen peroxide (H_2O_2)-producing lactobacilli whose absence is believed to be an early event in the disruption of the vaginal flora that characterizes this common syndrome.

In a cross-sectional study of 144 female commercial sex workers from Thailand, HIV seropositivity was significantly correlated with clinically diagnosed BV and with abnormal (BV-associated) vaginal flora on Gram stain, independent of other behavioral variables.[37] Similar findings were documented from a study of Ugandan women[28] in which the highest HIV seropositivity rates were found among the women with the most severe changes in their vaginal flora as documented by Gram stain, findings that suggested a "dose-response" relation between BV and the risk for HIV. Similar findings occurred in a study of pregnant women in North Carolina; in this cohort there was relatively low HIV prevalence, and the prevalence of HIV increased as the vaginal flora Gram stain score increased. The association of BV with HIV risk was independent of other demographic and behavioral variables.[39] Thus similar findings linking BV and HIV have been noted in diverse geographic settings with varied HIV prevalence. Cross-sectional studies do not prove cause and effect, however, and it is possible that the immunosuppression associated with HIV could lead to BV-associated changes in vaginal bacterial flora rather than the converse.

Two prospective longitudinal studies have been reported that further support the relation between BV and HIV risk. Taha et al., who followed 1196 HIV-seronegative women antenatally and postnatally in Malawi, Africa, found that bacterial vaginosis was significantly associated with HIV seroconversion, and that the risk increased in stepwise fashion as the vaginal flora disturbances increased in severity.[35] In a second Kenyan study, Martin et al.[35a] prospectively followed commercial sex workers with vaginal Gram stains and cultures for lactobacilli. They demonstrated that abnormal, BV-associated vaginal flora detected by Gram stain was significantly associated with HIV seroconversion. Additionally, they found that women without vaginal lactobacilli were at the greatest risk for HIV followed by women with lactobacilli that did not produce H_2O_2.

Although the above data strongly support a role for lactobacilli as being protective against HIV acquisition, other factors may have an influence. For example, Sturm-Ramirez et al. looked for tumor necrosis factor-α and interleukin-1β in cervical secretions and found high levels of these cytokines associated with BV. They suggested that cytokines could up-regulate HIV replication in the vagina through activation of the long terminal repeat promoter region.[40] Similarly, invitro, certain anaerobic bacteria (*Peptostreptococcus asaccharolyticus* and *Prevotella bivia*) associated with BV appear to stimulate HIV expression in monocytoid cells and T lymphocytes.[41]

Rates of BV are significantly higher than STD rates worldwide. Thus the attributable risk of BV with regard to HIV transmission is high.[42] Widespread control of BV has therefore been suggested as a possible means for decreasing the incidence of HIV, particularly in the developing world. However, current achievable cure rates combined with high recurrence rates makes this solution impractical. The recommended therapies for BV have cure rates of 70% to 80%, and recurrence rates are high.[43,44] In a study of controling STDs to prevent HIV in Uganda, therapy for BV was unable to reduce the rates of BV significantly in the treatment communities compared to the control communities. The same study also failed to show a difference in HIV acquisition between the two groups,[45] further supporting the theory that abnormal vaginal flora is a factor in HIV transmission.

Pelvic Inflammatory Disease

Pelvic inflammatory disease (PID) is the most common complication of bacterial STD in women and not infrequently leads to the need for operative intervention (drainage of tuboovarian abscesses, hysterectomy) and long-term sequelae such as chronic pelvic pain, increased risk for recurrent PID, infertility, and ectopic pregnancy. Several studies have reported increased rates of HIV seropositivity in women hospitalized for PID. In a San Francisco study Safrin and coworkers[46] found that HIV seroprevalence among women hospitalized for PID increased from 0 to 6.7% between 1985 and 1988 and suggested that, as for other STDs, a diagnosis of PID should be considered a cue for recommending HIV serologic counseling and testing. Sperling et al.[47] also found HIV seroprevalence to be elevated in New York women with PID. In their study, nearly 17% of women (5/30) hospitalized for PID during 1988–1989 were found to be HIV-seropositive, substantially more than the 2.7% seroprevalence described for obstetric patients in the same community.

More recent studies suggest that the presentation or response to therapy in HIV-infected women with PID differs from that of women who are HIV-seronegative. In a study of 116 women hospitalized for PID in Brooklyn, New York,[5] HIV-seropositive women (14% to 15% of the study population)—with the exception of less often having an elevated white blood cell (WBC) concentration at admission (40% of HIV-seropositive women vs. 89% of those who were HIV-seronegative)—had similar presentations and durations of hospitalization. Although the differences were not significant, there was a tendency for women with HIV to have tuboovarian abscess diagnosed more often than HIV-seronegative women (23% vs. 14%, respectively) and to require surgical intervention more often (27% vs. 8%, respectively; $P = 0.06$). Many of the observations regarding the presentation and management of PID among HIV-infected women were confirmed by a similar, retrospective study. In that San Francisco study, Korn et al.[6] found HIV-seropositive women who were hospitalized with PID to have significantly less abdominal tenderness and lower admission WBC counts than women who were HIV-seronegative. In addition, although tuboovarian and pelvic abscesses were actually less common among HIV-infected women (4%) than among HIV-seronegative women (13%), as in the Brooklyn, New York study, surgical intervention was more often necessary among HIV-infected women than among HIV-seronegative women (17% vs. 4%, respectively; $P < 0.05$).

Prospective studies underway in Nairobi, Kenya[7] have validated and extended the observations noted above. These studies also indicate that tuboovarian abscesses are significantly more common among HIV-infected women and that the likelihood of tuboovarian abscess increases among women with more profound immunosuppression, as indicated by lower CD4+ T-lymphocyte concentrations. In these studies, 33% of HIV-infected women had tuboovarian abscesses compared to 14% of HIV-seronegative women. When stratified by the CD4+ T-lymphocyte count, women with a CD4+ T-lymphocyte count of less than 200 cells/mm^3 had still more frequent abscesses (55% vs. 28% for women with counts of > 200 cells/mm^3).

Thus among women with PID, as for syphilis, HIV infection is associated with a change in clinical manifestations (increased frequency of tuboovarian abscess) that, although not modifying recommended therapy, necessitates more careful follow-up.[15]

▲ VIRAL STDs

Unlike bacterial STDs (which are largely amenable to therapy and are commonly acquired following infection with HIV), in many if not most instances infection with the most common viral STD agents (herpes simplex virus and human papillomavirus) often precedes HIV infection. In addition, given the important role of cellular immunity in the host response to these infections in modifying their presentation and natural history, it is not surprising that their management in HIV-infected persons is affected on multiple levels.

Genital Herpes Infections

Genital herpes is common in sexually active adults (see Chapter 41). Population-based serologic surveys indicate that by 1994 nearly 22% of sexually active American adults had serologic evidence of herpes simplex virus type 2 (HSV-2), the agent that causes more than 80% of genital herpes,[40] with considerably higher prevalence among populations identified as being at higher risk for HIV (MSM and African-Americans). A meta-analysis suggested that (frequently unrecognized) genital herpes is a major contributor to continuing HIV infections, accounting for up to 22% of the population's attributable risk for new HIV infections in the United States and far higher (up to 50%) risks in populations with a higher prevalence of this common infection, which is typically seen in developing nations.[49]

Although genital herpes is common in persons with HIV, in a small number the manifestations of infection may be particularly difficult to manage. Severe, unremitting episodes of anogenital herpes infections in homosexually active men were among the earliest descriptions of patients with acquired immunodeficiency syndrome (AIDS).[4] More recently, however, retrospective studies have indicated that although the prevalence of HSV is high in persons with HIV infection the frequency, duration, and severity of recurrence in most of these patients is not dramatically different from the natural history of the infection in persons without HIV infection.[50] Whether the frequency of recurrence or asymptomatic viral shedding is increased in HIV-infected persons as immunologic function declines with HIV progression is unknown.

At present, treatment for genital herpes in HIV-infected persons with thymidine kinase-inhibiting antiviral agents such as acyclovir, valacyclovir, or famciclovir is recommended using the same regimens as recommended for non-HIV-infected patients[15] (Table 49–1). The recommended dosage for each of these agents varies with the indications for treatment.[15] Chronic ingestion of acyclovir (and presumably valacyclovir and famciclovir) has been associated with the development of acyclovir-resistant HSV, which may cause severe, progressive, or slow-to-resolve recurrences.[51] Infections caused by acyclovir-resistant HSV can be treated with unrelated antiviral agents such as foscarnet or topical cidofovir.[15] (Topical cidofovir is not commercially available but can be formulated from the intravenous preparation.) Acyclovir-resistant HSV should be suspected when therapy does not lead to rapid clinical improvement. For such patients, repeat viral culture and antiviral susceptibility testing of isolates should be considered.

Human Papillomavirus Infections

Human papillomavirus (HPV) infections are common in persons with and without HIV infection.[52] HPV infection may manifest as visible genital warts or as subclinical infection seen as abnormalities on Papanicolaou smear screening. The diagnosis and management of HPV infections is discussed comprehensively in Chapter 47.

REFERENCES

1. Centers for Disease Control and Prevention. HIV Counseling and Testing in Publicly Funded Sites: 1993–1994 Summary Report. Atlanta, Centers for Disease Control and Prevention, 1996.
2. Johns DR, Tierney M, Felsenstein D. Alteration in the natural history of neurosyphilis by concurrent infection with the human immunodeficiency virus. N Engl J Med 316:1569, 1987.
3. Berry CD, Hooton TM, Collier AC, et al. Neurologic relapse after benzathine penicillin therapy for secondary syphilis in a patient with HIV infection. N Engl J Med 316:1587, 1987.
4. Siegal FP, Lopez C, Hammer GS, et al. Severe acquired immunodeficiency in male homosexuals, manifested by chronic perianal ulcerative herpes simplex lesions. N Engl J Med 305:1439, 1981.

5. Hoegsberg B, Abulafia O, Sedlis A, et al. Sexually transmitted diseases and human immunodeficiency virus infection among women with pelvic inflammatory disease. Am J Obstet Gynecol 163:1135, 1990.
6. Korn AP, Landers DV, Green JR, et al. Pelvic inflammatory disease in human immunodeficiency virus-infected women. Obstet Gynecol 82:765, 1993.
7. Bukusi E, Stevens CE, Cohen CR. Impact of HIV on acute pelvic inflammatory disease in a Nairobi out-patient clinic. In: Abstracts of the XIth International Conference on AIDS, Vancouver, 1996, abstract 1618.
8. Zenilman JM, Erickson B, Fox R, et al. Effect of HIV posttest counseling on STD incidence. JAMA 267:843, 1992.
9. Otten MW, Zaidi AA, Wroten JE, et al. Changes in sexually transmitted disease rates after HIV testing and posttest counseling, Miami, 1988–1989. Am J Public Health 83:529, 1993.
10. Bersoff-Matcha SJ, Horgan MM, Stoner BP. Sexually transmitted disease acquisition among HIV-infected women. In: Abstracts of the 35th Annual Meeting of the Infectious Diseases Society of America, San Francisco. Alexandria, VA Infectious Diseases Society of America, 1998, abstract 546.
11. Cohen MS, Hoffman IF, Royce RA, et al. Reduction of concentration of HIV-1 in semen after treatment of urethritis: implications for prevention of sexual transmission of HIV-1: AIDSCAP Malawi Research Group. Lancet 349:1868, 1997.
12. Royce RA, Sena A, Cates W Jr, et al. Sexual transmission of HIV. N Engl J Med 336:1072, 1997.
13. Levine WC, Pope V, Bhoomkar A, et al. Increase in endocervical CD4 lymphocytes among women with nonulcerative sexually transmitted diseases. J Infect Dis 177:167, 1998.
14. Grosskurth H, Mosha F, Todd J, et al. Impact of improved treatment of sexually transmitted diseases on HIV infection in rural Tanzania: randomized controlled trial. Lancet 346:530, 1995.
15. Centers for Diseases Control and Prevention. 1998 Guidelines for the treatment of sexually transmitted diseases. MMWR Morb Mortal Wkly Rep 47:1, 1998.
16. Centers for Disease Control and Prevention. HIV prevention through early detection and treatment of other sexually transmitted diseases—United States. MMWR Morb Mortal Wkly Rep 47:1, 1998.
17. Ruiz MS, Gable AR, Kaplan EH, et al (eds). No Time to Lose: Getting More From HIV Prevention. IOM. Washington, DC, National Academy Press, 2000.
18. Hays RB, Paul J, Ekstrand M, et al. Actual versus perceived HIV status, sexual behaviors and predictors of unprotected sex among young gay and bisexual men who identify as HIV-negative, HIV-positive and untested. AIDS 11:1495, 1997.
19. Ekstrand ML, Stall RD, Paul JP, et al. Gay men report high rates of unprotected anal sex with partners of unknown or discordant HIV status. AIDS 13:1525, 1999.
20. Centers for Disease Control and Prevention. Outbreak of syphlis among men who have sex with men—Southern California 2000. MMWR Morb Mortal Wkly Rep 50:117, 2001.
21. Centers for Disease Control and Prevention. Resurgent bacterial sexually transmitted disease among men who have sex with men—King County Washington, 1997–1999. MMWR Morb Mortal Wkly Rep 48:773, 1999.
22. Centers for Disease Control and Prevention. Primary and secondary syphilis—United States, 1999. MMWR Morb Mortal Wkly Rep 50:113, 2001.
23. Quinn TC, Cannon RO, Glasser D, et al. The association of syphilis with risk of human immunodeficiency virus infection in patients attending sexually transmitted disease clinics. Arch Intern Med 150:1297, 1990.
24. Division of STD Prevention. Sexually Transmitted Disease Surveillance, 1996. Atlanta, Centers for Disease Control and Prevention, 1997.
25. Hutchinson CM, Hook EW III, Shepherd M, et al. Altered clinical presentations and manifestations of early syphilis in patients with human immunodeficiency virus infection. Ann Intern Med 121:94, 1994.
26. Gourevitch M, Selwyn PA, Davenny K, et al. Effects of HIV infection on the serologic manifestations and response to treatment of syphilis in intravenous drug users. Ann Intern Med 118:350, 1993.
27. Rolfs RT, Joesoef MR, Hendershot EF, et al. A randomized trial of enhanced therapy for early syphilis in patients with and without human immunodeficiency virus infection: the Syphilis and HIV Study Group. N Engl J Med 337:307, 1997.
28. Hicks CB, Benson PM, Lupton GP, et al. Seronegative secondary syphilis in a patient infected with the human immunodeficiency virus (HIV) with Kaposi sarcoma: a diagnostic dilemma. Ann Intern Med 107:492, 1987.
29. Holtom PD, Larsen RA, Leal ME, et al. Prevalence of neurosyphilis in human immunodeficiency virus-infected patients with latent syphilis. Am J Med 93:9, 1992.
30. Malone JL, Wallace MR, Hendrick BB, et al. Syphilis and neurosyphilis in a human immunodeficiency virus type-1 seropositive population: evidence for frequent serologic relapse after therapy. Am J Med 99:55, 1995.
31. Lukehart SA, Hook EW III, Baker-Zander SA, et al. Invasion of the central nervous system by *Treponema pallidum*: implications for diagnosis and treatment. Ann Intern Med 109:855, 1988.
32. Wasserheit JN. Epidemiological synergy. interrelationships between human immunodeficiency virus infection and other sexually transmitted diseases. Sex Transm Dis 19:61, 1992.
33. Laga M, Manoka A, Kivuvu M, et al. Non-ulcerative sexually transmitted diseases as risk factors for HIV-1 transmission in women: results from a cohort study. AIDS 7:95, 1993.
34. Saigh JH, Sanders CC, Sanders WE Jr. Inhibition of *Neisseria gonorrhoeae* by aerobic and facultatively anaerobic components of the endocervical flora: evidence for a protective effect against infection. Infect Immun 19:704, 1978.
35. Taha TE, Hoover DR, Dallabetta GA, et al. Bacterial vaginosis and disturbances of vaginal flora: association with increased acquisition of HIV. AIDS 12:1699, 1998.
35a. Martin HL, Richardson B, Nyange PM, et al. Vaginal lactobacilli, microbial flora, and risk of human immunodeficiency virus type 1 and sexually transmitted disease acquisition. J, Infect Dis 180:1863, 1999.
36. Hillier SL. The vaginal microbial ecosystem and resistance to HIV. AIDS Res Hum Retroviruses 14 (suppl 1):S17, 1998.
37. Cohen CR, Duerr A, Pruithithada N, et al: Bacterial vaginosis and HIV seroprevalence among female commercial sex workers in Chiang Mai, Thailand. AIDS 9:1093, 1995.
38. Sewankambo N, Gray RH, Wawer MJ, et al. HIV-1 infection associated with abnormal vaginal flora morphology and bacterial vaginosis. Lancet 350:546, 1997.
39. Royce RA, Thorp J, Granados JL, et al. Bacterial vaginosis associated with HIV infection in pregnant women from North Carolina. J Acquir Immune Defic Syndr Hum Retrovirol 20:382, 1999.
40. Sturm-Ramirez K, Gaye-Diallo A, Eisen G, et al. High levels of tumor necrosis factor-α and interleukin-1β in bacterial vaginosis may increase susceptibility to human immunodeficiency virus. J Infect Dis 182:467, 2000.
41. Hashemi FB, Ghassemi M, Faro S, et al. Induction of human immunodeficiency virus type 1 expression by anaerobes associated with bacterial vaginosis. J Infect Dis 181:1574, 2000.
42. Schmid G, Markowitz L, Joesoef R, et al. Bacterial vaginosis and HIV infection. Sex Transm Infect 76:3, 2000.
43. Joesoef MR, Schmid GP, Hillier SL. Bacterial vaginosis: review of treatment options and potential clinical indications for therapy. Clin Infect Dis 28 (suppl 1):S57, 1999.
44. Blackwell AL, Fox AR, Phillips I, et al. Anaerobic vaginosis (nonspecific vaginitis): clinical, microbiological and therapeutic findings. Lancet 2:1379, 1982.
45. Waiver MJ, Seuankambo NK, Serwadda D. Control of sexually transmitted diseases for AIDS prevention in Uganda: a randomized community trial. Rakai Project Study Group. Lancet 353:513, 1999.
46. Safrin S, Dattel BJ, Hauer L, et al. Seroprevalence and epidemiologic correlates of human immunodeficiency virus infection in women with acute pelvic inflammatory disease. Obstet Gynecol 75:666, 1990.
47. Sperling RS, Friedman F Jr, Joyner M, et al. Seroprevalence of human immunodeficiency virus in women admitted to the hospital with pelvic inflammatory disease. J Reprod Med 36:122, 1991.
48. Fleming DT, McQuillan GM, Johnson RE, et al. Herpes simplex virus type 2 in the United States, 1976 to 1994. N Engl J Med 337:1105, 1997.

49. Wald A, Link K. Risk of human immunodeficiency virus infection in herpes simplex virus type 2-seropositive persons: a meta-analysis. J Infect Dis 185:45, 2002.
50. Safrin S, Ashley R, Houlihan C, et al. Clinical and serologic features of herpes simplex virus infection in patients with AIDS. AIDS 5:1107, 1991.
51. Erlich KS, Mills J, Chatis P, et al. Acyclovir-resistant herpes simplex virus infections in patients with the acquired immunodeficiency syndrome. N Engl J Med 320:293, 1989.
52. Baken LA, Koutsky LA, Kuypers J, et al. Genital human papillomavirus infection among male and female sex partners: prevalence and type-specific concordance. J Infect Dis 171:429, 1995.

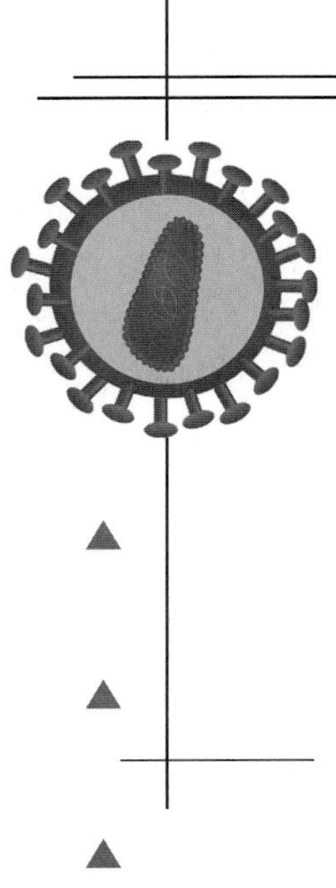

CHAPTER 50

Kaposi's Sarcoma

Susan E. Krown, MD

Kaposi's sarcoma (KS) was one of the first opportunistic diseases described in association with what would later be termed the acquired immune deficiency syndrome (AIDS).[1] Despite a decline in its incidence, which began before the introduction of human immunodeficiency virus-1 (HIV-1) protease inhibitors but which has accelerated since their introduction in 1996,[2] KS continues to be the most frequently diagnosed AIDS-associated neoplasm and a cause of significant morbidity and occasional mortality in HIV-infected patients. The rapid decline in KS incidence that followed the introduction of potent antiretroviral regimens for HIV and the occasional regression of established KS lesions after their use may be a consequence of a decrease in the production of KS-stimulatory cytokines and viral proteins associated with poorly controlled HIV infection. Alternatively or in addition, effective antiretroviral therapy might permit the development of an effective immune response against human herpesvirus 8 (HHV-8), the virus associated with KS. The emergence of drug-resistant HIV strains and intolerance or lack of adherence to effective antiviral regimens make it difficult to know whether the decreased incidence of KS in developed countries will continue. In addition, the incidence of KS remains high in parts of the world where effective antiretroviral therapy is not available and where HIV and HHV-8 incidence are both high.[3]

Kaposi's sarcoma most commonly presents with lesions on the skin that may be widely disseminated from the outset, although other sites may be initially involved. Although the course of KS is quite variable, in many patients KS not only disseminates in the skin but also involves the oral cavity and visceral organs, especially the lungs and gastrointestinal tract, and it is often complicated by lymphedema of the extremities, face, and genitalia. Depending on its location and severity, KS can cause serious functional disability. KS lesions of the feet may be painful and limit mobility. Oral KS may cause difficulty eating and speaking. Edema may be associated with ulceration, infection, pain, and reduced mobility. Gastrointestinal KS may be asymptomatic but sometimes causes bleeding, pain, and obstruction. Pulmonary KS can cause respiratory insufficiency; and untreated pulmonary KS was associated in one study with a median survival of only 2.1 months.[4] Even in the absence of symptomatic visceral disease or edema, KS often impairs the quality of life when it causes disfigurement, leads to social isolation, or serves as a visual reminder of an AIDS diagnosis.

Several treatment options are available for KS, and the choice is dictated by the extent of disease, the rate of disease progression, and the presence and severity of symptoms affecting function and quality of life. The choice of treatment may also be influenced by the severity of the underlying HIV infection and the presence of co-morbid opportunistic complications of HIV infection. KS usually presents multifocally, without a defined "primary" lesion, so staging according to a standard T(umor)/N(ode)/M(etastasis) classification is not appropriate. In addition to tumor extent, immune status and the presence of systemic manifestations of HIV infection are relevant to the prognosis of HIV-infected patients with KS. The most commonly applied staging classification for KS, which takes these factors into account, is the TIS system proposed in 1989 by the AIDS Clinical Trail Group (ACTG) Oncology Committee.[5] This staging system divides patients into good risk or poor risk groups according to extent of *t*umor, *i*mmune system status measured by CD4+ T-lymphocyte count, and severity of systemic HIV-associated illness. A prospective analysis of 294 patients entered into eight ACTG KS therapy trials between 1989 and 1995 showed that each of the TIS variables was significantly associated with survival.[6] Little information exists, however, about the factors predicting response to KS therapy or if TIS staging is a useful guide to the choice of therapy. Now that antiretroviral treatments are available that can effectively suppress the HIV burden, efforts are underway to determine whether the viral load adds to the predictive value of TIS staging with respect to survival or response to treatment.

▲ DIAGNOSIS

Although a presumptive diagnosis of KS is often based on visual identification of typical red or violaceous skin or oral lesions in a patient at risk, biopsy of at least one lesion is important for establishing the diagnosis and distinguishing KS from other pigmented skin lesions such as bacillary angiomatosis.[7] A diagnosis of gastrointestinal (GI) or pulmonary KS may be more difficult to establish. KS may occur throughout the GI tract and sometimes occurs in the absence of cutaneous or oral disease.[8] Although estimates of the frequency of GI KS range from 40% at the time of KS diagnosis to 80% in autopsy series,[9,10] it is frequently asymptomatic, and there is no evidence that the presence of asymptomatic GI lesions adversely affects prognosis or response to treatment. Therefore, it is generally recommended that patients be evaluated for the presence of GI KS only when symptoms (e.g., pain, occult or gross bleeding, dysphagia, obstructive signs) are present. Endoscopy is generally required for diagnosis, as KS lesions are often submucosal and not easily visualized on contrast radiographs or scans, which are nondiagnostic in any event. Upper or lower gastrointestinal endoscopy (or both) generally permits direct visualization of the red lesions in the esophagus, stomach, duodenum, or colon; digital rectal examination often discloses lesions in the anorectal area. Although endoscopic biopsy of typical KS lesions may confirm the diagnosis pathologically, superficial biopsies sometimes yield only normal mucosa, especially when the lesions are not ulcerated. In the presence of pathologically confirmed KS elsewhere in the body, however, the visual identification of typical lesions in the GI tract can be considered presumptive evidence of GI KS.

Pulmonary KS is generally seen as a late complication of KS, but on rare occasions the lung is the initial or sole site of KS. KS may occur on the pleural surfaces, in the lung parenchyma, and in the bronchial tree. Pulmonary KS usually, but not invariably, causes symptoms that may include dyspnea, cough, or hemoptysis, although gross bleeding is uncommon. The radiographic picture may include pleural effusions, diffuse interstitial or alveolar infiltrates, poorly defined nodules, or some combination of these features, although some patients with endobronchial lesions have normal plain films despite prominent respiratory symptoms.[11] Bronchoscopy is the diagnostic procedure of choice because it allows direct visualization of red endobronchial lesions (when present), and coexisting infectious diseases can be diagnosed or excluded. When endobronchial lesions are not present, however, a definitive diagnosis of KS may not be possible, as transbronchial biopsies often do not yield diagnostic tissue.[12] Gallium (or combined gallium-thallium) scanning has been advocated as a technique to distinguish pulmonary KS from other neoplastic or infectious conditions.[13] KS has been reported to be gallium-negative and thallium-positive, whereas infections or other inflammatory diseases of the lung typically show the opposite pattern. In practice, however, thallium scanning is not widely used, and false-negative gallium scans have been documented in patients with various opportunistic infections. A negative gallium scan alone is therefore not sufficient to exclude infectious causes of an abnormal radiograph, particularly in a febrile patient. In an afebrile patient with an established KS diagnosis, however, a negative gallium scan together with a negative infection workup (including bronchoscopy) and compatible radiographs may be accepted as presumptive evidence of pulmonary KS. Rarely, open lung biopsy or computed tomography (CT)-guided needle biopsy is required to establish a diagnosis of pulmonary KS, particularly when the differential diagnosis suggests other neoplasms or infections. CT scans may offer better definition of pulmonary nodules than plain radiographs[11] and may be helpful for following the response to treatment, especially in patients with poorly defined lesions on routine films.

▲ THERAPY OF AIDS-ASSOCIATED KAPOSI'S SARCOMA

Management of HIV Infection

A successful KS management strategy includes optimal antiretroviral therapy for the stage of HIV infection and prophylaxis for, and prompt recognition and treatment of, opportunistic infections. KS growth is stimulated by inflammatory cytokines,[14,15] whose production is increased in the setting of acute opportunistic infections and active HIV replication; it may also be stimulated by the HIV Tat protein, which has been shown in vitro to act synergistically with growth factors to increase KS cell proliferation.[16,17] The observation that KS sometimes regresses after initiation of protease inhibitor-containing antiretroviral regimens suggests that in some cases a decrease in immunosuppression, pathologic immune activation, and HIV replication may be sufficient to control KS. Therefore an attempt to optimize viral load suppression should be part of the management strategy for all patients presenting with KS who exhibit a high viral load; in the setting of a relatively low tumor burden and the absence of symptomatic lesions, a trial of antiretroviral therapy can be considered before specific anti-KS therapy is instituted. It should be emphasized, however, that successful control of HIV replication does not invariably lead to KS regression.

Local Therapy

For limited, relatively slowly progressive disease without life-threatening organ involvement, local therapy aimed at the control of individual lesions is suitable in some cases.

Local approaches are most appropriate for patients who have relatively few, small lesions but may also be suitable for patients with more widespread disease who have contraindications to systemic therapy but in whom control of certain lesions for cosmetic reasons is needed.

Several studies that investigated topical application of a 9-*cis*-retinoic acid (alitretinoin; Panretin) gel[18,19] provided the basis for U.S. Food and Drug Administration (FDA) approval of this agent for KS treatment. In one vehicle-controlled trial in which cutaneous lesions were treated two to four times daily, 35% of patients who received a 12-week course of 0.1% 9-*cis*-retinoic acid gel and 18% of patients treated with the vehicle gel showed an objective response ($P = 0.002$). The responses were partial in all but one patient. With longer treatment, additional responses were observed with 9-*cis*-retinoic acid gel. Application-site reactions (erythema, pain, pruritus, flaking, desquamation, crusting, swelling) were common but were rarely severe.[19]

Historically, the most commonly used local approaches were liquid nitrogen cryotherapy[20] and intralesional injections of vinblastine.[21] There are relatively few published studies on response rates or the characteristics of lesions best suited to local therapy. In one study[21] a single intralesional injection of vinblastine was administered to 33 lesions in 11 patients. The size of the treated lesions was not specified in the report. Of the 33 injected lesions, 20 (61%) showed complete clinical response, and 9 others (27%) showed partial regression. Raised (papular or nodular) lesions became macular after treatment, but nearly all the lesions healed with postinflammatory hyperpigmentation. Of 12 regressed lesions observed 4 to 7 months after treatment, 5 (42%) had relapsed, and three of four biopsy specimens from persistently "regressed" lesions showed histologic evidence of residual KS. Transient ($\leq$ 2 minutes) pain was associated with injection and was followed, after 6 to 48 hours, by more severe aching pain that was generally relieved by nonnarcotic analgesics. In another study[20] liquid nitrogen therapy was given to 61 lesions in 20 evaluable subjects. Each lesion received an average of three treatments (range one to eight) at 2- to 3-week intervals to allow for healing of local blisters. The average area of the treated lesions was relatively small, 68 mm^2 (range 10 to 230 mm^2). Based on the area of the residual tumor, 80% of the lesions showed a complete response, and 7% showed partial regression. An independent evaluation of pre- and posttreatment color slides for 44 lesions, however, was interpreted as complete absence of residual KS in 50% and partial response in 27% of lesions. Overall cosmetic results were scored as complete (normal skin) in 20.5% and partial (>50% improvement) in 50%. At a 6-month follow-up in 13 of the 20 subjects, only one showed progressive KS in a treated area. In addition to local blistering and crusting, no significant side effects were reported other than short-lived ($\leq$ 1 hour) local pain relieved by acetaminophen.

Several other locally injected agents have also been tested in small clinical trials, including recombinant interferon alfa,[22] recombinant granulocyte/macrophage colony stimulating factor,[23] recombinant platelet factor 4,[24] and human chorionic gonadotropin.[25] Although all of these agents have been shown to induce local KS regression, there are no convincing data to support their superiority over the more commonly used local agents. Local injections of vinblastine and the sclerosing agent Sotradecol[26] have also been reported to induce regression of oral KS lesions. Local treatments have the advantage of inducing few systemic side effects and can often be completed quickly, yielding acceptable cosmetic results in some patients. The benefits of local treatment are confined to the treated lesions, however, and there is no evidence that local lesion control inhibits the development of new lesions elsewhere. Lesions may recur at treated sites, and local side effects may include pain, eschar formation, and hyper- or hypopigmentation.

Radiation Therapy

Radiation therapy (RT) is frequently used to treat KS of the skin and oral cavity and less frequently to treat visceral KS. A review of the literature on RT for KS reveals no uniform "standard" approach.

In a prospectively randomized trial, Stelzer and Griffin[27] compared treatment of individual KS skin lesions with 6 MeV electrons given as 800 cGy in one fraction (a frequently recommended regimen[28]), 2000 cGy in 10 fractions over 2 weeks, or 4000 cGy in 20 fractions over 4 weeks to the palpable tumor with a 2 cm margin. Complete resolution of the palpable lesion was significantly better for the fractionated (2000 or 4000 cGy) regimens (79% and 83%) than for the single-dose (800 cGy) regimen (50%); and complete resolution of residual pigmentation was significantly better for the 4000 cGy regimen (43%) than for the 2000 or 800 cGy regimen (8% for each). The 4000 cGy regimen also led to a significantly longer median duration of lesion control (43 weeks) than 2000 cGy (26 weeks) or 800 cGy (13 weeks). Acute toxicity was somewhat higher in the 4000 cGy lesions, but this was limited to mild erythema, dry desquamation, local alopecia, and hyperpigmentation. These data suggest that the type of RT should be individualized based on the intent of treatment and the overall health status of the patient. If long-term cosmesis is the primary objective, a 4000 cGy regimen over a protracted course is optimal. However, for lesions of lesser cosmetic importance or for treating extremely ill or symptomatic patients who have limited mobility or a short overall life expectancy, a more rapid fractionation regimen may produce acceptable local results without the need for repeated treatment visits over many weeks. In addition, the 4000 cGy regimen was subsequently reported in one patient to be associated with a radiation recall reaction when bleomycin was administered, whereas there was no reaction in other lesions in the same patient that had been treated with 800 or 2000 cGy.[29] Thus for patients in whom a future need for systemic chemotherapy is anticipated, the more rapid fractionation regimens may be associated with a lower risk of recall reactions.

RT of more extensive KS, such as diffusely involved extremities, with or without edema, usually requires larger photon fields. Severe local reactions (skin erythema, pain, desquamation of the skin on the soles of the feet) were observed in five of seven patients who received 2000 cGy to the feet over 2 weeks.[30] Berson et al.[28] observed a lower incidence of high-grade local reactions with a single 800 cGy fraction to treat KS of the foot. Stelzer (personal communication) suggested, however, that lower doses per fraction and a planned rest period may allow delivery of higher total doses without severe acute reactions and may avoid later radiation-induced edema from subcutaneous fibrosis. Although KS-associated edema is often reduced with RT, its resolution is rarely complete.[28,30]

Although oral KS has also been treated successfully with RT, patients with HIV infection have sometimes been noted to have unusual radiation sensitivity of normal tissues. Oral radiation using 4 MeV photons at 180 cGy daily for 9 days (total 1620 cGy) was reported by Chak et al.[30] to be associated with severe mucositis, mouth dryness, and altered sense of taste, which was decreased but not eliminated by lowering the total dose to 1400 cGy. Berson et al.[28] also reported a high incidence of severe mucositis when the oropharynx was treated with high-dose fractions (180 to 400 cGy) to total doses of 2000 to 2400 cGy. The severity was decreased by using 150 cGy fractions to a total dose of 1500 cGy.[28] Stelzer (personal communication) has advocated using 150 cGy fractions 5 days a week for 10 doses to the oral cavity, followed by a 1-week scheduled break in therapy to reduce the risk of mucositis. Patients may then be given as many as five additional fractions, depending on tolerance. Tumor shrinkage is rapid with oral RT and is probably the treatment of choice when rapid relief of symptoms from bulky lesions is required. Systemic therapy is also effective for many patients with oral KS, so the decision to choose local RT or systemic therapy may depend on whether other indications for systemic KS treatment coexist with the oral disease.

Although chemotherapy is a more common approach to symptomatic lung or GI tract involvement, RT has also been used to treat selected patients with visceral KS. Berson et al.[28] reported responses in 88% of patients treated with involved field photons to GI lesions located mainly in the anorectum, and they described relief of obstructive symptoms in two patients with upper GI lesions. Rapid subjective improvement has also been reported[28,31] in patients with pulmonary KS who received whole-lung radiation, generally in 150 cGy fractions to total doses of 900 to 1500 cGy. Meyer[31] reported a significant reduction in hemoptysis and need for supplemental oxygen, but only 28% of patients with radiographic abnormalities showed a 50% or more reduction in measurable lesions.

Interferon Therapy

Interferons have the potential to influence many of the complex processes involved in the growth of KS[14,32] through their antiviral effects and multiple effects on cell growth and function. Recombinant interferons α2a (Roferon-A) and α2b (Intron-A) were approved for the treatment of certain patients with AIDS-associated KS on the basis of studies performed before the introduction of active antiretroviral drugs. The approved doses are therefore based on the results of studies of interferon (IFN) as a single agent in which extremely high doses (e.g., 36 million units daily, or 30 million units/m^2 three times a week) were required to achieve KS regression. The use of such doses was often complicated by fatigue, malaise, anorexia, and hepatotoxicity. In those early studies the overall tumor response rates were approximately 30%. Responses were usually observed only in patients with CD4+ T-lymphocyte counts of 200/μl or more who had no history of opportunistic infection and who lacked other signs and symptoms of advanced HIV infection. In patients with these "good risk" features, regression of extensive cutaneous, oral, or GI KS was sometimes observed.[33] Median response durations were 6 to 12 months for partial responders and up to 2 years among complete responders.

Today, IFN is generally administered in combination with other agents used to treat HIV infection and at lower doses. Although combined IFN and chemotherapy regimens have been poorly tolerated and have not yielded superior therapeutic results,[34–36] improved results have been described when IFNα was combined, at lower doses than those used for monotherapy, with nucleoside reverse transcriptase inhibitors (Table 50–1). Several Phase I studies of combined IFNα and zidovudine have demonstrated KS response rates exceeding 40% in patients treated with IFNα doses ranging from 4 million to 18 million IU/day.[37,38,42] These high response rates were confirmed in a Phase II trial of the combination, which used a daily IFN dose of 18

▲ **Table 50–1.** INTERFERON-α ± ZIDOVUDINE RESPONSE ACCORDING TO PRETREATMENT CD4 CELL COUNT

	% Complete and Partial Responses, by Pretreatment CD4 Count					
Parameter	IFNα2a without ZDV[34]	IFNα2a or IFNαn1 + ZDV[37]	IFNα2a or IFNαn1 + ZDV[38]	IFNα2a + ZDV[39]	IFNα2a + ZDV + GM-CSF[40]	IFNα2b + ZDV + GM-CSF[41]
IFN Dose(MU)	≥36	4.5–18.0	9–27	18	9	5–20
Pretreatment CD4 cell count (/μl)						
<100				27	19	
≥100				53	53	
<200	7	30	35			14
≥200	35	65	65			60
200–400	27	40				
>400	45	100				

GM-CSF, granulocyte/macrophage colony-stimulating factor; IFN, interferon; MU, million units; ZDV, zidovudine. α2a and α2b refer to recombinant IFNα species; αnl refers to IFNα induced in a human lymphoblastoid cell line.

million IU and a zidovudine dose of 100 mg every 4 hours.[39] The IFNα-zidovudine combination induced KS regression in 25% to 30% of patients with CD4+ T-lymphocyte counts less than 200/μl,[37,39] whereas fewer than 10% of such patients responded to high-dose IFNα monotherapy.[34] Although the dose-limiting neutropenia frequently seen with the combination[37–39,42] could be prevented or reversed by administration of granulocyte/macrophage colony stimulating factor (GM-CSF),[40,41] more recent trials have evaluated IFN in combination with less myelosuppressive antiretroviral therapy. In one such trial (ACTG 206) patients were randomly assigned to receive IFNα at a dose of either 1 million or 10 million IU/day together with standard doses of didanosine. Similar rates of objective tumor regression were observed in both dosage groups, but the lower dose was significantly better tolerated.[43] A Phase I study was conducted by the AIDS Malignancy Consortium (AMC 004) to evaluate the combination of varying doses of IFNα (0, 1 million, 5 million, or 10 million IU/day) with protease inhibitor-containing antiretroviral therapy. The overall response rate was 39% in this small study. Grade III hematologic toxicity was observed at IFN doses of 5 million or 10 million IU/day (J. VonRoenn, personal communication).

Maximal responses to IFNα, alone or combined with antiretroviral therapy, often require 6 months or more of treatment. Thus despite documented activity in some patients with visceral disease, IFN probably should not be considered for treating patients with rapidly progressive KS, particularly those with symptomatic visceral involvement. Because responses to IFN may persist for several years, however, it should be considered for patients with more slowly progressive KS when rapid relief of symptoms is not urgently required. It remains to be seen whether IFN combined with state-of-the-art antiretroviral therapy can induce higher response rates and faster times to response. Polyethylene glycol-conjugated (Pegylated) IFNα is being considered for trials in AIDS-associated KS. Because it has a long half-life and requires only infrequent (weekly) administration, it may prove more acceptable to patients who find it difficult to adhere to a frequent injection schedule.

Chemotherapy

Chemotherapy is indicated for patients with advanced or rapidly progressive KS that causes medical or functional impairment. This group includes patients with extensive or symptomatic cutaneous disease, extensive oral disease, symptomatic tumor-associated edema, pulmonary KS, or symptomatic gastrointestinal KS. The goals of such therapy are to induce durable regression of widespread, disfiguring, or disabling lesions; control or reverse life-threatening visceral disease; reduce functional impairment caused by edema or mucocutaneous disease; and achieve these benefits with agents that have an acceptable side effect profile. In addition, because the patients have an underlying HIV infection that is generally quite advanced, chemotherapy should not interfere with delivery of treatment with antiretroviral drugs or treatment and prophylaxis for other opportunistic complications of AIDS. It should be noted, however, that most trials of chemotherapeutic agents have been conducted in patients with extremely low CD4+ T-lymphocyte counts, and a low CD4+ T-lymphocyte count alone should not preclude systemic therapy when its use is otherwise warranted.

A wide variety of single chemotherapeutic agents and drug combinations have shown activity against AIDS-related KS. Only three such agents—liposomal daunorubicin (DaunoXome), liposomal doxorubicin (Doxil), paclitaxel (Taxol)—have been reviewed and approved by the FDA specifically for KS treatment.

In addition to the FDA-approved agents, which are discussed in detail later, other single agents with reported activity include etoposide,[44–48] vinblastine,[49] vincristine,[50] bleomycin,[50–53] and doxorubicin,[54–56] each of which has been studied alone or as part of combination regimens in multiple clinical trials. In addition, single clinical trials have indicated anti-KS activity for teniposide,[57] vinorelbine,[58] and epirubicin.[59] Reported results with these conventional agents in studies with a minimum of 14 evaluable patients are summarized in Table 50–2. Despite their demonstrated activity, disease control by these agents has often been limited by their toxicities, the most common of which are alopecia, mucositis, and neutropenia with etoposide and doxorubicin; neutropenia with vinblastine; peripheral neuropathy from vincristine; and fever and cutaneous and cumulative pulmonary toxicities from bleomycin. High cumulative doses of doxorubicin are also associated with cardiac toxicity. The reported response rates and response durations for these agents are difficult to interpret or compare, as patient characteristics and response definitions varied from study to study, the use of antiretroviral therapy and infection prophylaxis was inconsistent, the methods of disease documentation and response definitions were often ambiguous and inconsistently applied, and with rare exception the studies were not controlled.

Before the introduction of liposomal anthracyclines and the more recent introduction of paclitaxel, combination chemotherapy was generally considered to induce higher response rates than single agent therapy but at the expense of somewhat increased toxicity, which often limited long-term use. Nonetheless, by the early 1990s combination therapy was considered the standard of care, with the ABV regimen[55] consisting of doxorubicin (Adriamycin), bleomycin, and vincristine thought to be the most effective, at least in the United States. Several variations of the ABV regimen have been used, both with and without concomitant antiretroviral therapy and hematopoietic growth factor support,[55,56,60–64] but the most commonly used doses have been doxorubicin 20 mg/m^2, bleomycin 10 U/m^2, and vincristine 1 mg, administered every 2 weeks. Other frequently used combinations have included bleomycin and vincristine,[65–68] which has been more widely used as a standard regimen in Europe than in the United States, and a regimen that alternates vinblastine with vincristine on a weekly schedule.[69] Several more-intensive chemotherapy regimens have been tested,[70,71] but they have generally induced unacceptable toxicity without a corresponding increase in therapeutic activity or response duration. The results of trials with these chemotherapy combinations have been extensively reviewed elsewhere[32,72]; their use has

▲ **Table 50–2.** SINGLE-AGENT CHEMOTHERAPY FOR KS WITH CONVENTIONAL AGENTS

Drug	Schedule	No. Evaluable Patients	Response Rate (%)	Median Response Duration	Ref.
Etoposide					
150 mg/m² IV	d 1–3, q4wk	41	76	39 wk	44
150 mg/m² IV	d 1–3, q4wk	14	0	—	45
50 mg PO	d 1–21, q4–5wk	14	21	NA	48
25 mg/m² PO	d 1–7, bid q2wk	25	32	NA	47
150–400 mg PO	Once weekly	25	36	20 wk	46
Teniposide					
360 mg/m² IV	q3wk	25	40	9 wk	57
Vinblastine					
6 mg IV	Once weekly	38	26	13 wk	49
Vincristine					
2 mg/IV	q1–2wk	18	61	17 wk	50
Vinorelbine					
30 mg/m² IV	q2wk	27	44	8 mo (CR) 3 mo (PR)	58
Bleomycin					
5 mg IM	d 1–3, Q2–3wk	30[a]			
6 mg/m² CI	d 1–4, q4wk	30[a]	48[a]	37 wk[a]	52
5 mg IM	d 1–3, q2wk	70	74	20 wk	51
20 mg/m² CI	d 1–3, q3wk	17	65	13 wk	53
Doxorubicin					
15 mg/m² IV	Once weekly	50	10	13 wk	54
20 mg/m² IV	q2wk	29	48	NA	55
Epirubicin					
90 mg/m² IV	q2wk	26	42	22 wk	59

CI, continuous infusion; CR, Complete response; NA, not available; PR, partial response.
[a]Results are from pooled data from 60 patients treated with two regimens.

largely been supplanted over the past few years by the recently introduced liposomal anthracyclines and to some extent by paclitaxel. Table 50–3 shows the results of some combination chemotherapy regimens for AIDS-associated KS, each of which includes a minimum of 18 evaluable patients; the data were selected to illustrate the regimens used and the marked variation in reported response rates and response durations for similar regimens.

The first chemotherapeutic agents approved by the FDA specifically for treatment of advanced AIDS-related KS were liposomal doxorubicin (Doxil) and liposomal daunorubicin (DaunoXome) (Table 50–4). The liposomal formulation prolongs the circulating half-life of the anthracyclines (hours versus minutes for the unencapsulated drugs), increases drug concentrations in tumor tissue, and modifies toxicity.[85,87,88] Neutropenia is frequently induced by these agents,[73,74,77,78] but alopecia, nausea, and vomiting, which are common after administration of free doxorubicin, are uncommon with the liposomal agents.[73,89,90] Anthracycline-induced cardiac toxicity has been observed rarely after administration of high cumulative doses to patients with KS,[85,91,92] but maximum safe cumulative doses have not been defined. Doxil (but not DaunoXome) treatment has sometimes been associated with the hand-foot syndrome (palmar-plantar erythrodysesthesia).[93] This reaction, consisting of painful erythema and desquamation of the palms and soles, is generally associated with chemotherapeutic agents administered by continuous infusion. It is believed that the markedly increased serum half-life (approximately 48 hours) associated with the PEG-coated liposome used to formulate Doxil simulates a continuous drug infusion, whereas the uncoated liposome used to formulate DaunoXome has a $t_{1/2}$ of only about 4 hours. Both Doxil and DaunoXome administration, on occasion, have been complicated by acute infusional reactions characterized by back or chest pain, a sensation of choking, and intense flushing.[94] The latter reaction usually occurs within minutes of starting treatment and generally subsides quickly after stopping the drug infusion.

Doxil is approved for treatment of advanced KS after failure or intolerance of combination chemotherapy. According to the package insert, tumor response rates of 27% and 48%, respectively, were documented depending on whether a global disease assessment was used as the response criterion or the response was based on changes in selected indicator lesions. The median response durations were 2.4 and 2.3 months, respectively, from the time a partial response was recorded by these two assessment methods. Significantly, the lesions of some patients whose tumors had progressed on regimens containing conventional (unencapsulated) doxorubicin responded subsequently to Doxil. In practice, however, Doxil is often used as first-line chemotherapy. The recommended dose and treatment schedule for Doxil is 20 mg/m² as a slow (30 to 60 minute) intravenous infusion every 3 weeks. DaunoXome is approved for first-line chemotherapy of advanced KS based on a randomized comparison with a standard ABV regimen (described later). The labeled response rate is 23%, lasting a median of 3.7 months from the time a partial response was documented. The approved dose is 40 mg/m² every 2 weeks. Escalation to 60 mg/m² has sometimes induced responses in patients who did not respond or who relapsed after treatment at the lower dose. The 60 mg/m² dose has also proven effective for patients

▲ **Table 50–3.** COMBINATION CHEMOTHERAPY REGIMENS FOR KS

Drug	Dose[a]	Schedule[b]	No. Evaluable Patients	Response Rate (%)	Median Response Duration	Ref.
Doxorubicin Vinblastine Bleomycin Vincristine Dactinomycin Dacarbazine	20 mg/m² 4 mg/m² 15 U/m² 1.4 mg/m² 1 mg/m² 375 mg/m²	d 1, q3wk d 1, q3wk d 1, q3wk d 8, q3wk d 8, q3wk d 8, q3wk	18	83	2–3 mo	70
Doxorubicin Bleomycin Vinblastine	40 mg/m² 15 U 6 mg/m²	d 1, q4wk d 1 and 15, q4wk d 1, q4wk	31	84	8.5 mo (CR) 7.5 mo (PR)	44
Vincristine Vinblastine	2 mg 0.1 mg/kg	Alternating weekly	21	43	35+ wk	69
Doxorubicin Bleomycin Vincristine	20 mg/m² 10 mg/m² 1.4 mg/m²	q2wk q2wk q2wk	24	88	9.0 mo	55
Doxorubicin Bleomycin Vincristine	10 mg/m² 15 U 1 mg	q2wk q2wk q2wk	111	28	24.0 wk	73
Doxorubicin Bleomycin Vincristine	20 mg/m² 10 mg/m² 1 mg/m²	q2wk q2wk q2wk	110	25	14.0 wk	74
Doxorubicin Bleomycin Vincristine	20 mg/m² 10 U/m² 1 mg	q2wk q2wk q2wk	74	59	19–20 wk	64
Doxorubicin Bleomycin Vincristine	30 mg/m² 10 mg/m² 2 mg	q4wk q4wk q4wk	30	64[c]	3.5 wk[d]	60
Bleomycin Vincristine	15 U/m² 2 mg	q3wk q3wk	120	23	NA	68
Bleomycin Vincristine *or* Vinblastine[e]	30 mg 2 mg 2.5–5.0 mg	q3–4wk q3–4wk q3–4wk	46	57	6.4 mo	65
Bleomycin Vincristine	10 mg/m² 1.4 mg/m²	q2wk q2wk	18	72	8.0 wk	66
Bleomycin Vincristine	15 mg/m² 1.4 mg/m²	q2wk q2wk	45	64	12.3 wk	67

[a]All drugs given intravenously.
[b]Unless otherwise specified, all drugs given at the same time at the specified interval.
[c]Radiologic improvement in pulmonary KS.
[d]Duration of subjective improvement in dyspnea.
[e]Vinblastine substituted for vincristine if peripheral neuropathy occurred.

with pulmonary KS.[86] Objective response rates reported in the literature for these agents have varied widely. Some early reports in relatively small numbers of patients suggested that response rates might be as high as 70% to 90% even in previously treated patients.[75–79,82–85] Larger multicenter trials that applied strict response criteria, however, have documented response rates between 25% and 59%.[68,73,74,81] Although strictly defined response rates may be somewhat lower than originally believed, patients may experience palliation of KS-associated symptoms without achieving 50% tumor regression. At the time these studies were conducted, standard evaluation criteria for KS did not specifically address clinical benefits associated with tumor regression (e.g., pain relief, increased mobility associated with reduced edema). A joint National Cancer Institute (NCI)/FDA/AIDS Malignancy Consortium (AMC) initiative has attempted to address this gap. Revised evaluation criteria have been developed that quantitatively evaluate changes in KS-associated signs and symptoms that affect patient function and quality of life.[96] These clinical benefit assessments are now being tested prospectively in AMC clinical trials.

Several prospectively randomized studies have been conducted to compare liposomal anthracyclines with conventional combination chemotherapy. One study compared Doxil 20 mg/m² with ABV every 2 weeks. A significantly higher response rate was observed with Doxil (43%) than with ABV (25%).[74] A comparison of DaunoXome 40 mg/m² with ABV every 2 weeks yielded equivalent response rates of 25% and 28%, respectively.[73] A third study compared Doxil (20 mg/m²) with the combination of bleomycin (15 U/m²) and vincristine (2 mg).[68] Each regimen was given every 3 weeks. A significantly higher response rate was observed among patients who received Doxil (59%) than among those who received bleomycin and vincristine (23%).[68] In each of the three studies, patients who received the liposomal anthracycline showed a significantly lower incidence of peripheral neuropathy, nausea, and vomiting

▲ **Table 50–4.** LIPOSOMAL ANTHRACYCLINE CHEMOTHERAPY FOR KS

Dose (mg/m²)	Treatment Interval (weeks)	No. Evaluable Patients	Response Rate (%)	Median Response Duration (weeks)	Ref.
L-Dox					
20	2–3	16	69	14	75
10–20	2	15	73	NA	76
10–40	2	39	92	NA	77
20	3	34	74	9	78
10–40	2	238	81	NA[a]	79
20	2	62	79	NA	80
20	3	121	59	NA	68
20	3	53	38	18	81
20	2	118	43	15	74
L-Dauno					
40	2	10	40	4	82
40	2	24	63	12	83
50–60	2	22	95	NA	84
40	2	22	55	NA	85
40	2	116	25	25	73
60	2	53	35[b]	NA	86

L-Dauno, liposomal daunorubicin (Dauno Xome); L-Dox, Pegylated liposomal doxorubicin (Doxil); NA, not available.
[a]Median response duration approximately 13 weeks from graph in text.
[b]Pulmonary KS only. Response rate based on chest radiographs or CT scans. Functional response noted in 42%; symptomatic response noted in 48%.

than those who received combination therapy. Doxil induced more neutropenia than bleomycin and vincristine, and more mucositis than ABV, but it was less likely than ABV to cause significant alopecia and severe neutropenia. Response rates in each of these randomized trials were considerably lower than those reported previously for both the liposomal anthracyclines (in uncontrolled trials) and for the standard combination regimens (in both single-arm and randomized studies); but as noted before, objective response rates are not necessarily the equivalent of clinical benefit.

To determine if Doxil might be more effective as part of a combination chemotherapy regimen, a randomized, multicenter trial was conducted by the AIDS Clinical Trials Group (ACTG 286) to compare biweekly Doxil alone (at a dose of 20 mg/m²) to Doxil (at the same dose and schedule) in combination with bleomycin (10 U/m²) and vincristine (1 mg) in patients with advanced KS who had received no prior chemotherapy. The two regimens induced almost identical response rates of similar duration, but the combination regimen induced significantly more and earlier toxicity than Doxil alone and was associated with a more rapid decline in quality of life.[80]

Several studies have demonstrated that paclitaxel is highly active against KS. Paclitaxel is a mitotic spindle poison that promotes microtubulin formation[97] and leads to mitotic arrest.[98] Paclitaxel also inhibits cell chemotaxis and invasion induced by angiogenic factors.[99] HHV-8, the virus implicated in the development of KS, encodes a homologue of cellular bcl-2, an antagonist of apoptosis, and both viral and cellular bcl-2 mRNAs have been identified in KS biopsies.[100] Pertinently, paclitaxel has recently been shown to promote apoptosis and to down-regulate bcl-2 protein expression in KS cells in vitro and KS-like lesions in mice.[101] Two studies that used different doses and schedules of paclitaxel administration, but a similar planned dose intensity, were performed in patients with advanced, symptomatic KS, many of whom had visceral disease and tumor-associated edema.[102–104] Many of the patients had previously undergone systemic treatment for KS, and most had low CD4+ T-lymphocyte counts (median $\leq 20/\mu l$). Doses of 135 mg/m² every 3 weeks or 100 mg/m² every 2 weeks, each of which was administered as a 3-hour infusion, induced objective response rates of 69% and 59%, respectively, in a total of 85 patients, with median response durations of 7 to 10 months from the start of treatment. It should be noted that the methods used to measure response duration in these studies differed from those used in trials of the liposomal anthracyclines. In the latter studies, response duration was measured from the time a response was first achieved. Lesion regression was accompanied by alleviation of KS-associated edema and pain and an improved performance status; but treatment was complicated by significant myalgias, neutropenia, and alopecia in a high proportion of patients. Neutropenia was ameliorated by the use of granulocyte colony-stimulating factor (G-CSF). On the basis of these findings, the FDA approved paclitaxel as second-line chemotherapy for advanced AIDS-related KS. Currently, the Eastern Cooperative Oncology Group (ECOG) and the AMC are jointly conducting a randomized trial to compare Doxil and paclitaxel as first-line chemotherapy for AIDS-associated KS with respect to objective response rates and clinical benefit.

Investigational Therapy

Although several systemic and local approaches have proven effective in controlling the growth of KS lesions, a need still exists for more effective, less toxic therapeutic agents. Existing treatments are not invariably effective. In addition, KS may recur after effective treatment, and many of the available treatments are toxic or have the potential to interact pharmacologically with other drugs used to treat HIV infection and its nonneoplastic complications. Also, as the life expectancy of HIV-infected individuals increases, there is concern about the potential long-term consequences of treatment with cytotoxic drugs.

Recent advances in understanding the pathogenesis of KS and its relation to HIV infection have provided a framework for the rational development of more effective treatment strategies and underlie most current investigational approaches to this tumor. KS can be viewed as an angiogenic-inflammatory neoplasm that originates in vascular endothelial cells or their circulating precursors[105] that have been infected with HHV-8.[106] Infection with HHV-8 (also known as the KS-associated herpesvirus, or KSHV) precedes the development of KS and can be detected serologically.[107,108] The virus encodes an array of functional homologues of human cellular proteins that may contribute to neoplastic transformation.[109] In established KS lesions, latency-associated viral genes such as the viral *cyclin D* are expressed in most of the cells[110] and are thought to play a role in KS initiation or progression (or both).

Angiogenesis is a characteristic histologic feature of KS lesions. Spindle cells derived from KS lesions have been shown to express a variety of angiogenic/inflammatory cytokines and growth factors, which include vascular endothelial growth factor (VEGF), basic fibroblast growth factor (bFGF), interleukin-1 (IL-1), and IL-6, among others.[111,112] KS cells also express the relevant receptors for these cytokines, which can stimulate cell proliferation in an autocrine manner. KS cells also proliferate in response to exogenously administered cytokines, including IL-1, IFNγ, IL-6, and tumor necrosis factor (TNF), which are present in excess in the serum of patients with poorly controlled HIV infection.[113] KS cells also overexpress matrix metalloproteinases (MMPs),[114] which are enzymes involved in the destruction of extracellular matrix proteins required for angiogenesis, and express high levels of $\alpha_v\beta_3$, the vitronectin receptor,[115] which is strongly up-regulated on activated endothelium.

Although HIV infection is neither necessary nor sufficient to induce the development of KS, the presence of HIV infection is associated with an increased incidence of the tumor and alteration of its natural history. Acute HIV infection of CD4+ T cells results in extracellular release of the HIV transactivator protein Tat, which stimulates the growth of spindle cells derived from KS lesions.[116] KS-derived spindle cells become responsive to Tat's growth-promoting effects only in the presence of inflammatory cytokines and growth factors, which also stimulate spindle cell proliferation and migration.[115] In addition to their autocrine production by KS cells, the activated T cells and monocytes of individuals with poorly controlled HIV infection produce many of these factors. The Tat protein apparently mediates angiogenesis through two distinct regions: an RGD (Arg-Gly-Asp) region, which induces migration and invasion of KS by binding to integrins that are strongly expressed on KS-derived spindle cells, and a basic region, which allows release of a soluble form of bFGF that promotes vascular cell growth.[117] Tat also augments the angiogenesis-promoting activity of IFNγ on endothelial cells, transactivates the IL-6 promoter, induces phosphorylation of the Flk-1/KDR VEGF receptor, and increases MMP-9 expression by monocytes, which may facilitate breakdown of tissue matrix and permit migration of growing tumor and vascular endothelial cells.[116–119]

Various agents, acting by different mechanisms, have been described that may inhibit the complex processes involved in the development and progression of KS. Examples of some of the targets for a pathogenesis-driven approach to KS therapy and the agents that may influence them are shown in Table 50–5. Among the agents that have the potential to inhibit various steps in angiogenesis are synthetic retinoids[18,19,120,121]; thalidomide (which may limit angiogenesis through inhibition of TNF and through TNF-independent mechanisms)[14,122,123]; inhibitors of endothelial cell proliferation such as TNP-470[124,125] angiostatin,[126] and endostatin[127]; and inhibitors of matrix metalloproteinases.[128] Other targeted therapeutic approaches include agents that interfere with tyrosine kinase-mediated transmembrane receptor signals for angiogenic growth factors,[129] antisense oligonucleotides directed against these growth factors,[130] and agents directed against endothelial cell surface molecules expressed preferentially on proliferating vasculature, such as the $\alpha_v\beta_3$ integrin.[131] Some trials have provided preliminary evidence for anti-KS activity of thalidomide,[122,123] systemically administered 9-*cis*-retinoic acid,[132] COL-3 (an MMP inhibitor),[133] IL-12,[134] TNP-470,[123] and SU5416 (an inhibitor of the Flk-1/KDR VEGF receptor).[135] All of these agents have been associated with toxicities, however, and their ultimate role in KS management has yet to be defined. A preliminary clinical study has also indicated that IM862, an intranasally administered dipeptide

▲ **Table 50–5.** PATHOGENESIS-DIRECTED THERAPY FOR KS

Target	Therapeutic Agents that May Affect the Relevant Target
Inflammatory cytokines	Retinoids Thalidomide Interferons Receptor antagonists (e.g., IL-1RA)
VEGF	VEGF-receptor inhibitors (e.g., SU5416, PTK787/ZK 222584, anti-VEGF monoclonal antibodies) IL-12 Thalidomide Flavopiridol
bFGF	Antisense bFGF Interferons Thalidomide
Matrix metalloproteinases	MMPIs (e.g., COL-3, BMS-275291, Marimistat)
Integrin $\alpha_v\beta_3$	EMD121974 Vitaxin (humanized anti-$\alpha_v\beta_3$ monoclonal antibody)
Endothelial cell proliferation	TNP-470 Endostatin Angiostatin Interferons
Cyclin D	Flavopiridol
HHV-8	Ganciclovir and related agents Foscarnet Tenofovir Interferons
HIV Tat protein	Antiretroviral drugs

bFGF, basic fibroblast growth factor; HHV-8, human herpesvirus-8; IL-1RA, interleukin-1 receptor antagonist; VEGF, vascular endothelial growth factor.

with antiangiogenic properties, has activity against KS.[136] This agent is currently undergoing evaluation in a Phase III, placebo-controlled, randomized trial.

There is also considerable interest in evaluating the role of antiherpesvirus drugs in KS. Anecdotal reports that established KS regressed after treatment with foscarnet[137] and several studies that showed a decreased incidence of subsequent KS in patients treated with antiherpesvirus agents[138,139] suggest that under some circumstances inhibition of HHV-8 may also be of therapeutic or prophylactic value. Although the data supporting the use of antiherpesvirus drugs for treatment of established KS are not particularly compelling, it has been suggested that pharmacologic induction of HHV-8 lytic gene expression might render established KS susceptible to therapy with drugs that exert antiherpesvirus activity.[140] Flavopiridol, which has the potential to inhibit the activity of endogenous and HHV-8 cyclin/cdk complexes that regulate cell cycle progression,[141] has also been proposed as a potential therapeutic agent for KS. In addition to its cell cycle inhibitory effects, flavopiridol has been shown to block hypoxia-induced VEGF production[142] and to inhibit HIV replication,[143] but a reportedly high incidence of adverse events[144] may limit its clinical application. There is also considerable support for investigation of antiherpesvirus drugs as prophylactic agents in HHV-8-seropositive individuals at high risk for subsequent KS development. The role of more effective anti-HIV therapy in the treatment and prevention of KS also requires better definition. Finally, the combined administration of multiple therapeutic agents directed at various steps in the development of KS lesions remains to be explored.

Treatment Strategy

Regression and symptom palliation of KS can be achieved with many drugs and techniques. Although long-term tumor regression has been achieved in some cases, in most patients the benefits of treatment are temporary and treatment is not curative. The choice of therapy must be individualized. Factors to consider include the overall severity of the KS, the presence of specific KS-associated symptoms (e.g., edema, pain, dyspnea), the rate of KS progression, and the patient's treatment history. Individual patient goals and concerns (e.g., cosmetic issues or the desire to avoid particular treatment side effects) also require consideration. In addition, the degree to which the underlying HIV infection can be controlled, performance status, and the presence of concomitant conditions (e.g., neuropathy, wasting, chronic infections, abnormal hematologic, cardiac, hepatic or pulmonary function) may also influence the therapeutic approach. A successful KS treatment strategy requires intensive supportive care, including nutritional support, pain control, and adjunctive therapy for myelosuppression, in addition to standard treatments for HIV infection and its nonneoplastic complications. Although severe toxicity was observed unexpectedly when paclitaxel and delavirdine were combined,[145] chemotherapeutic agents and standard anti-HIV regimens have, for the most part, been safely combined. As a rule, KS treatment and state-of-the-art antiretroviral regimens should be used concurrently, as effective HIV control appears to be associated with a better KS outcome. Whenever possible, however, it is prudent to avoid zidovudine, which may cause excessive hematologic suppression and increase the need for hematopoietic growth factors. Table 50–6 outlines the major standard treatment options for various presentations of KS. It is intended as a general guide and excludes investigational approaches to KS treatment. Depending on the overall condition of the patient and the coexistence of multiple KS-related problems, various treatment approaches may have to be used sequentially or concomitantly.

Patients with AIDS-associated KS, like others with HIV infection, stand to derive long-term benefits from advances in antiretroviral therapy. Although improved antiretroviral therapy is welcome, it brings up several issues that must be considered when devising therapeutic plans and designing new treatment strategies. There is some uncertainty about the future incidence and clinical course of KS in patients who survive for many years with immunosuppression. Questions also remain about the best time to initiate KS therapy, the influence of concomitant antiretroviral ther-

Table 50–6. THERAPEUTIC OPTIONS FOR KS

KS Presentation	Main Treatment Options	Comments
Limited cutaneous	Optimize antiretroviral therapy Local therapy Radiation therapy Interferon-α + antiretrovirals	Choice depends on status of HIV infection, number and distribution of KS lesions, personal preference
Cosmetically unacceptable skin lesions	Local therapy Radiation therapy Systemic chemotherapy	Local therapy may be used alone or with chemotherapy, depending on extent of lesions
Extensive cutaneous	Interferon-α + antiretrovirals Systemic chemotherapy	Systemic chemotherapy best for symptomatic disease and/or poor HIV control. IFN favored for patients with good performance status and relatively asymptomatic KS
Bulky local skin or oral lesions	Systemic chemotherapy Radiation therapy	Chemotherapy probably superior as first-line therapy, particularly when diffuse skin lesions coexist with bulky local masses or edema
Tumor-associated edema (moderate to severe)	Systemic chemotherapy Radiation therapy	
Symptomatic visceral	Systemic chemotherapy	Radiation therapy may have limited application in palliating end-stage visceral disease

apy on the success of various KS treatment strategies, and the potential for untoward interactions between drugs used to treat KS and those used to treat HIV.[145] The latter subject is being addressed in several ongoing clinical trials. Moreover, as the life-span of patients with HIV infection and advanced KS increases, more concern is warranted about the potential long-term consequences of treatment with cytotoxic chemotherapy, including secondary neoplasms. In the long term, it is likely that early intervention with agents that influence the pathogenesis of this neoplasm will provide the most effective approach to KS treatment.

REFERENCES

1. Centers for Disease Control. Kaposi's sarcoma and Pneumocystis pneumonia among homosexual men—New York City and California. MMWR Morb Mortal Wkly Rep 30:305, 1981.
2. Jones JL, Hanson DL, Dworkin MS, et al. Incidence and trends in Kaposi's sarcoma in the era of effective antiretroviral therapy. J Acquir Immune Defic Syndr 24:270, 2000.
3. Chokunonga E, Levy LM, Bassett MT, et al. Cancer incidence in the African population of Harare, Zimbabwe: second results from the cancer registry 1993–1995. Int J Cancer 85:54, 2000.
4. Kaplan LD, Hopewell PC, Jaffe H, et al. Kaposi's sarcoma involving the lung in patients with the acquired immunodeficiency syndrome. J Acquir Immune Defic Syndr 1:23, 1988.
5. Krown SE, Metroka C, Wernz JC. Kaposi's sarcoma in the acquired immune deficiency syndrome: a proposal for uniform evaluation, response and staging criteria. J Clin Oncol 7:1201, 1989.
6. Krown WE, Testa MA, Huang J. AIDS-related Kaposi's sarcoma: prospective validation of the AIDS Clinical Trials Group staging classification. J Clin Oncol 15:3085, 1997.
7. Adal KA, Cockerell CJ, Petri WA Jr, et al. Cat scratch disease, bacillary angiomatosis, and other infections due to Rochalimaea. N Engl J Med 330:1509, 1994.
8. Barrison IG, Foster S, Harris JW, et al. Upper gastrointestinal Kaposi's sarcoma in patients positive for HIV antibody without cutaneous disease. BMJ 296:92, 1988.
9. Danzig JB, Brandt LJ, Reinus JF, et al. Gastrointestinal malignancy in patients with AIDS. Am J Gastroenterol 8:715, 1991.
10. Laine L, Amerian J, Rarick M, et al. The response of symptomatic gastrointestinal Kaposi's sarcoma to chemotherapy: a prospective evaluation using an endoscopic method of disease quantification. Am J Gastroenterol 85:959, 1990.
11. White DA. Pulmonary complications of HIV-associated malignancies. Clin Chest Med 17:755, 1996.
12. Meduri G, Stover D, Lee M, et al. Pulmonary Kaposi's sarcoma in the acquired immune deficiency syndrome: clinical, radiographic, and pathologic manifestations. Am J Med 81:11, 1986.
13. Lee V, Fuller J, O'Brien M, et al. Pulmonary Kaposi sarcoma in patients with AIDS: scintigraphic diagnosis with sequential thallium and gallium scanning. Radiology 180:409, 1991.
14. Karp JE, Pluda JM, Yarchoan R. AIDS-related Kaposi's sarcoma: a template for the translation of molecular pathogenesis into targeted therapeutic approaches. Hematol Oncol Clin North Am 10:1031, 1996.
15. Miles SA. Pathogenesis of AIDS-related Kaposi's sarcoma: evidence of a viral etiology. Hematol Oncol Clin North Am 10:1011, 1996.
16. Ensoli B, Barillari G, Salahuddin SZ, et al. Tat protein of HIV-1 stimulates growth of cells derived from Kaposi's sarcoma lesions of AIDS patients. Nature 345:84, 1990.
17. Ensoli B, Gendelman R, Markham P, et al. Synergy between basic fibroblast growth factor and HIV-1 Tat protein in induction of Kaposi's sarcoma. Nature 371:674, 1994.
18. Duvic M, Friedman-Kien AE, Looney DJ, et al. Topical treatment of cutaneous lesions of acquired immunodeficiency syndrome-related Kaposi sarcoma using alitretinoin gel: results of phase 1 and 2 trials. Arch Dermatol 136:1461, 2000.
19. Walmsley S, Northfelt DW, Melosky B, et al. Treatment of AIDS-related cutaneous Kaposi's sarcoma with topical alitretinoin (9-cis-retinoic acid) gel. J Acquir Immune Defic Syndr 22:235, 1999.
20. Tappero JW, Berger TG, Kaplan LD, et al. Cryotherapy for cutaneous Kaposi's sarcoma (KS) associated with acquired immune deficiency syndrome (AIDS): a phase II trial. J Acquir Immune Defic Syndr 4:839, 1991.
21. Boudreaux AA, Smith LL, Cosby CD, et al. Intralesional vinblastine for cutaneous Kaposi's sarcoma associated with acquired immunodeficiency syndrome: a clinical trial to evaluate efficacy and discomfort associated with injection. J Am Acad Dermatol 28:61, 1993.
22. Depuy J, Price M, Lynch G, et al. Intralesional interferon-alpha and zidovudine in epidemic Kaposi's sarcoma. J Am Acad Dermatol 28:966, 1993.
23. Boente P, Sampaio C, Brandáo MA, et al. Local perilesional therapy with rhGM-CSF for Kaposi's sarcoma. Lancet 341:1154, 1993.
24. Staddon A, Henry D, Bonnem E. A randomized dose finding study of recombinant platelet factor 4 (rPF4) in cutaneous AIDS-related Kaposi's sarcoma [abstract]. Proc Am Soc Clin Oncol 13:50, 1994.
25. Gill PS, Lunardi-Iskandar Y, Louie S, et al. The effects of preparations of human chorionic gonadotropin on AIDS-related Kaposi's sarcoma. N Engl J Med 335:1261, 1996.
26. Lucatoro FM, Sapp JP. Treatment of oral Kaposi's sarcoma with a sclerosing agent in AIDS patients: a preliminary study. Oral Surg Oral Med Oral Pathol 75:192, 1993.
27. Stelzer KJ, Griffin TW. A randomized prospective trial of radiation therapy for AIDS-associated Kaposi's sarcoma. Int J Radiat Oncol Biol Phys 27:1057, 1993.
28. Berson AM, Quivey JM, Harris JW, Wara WM. Radiation therapy for AIDS-related Kaposi's sarcoma. Int J Radiat Oncol Biol Phys 19:569, 1990.
29. Stelzer KJ, Griffin TW, Koh WJ. Radiation recall skin toxicity with bleomycin in a patient with Kaposi sarcoma related to acquired immune deficiency syndrome. Cancer 71:1322, 1993.
30. Chak LY, Gill PS, Levine AM, et al. Radiation therapy for acquired immunodeficiency syndrome-related Kaposi's sarcoma. J Clin Oncol 6:863, 1988.
31. Meyer JL. Whole-lung irradiation for Kaposi's sarcoma. Am J Clin Oncol 16:372, 1993.
32. Krown SE. Acquired immunodeficiency syndrome-associated Kaposi's sarcoma: biology and management. Med Clin North Am 81:471, 1997.
33. Real FX, Krown SE, Oettgen HF. Kaposi's sarcoma and the acquired immunodeficiency syndrome: treatment with high and low doses of recombinant leukocyte A interferon. J Clin Oncol 4:544, 1986.
34. Evans LM, Itri LM, Campion M, et al. Interferon-alpha 2a in the treatment of acquired immunodeficiency syndrome-related Kaposi's sarcoma. J Immunother 10:39, 1991.
35. Krigel RL, Slywotzky CM, Lonberg M, et al. Treatment of epidemic Kaposi's sarcoma with a combination of interferon-α2b and etoposide. J Biol Response Mod 7:359, 1988.
36. Shepherd FA, Evans WK, Garvey B, et al. Combination chemotherapy and α-interferon in the treatment of Kaposi's sarcoma associated with acquired immune deficiency syndrome. Can Med Assoc J 139:635, 1988.
37. Krown SE, Gold JWM, Niedzwiecki D, et al. Interferon-α with zidovudine: safety, tolerance, and clinical and virologic effects in patients with Kaposi's sarcoma associated with the acquired immunodeficiency syndrome (AIDS). Ann Intern Med 112:812, 1990.
38. Fischl MA, Uttamchandani R, Resnick L, et al. A phase I study of recombinant human interferon alfa-n1 and concomitant zidovudine in patients with AIDS-related Kaposi's sarcoma. J Acquir Immune Defic Syndr 4:1, 1991.
39. Fischl MA, Finkelstein DM, He W, et al. A phase II study of recombinant human interferon-α2a and zidovudine in patients with AIDS-related Kaposi's sarcoma. J Acquir Immune Defic Syndr Hum Retrovir 11:379, 1996.
40. Scadden DT, Bering HA, Levine JD, et al. Granulocyte-macrophage colony-stimulating factor mitigates the neutropenia of combined interferon alfa and zidovudine treatment of acquired immune deficiency syndrome-associated Kaposi's sarcoma. J Clin Oncol 9:802, 1991.
41. Krown SE, Paredes J, Bundow D, et al. Interferon-α, zidovudine and granulocyte-macrophage colony-stimulating factor: a phase I trial in patients with Kaposi's sarcoma associated with the acquired immunodeficiency syndrome (AIDS). J Clin Oncol 10:1344, 1992.
42. Kovacs JA, Deyton L, Davey R, et al. Combined zidovudine and interferon-α therapy in patients with Kaposi's sarcoma and the acquired immunodeficiency syndrome (AIDS). Ann Intern Med 111:280, 1989.

43. Krown SE, Li P, VonRoenn JH, et al. Randomized, open-label, phase II AIDS Clinical Trials Group study of two doses of interferon alfa-2b combined with didanosine in patients with AIDS-associated Kaposi's sarcoma: efficacy of daily low-dose interferon. J Interferon Cytokine Res (in press).
44. Laubenstein LJ, Krigel RL, Odajnyk CM, et al. Treatment of epidemic Kaposi's sarcoma with etoposide or a combination of doxorubicin, bleomycin and vinblastine. J Clin Oncol 2: 1115, 1984.
45. Bakker PJM, Danner SA, Lange JMA, Veenhof KHN. Etoposide for epidemic Kaposi's sarcoma: a phase II study. Eur J Cancer Clin Oncol 24:1047, 1988.
46. Paredes J, Kahn JO, Tong WP, et al. Weekly oral etoposide in patients with Kaposi's sarcoma associated with human immunodeficiency virus infection: a phase I multicenter trial of the AIDS Clinical Trials Group. J Acquir Immune Defic Syndr Hum Retrovirol 9:138, 1995.
47. Schwartsmann G, Sprinz E, Kromfield M, et al. Clinical and pharmacokinetic study of oral etoposide in patients with AIDS-related Kaposi's sarcoma with no prior exposure to cytotoxic therapy. J Clin Oncol 15:2118, 1997.
48. Bufill JA, Grace WR, Astrow AB. Phase II trial of prolonged, low-dose, oral VP-16 in AIDS-related Kaposi's sarcoma (KS) [abstract]. Proc Am Soc Clin Oncol 11:47, 1992.
49. Volberding PA, Abrams DI, Conant M, et al. Vinblastine therapy for Kaposi's sarcoma in the acquired immunodeficiency syndrome. Ann Intern Med 103:335, 1985.
50. Mintzer DM, Real FX, Jovino L, et al. Treatment of Kaposi's sarcoma and thrombocytopenia with vincristine in patients with acquired immunodeficiency syndrome. Ann Intern Med 102:200, 1985.
51. Caumes E, Guermonprez G, Katlama C, et al. AIDS-associated mucocutaneous Kaposi's sarcoma treated with bleomycin. AIDS 6:1483, 1992.
52. Lassoued K, Clauvel JP, Katlama C, et al. Treatment of the acquired immune deficiency syndrome-related Kaposi's sarcoma with bleomycin as a single agent. Cancer 66:1869, 1990.
53. Remick SC, Reddy M, Herman D, et al. Continuous infusion bleomycin in AIDS-related Kaposi's sarcoma. J Clin Oncol 12:1130, 1994.
54. Fischl MA, Krown SE, O'Boyle KP, et al. Weekly doxorubicin in the treatment of patients with AIDS-related Kaposi's sarcoma. J Acquir Immune Defic Syndr 6:259, 1993.
55. Gill PS, Rarick M, McCutchan JA, et al. Systemic treatment of AIDS-related Kaposi's sarcoma: results of a randomized trial. Am J Med 90:427, 1991.
56. Gill PS, Akil B, Colletti P, et al. Pulmonary Kaposi's sarcoma: clinical findings and results of therapy. Am J Med 87:57, 1989.
57. Schwartzmann G, Sprinz E, Kronfeld M, et al. Phase II study of teniposide in patients with AIDS-related Kaposi's sarcoma. Eur J Cancer 27:1637, 1991.
58. Nasti G, Errante D, Talamini R, et al. Vinorelbine is an effective and safe drug for AIDS-related Kaposi's sarcoma: results of a phase II study. J Clin Oncol 18:1550, 2000.
59. Shepherd FA, Burkes RL, Paul KE, Goss PE. A phase II study of 4′-epirubicin in the treatment of poor-risk Kaposi's sarcoma and AIDS. AIDS 5:305, 1991.
60. Cadranel JL, Kammoun S, Chevret S, et al. Results of chemotherapy in 30 AIDS patients with symptomatic pulmonary Kaposi's sarcoma. Thorax 49:958, 1994.
61. Gill PS, Rarick MU, Espina B, et al. Advanced acquired immune deficiency syndrome-related Kaposi's sarcoma: results of pilot studies using combination chemotherapy. Cancer 65:1074, 1990.
62. Gill PS, Miles SA, Mitsuyasu RT, et al. Phase I AIDS Clinical Trials Group (075) study of adriamycin, bleomycin and vincristine in the treatment of AIDS-related Kaposi's sarcoma. AIDS 8:1695, 1994.
63. Gill PS, Bernstein-Singer M, Espina BM, et al. Adriamycin, bleomycin and vincristine chemotherapy with recombinant granulocyte-macrophage colony-stimulating factor in the treatment of AIDS-related Kaposi's sarcoma. AIDS 6:1477, 1992.
64. Mitsuyasu RT, Gill P, Paredes J, et al. Combination chemotherapy, adriamycin, bleomycin, vincristine (ABV) with dideoxyinosine (ddI) or dideoxycytidine (ddC) in advanced AIDS-related Kaposi's sarcoma (ACTG 163) [abstract 822]. Proc Am Soc Clin Oncol 14:289, 1995.
65. Gompels MM, Hill A, Jenkins P, et al. Kaposi's sarcoma in HIV infection treated with vincristine and bleomycin. AIDS 6:1175, 1992.
66. Gill PS, Rarick M, Bernstein-Singer M. Treatment of advanced Kaposi's sarcoma using a combination of bleomycin and vincristine. Am J Clin Oncol 13:315, 1990.
67. Rizzardini G, Pastecchia C, Vigevani GM, et al. Stealth liposomal doxorubicin or bleomycin/vincristine for the treatment of AIDS-related Kaposi's sarcoma [abstract]. J Acquir Immune Defic Syndr Hum Retrovirol 14:A20, 1997.
68. Stewart JSW, Jablonowski H, Goebel FD, et al. Randomized comparative trial of pegylated liposomal doxorubicin versus bleomycin and vincristine in the treatment of AIDS-related Kaposi's sarcoma: International Pegylated Liposomal Doxorubicin Study Group. J Clin Oncol 16:683, 1998.
69. Kaplan L, Abrams D, Volberding P. Treatment of Kaposi's sarcoma in acquired immunodeficiency syndrome with an alternating vincristine-vinblastine regimen. Cancer Treat Rep 70:1121, 1986.
70. Gelmann EP, Longo D, Lane HC, et al. Combination chemotherapy of disseminated Kaposi's sarcoma in patients with the acquired immune deficiency syndrome. Am J Med 82:456, 1987.
71. Sloand E, Kumar PN, Pierce PF. Chemotherapy for patients with pulmonary Kaposi's sarcoma: benefit of filgrastim (G-CSF) in supporting dose administration. South Med J 86:1219, 1993.
72. Lee F-C, Mitsuyasu RT. Chemotherapy of AIDS-related Kaposi's sarcoma. Hematol Oncol Clin North Am 10:1051, 1996.
73. Gill PS, Wernz J, Scadden DT, et al. Randomized phase II trial of liposomal daunorubicin (DaunoXome) versus doxorubicin, bleomycin, vincristine (ABV) in AIDS-related Kaposi's sarcoma. J Clin Oncol 14:2353, 1996.
74. Northfelt DW, Dezube B, Thommes JA, et al. Pegylated liposomal doxorubicin versus doxorubicin, bleomycin, and vincristine in the treatment of AIDS-related Kaposi's sarcoma: results of a randomized phase III clinical trial. J Clin Oncol 16:2445, 1998.
75. Simpson JK, Miller RF, Spittle MF. Liposomal doxorubicin for treatment of AIDS-related Kaposi's sarcoma. Clin Oncol 5:372, 1993.
76. James ND, Coker RJ, Tomlinson D, et al. Liposomal doxorubicin (Doxil): an effective new treatment for Kaposi's sarcoma in AIDS. Clin Oncol 6:294, 1994.
77. Bogner JR, Kronawitter U, Rolinski B, et al. Liposomal doxorubicin in the treatment of advanced AIDS-related Kaposi's sarcoma. J Acquir Immune Defic Syndr 7:463, 1994.
78. Harrison M, Tomlinson D, Stewart S. Liposomal-entrapped doxorubicin: an active agent in AIDS-related Kaposi's sarcoma. J Clin Oncol 13:914, 1995
79. Goebel F-D, Goldstein D, Goos M, et al. Efficacy and safety of Stealth liposomal doxorubicin in AIDS-related Kaposi's sarcoma. Br J Cancer 73:989, 1996.
80. Mitsuyasu R, VonRoenn J, Krown S, et al. Comparison study of liposomal doxorubicin (Dox) alone or with bleomycin and vincristine (DBV) for treatment of advanced AIDS-associated Kaposi's sarcoma (AIDS-KS): AIDS Clinical Trial Group (ACTG) protocol 286 [abstract 191]. Proc Am Soc Clin Oncol 16:55a, 1997.
81. Northfelt DW, Dezube BJ, Thommes JA, et al. Efficacy of pegylated-liposomal doxorubicin in the treatment of AIDS-related Kaposi's sarcoma after failure of standard chemotherapy. J Clin Oncol 15:653, 1997.
82. Money-Kyrle JF, Bates F, Ready J, et al. Liposomal daunorubicin in advanced Kaposi's sarcoma: a phase II study. Clin Oncol (R Coll Radiol) 5:367, 1993.
83. Presant CA, Scolaro M, Kennedy P, et al. Liposomal daunorubicin treatment of HIV-associated Kaposi's sarcoma. Lancet 341:1242, 1993.
84. Chew T, Jacobs M, Huckabee M, et al. A phase II clinical trial of DaunoXome (VS103, liposomal daunorubicin) in Kaposi's sarcoma of AIDS patients [abstract WS-B15-3]. Int Conf AIDS 9:58, 1993.
85. Gill PS, Espina BM, Muggia F, et al. Phase I/II clinical and pharmacokinetic evaluation of liposomal daunorubicin. J Clin Oncol 13:996, 1995.
86. Tulpule A, Yung RC, Wernz J, et al. Phase II trial of liposomal daunorubicin in the treatment of AIDS-related pulmonary Kaposi's sarcoma. J Clin Oncol 16:3369, 1998.
87. Brenner DC. Liposomal encapsulation: making old and new drugs do new tricks. J Natl Cancer Inst 81:13, 1989.
88. Northfelt DW, Martin FJ, Working P, et al. Doxorubicin encapsulated in liposomes containing surface-bound polyethylene glycol: pharmacokinetics, tumor localization, and safety in patients with AIDS-related Kaposi's sarcoma. J Clin Pharmacol 36:55, 1996.
89. Cowens JW, Creaven PJ, Greco WR, et al. Initial clinical (phase I) trial of TLC D-99 (doxorubicin encapsulated in liposomes). Cancer Res 53:2796, 1993.
90. Wagner D, Kern WV, Kern P. Liposomal doxorubicin in AIDS-related Kaposi's sarcoma: long term experiences. Clin Invest 72:417, 1994.

91. Berry G, Billingham M, Alderman E, et al. The use of cardiac biopsy to demonstrate reduced cardiotoxicity in AIDS Kaposi's sarcoma patients treated with pegylated liposomal doxorubicin. Ann Oncol 9:711, 1998.
92. Ross M, Gill PS, Espina BM, et al. Liposomal daunorubicin (DaunoXome) in the treatment of advanced AIDS-related Kaposi's sarcoma: results of a phase II study [abstract PoB 3123]. Int Conf AIDS 8:B107, 1992.
93. Gordon KB, Tajuddin A, Guitart J, et al. Hand-foot syndrome associated with liposome-encapsulated doxorubicin therapy. Cancer 75:2169, 1995.
94. Uziely B, Jeffers S, Isaacson R, et al. Liposomal doxorubicin: antitumor activity and unique toxicities during two complementary phase I studies. J Clin Oncol 13:1777, 1995.
95. Dupont B, Pialoux G, Gonzalez G, et al. Phase II study of liposomal daunorubicin (DaunoXome) in AIDS-related Kaposi's sarcoma [abstract PoB 3119]. Int Conf AIDS 8:B106, 1992.
96. Feigal EG, VonRoenn J, Justice R, et al. Kaposi's sarcoma response criteria: issues identified by the National Cancer Institute, Food and Drug Administration, and the AIDS Malignancy Consortium [abstract 24]. J Acquir Immune Defic Syndr Hum Retrovirol 14:A22, 1997.
97. Schiff PB, Fant J, Horwitz SB. Promotion of microtubule assembly in vitro by Taxol. Nature 277:665, 1979.
98. Schiff PB, Horwitz SB. Taxol stabilizes microtubules in mouse fibroblast cells. Proc Natl Acad Sci USA 77:1561, 1980.
99. Belotti D, Vergani V, Drudis T, et al. The microtubule-affecting drug paclitaxel has antiangiogenic activity. Clin Cancer Res 2:1843, 1996.
100. Opalenik SR, Browning PJ. Human herpesvirus 8 (HHV-8) encodes a bcl-2 homologue that is expressed in Kaposi's sarcoma [abstract 42]. J Acquir Immune Defic Syndr Hum Retrovirol 14:A26, 1997.
101. Sgadari C, Toschi E, Palladino C, et al. Mechanism of paclitaxel activity in Kaposi's sarcoma. J Immunol 165:509, 2000.
102. Saville MW, Lietzau J, Pluda JM, et al. Treatment of HIV-associated Kaposi's sarcoma with paclitaxel. Lancet 346:26, 1995.
103. Welles L, Saville MW, Lietzau J, et al. Phase II trial with dose titration of paclitaxel for the therapy of human immunodeficiency virus-associated Kaposi's sarcoma. J Clin Oncol 16:1112, 1998.
104. Gill PS, Tulpule A, Espina BM, et al. Paclitaxel is safe and effective in the treatment of advanced AIDS-related Kaposi's sarcoma. J Clin Oncol 17:1876, 1999.
105. Browning PJ, Sechler JM, Kaplan M, et al. Identification and culture of Kaposi's sarcoma-like spindle cells from the peripheral blood of human immunodeficiency virus-1-infected individuals and normal controls. Blood 84:2711, 1994.
106. Davis MA, Sturzl MA, Blasig C, et al. Expression of human herpesvirus 8-encoded cyclin D in Kaposi's sarcoma spindle cells. J Natl Cancer Inst 89:1868, 1997.
107. Martin JN, Ganem DE, Osmond DH, et al. Sexual transmission and the natural history of human herpesvirus 8 infection. N Engl J Med 338:948, 1998.
108. Rabkin CS, Schulz TF, Whitby D, et al. Interassay correlation of human herpesvirus 8 serologic tests: HHV-8 Interlaboratory Collaborative Group. J Infect Dis 178:304, 1998.
109. Moore PS, Chang Y. Kaposi's sarcoma-associated herpesvirus-encoded oncogenes and oncogenesis. J Natl Cancer Inst Monogr 23:65, 1998.
110. Sturzl M, Ensoli B. Big but weak: how many pathogenic genes does human herpesvirus-8 need to cause Kaposi's sarcoma? Int J Oncol 14:287, 1999.
111. Ensoli B, Nakamura S, Salahuddin SZ, et al. AIDS Kaposi's sarcoma derived cells express cytokines with autocrine and paracrine growth effects. Science 243:223, 1989.
112. Miles SA, Rezai AR, Salazar-Gonzales JF, et al. AIDS Kaposi sarcoma-derived cells produce and respond to interleukin 6. Proc Natl Acad Sci USA 87:4068, 1990.
113. Samaniego F, Markham PD, Gendleman R, et al. Vascular endothelial growth factor and basic fibroblast growth factor present in Kaposi's sarcoma (KS) are induced by inflammatory cytokines and synergize to promote vascular permeability and KS lesion development. Am J Pathol 152:1433, 1998.
114. Meade-Tollin LC, Way D, Witte MH. Expression of multiple matrix metalloproteinases and urokinase type plasminogen activator in cultured Kaposi sarcoma cells. Acta Histochem 101:305, 1999.
115. Barillari G, Sgadari C, Palladino C, et al. Inflammatory cytokines synergize with the HIV-1 Tat protein to promote angiogenesis and Kaposi's sarcoma via induction of basic fibroblast growth factor and the alpha v beta 3 integrin. J Immunol 163:1929, 1999.
116. Fiorelli V, Barillari G, Toschi E, et al. IFN-gamma induces endothelial cells to proliferate and to invade the extracellular matrix in response to the HIV-1 Tat protein: implications for AIDS-Kaposi's sarcoma pathogenesis. J Immunol 162:1165, 1999.
117. Ganju RK, Munshi N, Nair BC, et al. Human immunodeficiency virus tat modulates the Flk-1/KDR receptor, mitogen-activated protein kinases, and components of focal adhesion in Kaposi's sarcoma cells. J Virol 72:6131, 1998.
118. Ambrosino C, Ruocco MR, Chen X, et al. HIV-1 Tat induces the expression of the interleukin-6 (IL6) gene by binding to the IL6 leader RNA and by interacting with CAAT enhancer-binding protein beta (NF-IL6) transcription factors. J Biol Chem 272:14883, 1997.
119. Kumar A, Dhawan S, Mukhopadhyay A, et al. Human immunodeficiency virus-1-tat induces matrix metalloproteinase-9 in monocytes through protein tyrosine phosphatase-mediated activation of nuclear transcription factor NF-kappaB. FEBS Lett 462:140, 1999.
120. Bonhomme L, Fredj G, Averous S, et al. Topical treatment of epidemic Kaposi's sarcoma with all-trans retinoic acid. Ann Oncol 2:234, 1991.
121. Bernstein ZP, Cohen P, Rios A, et al. A multicenter, phase II/III study of Atragen (Tretinoin Liposomal) in patients with AIDS-associated Kaposi's sarcoma [abstract 14]. J Acquired Immune Defic Syndr Hum Retrovirol 14:A19, 1997.
122. Little R, Wyvill K, Pluda JM, et al. Activity of thalidomide in AIDS-related Kaposi's sarcoma. J Clin Oncol 18:2593, 2000.
123. Fife K, Howard MR, Gracie F, et al. Activity of thalidomide in AIDS-related Kaposi's sarcoma and correlation with HHV8 titre. Int J STD AIDS 9:751, 1998.
124. Dezube BJ, VonRoenn JH, Holden-Wiltse J, et al. Fumagillin analog in the treatment of Kaposi's sarcoma: a phase I AIDS Clinical Trial Group study; AIDS Clinical Trial Group No. 215 Team. J Clin Oncol 16:1444, 1998.
125. Pluda JM, Wyvill KK, Lietzau J, et al. A phase I trial administering the angiogenesis inhibitor TNP-470 (AGM-1470) to patients (pts) with HIV-associated Kaposi's sarcoma (KS) [abstract 13]. J Acquir Immune Defic Syndr Hum Retrovirol 14:A19, 1997.
126. O'Reilly MS, Holmgren L, Shing Y, et al. Angiostatin: a novel angiogenesis inhibitor that mediates the suppression of metastases by a Lewis lung carcinoma. Cell 79:315, 1994.
127. O'Reilly MS, Boehm T, Shing Y, et al. Endostatin: an endogenous inhibitor of angiogenesis and tumor growth. Cell 88:277, 1997.
128. Heath EI, Grochow LB. Clinical potential of matrix metalloprotease inhibitors in cancer therapy. Drugs 59:1043, 2000.
129. Zhu Z, Witte L. Inhibition of tumor growth and metastasis by targeting tumor-associated angiogenesis with antagonists to the receptors of vascular endothelial growth factor. Invest New Drugs 17:195, 1999.
130. Ensoli B, Markham P, Kao V, et al. Block of AIDS-Kaposi's sarcoma (KS) cell growth, angiogenesis and lesion formation in nude mice by antisense oligonucleotide targeting basic fibroblast growth factor. J Clin Invest 94:1736, 1994.
131. Varner JA, Cheresh DA. Tumor angiogenesis and the role of vascular cell integrin $\alpha_v\beta_3$. Important Adv Oncol 69, 1996.
132. Miles SA, Dezube B, Lee JY, et al. Antitumor activity of oral 9-cis-retinoic acid in HIV infected patients with Kaposi's sarcoma: a multicenter trial of the AIDS Malignancy Consortium. AIDS 16:421, 2002.
133. Cianfrocca M, Cooley TP, Lee JY, et al. Matrix metalloproteinase inhibitor COL-3 in the treatment of AIDS-related Kaposi's sarcoma: a phase I AIDS Malignancy Consortium study. J Clin Oncol 20:153, 2002.
134. Little RF, Pluda JM, Wyvill K, et al. Interleukin 12 (IL-12) appears to be active in AIDS-associated Kaposi's sarcoma (KS): early results of a pilot study. Presented at the 7th Conference on Retroviruses and Opportunistic Infections 2000, San Francisco, abstract 5.
135. Arasteh K, Hannah A. The role of vascular endothelial growth factor (VEGF) in AIDS-related Kaposi's sarcoma. Oncologist 5 (suppl 1): 28, 2000.
136. Tulpule A, Scadden DT, Espina BM, et al. Results of a randomized study of IM862 nasal solution in the treatment of AIDS-related Kaposi's sarcoma. J Clin Oncol 18:716, 2000.

137. Morfeldt L, Torssander J. Long-term remission of Kaposi's sarcoma following foscarnet treatment in HIV-infected patients. Scand J Infect Dis 26:749, 1994.
138. Jones JL, Hanson DL, Chu SY, et al. AIDS-associated Kaposi's sarcoma [letter]. Science 267:1078, 1995.
139. Mocroft A, Youle M, Gazzard B, et al. Anti-herpesvirus treatment and risk of Kaposi's sarcoma in HIV infection: Royal Free/Chelsea and Westminster Hospitals collaborative group. AIDS 10:1101, 1996.
140. Shaw RN, Arbiser JL, Offermann MK. Valproic acid induces human herpesvirus 8 lytic gene expression in BCBL-1 cells [letter]. AIDS 14:899, 2000.
141. Senderowicz AM. Flavopiridol: the first cyclin-dependent kinase inhibitor in human clinical trials. Invest New Drugs 17:313, 1999.
142. Melillo G, Sausville EA, Cloud K, et al. Flavopiridol, a protein kinase inhibitor, down-regulates hypoxic induction of vascular endothelial growth factor expression in human monocytes. Cancer Res 59:5433, 1999.
143. Chao SH, Fujinaga K, Marion JE, et al. Flavopiridol inhibits P-TEFb and blocks HIV-1 replication. J Biol Chem 275:28345, 2000.
144. Stadler WM, Vogelzang NJ, Amato R, et al. Flavopiridol, a novel cyclin-dependent kinase inhibitor, in metastatic renal cancer: a University of Chicago phase II consortium study. J Clin Oncol 18:371, 2000.
145. Schwartz JD, Howard W, Scadden DT. Potential interaction of antiretroviral therapy with paclitaxel in patients with AIDS-related Kaposi's sarcoma [letter]. AIDS 13:283, 1999.

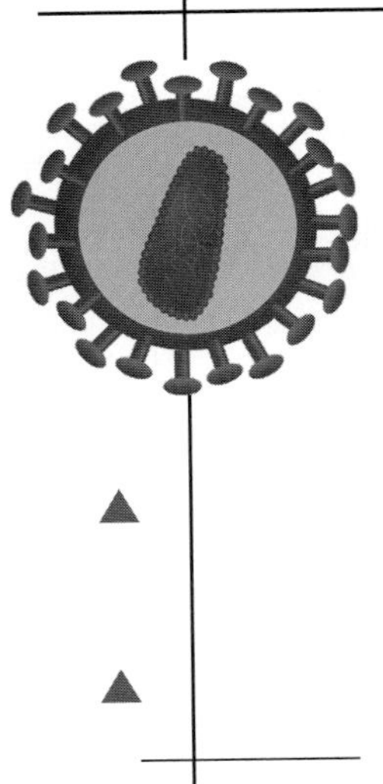

CHAPTER 51

Non-Hodgkin's Lymphoma

David T. Scadden, MD

Acquired immunodeficiency syndrome (AIDS)-related lymphoma (ARL) is the most lethal complication of AIDS.[1] However, recent advances in the care of patients with ARL coupled with the developments in antiretroviral therapy suggest that the nihilism previously surrounding this problem is no longer appropriate. The potential for meaningful, long-term remissions from ARL has been well demonstrated, and most patients should now be approached with curative rather than palliative intent. Multiple areas of investigation offer the potential for expanding curative outcomes to a broader range of patients. This chapter focuses on reviewing developments in understanding and treating ARL, and it highlights current standard treatment approaches and research directions.

The increased risk of developing lymphoma in the human immunodeficiency virus-1 (HIV-1)-infected population was noted early in the epidemic and was added to the definition of AIDS in 1985.[2] Unlike Kaposi's sarcoma, the risk of lymphoma is not restricted to particular subsets of patients with HIV disease, although a slightly higher risk has been reported for individuals with hemophilia.[3] The risk of lymphoma is related to the severity of immunosuppression, with a median CD4+ T-lymphocyte count of approximately 100 cells/mm^3 reported in several series and an annual risk estimated at 1.6% to 8.0% for patients with advanced immunosuppression.[4,5]

The advent of potent antiretroviral therapies has reduced the frequency of virtually all opportunistic diseases, including malignancies. Kaposi's sarcoma (KS) has been most markedly affected with reduction in frequency and regression of existing disease following highly active antiretroviral therapy (HAART) initiation.[6–10] The International Collaboration on HIV and Cancer documented a threefold decrease in risk (rate ratio 0.32) for KS when comparing incidence rates during 1992–1996 with those of 1997–1999.[11] The same study found a rate ratio of 0.58 for ARL, with primary central nervous system (CNS) lymphoma the most substantially reduced (rate ratio 0.42). It is of note that there were minor to no changes in the rates of Burkitt's lymphoma or Hodgkin's disease. Although this study is perhaps the most definitive, it should be noted that some studies show a continuing increase, a stable rate, or a decline in lymphoma incidence.[7–9,12–16]

The ARLs are almost exclusively of B cell origin, although rare T cell malignancies do occur. The T cell tumors are of particular interest in that some investigators have noted integration of HIV-1 into the host cell's genome upstream of the site of the c-*fes* oncogene, suggesting a potentially direct mechanism of transformation.[17] In general, however, HIV merely provides the backdrop against which malignant transformation occurs. HIV-1 itself is not found in most ARLs; rather, the immunodeficiency it induces appears to provide the appropriate milieu for lymphomatous outgrowth.

One potential means by which immune dysfunction may lead to malignancy is the loss of immunologic control of other, transforming virus infections. An example is the Epstein-Barr virus (EBV), which is found in a large proportion of ARLs. The association of EBV and ARL is most clearly seen in the primary CNS lymphoma of AIDS. This problem tends to occur in the most severely immunocompromised patients and is virtually uniformly associated with the presence of EBV in the tumor.[18] In this setting, the expression of EBV latency genes is identical with the profiles seen in lymphoproliferative disease complicating organ transplantation or congenital immunodeficiency. However, systemic

▲ **Table 51–1.** NON-HODGKIN'S LYMPHOMA: PATHOLOGY

Lymphoma Type	Knowles et al.[25]	Ziegler et al.[24]	Kaplan et al.[26]
Burkitt's	40%	36%	20%
Immunoblastic	25%	26%	46%
Diffuse large cell	25%	19%	34%

▲ **Table 51–2.** STAGE OF DISEASE FOR AIDS-RELATED LYMPHOMAS

No. of Patients	Stages I/II	Stages III/IV	Study
90	38 (42%)	52 (58%)	Ziegler et al.[24]
84	14 (17%)	69 (82%)	Kaplan et al.[26]
89	27 (30%)	57 (64%)	Knowles et al.[25]

ARL may or may not be associated with EBV, and variant viral latent gene expression patterns have been well described when EBV is present.[19] In addition, EBV is commonly seen in conjunction with another member of the herpesvirus family, human herpesvirus-8 (Kaposi's sarcoma herpesvirus), in the setting of the unusual subset of systemic lymphomas, primary effusion lymphoma, or body cavity lymphoma.[20] This rare tumor has a characteristic immunophenotype and generally presents as involvement of a compartmentalized body fluid without tumor mass. Thus the spectrum of virus-related ARL is continuing to evolve and, with it, understanding of the basis for lymphomatous transformation. Yet basic questions, such as why only a subset of patients develop lymphoma when infection with EBV is virtually ubiquitous in the population remain unanswered.

Other mechanisms for the development of B cell malignancies include the accumulation of genetic mutations in cells undergoing persistent stimulation. Chronic B cell activation in HIV disease is evident from the hypergammaglobulinemia and generalized lymphadenopathy often seen in infected individuals. The dysregulation of B cells has been attributed to direct antigenic stimulation or altered cytokine production by HIV-1-infected immune cells.[21] Whether such altered proliferation contributes directly to the transformation process remains conjectural, but it is hypothesized that polyclonal expansions of B cells may undergo mutations that permit the outgrowth of a malignant clone. Specific genetic lesions have been associated with particular histologic subsets of ARL.[21] For example, the germinal center-associated gene *BCL6* is mutated in 20% of diffuse large cell tumors, and c-*myc* is mutated in virtually all AIDS-related Burkitt's lymphomas, 60% of which also have disrupted *p53*.[22] In addition, genetic polymorphisms may be associated with the risk of lymphoma. Variant regulating regions of the chemokine SDF-1 have been rated to correlate with excess risk of Burkitt's lymphoma.[23]

In general, the tumors of ARL display a diffuse, aggressive B cell histology (Table 51–1). They can be divided into small-cell tumors (Burkitt's or Burkitt's-like lymphoma) or large-cell tumors. The large-cell category has in the past been subclassified as immunoblastic or histiocytic (diffuse large cell) and comprises about 60% of all ARLs. To put histologic characteristics in context, the frequency of small cell tumors is approximately 1000-fold increased in AIDS patients compared with that in the general population.[3] The clinical presentation of ARL can also be quite distinct from that of non-Hodgkin's lymphoma seen outside the setting of immunodeficiency (Table 51–2). There is a high frequency of extranodal involvement (74% to 98% in various reports) and of coincident systemic symptoms.[24–27] The favored sites for extranodal disease are bone marrow (23%), CNS (22%), gastrointestinal tract (21%), and liver (13%).[24–35] However, virtually every tissue has been reported to be involved with ARL, including otherwise extremely unusual infiltrations of the heart, bladder, gingiva, and anus (Table 51–3). About 20% to 40% of patients have leptomeningeal involvement at the time of diagnosis, and nearly half of such patients have no symptoms referable to the CNS. Systemic symptoms such as fever, night sweats, and weight loss are commonplace in the HIV-infected population but may be harbingers of ARL, in which they are seen virtually uniformly. When present in a patient diagnosed with ARL, a thorough microbiologic workup must be performed to exclude a coincident infectious process.

▲ SYSTEMIC LYMPHOMA

Diagnostic Workup and Staging

Patients presenting with fever or other B symptoms (night sweats, weight loss, anorexia) should be evaluated for a possible opportunistic infection (OI) such as those due to *Mycobacterium avium* complex or cytomegalovirus, acute EBV infection, toxoplasmosis, fungal infection, syphilis, or tuberculosis. Similarly, lymphadenopathy in the HIV setting may be related to HIV-associated lymphoid proliferation, Kaposi's sarcoma, or ARL. The diagnosis should be established by a tissue biopsy, which should undergo routine hematoxylin and eosin staining, staining for acid-fast bacilli and fungus, immunohistochemistry, flow cytometry, and culture. Inaccessible lesions may be approached by a fine-needle aspirate or core needle biopsy. Whenever possible, analysis for EBV in the tumor should be performed [preferably using EBER (EBV-encoded small nuclear RNAs) staining], as the presence of EBV has been correlated with a

▲ **Table 51–3.** SITES OF EXTRANODAL INVOLVEMENT FOR AIDS-RELATED HIGH-GRADE B CELL LYMPHOMAS

No. of Patients	% Extranodal	% CNS	% GI	% Marrow	% Liver	Study
90	98	42[a]	17	33	9	Ziegler et al.[24]
84	76	17	4	31	26	Kaplan et al.[26]
89	74	21	28	21	16	Knowles et al.[25]

[a]Meningeal and primary CNS involvement.

risk for CNS involvement.[36] Following confirmation of the lymphoma diagnosis, a staging workup should be undertaken and include the following.

1. Computed tomography (CT) scans of the chest, abdomen, and pelvis; and either CT or magnetic resonance imaging (MRI) of the head.
2. HIV RNA and CD4+ T-lymphocyte count.
3. Gallium or position-emission tomography (PET) scan in patients with disease that would be difficult to follow clinically, such as those with bulky intra-abdominal or intrathoracic tumors.
4. Bone marrow aspirate and biopsy (studies to include routine histopathology and flow cytometry).
5. Lumbar puncture and spinal fluid analysis (studies to include routine analysis, cytospin and flow cytometry, India ink stain, cryptococcal antigen, and EBV polymerase chain reaction if possible).
6. Blood cultures and serologies to exclude opportunistic infections in the presence of B symptoms or constitutional symptoms.

Therapy

The spectrum of opinions regarding ARL therapies is broad, ranging from intensive continuous infusion regimens to non-Hodgkin's lymphoma (NHL) regimens applied at half the standard dose intensity. The latter treatment strategy was driven by comparable clinical efficacy and reduced toxicity of low-dose chemotherapy noted in a Phase III trial comparing standard dose and modified (half-dose) m-BACOD (see Table 51–4 for the components).[28,29] This trial was performed prior to the availability of HAART, however, and is now generally reserved for patients who have advanced AIDS and have failed HAART. Concern has been raised in other HIV-infected populations owing to an inferior response rate noted in a Phase III trial in Europe.[34] Therefore most centers now use standard-dose CHOP (cyclophosphamide/hydroxydaunomycin/oncovin/prednisone) as the initial therapy for individuals with ARL. Studies using infusional regimens (EPOCH: etoposide/prednisone/vincristine/cyclophosphamide/doxorubicin) have reported highly encouraging activity levels that, if validated, could alter the standard of care. In addition, the monoclonal antibody Rituxan is being tested in conjunction with CHOP in patients with ARL and may ultimately be shown to be an advantageous addition to initial therapy.[27,32] Table 51–4 provides a listing of the commonly used regimens for ARL at the present time and results are discussed in more detail below.

Prognostic Factors

The prognosis for patients with ARL has been assessed in a number of clinical settings, most of which antedated the availability of HAART. The overall poor prognosis noted in these reports should be cautiously interpreted given the important effect of HAART on the risk from other HIV complications and on the tolerance of the chemotherapy itself. Long-term survival of both ARL and HIV are now realistic possibilities. Identifying individuals at greater risk from NHL is in part dictated by parameters of HIV disease and in part by parameters of the tumor.

In the phase III trial of 192 patients treated with either m-BACOD or modified m-BACOD, a CD4+ T-lymphocyte count of less than 100 cells/mm^3, age over 35 years, intravenous drug use (IVDU), and stage III/IV disease were noted as independent negative indicators of prognosis.[37] The overall survival in the setting of one or none of these factors was 46 weeks, of two factors 44 weeks, and of three or four factors 18 weeks.

The International Prognostic Index[38] [based on age, lactate dehydrogenase (LDH) level, tumor stage, performance status, number of extranodal sites] has not been systematically evaluated; but in a small study of 46 ARL patients it was a useful predictor of outcome.[39] Other studies have also identified an increased LDH level[40] or age over 40 years as factors independent of CD4+ T-lymphocyte counts. In a study of 101 ARL cases in France, poor outcome was associated with a CD4+ T-lymphocyte count of 50/mm^3 or less, hemoglobin 10 g/dl or less, or stage IV disease.[41] Prior AIDS-defining illness, Karnofsky performance status, and the presence of extranodal disease have also been reported to be predictive of risk.[26,28,42–44] Generally, histology has not been an important predictive factor. Despite the concern about Burkitt's and Burkitt's-like tumors, they have been shown to affect the prognosis adversely only inconsistently, and therefore histology-specific treatment trials have not been conducted. Favorable prognostic findings were identified by Kaplan and colleagues, who noted that the presence of polyclonality, particularly in the absence of EBV in the tumor and a CD4+ T-lymphocyte count of more than 300 cells/mm^3 positively affected outcome.[43]

Standard Dose Therapies

For patients responding to antiretroviral therapy, standard chemotherapy regimens such as CHOP (Table 51–5) have produced response rates slightly lower than that of the uninfected population.

The European Intergroup randomized ARL patients into three groups by prognostic risk factors: prior AIDS, CD4+ T-lymphocyte count less than 100/mm^3, and performance status of more than 1. The low risk patients (no adverse prognostic factors) were randomized to ACVB (see Table 51–4 for the compounds) and CHOP with granulocyte colony-stimulating factor (G-CSF) support. Complete response rates (63% for the ACVB group and 60% for the CHOP group) and survival were equivalent in the two arms. ARL patients with one poor prognostic factor (intermediate risk) were randomized to CHOP or modified CHOP (reduced by 50%). The complete response rates were 60% versus 39% for CHOP and reduced CHOP, respectively, though overall survival was no different between the treatment arms.[34]

Low-Dose Therapy

The aggressive nature of the lymphomas led early investigators to use intensive clinical approaches. The result was severe toxicity and frequent treatment-related death. In response, the modified (essentially half dose) m-BACOD regimen[29] was developed and tested in a Phase III trial comparing it directly with the full-dose regimen plus

Table 51–4. COMMONLY USED THERAPY REGIMENS FOR AIDS-RELATED LYMPHOMA

Therapy	Standard Regimen	Modified Regimen
M-BACOD		
Bleomycin	4 mg/m² IV, day 1	4 mg/m² IV, day 1
Doxorubicin	45 mg/m² IV, day 1	25 mg/m² IV, day 1
Cyclophosphamide	600 mg/m² IV, day 1	300 mg/m² IV, day 1
Vincristine sulfate	1.0 mg/m² IV, day 1	1.4 mg/m² IV (not to exceed 2 mg), day 1
Dexamethasone	6 mg/m² PO day 1–5	3 mg/m² PO, days 1, 5
Methotrexate	3000 mg/m² IV, day 14	500 mg/m² IV, day 15
Ara-C (CNS prophylaxis)	None	50 mg IT, days 1, 8, 21, 28
Whole-brain radiation prophylaxis or treatment	None	2400 cGy with marrow involvement; 4000 cGy with CNS involvement
Zidovudine	None	200 mg q4h for 1 year; starting after chemotherapy
Duration of treatment	10 cycles, every 21 days	4–6 cycles, every 28 days
m-BACOD		
Methotrexate (IV)	200 mg/m², day 15	200 mg/m², day 15[a]
Bleomycin (IV)	4 U/m², day 1	4 U/m², day 1
Doxorubicin (IV)	45 mg/m², day 1	25 mg/m², day 1
Cyclophosphamide (IV)	600 mg/m², day 1	300 mg/m², day 1
Vincristine (IV)	1.4 mg/m², day 1	1.4 mg/m², day 1
Dexamethasone (PO)	6 mg/m², days 1–5	3 mg/m², days 1–5
GM-CSF (SC)	5 μg/kg, days 4–13	5 μg/kg PRN, days 4–13
Meningeal lymphoma prophylaxis[b]	Cytarabine (50 mg IT), days 1, 8, 15, 22	
Pneumocystic prophylaxis	Trimethoprim-sulfamethoxazole, dapsone, or inhaled pentamidine	
CHOP		
Cyclophosphamide	750 mg/m² IVPB, day 1	375 mg/m², day 1
Doxorubicin	50 mg/m² IVPB, day 1	25 mg/m², day 1
Vincristine	1.4 mg/m² (not to exceed 2 mg) IVPB, day 1	1.4 mg/m² (max. 2 mg), day 1
Prednisone (each cycle q21–28d)	100 mg PO, days 1–5	50–100 mg PO, days 1–5
CHOP: Oral Regimen		
CCNU	100 mg/m² PO, day 1 (cycle 1, 3, 5)	
Etoposide	200 mg/m² PO, days 1–3	
Cyclophosphamide	100 mg/m² PO, days 22–31	
Procarbazine (each cycle q42d)	100 mg/m² PO, days 22–31	
CHOP: Continuous Infusion Regimen		
Cyclophosphamide	187.5 mg/m² CI, days 1–4	
Doxorubicin	12.5 mg/m² CI, days 1–4	
Etoposide	60 mg/m² CI, days 1–4	
ACVB Dose-Intensive Chemotherapy Regimen		
Induction[c]		
Adriamycin	75 mg/m², day 1	
Cyclophosphamide	1200 mg/m², day 1	
Vindescine	2 mg/m², days 1, 5	
Bleomycin	10 mg, days 1, 5	
Prednisolone	60 mg/m², days 1–5	
Consolidation		
Methotrexate (IV)	3 g/m², days 1, 5	
Folinic acid rescue (PO)	25 mg × 4, days 1–3, 15–17	
Ifosfamide (IV)	1.5 g/m², days 29, 33	
VP-16 (IV)	300 mg/m², days 29, 33	
L-Asparaginase (IM)	50,000 U/m², days 57, 64	
Ara-C (SC)	50 mg/m² q12h × 8, days 78, 92	
CNS Prophylaxis		
Methotrexate (IT)	12 mg, days 1, 15, 29	
CNS Treatment		
Methotrexate (IT)	12 mg 2 × weeks, for 5 wk	
Radiotherapy	2400 cGy	

CI, continuous infusion; IT, intensive therapy; IVPB, intravenous piggyback.

[a]This is a low-dose regimen.

[b]Prophylaxis was administered during cycle 1 only.

[c]Every 2 weeks for three cycles.

granulocyte/macrophage colony-forming factor (GM-CSF).[28] No statistically significant differences in the incidence of complete remission (50% vs. 46%), relapse after complete remission (19% vs. 23%), time to progression (22 vs. 28 weeks), overall median survival (31 vs. 34 weeks), death from AIDS (20 vs. 12 patients), or death from lymphoma (24 vs. 36 patients) were noted. The major difference between the two treatment arms was grade

▲ **Table 51–5.** ACTG 142 TREATMENT RESULTS: LOW-DOSE VERSUS STANDARD-DOSE m-BACOD

Regimen	CR (%)	Median Survival (weeks)	1-year Survival (%)	>2-year Survival (%)	Deaths due to AIDS (%)	Deaths due to Lymphoma (%)
LD m-BACOD	41	35	27	11	26	70
SD m-BACOD	52	31	24	7	30	57

There were three CNS relapses and 22% to 23% opportunistic infections in each arm.
Treatment-related mortality amounted to 1.5%.
There was less myelosuppression toxicity in the LD arm.
CR, complete remission; LD, low dose; SD, standard dose.
Data from Kaplan LD, Straus DJ, Testa MA, et al. Low-dose compared with standard-dose m-BACOD chemotherapy for non-Hodgkin's lymphoma associated with human immunodeficiency virus infection. National Institute of Allergy and Infectious Diseases AIDS Clinical Trials Group. N Engl J Med 336:1641, 1997. Copyright 1997 Massachusetts Medical Society.

4 neutropenia in patients receiving the standard-dose regimen despite the obligate use of GM-CSF by that treatment group. Due to the findings in a trial comparing m-BACOD and CHOP outside the context of HIV disease in which CHOP was found to be superior because of lower toxicity,[45] it was considered reasonable to use CHOP or modified CHOP rather than m-BACOD or modified m-BACOD. Using any modified therapy has been called into question, however, now that HAART has improved outcome and therapy tolerance. Furthermore, the European Intergroup found inferior treatment outcomes with the use of modified CHOP compared with full-dose CHOP (complete response rates 39% and 60%, respectively).[34] Therefore modified treatment regimens are generally reserved for patients with severe, advanced HIV disease (i.e., CD4 <50 cells/mm^3) in whom tolerance of chemotherapy is considered questionable.

Alternative Treatment Programs

Continuous infusion regimens have been tested for patients as first-line therapy. The CDE regimen (cyclophosphamide 800 mg/m^2/doxorubicin 50 mg/m^2/etoposide 240 mg/m^2, all daily doses for 4 days) to which didanosine (ddI) was added resulted in a complete response rate of 58% with a median response duration exceeding 18 months in a Phase II trial.[46] Perhaps the most encouraging results are from a study at the U.S. National Cancer Institute (NCI). Initial results from a trial there using infusional dose-adjusted EPOCH showed a 70% complete response rate[47] with no recurrence at 2 years.[48] Follow-up studies to validate the effect of EPOCH in a multiinstitutional setting are currently being developed.

Bower and colleagues reported the results of a weekly alternating chemotherapy for good prognosis ARL patients using bleomycin, etoposide, vincristine, methotrexate, prednisolonel, cyclophosamide, doxorubicin (BEMOP/CA). The complete response rate was 60% and the partial response rate 32%. The 2-year overall survival was 46%, and lymphoma-specific survival was 59%.[49] Although these results are encouraging, the apparent success of EPOCH suggests that it will be prioritized in follow-up multicenter trials.

Addition of Antiretroviral Therapy to Cytotoxic Chemotherapy

A trial of CHOP or modified CHOP plus indinivir, stavudine (d4T), and lamivudine (3TC) was conducted by the U.S. NCI-supported AIDS Malignancy Consortium. Combined cancer and antiretroviral therapy did not result in any usual toxicities or unexpectedly severe common toxicities. Pharmacokinetic data indicated that indinivir or doxorubicin clearance was as expected, but cyclophosphamide clearance was reduced by approximately 50%.[50] Although this study did not define a substantial risk of combining antiretroviral with antitumor therapy, a retrospective comparison of ARL patients treated prior to HAART with those receiving antiretrovirals found that the combination therapy group experienced more autonomic neuropathy (17% vs. 0%, $P = 0.002$) and neutropenia (7% vs. 33%; $P = 0.03$).[51] These increased toxicities were offset by a lower opportunistic infection rate (18% vs. 52%; $P = 0.05$) and mortality rate (38% vs. 85%; $P = 0.001$).

Because of the uncertainty of interactions between antiretroviral and antitumor therapies, the EPOCH study conducted by the intramural U.S. NCI program held all antiretroviral therapies during cancer treatment.[47] Preliminary results from this trial indicate that HIV RNA increases and CD4+ T-lymphocyte counts decline during cancer therapy, but a return to baseline occurs when antiretrovirals are resumed at the end of cancer treatment (typically 21 days following the last dose of chemotherapy). Given the wide range of antiretrovirals now available and the unpredictability of drug–drug interactions, this approach may be the most prudent for patients who are willing to consider an interruption in HAART and who can be followed carefully.

All patients following cytotoxic chemotherapy should be treated with antiretroviral drugs. One study found that such treatment was associated with improved survival.[41]

Investigational Approaches

The anti-CD20 humanized monoclonal antibody Rituxan has been shown to be active against aggressive lymphomas. Combining this therapy (which has a mechanism of action distinct from that of standard cytotoxic drugs) with cytotoxic agents has been encouraging in animal models and is being tested in multiple settings. The AIDS Malignancy Consortium is conducting a Phase III study comparing CHOP with CHOP plus Rituxan that is expected to be fully enrolled by mid-2002.

For patients with relapsed or refractory ARL, no therapies have been defined that have substantial activity. Autologous or miniallogeneic transplants are often undertaken outside the context of HIV disease. With the improved overall outlook and performance status of HIV-infected individuals due to the success of HAART, such aggressive approaches are now being considered for ARL. Trials are currently evaluating autologous or minimally myeloablative allogeneic transplantation in ARL patients. Two reports of autologous transplantation after either high-dose chemotherapy or total body irradiation plus chemotherapy have indicated the feasibility of performing this procedure during the HAART era.[52,53] Safety or engraftment did not appear to be adversely affected by the HIV infection setting in this small number of patients.

Supportive Care

It can be predicted that patients will experience a decline in CD4+ T-lymphocyte counts during chemotherapy and that the addition of steroids to most chemotherapy regimens will enhance immunosuppression. It is therefore our approach to treat all patients prophylactically against *Pneumocystis carinii* regardless of the CD4+ T-lymphocyte count on initiation of chemotherapy. Typically, trimethroprim/sulfamethoxazole (TMP-SMX) is used despite its myelotoxic potential. Patients with sulfa sensitivity are treated with dapsone, atovaquone, or aerosolized pentamidine. For patients who begin therapy with a CD4+ T-lymphocyte count of less than 100 cells/mm^3, additional prophylaxis may be considered, but no standard approach has been adopted.

It has been noted that patients with HIV disease have an unusual sensitivity to myelotoxic agents, and therefore hematopoietic growth factors are often used. A single randomized trial of CHOP versus CHOP plus GM-CSF found significant differences in the incidence of fever and neutropenia and days of hospitalization in patients receiving GM-CSF.[54] However, with the use of HAART, it is generally accepted that patients tolerate cytotoxic chemotherapy better. Therefore guidelines for growth factor used in the non-HIV population are often applied in ARL patients,[55] including patients who have had a prior episode of febrile neutropenia on chemotherapy or those on a regimen with a 40% risk of inducing severe neutropenia.[56]

The use of growth factors in the setting of HIV infection has raised concern about possible effects of the growth factor on viral replication.[57,58] GM-CSF has been of particular concern. Clinical data have indicated a rise in markers of viral load (HIV p24 at the time of these studies)[54,59] in some studies, whereas others have not seen an increase or only transient increases.[60–62] Moreover, data after G-CSF use have indicated some need for concern despite the fact that G-CSF is not able to induce increased HIV replication directly in vitro. G-CSF was shown to induce increases in HIV RNA in half the patients receiving it at doses sufficient for stem cell mobilization.[63] These increases were transient and returned to baseline following cessation of growth factor administration. The long-term consequences of growth factor use and its relation to the control of virus replication by antiretroviral drugs are not presently known. However, patients with strong indications for use of growth factors[55] should not be denied the therapy because of what appear to be minor, temporary viral load changes.

CNS Prophylaxis and Treatment of Leptomeningeal Lymphoma

The role of CNS prophylaxis has not been conclusively determined, but leptomeningeal seeding by systemic lymphoma appears to occur with increased frequency.[64] The risk of this complication has not been well defined, but factors associated with higher risk outside the setting of HIV disease (e.g., bone marrow, epidural or paranasal sinus, or small-cell histology) should be considered in this population. Because some studies early in the epidemic documented CNS involvement in most patients,[31] it has been debated as to whether all patients should receive CNS prophylaxis at the time of initial therapy.[28,29] This issue remains controversial and is unlikely to be answered by ongoing clinical trials. However, the results of Cingolani and colleagues[36] suggest that the presence of EBV in the tumor is highly associated with risk. EBV in the cerebrospinal fluid (CSF) of such patients was found to have a positive predictive value of 100% and a negative predicative value of 97.6% among the 50 patients studied.[36] When prophylaxis is used, it generally consists of intrathecal methotrexate (12 mg) or cytosine arabinoside (ara-C) (50 mg). There is no consistently employed treatment schedule. However, several trials have employed ara-C weekly for the first 4 weeks in patients without documented CNS involvement at diagnosis. Patients with bone marrow involvement in some studies have also received prophylactic cranial radiation therapy (24 Gy) upon completion of their systemic chemotherapy. Patients with overt CNS involvement receive intrathecal ara-C weekly until clearance of the CSF followed by cranial radiation therapy (40 Gy) upon completion of the systemic chemotherapy.

Others[27] have used methotrexate (MTX) given on the first day of each induction chemotherapy cycle as prophylaxis. For overt CNS disease, biweekly intrathecal MTX for 5 weeks or until clearing has been recommended followed by cranial radiation therapy (24 Gy) at completion of the systemic chemotherapy. A combination of MTX (12 mg) and ara-C (50 mg) with or without Solu-Cortef (100 mg) can be used biweekly in patients with overt leptomeningeal involvement, similar to what is recommended for leptomeningeal lymphoma in the non-AIDS population. Oral leucovorin (50 mg every 6 hours for four doses) is administered 24 hours after intrathecal MTX to avoid the myelosuppressive effect of frequent intrathecal MTX.

Primary CNS AIDS-Related Lymphoma

Patients who present with primary CNS ARL generally are at an advanced stage of HIV disease. Mean CD4 counts for this population have been reported as 30 cells/mm^3 compared with 189 cells/mm^3 for those with systemic lymphoma; prior OIs have been reported in approximately 75%.[18,44,65] Although histologic and genetic characteristics may vary among patients with systemic lymphoma, patients with primary CNS ARL uniformly present with large-cell or immunoblastic morphology and the virtually ubiquitous presence of EBV.

The presenting symptom complex for patients with primary CNS can be highly variable, and a high index of suspicion must be maintained for patients who present with neurologic or psychiatric changes in the setting of advanced immunosuppression. When a mass lesion is detected, the distinction between ARL and other infectious etiologies is problematic (Fig. 51–1). There are no radiographic guidelines to define ARL, but ARL is uncommon in the posterior fossa, tending to be periventricular and multifocal.[66–69] Like infectious processes, it may be ring-enhancing as a result of central necrosis; but unlike an infectious process, it can cross midline structures.

Tissue biopsy is the definitive diagnostic procedure and is strongly recommended. An alternative reasonable approach is to evaluate the serologic status of the patient for toxoplasmosis. If patients are positive, an empiric trial of anti-*Toxoplasma* therapy may be undertaken.[70] Alternatively, efforts to use the polymerase chain reaction (PCR) in

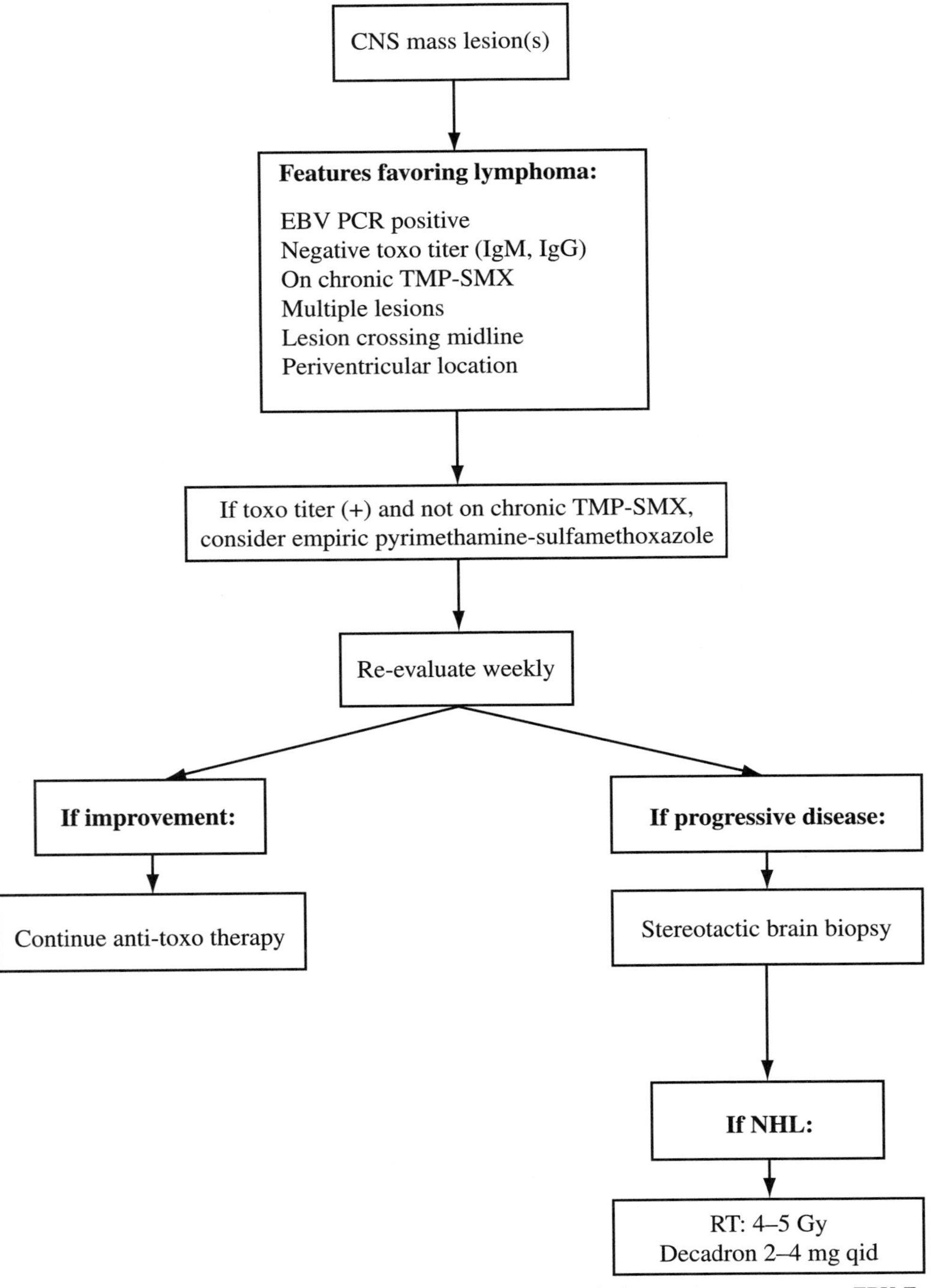

Figure 51–1. Evaluation algorithm for central nervous system mass lesions. CNS, central nervous system; EBV, Epstein-Barr virus; IgG, immunoglobulin G; NHL, non-Hodgkin's lymphoma; PCR, polymerase chain reaction; RT, radiotherapy; TMP-SMX, trimethoprim-sulfamethoxazole; toxo, toxoplasmosis.

CSF for EBV have been encouraging as a means of accurately determining the presence of EBV-related lymphoma.[71] Among patients with a focal brain lesion and AIDS in one large study, CSF positive for EBV by PCR had a sensitivity of 80% and a specificity of 100% for primary CNS lymphoma.[71] Other studies have reported 100% sensitivity and 98.5% specificity of EBV PCR for diagnosing primary CNS lymphoma.[72] Indeed, one report suggested that EBV PCR may precede and predict CNS lymphoma,[73] and another indicated that it may be used to follow the response.[74] Single-photon emission computed tomography (SPECT) thallium-201 scanning may also be useful. The increased lesion/contralateral scalp signal ratio (>0.90) had a sensitivity of 86% and a specificity of 83% for lymphoma.[75]

Patients documented to have lymphoma may be treated with a combination of high-dose corticosteroid therapy and radiation therapy. The duration of steroid treatment should be limited because of the underlying immunodeficiency, with an effort to taper the steroids completely by the end of radiation therapy based on patient tolerance. Radiation therapy remains the central modality for treating primary CNS lymphoma, and a clinical response has been reported in 75% of the patients in one series.[68] The durability of this response is highly variable, and the overall impact on survival has not been defined. High-dose MTX has also been used at 3 g/m^2 every 14 days with leucovorin rescue; the response rate was 47% with reasonable tolerability.[76] The prognosis for this disease is extremely poor, with median survival estimated at 2 to 5 months.[68,69,77,78] Many patients die of OIs rather than recurrent lymphoma. It is not yet clear if the era of improved antiretroviral therapy and better prophylactic control of secondary infections may affect these grim statistics. There is at least the potential for a better outcome for a subset of patients and for better tolerance of alternative or additional therapies.

Previous attempts to improve outcomes have included the addition of systemic chemotherapy to radiotherapy. Results of a clinical trial await final analysis, but the preliminary data are not encouraging. A number of clinical trials are in development to explore whether the underlying basis of tumor development may be exploited therapeutically.

Body Cavity Lymphoma

Body cavity lymphoma is an uncommon clinical presentation of a B cell malignancy in patients with AIDS.[79–81] Patients present with lymphomatous effusion in the absence of a discrete nodal or extranodal mass. The pleural, pericardial, and peritoneal cavities are most frequently involved; and patients present with symptoms resulting from the space-occupying accumulation in a restricted space: shortness of breath, ascites, and compromised cardiac function in the case of a large pericardial effusion. Histologically, the disease closely resembles immunoblastic lymphoma; and it occurs in older patients and in association with low CD4 counts.[80] It occasionally appears as a mass despite its proclivity for serosally lined spaces.[82] It is unique among the ARLs in that the tumor cells demonstrate an absence of cell surface markers for B or T cells. Rather, common leukocyte antigen (CD45) alone is present on the cell, and genetic analysis is required to demonstrate immunoglobulin locus rearrangement.[80,81,83] Of significant interest is the presence of the human herpesvirus-8 genome in all cases of body cavity lymphoma.[20,80] It is diagnosed by detecting malignant cells in an effusion in patients with AIDS presenting with associated symptoms. It may appear in the context of other HHV-8 diseases such as Castleman's disease or Kaposi's sarcoma.[84] The workup of patients with body cavity lymphoma is similar to that of other patients with systemic ARL, although detectable involvement is often restricted to a specific body space. Chemotherapy treatment programs similar to those for systemic ARL are generally used for such patients, but the likelihood of a clinical response remains unclear. Local radiotherapy may provide some symptomatic relief and reduction in effusion, especially in patients unable to tolerate chemotherapy and in whom the lymphoma is localized to the pleural or pericardial cavity.

▲ FUTURE TRENDS

There have been major shifts in the perspective of caring for AIDS patients generally and patients with AIDS-related malignancies specifically over the last half-decade. Well tolerated regimens providing durable remissions have been defined, shifting the focus to pursue a curative outcome more emphatically. However, the number of patients cured of ARL remains unacceptably small. The challenge of improving this number is being approached by combining antibody-based and standard cytotoxic chemotherapy, using infusional regimens to optimize the pharmacologic impact, and exploring autologous and allogeneic transplantation. Each of these modalities is being tested, but it is likely that combining the approaches—perhaps tailoring them to genomic subcategories of patients and lymphomas—may be required to affect the outlook maximally for patients with ARL.

REFERENCES

1. Selik RM, Chu SY, Ward JW. Trends in infectious diseases and cancers among persons dying of HIV infection in the United States from 1987 to 1992. Ann Intern Med 123:933, 1995.
2. Revision of the case definition of acquired immunodeficiency syndrome for national reporting—United States. Ann Intern Med 103:402, 1985.
3. Beral V, Peterman T, Berkelman R, et al. AIDS-associated non-Hodgkin lymphoma. Lancet 337:805, 1991.
4. Moore RD, Kessler H, Richman DD, et al. Non-Hodgkin's lymphoma in patients with advanced HIV infection treated with zidovudine. JAMA 265:2208, 1991.
5. Pluda JM, Yarchoan R, Jaffe ES, et al. Development of non-Hodgkin lymphoma in a cohort of patients with severe human immunodeficiency virus (HIV) infection on long-term antiretroviral therapy. Ann Intern Med 113:276, 1990.
6. Detels R, Munoz A, McFarlane G, et al. Effectiveness of potent antiretroviral therapy on time to AIDS and death in men with known HIV infection duration: Multicenter AIDS Cohort Study investigators. JAMA 280:1497, 1998.
7. Jacobson LP, Yamashita TE, Detels R, et al. Impact of potent antiretroviral therapy on the incidence of Kaposi's sarcoma and non-Hodgkin's lymphomas among HIV-1-infected individuals. Multicenter AIDS Cohort Study. J Acquir Immune Defic Syndr 21 (suppl 1):S34, 1999.

8. Rabkin CS, Testa MA, Huang J, et al. Kaposi's sarcoma and non-Hodgkin's lymphoma incidence trends in AIDS Clinical Trial Group study participants. J Acquir Immune Defic Syndr 21(suppl 1):S31, 1999.
9. Buchbinder SP, Holmberg SD, Scheer S, et al. Combination antiretroviral therapy and incidence of AIDS-related malignancies. J Acquir Immune Defic Syndr 21(suppl 1):S23, 1999.
10. Aboulafia D. Regression of AIDS-related pulmonary Kaposi's sarcoma after highly active antiretroviral therapy. Mayo Clin Proc 73:439, 1998.
11. Highly active antiretroviral therapy and incidence of cancer in human immunodeficiency virus-infected adults. J Natl Cancer Inst 92:1823, 2000.
12. Grulich AE. AIDS-associated non-Hodgkin's lymphoma in the era of highly active antiretroviral therapy. J Acquir Immune Defic Syndr 21(suppl 1):S27, 1999.
13. Sparano JA, Anand K, Desai J, et al. Effect of highly active antiretroviral therapy on the incidence of HIV- associated malignancies at an urban medical center. J Acquir Immune Defic Syndr 21(suppl 1):S18, 1999.
14. Jones JL, Hanson DL, Dworkin MS, et al. Effect of antiretroviral therapy on recent trends in selected cancers among HIV-infected persons: adult/adolescent spectrum of HIV Disease Project Group. J Acquir Immune Defic Syndr 21(suppl 1):S11, 1999.
15. Goedert JJ. The epidemiology of acquired immunodeficiency syndrome malignancies. Semin Oncol 27:390, 2000.
16. Matthews GV, Bower M, Mandalia S, et al. Changes in acquired immunodeficiency syndrome-related lymphoma since the introduction of highly active antiretroviral therapy. Blood 96:2730, 2000.
17. Shiramizu B, Herndier BG, McGrath MS. Identification of a common clonal human immunodeficiency virus integration site in human immunodeficiency virus-associated lymphomas. Cancer Res 54:2069, 1994.
18. MacMahon EM, Glass JD, Hayward SD, et al. Epstein-Barr virus in AIDS-related primary central nervous system lymphoma. Lancet 338:969, 1991.
19. Shibata D, Weiss LM, Hernandez AM, et al. Epstein-Barr virus-associated non-Hodgkin's lymphoma in patients infected with the human immunodeficiency virus. Blood 81:2102, 1993.
20. Cesarman E, Chang Y, Moore PS, et al. Kaposi's sarcoma-associated herpesvirus-like DNA sequences in AIDS-related body-cavity-based lymphomas. N Engl J Med 332:1186, 1995.
21. Knowles DM. Etiology and pathogenesis of AIDS-related non-Hodgkin's lymphoma. Hematol Oncol Clin North Am 10:1081, 1996.
22. Gaidano G, Carbone A, Dalla-Favera R. Genetic basis of acquired immunodeficiency syndrome-related lymphoma genesis. J Natl Cancer Inst Monogr 23:95, 1998.
23. Rabkin CS, Yang Q, Goedert JJ, et al. Chemokine and chemokine receptor gene variants and risk of non-Hodgkin's lymphoma in human immunodeficiency virus-1-infected individuals. Blood 93:1838, 1999.
24. Ziegler JL, Beckstead JA, Volberding PA. Non-Hodgkin's lymphoma in 90 homosexual men: relation to generalized lymphadenopathy and the acquired immunodeficiency syndrome. N Engl J Med 311:565, 1984.
25. Knowles DM, Chamulak GA, Subar M. Lymphoid neoplasia associated with the acquired immunodeficiency syndrome (AIDS): the New York University Medical Center experience with 105 patients. Ann Intern Med 108:744, 1988.
26. Kaplan LD, Abrams DI, Feigal E. AIDS-associated non-Hodgkin's lymphoma in San Francisco. JAMA 261:719, 1989.
27. Gisselbrecht C, Oksenhendler E, Tirelli U. Human immunodeficiency virus-related lymphoma: treatment with intensive combination chemotherapy. Am J Med 95:188, 1993.
28. Kaplan LD, Straus DJ, Testa MA, et al. Low-dose compared with standard-dose m-BACOD chemotherapy for non-Hodgkin's lymphoma associated with human immunodeficiency virus infection. National Institute of Allergy and Infectious Diseases AIDS Clinical Trials Group. N Engl J Med 336:1641, 1997.
29. Levine AM, Wernz JC, Kaplan L. Low-dose chemotherapy with central nervous system prophylaxis and zidovudine maintenance in AIDS-related lymphoma. JAMA 266:84, 1991.
30. Kalter SP, Riggs SA, Cabanillas F, et al. Aggressive non-Hodgkin's lymphomas in immunocompromised homosexual males. Blood 66:655, 1985.
31. Gill PS, Levine AM, Krailo M. AIDS-related malignant lymphoma: results of prospective treatment trials. J Clin Oncol 5:1322, 1987.
32. Bermudez MA, Grant KM, Rodvien R, et al. Non-Hodgkin's lymphoma in a population with or at risk for acquired immunodeficiency syndrome: indications for intensive chemotherapy. Am J Med 86:71, 1989.
33. Lowenthal DA, Straus DJ, Campbell SW, et al. AIDS-related lymphoid neoplasia: the Memorial Hospital experience. Cancer 61:2325, 1988.
34. Remick SC, McSharry JJ, Wolf BC. Novel oral combination chemotherapy in the treatment of intermediate-grade and high-grade AIDS-related non-Hodgkin's lymphoma. J Clin Oncol 11:1691, 1993.
35. Raphael M, Gentilhomme O, Tulliez M, et al. Histopathologic features of high-grade non-Hodgkin's lymphomas in acquired immunodeficiency syndrome: the French Study Group of Pathology for Human Immunodeficiency Virus-Associated Tumors. Arch Pathol Lab Med 115:15, 1991.
36. Cingolani A, Gastaldi R, Fassone L, et al. Epstein-barr virus infection is predictive of CNS involvement in systemic AIDS-related non-Hodgkin's lymphomas. J Clin Oncol 18:3325, 2000.
37. Straus DJ, Huang J, Testa MA, et al. Prognostic factors in the treatment of human immunodeficiency virus-associated non-Hodgkin's lymphoma: analysis of AIDS Clinical Trials Group protocol 142—low-dose versus standard-dose m-BACOD plus granulocyte-macrophage colony-stimulating factor: National Institute of Allergy and Infectious Diseases. J Clin Oncol 16:3601, 1998.
38. A predictive model for aggressive non-Hodgkin's lymphoma: the International Non-Hodgkin's Lymphoma Prognostic Factors Project. N Engl J Med 329:987, 1993.
39. Navarro JT, Ribera JM, Oriol A, et al. International prognostic index is the best prognostic factor for survival in patients with AIDS-related non-Hodgkin's lymphoma treated with CHOP: a multivariate study of 46 patients. Haematologica 83:508, 1998.
40. Vaccher E, Tirelli U, Spina M, et al. Age and serum lactate dehydrogenase level are independent prognostic factors in human immunodeficiency virus-related non-Hodgkin's lymphomas: a single-institute study of 96 patients. J Clin Oncol 14:2217, 1996.
41. Thiessard F, Morlat P, Marimoutou C, et al. Prognostic factors after non-Hodgkin lymphoma in patients infected with the human immunodeficiency virus: Aquitaine Cohort, France, 1986–1997: Groupe d'Epidemiologie Clinique du SIDA en Aquitaine (GECSA). Cancer 88:1696, 2000.
42. Tirelli U, Errante D, Dolcetti R, et al. Hodgkin's disease and human immunodeficiency virus infection: clinicopathologic and virologic features of 114 patients from the Italian Cooperative Group on AIDS and Tumors. J Clin Oncol 13:1758, 1995.
43. Kaplan LD, Shiramizu B, Herndier B, et al. Influence of molecular characteristics on clinical outcome in human immunodeficiency virus-associated non-Hodgkin's lymphoma: identification of a subgroup with favorable clinical outcome. Blood 85:1727, 1995.
44. Levine AM, Sullivan-Halley J, Pike MC, et al. Human immunodeficiency virus-related lymphoma: prognostic factors predictive of survival. Cancer 68:2466, 1991.
45. Fisher RI, Gaynor ER, Dahlberg S, et al. Comparison of a standard regimen (CHOP) with three intensive chemotherapy regimens for advanced non-Hodgkin's lymphoma. N Engl J Med 328:1002, 1993.
46. Sparano JA, Wiernik PH, Hu X, et al. Pilot trial of infusional cyclophosphamide, doxorubicin, and etoposide plus didanosine and filgrastim in patients with human immunodeficiency virus-associated non-Hodgkin's lymphoma. J Clin Oncol 14:3026, 1996.
47. Little R, Pearson D, Steinberg S, et al. Dose-adjusted EPOCH chemotherapy (CT) in previously untreated HIV-associated non-Hodgkin's lymphoma (HIV-NHL). Presented at the American Society of Clinical Oncology, 35th Annual Meeting. Atlanta, 1999, p 10a.
48. Little RF, Yarchoan R, Wilson WH. Systemic chemotherapy for HIV-associated lymphoma in the era of highly active antiretroviral therapy. Curr Opin Oncol 12:438, 2000.
49. Bower M, Stern S, Fife K, et al. Weekly alternating combination chemotherapy for good prognosis AIDS-related lymphoma. Eur J Cancer 36:363, 2000.
50. Ratner L, Lee J, Tang S, et al. Chemotherapy for human immunodeficiency virus-associated non-Hodgkin's lymphoma in combination with highly active antiretroviral therapy. J Clin Oncol 19:2171, 2001.
51. Vaccher E, Spina M, di Gennaro G, et al. Concomitant cyclophosphamide, doxorubicin, vincristine, and prednisone chemotherapy plus highly active antiretroviral therapy in patients with human

immunodeficiency virus-related, non-Hodgkin lymphoma. Cancer 91:155, 2001.
52. Gabarre J, Azar N, Autran B, et al. High-dose therapy and autologous haematopoietic stem-cell transplantation for HIV-1-associated lymphoma. Lancet 355:1071, 2000.
53. Molina A, Krishnan AY, Nademanee A, et al. High dose therapy and autologous stem cell transplantation for human immunodeficiency virus-associated non-Hodgkin lymphoma in the era of highly active antiretroviral therapy. Cancer 89:680, 2000.
54. Kaplan LD, Kahn JO, Crowe S. Clinical and virologic effects of recombinant human granulocyte-macrophage colony-stimulating factor in patients receiving chemotherapy for human immunodeficiency virus-associated non-Hodgkin's lymphoma: results of a randomized trial. J Clin Oncol 9:929, 1991.
55. Ozer H. American Society of Clinical Oncology guidelines for the use of hematopoietic colony-stimulating factors. Curr Opin Hematol 3:3, 1996.
56. Update of recommendations for the use of hematopoietic colony-stimulating factors: evidence-based clinical practice guidelines, 1997. *http://www.ASCO.org.*
57. Koyanagi Y, O'Brien WA, Zhao JQ. Cytokine alter the production of HIV-1 from primary mononuclear phagocytes. Science 241:1673, 1988.
58. Wang J, Rodriguez G, Oravecz T, et al. Cytokine regulation of human immunodeficiency virus type 1 entry and replication in human monocytes/macrophages through modulation of CCR5 expression. J Virol 72:7642, 1998.
59. Pluda JM, Yarchoan Y, Smith PD. Subcutaneous recombinant granulocyte-macrophage colony-stimulating factor used as a single agent and in alternating regimen with azidothymidine in leukopenia patients with severe human immunodeficiency virus infection. Blood 76:463, 1990.
60. Scadden DT, Bering HA, Levine JD. Granulocyte-macrophage colony-stimulating factor mitigates the neutropenia of combined interferon alfa and zidovudine treatment of acquired immunodeficiency syndrome associated Kaposi's sarcoma. J Clin Oncol 9:802, 1991.
61. Davey RT, Davey VJ, Metcalf JA. A phase I/II trial of zidovudine, interferon-alpha, and granulocyte-macrophage colony-stimulating factor in the treatment of human immunodeficiency virus type 1 infection. J Infect Dis 164:43, 1991.
62. Scadden DT, Pickus O, Hammer SM, et al. Lack of in vivo effect of granulocyte-macrophage colony-stimulating factor (GM-CSF) on human immunodeficiency virus-type 1 (HIV-1). AIDS Res Hum Retroviruses 12:1151, 1996.
63. Schooley RT, Mladenovic J, Sevin A, et al. Reduced Mobilization of CD34+ stem cells in advanced human immunodeficiency virus type 1 disease. J Infect Dis 181:148, 2000.
64. Van Besien K, Ha CS, Murphy S, et al. Risk factors, treatment, and outcome of central nervous system recurrence in adults with intermediate-grade and immunoblastic lymphoma. Blood 91:1178, 1998.
65. Meeker TC, Shiramizu B, Kaplan L, et al. Evidence for molecular subtypes of HIV-associated lymphoma: division into peripheral monoclonal, polyclonal and central nervous system lymphoma. AIDS 5:669, 1991.
66. Goldstein JD, Dickson DW, Moser FG, et al. Primary central nervous system lymphoma in acquired immune deficiency syndrome: a clinical and pathologic study with results of treatment with radiation. Cancer 67:2756, 1991.
67. Gill PS, Levine AM, Meyer PR, et al. Primary central nervous system lymphoma in homosexual men: clinical, immunologic, and pathologic features. Am J Med 78:742, 1985.
68. Baumgartner JE, Rachlin JR, Beckstead JH, et al. Primary central nervous system lymphomas: natural history and response to radiation therapy in 55 patients with acquired immunodeficiency syndrome. J Neurosurg 73:206, 1990.
69. So YT, Beckstead JH, Davis RL. Primary central nervous system lymphoma in acquired immune deficiency syndrome: a clinical and pathological study. Ann Neurol 20:566, 1986.
70. Mathews C, Barba D, Fullerton SC. Early biopsy versus treatment with delayed biopsy of non-responders in suspected HIV-associated cerebral toxoplasmosis: a decision analysis. AIDS 9:1243, 1995.
71. Cingolani A, De Luca A, Larocca LM, et al. Minimally invasive diagnosis of acquired immunodeficiency syndrome- related primary central nervous system lymphoma. J Natl Cancer Inst 90:364, 1998.
72. Cinque P, Brytting M, Vago L, et al. Epstein-Barr virus DNA in cerebrospinal fluid from patients with AIDS-related primary lymphoma of the central nervous system. Lancet 342:398, 1993.
73. Al-Shahi R, Bower M, Nelson MR, et al. Cerebrospinal fluid Epstein-Barr virus detection preceding HIV-associated primary central nervous system lymphoma by 17 months. J Neurol 247:471, 2000.
74. Antinori A, Cingolani A, De Luca A, et al. Epstein-Barr virus in monitoring the response to therapy of acquired immunodeficiency syndrome-related primary central nervous system lymphoma. Ann Neurol 5:259, 1999.
75. Skiest DJ, Erdman W, Chang WE, et al. SPECT thallium-201 combined with Toxoplasma serology for the presumptive diagnosis of focal central nervous system mass lesions in patients with AIDS. J Infect 40:274, 2000.
76. Jacomet C, Girard PM, Lebrette MG, et al. Intravenous methotrexate for primary central nervous system non-Hodgkin's lymphoma in AIDS. AIDS 11:1725, 1997.
77. Formenti SC, Gill PS, Lean E, et al. Primary central nervous system lymphoma in AIDS: results of radiation therapy. Cancer 63:1101, 1989.
78. Ling SM, Roach M III, Larson DA, et al. Radiotherapy of primary central nervous system lymphoma in patients with and without human immunodeficiency virus: ten years of treatment experience at the University of California San Francisco. Cancer 73:2570, 1994.
79. Ansari MQ, Dawson DB, Nador R, et al. Primary body cavity-based AIDS-related lymphomas. Am J Clin Pathol 105:221, 1996.
80. Carbone A, Tirelli U, Vaccher E, et al. A clinicopathologic study of lymphoid neoplasias associated with human immunodeficiency virus infection in Italy. Cancer 68:842, 1991.
81. Green I, Espiritu E, Ladanyi M, et al. Primary lymphomatous effusions in AIDS: a morphological, immunophenotypic, and molecular study. Mod Pathol 8:39, 1995.
82. Katano H, Suda T, Morishita Y, et al. Human herpesvirus 8-associated solid lymphomas that occur in AIDS patients take anaplastic large cell morphology. Mod Pathol 13:77, 2000.
83. Walts AE, Shintaku IP, Said JW. Diagnosis of malignant lymphoma in effusions from patients with AIDS by gene rearrangement. Am J Clin Pathol 94:170, 1990.
84. Ascoli V, Signoretti S, Onetti-Muda A, et al. Primary effusion lymphoma in HIV-infected patients with multicentric Castleman's disease. J Pathol 193:200, 2001.

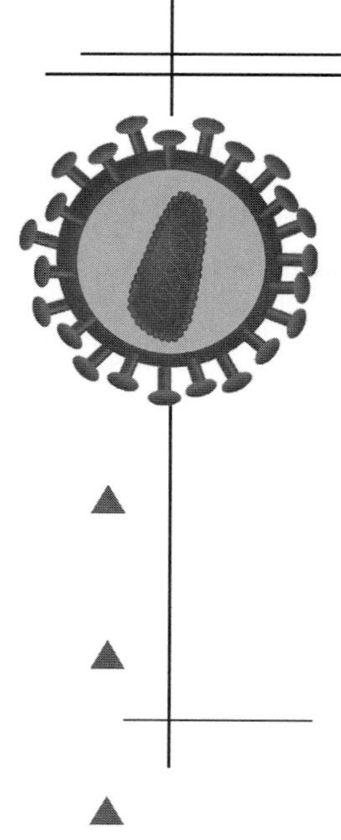

CHAPTER 52

Primary Care: Daily Management of HIV-Infected Patients

Kenneth H. Mayer, MD
Daniel E. Cohen, MD

Although specialists play an increasingly central role in the management of human immunodeficiency virus (HIV)-infected patients, well informed primary care providers are an essential part of any effective HIV prevention and treatment program. The prompt identification of HIV infection by primary care providers is vitally important, as they may be the first clinicians to have contact with at-risk individuals soon after they are infected. Multiple studies have demonstrated that earlier entry into care is associated with improved outcomes for HIV-infected patients.[1–3] Of the 750,000 to 900,000 Americans living with HIV infection, more than one-third are unaware of their infection, and an almost equal number who know they are HIV-infected may not receive state-of-the-art care.[4] Primary providers can play a vital role in identifying these individuals and either providing comprehensive care for them or triaging them to colleagues who can provide appropriate services.

In addition to identifying HIV-infected patients who are unaware of their serostatus, generalists can play a crucial role in HIV risk reduction and thus in slowing down the spread of the epidemic. Over the past few years, the rate of new HIV infections has plateaued at 30,000 to 50,000 new infections per year.[4] Most of the men and women in "high risk groups," are uninfected. Therefore clinical encounters with primary providers represent an educable moment, which may be used to convey information about the patient's risk of infection and hopefully to impart skills and motivation to help him or her reduce that risk.

▲ IDENTIFYING HIV-INFECTED PATIENTS

During the early years of the HIV epidemic in the United States the infection was detected primarily in specific populations, particularly intravenous drug users, men who had sex with men, hemophiliacs, and other blood product recipients, who were often described as "high risk groups."[5,6] This terminology implies that certain individuals could be less susceptible than others to infection. However, because HIV infection now affects persons from a wide spectrum of socioeconomic and cultural groups, it is more helpful to think in terms of "risk behaviors" rather than "risk groups" when deciding to screen patients for HIV. Identification of patients for HIV screening therefore means that the provider must discuss the individual patient's risk-taking behaviors and not rely on stereotypic assumptions. This determination depends on eliciting a thorough history of sexual practices and patterns of drug use (Table 52–1). Early manifestations of altered cell-mediated immunity, such as persistent thrush, in the absence of other underlying conditions should raise clinical suspicion and lead to HIV antibody screening, independent of the behavioral history. The patient's clinical history should be obtained in a detailed, nonjudgmental fashion. Persons of any age may be newly diagnosed with HIV infection, so this information should be obtained from all adult patients. Because several hundred thousand asymptomatic patients in the United States are unaware that they are HIV-infected, it is incumbent on the medical provider to recognize those who are infected or at increased risk and to provide counseling and recommend testing when appropriate. The rationale for the prompt detection of HIV infection is twofold: Infected people are more apt to benefit from antiretroviral therapy and opportunistic infection prophylaxis if they are identified early, and they are more amenable to protecting their partners if they are aware of their HIV status. A discussion of issues in the initiation of antiretroviral therapy is presented in Chapter 27.

▲ **Table 52–1.** INDICATIONS FOR HIV ANTIBODY SCREENING

Behaviors associated with increased risk
Men who have sex with men
People with multiple sexual partners
People with recent or prior sexually transmitted infections
Commercial sex workers and their partners
Travelers to areas of increased prevalence who were sexually active
Injection drug users
Sexual partners of at risk persons
Recipients of blood products between 1978 and 1985
Routine screening recommended to discover low risk persons with unanticipated infection
Pregnant women
Donors of blood products, semen, ova, or organs
Patients hospitalized in a center with more than 1/1000 HIV prevalence
Clinical conditions associated with increased risk behavior or occult immunocompromise
Sexually transmitted infection
Thrush or chronic/recurrent vulvovaginal candidiasis
Generalized lymphadenopathy
Recurrent herpes simplex or herpes zoster
Constitutional symptoms
Chronic diarrhea or wasting
Encephalopathy
Anemia, leukopenia, or thrombocytopenia
Opportunistic infections

Screening for HIV Infection

Because a large number of HIV-infected individuals are unaware of their infection, it is critical that all clinicians assess risk for HIV and offer testing when appropriate. Obtaining a thorough history, including nonjudgmental but specific questioning about sexual activity and drug use, has become even more important for identifying patients at risk for HIV infection. HIV testing should be performed for any patient who requests it. Other indications for voluntary testing include sexually transmitted diseases, pregnancy, and active tuberculosis (Table 52–1). Testing should be considered in young adults with shingles (herpes zoster) and women with refractory or recurrent vaginal candidiasis. Voluntary testing has been recommended for adults hospitalized in facilities where the HIV seroprevalence exceeds 1% or where the acquired immunodeficiency syndrome (AIDS) case rate exceeds 1 per 1000 discharges.[7] Finally, HIV testing should be considered in patients with generalized lymphadenopathy; unexplained dementia, aseptic meningitis, or peripheral neuropathy; chronic, unexplained fever, diarrhea, or weight loss; generalized herpes simplex infection or multidermatomal herpes zoster; unexplained cytopenias; B-lymphocyte lymphoma; or other opportunistic conditions suggestive of cell-mediated immunodeficiency.

All patients who are being tested for HIV antibodies should undergo counseling before the test is performed. This should include information about what the test is measuring (i.e., antibodies to HIV) and the significance of positive, negative, and indeterminate results. It is important to explain that if a person has recently engaged in risky behaviors HIV infection could be present without evidence of antibody formation because of a possible lag in the development of anti-HIV antibodies. However, within 1 month after a high risk exposure more than 90% of infected people do have a positive antibody test.[8] To be confident that HIV infection is truly not present in someone who engaged in recent high risk behavior, repeated testing should be offered approximately 6 months after the initial test. The patient must understand that the repeat test is most helpful if he or she has not had any additional potential exposures during that interval. For this reason, counseling around HIV testing must also address risk behaviors, and the patient must understand exactly when behaviors might expose him or her to infection. It is always best to be specific; many patients know that unprotected vaginal or anal intercourse may present a risk but are unaware that fellatio can also spread HIV. Likewise, patients may erroneously believe that sexual intercourse with penetration is only risky if ejaculation has occurred or that anal or vaginal intercourse is risky for the receptive but not for the insertive partner.

Acute HIV Infection

For many asymptomatic patients elucidation of a careful history of behavior associated with HIV acquisition may be the means by which their HIV infection is determined, but in others it may be due to an astute clinician identifying symptoms of acute HIV disease. The acute infection is symptomatic in a large proportion of patients.[9] The prevalence of symptomatic primary HIV infection, often referred to as acute retroviral syndrome, varies from series to series, but up to 90% of patients manifest some symptomatology if a clinician screens for HIV when an at-risk person manifests any of the classic symptoms (Table 52–2).[10] Because of a lack of awareness among susceptible patients and a low index of suspicion among health care providers, the syndrome is probably still underreported. Clinical manifestations of acute retroviral illness may appear within days to weeks of exposure to HIV, most commonly 2 to 6 weeks.[10] Common symptoms include fever (frequently in excess of 102°F), night sweats, headache, fatigue, and a nonpruritic erythematous maculopapular rash. This rash may be variable in appearance and evanescent; the patient may

▲ **Table 52–2.** SIGNS AND SYMPTOMS ASSOCIATED WITH ACUTE RETROVIRAL SYNDROME

Clinical Finding	Percent of Patients
Fever	> 80
Fatigue	> 70
Weight loss	70
Pharyngitis	50–70
Myalgia	50–70
Night sweats	50
Diarrhea	50
Rash	40–80
Lymphadenopathy	40–70
Headache	32–70
Nausea, vomiting	30–60
Aseptic meningitis	24
Oral or genital ulcers	10–20
Thrombocytopenia	45
Leukopenia	40
Elevated liver enzymes	21

Adapted from Kahn and Walker[9] and Schacker et al.[10]

▲ **Table 52–3.** DIFFERENTIAL DIAGNOSIS OF ACUTE RETROVIRAL
▲ SYNDROME

Infectious mononucleosis (Epstein-Barr virus or cytomegalovirus)
Toxoplasmosis
Streptococcal pharyngitis
Rubella
Secondary syphilis
Viral meningitis
Other viral infections (e.g., influenza)
Viral hepatitis
Disseminated gonococcal infection
Primary herpes simplex infection
Drug reaction

not even notice it. In dark-skinned individuals it may not be readily apparent. A mucosal enanthem, including oral ulcerations, may be seen. Other common findings include lymphadenopathy and pharyngitis, occasionally with exudates. The overall syndrome may be indistinguishable from infectious mononucleosis. Genital ulcers and oral candidiasis are occasionally seen. There may be neurologic findings, including a syndrome of aseptic meningitis.

Laboratory findings are generally nonspecific and may include lymphopenia, thrombocytopenia, anemia, and elevated liver enzymes. HIV antibody testing at this acute state may be negative. Occasionally there is an indeterminate HIV antibody result consisting of a reactive enzyme immunoassay and fewer than two reactive bands of the confirmatory Western blot test. The HIV p24 antigen assay is often positive within days to weeks after acute infection. Because of the nonspecific nature of the syndrome, the differential diagnosis for patients with acute retroviral syndrome can be broad (Table 52–3). Most frequently it includes infectious mononucleosis, streptococcal pharyngitis, and viral respiratory tract infections. Depending on the specific symptoms that predominate, acute HIV infection can be confused with secondary syphilis, acute toxoplasmosis, viral hepatitis, or viral meningitis. None of the initial clinical findings or laboratory results is pathognomonic for acute retroviral illness, and therefore acute HIV infection should be considered in any patient with a relevant risk history presenting with a compatible syndrome. One of the most important factors to consider when making the diagnosis is the identification of a potential HIV exposure during the preceding few weeks. Therefore, patients presenting with any similar illness should be questioned about any potential risk behaviors, particularly sexual activity or injection drug use, during the prior 6 to 8 weeks.

If suspicion is high based on this history, the diagnosis can be confirmed by testing plasma or serum for the presence of HIV RNA by one of the sensitive newer amplification techniques: the polymerase chain reaction (PCR), branched DNA assay, or nucleic acid sequence-based analysis (NASBA). HIV RNA testing is not recommended for screening low risk populations because nucleic acid amplification assays are costly and laborious, and they yield low-level false positive results if the prevalence of infection is low in a specific community.

After the acute retroviral syndrome HIV-infected patients may remain asymptomatic for years before the onset of immunodeficiency and symptomatic infection. They require careful medical follow-up to manage common co-morbidities (e.g., sexually transmitted diseases, tuberculosis, viral hepatitis) and to monitor immune and virologic function to determine when the use of antiretroviral and prophylactic antimicrobial therapy is indicated.

▲ NATURAL HISTORY OF HIV IN RELATION TO TREATMENT

The clinical course of untreated HIV infection has by now been well established.[11] In most cases HIV causes progressive loss of T-helper lymphocytes, which eventually renders the patient unable to mount an immune response against a variety of opportunistic pathogens. The time course of this decline is highly variable from one patient to another. Indeed, in a small number of cases no loss of immunologic function is detectable even after 10 years or more of untreated infection (so-called long-term nonprogressors). Antiretroviral drug therapy is generally not indicated for this population, as their immune system appears able to control HIV replication.

In most cases, however, T-helper lymphocyte counts in untreated individuals eventually decline to the point that clinical illness could be imminent if left untreated. The institution of highly active antiretroviral therapy (HAART) is based on an assessment of the likelihood of clinical progression. However, the clinical course of HIV disease is highly variable; that is, a decline may take place within 1 to 2 years or after more than 10 years of infection. One powerful predictor of the rate of eventual T-lymphocyte cell decline and subsequent risk of progression to AIDS is the initial plasma HIV RNA level observed in the patient prior to institution of antiretroviral therapy.[12] This value tends to be relatively stable after the acute HIV infection has been controlled by the host, when an equilibrium of sorts is established between viral replication on one hand and T-helper lymphocyte generation on the other. There is a fairly well defined correlation between a patient's T-helper lymphocyte count and the particular infections to which he or she may be susceptible[13,14] (Fig. 52–1). In general, more virulent bacterial pathogens such as *Mycobacterium tuberculosis* and *Streptococcus pneumoniae* may cause disease in patients with relatively high T-helper lymphocyte counts in excess of 300 cells per cubic millimeter. Other opportunistic

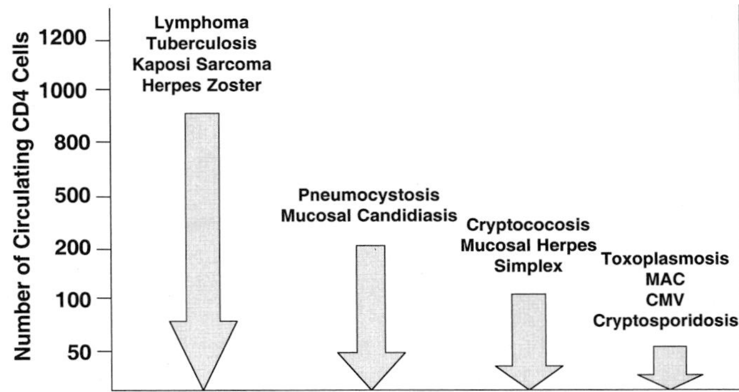

Figure 52–1. Typical relation of clinical manifestations to the CD4+ T-lymphocyte count in HIV-infected patients. CMV, cytomegalovirus; MAC, *Mycobacterium avium* complex.

pathogens, such as *Pneumocystis carinii*, seldom present a threat until counts are below 200 cells per cubic millimeter. Finally, organisms such as *Toxoplasma gondii* and *Mycobacterium avium* complex may be life-threatening when counts are below 100 cells per cubic millimeter.

▲ INITIAL MANAGEMENT OF THE HIV-INFECTED PATIENT

A typical flow sheet for initial management of the HIV-positive patient is presented in Figure 52–2.

Medical History

As part of the initial clinical management of a patient with HIV infection, the medical provider should review the date of the first positive HIV result, his last negative HIV test (if available), and any prior CD4+ T-lymphocyte counts and quantitative HIV RNA measurements that were obtained if the patient was previously in the care of another provider. It is helpful to obtain documentation of the patient's HIV status, as there have been cases of factitious HIV infection in which patients have sought to be identified as being HIV-infected for secondary gain (e.g., health

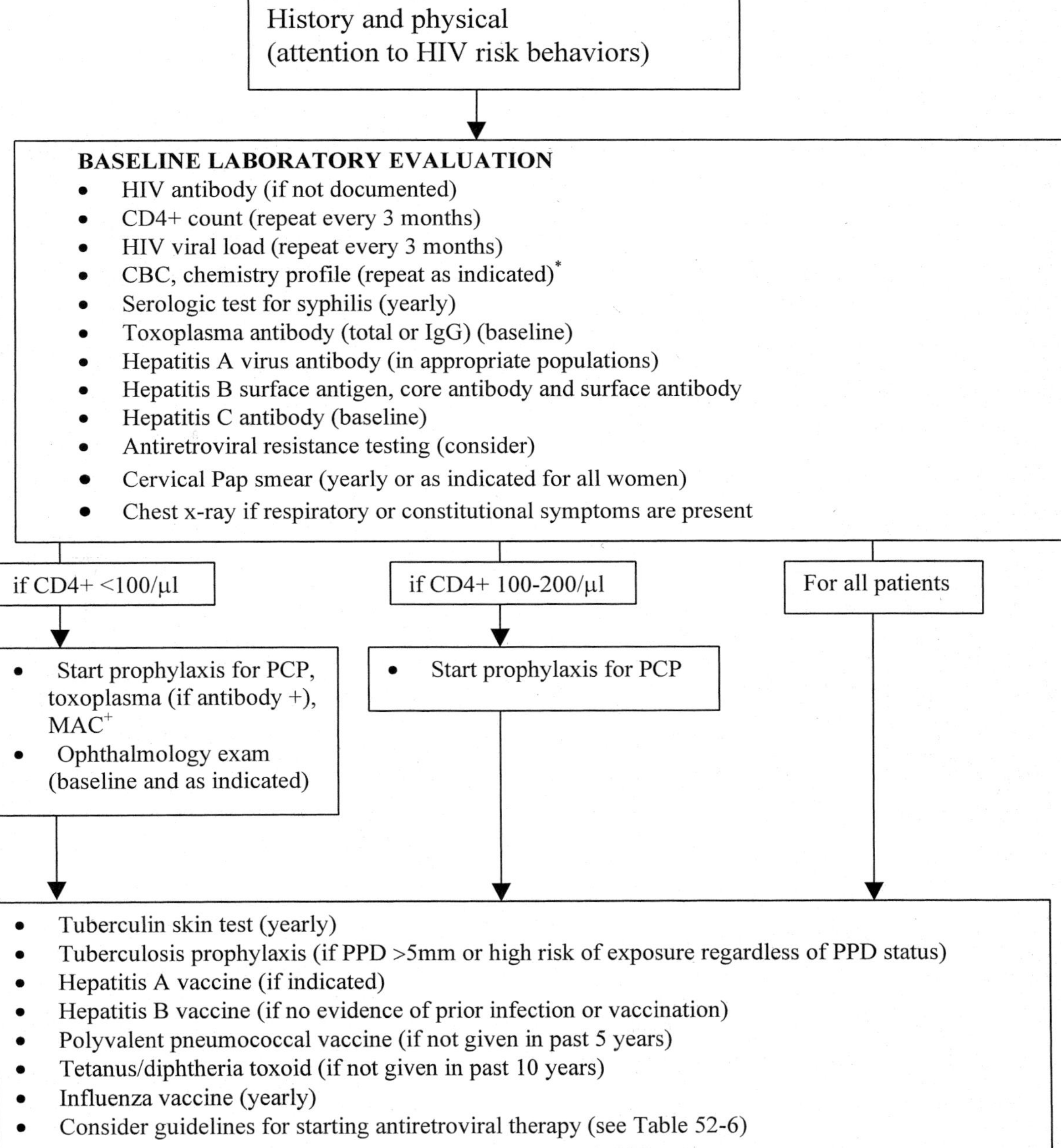

Figure 52–2. Flow chart for initial evaluation of the HIV-positive patient. *Include fasting triglyceride and cholesterol levels for those on antiretroviral therapy. +Some centers start MAC prophylaxis only when CD4+ T-lymphocyte counts are < 50 cells/μl.

insurance benefits, sympathy). It is also helpful to ascertain why the patient was tested, and what was the presumed mode of HIV acquisition. Occasionally, a patient does will not know how he or she became infected, and this can serve as an opportunity for educating him or her about methods of HIV transmission. When newly HIV-infected patients are identified, it is important to ask if they know or suspect the source of their infection, to ask the patients to notify their contacts, and to refer them for HIV counseling and testing as well.

Providers should initially review their patients' medical history and evaluate all of their symptoms and organ systems; but they should also focus on HIV-specific medical issues, including typical presenting symptoms that may be associated with HIV, such as fevers, night sweats, unanticipated weight loss, generalized lymphadenopathy, diarrhea, and oral candidiasis (Table 52–4). Questions should also address any history of opportunistic illnesses, especially including recurrent bacterial pneumonias, *Pneumocystis carinii* pneumonia, tuberculosis (including extrapulmonary disease), cryptococcal meningitis, herpes zoster infection, cytomegalovirus (CMV) infection, *Mycobacterium avium* infection, cervical cancer, and Kaposi sarcoma. A geographic history should be obtained, as regionally prevalent illnesses such as histoplasmosis, blastomycosis, and coccidioidomycosis may present as reactivation disease after an HIV-infected patient has left an endemic region. Because of the nature of HIV transmission, a detailed sexual history should also be included, and any history of specific sexually transmitted diseases should be elicited. Included in this category are viral hepatitides, which should be asked about specifically. Providers should also discuss whether patients have had a prior hepatitis A or B vaccination; and, if not, it should be offered to them if they are likely to engage in risk-taking behaviors.

▲ Table 52–4. RELEVANT CLINICAL HISTORY FOR HIV-INFECTED PATIENTS

Medical issues
Prior medical, surgical, or psychiatric conditions
Current medications
Drug allergies
Prior or current infection with tuberculosis, sexually transmitted infections, and/or viral hepatitis (A, B, or C)
Reproductive health history
Travel history
Immunizations
HIV-specific issues
Duration of infection
CD4+ T-lymphocyte counts
Plasma viral load measurements
History of opportunistic infections or neoplasms
Antiretroviral therapy history
Prophylactic medications
Nutritional history
Behavioral issues
Prior and current alcohol and other drug use
Cigarette and other nicotine use
Awareness of how HIV infection is transmitted, and current pattern of risk behaviors
Emotional status: presence of depression
Family and other primary support systems
Employment/insurance status
Community involvement

A detailed tuberculosis exposure history should be elicited, including any known exposure to tuberculosis, the family history, the date of the patient's last tuberculin skin test, and if there have been any reactive tuberculin skin tests. If the patient had a positive PPD, the duration of chemoprophylaxis (if any) and date of the last chest radiograph (if any) should be noted. If the patient had prior clinical tuberculosis, documentation of the adequacy of therapy and adherence to a full-course regimen is important. If the patient has undergone tuberculin skin testing, it is important to note whether control reagents were also used, and if the patient was anergic.

In settings where the presence of drug-resistant virus is suspected, genotypic or phenotypic resistance testing of the patient's virus should be considered (see Chapter 26).

Medication and Drug History

A thorough medication history is essential, especially if antiretroviral therapy is to be initiated. Patients should be asked about all medications they are currently taking, including over-the-counter drugs, complementary and alternative medications such as herbal preparations, and nutritional supplements. There is a tendency for many patients to consider herbal medications benign and not to mention their use; patients should be reminded that any pharmacologically active substance might have unwanted side effects or interactions with other medications. For example, St. John's wort, which is sold over the counter as an antidepressant, may alter the metabolism of protease inhibitors.[15] The use of tobacco, alcohol, and illicit drugs should be accurately ascertained in a nonjudgmental manner. The safety and efficacy of many alternative therapeutics is still not fully known but can be more carefully monitored if concomitant use of nonprescription medications is disclosed to the primary provider.

Physical Examination

A thorough physical examination should be done at the initial visit, focusing on organ systems likely to be affected by opportunistic illnesses. Height and weight should be measured at baseline; in particular, a change in weight can be a sensitive marker of systemic illness. With regard to vital signs, fever suggests infection or an inflammatory process, and hemodynamic instability suggests hypovolemia or adrenal insufficiency. A thorough skin examination should look for lesions suggestive of Kaposi sarcoma and other opportunistic illnesses. The ocular fundi should be visualized looking for retinal lesions, which may be associated with CMV, advanced HIV infection, toxoplasmosis, or atypical manifestations of other HIV-associated diseases. In the oropharynx, candidiasis and oral hairy leukoplakia are sensitive markers of immunosuppression. Kaposi sarcoma is often seen first in the mouth; and dental and gingival health should be carefully noted. An assiduous search should be made for enlarged lymph nodes in all palpable areas. Hepatomegaly or splenomegaly suggest a number of systemic infections, ranging from viral hepatitis to disseminated mycobacterial disease. A detailed anogenital examination is imperative, as many HIV-infected patients are also at risk for other sexually transmitted diseases. In the population of men who have sex with men (MSM), the anus should be closely examined for lesions of herpes simplex and human papillomavirus infection. Women should have a thorough pelvic examination with a Papanicolaou (Pap) smear and annual Pap smears thereafter; women with an abnormal Pap smear or a history of human papillomavirus infection should have more frequent examinations and should be referred for colposcopy.[16] Men who engage in anal sex should have anal Pap smears checked annually as well. A careful neurologic examination should also be done on all patients at baseline.

Routine Laboratory Screening

A baseline laboratory evaluation of a new HIV-positive patient (Fig. 52–2) should include a complete blood count and routine chemistries to assess liver and kidney function. These tests can help identify asymptomatic common comorbid problems such as viral hepatitis or HIV nephropathy, and they serve as a valuable indicator of clinical status prior to the initiation of antiretroviral therapy, which can affect these parameters. In addition, because antiretroviral therapy may be associated with new-onset glucose intolerance or hyperlipidemia,[17] new patients should also be screened with fasting blood glucose and lipid determinations.

Monitoring Immune Status

The CD4+ T-lymphocyte count, the most readily available quantitative measure of the status of the cell-mediated immune system, should be checked at baseline and periodically. The CD4+ T-lymphocyte count has a wide dynamic range in HIV-infected and HIV-uninfected persons; values between 2000 and 500 cells per cubic millimeter may be seen in noninfected persons. However, counts of less than 500 cells per cubic millimeter are atypical in HIV-uninfected persons. At counts between 500 and 350 cells per cubic millimeter, it is uncommon to find clinical manifestations of cell-mediated immune dysfunction. At counts below 350 cells per cubic millimeter, thrush, zoster, recurrent dermatoses, and other mucosal infections may connote impaired immune function, and patients with counts below 200 cells per cubic millimeter are at increased risk for life-threatening opportunistic infections.[14] Thus in an asymptomatic patient with a stable CD4+ T-lymphocyte count of 500 cells per cubic millimeter or more it is not necessary to check the count more than every 3 months, but in a patient whose count is showing a significant decline (i.e., more than 10% to 20%) repeating the test in a month makes sense, as a persistent trend may warrant the initiation of antiretroviral therapy or suggest the need to change medications in a treatment-experienced patient.

Measuring the Plasma Viral Load

A quantitative plasma HIV RNA assay should also be followed on a regular basis (see Chapter 1). There are three assays that can measure free plasma HIV RNA and offer comparable information: PCR, branched DNA (bDNA), and NASBA.[18] The HIV RNA level should be measured when a patient is first diagnosed, prior to any planned change in antiretroviral therapy, and at least every 4 weeks after a change until it has reached a stable level.[19] The goal of antiretroviral therapy is to achieve suppression so the virus cannot be detected with an ultrasensitive assay (cutoff $<$ 50 copies per milliliter). Measurements every 2 to 3 months thereafter are usually adequate if the patient is clinically stable. Because transient states of immune activation may elevate HIV RNA levels, they should not be measured within 4 weeks of receiving a vaccine or during an intercurrent illness unless there is concern that the illness is due to failure of antiretroviral therapy.[19]

Concomitant Infections

Newly diagnosed HIV-infected patients should also be tested for concomitant infections that may be transmitted by sexual or parenteral contact, such as hepatitis B, hepatitis C, and sexually transmitted infections such as syphilis, gonorrhea, and *Chlamydia* infection and those that present particular management problems among HIV-infected patients, such as tuberculosis and toxoplasmosis. As a minimum, baseline testing should include serologic screening for prior and active hepatitis B infection (hepatitis B surface antigen and antibody, and core antibody) and for hepatitis C antibodies. Patients who are not hepatitis B-seropositive should be given the hepatitis B vaccine series.[20] The MSM population and people who are exposed to unsanitary conditions can also benefit from hepatitis A vaccination if they are not already seropositive to hepatitis A (see Chapter 46).

Antibodies against *Toxoplasma gondii* should be measured at baseline.[20] This assay simply provides evidence of prior exposure, which would indicate a latent toxoplasmic infection and a risk for subsequent reactivation. Therefore, a single titer of total or immunoglobulin G (IgG) antibodies is adequate. This is in contrast with testing immunocompetent symptomatic patients for acute toxoplasmosis, in whom acute and convalescent antibodies or IgM antibodies are measured.

Syphilis

All HIV-infected patients should be tested for syphilis and treated if a confirmatory serologic test is reactive.[21] This population is at increased risk of complications from syphilis, including neurosyphilis, rapid progression of disease, and failure of treatment. For this reason a lumbar puncture should be strongly considered for all HIV-infected patients diagnosed with syphilis of unknown duration. The use of tetracyclines for treating syphilis in HIV-positive patients is discouraged because of their limited ability to cross the blood-brain barrier, and penicillin desensitization

▲ **Table 52–5.** IMMUNIZATIONS FOR HIV-INFECTED PATIENTS

Vaccine	Status	Dose/Regimen	Comments
Pneumococcal vaccine	Recommended	0.5 ml IM	Consider revaccination after 5 years
Hepatitis B vaccine	Recommended for HBsAg(-) pts	Engerix-B 20 μg or Recombivax HB 10 μg IM; give at 0, 1, 6 months	Test vaccinated pts for HBsAb after third dose; Nonresponders should get boosters.
Hepatitis A vaccine	Recommended for at-risk pts	1 ml IM with second vaccination at 6–12 months	Give to MSM, people who work in unsanitary conditions, pts with hepatitis B or C. Consider testing for HAV serostatus in older patients.
Influenza vaccine	Recommended	0.5 ml IM annually	Vaccine can ↑ HIV replication, so pt should be on suppressive anti-HIV therapy. Best response if CD4+ T-lymphocyte count > 200 cells/mm^3
Tetanus toxoid	Recommended	Td 0.5 ml IM	Same as for HIV(-); reboost every 10 years.
Haemophilus influenzae vaccine	See comments	0.5 ml IM	Only for asplenic pts and those with recurrent *H. influenzae* infections
Polio vaccine	IPV	0.5 ml SC in three doses for primary immunization series over 12 months	Routine immunization not necessary for adults residing in the U.S. IPV indicated for travel to endemic areas. OPV contraindicated.

HAV, hepatitis A virus; HBsAb, hepatitis B surface antibody; IM, intramuscular; IPV, enhanced inactivated polio vaccine; MSM, men who have sex with men; OPV, oral polio vaccine; pts, patients; SC, subcutaneous; Td, tetanus-diphtheria toxoid.

is preferred in penicillin-allergic individuals, as the spirochete tends to disseminate early to the central nervous system in the setting of HIV infection.

Tuberculosis

Tuberculin skin testing at baseline and annually should also be routine for HIV-infected patients.[22] Any HIV-positive patient with a reactive tuberculin skin test (at least 5 mm in diameter) should receive antituberculous prophylaxis for a year if previously untreated. Declining CD4+ T-lymphocyte counts are associated with an increased rate of anergy; therefore, in patients at particularly high risk of tuberculosis exposure (such as family members of infected persons) consideration should be given to antituberculous prophylaxis even in the absence of skin test reactivity.

Immunizations

There are several immunizations that carry little risk and are likely to benefit HIV-infected patients (Table 52–5).[20] Current recommendations suggest that all adult patients with a CD4+ T-lymphocyte count of 200 cells per cubic millimeter or more receive a single dose of the 23-valent pneumococcal vaccine if they have not received one in the prior 5 years. In patients with a CD4+ T-lymphocyte count of less than 200 cells per cubic millimeter, the likelihood of developing an effective humoral response to the vaccination is less; however, the vaccination is safe and should still be offered. Yearly influenza vaccinations are warranted for all HIV-infected patients, independent of their immune status. Investigators had been concerned because plasma HIV RNA measurements obtained immediately after influenza vaccination may show a transient rise in plasma viral load if the patient is not on effective suppressive antiretroviral therapy. However, there is no evidence that such transient "blips" lead to a sustained rise in viral load or to subsequent development of antiretroviral resistance; thus the risk of adverse consequences associated with influenza vaccination is negligible.[23]

HIV-infected patients should receive tetanus-diphtheria booster vaccinations every 10 years, in accordance with the recommendation for the general adult population. Vaccination against hepatitis B virus is recommended for all adults who do not have evidence of prior immunization or prior hepatitis B infection. Certain patient populations, such the MSM group and persons with chronic hepatitis C, should be immunized against hepatitis A. Younger patients are unlikely to have preexisting hepatitis A immunity, so it may be more cost-effective simply to vaccinate against hepatitis A virus (HAV) than to test for HAV antibodies.

Live virus vaccines should be avoided in HIV-positive adults, including oral polio vaccine, varicella-zoster vaccine, and vaccines for measles, mumps, and rubella. Furthermore, household members of an HIV-infected patient should not receive oral polio vaccine because of the risk of infection due to fecal shedding of live poliovirus. If someone in the patient's household has received oral polio vaccine, the patient should avoid contact with that person for the next month, while live virus may be excreted.

Prophylaxis for Opportunistic Infections

The 2001 U.S. Public Health Service/Infection Disease Society of America (USPHS/IDSA) guidelines for prophylaxis to prevent first-episode opportunistic infections in adults and adolescents infected with HIV are presented in Table 52–6 and those to prevent recurrence of opportunistic infections are presented in Table 52–7. Salient features of these recommendations are discussed below.

Pneumocystis carinii Pneumonia

Chemoprophylaxis against *Pneumocystis carinii* pneumonia (PCP) produces decreased HIV-associated mortality and should be strongly recommended in patients with a CD4+ T-lymphocyte count of less than 200 cells per cubic millimeter a CD4+ T-lymphocyte percentage less than 14%, oral thrush, or a history of PCP.[24] Trimethoprim-sulfamethoxazole is more

▲ **Table 52–6.** PROPHYLAXIS TO PREVENT FIRST EPISODE OF OPPORTUNISTIC DISEASE IN ADULTS AND ADOLESCENTS INFECTED WITH HIV

Pathogen	Preventive Regimens: Indication	First Choice	Alternatives
Strongly recommended as standard of care			
Pneumocystis carinii[a]	CD4+ T-lymphocyte count < 200/μl or oropharyngeal candidiasis	TMP-SMZ 1 DS PO qd (AI) TMP-SMZ 1 SS PO qd (AI)	Dapsone 50 mg PO bid *or* 100 mg PO qd (BI); dapsone 50 mg PO qd *plus* pyrimethamine 50 mg PO qw *plus* leucovorin 25 mg PO qw (BI); dapsone 200 mg PO *plus* pyrimethamine 75 mg PO *plus* leucovorin 25 mg PO qw (BI); aerosolized pentamidine 300 mg qm via Respirgard II nebulizer (BI); atovaquone 1500 mg PO qd (BI); TMP-SMZ 1 DS PO tiw (BI)
Mycobacterium tuberculosis Isoniazid-sensitive[b]	TST reaction ≥ 5 mm or prior positive TST result without treatment or contact with case of active tuberculosis regardless of TST result (BIII)	Isoniazid 300 mg PO *plus* pyridoxine 50 mg PO qd × 9 mo (AII) or isoniazid 900 mg PO *plus* pyridoxine 100 mg PO biw × 9 mo (BII); rifampin 600 mg *plus* pyrazinimide 15–20 mg/kg PO qd × 2 mo (AI)	Rifabutin 300 mg PO qd *plus* pyrazinamide 15–20 mg/kg PO qd × 2 mo (BIII); rifampin 600 mg PO qd = 4 mo (BIII)
Isoniazid-resistant	Same as above; high probability of exposure to isoniazid-resistant tuberculosis	Rifampin 600 mg *plus* pyrazinamide 15–20 mg/kg PO qd × 2 mo (AI)	Rifabutin 300 mg *plus* pyrazinamide 15–20 mg/kg PO qd × 2 mo (BIII); rifampin 600 mg PO qd × 4 mo (BIII); rifabutin 300 mg PO qd × 4 mo (CIII)
Multidrug (isoniazid and rifampin)-resistant	Same as above; high probability of exposure to multidrug-resistant tuberculosis	Choice of drugs requires consultation with public health authorities. Depends on susceptibility of isolate from source patient	—
Toxoplasma gondii[c]	IgG antibody to *Toxoplasma* and CD4+ count < 100/μl	TMP-SMZ, 1 DS PO qd (AII)	TMP-SMZ 1 SS PO qd (BIII); dapsone 50 mg PO qd *plus* pyrimethamine 50 mg PO qw *plus* leucovorin 25 mg PO qw (BI); atovaquone 1500 mg PO qd with or without pyrimethamine 25 mg PO qd *plus* leucovorin 10 mg PO qd (CIII)
Mycobacterium avium complex[d]	CD4+ count < 50/μl	Azithromycin 1200 mg PO qw (AI) or clarithromycin[e] 500 mg PO bid (AI)	Rifabutin, 300 mg PO qd (BI); azithromycin 1200 mg PO qw *plus* rifabutin 300 mg PO qd (CI)
Varicella zoster virus (VZV)	Significant exposure to chickenpox or shingles for patients who have no history of either condition or, if available, negative antibody to VZV	Varicella zoster immune globulin (VZIG), 5 vials (1.25 ml each) IM, administered ≤ 96 hr after exposure, ideally within 48 hr (AIII)	
Generally Recommended			
Streptococcus pneumoniae[f]	CD4+ count > 200/μl	23 Valent polysaccharide vaccine, 0.5 ml IM (BII)	None
Hepatitis B virus[g,h]	All susceptible (anti-HBc-negative) patients	Hepatitis B vaccine: 3 doses (BII)	None
Influenza virus[g,i]	All patients (annually, before influenza season)	Inactivated trivalent influenza virus vaccine one annual dose (0.5 ml) IM (BIII)	Oseltamivir 75 mg PO qd (influenza A or B) (CIII); rimantadine 100 mg PO bid (CIII) or amantadine 100 mg PO bid (CIII) (influenza A only)
Hepatitis A virus[g]	All susceptible (anti-HAV-negative) patients at increased risk for HAV infection (e.g., illicit drug users, men who have sex with men, hemophiliacs) or with chronic liver disease, including chronic hepatitis B or hepatitis C	Hepatitis A vaccine: two doses (BIII)	None

Table continued on following page

▲ **Table 52–6.** PROPHYLAXIS TO PREVENT FIRST EPISODE OF OPPORTUNISTIC DISEASE IN ADULTS AND ADOLESCENTS INFECTED WITH HIV *Continued*

Pathogen	Preventive Regimens		
	Indication	First Choice	Alternatives
Evidence for Efficacy But Not Routinely Indicated			None
Bacteria	Neutropenia	G-CSF 5–10 μg/kg SC qd × 2–4 wk or GM-CSF 250 μg/m² SC or IV qd × 2–4 wk (CII)	
Cryptococcus neoformans	CD4+ count < 50/μl	Fluconazole 100–200 mg PO qd (CI)	Itraconazone capsule 200 mg PO qd (CIII)
Histoplasma capsulatum[j]	CD4+ count < 100/μl, endemic geographic area	Itraconazole capsule 200 mg PO qd (CI)	None
Cytomegalovirus (CMV)[k]	CD4+ count < 50/μl and CMV antibody positivity	Oral ganciclovir 1g PO tid (CI)	None

From Centers for Disease Control and Prevention. 2001 USPHS/IDSA Guidelines for the prevention of opportunistic infections in persons infected with human immunodeficiency virus. MMWR (2002 in press).

Note: Information included in these guidelines might not represent Food and Drug Administration (FDA) approval or approved labeling for the particular products or indications in question. Specifically, the terms "safe" and "effective" might not be synonymous with the FDA-defined legal standards for product approval. The Respirgard II nebulizer is manufactured by Marquest, Englewood, Co. Letters and Roman numerals in parentheses after regimens indicate the strength of the recommendation and the quality of evidence supporting it (see Rating System below. Anti-HBc, antibody to hepatitis B core antigen; biw, twice a week; DS, double-strength tablet; GM-CSF, granulocyte/macrophage colony-stimulating factor; HAART, highly active antiretroviral therapy; HAV, hepatitis A virus; HIV, human immunodeficiency virus; qd, daily; qm, monthly; qw, weekly; SS, single-strength tablet; tiw, three times a week; TMP-SMZ, trimethoprim-sulfamethoxazole; TST, tuberculin skin test.

[a] Prophylaxis should also be considered for persons with a CD4+ T-lymphocyte percentage of < 14%, for persons with a history of an AIDS-defining illness and possibly for those with CD4+ T-lymphocyte counts of > 200 but < 250 cells/μl. TMP-SMZ also reduces the frequency of toxoplasmosis and some bacterial infections. Patients receiving dapsone should be tested for glucose-6-phosphate dehydrogenase deficiency. A dosage of 50 mg qd is probably less effective than 100 mg qd. The efficacy of parenteral pentamidine (e.g., 4 mg/kg/mo) is uncertain. Fansidar (sulfadoxine-pyrimethamine) is rarely used because of severe hypersensitivity reactions. Patients who are being administered therapy for toxoplasmosis with sulfadiazine-pyrimethamine are protected against *Pneumocystis carinii pneumonia* (PCP) and do not need additional prophylaxis against PCP.

[b] Directly observed therapy is recommended for isoniazid, e.g., 900 mg biw; isoniazid regimens should include pyridoxine to prevent peripheral neuropathy. If rifampin or rifabutin are adminstered concurrently with protease inhibitors or nonnucleoside reverse transcriptase inhibitors, careful consideration should be given to potential pharmacokinetic interactions exposure to multidrug-resistant tuberculosis might require prophylaxis with two drugs; consult public health authorities. Possible regimens include pyrazinamide plus either ethambutol or a fluoroquinolone.

[c] Protection against toxoplasmosis is provided by TMP-SMZ, dapsone plus pyrimethamine, and possibly by atovaquone. Atovaquone may be used with or without pyrimethamine. Pyrimethamine alone probably provides little if any protection.

[d] See "Disseminated Infection with *Mycobacterium avium* Complex for a discussion of drug interactions.

[e] During pregnancy azithromycin is preferred over clarithromycin because of the teratogenicity of clarithomycin in animals.

[f] Vaccination may be offered to persons who have a CD4+ T-lymphocyte count of < 200 cells/μl, although the efficacy is likely to be diminished. Revaccination 5 years after the first dose or sooner if the initial immunization was given when the CD4+ T-lymphocyte count was < 200 cells/μl and has increased to > 200 cells/μl on HAART is considered optional. Some authorities are concerned that immunizations might stimulate the replication of HIV.

[g] Data do not conclusively demonstrate a clinical benefit of these vaccines in this population, although it is logical to assume that those patients who develop antibody responses will derive some protection. Some authorities are concerned that immunizations might stimulate HIV replication, although for influenza vaccination a large observational study of HIV-infected persons in clinical care showed no adverse effect of this vaccine, including multiple doses, on patient survival (J. Ward, CDC, personal communication). Also this concern may less relevant in the setting of HAART. However, because of the theoretical concern that increases in HIV plasma RNA following vaccination during pregnancy might increase the risk of perinatal transmission of HIV, providers may wish to defer vaccination for such patients until after HAART in initiated.

[h] Hepatitis B vaccine has been recommended for all children and adolescents and for all adults with risk factors for hepatitis B virus (HBV).

[i] Oseltamivir is appropriate during outbreaks of influenza A or B. Rimantadine and amantadine are appropriate during outbreaks of influenza A (although neither rimantadine nor amantadine is recommended during pregnancy). Dosage reduction for antiviral chemoprophylaxis against influenza might be indicated for decreased renal or hepatic function and for persons with sezisure disorders. Physicians should consult the drug package inserts and the annual CDC inflenza guidelines for more specific information about adverse effects and dosage adjustments. For additional information regarding vaccination against hepatitis A and B and vaccination and antiviral therapy against influenza see the CDC: Prevention of hepatitis A through active or passive immunization: recommendations of the Advisory Committee on Immunization Practices (ACIP). *MMWR* 48 (No. RR-12): 1999; CDC. Hepatitis B virus: a comprehensive strategy for eliminating transmission in the United States through universal childhood vaccination: recommendations of the Advisory Committee on Immunization Practices (ACIP). *MMWR* 40 (No. RR-13): 1991; and CDC. Prevention and control of influenza: recommendations of the Advisory Committee on Immunization Practices (ACIP). For additional information about vaccination and antiviral therapy against influenza, see: CDC. Prevention and control of influenza: recommendations of the Advisory Committee on Immunization Practices (ACIP). *MMWR* 2000; 50 (No. RR-4).

[j] In a few unusual occupational or other circumstances, prophylaxis should be considered; consult a specialist.

[k] Acyclovir is not protective against CMV. Valacyclovir is not recommended because of an unexplained trend toward increased mortality observed in persons with AIDS who were being administered this drug for prevention of CMV disease.

System Used to Rate the Strength of Recommendations and Quality of Supporting Evidence

Rating	Criteria
Strength of the recommendation	
A	Strong evidence for efficacy and substantial clinical benefit support recommendation for use. Should always be offered.
B	Moderate evidence for efficacy—or strong evidence for efficacy but only limited clinical benefit—supports recommendation for use. Should generally be offered.

▲ **Table 52–6.** PROPHYLAXIS TO PREVENT FIRST EPISODE OF OPPORTUNISTIC DISEASE IN ADULTS AND ADOLESCENTS INFECTED WITH HIV *Continued*

Rating	Criteria
C	Evidence for efficacy is insufficient to support a recommendation for or against use, or the evidence might not outweigh adverse consequences (e.g., drug toxicity, drug interactions) or cost of the chemoprophylaxis or alternative approaches. Optional.
D	Moderate evidence for lack of efficacy or for adverse outcome supports a recommendation against use. Should generally not be offered.
E	Good evidence for lack of efficacy or for adverse outcome supports a recommendation against use. Should never be offered.
Quality of evidence supporting the recommendation	
I	Evidence from at least one properly randomized, controlled trial.
II	Evidence from at least one well designed clinical trial without randomization, from cohort or case-controlled analytic studies (preferably from more than one center), or from multiple time series studies; or dramatic results from uncontrolled experiments.
III	Evidence from opinions of respected authorities based on clinical experience, descriptive studies, or reports of expert committees.

efficacious than other preventive therapies (dapsone, atovaquone, inhaled pentamidine) and should be used whenever possible. Patients who develop a mild nonurticarial skin rash from sulfonamides should be advised to continue the medication and to use antihista-mines as needed, as the rash frequently abates. In patients with more severe reactions to sulfonamides, an oral desensitization regimen can be considered. Trimethoprim-sulfamethoxazole also provides some protection against bacterial pneumonia and sinusitis, as well as toxoplasmic encephalitis.

Mycobacterium Avium Complex

Use of macrolides for primary prophylaxis against *Mycobacterium avium* complex disease is recommended for patients with a CD4+ T-lymphocyte count of less than 100 cells per cubic millimeter.[20] Azithromycin or clarithromycin likely also provide some protection against community-acquired pneumonia.

Other Opportunistic Infections

The HIV-infected patients with severely compromised immune systems may have recurrent infections with *Candida albicans* (thrush, or vaginitis in women) and may require chronic suppressive antifungal therapy.[14] Likewise, the patients with recurrent herpes simplex infections may require acyclovir as prophylaxis to decrease the frequency of recurrences. In both situations the need for chronic suppressive therapy may be obviated by the restoration of immunocompetence through the institution of HAART.

Management of Advanced HIV Infected Patients

The care of HIV-infected individuals has become increasingly complex as newer antiretroviral therapies have become available. Natural history studies suggest that patients are likely to progress clinically and develop opportunistic infections if their CD4+ T-lymphocyte counts are less than 200 cells per cubic millimeter; but they are more apt to benefit from antiretroviral therapy if it is initiated when the counts are above 200 cells per cubic millimeter.[25] The most recent guidelines have cautioned clinicians regarding starting therapy when the CD4+ T-lymphocyte count is 350 to 500 cells per cubic millimeter because of the increasing reports of antiretroviral medication-associated morbidities.[19] The recommendations suggest that waiting until the count is 350 cells per cubic millimeter or lower and the plasma viral load is in the range of 30,000 to 50,000 copies per milliliter is justifiable. Moreover, it may decrease cost, and morbidity and improve adherence while delaying the onset of drug resistance (see Chapter 27).

▲ MEDICATION ADHERENCE

Antiretroviral therapy and prophylactic medicines to prevent the onset of opportunistic infections cannot be effective if patients do not adhere to the regimen, as current treatment is capable of suppressing, but not curing, HIV-associated immunodeficiency. Suboptimal adherence to antiretroviral therapy has been associated with less durable viral suppression and increased risk of clinical progression.[26] Providers should feel comfortable discussing strategies to optimize adherence with their patients and should take into consideration patient preferences (e.g., decreased pill burden, frequency of dosing, relation of meals to when the medications are to be taken) when choosing an antiretroviral regimen.

▲ PRIMARY CARE FOR HIV-INFECTED WOMEN

Women who are HIV-infected have unique clinical and psychological issues that should be addressed as part of their comprehensive care.[27] They are more apt to have recurrent candidal vaginitis and may frequently have bacterial vaginosis and *Trichomonas*-induced vaginitis. Hence comprehensive, accessible gynecologic services are a vital part of the care of HIV-infected women.[28] They may also develop the complications of pelvic inflammatory disease (e.g., tuboovarian abscesses) more readily than HIV-uninfected women and thus require careful monitoring for this serious condition if they present with pelvic pain, discharge, or both.

Table 52–7. PROPHYLAXIS TO PREVENT RECURRENCE OF OPPORTUNISTIC DISEASE IN ADULTS (AFTER CHEMOTHERAPY FOR ACUTE DISEASE) IN ADULTS AND ADOLESCENTS INFECTED WITH HIV

Pathogen	Preventive Regimens		
	Indication	First Choice	Alternatives
Recommended as standard of care			
Pneumocystis carinii	Prior PCP	TMP-SMZ 1 DS PO qd (AI); TMP-SMZ 1 SS PO qd (AI)	Dapsone 50 mg PO bid or 100 mg PO qd (BI); dapsone 50 mg PO qd plus pyrimethamine 50 mg PO qw plus leucovorin 25 mg PO qw (BI); dapsone 200 mg PO plus pyrimethamine 75 mg PO plus leucovorin 25 mg PO qw (BI); aerosolized pentamidine 300 mg qm via Respirgard II nebulizer (BI); atovaquone 1500 mg PO qd (BI); TMP-SMZ 1 DS PO tiw (CI)
Toxoplasma gondii[a]	Prior toxoplasmic encephalitis	Sulfadiazine 500–1000 mg PO qid, *plus* pyrimethamine 25–50 mg PO qd *plus* leucovorin 10–25 mg PO qd (AI)	Clindamycin 300–450 mg PO q6–8h plus pyrimethamine 25–50 mg PO qd plus leucovorin 10–25 mg PO qd (BI); atovaquone 750 mg PO q6–12h with or without pyrimethanine 25 mg PO qd plus leucovorin 10 mg PO qd (CIII)
Mycobacterium avium complex[b]	Documented disseminated disease	Clarithromycin[c] 500 mg PO bid (AI) plus ethambutol 15 mg/kg PO qd (AII); with or without rifabutin 300 mg PO qd (CI)	Azithromycin 500 mg PO qd (AII) plus ethambutol, 15 mg/kg PO qd (AII); with or without rifabutin, 300 mg PO qd (CI)
Cytomegalovirus	Prior end-organ disease	Ganciclovir 5–6 mg/kg/day IV 5–7 days/wk or 1000 mg PO tid (AI); *or* foscarnet 90–120 mg/kg IV qd (AI); *or* (for retinitis) ganciclovir sustained-release implant q6–9 mo *plus* ganciclovir 1.0–1.5 g PO tid (AI) or Valganciclovir 900 mg PO qd (AIII)	Cidofovir 5 mg/kg IV qow with probenecid 2 g PO 3 hours before the dose or by 1 g PO 2 hours after the dose, and 1 g PO 8 hours after the dose (toral 4 g) (AI); fomivirsen 1 vial (330 μg) injected into the vitreous, then repeated every 2–4 wk with ganciclovir 1.0–1.5 g PO TID (AI) or valganciclovir 900 mg PO qd (BI)
Cryptococcus neoformans	Documented disease	Fluconazole 200 mg PO qd (AI)	Amphotericin B 0.6–1.0 mg/kg IV qw–tiw (AI); itraconazole 200 mg PO qd (BI)
Histoplasma capsulatum	Documented disease	Itraconazole capsule 200 mg PO bid (AI)	Amphotericin B 1.0 mg/kg IV qw (AI)
Coccidioides immitis	Documented disease	Fluconazole 400 mg PO qd (AII)	Amphotericin B 1.0 mg/kg IV qw (AI); itraconazole 200 mg capsule PO bid (AII)
Salmonella species, (non-typhi)[d]	Bacteremia	Ciprofloxacin 500 mg PO bid for several months (BII)	Antibiotic chemoprophylaxis with another active agent (CIII)
Recommended only if subsequent episodes are frequent or severe			
Herpes simplex virus	Frequent/severe recurrences	Acyclovir 200 mg PO tid or 400 mg PO bid (AI) Famciclovir 500 mg PO bid (AI)	Valacyclovir 500 mg PO bid (CIII)
Candida (oropharyngeal or vaginal)	Frequent/severe recurrences	Fluconazole 100–200 mg PO qd (CI)	Itraconazole solution 200 mg PO qd (CI)
Candida (esophageal)	Frequent/severe recurrences	Fluconazole 100–200 mg PO qd (BI)	Itraconazole solution 200 mg PO qd (BI)

From Centers for Disease Control and Prevention. 2001 USPHS/IDSA guidelines for the prevention of opportunistic infections in persons infected with human immunodeficiency virus. MMWR (2002, in press).

Note: Information included in these guidelines might not represent Food and Drug Administration (FDA) approval or approved labeling for the particular products or indications in question. Specifically, the terms "safe" and "effective" might not be synonymous with the FDA-defined legal standards for product approval. The Respirgard II nebulizer is manufactured by Marquest, Englewood, Colorado. Letters and Roman numerals in parentheses after regimens indicate the strength of the recommendation and the quality of evidence supporting it (as in Table 27–6). bid, twice a day; DS, double-strength tablet; PCP, Pneumocystis Carinii pneumonia; qd, daily; qm, monthly; qw, weekly; qow, every other week; SS, single-strength tablet; tid, three times a day; tiw, three times a week; TMP-SMZ, trimethoprim-sulfamethoxazole.

[a]Pyrimethamine-sulfadiazine confers protection against PCP as well as toxoplasmosis; clindamycin-pyrimethamine does not offer protection against PCP.

[b]Many multiple-drug regimens are poorly tolerated. Drug interactions (e.g., those seen with clarithromycin and rifabutin) can be problematic; rifabutin has been associated with uveitis, especially when administered at daily doses of > 300 mg or concurrently with fluconazole or clarithromycin.

[c]During pregnanacy, azithromycin is recommended instead of clarithromycin because clarithromycin is teratogenic in animals.

[d]Efficacy for eradication of *Salmonella* been demonstrated only for ciprofloxacin.

Infection with human papillomavirus (HPV) is common among HIV-infected women, putting them at increased risk for cervical neoplasia.[29] Although cervical cancer is more common among HIV-infected women than HIV-uninfected women, routine Pap smear screening has been associated with limiting morbidity and mortality. A full pelvic examination and Pap smear test should be performed as part of the initial evaluation of all HIV-infected women and should be repeated 6 months later. If it is normal, the subsequent pelvic examinations can be performed yearly. If any abnormalities are detected, colposcopy should be promptly instituted and atypical regions biopsied. HPV disease may manifest as lesions in the vulva and vagina, as well as the cervix, so clinical examinations and colposcopy should be thorough. Women and men who engage in anal intercourse are at risk for anal HPV and neoplasia and should undergo routine Pap smears examination of the area (see Chapter 45).

Women living with HIV often have other unique concerns, such as being the sole support of a family unit that may include dependent children or elders. Programs that care for these women need to develop social service supports, such as the availability of an on-site case manager who can assist the women and their families to find stable, safe housing, deal with substance use concerns, and address related issues that may affect a woman's ability to adhere to a complex antiretroviral regimen.

▲ PREGNANCY

The incidence of HIV among women has increased 20-fold since 1981, so 1 in 1000 women of childbearing age in the United States is thought to be HIV-infected. Most HIV-infected women make decisions about pregnancy similar to these of their demographically matched peers. Thus the clinician must be able to educate prospective HIV-infected mothers about the relative risks and benefits of pregnancy. Optimal management of HIV-infected pregnant women should include general prenatal care, optimizing antiretroviral and prophylactic therapies in the mother, and careful monitoring for disease progression. Further discussion of the care of HIV-infected pregnant women is covered in Chapter 28.

▲ MENTAL HEALTH CONCERNS

People living with HIV may manifest a variety of psychological problems, some of which predispose them to HIV risk-taking behavior and others that reflect adaptation to the diagnosis.[30] Common diagnostic categories include adjustment disorders, major depression, anxiety, sleep disorders, and problems with substance abuse. In HIV-infected patients with advanced disease, the possibility of concomitant organic brain disease must also be considered; it requires careful evaluation, including neuroradiographic imaging. Optimal management of patients manifesting new behavioral problems involves a team approach in which a primary care physician works closely with a neuropsychiatrist and a social worker. For example, the differential diagnosis of sudden withdrawal, apathy, and decreased mental activity could range from HIV encephalopathy to an opportunistic infection to a major depression.

Adjustment disorders after learning of a new HIV diagnosis may be associated with anxious or depressed affect (or both), and the patient may benefit from referral for psychotherapy, pharmacologic management, or both. Precipitants may include a nonspecific response to the new stress of confronting a potentially life-threatening illness, dealing with the stigma associated with HIV disease, anxiety about the course of the illness, and difficulty navigating the social insurance system or concerns about finances. It is important to identify a neuropsychiatrist who is familiar with potential interactions between psychotropic medications and antiretroviral therapy, as many drugs from both groups are metabolized by the hepatic cytochrome P_{450} system, and various drugs may inhibit or induce enzymatic activity. Drug interactions may require altering doses of these medications (see Chapter 66).

In addition to providing psychotherapy and pharmacologic management of HIV-related mental health conditions, therapists should be knowledgeable about local supportive services. For many patients, access to peer-run AIDS service organizations can help them adapt to living with a chronic, serious infection. Services include peer "buddies," support groups, and information sessions with professionals, all of which are helpful for optimal coping. Adjunctive mental health services, including counseling, may be helpful for optimizing adherence to antiretroviral therapy.

▲ SOCIAL CONCERNS

As HIV becomes a more chronic, complex infection, the long-term success of any therapeutic regimen will depend on the patient's ability to maintain a stable home and work environment and to achieve trust with one's care team. Relevant concerns include the high prevalence of substance use among HIV-infected persons. The stress of HIV disease may lead to relapse of substance abuse, so clinicians should anticipate this eventuality when working with high risk patients; access to good substance use treatment resources is vital. Having case workers integrated into the clinical team is vital, so personal financial issues, legal issues, and partner or family issues can be appropriately addressed.

▲ SAFE SEX COUNSELING

The Centers for Disease Control and Prevention has estimated that there are 30,000 to 40,000 new HIV infections annually in the United States. Medical professionals who provide primary care for HIV-infected patients have an optimal opportunity to inculcate and reinforce norms of safer sexual practices with their patients, as they have frequent contact with such patients. [31] When discussing issues relating to potential HIV transmission, it is important to convey the concept of relative risk. Often when patients are counseled about the inadvisability of "high risk" behaviors, they perceive a message that most of the activities they enjoy are dangerous and hence forbidden. This may instill a sense that nothing short of complete abstinence is of any benefit, which can undermine the patient's will to avoid risk. A more profitable strategy is to discuss the fact that some behaviors (e.g., unprotected anal intercourse) are associated with a high risk of transmitting infection, others (e.g., intercourse with a latex condom) are much less risky, and still others (e.g., fellatio) present intermediate risk.

The actual per-contact rates of HIV transmission are not well established, and ethical and logistical issues complicate determinations of the efficiency of specific practices to spread HIV infection. Cohort studies suggest that the average per-contact rate may vary from less than 1 per 1000 contacts to more than a 10% risk of transmission for unprotected anal or unprotected vaginal intercourse.[32] A circumcised infected man is four times more likely to transmit HIV to his female partner than vice versa; but uncircumcised men have a risk of HIV acquisition comparable to that of women in serodiscordant couples.[33] Men engaging in receptive anal intercourse are far more likely to acquire HIV from their insertive partner than the reverse. The reasons for the variability include the fact that certain tissues (e.g., foreskin, cervix, rectal mucosa) are more susceptible to HIV infection, because of the numbers and types of cells present that can bind or transmit HIV. Other factors may alter HIV susceptibility or infectiousness, including the presence of concomitant genital tract infections, sexual trauma, the HIV level in the infected partners' genital secretions, and the strain of the virus to which one is exposed. One additional factor that can play a role in HIV susceptibility is whether a woman is prepubescent or postmenopausal (estrogen thickens the cervicovaginal epithelium and protects against HIV). Lastly, oral exposure to HIV appears to be much less risky than anal or vaginal intercourse,[34] possibly because of endogenous anti-HIV substances that are present in the oropharynx. However, it is important to note that there are several well documented case reports describing HIV infection after oral exposure to ejaculate; so although fellatio is not as risky as unprotected anal or vaginal intercourse, it is not risk-free.[35] It is up to the well informed patient to make his or her own decision regarding how much risk he or she is willing to accept with partners, and providers should serve as nonjudgmental advisors. However, health professionals should remind patients that even if their plasma viral load is undetectable they can still transmit a virus that is incurable despite treatment advances. Recent reports of the sexual transmission of multiresistant HIV by a patient taking antiretroviral therapy underscore the need for medical providers to continue to emphasize safer sexual practices with their infected patients.[36,37] Any attempt to assign specific numerical values to the risk associated with a single act are not likely to be helpful, and the patient may be left with the impression that the physician has given him or her permission to engage in certain behaviors because the individual risk is low.

Patients at risk for HIV infection may be from relatively stigmatized groups, including injection drug users and the MSM group. An accurate assessment of HIV risk and appropriate counseling for risk reduction depend on complete reporting of all potential risk behaviors. This includes activities that may be socially unacceptable or illegal, or which the clinician may find personally objectionable. In such circumstances, it is essential for the clinician to remain absolutely objective while questioning the patient. Such marginalized patients are not forthcoming with accurate information if they believe that their medical provider disapproves of specific behaviors or is inclined to judge them based on what they relate about themselves. Conversely, once a bond of trust has been established between physician and patient, the patient is more likely to discuss high risk behavior frankly and to accept the physician's counseling regarding risk reduction.

▲ CONCLUSIONS

It is clear that the management of HIV infection has become increasingly complex as people with HIV are living longer and require more complex regimens with their associated toxicities. Thus during the current era it is recommended that all primary care providers familiarize themselves with the recognition of HIV infection and be comfortable with pretest and posttest counseling for persons at risk. It is also clear that people living with HIV tend to have better outcomes if managed by a clinician who has extensive clinical experience and undergoes HIV-specific continuing medical education. The provider should either be trained in infectious diseases or be a generalist who has then focused on AIDS medicine or who has extensive experience caring for HIV-infected individuals. One of the important activities that nonspecialized primary providers can do in relation to HIV care is to identify the individuals in their community who can serve as referrals or partners in the care of HIV-infected persons. With more effective identification of infected persons at earlier stages of their infection by primary providers and through effective triage to specialized clinicians for chronic management, the care of people living with HIV will be optimized.

REFERENCES

1. De Wolf F, Spijkerman I, Schellekens P, et al. AIDS prognosis based on HIV-1 RNA, CD4+ T-cell count and function: markers with reciprocal predictive value over time after seroconversion. AIDS 11:1799–1806, 1997.
2. Miller V, Mocroft A, Reiss P, et al. Relations among CD4 lymphocyte count nadir, antiretroviral therapy, and HIV-1 disease progression: results from the EuroSIDA study. Ann Intern Med, 130:570–577, 1999.
3. Hanson D, Horsburgh CJ, Fann S, et al. Survival prognosis of HIV-infected patients. J Acquir Immune Defic Syndr, 6:624–629, 1993.
4. Centers for Disease Control and Prevention. HIV/AIDS Surveillance Report. 2000.
5. Centers for Disease Control and Prevention. Kaposi's sarcoma and *Pneumocystis* pneumonia among homosexual men—New York City and California. MMWR Morb Mortal Wkly Rep 30:305–308, 1981.
6. Masur H, Michelis MA, Greene JB, et al. An outbreak of community-acquired *Pneumocystis carinii* pneumonia: initial manifestation of cellular immune dysfunction. N Engl J Med 305:1431–1438, 1981.
7. Owens DK, Nease RF Jr, Harris RA. Cost-effectiveness of HIV screening in acute care settings. Arch Intern Med 156:394–404, 1996.
8. Busch MP, Satten GA. Time course of viremia and antibody seroconversion following human immunodeficiency virus exposure. Am J Med 102:117–126, 1997.
9. Kahn JO, Walker BD. Acute human immunodeficiency virus type 1 infection. N Engl J Med 339:33–39, 1998.
10. Schacker T, Collier AC, Hughes J, et al. Clinical and epidemiologic features of primary HIV infection. Ann Intern Med 125:257–264, 1996. Erratum. Ann Intern Med 126:74, 1997.
11. Phair JP. Determinants of the natural history of human immunodeficiency virus type 1 infection. J Infect Dis 179 (suppl 2):S384–S386, 1999.
12. Lyles RH, Munoz A, Yamashita TE, et al. Natural history of human immunodeficiency virus type 1 viremia after seroconversion and

proximal to AIDS in a large cohort of homosexual men: Multicenter AIDS Cohort Study. J Infect Dis 181:872–880, 2000.

13. Masur H, Ognibene F, Yarchoan R, et al. CD4 counts as predictors of opportunistic pneumonias in human immunodeficiency virus (HIV) infection. Ann Intern Med 111:223–231, 1989.
14. Crowe SM, Carlin JB, Stewart KI, et al. Predictive value of CD4 lymphocyte numbers for the development of opportunistic infections and malignancies in HIV-infected persons. J Acquir Immune Defic Syndr 4:770–776, 1991.
15. Piscitelli SC, Burstein AH, Chaitt D, et al. Indinavir concentrations and St. John's wart. Lancet 355:547–548, 2000.
16. Frankel R, Selwyn P, Mezger J, Andrews S. High prevalence of gynecologic disease among hospitalized women with human immunodeficiency virus infection. Clin Infect Dis 25:706–712, 1997.
17. Hadigan C, Meigs J, Corcoran C, et al. Metabolic abnormalities and cardiovascular disease risk factors in adults with human immunodeficiency virus infection and lipodystrophy. Clin Infect Dis 32:130–139, 2001.
18. Parekh B, Phillips S, Granade T, et al. Impact of HIV type 1 subtype variation on viral RNA quantitation. AIDS Res Hum Retroviruses 15:133–142, 1999.
19. Carpenter C, Cooper D, Fischl M, et al. Antiretroviral therapy in adults: updated recommendations of the International AIDS Society—USA Panel. JAMA 283:381–390, 2000.
20. Centers for Disease Control and Prevention. 2001 USPHS/IDSA guidelines for the prevention of opportunistic infections in persons infected with human immunodeficiency virus. MMWR Morb Mortal Wkly Rep (in press; draft available at http://www.hivatis.org).
21. Centers for Disease Control and Prevention. Sexually transmitted diseases treatment guidelines. MMWR Morb Mortal Wkly Rep 51(RR-6):1–80, 2002.
22. Centers for Disease Control and Prevention. Prevention and treatment of tuberculosis among patients infected with human immunodeficiency virus: principles of therapy and revised recommendations MMWR Morb Mortal Wkly Rep 47:1–58, 1998.
23. Gunthard HF, Wong JK, Spina CA, et al. Effect of influenza vaccination on viral replication and immune response in persons infected with human immunodeficiency virus receiving potent antiretroviral therapy. J Infect Dis 181:522–531, 2000.
24. Chaisson, RE, Keruly J, Richman DD, Moore RD. *Pneumocystis* prophylaxis and survival in patients with advanced human immunodeficiency virus infection treated with zidovudine: the Zidovudine Epidemiology Group. Arch Intern Med 152:2009–2013, 1992.
25. Deeks SG, Determinants of virological response to antiretroviral therapy: implications for long-term strategies. Clin Infect Dis 30 (suppl 2): S177–S184, 2000.
26. Paterson DL, Swindells S, Mohr J, et al. Adherence to protease inhibitor therapy and outcomes in patients with HIV infection. Ann Intern Med 133:21–30, 2000.
27. Klirsfeld D. HIV disease and women. Med Clin North Am 82:335–357, 1998.
28. Sobel J. Gynecologic infections in human immunodeficiency virus-infected women. Clin Infect Dis 31:1225–1233, 2000.
29. Ellerbrock TV, Chiasson MA, Bush TJ, et al. Incidence of cervical squamous intraepithelial lesions in HIV-infected women. JAMA 283:1031–1037, 2000.
30. Searight H, McLaren A. Behavioral and psychiatric aspects of HIV infection. Am Fam Physician 55:1227–1237, 1241–1242, 1997.
31. Kelly J, Hoffman R, Rompa D, Gray M. Protease inhibitor combination therapies and perceptions of gay men regarding AIDS severity and the need to maintain safer sex. AIDS 12:F91–95, 1998.
32. Gray RB, Wawer MJ, Brookmeyer R, et al. The probability of HIV-1 transmission per coital act in monogamous HIV-discordant couples, Rakai, Uganda. Lancet 357:1149–1153, 2001.
33. Gray RH, Kiwanuka N, Quinn TC, et al. Male circumcision and HIV acquisition and transmission: cohort studies in Rakai, Uganda: Rakai project team. AIDS 14: 2371–2381, 2000.
34. Vittinghoff F, Douglas J, Judson F, et al. Per-contact risk of human immunodeficiency virus transmission between male sexual partners. Am J Epidemiol 150: 306–311, 1999.
35. Dillon BH, Hecht FM, Swanson M, et al. Primary HIV Infections associated with oral transmission. Presented at the 7th Annual Conference on Retroviruses and Opportunistic Infections, San Francisco, 2000.
36. Salomon H, Wainberg M, Brenner B, et al. Prevalence of HIV-1 resistant to antiretroviral drugs in 81 individuals newly infected by sexual contact or injecting drug use: investigators of the Quebec Primary Infection Study. AIDS 14: F17–F23, 2000.
37. Hecht FM, Grant RM, Petropoulos CJ, et al. Sexual transmission of an HIV-1 variant resistant to multiple reverse-transcriptase and protease inhibitors. N Engl J Med 339:307–311, 1998.

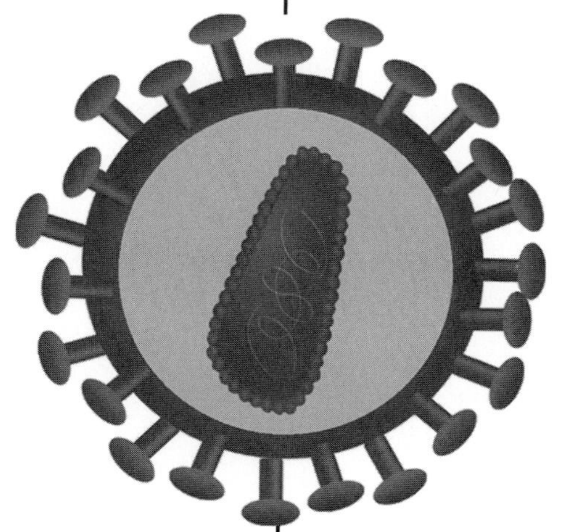

SECTION VII

Approach to Specific Syndromes

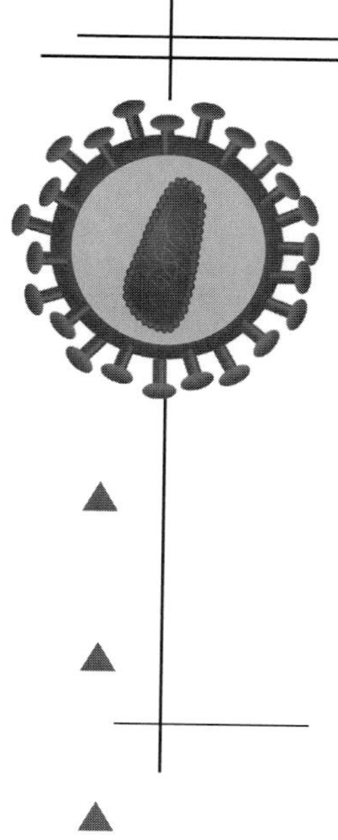

CHAPTER 53
Wasting Syndrome

Jamie H. Von Roenn, MD
Kathleen Mulligan, PhD

Body wasting was designated by the U.S. Centers for Disease Control and Prevention (CDC) as an acquired immunodeficiency syndrome (AIDS)-defining condition in 1987. With advances in antiretroviral therapy, the frequency of opportunistic infections and malignancies is decreasing, but the incidence of the wasting syndrome appears unchanged.[1–3] In 1997 wasting was the second most frequent AIDS-indicating condition in cases reported to the CDC and accounted for 18% of all reports.[4] In a paper comparing trends in patients followed at the Johns Hopkins AIDS Service in 1994 with those in 1998, wasting, along with lymphoma and cervical cancer, were the only complications that did not decline in incidence over that time.[3] Using data from an ongoing natural history study of more than 600 adults with HIV at Tufts University, Wanke et al.[5] suggested that the incidence of wasting was not significantly affected by using highly active antiretroviral treatment (HAART). Among patients on a HAART regimen, approximately 13% (633 patients) met the study's criteria for wasting after initiation of HAART.

The CDC definition of the "wasting syndrome" requires a weight loss of at least 10% in the presence of diarrhea (two or more loose stools per day) or chronic weakness and documented fever (intermittent or constant) for at least 30 days that is not attributable to a concurrent condition other than the HIV infection itself.[6] In practice, an involuntary *net* weight loss of this magnitude in the absence of an acute secondary infection is identified as wasting. Surveys of large population databases indicate that wasting occurs with equal frequency in men and women.[7,8]

Weight loss with HIV infection tends to be episodic[9,10] and is characterized by depletion of both fat and lean tissue.[11–20] Rapid weight loss is typically associated with acute systemic infections,[9,10] whereas more gradual weight loss occurs in individuals with malabsorptive disorders.[10] A common pattern of weight loss in individuals with HIV infection features periods of rapid weight loss during infection and failure to regain the weight fully during the subsequent recovery phase.[21]

Numerous prospective and retrospective studies have demonstrated significant relations between loss of weight[22–28] or body cell mass (BCM)[13,22,29] and mortality in HIV-infected individuals, independent of other survival factors. This relation persists during the current treatment era.[30] Notably, loss of weight of as little as 5% has been associated with decreased survival and should trigger evaluation and intervention.[28] Kotler et al.[22] reported extrapolated values for body weight and BCM at the time of death of 66% and 54% of normal, respectively, and observed that death from malnutrition in patients with AIDS occurred at the same degree of depletion as was seen in historical reports of death from starvation.[30,31] In addition to affecting survival, wasting is associated with accelerated disease progression[24,28] and impairment of physical functioning in patients with HIV infection.[32,33]

▲ PATHOPHYSIOLOGY

Factors demonstrated or hypothesized to contribute to wasting are anorexia, metabolic abnormalities, endocrine dysfunction, malabsorption, and cytokine dysregulation. In most cases a combination of factors or failed compensatory responses contribute to the wasting process.

Although increased resting energy expenditure (REE) is a common finding in patients with HIV infection,[9,34–39] particularly in patients with systemic secondary infections,[9,35,40] not all patients with HIV infection are hypermetabolic.[14,40] There is no convincing causal relation between REE and wasting. Instead, decreased energy intake has been found to be the primary contributor to wasting, particularly during periods of rapid weight loss.[9,38,41] Elevated REE may serve as a cofactor in accelerating weight loss and provides evidence of failure to compensate for decreased energy intake. Studies using stable isotope techniques have demonstrated that total energy expenditure (TEE) is not elevated in weight-stable patients with HIV infection when compared with estimates of TEE in other studies of healthy adults.[38,41] Notably, TEE is *decreased* during weight-losing episodes, despite elevated rates of REE, indicative of a voluntary reduction in activity levels.[38] Although a decrease in physical activity can narrow the gap between energy intake and expenditure, reduced activity levels can result in loss of lean tissue and impaired quality of life and cannot be considered an appropriate adaptation to reduced energy intake.

A variety of other metabolic alterations have been described in individuals across the spectrum of HIV infection, including increased[39] and decreased[42] rates of protein turnover; increased rates of *de novo* hepatic lipogenesis,[43] circulating triglycerides,[44] and lipid flux and oxidative and nonoxidative lipid disposal[37]; and decreased in lipid clearance and lipoprotein lipase activity.[9] However, no quantitative causal relation has been demonstrated between these or other metabolic alterations and wasting.

Endocrine disturbances resulting in decreased production or activity (or both) of endogenous anabolic substances may also contribute to HIV-related weight loss. Serum testosterone levels are decreased in 30% to 50% of HIV-infected men and have been associated with progressive immunodeficiency, decreased CD4+ T-lymphocyte counts, and poor survival.[45–47] In hypogonadal men with AIDS-related wasting, androgen levels have been correlated with weight loss, BCM, and exercise functional capacity.[45,48] The decrease in serum testosterone is most frequently secondary to the effects of systemic illness, medications or undernutrition.[46,49–52] About 25% of HIV-infected men with hypogonadism have primary hypogonadism, which is most often idiopathic. The role of serum dihydrotestosterone (DHT) in the etiology of weight loss is unclear. Some investigators have suggested that a defect in DHT synthesis contributes to weight loss in HIV-infected men,[53a] but it is unclear whether the reduced serum DHT levels are causally related to AIDS wasting or secondary to the weight loss. The latter is likely the explanation, as serum total testosterone and DHT levels are highly correlated with each other. However, serum DHT levels are not significantly correlated with a change in fat-free mass when the change in serum testosterone is taken into account.[54a]

Growth hormone (GH) has direct effects on nitrogen balance and muscle protein synthesis. Although disturbances in the GH–insulin-like growth hormone (IGF-1) axis have been described in HIV-seropositive subjects, their relation to involuntary weight loss is incompletely defined. Elevated GH and reduced IGF-1 levels, both abnormal and normal GH secretory dynamics, and normal IGF-1 levels have been described in HIV-seropositive subjects with weight loss.[37,53,54] A blunted IGF-1 response to GH stimulation was seen in two studies in patients with HIV-associated weight loss.[37,55] Whether these discrepancies are a result of differences in the patient populations studied (e.g., active weight loss versus stable weight, co-morbid conditions) or as yet unidentified factors is unclear.

Malabsorption of carbohydrates, fats, and micronutrients have been observed in patients at all stages of HIV infection without a direct correlation with diarrhea or weight loss.[27,55–57] One study suggested that loss of intestinal absorptive surface may be present at an early stage of HIV infection and progress as the HIV disease progresses. Abnormal D-xylose absorption tests, abnormal Schilling tests, and abnormal small intestinal biopsies have been noted in HIV-seropositive adults in the absence of clinically significant diarrhea.[55,56,58]

Diarrhea is a frequent gastrointestinal complaint of patients with HIV infection, occurring in up to 80% of AIDS patients from North America and Europe and in nearly 100% of those in developing countries.[59–61] For most patients, a diagnostic evaluation yields a specific pathogen to explain the diarrhea.[62] Most patients with persistent diarrhea are infected with a protozoon, primarily *Cryptosporidium parvum*, microsporidia, or other pathogens.[62] Geographic location determines the relative frequency of infection with the various diarrhea-causing enteral pathogens.[63] The clinical presentations of these pathogens vary. Patients with cryptosporidiosis generally have greater malnutrition than those with microsporidiosis, and patients with microsporidiosis are at greater risk for malnutrition than are those without an identified enteric pathogen.[64–67] Although gastrointestinal diarrheal diseases with malabsorption are most frequently associated with chronic progressive weight loss, the fraction of patients with the wasting syndrome who have diarrhea, clinically significant malabsorption, or both is unknown. In a multivariate analysis, only a weak association between loss of lean body mass and diarrhea was observed in patients in the Multicenter AIDS Cohort Study.[68]

A small but significant number of patients with severe diarrhea have no identifiable pathogen despite an extensive evaluation. The etiology of the malabsorption, weight loss, and diarrhea in these patients is unclear. Localization of HIV to the intestinal epithelium or indirect effects of HIV or local cytokines as a cause of small intestinal mucosal damage has been postulated.[58,69,70] Although many abnormalities in gastrointestinal structure and function have been identified in HIV-seropositive subjects, they may occur in the absence of weight loss or diarrhea, making it unclear what role these abnormalities play in the pathogenesis of HIV-related weight loss.

Dysregulation of the cytokine network is a prominent feature of advanced HIV infection. Experimental therapy in animals with cytokines including interferon-γ tumor (IFNγ) necrosis factor-α (TNFα), interleukin-6 (IL-6), and IL-1β, can produce striking anorexia and weight loss.[71,72] Though frequently cited as a causative factor of anorexia, TNFα levels are not consistently elevated in the serum of patients with cancer cachexia or HIV-related weight loss.[21,44,73] No correlation between TNFα levels and the degree of weight loss in HIV-infected patients has been identified.[44]

Elevations in IL-1β are seen in response to opportunistic infections and can produce clinical and biochemical abnormalities associated with cachexia.[74] Furthermore, elevated circulating levels of the IL-1 receptor antagonist (IL-1Ra), reported in a variety of inflammatory conditions, have been correlated with HIV-related weight loss independent of HIV stage or the CD4+ T-lymphocyte count.[75] In addition to the anorexia that may result from the abnormal cytokine milieu of advanced HIV infection, interactions between multiple cytokines (IL-1β, TNFα, IFNα, IFNγ, IL-6) and cytokine disturbances have been implicated in the metabolic abnormalities seen in patients with HIV infection. There are few data to support that chronic elevation of one or more cytokines causes wasting.

▲ APPROACH TO THERAPY

Weight History

Many factors must be considered during the initial evaluation of weight loss, beginning with an assessment of the amount and rate of weight loss (Table 53–1). A useful technique for monitoring the nutritional status of patients is the simple plotting of weight trends.[76] Although weight is often determined routinely as part of a medical examination, its utility as a diagnostic tool can be improved if serial weights are measured under standardized conditions. Calculation of the body mass index (BMI: weight in kilogram divided by the height in square meters) is a simple means of comparing a patient's current weight with population norms. A BMI of less than 20 kg/m^2 in adult men or women with HIV infection puts them at greater risk for complications. Weight for height tables, such as the Metropolitan Life Insurance tables,[77] provide another means of comparing an individual's value with population standards. In the absence of such tables, the following formulas provide a simple approximation of ideal weight for height in adults: For men it is 106 pounds for the first 5 feet plus 6 pounds for each additional inch; for women it is 100 pounds for the first 5 feet plus 5 pounds for each additional inch.

Body Composition

Because mortality is related not just to loss of weight but also to depletion of lean tissue, there has been considerable interest in measuring body composition in patients with HIV infection. Two simple techniques, bioelectrical impedance analysis (BIA) and anthropometry, are available to many practitioners and can be used in conjunction with well maintained weight records to monitor changes and, when indicated, characterize an individual's response to various medical or nutritional interventions. More accurate assessment of body composition is provided by underwater weighing, dual-energy x-ray absorptiometry (DEXA), estimation of total body water and extracellular water by dilution techniques, total body electrical conductivity (TOBEC), and whole-body counting of potassium, nitrogen, and other elements. Unfortunately, these techniques are impractical outside a research setting.

Bioimpedance Analysis

Bioimpedance analysis is based on the differential resistance to a low-intensity electrical current by the fat and lean compartments of the body. Measured values of resistance and reactance obtained by BIA can be used in regression equations[78] to estimate fat and lean tissue as well as total body water content. Equations have also been developed to calculate the body cell mass and extracellular and intracellular fluid content from BIA measurements, although there is less consensus regarding the ability of BIA

▲ **Table 53–1.** INITIAL EVALUATION OF WEIGHT LOSS

Evaluation	Comments
Weight history: extent and rate of weight loss	Acute weight loss suggests an opportunistic illness
Body composition	
Bioelectric impedance analysis (BIA)	BIA is useful for monitoring change in whole body lean mass and fat mass
Anthropometry	Surrogate for muscle mass but need serial measurements by a trained clinician
Dietary assessment	Careful appetite assessment may direct therapeutic recommendations Assess nutrient requirements, current dietary intake, height, weight, ideal body weight
Review of clinical history	
HIV history: viral load, acute or chronic opportunistic diseases.	
Identify symptoms that interfere with oral intake	Examples include treatment of early satiety with metoclopramide, use of antiemetics for nausea
Psychosocial evaluation	Depression or financial constraints may interfere with nutritional intake
Medication side effects and drug interventions	Change in taste, nausea and vomiting from multiple medications, and potential changes in drug choices should be considered.
Signs and symptoms of gonadal dysfunction: hair loss, sexual dysfunction	If present, check total and free testosterone
Malabsorption/diarrhea	Check stool for ova and parasites, enteric pathogens
Fever	Rule out opportunistic infection; specifically consider CMV and MAC.

CMV, cytomegalovirus; MAC, *mycobacterium avium* complex.

to estimate these compartments reliably. The BIA equipment is relatively inexpensive and portable; a measurement takes only approximately 10 minutes and involves no pain or discomfort for the patient. Accurate estimates of body composition using this technique are highly dependent on accurate measurement of weight and height, as well as correct and consistent positioning of electrodes. Currently, there are no population standards for fat or lean tissue measured by BIA, but this technique can be useful for monitoring change over time in individuals. The accuracy of BIA for measuring total fat and lean body mass in patients with abnormal fat distribution has not been established.

Anthropometry

Sequential measurements of midarm circumference using a tape measure and triceps skinfolds using calipers can be used as surrogate indicators of the change in arm muscle mass. Although anthropometric measurements can also be used to estimate whole-body composition, the regression equations used for such calculations were developed from studies in healthy people and may not be relevant to those with HIV-associated wasting or syndromes of abnormal fat distribution. To optimize the usefulness of anthropometric measures, duplicate measurements should be obtained by a trained clinician and serial measurements by the same individual whenever possible.

Dietary History and Clinical Assessment

A comprehensive dietary assessment includes estimation of current energy intake, weight history, current disease state, tests of malabsorption when appropriate, and identification of factors that might interfere with food intake. Quantitative estimation of daily intake of energy, along with macro- and micronutrients, should be obtained by a trained dietitian using techniques such as diet history, 24-hour recall, or prospective food intake diaries.

A direct effect of HIV as a cause of weight loss secondary to metabolic disturbances or cytokine dysregulation has been postulated. The observed weight gain of 2 to 4 kg after treatment with antiretroviral agents lends support to this contention.[79,80] However, plasma HIV-1 viral load has not been correlated with nutritional status in asymptomatic HIV-seropositive individuals[81,82] and variation of body weight after initiation of HAART does not correlate with changes in plasma viral load.[82] Furthermore, although few data are available, the composition of the weight gain after the initiation of protease inhibitor-based antiretroviral therapy appears variable.[83–85]

Although the etiologies of both classic wasting and the more recently noted abnormalities of fat distribution have not yet been fully described, there are undoubtedly many aspects that are different. Thus it is critical to be able to distinguish between these syndromes so the appropriate management strategies can be identified. For example, classic wasting may be more likely to occur in the context of virologic or immunologic failure, a secondary infection, or in the presence of clinically significant diarrhea. One cross-sectional study suggested that in patients with classic wasting fat is reduced in both central and peripheral regions, but fat distribution is no different from that in patients without wasting who are on comparable antiretroviral regimens.[86] In contrast, in patients with evidence of fat loss in the appendices, buttocks, or face but not in the central region, malnutrition per se is unlikely to be the primary factor.

Bioavailable testosterone may decrease early in the course of HIV-related involuntary weight loss.[53] Although testosterone and free testosterone levels have been highly correlated in HIV-seropositive individuals with weight loss, free testosterone levels are reduced almost twice as frequently as total testosterone concentration.[48] As total testosterone is protein-bound, measurement of total testosterone concentration in the face of weight loss and protein depletion may not accurately reflect the level of functionally available testosterone.[87] Without symptoms to suggest thyroid disease or adrenal dysfunction, routine evaluation of cortisol levels and thyroid function are not warranted.

A thorough history and physical examination with special attention to symptoms and treatment regimens that interfere with oral intake may identify readily reversible, easily treated problems. Many of the medications frequently prescribed to HIV-infected individuals are associated with gastrointestinal side effects. Simple interventions such as decreasing the rate of a foscarnet infusion or premedication with antiemetics may alleviate drug-associated side effects (nausea, vomiting) and improve oral intake.

Oral manifestations of HIV infection may interfere with oral intake. Early satiety from ascites, hepatomegaly, or massive splenomegaly due to organ infiltration by opportunistic organisms such as cytomegalovirus (CMV) or *mycobacterium avium* complex (MAC) may further compromise intake, as may progressive malignancy. Anorexia associated with early satiety may benefit from a trial of metoclopramide.

Gastrointestinal dysfunction and malabsorption are highly prevalent in those with advanced HIV disease. The optimal diagnostic strategy for the patient with HIV-associated diarrhea and weight loss is unclear. Most enteric pathogens in patients with AIDS-related diarrhea are identified by stool studies, suggesting that the initial diagnostic evaluation should include three stool cultures for ova, parasites, and enteric pathogens. Definitive diagnosis of microsporidia generally requires small bowel biopsy and electron microscopy; and polymerase chain reaction (PCR)-based analyses of stool specimens may improve microsporidia detection.[88] If patients have no associated fever and no specific pathogen is identified, symptomatic treatment with an antimotility agent may be a first step. Somatostatin analogues and enkephalinase inhibitors have proven useful for refractory diarrhea.[89] For patients who do not respond to symptomatic therapy, the diagnostic evaluation should proceed to sigmoidoscopy with biopsy of the colon, primarily to identify CMV infection. The diagnostic yield of esophageal gastroduodenoscopy (EGD) is relatively low.[90,91] For pathogen-negative diarrhea, an alternative treatment consideration is dietary modification, with prescription of a low-fat simple-carbohydrate diet.

Weight loss associated with fever demands a workup for systemic opportunistic infection. Acute severe weight loss accompanied by anorexia is most often associated with systemic opportunistic diseases.[10] Treatment of the secondary infection may lead to maintenance or replenishment of lean body mass as documented with treatment of CMV colitis.[92] A marked reduction in oral intake may precede the specific signs and symptoms of an opportunistic infection by weeks.

▲ TREATMENT

Nutritional Interventions

Decreased energy intake has been identified as a primary contributor to weight loss, so strategies for intervening to forestall or reverse wasting must include means of maintaining or increasing energy intake. Metabolic ward studies have shown that patients with HIV infection are capable of increasing their protein synthesis rates[38] and improving nitrogen balance[93] during feeding. However, nutritional supplementation alone has not fully restored weight or consistently replenished lean tissue in patients with HIV infection; and in weight-stable, HIV-infected adults, caloric supplements do not promote weight gain or an increase in body cell mass.[94]

At present, there are no universally accepted HIV-specific recommendations for intake of energy or macronutrients. Total energy expenditure in weight-stable HIV-infected individuals is comparable to that seen in healthy subjects,[38,41] so the target ranges of energy intakes derived from the Recommended Dietary Allowances for adults (age 23 to 50 years) might be 33 to 44 and 29 to 44 kcal/kg in men and women, respectively.[95] However, individual requirements may vary widely for persons with HIV infection owing to the variable presence of increased rates of REE or reduced activity levels. Although the recommended level of protein intake in healthy adults is 0.8 g/kg, protein requirements in patients with HIV infection have not been defined. A target protein intake of 1.5 g/kg has been frequently recommended for patients with HIV infection. The effects of dietary fat and carbohydrate on insulin resistance and hyperlipidemia during the current treatment era have not yet been studied. In the absence of evidence of specific nutrient deficiencies, patients should be advised only to use a generic, low-cost, daily multivitamin and mineral supplement.

Net daily energy intake can be increased in individuals using oral supplements despite some compensatory decrease in food consumption. Such supplements can be useful in individuals for whom inability or unwillingness to prepare or consume meals becomes an impediment to oral intake. A variety of liquid and solid oral supplements are available, including conventional preparations and specialized formulas for patients with specific intolerances (e.g., fat malabsorption or lactose intolerance). Elemental formulas provide another option for individuals with malabsorptive disorders. Some studies suggest an increased benefit from preparations specifically designed for people with HIV infection.[96–98] Such benefits can be confirmed. The primary criteria for selecting a specific supplement should be cost, palatability, and tolerability.

Repletion or maintenance of weight by the enteral or parenteral route might be considered in individuals who are unable to meet nutritional goals with oral intake because of profound anorexia, nausea, oral or esophageal lesions, diarrhea, or neurologic disorders but in whom there is potential for stabilization or improvement. Studies employing enteral and parenteral feeding in patients with HIV-associated wasting have demonstrated weight increases[99,100]; lean tissue increases occur less consistently.[99,101,102] Notably, two studies have suggested that survival may be increased in patients who received enteral or parenteral nutritional support compared with those receiving standard counseling[103] or who declined to receive supplemental feeding.[100] The choice of specific nonvolitional feeding techniques should be guided by the goal of using the gastrointestinal tract to the greatest extent possible.

Individuals with full or only mildly impaired gut function might be candidates for short-term nasogastric tube feeding; for longer periods, percutaneous endoscopic gastrostomy (PEG) or jejunostomy is recommended. Standard or elemental enteral formulas can be used, so the cost of the nutrition itself is considerably less than for parenteral feeding. PEG is a relatively simple procedure, and routine care and maintenance can be performed by the patient at home. The most common complication is superficial skin infection; other potential complications are aspiration, necrotizing fasciitis, and colocutaneous fistulas.

Provision of central or peripheral parenteral nutrition may nutritionally stabilize and maintain hydration in patients who experience a loss of gastrointestinal function. The costs and risks of this therapeutic maneuver are greater than for enteral approaches, and there is no widespread consensus regarding the appropriate use of this technique in individuals with advanced HIV infection.

Pharmacologic Treatments

Appetite Stimulants

The recognized importance of decreased energy intake as a contributing factor to HIV-associated weight loss has led to the evaluation of a variety of pharmacologic agents to stimulate appetite. Corticosteroids, used anecdotally for the treatment of HIV-related anorexia, have been evaluated as a therapeutic intervention for cancer-associated anorexia and cachexia in multiple placebo-controlled trials.[104,105] In the setting of cancer-related weight loss, corticosteroids result in significant, though short-term (about 4 weeks), stimulation of appetite, but it does not translate into increased body weight. The potential side effects of steroids, including proximal muscle wasting, gastric irritation, fluid retention, and glucose intolerance, suggest that corticosteroids may have a therapeutic role only as a palliative maneuver for end-of-life care.

Cyproheptadine is an antihistaminic, antiserotonergic agent reported to stimulate appetite and weight gain in geriatric patients, adults with essential anorexia, and adolescents with anorexia nervosa. A single small randomized trial of megestrol acetate versus cyproheptadine (12 mg/day) in HIV-seropositive patients with weight loss of 5 kg or more reported weight gain in three of the seven patients treated with cyproheptadine for 3 months.[106] Weight gain was associated with an increase in daily caloric intake and a mean weight increase of 3.1 kg. Body composition data are unavailable from this trial.

Cannabinoids

Dronabinol (Δ^9-tetrahydrocannabinol), the primary psychoactive component of marijuana, produced patient-reported appetite enhancement in a series of small Phase II trials in patients with HIV-related weight loss.[107,108] A randomized placebo-controlled Phase III trial in patients with AIDS-related weight loss enrolled 139 patients, 88 of whom (63%) were evaluable for efficacy.[109] Dronabinol, compared to placebo, produced improved patient-reported appetite ($P = 0.01$), a trend toward weight gain after 6 weeks of therapy (+0.1 kg and −0.4 kg, respectively, $P = 0.21$), improved mood ($P = 0.005$), and decreased occurrence of nausea ($P = 0.05$). Altogether, 43% of the dronabinol-treated patients and 13% of the placebo-treated patients ($P < 0.001$) experienced treatment-related toxicity. This difference was largely due to neurologic toxicity, which occurred in 35% of patients in the dronabinol-treated group and 9% of the placebo-treated patients ($P < 0.001$). Of the dronabinol-treated patients, 18% required dose reductions because of neurologic toxicity characterized primarily by euphoria, dizziness, thinking abnormalities, and somnolence. After completion of the 6-week randomized study, patients were eligible to continue on open-label dronabinol for up to 1 year. Of the 90 patients for whom data are available from the unblinded study extension, patient reported appetite stimulation was maintained for at least 6 months and was associated with an increase in body weight of at least 2 kg in 39% of patients.[110] The lack of objective measures of appetite improvement (e.g., changes in calorie intake) or evidence of weight gain in most of the dronabinol-treated patients suggests limited usefulness for this agent. Significant weight gain was reported in HIV-infected subjects on protease inhibitors who were randomized to receive dronabinol or smoke marijuana in a 3-week inpatient study of the safety of cannabinoids.[111] Wasting was not an eligibility criterion for enrollment in this study.

Megestrol Acetate

Megestrol acetate is an oral synthetic progestational agent used widely for the treatment of hormone responsive malignancies.[112] With conventional doses, 160 mg/day, megestrol acetate results in stimulation of appetite and weight gain in about 30% of advanced breast cancer patients.[112] Phase I/II studies of megestrol acetate at doses up to 1600 mg/day in patients with advanced breast cancer reported a marked increase in appetite and weight gain with treatment.[113] Multiple randomized, double-blind, placebo-controlled trials have demonstrated the benefit of megestrol acetate for cancer cachexia.[114,115] A pilot study of megestrol acetate (320 to 640 mg/day) for the treatment of HIV-related cachexia noted weight gain in 21 of 22 treated patients.[116]

Two double-blind, randomized, placebo-controlled trials of megestrol acetate in patients with AIDS-related weight loss compared the efficacy of megestrol acetate oral suspension, 800 mg versus placebo, for its effect on caloric intake, appetite, body weight, body composition, and overall sense of well-being in patients with AIDS-associated weight loss.[117,118] The first study randomized patients to receive megestrol acetate oral suspension 100, 400, or 800 mg/day versus placebo (four-arm trial), and the second compared megestrol acetate oral suspension, 800 mg, with placebo (two-arm trial).

A total of 270 patients were enrolled, of whom 195 were evaluable for efficacy in the four-arm trial.[118] In the two-arm trial, 100 patients were enrolled and received the study medication, and 65 were evaluable for efficacy.[117] In the latter trial, food intake, patient-reported sense of well-being, and mean weight change were greater with megestrol acetate 800 mg than with placebo. In the four-arm trial, megestrol acetate 800 mg/day resulted in a weight gain of more than 2.27 kg in 64.2% but in only 21.4% of the placebo-treated patients ($P < 0.001$). An intent-to-treat analysis showed significant differences between the placebo group and the megestrol acetate 800 mg group with respect to mean change in lean body mass (−1.7 vs. +2.5 pounds; $P < 0.001$), patient-reported improvement in overall sense of well-being, caloric intake (−107 vs. +645.6 calories/day; $P = 0.001$), and appetite grade ($P < 0.001$). Although most of the patients treated with megestrol acetate (800 mg/day) gained weight, a significant proportion of the observed weight gain (about two-thirds) was fat mass rather than lean tissue. It has been hypothesized that the excess fat accrual in male patients treated with megestrol acetate may be a result of decreased androgen levels, setting the stage for trials of combination therapy with megestrol acetate and testosterone.

The effect of testosterone on the response to megestrol acetate in patients with HIV-associated wasting was evaluated in a randomized double-blind placebo-controlled trial (ACTG 313).[119] A total of 81 HIV-positive patients (79 men, 2 women) with 5% or more weight loss were randomized to receive megestrol acetate (MA) oral suspension 800 mg daily and either testosterone enanthate (T) (200 mg IM every 2 weeks in men, 100 mg IM every 2 weeks in women) or placebo (P) injections for 12 weeks. Altogether, 63 (80%) of the men completed 12 weeks of treatment. Weight gain (5.3 kg in MA+T versus 7.3 kg in MA+P) and accrual of lean body mass (3.3 kg in both groups) did not differ significantly by treatment group. Serum testosterone level and sexual functioning decreased significantly in the placebo-treated group but not in the testosterone-treated patients. The study team concluded that megestrol acetate, with or without testosterone, results in robust weight gain and accrual of lean body mass. Although a conventional testosterone replacement dose preserved sexual function during megestrol acetate treatment, it did not increase the proportion of weight gained as lean body mass.

The most common megestrol acetate-related toxicity is dose-related, reversible impotence. An analysis of serum testosterone levels from patients enrolled in the ACTG trial of megestrol acetate plus or minus testosterone documented a significant decrease in serum testosterone levels in the megestrol acetate plus placebo-treated patients compared to those treated with megestrol acetate plus testosterone (−360 vs. −160 ng/dl, $P = 0.013$).[119] As experience with high-dose megestrol acetate (800 mg/day) for the treatment of AIDS-related weight loss has increased, a variety of adverse endocrinologic side effects have been reported. Megestrol acetate has weak glucocorticoid activity and may suppress the pituitary adrenal axis, resulting in reversible adrenal suppression, diabetes mellitus, and a steroid withdrawal syndrome that requires close monitoring of patients when megestrol acetate is discontinued.[119–122] In the ACTG trial, cortisol levels decreased to nearly undetectable levels in virtually all patients in whom plasma megestrol acetate levels were more than 150 ng/ml.[119] The frequency of endocrinologic toxicity appears related to total drug exposure; higher doses over a more prolonged treatment period leads to greater risk.

Combination therapy with two appetite stimulants, megestrol acetate and dronabinol, offers no advantage over treatment with megestrol acetate alone.[123] In an open-label randomized trial in 52 patients with HIV-associated weight loss, patients were randomized to treatment with (1) dronabinol 2.5 mg twice daily; (2) or megestrol acetate 750 mg daily; (3) megestrol acetate 750 mg daily/dronabinol 2.5 mg twice daily; or (4) megestrol acetate 250 mg daily/dronabinol 2.5 mg twice daily. A significant increase in weight was seen only in the patients receiving megestrol acetate 750 mg daily, whether alone or in combination with dronabinol. The mean weight change observed over the 12-week study period were gains of 6.5 ± 0.1 kg and 6.0 ± 1.0 kg in the treatment groups receiving the high-dose megestrol acetate, whereas the mean weight changes were a losses of 2.0 ± 1.0 kg and 0.3 ± 1.0 kg for the dronabinol alone and the low-dose combination therapy, respectively. Megestrol acetate is clearly the most potent of the available appetite stimulants. Unfortunately, replacement or supplementation of calories alone appears inadequate to restore lean body mass for most patients with AIDS-related wasting.

Protein Anabolic Agents

Recombinant Human Growth Hormone

Pharmacologic doses of recombinant human growth hormone (rhGH) caused weight gain and retention of nitrogen and potassium during a short-term metabolic ward study[37] and increases in weight and lean body mass (LBM) in a small, 3-month open-label study.[124] In a randomized, double-blind, placebo-controlled trial in 178 patients with HIV-associated wasting, treatment with rhGH (0.1 mg/kg/day sc) for 3 months produced sustained, significant ($P < 0.001$ vs. placebo) increases in weight (1.6 ± 3.7 kg) and LBM (3.0 ± 3.0 kg) that were accompanied by decreases in fat (1.7 ± 1.7 kg).[125] Treadmill work output at volitional exhaustion increased significantly in patients treated with rhGH, and changes in work output and time to exhaustion were significantly and positively correlated with changes in LBM. Side effects (i.e., arthralgias, myalgia, puffiness, diarrhea) were generally mild to moderate in severity and resolved spontaneously or with dose reduction. All patients were required to be maintained on antiretroviral therapy throughout the study, and rhGH did not increase the plasma HIV RNA levels. Short-term (2 weeks) treatment with rhGH the increased the LBM and decreased rates of protein breakdown in a placebo-controlled study in HIV-infected patients with newly diagnosed secondary infections,[126] suggesting that short-term use of this agent might mitigate wasting during periods of rapid weight loss. Overall, the cost of this recombinant agent may limit its accessibility for many patients, and the optimal therapeutic and maintenance dosing regimens have not been identified.

Recombinant Human Insulin-like Growth Factor-I

Infusions of recombinant human IGF-1 (rhIGF-1) produced significant but transient nitrogen retention during a metabolic ward study in patients with HIV-associated wasting.[55] Subcutaneous injections of 10 mg rhIGF-1 daily failed to increase weight or LBM significantly over a 12-week period in a placebo-controlled trial.[127] In two placebo-controlled trials, combinations of pharmacologic doses of rhIGF-1 (total 10 mg/day) with smaller doses of rhGH (total 1.4 or 0.7 mg/day) produced increases in LBM that averaged approximately 3.2 and 1.0 kg, respectively, at the end of a 12-week study period.[128] These results provide little justification for using a combination of two costly recombinant drugs, requiring three or four subcutaneous injections daily, in preference to a single pharmacologic dose of rhGH alone.

Anabolic Steroids

Testosterone

Testosterone replacement by injection (300 mg IM q3wk)[129] increased LBM in one placebo-controlled study in hypogonadal HIV-infected men with wasting.[129] However, their weight did not increase significantly in this study or in another placebo-controlled study using a comparable dose of testosterone (200 mg IM q2wk).[130] Testosterone administered by transdermal patch (5 to 6 mg/day) has had variable effects on LBM in placebo-controlled studies in hypogonadal men with wasting. In one study that used nongenital patches designed to deliver 5 mg/day,[131] LBM increased significantly. However, use of a transscrotal patch designed to deliver 6 mg/day failed to increase LBM or weight, despite normalizing the serum testosterone levels.[132] Two placebo-controlled studies of testosterone with and without resistance exercise have also been performed in HIV-infected men with wasting. In one, men with a 5% weight loss and low serum testosterone levels experienced significant increases in LBM, muscle mass, and muscle strength with either a replacement dose of testosterone (100 mg/week IM) or resistance exercise, but the effects were not additive.[133] The other, eugonadal men with a 10% weight loss who were randomized to receive either a supraphysiologic dose of testosterone (200 mg/week IM) or resistance training experienced significant increases in muscle mass and strength, but there was no interaction between the two interventions regarding their effects on muscle mass.[134] High density lipoprotein (HDL) cholesterol decreased with testosterone but increased with exercise.

Taken together, these studies suggest that physiologic testosterone replacement can be used to increase LBM, muscle mass, and function in hypogonadal men with wasting; and a pharmacologic dose can similarly improve lean tissue in eugonadal men with wasting. The effects of testosterone on weight and quality of life are more variable, and the safety profile of pharmacologic doses warrants attention. Testosterone enanthate or cypionate is administered by intramuscular injection. Transdermal preparations (by patch or gel) are also available.

Nandrolone Decanoate

Nandrolone decanoate, an injectable testosterone derivative with a relatively long half-life, has been shown to increase LBM in two open-label studies in men with HIV-associated weight loss in doses ranging from 100 to 200 mg/week.[135] In an open-label study in eugonadal men with no history of weight loss, use of a higher dose of nandrolone (600 mg/week) produced increases in LBM comparable in magnitude to those achieved with lower doses.[136] In the latter study, concurrent resistance exercise produced significantly greater increases in LBM than nandrolone alone. Nandrolone decanoate is currently approved only for anemia associated with chronic renal failure.

Oxandrolone

Oxandrolone, an oral agent, is approved by the U.S. Food and Drug Administration (FDA) as a treatment for weight loss incurred in conjunction with surgery, chronic infection, trauma, or prolonged use of corticosteroids, but there is no HIV-specific indication. At the approved dosing level (5 to 20 mg/day), there appears to be less potential for virilizing effects and hepatic toxicity than has been seen with other oral agents. In a placebo-controlled study in 63 HIV-infected men with more than 10% weight loss, patients randomized to receive oxandrolone in a dose of 15 mg/day gained an average of 0.6 kg at the end of the 16-week study period, whereas those who received placebo lost 1.1 kg.[137] These changes were not statistically significant, and the composition of the weight changes was not measured. The concurrent use of oxandrolone (20 mg/day) in men on testosterone (100 mg/week) who were undergoing progressive resistance exercise produced significant increases in LBM when compared to results in men on exercise and testosterone alone.[138] However, HDL cholesterol decreased significantly in those randomized to receive oxandrolone.

Oxymetholone

In an open-label study, treatment with oxymetholone (50 mg PO three times daily) produced weight gain (mean 5.7 kg) and improvements in the Karnofsky score in patients with HIV-associated weight loss.[139] This agent is currently approved as a treatment for anemia.

Anabolic/androgenic steroids have been used in women with HIV-associated wasting. In view of evidence of decreased testosterone levels in HIV-infected women with wasting,[140] a placebo-controlled trial of testosterone therapy was performed using a specially prepared patch designed to deliver physiologic or supraphysiologic daily doses of testosterone (150 and 300 μg/day, respectively).[141] Weight, but not LBM, increased with the lower dose of testosterone, whereas the higher dose was not associated with improvements in body composition or quality of life. In a randomized, double-blind, placebo-controlled study of nandrolone decanoate in women with HIV-associated weight loss (ACTG 329), those randomized to nandrolone (100 mg every other week) experienced highly significant increases in weight and LBM with no change in fat mass.[142] Virilizing effects, predominantly hoarseness and hirsutism, were reported in some women randomized to nandrolone, although these changes had no apparent effect on the study completion rate.

Cytokine Modulation

Thalidomide

Thalidomide, which suppresses TNFα production in vitro,[143] has been evaluated for its effects on wasting in three placebo-controlled studies. In one, treatment with thalidomide at a dose of 300 mg/day was associated with a 4% increase in weight in patients with HIV infection and, in those co-infected with tuberculosis, a weight increase of 8%.[144] There was a high incidence of side effects at this dosing level, however. In another study, patients with HIV-associated wasting who were treated with thalidomide (100 mg four times daily for 12 weeks) experienced a median weight gain of 4.05 kg ($P = 0.0001$ vs. placebo).[145] Muscle mass, estimated by anthropometry, increased by 1.01 kg ($P = 0.001$). More recently, in an 8-week, randomized, double-blind, multicenter trial, patients randomized to thalidomide at a dose of 100 mg/day experienced significant weight gain (3.0%, approximately half of which was LBM).[146] In this trial, a dose of 200 mg/day did not produce greater weight gain and was associated with more side effects. Levels of HIV RNA increased modestly but significantly in both thalidomide groups but not in those who received placebo. The mechanism and clinical significance of this increase is not understood. Thalidomide has also produced a dramatic reversal of HIV-associated oral aphthous ulcers[147] and reduced stool frequency in patients with chronic diarrhea.[148] In each case, weight increases accompanied symptom alleviation.

Thalidomide is approved by the FDA for the treatment of cutaneous manifestations of erythema nodosum leprosum. The recommended initial dose is 100 mg to be taken daily at bedtime. Because of the potential for teratogenic effects, women of childbearing potential must be advised to use at least two methods of contraception while taking thalidomide, and all patients must be specifically advised not to share their drug with any other person. The most prevalent side effects of thalidomide in patients with HIV-associated wasting have been somnolence, potentially irreversible peripheral neuropathy, hypersensitivity, and neutropenia.

Other Cytokine Suppressors

A variety of other weak cytokine suppressors, including pentoxifylline,[149,150] n-3 fatty acids (fish oil),[151] and ketoifen,[139,152] have been studied with modest results. Use of these agents for anabolic therapy is not supported by current data. Table 53–2 summarizes the results of the major

Table 53–2. PHARMACOLOGIC AGENTS FOR AIDS-RELATED WASTING: DATA FROM PHASE III TRIALS

Intervention and Study	No.	Study Duration (weeks)	Weight (mean change)	Lean Body Mass (mean change)	Appetite	Major Adverse Events
Megestrol acetate (800 mg qd)						
Von Roenn et al.[118]	195	12	+3.5 kg	+1.1 kg[a]	↑	Hypogonadism and other endocrine abnormalities
Oster et al.[117]	65	12	+4.2 kg	No change	↑	
Summerbell et al. (160 mg/d)[106 b]	14	12	+3.6 kg	N/a	↑	
Timpone et al.[123] (750 mg/d)[b] (± dronabinol)[c]	52	12	+6.5 kg	N/a	↑	
Schambelan et al.[119] (± testosterone)	81	12	+6.3 kg	+3.3 kg[a]	N/a	Hypocortisolemia; decreased testosterone and sexual functioning in the absence of testosterone replacement
Dronabinol (2.5 mg bid)						
Beal et al.[110]	89	6	No change	N/a	↑	Euphoria, dizziness, thinking abnormalities[d]
Timpone et al.[123b]	52	12	−2.0 kg	N/a		
Cyproheptadine (12 mg/d)[106]						
Summerbell et al.[b]	14	12	+3.1 kg	N/a	↑	None
rhGH (0.1 mg/kg/d sc)[125]	178	12	+1.6 kg	+3.0 kg[e]	—[f]	Arthralgias, myalgias, puffiness, diarrhea
Oxandrolone (15 mg/d)[137]	63	16	+0.6 kg	N/a	↑	Well tolerated
Thalidomide						
Reyes-Teran et al.[145] (100 mg qid)	28	12	+4.1 kg[g]	+1.0 kg[h]	N/a	Somnolence, peripheral neuropathy, neutropenia, hypersensitivity[i]
Kalpan[146] (100 vs. 200 mg/d)	99	8	+2.0 kg (100 mg) +0.9 kg (200 mg)	+1.2 kg[a] +0.6 kg	—[f] —[f]	
Testosterone in hypogonadal men						
Transdermal						
Dobs[132] (6 mg/d)	133	12	+0.8 kg[j]	0.3 kg[j,k]	N/a	Well tolerated
Bhasin[131] (5 mg/d)	41	12	+0.6 kg	1.3 kg[e,j]	N/a	Some irritation with nonscrotal patch
Injections						
Grinspoon[129] (300 mg q3wk)	51	26	No change	+1.9 kg[e]	N/a	Well tolerated
Bhasin[133] (100 mg weekly) (± exercise)	61	16	+2.6 kg	+2.9 kg[e,l]	—[f]	
Coodley[130] (200 mg q2wk)	39	12	No change	N/a	N/a	
Testosterone in eugonadal men						
Grinspoon[134] (200 mg/wk IM) (± exercise)	54	12	+2.6 kg	+4.4 kg[e,l]	—[f]	Well tolerated
Testosterone in women (transdermal)						
Miller[141] (150 vs. 300 μg/d)	53	12	+1.9 kg (150 μg/d) No change (300 μg/d)	No change[e] 0.5 kg[e]	—[f]	Virilizing effects in some women
Nandrolone in women (injections)						
Mulligan[142] (100 mg q2wk)	38	12	+4.6 kg[g]	+3.5[a,g]	N/a	Virilizing effects in some women

N/a, not available; rhGH, recombinent human growth hormone. [a]Measured by bioelectrical impedance analysis. [b]No placebo arm in these trials. [c]Results unchanged by addition of dronabinol. [d]Side effects may improve with dose reduction to 2.5 mg/day. [e]Measured by dual energy x-ray absorptiometry training. [f]No increase in energy intake in patients who kept food diaries. [g]Median (mean not reported). [h]Measured by anthropometry. [i]Teratogenic; pregnancy must be avoided in patients using this agent. [j]Change not significant compared with placebo. [k]Reported as body cell mass by BIA; LBM not available. [l]Comparable increases achieved with resistance exercise.

published trials of the pharmacologic agents evaluated for the treatment of AIDS-related wasting.

Exercise

Because inactivity is associated with significant loss of muscle mass and studies of exercise interventions have produced favorable results in other populations with decreased lean tissue and functional capacity,[153] there is increasing interest in physical activity and supervised exercise as a means of maintaining or restoring lean tissue in patients with HIV infection. In early studies in subjects with HIV infection, progressive resistance training was reported to increase upper and lower body strength and weight in individuals recovering from acute Pneumocystis carinii pneumonia,[154] and combinations of aerobic and resistance training were associated with increases in fitness level with no apparent acceleration in the decline of indices of immune function in patients with HIV infection.[155,156] Body composition was not measured in these latter studies. More recently, HIV-seropositive patients with no history of significant weight loss who underwent an 8-week course of progressive resistance training gained weight and LBM.[157] An acute bout of exercise does not increase viral load.[158] As discussed earlier, studies of exercise with and without concurrent use of anabolic steroids have demonstrated significant improvements in muscle mass and function.[130,131,133]

▲ CONCLUSIONS

The multifactorial nature of HIV-associated wasting and our incomplete understanding of its pathogenesis pose difficulties when designing a therapeutic blueprint. Figure 53–1 presents an algorithm for an overall approach to the management of HIV-related wasting. Therapeutic options with doses and toxicities are listed in Table 53–3. Identification and treatment of readily reversible symptoms that interfere with oral intake, opportunistic diseases (e.g., fever, visual disturbances), and changes in medications with gastrointestinal side effects are the initial steps in treating involuntary weight loss. Although treatment of opportunistic diseases may result in replenishment of weight, the weight gain is often incomplete. Recognizing the decrease in energy intake associated with acute opportunistic infections (OIs), an appetite stimulant or anabolic agent (or both) may be considered as an adjuvant to specific OI therapy.

For patients with adequate oral intake, a gastrointestinal evaluation to rule out significant malabsorption (with or

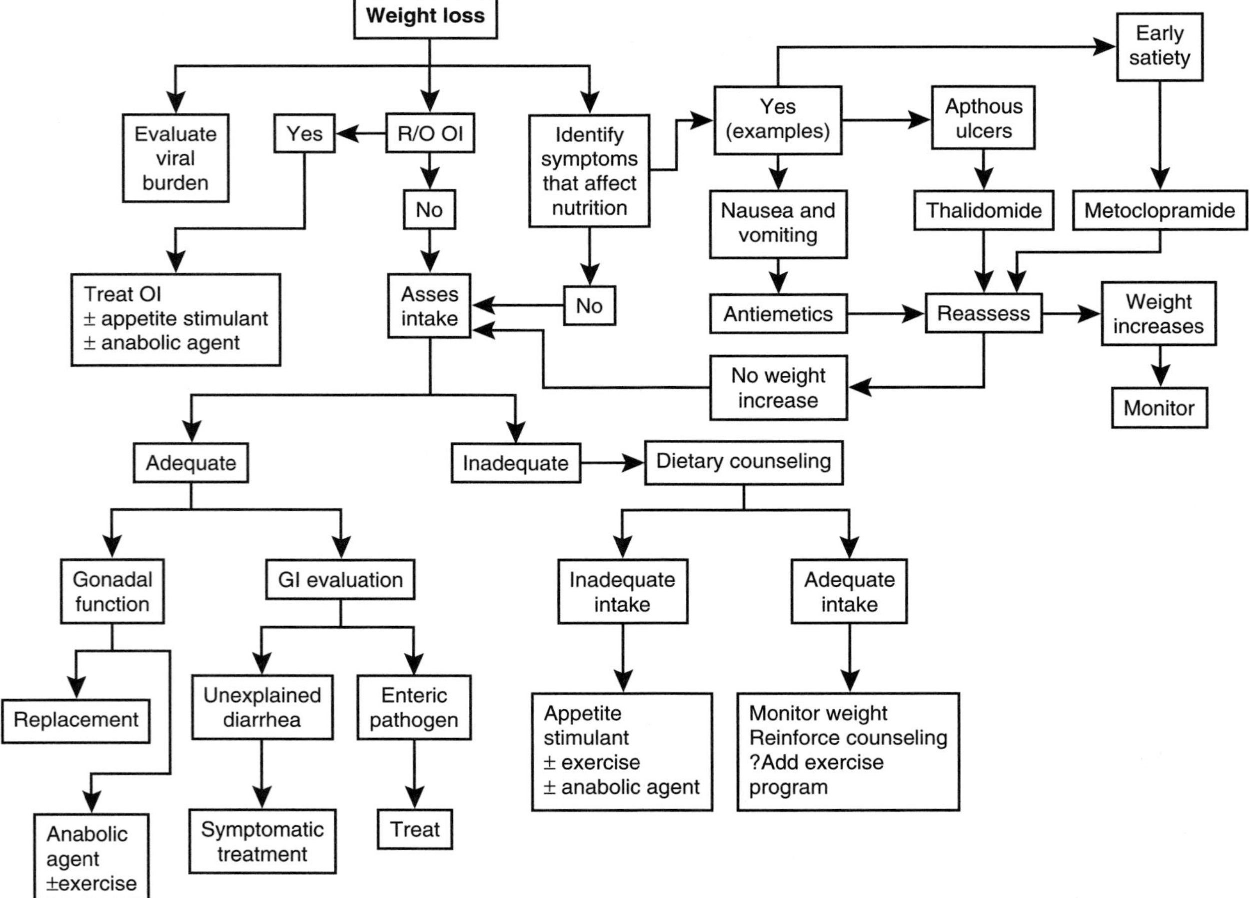

Figure 53–1. Algorithm for evaluation and treatment of HIV-related weight loss.

▲ **Table 53–3.** THERAPEUTIC OPTIONS

Drug	Dose	Major Toxicities
Dronabinol	2.5 mg bid	Neurologic toxicity (euphoria, dizziness, somnolence, decreased concentration)
Megestrol acetate (oral suspension)	400–800 mg/d	Impotence, bloating, endocrinologic side effects
rhGH	0.1 mg/kg/d	Arthralgias, myalgias, puffiness, diarrhea, insulin resistance
Testosterone cypionate or enanthate	200–400/mg IM q2wk[a]	Virilizing effects, hepatic toxicity, mood changes, decreased HDL cholesterol with pharmacologic doses
Nandrolone decanoate	100 mg IM q2wk[a]	Virilizing effects, mood changes
Oxandrolone	20 mg/day[b]	Well tolerated at this dosing level; decreased HDL cholesterol
Thalidomide	100 mg qid[a]	Teratogenic effects, somnolence, potentially irreversible peripheral neuropathy, hypersensitivity, neutropenia

HDL, high density lipoprotein.
[a]This is an unapproved use of this agent.
[b]Higher doses are currently under evaluation.

without the presence of diarrhea) should be undertaken. If oral intake is adequate and the gastrointestinal evaluation is unremarkable, an evaluation of gonadal function may identify an easily treated factor contributing to weight loss. Testosterone replacement should be considered for patients with low-normal levels of testosterone and for frankly hypogonadal men. For the patient with adequate oral intake without gastrointestinal or gonadal dysfunction, the pathogenesis of the weight loss and its therapy are not clearly defined. Anabolic agents, with or without a well planned exercise program, are a reasonable recommendation.

For those with inadequate caloric intake, nutritional counseling may improve energy intake for a substantial number of patients.[93,93a] For the patients who fail to gain weight after dietary counseling, gastrointestinal abnormalities should be considered. If gastrointestinal abnormalities are not present, an appetite stimulant, with or without an anabolic agent and exercise, can be recommended.

Patients with HIV-related weight loss are a heterogeneous group. Numerous factors may contribute to weight loss in an individual patient. Although the algorithm offers a general approach to the treatment of involuntary weight loss, treatment and evaluation of a patient may proceed along multiple pathways. Frequent reassessment and ultimately better definition of pathogenesis-based patient subgroups will determine optimal, individualized treatment of wasting.

REFERENCES

1. Palella FJ, Delaney KM, Moorman AC, et al. Declining morbidity and mortality among patients with advanced human immunodeficiency virus infection: HIV Outpatient Study Investigators. N Engl J Med 338:853, 1998.
2. Weiss PJ, Wallace MR, Olson PE, Rossetti R. Change in the mix of AIDS-defining conditions. N Engl J Med 329:1962, 1993.
3. Moore RD, Chaisson RE. Natural history of HIV infection in the era of combination antiretroviral therapy. AIDS 13:1933, 1999.
4. Centers for Disease Control. HIV/AIDS surveillance report. MMWR 9:18, 1997.
5. Wanke C, Silva M, Knox T, et al. Weight loss and wasting remain common complications in individuals infected with HIV in the era of highly active antiretroviral therapy. Clin Infect Dis 31:803, 2000.
6. Centers for Disease Control. Revision of the CDC surveillance case definition of acquired immunodeficiency syndrome. MMWR Morb Mortal Wkly Rep 36(suppl 1):3S, 1987.
7. Nahlen BL, Chu SY, Nwanyanwu OC, et al. HIV wasting syndrome in the United States. AIDS 7:183, 1993.
8. Melnick SL, Sherer R, Louis TA, et al. Survival and disease progression according to gender of patients with HIV infection. JAMA 272:1915, 1994.
9. Grunfeld C, Pang M, Shimizu L, et al. Resting energy expenditure, caloric intake and short-term weight change in human immunodeficiency virus infection and the acquired immunodeficiency syndrome. Am J Clin Nutr 55:455, 1992.
10. Macallan DC, Noble C, Baldwin C, et al. Prospective analysis of patterns of weight change in stage IV HIV infection. Am J Clin Nutr 58:417, 1993.
11. Kotler DP, Wang J, Pierson RN Jr. Body composition studies in patients with the acquired immunodeficiency syndrome. Am J Clin Nutr 42:1255, 1985.
12. Ott M, Lembcke B, Fischer H, et al. Early changes of body composition in human immunodeficiency virus-infected patients: tetrapolar body impedance analysis indicates significant malnutrition. Am J Clin Nutr 57:15, 1993.
13. Suttmann U, Ockenga J, Selberg O, et al. Incidence and prognostic value of malnutrition and wasting in human immunodeficiency virus-infected patients. J Acquir Immune Defic Syndr 8:239, 1995.
14. Suttmann U, Ockenga J, Hoogestraat L, et al. Resting energy expenditure and weight loss in human immunodeficiency virus-infected patients. Metabolism 42:1173, 1993.
15. Sharkey SJ, Sharkey KA, Sutherland LR, Church DL. Nutritional status and food intake in human immunodeficiency virus infection. J Acquir Immune Defic Syndr 5:1091, 1992.
16. Grady C, Ropka M, Anderson R, Lane H. Body composition in clinically stable men with HIV infection. J Assoc Nurses AIDS Care 7:29, 1996.
17. Schwenk A, Burger B, Wessel D, et al. Clinical risk factors for malnutrition in HIV-1-infected patients. AIDS 7:1213, 1993.
18. Paton N, Macallan D, Jebb S, et al. Longitudinal changes in body composition measured with a variety of methods in patients with AIDS. J Acquir Immune Defic Syndr 14:119, 1997.
19. Sharpstone D, Murray C, Ross H, et al. Energy balance in asymptomatic HIV infection. AIDS 10:1377, 1996.
20. Mulligan K, Tai VW, Schambelan M. Cross-sectional and longitudinal evaluation of body composition in men with HIV infection. J Acquir Immune Defic Syndr 15:43, 1997.
21. Grunfeld C, Feingold KR. Metabolic disturbances and wasting in the acquired immunodeficiency syndrome. N Engl J Med 327:329, 1992.
22. Kotler DP, Tierney AR, Wang J, Pierson RN Jr. Magnitude of body-cell-mass depletion and the timing of death from wasting in AIDS. Am J Clin Nutr 50:444, 1989.
23. Chlebowski RT, Grosvenor MB, Bernhard NH, et al. Nutritional status, gastrointestinal dysfunction, and survival in patients with AIDS. Am J Gastroenterol 84:1288, 1989.
24. Guenter P, Muurahainen N, Kosok A, et al. Relationships among nutritional status, disease progression, and survival in HIV infection. J Acquir Immune Defic Syndr 6:1130, 1993.
25. Palenicek JG, Graham NMH, He YD, et al. Weight loss prior to clinical AIDS as a predictor of survival. J Acquir Immune Defic Syndr 10:366, 1995.

26. Semba R, Caiaffa W, Graham N, et al. Vitamin A deficiency and wasting as predictors of mortality in human immunodeficiency virus-infected injection drug users. J Infect Dis 171:1196, 1995.
27. Ehrenpreis ED, Ganger DR, Kochvar GT, et al. D-Xylose malabsorption: characteristic finding in patients with AIDS wasting syndrome and chronic diarrhea. J Acquir Immune Defic Syndr 5:1047, 1992.
28. Wheeler DA, Gibert C, Muurahainen N, et al. Weight loss as a predictor of survival and disease progression in HIV infection. J Acquir Immune Defic Syndr 18:80, 1998.
29. Ott M, Fischer H, Polat H, et al. Bioelectrical impedance analysis as a predictor of survival in patients with human immunodeficiency virus infection. J Acquir Immune Defic Syndr 9:20, 1995.
30. Schwenk A, Beisenherz A, Romer K, et al. Phase angle from bioelectrical impedance analysis remains an independent predictive marker in HIV-infected patients in the era of highly active antiretroviral treatment. Am J Clin Nutr 72:496, 2000.
31. Fliederbaum J. Clinical aspects of hunger disease in adults. In: Winick M (ed) Hunger Disease: Studies by the Jewish Physicians in the Warsaw Ghetto. New York, Wiley, 1979, p 11.
32. Wilson IB, Cleary PD. Clinical predictors of declines in physical functioning in persons with AIDS: results of a longitudinal study. J Acquir Immune Defic Syndr 16:343, 1997.
33. Grinspoon S, Corcoran C, Rosenthal D, et al. Quantitative assessment of cross-sectional muscle area, functional status and muscle strength in men with the AIDS wasting syndrome. J Clin Endocrinol Metab 84:201, 1999.
34. Melchior J-C, Salmon D, Rigaud D, et al. Resting energy expenditure is increased in stable, malnourished HIV-infected patients. Am J Clin Nutr 53:437, 1991.
35. Melchior J-C, Raguin G, Boulier A, et al. Resting energy expenditure in human immunodeficiency virus-infected patients: comparison between patients with and without secondary infections. Am J Clin Nutr 57:614, 1993.
36. Hommes MJT, Romijn JA, Endert E, Sauerwein HP. Resting energy expenditure and substrate oxidation in human immunodeficiency virus (HIV)-infected asymptomatic men: HIV affects host metabolism in the early asymptomatic stage. Am J Clin Nutr 54:311, 1991.
37. Mulligan K, Grunfeld C, Hellerstein MK, et al. Anabolic effects of recombinant human growth hormone in patients with wasting associated with human immunodeficiency virus infection. J Clin Endocrinol Metab 77:956, 1993.
38. Macallan DC, Noble C, Baldwin C, et al. Energy expenditure and wasting in human immunodeficiency virus infection. N Engl J Med 333:83, 1995.
39. Macallan DC, McNurlan MA, Milne E, et al. Whole-body protein turnover from leucine kinetics and the response to nutrition in human immunodeficiency virus infection. Am J Clin Nutr 61:818, 1995.
40. Sharpstone DR, Ross HM, Gazzard BG. The metabolic response to opportunistic infections in AIDS. AIDS 10:1529, 1996.
41. Sheehan LA, Macallan DC. Determinants of energy intake and energy expenditure in HIV and AIDS. Nutrition 16:101, 2000.
42. Stein TP, Nutinsky C, Condoluci D, et al. Protein and energy substrate metabolism in AIDS patients. Metabolism 39:876, 1990.
43. Hellerstein MK, Grunfeld C, Wu K, et al. Increased de novo hepatic lipogenesis in human immunodeficiency virus infection. J Clin Endocrinol Metab 76:559, 1993.
44. Grunfeld C, Pang M, Doerrler W, et al. Lipids, lipoproteins, triglyceride clearance, and cytokines in human immunodeficiency virus infection and the acquired immunodeficiency syndrome. J Clin Endocrinol Metab 74:1045, 1992.
45. Coodley CO, Loveless MO, Nelson HD, Coodley MK. Endocrine function in the HIV wasting syndrome. J AIDS 7:45, 1994.
46. Dobs AS, Dempsey MA, Landensen PW, Polk BF. Endocrine disorders in men infected with human immunodeficiency virus. Am J Med 84:611, 1988.
47. Wagner G, Rabkin JG, Rabkin R. Illness stage, concurrent medications, and other correlates of low testosterone in men with HIV illness. J Acquir Immune Defic Syndr Hum Retrovirol 8:204, 1995.
48. Grinspoon S, Corcoran C, Lee K, et al. Loss of lean body and muscle mass correlates with androgen levels in hypogonadal men with acquired immunodeficiency syndrome and wasting. J Clin Endocrinol Metab 81:4051, 1996.
49. Lefrere JJ, Laplanche JL, Vitecoq D, et al. Hypogonadism in AIDS. AIDS 2:135, 1988.
50. Croxson RS, Chapman WE, Miller KL, et al. Changes in the hypothalamic-pituitary-gonadal axis in human deficiency virus-infected homosexual men. J Clin Endocrinol Metab 68:317, 1989.
51. Smith CG, Asch RH. Drug abuse and reproduction. Fertil Steril 48:355, 1987.
52. Woolf PD, Hamill RW, McDonald JV, et al. Transient hypogonadotrophic hypogonadism caused by critical illness. J Clin Endocrinol Metab 60:444, 1985.
53. Dobs AS, Few WL III, Blackman MR, et al. Serum hormones in men with human immunodeficiency virus-associated wasting. J Clin Endocrinol Metab 81:4108, 1996.
53a. Sattler F, William B, Antonipillai I, et al. Low dihydrotestosterone and weight loss in the AIDS wasting syndrome. J AIDS Hum Retrovir 18:246, 1998.
54. Salbe AD, Kotler DP, Tierney AR, et al. Correlation between serum insulin-like growth factor (IFG-1) concentrations and nutritional status in HIV seropositive individuals. Nutr Res 14:1437, 1995.
54a. Arver S, Sinha-Hikim I, Beall G, et al. Serum dihydrotestosterone and testosterone concentrations in human immunodeficiency virus-infected men with and without weight loss. J Androl 20:611, 1999.
55. Lieberman SA, Butterfield GE, Harrison D, Hoffman AR. Anabolic effects of recombinant insulin-like growth factor-I in cachectic patients with the acquired immunodeficiency syndrome. J Clin Endocrinol Metab 78:404, 1994.
56. Pernet P, Vittecoq D, Kodjo A, et al. Intestinal absorption and permeability in human immunodeficiency virus-infected patients. Scand J Gastroenterol 34:29, 1999.
57. Lim SG, Menzies IS, Lee CA, et al. Intestinal permeability and function in patients infected with human immunodeficiency virus. Scand J Gastroenterol 28:573, 1993.
58. Ehrenpreis ED, Ganger DR, Kochvar et al. D-Xylose malabsorption: characteristic finding in patients with the AIDS wasting syndrome and chronic diarrhea. J Acquir Immune Defic Syndr 5:1047, 1992.
59. Dworkin B, Wormster GP, Rosenthal WS, et al. Gastrointestinal manifestations of the acquired immunodeficiency syndrome. Am J Gastroenterol 80:774, 1985.
60. May GR, Gill MJ, Church DL, Sutherland LR. Gastrointestinal symptoms in ambulatory HIV-infected patients. Dig Dis Sci 38:1388, 1993.
61. Quinn TC, Piot P, McCormick JB, et al. Serologic and immunologic studies in patients with AIDS in North America and Africa. JAMA 257:2617, 1987.
62. Beaugerie L, Carbonnel F, Carrot F, et al. Factors of weight loss in patients with HIV and chronic diarrhea. J Acquir Immune Defic Syndr 19:34, 1998.
63. Farthing MJG, Kelly PM, Veitch AM. Recently recognized microbial enteropathies and HIV infections. J Antimicrob Chemother 37(suppl):61, 1996.
64. Carbonnel F, Beaugerie L, Rached AA, et al. Macronutrient intake and malabsorption in HIV infection: a comparison with other malabsorptive states. Gut 41:805, 1997.
65. Sharpstone D, Neild P, Crane R, Taylor C. Small intestinal transit, absorption, and permeability in patients with AIDS with and without diarrhoea. Gut 45:70, 1999.
66. Lumadue JA, Manabe YC, Moore RD, et al. A clinicopathologic analysis of AIDS-related cryptosporidiosis. AIDS 12:2459, 1998.
67. Manabe YC, Clark DP, Moore RD, et al. Cryptosporidiosis in patients with AIDS: correlates of disease and survival. Clin Infect Dis 27:536, 1998.
68. Graham NHM, Munoz A, Bacellar H, et al. Clinical factors associated with weight loss related to infection with the human immunodeficiency virus type 1 in the multicenter AIDS cohort study. Am J Epidemiol 137:439, 1993.
69. Fox CH, Kotler D, Tierney A, et al. Detection of HIV-r RNA in the lamina propria of patients with AIDS and gastrointestinal disease. J Infect Dis 159:467, 1989.
70. Kotler DP, Francisco A, Clayton F, et al. Small intestinal injury and parasitic infections in AIDS. Ann Intern Med 113:444, 1990.
71. Hellerstein MK, Meydani SN, Meydani M, et al. Interleukin-1 inducted anorexia in the rat: influence of prostaglandins. J Clin Invest 84:228, 1989.
72. Tracey KJ, Cerami A. The role of cachectin/tumor necrosis factor in AIDS. Cancer Cells 1:62, 1989.

73. Lahdevirta J, Maury CPJ, Teppo AM, Repo H. Elevated levels of circulating cachectin/tumor necrosis factor in patients with acquired immunodeficiency syndrome. Am J Med 85:289, 1988.
74. Feingold KR, Grunfeld C. Role of cytokines in inducing hyperlipidemia. Diabetes 41(suppl 2):97, 1992.
75. Rimaniol AC, Zylberberg H, Zavala F, Viard JP. Inflammatory cytokines and inhibitors in HIV infection: correlation between interleukin-1 receptor antagonist and weight loss. AIDS 10:1349, 1996.
76. Grunfeld C, Feingold KR. Body weight as essential data in the management of patients with human immunodeficiency virus infection and the acquired immunodeficiency syndrome. Am J Clin Nutr 58:317, 1993.
77. Society of Actuaries and Association of Life Insurance Medical Directors of America. 1979 Build Study. New York, Metropolitan Life Insurance, 1989.
78. Kotler DP, Burastero S, Wang J, Pierson RN Jr. Prediction of body cell mass, fat-free mass, and total body water with bioelectrical impedance analysis: effects of race, sex, and disease. Am J Clin Nutr 64(suppl):489S, 1996.
79. Yarchoan R, Weinhold KJ, Lyerly HK, et al. Administration of 3′-azido-3′deoxythymidine, an inhibitor of HTLV/LAV replication, to patients with AIDS or AIDS-related complex. Lancet 2:575, 1986.
80. Force G, Jockey C, Tugler MH, et al. Characteristics of change in body composition with efficiency of antiretroviral treatment in AIDS patients [abstract]. Nutrition 12:290, 1997.
81. Zucman D, Teixeira A, Olivieri MP, et al. Correlation between body composition, caloric intake and plasma viral load in HIV-infected patients [abstract]. Nutrition 13:292, 1997.
82. Teixerra A, Leu JC, Honderlick P, et al. Variation in body weight and plasma viral load in HIV patients related with tritherapy including a protease inhibitor [abstract]. Nutrition 13:269, 1997.
83. Silva M, Skolnik P, Gorbach S, et al. The effect of protease inhibitors on weight and body composition in HIV-infected patients. AIDS 12:1645, 1998.
84. Schwenk A, Kremer G, Cornely O, et al. Body weight changes with protease inhibitor treatment in undernourished HIV-infected patients. Nutrition 15:453, 1999.
85. Pernerstorfer-Schoen H, Schindler K, Parschalk B, et al. Beneficial effects of protease inhibitors on body composition and energy expenditure: a comparison between HIV-infected and AIDS patients. AIDS 13:2389, 1999.
86. Mulligan K, Tai VW, Algren H, et al. Altered fat distribution in HIV-positive men on nucleoside analog reverse transcriptase inhibitors. J Acquir Immune Defic Syndr Retrovirol 26:443, 2001.
87. Martin ME, Benassayag C, Amiel C, et al. Alterations in the concentrations and binding properties of sex steroid binding protein and corticosteroid-binding globulin in HIV^+ patients. J Endocrinol Invest 15:597, 1992.
88. Talal AH, Kotler DP, Orenstein JM, Weiss LM. Detection of Enterocytozoon bieneusi in fecal specimens by polymerase chain reaction analysis with primers to the small-subunit rRNA. Clin Infect Dis 26:673, 1998.
89. Beaugerie L, Baumer P, Chaussade S, et al. Treatment of refractory diarrhoea in AIDS with acetorphan and octreotide: a randomized crossover study. Eur J Gastroenterol Hepatol 8:485, 1996.
90. Johanson JF. To scope or not to scope: the role of endoscopy in the evaluation of AIDS-related diarrhea. Am J Gastroenterol 91:2261, 1996.
91. Brown JW, Savides TJ, Mathews C, et al. Diagnostic yield of duodenal biopsy and aspirate in AIDS-associated diarrhea. Am J Gastroenterol 91:2289, 1996.
92. Kotler DP, Tierney AR, Atilio D, et al. Body mass depletion during ganciclovir therapy of cytomegalovirus infections in patients with the acquired immunodeficiency syndrome. Arch Intern Med 149:901, 1989.
93. Selberg O, Suttmann U, Melzer A, et al. Effect of increased protein intake and nutritional status on whole-body protein metabolism of AIDS patients with weight loss. Metabolism 44:1159, 1995.
93a. Rabeneck L, Palmer A, Knowles JB, et al. A randomized controlled trial evaluating nutrition counseling with or without oral supplementation in malnourished HIV-infected patients. J Am Diet Assoc 98:434, 1999.
94. Gibert CL, Wheeler DA, Collins G, et al. Randomized, controlled trial of caloric supplements in HIV infection. J Acquir Immune Defic Syndr 22:253, 1999.
95. Subcommittee on the Tenth Edition of the RDAs, Food and Nutrition Board, Commission on Life Sciences, National Research Council. Recommended Dietary Allowances, 10th ed. Washington, DC, National Academy Press, 1989.
96. Chlebowski RT, Beall G, Grosvenor M, et al. Long-term effects of early nutritional support with new enterotropic peptide-based formula vs. standard enteral formula in HIV-infected patients: randomized prospective trial. Nutrition 9:507, 1993.
97. Shabert JK, Winslow C, Lacey JM, Wilmore DW. Glutamine-antioxidant supplementation increases body cell mass in AIDS patients with weight loss: a randomized, double-blind controlled trial. Nutrition 15:860, 1999.
98. Suttmann U, Ockenga J, Schneider H, et al. Weight gain and increased concentrations of receptor proteins for tumor necrosis factor after patients with symptomatic HIV infection received fortified nutrition support. J Am Diet Assoc 96:565, 1996.
99. Kotler DP, Tierney AR, Ferraro R, et al. Enteral alimentation and repletion of body cell mass in malnourished patients with acquired immunodeficiency syndrome. Am J Clin Nutr 53:149, 1991.
100. Ockenga J, Sutman U, Selberg O, et al. Percutaneous endoscopic gastrostomy in AIDS and control patients: risks and outcome. Am J Gastroenterol 91:1817, 1996.
101. Kotler DP, Tierney AR, Culpepper-Morgan JA, et al. Effect of home total parenteral nutrition on body composition in patients with acquired immunodeficiency syndrome. J Parenter Ent Nutr 14:454, 1990.
102. Melchior J, Chastang C, Gelas P, et al. Efficacy of 2-month total parenteral nutrition in AIDS patients: a controlled randomized prospective trial. AIDS 10:379, 1996.
103. Melchior J, Gelas P, Carbonnel F, et al. Improved survival by home total parenteral nutrition in AIDS patients: follow up of a controlled randomized prospective trial [abstract]. Nutrition 13:272, 1997.
104. Wilcox J, Corr J, Shaw J. Prednisone as an appetite stimulant in patients with cancer. BMJ 200:37, 1984.
105. Robustelli D, Cuna G, Pellegrini A, et al. Effect of methylprednisolone in terminal cancer patients: a placebo-controlled, multi-center study. Eur J Cancer Clin Oncol 25:1817, 1989.
106. Summerbell CD, Youle M, McDonald V, et al. Megestrol acetate versus cyproheptadine in the treatment of weight loss associated with HIV infection. Int J STD AIDS 3:278, 1992.
107. Gorter R, Seefried M, Volberding P. Dronabinol effects on weight in patients with HIV infection. AIDS 6:127, 1992.
108. Struwe M, Kaempfer SH, Geiger CJ, et al. The effect of dronabinol on nutritional status in HIV infection. Ann Pharmacother 27:827, 1993.
109. Beal JE, Olson R, Laubenstein L, et al. Dronabinol as a treatment for anorexia associated with weight loss in patients with AIDS. J Pain Symptom Manage 10:89, 1995.
110. Beal J, Olson R, Lefkowitz L, et al. Long term efficacy and safety of dronabinol for acquired immunodeficiency syndrome-associated anorexia. J Pain Symptom Manage 14:7, 1997.
111. Abrams DI, Leiser RJ, Shade SB, et al. Short-term effects of cannabinoids on HIV-1 viral load. Presented at the 13th International AIDS Conference, Durban, 2000, abstract LbPeB7053.
112. Gregory EJ, Cohen SC, Oives DW. Megestrol acetate therapy for advanced breast cancer. J Clin Oncol 3:155, 1985.
113. Tchekmedyian NS, Tait N, Moody M, Aisner J. High dose megestrol acetate: a possible treatment for cachexia. JAMA 9:1195, 1987.
114. Bruera E, MacMillan K, Kuehn N, et al. A controlled trial of megestrol acetate on appetite, caloric intake, nutritional status and other symptoms in patients with advanced cancer. Cancer 66:1279, 1990.
115. Loprinzi CL, Ellison NM, Schaid DJ, et al. Controlled trial of megestrol acetate for the treatment of cancer anorexia and cachexia. J Natl Cancer Inst 82:1127, 1990.
116. Von Roenn JH, Murphy RL Weber KM, et al. Megestrol acetate for the treatment of cachexia associated with human immunodeficiency virus (HIV) infection. Ann Intern Med 109:840, 1988.
117. Oster MH, Enders SR, Samuels SJ, et al. Megestrol acetate in patients with AIDS-related cachexia. Ann Intern Med 121:393, 1994.
118. Von Roenn JH, Armstrong D, Kotler DP, et al. Megestrol acetate in patients with AIDS-related cachexia. Ann Intern Med 121:393, 1994.
119. Schambelan M, Zackin R, Mulligan K, et al. Effect of testosterone (T) on the response to megestrol acetate (MA) in patients with HIV-associated wasting: a randomized, double-blind placebo-controlled trial (ACTG 313) [abstract]. Presented at the 8th Conference on Retroviral Opportunistic Infections, 2001.

120. Loprinzi CL, Jensen MD, Jiang NS, Schaid DJ. Effect of megestrol acetate on the human pituitary-adrenal axis. Mayo Clin Proc 67:1160, 1992.
121. Henry K, Rathigaber S, Sullivan C, McCabe K. Diabetes mellitus induced by megestrol acetate in a patient with AIDS and cachexia. Ann Intern Med 116:53, 1992.
122. Leinung MC, Liporoce R, Miller CH. Induction of adrenal suppression by megestrol acetate in patients with AIDS. Ann Intern Med 122:843, 1995.
123. Timpone JG, Wright D, Li N, et al. The safety and pharmacokinetics of single agent and combination therapy with megestrol acetate and dronabinol for the treatment of HIV-wasting syndrome. AIDS Res Hum Retroviruses 13:305, 1997.
124. Krentz AJ, Koster FT, Crist DM, et al. Anthropometric, metabolic, and immunological effects of recombinant human growth hormone in AIDS and AIDS-related complex. J Acquir Immune Defic Syndr 6:245, 1993.
125. Schambelan M, Mulligan K, Grunfeld C, et al. Recombinant human growth hormone in patients with HIV-associated wasting: a randomized, placebo-controlled trial. Ann Intern Med 125:873, 1996.
126. Paton N, Newton P, Sharpstone D, et al. Short-term growth hormone administration at the time of opportunistic infections in HIV-positive people. AIDS 13:1995, 1999.
127. Waters D, Danska J, Hardy K, et al. Recombinant human growth hormone, insulin-like growth factor I, and combination therapy in AIDS-associated wasting: a randomized, double-blind, placebo-controlled trial. Ann Intern Med 125:865, 1996.
128. Lee PDK, Pivarnik JM, Bukar JG, et al. A randomized, placebo-controlled trial of combined insulin-like growth factor I and low dose growth hormone therapy for wasting associated with human immunodeficiency virus infection. J Clin Endocrinol Metab 81:2968, 1996.
129. Grinspoon S, Corcoran C, Askari H, et al. Effects of androgen administration in men with AIDS wasting: a randomized, placebo-controlled trial. Ann Intern Med 129:18, 1998.
130. Coodley GO, Coodley MK. A trial of testosterone therapy for HIV-associated weight loss. AIDS 11:1347, 1997.
131. Bhasin S, Storer T, Asbel-Sethi N, et al. Effects of testosterone replacement with a nongenital, transdermal system, Androderm, in human immunodeficiency virus-infected men with low testosterone levels. J Clin Endocrinol Metab 83:3155, 1998.
132. Dobs AS, Cofrancesco J, Nolten WE, et al. The use of a transscrotal testosterone delivery system in the treatment of patients with weight loss related to human immunodeficiency virus infection. Am J Med 107:126, 1999.
133. Bhasin S, Storer T, Javanbakht M, et al. Testosterone replacement and resistance exercise in HIV-infected men with weight loss and low testosterone levels. JAMA 283:763, 2000.
134. Grinspoon S, Corcoran C, Parlman K, et al. Effects of testosterone and progressive resistance training in eugonadal men with AIDS wasting. Ann Intern Med 133:34, 2000.
135. Strawford A, Barbieri T, Neese R, et al. Effects of nandrolone decanoate therapy in borderline hypogonadal men with HIV-associated weight loss. J Acquir Immune Defic Syndr Hum Retrovirol 20:137, 1999.
136. Sattler FR, Jaque SV, Schroeder ET, et al. Effects of pharmacological doses of nandrolone decanoate and progressive resistance training in immunodeficient patients infected with human immunodeficiency virus. J Clin Endocrinol Metab 84:1268, 1999.
137. Berger J, Pall L, Hall C, et al. Oxandrolone in AIDS-wasting myopathy. AIDS 10:1657, 1996.
138. Strawford A, Barbieri T, Van Loan M, et al. Resistance exercise and supraphysiologic androgen therapy in eugonadal men with HIV-related weight loss. JAMA 281:1282, 1999.
139. Hengge UR, Baumann M, Maleba R, et al. Oxymetholone promotes weight gain in patients with advanced human immunodeficiency virus (HIV-1) infection. Br J Nutr 75:129, 1996.
140. Grinspoon S, Corcoran C, Miller K, et al. Body composition and endocrine function in women with acquired immunodeficiency syndrome wasting. J Clin Endocrinol Metab 82:1332, 1997.
141. Miller K, Corcoran C, Armstrong C, et al. Transdermal testosterone administration in women with acquired immunodeficiency syndrome wasting: a pilot study. J Clin Endocrinol Metab 83:2717, 1998.
142. Mulligan K, Zackin R, Clark RA, et al. Nandrolone decanoate increases weight and lean body mass in HIV-infected women with weight loss: a randomized, double-blind, placebo-controlled, multicenter trial. Presented at the 8th Conference on Retroviruses and Opportunistic Infections, Chicago, 2001.
143. Sampaio EP, Euzenir EN, Galilly R, et al. Thalidomide selectivity inhibits tumor necrosis factor α production by stimulated human monocytes. J Exp Med 173:699, 1991.
144. Klausner JD, Makonkawkeyoon S, Akarasewi P, et al. The effect of thalidomide on the pathogenesis of human immunodeficiency virus type 1 and M. tuberculosis infection. J Acquir Immune Defic Syndr 11:247, 1996.
145. Reyes-Teran G, Sierra-Madero JG, del Cerro VM, et al. Effects of thalidomide on HIV-associated wasting syndrome: a randomized, double-blind, placebo-controlled clinical trial. AIDS 10:1501, 1996.
146. Kaplan G, Thomas S, Fierer DS, et al. Thalidomide for the treatment of AIDS-associated wasting. AIDS Res Hum Retroviruses 16:1345, 2000.
147. Jacobson J, Greenspan J, Spritzler J et al. Thalidomide for the treatment of oral aphthous ulcers in patients with human immunodeficiency virus infection. N Engl J Med 336:1487, 1997.
148. Quinones F, Sierra-Madero J, Calva-Mercado JJ, Ruiz-Palacios, GM. Thalidomide in patients with HIV infection and chronic diarrhea: double blind placebo controlled trial [abstract]. Presented at the 4th Conference on Retroviral Opportunistic Infections, 1997.
149. Dezube BJ, Pardee AB, Chapman B, et al. Pentoxifylline decreases tumor necrosis factor expression and serum triglycerides in people with AIDS: NIAID AIDS clinical trials group. J Acquir Immune Defic Syndr 6:787, 1993.
150. Landman D, Sarai A, Sathe SS. Use of pentoxifylline therapy for patients with AIDS-related wasting: pilot study. Clin Infect Dis 18:97, 1994.
151. Hellerstein MK, Wu K, McGrath M, et al. Effects of dietary n-3 fatty acid supplementation in men with weight loss associated with the acquired immune deficiency syndrome: relation to indices of cytokine production. J Acquir Immune Defic Syndr Hum Retrovirol 11:258, 1996.
152. Ockenga J, Rohde F, Suttmann U, et al. Ketotifen in HIV-infected patients: effects on body weight and release of TNF-α. Eur J Clin Pharmacol 50:167, 1996.
153. Fiatarone M, O'Neill E, Ryan N, et al. Exercise training and nutritional supplementation for physical frailty in very elderly people. N Engl J Med 330:1769, 1994.
154. Spence DW, Galantino MLA, Mossberg KA, Zimmerman SO. Progressive resistance exercise: effect on muscle function and anthropometry of a select AIDS population. Arch Phys Med Rehabil 71:644, 1990.
155. Rigsby LW, Dishman RK, Jackson AW, et al. Effects of exercise training on men seropositive for the human immunodeficiency virus-1. Med Sci Sports Exerc 24:6, 1992.
156. Macarthur RD, Levine SD, Birk TJ. Supervised exercise training improves cardiopulmonary fitness in HIV-infected persons. Med Sci Sports Exerc 25:684, 1993.
157. Roubenoff R, McDermott A, Weiss L, et al. Short-term progressive resistance training increases strength and lean body mass in adults infected with human immunodeficiency virus. AIDS 13:231, 1999.
158. Roubenoff R, Skolnik PR, Shevitz A, et al. Effect of a single bout of acute exercise on plasma human immunodeficiency virus RNA levels. J Appl Physiol 86:1997, 1999.

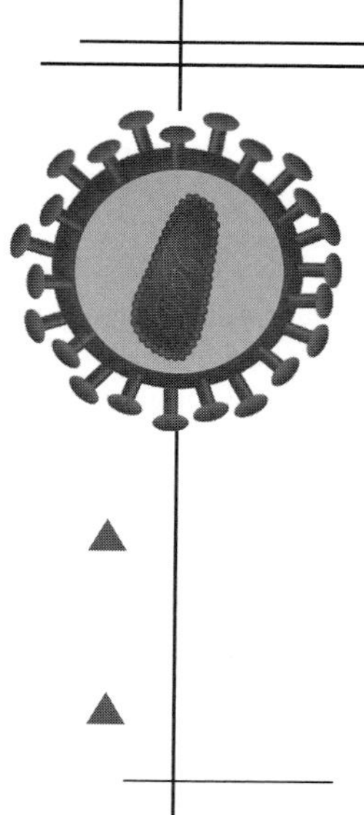

CHAPTER 54
Neurologic Disease

Richard W. Price, MD

Human immunodeficiency virus-1 (HIV-1) infection, particularly its late stage of severe immunodeficiency (AIDS), renders the nervous system susceptible to an array of neurologic disorders. In the aggregate, these disorders can afflict virtually every component of the nervous system, manifest in a variety of clinical syndromes, and contribute importantly to morbidity and mortality. This chapter provides a general view of the diagnostic approach to these disorders. Because several of the specific neurologic diseases are discussed in detail in other chapters of this volume, individual disorders are considered here chiefly in relation to issues of differential diagnosis, with greater detail confined to some of the disorders not considered elsewhere. Several recent and older reviews also discuss the individual neurologic complications in more detail and provide useful, more extensive reference sections.[1–7] Likewise, discussion of specific therapies is largely avoided to reduce redundancy.

The frequency of neurologic complications of HIV-1 infection has changed considerably since the mid-1990s, at least in the developed world, where there has been a marked reduction related to the widespread use of highly active antiretroviral therapy (HAART) and other measures.[8–15] Despite this overall decrease in incidence, the spectrum of disorders afflicting those who progress to severe immunosuppression is largely the same as was recorded earlier in the epidemic, with some exceptions. This chapter maintains its principal focus on these "late-stage" HIV-1-infected patients who continue with these susceptibilities. However, it should be kept in mind that as clinics follow increasing numbers of HIV-1-infected patients who do not progress to this stage of susceptibility the frequency of encountering more "ordinary" neurologic diseases similar to those affecting patients' HIV-1 uninfected peers will rise. For these patients, the approach to the neurologic diagnosis follows that of the general neurology text, rather than the algorithms presented here, which most often assume this late-stage susceptibility. Additionally, these algorithms should be followed with the usual caution that the diagnosis must also be carefully individualized, not only with respect to variability of presenting symptoms and signs but also recognizing that such simple formulas can hardly be comprehensive or able to deal with the "oddball" patient who presents with an unusual manifestation of a common disease or a truly rare condition. Also, these algorithms necessarily present diagnostic pathways as if they are linear when, in fact, parallel processing of several avenues is commonplace, indeed the rule.

GENERAL APPROACH TO DIAGNOSIS

Despite the variety of neurologic diseases in those with HIV-1 infection, a diagnostic approach based on three principal variables—neuroanatomic localization of the lesion(s), temporal course of the onset and evolution, and the constellation of background risks—affords a firm starting point and logical evaluation sequence that usually leads to a timely, precise diagnosis. The first of these variables, neuroanatomic localization, also provides the organizing principal of this chapter, with individual conditions considered within anatomic categories. This follows the time-tested, empiric approach of the neurologist to most diseases of the nervous system. The value of this approach rests on two central considerations. First, disease processes, including opportunistic infections, have a predilection to damage particular structures within the nervous system—

the principle of selective vulnerabilities—in predictable patterns and thus cause anatomically defined syndromes. Second, anatomic localization guides further diagnostic evaluation, most importantly neuroimaging in the case of the central nervous system (CNS) and electrophysiologic testing for diseases of the peripheral nervous system (PNS).

Figure 54–1 outlines the first steps in this anatomic approach. The clinical history usually provides a first approximation of the *neuoranatomic localization* (e.g., language difficulty related to dysfunction of the dominant cerebral hemisphere or numbness of both feet suggesting polyneuropathy) and the formulation of an initial neuroanatomic hypothesis. This is then tested by the neurologic examination. The combination of these two bedside components usually allows not only tentative localization but also initial consideration of the most likely diagnoses. These evaluations usually distinguish between CNS and PNS disease (and diseases of muscle, which in Figures 54–1 through 54–4 are grouped with those of the PNS). CNS disease can be further subdivided into those affecting the brain or the spinal cord.

The second diagnostic element—the *time course* of the evolution of symptoms and signs—though not included in any of the algorithms outlined here, is also often critical to the diagnosis and management. The utility of this variable also has a pathobiologic basis, as individual disease processes evolve over characteristic time frames. Hence the temporal profile narrows the possibilities. It also importantly guides the pace of diagnostic evaluation and therapeutic intervention. For example, 5 months of gradually worsening gait in a patient who walks comfortably but stiffly (as seen with the vacuolar myelopathy variant of the AIDS dementia complex) may warrant either no or only elective spinal magnetic resonance imaging (MRI). By contrast, 3 days of back pain and 4 hours of leg weakness, as might accompany a spinal epidural abscess, demands emergency imaging. As outlined below, the three most common causes of focal brain lesions tend to evolve at different, although overlapping, rates. This relates to the time scales of the replication of the invading organisms or of tumor cells in concert with the tempo and strength of immune responses, and it can provide an initial clue to which is most likely. Exceptions to the subacute progression of most of AIDS-related CNS diseases can relate to secondary developments, such as seizures, which can dramatically punctuate the course of macroscopic or microscopic brain diseases. Hemorrhage into focal brain lesions, although far less common, can also accelerate presentation. For these reasons it is always important to define the time course of the illness and be certain that it is explained by the diagnoses being considered.

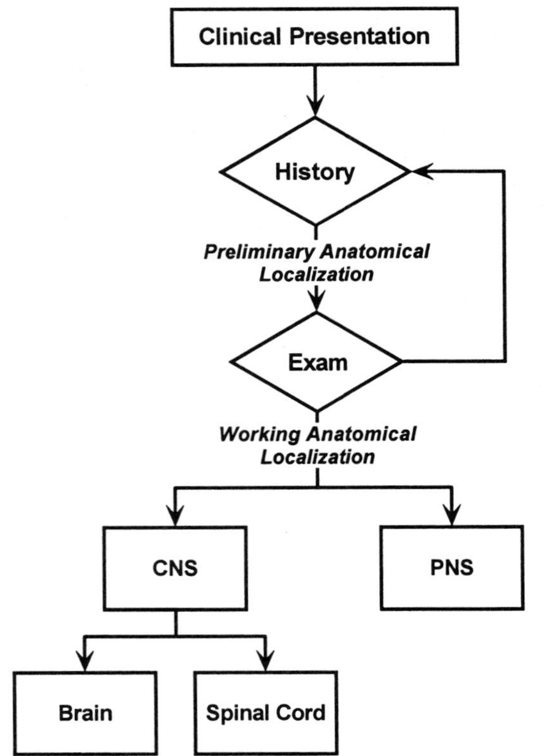

Figure 54–1. Initial approach to neurologic diagnosis in those with an HIV-1 infection. PNS, peripheral nervous system.

The patient's *risk background* is the third important variable for determining probability in the differential diagnosis. The most important variable in this category is the stage of the systemic HIV-1 infection and resultant immunosuppression as alluded to earlier. Severe compromise of cell-mediated immunity so importantly increases vulnerability to a particular group of disorders that they come to dominate the course of late infection and hence the diagnostic probabilities. If patients presenting with subacute onset of focal cerebral dysfunction have less than 50 CD4+ T-lymphocytes/mm^3 in blood, more than 90% of the patients have one of three diagnoses: CNS toxoplasmosis, primary CNS lymphoma (PCNSL), or progressive multifocal leukoencephalopathy (PML). Earlier stages of HIV-1 infection may result in a higher risk of certain autoimmune disorders, including demyelinating peripheral neuropathies. Other background factors in patients with HIV-1 infection (including the risks that led to acquisition of HIV-1 infection) may also confer different risks that "compete," particularly at early stages of HIV-1 infection when immunosuppression is milder and opportunistic disease vulnerability is far less. This includes, for example, the development of pyogenic infections, including bacterial endocarditis with septic cerebral emboli, in the active intravenous drug abuser. For this reason, it is important to define both the stage of HIV-1 infection and other background risks in each patient who presents with neurologic disease. The importance of "non-HIV-1-related" neurologic diseases in those with preserved immunity was emphasized earlier. Another potential implication of the larger number of treated patients with preserved immunity is that clinicians may encounter major opportunistic infections or the AIDS dementia complex at CD4+ T-lymphocyte counts higher than those reported for most such patients during earlier eras. In part, this simply relates to the development of this expanding population: Despite continued low probabilities, the susceptible (denominator) group is larger. Some differences may also relate to recovery of immune function after antiretroviral therapy. On the one hand, restoration of CD4 counts may not be followed by reconstitution of protective immunity against some opportunistic diseases; although it is becoming clear that this is not a major threat with some of the common infections, data relevant to some of the neurologic diseases are limited. On the other hand, effective restoration of immunity may affect the disease phenotype if vigorous host responses cause immunopathologic injury. Although defined in other settings, the exacerbating impact of immunologic reconstitution on the neurologic infections discussed in this chapter remains less clear. Nonetheless, it is likely that in certain patients the introduction of antiretroviral therapy in the presence of recognized or unrecognized pathogens in the nervous symptoms causes symptoms and signs and alters the neuroimaging findings in surprising ways. Hence clinicians should be alert to the potential for unusual manifestations in this therapeutic setting.

▲ NONFOCAL BRAIN DISEASES

Figure 54–2 depicts a general algorithm for diagnosis of brain disease in AIDS patients. The upper third of this figure concentrates on disorders that characteristically lack focal features. These conditions present with "diffuse" alterations in cognition and symmetrical motor dysfunction that is not readily explained by one or a few macroscopic focal brain lesions. There is no aphasia, apraxia, or agnosia to provide discrete cortical localization, nor is there hemiparesis or dysmetria to point to a lesion in a cerebral or cerebel-

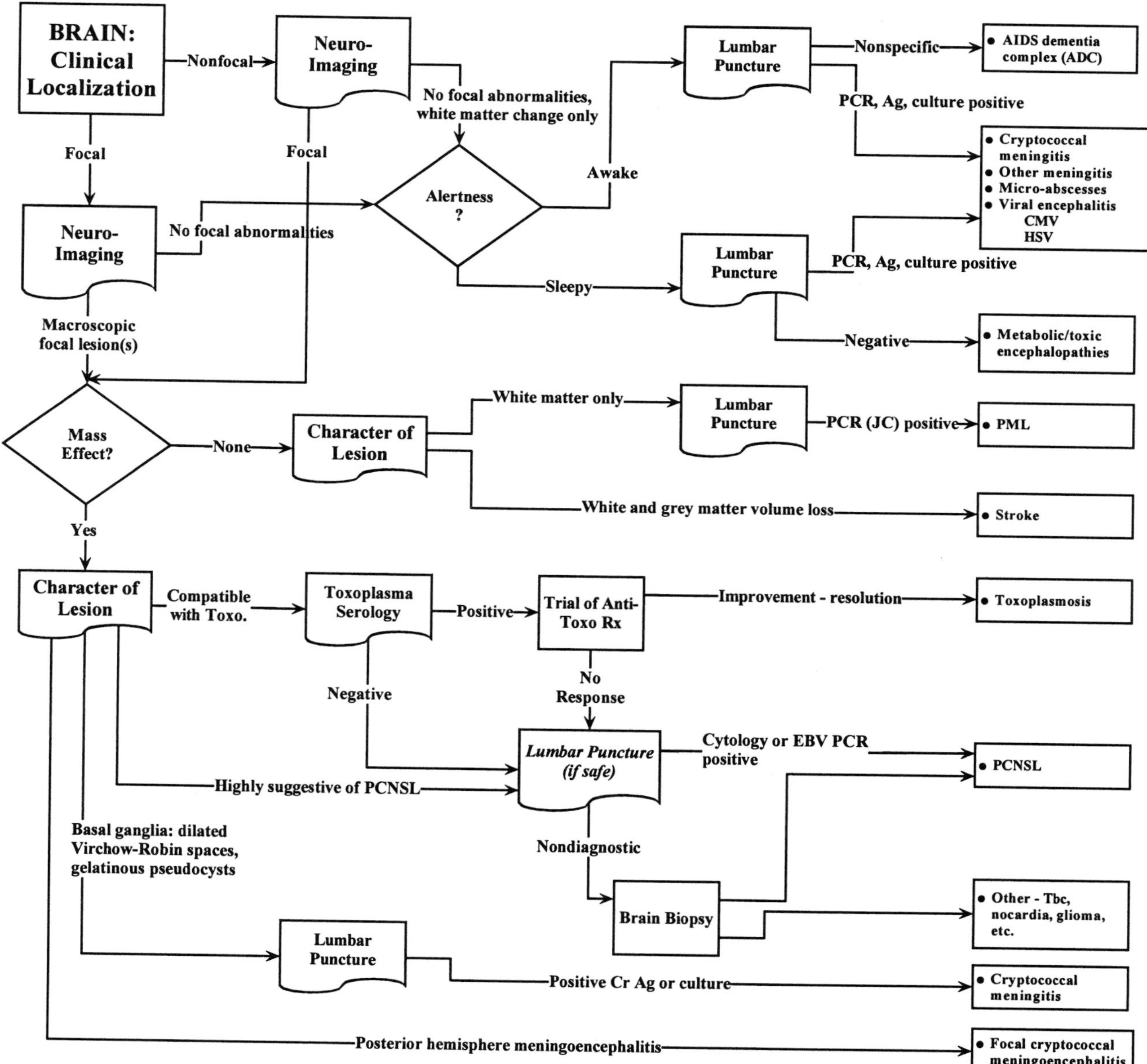

Figure 54–2. Diagnostic approach to brain diseases in those with a late HIV-1 infection. Ag, antigen; CMV, cytomegalovirus; Cr Ag, cryptococcal antigen; HSV, herpes simplex virus; PCR, polymerase chain reaction; PML, progressive multifocal leukoencephalopathy; PCNSL, primary central nervous system lymphoma; Tbc, tuberculosis.

lar hemisphere. Sensory abnormalities are usually absent or reflect coincident neuropathy. These *nonfocal* disorders can be further segregated clinically into those in which cognition is altered in the face of preserved alertness and those in which these two elements are altered in parallel. The most important disorder in the first category is the AIDS dementia complex (ADC).

AIDS Dementia Complex

A syndrome of cognitive and motor dysfunction, ADC has also been designated several other names, including HIV-associated cognitive-motor complex and the shorter terms AIDS dementia or HIV dementia.[16,17] Its pediatric counterpart, which is not discussed in detail here, is most often called HIV encephalopathy.[18,19] I prefer the term AIDS dementia complex for the adult form because it is simple and emphasizes that cognitive impairment is the predominating difficulty, but it also implies that this is not the only clinical manifestation and it is usually accompanied by abnormal motor function and, at times, characteristic behavioral abnormalities as well.[2,20]

It is believed to be caused by HIV-1 itself, rather than by an opportunistic organism, although the detailed mechanistic links between the virus and brain injury remain speculative.[21-28] It is characteristically a late complication of HIV-1 infection and, particularly in its more severe form, occurs in the same context as the major clinical AIDS-defining opportunistic infections. Table 54–1 outlines the ADC staging scheme used to describe patients' disease severity based on their functional capacity in cognitive and motor spheres.[29,30]

On the basis of its central clinical features, which include impaired attention and concentration, slowed mental speed and agility, concomitantly slowed motor speed, and apathetic behavior, ADC has been classified among the subcortical dementias.[31-34] More detailed description of its clinical features is available elsewhere.[20,35,36] Although Figure 54–2 depicts the process of diagnosis as being largely exclusionary (nonfocal neuroimaging and nonspecific lumbar puncture findings), the diagnosis should be pursued principally on the basis of its positive features, which include characteristic mental and motor findings. Additionally, although the character of the clinical abnormalities is consistent through the spectrum of its severity, it is useful to segregate the approach to diagnosis: those with mild (stage 0.5 or 1) ADC from those with more severe (stages 2 to 4) affliction. The major differential diagnoses often diverge in these two settings.

Mild ADC

Patients with mild ADC usually complain of difficulties with concentration and attention. They lose their train of thought in conversation or need to reread paragraphs of a book. More complex tasks formerly performed "reflexively" now are more labored and take longer. Patients must keep lists of formerly routine daily chores. These difficulties become intrusive and require compensatory strategies or changes in activities. Although most often ADC patients are not dysphoric, these complaints can be similar to those of depression or hypochondriasis. Diagnosis of these milder cases can, as a result, center on the question of whether there is indeed "organic" brain disease, rather than pursuit of the other nonfocal diagnoses shown in Figure 54–2. The presence of motor symptoms or, more commonly, motor signs may help support the diagnosis of ADC. These patients often have slowing of rapid finger movements (e.g., repeated opposing of the thumb and index tips), toe tapping, and walking, along with hyperactive deep tendon reflexes and the development of "release" reflexes, most notably a snout response. If there is any doubt regarding either the presence or pattern of cognitive changes, formal evaluation by a neuropsychologist familiar with this condition may be helpful.[37]

Table 54–1. AIDS DEMENTIA COMPLEX STAGING

ADC Stage	Characteristics
0 (normal)	Normal mental and motor function.
0.5 (equivocal/ subclinical)	Minimal or equivocal symptoms of cognitive or motor dysfunction characteristic of AIDS dementia complex, or mild signs (snout response, slowed extremity movements) but without impairment of work or capacity to perform activities of daily living (ADL). Gait and strength are normal.
1 (mild)	Unequivocal evidence (symptoms, signs, neuropsychological test performance) of functional intellectual or motor impairment characteristic of ADC but able to perform all but the more demanding aspects of work or ADL. Can walk without assistance.
2 (moderate)	Cannot work or maintain the more demanding aspects of daily life but able to perform basic activities of self-care. Ambulatory but may require a single prop.
3 (severe)	Major intellectual incapacity (cannot follow news or personal events, cannot sustain complex conversation, considerable slowing of all output) or motor disability (cannot walk unassisted, requiring walker or personal support, usually with slowing and clumsiness of arms as well).
4 (end-stage)	Nearly vegetative. Intellectual and social comprehension and responses are at a rudimentary level. Nearly or absolutely mute. Paraparetic or paraplegic with double incontinence.

Adapted from Price R, Brew B. The AIDS dementia complex. J Infect Dis 158:1079, 1988; and Sidtis JJ, Price RW. Early HIV-1 infection and the AIDS dementia complex. Neurology 40:323, 1990.

Severe ADC

In patients with more severe ADC (stage 2 or above), neurologic abnormalities are more distinct. These patients cannot live comfortably without some help from others. They are usually clearly mentally slow and have trouble performing tasks requiring concentration (reversing a five-letter word or subtracting serial sevens) with either slowed performance or inaccuracy. Motor findings are also more evident and may now include more marked slowing or unsteadiness of gait. Abnormal reflexes are also more prevalent. When alertness is completely preserved, the diagnosis is usually evident unless there is concern that cognitive difficulty relates to earlier, static brain disease. However, manifestations of some other conditions may overlap, and for this reason neuroimaging is usually justified to screen for other disorders that may present similarly. For example, primary CNS lymphoma that involves the frontal white matter bilaterally may cause cognitive slowing without notable focal or lateralizing signs. Cytomegalovirus (CMV) encephalitis can also be confused with ADC as described later.

Laboratory Diagnosis

Fundamentally a clinical diagnosis, it relies on recognizing the characteristic profile of cognitive and motor impairment in the absence of confounding causes. Laboratory tests are performed chiefly to rule out other conditions, though certain findings provide evidence that suggests an ADC diagnosis. Most important in this regard are neuroimaging and cerebrospinal fluid (CSF) examination.

Although neuroimaging is usually performed to detect evidence of alternative diagnoses (e.g., mass lesions, hydrocephalus, prior trauma), it is sometimes helpful for supporting an ADC diagnosis. Probably the most common neuroimaging finding in ADC is brain atrophy, detected by computed tomography (CT) or MRI.[38,39] Unfortunately, it is not diagnostically specific and less than 100% sensitive. Most ADC patients have some degree of atrophy, but this is also found in those without clinical ADC and is common in certain risk groups more broadly, such as substance abusers. Nonetheless, those with more severe and protracted ADC usually have marked brain atrophy, which sets them apart. The exception may be the patient with more severe ADC who presents with a brief, subacute course in whom atrophy is inconspicuous or absent. Somewhat more characteristic are changes in white matter with increased water content noted on T2-weighted, proton density or FLAIR sequences.[40] Most common are regional changes in the white matter signal, ranging from diffuse to more circumscribed "fluffy" patches of increased signal. Although helpful when present, they tend to be more common with severe disease and thus less useful for mild ADC. Moreover, they are not always present even with severe disease. More recently, magnetic resonance spectroscopy (MRS) has revealed abnormalities in ADC that may eventually prove useful for diagnosing and characterizing ADC.[41–45] This method has not yet been tested for individual case diagnosis; rather, it has been used in clinical trials to characterize patient groups. Hence the sensitivity and specificity for clinical application awaits further study.

Examination of the CSF has much the same purpose as neuroimaging: primarily to screen for such disorders as cryptococcal and other meningitides, neurosyphilis, or viral encephalitis using cultures, tests for antigens, and polymerase chain reaction (PCR) amplifications. As with MRS, it would be helpful if CSF tests could be used to confirm an ADC diagnosis. Unfortunately, this is not yet the case. Although CSF findings are often abnormal, the abnormalities are not diagnostically specific. Among routine assessments, the CSF protein and cell counts are frequently elevated, but in fact these abnormalities are common in early asymptomatic systemic HIV-1 infection. Thus elevated protein or cell counts in ADC patients is not diagnostically specific. Similarly, a number of markers of macrophage activation have been observed to be elevated in ADC but also are not diagnostically specific. Thus early studies showed elevations in neopterin, β_2-microglobulin, and quinolinic acid.[46–50] More recent reports show elevations of monocyte chemoattractant protein-1 (MCP-1), other cytokines, and related inflammatory markers[51,52]; but these factors are also elevated in other conditions, and their practical application to the clinical diagnosis has not been carefully evaluated. One can think of situations where they might be useful (e.g., for diagnosing stage 1 ADC or distinguishing active ADC from residual injury or other static encephalopathy), but diagnostic guidelines using these tests have not been defined.

Initial application of quantitative HIV-1 nucleic acid amplification to CSF suggested that viral load measurement in this compartment might help with the diagnosis.[53] Though there may be a correlation of CSF HIV-1 concentration with ADC severity and HIV encephalitis pathologically,[54] this correlation applies only to patients with advanced immunosuppression.[55–57] In those with high CD4+ T-lymphocyte counts, CSF viral loads may also be elevated without neurologic abnormalities; additionally, CNS opportunistic infections may be accompanied by an increased CSF viral load.[53] Thus interpretations regarding CSF HIV-1 concentrations are not simple, and certainly the CSF viral load cannot be used by itself for ADC diagnosis. Like the macrophage markers, there may be situations where CSF HIV-1 measurement may be useful for diagnosis (e.g., in the presence of a low CD4+ T-lymphocyte count or when the CSF viral load is higher than that of plasma) or for tracking responses to therapy. However, clear guidelines have not yet been defined, and so the CSF viral load is not yet a part of clinical practice.

Treatment

Optimal treatment for ADC has not yet been established, but it is clear from epidemiologic studies that antiretroviral therapy can prevent ADC and from limited coordinated trials and individual case experience that treatment can arrest or reverse the condition.[58–68] Early studies demonstrated that zidovudine monotherapy had both therapeutic and preventive effects on ADC. Because formal clinical trials of ADC are now difficult to implement, reports describing responses to contemporary combination antiretroviral therapy are largely anecdotal. Nonetheless, there is a reasonable basis for considering HAART to be an effective avenue of treatment for ADC if one: (1) uses the early experience with monotherapy as proof of concept; (2) extends the advantage of multidrug therapy on systemic disease to treating the CNS; (3) extrapolates from the therapeutic reduction of CSF viral load to effects on brain parenchymal infection (assuming that ADC is indeed caused by this direct brain infection); and (4) calls on the anecdotal (including my own personal) experience. More at issue now are refinements of therapy to target the CNS better, particularly the question of whether it is necessary that each of the components of a multidrug regimen penetrate well into the brain. Whereas several of the current nucleoside (including zidovudine, abacavir, and stavudine) and nonnucleoside (nevirapine) reverse transcriptase inhibitors seem to penetrate relatively well (though with extracellular fluid exposures that may still be only about one-third that of plasma), most of the protease inhibitors do not.[69–83] Indinavir may be an exception, with exposure also aided by combination with ritonavir. On the other hand, judging from CSF HIV responses, patients seem to respond to regimens with one or more poorly penetrating drugs, and the need for such drug penetration may vary among patient. Also, drug levels in CSF do not necessarily indicate exposure and an effect on the critical target cells, including particularly brain macrophages. As a result, in the absence of clearer guidelines, I recommend that drugs for symptomatic ADC patients be selected with the following general priorities: (1) ensure susceptibility of virus isolates to the individual drugs just as when treating systemic infection, including susceptibility to CSF isolates in cases with prior drug exposure and suspected "compartmentalized" infection; (2) use an aggressive regimen; and finally (3) when possible, choose drugs with favorable CNS penetration, including those listed above.

Additional approaches to treating ADC can be grouped under the category *adjuvant* treatments. These range from various forms of symptom management (e.g., cautious use of neuroleptics or mood stabilizers to relieve behavioral symptoms and signs) to efforts to attenuate the disease process by interfering with various endogenous neurotoxic pathways. The latter has led to clinical trials of candidate neuroprotective agents without firm evidence of efficacy.[84–86]

Other Nonfocal Brain Disorders

Most nonfocal brain disorders complicating HIV-1 infection other than ADC are accompanied by concomitant depression of both alertness and cognition. Overall, the most common in this category are the toxic encephalopathies related to sedative, narcotic, and other CNS-acting medications. Metabolic encephalopathies are also common and relate to failure of systemic organs, such as hypoxia and renal or hepatic failure.

Among opportunistic infections, the most common "nonfocal" infection causing general confusion with a picture similar to metabolic encephalopathy is CMV encephalitis.[87–94] Like other organ afflictions with this herpesvirus, CMV encephalitis is becoming rare in patients taking HAART. Additionally, its clinical limits have not been sharply defined. Autopsy studies earlier in the AIDS epidemic showed histologic evidence of CMV infection in about one-fourth of brains.[95–98] However, the extent to which these lesions, some quite mild, contribute to clinical abnormalities is uncertain in many cases. On the other hand, it is also clear that some patients develop severe CMV encephalitis with distinct morbidity and mortality. Thus the key issue is not whether CMV caused symptomatic brain infection in AIDS patients but, rather, what was the importance of the milder end of the spectrum. Also, CMV infection can coincide with ADC, and it may be difficult to discern which process is responsible for particular clinical manifestations. Clinicopathologic studies have pointed out certain features that associate with CMV encephalitis, including subacute onset, frank confusion or delirium, hyponatremia, and more specifically periventricular abnormalities on MRI (increased water signal or enhancement with contrast). Some patients have distinct focal features, including nystagmus, ataxia, and ocular motor palsies, indicating brain stem involvement; seizures are likely to be more common than with ADC. Unusual cases of CMV infection have more prominent focal features and may even have focal lesions detected on neuroimaging that exceed 1 cm in diameter.[99] CSF may vary from a bland fluid to one with pleocytosis with polymorphonuclear or mononuclear predominance and high protein content. The diagnosis has been revolutionized by nucleic acid amplification techniques, and detection of CMV DNA provides a sensitive test.[94,100–104] Most but not all patients have CMV disease in other organs, which often supports the diagnosis. Therapy is with one or more of the anti-CMV drugs discussed elsewhere in this volume (see Chapter 43).

Other diseases that cause widespread microscopic pathology may present a similar picture. This includes disseminated intravascular coagulation in the septic or otherwise gravely ill patient. It also includes the so-called encephalitic form of cerebral toxoplasmosis that presents without distinct focality and sometimes a CT scan that appears normal or nearly normal.[105,106] The latter is usually a fulminant infection associated with multiple microabscesses; there may be little inflammatory or tissue reaction. In cases of rapid-onset encephalitis of this type, empiric anti-*Toxoplasma* therapy may be justified while the diagnostic evaluation is underway. Herpes simplex encephalitis in the AIDS patient may also present as a diffuse encephalopathy and differ from the characteristic focal encephalitis of the nonimmunosuppressed patient, although the frequency and range of presentations has never been clearly characterized.[102,107–110] Neuroimaging in these cases may be negative, although it may be improved by some of the newer sequencing techniques. PCR amplification of HSV in the CSF is probably the most sensitive diagnostic tool, but test results are often delayed; if this diagnosis is suspected, empiric therapy with intravenous acyclovir may be warranted until results are available.

Meningitis and Headache

As in other settings, meningitis in AIDS patients may present with confusion and altered consciousness as the predominant manifestations. In the case of the uncommon bacterial meningitis caused by *Listeria monocytogenes* or *Streptococcus pneumoniae*, headache and stiff neck are usually present and push the clinician to perform a lumbar puncture. However, these findings may be less conspicuous or even absent at the onset of cryptococcal meningitis, the most common meningitis in this setting (see Chapter 36).[111] Hence, even relatively low suspicion of the latter calls for lumbar puncture and analysis for cryptococcal antigen, along with diagnostic studies for bacteria and other fungi, particularly when the CD4+ T-lymphocyte count is low.

Headache is a common symptom of AIDS, but most patients with this complaint do not suffer bacterial or fungal infections.[112–118] As already discussed, in some individuals with HIV-1 infection lumbar puncture detects a pleocytosis sufficient to warrant the designation "aseptic meningitis." Use of this term for a relatively common laboratory finding in otherwise asymptomatic individuals can be problematic, however, and one should probably distinguish patients who develop meningitic symptoms and exhibit such CSF findings from those in whom they are incidental. In an earlier report, Hollander and Stringari divided patients who presented with headache and CSF pleocytosis into two groups: those with acute presentation and those with a more chronic course.[119] However, because of the high prevalence of asymptomatic pleocytosis in HIV-1 infection, the relation between these CSF cells and headache is not always clear; and in some the headache and the laboratory finding may indeed be unrelated.[120] In our own studies of treatment interruption in which we noted a resurgence of the HIV-1 load in CSF accompanying that in plasma, we were struck not only by the robust lymphocytic cell response but also by the fact that this response is clinically silent.[121] No formal study has addressed the question of whether headache associated with HIV-1 infection responds to HAART, though pleocytosis without other causes characteristically resolves after institution of HAART in parallel with clearing of the virus in the CSF.[122] Further complicating this issue is the fact that a clinically similar headache can manifest in HIV-1-infected patients in the absence of pleocytosis; this situation is common enough to have been designated "HIV headache."[123,124] In some it has a migrainous quality with periodicity, photophobia, and nausea. Treatment is empiric and may include agents active in prophylaxis of migraine, such as anticonvulsants, tricyclics, or calcium channel blockers, although evidence of efficacy is anecdotal in this setting.

▲ FOCAL BRAIN DISEASES

The diagnosis of a macroscopic brain disorder begins with clinical recognition of symptoms and signs that indicate the presence of focal brain dysfunction. They include hemispheric dysfunction (hemiparesis, hemianopsia, aphasia, apraxia) or brain stem-cerebellar dysfunction (e.g., vertigo, ataxia, diplopia, bilateral pyramidal signs). Symptoms and signs may be prominent or subtle, and more than one focal lesion affecting "eloquent" brain structures may confuse the exact site. The first step in evaluation is usually neuroimaging to confirm the presence of detectable focal lesions and to define their character (see the lower two-thirds of Fig. 54–2). Only rarely do focal lesions escape detection by MRI; in such patients either the imaging is done too early to discern abnormalities, such as the rare patient with progressive multifocal leukoencephalopathy (PML) at its earliest stage, or, more commonly, the abnormalities are microscopic and below the limit of image detection. Such false-negative results are now less common as newer pulse sequences are added to MRI protocols. Some metabolic disorders present with focal features (e.g., nonketotic, hyperglycemic hyperosmolar encephalopathy). Perhaps more commonly, microscopic disease can cause seizures that transiently expand the zone of physiologic dysfunction beyond that caused by the lesion itself. Examples include CMV encephalitis, the encephalitic form of toxoplasmosis, other viral encephalitides, including those caused by herpes simplex virus-1 (HSV-1) or HSV-2. Cryptococcal or other meningitides may also cause seizures with residual focal deficits that are slow to clear.

Among the focal brain disorders afflicting AIDS patients, three stand out as most common: primary CNS lymphoma: (PCNSL), cerebral toxoplasmosis, and PML. As a result, most diagnostic efforts relate to distinguishing these three diseases. Fortunately, this is not difficult in most patients. Because neurologic symptoms and signs are determined by site, the particular deficits are not helpful for their distinction. However, each of the three tends to have a different temporal profile, although with overlap. In general, toxoplasmosis evolves most rapidly, presenting within a few days after the onset of symptoms. PCNSL usually evolves somewhat slower, with one or a few weeks separating the onset of symptoms and presentation to the physician. PML advances even more slowly and may take several weeks to a few months before the patient seeks medical evaluation. Associated constitutional symptoms also tend to differ. Patients with toxoplasmosis are more often febrile, appear generally ill, and are lethargic or sleepy; they also more commonly complain of headache. This contrasts with both the PCNSL and PML patients, who are otherwise well unless they suffer an additional overt infection.

Progressive Multifocal Leukoencephalopathy

Despite clinical differences, neuroimaging is needed to define the diagnosis of focal disorders. MRI usually readily identifies PML.[125–128] This viral infection causes neither the mass effect nor surrounding edema characteristic of toxoplasmosis and PCNSL. PML lesions usually lack the contrast enhancement seen with these other two diseases. PML, caused by JC virus brain infection, is characterized by demyelination and loss of tissue rather than an expanding mass effect.[129,130] Areas of demyelination that follow the death of infected oligodendrocytes coalesce to leave behind areas of lost white matter and even cavitation. PML lesions usually begin as small foci that expand concentrically, singly or in several sites. Inflammation is usually absent or scant, and consequently the typical MRI of PML shows one or more lesions afflicting the white matter predominantly or exclusively in which there is increased signal (white) on T2-weighted images but diminished signal (black) on T1-weighted images. Lesions have a predilection to involve the white matter adjacent to the cortex but can be located anywhere. When contrast enhancement is present (likely in fewer than 10% of cases), it tends to have a delicate, lacy appearance. There are two principal differential diagnoses to consider with this type of scan, both of which are usually easily eliminated by correlation with the clinical presentation and by observing their evolution over time. The first is ADC, which can be associated with focal white matter changes. However, ADC characteristically involves deeper white matter, lesions usually are not black on T1-

weighted images, and most importantly localized image abnormalities are not accompanied by corresponding focal neurologic deficits. The second is cerebral infarction. However, in the latter the gray matter is also affected, the distribution of the lesion follows a vascular territory, and of course the clinical evolution occurs in hours rather than weeks.

A common clinical question in these patients is, "What level of diagnostic certainty is necessary for clinical management of PML?" For typical cases where MRI shows the abnormalities already outlined (confirmed by an experienced neuroradiologist) and these imaging findings can be correlated with the clinical picture (with the time of evolution and the location of deficits), a clinical diagnosis of PML is highly probable and may not require further diagnostic testing. CSF examination should probably be done routinely to eliminate diagnostic surprises (e.g., neurosyphilis or vasculitis) depending on the patient's findings. PCR confirmation of local JC virus infection in the CSF has about 75% sensitivity but high specificity for PML in this setting.[131–135] If other measures fail and the case is atypical, brain biopsy should be undertaken for final confirmation.

There is no proven specific treatment for PML, although remission has been clearly documented. Early in the AIDS epidemic Berger and Mucke[136] noted spontaneous remission in the absence of treatment; and following a number case reports documenting remission in PML patients treated with HAART, retrospective studies comparing the outcome of this opportunistic infection before and after HAART demonstrated that about half of the PML patients do well after starting HAART, with arrest of progression and an element of improvement in some.[137–142] Radiographic improvement has also been documented by MRI. The theoretical interpretation of this response, which is in keeping with earlier reports of PML remission in non-AIDS patients, is that HAAART restores the host's capacity to mount an effective immune response to the JC virus. The current standard of therapy for PML therefore begins with institution or modification of HAART, which is then assessed by the standard measures of viral load reduction and CD4+ cell increase.

For the cases that fail to respond, the remaining treatment options are experimental. Unfortunately, the history of PML includes reports of several therapies that initially showed promise but failed when examined prospectively in a larger trial.[143] Most recently, interest has focused on the use of cidofovir, an antiviral agent active against CMV. Unfortunately, studies of this drug in PML have been uncontrolled, and the results are conflicting[144–146] (see Chapter 48).

Cerebral Toxoplasmosis and PCNSL

The other two common focal brain lesions, cerebral toxoplasmosis and PCNSL, in contrast to PML, usually are defined radiologically as having a mass effect (an expansion of tissue) with surrounding edema. Figure 54–2 outlines an approach to the diagnosis of focal mass lesions; it is aimed particularly at the early diagnosis of brain lesions other than toxoplasmosis. Because cerebral toxoplasmosis is nearly always due to reactivated *Toxoplasma gondii* infection, more than 95% of such patients have detectable serum antibody to this organism.[105,147–149] Hence if the radiographic character of the lesion(s) is compatible with toxoplasmosis and the blood serology is positive, I subject patients to a trial of anti-*Toxoplasma* therapy. If they improve clinically within days to (at most) 2 weeks, followed with radiographic documentation, I am satisfied with this diagnosis. Typically, neuroimaging shows contrast-enhancing lesions (usually multiple, but they can be single) involving the cortex or deep gray nuclei (basal ganglia and thalamus); the lesions often have a ring of strong contrast enhancement, and there may be an "eccentric target" sign.[150,151] Because prophylaxis against *Pneumocystis carinii* pneumonia with trimethoprim-sulfamethoxazole is also active in preventing cerebral toxoplasmosis, this variable is considered in the probability of this diagnosis.[134] Indeed, its widespread use and more recently the use of HAART has markedly reduced the incidence of toxoplasmosis.[11] In my consultation practice, cerebral toxoplasmosis is now an uncommon disease, and the few cases seen have developed chiefly in individuals who have not been receiving ongoing medical care.

Because the outcome of PCNSL is likely influenced by how early it is diagnosed and treatment started, it is important to pursue this diagnosis aggressively. In this respect, it is not reasonable to apply a trial of toxoplasmosis therapy to all AIDS patients with mass lesions, as had been recommended by some in the past. Hence in patients with either negative *Toxoplasma* blood serology or with neuroimaging abnormalities that suggest PCNSL, I advocate immediate brain biopsy, though usually after CSF examination if a lumbar puncture is judged to be safe. The imaging abnormalities that favor PCNSL are deep lesions involving the white matter, including the corpus callosum; subependymal extension of lesions along the ventricular walls; and diffuse or weak contrast enhancement rather than the ring-like appearance of toxoplasmosis.[150,152] In most settings, brain biopsy is necessary for a certain diagnosis of PCNSL. PCR detection of Epstein-Barr virus (EBV) DNA sequences in CSF has been reported to enhance the diagnosis, perhaps to the point of substituting this test for a biopsy.[6,134,153,154] However, its sensitivity and specificity must be confirmed by more extensive experience, including results from various commercial laboratories. Conventional cytology is commonly much less helpful.[155]

A number of more recent reports have also shown the potential utility of metabolic imaging of focal CNS lesions using several methods including (1) positron emission tomography (PET) scanning with labeled deoxyglucose to measure active tissue metabolism; (2) single-photon emission computed tomography (SPECT) scanning to detect metabolically linked cerebral blood flow; and (3) most recently, MRS to detect different tissue metabolite profiles.[42,134,156–163] As seen by PET and SPECT, PCNSLs are characteristically "active" with increased uptake of the tracer, whereas toxoplasmosis lesions characteristically appear "cold" by these techniques. Although the results of these scanning techniques can be impressive in the individual case, specificity is not absolute, and these tests may not add greatly to the findings of anatomic imaging. Because of the widespread deployment of MRI, the increasing interest in MRS, and the fact that MRS can be performed in the same facility as MRI, MRS perhaps holds greater potential for broad application. At this time, reports of case series show promise, but further study defining the characteristics of the different focal lesions and evaluating sensitivity and specificity are needed before it is known if MRS analysis can obviate the need for biopsy.

Other Focal Lesions

There are other, miscellaneous causes of focal brain lesions. The general approach to their diagnosis usually includes a search for particularly susceptibilities or involvement of other organs more easily accessible to culture or biopsy. When this fails, brain biopsy should be considered. This modality remains an essential tool for diagnosis of unusual focal brain lesions as well as in most cases of PCNSL, and it is often the fastest and surest approach to such uncommon CNS focal disorders as *Mycobacterium tuberculosis* infection,[5,164,165] *Nocardia* infection,[166,167] glioma,[168,169] macronodular CMV lesions,[170] or *Aspergillus* infection,[171,172] when disease is not identified at other sites. It is my impression that many clinicians are unduly wary of resorting to brain biopsy. However, when used selectively, its morbidity is low[173–175] and the most frequent disappointment is failure of biopsy to establish a diagnosis.

Cryptococcal meningitis can also be complicated by focal brain lesions of several types. One of these relates to dilatation of the perivascular (Virchow-Robin) spaces at the base of the brain by organisms and capsular debris. Such debris may be small and give rise to a mottled appearance of the diencephalon on MRI, particularly with T2 weighting.[176] Larger lesions justify the term *gelatinous pseudocysts* and may range from a solitary cystic appearance to bubbly lesions that encompass the entire basal ganglia.[177] Because they are not associated with inflammation, these lesions do not elicit contrast enhancement, and they resolve with treatment of the meningitis. Although cryptococcal granulomas (cryptococcomas) are unusual in AIDS patients, we have encountered six patients with another characteristic type of inflammatory lesion that develops as a delayed complication of cryptococcal meningitis.[178] Patients characteristically present with focal seizures and subsequently focal neurologic deficits. MRI shows a characteristic pattern of linear deep sulcal enhancement and underlying edema that extends into the white matter. There is a predilection for the posterior hemispheres: the parietal and occipital lobes. Biopsy has shown cortical invasion by the cryptococci and local inflammation. However, the MRI findings are sufficiently distinct in this setting to allow a clinical diagnosis without biopsy. This complication can occur while patients are on maintenance therapy, and the CSF cryptococcal antigen titer is usually lower than at the time of the patient's initial presentation with meningitis. Although four of the six patients responded well to changes in therapy, two of the lesion progressed despite all therapeutic efforts.

Stroke is unusual in those with HIV-1 infection,[179–181] although it may become more common as the infected population survives to a more susceptible age and if the lipid abnormalities accompanying therapy predispose to cerebrovascular disease. This diagnosis is suspected when the onset of the neurologic deficit is acute.[182,183] In younger AIDS patients who are otherwise well, the causes of stroke include miscellaneous relatively uncommon conditions.[184] Cerebral vasculitis can complicate varicella-zoster virus (VZV) infection, usually manifesting as delayed hemiplegia contralateral to trigeminal herpes zoster, although other distributions of both rash and cerebral infarction can occur.[185–188] The diagnosis is suspected by the setting of recent zoster and supported by the finding of cerebral infarction and vascular occlusion or narrowing on magnetic resonance or conventional angiography. CSF PCR may also be helpful.[189,190] The effect of treatment is uncertain, although usually anti-VZV therapy is given alone or in combination with anticoagulants or corticosteroids. Septic embolism, invasive fungal vasculitis (most commonly caused by *Aspergillus*), and neurosyphilis can also occur in this setting; and patients may develop the more common cerebrovascular diseases that afflict the general population. For those still using illicit drugs, cocaine and amphetamines may cause infarction or cerebral hemorrhage. When patients are more systemically ill, nonbacterial thrombotic endocarditis and other coagulopathic strokes may occur. Although AIDS patients frequently exhibit laboratory abnormalities that may predispose to stroke (e.g., protein S deficiency), the role of these serologic abnormalities in clinical stroke is uncertain.[191]

▲ MYELOPATHIES

Diagnostic considerations of myelopathies echo those of brain diseases. The starting point is recognizing that the site of disease is the spinal cord; and the next step involves distinguishing nonsegmental from focal myelopathies (Fig. 54–3).

Vacuolar and Other Nonsegmental Myelopathies

The nonsegmental myelopathies are distinguished by their "diffuse," rather than focal, character. In these patients there is no discrete level below which abnormalities are distinct and above which signs are absent. Rather, there is gradual shading toward increasing abnormality caudally; hence the legs are more affected than the arms. Motor abnormalities tend to predominate, and when sensory symptoms or signs are present they involve distal loss of sensation, usually without any changes over the trunk. Right–left asymmetries are usually minor or absent. Bladder and bowel dysfunction tend to occur late.

The most common myelopathy of this type in AIDS patients is vacuolar myelopathy, which was defined as a component of ADC.[192–194] The reason this myelopathy is included within the larger ADC syndrome relates to the frequency with which clinical myelopathy and cognitive deficits coexist, and the observation that abnormalities may not be confined to the spinal cord even in patients in whom cognition is spared; for example, a brisk jaw jerk is com-

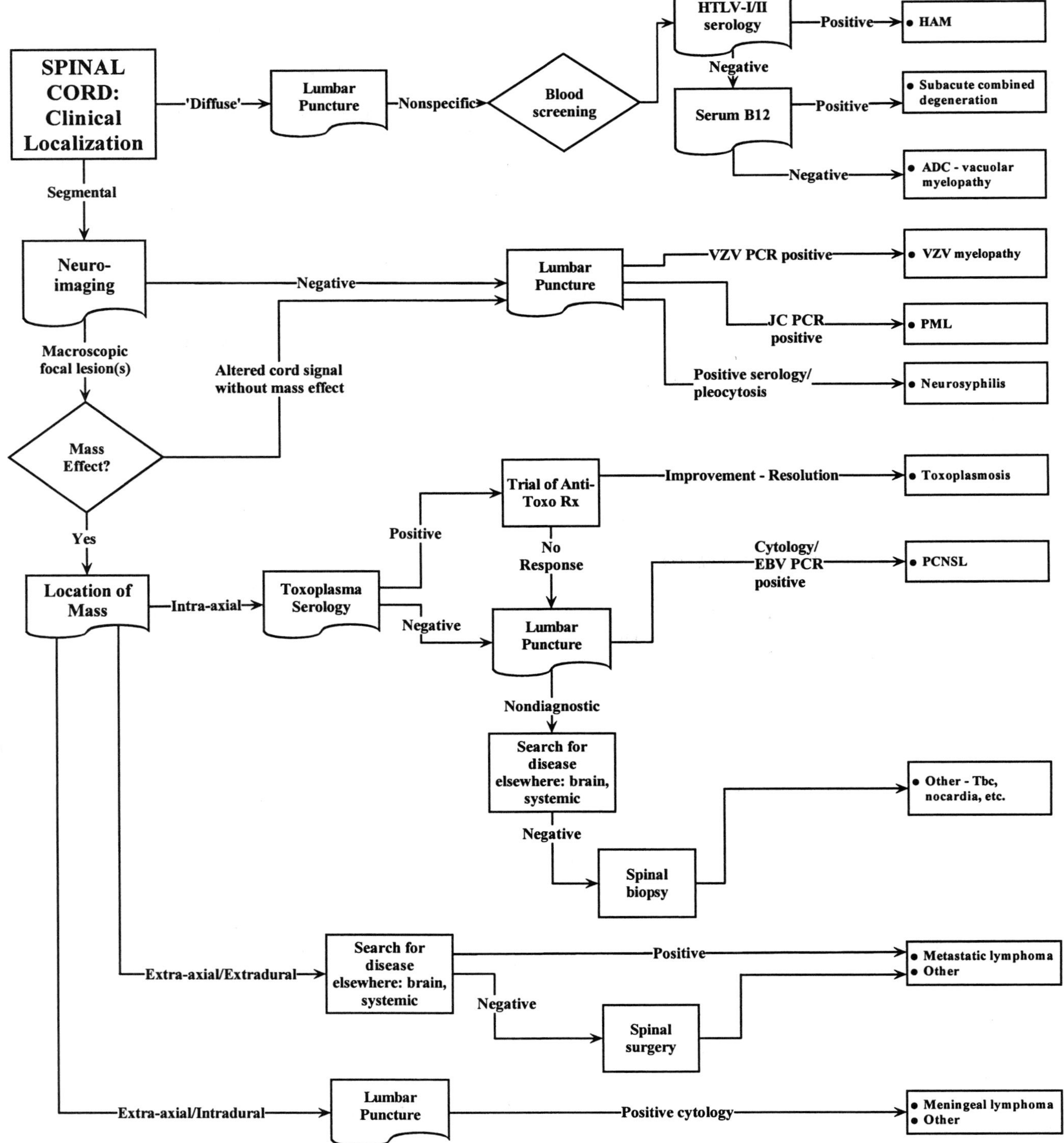

Figure 54–3. Diagnostic approach to spinal cord diseases in those with late HIV-1 infection. HAM, HTLV-1B-associated myelopathy; Tbc, tuberculosis; VZV, varicella-zoster virus.

mon with vacuolar myelopathy. Despite this overlap, many patients present with a strongly predominating picture of spastic or spastic-ataxic gait that may progress to paraparesis or paraplegia with minor or no cognitive deficit. Pathologically, the spinal cord shows a characteristic vacuolated or foamy appearance of the white matter, most notably affecting the lateral and posterior columns. This pathology is indistinguishable from that of subacute combined degeneration caused by vitamin B_{12} deficiency, although AIDS patients with this complication usually have normal levels of this vitamin in the blood; although it develops in the setting of advanced HIV infection, vacuolar changes do not correlate with productive spinal cord infection.[195–200] Thus the etiology and pathogenesis of vacuolar myelopathy remain a matter of speculation.[201]

Vacuolar myelopathy is (or *was* before HAART) common in late AIDS as an overt, symptomatic disease or as a milder, subclinical form evidenced by hyperactive knee jerks and mildly slow or clumsy walking. The ankle jerks are less brisk in some patients because concomitant neuropathy is common. The disorder is usually gradually progressive and may exacerbate with severe coincident infections, resolving partially afterward. Because there is no distinct laboratory marker, the diagnosis is a clinical one. MRI is usually normal or detects only spinal cord atrophy, and therefore in typical cases I do not routinely pursue diagnostic neuroimaging.[202] However, if there is reason to suspect a segmental lesion (e.g., cervical spinal cord compression), MRI should be done. Lumbar puncture is performed to rule out other conditions rather than to confirm the diagnosis and is usually unrewarding. Among the principal differential diagnoses to be considered are the myelopathies associated with the human T cell lymphoma virus type I (HTLV-I), called HTLV-I-associated myelopathy (HAM), tropical spastic paraparesis (TSP), combined HAM/TSP, and HTLV-II myelopathy.[203–210] Except for cases of more rapid onset following transfusion, HAM is clinically similar to vacuolar myelopathy, although spasticity can be more severe early in the course and low back pain more frequent. The diagnosis usually relies on serologic studies showing antibodies to these other retroviruses in blood and CSF. Unlike vacuolar myelopathy, HVLV-I/II myleopathies are not associated with low blood CD4 cells. Treatment with interferon has shown some effect in the non-AIDS HAM patient, but there are no clear studies of treatment-induced improvement in co-infected patients. Vitamin B_{12} deficiency should be ruled out.

There is some controversy regarding whether vacuolar myelopathy responds to antiretroviral therapy in a fashion similar to the cognitive impairment of ADC. Because vacuolar pathology does not correlate with local productive HIV-1 infection of the spinal cord, there is also theoretical reason to suspect that this mode of treatment would not be effective.[211,212] However, the lack of seeming efficacy in past experience might relate to the low potency of antiviral therapies available at the time. This issue needs to be reexamined during the current era of HAART. I have seen patients with a clinical diagnosis of vacuolar myelopathy and recent onset who have improved markedly following contemporary combination antiviral drug treatment. Although this therapeutic issue needs careful study, in the absence of conclusive data I pursue the optimistic path of treating such patients aggressively with antiviral drug combinations as discussed for ADC in general.

Focal (Segmental) Myelopathies

Focal myelopathies are much less common than vacuolar myelopathy. Although most of these myelopathies are caused by the same diseases that cause focal lesions in brain, there are a few causes that are more specific or common to the spinal cord in HIV-1-infected patients. The most common of these is VZV infection, which characteristically complicates cutaneous herpes zoster after a variable delay (days to a week or two, rarely several weeks or months).[213,214] The focal myelopathy, usually centered at or near the spinal cord segment corresponding to the dermatomal zoster rash, is caused by direct viral infection that enters at the dorsal root entry zone and then extends centrifugally. This explains localization in some to a partial or complete hemicord (Brown-Sequard) syndrome. Pathologically, there may be both parenchymal infection and infectious vasculitis with infarction. The latter likely accounts for the abruptness of onset in many cases. The diagnosis is usually suspected on the basis of the combined temporal and spatial (spinal segment) relation to the rash. Clinical severity varies from transverse myelitis to subclinical hyperactive reflexes and Babinski sign on the side of the rash. Because of the rapid evolution of the condition and its rarity, the effects of treatment are not well established. However, in the absence of adequate data, aggressive anti-VZV treatment seems appropriate. Spinal MRI may show a focal cord lesion with little or no mass effect but with focal edema that extends above and below the central location of the pathology. CSF may exhibit a mononuclear pleocytosis, although this can also be present with uncomplicated herpes zoster. PCR detection of VZV DNA sequences in CSF may also be helpful,[215,216] although again interpretation may be tainted by recent cutaneous herpes zoster, which might also cause a positive CSF PCR. Thus the clinical presentation is the principal basis of the diagnosis, and laboratory tests are of ancillary value.

The diagnostic approach to the other focal myelopathies is similar to that of their counterparts in the brain. It relies heavily on neuroimaging, chiefly spinal MRI.[217,218] As outlined in Figure 54–3, the cross-sectional location of the mass lesion divides the major diagnostic categories into three anatomic groups: intra-axial, extra-axial/intradural, and extra-axial/extradural. Although intra-axial lesions (within the spinal cord) are uncommon and toxoplasmosis and PCNSL are the most frequent,[219–221] the diagnostic evaluation follows the same path as for brain lesions. Because both may be part of a multifocal process, brain imaging may be helpful for revealing clinically silent lesions that may be more characteristic or accessible by imaging. These diseases usually show contrast enhancement. In *Toxoplasma*-seropositive patients a trial of therapy may establish the diagnosis, whereas cytologic assessment or PCR detection of EBV sequences may confirm the presence of PCNSL. When these measures fail, direct biopsy may be required.

The most common extra-axial/extradural lesions in HIV-1-infected patients are caused by metastatic lymphoma.[222,223] This diagnosis is usually established by tissue sampling from another site. Without this method, needle or open biopsy is required. An important item in the differential diagnosis in the intravenous drug user is pyogenic epidural abscess. This infection requires rapid evaluation, rapid commencement of antibiotic therapy, and usually surgical drainage. These patients generally present with an acute (hours) or subacute (days) history, back pain, and leukocytosis or elevated erythrocyte sedimentation rate, although these elements are minor or absent in some patients. Neuroimaging usually distinguishes these diseases.

Metastatic lymphoma can also present with primary meningeal involvement, causing back pain, patchy or ascending radiculopathies, or cranial nerve palsies; in some of these cases compressive or invasive myelopathy is part of the picture.[224] Spinal MRI reveals thickened nerve roots and nodular enhancing lesions within the dura. CSF cytology usually establishes the diagnosis. CMV polyradiculopathy may also be accompanied by spinal cord involvement and clinical myelopathy, and even an MRI picture similar to that seen with enlarged nerve roots.[225] The CSF profile is usually different, however.

▲ NEUROPATHIES

Figure 54–4 outlines a diagnostic approach to the more common neuropathies that complicate HIV-1 infection. The starting point, again, is clinical localization based on the history and examination. Anatomic localization can divide patients into four groups, the first two relating to polyneuropathies with sensory or motor abnormalities predominating and the third and fourth encompassing more focal processes: sacral ascending polyradiculopathy and asymmetrical radiculopathies and neuropathies. Myopathies are included with motor localization in Figure 54–4, but they are discussed in a separate section later in the chapter.

Sensory Polyneuropathies

The sensory polyneuropathies are the most common neuropathies complicating AIDS.[226,227] They characteristically present with distal sensory symptoms: paresthesias, numbness, or pain that begins in the toes or feet and extends proximally. With greater severity the fingertips and hands may be included. These symptoms are usually symmetrical or show only minor asymmetries; and they evolve in a length-dependent fashion. Initial symptoms indicate preferential affliction of the most distal portions of the longest nerves.

The most important neuropathy of this type is distal sensory polyneuropathy (DSP), which appears to be caused in some way by the retrovirus itself and is referred to as HIV-related DSP, among other terms.[228,229] Its pathogenesis is still a matter of speculation because it does not clearly result from direct viral infection of the nerves themselves. A cytokine-mediated toxic pathway has been hypothesized in this disorder similar to that invoked to explain brain injury in ADC.[230] The principal targets of this pathogenetic process are the axon and sensory ganglion cell body rather than the myelin sheath. Hence it is classified among the axonal neuropathies.

Although severity may vary, the presentation of HIV-related DSP is fairly stereotyped. Symptoms of paresthesias and pain usually markedly overshadow disability caused by loss of either sensory or motor function. Thus unless pain is severe, patients walk normally and suffer little or no evident imbalance despite the demonstration of mildly impaired distal sensation (cold, pin, scratch, vibration, position) and depressed or absent ankle jerks. These deficits are thus sufficiently mild that they do not translate into functional incapacity. Characteristically, the earliest sensory symptoms are perceived in the toes or over the anterior plantar surface (the ball) of the foot. With progression the level rises to the foot, the ankle, or beyond. The degree of accompanying pain is curiously variable; patients with equal degrees of sensory loss may have different levels of pain. Most frequently the pain is described as "burning" or "tingling" in type, but sometimes "tightness" is noted. When severe, all skin contact in the affected zone is abhorrent, and patients may not be able to wear shoes, tolerate foot contact with bedclothes, or walk. Some patients also experience superimposed, intermittent "shooting" or "electric" pains.

Treatment usually focuses on symptom relief. The general impression has been that antiretroviral therapy has had little impact on this neuropathy, particularly in alleviating it once it develops. However, as more individuals are being maintained on successful antiviral therapy without viremia or progressive immunosuppression, the incidence is declining, though this issue requires additional study.[12] Another exception to the purely symptomatic approach has been the use of recombinant human nerve growth factor (NGF), a trophic factor involved in the development and maintenance of sensory nerves; results of an initial trial suggest that NGF may have afforded some symptomatic benefit, but the trial failed to document nerve regeneration as assessed by cutaneous nerve density in skin biopsies.[231]

At present the first approach to symptom relief has been with gabapentin given three times a day in escalating dosage.[232–234] Next in line for longer-term management are the tricyclic antidepressants, generally started at low doses (e.g., 10 to 25 mg of amitriptyline at bedtime) and gradually increased; this conservative dosing approach avoids early experience of side effects, which may lead patients to abandon treatment before an adequate trial.[235] Beyond these measures, treatment is more difficult. Some of those with prominent shooting pains benefit from carbamazapine or phenytoin. For others, narcotic analgesics may be necessary.

The second most frequent sensory polyneuropathy is that caused by a group of the antiretroviral nucleosides: zalcitabine, didanosine, and stavudine, in descending order of neurotoxic frequency.[236–242] Whereas some patients with this type of toxic neuropathy complain of "aching" or "deep" pain across the top of the foot rather than the tingling or burning pain of HIV-related DSP, most describe symptoms that are indistinguishable from the latter. This is not surprising because this toxic neuropathy also targets axons. Because of these similar symptoms, the diagnosis may rely on a clear history either of the onset temporally linked to initiation of one of these drugs or of clinical improvement after their discontinuation, perhaps after an initial period of "coasting." The distinction between spontaneous HIV-related DSP and nucleoside neuropathy is of major importance in some patients for whom the toxic neuropathy precludes use of one or more of these active nucleosides as part of drug combinations when alternatives are limited. It is my impression that neuropathy is attributed to these nucleosides by patients and even their clinicians more often than is justified, although there is no doubt that a

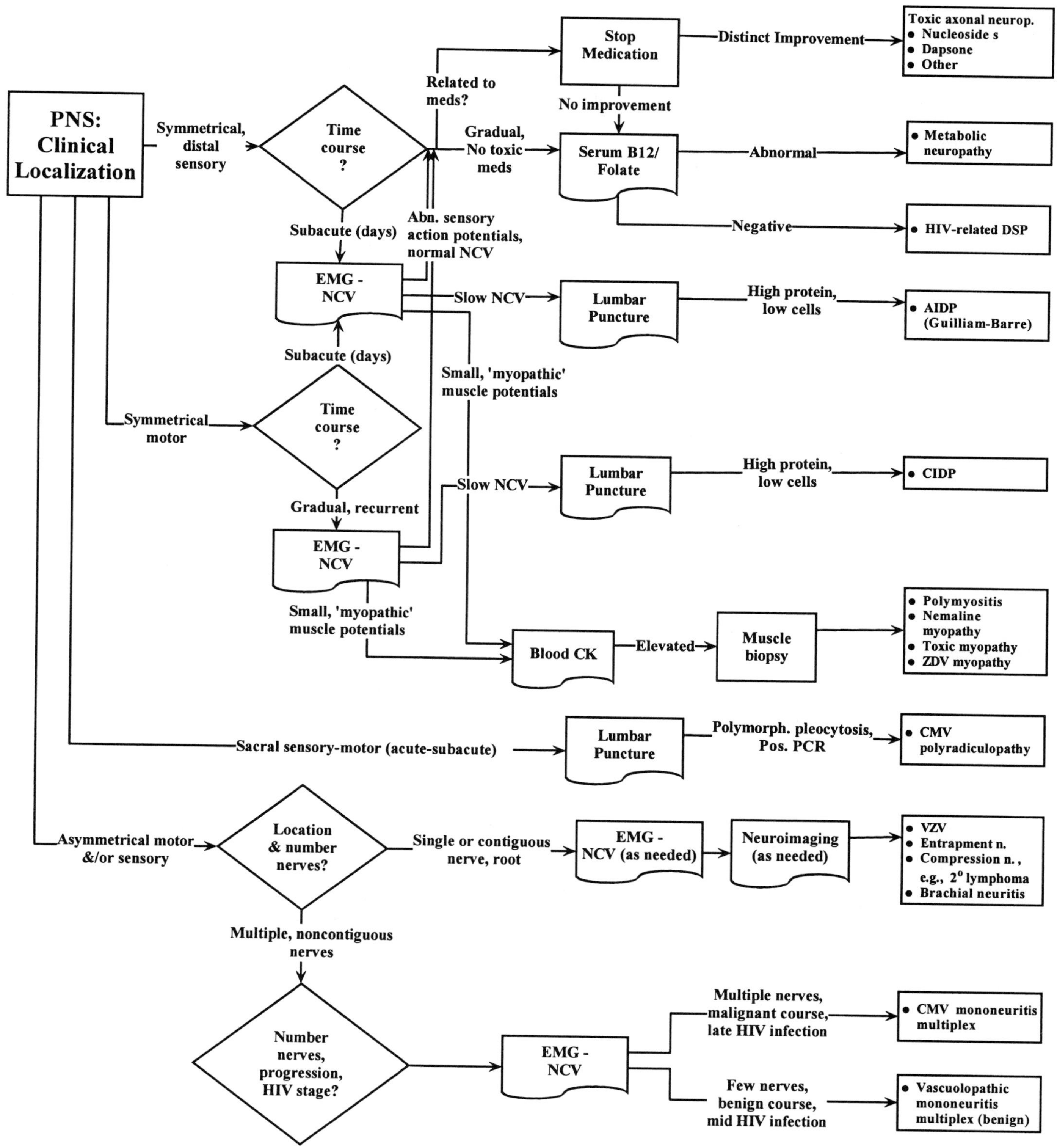

Figure 54–4. Diagnostic approach to peripheral nervous system and muscle diseases in those with an HIV-1 infection. AIDP, acute idiopathic demyelinating polyneuropathy; CIDP, chronic idiopathic demyelinating polyneuropathy; CK, creatine kinase; DSP, distal sensory polyneuropathy; EMG, electromyography; NCV, nerve conduction velocity.

substantial number of patients also have major difficulty with these drugs. Other than stopping the offending drug, symptomatic management is the same as for HIV-related DSP. Among other drugs commonly prescribed for AIDS patients, dapsone can also cause toxic neuropathy, but this usually occurs after longer exposure and affects motor more than sensory function.[243] Thalidomide is also complicated by toxic neuropathy.[244] Patients therefore must be queried regarding their orthodox and supplementary medications; high doses of vitamin B_6, arsenicals, and other substances can rarely underlie the neuropathies in these patients. A vasculitic neuropathy responsive to corticosteroids may present in a manner similar to axonal polyneuropathy.[245] Painful polyneuropathy can also complicate the diffuse infiltrative lymphocytosis syndrome; this syndrome includes Sjögren-like manifestations and may improve with antiretroviral therapy.[246]

In general, electrodiagnostic studies (electromyography and nerve conduction studies) are not necessary for routine diagnosis of these axonal neuropathies. They do not help distinguish HIVR-DSPN from nucleoside toxicity. However, if there is any question of whether complaints of distal extremity pain do or do not relate to neuropathy, or if there are atypical features such as motor weakness, functionally important sensory loss, or major asymmetries in symptoms or signs, electromyography and nerve conduction studies may be helpful.

Motor Polyneuropathies

Because the common axonal neuropathies of HIV-1 infection rarely cause motor impairment, when patients present with weakness other diagnoses must be pursued. The most common types of polyneuropathy causing symmetrical motor weakness relate to underlying demyelination.[226] Presentation may be acute/subacute (Guillain-Barré syndrome or acute idiopathic demyelinating polyneuropathy) or chronic (chronic idiopathic demyelinating polyneuropathy).[247,248] Typically these disorders manifest with weakness that begins distally, most often in the feet. Reflexes are lost, although they may be preserved at initial presentation of acute idiopathic demyelinating polyneuropathy despite weakness, and sensory abnormalities are absent or inconspicuous in relation to the degree of weakness. When severe, these neuropathies can eventuate in ventilatory compromise and may also be accompanied by autonomic instability. Electrodiagnostic studies, when performed after a few weeks, show the characteristic decline in nerve conduction velocity. It is generally thought that these neuropathies have an autoimmune basis and resemble counterparts that occur in the absence of HIV-1 infection. One atypical feature that has been emphasized is the presence of more frequent CSF pleocytosis in the HIV-1 setting; but whether this suggests a pathogenetic difference or simply reflects the high background incidence of pleocytosis accompanying HIV-1 infection generally is uncertain. Although these neuropathies characteristically occur during the early phase of HIV-1 infection, when the CD4+ T-lymphocyte count is above 200/mm^3, they can also complicate more advanced infection. Treatment follows guidelines for non-HIV-associated demyelinating neuropathies and includes intravenous immunoglobulin and plasma exchange, along with supportive therapies.[226,249,250]

Sacral Ascending Polyradiculopathy

One of the most dramatic and devastating neuropathies complicating HIV-1 is the ascending polyradiculitis caused by CMV infection.[87,225,251,252] It characteristically begins abruptly, evolves relatively rapidly (over days), and is often fatal if not treated. Most commonly the initial abnormalities localize to sacral and lumbar nerve roots with sensory, motor, and autonomic dysfunction. Back pain is also common. Patients develop impaired bladder and bowel function, sacral sensory loss, and ascending leg weakness and sensory loss early in the course. These abnormalities then progress rostrally to involve the trunk and arms. Pathologically, the nerve roots and then the spinal cord are involved in CMV infection and inflammatory reaction. The CSF shows a characteristic, and indeed virtually pathognomonic, neutrophil-predominant pleocytosis—a pattern otherwise rare with AIDS. CMV can also be cultured and its nucleic acid sequences detected by amplification techniques in CSF.

Treatment should be started based on clinical grounds and not delayed until these specialized results are available because the outcome depends on how soon treatment starts. Spinal MRI is usually not necessary but when done may show inflammatory arachnoiditis with contrast enhancement and thickening of the nerve roots.[225] This disease most commonly complicates CMV infection that has manifested clinically elsewhere (e.g., the eye or gastrointestinal tract) but can occur as the first clinical presentation of CMV disease. Like other manifestations of CMV infection, the incidence of this condition has decreased markedly. Although the optimal treatment is uncertain and in most cases must take into account previous or ongoing treatment of CMV infection of other organs, most now recommend some type of combined drug therapy (e.g., ganciclovir plus foscarnet). Those treated successfully may not only stop progressing but experience a degree of recovery.[253]

Focal Radiculopathies and Neuropathies

Through the course of its evolution HIV-1 infection can be complicated by a variety of focal neuropathies and radiculopathies. They present with asymmetrical motor and sensory symptoms and signs. Diagnostic evaluation depends on their localization and their pattern of deficits. This begins with clear delineation of whether abnormalities can be attributed to involvement of a single nerve or nerve root or several contiguous or spatially separate nerves are afflicted. This may be evident from the history and examination or may require electrodiagnostic studies for additional clarification and precision. As with other neurologic complications, the stage of HIV-1 infection is an important variable because early in infection the diagnostic probabilities, with a few relatively uncommon exceptions, parallel those of the general population, whereas in late-stage disease complications of HIV-1 assume increasing importance. Cervical and lumbar radiculopathies complicating cervical and lumbar spine degeneration and disc herniation as well as entrapment neuropathies such as carpel tunnel syndrome may occur in the HIV-1-infected patient just as in the noninfected patient.

Among the neuropathic complications occurring earlier in infection that are more specific to patients with HIV-1 infection are brachial neuritis and metastatic systemic lymphoma. The first of these is thought to be an autoimmune disorder but is otherwise pathogenetically obscure. It may complicate or follow shortly upon primary infection and seroconversion or occur later during the "asymptomatic" phase.[254] Onset and evolution are subacute, and the disorder is usually unilateral, presenting as painful weakness in a distribution beyond that of a single root or nerve. Systemic lymphoma complicating early HIV-1 infection can cause a variety of nerve dysfunctions. Just as with systemic lymphoma in the non-AIDS patient, this cancer can compress nerve roots by epidural extension from bony disease or by infiltration into neural foramina and the epidural space.[255,256] Most frequently there is sequential development of local or radicular pain followed by segmental nerve deficit and finally spinal cord compression. It is important to establish the diagnosis during the early phases to prevent irreparable nerve or spinal cord injury and more specifically to relieve pain. Neuroimaging is usually an essential component of diagnosis. Meningeal lymphomatosis may present with radicular or cranial nerve dysfunction.[257]

Recurrent VZV infection (herpes zoster) is perhaps the most common radiculopathy seen during the midphase of HIV-1 infection, but it usually remains a diagnostic question only for the period between the onset of discomfort and appearance of the characteristic rash. Although radicular pain may develop without a rash (zoster sine herpete), it is highly unusual. Cutaneous zoster can also be complicated by myelopathy, as described earlier. Treatment of herpes zoster is described elsewhere in this volume (see Chapter 42).

Isolated unilateral or bilateral facial palsy was recognized as a complication of AIDS early in the epidemic.[223] It may occur in the presence or absence of CSF pleocytosis, and examples have been reported during both the early and late phases of HIV-1 infection. The course appears to be similar to that in individuals without HIV infection.[258–260]

Also important among the focal neuropathies associated with HIV-1 are at least two types of mononeuritis multiplex (a disorder afflicting multiple independent peripheral nerves).[261] One occurs early (CD4+ T-lymphocyte count >200 cells/mm^3) in the course of HIV-1 infection, results in less severe deficits, and appears to be self-limiting.[262] It is presumed to have an immunopathologic basis, and it involves microvascular occlusions. Cryoglobulinemia has also been reported to be associated with vasculitic mononeuritis multiplex in an HIV-infected patient.[263] The more severe type of mononeuritis multiplex occurs later when CD4+ T-lymphocyte counts are low (usually <50 cells/mm^3), assumes a more malignant course, and is caused by CMV infection.[251,264,265] This disease has a penchant for affecting nerves supplying proximal muscles of the shoulder girdle. In the absence of treatment, it is often fatal. The diagnosis is usually based on clinical grounds; and treatment is with anti-CMV therapy using one or more drugs depending on previous CMV infections and treatments. Because the diagnosis may be difficult or slow, patients should be treated aggressively on the basis of the clinical presentation alone.

▲ MYOPATHIES

Several myopathies have been noted to complicate AIDS. They may have inflammatory (polymyositis) and noninflammatory pathology, including nemaline rod myopathy.[266–271] In both instances patients usually present with progressive proximal muscle weakness. Corticosteroid treatment has been the principal treatment of inflammatory myopathy and has been advocated by some for noninflammatory myopathy as well. Zidovudine used to be the most common cause of myopathy in AIDS patients, but this now seems to be uncommon at current dosing and treatment duration.[272–278] The pathogenesis likely relates to an effect of this nucleoside on muscle mitochondria, and some biopsies show ragged red fibers with abnormal-appearing mitochondria. A diagnosis of myopathy is established by the clinical features (pattern of proximal weakness, preservation of reflexes), laboratory findings (elevated creatinine kinase levels in blood), electrodiagnostic studies (small, brief "myopathic" potentials), and histologic analyses. The tests performed and their interpretation depend on the clinical setting, severity, and correlations among these findings. Pyogenic infection, usually caused by *Staphylococcus aureus,* may cause severe myositis; and several other opportunistic infections, including *Toxoplasma gondii, Cryptococcus neoformans,* and *Mycobacterium avium,* have been reported to involve muscle, but usually with less severe or silent clinical manifestations.[226,279]

▲ CONCLUSIONS

On first consideration, the array of neurologic diseases complicating HIV-1 infection and AIDS appears overwhelmingly complex. Although the algorithms outlined in Figures 54–1 through 54–4 may also give this initial impression, with crossing lines and multiple tests, the range of common disorders is actually relatively narrow, and, the diagnosis is straightforward. Following a route from anatomic diagnosis through targeted laboratory testing leads to a confirmed or high-probability presumptive diagnosis to guide therapy in perhaps 90% or more of cases, which are comprised largely of the common diseases discussed here. In the remaining 10% or so, diagnosis may be more difficult either because the clinical presentation is atypical or because the patient actually has a rarer condition. Finally, in a few patients the diagnosis is something previously unreported or it eludes all efforts because the complete map of neurologic diseases complicating HIV-1 has not been drawn in detail. This should lead the clinician to a continuous sense of discovery and challenge in these patients, for whom an exact diagnosis may importantly prolong the duration and quality of life. Even when treatment is not available, an informed prognosis allows patients, their families, and their caregivers to plan the future. Although neurologic disability often leads to therapeutic nihilism because of the patient's momentary incapacity, this is not always justified and should not take place in the face of diagnostic ignorance.

REFERENCES

1. Harrison MJG, McArthur JC. AIDS and Neurology. New York, Churchill Livingstone, 1995.
2. Price RW. Management of the neurological complications of HIV-1 and AIDS. In: Sande MA, Volberding PA (eds) The Medical Management of AIDS, 6th ed. Philadelphia, WB Saunders, 1999, p 217.
3. Berger JR, Levy RM. AIDS and the Nervous System, 2nd ed. Philadelphia, Lippincott-Raven, 1997.
4. Gendelman HE, Lipton SA, Epstein L, et al. The Neurology of AIDS. New York: Chapman & Hall, 1998.
5. Marra CM. Bacterial and fungal brain infections in AIDS. Semin Neurol 19:177, 1999.
6. Ammassari A, Cingolani A, Pezzotti P, et al. AIDS-related focal brain lesions in the era of highly active antiretroviral therapy. Neurology 55:1194, 2000.
7. Brew BJ. HIV Neurology, vol 61. New York, Oxford University Press, 2001.
8. Detels R, Tarwater P, Phair JP, et al. Effectiveness of potent antiretroviral therapies on the incidence of opportunistic infections before and after AIDS diagnosis. AIDS 15:347, 2001.
9. Lee LM, Karon JM, Selik R, et al. Survival after AIDS diagnosis in adolescents and adults during the treatment era, United States, 1984–1997. JAMA 285:1308, 2001.
10. Berrey MM, Schacker T, Collier AC, et al. Treatment of primary human immunodeficiency virus type 1 infection with potent antiretroviral therapy reduces frequency of rapid progression to AIDS. J Infect Dis 183:1466, 2001.
11. Sacktor N, Lyles RH, Skolasky R, et al. HIV-associated neurologic disease incidence changes: Multicenter AIDS Cohort Study, 1990–1998. Neurology 56:257, 2001.
12. Maschke M, Kastrup O, Esser S, et al. Incidence and prevalence of neurological disorders associated with HIV since the introduction of highly active antiretroviral therapy (HAART). J Neurol Neurosurg Psychiatry 69:376, 2000.
13. D'Arminio Monforte A, Duca PG, Vago L, et al. Decreasing incidence of CNS AIDS-defining events associated with antiretroviral therapy. Neurology 54:1856, 2000.
14. Brew BJ, Dore G. Decreasing incidence of CNS AIDS defining events associated with antiretroviral therapy. Neurology 55:1424, 2000.
15. Lanska DJ. Epidemiology of human immunodeficiency virus infection and associated neurologic illness. Semin Neurol 19:105, 1999.
16. Janssen RS, Cornblath DR, Epstein LG, et al. Human immunodeficiency virus (HIV) infection and the nervous system: report from the American Academy of Neurology AIDS Task Force. Neurology 39:119, 1989.
17. Organization WH. 1990 World Health Organization consultation on the neuropsychiatric aspects of HIV-1 infection. AIDS 935, 1990.
18. Belman AL. Infants, children and adolescents. In: Berger JR, Levy RM (eds) AIDS and the Nervous System, 2nd ed. Philadelphia, Lippincott-Raven, 1997, pp 223.
19. Mintz M. Clinical features and treatment interventions for human immunodeficiency virus-associated neurologic disease in children. Semin Neurol 19:165, 1999.
20. Navia B, Jordan B, Price R. The AIDS dementia complex. I. Clinical features. Ann Neurol 19:517, 1986.
21. Price R, Brew B, Sidtis J, et al. The brain in AIDS: central nervous system HIV-1 infection and AIDS dementia complex. Science 239:586, 1988.
22. Price R. Neurological complications of HIV infection. Lancet 348:445, 1996.
23. Epstein LG, Gendelman HE. Human immunodeficiency virus type 1 infection of the nervous system: pathogenetic mechanisms. Ann Neurol 33:429, 1993.
24. Zheng J, Gendelman HE. The HIV-1 associated dementia complex: a metabolic encephalopathy fueled by viral replication in mononuclear phagocytes. Curr Opin Neurol 10:319, 1997.
25. Wesselingh SL, Thompson KA. Immunopathogenesis of HIV-associated dementia. Curr Opin Neurol 14:375, 2001.
26. Thompson KA, McArthur JC, Wesselingh SL. Correlation between neurological progression and astrocyte apoptosis in HIV-associated dementia. Ann Neurol 49:745, 2001.
27. Nath A, Haughey NJ, Jones M, et al. Synergistic neurotoxicity by human immunodeficiency virus proteins Tat and gp120: protection by memantine. Ann Neurol 47:186, 2000.
28. Kaul M, Garden GA, Lipton SA. Pathways to neuronal injury and apoptosis in HIV-associated dementia. Nature 410:988, 2001.
29. Price R, Brew B. The AIDS dementia complex. J Infect Dis 158:1079, 1988.
30. Sidtis JJ, Price RW. Early HIV-1 infection and the AIDS dementia complex. Neurology 40:323, 1990.
31. Benson D. The spectrum of dementia: a comparison of the clinical features of AIDS dementia and dementia of the Alzheimer's type. Alzheimer Dis Assoc Dis 1:217, 1987.
32. Gray F. [Dementia and human immunodeficiency virus infection.] Rev Neurol (Paris) 154(suppl 2):S91, 1998.
33. Lopez OL, Smith G, Meltzer CC, et al. Dopamine systems in human immunodeficiency virus-associated dementia. Neuropsychiatry Neuropsychol Behav Neurol 12:184, 1999.
34. Castellon SA, Hinkin CH, Myers HF. Neuropsychiatric disturbance is associated with executive dysfunction in HIV-1 infection. J Int Neuropsychol Soc 6:336, 2000.
35. McArthur JC, Selnes OA. Human immunodeficiency virus-associated dementia. In: Berger JR, Levy RM (eds) AIDS and the Nervous System, 2nd ed. Philadelphia, Lippincott-Raven, 1997, p 527.
36. Price RW. The AIDS dementia complex and human immunodeficiency virus type 1 infection of the central nervous system. In: Aminoff MJ, Goetz CG (eds) Handbook of Clinical Neurology, Systemic Diseases, Part III vol 71. Amsterdam, Elsevier Science, 1998, pp 235–260.
37. Sidtis JJ. Evaluation of the AIDS dementia complex in adults. Res Pub Assoc Res Nerv Mental Dis 72:273, 1994.
38. Dal Pan GJ, McArthur JH, Aylward E, et al. Patterns of cerebral atrophy in HIV-1-infected individuals: results of a quantitative MRI analysis. Neurology 42:2125, 1992.
39. Gelman B, Guinto FJ. Morphometry, histopathology, and tomography of cerebral atrophy in the acquired immunodeficiency syndrome. Ann Neurol 31:32, 1992.
40. Post MJ. Fluid-attenuated inversion-recovery fast spin-echo MR: a clinically useful tool in the evaluation of neurologically symptomatic HIV- positive patients. AJNR Am J Neuroradiol 18:1611, 1997.
41. Tracey I, Carr CA, Guimaraes AR, et al. Brain choline-containing compounds are elevated in HIV-positive patients before the onset of AIDS dementia complex: a proton magnetic resonance spectroscopic study. Neurology 46:783, 1996.
42. Ernst T, Itti E, Itti L, et al. Changes in cerebral metabolism are detected prior to perfusion changes in early HIV-CMC: a coregistered ^{1}H MRS and SPECT study. J Magn Reson Imaging 12:859, 2000.
43. Chang L, Ernst T, Leonido-Yee M, et al. Cerebral metabolite abnormalities correlate with clinical severity of HIV-1 cognitive motor complex. Neurology 52:100, 1999.
44. Chang L, Ernst T, Leonido-Yee M, et al. Highly active antiretroviral therapy reverses brain metabolite abnormalities in mild HIV dementia. Neurology 53:782, 1999.
45. Moller HE, Vermathen P, Lentschig MG, et al. Metabolic characterization of AIDS dementia complex by spectroscopic imaging. J Magn Reson Imaging 9:10, 1999.
46. Brew B, Bhalla R, Paul M, et al. Cerebrospinal fluid neopterin in human immunodeficiency virus type 1 infection. Ann Neurol 28:556, 1990.
47. Griffin DE, McArthur JC, Cornblath DR. Neopterin and interferon-gamma in serum and cerebrospinal fluid of patients with HIV-associated neurologic disease. Neurology 41:69, 1991.
48. Brew BJ, Bhalla RB, Paul M, et al. Cerebrospinal fluid beta 2-microglobulin in patients with AIDS dementia complex: an expanded series including response to zidovudine treatment. AIDS 6:461, 1992.
49. Heyes MP, Brew BJ, Saito K, et al. Inter-relationships between quinolinic acid, neuroactive kynurenines, neopterin and beta 2-microglobulin in cerebrospinal fluid and serum of HIV-1-infected patients. J Neuroimmunol 40:71, 1992.
50. McArthur JC, Nance-Sproson TE, Griffin DE, et al. The diagnostic utility of elevation in cerebrospinal fluid beta 2-microglobulin in HIV-1 dementia: Multicenter AIDS Cohort Study. Neurology 42:1707, 1992.
51. Kelder W, McArthur JC, Nance-Sproson T, et al. Beta-chemokines MCP-1 and RANTES are selectively increased in cerebrospinal fluid of patients with human immunodeficiency virus-associated dementia. Ann Neurol 44:831, 1998.
52. Conant K, McArthur JC, Griffin DE, et al. Cerebrospinal fluid levels of MMP-2, 7, and 9 are elevated in association with human immunodeficiency virus dementia. Ann Neurol 46:391, 1999.

53. Brew B, Pemberton L, Cunningham P, et al. Levels of human immunodeficiency virus type 1 RNA in cerebrospinal fluid correlate with AIDS dementia stage. J Infect Dis 175:963, 1997.
54. Cinque P, Vago L, Ceresa D, et al. Cerebrospinal fluid HIV-1 RNA levels: correlation with HIV encephalitis. AIDS 12:389, 1998.
55. Ellis RJ, Hsia K, Spector SA, et al. Cerebrospinal fluid human immunodeficiency virus type 1 RNA levels are elevated in neurocognitively impaired individuals with acquired immunodeficiency syndrome: HIV Neurobehavioral Research Center Group. Ann Neurol 42:679, 1997.
56. McArthur JC, McClernon DR, Cronin MF, et al. Relationship between human immunodeficiency virus-associated dementia and viral load in cerebrospinal fluid and brain. Ann Neurol 42:689, 1997.
57. Price RW, Staprans S. Measuring the "viral load" in cerebrospinal fluid in human immunodeficiency virus infection: window into brain infection [editorial]? Ann Neurol 42:675, 1997.
58. Schmitt F, Bigleg J, McKinnis R, et al. Neuropsychological outcome of azidothymidine (AZT) in the treatment of AIDS and AIDS-related complex: a double blind, placebo-controlled trial. N Engl J Med 319:1573, 1988.
59. Sidtis JJ, Gatsonis C, Price RW, et al. Zidovudine treatment of the AIDS dementia complex: results of a placebo-controlled trial: AIDS Clinical Trials Group. Ann Neurol 33:343, 1993.
60. Brouwers P, Moss H, Wolters P, et al. Effect of continuous-infusion zidovudine therapy on neuropsychologic functioning in children with symptomatic human immunodeficiency virus infection. J Pediatr 116:980, 1990.
61. Gray F, Belec L, Keohane C, et al. Zidovudine therapy and HIV encephalitis: a 10-year neuropathological survey. AIDS 8:489, 1994.
62. Galgani S, Balestra P, Narciso P, et al. Nimodipine plus zidovudine versus zidovudine alone in the treatment of HIV-1-associated cognitive deficits [letter]. AIDS 11:1520, 1997.
63. Chiesi A, Vella S, Dally LG, et al. Epidemiology of AIDS dementia complex in Europe: AIDS in Europe Study Group. J Acquir Immune Defic Syn Hum Retrovirol 11:39, 1996.
64. Baldeweg T, Catalan J, Lovett E, et al. Long-term zidovudine reduces neurocognitive deficits in HIV-1 infection. AIDS 9:589, 1995.
65. Portegies P. Review of antiretroviral therapy in the prevention of HIV-related AIDS dementia complex ADC. Drugs 49 (suppl): 125, 1995.
66. Sacktor NC, Lyles RH, Skolasky RL, et al. Combination antiretroviral therapy improves psychomotor speed performance in HIV-seropositive homosexual men: Multicenter AIDS Cohort Study (MACS). Neurology 52:1640, 1999.
67. Filippi CG, Sze G, Farber SJ, et al. Regression of HIV encephalopathy and basal ganglia signal intensity abnormality at MR imaging in patients with AIDS after the initiation of protease inhibitor therapy. Radiology 206:491, 1998.
68. Price R. Management of AIDS dementia complex and HIV-1 infection of the nervous system. AIDS 9(suppl A):S221, 1995.
69. Burger D, Kraaijeveld C, Meenhorst P, et al. Penetration of zidovudine into the cerebrospinal fluid of patients infected with HIV. AIDS 7:1581, 1993.
70. Foudraine N, De Wolf F, Hoetelmans R, et al. CSF and serum HIV-RNA levels during AZT/3TC and d4T/3TC treatment. Presented at the 4th Conference on Retroviruses and Opportunistic Infections, Washington, DC, 1997.
71. Collier A, Marra C, Coombs R. Cerebrospinal fluid (CSF) HIV RNA levels in patients on chronic indinavir therapy [abstract 22]. In: Abstracts of the Infectious Diseases Society of America, 35th Annual Meeting, San Francisco, 1997.
72. Zhang L, Price R, Aweeka F, et al. Making the most of sparse clinical data by using a predictive-model-based analysis, illustrated with a stavudine pharmacokinetic study. Eur J Pharm Sci 12:377, 2001.
73. Lanier ER, Sturge G, McClernon D, et al. HIV-1 reverse transcriptase sequence in plasma and cerebrospinal fluid of patients with AIDS dementia complex treated with abacavir. AIDS 15:747, 2001.
74. Van Praag RM, Weverling GJ, Portegies P, et al. Enhanced penetration of indinavir in cerebrospinal fluid and semen after the addition of low-dose ritonavir. AIDS 14:1187, 2000.
75. Gisolf EH, Enting RH, Jurriaans S, et al. Cerebrospinal fluid HIV-1 RNA during treatment with ritonavir/saquinavir or ritonavir/saquinavir/stavudine. AIDS 14:1583, 2000.
76. Enting RH, Foudraine NA, Lange JM, et al. Cerebrospinal fluid beta2-microglobulin, monocyte chemotactic protein-1, and soluble tumour necrosis factor alpha receptors before and after treatment with lamivudine plus zidovudine or stavudine. J Neuroimmunol 102:216, 2000.
77. Albright AV, Erickson-Viitanen S, O'Connor M, et al. Efavirenz is a potent nonnucleoside reverse transcriptase inhibitor of HIV type 1 replication in microglia in vitro. AIDS Res Hum Retroviruses 16:1527, 2000.
78. Sawchuk RJ, Yang Z. Investigation of distribution, transport and uptake of anti-HIV drugs to the central nervous system. Adv Drug Deliv Rev 39(1-3):5, 1999.
79. Thomas SA, Segal MB. The transport of the anti-HIV drug, 2′,3′-didehydro-3′-deoxythymidine (d4T), across the blood-brain and blood-cerebrospinal fluid barriers. Br J Pharmacol 125:49, 1998.
80. Gisslen M, Svennerholm B, Fuchs D, et al. Neurological efficacy of stavudine, zidovudine, and lamivudine. Lancet 352:402, 1998.
81. Foudraine NA, Hoetelmans RM, Lange JM, et al. Cerebrospinal-fluid HIV-1 RNA and drug concentrations after treatment with lamivudine plus zidovudine or stavudine. Lancet 351:1547, 1998.
82. Brew BJ. Neurological efficacy of stavudine, zidovudine, and lamivudine. Lancet 352:402, 1998.
83. Portegies P. HIV-1, the brain, and combination therapy. Lancet 346:1244, 1995.
84. Clifford DB. Human immunodeficiency virus-associated dementia. Arch Neurol 57:321, 2000.
85. Navia BA, Dafni U, Simpson D, et al. A phase I/II trial of nimodipine for HIV-related neurologic complications. Neurology 51:221, 1998.
86. A randomized, double-blind, placebo-controlled trial of deprenyl and thioctic acid in human immunodeficiency virus-associated cognitive impairment: Dana Consortium on the Therapy of HIV Dementia and Related Cognitive Disorders. Neurology 50:645, 1998.
87. Fuller GN. Cytomegalovirus and the peripheral nervous system in AIDS. J Acquir Immune Defic Syndr 5:S33, 1992.
88. Holland NR, Power C, Mathews VP, et al. Cytomegalovirus encephalitis in acquired immunodeficiency syndrome (AIDS). Neurology 44:507, 1994.
89. Kalayjian RC, Cohen ML, Bonomo RA, et al. Cytomegalovirus ventriculoencephalitis in AIDS: a syndrome with distinct clinical and pathologic features. Medicine 72:67, 1993.
90. Cohen B, Dix R. Cytomegalovirus and other herpesviruses. In: Berger J, Levy R (eds) AIDS and the Nervous System, 2nd ed. Philadelphia, Lippincott-Raven, 1997, p 595.
91. McCutchan JA. Clinical impact of cytomegalovirus infections of the nervous system in patients with AIDS. Clin Infect Dis 21(suppl 2):S196, 1995.
92. Setinek U, Wondrusch E, Jellinger K, et al. Cytomegalovirus infection of the brain in AIDS: a clinicopathological study. Acta Neuropathol (Berl) 90:511, 1995.
93. Salazar A, Podzamczer D, Rene R, et al. Cytomegalovirus ventriculoencephalitis in AIDS patients. Scand J Infect Dis 27:165, 1995.
94. Cinque P, Cleator GM, Weber T, et al. Diagnosis and clinical management of neurological disorders caused by cytomegalovirus in AIDS patients: European Union Concerted Action on Virus Meningitis and Encephalitis. J Neurovirol 4:120, 1998.
95. Petito C, Cho E-S, Lemann W, et al. Neuropathology of acquired immunodeficiency syndrome (AIDS): an autopsy review. J Neuropathol Exp Neurol 45:635, 1986.
96. Gray F, Belec L, Geny C, et al. [Diagnosis of diffuse encephalopathies in adults with HIV infection. I.] Presse Med 22:1226, 1993.
97. Bell JE. The neuropathology of adult HIV infection. Rev Neurol (Paris) 154:816, 1998.
98. Miller RF, Lucas SB, Hall-Craggs MA, et al. Comparison of magnetic resonance imaging with neuropathological findings in the diagnosis of HIV and CMV associated CNS disease in AIDS. J Neurol Neurosurg Psychiatry 62:346, 1997.
99. Masdeu JC, Small CB, Weiss L, et al. Multifocal cytomegalovirus encephalitis in AIDS. Ann Neurol 23:97, 1988.
100. Gozlan J, el Amrani M, Baudrimont M, et al. A prospective evaluation of clinical criteria and polymerase chain reaction assay of cerebrospinal fluid for the diagnosis of cytomegalovirus-related neurological diseases during AIDS. AIDS 9:253, 1995.
101. Arribas JR, Clifford DB, Fichtenbaum CJ, et al. Level of cytomegalovirus CMV DNA in cerebrospinal fluid of subjects with AIDS and CMV infection of the central nervous system. J Infect Dis 172:527, 1995.

102. Cinque P, Vago L, Dahl H, et al. Polymerase chain reaction on cerebrospinal fluid for diagnosis of virus-associated opportunistic diseases of the central nervous system in HIV-infected patients. AIDS 10:951, 1996.
103. Bestetti A, Pierotti C, Terreni M, et al. Comparison of three nucleic acid amplification assays of cerebrospinal fluid for diagnosis of cytomegalovirus encephalitis. J Clin Microbiol 39:1148, 2001.
104. Zhang F, Tetali S, Wang XP, et al. Detection of human cytomegalovirus pp67 late gene transcripts in cerebrospinal fluid of human immunodeficiency virus type 1-infected patients by nucleic acid sequence-based amplification. J Clin Microbiol 38:1920, 2000.
105. Navia B, Petito C, Gold J, et al. Cerebral toxoplasmosis complicating the acquired immune deficiency syndrome: clinical and neuropathological findings in 27 patients. Ann Neurol 19:224, 1986.
106. Gray F, Gherardi R, Wingate E, et al. Diffuse "encephalitic" cerebral toxoplasmosis in AIDS: report of four cases. J Neurol 236:273, 1989.
107. Chrâetien F, Bâelec L, Hilton DA, et al. Herpes simplex virus type 1 encephalitis in acquired immunodeficiency syndrome. Neuropathol Appl Neurobiol 223:394, 1996.
108. Hamilton RL, Achim C, Grafe MR, et al. Herpes simplex virus brainstem encephalitis in an AIDS patient. Clin Neuropathol 14:45, 1995.
109. Chretien F, Belec L, Wingerstmann L, et al. [Central nervous system infection due to herpes simplex virus in AIDS.] Arch Anat Cytol Pathol 45:153, 1997.
110. Cinque P, Vago L, Marenzi R, et al. Herpes simplex virus infections of the central nervous system in human immunodeficiency virus-infected patients: clinical management by polymerase chain reaction assay of cerebrospinal fluid. Clin Infect Dis 27:303, 1998.
111. Saag MS, Graybill RJ, Larsen RA, et al. Practice guidelines for the management of cryptococcal disease: Infectious Diseases Society of America. Clin Infect Dis 30:710, 2000.
112. Lipton RB, Feraru ER, Weiss G, et al. Headache in HIV-1-related disorders. Headache 31:518, 1991.
113. Lorenz KA, Shapiro MF, Asch SM, et al. Associations of symptoms and health-related quality of life: findings from a national study of persons with HIV infection. Ann Intern Med 134:854, 2001.
114. Graham IC, Wippold IF. Headache in the HIV patient: a review with special attention to the role of imaging. Cephalalgia 21:169, 2001.
115. Gifford AL, Hecht FM. Evaluating HIV-infected patients with headache: who needs computed tomography? Headache 41:441, 2001.
116. Hewitt DJ, McDonald M, Portenoy RK, et al. Pain syndromes and etiologies in ambulatory AIDS patients. Pain 70:117, 1997.
117. Singer EJ, Kim J, Fahy-Chandon B, et al. Headache in ambulatory HIV-1-infected men enrolled in a longitudinal study. Neurology 47:487, 1996.
118. Berger JR, Stein N, Pall L. Headache and human immunodeficiency virus infection: a case control study. Eur Neurol 36:229, 1996.
119. Hollander H, Stringari S. Human immunodeficiency virus-associated meningitis: clinical course and correlations. Am J Med 83:813, 1987.
120. Hollander H, McGuire D, Burack JH. Diagnostic lumbar puncture in HIV-infected patients: analysis of 138 cases. Am J Med 96:223, 1994.
121. Price RW, Paxinos EE, Grant RM, et al. Cerebrospinal fluid response to structured treatment interruption after virological failure. AIDS 15:1251, 2001.
122. Staprans S, Marlowe N, Glidden D, et al. Time course of cerebrospinal fluid responses to antiretroviral therapy: evidence for variable compartmentalization of infection. AIDS 13:1051, 1999.
123. Brew BJ, Miller J. Human immunodeficiency virus-related headache. Neurology 43:1098, 1993.
124. Holloway RG, Kieburtz KD. Headache and the human immunodeficiency virus type 1 infection. Headache 35:245, 1995.
125. Trotot PM, Vazeux R, Yamashita HK, et al. MRI pattern of progressive multifocal leukoencephalopathy (PML) in AIDS: pathological correlations. J Neuroradiol 17:233, 1990.
126. Thurnher MM, Thurnher SA, Meuhlbauer B, et al. Progressive multifocal leukoencephalopathy in AIDS: initial and follow-up CT and MRI. Neuroradiology 39:611, 1997.
127. Von Giesen HJ, Neuen-Jacob E, Dorries K, et al. Diagnostic criteria and clinical procedures in HIV-1 associated progressive multifocal leukoencephalopathy. J Neurol Sci 147:63, 1997.
128. Post MJ, Yiannoutsos C, Simpson D, et al. Progressive multifocal leukoencephalopathy in AIDS: are there any MR findings useful to patient management and predictive of patient survival? AIDS Clinical Trials Group, 243 Team. AJNR Am J Neuroradiol 20:1896, 1999.
129. Berger J, Lorraine P, Lanska D, et al. Progressive multifocal leukoencephalopathy in patients with HIV infection. J Neurovirol 4:59, 1998.
130. Tornatore C, Berger JR, Houff SA, et al. Detection of JC virus DNA in peripheral lymphocytes from patients with and without progressive multifocal leukoencephalopathy. Ann Neurol 31:454, 1992.
131. Hammarin AL, Bogdanovic G, Svedhem V, et al. Analysis of PCR as a tool for detection of JC virus DNA in cerebrospinal fluid for diagnosis of progressive multifocal leukoencephalopathy. J Clin Microbiol 34:2929, 1996.
132. Matsiota-Bernard P, De Truchis P, Gray F, et al. JC virus detection in the cerebrospinal fluid of AIDS patients with progressive multifocal leucoencephalopathy and monitoring of the antiviral treatment by a PCR method. J Med Microbiol 46:256, 1997.
133. Garcia de Viedma D, Alonso R, Miralles P, et al. Dual qualitative-quantitative nested PCR for detection of JC virus in cerebrospinal fluid: high potential for evaluation and monitoring of progressive multifocal leukoencephalopathy in AIDS patients receiving highly active antiretroviral therapy. J Clin Microbiol 37:724, 1999.
134. Antinori A, Ammassari A, De Luca A, et al. Diagnosis of AIDS-related focal brain lesions: a decision-making analysis based on clinical and neuroradiologic characteristics combined with polymerase chain reaction assays in CSF. Neurology 48:687, 1997.
135. Yiannoutsos CT, Major EO, Curfman B, et al. Relation of JC virus DNA in the cerebrospinal fluid to survival in acquired immunodeficiency syndrome patients with biopsy-proven progressive multifocal leukoencephalopathy. Ann Neurol 45:816, 1999.
136. Berger J, Mucke L. Prolonged survival and partial recovery in AIDS-associated progressive multifocal leukoencephalopathy. Neurology 38:1060, 1988.
137. Garrels K, Kucharczyk W, Wortzman G, et al. Progressive multifocal leukoencephalopathy: clinical and MR response to treatment. AJNR Am J Neuroradiol 17:597, 1996.
138. Berger JR, Concha M. Progressive multifocal leukoencephalopathy: the evolution of a disease once considered rare. J Neurovirol 1:5, 1995.
139. Domingo P, Guardiola JM, Iranzo A, et al. Remission of progressive multifocal leucoencephalopathy after antiretroviral therapy [letter]. Lancet 349:1554, 1997.
140. Baldeweg T, Catalan J. Remission of progressive multifocal leucoencephalopathy after antiretroviral therapy [letter]. Lancet 349:1554, 1997.
141. Elliot B, Aromin I, Gold R, et al. 2.5 Year remission of AIDS-associated progressive multifocal leukoencephalopathy with combined antiretroviral therapy [letter]. Lancet 349:850, 1997.
142. Albrecht H, Hoffmann C, Degen O, et al. Highly active antiretroviral therapy significantly improves the prognosis of patients with HIV-associated progressive multifocal leukoencephalopathy. AIDS 12:1149, 1998.
143. Hall CD, Dafni U, Simpson D, et al. Failure of cytarabine in progressive multifocal leukoencephalopathy associated with human immunodeficiency virus infection: AIDS Clinical Trials Group 243 Team. N Engl J Med 338:1345, 1998.
144. Houston S, Roberts N, Mashinter L. Failure of cidofovir therapy in progressive multifocal leukoencephalopathy unrelated to human immunodeficiency virus. Clin Infect Dis 32:150, 2001.
145. Happe S, Besselmann M, Matheja P, et al. [Cidofovir (vistide) in therapy of progressive multifocal leukoencephalopathy in AIDS: review of the literature and report of 2 cases.] Nervenarzt 70:935, 1999.
146. De Luca A, Fantoni M, Tartaglione T, et al. Response to cidofovir after failure of antiretroviral therapy alone in AIDS-associated progressive multifocal leukoencephalopathy. Neurology 52:891, 1999.
147. Israelski DM, Chmiel JS, Poggensee L, et al. Prevalence of Toxoplasma infection in a cohort of homosexual men at risk of AIDS and toxoplasmic encephalitis. J Acquir Immune Defic Syndr 6:414, 1993.
148. Grant I, Gold J, Rosemblum M, et al. Toxoplasma gondii serology in HIV-infected patients: the development of central nervous system toxoplasmosis in AIDS. AIDS 4:519, 1990.
149. Belanger F, Derouin F, Grangeot-Keros L, et al. Incidence and risk factors of toxoplasmosis in a cohort of human immunodeficiency virus-infected patients: 1988–1995; HEMOCO and SEROCO study groups. Clin Infect Dis 28:575, 1999.
150. Laissy JP, Soyer P, Tebboune J, et al. Contrast-enhanced fast MRI in differentiating brain toxoplasmosis and lymphoma in AIDS patients. J Comput Assist Tomogr 18:714, 1994.

151. Brightbill TC, Post MJ, Hensley GT, et al. MR of Toxoplasma encephalitis: signal characteristics on T2-weighted images and pathologic correlation. J Comput Assist Tomogr 20:417, 1996.
152. Hawkins CP, McLaughlin JE, Kendall BE, et al. Pathological findings correlated with MRI in HIV infection. Neuroradiology 35:264, 1993.
153. D'Arminio Monforte A, Cinque P, Vago L, et al. A comparison of brain biopsy and CSF-PCR in the diagnosis of CNS lesions in AIDS patients. J Neurol 244:35, 1997.
154. Antinori A, De Rossi G, Ammassari A, et al. Value of combined approach with thallium-201 single-photon emission computed tomography and Epstein-Barr virus DNA polymerase chain reaction in CSF for the diagnosis of AIDS-related primary CNS lymphoma. J Clin Oncol 17:554, 1999.
155. DeAngelis L. Primary CNS lymphoma: a new clinical challenge. Neurology 41:619, 1991.
156. Hoffman JM, Waskin HA, Schifter T, et al. FDG-PET in differentiating lymphoma from nonmalignant central nervous system lesions in patients with AIDS. J Nucl Med 34:567, 1993.
157. Lorberboym M, Estok L, Machac J, et al. Rapid differential diagnosis of cerebral toxoplasmosis and primary central nervous system lymphoma by thallium-201 SPECT. J Nucl Med 37:1150, 1996.
158. Catafau AM, Sola M, Lomena FJ, et al. Hyperperfusion and early technetium-99m-HMPAO SPECT appearance of central nervous system toxoplasmosis. J Nucl Med 35:1041, 1994.
159. Skiest DJ, Erdman W, Chang WE, et al. SPECT thallium-201 combined with Toxoplasma serology for the presumptive diagnosis of focal central nervous system mass lesions in patients with AIDS. J Infect 40:274, 2000.
160. Simone IL, Federico F, Tortorella C, et al. Localised ^{1}H-MR spectroscopy for metabolic characterisation of diffuse and focal brain lesions in patients infected with HIV. J Neurol Neurosurg Psychiatry 64:516, 1998.
161. Lorberboym M, Wallach F, Estok L, et al. Thallium-201 retention in focal intracranial lesions for differential diagnosis of primary lymphoma and nonmalignant lesions in AIDS patients. J Nucl Med 39:1366, 1998.
162. Chang L, Ernst T. MR spectroscopy and diffusion-weighted MR imaging in focal brain lesions in AIDS. Neuroimaging Clin North Am 7:409, 1997.
163. Ernst TM, Chang L, Witt MD, et al. Cerebral toxoplasmosis and lymphoma in AIDS: perfusion MR imaging experience in 13 patients. Radiology 208:663, 1998.
164. Farrar DJ, Flanigan TP, Gordon NM, et al. Tuberculous brain abscess in a patient with HIV infection: case report and review. Am J Med 102:297, 1997.
165. Folgueira L, Delgado R, Palenque E, et al. Polymerase chain reaction for rapid diagnosis of tuberculous meningitis in AIDS patients. Neurology 44:1336, 1994.
166. Kim J, Minamoto GY, Grieco MH. Nocardial infection as a complication of AIDS: report of six cases and review. Rev Infect Dis 13:624, 1991.
167. Jones N, Khoosal M, Louw M, et al. Nocardial infection as a complication of HIV in South Africa. J Infect 41:232, 2000.
168. Neal JW, Llewelyn MB, Morrison HL, et al. A malignant astrocytoma in a patient with AIDS: a possible association between astrocytomas and HIV infection. J Infect 33:159, 1996.
169. Vannemreddy PS, Fowler M, Polin RS, et al. Glioblastoma multiforme in a case of acquired immunodeficiency syndrome: investigation a possible oncogenic influence of human immunodeficiency virus on glial cells: case report and review of the literature. J Neurosurg 92:161, 2000.
170. Dyer JR, French MA, Mallal SA. Cerebral mass lesions due to cytomegalovirus in patients with AIDS: report of two cases. J Infect 30:147, 1995.
171. Mylonakis E, Paliou M, Sax PE, et al. Central nervous system aspergillosis in patients with human immunodeficiency virus infection: report of 6 cases and review. Medicine 79:269, 2000.
172. Stevens DA. Management of systemic manifestations of fungal disease in patients with AIDS. J Am Acade Dermatol 31:S64, 1994.
173. Viswanathan R, Ironside J, Bell JE, et al. Stereotaxic brain biopsy in AIDS patients: does it contribute to patient management? Br J Neurosurg 8:307, 1994.
174. Nielsen CJ, Gjerris F, Pedersen H, et al. Brain biopsy in AIDS: diagnostic value and consequence. Acta Neurochir (Wien) 127:99, 1994.
175. Andrews BT, Kenefick TP. Neurosurgical management of the acquired immunodeficiency syndrome: an update. West J Med 158:249, 1993.
176. Miszkiel KA, Hall-Craggs MA, Miller RF, et al. The spectrum of MRI findings in CNS cryptococcosis in AIDS. Clin Radiol 51842, 1996.
177. Garcia CA, Weisberg LA, Lacorte WS. Cryptococcal intracerebral mass lesions: CT-pathologic considerations. Neurology 35731, 1985.
178. McGuire D, Bromley E, Aberg J, et al. Focal posterior hemisphere invasive cryptococcal encephalitis: a distinct neuroimaging entity complicating cryptococcal meiningitis in AIDS [abstract]. Ann Neurol 41:467, 1997.
179. Berger JR, Harris JO, Gregorios J, et al. Cerebrovascular disease in AIDS: a case-control study. AIDS 4:239, 1990.
180. Davies J, Everall IP, Weich S, et al. HIV-associated brain pathology in the United Kingdom: an epidemiological study. AIDS 11:1145, 1997.
181. Connor MD, Lammie GA, Bell JE, et al. Cerebral infarction in adult AIDS patients: observations from the Edinburgh HIV Autopsy Cohort. Stroke 31:2117, 2000.
182. Engstrom JW, Lowenstein DH, Bredesen DE. Cerebral infarctions and transient neurologic deficits associated with acquired immunodeficiency syndrome. Am J Med 86:528, 1989.
183. Gillams AR, Allen E, Hrieb K, et al. Cerebral infarction in patients with AIDS. AJNR Am J Neuroradiol 18:1581, 1997.
184. Roquer J, Palomeras E, Knobel H, et al. Intracerebral haemorrhage in AIDS. Cerebrovasc Dis 8:222, 1998.
185. Eidelberg D, Sotrel A, Horopian D, et al. Thrombotic cerebral vasculopathy associated with herpes zoster. Ann Neurol 19:7, 1986.
186. Hilt D, Bucholz D, Krumholz A, et al. Herpes zoster ophthalmicus and delayed contralateral hemiparesis caused by cerebral angiitis: diagnosis and management approaches. Ann Neurol 14:543, 1983.
187. Morgello S, Block G, Price R, et al. Varicella-zoster virus leukoencephalitis and cerebral vasculopathy. Arch Pathol Lab Med 112:173, 1988.
188. Picard O, Brunereau L, Pelosse B, et al. Cerebral infarction associated with vasculitis due to varicella zoster virus in patients infected with the human immunodeficiency virus. Biomed Pharmacother 51:449, 1997.
189. Gilden DH, Kleinschmidt-DeMasters BK, Wellish M, et al. Varicella zoster virus, a cause of waxing and waning vasculitis: the New England Journal of Medicine case 5-1995 revisited. Neurology 47:1441, 1996.
190. Kleinschmidt-DeMasters BK, Amlie-Lefond C, Gilden DH. The patterns of varicella zoster virus encephalitis. Hum Pathol 27:927, 1996.
191. Thirumalai S, Kirshner HS. Anticardiolipin antibody and stroke in an HIV-positive patient [letter]. AIDS 8:1019, 1994.
192. Petito C, Navia B, Cho E, et al. Vacuolar myelopathy pathologically resembling subacute combined degeneration in patients with acquired immunodeficiency syndrome (AIDS). N Engl J Med 312:874, 1985.
193. Navia B, Cho E-W, Petito C, et al. The AIDS dementia complex. II. Neuropathology. Ann Neurol 19:525, 1986.
194. Di Rocco A. Diseases of the spinal cord in human immunodeficiency virus infection. Semin Neurol 19:151, 1999.
195. Tan SV, Guiloff RJ, Scaravilli F. AIDS-associated vacuolar myelopathy: a morphometric study. Brain 118:1247, 1995.
196. Schmidbauer M, Budka H, Okeda R, et al. Multifocal vacuolar leucoencephalopathy: a distinct HIV-associated lesion of the brain. Neuropathol Appl Neurobiol 16:437, 1990.
197. Rosenblum M, Scheck A, Cronin K, et al. Dissociation of AIDS-related vacuolar myelopathy and productive human immunodeficiency virus type 1 (HIV-1) infection of the spinal cord. Neurology 39:892, 1989.
198. Petito CK, Vecchio D, Chen YT. HIV antigen and DNA in AIDS spinal cords correlate with macrophage infiltration but not with vacuolar myelopathy. J Neuropathol Exp Neurol 53:86, 1994.
199. Dal Pan GJ, Glass JD, McArthur JC. Clinicopathologic correlations of HIV-1-associated vacuolar myelopathy: an autopsy-based case-control study. Neurology 44:2159, 1994.
200. Shepherd EJ, Brettle RP, Liberski PP, et al. Spinal cord pathology and viral burden in homosexuals and drug users with AIDS. Neuropathol Appl Neurobiol 25:2, 1999.
201. Di Rocco A. Diseases of the spinal cord in human immunodeficiency virus infection. Semin Neurol 19:151, 1999.

202. Chong J, Di Rocco A, Tagliati M, et al. MR findings in AIDS-associated myelopathy. AJNR Am J Neuroradiol 20:1412, 1999.
203. Kitze B, Brady JN. Human T cell lymphotropic retroviruses: association with diseases of the nervous system. Intervirology 40:132, 1997.
204. Izumo S, Umehara F, Kashio N, et al. Neuropathology of HTLV-1-associated myelopathy HAM/TSP. Leukemia 11(suppl):382, 1997.
205. Murphy EL, Fridey J, Smith JW, et al. HTLV-associated myelopathy in a cohort of HTLV-I and HTLV-II-infected blood donors: the REDS investigators. Neurology 48:315, 1997.
206. Heollsberg P. Pathogenesis of chronic progressive myelopathy associated with human T-cell lymphotropic virus type I. Acta Neurol Scand Suppl 169:86, 1997.
207. Lehky TJ, Flerlage N, Katz D, et al. Human T-cell lymphotropic virus type II-associated myelopathy: clinical and immunologic profiles. Ann Neurol 40:714, 1996.
208. Nakagawa M, Nakahara K, Maruyama Y, et al. Therapeutic trials in 200 patients with HTLV-I-associated myelopathy/tropical spastic paraparesis. J Neurovirol 2:345, 1996.
209. Kitze B, Puccioni-Sohler M, Scheaffner J, et al. Specificity of intrathecal IgG synthesis for HTLV-1 core and envelope proteins in HAM/TSP. Acta Neurol Scand 92:213, 1995.
210. Nakagawa M, Izumo S, Ijichi S, et al. HTLV-I-associated myelopathy: analysis of 213 patients based on clinical features and laboratory findings. J Neurovirol 1:50, 1995.
211. Geraci A, Di Rocco A, Liu M, et al. AIDS myelopathy is not associated with elevated HIV viral load in cerebrospinal fluid. Neurology 55:440, 2000.
212. Di Rocco A, Tagliati M. Remission of HIV myelopathy after highly active antiretroviral therapy. Neurology 55:456, 2000.
213. Devinsky O, Cho E, Petito C, et al. Herpes zoster myelitis. Brain 114:1181, 1991.
214. Gray F, Belec L, Lescs MC, et al. Varicella-zoster virus infection of the central nervous system in the acquired immune deficiency syndrome. Brain 117:987, 1994.
215. Cinque P, Bossolasco S, Vago L, et al. Varicella-zoster virus VZV DNA in cerebrospinal fluid of patients infected with human immunodeficiency virus: VZV disease of the central nervous system or subclinical reactivation of VZV infection? Clin Infect Dis 25:634, 1997.
216. Burke DG, Kalayjian RC, Vann VR, et al. Polymerase chain reaction detection and clinical significance of varicella-zoster virus in cerebrospinal fluid from human immunodeficiency virus-infected patients. J Infect Dis 176:1080, 1997.
217. Thurnher MM, Post MJ, Jinkins JR. MRI of infections and neoplasms of the spine and spinal cord in 55 patients with AIDS. Neuroradiology 42:551, 2000.
218. Quencer RM, Post MJ. Spinal cord lesions in patients with AIDS. Neuroimaging Clin North Am 7:359, 1997.
219. Fairley CK, Wodak J, Benson E. Spinal cord toxoplasmosis in a patient with human immunodeficiency virus infection. Int J STD AIDS 3:366, 1992.
220. Henin D, Smith TW, De Girolami U, et al. Neuropathology of the spinal cord in the acquired immunodeficiency syndrome. Hum Pathol 23:1106, 1992.
221. Resnick DK, Comey CH, Welch WC, et al. Isolated toxoplasmosis of the thoracic spinal cord in a patient with acquired immunodeficiency syndrome: case report. J Neurosurg 82:493, 1995.
222. Levy RM, Bredesen DE, Rosenblum ML. Neurological manifestations of the acquired immunodeficiency syndrome (AIDS): experience at UCSF and review of the literature. J Neurosurgery 62:475, 1985.
223. Snider W, Simpson D, Nielson S, et al. Neurological complications of acquired immune deficiency syndrome: analysis of 50 patients. Ann Neurol 14:403, 1983.
224. Chamberlain MC, Dirr L. Involved-field radiotherapy and intra-Ommaya methotrexate/cytarabine in patients with AIDS-related lymphomatous meningitis. J Clin Oncol 11:1978, 1993.
225. Eidelberg D, Sotrel A, Vogel H, et al. Progessive polyradioculopathy in acquired immune deficiency syndrome. Neurology 36:912, 1986.
226. Simpson D, Tagliati M. Neuromuscular syndromes in human immunodeficiency virus disease. In: Berger J, Levy R (eds) AIDS and the Nervous System, 2nd ed. Philadelphia, Lippincott-Raven, 1997, p 189.
227. Verma A. Epidemiology and clinical features of HIV-1 associated neuropathies. J Peripher Nerv Syst 6:8, 2001.
228. Cornblath D, McArthur J. Predominantly sensory neuropathy in patients with AIDS and AIDS-related complex. Neurology 38:794, 1988.
229. Rizzuto N, Cavallaro T, Monaco S, et al. Role of HIV in the pathogenesis of distal symmetrical peripheral neuropathy. Acta Neuropathol (Berl) 90:244, 1995.
230. Wesselingh SL, Glass J, McArthur JC, et al. Cytokine dysregulation in HIV-associated neurological disease. Adv Neuroimmunol 4:199, 1994.
231. McArthur JC, Yiannoutsos C, Simpson DM, et al. A phase II trial of nerve growth factor for sensory neuropathy associated with HIV infection: AIDS Clinical Trials Group Team 291. Neurology 54:1080, 2000.
232. Newshan G. HIV neuropathy treated with gabapentin [letter]. AIDS 12:219, 1998.
233. Nicholson B. Gabapentin use in neuropathic pain syndromes. Acta Neurol Scand 101:359, 2000.
234. Tremont-Lukats IW, Megeff C, Backonja MM. Anticonvulsants for neuropathic pain syndromes: mechanisms of action and place in therapy. Drugs 60:1029, 2000.
235. Max MB. Treatment of post-herpetic neuralgia: antidepressants. Ann Neurol 35(suppl):S50, 1994.
236. Berger AR, Arezzo JC, Schaumburg HH, et al. 2′,3′-dideoxycytidine (ddC) toxic neuropathy: a study of 52 patients. Neurology 43:358, 1993.
237. Rana KZ, Dudley MN. Clinical pharmacokinetics of stavudine. Clin Pharmacokinet 33:276, 1997.
238. Adkins JC, Peters DH, Faulds D. Zalcitabine: an update of its pharmacodynamic and pharmacokinetic properties and clinical efficacy in the management of HIV infection. Drugs 53:1054, 1997.
239. Blum AS, Dal Pan GJ, Feinberg J, et al. Low-dose zalcitabine-related toxic neuropathy: frequency, natural history, and risk factors. Neurology 46:999, 1996.
240. Fichtenbaum CJ, Clifford DB, Powderly WG. Risk factors for dideoxynucleoside-induced toxic neuropathy in patients with the human immunodeficiency virus infection. J Acquir Immune Defic Syndr Hum Retrovirol 10:169, 1995.
241. Simpson DM, Tagliati M. Nucleoside analogue-associated peripheral neuropathy in human immunodeficiency virus infection. J Acquir Immune Defic Syndr and Hum Retrovirol 9:153, 1995.
242. Moyle GJ, Sadler M. Peripheral neuropathy with nucleoside antiretrovirals: risk factors, incidence and management. Drug Saf 19:481, 1998.
243. Waldinger TP, Siegle RJ, Weber W, et al. Dapsone-induced peripheral neuropathy: case report and review. Arch Dermatol 120:356, 1984.
244. Molloy FM, Floeter MK, Syed NA, et al. Thalidomide neuropathy in patients treated for metastatic prostate cancer. Muscle Nerve 24:1050, 2001.
245. Bradley WG, Verma A. Painful vasculitic neuropathy in HIV-1 infection: relief of pain with prednisone therapy. Neurology 47:1446, 1996.
246. Moulignier A, Authier FJ, Baudrimont M, et al. Peripheral neuropathy in human immunodeficiency virus-infected patients with the diffuse infiltrative lymphocytosis syndrome. Ann Neurol 41:438, 1997.
247. Cornblath D, McArthur J, Kennedy P, et al. Inflammatory demylinating peripheral neuropathies associated with human T-cell lymphotropic virus type III infection. Ann Neurol 21:32, 1986.
248. Cornblath D, Chaudhry V, Griffin J. Treatment of chronic inflammatory demyelinating polyneuropathy with intravenous immunoglobin. Ann Neurol 30:104, 1991.
249. Lindenbaum Y, Kissel JT, Mendell JR. Treatment approaches for Guillain-Barré syndrome and chronic inflammatory demyelinating polyradiculoneuropathy. Neurol Clin 19:187, 2001.
250. Saperstein DS, Katz JS, Amato AA, et al. Clinical spectrum of chronic acquired demyelinating polyneuropathies. Muscle Nerve 24:311, 2001.
251. Said G, Lacroix C, Chemouilli P, et al. CMV neuropathy in AIDS: a clinical and pathological study. Ann Neurol 29:139, 1991.
252. Kolson DL, Gonzalez-Scarano F. HIV-associated neuropathies: role of HIV-1, CMV, and other viruses. J Peripher Nerv Syst 6:2, 2001.
253. So YT, Olney RK. Acute lumbosacral polyradiculopathy in acquired immunodeficiency syndrome: experience with 23 patients. Ann Neurol 35:53, 1994.
254. Calabrese L, Proffitt M, Levin K, et al. Acute infection with the human immunodeficiency virus (HIV) associated with acute brachial neuritis and exanthematous rash. Ann Intern Med 107:849, 1987.
255. Berger JR, Flaster M, Schatz N, et al. Cranial neuropathy heralding otherwise occult AIDS-related large cell lymphoma. J Clin Neuroophthalmol 13:113, 1993.

256. Levy RM, Bredesen DE, Rosenblum ML. Neurological manifestations of the acquired immunodeficiency syndrome (AIDS): experience at UCSF and review of the literature. J Neurosurg 62:475, 1985.
257. Enting RH, Esselink RA, Portegies P. Lymphomatous meningitis in AIDS-related systemic non-Hodgkin's lymphoma: a report of eight cases. J Neurol Neurosurg Psychiatry 57:150, 1994.
258. Murr AH, Benecke JE Jr. Association of facial paralysis with HIV positivity. Am J Otol 12:450, 1991.
259. Casanova-Sotolongo P, Casanova-Carrillo P. [Association of peripheral facial paralysis in patients with human immunodeficiency virus infection.] Rev Neurol 32:327, 2001.
260. Schot LJ, Devriese PP, Hadderingh RJ, et al. Facial palsy and human immunodeficiency virus infection. Eur Arch Otorhinolaryngol Suppl S498, 1994.
261. So Y, Olney R. The natural history of mononeuropathy multiplex and simplex in patients with HIV infection [abstract]. Neurology 41(suppl)374, 1991.
262. Lipkin W, Parry G, Kiprov D, et al. Inflammatory neuropathy in homosexual men with lymphadenopathy. Neurology 35:1479, 1985.
263. Stricker RB, Sanders KA, Owen WF, et al. Mononeuritis multiplex associated with cryoglobulinemia in HIV infection. Neurology 42:2103, 1992.
264. Roullet E, Assuerus V, Gozlan J, et al. Cytomegalovirus multifocal neuropathy in AIDS: analysis of 15 consecutive cases. Neurology 44:2174, 1994.
265. Robert ME, Geraghty JD, Miles SA, et al. Severe neuropathy in a patient with acquired immune deficiency syndrome (AIDS):evidence for widespread cytomegalovirus infection of peripheral nerve and human immunodeficiency virus-like immunoreactivity of anterior horn cells. Acta Neuropathol (Berl) 79:255, 1989.
266. Nordstrom DM, Petropolis AA, Giorno R, et al. Inflammatory myopathy and acquired immunodeficiency syndrome. Arthritis Rheum 32:475, 1989.
267. Simpson DM, Bender AN. Human immunodeficiency virus-associated myopathy: analysis of 11 patients. Ann Neurol 24:79, 1988.
268. Gherardi RK. Skeletal muscle involvement in HIV-infected patients. Neuropathol Appl Neurobiol 20:232, 1994.
269. Bailey RO, Turok DI, Jaufmann BP, et al. Myositis and acquired immunodeficiency syndrome. Hum Pathol 18:749, 1987.
270. Wulff EA, Simpson DM. Neuromuscular complications of the human immunodeficiency virus type 1 infection. Semin Neurol 19:157, 1999.
271. Mió O, Grau JM, Pedrol E. Distinct light microscopic changes in HIV-associated nemaline myopathy [letter]. Neurology 53:241, 1999.
272. Dalakas M, Illa I, Pezeshkpour G, et al. Mitochondrial myopathy caused by long term zidovudine therapy. N Engl J Med 322:1098, 1990.
273. Arnaudo E, Dalakas M, Shanske S, et al. Depletion of muscle mitochondrial DNA in AIDS patients with zidovudine-induced myopathy. Lancet 337:508, 1991.
274. Casademont J, Barrientos A, Grau JM, et al. The effect of zidovudine on skeletal muscle mtDNA in HIV-1 infected patients with mild or no muscle dysfunction. Brain 119:1357, 1996.
275. Manji H, Harrison MJ, Round JM, et al. Muscle disease, HIV and zidovudine: the spectrum of muscle disease in HIV-infected individuals treated with zidovudine. J Neurol 240:479, 1993.
276. Masanaes F, Pedrol E, Grau JM, et al. Symptomatic myopathies in HIV-1 infected patients untreated with antiretroviral agents—a clinico-pathological study of 30 consecutive patients. Clin Neuropathol 15:221, 1996.
277. Morgello S, Wolfe D, Godfrey E, et al. Mitochondrial abnormalities in human immunodeficiency virus-associated myopathy. Acta Neuropathol (Berl) 90:366, 1995.
278. Peters BS, Winer J, Landon DN, et al. Mitochondrial myopathy associated with chronic zidovudine therapy in AIDS. Q J Med 86:5, 1993.
279. Gherardi R, Baudrimont M, Lionnet F, et al. Skeletal muscle toxoplasmosis in patients with acquired immunodeficiency syndrome: a clinical and pathological study. Ann Neurol 32:535, 1992.

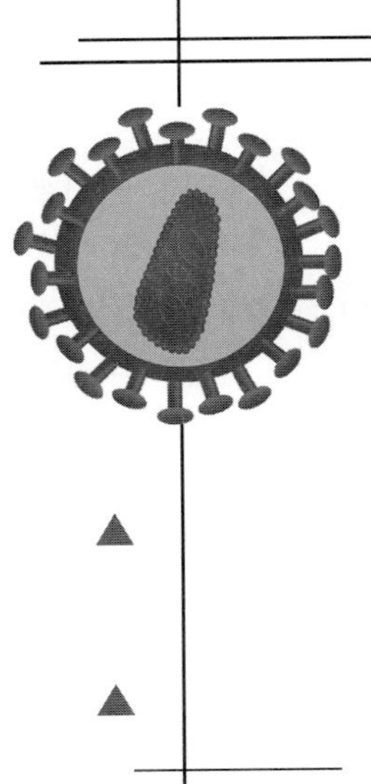

CHAPTER 55

Dermatologic Disease

Richard A. Johnson, MD

Cutaneous disorders occur nearly universally during the course of human immunodeficiency virus (HIV) disease as a result of either the acquired immunodeficiency or treatment. Management of dermatologic conditions in HIV disease is a broad subject, overlapping many other medical specialties.[1] Individuals who have access to highly active antiretroviral therapy (HAART)—in most cases those living in North America, Western Europe, and Australia—have a markedly altered course of HIV disease if immune restoration is achieved. In most cases there is a marked reduction in the incidence of opportunistic infections and neoplasms. Globally, however, more than 95% of HIV-infected individuals have no access to any medical interventions, and consequently many of the cutaneous manifestations associated with HIV disease become chronic and progressive.

▲ DIAGNOSIS

Clinical findings are often adequate for diagnosing most cutaneous disorders in HIV-infected persons. With more advanced immunodeficiency, the clinical value of the gross appearance of a cutaneous lesion may be limited. Lesional skin biopsy is often the most rapid, sensitive method for diagnosing any dermatosis. Infectious agents can be detected both histologically and immunologically by appropriate cultures and stains. A 6- or 8-mm punch biopsy is usually adequate. An adequate portion of the tissue is sent for histopathologic evaluation using routine methods and special stains for fungi, mycobacteria, and bacteria. When indicated, the remaining tissue can be cultured for aerobic and anaerobic bacteria, mycobacteria, and fungi.

▲ ACUTE HIV INFECTION (PRIMARY RETROVIRAL SYNDROME)

Mucocutaneous findings in acute HIV infection include "rash" (50% to 60%), oral candidiasis (17%), oral ulcers (10% to 20%), and genital ulcers (5% to 15%).[2,3] Individuals with a problematic rash or ulceration(s) should be treated symptomatically as well as with HAART. Symptomatic candidiasis can be treated with topical or systemic anticandidal therapy (see Cutaneous Candidiasis, below; see also Chapter 24).

▲ CUTANEOUS DISORDERS OCCURRING WITH HIV DISEASE

Pruritus and Pruritic Eruptions

Pruritus, a common complaint in patients with late symptomatic and advanced HIV disease, is a surrogate cutaneous marker for disease progression, occurring commonly in patients with CD4+ T-lymphocyte counts of less than 50 cells/μl compared with those whose counts are more than 250 cells/μl.[4] In most cases primary or secondary dermatoses rather than metabolic disorders are the cause of pruritus.[5] The differential diagnosis of primary pruritic skin disorders includes eosinophilic folliculitis, adverse cutaneous drug eruptions, atopic dermatitis, xerosis, dermatographism, allergic contact dermatitis, scabies, and insect bites.[6] Much less commonly, systemic and metabolic disorders, such as lymphoma, renal failure, viral hepatitis (B or C), or obstructive liver disease, are associated with pruritus in the absence of cutaneous findings (i.e., "metabolic" pruritus).[7]

An atopic diathesis (characterized by a personal or family history of atopic dermatitis, asthma, and allergic rhinitis), which exists in 20% of the general population, may manifest in individuals with advanced HIV disease and pruritus. Changes secondary to chronic rubbing and scratching include excoriations, atopic dermatitis, lichen simplex chronicus, and prurigo nodularis. Up to 50% of HIV-infected individuals are nasal carriers of *Staphylococcus aureus.* Secondary *S. aureus* infection (impetiginization, furunculosis, cellulitis) is common in any of these traumatized lesions. Ichthyosis vulgaris and xerosis are common in patients with advanced HIV disease and may be associated with mild pruritus.

The protease inhibitors (especially indinavir) frequently cause xerosis with or without eczematous dermatitis, which may be associated with mild or moderate pruritus (see Adverse Cutaneous Drug Reactions). These changes occur relatively soon after initiation of therapy, presenting as xerosis (dry skin) with or without eczematous dermatitis or nummular eczema. Exanthematous drug eruptions such as those caused by trimethoprim-sulfamethoxazole occur relatively suddenly and usually are associated with a newly prescribed drug.

Scabies can present with significant pruritus with few cutaneous findings during HIV disease early in the course of infestation (see below). Conversely, in individuals with advanced disease, pruritus may be minimal, resulting in delayed diagnosis. In these cases the clinical presentation is of a generalized eczematous or psoriasiform dermatosis, that is, hyperkeratotic or crusted (Norwegian) scabies.

Insect bites, especially those of mosquitos, can become extremely large, 1 to 2 cm, presenting as a few or multiple pruritic papules or nodules on exposed skin sites. Severely symptomatic insect bites may require corticosteroid therapy applied topically or given intralesionally or orally (usually a 1-week tapered course).

Control of pruritus is important in that scratching or rubbing the skin both causes and compounds the eczematous dermatitis. Oral doxepin is an excellent antipruritic agent taken at bedtime, the adult dosing varying from 10 to 200 mg. Many other less sedating antihistaminic agents are also effective for daytime or bedtime dosing.

Eosinophilic Folliculitis

Eosinophilic folliculitis (EF) is a chronic dermatosis occurring in persons with advanced HIV disease or in those with immune restoration associated with HAART. "Pruritic papular eruption of HIV disease" previously described in the literature appears to be the same entity as EF. The etiology and pathogenesis are unknown. Symptoms of EF usually occur when the CD4+ T-lymphocyte count is less than 100 cells/μl; however, with HAART, EF occurs initially, recurs, or flares as immune restoration occurs and the viral load diminishes.

The pruritus associated with EF is often intense, more so in individuals with an atopic diathesis. Even early in the course of EF, with few lesions present, pruritus can be the most bothersome symptom, especially because of disturbed sleep. Clinically, small pink-to-red, edematous, folliculocentric papules (and, much less commonly, pustules) occur symmetrically above the nipple line on the chest, proximal arms, head, and neck. The lesions have the appearance of small insect bites (papular urticaria). Rubbing, scratching, and excoriation soon alter primary lesions, with the appearance of excoriations, excoriated papules, lichen simplex chronicus, and prurigo nodularis. In individuals with darker skin, postinflammatory hyperpigmentation often produces significant cosmetic disfigurement. Any of these secondary changes can become infected with *S. aureus*, or less commonly, group A streptococcus. Once significant immune restoration has been achieved with HAART, the EF resolves.

Although subjective and objective findings of early EF are nearly pathognomonic, subacute or chronic EF may have many secondary changes, which make a clinical diagnosis tentative. In these cases, diagnosis of EF should be confirmed by the histologic findings. Peripheral eosinophilia is common in HIV-associated EF, in some cases up to 35%.[8]

The most effective therapy for EF is prednisone. Beginning with an initial dose of 70 mg PO, prednisone is tapered by 10 or 5 mg over 7 or 14 days; established lesions resolve, new lesions do not occur, and the pruritus resolves. In most persons with successfully treated EF, lesions and pruritus recur within a few weeks after prednisone has been discontinued. In those with severe symptoms, prednisone can be given on alternate days or weekly.

Several orally administered agents have been reported to be effective for treating EF. Oral isotretinoin is effective and safe for this purpose; the dosage is usually 40 mg bid until lesions and symptoms resolve, tapered to 40 mg daily for several weeks, and then to 20 mg daily or 40 mg qod.[9] Isotretinoin can raise serum triglyceride levels, which are often high in HIV-infected persons; serum lipids should be monitored regularly. Isotretinoin (and protease inhibitors) commonly causes cheilitis, eczematous dermatitis, and xerosis; these adverse effects can usually be managed with "moisturizing" agents and corticosteroid ointment.

Oral itraconazole 200 mg/day has been reported to be an effective therapy, with symptomatic relief occurring within 2 weeks of therapy; if the response is not significant, the dose is increased up to 400 mg/day. The incidence of adverse cutaneous drug reactions to itraconazole is approximately 15% in patients with HIV disease compared with 2% in non-HIV-infected persons.

Phototherapy with ultraviolet radiation (UVR), using ultraviolet A (UVA), or UVB with or without topical or systemic psoralen is considered a safe topical treatment modality in HIV-infected persons.[10] UVR does not appear to have a significant deleterious effect on the HIV viral load.[11] UVB phototherapy of EF, given by skilled technicians to compliant patients, is effective in suppressing both lesions and symptoms. Compliance is an issue for many individuals in that treatment is usually given three times per week for 4 to 8 weeks, subsequently reducing the frequency of treatment as the skin clears.

High-potency topical corticosteroid preparations may reduce the formation of new EF lesions and cause established lesions to resolve, thereby providing symptomatic relief. New lesions occur once corticosteroids are discontinued. There is a significant risk of cutaneous atopy if corticosteroids are applied chronically. Tacrolimus ointment 0.1% or pimecrolimus cream may be effective in a case report of non-HIV EF.[11]

Sedating antihistamines such as doxepin are most effective for symptomatic control of nocturnal pruritus. Nonsedating antihistamines are ineffective for controlling pruritus.

Atopic Dermatitis (Eczematous Dermatitis)

Eczematous dermatitis is managed by treating underlying causes such as xerosis, adverse cutaneous drug reactions, scabies, or metabolic pruritus. Potent corticosteroids or tacrolimus 0.1% ointment or pimecrolimus cream may be the most effective topical agents for treatment of eczematous dermatitis. High potency, short-term dosing usually minimizes the use of topical corticosteroid preparations. In more severe cases, a 1- to 2-week tapered course of prednisone is indicated, beginning at an initial dose of 70 mg in adults. For patients with dermatitis recurring after prednisone, phototherapy is effective and safe (see Pruritus and Pruritic Eruptions, above).[12]

Psoriasis Vulgaris

The prevalence of psoriasis vulgaris in HIV-infected individuals may be somewhat higher than that of the general population. Psoriatic arthritis, however, is present more frequently in HIV-infected patients and correlates with the presence of HLA-B27. The onset of psoriatic lesions may be prior to or following HIV infection. Onset of psoriasis in an individual at risk for HIV disease may be an indication for HIV serotesting. Psoriasis and Reiter syndrome may coexist in the same patient, suggesting that the two disorders are part of the spectrum of clinical manifestations of one disease. Psoriasis with onset following HIV infection has been observed to improve more with HAART than psoriasis with its onset prior to HIV infection.

In a cohort of 50 HIV-infected individuals with psoriasis, one-third of psoriasis cases were presumed to have occurred prior to the HIV infection (group I) and two-thirds after it (group II). Group I had a lower mean age of onset (19 vs. 36 years) and more commonly had a family history of psoriasis. The clinical patterns of psoriasis were reported to be plaque type (78%), inverse (37%), guttate (29%), palmoplantar (8%), erythrodermic (14%), and pustular (8%). Palmoplantar and inverse pattern psoriasis were more common in group II; severe psoriasis occurred in one-fourth of these patients. Psoriasis tended to become more severe as the degree of immunodeficiency increased, but it did not affect survival.

Topical agents may be effective for managing limited psoriasis (i.e., corticosteroids, calcipotriene, retinoids). Tacrolimus ointment may be effective for psoriasis that occurs in naturally occluded skin (inverse-pattern psoriasis), such as in the axilla, submammary region, and anogenital sites. Subacute or chronic use of corticosteroids to these sites causes cutaneous atrophy, striae, or erosions.

For more widespread disease, phototherapy with UVB, narrow-band UVB (311 nm), or psoralen UVA (PUVA) is safe and effective (see Eosinophilic Folliculitis, above). Photosensitizing agents such as sulfa drugs can cause a phototoxic or photoallergic reaction in individuals being treated with phototherapy.

Oral therapy with retinoids such as acitretin, methotrexate, and cyclosporin is indicated for persons with psoriasis unresponsive to topical and phototherapy. Oral or intramuscular methotrexate given weekly is effective for psoriatic arthritis. Ascomycin is a relatively new agent (of the same class as cyclosporin and tacrolimus) that is effective both topically and systemically for psoriasis, producing little if any systemic immunosuppression.

Erythroderma

Erythroderma in HIV disease may be related to drug hypersensitivity, atopic dermatitis, psoriasis vulgaris, photosensitivity dermatitis, the hypereosinophilic syndrome, coexistent human T-cell leukemia virus type 1 (HTLV-1) infection, and cutaneous T-cell lymphoma.

Xerosis and Ichthyosis

Xerosis and acquired ichthyosis are common in HIV-infected individuals, occurring in up to 30% of those with advanced disease. These disorders are more common during the winter months and are associated with low relative humidity. Several factors are involved in the pathogenesis, including chronic illness, malnutrition, atopic diathesis with ichthyosis vulgaris, wasting syndrome, protease inhibitor therapy, or the HIV infection itself. Xerosis is best treated by applying "moisturizing" creams after bathing. Products with hydroxy acids are keratolytic and hydrophilic. In persons with chronic xerosis, eczematous dermatitis can occur within fissures in areas of hyperkeratosis (i.e., eczema craquelé or asteatotic eczema) (see Atopic Dermatitis).

Photosensitivity

Idiopathic photosensitivity is a rare phenomenon in HIV disease but may be the presenting complaint.[13,14] The most common types of photosensitivity seen in HIV disease are related to drug therapy. Drug-induced photosensitivity manifests two types of reaction: phototoxic (occurs in all individuals and is essentially an exaggerated sunburn response, such as erythema, edema, vesicles) (e.g., trimethoprim-sulfamethoxazole) and photoallergic, which involves an immunologic response and in which the eruption is papular, vesicular, and eczema-like and occurring only in previously sensitized individuals. Drug-induced photosensitivity reactions are most commonly caused by UVA and to a much lesser extent UVB. Photosensitivity in HIV disease appears to be a manifestation of advanced disease.[15] (see Porphyria Cutanea Tarda and pseudoporphyria, below).

Three phototoxic reaction patterns occur: (1) immediate erythema and urticaria; (2) delayed sunburn-type pattern developing within 16 to 24 hours or later (48 to 72 hours); or (3) delayed (72 to 96 hours) melanin pigmentation. Clinically, phototoxic reactions are an "exaggerated sunburn," presenting as erythema, edema, and blister formation (e.g., pseudoporphyria). Marked brown epidermal melanin pigmentation may occur during the course of the eruption; a gray dermal melanin pigmentation develops with certain drugs (chlorpromazine and amiodarone). After repeated exposure, some scaling and lichenification can develop. The reaction is confined exclusively to areas exposed to light.

With photoallergic drug hypersensitivity, the drug present in the skin absorbs protons and forms a photodrug, which then binds to a soluble or membrane-bound protein to form an antigen. Because photoallergy depends on individual immunologic reactivity, it develops in only a small percentage of persons exposed to drugs and light. Clinically, acute photoallergic reactions present as eczematous dermatitis or as lichen planus-like (lichenoid) eruptions. With chronic drug photoallergy, marked scaling, lichenification (thickening), and pruritus/scratching mimic atopic dermatitis or chronic allergic contact dermatitis. Photoallergic eruptions are confined primarily to areas exposed to light but may spread to adjacent nonexposed skin; therefore they are not as circumscribed as phototoxic reactions.

For management of photosensitivity, the photosensitizing agent should be identified and removed or discontinued if possible. If the offending drug cannot be discontinued, sunlight should be avoided and sunscreen and protective clothing used. Phototoxic drug reactions disappear after cessation of the drug. Photoallergic drug reactions can persist for months or years after the drug is discontinued (known as persistent light reaction or chronic actinic dermatitis). In severe cases of photoallergic dermatitis, topical or systemic corticosteroids or other agents such as nonsteroidal antiinflammatory drugs (NSAIDs) or pentoxifylline are indicated.[16]

Pigmentary Disorders

Postinflammatory hyper- and hypopigmentation is the most common disorder affecting HIV-infected individuals. With the exception of light-skinned individuals of northern European heritage, significant lightening or darkening of skin color occurs following any type of inflammatory dermatosis or infection. In addition to pigmentary alterations, significant atrophic or hypertrophic scarring can follow herpes zoster. This alteration in normal skin color results in significant cosmetic disfigurement, especially when it occurs on highly visible sites such as the face, neck, and upper extremities. If the dermatosis is chronic, the pigmentary change can become persistent and progressive. If the dermatosis resolves, the pigmentary disorder can take months to years to fade gradually to uniform pigmentation.

The primary goal in the management of these pigmentary disorders is to treat the primary skin disorder. Topical preparations containing 4% hydroquinone may be helpful for treating postinflammatory hyperpigmentation.

▲ APHTHOUS ULCERS
See Chapter 56.

Recurrent or persistent aphthous ulcers (AUs) that arise in the mouth, oropharynx, and esophagus complicate advanced HIV disease. Aphthous ulcer-like lesions occur on the external genitalia during the course of acute HIV infections. AUs of the upper mouth and esophagus frequently cause moderate to severe pain, impairing eating and speaking; and they are associated with significant weight loss. The incidence appears to be reduced with HAART. Individual AUs of the anterior mouth and oropharynx usually respond to intralesional triamcinolone injection; deeper lesions, however, cannot be treated with this effective, low risk modality. Oral prednisone is usually quite effective for treating persistent AUs; most AUs resolve with an initial dose of 70 mg tapered by 10 or 5 mg/day. In persons in whom prednisone is contraindicated or ineffective, thalidomide 50 to 200 mg hs is an effective alternative medication.[17] The most common adverse events occurring with thalidomide are neutropenia, rash, and peripheral sensory neuropathy.

▲ CUTANEOUS MANIFESTATIONS OF SYSTEMIC DISORDERS SEEN WITH HIV DISEASE

Porphyria Cutanea Tarda and Pseudoporphyria

Porphyria cutanea tarda (PCT) in HIV disease is most often associated with an underlying hepatopathy [hepatitis C virus (HCV) infection, alcoholism, or hepatitis B virus (HBV) infection].[18] In one study about 40% of patients (n = 33) with advanced HIV disease had increased urinary porphyrin excretion; 31 patients were HCV-seropositive, and 4 had urine and stool porphyrin excretion patterns that were classic for PCT.[19] No study patient, however, had clinical evidence of PCT. Porphyrin studies are recommended for HIV-infected individuals with photosensitivity. Clinically, PCT presents with blisters, erosions, crusts, and milia on the dorsum of the hands as a manifestation of photosensitivity. Hyperpigmentation and hypertrichosis often occur on the face. PCT is managed by removing the hepatotoxic agents, especially alcohol. Biochemical remission can be achieved by depleting iron stores via weekly or biweekly phlebotomy of 500 ml of blood until the hemoglobin is reduced to 10 g. Chloroquine can be effective in persons with anemia.

Pseudoporphyria (pseudo-PCT) occurs in the absence of abnormalities of porphyrin metabolism; it is usually drug-induced and is characterized clinically by blisters or erosions on the dorsum of the hands. The most common drugs associated with pseudo-PCT are NSAIDs such as naproxen, ibuprofen, oxaprozin, and nabumetone. Other drugs implicated include tetracyclines, nalidixic acid, dapsone, amiodarone, bumetanide, cyclosporine, furosemide, chlorthalidone, hydrochlorothiazide, and pyridoxine. The UVA used for phototherapy or in tanning beds can induce pseudoporphyria. Pseudo-PCT also occurs in the setting of chronic renal failure with hemodialysis.

Vasculitis

Cutaneous and systemic vasculitis of many etiologies have been reported to occur with HIV disease. Etiologies include adverse cutaneous drug reaction, cytomegalovirus (CMV) infection, HBV or HCV infection, polyarteritis nodosa, lymphomatoid granulomatosis, and possibly the HIV infection itself.[20] Causative drugs should be discontinued if possible. Most other causes are not specifically treatable. Systemic immunosuppressive therapy is indicated in some cases.

▲ OPPORTUNISTIC CUTANEOUS INFECTIONS IN HIV DISEASE

Bacterial Infections

Staphylococcus aureus causes most pyodermas and soft tissue infections. Colonization of the anterior nares occurs in more than 50% of HIV-infected individuals. Mupirocin ointment is effective in eradicating colonizing *S. aureus*. Benzoyl peroxide used as a wash is effective for treating colonized cutaneous sites or lesions. Systemic therapy with antibiotics such as dicloxacillin, cephalexin, or clindamycin is indicated for superficial or invasive cutaneous infections. Intravascular catheters and cutaneous infections are the most common sources of *S. aureus* bacteremia.

Helicobacter cinaedi causes a syndrome characterized by fever, bacteremia, and recurrent or chronic cellulitis (resembling erythema nodosum) in compromised patients.[21–23] The organism is carried as bowel flora in 10% of homosexual men (no carriage in other groups). It is diagnosed by considering it in immunocompromised individuals, demonstrating cellulitis on a lesional biopsy (excluding panniculitis), and failing to isolate other pathogens. Bacteremia is intermittent; the organism is difficult to isolate, requiring hydrogen in the culture vial. Ciprofloxacin 500 mg bid or clarithromycin 500 mg bid is effective, given for 6 to 8 weeks to prevent relapse.

In developing countries, tuberculosis is the most common opportunistic infection associated with HIV disease; however, cutaneous tuberculosis is relatively uncommon. In non-HIV-infected persons with tuberculosis, the incidence of extrapulmonary tuberculosis is 15%; in those with HIV disease it is 20% to 40%. In those with advanced HIV disease, the incidence of extrapulmonary disease increases to 70% (see Chapter 33).

Bacillary angiomatosis (BA) and bacillary peliosis (BAP), caused by the genus *Bartonella* (*B. henselae* and *B. quintana*), occur most commonly in the setting of HIV-induced immunodeficiency. They are characterized by angioproliferative lesions resembling cherry hemangiomas, pyogenic granulomas, or Kaposi sarcoma.[24,25] Currently, the prevalence of BA in North America and western Europe[26] is low because of improved immune function with HAART and the prophylaxis given for infections such as *Mycobacterium avium* complex (MAC) (see Chapter 35).

Fungal Infections

Cutaneous fungal infections occur as superficial infections (dermatomycoses), invasive fungal infections, or hematogenous dissemination of systemic fungal infection to the skin. The two most common dermatomycoses are dermatophytoses and candidiasis; both of these infections occur with increased frequency in the setting of compromised local or systemic immunity.

Dermatophytoses

Dermatophytes, especially *Trichophyton rubrum,* can infect any keratinized epidermal structure: epidermis (tinea pedis, tinea cruris, tinea manuum, tinea corporis, tinea facialis, tinea incognito), nails (tinea unguium or onychomycosis),[27] and hair (tinea capitis, tinea barbae, dermatophytic folliculitis).[28,29] Dermatophytes infect nonviable tissue in otherwise healthy individuals, although in the compromised host direct invasion of the dermis may occur. Dermatophytoses are of importance for three reasons: (1) the morbidity and disfigurement caused by the dermatophyte infection itself, which can be extensive; (2) the breakdown in the integrity of the skin, providing a portal of entry for other pathogens, particularly *S. aureus*; and (3) clinical manifestations that mimic other dermatologic conditions.[30] Dermatophyte infections in the compromised host are more frequent, often widespread, atypical in appearance, and invasive.[31]

Trichophyton rubrum causes proximal subungual onychomycosis (PSO), an infection of the undersurface of the proximal nail plate. PSO occurs most often in HIV-infected individuals; the diagnosis is an indication for HIV testing. Unless immunocompetence is restored, dermatophyte infections are chronic and recurrent.[32]

The HIV-infected patients who are taking oral imidazoles such as fluconazole or itraconazole for candidiasis or cryptococcosis are also being inadvertently treated for dermatophytoses. Terbinafine, which is highly efficacious for dermatophytic infection, is not predictably effective for nondermatophytic fungal infections.

Dermatophyte infections are managed with systemic and topical antifungal agents (Table 55–1). Infections of the epidermis (Table 55–1), nail apparatus (Table 55–2), and hair shaft/hair follicle (Table 55–3) cannot be cured by topical agents alone, especially in the setting of immunocompromise.

Cutaneous Candidiasis

Cutaneous *Candida* infections such as intertrigo are relatively uncommon in adults with HIV disease (Table 55–4); concomitant diabetes mellitus associated with HAART may increase the prevalence. Candidiasis of moist, keratinized cutaneous sites such as the anogenital region occurs with some frequency. Candidal angular cheilitis occurs at the corners of the mouth as an intertrigo, unilaterally or bilaterally, and is more common in edentulous patients; it may occur in conjunction with oropharyngeal or esophageal disease or as the only manifestation of candidal infection. Children with HIV infection commonly experience candidiasis in the diaper area and intertrigo in the axillae and neck fold. Fingernail chronic *Candida* paronychia with secondary nail dystrophy (onychia) is common in HIV-infected children.[33] Topical therapy is usually adequate, but a systemic agent may be required in the setting of advanced immunocompromise (Tables 55–5, 55–6).

▲ **Table 55–1.** AGENTS USED IN THE MANAGEMENT OF DERMATOPHYTE INFECTIONS

Parameter	Comments
Prevention	Immune restititution with HAART markedly reduces the incidence of dermatophyte infections. Apply powder containing miconazole or tolnaftate to areas prone to fungal infection after bathing.
Topical antifungal preparations	These preparations may be effective for treatment of dermatophytoses of skin but not for those of hair or nails. Topical agents should be continued for at least 1 week after lesions have cleared. Apply at least 3 cm beyond advancing margin of lesion. These agents are comparable. Differentiated by cost, base, vehicle, and antifungal activity. Preparation is applied twice a day to involved area optimally for 4 weeks.
Imidazoles	Clotrimazole (Lotrimin, Mycelex) Miconazole (Micatin) Ketoconazole (Nizoral) Econazole (Spectazole) Oxiconazole (Oxistat) Sulconazole (Exelderm)
Allylamines	Naftifine (Naftin) Terbinafine (Lamisil)
Naphthiomates	Tolnaftate (Tinactin)
Substituted pyridone	Ciclopiroxolamine (Loprox)
Systemic antifungal agents	For infections of keratinized skin: use if lesions are extensive or if infection has failed to respond to topical preparations. Usually required for treatment of tinea capitis and tinea unguium. Also may be required for inflammatory tineas and hyperkeratotic moccasin-type tinea pedis.
Terbinafine	250 mg tablet. Allylamine.
Azole/imidazoles	Itraconazole and ketoconazole have potential clinically important interactions when administered with calcium channel antagonists, warfarin, cyclosporin A, tacrolimus, oral hypoglycemic agents, phenytoin, protease inhibitors, terfenadine, theophylline, trimetrexate, and rifampin.
Itraconazole	Capsules (100 mg); oral solution (10 mg/ml); intravenous iriazole. Needs acid gastric pH for dissolution of capsule.
Fluconazole	Tablets (100, 150, 200 mg); oral suspension (10 or 40 mg/ml); 400 mg IV.
Ketoconazole	Tablets (200 mg) (little used currently).

Mucosal candidiasis is discussed in Chapter 39.

Invasive Fungal Infections

Latent pulmonary fungal infections such as cryptococcosis, histoplasmosis, coccidioidomycosis, sporotrichosis, or penicilliosis can reactivate and disseminate to various organs including meninges and skin in persons with advanced HIV disease. The cutaneous findings most commonly resemble multiple molluscum contagiosum-like lesions, which occur most often on the face and upper trunk.[34] Disseminated deep mycoses are much less common during the era of HAART (see Chapters 36, 37, 38).

Viral Infections

Viruses are major pathogens causing opportunistic infections (OIs) in HIV disease, many of which are manifested at mucocutaneous sites, ranging from cosmetically disfiguring facial molluscum contagiosum (MCV) to extensive common or genital warts to life-threatening/invasive human papillomavirus (HPV)-induced squamous cell carcinoma. In most cases viral OIs represent activation of subclinical infection (HPV, MCV) or of a latent infection [human herpesviruses: herpes simplex virus-1 (HSV-1) and HSV-2; varicella-zoster virus (VZV); cytomegalovirus (CMV); Epstein-Barr virus (EBV); HHV-8 (Kaposi sarcoma-associated virus)].

HSV-1 and HSV-2 Infections
See Chapter 41.

With advanced immunocompromise, lesions tend to be subacute or chronic, indolent, and atypical; and they respond less promptly to oral antiviral therapy. Chronic herpetic ulcers of more than 1 month's duration are an AIDS-defining condition. Clinically, reactivated latent infections (ulcers) are larger and deeper than the primary lesions. Ulcerated, crusted lesions at perioral, anogenital, or digital locations are usually HSV in etiology despite atypical clinical appearances. With increasing immunocompromise, recurrent HSV infection may become persistent and progressive. Erosions occurring at typical sites (perioral, anogenital, digital) enlarge and deepen into painful ulcers. In addition to ulceration, chronic HSV infections can also present as proliferative lesions of the epidermis with or without scale.

Currently, three drugs are available for oral therapy of HSV infections: famciclovir[35] valacyclovir, and acyclovir. Acyclovir and famciclovir are approved for treatment of the primary infection (Table 55–7); and all three are approved for reactivated infection or to suppress reactivation. For the management of chronic herpetic ulcers, immunocompromise should be corrected if possible. Chronic oral antiviral therapy has been advocated for HSV infections in HIV disease, as HIV viral loads have been reported to increase with reactivation of latent HSV infection.[36] Oral acyclovir is effective for suppressing recurrences of HSV in HIV-infected persons; a dosage of 600 mg/day is more effi-

▲ **Table 55–2.** MANAGEMENT OF DERMATOPHYTIC INFECTIONS OF THE NAIL APPARATUS

Agent	Comments
Débridement	Dystrophic nails should trimmed. In DLSO the nail and the hyperkeratotic nail bed should be removed with nail clippers. In SWO the abnormal nail can be débrided with a curette.
Topical agents	Available as lotions and lacquer. Usually not effective except for early DLSO and SWO after prolonged use (months). Amorolfine nail lacquer: reported to be effective when applied >12 months (available in Europe). Penlac: monthly professional nail débridement recommended.
Systemic agents	During systemic treatment of onychomycosis, nails usually do not appear normal after the treatment times recommended because of slow growth of nail. If cultures and KOH preparations are negative after these time periods, medication can nonetheless be stopped and the nail usually regrows normally.
Allylamines	Most effective against dermatophyte infections; also efficacious against select other fungi.
Terbinafine	Dose: 250 mg/day for 6 weeks for fingernails and 12 weeks for toenail.
Azoles	Drugs in this category are usually effective for treating nail infections caused by dermatophytes, yeasts, and molds.
Itraconazole[a]	Continuous therapy with 200 mg daily for 6 weeks (fingernails) or 12 weeks (toenails). Dose: 200 mg bid for first 7 days of each month for 2 months (fingernails) (pulse dosing). Although not approved for toenail onychomycosis, pulse dosing is used for 3–4 months.
Fluconazole[a]	Reported effective at dosing of 150–400 mg 1 day per week or 100–200 mg daily until the nails grow back normally. Effective against yeasts and less so for dermatophytes.
Secondary prophylaxis	Recommended for all patients. The entirety of both feet should be treated. Prophylaxis should be simple to use and inexpensive. Benzoyl peroxide bar for washing feet when bathing Antifungal cream daily Zeaborb (miconazole) AF lotion/powder on feet Antifungal sprays or powders in shoes

DLSO, distal and lateral subungual onychomycosis; SWO, superficial white onychomycosis.
[a]Effective against dermatophytes and *Candida*.

cacious than 400 mg/day.[37] Although data in HIV-infected patients are lacking, many clinicians prefer the use of a valacyclovir or famciclovir because of improved pharmacokinetics or convenience of administration. Foscarnet and cidofovir are administered intravenously for infections caused by acyclovir-resistant HSV.[38] Cidofovir gel has been effective for topical treatment of acyclovir-resistant HSV infections, although it is not available commercially and must be made up by the pharmacist.[39] Imiquimod 5% cream is also an effective topical treatment for cutaneous herpetic infections, including those caused acyclovir-resistant HSV strains. Imiquimod 5% cream is applied to the lesion(s) at bedtime daily or every other day if irritation occurs.[40]

Varicella-Zoster Virus Infections See Chapter 42.

Primary VZV infection manifests as varicella (chickenpox); reactivation of VZV from a dorsal root ganglion or cranial nerve ganglion manifests as herpes zoster (HZ). In the

▲ **Table 55–3.** MANAGEMENT OF DERMATOPHYTIC INFECTIONS OF THE HAIR SHAFT/HAIR FOLLICLE

Parameter	Comments
Prevention	Important to examine home and school contacts of affected children for asymptomatic carriers and mild cases of tinea capitis. Ketoconazole or selenium sulfide shampoo may be helpful for eradicating the asymptomatic carrier state.
Topical antifungal agents	Topical agents are ineffective for management of tinea capitis. Duration of treatment should be extended until symptoms have resolved and fungal cultures negative.
Oral antifungal agents	Of the systemic antifungals available, terbinafine and itraconazole are superior to ketoconazole, and all three are superior to griseofulvin. Side effects in increasing order: terbinafine < itraconazole < ketoconazole < griseofulvin
Terbinafine	Dose: 250 mg qd. Reduce dosing according to weight in pediatric patients.
Itraconazole	Dose: 100 mg capsules or oral solution (10 mg/ml). Treatment duration: 4–8 weeks. Pediatric dose 5 mg/kg/day; adult dose 200 mg/day.
Fluconazole	Tablets (100, 150, 200 mg); oral solution (10 and 40 mg/ml). Dosage: 6–8 mg/kg/d. Treatment duration 3–4 weeks. Pediatric dose 6 mg/kg/d for 2 wks; repeat at 4 wks if indicated; adult dose 200 mg/day.
Ketoconazole	Tablets (200 mg). Treatment duration 4–6 weeks (little used currently). Pediatric dose 5 mg/kg/d; adult dose 200–400 mg/d.
Adjunctive therapy	
Prednisone	Dose: 1 mg/kg/d for 14 days for children with severe, painful kerion.
Systemic antibiotics	For secondary *S. aureus* or group A streptococcal infection: clindamycin, dicloxacillin, or cephalexin.
Surgery	Drain pus from kerion lesions.

▲ **Table 55–4.** CLASSIFICATION OF CANDIDIASIS INVOLVING SKIN AND MUCOSA

Type	Site	Clinical Presentation
Occluded site (occurs where occlusion and maceration create warm, moist microecology)	Body folds	Axillae, inframammary, groins, intergluteal, abdominal panniculus
		Webspace: hands (erosio interdigitalis blastomycetica), feet
		Angular cheilitis; often associated with oropharyhgeal candidiasis
	Genitalia	Balanitis, balanoposthitis
		Vulvitis
	Occluded skin	Under occlusive dressing, under cast, back in hospitalized patient
	Folliculitis	Back in hospitalized patient
	Area occluded under diaper	Diaper dermatitis
Nail apparatus	Paronychium	Chronic paronychia
	Nail plate	Onychia
	Hyponychium	Onycholysis
Chronic mucocutaneous	Extensive, multiple or 20 nails	In HIV-infected children, persistent or recurrent mucosal, cutaneous, and/or paronychial/nail infections
Genital	Vulva, vagina; preputial sac	Erythema, erosions, white plaques of candidal colonies
Mucosal	Oropharynx	Thrush; atrophic candidiasis; hyperplastic candidiasis
	Esophagus	Inflamed, eroded plaques
	Trachea, bronchi	Inflamed, eroded plaques
Candidemia	Skin, viscera	Skin: erythematous papules ± hemorrhage

compromised host, VZV infection can present as severe varicella, persistent varicella,[41] dermatomal HZ, disseminated HZ (sometimes without dermatomal HZ), and chronic or recurrent HZ. Disseminated HZ is defined as cutaneous involvement by more than three contiguous dermatomes, more than 20 lesions scattered outside the initial dermatome, or systemic infection (hepatitis, pneumonitis, encephalitis). Disseminated VZV infection in an individual harboring latent VZV can present with a clinical pattern of scattered vesicles in the absence of dermatomal HZ. In immunocompetent individuals, the main complication of zoster is postherpetic neuralgia (defined as pain persisting more than 6 weeks after the development of cutaneous lesions).

Individuals infected with HIV who are seronegative for VZV and hence are at risk for primary infection should promptly receive zoster immune globulin on exposure to the virus, with high-dose intravenous acyclovir (10 mg/kg q8h) instituted at the earliest signs of primary infection.

Administration of varicella vaccine during early HIV disease in children appears safe and beneficial. HIV-infected children exposed to VZV, whether varicella or zoster, may benefit by prophylaxis with varicella-zoster immune globulin and by treatment with acyclovir if chickenpox develops. Most persons with zoster that occurs during early HIV disease do well without antiviral therapy. The same drugs approved for treatment of HSV are approved for treatment of VZV infection: famciclovir, valacyclovir, and acyclovir. Intravenous acyclovir (10 mg/kg q8h) is given for severe infections. Intravenous acyclovir is usually given because of the risk of visual impairment following ophthalmic zoster. As with HSV infections, acyclovir-resistant strains can emerge following prolonged acyclovir treatment; most of these resistant strains respond to foscarnet therapy. Suppressive therapy is usually not indicated after the VZV infection resolves.

The management of VZV infections in patients with mild to moderate immunocompromise is identical to that in the immunocompetent host (see Chapter 42).[42] The cornerstone of treatment for severe VZV infection or VZV infection in the severely immunocompromised host is intra-

▲ **Table 55–5.** MANAGEMENT OF CUTANEOUS CANDIDIASIS

Management	Comments
HAART	With immune restitution, candidiasis resolves and/or does not occur.
Prevention	Keep intertriginous areas dry (often difficult).
	Washing with benzoyl peroxide bar may reduce *Candida* colonization.
	Powder with miconazole applied daily.
Topical treatment	
Castellani's paint	Brings almost immediate relief of symptoms (i.e., candidal paronychia)
Corticosteroid preparation	Judicious short-term use speeds resolution of symptoms.
Topical antifungal agents	Antifungal preparation: nystatin, azole, or imidazole cream bid or more often with diaper dermatitis. Telnaftate not effective for candidiasis. Terbinafine may be effective.
Nystatin cream	Effective for *Candida* only. Not effective for dermatophytosis.
Azole creams	Effective for candidiasis, dermatophytosis, and pityriasis versicolor.
Oral antifungal agents	Eliminate bowel colonization. Azoles treat cutaneous infection.
Nystatin (suspension, tablet, pastille)	Not absorbed from the bowel. Eradicates bowel colonization. May be effective for recurrent candidiasis of diaper area, genitalia, or intertrigo.
Systemic antifungal agents	See Table 55–6 and Chapter 39.

▲ **Table 55–6.** MANAGEMENT OF OROPHARYNGEAL CANDIDIASIS

Management	Comments
HAART	With immune restitution, candidiasis resolves and/or does not occur.
Topical agents	Effective in most cases.
Nystatin	Vaginal tablets: 100,000 units qid dissolved slowly in the mouth. Oral suspension: 1–2 teaspoons held in mouth for 5 minutes and then swallowed.
Clotrimazole	Oral tablets (troche), 10 mg: one tablet 5 times daily.
Systemic therapy	Systemic therapy indicated if OPC fails to respond to topical agents.
Fluconazole	Oral: 200 mg PO once followed by 100 mg daily for 2–3, weeks, then discontinue. Increase the dose to 400–800 mg in resistant infection. IV also available.
Itraconazole	Capsules or oral solution: 100–200 mg PO 100 mg PO qd or bid for 2 weeks. Increase dose with resistant disease.
Ketoconazole	200 mg PO qd to bid for 1–2 weeks (little used currently).
Voriconazole	Investigational; may be useful for *Candida* species with relatively high MIC.
Fluconazole-resistant candidiasis	Defined as clinical persistence of infection following treatment with fluconazole 100 mg/day PO for 7 days. Occurs most commonly in HIV-infected individuals with CD4+ lymphocyte counts < 50/mm^3 who have had prolonged fluconazole exposure. Chronic low-dose fluconazole treatment (50 mg/d) facilitates emergence of resistant strains.
Amphotericin B	For severe resistant disease. New liposomal preparations are effective and less toxic.

MIC, minimal inhibitory concentration; OPC, oropharyngeal candidiasis.

venous acyclovir. As with HSV infection, acyclovir-resistant VZV has been reported following chronic acyclovir therapy for persistent or recurrent VZV infection.[43,44]

Oral Hairy Leukoplakia See Chapter 45.

Epstein-Barr virus selectively infects certain types of squamous epithelium producing oral hairy leukoplakia (OHL). OHL presents as a white plaque on the lateral aspects of the tongue and is nearly pathognomonic for HIV disease; its occurrence correlates with moderate to advanced HIV-induced immunodeficiency.[45–49] OHL typically presents as hyperplastic, verrucous, whitish, epithelial plaques on the lateral aspects of the tongue, frequently extending onto the contiguous dorsal or ventral surfaces.[50] Usually, a single lesion or three to six discrete plaques separated by normal-appearing mucosa are observed. Although described as hairy, the most frequently noted appearance of the lesion on the tongue is a corrugated appearance, with parallel white rows arranged nearly vertically.

For the most part, OHL is asymptomatic, but its presence may be associated with some degree of anxiety. Patients should be reassured and advised that OHL is not thrush. When treated with HAART, the OHL may resolve without additional interventions.[51–53] Topically applied podophyllin in benzoin is effective in concerned patients with persistent lesions, although recurrence within weeks to months is common. Topical tretinoin or imiquimod cream can also be considered. Acyclovir, valacyclovir, famciclovir, ganciclovir, or foscarnet given for other indications are often effective therapies for OHL.

Molluscum Contagiosum

Molluscum contagiosum virus (MCV) commonly infects keratinized skin subclinically and can cause lesions at sites of minor trauma and in the infundibular portion of the hair follicle.[54] The clinical course of MCV infection in patients with HIV disease differs significantly from that in the normal host, and it is an excellent clinical marker of the degree of immunodeficiency.[55] Large, confluent lesions cause significant morbidity and disfigurement. Prior to HAART, MCV infections were detected in 10% of individuals with HIV disease and in 30% of those with CD4+ T-lymphocyte counts of less than 100 cells/mm^3, the number of lesions being inversely related to the CD4+ T-lymphocyte count.[56] In HIV-infected individuals, MCV infection tends to be progressive and is recurrent after the usual therapies. With response to HAART, MCV infections regress, resolve completely, or do not occur; and beneficial effects on MCV infections are associated with increased CD4+ T-lymphocyte counts and a reduced viral load.[57]

Therapeutically, the most efficacious approach to MCV infection is to correct the underlying immunodeficiency; if this can be accomplished, lesions regress. If correction of immunodeficiency is not possible, treatment is directed at controlling the numbers and bulk of cosmetically disturbing lesions rather than eradicating all lesions (Table 55–8). Liquid nitrogen cryospray is the most convenient therapy and usually must be repeated every 2 to 4 weeks. Simple curettage is effective for small lesions but not practical for larger, more numerous lesions. Electrosurgery is more effective than cryosurgery; local anesthesia is required by most subjects with either injected lidocaine or EMLA cream. CO_2 or pulse-dye laser ablation is also effective but relatively costly. Imiquimod 5% cream applied three times a week is an effective patient-administered therapy for children and adults.[58,59] Cidofovir, a nucleotide analogue with activity against several DNA viruses that is given either intravenously or topically as a cream (unavailable commercially), may be an effective therapy.[60–62]

Human Papillomavirus Infections

Subclinical infection with HPV is nearly universal in humans. With immunocompromise, cutaneous or mucosal HPV infections (or both) (re)emerge from latency, presenting clinically on keratinized epithelium as verrucae and on nonkeratinized or poorly keratinized mucosa as mucosal

▲ **Table 55–7.** MANAGEMENT OF CUTANEOUS HSV INFECTIONS

Management	Comments
Scope	Lesions caused by HSV are relatively common among HIV-infected persons. For severe disease, IV acyclovir therapy may be required. If lesions persist among patients undergoing acyclovir treatment, resistance to acyclovir should be suspected.
HAART	With immune restitution, the incidence and severity of HSV infections are markedly reduced.
Oral antiviral therapy	Currently, anti-HSV agents are approved for use in genital herpes. Presumably, similar dosing regimens are effective for nongenital infections. Drugs for oral HSV therapy include acyclovir, valacyclovir, and famciclovir. Valacyclovir, the prodrug of acyclovir, has better bioavailability and is nearly 85% absorbed after oral administration. Famciclovir is equally effective for cutaneous HSV infections.
First episode	Primary infections are more severe and prolonged.
Acyclovir	Dose: 400 mg tid or 200 mg 5×/d × 7–10 d.
Valacyclovir	Dose: 1 g bid × 7–10 d (not approved for first-episode disease).
Famciclovir	Dose: 250 mg tid × 5–10 d.
Recurrences	For severe recurrent disease, patients who start therapy at the beginning of the prodrome or within 2 days after onset of lesions may benefit from therapy by shortening and reducing severity of eruption. Recurrences cannot be prevented by intermittent therapy.
Acyclovir	Dose: 400 mg PO tid for 5 d *or* 800 mg PO bid for 5 d.
Valacyclovir	Dose: 500 mg bid × 5 d *or* 2 g bid for day 1, then 1 g bid on day 2.
Famciclovir	Dose: 125 mg bid for 5 d.
Chronic suppression	Decreases frequency of symptomatic recurrences and asymptomatic HSV shedding. After 1 year of continuous daily suppressive therapy, acyclovir should be discontinued to determine the recurrence rate.
Acyclovir	Dose: 400 mg bid.
Valacyclovir	Dose: 500–1000 mg qd.
Famciclovir	Dose: 250 mg bid.
Mucocutaneous HSV infections in advanced HIV disease	Neither the need for nor the proper increased dosage of acyclovir has been established conclusively. Patients with herpes simplex who do not respond to the recommended dose of acyclovir may require a higher oral dose of acyclovir, IV acyclovir, or be infected with an acyclovir-resistant HSV strain, requiring IV foscarnet. The roles of valacyclovir and famciclovir are not yet established.
Acyclovir	Dose: 5 mg/kg IV q8h for 7–14 d *or* 400 mg 5×/d × 7–14 d.
Valacyclovir *or* famciclovir	Reduces the necessity for IV acyclovir therapy.
Acyclovir resistance	Usually occurs in individuals with long-standing HIV disease and chronic treatment with oral anti-HSV drugs. Chronic HSV infections are mucocutaneous, rarely invasive. Resistant HSV strains are thymidine-kinase deficient. Alternative drugs: foscarnet, cidofovir.
Foscarnet	For severe disease caused by proven or suspected acyclovir-resistant strains, hospitalization should be considered. Forscarnet, 40 mg/kg body weight until q8h clinical resolution is attained, appears to be the best available treatment.

HSV, herpes simplex virus.

warts (condyloma acuminatum), squamous intraepithelial lesions, or invasive squamous cell carcinoma.[63]

Common Warts (Verruca Vulgaris, Verruca Plana, Verruca Plantaris), In Situ and Invasive Squamous Cell Carcinoma

The verrucae in HIV-infected individuals are not unusual in morphology, number, or response to treatment; with advancing disease, however, verrucae can enlarge, become confluent, and be unresponsive to therapy.[64] HPV-5 can cause an unusual pattern of extensive verruca plana and pityriasis (tinea) versicolor-like warts, similar to the pattern seen in epidermodysplasia verruciformis. With moderate or advanced immunodeficiency, warts may become much more numerous, confluent, and refractory to the usual treatment modalities. Precancerous lesions identical to mucosal lesions, namely squamous itraepithalial lesions (SILs) and squamous cell carcinoma in situ (SCCIS), can occur periungually on the fingers. In some cases, invasive SCCs arise at one or multiple sites on the fingers and nail bed. These tumors are aggressive and invade to the underlying periosteum and bone relatively early owing to the proximity of the underlying bony structures. Despite immune restitution with HAART, HPV infections often persist and progress, unlike other opportunistic viral infections.

Verrucae in HIV-infected individuals are usually asymptomatic, with the most common complaint being a cosmetic one, although warts on the plantar aspect of the foot can become large and painful. Verruca vulgaris and verruca

▲ **Table 55–8.** MANAGEMENT OF MOLLUSCUM CONTAGIOSUM

Management	Comments
Prevention	Avoid skin-to-skin contact with individual having molluscum lesions. HIV-infected individuals with molluscum lesions in the beard area should be advised to minimize shaving facial hair or grow a beard.
HAART	With immune restitution, molluscum lesions resolve and/or do not occur.
Treatment of lesions	
Topical patient-directed therapy	Aldara cream (5% imiquimod) applied hs three times/wk for up to 1–3 months
Clinician directed therapy (office)	These procedures are painful and traumatic, especially for young children. EMLA cream applied to lesions 1 hour prior to therapy may reduce/eliminate pain.
Curettage	Small molluscum lesions can be removed with a small curette with little discomfort or pain.
Cryosurgery	Freezing lesions for 10–15 seconds is effective and minimally painful using either a cotton-tipped applicator or liquid nitrogen spray.
Electrodesiccation	For molluscum lesions refractory to cryosurgery, especially in HIV-infected individuals with numerous and/or large lesions, electrodesiccation or laser surgery is the treatment of choice. Large lesions usually require injected lidocaine anesthesia. Giant lesions may require several cycles of electrodesiccation and curettage to remove the large bulk of lesions; these lesions may extend through the dermis into the subcutaneous fat.

plantaris appear as well demarcated keratotic papules or nodules, usually with multiple tiny red-brown dots representing thrombosed capillaries; palmar and plantar warts characteristically interrupt the normal dermatoglyphics. They may be numerous and confluent, giving the appearance of a mosaic. Verruca plana appears as a well demarcated, flat-topped papule that lacks the dots seen in other types of verrucae.[65,66] When present in the beard area, hundreds of flat warts may be present. All types of verruca may have a linear arrangement due to Koebner's phenomenon or autoinoculation.

The efficacy of treatment of verruca vulgaris (Table 55–9) and condyloma acuminatum in HIV disease varies with the degree of immunocompromise. In patients with early disease, these lesions should be managed as in the normal host. In patients with advanced HIV-induced immunodeficiency, complete eradication of benign HPV-induced lesions is often not possible, and aggressive treatment is contraindicated.[67] Cytologic smears, lesional biopsies, or both should be undertaken to monitor the evolution of benign neoplasia to dysplasia (SIL) to invasive SCC.

Condyloma Acuminatum

See Chapter 47.

Most sexually active individuals are or have been subclinically infected with one or multiple HPV types. HPV-6 and HPV-11 infect nonkeratinized or scantily keratinized epithelium (e.g., anogenital sites and the oropharynx) and cause genital warts (condyloma acuminatum); HPV-16 and HPV-18 cause such precancerous lesions as low-grade SILs (LSILs) and high-grade SILs (HSILs) as well as invasive SCC. Oropharyngeal HPV-induced lesions resemble anogenital condyloma; they are pink or white but never the tan to brown of some genital lesions. Extensive intraoral condyloma acuminatum (oral florid papillomatosis) presents as multiple large plaques, analogous to anogenital giant

▲ **Table 55–9.** MANAGEMENT OF HPV INFECTIONS OF KERATINIZED SKIN: CUTANEOUS WARTS (VERRUCAE)

Management	Comments
HAART	Unlike other viral opportunistic infections, HPV infections may persist despite immune restitution.
Patient-initiated therapy	Minimal cost; no/minimal pain.
For small lesions	Salicylic acid (10%–20%) and lactic acid in collodion.
For large lesions	Salicylic acid (40%) plaster for 1 week, then application of salicylic acid–lactic acid in collodion.
Aldara cream	At sites that are not thickly keratinized, apply with hs 3×/wk. Persistent warts may require occlusion. Hyperkeratotic lesions on palms/soles should be débrided frequently; Aldara used alternately with a topical retinoid such as tazarotene topical gel may be effective.
Clinician-initiated therapy	Costly, painful.
Cryosurgery	If patients have tried home therapies and liquid nitrogen is available, light cryosurgery using a cotton-tipped applicator or cryospray, freezing the wart and 1 to 2 mm of surrounding normal tissue for approximately 30 seconds, is quite effective. Freezing kills the infected tissue but not HPV. Cryosurgery is usually repeated about every 4 weeks until the warts have disappeared. Painful.
Electrosurgery	More effective than cryosurgery but also associated with a greater chance of scarring. EMLA cream can be used for anesthesia for flat warts. Lidocaine injection is usually required for thicker warts, especially palmar/plantar lesions.
CO_2 laser surgery	May be effective for recalcitrant warts but no better than cryosurgery or electrosurgery in the hands of experienced clinicians.
Surgery	Single, nonplantar verruca vulgaris: curettage after Freon freezing; surgical excision of cutaneous HPV infections is not indicated in that these lesions are epidermal infections.
Intralesional bleomycin	Highly effective in the hands of experienced clinician.

HPV, human papillomavirus.

condylomata acuminata of Buschke-Löwenstein; and they can transform to verrucous carcinoma.

Management of external genital warts can be office-based or patient-initiated. For a discussion of treatment modalities, see Chapter 47.

Low-Grade and High-Grade Squamous Intraepithelial Lesions, Squamous Cell Carcinoma In Situ, Invasive Squamous Cell Carcinoma

The natural history of external anogenital HPV-induced dysplasia is not known. Prolonged, severe immunodeficiency provides the necessary milieu for the emergence of HPV-induced anogenital neoplasia. The incidence of transformation of squamous cell carcinoma in situ (SCCIS) to invasive SCC appears to be low. The relative risk for HPV-related anal invasive SCC is much higher in HIV-infected than in non-HIV-infected homosexual men and is more likely with advanced HIV disease. The most common sites for HPV-induced squamous intraepithelial lesions (SILs, SCCIS, and invasive SCC are the cervix, anus, perineum, vulva, penis, oropharynx/tongue, conjunctivae, and nail apparatus.[68]

Anogenital neoplasias are likely to become more common manifestations of HIV disease as patients with profound immunodeficiency, who would previously have succumbed to opportunistic infections, are now surviving for extended periods because of HAART.[69] Cervical, anal, and external anogenital low- and high-grade SIL and invasive SCC have become more common in long-term survivors of HIV disease. Invasive SCC arising on external anogenital sites is usually detected earlier and is less aggressive than that arising on the cervix or anal canal.

Management of external anogenital HPV infection in HIV-infected individuals is directed at identifying high-grade SIL before progression to invasive SCC has occurred. All HIV-infected individuals should be examined annually for evidence of HPV infection, especially those with prior HPV infections. Because HPV-induced neoplasia may extend to the cervix or anus (or both), direct examination by speculum and anoscope should also be performed and samples for cytology obtained using a cervical brush and Cytofix solution during the examination. High-resolution anoscopy and biopsy are done on individuals with high-grade SIL.[69] Individuals with documented external anogenital SIL should be followed by periodic follow-up examinations (every 4 to 6 months), noting the appearance of new lesions at these sites or an enlarging nodule or ulcerated site; biopsy of these sites is recommended.

Low-grade and high-grade SILs of the external anogenital epithelium can be treated by several methods: topical chemotherapy (5% 5-fluorouracil or imiquimod 5% cream, especially for extensive multifocal lesions)[70]; surgical excision of single or several lesions; focal destruction of lesions by cryosurgery, electrosurgery, or laser surgery. Unlike topical 5-fluorouracil or imiquimod, surgical modalities treat only clinically detectable lesions, not subclinical infection.

For minimally invasive SCCs arising on the anal verge (nonkeratinized to keratinized epithelium) or on external anogenital sites (penis, vulva, perineum), surgical excision is recommended with adequate borders around the lesion. Invasive SCC of the anus (transformation zone) is treated by radiation therapy and chemotherapy. The prognosis for invasive anal SCC is better in those with higher CD4+ T-lymphocyte counts at the time of diagnosis.[71]

▲ CRUSTED (NORWEGIAN) SCABIES

Crusted (hyperkeratotic, Norwegian) scabies occurs in immunocompromised hosts. Currently in the United States, HIV disease is the most common associated immunocompromised state. In obtunded or compromised individuals, pruritus may be diminished or absent in crusted scabies. Scabetic infestation can be severe, with millions of mites infesting the skin, presenting as a hyperkeratotic dermatitis but resembling atopic erythroderma, psoriasis vulgaris, keratoderma blennorrhagicum, keratosis follicularis (Darier's disease), or seborrheic dermatitis (in infants).[72] Thickly crusted plaques occur on the ears, buttocks, and extensor surfaces of the extremities, palms, and soles. Heavy infestation occurs around the nails with nail dystrophy and subungual and periungual scale-crust.[73,74] Scabetic infestation, which usually spares the head and neck in adults, can be generalized. *Staphylococcus aureus* and gram-negative superinfection can occur, sometimes complicated by septicemia and death.[75–77] Because of the number of organisms in crusted scabies, recurrences are common, and hospital epidemics may occur.

Use of potent topical corticosteroids for such previously diagnosed pruritic conditions may mask the presence of scabetic infestation. Eradication of the infestation is difficult because of the number of organisms. Topical treatment with gamma benzene hexachloride (lindane), permethrin lotion, or 10% sulfur ointment is effective; total-body application is required. Keratolytic agents are needed to débride hyperkeratotic areas in conjunction with débridement of involved nails. Orally administered ivermectin 200 μg/kg given as a single dose has been reported to be highly effective for common as well as crusted scabies.[78–80] Two or three doses separated by 1 to 2 weeks are usually required for heavy infestation or in those with advanced immunocompromise.

▲ OPPORTUNISTIC NEOPLASMS IN HIV DISEASE

General Information

The prevalence of the "opportunistic neoplasms"—Kaposi sarcoma (KS), HPV-induced neoplasia (SIL; SCCIS; invasive SCC of the cervix, external anogenitalia, and perineum), undifferentiated non-Hodgkin B-cell lymphoma (NHL), primary central nervous system (CNS) lymphoma—is increased in individuals with HIV disease. The incidence of nonmelanoma skin cancer, HPV-induced invasive SCC of the cervix and anus, Hodgkin lymphoma, T-cell lymphomas, and seminoma may also be increased. Many of these opportunistic neoplasms (NHL, KS, and anogenital in situ and invasive SCCIS) are associated with human viruses (EBV, HHV-8, HPV) and diminished immune-mediated tumor surveillance.

Basal Cell Carcinoma and Squamous Cell Carcinoma

The prevalence of ultraviolet radiation (UVR)-induced SCC appears to be increased in HIV disease as it is in immunosuppressed renal transplant recipients. As with transplant recipients, UVR-induced SCC in HIV disease may be more aggressive than in the immunocompetent host. In a report from San Francisco, 33 HIV-infected individuals with 97 SCCs were compared with 24 HIV-infected persons with 70 basal cell carcinomas (BCCs).[81] Risk factors for the development of both types of carcinoma were fair skin and excessive sun exposure (> 6 hours per day during the previous 10 years). Those with SCCs tended to have outdoor occupations. SCCs occurred more often on the head and neck, whereas BCCs were seen on the trunk. SCCs were diagnosed more commonly in individuals with advanced HIV disease than were BCCs. HPV was not an oncogenic factor in the development of these cutaneous tumors; *p53* overexpression was hypothesized to play an etiologic role.

Response to therapy in most cases is the same as for the general population; however, aggressive SCCs or BCCs, both UVL- and HPV-induced, have been reported. Frequent follow-up examinations (every 4 to 6 months) for individuals with UVL-associated SCCs or BCCs is recommended to detect recurrence of treated tumors or the development of new lesions.

▲ ADVERSE CUTANEOUS DRUG REACTIONS

The incidence of adverse cutaneous drug eruptions (ACDEs) in response to a variety of drugs is high in HIV disease (100 times more common than in the general population) and increases with advancing immunodeficiency.[82] Drug hypersensitivity complicated 3% to 20% of all prescriptions in one large series.[83]

The pathogenesis of the high rates of ACDE in HIV disease is unknown; pathogenetic factors include immune dysregulation with increased B-cell activity with immunoglobulin E (IgE) and IgA hyperimmunoglobulinemia and hypereosinophilia, The diagnosis can often be made based on clinical findings; lesional skin biopsy is helpful is some cases, differentiating an exanthematous reaction from a drug-induced vasculitis.

In a report of 974 HIV-infected individuals followed for 46 months, 283 ACDEs occurred in 201 patients.[84] ACDEs were noted more commonly in white than black people. Acute or reactivated EBV or CMV infections were significantly more common in patients with an ACDE. The onset of most of ACDEs is within 6 to 14 days of initiating therapy. Trimethoprion-sulfamathoxezole (TMP-SMZ), other sulfonamide drugs, and penicillins were the causative agents in 75% of cases of ACDE. Exanthematous (morbilliform) eruptions were by far the most commonly occurring ACDE, occurring in 95% of cases; other ACDEs observed were urticaria (4 cases), erythema multiforme (EM) [8 cases: EM major 2 cases, EM minor 6 cases], a lichenoid eruption (1 case), and fixed drug eruption (2 cases). Systemic symptoms were reported in 20% of cases, including fever, headache, myalgia, and arthralgia.

Most ACDEs are mild and are accompanied by pruritus, resolving promptly after the offending drug is discontinued. However, severe, life-threatening adverse cutaneous drug reactions (ACDRs) do occur and are unpredictable. Drug eruptions can mimic virtually all the morphologic expressions in dermatology and must be first on the differential diagnosis list at the appearance of a sudden symmetrical eruption. Drug eruptions are caused by immunologic or nonimmunologic mechanisms and are provoked by systemic or topical administration of a drug. Most are based on a hypersensitivity mechanism and may be of type I, II, III, or IV (Table 55–10).

Nonimmunologic ACDEs are classified in the following categories: (1) idiosyncratic sensu strictiori (reactions due to hereditary enzyme deficiencies); (2) cumulation (depends on the total amount of drug ingested: pigmentation, (i.e., gold, amiodarone, minocycline); (3) reactions due to the combination of a drug with ultraviolet irradiation [i.e., photosensitivity with either a toxic or immunologic (allergic) pathogenesis]; (4) irritance/toxicity of a topically applied drug (5-fluorouracil, imiquimod, podophyllotoxin, imiquimod), individual idiosyncrasy to a topical or systemic drug, or unknown mechanisms.

Guidelines for the assessment of possible ACDR include the following: (1) Alternative causes should be excluded, especially infections, in that many infections (especially viral) are difficult to distinguish clinically from the adverse effects of drugs used to treat infections. (2) The interval between introducing a drug and the onset of the reaction should be examined. (3) Any improvement after drug withdrawal should be noted. (4) The caregiver should determine whether similar reactions have been associated with the same compound. (5) Any reaction on readministration of the drug should be noted. Clinical patterns of ACDR vary widely and should be ruled out in the presence of a change in the clinical status of the patient (Table 55–10).

Skin findings that indicate possible life-threatening ACDRs include confluent skin pain, erythema, urticaria, facial edema or central facial involvement, palpable purpura (vasculitis), skin necrosis, blisters of epidermal detachment, or a positive Nikolsky's sign (epidermis separates readily from the dermis with lateral pressure). Mucosal findings correlating with a serious ACDR include mucous membrane erosions and swelling of the tongue. Systemic findings indicating possible serious adverse drug reaction include high fever (temperature ≥ 40°C), hypotension, shortness of breath, wheezing, enlarged lymph nodes, arthralgias, and arthritis.

In most cases the implicated or suspected drug should be discontinued. In some, such as with morbilliform eruptions, the offending drug can be continued, and the eruption may resolve. In cases of urticaria/angioedema or early Stevens-Johnson syndrome/toxic epidermonecrolysis, the ACDR can be life-threatening, and the drug should be discontinued.

Antiretroviral Agents

Drug hypersensitivity commonly occurs with the nonnucleoside reverse transcriptase inhibitors (NNRTIs) nevirapine,

▲ **Table 55–10.** TYPES OF ALLERGIC CUTANEOUS DRUG REACTIONS

Reaction	Comments
Exanthematous (morbilliform) reactions	Most common type of ACDR. Can occur with nearly any drug. Onset: < 14 days after drug therapy initiated. Same reaction recurs shortly after rechallenge with the sensitizing agent.
Urticaria/angioedema	Urticaria is the second most common type of ACDR after exanthematous reaction; in some cases, angioedema also occurs. Onset: usually within 36 hours after initial exposure; within minutes after rechallenge. Agents: aspirin and NSAIDs are common causes; also codeine, penicillin, blood transfusion. Drugs that release mast cell mediator(s): opiates, codeine, amphetamine, polymyxin B, atropine, hydralazine, pentamidine, quinine, radiocontrast media. Drug that may cause urticaria/angioedema by pharmacologic mechanisms: cyclooxygenase inhibitors (aspirin, indomethacin).
Angioedema	Uncommon. Characterized by edema of deep dermis and subcutaneous and submucosal areas.
Anaphylaxis and anaphylactoid reactions	Most serious type of adverse drug reaction. Occurs within minutes or hours after administration of drug. May be systemic life-threatening reaction. Agents: radiographic contrast media, antibiotics, extracts of allergens. More common with parenteral than oral administration. Intermittent administration may predispose to anaphylaxis.
Serum sickness	Onset: 5–21 days after initial exposure. Minor form: fever, urticaria, arthralgia. Major (complete) form: fever, urticaria, angioedema, arthralgia, arthritis, lymphadenopathy, eosinophilia, ± nephritis, ± endocarditis. Agents: IV immunoglobulin G (IVIG), antibiotics, and bovine serum albumin (used oocyte retrieval during in vitro fertilization).
Erythema multiforme	Most cases considered to be associated with reactivated HSV infection.
Stevens-Johnson syndrome	Moderate mucocutaneous and systemic reaction. With more severe mucocutaneous and systemic involvement, clinical findings merge into toxic epidermal necrolysis.
Toxic epidermal necrolysis	Severe, life-threatening mucocutaneous and systemic reaction.
Fixed drug eruptions	Appears 0.5–1.0 hours after readministration in sensitized individuals. Lesions often solitary, recurring at same site; may be multiple. More numerous lesions occur after repeated administration; multiple bullous lesions can mimic those of TEN.
Lichenoid eruptions	Onset: weeks to months after initiation of drug therapy; may progress to exfoliative dermatitis. May be extensive. Adnexal involvement may result in alopecia, anhidrosis. Oral involvement occurs with some drugs. Resolution after discontinuation slow, 1–4 months; up to 24 months after gold. May be photodistributed or bullous.
Photosensitivity	Classified as phototoxic (occurring in all individuals if dosing high enough, only at sites of light exposure), photoallergic (may be eczematous or lichenoid), or photocontact reactions. Some drugs cause both phototoxic and photoallergic reactions.
Porphyria cutanea tarda (PCT), pseudoporphyria, and photosensitivity	May be precipitated by drugs in sunexposed sites. Pseudo-PCT with bulla formation can also be a drug-induced reaction
Purpura (petechiae, ecchymoses)	Thrombocytopenia: allergic or cytotoxic; results in petechiae/ecchymoses if platelet counts are < 30,000/μl. Hemorrhage into a morbilliform ACDR occurs not uncommonly on the legs. Oral, inhalation, and topical corticosteroid usage are associated with ecchymoses, usually on the extremities in areas of dermatoheliosis. Progressive pigmented purpura has also been reported to associated with drug therapy.
Acneiform eruptions	Folliculocentric pustules, usually without comedones. Drugs: anabolic steroids/testosterone (replacement) corticosteroids (parenteral, topical), ACTH, anabolic steroids, oral contraceptives, halogens (iodides, bromides), isoniazid, danazol, lithium, azathioprine.
Pustular eruptions	Toxic pustuloderma, acute generalized exanthematous pustulosis. Must be differentiated from pustular psoriasis. Eosinophil in the infiltrate suggests ACDR. Drugs: ampicillin, amoxicillin, macrolides, tetracyclines.
Psoriasiform reactions	Drugs reported to exaccerbate psoriasis: antimalarials; β-blockers; lithium salts; NSAIDs (ibuprofen, indomethacin); miscellaneous (captopril, cimetidine, clonidine, gemfibrozil, interferon, methyldopa, penicillamine, trazadone).

Table continued on following page

▲ **Table 55–10.** TYPES OF ALLERGIC CUTANEOUS DRUG REACTIONS *Continued*

Reaction	Comments
Eczematous eruptions	Systemic administration of a drug to an individual who has been previously sensitized to the drug by topical application can experience widespread eczematous dermatitis (systemic contact-type dermatitis medicamentosa) or urticaria. Systemically administered drugs that reactivate allergic contact dermatitis to related topical agents (systemic drug/topical agent): ethylenediamine antihistamines, aminophylline/aminophylline suppositories, ethylenediamine HCl; procaine/benzocaine; iodides, iodinated organic compounds, radiographic contrast media/iodine; streptomycin, kanamycin, paramomycin, gentamicin/neomycin sulfate; nitroglycerin tablets/nitroglycerin ointment; disulfuram/thiuram.
Exfoliative dermatitis and erythroderma	This widespread or generalized reaction may follow an exanthematous ACDR or begin with erythema and exudation in body folds and progress to become generalized. In individuals previously sensitized by topical administration of a drug, systemic administration of the sensitizing agent (or closely related compound) may cause a generalized eczematous dermatitis. The most commonly implicated drugs are sulfonamides, antimalarials, phenytoin, and penicillin.

ACDR, allergic cutaneous drug reaction; TEN, toxic epidermal necrolysis.

delavirdine, and efavirenz; the nucleoside reverse-transcriptase inhibitor (NRTI) abacavir; and the protease inhibitor amprenavir.[82] HIV drug hypersensitivity is characterized principally by morbilliform/maculopapular/exanthematous rash, fever (often precedes rash), myalgias/fatigue, and mucosal ulcerations, as well as less common features (< 5%) such as Stevens-Johnson syndrome, toxic epidermal necrolysis, anicteric hepatitis, hypotension, acute interstitial nephritis, and acute interstitial pneumonitis. Nearly 20% of nevirapine-treated patients experience rash, most commonly an exanthematous eruption and less commonly Stevens-Johnson syndrome,[85] requiring drug discontinuation.[82] About 18% to 50% of delavirdine-treated patients experience rash.

Approximately half of the cases of antiretroviral hypersensitivity resolve despite continuation of therapy. Drug therapy should be discontinued if the following occur: mucosal involvement, blistering, exfoliation, clinically significant hepatic dysfunction, fever higher than 39°C, or intolerable fever or pruritus.[86] Rechallenge with abacavir has been associated with several deaths.

Indinavir, which has a retinoid-like effect, causes cheilitis (57%), diffuse dryness and pruritus (41%), asteatotic dermatitis on the trunk, arms, and thighs (12%), and scalp defluvium (12%)[87]; pyogenic granulomas, single or multiple, have also been reported. Symptoms resolved when the indinavir was discontinued. Peripheral lipodystrophy syndrome occurs in 14% of subjects.

Longitudinal melanonychia, brown-black longitudinal streaks in the nail plate, occur in up to 40% of zidovudine (ZDV)-treated individuals, more commonly in Blacks than in Latinos or Whites. The pigmentary changes are usually noted in the fingernails or toenails (or both) within 4 to 8 weeks after initiating ZDV therapy but may occur as long as 1 year later. ZDV pigmented macules of mucous membranes is also common, occurring more commonly in more heavily melanized individuals. Diffuse hyperpigmentation mimicking primary adrenal insufficiency has been reported. Melanonychia and mucocutaneous pigmentation has also been reported with hydroxyurea in HIV disease.[88]

Trimethoprim-Sulfamethoxazole

Approximately 50% to 60% of HIV-infected individuals treated with intravenous TMP-SMZ develop an exanthematous eruption (often associated with fever) 1 to 2 weeks after starting therapy, an incidence 10 times greater than that in the general population.[89] Successful desensitization has been accomplished in patients with prior exanthematous or urticarial reactions to TMP-SMZ, sulfadiazine, and dapsone.[90–92] Desensitization in patients with prior Stevens-Johnson syndrome has also been reported.[93] Co-administration of corticosteroids with TMP-SMX reduced the incidence of adverse cutaneous reactions from 47% to 13%.[94] The occurrence of adverse reactions to TMP-SMZ has also been noted to be associated with a more rapid decline in CD4+ T-lymphocyte counts.[95]

Severe bullous eruptions appear to be common with HIV disease. In a report of six cases of erythema multiforme major and six of toxic epidermal necrolysis (TEN), all adverse reactions were to sulfonamide: sulfadiazine (six cases), TMP-SMZ (two cases), and sulfadoxine-pyrimethamine (Fansidar) (two cases).[96] Of 14 cases of TEN over a 6-year period (1984–1989), sulfa drugs were the most common causative agents.[96] The number of cases of TEN was 375 times that expected. TEN occurred in patients with advanced HIV disease and was associated with a 21% mortality rate.

Oral Corticosteroids

Oral corticosteroid therapy in HIV-infected individuals raises concerns regarding increased immunosuppression with exacerbations of opportunistic infections and neoplasms such as Kaposi sarcoma or HSV infections. A cohort of 44 asymptomatic HIV-infected individuals (CD4+ T-lymphocyte count of 200 to 799 cells/mm^3) were treated with oral prednisolone (0.5 mg/kg for 6 months; 0.3 mg/kg thereafter).[97] After 1 year of prednisolone therapy, no major side effects or HIV disease-related events had occurred.

Serum p24 antigen and HIV RNA levels remained stable; CD4+ T-lymphocyte counts increased significantly at all time points (median increase at 1 year was 119 cells/mm^3). A more recent study concluded that short-term prednisone was well tolerated and reasonably safe.[98] Short-term oral corticosteroid therapy appears to be safe in most HIV-infected individuals.

Foscarnet

Foscarnet (trisodium phosphonoformate) causes painful, penile erosions or ulcers (or both) in 30% of patients undergoing high-dose induction therapy for CMV retinitis 7 to 24 days after starting treatment. The ulcers are caused by high urinary concentrations of the urinary metabolites of foscarnet. Hyperhydration reduces the risk of ulceration; in some cases the drug must be discontinued for the ulcers to heal.

REFERENCES

1. Rico MJ, Myers SA, Sanchez MR. Guidelines of care for dermatologic conditions in patients infected with HIV: Guidelines/Outcomes Committee. American Academy of Dermatology. J Am Acad Dermatol 37:450, 1997.
2. Kahn JO, Walker BD. Acute human immunodeficiency virus type 1 infection. N Engl J Med 339:33, 1998.
3. Vanhems P, Dassa C, Lambert J, et al. Comprehensive classification of symptoms and signs reported among 218 patients with acute HIV-1 infection. J Acquir Immune Defic Syndr 21:99, 1999.
4. Boonchai W, Laohasrisakul R, Manonukul J, Kulthanan K. Pruritic papular eruption in HIV seropositive patients: a cutaneous marker for immunosuppression. Int J Dermatol 38:348, 1999.
5. Rodwell GE, Berger TG. Pruritus and cutaneous inflammatory conditions in HIV disease. Clin Dermatol 18:479, 2000.
6. Gelfand JM, Rudikoff D. Evaluation and treatment of itching in HIV-infected patients. Mt Sinai J Med 68:298, 2001.
7. Bonacini M. Pruritus in patients with chronic human immunodeficiency virus, hepatitis B and C virus infections. Dig Liver Dis 32:621, 2000.
8. Milazzo F, Piconi S, Trabattoni D, et al. Intractable pruritus in HIV infection: immunologic characterization. Allergy 54:266, 1999.
9. Otley CC, Avram MR, Johnson RA. Isotretinoin treatment of human immunodeficiency virus-associated eosinophilic folliculitis: results of an open, pilot trial. Arch Dermatol 131:1047, 1995.
10. Lim HW, Vallurupalli S, Meola T, Soter NA. UVB phototherapy is an effective treatment for pruritus in patients infected with HIV. J Am Acad Dermatol 37:414, 1997.
11. Gelfand JM, Rudikoff D, Lebwohl M, Klotman ME. Effect of UV-B phototherapy on plasma HIV type 1 RNA viral level: a self-controlled prospective study. Arch Dermatol 134:940, 1998.
12. Corominas M, Garcia JF, Mestre M, et al. Predictors of atopy in HIV-infected patients. Ann Allergy Asthma Immunol 84:607, 2000.
13. Schreckenberg C, Lipsker D, Petiau P, et al. [Photosensitivity as presenting sign of HIV infection: control with triple antiretroviral therapy.] Ann Dermatol Venereol 125:516, 1998.
14. Meola T, Sanchez M, Lim HW, et al. Chronic actinic dermatitis associated with human immunodeficiency virus infection. Br J Dermatol 137:431, 1997.
15. Vin-Christian K, Epstein JH, Maurer TA, et al. Photosensitivity in HIV-infected individuals. J Dermatol 27:361, 2000.
16. Smith KJ, Skelton HG, Yeager J, et al. Pruritus in HIV-1 disease: therapy with drugs which may modulate the pattern of immune dysregulation. Dermatology 195:353, 1997.
17. Jacobson JM, Greenspan JS, Spritzler J, et al. Thalidomide in low intermittent doses does not prevent recurrence of human immunodeficiency virus-associated aphthous ulcers. J Infect Dis 183:343, 2001.
18. Cribier B, Rey D, Uhl G, et al. Abnormal urinary coproporphyrin levels in patients infected by hepatitis C virus with or without human immunodeficiency virus: a study of 177 patients. Arch Dermatol 132:1448, 1996.
19. O'Connor WJ, Murphy GM, Darby C, et al. Porphyrin abnormalities in acquired immunodeficiency syndrome. Arch Dermatol 132:1443, 1996.
20. Gisselbrecht M, Cohen P, Lortholary O, et al. Human immunodeficiency virus-related vasculitis: clinical presentation of and therapeutic approach to eight cases. Ann Med Interne (Paris) 149:398, 1998.
21. Hung CC, Hsueh PR, Chen MY, et al. Bacteremia caused by *Helicobacter cinaedi* in an AIDS patients. J Formos Med Assoc 96:558, 1997.
22. Sullivan AK, Nelson MR, Walsh J, Gazzard BG. Recurrent *Helicobacter cinaedi* cellulitis and bacteraemia in a patient with HIV Infection. Int J STD AIDS 8:59, 1997.
23. Burman WJ, Cohn DL, Reves RR, Wilson ML. Multifocal cellulitis and monoarticular arthritis as manifestations of *Helicobacter cinaedi* bacteremia. Clin Infect Dis 20:564, 1995.
24. Wong R, Tappero J, Cockerell CJ. Bacillary angiomatosis and other *Bartonella* species infections. Semin Cutan Med Surg 16:188, 1997.
25. Gazineo JL, Trope BM, Maceira JP, et al. Bacillary angiomatosis: description of 13 cases reported in five reference centers for AIDS treatment in Rio de Janeiro, Brazil. Rev Inst Med Trop Sao Paulo 43:1, 2001.
26. Plettenberg A, Lorenzen T, Burtsche BT, et al. Bacillary angiomatosis in HIV-infected patients—an epidemiological and clinical study. Dermatology 201:326, 2000.
27. Gupta AK, Taborda P, Taborda V, et al. Epidemiology and prevalence of onychomycosis in HIV-positive individuals. Int J Dermatol 39:746, 2000.
28. Johnson RA. Dermatophyte infections in human immune deficiency virus (HIV) disease. J Am Acad Dermatol 43(suppl 5):S135, 2000.
29. Korting HC, Blecher P, Stallmann D, Hamm G. Dermatophytes on the feet of HIV-infected patients: frequency, species distribution, localization and antimicrobial susceptibility. Mycoses 36:271, 1993.
30. Almeida L, Grossman M. Widespread dermatophyte infections that mimic collagen vascular disease. J Am Acad Dermatol 23:855, 1990.
31. Elewski BE, Sullivan J. Dermatophytes as opportunistic pathogens. J Am Acad Dermatol 30:1021, 1994.
32. Wright DC, Lennox JL, James WD, et al. Generalized chronic dermatophytosis in patients with human immunodeficiency virus type I infection and CD4 depletion [letter]. Arch Dermatol 127:265, 1991.
33. Prose NS. HIV infection in children. J Am Acad Dermatol 22:1223, 1990.
34. Kantipong P, Walsh DS. Oral penicilliosis in a patient with human immunodeficiency virus in northern Thailand. Int J Dermatol 39:926, 2000.
35. Schacker T, Hu HL, Koelle DM, et al. Famciclovir for the suppression of symptomatic and asymptomatic herpes simplex virus reactivation in HIV-infected persons: a double-blind, placebo-controlled trial. Ann Intern Med 128:21, 1998.
36. Conant M. Current clinical issues in the management of herpes simplex virus infections in patients with HIV. Dermatology 194:93, 1997.
37. Chang E, Absar N, Beall G. Prevention of recurrent herpes simplex virus (HSV) infections in HIV-infected persons. AIDS Patient Care 9:252, 1995.
38. Saint-Leger E, Fillet AM, Malvy D, et al. [Efficacy of cidofovir in an HIV infected patient with an acyclovir and foscarnet resistant herpes simplex virus infection.] Ann Dermatol Venereol 128:747, 2001.
39. Lalezari J, Schacker T, Feinberg J, et al. A randomized, double-blind, placebo-controlled trial of cidofovir gel for the treatment of acyclovir-unresponsive mucocutaneous herpes simplex virus infection in patients with AIDS. J Infect Dis 176:892, 1997.
40. Gilbert J, Drehs M, Weinberg J, et al. Topical imiquimod for acyclovir-unresponsive herpes simplex virus 2 infection. Arch Dermatol 127:1015, 2001.
41. Zampogna JC, Flowers FP. Persistent verrucous varicella as the initial manifestation of HIV infection. J Am Acad Dermatol 44(suppl 2):391, 2001.
42. Leautez S, Billaud E, Milpied B, Raffi F. [Varicella zoster virus infection area in 39 HIV-infected patients: therapeutic management.] Presse Med 28:473, 1999.
43. Safrin S, Berger TG, Gilson I, et al. Foscarnet therapy in five patients with AIDS and acyclovir-resistant varicella-zoster virus infection. Ann Intern Med 115:19, 1991.
44. Safrin S, Assaykeen T, Follansbee S, Mills J. Foscarnet therapy for acyclovir-resistant mucocutaneous herpes simplex virus infection in 26 AIDS patients: preliminary data. J Infect Dis 161:1078, 1990.

45. Patton LL, McKaig R, Strauss R, et al. Changing prevalence of oral manifestations of human immunodeficiency virus in the era of protease inhibitor therapy. Oral Surg Oral Med Oral Pathol Oral Radiol Endod 89:299, 2000.
46. Patton LL. Sensitivity, specificity, and positive predictive value of oral opportunistic infections in adults with HIV/AIDS as markers of immune suppression and viral burden. Oral Surg Oral Med Oral Pathol Oral Radiol Endod 90:182, 2000.
47. Greenspan D, Komaroff E, Redford M, et al. Oral mucosal lesions and HIV viral load in the Women's Interagency HIV Study (WIHS). J Acquir Immune Defic Syndr 25:44, 2000.
48. Greenspan D, Greenspan JS, Hearst NG, et al. Relation of oral hairy leukoplakia to infection with the human immunodeficiency virus and the risk of developing AIDS. J Infect Dis 155:475, 1987.
49. Greenspan D, Greenspan JS. Oral manifestations of HIV infection. Dermatol Clin 9:517, 1991.
50. Alessi E, Berti E, Cusini M, et al. Oral hairy leukoplakia. J Am Acad Dermatol 22:79, 1990.
51. Eyeson JD, Warnakulasuriya KA, Johnson NW. Prevalence and incidence of oral lesions—the changing scene. Oral Dis 6:267, 2000.
52. Logan RM, Coates EA, Pierce AM, Wilson DF. A retrospective analysis of oral hairy leukoplakia in South Australia. Aust Dent J 46:108, 2001.
53. Ceballos-Salobrena A, Gaitan-Cepeda LA, Ceballos-Garcia L, Lezama-Del Valle D. Oral lesions in HIV/AIDS patients undergoing highly active antiretroviral treatment including protease inhibitors: a new face of oral AIDS? AIDS Patient Care STDS 14:627, 2000.
54. Weinberg JM, Mysliwiec A, Turiansky GW, et al. Viral folliculitis: atypical presentations of herpes simplex, herpes zoster, and molluscum contagiosum. Arch Dermatol 133:983, 1997.
55. Myskowski PL. Molluscum contagiosum: new insights, new directions [editorial]. Arch Dermatol 133:1039, 1997.
56. Koopman RJ, van Merrienboer FC, Vreden SG, Dolmans WM. Molluscum contagiosum; a marker for advanced HIV infection [letter]. Br J Dermatol 126:528, 1992.
57. Hicks CB, Myers SA, Giner J. Resolution of intractable molluscum contagiosum in a human immunodeficiency virus-infected patient after institution of antiretroviral therapy with ritonavir. Clin Infect Dis 24:1023, 1997.
58. Strauss RM, Doyle EL, Mohsen AH, Green ST. Successful treatment of molluscum contagiosum with topical imiquimod in a severely immunocompromised HIV-positive patient. Int J STD AIDS 12:264, 2001.
59. Liota E, Smith KJ, Buckley R, et al. Imiquimod therapy for molluscum contagiosum. J Cutan Med Surg 4:76, 2000.
60. Toro JR, Wood LV, Patel NK, Turner ML. Topical cidofovir: a novel treatment for recalcitrant molluscum contagiosum in children infected with human immunodeficiency virus 1. Arch Dermatol 136:983, 2000.
61. Calista D. Topical cidofovir for severe cutaneous human papillomavirus and molluscum contagiosum infections in patients with HIV/AIDS: a pilot study. J Eur Acad Dermatol Venereol 14:484, 2000.
62. Meadows KP, Tyring SK, Pavia AT, Rallis TM. Resolution of recalcitrant molluscum contagiosum virus lesions in human immunodeficiency virus-infected patients treated with cidofovir. Arch Dermatol 133:987, 1997.
63. Cohen LM, Tyring SK, Rady P, Callen JP. Human papillomavirus type 11 in multiple squamous cell carcinomas in a patient with subacute cutaneous lupus erythematosus. J Am Acad Dermatol 26:840, 1992.
64. Viac J, Chardonnet Y, Euvrard S, et al. Langerhans cells, inflammation markers and human papillomavirus infections in benign and malignant epithelial tumors from transplant recipients. J Dermatol 19:67, 1992.
65. Berger TG, Sawchuk WS, Leonardi C, et al. Epidermodysplasia verruciformis-associated papillomavirus infection complicating human immunodeficiency virus disease. Br J Dermatol 124:79, 1991.
66. Prose NS, von Knebel-Doeberitz C, Miller S, et al. Widespread flat warts associated with human papillomavirus type 5: a cutaneous manifestation of human immunodeficiency virus infection. J Am Acad Dermatol 23:978, 1990.
67. Beck DE, Jaso RG, Zajac RA. Surgical management of anal condylomata in the HIV-positive patient. Dis Colon Rectum 33:180, 1990.
68. Poblet E, Alfaro L, Fernander-Segoviano P, et al. Human papillomavirus-associated penile squamous cell carcinoma in HIV-positive patients. Am J Surg Pathol 23:1119, 1999.
69. Goldstone SE, Winkler B, Ufford LJ, et al. High prevalence of anal squamous intraepithelial lesions and squamous-cell carcinoma in men who have sex with men as seen in a surgical practice. Dis Colon Rectum 44:690, 2001.
70. Pehoushek J, Smith KJ. Imiquimod and 5% fluorouracil therapy for anal and perianal squamous cell carcinoma in situ in an HIV-1-positive man. Arch Dermatol 137:14, 2001.
71. Place RJ, Gregorcyk SG, Huber PJ, Simmang CL. Outcome analysis of HIV-positive patients with anal squamous cell carcinoma. Dis Colon Rectum 44:506, 2001.
72. Donabedian H, Khazan U. Norwegian scabies in a patient with AIDS. Clin Infect Dis 14:162, 1992.
73. Portu JJ, Santamaria JM, Zubero Z, et al. Atypical scabies in HIV-positive patients. J Am Acad Dermatol 34:915, 1996.
74. Arico M, Noto G, La Rocca E, et al. Localized crusted scabies in the acquired immunodeficiency syndrome. Clin Exp Dermatol 17:339, 1992.
75. Hulbert TV, Larsen RA. Hyperkeratotic (Norwegian) scabies with gram-negative bacteremia as the initial presentation of AIDS [letter]. Clin Infect Dis 14:1164, 1992.
76. Glover A, Young L, Goltz AW. Norwegian scabies in acquired immunodeficiency syndrome: report of a case resulting in death from associated sepsis [letter]. J Am Acad Dermatol 16:396, 1987.
77. Glover RA, Piaquadio DJ, Kern S, Cockerell CJ. An unusual presentation of secondary syphilis in a patient with human immunodeficiency virus infection: a case report and review of the literature. Arch Dermatol 128:530, 1992.
78. Alberici F, Pagani L, Ratti G, Viale P. Ivermectin alone or in combination with benzyl benzoate in the treatment of human immunodeficiency virus-associated scabies. Br J Dermatol 142:969, 2000.
79. Meinking TL, Taplin D, Hermida JL, et al. The treatment of scabies with ivermectin. N Engl J Med 333:26, 1995.
80. Taplin D, Meinking TL. Treatment of HIV-related scabies with emphasis on the efficacy of ivermectin. Semin Cutan Med Surg 16:235, 1997.
81. Maurer TA, Christian KV, Kerschmann RL, et al. Cutaneous squamous cell carcinoma in human immunodeficiency virus-infected patients: a study of epidemiologic risk factors, human papillomavirus, and p53 expression. Arch Dermatol 133:577, 1997.
82. Carr A, Cooper DA. Adverse effects of antiretroviral therapy. Lancet 356:1423, 2000.
83. Coopman SA, Johnson RA, Platt R, Stern RS. Cutaneous disease and drug reactions in HIV infection. N Engl J Med 328:1670, 1993.
84. Smith KJ, Skelton HG, Yeager J, et al. Increased drug reactions in HIV-1-positive patients: a possible explanation based on patterns of immune dysregulation seen in HIV-1 disease: the Military Medical Consortium for the Advancement of Retroviral Research (MMCARR). Clin Exp Dermatol 22:118, 1997.
85. Metry DW, Lahart CJ, Farmer KL, Hebert AA. Stevens-Johnson syndrome caused by the antiretroviral drug nevirapine. J Am Acad Dermatol 44(suppl 2):354, 2001.
86. Max B, Sherer R. Management of the adverse effects of antiretroviral therapy and medication adherence. Clin Infect Dis 30(suppl 2):S96, 2000.
87. Calista D, Boschini A. Cutaneous side effects induced by indinavir. Eur J Dermatol 10:292, 2000.
88. Laughon SK, Shinn LL, Nunley JR. Melanonychia and mucocutaneous hyperpigmentation due to hydroxyurea use in an HIV-infected patient. Int J Dermatol 39:928, 2000.
89. Roudier C, Caumes E, Rogeaux O, et al. Adverse cutaneous reactions to trimethoprim-sulfamethoxazole in patients with the acquired immunodeficiency syndrome and *Pneumocystis carinii* pneumonia. Arch Dermatol 130:1383, 1994.
90. Absar N, Daneshvar H, Beall G. Desensitization to trimethoprim/-sulfamethoxazole in HIV-infected patients. J Allergy Clin Immunol 93:1001, 1994.
91. Gluckstein D, Ruskin J. Rapid oral desensitization to trimethoprim-sulfamethoxazole (TMP-SMZ): use in prophylaxis for *Pneumocystis carinii* pneumonia in patients with AIDS who were previously intolerant to TMP-SMZ. Clin Infect Dis 20:849, 1995.
92. Yoshizawa S, Yasuoka A, Kikuchi Y, et al. A 5-day course of oral desensitization to trimethoprim/sulfamethoxazole (T/S) in patients with human immunodeficiency virus type-1 infection who were previously intolerant to T/S. Ann Allergy Asthma Immunol 85:241, 2000.
93. Douglas R, Spelman D, Czarny D, O'Hehir RE. Successful desensitization of two patients who previously developed Stevens-Johnson syn-

drome while receiving trimethoprim-sulfamethoxazole. Clin Infect Dis 25:1480, 1997.

94. Caumes E, Roudier C, Rogeaux O, et al. Effect of corticosteroids on the incidence of adverse cutaneous reactions to trimethoprim-sulfamethoxazole during treatment of AIDS-associated *Pneumocystis carinii* pneumonia. Clin Infect Dis 18:319, 1994.
95. Veenstra J, Veugelers PJ, Keet IP, et al. Rapid disease progression in human immunodeficiency virus type 1-infected individuals with adverse reactions to trimethoprim-sulfamethoxazole prophylaxis. Clin Infect Dis 24:936, 1997.
96. Roujeau JC, Chosidow O, Saiag P, Guillaume JC. Toxic epidermal necrolysis (Lyell syndrome). J Am Acad Dermatol 23:1039, 1990.
97. Andrieu JM, Lu W, Levy R. Sustained increases in CD4 cell counts in asymptomatic human immunodeficiency virus type 1-seropositive patients treated with prednisolone for 1 year. J Infect Dis 171:523, 1995.
98. McComsey GA, Whalen CC, Mawhorter SD, et al. Placebo-controlled trial of prednisone in advanced HIV-1 infection. AIDS 15:321, 2001.

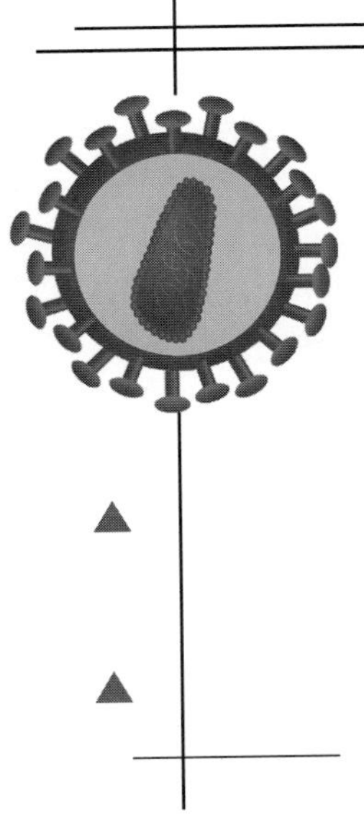

CHAPTER 56
Oropharyngeal Disease

Jeffery D. Hill, DMD

Oral lesions are common throughout the course of human immunodeficiency virus (HIV) infection. They may represent the initial signs of infection in the undiagnosed individual, or they may occur in patients with well established disease. Severe pain as a result of oral disease processes can significantly alter the patient's ability to sustain proper nutritional intake, take oral medications, and communicate effectively. Although the use of highly active antiretroviral therapy (HAART) has significantly reduced the incidence of opportunistic infections in general, oral lesions continue to occur.

▲ FUNGAL INFECTIONS

Oropharyngeal Candidiasis

Oropharyngeal candidiasis is the most common intraoral lesion among HIV-infected individuals. Reports indicate a prevalence of approximately 50% in adults living with HIV and as high as 96% in those with acquired immunodeficiency syndrome (AIDS).[1] Predominantly caused by *Candida albicans*,[2] this localized fungal infection is often a presenting sign of HIV infection. It is a marker for progression of HIV disease to AIDS and indicates that the risk of an AIDS diagnosis is higher during a candidiasis episode.[3]

Four distinct clinical presentations of oral candidiasis may be seen: pseudomembranous, erythematous, chronic or hyperplastic, angular cheilitis (Table 56–1). The diagnosis is based on the clinical appearance of the lesions and may be confirmed by the presence of hyphae on a potassium hydroxide smear if necessary. Some species of *Candida*, such as *C. lusitania* and *C. glabrata*, are inherently drug-resistant or respond poorly to certain azoles. However, identification of species by culture is not indicated except in nonresponsive cases where lesions fail to resolve with appropriate therapy.

Pseudomembranous candidiasis presents as a creamy-white plaque that can be scraped off with a tongue blade or cotton gauze, often leaving an erythematous surface underneath. Patients may complain of a mild burning sensation or a foul or metallic-like taste. The most common sites are the buccal mucosa, ventral tongue or floor of the mouth, and palate; but the lesions may appear anywhere in the oral cavity. Severe cases may lead to difficulty speaking, eating, or swallowing.

Erythematous candidiasis may be seen as a red macular lesion of the dorsal tongue, posterior hard palate, or buccal mucosa. Occasionally this form of oral candidiasis appears as an erythematous, atrophic or "bald" area of the midline posterior dorsum of the tongue, which may be asymptomatic. It represents a loss of filiform papillae, which should regenerate with proper treatment.

Chronic or hyperplastic candidiasis is a diffuse white or yellowish plaque that cannot be wiped off. These lesions may appear on any mucosal surface, often with multiple surfaces being affected at once. The plaque cannot be easily removed because the long-standing infection has allowed the candidal hyphae to become anchored deep in the mucosa. Chronic candidiasis may clinically resemble leukoplakia and may be associated with painful ulcerations of the affected mucosa. This type of candidal infection is most often seen with advanced HIV disease.

Angular cheilitis presents as erythematous, fissured, scaly patches at the angles of the mouth, usually with a pseudomembranous covering. The lesions may appear

▲ **Table 56–1.** COMMON ORAL LESIONS ASSOCIATED WITH HIV

Lesion	Clinical Appearance	Treatment
Fungal Infections		
Pseudomembranous candidiasis	White plaque; can be scraped off; any mucosal surface	Topical or systemic antifungal
Erythematous candidiasis	Red, macular; hard/soft palate; "bald" area, dorsum of tongue	Topical or systemic antifungal
Hyperplastic candidiasis	Diffuse white/yellow plaque; cannot be wiped off; multiple mucosal surfaces	Systemic or IV antifungal
Angular cheilitis	Red, fissured; corner of mouth; pseudomembranous covering	Topical antifungal
Viral Infections		
Herpes simplex virus	Painful ulcers; raised yellow border with red center; keratinized mucosa	Acyclovir; valacyclovir
Herpes labialis	Cluster of vesicles; rupture, crust over; outer border of lip; prodromal phase	Acyclovir; valacyclovir
Varicella-zoster virus	Extremely painful; cluster of vesicles; rupture, ulcerate, crust over; along distribution of trigeminal nerve; bound or movable mucosa; prodromal phase	Acyclovir; valacyclovir
Human papillomavirus	Any mucosal surface	
Oral papilloma	Exophytic, pedunculated; finger-like surface projections; whitish surface	Surgical excision; cryotherapy
Condyloma	Exophytic, sessile; short, blunted surface projections; pink; multiple, clustered; larger than papilloma	Surgical excision; cryotherapy
Focal epithelial hyperplasia	Multiple flat-topped papules or papillary areas; normal mucosal color	Surgical excision; cryotherapy
Epstein-Barr virus		
Oral hairy leukoplakia	White vertical streaks along lateral border of tongue; does not rub off	No treatment; acyclovir
Bacterial Infections		
Linear gingival erythema	Red band at gingival margin	Dental prophylaxis; 10% povidone-iodine irrigation; 0.12% chlorhexidine rinse; frequent follow-up; antifungals?
Acute necrotizing ulcerative gingivitis	Interproximal gingival necrosis; bleeding, pain, halitosis	Débridement of necrotic tissue; 10% povidone-iodine irrigation; 0.12% chlorhexidine rinse; frequent follow-up
Necrotizing ulcerative gingivitis/necrotizing ulcerative periodontitis	Intense, deep-seated, nongingival pain; spontaneous bleeding; rapid destruction of tissue; loose teeth; fetid breath; localized area	Débridement of necrotic tissue; scaling and root planing; 10% povidine-iodine irrigation; 0.12% chlorhexidine rinse; systemic antibiotics; pain medication; frequent follow-up
Neoplasms		
Kaposi's sarcoma	Initial lesion appears as diffuse, macular, red-purplish area; advanced lesions become nodular, dark purplish-brown; may ulcerate; any mucosal surface, most often hard or soft palate	Intralesional injection of vinblastine sulfate; surgical excision; cryotherapy; chemotherapy; radiation therapy
Non-Hodgkin's lymphoma	Rapidly growing red-purplish mass of the gingiva, posterior buccal vestibule, or retromolar area; ulceration, necrosis; mobility/loss of teeth; diffuse, slightly tender swelling of posterior hard palate; in the mandible, may produce paresthesia or vague tooth pain, followed by soft tissue eruption	Polychemotherapy; radiation therapy
Nonspecific Lesions		
Recurrent aphthous ulcers	Painful; yellow/gray pseudomembrane with red halo; nonkeratinized mucosa	
Herpetiform aphthae	Less than 3 mm diameter; multiple; may coalesce into larger, irregular ulcerations	Heal in about 10 days without treatment
Minor aphthae	Round; 3–10 mm diameter; superficial erosion	Heal in 7–14 days without treatment
Major aphthae	Extremely painful; 1–3 cm diameter; crater-like ulceration, may extend onto keratinized mucosa; persists 2–6 weeks or more; no spontaneous healing; may have fungal suprainfection	Topical and/or systemic glucocorticosteroids; thalidomide; pain medication; antifungals
Xerostomia	Dry or pasty mouth; bad breath; cervical caries	Eliminate causative factor; sugarless gum/candy; salivary substitutes/oral moisturizers; frequent water; prescription fluoride

unilaterally or bilaterally and most often in conjunction with intraoral candidiasis.

A variety of topical and systemic antifungal agents are available. When selecting the appropriate therapy, consideration should be given to the patient's history of oral candidiasis outbreaks, other current medications, and patient adherence factors. Topical therapy can be used to treat initial or recurring episodes in which there is no esophageal involvement, the CD4+ T-lymphocyte cell count is higher than 50 cells/mm^3, and the patient is currently receiving or expecting to undergo HAART.[4] The patient should be evaluated for saliva sufficient to dissolve topical agents and the ability to comply with the proper dosing regimen, providing sufficient contact between the drug and oral mucosa. It is also suggested that, because of the high sugar content of some topical preparations, the use of daily fluoride rinses should be employed to help reduce the risk of caries. Effective topical agents include clotrimazole (10 mg) oral troches, nystatin (200,000 U) oral pastilles, or nystatin (100,000 U) vaginal troches, which have the advantage of not containing sugars. Each should be administered as one troche or pastille dissolved slowly in the mouth four or five times a day for 10 to 14 days. Nystatin is also available as an oral suspension (500,000 U/5 ml), to be swished 5 ml four times a day for 5 minutes and then swallowed. For the treatment of angular cheilitis, clotrimazole cream (1%), nystatin ointment (100,000 U), or ketoconazole cream (2%) applied to the affected area three or four times a day may be used in conjunction with topical therapy for intraoral candidiasis.

Systemic therapy with oral azoles is more convenient for most patients and is especially recommended for those who have oropharyngeal candidiasis with esophageal involvement, or where the patient has a CD4+ T-lymphocyte count of less than 50 cells/mm^3, a high viral load, and is not receiving or anticipating HAART.[4] Systemic treatment is warranted in cases where lesions are nonresponsive to topical therapy following a review to verify the proper regimen and patient compliance. Although the advantage of once-daily dosing of the oral azoles may translate into increased compliance, consideration must be given to possible important drug interactions and side effects of the systemic agents. Commonly reported side effects include headache, nausea, vomiting, diarrhea, abdominal pain, and skin rash. Long-term use has been associated with hepatotoxicity, and liver function should be monitored accordingly.[5] The recommended treatment duration is 14 days. Chronic suppressive therapy should be avoided.

Ketoconazole is still used on rare occasions. It is given as 200 mg tablets: two tablets taken the first day, then one tablet each day thereafter. The absorption of ketoconazole is affected by gastric pH and may have reduced bioavailability in patients suffering from hypochlorhydria. The tablets should be taken with food or fruit juice, or they may be dissolved in a carbonated soft drink prior to ingestion. Itraconazole or fluconazole are preferred over ketoconazole. Itraconazole is available as tablets or a suspension. It can be given as two 100 mg tablets once daily with food or as the oral solution (10 mg/ml), with 20 ml swished and swallowed once a day on an empty stomach. Fluconazole has been used as an effective antifungal agent for many years. It is available as 50, 100, 150, or 200 mg tablets. The recommended dosage is 50 to 400 mg once a day. If using the oral suspension (50 mg/5 ml or 200 mg/5 ml), patients should swish and swallow 5 ml once a day. Voriconazole appears to be highly effective as well.

Fluconazole-refractory oral candidiasis (FROC) had become increasingly problematic before the widespread use of HAART. FROC is defined as cases that fail to resolve within 14 days with treatment of 200 mg fluconazole per day. Factors associated with the development of FROC include profound immunosuppression (CD4+ T-lymphocyte count <50 cells/mm^3), frequency of oral or esophageal candidiasis episodes, chronic use of trimethoprim-sulfamethoxazole (TMP-SMX) as prophylaxis for PCP, and prior occurrence of *Mycobacterium avium* complex (MAC). Higher daily doses and continuous use of fluconazole can also lead to FROC. However, intermittent usage and the total dose of fluconazole are not significantly associated with the development of refractory infection.[6] FROC has been effectively treated with itraconazole solution (40 mg/ml), 2.5 to 5.0 ml swished and swallowed twice a day.[7] For patients with severe oral infection or esophageal involvement, parenteral amphotericin B (0.5 to 1.0 mg/kg/day) administered intravenously once a day is the treatment of choice. Relapse rates are high, and maintenance therapy is often required.

Oral Lesions Associated with Systemic Mycoses

Aspergillus species, *Mucor*, *Cryptococcus*, and *Histoplasma* occasionally cause local invasion of oropharyngeal and nasopharyngeal structures, and these fungi can then disseminate. Diagnosis is established by identifying characteristic organisms through histologic examination or by culture. Cryptococcosis may present as a crater-like, nonhealing ulcer that is tender to palpation. Histoplasmosis is caused by the organism *Histoplasma capsulatum*.[8,9] This lesion appears as a solitary, painful ulceration of several weeks' duration and firm, rolled margins. Some lesions present as white or erythematous areas with an irregular surface. The tongue, palate, and buccal mucosa are the most commonly affected sites.

Zygomycosis can manifest as maxillary alveolar or palatal swelling (or both) that may result in a black, necrotic ulceration if left untreated. *Geotrichum candidum* is the causative pathogen of geotrichosis, which appears as a mucosal lesion with a pseudomembranous covering or as an esophageal ulceration.[10] Aspergillosis is most commonly caused by the *Aspergillus* species *A. fumigatus* and *A. flavus*, the most frequent fungus cultured in the maxillary sinus of the immunocompromised patient.[11] Tissue damage to the maxillary sinus following tooth extraction or endodontic procedures, especially in the maxillary posterior region, can provide an opportunity for infection. This invasive fungal disease may initially present as localized pain and tenderness accompanied by nasal discharge. Aspergillosis can result in necrotic palatal perforation, which may present clinically as a yellow or black ulcer and facial swelling. Treatment for deep-seated fungal infections is detailed in Chapter 40.

▲ VIRAL INFECTIONS

Herpes Simplex Virus

Recurrent herpes simplex virus (HSV) infections are common among HIV-infected patients[12,13] (Table 56–1). Lesions are often multiple and widespread. These large, extremely painful ulcerations can persist for months, resulting in a high degree of morbidity. Oral mucosal involvement usually begins on keratinized mucosa but may spread onto nonkeratinized tissue, thus presenting in an atypical pattern for oral HSV. The lesions begin as an area of necrotic epithelium, then spread laterally to form a zone of erosion with a circinate, raised, yellow border. Multiple smaller lesions may coalesce, forming an irregular pattern. Intraoral lesions usually appear in conjunction with herpes labialis. HSV infection can be presumptively diagnosed based on its clinical appearance and the diagnosis verified with cytologic smears or tissue biopsy, if necessary.

Treatment consists of acyclovir 200 to 400 mg PO taken five times per day; valacyclovir 500 mg PO twice a day; or famciclovir 125 to 250 mg PO twice daily. Generally, treatment is given for 5 to 7 days. Severe cases may require 14 days of therapy or more. Intravenous acyclovir (5 mg/kg q8h for 10 to 14 days) may be instituted initially for severe cases but can be switched to oral therapy as soon as a favorable clinical response is noted. Patients with frequent recurrences or with advanced HIV infection often need chronic suppressive therapy with oral acyclovir 200 mg three times a day or 400 mg twice a day; valacyclovir 500 mg once a day; or famciclovir 125 mg twice a day. Acyclovir-resistant cases have been successfully treated with intravenous foscarnet.[14]

Varicella-Zoster Virus

Recurrent varicella-zoster virus (VZV), or herpes zoster, occurs with increased frequency in HIV-infected individuals[15] (Table 56–1). The disease is much more severe and persistent in the compromised host and may manifest at an earlier age than in immunocompetent patients. Lesions appear along the distribution of one or more branches of the trigeminal nerve as painful clusters of vesicles on an erythematous base. Cutaneous dissemination beyond the classic dermatomal distribution is uncommon. Oral lesions may appear on bound or movable mucosa. The vesicles rupture and ulcerate, with crusts developing after several days. The appearance of the lesions is usually preceded by prodromal pain, itching, or tingling that may be accompanied by fever, malaise, and headache. During the prodromal phase, pain may present as sensitive or aching teeth that appear otherwise healthy. Herpes zoster most often can be diagnosed based on the clinical presentation and confirmed with cytologic smears or cultures.

Treatment consists of acyclovir, 800 mg taken five times daily for 7 to 10 days or until the lesions are healed. Famciclovir 500 mg PO or valacyclovir 1.0 g PO, given every 8 hours until healing occurs, is a more convenient but more expensive alternative. For more severe cases, acyclovir may be given intravenously (10 mg/kg q8h for 7 to 10 days). Foscarnet has been effective in treating acyclovir-resistant infection.[16]

Cytomegalovirus

Disseminated cytomegalovirus (CMV) disease can manifest as painful, nonhealing mucosal ulcerations.[17] Such lesions may be the first sign of CMV infection.[18] The ulcers may appear anywhere in the oral cavity, with the gingiva, buccal mucosa, and palate being the most common sites. CMV-associated ulcers have a clinical appearance similar to that of major aphthous ulcerations, non-Hodgkin's lymphoma, and necrotizing ulcerative periodontitis. Therefore biopsy with histologic verification is necessary for a definitive diagnosis. The oral lesions usually resolve with intravenous ganciclovir therapy.

Human Papillomavirus

Certain "high risk" types of human papillomavirus (HPV), such as HPV 16, 18, and 33, have been shown to be associated with the development of invasive oral carcinomas[19,20] (Table 56–1). The potential for malignant transformation correlates with the presence of HPV DNA, the extent of the disease, and the degree of immunosuppression. Patients with a CD4+ T-lymphocyte count of less than 200 cells/mm^3 are at greatest risk.[21] HPV-associated oral lesions present as oral papillomas, condylomas, and focal epithelial hyperplasia. The lesions are usually multiple and may appear on any mucosal surface, most commonly the labial and buccal mucosa, tongue, and gingiva. The vermilion border and labial commissures may also be involved. Lesions may be white, slightly erythematous, or normal in color. Clinical presentations vary from a pedunculated, exophytic lesion with numerous finger-like surface projections (papilloma) to multiple inconspicuous flat-topped papules or papillary areas (focal epithelial hyperplasia). Condylomas present as sessile, pink, exophytic masses with short, blunted surface projections. They are usually larger than papillomas and are typically multiple and clustered. Biopsy is often necessary because the clinical appearance of some HPV-associated lesions is nonspecific. Efforts to eliminate HPV infection have been ineffective. Treatment therefore should be directed at removing the associated lesions. Treatment consists of removal by electrosurgery, cryotherapy, or scalpel excision. The recurrence rate is high, and repeated treatment is often necessary.

Oral Hairy Leukoplakia

Oral hairy leukoplakia (OHL) is an Epstein-Barr virus (EBV)-associated lesion that is clearly related to HIV disease progression (Table 56–1). It has been associated with the development of AIDS within 2 years of the appearance of the lesions.[22,23] It has also been documented in patients with other types of immunosuppression.[24] Although the prevalence of OHL in the HIV-positive population has decreased dramatically with the widespread use of HAART, it is still seen in approximately 12% of patients.[25] OHL occurs most often on the lateral borders of the tongue but can extend to the dorsal surface and other mucosal surfaces. The lesions range in appearance from faint, white, vertical streaks to thickened corrugated areas of leukoplakia, with a shaggy, or "hairy," keratotic surface. The white plaques typically do not rub off, and extralingual or sublingual involvement is usually without the characteristic corrugations. Heavy candidal infestation is not uncommon and should be eliminated with antifungal therapy. The diagnosis is established by its clinical appearance or by lack of response to antifungal therapy in less characteristic presentations. Lesions that fail to clear with antifungal therapy are treated empirically with acyclovir. If the lesion persists, demonstration of EBV in the lesion is a definitive diagnostic requirement.

Treatment for OHL is not always necessary but may be instituted owing to patient discomfort or esthetic concerns. In many cases the lesions resolve spontaneously. If required, oral acyclovir (800 mg) may be taken four times a day for 2 weeks or until the lesions disappear. Other antiviral drugs, such as valacyclovir and famciclovir, as well as topical applications of podophyllin resin and tretinoin are also effective against OHL. The recurrence rate is extremely high when treatment is discontinued. If necessary, maintenance therapy with acyclovir 200 mg PO four times a day may be instituted.

▲ BACTERIAL INFECTIONS

Gingivitis and Periodontitis

It has been demonstrated that there is no difference in the periodontal flora of HIV-positive versus HIV-negative individuals with gingivitis or adult periodontitis,[26] and there appears to be no increased incidence of conventional periodontal disease in HIV patients. However, severe and rapidly progressive forms of gingivitis and periodontitis can be seen in HIV-seropositive patients, especially those who are severely immunocompromised.[27] Additionally, studies have indicated a more rapid loss of periodontal attachment among patients with HIV and preexisting periodontal disease, as well as an increased incidence of attachment loss with the progression of HIV disease.[28]

Linear gingival erythema (LGE) presents as a distinctive linear band of erythema at the free gingival margin, extending 2 to 3 mm apically. Petechial patches may be seen on the attached gingiva and adjacent alveolar mucosa. Mild pain and occasional bleeding are often reported. Linear gingival erythema can be distinguished from conventional gingivitis in its failure to respond to routine plaque control measures and proper home care maintenance. Thorough prophylaxis and irrigation with 10% povidone-iodine solution should be undertaken, followed by a 0.12% chlorhexidine gluconate rinse twice daily for 2 weeks. Frequent follow-ups and a maintenance dose of 0.12% chlorhexidine gluconate may be required. Studies have associated linear gingival erythema with intraoral *Candida* infection.[29] Therefore persistent lesions should be biopsied and the appropriate antifungal therapy instituted if necessary.

Necrotizing ulcerative gingivitis (NUG) and necrotizing ulcerative periodontitis (NUP) have similar clinical characteristics, differing in that patients with necrotizing ulcerative periodontitis demonstrate a loss of gingival attachment and alveolar bone at affected sites. Acute necrotizing ulcerative gingivitis (ANUG) is differentiated by interproximal gingival necrosis, bleeding, pain, and halitosis. The appearance of necrotizing ulcerative periodontitis is more closely associated with severe immune deterioration.[30] It is distinguished by the presence of intense, deep-seated (nongingival) pain, spontaneous bleeding, and rapid destruction of soft tissue and supporting bone with minimal pocketing. This is often accompanied by loose teeth and fetid breath. The defects are usually localized, not in the diffuse pattern of routine periodontitis; and necrotizing ulcerative periodontitis does not respond well to conventional periodontal therapy.

Treatment for necrotizing ulcerative periodontitis consists of thorough debridement of necrotic tissues and scaling and root planing of affected teeth to remove all accumulated plaque, calculus, and debris. The area should be irrigated with 10% povidone-iodine solution and rinsed with 0.12% chlorhexidine gluconate. Frequent follow-up appointments every 1 to 3 days for the débridement of additional affected tissues may be necessary during the first 2 to 3 weeks, depending on patient response. Diligent home care is extremely important and should include oral rinses with 0.12% chlorhexidine gluconate twice a day during the initial procedure, which may be helpful for long-term maintenance as well. Systemic antibiotics, such as metronidazole (250 mg four times a day), amoxicillin/clavulanic acid (250 mg three times a day), or clindamycin (300 mg three times a day), for 4 to 5 days are usually indicated. Difficulty chewing is a common complication, and pain medication is often required for the first few days. Nutritional supplements should be considered as well. Monthly root planing and curettage are necessary until the patient's overall periodontal condition has stabilized. Evaluation every 3 months thereafter is recommended.

Other Intraoral Bacterial Infections

Mycobacterium tuberculosis, *Mycobacterium avium-intracellulare*, *Klebsiella pneumoniae*, *Enterobacter cloacae*, *Actinomycosis*, *Escherichia coli*, *Neisseria gonorrhoeae*, and *Treponema pallidum* have each been associated with nonhealing oral ulcerations.[31–38] Whether these bacteria are the primary causative pathogens of the lesions or are the result of secondary infection is difficult to determine.

Bacillary angiomatosis is caused by *Bartonella henselae* and *Bartonella qiuntana*.[39] Oral lesions of bacillary angiomatosis clinically resemble Kaposi's sarcoma.[40] The diagnosis may be confirmed by biopsy and Warthin-Starry silver staining. Erythromycin, 500 mg four times a day for 2 to 4 weeks, is the treatment of choice (see Chapter 35).

▲ NEOPLASMS

Kaposi's Sarcoma

Kaposi's sarcoma (KS) is the most common intraoral neoplasm seen in AIDS patients, occurring in 15% to 20% of that population. Intraoral lesions comprise the initial presentation in up to 60% of these cases.[41] Intraoral KS has a higher predilection for homosexual and bisexual men; it is rarely found in HIV-infected women.[42,43] Progression of the lesions is often associated with increased immunosuppression.[19] Depending on the severity and location, oral KS lesions can cause pain, bleeding, and functional interferences, leading to difficulty speaking, eating, and swallowing. Some lesions pose an aesthetic concern as well.

Intraoral KS is seen most often on the hard or soft palate but may appear anywhere in the oral cavity. Initial lesions appear as nonpainful diffuse, macular red or purplish patches that may resemble physiologic pigmentation (Table 56–1). More advanced lesions become nodular, with a darker purplish-brown appearance. Long-standing lesions may cover large areas and develop painful ulcerations that can become suprainfected by fungal or bacterial organisms. Multiple sites may be affected at once. Lesions involving the gingiva can be further complicated by the accumulation of plaque and debris. Therefore frequent cleanings and good oral hygiene should be stressed. Clinically, KS may resemble normal melanotic pigmentation, bacillary angiomatosis, or malignant lymphomas. A definitive diagnosis can be established through biopsy and histopathologic verification.

Therapy for intraoral lesions is directed at reducing the size and number of lesions. Lesions may recur at the same site or in different areas, and they may be treated more than once and with different treatment approaches. Small intraoral lesions may be treated with intralesional injections of vinblastine sulfate (up to 0.1 mg/cm^2) or the sclerosing solution sodium tetradecyl sulfate (up to 0.1 ml/cm^2) (see Chapter 50). Painful ulcerations and areas of necrosis may develop at the injection site but are usually short-lived. Surgical excision, cryotherapy, and removal with the carbon dioxide laser are also effective treatments. Large, bulky lesions usually require systemic chemotherapy or radiation therapy. The latter may be administered as a single, high-dose (800 cGy) regimen,[44] although the use of fractionated therapy (2000 cGy in 10 fractions over 2 weeks) has been shown to be more successful for complete resolution of palpable lesions.[45] Complications of xerostomia, altered sense of taste, and severe mucositis associated with radiation therapy to the oral cavity may be decreased using 150 cGy fractions to a total of 1500 cGy.[44] For patients in whom systemic therapy is indicated, effective chemotherapeutic agents include paclitaxel[46] and the liposomal anthracyclines daunorubicin[47] and doxorubicin.[48]

Non-Hodgkin's Lymphoma

Non-Hodgkin's lymphoma (NHL) is the second most common malignancy and neoplasm in HIV-infected patients. The head and neck region is the most commonly involved site, and most presentations are extranodal.[49] Intraoral NHL is the initial presentation in approximately 5% of reported cases[50] (Table 56–1). Most lymphomas seen in AIDS patients are of the high-grade, large-cell immunoblastic type, and almost all are of B cell origin, although rare T cell tumors have been reported (see Chapter 51). Plasmablastic lymphoma, a novel subtype of AIDS-related NHL, may be confused with nonlymphoid malignancies owing to its unusual morphologic and immunophenotypic profile. These lymphomas are generally limited to the oral cavity at the time of diagnosis and display a peculiar immunophenotypic pattern that is negative for the most common B cell-associated surface antigens but consistently expresses high levels of plasma cell-associated markers, such as VS38c.[51] The risk of developing NHL is related to the severity of immunosuppression, and there is an association with the presence of Epstein-Barr virus.[52–54]

Intraoral NHL presents as a rapidly growing mass of the gingiva, posterior buccal vestibule, or retromolar area. The lesions usually appear erythematous or purplish and may ulcerate. NHL may also be seen as a nontender, diffuse swelling of the posterior hard palate. Gingival lesions, which may be initially diagnosed as periodontal disease, can cause extensive necrosis of affected tissues and lead to severe mobility or loss of involved teeth. In some cases NHL originates in the jawbone, producing paresthesia and a vague pain or "toothache." The tumor may cause expansion of the bone, perforate the cortical plate, and arise as a soft tissue swelling, usually without significant associated pain. This unusual presentation can be mistaken for a common dental abscess. The clinical appearance of intraoral NHL may often mimic other, more common lesions. Therefore a biopsy should be obtained for a definitive diagnosis, especially if the lesion fails to clear with the appropriate standard therapy for the initial diagnosis. Treatment for NHL consists of polychemotherapy for disseminated disease and radiation therapy for localized lesions.

Squamous Cell Carcinoma

Although there have been documented cases of intraoral squamous cell carcinoma in HIV-positive patients, there is no strong evidence suggesting increased prevalence in the HIV population. However, intraoral squamous cell carcinoma is often more aggressive, is not always associated with the typical risk factors, and can manifest at an earlier age in patients with HIV than in individuals without HIV. Intraoral squamous cell carcinoma has a varied clinical presentation, including an exophytic, ulcerating, leukoplakic, erythroplakic, or erythroleukoplakic appearance. There is minimal pain during the early growth phase, which may allow the lesion to go unnoticed by the patient or cause a delay in seeking professional care. Given the increased prevalence of HPV in the HIV-positive population and the apparent involvement of HPV in oral carcinogenesis,[20] clinicians should routinely perform visual oral screenings and maintain a high index of suspicion of any abnormal soft tissue changes.

▲ OTHER LESIONS

Recurrent Aphthous Ulcers

Recurrent aphthous ulcers are not uncommon among persons with HIV.[55] Minor, major, and herpetiform variants may be seen. In HIV-positive patients, most of these lesions are the usually less common major and herpetiform types. A correlation between outbreaks and a decrease in the CD4+/CD8+ T-lymphocyte ratio has been demonstrated in patients with aphthae,[56] but the exact etiology of recurrent aphthous ulcers remains uncertain. The lesions are intensely painful and in severe cases can be quite debilitating, interfering with the patient's ability to speak, eat, or take medications. Recurrent aphthous ulcers arise almost exclusively on nonkeratized movable mucosa (Table 56–1). The labial and buccal mucosa is affected most often, but lesions may occur on the ventral tongue, soft palate, floor of the mouth, and oropharynx. Aphthous ulcers are covered by a yellowish-gray pseudomembrane and are surrounded by an erythematous halo. This is in contrast to herpetic lesions, which usually have a red center surrounded by a raised yellow or white border.

Minor aphthae do not occur more often among HIV-positive patients,[57] but they are more severe and persistent. The lesions are usually round, measuring 3 to 10 mm in diameter; and they may occur singly or in groups of one to five during each episode. Associated pain is often disproportionate for the size of the ulceration. Surface erosion is largely superficial, and healing occurs within 7 to 14 days without treatment and without scarring. The herpetiform variant produces the largest number of lesions with the most frequent recurrences. The individual lesions are usually less than 3 mm in diameter, and as many as 100 can be present in a single recurrence. Smaller lesions may coalesce, forming large, irregular ulcerations. The lesions usually heal within 10 days without treatment, but recurrences tend to be closely spaced.

Major aphthous ulcerations pose the greatest threat to patients living with HIV and appear to be associated with severe immune deterioration. One study reported an average CD4+ T-lymphocyte count of less than 50/mm^3 in HIV-infected persons presenting with this type of recurrent aphthous ulcer.[55] Major aphthous ulcers can be much larger than the other variants, sometimes exceeding 3 cm in diameter. They may extend onto keratinized mucosa, thus presenting in an irregular and atypical pattern for aphthae. Ulcerations are crater-like with a deeply eroded base and are extremely painful, interfering with speech and swallowing. The lesions rarely undergo spontaneous healing and may persist 2 to 6 weeks or more. Multiple ulcers may be present simultaneously, and resolution of the lesions is often associated with scarring of the affected tissues. Fungal superinfections are common and should be managed appropriately. Some large ulcers may clinically resemble other intraoral lesions, such as NHL or squamous cell carcinoma, so biopsy is necessary to rule out these causes prior to instituting systemic therapy.

Treatment for major aphthous ulcers usually involves administration of glucocorticosteroids given topically or systemically, depending on the severity of the lesions. Topical applications include fluocinomide ointment 0.05% or clobetasol ointment 0.05% mixed equally with Orabase and applied directly to the lesions four to six times a day. For multiple or difficult to reach lesions, dexamethasone elixir (0.5 mg/5 ml), 1 tablespoon swished for at least 1 minute and expectorated, may be used four times a day. Soothe-N-Seal is an over-the-counter product that has received U.S. Food and Drug Administration (FDA) approval for intraoral use. This cyanoacrylate bioadhesive provides a protective barrier against trauma and irritation during eating and speaking, thereby reducing pain and promoting faster healing. The gel is applied directly to the lesion several times a day and its effect lasts up to 6 hours. Systemic therapy may be warranted for severe cases that do not respond to topical treatment. Prednisone 10 mg six times a day may be used for up to 1 week. Thalidomide may be used for an 8 week course, with an initial dosage of 400 mg per day for 1 week followed by 200 mg per day for 7 weeks.[58] Pregnancy must be excluded in women because of the well known teratogenicity of the compound. The most common side effect is skin rash. Other side effects include drowsiness, neuropathy, and teratogenic changes. In refractory cases, levamisole, an antineoplastic immunomodulator, has been shown to be beneficial.[59] Patients given levamisole should be monitored for agranulocytosis. Until healing occurs, viscous lidocaine may be swished and expectorated several times a day to assist patients in taking their medications and to allow nutritional intake.

Necrotizing Stomatitis

Necrotizing stomatitis is a localized acute, highly destructive ulceronecrotic lesion that affects mucosal tissue and underlying osseous structures. It begins as a mildly to moderately painful gingival lesion and progresses rapidly to an intensely painful involvement of contiguous tissues. Without prompt treatment, necrotizing stomatitis may result in the exposure and sequestration of alveolar bone with subsequent spontaneous exfoliation of affected teeth. In a study of HIV-seropositive patients, necrotizing stomatitis was classified as an inflammatory disease.[60] As with recurrent aphthous ulcers, however, no specific causative pathogen has been identified. Necrotizing stomatitis is histopathologically similar to aphthous ulcers and may clinically resemble localized periodontal disease.

Treatment should begin with thorough débridement of necrotic tissues, plaque, and calculus. A combination of topical and systemic antibacterial and corticosteroid therapy may be necessary to gain control of the lesion. Effective regimens have included the use of fluocinomide or clobetasol (0.05%) ointment, mixed in equal parts with Orabase and applied three or four times daily, plus metronidazole (250 mg) four times a day. Treatment should continue for 5 to 7 days with appropriate follow-up appointments.

Xerostomia

Xerostomia, or dry mouth, is a common complaint among HIV-positive individuals (Table 56–1). It may be associated with salivary gland disease of the parotid or submandibular glands,[61] or it may be a consequence of tobacco, alcohol, or illicit drug abuse. Radiation therapy to the head and neck region may also be a cause of dry mouth. Xerostomia is a side effect of a number of commonly prescribed medications, including antianxiolytics, anticholinergics, antidepressants, antihistamines, antihypertensives, decongestants, didanosine, foscarnet, meperidine, and zidovudine. Diuretics, including caffeinated beverages, may also cause dry mouth. Decreased salivary flow contributes to the rampant development of caries, especially in the cervical region, and enhances the growth of fungal infections. Oral dryness may be alleviated by reducing or eliminating the causative factor, or it can be managed with the use of sialagogues and artificial salivary substitutes. Salivary flow can be stimulated by chewing sugarless gum or sucking on sugarless candies. The mouth can be kept moist with frequent sips of water or by eating crushed ice. Sodas, diet sodas, juices, sports drinks, alcohol, tea, and coffee should not be used in an effort to alleviate dryness. Although seemingly helpful, because of the sugar and acid content these products only exacerbate the situation. Mouthwashes containing alcohol should also be avoided. Pilocarpine (2.5 mg to 7.5 mg three times a day) has been effective in increasing salivation.[62] Patients given this type of medication should be monitored for side effects including nausea, excess sweating, and cardiovascular complications. Over-the-counter oral comfort products, such as Biotene (toothpaste, mouthwash, chewing gum) and Oralbalance gel may also be of benefit to patients suffering from xerostomia.[63]

Intraoral Pain

Intraoral pain is associated with increased morbidity in patients living with HIV, interfering with normal daily functions such as talking, eating, and swallowing. Consequently, patients may experience a decrease in oral nutritional intake with subsequent weight loss as well as difficulty taking oral medications. Many factors can contribute to the pain in the oral cavity, and a proper diagnosis is essential for managing these conditions. Oral pain may be of odontogenic origin, such as tooth-related (pulpitis), periapical pathology, gingivitis, periodontitis, pericoronitis, alveolar osteitis, or ill-fitting dentures. These conditions are usually acute and are readily treated by general dentists. Neurologic or myofascial disorders may also contribute to oral pain but are often chronic and more difficult to diagnose and treat. Such conditions include temporomandibular joint disorder, postherpetic and trigeminal neuralgia, myofascial pain, and drug-induced or idiopathic neuropathy. Finally, mucosal and soft tissue lesions, such as ulcers, fungal infections, mucositis, and xerostomia are the most common causes of intraoral pain in HIV-positive patients. These conditions are disease-specific and treated accordingly or are managed symptomatically with topical analgesics and mucosal protectives.[64]

REFERENCES

1. Samaranayake LP. Oral mycosis in HIV infection. Oral Surg Oral Med Oral Pathol 73:171, 1992.
2. Franker CK, Lucartorto FM, Johnson BS, et al. Characterization of the mycoflora from oral mucosal surfaces of some HIV-infected patients. Oral Surg Oral Med Oral Pathol 69:683, 1990.
3. Hilton JF. Functions of oral candidiasis episodes that are highly prognostic for AIDS. Stat Med 19:989, 2000.
4. Powderly WG, Gallant JE, Ghannoum MA, et al. Oropharyngeal candidiasis in patients with HIV: suggested guidelines for therapy. AIDS Res Hum Retroviruses 15:1619, 1999.
5. Munoz P, Moreno S, Berengeur J, et al. Fluconazole-related hepatotoxicity in patients with acquired immunodeficiency syndrome. Arch Intern Med 151:1020, 1991.
6. Fichtenbaum CJ, Koletar S, Yiannoutsos C, et al. Refractory mucosal candidiasis in advanced human immunodeficiency virus infections. Clin Infect Dis 30:749, 2000.
7. Saag MS, Fessel WJ, Kaufman CA, et al. Treatment of fluconazole-refractory oropharyngeal candidiasis with itraconazole oral solution in HIV-positive patients. AIDS Res Hum Retroviruses 15:1413, 1999.
8. Glick M, Cohen SG, Cheney RT, et al. Oral manifestations of disseminated Cryptococcus neoformans in a patient with acquired immunodeficiency syndrome. Oral Surg Oral Med Oral Pathol 64:454, 1987.
9. Heinic GS, Greenspan D, MacPhail LA, et al. Oral Histoplasma capsulatum infection in association with HIV infection: a case report. J Oral Pathol Med 21:85, 1992.
10. Heinic GS, Greenspan D, MacPhail LA, et al. Oral Geotrichum candidus infection associated with HIV infection. Oral Surg Oral Med Oral Pathol 73:726, 1992.
11. Shannon MT, Sclaroff A, Cohen SJ. Invasive aspergillosis of the maxilla in an immunocompromised patient. Oral Surg Oral Med Oral Pathol 70:425, 1990.
12. Severson JL, Tyring SK. Relationship between herpes simplex viruses and human immunodeficiency virus infections. Arch Dermatol 135:1393, 1999.
13. Wutzler P, Doerr HW, Farber I, et al. Seroprevalence of herpes simplex virus type 1 and type 2 in selected German populations: relevance for the incidence of genital herpes. J Med Virol 61:201, 2000.
14. Hardy WD. Foscarnet treatment of acyclovir-resistant herpes simplex virus infection in patients with the acquired immuno-deficiency syndrome: preliminary results of a controlled, randomized, regimen-comparative trial. Am J Med 92(suppl 2A):305, 1992.
15. Stewart JA, Reef SE, Pellet PE, et al. Herpesvirus infections in persons infected with human immunodeficiency virus. Clin Infect Dis 21(suppl 1):5114, 1995.
16. Safrin S, Berger TG, Gilson I, et al. Foscarnet therapy in five patients with AIDS and acyclovir-resistant varicella-zoster virus infection. Ann Intern Med 115:19, 1991.
17. Jones AC, Freedman PD, Phelan JA, et al. Cytomegalovirus infections in the oral cavity: a report of six cases and review of the literature. Oral Surg Oral Med Oral Pathol 75:76, 1993.
18. Glick M, Muzyka BC, Lurie D, et al. Oral manifestations associated with HIV disease as markers for immune suppression and AIDS. Oral Surg Oral Med Oral Pathol 77:344, 1994.
19. Womack SD, Chirenje ZM, Gaffikin L, et al. HPV-based cervical cancer screening in a population at high risk for HIV infection. Int J Cancer 85:206, 2000.
20. Bouda M, Gorgoulis VG, Kastrinakis NG, et al. "High risk" HPV types are more frequently detected in potentially malignant and malignant oral lesions, but not in normal oral mucosa. Mod Pathol 13:644, 2000.
21. Chopra KF, Tyring SK. The impact of human immunodeficiency virus on the human papillomavirus epidemic. Arch Dermatol 133:829, 1997.
22. Greenspan JS, Greenspan D, Lennette ET, et al. Replication of Epstein-Barr virus within the epithelial cells of oral "hairy" leukoplakia, on AIDS-associated lesion. N Engl J Med 313:1564, 1985.
23. Greenspan D, Greenspan JS, Overby G, et al. Risk factors for rapid progression from hairy leukoplakia to AIDS: a nested case-control study. J Acquir Immune Defic Syndr 4:652, 1991.
24. Syrjaren S, Laire P, Happoren R-P, et al. Oral hairy leukoplakia is not a specific sign of HIV-infection but related to immunosuppression in general. J Oral Pathol Med 18:28, 1989.
25. Patton LL, McKaig R, Strauss R, et al. Changing prevalence of oral manifestations of human immuno-deficiency virus in the era of pro-

tease inhibitor therapy. Oral Surg Oral Med Oral Pathol Oral Radiol Endod 89:299, 2000.
26. Moore LVH, Moore WEC, Riley C, et al. Periodontal microflora of HIV positive subjects with gingivitis or adult periodontitis. J Periodontol 64:48, 1993.
27. Glick M, Muzyka BC, Salkin LM, et al. Necrotizing ulcerative periodontitis: a marker for immune deterioration and a predictor for the diagnosis of AIDS. J Periodontol 65:393, 1994.
28. Yeung SCH, Stewart GJ, Cooper DA. Progression of periodontal disease in HIV seropositive patients. J Periodontol 64:651, 1993.
29. Velegraki A, Nicolatou O, Theodoridou M, et al. Paedeatric AIDS-related linear gingival erythema: a form of erythematous candidiasis? J Oral Pathol Med 28:178, 1999.
30. Winkler JR, Murray PA, Grassi M, et al. Diagnosis and management of HIV-associated periodontal lesions. J Am Dent Assoc 119(suppl):25, 1989.
31. Volpe F, Schwimmer A, Barr C. Oral manifestations of disseminated Mycobacterium avium-intracellulare in a patient with AIDS. Oral Surg Oral Med Oral Pathol 60:567, 1985.
32. Barone R, Ficarra G, Gaglioti D, et al. Prevalence of oral lesions among HIV-infected intravenous drug abusers and other risk groups. Oral Surg Oral Med Oral Pathol 69:169, 1990.
33. Greenspan D, Schiodt M, Greenspan JS, et al. AIDS and the Mouth. Copenhagen, Munksgaard, 1990.
34. Ficarra G, Shillitoe EJ. HIV-related infections of the oral cavity. Crit Rev Oral Biol Med 3:207, 1992.
35. Graden JD, Timpone JG. Emergence of unusual opportunistic pathogens in AIDS: a review. Clin Infect Dis 15:134, 1992.
36. Schmidt-Westhausen A, Fehrenbach FJ, Reichart PA. Oral Enterobacteriaceae in patients with HIV infection. J Oral Pathol Med 19:229, 1990.
37. Ficarra G, Zaragoza AM, Stendardi L, et al. Early oral presentation of lues maligna in a patient with HIV infection: a case report. Oral Surg Oral Med Oral Pathol 75:728, 1993.
38. Yeager BA, Hoxie J, Weisman RA, et al. Actinomycosis in the acquired immunodeficiency syndrome-related complex. Arch Otolaryngol Head Neck Surg 112:1293, 1986.
39. Gasquet S, Maurin M, Brouqui P, et al. Bacillary angiomatosis in immunocompromised patients. AIDS 12:1793, 1998.
40. Glick M, Cleveland DB. Oral mucosal bacillary (epithelioid) angiomatosis in a patient with AIDS associated with rapid alveolar bone loss: report of a case. J Oral Pathol Med 22:235, 1993.
41. Weinert M, Grimes RM, Lynch DP. Oral manifestations of HIV infection. Ann Intern Med 125:485, 1996.
42. Beral V, Peterman TA, Berkelmann RL, et al. Kaposi's sarcoma among persons with AIDS: a sexually transmitted infection? Lancet 335:123, 1990.
43. Dodd CL, Greenspan D, Greenspan JS. Oral Kaposi's sarcoma in a woman as a first indication of HIV infection. J Am Dent Assoc 122:61, 1991.
44. Berson AM, Quivey JM, Harris JW, et al. Radiation therapy for AIDS-related Kaposi's sarcoma. Int J Radiat Oncol Biol Phys 19:569, 1990.
45. Stelzer KJ, Griffin TW. A randomized prospective trial of radiation therapy for AIDS-associated Kaposi's sarcoma. Int J Radiat Oncol Biol Phys 27:1057, 1993.
46. Saville MW, Lietzau J, Pluda JM, et al. Treatment of HIV-associated Kaposi's sarcoma with paclitaxel. Lancet 346:26, 1995.
47. Presant CA, Scolaro M, Kennedy P, et al. Liposomal daunorubicin treatment of HIV-associated Kaposi's sarcoma. Lancet 341:1242, 1993.
48. Goebel F-D, Goldstein D, Goos M, et al. Efficacy and safety of stealth liposomal doxorubicin in AIDS-related Kaposi's sarcoma. Br J Cancer 73:989, 1996.
49. Singh B, Poluri A, Shaha AR, et al. Head and neck manifestations of non-Hodgkin's lymphoma in human immunodeficiency virus-infected patients. Am J Otolaryngol 21:10, 2000.
50. Ziegler JL, Beckstead JA, Volberding PA, et al. Non-Hodgkin's lymphoma in 90 homosexual men: relation to generalized lymphadenopathy and the acquired immunodeficiency syndrome. N Engl J Med 311:565, 1984.
51. Carbone A, Gaidano G, Gloghini, A, et al. AIDS-related plasmablastic lymphomas of the oral cavity and jaws: a diagnostic dilemma. Ann Otol Rhinol Laryngol 108:95, 1999.
52. Shibata D, Weiss LM, Hernandez AM, et al. Epstein-Barr virus associated with non-Hodgkin's lymphoma in patients infected with the human immunodeficiency virus. Blood 81:2102, 1993.
53. Vilchez R, Shahab I, Kozinetz C, et al. The association of polyomavirus with AIDS-related systemic non-Hodgkin's lymphoma. In: Abstracts of the 8th Conference on Retroviruses and Opportunistic Infections, Chicago, 2001, abstract 594.
54. Rabkin C, Gamache C, El-Omar E. Interleukin-6 (IL-6) promoter polymorphism associated with increased risk of AIDS-related non-Hodgkin's lymphoma. In: Abstracts of the 8th Conference on Retroviruses and Opportunistic Infections, Chicago, 2001, abstract 593.
55. Muzyka BC, Glick M. Major aphthous ulcers in patients with HIV disease. Oral Surg Oral Med Oral Pathol 77:116, 1994.
56. Pedersen A, Hougen HP, Kenrad B. T-lymphocyte subsets in oral mucosa of patients with recurrent aphthous ulceratus. J Oral Pathol Med 21:176, 1992.
57. Epstein JB, Silverman S Jr. Head and neck malignancies associated with HIV infection. Oral Surg Oral Med Oral Pathol 73:193, 1992.
58. Ramirez-Amador VA, Esquivel-Pedraza L, Ponce-de-Leon S, et al. Thalidomide as therapy for human immunodeficiency virus-related oral ulcers: a double-blind placebo controlled clinical trial. Clin Infect Dis 28:892, 1999.
59. Glick M, Muzyka BC. Alternate treatment for major aphthous ulcerations in patients with AIDS. J Am Dent Assoc 123:61, 1992.
60. Jones AC, Gulley ML, Freedman PD. Necrotizing ulcerative stomatitis in human immunodeficiency virus-seropositive individuals: a review of the histopathologic, immunohistochemical, and virologic characteristics of 18 cases. Oral Surg Oral Med Oral Pathol Oral R Endod 89:323, 2000.
61. Schiodt M, Dodd CL, Greenspan D, et al. Natural history of HIV-associated salivary gland disease. Oral Surg Oral Med Oral Pathol 74:326, 1992.
62. Ferguson MM. Pilocarpine and other cholinergic drugs in the management of salivary gland dysfunction. Oral Surg Oral Med Oral Pathol 75:186, 1993.
63. Warde P, Kroll B, O'Sullivan B, et al. A phase II study of Biotene in the treatment of postradiation xerostomia in patients with head and neck cancer. Support Care Cancer 8:203, 2000.
64. Glick M. Dental Management of Patients with HIV. Chicago, Quintessence Publishing, 1994, p 175.

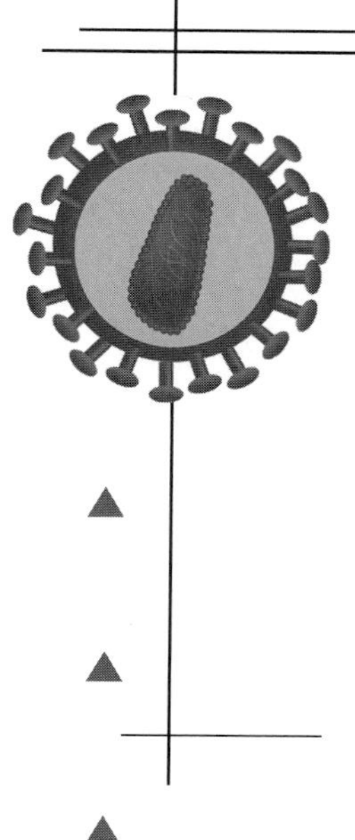

CHAPTER 57

Ophthalmologic Disease

Douglas A. Jabs, MD
Jennifer E. Thorne, MD

Ocular manifestations are common in patients with acquired immunodeficiency syndroma (AIDS); during the era before highly active antiretroviral therapy (HAART) most patients with AIDS developed some form of ocular involvement during the course of their disease[1] (Table 57–1). The most frequently encountered ocular manifestation was microangiopathy, most often recognized in the retina and often referred to as "AIDS retinopathy," "human immunodeficiency virus (HIV) retinopathy," or "noninfectious HIV retinopathy." Opportunistic ocular infections, particularly cytomegalovirus (CMV) retinitis, were common and a substantial cause of visual morbidity. Ocular structures also may be affected by those neoplasms seen in patients with AIDS (e.g., Kaposi's sarcoma or lymphoma), by neuro-ophthalmic lesions, or by adverse drug side effects.

Most ocular symptoms are nonspecific, and any patient with visual symptoms should be referred to an ophthalmologist for evaluation. Most diagnoses can be made by an ophthalmologist on examination; only occasionally are ancillary laboratory or imaging tests necessary. For example, a review of The Johns Hopkins Medical Institutions' experience with CMV retinitis suggests that CMV retinitis can be diagnosed accurately on the first evaluation by an experienced ophthalmologist using indirect ophthalmoscopy in more than 95% of cases. With the exception of syphilis, serologic tests (e.g., for *Toxoplasma gondii,* CMV) are not needed. Occasionally, corneal cultures for keratitis and vitreous cultures or molecular diagnostic techniques (via vitreous aspirate or diagnostic vitrectomy) are used to diagnose bacterial endophthalmitis.

▲ OCULAR MICROANGIOPATHY

Ocular microangiopathy is the most common ophthalmologic finding in patients with AIDS.[1–8] The most often recognized manifestation of this microangiopathy is retinopathy, consisting of cotton wool spots (Fig. 57–1) and less frequently intraretinal hemorrhages.[1–5] Cotton wool spots are microinfarcts of the nerve fiber layer of the retina and are due to occlusion of the retinal capillaries. During the pre-HAART era retinal microangiopathy was recognized clinically in about one-half of patients with AIDS but substantially less frequently in earlier stages of HIV infection.[1,5] Clinically evident HIV retinopathy is associated with low CD4+ T-lymphocyte counts, particularly less than 100 cells/μl.[6,7] Fluorescein angiographic studies and autopsy studies[3,4] have suggested that there was an even higher frequency of microangiopathic changes. Although conjunctival changes were reported less frequently, one study suggested that conjunctival vascular changes also were common in patients with AIDS.[8]

The pathogenesis of ocular microangiopathy is unknown; hypotheses have included (1) circulating immune complex disease[2–4]; (2) infection of the retinal vasculature by HIV[9]; and (3) hemorheologic abnormalities.[10] Polyclonal B cell activation is present in patients with AIDS,[11] circulating immune complexes have been reported,[2,12] and immunoglobulin deposition has been demonstrated in the retinal capillaries,[4] suggesting that immune complex deposition disease may account for the microangiopathy.[3] Alternatively, HIV infection of the retinal vascular endothe-

▲ **Table 57–1.** FREQUENCY OF OCULAR MANIFESTATIONS OF AIDS DURING THE PRE-HAART ERA

Lesion	Frequency (%)
Microangiopathy	
Conjunctival	75
Retinal	50–67
Opportunistic ocular infections	
Cytomegalovirus retinitis	30
Varicella-zoster virus (VZV)	
Herpes zoster ophthalmicus	3–4
VZV retinitis	<1
Toxoplasmic retinitis	1–3
Pneumocystis choroidopathy	<1
Microsporidial keratitis	<1
Ocular syphilis	<1
Ocular neoplasms	
Kaposi's sarcoma (lids, conjunctiva)	1–4
Lymphoma (orbital, intraocular)	<1
Neuro-ophthalmic lesions	5–10

lial cells has been demonstrated,[9] although some have argued that the amount of HIV infection of the retinal vascular endothelial cells is inadequate to account for the retinal vasculopathy.[13]

Although HIV retinopathy generally is clinically silent,[1] ocasional patients have larger-vessel retinal disease, such as a branch vein occlusion or central retinal vein occlusion.[1] Subtle abnormalities of visual function, including color vision and contrast sensitivity, have been reported in patients with AIDS[14,15]; and autopsy studies have reported a loss of optic nerve fibers.[16] It has been speculated that this loss is due to either a cumulative insult from the microinfarcts of the nerve fiber or a direct HIV-related toxic effect on the optic nerve.

Although microangiography is the most common ocular involvement in patients with AIDS, opportunistic ocular infections, particularly CMV retinitis, account for most of the ocular morbidity.

▲ CYTOMEGALOVIRUS RETINITIS

Epidemiology

Disease caused by CMV is among the most common opportunistic infections in patients with AIDS.[17,18] During the era before HAART, CMV disease affected an estimated 45% of patients.[18] Infection of the retina with CMV accounted for 75% to 85% of all CMV disease,[19,20] and it was estimated that 30% of patients with AIDS would develop CMV retinitis sometime between the diagnosis of AIDS and death.[20] CMV retinitis is a late-stage manifestation of AIDS, typically associated with CD4+ T-lymphocyte counts under 50 cells/μl.[19–21] The incidence of CMV retinitis among patients with CD4+ T-lymphocyte counts under 100 cells/μl was approximately 10% per year prior to the widespread use of HAART, and that among patients with a CD4+ T-lymphocyte count under 50 cells/μl was approximately 20% per year.[19,21] HAART has resulted in a 55% to 95% decrease in the number of new cases of CMV retinitis at major urban medical centers throughout the United States since 1995.[22–24] This decline is due to a decrease in the cohort of patients with low CD4+ T-lymphocyte counts and low viral loads (i.e., patients at risk for CMV retinitis) and has occurred as a result of the improved immune function seen in patients treated with HAART. A similar but much more modest and short-lived drop in the incidence of CMV retinitis was seen when zidovudine was first introduced,[22] an observation consistent with this premise and the more modest effect of monotherapy with zidovudine on HIV. Data suggest that the incidence of CMV retinitis now has stabilized at approximately 25% of that during the era prior to HAART, and that most new cases are seen in patients who are HAART-naive or have failed at least one HAART regimen.[25,26]

Diagnosis and Natural History

Retinitis due to CMV can be diagnosed reliably by an experienced ophthalmologist based on its clinical appearance (Fig. 57–2). CMV retinitis typically is described as a focal

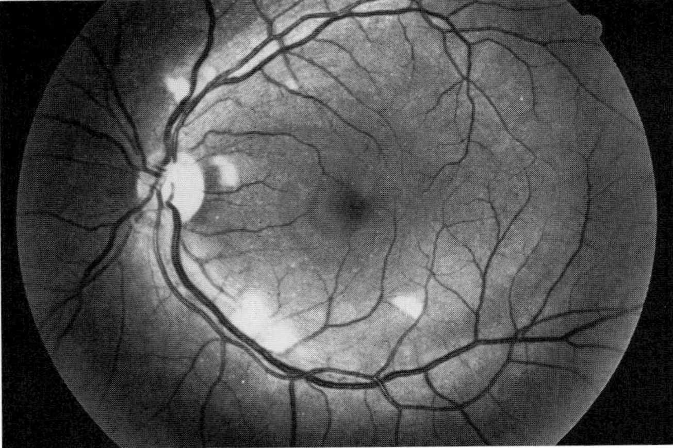

Figure 57–1. Noninfectious retinal microangiopathy ("HIV retinopathy") in a patient with AIDS, manifested by cotton wool spots. (From Jabs DA. Ocular manifestations of HIV infection. Trans Am Ophthalmol Soc 93:623, 1995, with permission.)

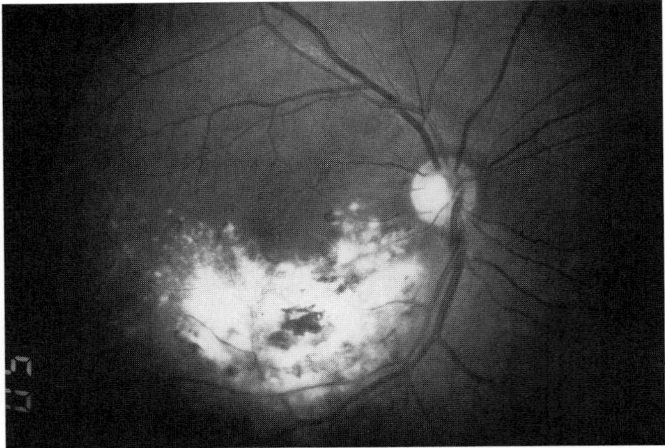

Figure 57–2. Cytomegalovirus retinitis in a patient with AIDS. (From Jabs DA. Ocular manifestations of HIV infection. Trans Am Ophthalmol Soc 93:623, 1995, with permission.)

necrotizing retinitis that may or may not be hemorrhagic. Unless there is immune reconstitution, untreated CMV retinitis spreads throughout the retina over a period of a few months, resulting in total retinal destruction and irreversible blindness.[27] The symptoms of CMV retinitis are nonspecific and include floaters, flashing lights, loss of visual field, or a vague sense of visual loss. CMV retinitis often is asymptomatic, and two studies estimated the prevalence of asymptomatic and undiagnosed CMV retinitis at 13% to 15% of patients with CD4+ T-lymphocyte counts under 50 cells/μl.[7,28] This fact led some experts to recommend routine evaluation of patients at high risk for CMV retinitis by an ophthalmologist using dilated indirect ophthalmoscopy to detect asymptomatic CMV retinitis. Although not universally accepted, and although no long-term outcome studies have been performed to validate this approach, a typical recommendation was that patients with CD4+ T-lymphocyte counts less than 50 cells/μl be seen every 3 to 4 months. Patients with CD4+ T-lymphocyte counts more than 100 cells/μl are at low risk for developing CMV retinitis and generally are seen annually. Patients with CD4+ T-lymphocyte counts of 50 to 100 cells/μl are often seen twice annually. Ophthalmoscopy using the direct ophthalmoscope through an undilated pupil evaluates only 10% of the retinal area and is inadequate for either the diagnosis or the routine evaluation of patients for CMV retinitis.

The use of virologic assays of peripheral blood [culture, antigen detection, or polymerase chain reaction (PCR)] usually is unnecessary for establishing a diagnosis. In unusual cases a diagnostic study of the peripheral blood, vitreous, or retina may be useful.

Treatment

The goal of treatment of CMV retinitis is to arrest progression of the disease, prevent further spread of infection in the retina, and preserve visual function. Treatment with anti-CMV agents suppresses viral replication in the eye but does not eliminate the virus.[29] Discontinuation of therapy in patients who have not had immune reconstitution is associated with prompt relapse of the retinitis.[30] Each relapse of retinitis is associated with retinal destruction and loss of visual field. One study of 287 patients treated with intravenous ganciclovir or foscarnet (or both) reported that the median time to bilateral visual acuity of 20/50 or worse was 16 months (a visual acuity of 20/40 or better in at least one eye is required for permission to drive a car). In this study, the median time to bilateral visual acuity of 20/200 or worse ("legal blindness") was 21 months.[1] Therefore unless there is immune recovery from antiretroviral therapy, long-term suppressive anti-CMV therapy is required.

Treatment options for CMV retinitis are outlined in Table 57–2. When systemically administered anti-CMV drugs are used, the treatment of CMV retinitis generally is performed in a two-step fashion. Initially a high dose of an anti-CMV drug is given to control the infection (induction) with a subsequent lower dose to prevent relapse (maintenance therapy or secondary prophylaxis). As of May 2001, four drugs were approved by the U.S. Food and Drug Administration (FDA) for the treatment of CMV retinitis: ganciclovir (Cytovene), foscarnet (Foscavir), cidofovir (Vistide), and fomivirsen (Vitravene). Ganciclovir is available as intravenous and oral formulations and as a surgically placed slow-release implant (Vitrasert). A prodrug of ganciclovir, valganciclovir (Valcyte), with good oral bioavailability was approved by the FDA in April 2001. Foscarnet and cidofovir are available only as intravenous formulations. Intravenous ganciclovir and intravenous foscarnet therapy require twice-daily intravenous infusions for induction therapy and once-daily intravenous infusions for maintenance therapy. Both require placement of a permanent indwelling central venous catheter. Fomivirsen is available for intravitreous injection only.[31] The intravenous formulations of ganciclovir, foscarnet, and cidofovir may be used for intravitreous injections as well.

Despite the use of chronic maintenance therapy with systemically administered drugs, relapse of CMV retinitis in patients without immune reconstitution is typical and occurs in almost all such patients given sufficient time.[1]

▲ **Table 57–2.** TREATMENT OF CMV RETINITIS

Initial Therapy	Maintenance Therapy	Monitor
Ganciclovir implant plus oral ganciclovir 1 g tid[a]	Replace implant every 6–8 months plus oral ganciclovir 1 g tid[a]	CBC, creatinine
or	*or*	
Oral valganciclovir 900 mg bid for 14–21 days	Valganciclovir 900 mg qd	CBC, creatinine
or	*or*	
Intravenous ganciclovir 5 mg/kg bid for 14–21 days	Intravenous ganciclovir 5 mg/kg qd or oral ganciclovir 1 g tid[a,b]	CBC, creatinine
or	*or*	
Intravenous foscarnet 60 mg/kg tid or 90 mg/kg bid for 14–21 days	Intravenous foscarnet 90–120 mg/kg qd	CBC, creatinine, electrolytes, calcium, magnesium
or	*or*	
Intravenous cidofovir 5 mg/kg once weekly × 2	Intravenous cidofovir 5 mg/kg every other week	CBC, creatinine, urinalysis

Note: In patients with immune recovery (CD4+ T-lymphocyte count > 100–150 cells/L) due to HAART for more than 3–6 months, maintenance therapy may be discontinued but should be restarted if there is a drop in the CD4+ T-lymphocyte count to less than 50 cells/L.

CBC, complete blood count; CMV, cytomegalovirus; HAART, highly active antiretroviral therapy.

[a]May substitute valganciclovir 900 mg qd for oral ganciclovir.

[b]Oral ganciclovir is less effective than intravenous ganciclovir and is not as good a choice for zone 1 disease.

Therefore the efficacy of an anti-CMV drug has been evaluated based on its ability to prolong the time to relapse, typically defined as the time to progression. Progression is the movement of the border of a CMV lesion a specified distance, typically 750 μm, along a specified distance of the front.[32,33] The comparative efficacy of two drugs is determined by their relative ability to prolong the time to progression.[33] The efficacy of a new anti-CMV drug is evaluated by comparing the ability of that drug to prolong the time to progression versus observation. This approach has been used to demonstrate the efficacy of intravenous ganciclovir, intravenous foscarnet, intravenous cidofovir, the ganciclovir implant, and intravitreous fomivirsen.[31,34–38]

The posterior pole of the retina (also referred to as the macula) contains the vital ocular structures (optic nerve and fovea) responsible for good reading acuity. Lesions adjacent to the optic nerve or fovea are immediately vision-threatening. For clinical trial purposes, the retina has been arbitrarily divided into three zones. Zone 1 encompasses a region 3000 μm from the center of the fovea and 1500 μm from the edge of the optic nerve. Lesions in zone 1 are immediately vision-threatening. Zone 2 goes from the edge of zone 1 to the equator of the eye, and zone 3 extends anteriorly from the equator to the pars plana of the retina. Lesions in zones 2 and 3 become vision-threatening given sufficient time but are not immediately 50. Therefore patients with small "peripheral" lesions located entirely in zone 2 or 3 may be observed for a short time without increased risk of loss of visual acuity.[36]

Ganciclovir

Ganciclovir was the first drug approved by the FDA for the treatment of CMV retinitis in immunocompromised patients. It is a nucleoside analogue that is taken up by the virally infected cells and triphosphorylated; it inhibits viral replication through its effect on the viral DNA polymerase. The first phosphorylation step is performed by a virally encoded phosphotransferase, whereas the next two phosphorylation steps are performed by cellular enzymes. Ganciclovir induction is continued for 2 to 3 weeks at a dose of 5 mg/kg every 12 hours. Maintenance therapy is given at 5 mg/kg IV once daily. Ganciclovir has been demonstrated to be effective treatment for CMV retinitis in controlled studies.[27,34] The most frequently encountered side effect of ganciclovir is a reversible granulocytopenia. An absolute neutrophil count of less than 500 cells/μl occurs in approximately one-third of patients treated for 6 months with intravenous ganciclovir.[39] The granulocytopenia promptly reverses with discontinuation of the drug and typically is treated with hematologic growth factors, such as granulocyte colony-stimulating factor (G-CSF; filgrastim, Neupogen). Clinically significant thrombocytopenia occurs in fewer than 10% of patients and is reversible with discontinuation of the drug.

An oral formulation of ganciclovir is FDA-approved for maintenance therapy after induction with intravenous ganciclovir. The oral formulation has poor bioavailability because of its limited absorption from the gastrointestinal tract.[40] The dose of oral ganciclovir for maintenance therapy is 1 g three times daily. Although two studies suggested that oral ganciclovir is equivalent to intravenous ganciclovir as maintenance therapy for CMV retinitis,[41,42] more recent data have demonstrated that oral ganciclovir is less effective than intravenous ganciclovir as maintenance therapy.[43] Therefore oral ganciclovir maintenance appears to be a poor choice for patients with immediately vision-threatening disease (zone 1) especially those not on HAART or who have failed HAART. For patients with peripheral retinitis, who likely can tolerate a relapse of the retinitis without loss of visual acuity, oral ganciclovir may be an appropriate choice. An oral ganciclovir prodrug, valganciclovir, was approved by the FDA in April 2001. It appears to produce blood levels similar to that seen with intravenous ganciclovir,[44] but few data have been published, and there have been no studies on its comparative efficacy long term. The induction dose is 900 mg PO twice daily for 21 days; the maintenance dose is 900 mg PO once daily.

Foscarnet

Foscarnet is a pyrophosphate analogue that inhibits the CMV DNA polymerase. The FDA-approved dose of foscarnet for treating CMV retinitis is 60 mg/kg every 8 hours as induction therapy and 90 to 120 mg/kg once daily for maintenance. In clinical practice a dose of 90 mg/kg twice daily generally is used for induction therapy.[45] A randomized controlled clinical trial demonstrated that foscarnet is effective for controlling CMV retinitis,[35] and the Foscarnet-Ganciclovir Cytomegalovirus Retinitis Trial demonstrated that intravenous ganciclovir and intravenous foscarnet were equally effective for controlling CMV retinitis.[46] The most important side effect of foscarnet is reversible nephrotoxicity, which occurs in approximately 13% of patients treated for 6 months.[39] The serum creatinine and electrolytes (including potassium, calcium, and magnesium) must be monitored twice weekly during induction therapy and once weekly during maintenance therapy; frequent dosage adjustments often are required. Other important side effects include metabolic abnormalities; and potassium, magnesium, and calcium supplementation often are required.[39] Much less common side effects include genital ulcers and infusion-related nausea.[39]

Cidofovir

Cidofovir is a nucleotide analogue whose intracellular activation requires two phosphorylation steps, which are mediated by cellular enzymes. Cidofovir has a prolonged duration of effect and can be given as an intermittent intravenous infusion. Cidofovir induction is given as 5 mg/kg once weekly for 2 weeks, and maintenance therapy is given once every 2 weeks at a 5 mg/kg dose. Because of its potential nephrotoxicity, cidofovir is given in conjunction with probenecid and saline hydration.[47] Two studies comparing cidofovir to observation in patients with small peripheral CMV lesions have demonstrated that cidofovir is effective for the treatment of CMV retinitis.[36,37]

Cidofovir's major side effect is nephrotoxicity, which is not always reversible.[46] Because proteinuria appears to predate a rise in serum creatinine, all patients are monitored for proteinuria and serum creatinine prior to each cidofovir infusion. Persistent proteinuria of 3+ or more that does not clear with hydration is an indication to discontinue cidofovir therapy. Proteinuria of 2+ or more occurs at a rate of 1.22 per person-year. Other indications for discontinuing cidofovir include a serum creatinine of 2.0 mg/dl or higher or a rise in the serum creatinine by 0.5 mg/dl or more. Withdrawal of cidofovir resolves the proteinuria in 90% of cases.[48] Intravenous cidofovir also may cause uveitis or hypotony (low intraocular pressure), which may cause visual loss. A long-term follow-up study of patients with CMV retinitis treated with cidofovir reported the incidence of cidofovir-related uveitis as 0.20 per person-year. Regular ophthalmologic monitoring for the development of cidofovir-related ocular side effects is necessary.

Despite the use of systemically administered anti-CMV drugs as maintenance therapy, relapse of CMV retinitis is a nearly universal phenomenon unless there is immune reconstitution. Although reinduction with the same drug may control the retinitis, the interval between the relapses successively declines, suggesting a decreasing ability of single-agent monotherapy to control CMV retinitis over time.[1,46] The primary reason for relapse appears to be the limited intraocular penetration of systemically administered anti-CMV drugs.[49–51] The efficacy of the ganciclovir implant, which delivers high levels of ganciclovir to the eye and effectively suppresses retinitis in patients with newly diagnosed CMV until it runs out of drug,[38] supports this idea. The Cytomegalovirus Retinitis Retreatment Trial evaluated treatment strategies for patients who had relapsed.[47,52] In this trial, combination intravenous ganciclovir and foscarnet were substantially more effective than either monotherapy with ganciclovir alone or foscarnet alone in patients with relapsed retinitis. Although not more toxic and not associated with any greater impact on general health or mental health, combination therapy did have a greater negative treatment impact on quality of life because it required two intravenous infusions rather than one. In this trial, switching from one monotherapy to another was no more effective than staying on the same monotherapy for the treatment of relapsed retinitis.[52] Given the in vitro synergy of foscarnet and ganciclovir, the superiority of combination therapy perhaps is not surprising. More recently other approaches to combination therapy, including use of the ganciclovir implant and intravenous foscarnet, oral ganciclovir and intravenous foscarnet, and intravitreal foscarnet combined with another mode of ganciclovir therapy, have been used and appear to have merit for treating frequently relapsing retinitis.

Ganciclovir Implant

The ganciclovir implant contains a reservoir of ganciclovir that is surgically implanted into the eye. The implant slowly releases ganciclovir and obtains sustained intraocular levels of ganciclovir four to five times those achievable with systemically administered drugs. In patients with newly diagnosed retinitis, the implant suppresses retinitis for 6 to 8 months until it runs out of drug.[38] Scheduled replacement of the implant every 6 to 7 months appears to suppress the retinitis effectively in patients with newly diagnosed disease and to prevent its relapse. The implant appears to be less effective in patients with relapsed disease who were previously treated with ganciclovir. Approximately 75% to 85% of relapsed patients respond.[53,54] Because placement of the ganciclovir implant requires an intraocular surgical procedure, it is associated with the typical complications of ocular surgery (including bacterial endophthalmitis) and vitreous hemorrhage. Severe vision-threatening complications occur in fewer than 5% of patients. Although there were concerns that the implant could increase the retinal detachment rate in patients with CMV retinitis, studies have shown no increase in the rate of retinal detachment between eyes with CMV retinitis treated with systemic therapy and those treated with the ganciclovir implant.[55,56] The surgical procedure is associated with transient mild blurring of the patient's vision during the immediate postoperative period caused by a refractive change while the eye heals. However, the vision typically returns to normal within 1 to 2 weeks.[38] The primary disadvantage of the ganciclovir intraocular device is that it provides no systemic therapy for patients with CMV retinitis. Most patients with CMV retinitis have positive blood or urine cultures (or both) for CMV.[1,27] Prior to HAART the use of the ganciclovir implant alone was associated with an incidence of contralateral ocular disease of 50% at 6 months and visceral disease of 31%,[38] rates higher than those seen in patients treated with systemically administered drugs.[46] As such, most patients treated with the ganciclovir implant also are given oral ganciclovir to decrease the probability of involvement of the second eye or the viscera. A clinical trial comparing implant plus oral ganciclovir to the implant alone and to intravenous ganciclovir showed that the use of oral ganciclovir decreased the incidence of contralateral ocular and visceral disease when compared to the implant alone.[55] With the advent of HAART and immune recovery, oral ganciclovir still is used as adjunctive therapy following placement of a ganciclovir implant in patients who are not taking HAART or have failed HAART and whose CD4+ T-lymphocyte counts remain below 100 cells/μl. For patients taking HAART who have immune recovery, oral ganciclovir therapy typically is discontinued after 3 to 6 months (see below).

The Ganciclovir Cidofovir Cytomegalovirus Retinitis Trial compared the regimen of the ganciclovir implant plus oral ganciclovir to a regimen of intravenous cidofovir. This trial was performed during the HAART era and detected no difference in the rate of relapse of the retinitis for the two regimens.[57] In this trial the rate of progression in the cidofovir group was substantially less than that seen in patients treated with systemic-only therapies during the era before HAART. These data suggest that HAART may have had an effect on retinitis progression, even though it did not have sufficient effect to prevent CMV retinitis.[57]

An alternative approach to the use of intraocular therapy for the treatment of CMV retinitis has been repetitive intravitreous injections.[58–62] The dose of intravitreous ganciclovir has ranged from 200 g to 2 mg given two or three times weekly as induction therapy and once weekly as maintenance therapy[58–60]; typically, the 2 mg dose is used. The dose of intravitreous foscarnet is 2.4 mg given two or three times weekly for 2 to 3 weeks as induction therapy and once weekly as maintenance therapy.[61] Because of its prolonged duration of effect, intravitreous cidofovir can be given as a 20 g injection once every 5 to 6 weeks.[62,63] Uveitis and hypotony are potential ocular complications of intravitreous cidofovir. Intravitreous injections of ganciclovir and foscarnet are used in clinical practice, but intravitreous cidofovir is still only investigational. The package insert for intravenous cidofovir states that it is not for intravitreous use.

Fomivirsen

Fomivirsen was approved by the FDA in 1998 for treating CMV retinitis. It is a 21-nucleoside phosphorothiolate oligonucleotide that hybridizes to complementary mRNA, which encodes the proteins of the major immediate to early region (IE_2) of CMV.[31] The mechanism of action is an antisense one in which the affected mRNA site shuts down the translation and production of specific proteins. Fomivirsen does not cross the blood-ocular barrier and therefore is given as an intravitreous injection only. The induction dose of fomivirsen is 330 g in a single dose every 2 weeks for two cycles. The maintenance dose is one 330 g intravitreal injection once every 4 weeks. Fomivirsen was shown in a randomized, controlled, clinical trial to be effective treatment for CMV retinitis.[31] No systemic side effects attributable to fomivirsen have been found in patients receiving the drug. Ocular effects have included intraocular inflammation, cataract, and increased intraocular pressure.[31,64]

Intravitreous injections generally are used as an adjunct to therapy (e.g., intravitreous injections of foscarnet with the ganciclovir implant) in patients with relapsed disease or as initial induction therapy until the ganciclovir implant can be placed. They also are used in areas where the implant is not readily available. With the exception of fomivirsen, most of the data on intravitreous injection therapy comes from case series and not from controlled clinical trials.

Management Strategy

Management of the patient with CMV retinitis requires close cooperation between the ophthalmologist and the patient's primary care provider or infectious disease physician (or both). Ophthalmologic examination, including dilated indirect ophthalmoscopy, should be performed at the time of the diagnosis of retinitis, after completion of induction therapy (typically 2 weeks after the initiation of therapy), 1 month after the initiation of therapy, and monthly thereafter. For patients who are treated with the ganciclovir implant, typical postoperative follow-up is 1 day, 1 week, and 1 month after the surgical procedure. Routine (monthly) fundus photographs using a standardized photographic technique that documents the entire photographic area of the retina provides the optimal method for following patients.[33,46] The ophthalmologist can then compare the patient's current appearance to that in previous photographs and detect early relapse of the retinitis. The use of photographs is superior to ophthalmoscopy alone or ophthalmoscopy and retinal drawings.

Because of the toxicity of systemically administered drugs, routine long-term monitoring for toxicity is an important part of managing these patients. For patients on intravenous ganciclovir or oral valganciclovir, weekly complete blood counts and monthly chemistries (for creatinine) should be performed. The complete blood count monitors for ganciclovir toxicity, and the serum creatinine assay evaluates renal function to adjust the ganciclovir dose appropriately. During induction therapy with intravenous ganciclovir, twice-weekly complete blood counts and weekly chemistries are appropriate. For patients being treated with oral ganciclovir maintenance therapy, a complete blood count every 2 to 4 weeks may be adequate because of the lower incidence of toxicity with oral ganciclovir. During foscarnet induction, patients should have serum chemistries, particularly creatinine, calcium, magnesium, and potassium, checked twice weekly and during maintenance therapy once weekly. Because foscarnet is eliminated by the kidney and because its toxicity is primarily renal, frequent dose adjustments are necessary to avoid substantial nephrotoxicity. For patients being treated with foscarnet, a monthly complete blood count is probably adequate. For patients being treated with cidofovir, because of its intermittent mode of administration laboratory monitoring is done prior to each dose. Typically this monitoring consists of chemistries, primarily serum creatinine, and urinalysis. Because proteinuria appears to precede significant nephrotoxicity, persistent proteinuria that does not clear with hydration should result in discontinuation of cidofovir. In addition, patients receiving cidofovir therapy require regular ophthalmologic evaluation for the occurrence of cidofovir-associated uveitis. No systemic adverse events have been reported with intravitreous therapy, and no laboratory abnormalities have been attributed to its use. Therefore there are no specific recommendations for routine laboratory monitoring for patients treated only with intravitreous therapy.

Viremia with CMV is predictive of CMV disease in patients with AIDS and CD4+ T-lymphocyte counts under 50 cells/μl.[2-4] Several studies have shown a correlation between increased levels of CMV DNA in the blood and new-onset CMV retinitis.[65-71] With the decline in the incidence of CMV retinitis as a consequence of HAART, there has been little further development of CMV viral load assays for predicting the occurrence of retinitis or for assessing the adequacy of therapy.[68]

Resistance

Patients with CMV retinitis treated with long-term maintenance therapy may develop CMV resistant to ganciclovir, foscarnet, or cidofovir.[72-79] After 6 months of ganciclovir therapy, approximately 11% to 12% of patients develop a ganciclovir-resistant isolate from blood or urine; and after 9 months of therapy, approximately 27% to 28% develop a ganciclovir-resistant isolate.[75,76] The detection of a ganciclovir-resistant isolate from either the blood or urine is associated with poorly controlled disease.[77,78] Even in patients who do not develop a fully resistant isolate as evidenced by a 50% inhibitory concentration above a certain threshold (e.g., for ganciclovir it is 6 M), there appears to be a declining susceptibility to drug over time.[79] It may be that this declining susceptibility accounts for the accelerating pace of relapse over time. Reported data, although from small numbers of patients, suggest that foscarnet and cidofovir resistance occur at rates similar to that for ganciclovir resistance.[80]

The primary mechanism of ganciclovir resistance is a mutation in the CMV *UL97* gene. This gene encodes for the phosphotransferase that catalyzes the first phosphorylation step of ganciclovir to ganciclovir triphosphate.[81–84] Although 80% to 90% of ganciclovir-resistant CMV isolates have a mutation in the CMV *UL97* gene,[81,82,85] mutations in the *UL54* gene, the DNA polymerase gene, also contribute to ganciclovir resistance.[85,86] Mutations in both the *UL97* and *UL54* genes appear to be responsible for high-level ganciclovir resistance, as well as cross resistance to cidofovir.[85] Culture and susceptibility methods for detecting phenotypic antiviral resistance are labor-intensive and not used routinely in clinical practice. Should rapid methods for the detection of resistant CMV prove to be clinically useful, resistance testing may become more readily available.

Retinal Detachments

During the era prior to HAART, retinal detachments were a common complication of CMV retinitis.[1,46,87–89] In long-term studies conducted before 1995, the incidence of a retinal detachment in either eye of a patient with CMV retinitis was approximately 25% at 6 months after diagnosis of retinitis and 50% to 60% at 1 year.[1,46,88] The detachment rate in an eye involved by CMV retinitis was 38% by 1 year,[90] and a patient with a CMV retinitis-related retinal detachment in one eye would have a 28% to 46% chance of developing a detachment in the other eye.[1,91] In a study of the incidence of retinal detachment in 773 eyes with CMV retinitis from 511 patients with AIDS during both the pre-HAART and HAART eras, patients treated with HAART had a 60% reduction in the retinal detachment rate compared to that for patients not taking HAART. Prior to HAART, CMV retinitis-related retinal detachments typically were repaired by a vitrectomy surgical technique with silicone oil injection. Surgical repair without the use of silicone oil was associated with unacceptably high failure rates for retinal reattachment.[88] Although early reports suggested poor visual acuity results in patients undergoing retinal reattachment surgery for CMV retinitis-related retinal detachments, more recent reports suggested that 75% to 85% of patients achieved ambulatory visual acuity.[91,92] Long-term retinal reattachment repair using silicone oil often is associated with cataract formation, necessitating cataract surgery in these patients. Delimiting laser photocoagulation has been used to check the spread of small peripheral retinal detachments.[93] Most, if not all, of these detachments will ultimately break through the laser barrier, but some patients may be spared vitreoretinal surgery, and the approach is useful in some patients. With the improved control of CMV retinitis in patients treated with HAART, surgical repair without silicone oil is being used more often, although the reported experience remains limited.

Prophylaxis

Two studies have evaluated oral ganciclovir as prophylaxis to prevent the occurrence of CMV disease in patients at high risk for the development of CMV retinitis. Spector et al.[94] reported that oral ganciclovir prophylaxis resulted in a 49% reduction in the incidence of CMV disease, primarily retinitis. In contrast, Brosgart et al.[95] used a similar but not identical study design and reported that oral ganciclovir was ineffective as primary prophylaxis: The relative risk for CMV disease among those receiving oral ganciclovir prophylaxis was 0.92. The study reported by Spector et al.[94] used routine ophthalmologic examination to detect CMV disease. In the study reported by Brosgart et al.,[95] patients were seen only if symptomatic or if their primary care physician referred them. Despite the reduction in the number of outcomes incurred by the lack of routine screening for CMV retinitis in the Brosgart et al. study,[95] the absence of any demonstrable effect for oral ganciclovir prophylaxis remains unexplained.

Because of the expense of oral ganciclovir as CMV primary prophylaxis,[96] the conflicting results of the two studies, and the decreased incidence of CMV disease as a consequence of HAART, primary prophylaxis for CMV disease is not widely used, nor is it recommended in the U.S. Public Health Service–Infections Disease Society of America (USPHS-IDSA) guidelines. One goal of current research is to better define a subpopulation of patients with HIV infection who are at high risk of developing CMV disease and thereby target them for primary prophylaxis. This approach has detected CMV DNA in the blood of patients with the polymerase chain reaction (PCR) or branched-chain DNA technique to better define a subset of patients at high risk for CMV disease[65,68,69,97,98] for whom prophylaxis might be appropriate.

CMV Retinitis During the HAART Era

Highly active antiretroviral therapy has changed the incidence, natural history, and management of CMV retinitis. Immune reconstitution secondary to HAART typically restores specific CMV immunity, reduces the population of patients with AIDS at risk for CMV disease, and has led to a decline in the incidence of CMV retinitis.

With restoration of specific CMV immunity as a consequence of HAART, it has become possible to discontinue anti-CMV maintenance therapy. Several case series of successful discontinuation of anti-CMV therapy in patients with immune reconstitution have been reported.[99–105] In these case series, the CD4+ T-lymphocyte count typically has increased to levels above 100 to 150 cells/μl, and the increase has been sustained for 6 months or more. So long as the CD4+ T-lymphocyte count remains above 50 cells/μl, relapse of the retinitis has occurred only rarely.[104,106,107] The USPHS-IDSA guidelines recommend that maintenance therapy be stopped if patients have inactive disease, have had a CD4+ T-lymphocyte count above 100 to 150 cells/μl for 6 to 12 months, and can have regular ophthalmologic follow-up.

There is a lag between the restoration of specific CMV immunity and a rise in the CD4+ T-lymphocyte count. Patients have been reported with a diagnosis of CMV retinitis within the first 2 months after initiation of HAART despite a rise in the CD4+ T-lymphocyte count.[108–110] Therefore most experts recommend that the CD4+ T-lymphocyte count be increased to higher than 100 to 150 cells/μl, and that this increase be sustained for 3 to 6 months before discontinuing anti-CMV therapy. Although there have been occasional case reports of CMV retinitis entering remission during treatment with HAART without specific anti-CMV therapy,[111,112] many of the ocular complications of CMV retinitis are related to the size of the lesion. Therefore HAART-naive patients with CMV retinitis should be treated with specific anti-CMV therapy and started on HAART until there has been an immune recovery for 3 to 6 months. At that time, discontinuing the anti-CMV therapy can be considered.

Immune Recovery Uveitis

Prior to HAART, CMV retinitis rarely was associated with substantial intraocular inflammation. Since the introduction of HAART, a new ocular inflammatory disorder termed HAART-induced immune recovery uveitis (IRU) has been described in patients with CMV retinitis and immune recovery.[113–118] IRU also is known as immune recovery vitritis and is characterized by increasing (or new-onset) vitritis in conjunction with immune reconstitution. IRU may occur soon after initiating HAART (<1 month) but also has been reported to occur as long as 33 months after starting HAART.[115–117] The most common complications of IRU are cystoid macular edema and epiretinal membrane formation. Other reported complications of IRU include anterior uveitis, optic disc edema, cataract, and retinal neovascularization. The complications of IRU may result in a substantial decrease in vision. IRU typically has been treated with topical or periocular corticosteroids or short courses of oral corticosteroids. Approximately 50% of patients treated have a decrease in IRU and improved vision. It is unproven whether this improvement rate is better than for patients who receive no antiinflammatory therapy.

The pathogenesis of IRU is an immune response to CMV antigen present in the retina or to low-level viral replication in the retina.[107,113,115] Consistent with this hypothesis is the observation that the method of treatment of CMV retinitis may influence the rate of IRU development.[102] Patients treated with the ganciclovir implant, which delivers intraocular levels of ganciclovir five times higher than that of intravenous ganciclovir,[38] appear to be less likely to develop IRU. The reported incidence of IRU has ranged from 0.11 per person-year to 0.83 per person-year.[114,115] The higher rates come from series with little implant use and the lower rates from series with substantially more implant use. This result supports the concept that aggressive therapy of CMV retinitis to minimize the quantity of retinal virus may be a useful strategy for minimizing the likelihood that IRU will occur.

▲ OTHER OCULAR INFECTIONS

The advent of HAART has substantially decreased the incidence of other opportunistic ocular infections in patients with AIDS, as well as that of CMV retinitis.

Varicella-Zoster Virus

Varicella-zoster virus (VZV) is the second most common ocular pathogen in patients with HIV infection. Prior to HAART, herpes zoster ophthalmicus occurred in 3% to 4% of patients with HIV infection. A diagnosis of herpes zoster ophthalmicus, which can occur at all stages of HIV infection,[1,119,120] is suggested by the occurrence of typical zosteriform lesions over the distribution of the ophthalmic branch of the V cranial nerve. Disseminated cutaneous disease may be more common in immunocompromised patients. The diagnosis can be confirmed by obtaining a Tzank preparation of a lesion to demonstrate typical inclusion bodies or by demonstrating virus by culture or immunofluorescence techniques. Because of the high frequency of ocular complications in patients with herpes zoster ophthalmicus and the association of zoster retinitis, patients with herpes zoster ophthalmicus should undergo prompt ophthalmologic examination, including dilated indirect ophthalmoscopy. Ocular complications occur in 49% of HIV-infected patients with herpes zoster ophthalmicus, the most common of which are keratitis, uveitis, and scleritis, occurring in 26%, 23%, and 6% of patients, respectively. Other reported complications are less common and include VI cranial nerve palsies, conjunctivitis, and ischemic neuropathy (an infarct of the optic nerve).[1] In HIV-infected patients with immunodeficiency, herpes zoster ophthalmicus can cause a widespread necrotizing and destructive cutaneous lesion that damages the eyelids, resulting in long-term problems with corneal exposure.

Herpes zoster ophthalmicus in HIV-infected patients responds to standard treatments for VZV infection, including oral or intravenous acyclovir, oral valacyclovir, and oral famciclovir. However, HIV-infected patients may require intravenous acyclovir, rather than oral acyclovir, for severe ocular involvement; and chronic suppressive therapy is required unless there is immune reconstitution.

Retinitis due to VZV was estimated to occur in 0.6% of patients with AIDS during the pre-HAART era.[1] In HIV-infected patients, VZV retinitis may occur in one of two clinical syndromes. The first is the acute retinal necrosis syndrome, which also may be seen in immunologically normal hosts.[121,122] Acute retinal necrosis, which can occur at any stage of HIV infection, is characterized by prominent anterior chamber reaction, vitritis, occlusive retinal vasculitis, and full-thickness retinal necrosis (Fig. 57–3). Typically, the retinal lesions begin peripherally and extend circumferentially. Retinal detachment occurs in 66% to 80% of patients. Affected patients may have a history of cutaneous herpes zoster preceding or simultaneously with the retinitis. The acute retinal necrosis syndrome can be managed successfully with intravenous acyclovir at a dose of 500 mg/m^2 every 8 hours for 10 to 14 days followed by long-term suppression with oral acyclovir, valacyclovir, or famciclovir.

The second clinical syndrome occurs in patients with low CD4+ T-lymphocyte counts, typically less than 50 cells/μl, and it is sometimes known as the progressive outer retinal necrosis syndrome.[123–127] This variant is characterized by multifocal retinal opacification that progresses rapidly and is associated with little or no ocular inflammation. Approximately two-thirds of patients develop bilateral disease and,

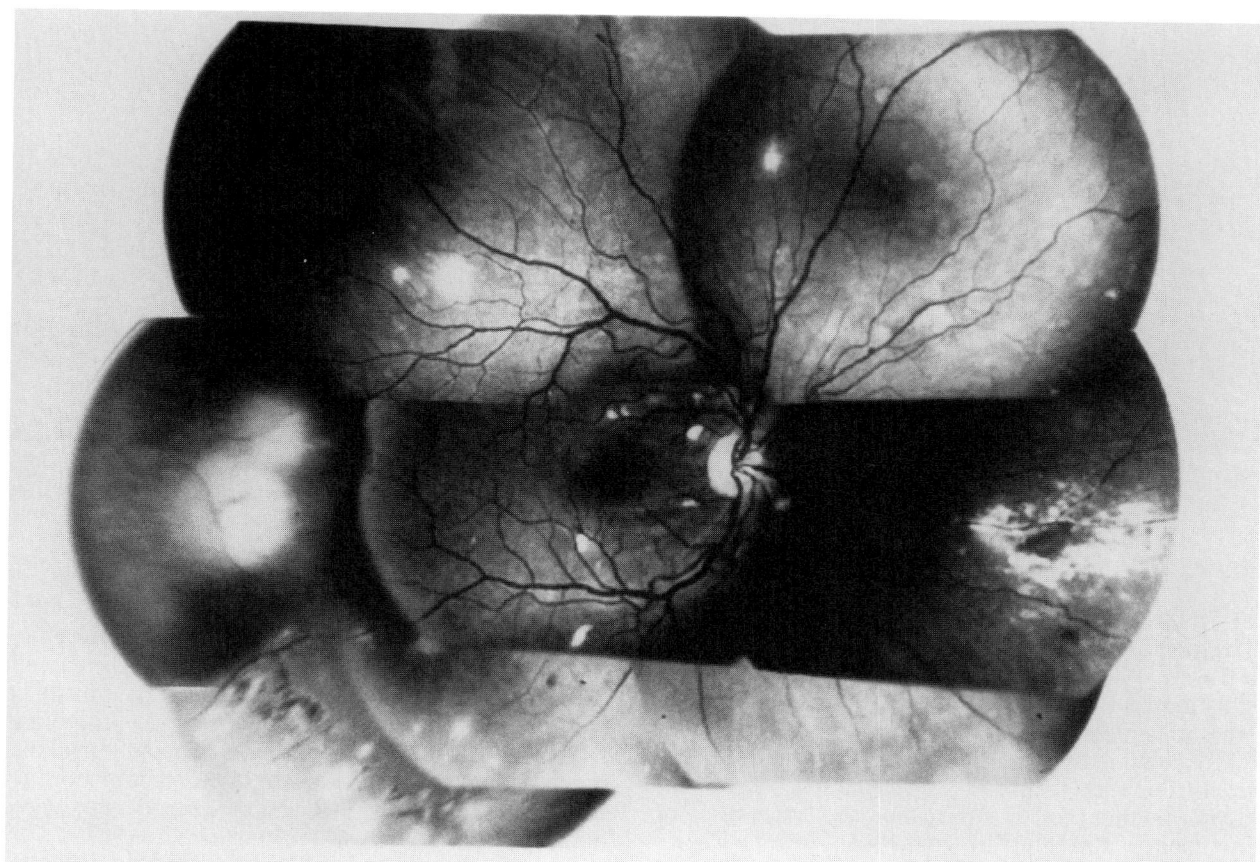

Figure 57–3. Varicella-zoster retinitis in a patient with AIDS. The patient also had a small area of cytomegalovirus retinitis nasally. (From Jabs DA. Ocular manifestations of HIV infection. Trans Am Ophthalmol Soc 93:623, 1995, with permission.)

in contrast to the acute retinal necrosis syndrome, the progressive outer retinal necrosis syndrome often begins in the posterior pole and can involve the optic nerve.[123–126] Medical therapy of the progressive outer retinal necrosis syndrome is problematic. This variant of VZV retinitis does not appear to respond to intravenous acyclovir or other forms of monotherapy.[1,125–127] Anecdotal reports have suggested that combination foscarnet and intravenous acyclovir may be effective in controlling the retinitis,[1] although retinal detachments occur in approximately 70% of patients with this syndrome and often result in poor vision.[125,126]

Ocular Toxoplasmosis

In the United States, infection of the eye by *Toxoplasma gondii* occurred in approximately 1% of patients with AIDS prior to HAART.[1] In other countries, where the baseline seroprevalence of antibodies to *T. gondii* was higher, ocular toxoplasmosis was seen more often in patients with AIDS; in France the frequency was 3%.[128] Although ocular toxoplasmosis may occur in immunologically normal hosts and at any stage of HIV infection, ocular toxoplasmosis is seen most often in patients with CD4+ T-lymphocyte counts of less than 100 cells/μl.[128] Concurrent toxoplasmic encephalitis occurs in 29% to 56% of patients with ocular toxoplasmosis and AIDS,[1,128] suggesting that patients with ocular toxoplasmosis and AIDS should be considered for neuroimaging. Unlike immunocompetent patients, who generally develop ocular toxoplasmosis as a result of reactivation of a congenitally acquired ocular infection, patients with AIDS may develop ocular toxoplasmosis owing to primary infection or to reactivation of latent disease.[127,128] In one large series of patients with ocular toxoplasmosis, only 4% of HIV-infected patients with toxoplasmic retinitis had retinal scars suggesting local reactivation.[128]

The clinical appearance of ocular toxoplasmosis in patients with AIDS (Fig. 57–4) is variable; although a focal white, full-thickness necrotizing retinitis similar to those lesions seen in immunocompetent patients may be present, patients may also have a diffuse necrotizing retinitis, which could be mistaken for CMV infection, or a multifocal disease with a "miliary" appearance.[129–132] Vitritis and anterior uveitis are common but are not required for the diagnosis. The disease is primarily unilateral, although it may be bilateral.

The diagnosis is generally established on the basis of the clinical appearance of the lesion. Patients with ocular toxoplasmosis should have a positive serum immunoglobulin G (IgG) test for toxoplasmosis, although many laboratories use relatively insensitive assays that may yield false-negative results if patients have low titers. Occasionally, IgM tests are helpful, particularly for those with acquired disease (12% of ocular toxoplasmosis in patients with AIDS).[128]

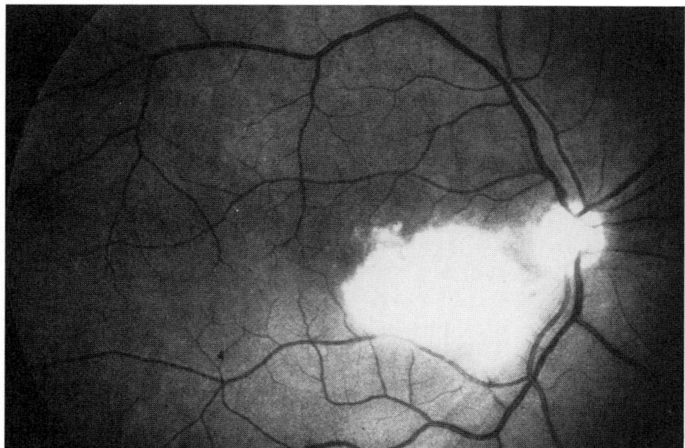

Figure 57–4. Ocular toxoplasmosis in a patient with AIDS. (From Jabs DA. Ocular manifestations of HIV infection. Trans Am Ophthalmol Soc 93:623, 1995, with permission.)

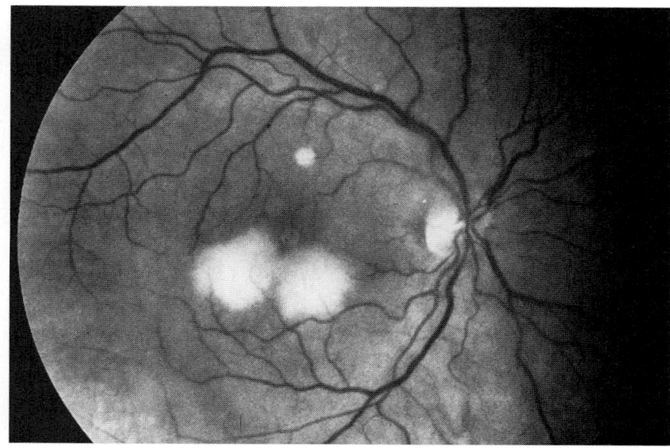

Figure 57–5. *Pneumocystis* choroidopathy in a patient with AIDS. (From Jabs DA. Ocular manifestations of HIV infection. Trans Am Ophthalmol Soc 93:623, 1995, with permission.)

Most cases of toxoplasmic retinitis in patients with AIDS respond to standard anti-*Toxoplasma* treatment within 6 weeks. Regimens typically include pyrimethamine plus sulfadiazine with or without clindamycin. Atovaquone may have value in patients intolerant of other drugs. Prior to HAART, long-term maintenance therapy typically was required to prevent relapse.[128,129] There are few data currently available that provide information about the safety of stopping maintenance therapy in patients who have responded immunologically to HAART. Oral corticosteroid therapy, often given to immunocompetent hosts with ocular toxoplasmosis to reduce the "innocent bystander" damage to the retina, was not needed in patients with AIDS and ocular toxoplasmosis because the infection responded to antibiotics alone.

Pneumocystis carinii Choroidopathy

Choroidal infection with *Pneumocystis carinii* is uncommon clinically, occurring in fewer than 1% patients with AIDS.[1] Choroidal pneumocystosis, however, accounted for 22% of infectious choroidopathies identified in one autopsy series during the pre-HAART era.[133–136] Most, but not all, patients with *P. carinii* choroiditis have a history of *P. carinii* pneumonia[1,136]; and in an aggregate series from several centers[136] 86% of patients with *P. carinii* choroidopathy had received aerosolized pentamidine as *Pneumocystis* prophylaxis. *P. carinii* choroidopathy typically was associated with other extrapulmonary lesions, but it may be the initial or only sign of disseminated disease.

Clinically, the lesions are one-third to two disc diameters in size, creamy yellow to white, round or oval, and located at the level of the choroid (Fig. 57–5).[133,134] They usually are multifocal and bilateral[135,136] and are generally found in the posterior pole or midperiphery of the retina.[136] Over time the lesions can become confluent and appear multilobulated.[136] There is no overlying vitritis.[133–136] The lesions generally are asymptomatic, although an occasional patient complains of blurred vision.[133–136] Pathologically, an eosinophilic, amorphic, acellular, foamy infiltrate is identified in the inner choroid and choriocapillaris,[133–136] and organisms can be identified with electron microscopy. *P. carinii* choroidopathy responds to systemic trimethoprim-sulfamethoxazole, pentamidine, or dapsone alone or in combination. During the pre-HAART era, lifelong maintenance was necessary to prevent recurrence.[133–136]

With the widespread use of trimethoprim-sulfamethoxazole as prophylaxis for *P. carinii* pneumonia, the frequency of *Pneumocystis* choroidopathy decreased. Moreover, HAART appears to have further reduced the incidence of *Pneumocystis* choroidopathy.

Bacterial Infections Including Mycobacterial Lesions

Before the advent of HAART mycobacterial infection of the choroid with *Mycobacterium avium* complex or *Mycobacterium tuberculosis* were demonstrated at autopsy[5,133] but were uncommon clinically. Although there are case reports of choroidal granulomas caused by *M. tuberculosis* producing clinical disease,[137,138] one study estimated that only 5% of patients with active tuberculosis and HIV infection had clinical ocular lesions that produced signs or symptoms.[1]

The most common bacterial eye infection in HIV-infected patients is ocular syphilis, which may occur at any stage of HIV infection.[1] Ocular manifestations of syphilis include iridocyclitis, retinitis, neuroretinitis, panuveitis, papillitis, optic perineuritis, and retrobulbar optic neuritis.[139–143] In one study 90% of HIV-infected patients presented with uveitis.[143] Patients with suspected syphilitic uveitis should undergo the fluorescent treponemal antibody-absorbed (FTA-Abs) test regardless of the results of nonspecific testing [rapid plasma reagen (RPR) or Venereal Disease Research Laboratory (VDRL) test], as one-third of patients with syphilitic uveitis have a negative nonspecific test.[144] Although many patients with ocular syphilis were staged clinically as having secondary syphilis, approximately two-thirds of the patients had a positive cerebrospinal fluid VDRL test and neurologic disease.[139–143] Therefore, all patients with syphilitic uveitis should undergo a lumbar puncture and be treated with an antibiotic regimen for neurosyphilis (e.g., 12 million to 24 million units of penicillin per day intravenously for 10 to 14 days).

Fungal Infections

Intraocular infection with *Cryptococcus neoformans* is rare, reportedly occurring in fewer than 1% of patients with AIDS,[2] 2.5% of patients with systemic cryptococcosis, and 6% of patients with cryptococcal meningitis during the pre-HAART era.[1,145–147] Cryptococcal choroiditis is nearly always diagnosed in the presence of cryptococcal meningitis. The route of ocular infection is presumably hematogenous dissemination to the eye.[1,145] Clinically, cryptococcal lesions of the choroid clinically appear to be deep, hypopigmented or yellow-white, often with multifocal spots; they range from one-fifth to one disc diameter in size.[1,133,145,146] Treatment of cryptococcal infection typically is amphotericin B or fluconazole, and choroidal lesions have been reported to decrease in size and fade in coloration with adequate treatment.[5,133,145] Isolated cases of choroidal infection with *Histoplasma capsulatum* and *Aspergillus fumigatus* have been reported but are rare.[133,148,149] *Candida* retinitis and endophthalmitis are uncommon in patients with AIDS and are reported to occur in fewer than 1% of patients with AIDS.[1] Most HIV-infected patients with *Candida* endophthalmitis are injection drug users, and the candidal infection was related to the injection drug use rather than the HIV infection.

Other Ocular Infections

Other ocular infections reported in patients with AIDS include corneal ulcers, molluscum contagiosum, and microsporidial keratoconjunctivitis.[1,150–153] Herpes simplex virus keratitis has not been shown to be more common in HIV-infected patients than in the general population; however, when it does occur, it may be atypical, more severe, and take longer to heal.[1] Microsporidial keratoconjunctivitis (see Chapter 32), caused by eukaryotic obligate intracellular protozoa of the *Encephalitozoon* species, usually *E. hellum* or *E. cuniculi,*[150–153] occurs in fewer than 1% of patients with AIDS.[1] It is characterized by a fine to coarse corneal punctate epitheliopathy with associated conjunctival hyperemia with or without conjunctival staining with fluorescein. Agents with activity against these parasites include fumagillin, itraconazole, propamidine isethionate, and the benzimidazoles. Topical fumagillin (Fumadil B) 3 mg/ml instilled hourly for 1 week and then tapered over several weeks appears to be effective. The required duration of therapy remains undefined, but given the persistence of spores with therapy indefinite suppressive therapy may be needed.

▲ OCULAR NEOPLASMS

Prior to the HAART era ocular involvement by Kaposi's sarcoma was reported in 2% of patients with AIDS and in 15% to 22% of patients with AIDS and Kaposi's sarcoma involving their other organs or skin.[1,154,155] The eyelids or the conjunctiva could be involved. Conjunctival Kaposi's sarcoma may not require treatment. The lesions are slow-growing, do not invade the eye, and often do not compromise vision. When removal is necessary, small, early lesions of the conjunctiva do well with surgical excision with a clear margin.[156] Larger lesions of the conjunctiva often recur with simple excision.[156] Eyelid involvement by Kaposi's sarcoma may require therapy if it causes functional problems with the eyelid. Local excision, cryotherapy, radiation therapy, and local or systemic chemotherapy have all been reported to produce a good response in some patients.[154–157]

In patients with HIV infection, high-grade lymphoma is an AIDS-defining disorder. Orbital and intraocular involvement by lymphoma have been reported,[158–161] but it occurs in fewer than 1% of patients with AIDS.[1] The clinical appearance of intraocular lymphoma is that of multifocal, yellow-white chorioretinal lesions associated with vitritis, retinal vascular disease, and disc edema. Intraocular lymphoma may be associated with central nervous system (CNS) lymphoma.

▲ NEURO-OPHTHALMOLOGIC DISEASE

Before the advent of HAART neuro-ophthalmic lesions were reported in 5% to 10% of patients with AIDS.[1,5] Reported lesions included cranial nerve palsies, papilledema, optic neuropathy, hemianopsias, and cortical blindness.[1,162–172] The most common etiology for a neuro-ophthalmic lesion in a patient with AIDS was cryptococcal meningitis, accounting for up to 54% of these lesions.[1,145] Of patients with AIDS and cryptococcal meningitis, approximately 25% would have a neuro-ophthalmic lesion.[1] Papilledema is the most common finding in patients with cryptococcal meningitis; other findings include cranial nerve palsies and optic nerve damage.[1,145] Visual loss from cryptococcal meningitis was reported in 1% to 9% of patients as a result of direct invasion of the optic nerve by *Cryptococcus neoformans,* elevated intracranial pressure, or adhesive arachnoiditis.[1,165–167] Other causes of neuro-ophthalmic lesions include herpes zoster ophthalmicus, syphilis, viral encephalitis, and CNS lymphoma.[1] Subtle ocular motility defects also can be detected in patients with AIDS by eye movement recordings using infrared oculography. These defects include slowed saccades, fixational instability, and abnormal pursuit. They appear to be related to HIV infection itself rather than to opportunistic ocular or neurologic infections, and they may correlate with the severity of the AIDS dementia complex.[168–170] Although lacking definitive proof, HIV may be responsible for some cases of optic neuritis or optic neuropathy. Case reports of optic neuropathies in the setting of HIV infection but without another identified cause have been described.[1,171,172]

▲ DRUG-INDUCED OCULAR SIDE EFFECTS

Several drugs used to treat HIV and its complications have been associated with adverse ocular effects. Clofazimine, used to treat *Mycobacterium avium* complex infections, has been associated with a bull's-eye maculopathy.[173] Didanosine, used to treat HIV, has been reported to cause well circumscribed areas of retinal pigment epithelial atrophy in 7% of children treated with high-dose therapy,[174] but no such ocular toxicity has been reported in adults. Rifabutin, an antimycobacterial agent, has been linked to the development of a fulminant anterior uveitis that may mimic infectious endophthalmitis.[175–180] This uveitis may be seen in association with the rifabutin polyarthralgia/polyarthritis syndrome but may also develop on its own. The use of concurrent fluconazole or clarithromycin (or both) has been suggested as a cofactor for rifabutin-associated uveitis because of the pharmacokinetic effect of raising serum levels of rifabutin. Rifabutin uveitis responds well to topical steroids and discontinuing rifabutin or reducing the dose. Of 59 patients randomized to receive rifabutin 600 mg/day, clarithromycin, and ethambutol for the treatment of *M. avium* complex infections as part of one study, 39% developed iridocyclitis.[175] The incidence appears to be lower with lower doses, such as 300 mg/day. This uveitis may be unilateral or bilateral, and 55% to 100% of the patients reported presented with a hypopyon.

Intravitreous cidofovir injections often are associated with uveitis, and the frequency is dose-related.[36,48] Complications of cidofovir uveitis include hypotony (low intraocular pressure) and decreased vision. Uveitis also has been described in patients given parenteral cidofovir, with the rate estimated at 0.20 to 0.24 per person-year.[36,48] As such, all patients receiving cidofovir therapy for CMV retinitis should undergo regular ocular examinations, even if the retinitis is well controlled, and such examinations should include measurement of the intraocular pressure. Fomivirsen also may cause uveitis, elevated intraocular pressure, cataract, and possibly a peripheral pigmentary retinopathy.[31,64] Drugs associated with ocular toxicity used in nonimmunosuppressed patients, such as ethambutol, are likely to have similar toxicity profiles in patients with HIV infection.

REFERENCES

1. Jabs DA. Ocular manifestations of HIV infection. Trans Am Ophthalmol Soc 93:623, 1995.
2. Holland GN, Pepose JS, Pettit TH, et al. Acquired immune deficiency syndrome: ocular manifestations. Ophthalmology 90:859, 1983.
3. Newsome DA, Green WR, Miller ED, et al. Microvascular aspects of acquired immune deficiency syndrome retinopathy. Am J Ophthalmol 98:590, 1984.
4. Pepose JS, Holland GN, Nestor MS, et al. Acquired immune deficiency syndrome: pathogenic mechanisms of ocular disease. Ophthalmology 92:472, 1985.
5. Jabs DA, Green WR, Fox R, et al. Ocular manifestations of acquired immune deficiency syndrome. Ophthalmology 96:1092, 1989.
6. Freeman WR, Chen A, Henderly DE, et al. Prevalence and significance of acquired immunodeficiency syndrome-related retinal microvasculopathy. Am J Ophthalmol 107:229, 1989.
7. Kuppermann BD, Petty JG, Richman DD, et al. Correlation between CD4$^+$ counts and prevalence of cytomegalovirus retinitis and human immunodeficiency virus-related noninfectious retinal vasculopathy in patients with acquired immunodeficiency syndrome. Am J Ophthalmol 115:575, 1993.
8. Teich SA. Conjunctival vascular changes in AIDS and AIDS-related complex. Am J Ophthalmol 103:332, 1987.
9. Pomerantz RJ, Kuritzkes R, Monte M, et al. Infection of the retina by human immunodeficiency virus type I. N Engl J Med 317:1643, 1987.
10. Engstrom RE, Holland GN, Hardy WD, et al. Hemorheologic abnormalities in patients with human immunodeficiency virus infection and ophthalmic microvasculopathy. Am J Ophthalmol 109:153, 1990.
11. Lane HC, Masur H, Edgar LC, et al. Abnormalities of B-cell activation and immunoregulation in patients with the acquired immunodeficiency syndrome. N Engl J Med 309:453, 1983.
12. Gupta S, Licorish K. Circulating immune complexes in AIDS. N Engl J Med 310:1530, 1984.
13. Faber DW, Wiley CA, Lynn GB, et al. Role of HIV and CMV in the pathogenesis of retinitis and retinal vasculopathy in AIDS patients. Invest Ophthalmol Vis Sci 33:2345, 1992.
14. Quiceno JI, Capparelli E, Sadun AA, et al. Visual dysfunction without retinitis in patients with acquired immunodeficiency syndrome. Am J Ophthalmol 113:8, 1992.
15. Geier SA, Hammel G, Bogner JR. HIV-related ocular microangiopathic syndrome and color contrast sensitivity. Invest Ophthalmol Vis Sci 35:3011, 1994.
16. Tenhula WN, Xu S, Madigan MC, et al. Morphometric comparisons of optic nerve loss in acquired immunodeficiency syndrome. Am J Ophthalmol 113:14, 1992.
17. Moore RD, Chaisson RE. Natural history of opportunistic disease in an HIV-infected urban clinic cohort. Ann Intern Med 124:633, 1996.
18. Hoover DR, Saah J, Bacellar H, et al. Clinical manifestations of AIDS in the era of Pneumocystis prophylaxis. N Engl J Med 329:1922, 1993.
19. Gallant JE, Moore RD, Richman DD, et al. Incidence and natural history of cytomegalovirus disease in patients with advanced human immunodeficiency virus disease treated with zidovudine: the Zidovudine Epidemiology Group. J Infect Dis 166:1223, 1992.
20. Hoover DR, Peng Y, Saah A, et al. Occurrence of cytomegalovirus retinitis after human immunodeficiency virus immunosuppression. Arch Ophthalmol 114:821, 1996.
21. Pertel P, Hirschtick JP, Phair J, et al. Risk of developing cytomegalovirus retinitis in persons infected with the human immunodeficiency virus. J Acquir Immune Defic Syndr 5:1069, 1992.
22. Jabs DA, Bartlett JG. AIDS and ophthalmology: a period of transition. Am J Ophthalmol 124:227, 1997.
23. Palella FJ, Delaney KM, Moorman AC, et al. Declining morbidity and mortality among patients with advanced human immunodeficiency virus infection. N Engl J Med 338:853, 1998.
24. Holtzer DC, Jacobson MA, Hadley WK, et al. Decline in the rate of specific opportunistic infections at San Francisco General Hospital. AIDS 12:1931, 1998.
25. Jacobson MA, Stanley H, Holtzer C, et al. Natural history and outcome of new AIDS-related cytomegalovirus retinitis diagnosed in the era of highly active antiretroviral therapy. Clin Infect Dis 30:231, 2000.
26. Wohl DA, Pedersen S, van der Horst CM. Routine ophthalmologic screening for cytomegalovirus retinitis in patients with AIDS. J Acquir Immune Defic Syndr 23:438, 2000.
27. Jabs DA, Enger C, Bartlett JG. Cytomegalovirus retinitis and acquired immunodeficiency syndrome. Arch Ophthalmol 107:75, 1989.
28. Baldassano V, Dunn JP, Feinberg J, et al. Cytomegalovirus retinitis and low CD4$^+$ T-lymphocyte counts. N Engl J Med 333:670, 1995.
29. Pepose JS, Newman C, Bach MC, et al. Pathologic features of cytomegalovirus retinopathy after treatment with the antiviral agent ganciclovir. Ophthalmology 94:414, 1987.
30. Jacobson MA, O'Donnell JJ, Brodie HR, et al. Randomized prospective trial of ganciclovir maintenance therapy for cytomegalovirus retinitis. J Med Virol 25:339, 1988.
31. De Smet MD, Meenken C, van den Horn GJ. Fomivirsen: a phosphorothioate oligonucleotide for the treatment of CMV retinitis. Ocul Immunol Inflamm 7:189, 1999.
32. Holland GN, Buhles WC, Mastre B, et al. A controlled retrospective study of ganciclovir treatment for cytomegalovirus retinopathy: use

of a standardized system for the assessment of disease outcome. Arch Ophthalmol 107:1759, 1989.
33. Studies of ocular complications of AIDS Research Group, in collaboration with the AIDS Clinical Trials Group. Studies of ocular complications of AIDS foscarnet-ganciclovir cytomegalovirus retinitis trial: rationale, design, and methods. Control Clin Trials 13:22, 1992.
34. Spector SA, Weingeist T, Pollard RB, et al. A randomized, controlled study of intravenous ganciclovir therapy for cytomegalovirus peripheral retinitis in patients with AIDS. J Infect Dis 168:557, 1993.
35. Palestine AG, Polis MA, DeSmet MD, et al. A randomized, controlled trial of foscarnet in the treatment of cytomegalovirus retinitis in patients with AIDS. Ann Intern Med 115:665, 1991.
36. Studies of ocular complications of AIDS Research Group in Collaboration with the AIDS Clinical Trial Group. Parenteral cidofovir for cytomegalovirus retinitis in patients with AIDS: the HPMPC peripheral cytomegalovirus retinitis trial. Ann Intern Med 126:264, 1997.
37. Lalezari JP, Stagg RJ, Kuppermann BD, et al. Intravenous cidofovir for peripheral cytomegalovirus retinitis in patients with AIDS: a randomized, controlled trial. Ann Intern Med 126:257, 1997.
38. Martin DF, Parks DJ, Mellow SD, et al. Treatment of cytomegalovirus retinitis with an intraocular sustained-release ganciclovir implant: a randomized controlled clinical trial. Arch Ophthalmol 112:1531, 1994.
39. Studies of ocular complications of AIDS Research Group, in collaboration with the AIDS Clinical Trials Group. Morbidity and toxic effects associated with ganciclovir and foscarnet therapy in a randomized cytomegalovirus retinitis trial. Arch Intern Med 155:65, 1995.
40. Spector SA, Busch DF, Follansbee S, et al. Pharmacokinetic, safety and antiviral profiles of oral ganciclovir in persons infected with human immunodeficiency virus: a phase I/II study. J Infect Dis 171:1431, 1995.
41. Oral Ganciclovir European and Australian Cooperative Study Group. Intravenous versus oral ganciclovir: European/Australian comparative study of efficacy and safety in the prevention of cytomegalovirus retinitis recurrence in patients with AIDS. AIDS 9:471, 1995.
42. Drew WL, Ives D, Lalezari JP, et al. Oral ganciclovir as maintenance treatment for cytomegalovirus retinitis in patients with AIDS. N Engl J Med 333:615, 1995.
43. Lalezari J, Friedberg D, Bisset J, et al. A comparison of the safety and efficacy of 3 g, 4.5 g, and 6 g doses of oral ganciclovir vs IV ganciclovir for maintenance treatment of CMV retinitis. In: Abstracts of the XIth International Conference on AIDS, Vancouver, vol 2, 1996, p 225.
44. Hoffman VF, Skiest DJ. Therapeutic developments in cytomegalovirus retinitis. Expert Opin Invest Drugs 9:207, 2000.
45. Katlama C, Dohin E, Caumes E, et al. Foscarnet induction therapy for cytomegalovirus retinitis in AIDS: comparison of twice-daily and three-times-daily regimens. J Acquir Immune Defic Synd 5(suppl 5):S18, 1992.
46. Studies of ocular complications of AIDS Research Group, in collaboration with the AIDS Clinical Trials Group. Foscarnet-ganciclovir cytomegalovirus retinitis trial. 4. Visual outcomes. Ophthalmology 101:1250, 1994.
47. Lalezari JP, Drew WL, Glutzer E, et al. (S)-1-[3-Hydroxy-2-(phosphonylmethoxy) propyl] cytosine (cidofovir): results of a phase I/II study of a novel antiviral nucleotide analogue. J Infect Dis 171:788, 1995.
48. Studies of ocular complications of AIDS Research Group, in collaboration with the AIDS Clinical Trials Group. Long-term follow-up of patients with AIDS treated with parenteral cidofovir for CMV retinitis: the HPMPC peripheral CMV retinitis trial. AIDS 14:1571, 2000.
49. Jabs DA, Wingard JR, de Bustros S, et al. BW B759U for cytomegalovirus retinitis: intraocular drug penetration. Arch Ophthalmol 104:1436, 1986.
50. Kupperman BD, Quiceno JI, Flores-Aguilar M, et al. Intravitreal ganciclovir concentration after intravenous administration in AIDS patients with cytomegalovirus retinitis: implications for therapy. J Infect Dis 168:1506, 1993.
51. Arevalo JF, Gonzalez C, Capparelli EV, et al. Intravitreous and plasma concentrations of ganciclovir and foscarnet after intravenous therapy in patients with AIDS and cytomegalovirus retinitis. J Infect Dis 172:951, 1995.
52. Studies of the ocular complications of AIDS Research Group, in collaboration with the AIDS Clinical Trials Group. Combination foscarnet and ganciclovir therapy vs monotherapy for the treatment of relapsed cytomegalovirus retinitis in patients with AIDS: the cytomegalovirus retreatment trial. Arch Ophthalmol 114:23, 1996.
53. Marx JL, Kapusta MA, Patel SS, et al. Use of the ganciclovir implant in the treatment of recurrent cytomegalovirus retinitis. Arch Ophthalmol 114:815, 1996.
54. Hatton MR, Duker JS, Reichel E, et al. Treatment of relapsed cytomegalovirus retinitis with the sustained-release ganciclovir implant. Retina 18:50, 1998.
55. Martin DF, Kupperman BD, Wolitz RA, et al. Oral ganciclovir for patients with cytomegalovirus retinitis treated with a ganciclovir implant. N Engl J Med 340:1063, 1999.
56. Kempen JH, Jabs DA, Dunn JP, et al. Retinal detachment risk in cytomegalovirus retinitis related to the acquired immune deficiency syndrome. Arch Ophthalmol 119:33, 2001.
57. Studies of ocular complications of AIDS Research Group, in collaboration with The AIDS Clinical Trials Group. The ganciclovir implant plus oral ganciclovir versus parenteral cidofovir for the treatment of cytomegalovirus retinitis in patients with AIDS: the Ganciclovir Cidofovir Retinitis Trial. Am J Ophthalmol 131:457, 2001.
58. Heinemann MH. Long-term intravitreal ganciclovir therapy for cytomegalovirus retinopathy. Arch Ophthalmol 107:1767, 1989.
59. Cochereau-Massin I, Lehoang P, Lautier-Frau M, et al. Efficacy and tolerance of intravitreal ganciclovir in cytomegalovirus retinitis in acquired immune deficiency syndrome. Ophthalmology 98:1348, 1992.
60. Young SH, Morlet N, Heery S, et al. High dose intravitreal ganciclovir in the treatment of cytomegalovirus retinitis. Med J Aust 157:370, 1992.
61. Diaz-Llopis M, Espana E, Munoz G, et al. High dose intravitreal foscarnet in the treatment of cytomegalovirus retinitis in AIDS. Br J Ophthalmol 78:120, 1994.
62. Kirsch LS, Arevalo JF, DeClercq E, et al. Phase I/II study of intravitreal cidofovir for the treatment of cytomegalovirus retinitis in patients with the acquired immunodeficiency syndrome. Am J Ophthalmol 119:466, 1995.
63. Rahhal FM, Arevalo JF, Chavez de la Paz E, et al. Treatment of cytomegalovirus retinitis with intravitreous cidofovir in patients with AIDS: a preliminary report. Ann Intern Med 125:98, 1996.
64. Boyer DS, Muccioli C, Leiberman RM, et al. Phase 3 results of the efficacy and safety of fomivirsen in the treatment of CMV retinitis. Ophthalmology 152S:167, 1998.
65. Dronet E, Boibieux A, Michelson S, et al. Polymerase chain reaction detection of cytomegalovirus DNA in peripheral blood leukocytes as a direction of cytomegalovirus disease in HIV-infected patients. AIDS 7:665, 1993.
66. Hansen KK, Rickstent A, Hofmann B, et al. Detection of cytomegalovirus DNA in serum correlates with clinical cytomegalovirus retinitis in AIDS. J Infect Dis 170:1271, 1994.
67. Gerard L, Leport C, Flander P, et al. Cytomegalovirus (CMV) viremia and the $CD4^+$ lymphocyte count as predictors of CMV disease in patients infected with human immunodeficiency virus. Clin Infect Dis 24:836, 1997.
68. Bowen EF, Sabin CA, Wilson P, et al. Cytomegalovirus (CMV) viremia detected by polymerase chain reaction identifies a group of HIV-positive patients at high risk of CMV disease. AIDS 11:889, 1997.
69. Shinkai M, Bozzette SA, Powderly W, et al. Utility of urine and leukocyte cultures and plasma DNA polymerase chain reaction for identification of AIDS patients at risk for developing human cytomegalovirus disease. J Infect Dis 175:302, 1997.
70. Bowen EF, Emery VC, Wilson P, et al. Cytomegalovirus polymerase chain reaction viraemia in patients receiving ganciclovir maintenance therapy for retinitis. AIDS 12:605, 1998.
71. Tufail A, Moe AA, Miller ME, et al. Quantitative cytomegalovirus DNA level in the blood and its relationship to cytomegalovirus retinitis in patients with acquired immune deficiency syndrome. Ophthalmology 106:133, 1999.
72. Drew WL, Miner RC, Busch DF. Prevalence of resistance in patients receiving ganciclovir for serious cytomegalovirus infection. J Infect Dis 163:716, 1991.
73. Drew WL, Miner RC, Saleh E. Antiviral susceptibility of cytomegalovirus: criteria for detecting resistance to antivirals. Clin Diagn Virol 1:179, 1993.

74. Jabs DA, Dunn JP, Enger C, et al. Cytomegalovirus retinitis and viral resistance: prevalence of resistance at diagnosis, 1994. Arch Ophthalmol 114:809, 1996.
75. Jabs DA, Enger C, Dunn JP, et al. Cytomegalovirus retinitis and viral resistance. 4. Ganciclovir resistance. J Infect Dis 177:770, 1998.
76. Jabs DA, Enger C, Dunn JP, et al. Cytomegalovirus retinitis and viral resistance. 3. Culture results. Am J Ophthalmol 126:543, 1998.
77. Erice A, Chou S, Biron KK, et al. Progressive disease due to ganciclovir-resistant cytomegalovirus in immunocompromised patients. N Engl J Med 320:289, 1989.
78. Dunn JP, MacCumber MW, Forman MS, et al. Viral sensitivity testing in patients with cytomegalovirus retinitis clinically resistant to foscarnet or ganciclovir. Am J Ophthalmol 119:587, 1995.
79. Studies of ocular complications of AIDS (SOCA) in collaboration with the AIDS Clinical Trial Group. Cytomegalovirus (CMV) culture results, drug resistance, and clinical outcome in patients with AIDS and CMV retinitis treated with foscarnet or ganciclovir. J Infect Dis 176:50, 1997.
80. Jabs DA, Enger C, Forman M, et al. Incidence of foscarnet resistance and cidofovir resistance in patients treated for cytomegalovirus retinitis. Antimicrob Agents Chemother 42:2240, 1998.
81. Chou S, Erice A, Jordan MC, et al. Analysis of the UL97 phosphotransferase coding sequence in clinical cytomegalovirus isolates and identification of mutations conferring ganciclovir resistance. J Infect Dis 171:576, 1995.
82. Chou S, Guentzel S, Michels KR, et al. Frequency of UL97 phosphotransferase mutations related to ganciclovir resistance in clinical cytomegalovirus isolates. J Infect Dis 172:239, 1995.
83. Hanson MN, Preheim LC, Chou S, et al. Novel mutation in the UL97 gene of a clinical cytomegalovirus strain conferring resistance to ganciclovir. Antimicrob Agents Chemother 39:1204, 1995.
84. Wolf DG, Smith IL, Lee DJ, et al. Mutations in human cytomegalovirus UL97 gene confer clinical resistance to ganciclovir and can be detected directly in patient plasma. J Clin Invest 95:257, 1995.
85. Smith IL, Cherrington JM, Jiles RE, et al. High-level resistance of cytomegalovirus to ganciclovir is associated with alterations in both the UL97 and DNA polymerase genes. J Infect Dis 176:69, 1997.
86. Lurain NS, Thompson KD, Holmes EW, et al. Point mutations in the DNA polymerase gene of human cytomegalovirus that result in resistance to antiviral agents. J Virol 66:7146, 1992.
87. Freeman WR, Henderly DE, Wan WL, et al. Prevalence, pathophysiology, and treatment of rhegmatogenous retinal detachment in treated cytomegalovirus retinitis. Am J Ophthalmol 103:527, 1987.
88. Jabs DA, Enger C, Haller J, et al. Retinal detachments in patients with cytomegalovirus retinitis. Arch Ophthalmol 109:794, 1991.
89. Freeman WR, Friedberg DN, Berry C, et al. Risk factors for development of rhegmatogenous retinal detachment in patients with cytomegalovirus retinitis. Am J Ophthalmol 116:713, 1993.
90. Studies of ocular complications of AIDS Research Group, in collaboration with the AIDS Clinical Trials Group. Rhegmatogenous retinal detachment in patients with cytomegalovirus retinitis: the Foscarnet-Ganciclovir CMV Retinitis Trial. Am J Ophthalmol 124:61, 1997.
91. Freeman WR, Quiceno JI, Crapotta JA, et al. Surgical repair of rhegmatogenous retinal detachment in immunosuppressed patients with cytomegalovirus retinitis. Ophthalmology 99:466, 1992.
92. Lim JI, Enger C, Haller JA, et al. Improved visual results after surgical repair of cytomegalovirus-related retinal detachments. Ophthalmology 101:264, 1994.
93. McCluskey P, Grigg J, Playfair TJ. Retinal detachments in patients with AIDS and CMV retinopathy: a role for laser photocoagulation. Br J Ophthalmol 79:153, 1995.
94. Spector SA, McKinley GF, Lalezari JP, et al. Oral ganciclovir for the prevention of cytomegalovirus disease in persons with AIDS. N Engl J Med 334:1491, 1996.
95. Brosgart C, Louis TA, Hillman DW, et al. A randomized, placebo-controlled trial of the safety and efficacy of oral ganciclovir for prophylaxis of cytomegalovirus disease in HIV-infected individuals: Terry Beirn community programs for clinical research on AIDS. AIDS 12:269, 1998.
96. Moore RD, Chaisson RE. Cost-utility analysis of prophylactic treatment with oral ganciclovir for cytomegalovirus retinitis. J Acquir Immune Defic Syndr Hum Retrovirol 16:15, 1997.
97. Rasmussen L, Morris S, Zipeto D, et al. Quantitation of human cytomegalovirus DNA from peripheral blood cells of human immunodeficiency virus-infected patients could predict cytomegalovirus retinitis. J Infect Dis 171:177, 1995.
98. Zipeto D, Morris S, Hong C, et al. Human cytomegalovirus (CMV) DNA in plasma reflects quantity of CMV DNA present in leukocytes. J Clin Microbiol 33:2607, 1995.
99. Whitcup SM, Fortin E, Lindblad AS, et al. Discontinuation of anticytomegalovirus therapy in patients with HIV infection and cytomegalovirus retinitis. JAMA 282:1633, 1999.
100. Tural C, Romeu J, Sirera G, et al. Long-lasting remission of cytomegalovirus retinitis without maintenance therapy in human immunodeficiency virus-infected patients. J Infect Dis 177:1080, 1998.
101. Macdonald JC, Torriani FJ, Morse LS, et al. Lack of reactivation of cytomegalovirus (CMV) retinitis after stopping CMV maintenance therapy in AIDS patients with sustained elevations in CD4 T cells in response to highly active antiretroviral therapy. J Infect Dis 177:1182, 1998.
102. Jabs DA, Bolton SG, Dunn JP, et al. Discontinuing anti-cytomegalovirus therapy in patients with immune reconstitution after combination antiretroviral therapy. Am J Ophthalmol 126:817, 1998.
103. Vrabec TR, Baldassano VF, Whitcup SM. Discontinuation of maintenance therapy in patients with quiescent cytomegalovirus retinitis and elevated $CD4^+$ counts. Ophthalmology 105:1259, 1998.
104. Macdonald JC, Karavellas MP, Torriani FJ, et al. Highly active antiretroviral therapy-related immune recovery in AIDS patients with cytomegalovirus retinitis. Ophthalmology 197:877, 2000.
105. Uthayakumar S, Birthistle J, Hay PE. Cytomegalovirus retinitis after initiation of highly active antiretroviral therapy [letter]. Lancet 350:588, 1997.
106. Torriani FJ, Freeman WR, Macdonald JC, et al. CMV retinitis recurs after stopping treatment in virological and immunological failure of potent antiretroviral therapy. AIDS 14:173, 2000.
107. Nussenblatt RB, Lane HC. Perspective—human immunodeficiency virus disease: changing patterns of intraocular inflammation. Am J Ophthalmol 125:374, 1998.
108. Jacobson MA, Zegans M, Pavan PR, et al. Cytomegalovirus retinitis after initiation of highly active antiretroviral therapy. Lancet 349:1443, 1997.
109. Gilquin J, Piketty C, Thomas V, et al. Acute cytomegalovirus infection in AIDS patients with CD4 counts above 100×10^6 cells/l following combination antiretroviral therapy including protease inhibitors [letter]. AIDS 111:1659, 1997.
110. Van den Horn GJ, Meenken C, Danner SA, et al. Effects of protease inhibitors on the course of CMV retinitis in relation to $CD4^+$ lymphocyte responses in HIV patients. Br J Ophthalmol 82:998, 1998.
111. Reed JB, Schwab IR, Gordon, et al. Regression of cytomegalovirus retinitis associated with pretease inhibitor treatment in patients with AIDS. Am J Ophthalmol 124:199, 1997.
112. Whitcup SM, Cunningham ET, Polis MA, et al. Spontaneous and sustained resolution of CMV retinitis in patients receiving highly active antiretroviral therapy [letter]. Br J Ophthalmol 82:845, 1998.
113. Karavellas MP, Lowder CY, Macdonald C, et al. Immune recovery vitritis associated with inactive cytomegalovirus retinitis: a new syndrome. Arch Ophthalmol 116:169, 1998.
114. Nguyen QD, Kempen JH, Bolton SG, et al. Immune recovery uveitis in patients with AIDS and cytomegalovirus retinitis after highly active antiretroviral therapy. Am J Ophthalmol 129:634, 2000.
115. Karavellas MP, Plummer DJ, Macdonald JC, et al. Incidence of immune recovery vitritis in cytomegalovirus retinitis patients following institution of successful highly active antiretroviral therapy. J Infect Dis 179:697, 1999.
116. Zegans ME, Walton RC, Holland GN, et al. Transient vitreous inflammatory reactions associated with combination antiretroviral therapy in patients with AIDS and cytomegalovirus retinitis. Am J Ophthalmol 125:292, 1998.
117. Robinson MR, Reed G, Csaky KG, et al. Immune-recovery uveitis in patients with cytomegalovirus retinitis taking highly active antiretroviral therapy. Am J Ophthalmol 130:49, 2000.
118. Karavellas MP, Song M, Macdonald JC, et al. Long-term posterior and anterior segment complications of immune recovery uveitis associated with cytomegalovirus retinitis. Am J Ophthalmol 130:57, 2000.

119. Cole EL, Meisler DM, Calabrese LH, et al. Herpes zoster ophthalmicus and acquired immune deficiency syndrome. Arch Ophthalmol 102:1027, 1984.
120. Sandor EV, Millman A, Croxson S, et al. Herpes zoster ophthalmicus in patients at risk for the acquired immune deficiency syndrome (AIDS). Am J Ophthalmol 101:153, 1986.
121. Jabs DA, Schachat AP, Liss R, et al. Presumed varicella zoster retinitis in immunocompromised patients. Retina 7:9, 1987.
122. Sellitti TP, Huang AJW, Schiffman J, et al. Association of herpes zoster ophthalmicus with acquired immunodeficiency syndrome and acute retinal necrosis. Am J Ophthalmol 116:297, 1993.
123. Forster DJ, Dugel PU, Frangieh GT, et al. Rapidly progressive outer retinal necrosis in the acquired immunodeficiency syndrome. Am J Ophthalmol 110:341, 1990.
124. Johnston WH, Holland GN, Engstrom RE, et al. Recurrence of presumed varicella-zoster virus retinopathy in patients with acquired immunodeficiency syndrome. Am J Ophthalmol 116:42, 1993.
125. Margolis TP, Lowder CY, Holland GN, et al. Varicella-zoster virus retinitis in patients with the acquired immunodeficiency syndrome. Am J Ophthalmol 112:119, 1991.
126. Engstrom RE Jr, Holland GN, Margolis TP, et al. The progressive outer retinal necrosis syndrome: a variant of necrotizing herpetic retinopathy in patients with AIDS. Ophthalmology 101:1488, 1994.
127. Morley MG, Duker JS, Zacks S. Successful treatment of rapidly progressive outer retinal necrosis in the acquired immunodeficiency syndrome. Am J Ophthalmol 117:264, 1994.
128. Cochereau-Massin I, Lehoang P, Lautier-Frau M, et al. Ocular toxoplasmosis in human immunodeficiency virus-infected patients. Am J Ophthalmol 114:130, 1992.
129. Holland GN, Engstrom RE, Glasgow BJ, et al. Ocular toxoplasmosis in patients with the acquired immunodeficiency syndrome. Am J Ophthalmol 106:653, 1988.
130. Parke DW, Font RL. Diffuse toxoplasmic retinochoroiditis in a patient with AIDS. Arch Ophthalmol 104:571, 1986.
131. Weiss A, Margo CE, Ledford DK, et al. Toxoplasmic retinochoroiditis as an initial manifestation of the acquired immune deficiency syndrome. Am J Ophthalmol 101:248, 1987.
132. Berger BB, Egwuagu CE, Freeman WR, et al. Miliary toxoplasmic retinitis in acquired immunodeficiency syndrome. Arch Ophthalmol 111:373, 1993.
133. Morinelli EN, Dugel PU, Riffenburgh R, et al. Infectious multifocal choroiditis in patients with acquired immune deficiency syndrome. Ophthalmology 100:1014, 1993.
134. Rao NA, Zimmerman PL, Boyer D, et al. A clinical, histopathologic, and electron microscopic study of Pneumocystis carinii choroiditis. Am J Ophthalmol 107:218, 1989.
135. Dugel PU, Rao NA, Forster DJ, et al. Pneumocysitis carinii choroiditis after long-term aerosolized pentamidine therapy. Am J Ophthalmol 110:113, 1990.
136. Shami MJ, Freeman W, Friedberg D, et al. A multicenter study of Pneumocystis choroidopathy. Am J Ophthalmol 112:15, 1991.
137. Croxatto JO, Mestre C, Puente S, et al. Nonreactive tuberculosis in a patient with acquired immune deficiency syndrome. Am J Ophthalmol 105:659, 1986.
138. Blodi BA, Johnson MW, McLeish WM, et al. Presumed choroidal tuberculosis in a human immunodeficiency virus infected host. Am J Ophthalmol 108:605, 1989.
139. Passo MS, Rosenbaum JT. Ocular syphilis in patients with human immunodeficiency virus infection. Am J Ophthalmol 106:1, 1988.
140. Carter JB, Hamill RJ, Matoba AY. Bilateral syphilitic optic neuritis in a patient with a positive test for HIV. Arch Ophthalmol 105:1485, 1987.
141. Becerra LI, Ksiazek SM, Savino PJ, et al. Syphilitic uveitis in human immunodeficiency virus-infected and noninfected patients. Ophthalmology 96:1727, 1989.
142. McLeish WM, Pulido JS, Holland S, et al. The ocular manifestations of syphilis in the human immunodeficiency virus type 1-infected host. Ophthalmology 97:196, 1990.
143. Shalaby IA, Dunn JP, Semba RD, et al. Syphilitic uveitis in human immunodeficiency virus-infected patients. Arch Ophthalmol 115:469, 1997.
144. Tamesis RR, Foster CS. Ocular syphilis. Ophthalmology 97:1281, 1990.
145. Kestelyn P, Taelman H, Bogaerts J, et al. Ophthalmic manifestions of infections with Cryptococcus neoformans in patients with the acquired immunodeficiency syndrome. Am J Ophthalmol 116:721, 1993.
146. Carney MD, Coombs JL, Waschler W. Cryptococcal choroiditis. Retina 10:27, 1990.
147. Charles NC, Boxrud CA, Small EA. Cryptococcosis of the anterior segment in acquired immune deficiency syndrome. Ophthalmology 99:813, 1992.
148. Specht CS, Mitchell KT, Bauman AE, et al. Ocular histoplasmosis with retinitis in a patient with acquired immune deficiency syndrome. Ophthalmology 98:1356, 1991.
149. Macher A, Rodrigues MM, Kaplan W, et al. Disseminated bilateral chorioretinitis due to Histoplasma capsulatum in a patient with the acquired immunodeficiency syndrome. Ophthalmology 92:1159, 1985.
150. Friedberg DN, Stenson SM, Orenstein JM, et al. Microsporidial keratoconjunctivitis in acquired immunodeficiency syndrome. Arch Ophthalmol 108:504, 1990.
151. Lowder CY, Meisler DM, McMahon JT, et al. Microsporidia infection of the cornea in a man seropositive for human immunodeficiency virus. Am J Ophthalmol 109:242, 1990.
152. Metcalfe TW, Doran RML, Rowlands PL, et al. Microsporidial keratoconjunctivitis in a patient with AIDS. Br J Ophthalmol 76:177, 1992.
153. Rastrelli PD, Didier E, Yee RW. Microsporidial keratitis. Ophthalmol Clin North Am 7:617, 1994.
154. Schuler JD, Holland GN, Miles SA, et al. Kaposi sarcoma of the conjunctiva and eyelids associated with the acquired immunodeficiency syndrome. Arch Ophthalmol 107:858, 1989.
155. Dugel PU, Gill PS, Frangieh GT, et al. Ocular adnexal Kaposi's sarcoma in acquired immunodeficiency syndrome. Am J Ophthalmol 119:500, 1990.
156. Dugel PU, Gill PS, Frangieh GT, et al. Treatment of ocular adnexal Kaposi's sarcoma in acquired immunodeficiency syndrome. Ophthalmology 99:1127, 1992.
157. Ghabrial R, Quivey JM, Dunn JP Jr, et al. Radiation therapy of acquired immunodeficiency syndrome-related Kaposi's sarcoma of the eyelids and conjunctiva. Arch Ophthalmol 110:1423, 1992.
158. Schanzer MC, Font RL, O'Malley RE. Primary ocular malignant lymphoma associated with the acquired immune deficiency syndrome. Ophthalmology 98:88, 1991.
159. Antle CM, White VA, Horsman DE, et al. Large cell orbital lymphoma in a patient with acquired immune deficiency syndrome: case report and review. Ophthalmology 97:1494, 1990.
160. Stanton CA, Sloan DB III, Slusher MM, et al. Acquired immunodeficiency syndrome-related primary intraocular lymphoma. Arch Ophthalmol 110:1614, 1992.
161. Matzkin DC, Slamovits TL, Rosenbaum PS. Simultaneous intraocular and orbital non-Hodgkin lymphoma in the acquired immune deficiency syndrome. Ophthalmology 101:850, 1994.
162. Keane JR. Neuro-ophthalmologic signs of AIDS: 50 patients. Neurology 41:841, 1991.
163. Mansour AM. Neuro-ophthalmic findings in acquired immunodeficiency syndrome. J Clin Neuroophthalmol 10:167, 1990.
164. Winward KE, Hamed LM, Glaser JS. The spectrum of optic nerve disease in human immunodeficiency virus infection. Am J Ophthalmol 107:373, 1989.
165. Lipson BK, Freeman WR, Beniz J, et al. Optic neuropathy associated with cryptococcal arachnoiditis in AIDS patients. Am J Med 107:523, 1989.
166. Rex JH, Larsen RA, Dismukes WE, et al. Catastrophic visual loss due to Cryptococcus neoformans meningitis. Medicine 72:207, 1993.
167. Cohen DB, Glasgow BJ. Bilateral optic nerve cryptococcosis in sudden blindness in patients with acquired immune deficiency syndrome. Ophthalmology 100:1689, 1993.
168. Hamed LM, Schatz NJ, Galetta SL. Brainstem ocular motility defects in AIDS. Am J Ophthalmol 106:437, 1988.
169. Nguyen N, Rimmer S, Katz B. Slowed saccades in the acquired immunodeficiency syndrome. Am J Ophthalmol 107:356, 1989.
170. Currie J, Benson E, Ramsden B, et al. Eye movement abnormalities as a predictor of the acquired immunodeficiency syndrome dementia complex. Arch Neurol 45:949, 1988.
171. Sweeney BJ, Manji H, Gilson RJC, et al. Optic neuritis and HIV-1 infection. J Neurol Neurosurg Psychiatry 567:705, 1993.

172. Newman NJ, Lessell S. Bilateral optic neuropathies with remission in two HIV-1 positive men. J Clin Neuroophthalmol 12:1, 1992.
173. Cunningham CA, Friedberg DN, Carr RE. Clofazimine-induced generalized retinal degeneration. Retina 10:131, 1990.
174. Whitcup SM, Butler KM, Caruso R, et al. Retinal toxicity in human immunodeficiency virus-infected children treated with 2,3-dideoxyinosine. Am J Ophthalmol 113:1, 1992.
175. Shafran SD, Deschenes J, Miller M, et al. The MAC Study Group of the Canadian HIV Trials Network: uveitis and pseudojaundice during a regimen of clarithromycin, rifabutin and ethambutol. N Engl J Med 330:438, 1994.
176. Jacobs DS, Piliero PJ, Kuperwaser MG, et al. Acute uveitis associated with rifabutin use in patients with human immunodeficiency virus infection. Am J Ophthalmol 118:716, 1994.
177. Rifai A, Peyman GA, Daun M, et al. Rifabutin-associated uveitis during prophylaxis for Mycobacterium avium complex infection. Arch Ophthalmol 113:707, 1995.
178. Karbassi M, Nikou S. Acute uveitis in patients with acquired immunodeficiency syndrome receiving prophylactic rifabutin. Arch Ophthalmol 113:699, 1995.
179. Saran BR, Maguire AM, Nichols C, et al. Hypopyon uveitis in patients with acquired immunodeficiency syndrome treated for systemic Mycobacterium avium complex infection with rifabutin. Arch Ophthalmol 112:1159, 1994.
180. Siegal FP, Eilbott D, Burger H, et al. Dose-limiting toxicity of rifabutin in AIDS-related complex: syndrome of arthralgia/arthritis. AIDS 4:433, 1990.

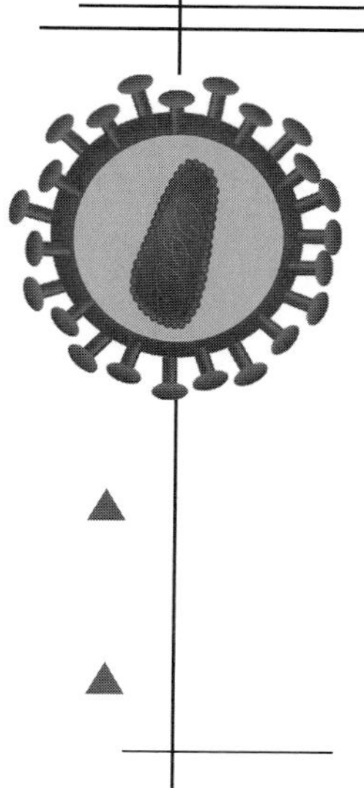

CHAPTER 58

Hematologic Disease

Ronald Mitsuyasu, MD

Hematologic abnormalities are widely recognized and are of significant clinical importance in the management of patients with human immunodeficiency virus (HIV) infection. Infection with HIV results in multiple disturbances of immune function and multilineage hematologic defects. Cytopenias were some of the first recognized signs of HIV infection, and myelosuppression is a major dose-limiting toxicity for a number of therapeutic agents used to treat HIV infection and its associated diseases.

The underlying causes of these various hematologic abnormalities are multiple, but HIV infection of lymphocytes, monocytes, and macrophages is believed to induce abnormalities in cytokine production that in turn have marked effects on the regulation of both the hematopoietic and immune systems. In addition to ineffective hematopoiesis, rapid apoptosis of blood cells and myelosuppression resulting from drugs, infections, and malignancies contribute to a higher incidence of cytopenia in patients with HIV.

Correction of these defects involves inhibition of HIV replication, treatment of infections and tumors, discontinuation or reduction in dosages of myelosuppressive medications, correction of nutritional or other deficiencies, and augmentation with hematopoietic growth factors to facilitate the proliferation, maturation, and differentiation of mature blood cells. Studies of recombinant hematopoietic growth factors in patients with HIV disease have proven their overall effectiveness in increasing blood cell numbers and correcting cytopenias. These agents provide important means of correcting cytopenias and allowing continued use of important myelosuppressive antibiotics and antitumor drugs in HIV-infected individuals.

▲ SPECIFIC CYTOPENIAS

The presence of isolated or multilineage cytopenias is frequently seen in patients with HIV infection. Anemia, neutropenia, and thrombocytopenia occur in up to 17%, 8%, and 13%, respectively, of asymptomatic HIV-infected individuals, with higher percentages seen in those with more advanced HIV disease.[1] These hematologic abnormalities may also be responsible for some of the morbidity associated with acquired immunodeficiency syndrome (AIDS) because they may hinder therapy directed at HIV and the secondary infections and neoplasms of AIDS.[2–4] The need to reduce doses or interrupt therapy because of poor hematologic tolerance may also result in emergence of drug-resistant organisms and progression of malignancies.[5,6]

Anemia

Anemia is the most common hematologic abnormality seen in patients with HIV infection (Figs. 58–1, 58–2). At the time of HIV disease presentation, 10% to 20% of patients are anemic, and eventually 66% to 85% become anemic with overt AIDS.[7–9] Anemia, particularly if it does not resolve, is associated with shorter survival in patients infected with HIV.[10,11]

The major cause of anemia in HIV-infected patients is impaired erythropoiesis, either as a direct consequence of HIV infection of erythrocyte precursors or, more likely, as a result of inappropriate release of inflammatory cytokines such as tumor necrosis factor (TNF), a potent inhibitor of

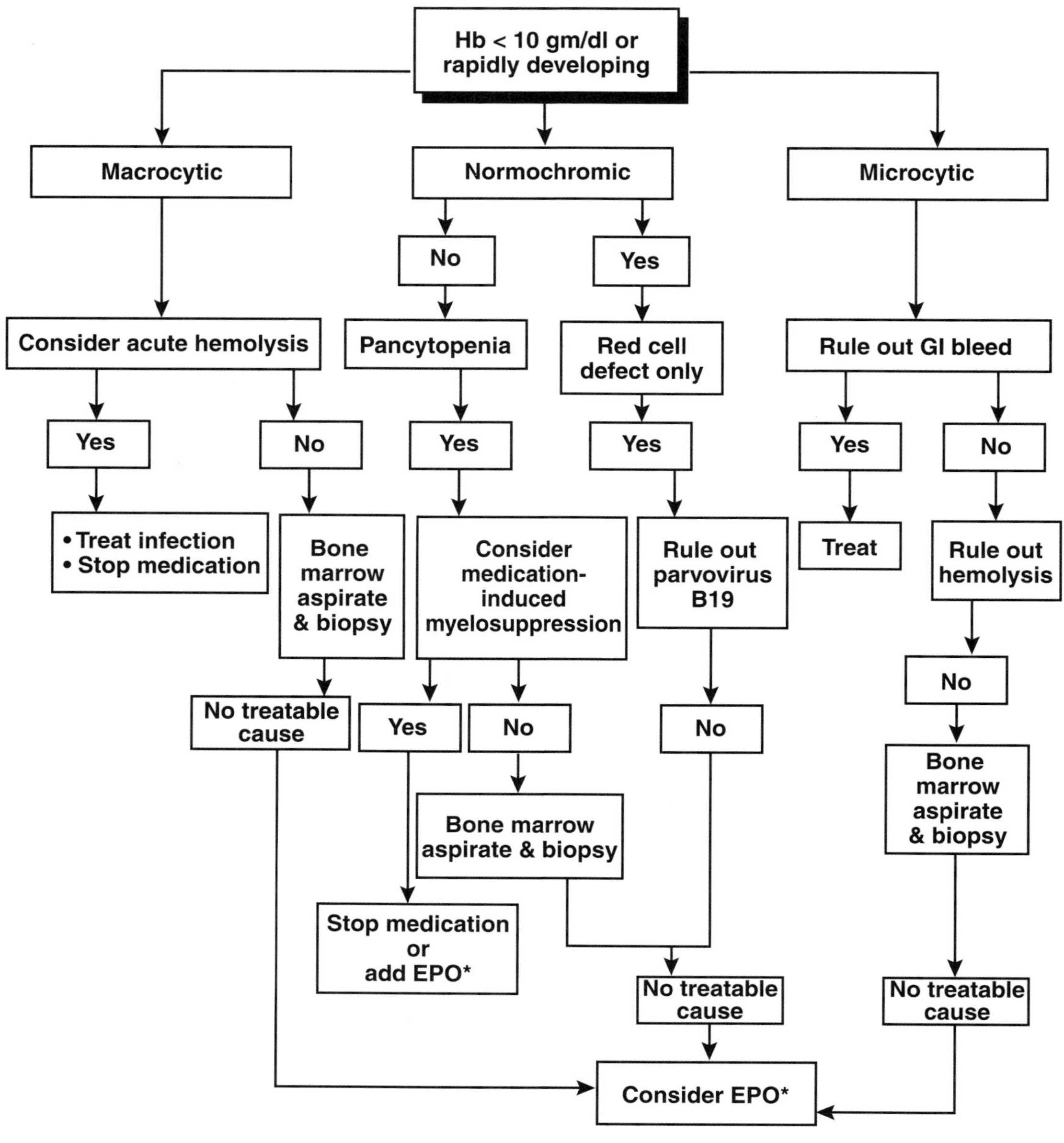

Figure 58–1. Evaluation of rapidly developing anemia in HIV infection. EPO, erythropoietin; GI, gastrointestinal; Hb, hemoglobin.

erythroid maturation in vitro.[12,13] The anemia is typically normochromic/normocytic and is associated with an inappropriately low reticulocyte count. Macrocytosis is unusual except in patients treated with zidovudine.[14] The anemia is typically classified as an anemia of chronic disease and is characterized by an elevated ferritin level but adequate iron stores in the bone marrow. This anemia may diminish with highly active antiretroviral therapy (HAART)[15] but the hemoglobin often does not return to completely normal levels.

Some common causes of anemia in patients with HIV infection are infiltrative diseases of the bone marrow, such as that caused by *Mycobacterium avium* complex (MAC) in patients with advanced HIV disease.[16] Patients with MAC infections often have profound anemias with hematocrits as low as 15% to 20%. Fungal infections and lymphomas can also infiltrate bone marrow and may cause profound anemia, often with associated neutropenia and thrombocytopenia.

Persistent infection with B19 parvovirus has also been associated with intractable anemia in immunosuppressed patients.[17,18] Parvovirus B19 can selectively infect actively replicating erythroid progenitors, resulting in loss of red blood cells and erythroid hypoplasia. Control of this infection is mediated by an intact humoral immune response; therefore immunocompromised patients may fail to clear this infection because they are unable to maintain

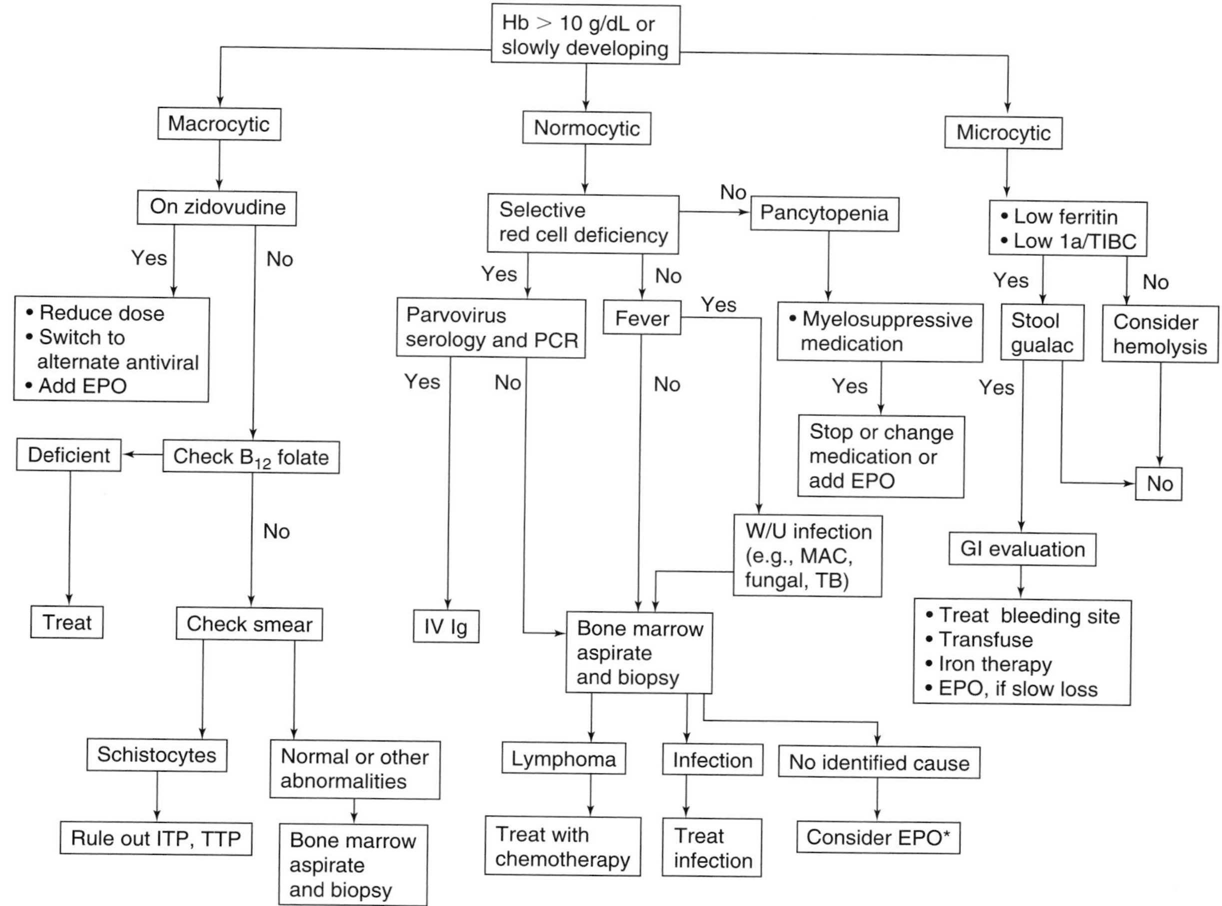

Figure 58–2. Evaluation of slowly developing anemia in HIV infection. EPO, erythropoietin; fe/TIBC, iron/total iron-binding capacity; GI, gastrointestinal; Hb, hemoglobin; ITP, idiopathic thrombocytopenic purpura; IV Ig, intravenous immunoglobulin; MAC, *Mycobacterium avium* complex; PCR, polymerase chain reaction; rEPO, recombinant erythropoietin; TB, tuberculosis; TTP, thrombotic thrombocytopenic purpura; W/U, workup.

an adequate antibody response to this virus.[18–20] The B19 parvovirus infection is usually diagnosed by serologic or genotypic detection of parvovirus infection in blood or bone marrow. In general, detection of B19 parvovirus DNA by the polymerase chain reaction (PCR) is highly specific for infection even when immunoglobulin M (IgM) antibodies are absent. The presence of giant, abnormal pronormoblasts is also pathognomonic for parvovirus infection. Treatment of this infection and resultant anemia involves a course of intravenous immunoglobulin (IVIG) over several days. Generally a dose of 400 mg/kg/d is given for 5 days and is effective in more than 75% of patients. Repeat administration of a course of IVIG may be necessary in patients with severe immune deficiencies who are unable to generate their own antibody response to B19 parvovirus infection. Some patients require maintenance IVIG of 30 g per month to maintain red blood cell counts. Treatment with folate and other hematinics may also be necessary to sustain an erythropoietic response.

Nutritional deficiencies have been described in patients with HIV infection and may include disorders of iron metabolism or iron deficiency as well as vitamin B_{12} deficiency, which occurs in up to 20% of HIV-infected patients.[2,8,21] Patients usually do not have other manifestations of vitamin B_{12} deficiency and often do not improve markedly with parenteral repletion.[22] The low vitamin B_{12} levels may result from abnormalities in vitamin B_{12}-binding proteins and decreased serum transport of vitamin B_{12}[23]; however, abnormal absorption of vitamin B_{12} may also occur in patients with advanced HIV infection.[24–26] Folate deficiency does not appear to be prevalent in this patient population. Iron deficiency may result from chronic blood loss from Kaposi sarcoma, lymphoma of the gastrointestinal tract, or various infectious enterocolitides. Replacement therapy with iron or folic acid is useful in patients with true deficiencies in these nutrients.

Although some patients have direct Coombs' test positivity, it is usually nonspecific, and antibody-mediated hemolysis is rare in patients with HIV infection. Between 20%

and 44% of asymptomatic HIV-infected patients are Coombs' test-positive, with the numbers increasing up to 85% in those with frank AIDS.[27,28] Although these antibodies may be reactive with specific minor antigens on erythrocytes, in most cases nonspecific binding of anti-phospholipid antibodies or deposition of immune complexes on erythrocytes are responsible for these positive Coombs' tests.[29] Circulating anti-erythropoietin antibodies have also been correlated with anemia in a subset of patients with HIV.[30]

Neutropenia

Infection with HIV affects lymphocytes, neutrophils, and macrophages/monocytes (Fig. 58–3). The hallmark of HIV infection is progressive and profound depletion of CD4+ T-lymphocytes, presumably through direct viral invasion of these cells and enhanced cytolysis and apoptosis.[12,31] Infection of macrophages and monocytes also occurs and may result in significant perturbation of the complex network of growth factor and cytokine generation seen with HIV infection. Granulocytopenia can increase the risk of severe bacterial and fungal infection in HIV.[32]

Granulocytopenia often occurs concomitantly with anemia. Among patients with early symptomatic HIV infection, 10% to 30% are neutropenic, and this may progress to 75% of those with frank AIDS.[1,2] Myelotoxic medications, including various antiretroviral drugs and drugs used to treat opportunistic infections and malignancies, are the major cause of neutropenia in patients with HIV infection. In addition, impaired myelopoiesis has been described in patients with leukopenia and HIV infection.[33,36] Deficiencies in granulocyte colony-stimulating factor (G-CSF) production in response to neutropenia has been described in patients with HIV infection, although the G-CSF response to infection and febrile episodes appears to be normal.[34] About one-third of patients have anti-neutrophil antibodies, but their presence does not appear to correlate with the incidence or severity of neutropenia.[8,35] Accelerated neutrophil apoptosis has also been described in patients with HIV.[37]

Defects in qualitative functions of neutrophils, such as chemotaxis, deficient degranulation responses, inhibition of leukocyte migration, ineffective killing of pathogens, and deficient superoxide generation, have been described in neutrophils from patients with HIV infection.[38,39] The clinical importance of these functional neutrophil defects in terms of host defense among HIV-infected individuals is

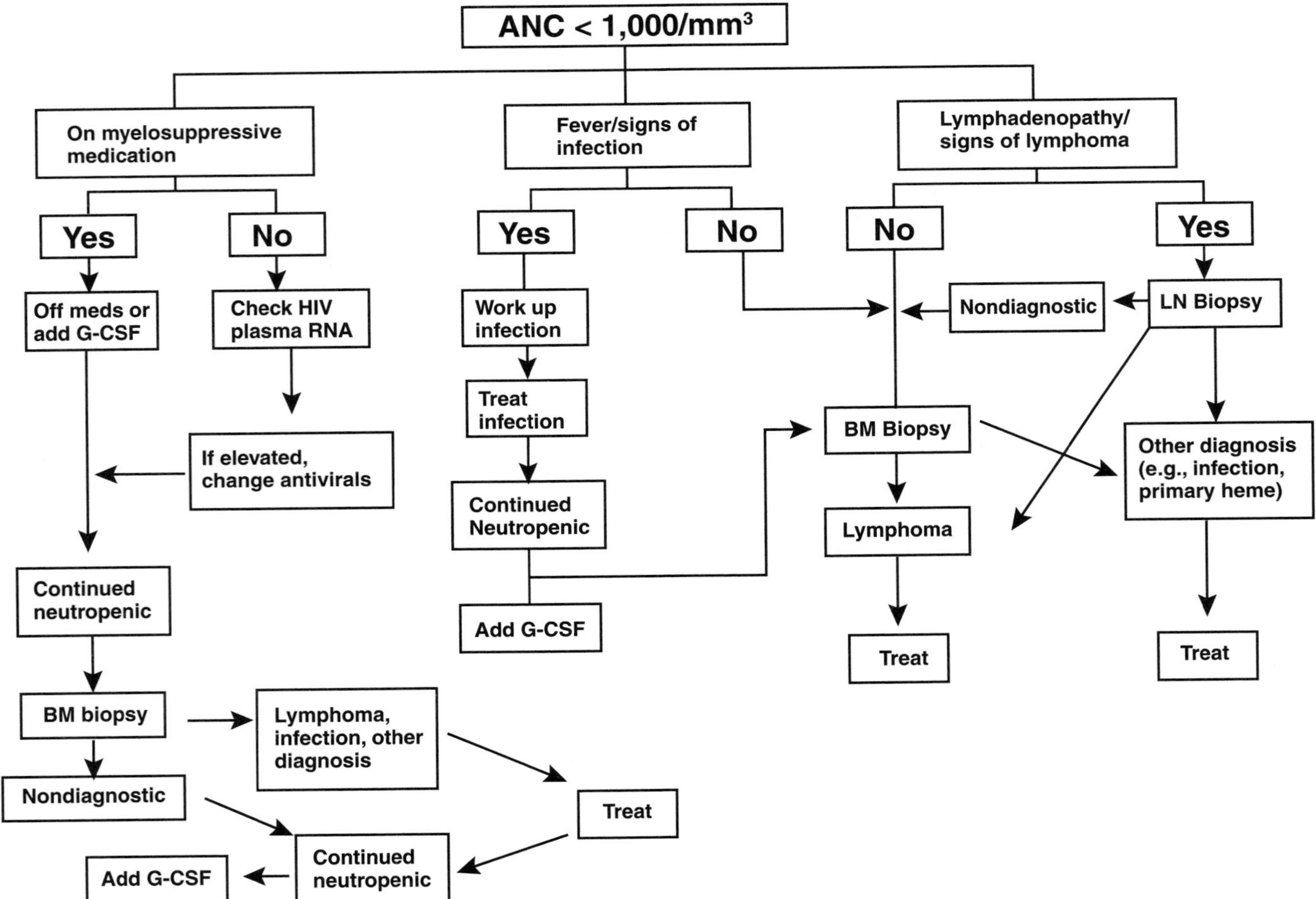

Figure 58–3. Evaluation of neutropenia in HIV infection. ANC, absolute neutrophil count; BM, bone marrow; G-CSF, granulocyte colony-stimulating factor; LN, lymph node.

unclear, although an increasing incidence of bacterial infections such as sinusitis and pneumonia does occur in patients with advanced HIV disease. In a similar way, HIV-infected monocytes have also been shown to exhibit marked reduction in chemotaxis and phagocytosis in some in vitro studies.[31]

Thrombocytopenia

Although granulocytopenia and anemia may occur concomitantly and their severity appears to parallel the course of HIV infection, thrombocytopenia (Fig. 58–4) can occur independently of other cytopenias and at all stages of HIV infection.[2,8,40] Thrombocytopenia to one degree or another occurs in 30% to 60% of HIV-infected patients.[40–42] Unlike anemia, thrombocytopenia is not directly correlated with the stage or prognosis of the HIV infection.[43]

Most patients with HIV-related immune thrombocytopenia have only minor submucosal bleeding, characterized by petechiae, ecchymosis, and occasional epistaxis. Rare patients have gastrointestinal blood loss. Splenomegaly occurs in some individuals with HIV-associated thrombocytopenia. Laboratory findings include isolated thrombocytopenia with typically normal peripheral blood smears and nonspecific bone marrow findings except for increased numbers of megakaryocytes.

Etiology

The causes of thrombocytopenia in HIV include reduced bone marrow production and immune and nonimmune pe-

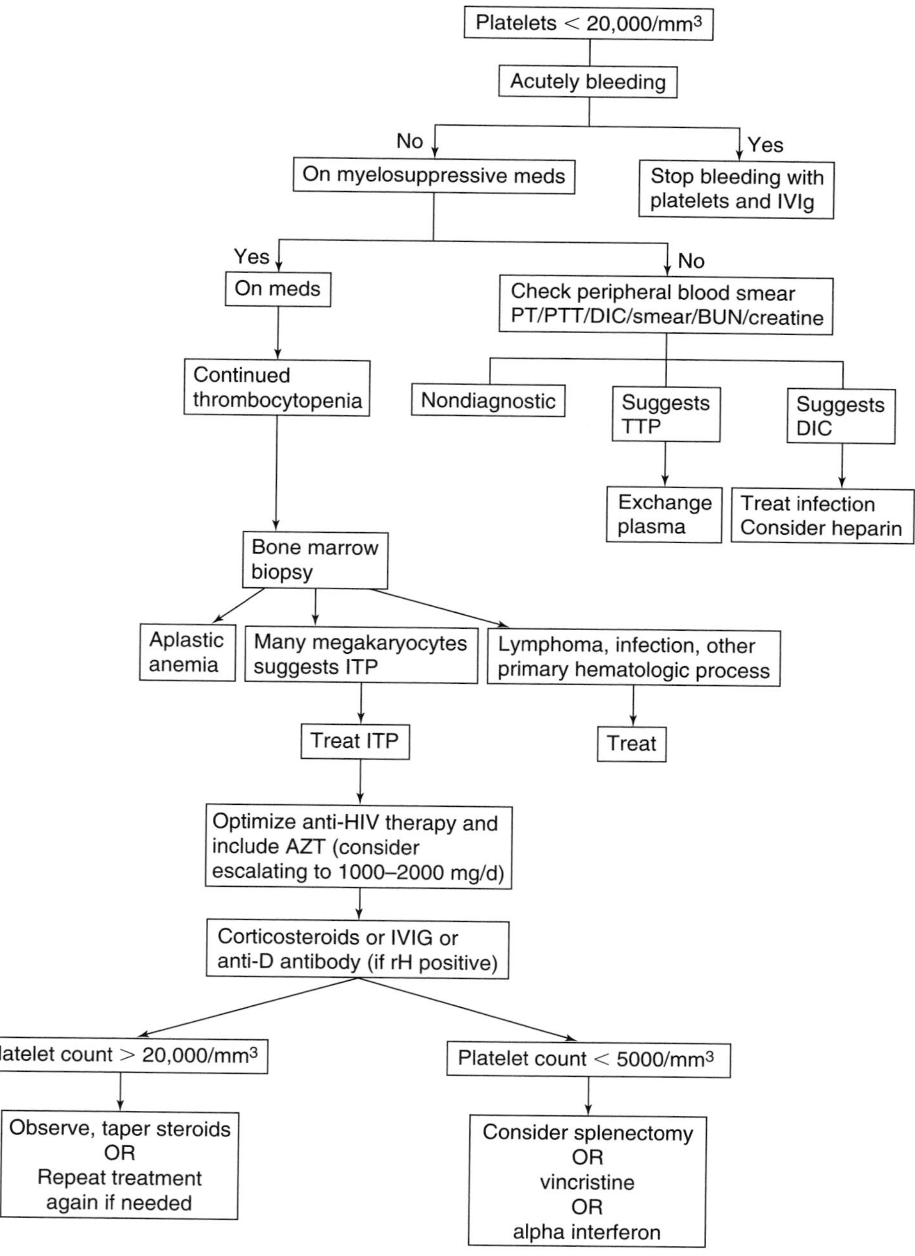

Figure 58–4. Evaluation of thrombocytopenia in HIV infection. AZT, zidovudine; BUN, blood urea nitrogen; DIC, disseminated intravascular coagulation; ITP, idiopathic thrombocytopenic purpura; PT, prothrombin time; PTT, partial thromboplastin time; TTP, thrombotic thrombocytopenic purpura.

ripheral destruction of platelets. Reduction in the productive capacity of megakaryocytes may be due to direct suppression of platelet production by HIV because megakaryocytes are potential targets of infection for the virus.[44] Subpopulations of megakaryocytes express CD4[45,46] and CXCR-4.[47,48] HIV may also indirectly suppress platelet production by exposing or altering antigen expression on the surface of megakaryocytes, which renders them targets of anti-platelet antibodies.[49] Alteration in cytokine and growth factor production during HIV infection may also modify platelet production.[44]

Peripheral destruction of platelets occurs as a result of infections and fevers that reduce the life span of circulating platelets as well as other nonimmune destruction of circulating platelets such as occurs with hemolytic uremia and thrombotic thrombocytopenic purpura, which have been described in patients with HIV.[40,50–52]

Immune destruction of platelets is the major cause of thrombocytopenia in HIV patients. In many patients with HIV infection antibodies coat the platelets.[53–61] Nonspecific binding of immune complexes to platelets and more specific molecular mimicry between gp160/120 antigens of HIV and the gpIIb/IIIa of platelets lead to specific platelet-associated antibodies.[49,53–55] Another hypothesis holds that a specific IgG anti-platelet antibody binds to a 25 kDa antigen on the platelet membrane, resulting in platelet destruction.[40] Nonspecific binding of anti-HIV immune complexes to the platelet Fc receptor may make platelets more susceptible to phagocytosis by macrophages.[62,63] There is no direct correlation between the presence of platelet-associated antibodies and the platelet count because of additional defective reticuloendothelial clearance of platelets in HIV-infected patients.[57]

Treatment

Most evaluations of various treatments for HIV-associated thrombocytopenia are hampered by the relative lack of well controlled, prospectively randomized trials of various treatment options for HIV-associated thrombocytopenia. Spontaneous remissions have been reported in 1% to 20% of patients.[58] In many with sustained decreases of platelet counts, therapy is not always necessary because the incidence of significant bleeding is low despite low platelet counts.[40,58] It is difficult to predict the risk of bleeding based solely on platelet counts.[58,59]

Thrombocytopenia associated with HIV infection may be corrected with the administration of zidovudine. Zidovudine elevates the platelet count in a minimum of 30% treatment-naive patients within 12 weeks of initiating therapy in placebo-controlled, crossover studies.[60,61] Anecdotal responses have also been seen with didanosine and other effective antiretroviral treatments.[64–66] Although there are no reported prospective, randomized controlled trials of HAART, two small retrospective studies show that HAART is beneficial in correcting the thrombocytopenia of HIV.[65,66] Dapsone may also elevate platelet counts in a small number of patients within 3 weeks of initiating therapy.[6] The mechanism by which zidovudine increases platelet counts is unknown; dapsone may act by reducing monocyte/macrophage-mediated cytotoxicity.[67]

Corticosteroids and immunoglobulin therapy can be initiated for patients needing immediate restoration of platelet counts. Corticosteroids elevate platelet counts in 40% to 80% of patients with HIV-associated thrombocytopenia, although long-term remission occurs in only 10% to 20% of patients.[40,59] Although chronic low-dose corticosteroids may be effective in maintaining an acceptable platelet count,[59] side effects of long-term corticosteroid use preclude their routine use. Infusion of gamma globulin (400 mg/kg/d for 4 to 5 days) may be used to increase the platelet count rapidly, although its effect is transient, lasting 2 to 3 weeks.[68] Acute response rates of 70% to 90% have been reported,[40,69] although sustained remission from a single course of such therapy occurs in fewer than 10% of patients.[40] The probable mechanism of its effect is blockage of the reticuloendothelial system by saturation of Fc receptors. The high cost and transient nature of immunoglobulin therapy limit its use to situations of acute bleeding or as a preoperative intervention for patients undergoing splenectomy, when rapid elevation of platelet count is necessary.

A similar response has been seen with anti-D (anti-Rh) antibody, which produces a short-term response of 75% and a more sustained platelet response than with IVIG.[70] As with gamma globulin infusion, readministration is effective in elevating the platelet count in patients who respond initially.[40,71] A slightly longer response time is seen, and there may be some hemolysis. Anti-D antibody is generally not effective with splenectomized patients or those who are Rh-negative. Immunoglobulin infusion and anti-D antibody may also work by increasing the production of thrombopoietic cytokines, such as interleukin-6 (IL-6), from cells of the reticuloendothelial system in addition to decreasing platelet destruction.[72] Anti-RhD has the advantage of requiring lesser amounts of antibody to be administered than IVIG.[73]

Splenectomy is also a successful therapeutic intervention for patients who fail to respond to corticosteroid therapy and is generally not associated with greater morbidity or mortality than in patients with non-HIV-associated thrombocytopenia.[74,75] This procedure has a short-term response rate of 60% to 100%, with durable responses occurring in 40% to 60% of patients.[40] No demonstrated detrimental effects of splenectomy have been seen on HIV progression.[76] This procedure can, however, result in artificial elevation of CD4+ T-lymphocyte counts because of peripheral lymphocytosis.[76] A small uncontrolled study of splenic irradiation as an alternative to splenectomy has also demonstrated a short-term response rate of 70% with a durable response occurring in 40% of small numbers of patients.[77,78] The total dose used is 900 to 1000 cGy administered over the course of a month.

For patients who do not require immediate increases in platelet count, the institution of or alteration in antiretroviral therapy is warranted to decrease the viral load to less than 50 copies/μl. Other modalities of treatment include vincristine and anabolic steroids, with an overall response rate of about 10%.[79,80] Interferon-α has also been shown in controlled trials to have some efficacy in zidovudine-resistant HIV-associated thrombocytopenia.[81] One potential mechanism by which interferon-α restores platelet production may be by increasing the levels of IL-6, a cytokine with trophic effects on megakaryocytes.[82] Partial responses to interferon-α appear to be more common than complete normalization of the platelet count, and the drug is generally well tolerated at doses of 3 million units given subcutaneously three times a week.[83,84]

The nonandrogenizing testosterone danazole (Danocrine), initially thought to reverse HIV-related thrombocytopenia, has not proved efficacious in large-scale trials.[79]

The potential use of pegylated recombinant human megakaryocyte growth and development factor (PEG-rHuMGDF) and recombinant human thrombopoietin (rHu-TPO) in patients with HIV-inducted thrombocytopenia has become of interest. PEG-rHuMGDF has been given twice weekly to HIV-positive throbocytopenic patients, and their platelet counts rose 10-fold within 14 days and were sustained for the 16 weeks of the study before falling to baseline levels within 14 days of discontinuing therapy.[85,86]

▲ BONE MARROW ABNORMALITIES

Bone marrow in most patients with HIV infection exhibits morphologic abnormalities[7,87,88] that increase with progression of HIV infection.[8,89] These abnormalities, however, are nonspecific and are seen in other diseases as well.[89,90] Hypercellularity occurs in 50% to 60% of patients and does not seem to correlate with peripheral cell counts or with the stage of HIV infection.[87,89] The myeloid/erythroid cell ratio tends to be normal or to exhibit a mild myeloid predominance. Hypocellularity of the marrow is rare, occurring in fewer than 5% of cases; it is usually a manifestation of advanced HIV disease.[3,8] Atrophy or necrosis of the bone marrow may be seen in the late stages of HIV infection.[89]

Dysplasia of one or more cell lines occurs in 30% to 70% of HIV-infected patients.[91,92] This dysplasia may be indistinguishable from myelodysplastic syndrome.[9,90] Dysplasia of the granulocyte series is most common, with vacuolation of peripheral neutrophils and granulocyte precursors in the marrow often seen.[91] The degree of dysplastic changes in the bone marrow increases with progression of HIV infection and with concurrent opportunistic infections.

Other common abnormalities in the bone marrow include lymphoid aggregates, which are encountered in 20% of patients and may be seen in patients even with peripheral lymphopenia.[91] About 20% of patients with advanced HIV infection have focal or diffuse increases in reticulin deposits in the marrow. Marrow involvement with fungal or mycobacteria organisms may also result in marrow fibrosis. Other nonspecific morphologic changes seen in the bone marrow with HIV infection include eosinophilia, plasmacytosis, and histiocytic erythrophagocytosis.[8,88,91,93,94]

The bone marrow is also involved in about one-third of patients with AIDS-related lymphoma. The extent of bone marrow replacement by these malignant cells does not correlate well with peripheral blood counts.[95] Several opportunistic infections can also involve the bone marrow and contribute to bone marrow failure. Bone marrow may reveal disseminated mycobacterial or fungal infections long before other indications of the infection become apparent in the AIDS patient.[96,97] Special stains and cultures of the bone marrow for these organisms are helpful and may be positive before peripheral cultures turn positive. Small studies have shown that bone marrow examination or cultures are positive for mycobacteria or fungi in at least 75% of patients who are subsequently found to have these infections.[96–98] The most common manifestation of these infections is diffuse infiltration of bone marrow with the organisms, with loose aggregates and clusters of macrophages. These cells may organize into granulomas, which are less prominent in the presence of more advanced disease. Pseudo-Gaucher cells may also be a manifestation of these infections.[99] Cytomegalovirus (CMV) can also infect bone marrow progenitor cells and render them less responsive to colony-stimulating factors.[100] CMV can affect the bone marrow stromal cells as well, interfering with their hematopoietic supporting function largely by decreasing local growth factor production by these cells.[100] CMV does not, however, cause distinctive histologic changes of the bone marrow. It is best cultured from the buffy coat of blood and not from the bone marrow itself.

Human herpesvirus-6 (HHV-6) targets CD4+ T-lymphocytes and monocytes.[101,102] Immunosuppression as a result of HIV infection may result in loss of latency of this virus. Subsequent exposure of bone marrow precursor cells to this virus may inhibit their ability to respond to growth factors. Infection of T lymphocytes by this virus may also cause further suppression of T-cell function. Despite these laboratory observations, the clinical relevance of HHV-6 in this population and the benefits of treating HHV-6 are unclear.

▲ HIV INFECTION AND BONE MARROW PROGENITOR CELLS

Studies involving HIV infection of bone marrow progenitor cells have been somewhat conflicting.[8,87,103] Although there are data indicating that progenitor cells may be the target of HIV infection, other findings have revealed that CD34+ bone marrow progenitor cells are infrequently infected with HIV.[104–107] Some investigators have shown that progenitor cells in the bone marrow and in peripheral blood are decreased with HIV infection,[104,108] whereas others have shown no significant differences in the number of these cells in HIV-infected patients compared to uninfected controls.[109] Similarly, some studies have revealed HIV RNA in protein products in committed myeloid and erythroid progenitor cells,[108] whereas other studies have not been able to detect HIV in these cells.[109]

These conflicting results may be due to a number of factors. Some CD34+ progenitor cells in the marrow are also CD4+ or express HIV-1 co-receptors, CXCR4 or CCR5, and they may be targets for HIV.[104,106] The presence or absence of accessory cells in the bone marrow can also influence hematopoiesis through the local production of growth factors.[110] These accessory T cells, monocytes, and fibroblasts are targets for HIV and may serve as a reservoir for virus in the marrow. These HIV-infected accessory cells may be less able to produce local hematopoietic growth factors, which in turn may slow normal hematopoiesis or facilitate apoptosis.[111,112] These accessory cells may also produce inhibitors of hematopoiesis such as transforming growth factor-β and TNFα.[113–116] HIV protein products such as the gp120 and gp160 envelope proteins, or antibodies to these HIV protein products, may suppress normal hematopoiesis by either inducing other cells to produce TNF or other hematopoietic suppressive cytokines. HIV may also inhibit the hematopoietic process more directly, such as with antibodies to gp120 or through functioning of accessory genes.[117,118] The presence of antiretroviral drugs may influence hematopoiesis by decreasing these various inhibitory processes. Therefore administration of effective antiretroviral therapy becomes critical to any strategy to alleviate cytopenias in patients with HIV.

▲ USE OF HEMATOPOIETIC GROWTH FACTORS IN HIV INFECTION

The colony-stimulating factors include G-CSF, granulocyte/macrophage colony-stimulating factor (GM-CSF), interleukin-3 (IL-3), macrophage colony-stimulating factor (M-CSF), stem cell factor, and erythropoietin (EPO).[119] These glycoproteins regulate the production of various hematopoietic cells and the process of terminal differentiation and maturation. They also suppress apoptosis,[120] and many can enhance the function of terminally differentiated hematopoietic and other cells.[119] Production of G-CSF, GM-CSF, and M-CSF is increased during the early phases of HIV infection.[121] This increase is stimulated by the effects of IL-1 and other inflammatory cytokines on the cells in the bone marrow, as well as by T cells, monocytes, and fibroblasts. The latter cells, when infected by HIV, have progressively impaired ability to produce growth factors. Exogenous administration of growth factors offers the potential of ameliorating some of the adverse effects of HIV infection on normal hematopoiesis and may allow continued or heightened use of myelosuppressive antibiotics and other drugs necessary to control HIV and its related complications.

Granulocyte Colony-Stimulating Factor

Granulocyte colony-stimulating factor is produced by activated, monocyte-stimulated endothelial cells and fibroblasts. Studies of G-CSF in patients with HIV infection have demonstrated that it can increase neutrophil counts, improve neutrophil function, and reverse severe neutropenia in patients with HIV infection. Open-label studies of G-CSF for the treatment of neutropenia in patients with HIV have shown almost universal correction of neutropenia that is maintained for long periods of time with induction doses of 1 to 4 μg/kg/d followed by a maintenance dose of 300 μg one to seven times a week.[122] In these studies, no significant changes in CD4+ or CD8+ cell counts or in HIV replication were seen.

With advanced HIV infection, interruption of HIV therapy as a result of neutropenia may be associated with loss of disease control and poor prognosis. By supporting delivery of essential medications used to treat HIV or CMV infection, *Pneumocystis carinii* pneumonia, toxoplasmosis, and malignancies, G-CSF may improve the quality of life and help avoid the potential serious clinical consequences associated with dose reduction or discontinuation of critical medications. Clinical studies have shown that G-CSF allows myelosuppressive medications to be given as scheduled and permits additional myelosuppressive drugs to be added when necessary.[122–124] In a large, multicenter trial that included more than 200 neutropenic HIV-infected patients, G-CSF reversed neutropenia in 98%, with a mean time of 2 days to reversal. G-CSF also allowed more than 84% of patient to increase or maintain doses of myelosuppressive medications or add them to their therapy.[122] G-CSF may also reduce infectious complications associated with neutropenia, including the need for hospitalization and the use of intravenous antibiotics. Survival may also be enhanced.[125]

In another large prospective, randomized study, the use of G-CSF to prevent severe neutropenia [absolute neutrophil count (ANC) < 500 cells/mm^3] was studied in 258 moderately neutropenic (ANC 750 to 1000 cells/mm^3) HIV-infected individuals with CD4+ T-lymphocyte counts of less than 200 cells/mm^3.[126,127] Patients were randomized to receive subcutaneous G-CSF (either 1.0 μg/kg/d or 300 μg two to five times per week, titrated to maintain the ANC between 2000 and 10,000 cells/mm^3) or to an observational control group. The incidence of severe neutropenia was significantly lower during the 24-week study period in the groups of patients receiving G-CSF (1.7%) compared with controls (22%) ($P < 0.001$). The incidence of all bacterial infections was 31% lower in the G-CSF-treated group (2.93/1000 vs. 4.24/1000 patient-days). G-CSF-treated patients also had 54% fewer severe bacterial infections and required less frequent use of intravenous antibiotics than control patients. No difference in plasma HIV-1 RNA levels were seen between the groups. This suggests that G-CSF is effective in preventing severe neutropenia and reducing the incidence of bacterial infection in HIV-infected individuals.[126]

Improvement in neutrophil function has also been demonstrated in patients receiving G-CSF. Improvements in chemotaxis, superoxide generation, and neutrophil killing of bacterial pathogens have been demonstrated with G-CSF.[128] Reduction in accelerated apoptosis of neutrophils with HIV was also seen with G-CSF.[129] Improvements in survival have been seen in HIV-infected patients receiving G-CSF compared to those not receiving this agent in retrospective studies of patients with advanced HIV disease in general and in HIV patients with MAC infections.[125,130] In one study in advanced HIV patients, G-CSF was associated with significantly prolonged survival, 397 days, compared to 165 days in those not treated with G-CSF.[125] G-CSF may also be important in increasing the number of CD34+ hematopoietic progenitor cells and can be used to mobilize CD34+ cells for autologous stem cells transplants or for gene therapy studies.[131,132]

Granulocyte/Macrophage Colony-Stimulating Factor

The growth factor GM-CSF is produced primarily by stimulated fibroblasts and endothelial cells, although it is also produced by T cells. Administration of GM-CSF, as with G-CSF, results in a dose-dependent elevation in neutrophils. The kinetic basis of the elevation in neutrophils differs from that of G-CSF in that GM-CSF prolongs the circulating half-life of neutrophils rather than decreasing the production time.[133] Unlike G-CSF, GM-CSF results in a significant increase in eosinophils and monocytes.[133] Correction of granulocyte and macrophage/monocyte functional defects have been noted in patients receiving this drug where deficiencies have been observed.[134] Additionally, enhancement of antimicrobial function of leukocytes have been demonstrated in several in vitro studies. Use of this agent in combination with myelosuppressive chemotherapy for non-Hodgkin lymphoma and Kaposi sarcoma and with myelosuppressive antibiotics for opportunistic infections, such as ganciclovir treatment for CMV retinitis, have demonstrated that the use of this agent may allow continued administration of important medications for HIV-related diseases.

Factors GM-CSF and G-CSF have different effects on HIV-infected cells.[133,135–137] Whereas G-CSF does not seem to alter HIV replication in cells that are targets for the growth factor, GM-CSF can stimulate HIV replication in vitro in infected monocytes.[137–139] In addition, activation by HIV of monocytes induces production of GM-CSF and stimulates T cells, endothelial cells, and fibroblasts to produce this growth factor, which in turn augments HIV replication. When GM-CSF is administered in conjunction with zidovudine, the result is enhanced antiviral effects seen in vitro, perhaps because of an increase in the concentration of the phosphorylated active form of the drug in monocytes.[137] Studies of GM-CSF in HIV-infected individuals refractory to antiretroviral therapy have demonstrated some enhancement of the antiretroviral effect of protease inhibitors.[140] A further randomized, controlled study of GM-CSF in HIV-infected patients with elevated HIV plasma viremia is in progress (ACTG 5041).

Erythropoietin

Most HIV-infected patients with anemia have adequate erythropoietic capacity but are unable to augment it during periods of demand in large part because of relatively inadequate EPO levels.[141] Inappropriately low endogenous levels (< 500 mU/ml) of serum EPO are seen in most AIDS patients with anemia.[141,142] In addition, cytokines that are produced in response to HIV infection, such as IL-1 and TNFα, blunt the normal rise in hematocrit with rising serum EPO levels.[143] In patients who become anemic after receiving zidovudine, the EPO level may continue to be inadequately low or it may be increased; however, it does not prevent anemia. This observation has suggested that zidovudine-related anemia is probably not due solely to EPO deficiency. Two forms of anemia appear to result from zidovudine therapy that may respond differently to zidovudine dose adjustment. The most common is megaloblastic anemia, which corrects with dose adjustment of zidovudine. The other, less frequent form is more similar to red blood cell aplasia and usually does not respond to zidovudine dose reduction; it may be due to an increased sensitivity of erythroid progenitor cells to the myelosuppressive effects of this drug.

Placebo-controlled trials have shown that small amounts of recombinant human EPO (epoietin-α) can increase hemoglobin and significantly reduce transfusion requirements of patients with HIV infection and anemia.[144,145] In several placebo-controlled clinical trials, erythropoietin significantly reduced transfusion requirements, increased the hematocrit, and improved the quality of life of patients with HIV infection and anemia. The elevation in erythrocyte count appeared to be dose-dependent.[144] Patients were retrospectively divided into two groups based on entry-level endogenous EPO levels. Patients whose EPO levels were less than 500 mU/ml had statistically significant reductions in red blood cell transfusions and increases in hematocrit compared to placebo-treated patients after 6 to 8 weeks of therapy. Patients with endogenous EPO levels of more than 500 mU/ml did not experience significant increases in hematocrit or reduction in transfusion requirements when compared to placebo-treated patients.[144] Stem cell exhaustion or lineage diversion was not seen. EPO neither promoted nor prevented HIV replication.[144] Approximately 25% of patients on zidovudine did not have a significant elevation in their hematocrit with concurrent administration of EPO.[135,144] Opportunistic infections rendered patients relatively resistant to the effects of exogenous EPO. The drug was well tolerated. The use of iron and hematinics is recommended for patients on long-term EPO therapy. EPO is approved for use in patients with anemia as a result of zidovudine therapy, and the initial recommended dose is 100 IU/kg three times weekly. Failure to respond to this treatment after 6 to 8 weeks would warrant increasing the dose and possibly performing a bone marrow aspiration and biopsy to exclude other possible causes of myelosuppression. EPO may be combined with myeloid hematopoietic growth factors such as G-CSF in patients with both neutropenia and anemia with good multilineage effects.[135] EPO is also effective in a once-a-week dosing schedule of 40,000 IU.[146] Many HIV-treating physicians now would consider treatment of anemia to maintain the hemoglobin level above 12 g/dl for men and above 11 g/dl for women.[146]

A randomized controlled study of epoetin alfa (100 to 300 IU/kg SC three times per week) in anemic HIV-infected patients in the community setting showed significant increases in hemogloblin levels that were independent of the baseline CD4+ T-lymphocyte counts. The mean quality of life score, as measured by the Functional Assessment of HIV Infection (FAHI) scale, improved significantly, with increases in hemoglobin after epoetin alfa use.[145]

Administration of EPO offers an alternative to transfusions and their potential morbidity and mortality. Transfusions may be immunosuppressive,[147] and the time to progression to AIDS is shorter in those who are given transfusions.[148] Data suggest an increase in HIV replication in those receiving red blood cell transfusions as well.[149] There is a risk of exposure to new infectious agents with transfusions and a risk of transfusion reactions despite the immunodeficiency caused by HIV.[89] If one does need to transfuse red blood cells in an HIV patient, however, results from the Viral Activation Transfusion Study did not show any advantage to using leukocyte-reduced red blood cells in a large prospective randomized controlled study.[150]

▲ COAGULATION ABNORMALITIES ASSOCIATED WITH HIV INFECTION

Coagulation abnormalities are frequently encountered in patients with HIV infection. The most common is the lupus anticoagulant, which is one of several antibodies to acidic phospholipids that can occur as a result of the abnormal immune responses seen with HIV infection. An incidence of 20% to 66% has been reported for the lupus anticoagulant in patients with HIV infection.[151–155] The IgG or IgM antibody titer increases with active opportunistic infections. The presence of this anti-phospholipid antibody is established by the use of phospholipid-dependent coagulation assays such as the activated partial thromboplastin time (aPTT) or the Russell viper venom clotting time; or it is confirmed on an enzyme-linked immunosorbent assay.[153–157] These antibodies may give false-positive test results for the Venereal Disease Research Laboratory and anti-cardiolipin antibody assays. The most commonly seen abnormality is an elevation in the aPTT that is not corrected with 1:1 mixing of normal and patient plasma. The prothrombin time may be prolonged to a mild degree in about 10% of patients who have the lupus anticoagulant. Also abnormal is the dilute thromboplastin inhibition assay and the Russell viper venom clotting time. Once thought to be clinically insignificant, the lupus anticoagulant in HIV-infected patients may be associated with major thromboembolic events.[156,157] Prolonged bleeding after surgery is seldom seen.

The incidence of thrombotic disease does appear to be increased in HIV-infected individuals,[158] but the exact reason for it is unknown. Thromboembolic events may also occur as a result of reduced production of active protein S. This peptide is a cofactor for protein C by localizing active protein C to the phospholipid surface. Free protein S levels are statistically lower in HIV-infected patients with or without thrombosis than in healthy controls.[159]

The total protein S level does not correlate with the CD4+ T-lymphocyte count or the stage of the HIV infection. Protein S binds to C4b-binding protein. The chronic inflammatory state encountered with HIV infection results in increased C4b-binding protein and more binding of protein S by C4b-binding protein, so less is available to prevent abnormal thrombotic events.[159] In addition, higher levels of anti-protein S antibodies have been detected that may bind protein C.[160] Anticoagulant therapy is appropriate in patients with documented deficiencies of protein S.

In addition, infection with CMV and herpes simplex virus types 1 and 2 may affect normal vascular endothelial cells and their procoagulant expression. Alterations of the surface phospholipid expression may activate the coagulation system locally and result in microangiopathies, such as thrombotic thrombocytopenic purpura and other localized coagulation defects.[50,51,161]

Acknowledgments. This work was supported in part by a grant from the State of California University-wide AIDS Research Program to the UCLA AIDS Clinical Research Center (CC99-LA002) and grants from the U.S. Public Health Service, National Institutes of Health, (AI27660, CA70080, and RR00865).

REFERENCES

1. Zon L, Groopman J. Hematologic manifestations of the human immune deficiency virus. Semin Hematol 25:208, 1988.
2. Evans RH, Scadden DT. Haematological aspects of HIV infection. Ballieres Clin Haematol 13:215, 2000.
3. Mir N, Costello C, Luckitt J, et al. HIV disease and bone marrow changes: a study of 60 cases. Eur J Haematol 42:339, 1989.
4. Perkocha L, Rodgers G. Hematologic aspects of human immunodeficiency virus infection: laboratory and clinical considerations. Am J Hematol 29:94, 1988.
5. Doweiko JP. Hematologic aspects of HIV infection. AIDS 7:753, 1993.
6. Harbol AW, Liesveld JL, Simpson-Haidaris PJ, et al. Mechanisms of cytopenia in human immunodeficiency virus infection. Blood Rev 8:241, 1994.
7. Hambleton J. Hematologic complications of HIV infection. Oncology 10:671, 1996.
8. Scadden DT, Zon LI, Groopman GE. Pathophysiology and management of HIV-associated hematologic disorders. Blood 74:1455, 1989.
9. Ganser A. Abnormalities of hematopoiesis in the acquired immunodeficiency syndrome. Blut 56:49, 1988.
10. Sullivan PS, Hanson DL, Chu SY, et al. Epidemiology of anemia in human immunodeficiency virus (HIV)-infected persons: results from the Multi-state Adult and Adolescent Spectrum of HIV Disease Surveillance Project. Blood 91:301, 1998.
11. Moore RD, Keruly JC, Chaisson RE. Anemia and survival in HIV infection. J Acquir Immune Defic Syndr Hum Retrovirol 19:29, 1998.
12. Fauci A, Schnittman S, Poli G. Immunopathogenic mechanisms in human immunodeficiency virus (HIV) infection. Ann Intern Med 114:678, 1991.
13. Zhang Y, Harada A, Bluethmann H, et al. Tumor necrosis factor (TNF) is a physiologic regulator of hematopoietic cells: increase of early hematopoietic cells in TNF receptor p55-deficient mice in vivo and potent inhibition of progenitor cell proliferation by TNF in vitro. Blood 86:2930, 1995.
14. Richman DD, Fischl MA, Grieco MH, et al. The toxicity of azidothymidine (AZT) in the treatment of patients with AIDS and AIDS-related complex. N Engl J Med 317:192, 1987.
15. Semba RD, Shah N, Vlahov D. Improvement of anemia among HIV-infected injection drug users receiving highly active antiretroviral therapy. J Acquir Immune Defic Syndr Hum Retrovirol 26:315, 2001.
16. Gascom P, Sathe S, Rameshwar P. Impaired erythropoiesis in the acquired immunodeficiency syndrome with disseminated *Mycobacterium avium* complex. Am J Med 94:41, 1993.
17. Gyllensten K, Sponnerborg A, Jorup-Ronstrom C, et al. Parvovirus B19 infection in HIV-1 infected patients with anemia. Infection 22:356, 1994.
18. Chernak E, Dubin G, Henry D, et al. Infection due to parvovirus B19 in patients infected with human immunodeficiency virus. Clin Infect Dis 20:170, 1995.
19. Naides S, Howard EJ, Swack NS, et al. Parvovirus B19 infection in HIV type 1-infected persons failing or intolerant to zidovudine therapy. J Infect Dis 168:101, 1993.
20. Bremner J, Beard B, Cohen A. Secondary infection with parvovirus B19 in an HIV-positive patient. AIDS 7:1131, 1993.
21. Gupta S, Inman A, Licorish K. Serum ferritin in acquired immune deficiency syndrome. J Clin Lab Immunol 20:11, 1986.
22. Remacha AF, Riera A, Cadafalch J, et al. Vitamin B_{12} abnormalities in HIV-infected patients. Eur J Haematol 47:60, 1991.
23. Remacha AF, Cadafalch J. Cobalamin deficiency in patients infected with the human immunodeficiency virus. Semin Hematol 36:75, 1999.
24. Beach RS, Mantero-Atienza E, Shor-Posner G, et al. Specific nutrient abnormalities in asymptomatic HIV-1 infection. AIDS 6:701, 1991.
25. Ehrenpreis E, Carlson SJ, Boorstein HL, et al. Malabsorption and deficiency of vitamin B_{12} in HIV-infected patients with chronic diarrhea. Dig Dis Sci 39:2159, 1994.

26. Paltiel O, Falutz J, Veilleux M, et al. Clinical correlates of subnormal vitamin B_{12} levels in patients infected with the human immunodeficiency virus. Am J Hematol 49:318, 1995.
27. Saif MW. HIV-associated autoimmune hemolytic anemia: an update. AIDS Patient Care STDs 15:217, 2001.
28. Toy P, Reid M, Burns M. Positive direct antiglobulin test associated with hyperglobulinemia in acquired immunodeficiency syndrome. Am J Hematol 19:145, 1985.
29. McGinniss M, Macher A, Rook A, et al. Red cell autoantibodies in patients with acquired immune deficiency syndrome. Transfusion 26:405, 1986.
30. Sipas NV, Kokori SI, Ioannidis JP, et al. Circulating autoantibodies to erythropoietin are associated with human immunodeficiency virus type 1-related anemia. J Infect Dis 180:2044, 1999.
31. Brizzi M, Porcu P, Porteri A, et al. Haematologic abnormalities in the acquired immunodeficiency syndrome. Haematologica 75:454, 1990.
32. Hermans P, Sommereijns B, Van Cutsen N, Clumeck N. Neutropenia in patiens with HIV infection: a case control study in a cohort of 1403 patients between 1982 and 1993. J Hematother Stem Cell Res 1(suppl 8):S23, 1999.
33. Israel D, Plaisance K. Neutropenia in patients infected with human immunodeficiency virus. Clin Pharm 10:268, 1990.
34. Mauss S, Steinmetz HT, Willers R, et al. Induction of granulocyte colony-stimulating factor by acute febrile infection but not by neutropenia in HIV-seropositive individuals. J Acquir Immune Defic Syndr Hum Retrovirol 14:430, 1997.
35. Donahue R, Johnson M, Zon L. Suppression of in vitro hematopoiesis following human immunodeficiency virus infection. Nature 326:200, 1987.
36. Leiderman I, Greenberg M, Adlesberg B, et al. A glycoprotein inhibitor of in vitro granulopoiesis associated with AIDS. Blood 70:1267, 1987.
37. Pitrak DL, Mullane KM, Bilek ML, et al. Impaired phagocyte oxidative capacity in patients with human immunodeficiency virus infection. J Lab Clin Med 132:284, 1998.
38. Murphy P, Lane C, Fauci A, et al. Impairment of neutrophil bactericidal capacity in patients with AIDS. J Infect Dis 158:627, 1988.
39. Valone F, Payan D, Abrams D, et al. Defective polymorphonuclear leukocyte chemotaxis in homosexual men with persistent lymph node syndrome. J Infect Dis 150:267, 1984.
40. Stricker RB. Hemostatic abnormalities in HIV disease. Hematol Oncol Clin North Am 5:249, 1991.
41. Perkocha LA, Rodgers GM. Hematologic aspects of human immunodeficiency virus infection: laboratory and clinical considerations. Am J Hematol 29:94, 1988.
42. Sullivan PS, Hanson DL, Chu SY, et al. Surveillance for thrombocytopenia in persons infected with HIV: results from the multistate Adult and Adolescent Spectrum of Disease Project. J Acquir Immune Defic Syndr Hum Retrovirol 14:374, 1997.
43. Holzman RS, Walsh CM, Karpatkin S. Risk for the acquired immunodeficiency syndrome among thrombocytopenic and nonthrombocytopenic homosexual men seropositive for the human immunodeficiency virus. Ann Intern Med 106:383, 1987.
44. Bellem PJ, Belzberg A, Devine DV, et al. Kinetic studies of the mechanisms of thrombocytopenia in patients with human immunodeficiency virus infection. N Engl J Med 327:1779, 1992.
45. Basch RS, Louri YH, Karpatkin S. Expression of CD4 by human megakaryocytes. Proc Nati Acad Sci USA 87:8085, 1990.
46. Kouri YH, Borkowsky W, Nardi M, et al. Human megakaryocytes have a CD4 molecule capable of binding human immunodeficiency virus-1. Blood 81:2664, 1993.
47. Wang JF, Liu ZY, Groopman JE. The alpha-chemokine receptor CXCR4 is expressed on the megakaryocytic lineage from progenitor to platelets and modulates migration and adhesion. Blood 92:756, 1998.
48. Riviere C, Subra F, Cohen-Solal K, et al. Phenotypic and functional evidence for the expression of CXCR4 receptor during megakaryocytopoiesis. Blood 93:1511, 1999.
49. Dominguez A, Gamallo G, Garcia R, et al. Pathophysiology of HIV related thrombocytopenia: an analysis of 41 patients. J Clin Pathol 47:999, 1994.
50. Leaf AN, Laubenstein LH, Raphael B, et al. Thrombotic thrombocytopenic purpura associated with human immunodeficiency virus type 1 (HIV-1) infection. Ann Intern Med 109:194, 1988.
51. Thompson CE, Damon LE, Ries CA, et al. Thrombotic micro-angiopathies in the 1980s: clinical features, response to treatment, and the impact of the human immunodeficiency virus epidemic. Blood 80:1890, 1992.
52. Badesha PS, Saklayen MG. Hemolytic uremic syndrome as a presenting form of HIV infection. Nephron 72:472, 1996.
53. Bettaieb A, Fromont P, Louache F, et al. Presence of cross-reactive antibody between human immunodeficiency virus (HIV) and platelet glycoproteins in HIV-related immune thrombocytopenic purpura. Blood 80:162, 1992.
54. Stanworth DR, Solder B, Lewin IV, et al. Related epitopes in HIV viral coat protein and human IgG. Lancet 1:1458, 1989.
55. Gonzalez-Conejero R, Rivera J, Rosillo MC, et al. Antibodies against platelet glycoproteins Ib/IX and IIb/IIIa, and platelet reactive anti-HIV antibodies in thrombocytopenic narcotic addicts. Br J Hematol 93:464, 1996.
56. Nardi M, Karpatkin S. Anti-idiotype antibody against platelet anti-GPIIIa contributes to the regulation of thrombocytopenia in HIV-1-ITP patients. J Exp Med 191:2093, 2000.
57. Bender BS, Quinn TC, Spival JL. Homosexual men with thrombocytopenia have impaired reticuloendothelial system Fc receptor specific clearance. Blood 70:392, 1987.
58. Walsh C, Kriegel R, Lennette E, et al. Thrombocytopenia in homosexual patients. Ann Intern Med 103:542, 1985.
59. Karpatkin S. Immunologic thrombocytopenic purpura in HIV-seropositive homosexuals, narcotic addicts and hemophiliacs. Semin Hematol 25:219, 1988.
60. Oksenhendler E, Bierling P, Ferchal F. Zidovudine for thrombocytopenia purpura related to human immunodeficiency virus infection. Ann Intern Med 110:365, 1989.
61. Swiss Group for Clinical Studies on AIDS. Zidovudine for the treatment of thrombocytopenia associated with human immunodeficiency virus. Ann Intern Med 209:718, 1988.
62. Walsh C, Nardi MA, Karpatikin S. On the mechanism of thrombocytopenic purpura in sexually active homosexual men. N Engl J Med 311:635, 1984.
63. Dominguez A, Gamallo G, Garcia R, et al. Pathophysiology of HIV related thrombocytopenia: an analysis of 41 patients. J Clin Pathol 47:999, 1994.
64. Piketty C, Gilguin J, Kazatchkine M, et al. Successful treatment of HIV-related thrombocytopenia with didanosine. J Acquir Immune Defic Syndr 7:521, 1994.
65. Maness LJ, Blair DC, Newman N, et al. Elevation of platelet counts associated with indinavir treatment in human immunodeficiency virus-infected patients. Clin Infect Dis 26:207, 1998.
66. Arranz Caso JA, Sanchez MC, Garcia TJ. Effect of highly active antiretroviral therapy on thrombocytopenia in patients with HIV infection [letter]. N Engl J Med 341:1239, 1999.
67. Durand JM, Lefevre P, Hovette P, et al. Dapsone for thrombocytopenic purpura related to human immunodeficiency virus infection. Am J Med 90:675, 1991.
68. Yap PL, Todd AAM, William PE, et al. Use of intravenous imunoglobulin in acquired immune deficiency syndrome. Cancer 68:1440, 1991.
69. Pollak AN, Jaminis J, Green D. Successful intravenous immune globulin therapy for human immunodeficiency virus-associated thrombocytopenia. Arch Intern Med 148:695, 1988.
70. Oskenhendler E, Bierling P, Brossard, et al. Anti-Rh immunoglobulin therapy for human immunodeficiency virus-related immune thrombocytopenia. Blood 71:1499, 1989.
71. Biniek R, Malessa R, Brochmeyer NH, et al. Anti-Rh(D) immunoglobulin for AIDS-related thrombocytopenia. Lancet 2:627, 1986.
72. Than S, Oyaizu N, Pahwa RN. Effect of human immunodeficiency virus type-1 envelope glycoprotein gp120 on cytokine production from cord-blood T cells. Blood 84:184, 1994.
73. Gringeri A, Cattaneo M, Santagostino E, Mannucci PM. Intramuscular anti-D immunoglobulins for home treatment of chronic immune thrombocytopenic purpura. Br J Haematol 80:337, 1992.
74. Oksenhendler E, Bierling P, Chevret S, et al. Splenectomy is safe and effective in HIV-related immune thrombocytopenia. Blood 82:29, 1993.
75. Schneider P, Abrams D, Rayneret A, et al. Immunodeficiency-associated thrombocytopenic purpura: response to splenectomy. Arch Surg 122:1175, 1987.

76. Zambello R, Trentin L, Agostini C, et al. Persistent polyclonal lymphocytosis in human immunodeficiency virus-1 infected patients. Blood 81:3015, 1993.
77. Calverley DC, Jones GW, Kelton JG. Splenic radiation for corticosteroid-resistant immune thrombocytopenia. Ann Intern Med 116:977, 1992.
78. Blauth J, Fisher S, Henry D, Nichini F. The role of splenic irradiation in treating HIV-associated immune thrombocytopenia. Int J Radiat Oncol Biol Phys 45:457, 1999.
79. Ahn YS. Efficacy of danazol in hematologic disorders. Acta Haematol 84:122, 1990.
80. Minter DM, Real FX, Jovino L, et al. Treatment of Kaposi's sarcoma and thrombocytopenia with vincristine in patients with the acquired immunodeficiency syndrome. Ann Intern Med 102:200, 1985.
81. Marroni M, Gresele P, Landonio G, et al. Interferon-alpha is effective in the treatment of HIV-1-related, severe, zidovudine-resistant thrombocytopenia: a prospective, placebo-controlled, double-blind trial. Ann Intern Med 121:423, 1994.
82. Zauli G, Re MC, Gugliotta L, et al. The elevation of circulating platelets after IFN-alpha therapy in HIV-seropositive thrombocytopenic patients correlates with increased plasma levels of IL-6. Microbiologica 16:27, 1993.
83. Stellini R, Rossi G, Paraninfo G. Interferon therapy in intravenous drug-users with HIV-associated idiopathic thrombocytopenic purpura. Haematologica 77:418, 1992.
84. Vianelli N, Cantai L, Gugliotta L. Recombinant alpha interferon 2b in the therapy of HIV-related thrombocytopenia. AIDS 7:823, 1993.
85. Harker LA. Physiology and clinical application of platelet growth factors. Curr Opin Hematol 6:127, 1999.
86. Harker LA, Carter RA, Marzec UM, et al. Correction of thrombocytopenia and ineffective platelet production in patients infected with human immunodeficiency virus by PEG-rHuMGDF therapy. Blood 92(suppl 1):707a, 1998.
87. Calenda V, Chermann JC. The effects of HIV on hematopoiesis. Eur J Haematol 48:181, 1992.
88. Harris C, Biggs, JC, Concannon AJ, et al. Peripheral blood and bone marrow findings in patients with acquired immune deficiency syndrome. Pathology 22:206, 1990.
89. Perkocha LA, Rodgers GM. Hematologic aspects of human immunodeficiency virus infection. Am J Hematol 29:94, 1992.
90. Goasguen JE, Bennett JM. Classification and morphologic features of myelodysplastic syndromes. Semin Oncol 19:4, 1992.
91. Candido A, Rossi P, Menichella G, et al. Indicative morphological myelodysplastic alterations of bone marrow in overt AIDS. Haematologica 75:327, 1990.
92. Katsarou O, Terpos E, Patsouris E, et al. Myelodysplastic features in patients with long-term HIV infection and haemophilia. Haemophilia 7:47, 2001.
93. Abrams D, Chinn E, Lewis B. Hematologic manifestations in homosexual men with Kaposi's sarcoma. Am J Clin Pathol 81:13, 1984.
94. Sasadeusz J, Buchanan M, Speed B. Reactive haemophagocytic syndrome in human immunodeficiency virus infection. J Infect 20:65, 1990.
95. Seneviratne LS, Tulpule A, Mummaneni M, et al. Clinical, immunological and patholgic correlates of bone marrow involvment in 253 patients with AIDS-related lymphoma. Blood 92(suppl 1):244A, 1998.
96. Poropatich CO, Labriola AM, Tuazon CU. Acid-fast smear and culture of respiratory secretions, bone marrow and stools as predictors of disseminated *Mycobacterium avium* complex infection. J Microbiol 25:929, 1987.
97. Neubauer MA, Bodensteiner DC. Disseminated histoplasmosis in patients with AIDS. South Med J 85:1166, 1992.
98. Cohen RJ, Samoszul MK, Busch D, et al. Occult infections with *M. intracellulare* in bone marrow biopsy specimens from patients with AIDS. N Engl J Med 308:1475, 1983.
99. Solis OC, Belmonte AH, Ramaswamy G. Pseudo-Gaucher cells in *Mycobacterium avium intracellulare* infection in the acquired immune deficiency syndrome (AIDS). Am J Clin Pathol 85:233, 1986.
100. Maciejewski JP, Bruening EE, Donahue RE, et al. Infection of hematopoietic progenitor cells by human cytomegalovirus. Blood 80:170, 1992.
101. Flamand L, Gosselin J, Stefanescu I, et al. Immunosuppressive effect of human herpesvirus 6 on T-cell functions: suppression of interleukin-2 synthesis and cell proliferation. Blood 85:1263, 1995.
102. Carrigan DR, Knox KK. Human herpesvirus 6 (HHV-6) isolated from bone marrow: HHV-6 bone marrow suppression in bone marrow transplant patients. Blood 84:3307, 1994.
103. Sugiura K, Oyaizu N, Pahwa R. Effect of human immunodeficiency virus-1 envelope glycoprotein on in vitro hematopoiesis of umbilical cord blood. Blood 80:1463, 1992.
104. Louache F, Debili N, Marandin A, et al. Expression of CD4 by human hematopoietic progenitors. Blood 84:3344, 1994.
105. Zauli G, Furlini G, Vitale M, et al. A subset of human CD34+ hematopoietic progenitors express low levels of CD4, the high-affinity receptor for human immunodeficiency virus-type 1. Blood 84:1896, 1994.
106. Deichmann M, Kronenwett R, Haas R. Expression of the human immunodeficiency virus type-1 coreceptors CXCR-4 (fusin, LESTR) and CCR5 in CD34+ hematopoietic progenitor cells. Blood 89:3522, 1997.
107. Shen H, Cheng T, Preffer FI, et al. Intrinsic human immunodeficiency virus type 1 resistance of hematopoietic stem cells despite coreceptor expression. J Virol 73:728, 1999.
108. Bagnara G, Zauli G, Gionvannini M, et al. Early loss of circulating hematopoietic progenitor in human immunodeficiency virus I infected cells. Exp Hematol 18:426, 1990.
109. Molina JS, Scadden DT, Sakaguchi M, et al. Lack of evidence for infection of or effect on growth of hematopoietic progenitor cells after in vivo or in vitro exposure to human immunodeficiency virus. Blood 76:2476, 1990.
110. Moses AV, Williams S, Heneveld ML, et al. Human immunodeficiency virus infection of human bone marrow endothelium reduces induction of stromal hematopoietic growth factors. Blood 87:919, 1996.
111. Re MC, Zauli G, Furlini G, et al. GM-CSF production by CD4+ T-lymphocytes is selectively impaired during the course of HIV-1 infection: a possible indication of a preferential lesion of a specific subset of peripheral blood CD4+ T-lymphocytes. Microbiologica 15:265, 1992.
112. Re MC, Zauli G, Gibellini D, et al. Uninfected haematopoietic progenitor (CD34+) cells purified from the bone marrow of AIDS patients are committed to apoptotic cell death in culture. AIDS 7:1049, 1993.
113. Dubois CM, Ruscetti RW, Stankova J, et al. Transforming growth factor-beta regulates c-kit message stability and cell surface protein expression in hematopoietic progenitors. Blood 83:3138, 1994.
114. Scadden DT, Zeira M, Woon A, et al. Human immunodeficiency virus infection of human bone marrow stromal fibroblasts. Blood 76:317, 1990.
115. Maiejewski JP, Weichold FF, Young NS. HIV-1 suppression of hematopoiesis in vitro mediated by envelope glycoprotein and TNF-α. J Immunol 153:4304, 1994.
116. German MA, Zaldivar F Jr, Imfeld KL, et al. HIV-1 infection of macrophages promotes long-term survival and sustained release of interleukins 1-α and 6. AIDS Res Hum Retroviruses 10:529, 1994.
117. Zauli G, Re MC, Furlini G, et al. Human immunodeficiency virus type 1 envelope glycoprotein gp120-mediated killing of human haematopoietic progenitors (CD34+ cells). J Gen Virol 73:417, 1992.
118. Kulkosky J, Laptev A, Shetty S, et al. Human immunodeficiency virus type 1 Vpr alters bone marrow cell function. Blood 93:1906, 1999.
119. Groopman J, Feder D. Hematopoietic growth factors in AIDS. Semin Oncol 19:408, 1992
120. Williams GT, Smith CA, Spooncer E, et al. Haematopoietic colony stimulating factors promote cell survival by suppressing apoptosis. Nature 343:76, 1990.
121. Re MC, Furlini G, Zauli G, et al. Human immunodeficiency virus type 1 (HIV-1) and human hematopoietic progenitor cells. Arch Virol 1:137, 1994.
122. Hermans P, Rozenbaum W, Jou A, et al. Filgrastim (r-metG-CSF) to treat neutropenia and support myelosuppressive medication dosing in HIV infection. AIDS 10:1627, 1996.
123. Jacobson MA, Kramer F, Bassiakes Y, et al. Randomized phase I trial of two different combination foscarnet and ganciclovir chronic maintenance therapy regimens for AIDS patients with CMV retinitis: ACTG 151. J Infect Dis 170:189, 1994.
124. Dubreuil-Lemaire MK, Gori A, Vittecoq D, et al. Lenograstim for the treatment of neutropenia in patients receiving ganciclovir for cytomegalovirus infection: a randomized placebo-controlled trial in AIDS patients: GCS309 European study group. Eur J Haematol 65:337, 2000.

125. Keiser P, Rademacher S, Smith JW, et al. Granulocyte colony-stimulating factor use is associated with decreased bacteremia and increased survival in neutropenic HIV-infected patients. Am J Med 104:48, 1998.
126. Kuritzkes DR, Parenti D, Ward DJ, et al. Filgrastim prevents severe neutropenia and reduces infective morbidity in patients with advanced HIV infection: results of a randomized, multicenter, controlled trial: G-CSF 930101 study group. AIDS 12:65, 1998.
127. Kuritzkes DR. Neutropenia, neutrophil dysfunction and bacterial infection in patients with human immunodeficiency virus disease: the role of granulocyte colony-stimulating factor. Clin Infect Dis 30:256, 2000.
128. Pitrak DL, Bak P, DeMarais P, et al. Depressed neutrophil superoxide production in HIV infection. J Infect Dis 167:1406, 1993.
129. Pitrak DL. Filgrastim treatment of HIV-infected patients improves neutrophil function. AIDS 13(suppl 2):S25, 1999.
130. Keiser P, Rademacaher S, Smith J, Skiest D. G-CSF association with prolonged survival in HIV-infected patients with disseminated *Mycobacterium avium* complex infection. Int J STD AIDS 9:394, 1998.
131. Nielsen SD, Sorensen TU, Aladdin H, et al. The effect of long-term treatment with granulocyte colony-stimulating factor on hematopoiesis in HIV-infected individuals. Scand J Immunol 52:298, 2000.
132. Schooley RT, Mladenovic J, Sevin A, et al. Reduced mobilization of CD34+ stem cells in advanced human immunodeficiency virus type 1 disease. J Infect Dis 181:148, 2000.
133. Lieschke GJ, Burgess AW. Granulocyte colony-stimulating factor and granulocyte-macrophage colony-stimulating factor (first of two parts). N Engl J Med 327:28, 1992.
134. Baldwin C, Gasson J, Quan S. Granulocyte-macrophage colony-stimulating factor enhances neutrophil function in acquired immunodeficiency syndrome patients. Proc Natl Acad Sci USA 85:2763, 1988.
135. Miles SA, Mitsuyasu RT, Moreno J, et al. Combined therapy with recombinant granulocyte colony-stimulating factor and erythropoietin decreases hematologic toxicity from zidovudine. Blood 77:2109, 1991.
136. Pluda JM, Yarchoan R, Smith PH, et al. Subcutaneous recombinant granulocyte-macrophage colony-stimulating factor used as a single agent and in an alternating regimen with azidothymidine in leukopenic patients with severe human immunodeficiency virus infection. Blood 76:463, 1990.
137. Perno CF, Cooney DA, Gao W-Y, et al. Effects of bone marrow stimulatory cytokines on human immunodeficiency virus replication and the antiviral activity of dideoxynucleosides in cultures of monocyte/macrophages. Blood 80:995, 1992.
138. Hammer SM, Gillis JM, Pinkston P, et al. Effect of zidovudine and granulocyte-macrophage colony-stimulating factor on human immunodeficiency virus replication in alveolar macrophages. Blood 75:1215, 1990.
139. Koyanagi Y, O'Brien WA, Zhao JQ, et al. Cytokines alter production of HIV-1 from primary mononuclear phagocytes. Science 241:1673, 1988.
140. Skowron G, Stein D, Drusano G, et al. The safety and efficacy of granulocyte-macrophage colony-stimulating factor (sargramostim) added to indinavir- or ritonavir-based antiretroviral therapy: a randomized double-blind, placebo controlled trial. J Infect Dis 180:1064, 1999.
141. Spivak J, Barnes DC, Fuchs E, et al. Serum immunoreactive erythropoietin in HIV-infected patients. JAMA 261:3104, 1989.
142. Fischl M, Galpin JE, Levine JD, et al. Recombinant human erythropoietin for patients with AIDS treated with zidovudine. N Engl J Med 322:1488, 1990.
143. Erslev A. Erythropoietin. N Engl J Med 324:1339, 1991.
144. Henry D, Beall G, Benson C. Recombinant human erythropoietin in the therapy of anemia associated with HIV infection and zidovudine therapy: overview of four clinical trials. Ann Intern Med 117:739, 1992.
145. Abrams DI, Steinhart C, Frascino R. Epoetin alfa therapy for anemia in HIV-infected patients: impact on quality of life. Int J STD AIDS 11:659, 2000.
146. Volberding P. Consensus statement: anemia in HIV infection—current trends, treatment options, and practice strategies: anemia in HIV working group. Clin Ther 22:1004, 2000.
147. Brunson ME, Alexander JW. Mechanisms of transfusion-induced immunosuppression. Transfusion 30:651, 1990.
148. Vamvakas E, Kaplan HS. Early transfusion and length of survival in acquired immune deficiency syndrome: experience with a population receiving medical care at a public hospital. Transfusion 33:111, 1993.
149. Mudido PM, Georges D, Dorazio D, et al. Human immunodeficiency virus type 1 activation after blood transfusion. Transfusion 36:860, 1996.
150. Collier AC, Kalish LA, Busch MP, et al. Leukocyte-reduced red blood cell transfusion in patients with anemia and human immunodeficiency virus infection: the Viral Activation Transfusion Study: a randomized controlled trial. JAMA 285:1592, 2001.
151. Cohen AJ, Phillips TM, Kessler CM. Circulating coagulation inhibitors in the acquired immunodeficiency syndrome. Ann Intern Med 104:175, 1986.
152. Gold JE, Haubenstock A, Zalusky R. Lupus anticoagulant and AIDS. N Engl J Med 314:1252, 1986.
153. Bloom EJ, Abrams DI, Rodgers GM. Lupus anticoagulant in the acquired immunodeficiency syndrome. JAMA 256:491, 1986.
154. Cohen AJ, Philips TM, Kessler CM. Circulating coagulant inhibitors in the acquired immunodeficiency syndrome. Ann Intern Med 104:175, 1986.
155. Cohen H, Mackie IJ, Anagnostopoulos N, et al. Lupus anticoagulant, anticardiolipin antibodies, and human immunodeficiency virus in haemophilia. J Clin Pathol 42:629, 1989.
156. Cappell MS, Simon T, Tiku M. Splenic infarction associated with anticardiolipin antibodies in a patient with acquired immunodeficiency syndrome. Dig Dis Sci 38:1152, 1993.
157. Roubey RAS. Autoantibodies to phospholipid-binding plasma proteins: a new view of lupus anticoagulants and other "antiphospholipid" autoantibodies. Blood 84:2854, 1994.
158. Sullivan PS, Dworkin MS, Jones JF, Hooper WC. Epidemiology of thrombosis in HIV-infected individuals. AIDS 14:321, 2000.
159. Stahl CP, Sideman CS, Spira TJ, et al. Protein S deficiency in men with long-term human immunodeficiency virus infection. Blood 81:1801, 1993.
160. Lafeuillade A, Sorice M, Griggi T, et al. Role of autoimmunity in protein S deficiency during HIV-1 infection. Infection 22:201, 1994.
161. Nair J, Bellevue R, Bertoni M, et al. Thrombotic thrombocytopenic purpura in patients with the acquired imunodeficiency syndrome-related complex. Ann Intern Med 109:209, 1988.

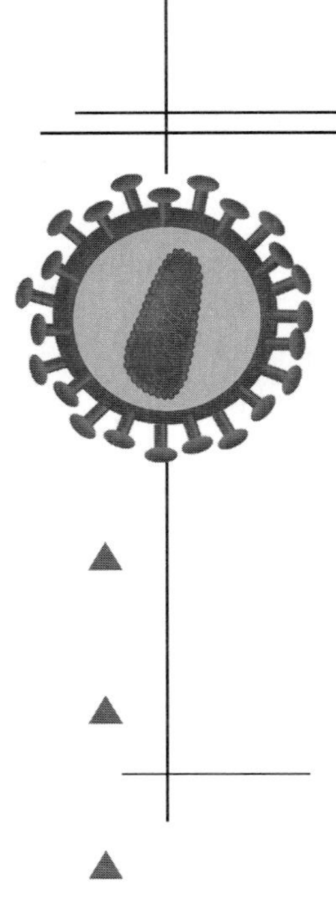

CHAPTER 59

Cardiac Disease

Stacy D. Fisher, MD
Steven E. Lipshultz, MD

Cardiovascular abnormalities are becoming more common in human immunodeficiency virus (HIV)-infected individuals as life expectancy increases with highly active antiretroviral therapy (HAART). Clinicians need to be aware of cardiac diseases that are directly related to HIV infection and its sequelae (Table 59–1) as well as those caused by atherosclerosis, immunopathologic processes, or drug toxicities.[1–6]

LEFT VENTRICULAR DYSFUNCTION

One prospective study of asymptomatic HIV-infected adults with initial CD4+ T-lymphocyte counts higher than 400 cells/ml found that 76 of 952 patients (8%) already had or developed significant left ventricular dysfunction over 60 months of observation.[7] Almost all had a CD+ T-lymphocyte count of less than 400 cells/ml at the time their cardiomyopathy was diagnosed. Cardiac complications of HIV infection ranged from subclinical electrocardiographic (ECG) changes to cardiomyopathy and sudden death.

Left ventricular dysfunction is also a common consequence of HIV infection in children. In a study of 205 vertically HIV-infected children enrolled at a median age of 22 months and followed with echocardiography every 4 to 6 months and by ECG, Holter monitoring, and chest radiograph every year, the prevalence of decreased left ventricular function was 5.7%. The 2-year cumulative incidence was 15.3%.[1] The cumulative incidence of symptomatic congestive heart failure or the use of cardiac medications (or both) was 10% over 2 years.[1] A variety of potential etiologies have been postulated for HIV-related cardiomyopathy (Table 59–1).

Myocarditis

Myocarditis is perhaps the best studied of the possible causes of cardiac abnormalities. Dilated cardiomyopathy may be related to a direct action of HIV on the myocardial tissue or to an autoimmune process induced by HIV itself or by HIV in conjunction with co-infecting viruses.[2] Right ventricular biopsy performed on 76 patients within 1 month of the diagnosis of cardiomyopathy revealed 63 patients with histopathologic evidence of myocarditis, of whom 36 had active myocarditis, and 58 patients had HIV nucleic acid sequences detected in cardiac myocytes.[2] In the 36 patients with active myocarditis, 9 had coexisting viral infections [coxsackievirus group B ($n = 6$), cytomegalovirus ($n = 2$), or Epstein-Barr virus ($n = 1$)].[2] Other biopsy studies have also implicated the above co-infecting viruses and *Toxoplasma gondii* or adenovirus.[8]

Autopsy and biopsy results have revealed scant and patchy inflammatory cell infiltrates in the myocardium.[7] HIV virions appear to infect myocardiocytes in patchy distributions. The infected cells are not surrounded by an inflammatory response, and no clear association has been made between the infection and cardiac myocyte dysfunction. Endocardial biopsy has infrequently revealed a treatable cause of myocarditis but on occasion may be clinically helpful by revealing lymphocytic infiltrates suggesting myocarditis or opportunistic infections (by special stains), which can lead to aggressive therapy of an underlying pathogen.[7–9] Notably, HIV-related cardiomyopathy is often not associated with any specific opportunistic infection, and approximately 40% of patients have not experienced any opportunistic infection before the onset of cardiac symptoms.[9]

▲ **Table 59–1.** HIV-ASSOCIATED CARDIOVASCULAR ABNORMALITIES

Abnormality	Frequency	Possible Etiologies and Associations
Dilated cardiomyopathy	Estimated 15.9 patients/1000 asymptomatic HIV-infected persons[1]	Infectious HIV, *Toxoplasma gondii,* coxsackievirus group B, Epstein-Barr virus, CMV, adenovirus infections Autoimmune response to infection Drug-related Cocaine, possibly nucleoside analogues, IL-2, doxorubicin, interferon Metabolic/endocrine Nutritional deficiency/wasting selenium, vitamin B_{12}, carnitine, thyroid hormone, growth hormone, adrenal insufficiency Hyperinsulinemia Hypothermia Hyperthermia Autonomic insufficiency Encephalopathy
Pericardial effusion	11%/year[25] Spontaneous resolution in up to 42% of affected patients[14,25]	Idiopathic Infectious Viral (HIV, enteroviruses, CMV, HSV) Bacterial (pyogenic, mycobacteria) Fungal (*Cryptococcus, Histoplasma*) *Toxoplasma* Malignancy (lymphoma, KS) Malnutrition Hypothyroidism
Isolated right ventricular and pulmonary disease		Recurrent bronchopulmonary infections, pulmonary arteritis, microvascular pulmonary emboli due to thrombus or drug injection
Primary pulmonary hypertension	0.5% Incidence[30,31]	Plexogenic pulmonary arteriopathy Mediator release from endothelium
Nonbacterial thrombotic endocarditis (generally tricuspid valve)	Rare	Underlying valvular endothelial damage, vitamin C deficiency, valvular injury secondary to catheters or injected impurities (intravenous drug use), disseminated intravascular coagulation, hypercoagulable state, malnutrition, wasting, prolonged acquired immunodeficiency
Malignancy	1% Incidence (3/440)	KS Non-Hodgkin lymphoma Leiomyosarcoma
Vasculitis	Case reports	Systemic necrotizing vasculitis Hypersensitivity Schönlein-Henoch purpura Lymphomatoid granulomatosis Primary CNS angiitis
Accelerated atherosclerosis, coronary artery disease, cerebrovascular disease	Up to 8% prevalence by autopsy and case reports	Protease inhibitor therapy, atherogenesis by virus-infected macrophages, chronic inflammation
Arrhythmias		Drug therapy interactions Autonomic dysfunction

CMV, cytomegalovirus; HSV, herpes simplex virus; IL-2, interleukin-2; KS, Kaposi sarcoma.

Nutritional Deficiencies

Nutritional deficiencies are common with HIV infection, particularly late-stage disease. Poor absorption and diarrhea both lead to electrolyte imbalances and deficiencies in elemental nutrients. Deficiencies of trace elements have occasionally been associated directly or indirectly with cardiomyopathy.[10] For example, selenium deficiency increases the virulence of coxsackie virus to cardiac tissue.[11] Selenium replacement reverses cardiomyopathy and restores left ventricular function in nutritionally depleted patients.[11,12] Levels of vitamin B_{12}, carnitine, growth hormone, and thyroid hormone may also be altered in HIV disease; all have been associated with left ventricular dysfunction.

Course of Disease/Prognosis

Cardiomyopathy that is HIV-related has a grave prognosis, even when compared to idiopathic cardiomyopathy.[9,13,14] The median survival of patients with HIV-associated cardiomyopathy was 11 months compared to 19 months for patients with idiopathic dilated cardiomyopathy.[13,15]

Mortality in HIV-infected patients with cardiomyopathy is increased independently of CD4+ T-lymphocyte count, age, gender, and risk group. The median survival to acquired immunodeficiency syndrome (AIDS)-related death was 101 days in patients with left ventricular dysfunction and 472 days in patients with a normal heart, at similar infection stages.[2] Isolated right ventricular dysfunction or borderline left ventricular dysfunction did not place patients at risk for death.

In the multicenter Pulmonary and Cardiac Complications of HIV study (P^2C^2 HIV), children with vertically transmitted HIV infection (median age 2.1 years), had a 5-year cumulative survival of 64%.[16] Mortality was higher in children with baseline depressed left ventricular fractional shortening or increased left ventricular dimension, thickness, mass, wall stress, heart rate, or blood pressure.[14,16]

Rapid-onset congestive heart failure has a grim prognosis in HIV-infected adults and children, and more than half of such patients die from primary cardiac failure within 6 to 12 months of presentation.[9,14] Chronic-onset heart failure may respond better to medical therapy in this patient population.[9]

Therapy

Therapy for dilated cardiomyopathy associated with HIV infection is generally similar to therapy for nonischemic cardiomyopathy. It includes diuretics, digoxin, and angiotension-converting enzyme (ACE) inhibitors.

Intravenous immunoglobulins have been used with some success for treating acute congestive cardiomyopathy and nonspecific myocarditis in patients without HIV infection.[17] Immunoglobulin therapy is beneficial in Kawasaki disease, an immunologically mediated illness with cardiac dysfunction resembling that seen with HIV disease.[18,19]

Immunoglobulin therapy has been shown in murine models to suppress myocarditis induced by coxsackievirus B3[20–22] and encephalomyocarditis virus (not infectious to humans)[23] at least in part by neutralizing the virus itself. Monthly immunoglobulin infusions in HIV-infected pediatric patients have been associated with minimized left ventricular dysfunction, an increase in left ventricular wall thickness, and a reduction in peak left ventricular wall stress, suggesting that both impaired myocardial growth and left ventricular dysfunction may be immunologically mediated (Fig. 59–1).[23]

The apparent efficacy of immunoglobulin therapy may be the result of immunoglobulins inhibiting cardiac autoantibodies by competing for Fc receptors or dampening the secretion or effects of cytokines and cellular growth factors. Immunomodulatory therapy may be helpful in HIV-infected adults and children with declining left ventricular function, but definitive studies of the efficacy of this approach have not been carried out.

Opportunistic or other infections should be sought and treated aggressively in HIV-infected patients with cardiomyopathy. Patients should be evaluated for nutritional status, and any with deficiencies should receive supplements. Supplementation with selenium, carnitine, multivitamins, or all three may be helpful, especially in anorexic patients or those with wasting or diarrheal syndromes.

Animal Models

Chronic pathogenic simian immunodeficiency virus (SIV) infection in rhesus macaques has resulted in depressed left ventricular systolic function and extensive coronary arteriopathy suggestive of injury due to cell-mediated immune response.[24] Two-thirds of chronically infected macaques that died of SIV had related myocardial effects. Coronary arteriopathy was extensive, with evidence of vessel occlusion and recanalization, as well as related regions of myocardial necrosis. At necropsy two of nine animals had marantic endocarditis, and one had a left ventricular mural thrombus. Macaques with cardiac pathology were emaciated to a greater extent than macaques with SIV and similar periods of infection that did not experience cardiac pathology.[24]

▲ CARDIOVASCULAR LABORATORY TESTING

Routine physical examination alone is unreliable for the diagnosis and follow-up of cardiovascular illness; therefore judicious use of the cardiovascular laboratory is warranted (Fig. 59–2). Echocardiography may be particularly useful for following HIV-infected patients with cardiovascular problems.[25–33] Echocardiography has been especially helpful for identifying left ventricular systolic dysfunction and inappropriately increased left ventricular hypertrophy.[6,14] In previous multivariate analyses the development of either of these abnormalities in an HIV-infected infant or child is an

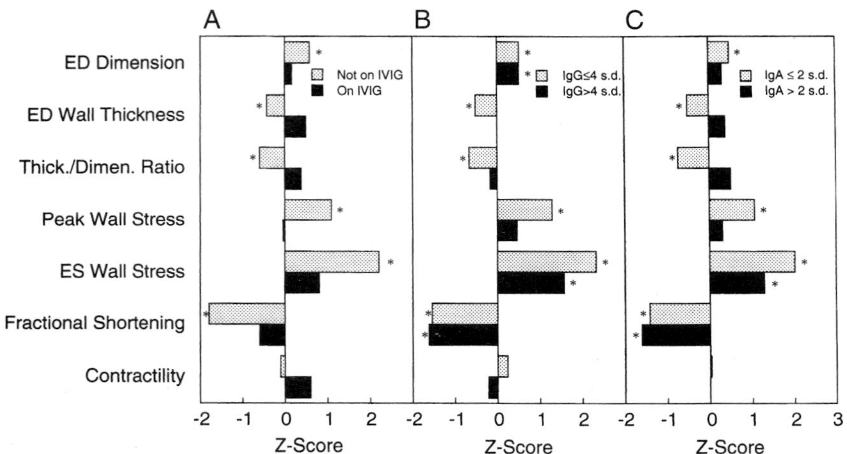

Figure 59–1. Monthly intravenous immunoglobulin (IVIG) therapy is associated with more normal left ventricular structure and function in HIV-infected patients without congestive heart failure.[23] Echocardiographic measurements of left ventricular structure and function in HIV-infected patients without heart failure who received monthly IVIG therapy (black bars) and who did not not receive IVIG therapy (shaded bars). Z-scores indicate number of standard deviations above or below normal (z-score = 0) for each parameter. Asterisks indicate that the parameter was significantly different from normal. Dimen., left ventricular dimension; ED, end-diastolic; ES, end-systolic; Thick., left ventricular thickness. (From Lipshultz SE, Orav EJ, Sanders SP, Colan SD. Immunoglobulins and left ventricular structure and function in pediatric HIV infection. Circulation 92: 2220, 1995, with permission.)

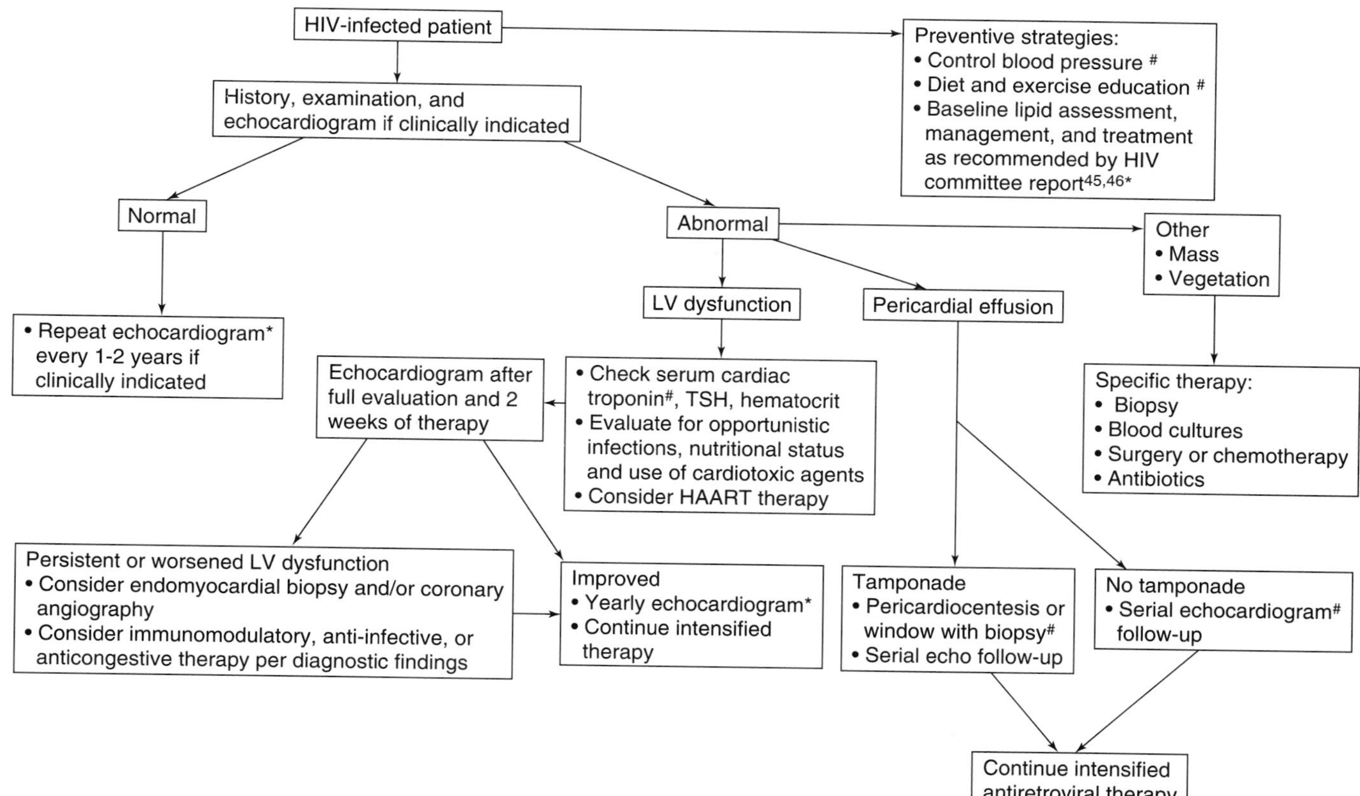

Figure 59–2. Screening and treatment strategies for cardiac dysfunction in HIV infection. Cardiac dysfunction is common in this population and predicts all-cause mortality. Echocardiography should be used during the initial evaluation. *Evidence-based. #Non-HIV standard of care data. HAART, highly active antiretroviral therapy; LV, left ventricular; TSH, thyroid-stimulating hormone.

independent predictor of all-cause mortality, even when wasting, encephalopathy, CD4+ T-lymphocyte count, HIV viral load, and other risk factors are taken into account.[16] Left ventricular diastolic dysfunction is common in HIV-infected children, but the clinical significance of this dysfunction in these patients is not entirely clear.

Conditions detectable by ECG are common among HIV-infected patients, and such studies may be helpful in high risk patients. Abnormalities of intraventricular conduction and rhythm appear to be more common in HIV-infected individuals than the general population.[6] Autonomic dysfunction is also common in this population (Fig. 59–3),[34] and sinus tachycardia is frequently found in HIV-infected patients. In addition, many medications given to HIV-infected patients may result in QT prolongation; and ECG algorithms addressing the baseline QTc interval and change in the QTc interval with medications have been proposed to reduce the risk of developing pentamidine-associated torsades de pointes.[35,36] Medications with QT-prolonging effects are reported and updated regularly on the internet (www.torsades.org).

Electrocardiographic or Holter monitoring of HIV-infected patients may be useful for HIV-infected patients with palpitations, syncope, near-syncope, unexplained stroke, or known autonomic dysfunction. It is also useful for those who are starting or receiving medications known to be arrhythmogenic or to affect repolarization (Table 59–2).

Exercise stress testing may be helpful in selected HIV-infected patients, and indications for the performance of such tests are similar to those in HIV-uninfected patients. Premature atherosclerosis has been described in HIV-infected patients, particularly those receiving HAART therapy (see Chapter 62), and stress testing may be helpful for assessing chest pain and diagnosing ischemia in those determined to be at increased risk clinically. Indium-111 anti-myosin antibody scanning may be useful for detecting myocarditis in HIV-infected patients and for distinguishing acute coronary syndromes from myocarditis in patients with clinical symptoms.[35]

For HIV-infected patients with congestive heart failure of unclear etiology that has not responded to 2 weeks of anticongestive therapy, cardiac catheterization with endomyocardial biopsy may provide useful information.[36–38] The finding of cytomegalovirus (CMV) inclusions or other histologic evidence of infection may help direct therapy. The presence of abnormal mitochondria suggests the need for a drug holiday from antiretroviral therapy. The presence of active inflammation suggests the need to consider immunomodulatory therapy.[39] Positive results on a viral polymerase chain reaction (PCR) suggests myocardial infections not apparent histologically.[39]

▲ PERICARDIAL DISEASE

Pericardiocentesis in an HIV-infected patient with a pericardial effusion leads to a diagnosis in up to 50% of cases, particularly if the effusion is large; and it may therefore be

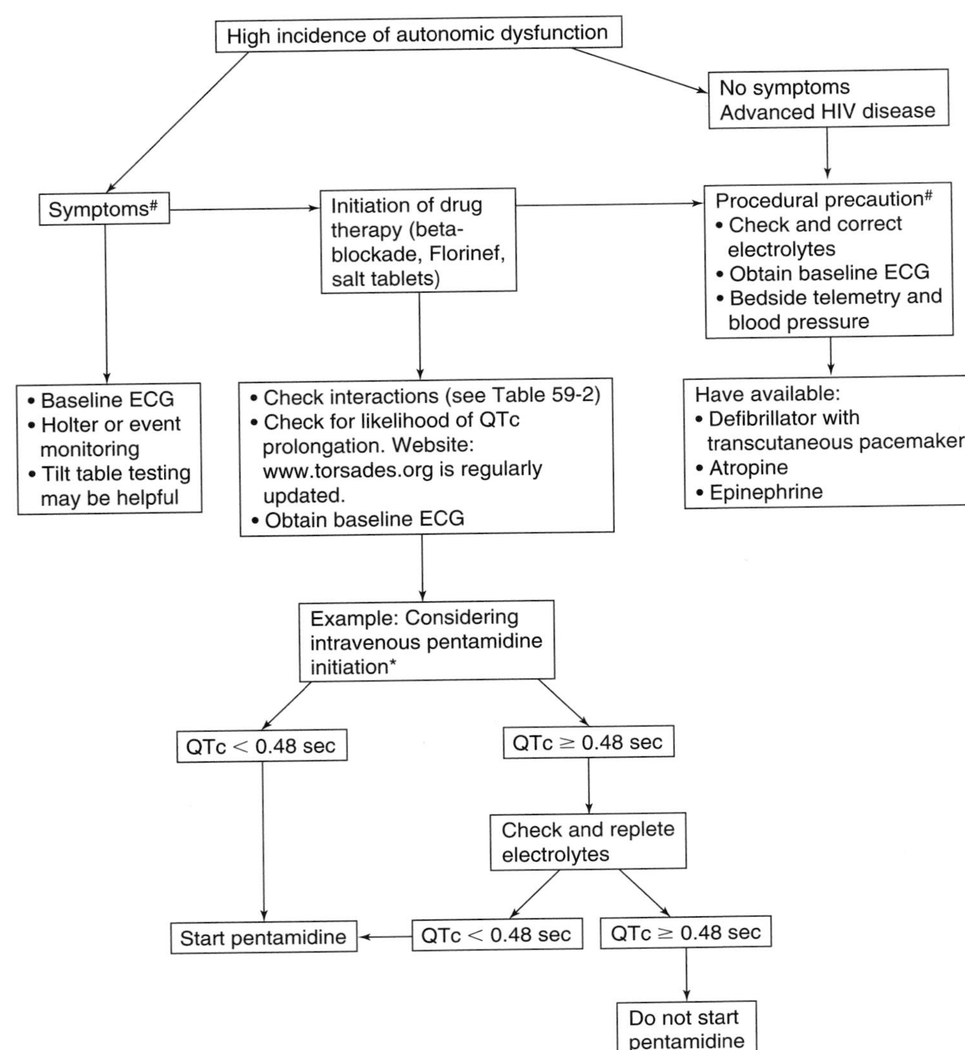

Figure 59–3. Diagnostic and treatment strategies for autonomic dysfunction. Because autonomic dysfunction is so common with HIV disease, precautions should be considered when initiating drug therapy associated with cardiac abnormalities, including conscious sedation or anesthesia. ECG, electrocardiogram.

useful diagnostically as well as therapeutically.[25,26] Patients with pericardial effusion without tamponade should be evaluated for treatable opportunistic infections (e.g., tuberculosis) and malignancy. HAART should be initiated if antiretroviral therapy has not yet begun. Repeat echocardiography is recommended after 1 month or sooner if clinically indicated.

▲ MYOCARDIAL INJURY AND INFLAMMATION

Serum cardiac troponin T (cTnT), a biomarker of active myocardial injury, may help identify myocarditis, unstable angina, or acute myocardial infarction.[40,41] This can then lead to additional tests for myocarditis,[4] such as endomyocardial biopsy including viral PCR studies for suspected myocarditis, exercise stress tests, and angiographic studies for suspected acute coronary syndromes. In non-HIV-infected patients, the assessment of brain natriuretic peptides (BNPs) in the blood is becoming useful for detecting being at high risk for morbidity or mortality from left ventricular dysfunction.[42–44] Assays for NP and N terminal pro-BNP (NT-proBNP) should be considered in HIV patients to assess the severity of damage during congestive heart failure.

Elevations of markers of inflammation have been shown to be predictive of increased subsequent coronary events in non-HIV-infected patients. Inflammation has emerged as an important factor contributing to the formation of atherosclerotic plaques, and this mechanism may have an even greater role in HIV disease.[45] Markers of inflammation have not been formally studied in HIV-infected patients. Potential biochemical surrogates, such as highly sensitive C-reactive protein (hsCRP),[45–50] serum amyloid A, and fibrinogen do not have a clear predictive role in HIV-related heart disease at this time.

▲ LIPID DISORDERS

Long-term therapy with protease inhibitors and HAART, although effective in prolonging life and disease-free survival, can be associated with dyslipidemia and premature

▲ **Table 59–2.** CARDIOVASCULAR ACTIONS/INTERACTIONS OF DRUGS COMMONLY USED FOR HIV THERAPY

Class	Cardiac Drug Interactions	Cardiac Side Effects
Antiretroviral Agents		Rare: lacticacidosis hypotension
Nucleoside reverse transcriptase inhibitors	Zidovudine and dipyridamole	Zidovudine: skeletal muscle myopathy, ?myocarditis, dilated cardiomyopathy Zalcitabine: short-term free radical cardiotoxicity
Nonnucleoside reverse transcriptase inhibitors	Calcium channel blockers, warfarin, β-blockers, nifedipine, quinidine, steroids, theophylline Delavirdine can cause serious toxic effects if given with antiarrhythmia drugs and calcium channel blockers	Delavirdine and vasocontrictors can cause ischemia
Protease inhibitors (PIs)	Metabolized by cytochrome P_{450} and interact with: antimycobacterials, antifungals, macrolide and quinolone antibacterials, antihistamines, psychotropic drugs, antiarrhythmics, cisapride, statins, antiepileptics, antineoplastic alkaloids to produce cardiotoxic effects including QT prolongation and torsades de pointes. Sildenafil, amiodarone, lidocaine, quinidine, warfarin (increased levels), 3-hydroxy-3-methylglutaryl coenzyme A (HMG CoA) reductase inhibitors: lovastatin and simvastatin). Bepridil and PIs should be avoided. Potentially dangerous interactions that require close monitoring or dose adjustment can occur between PIs and amiodarone, disopyramide, flecainide, lignocaine, mexiletine, propafenone, and quinidine. Co-administration of PIs with astemizole, terfenadine or cisapride is contraindicated to owing to life-threatening arrhythmias. Many antipsychotic, antidepressant, and anticonvulsant drugs interact with PIs. Some of these interactions are clinically relevant and contraindicate concomitant use or require dose adjustment. Ritonavir is most potent cytochrome activity (CYP3A) inhibitor and is most likely to interact. Indinavir, amprenavir, and nelfinavir are moderate. Saquinavir has the lowest probability. Some: calcium channel blockers, prednisone, quinine, β-blockers (1.5- to 3.0-fold increase). Decreases theophylline concentrations	Implicated in premature atherosclerosis, dyslipidemia, insulin resistance, diabetes mellitus, fat wasting, redistribution
Antiinfective Agents		
Antibiotics	Rifampin: reduces digoxin therapeutic effect by induction of intestinal P-glycoprotein Erythromycin: cytochrome P_{450} metabolism and drug interactions Trimethoprim-sulfamethoxazole (Bactrim) increases warfarin effects	Erythromycin: orthostatic hypotension, ventricular tachycardia, bradycardia, torsades (with drug interactions) Clarithromycin: QT prolongation and torsades de pointes Trimethoprim/sulfamethoxazole: orthostatic hypotension, anaphylaxis, QT prolongation, torsades de pointes, hypokalemia Sparfloxacin (fluoroquinolones): QT prolongation
Antifungal agents	Amphotericin B: digoxin toxicity Ketoconazole or itraconazole: cytochrome P_{450} metabolism and drug interactions: increased levels of sildenafil, warfarin, HMG CoA reductase inhibitors, nifedipine, digoxin	Amphotericin B: hypertension, arrhythmia, renal failure, hypokalemia, thrombophlebitis, bradycardia, angioedema, dilated cardiomyopathy. Liposomal formulations still have the potential for electrolyte imbalance and QT prolongation Ketoconazole, fluconazole, itraconazole: QT prolongation and torsades de pointes
Antiviral agents	Ganciclovir, zidovudine	Foscarnet: reversible cardiac failure, electrolyte abnormalities Ganciclovir: ventricular tachycardia, hypotension
Antiparasitic agents		Pentamidine: hypotension, QT prolongation, arrhythmias (torsades de pointes), ventricular tachycardia, hyperglycemia, hypoglycemia, sudden death. These effects are enhanced by hypomagnesemia and hypokalemia

Table continued on following page

▲ **Table 59–2.** CARDIOVASCULAR ACTIONS/INTERACTIONS OF DRUGS COMMONLY USED FOR HIV THERAPY *Continued*

Class	Cardiac Drug Interactions	Cardiac Side Effects
Chemotherapy Agents	Vincristine, doxorubicin: decrease digoxin level	Vincristine: arrhythmia, myocardial infarction, cardiomyopathy, cardiac autonomic neuropathy Recombinant human interferon-α: hypertension, hypotension, tachycardia, ischemic heart disease, acute coronary events including myocardial infarction, dilated cardiomyopathy, ventricular and supraventricular arrhythmias, sudden death, atrioventricular block, periperal vasodilation, increased cardiac work load. Contraindicated in patients with unstable angina or myocardial infarction Interleukin-2: hypotension, arrhythmia, sudden death, myocardial infarction, dilated cardiomyopathy, cardiac failure, myocardial stunning, capillary leak, thyroid alterations Anthracyclines (doxorubicin, daunorubicin, mitoxantrone): myocarditis, cardiomyopathy, cardiac failure Liposomal anthracyclines: as above for doxorubicin but also vasculitis
Other Agents		
Systemic corticosteroids	Corticosteroids: decrease salicylate levels and increase gastric ulceration in combination with salicylates	Ventricular hypertrophy, cardiomyopathy, hyperglycemia
Pentoxifylline		Decreased triglyceride levels, arrhythmias, chest pain
Growth hormone		Ventricular hypertrophy, activation of the renal angiotension system (hypertension)
Megace		Edema, thrombophlebitis, hyperglycemia
Epoetin alfa (erythropoietin)		Hypertension, ventricular dysfunction, thrombotic events including myocardial infarction
Antihistamines (terfenadine, astemizole)		QT prolongation, torsades de pointes, sudden death
Cisapride		Torsades de pointes
Tricyclic antidepressants (amitriptyline, doxepine, desipramine, imipramine, clomipramine)		QT prolongation in all. Sudden death with desipramine, clomipramine, and imipramine
Antipsychotic agents (butyrophenone and phenotiazine classes including thioridazine, chlorpromazine, pimozide, sertindole, haloperidol)		QT prolongation and torsades de pointes

atherosclerosis. The mechanism of HAART-associated premature atherosclerosis is unclear, as is its incidence and severity.[51] A fasting blood glucose level and lipid profile should be obtained before and at approximately 3-month intervals during HAART therapy. Low density lipoprotein (LDL) cholesterol is currently the primary therapeutic target for cardiovascular disease, but other lipoproteins [high density lipoprotein (HDL), apolipoprotein B, and lipoprotein(a)] may also be useful for stratifying non-HIV-infected patients by risk for cardiovascular disease.[52]

As with any patient, long-term cardiovascular risk factors should be addressed in HIV-infected patients.[53] These risk factors include a history of tobacco use, a family history of premature atherosclerosis, poor diet, high alcohol intake, lack of physical exercise, older age, diabetes, dyslipidemia, hypertriglyceridemia, hypertension, menopausal status, cocaine use, and heroin use. Other important risk factors are a family or patient history of hypothyroidism, renal disease, liver disease, or hypogonadism in the patient or the family.

▲ HYPERTENSION

Routine assessment of blood pressure in HIV-infected patients may be particularly important because these patients seem to be at higher risk to develop hypertension and may develop hypertension at a younger age than the general population.[54] Predisposing conditions include vasculitis, acquired glucocorticoid resistance, acute and chronic renal failure, atherosclerosis, and drug interactions (e.g., the interaction between indinavir and stavudine-phenylpropanolamine).[54,55] The true prevalence of hypertension in HIV-infected patients is unknown. Echocardiography is useful for assessing increased left ventricular mass in patients with systemic hypertension or right ventricular pressure in a patient with suspected pulmonary hypertension.

▲ HEART FAILURE

Nonpharmacologic treatments for heart failure, including exercise, should be emphasized. Multidisciplinary care addressing nutrition, patient counseling, and patient education reduces hospital admissions for heart failure, may improve quality of life and enhances patient knowledge.[56] However, other data suggest that multidisciplinary follow-up increases readmission rates.[56]

Prescribed exercise training improves functional capacity and quality of life and reduces the rate of adverse cardiac events.[57–60] Patients should start slowly and gradually work to a goal of 20 to 30 minutes at least three times weekly for cardiovascular conditioning. Low-intensity training such as walking around the block is beneficial both physiologically and in terms of quality of life. A stress test can establish the patient's baseline and may provide confidence that the exercise can proceed safely. People with systolic dysfunction can undergo exercise training safely without exacerbation of arrhythmia and other problems. American Heart Association endorsement of exercise for these patients is expected.

Pharmacotherapy for heart failure improves survival, but patients continue to deteriorate over time. Not every drug that helps initially is necessarily a good long-term treatment. Five agents that are components of standard polypharmacy therapy for heart failure are digoxin, loop diuretics, ACE inhibitors, aldosterone antagonists, and β-blockers. A detailed discussion of individual agents is beyond the scope of this chapter, and the reader is referred to excellent reviews of this subject.[61–85] There is no evidence that using ACE inhibitors to treat heart failure due to AIDS is beneficial, but the universal benefit of these agents in most other forms of heart failure is well demonstrated. HIV-infected patients with nephropathy should receive extra care when treated with ACE inhibitor therapy, as deterioration of renal function and hyperkalemia are known side effects that may require cessation of therapy.

▲ PRIMARY PREVENTION OF CORONARY HEART DISEASE

Aggressive modification of risk factors is recommended for patients without HIV infection who are at high risk of developing coronary heart disease (CHD).[86] Evidence that such measures are effective in HIV-infected patients is generally lacking, and the application of these measures may pose particular problems in such patients. In this section, we list recommendations for primary prevention in patients without HIV infection. Clinicians must determine the relative benefits and risks of specific recommendations on an individual basis in HIV-infected patients.

Exercise

Moderate to strenuous physical activity reduces the risk of CHD and stroke.[86–102] Sudden death after strenuous exercise is rare, is more common in sedentary people, and does not outweigh the benefits of exercise. Regular exercise programs decrease the rates of cardiovascular disease,[103] decrease the frequency of osteoporosis in women,[104] improve the functioning of those with rheumatoid arthritis,[105] and lower the risk of diabetes.[106]

The effects of exercise on the immune system vary with its intensity. Moderate activity apparently stimulates the immune system, but strenuous activity suppresses natural killer (NK) cell function, lymphocyte proliferation, immunoglobulin production, and cytokine cascade activation.[107–109] Prolonged strenuous exercise, such as long-distance running, causes leukocytosis, with an increase in neutrophils and depression of lymphocytes that can persist for up to 6 hours.[110] In many clinical conditions, the biologic effect of exercise on the immune system is unclear, but it appears to be safe in controlled training situations.[111] Exercise should be intense enough and should last long enough to provide benefits for the heart, lungs, and skeletal muscle but must not be so strenuous as to induce injury.

Chronic illness, such as HIV infection, is likely to result in decreased physical activity, poor muscle strength, decreased aerobic capacity, and overall deconditioning. Pulmonary function studies of adults with HIV infection have shown a lower workload, lower anaerobic threshold, and decreased oxygen utilization compared to an age-matched control group.[112] These conditions appear to be reversible; oxygen utilization improves with aerobic training in HIV-infected adults.[113] A retrospective study of self-reported exercise patterns in 415 adults with HIV and controls suggested that exercise three or four times per week had a significant protective effect on HIV disease progression.[114] Studies of progressive resistance and aerobic training in HIV-infected adults have been limited, but current data show that exercise helps patients gain lean weight.[115,116] Furthermore, controlled training programs in HIV-infected patients have not produced decreases in CD4+ T-lymphocyte counts or increased cytokine activation.[117–119] Strength-resistance training can decrease truncal adiposity, which is part of the fat redistribution syndrome that develops in many HAART-treated patients. In a small pilot study of 10 men, 16 weeks of resistance training significantly improved strength and decreased fat mass, particularly in the trunk.[120]

Encouraging lifelong physical activity programs appears to be even more important as HIV infection becomes a chronic disease. Because HAART may predispose patients to the chronic problems of abnormal lipid metabolism, fat redistribution, insulin resistance, and premature cardiovascular disease, it is important to determine if exercise programs that benefit people without HIV infection are practical and effective in patients with HIV. Because of the strong association between smoking and overall mortality and ischemic vascular disease,[121–125] smoking cessation should also be encouraged. Control of hypertension is an important part of cardiovascular risk reduction in HIV-infected patients.[126–133]

Standard treatment based on guidelines from the Joint National Commission (JNC) should be followed in HIV-infected patients with hypertension, as there are no specific subpopulation studies at this time.

Lowering Cholesterol

Lipid abnormalities in HIV-infected patients predate HAART therapy and have included increased serum triglyceride and cholesterol levels.[51,134–142] HIV infection is associated with low high density lipoprotein cholesterol (HDL-C) and low density lipoprotein cholesterol (LDL-C), lower triglyceride clearance, increased lipoprotein(a), and higher LDL-B phenotype (small, dense LDL-C). Zidovudine therapy has been reported to lower serum triglyceride levels. Protease inhibitors and nonnucleoside reverse transcriptase inhibitors are both associated with increased serum triglyceride and cholesterol levels. In one study, HAART therapy was associated with 47% of patients having serum cholesterol levels in the elevated but treatable range. The chronic abnormalities in lipids and other cardiovascular risk factors associated with HAART may mean that the therapy is linked to premature cardiovascular events, but definitive studies are lacking.

Because pharmacologic treatment to reduce cholesterol in HIV-infected patients is complicated by drug interactions, nondrug therapies such as modification of CHD risk factors should be emphasized.[51] The 1994 National Cholesterol Education Program (NCEP) guidelines were recommended as a starting point for HIV-infected patients.[51] More recent NCEP guidelines have been established and should also be considered (www.nhlbi.nih.gov and *JAMA* 285:2486, 2001). The new guidelines place increased emphasis on therapy for "metabolic syndrome" (i.e., obesity, physical inactivity, high blood pressure, high triglycerides, high blood sugar, high concentrations of LDL-C, low concentrations of HDL-C, insulin resistance, diabetes). The "metabolic syndrome" is as strong a contributor to early heart disease as cigarette smoking and should be treated with intensive lifestyle changes including weight control, physical activity, and medication. The Guidelines define optimal HDL-C as more than 40 mg dl and optimal LDL-C less than 100 mg/dl.

The combined use of a cholesterol-lowering diet and lipid-lowering drugs reduces the cholesterol concentration more than lifestyle interventions alone. In the HIV-infected population, a bile acid sequestrant may have fewer side effects than 3-hydroxy-3-methylglutaryl coenzyme A (HMG CoA) reductase inhibitors because it is less likely to cause drug interactions. However, cholestyramine and colestipol may be associated with increased triglyceride levels, and their effect on antiviral drug absorption has not been studied. Colesevelam lowers plasma LDL cholesterol and has an additive effect when taken with a statin.[142] It has fewer gastrointestinal side effects and causes less interference with intestinal absorption of vitamins and drugs than other sequestrants.

When exercise, colesevelam, and diet are not enough, certain statin drugs may be added to a dietary regimen to lower LDL cholesterol, raise HDL cholesterol, extend life by reducing the frequency of first and second heart attacks and of bypass surgery and angioplasty, and reduce the risk of stroke and slow progression of atherosclerosis for people with heart attacks or coronary heart disease. Unfortunately, the use of these agents is problematic in HIV-positive patients because of side effects, which include muscle weakness, muscle pain, and elevated hepatic enzymes, and because they may interact with protease inhibitors.

Statins may also have immunomodulatory effects. In human endothelial cells and macrophages atorvastatin, lovastatin, and pravastatin suppressed the induction of major histocompatibility complex class II expression by interferon-γ in a dose-dependent fashion. In addition, statin pretreatment of human endothelial cells and monocytemacrophages reduced subsequent proliferation of T lymphocytes, suggesting that statins can modulate T-cell activation.[143,144]

For HIV-infected patients with dyslipidemia, drug therapy to lower cholesterol may be useful if antiretroviral therapy cannot be changed, interrupted, or delayed.[145–147] Preliminary recommendations for the management of dyslipidemia in patients with HIV infection have been devised by the U.S.-based Adult AIDS Clinical Trial Group Cardiovascular Disease Focus Group (see Chapter 62).[51] For protease inhibitor-treated HIV-infected patients with hypercholesterolemia, treatment with low-dose pravastatin (initial dosage 20 mg/day) or atorvastatin (10 mg/day) is recommended. Careful monitoring of virologic status and creatine kinase values is recommended for patients on these therapies. Fluvastatin is an acceptable alternative, but data are not available on potential interactions with protease inhibitors. Lovastatin or simvastatin therapy should be avoided because of interactions with protease inhibitors. When treatment with HMG CoA reductase inhibitors (statins) is not appropriate or when patients do not respond to these agents, gemfibrozil (600 mg twice daily) or fenofibrate (200 mg once daily) are reasonable alternatives. Concomitant use of fibrates and statins may increase the risk of skeletal muscle toxicity.

Nondrug therapy (diet and exercise) is recommended for patients with fasting serum triglyceride levels of more than 200 mg/dl.[51] Dietary and exercise interventions have been successful at reducing serum triglycerides in HIV-infected patients. Recommended actions include consultation with a dietitian, smoking cessation, regular aerobic exercise, weight reduction, decreasing fat intake without excess increases in carbohydrate intake, and replacement of some saturated fat with monounsaturated fat. Severe hypertriglyceridemia requires an extremely low-fat diet, avoidance of free sugars, and decreased alcohol intake. Omega-3 fatty acids as oil or supplements may be helpful.

The cutoff at which isolated hypertriglyceridemia in this population should be treated with drugs is not known. In the absence of CHD risk factors or hypercholesterolemia, patients with elevations above 1000 mg/dl should be considered for treatment to reduce the risk of pancreatitis. This threshold may be even lower in a patient with a history of pancreatitis. Fibric acid analogues such as gemfibrozil and fenofibrate decrease serum triglycerides. These agents individually or in combination have been tested only in a preliminary fashion in HIV-infected patients with dyslipidemia but seem effective. Gemfibrozil (adults: 600 mg twice a day 30 minutes before the morning and evening meals) and micronized fenofibrate (adults: 200 mg once daily) are recommended for patients with hypertriglyceridemia who require drug therapy; these agents are also considered reasonable initial treatment choices for patients with combined hyperlipidemia. Statins are not generally recommended as first-line therapy for isolated hypertriglyceridemia, but cautious addition of a statin may be considered when fibrate therapy does not adequately lower triglyceride levels or when LDL cholesterol levels remain elevated.[51] Niacin, although likely to be effective at reducing elevated triglycerides, is not recommended as a first-line agent because of the frequency of side effects, such as cutaneous flushing, pruritus, and insulin resistance.

▲ HAART AND PREVENTION OF CARDIOVASCULAR DISEASE

HAART has been associated with a lipodystrophy syndrome, and considerations when initiating HAART should include cardiovascular risk assessment (see Chapter 62). Any modifiable risk factors should be addressed as above. Fasting serum glucose and lipid levels should be checked. If serum studies are abnormal, dietary adjustments, exercise, and possibly medical therapy should be instituted along with HAART. During therapy, nutritional counseling, aerobic exercise, and close monitoring for drug interactions are recommended. In patients with a high baseline triglyceride level, the assay should be repeated after 1 to 2 months. In all HAART patients, the fasting lipid profile and serum glucose should be rechecked every 3 to 4 months during therapy.

▲ CONCLUSIONS

Cardiovascular disease is common in HIV-infected patients, and physical examination may not be reliable for diagnosis and follow-up. Echocardiographic examination should be considered for detecting of early disease and identifying patients who would benefit from early intervention and aggressive early antiretroviral therapy. Prevention of cardiovascular disease in HIV-infected patients should be the goal rather than merely treatment of cardiovascular disease when it is encountered. HIV-specific preventive cardiovascular strategies for HIV-infected patients have not been developed, but evidence-based recommendations can be extrapolated from those recommended for the general population. However, because of medication interactions and side effects, therapy with cardiovascular and lipid-modifying drugs in HIV-infected patients must be individualized.

Acknowledgments. This work was supported in part by research grants from the National Institutes of Health (HL53392, HL59837, HL07937, HD34568, CA68484, CA79060, HD34568).

REFERENCES

1. Starc TJ, Lipshultz SE, Kaplan S, et al. Cardiac complications in children with human immunodeficiency virus infection. Pediatrics 104:e14, 1999; URL: http://www.pediatrics.org/cgi/content/full/104/2/e14; HIV, cardiac disease, pediatrics.
2. Barbaro G, Di Lorenzo G, Grisorio B, Barbarini G. Cardiac involvement in the acquired immunodeficiency syndrome: a multicenter clinical-pathological study. AIDS Res 14:1071, 1998.
3. Acierno LJ. Cardiac complications in acquired immunodeficiency syndrome (AIDS): a review. J Am Coll Cardiol 13:1144, 1989.
4. Rerkpattanapipat P, Wongpraparut N, Jacobs LE, Kotler MN. Cardiac manifestations of acquired immunodeficiency syndrome. Arch Intern Med 160:602, 2000.
5. Luginbuhl LM, Orav EV, Mclntosh K, Lipshultz SE. Cardiac morbidity and related mortality in children with HIV infection. JAMA 269:2869, 1993.
6. Barbaro G, Barbarini G, Di Lorenzo G. Early impairment of systolic and diastolic function in asymptomatic HIV-positive patients: a multicenter echocardiographic and echo-Doppler study. AIDS Res 12:1559, 1996.
7. Fisher SD, Lipshultz SE. Epidemiology of cardiovascular involvement in HIV disease and AIDS. Ann N Y Acad Sci 946:13, 2001.
8. Herskowitz A. Cardiomyopathy and other symptomatic heart diseases associated with HIV infection. Curr Opin Cardiol 11:325, 1996.
9. Herskowitz A, Willoughby SB, Vlahov D, et al. Dilated heart muscle disease associated with HIV infection. Eur Heart J 16(suppl O): 50, 1995.
10. Fisher SD, Lipshultz SE. Cardiovascular disease in HIV-infected individuals. In: Braunwald E et al. (eds) The Heart, 6th ed. Philadelphia, WB Saunders, 2000, pp 2211–2222.
11. Hoffman M, et al. Malnutrition and cardiac abnormalities in the HIV-infected patient. In: Miller TL, Gorbachs (eds) Nutritional Aspects of HIV Infection. London, Arnold, 1999, pp 133–139.
12. Miller TL, Orav EJ, Colan SD, Lipshultz SE. Nutritional status and cardiac mass and function in children infected with the human immunodeficiency virus. Am J ClinNutr 66:660, 1997.
13. Felker GM, Thompson RE, Hare JM, et al. Underlying causes and long-term survival in patients with initially unexplained cardiomyopathy. N Engl J Med 342:1077, 2000.
14. Lipshultz SE, Easley KA, Orav J, et al. Left ventricular structure and function in children infected with human immunodeficiency virus: the prospective P^2C^2 HIV multicenter study. Circulation 97:1246, 1998.
15. Blanchard DG, Hagenhoff C, Chow LC, et al. Reversibility of cardiac abnormalities in human immunodeficiency virus (HIV)-infected individuals: a serial echocardiographic study. J Am Coll Cardiol 17:1270, 1991.
16. Lipshultz SE, Easley KA, Orav EJ, et al. Cardiac dysfunction and mortality in HIV-infected children: the prospective P^2C^2 HIV multicenter study. Circulation 102:1542, 2000.
17. McNamara DM, Rosenblum WD, Janosko KM, et al. Intravenous immune globulin in the therapy of myocarditis and acute cardiomyopathy. Circulation 95:2476, 1997.
18. Newburger JW, Takahashi M, Beiser AS, et al. A single intravenous infusion of gamma globulin as compared with four infusions in the treatment of acute Kawasaki syndrome. N Engl J Med 324:1633, 1991.
19. Martino TA, Liu P, Sole MJ. Viral infection and the pathogenesis of dilated cardiomyopathy. Circ Res 74:182, 1994.
20. Fujioka S, Kitaura Y, Ukimura A, et al. Evaluation of viral infection in the myocardium of patients with idiopathic dilated cardiomyopathy. J Am Coll Cardiol 36:1920, 2000.
21. Takada H, Kishimoto C, Hiraoka Y. Therapy with immunoglobulin suppresses myocarditis in a murine coxsackievirus B3 model: antiviral and antiinflammatory effects. Circulation 92:1604, 1995.
22. Kishimoto C, Takamatsu N, Kawamata H, et al. Immunoglobulin treatment ameliorates murine myocarditis associated with reduction of neurohumoral activity and improvement of extracellular matrix change. J Am Coll Cardiol 36:1979, 2000.
23. Lipshultz SE, Orav EJ, Sanders SP, Colan SD. Immunoglobulins and left ventricular structure and function in pediatric HIV infection. Circulation 92:2220, 1995.
24. Shannon RP, Simon MA, Mathier MA, et al. Dilated cardiomyopathy associated with simian AIDS in nonhuman primates. Circulation 101:185, 2000.
25. Heidenreich PA, Eisenberg MJ, Kee LL, et al. Pericardial effusion in AIDS: incidence and survival. Circulation 92:3229, 1995.
26. Silva-Cardoso J, Moura B, Martins L, et al. Pericardial involvement in human immunodeficiency virus infection. Chest 115:418, 1999.
27. Currie PF, Sutherland GR, Jacob AJ, et al. A review of endocarditis in acquired immunodeficiency syndrome and human immunodeficiency virus infection. Eur Heart J 16(B):15, 1995.
28. Nahass RG, Weinstein MP, Bartels J, Gocke DJ. Infective endocarditis in intravenous drug users: a comparison of human immunodeficiency virus type 1-negative and-positive patients. J Infect Dis 162:967, 1990.

29. Jenson HB, Pollock BH. Cardiac cancers in HIV-infected patients. In: Lipshultz SE (ed) Cardiology in AIDS. New York, Chapman & Hall, 1998, pp 255–263.
30. Saidi A, Bricker JT. Pulmonary hypertension in patients infected with HIV. In Lipshultz SE (ed) Cardiology in AIDS. New York, Chapman & Hall, 1998, pp 187–193.
31. Himelman RB, Dohrmann M, Goodman P, et al. Severe pulmonary hypertension and cor pulmonale in the acquired immunodeficiency syndrome. Am J Cardiol 64:1396, 1989.
32. Aarons EJ, Nye FJ. Primary pulmonary hypertension and HIV infection. AIDS 5:1276, 1991.
33. Coplan NL, Shimony RY, Ioachim HL, et al. Primary pulmonary hypertension associated with human immunodeficiency viral infection. Am J Med 89:96, 1990.
34. Freeman R, Roberts MS, Friedman LS, Broadbridge C. Autonomic function and human immunodeficiency virus infection. Neurology 40:575, 1990.
35. Sarda L, Colin P, Boccara F, et al. Myocarditis in patients with clinical presentation of myocardial infarction and normal coronary angiograms. J Am Coll Cardiol 37:786, 2001.
36. Moorthy LN, Lipshultz SE. Cardiovascular monitoring of HIV-infected patients. In: Lipshultz SE (ed) Cardiology in AIDS. New York, Chapman & Hall, 1998, pp 345–386.
37. Giantris A, Lipshultz SE. Cardiac therapeutics in HIV-infected patients. In: Lipshultz SE (ed) Cardiology in AIDS. New York, Chapman & Hall, 1998, pp 387–422.
38. Giantris A, Lipshultz SE. Cardiac disease. In: Dolin R, Masur H, Saag MS (eds) AIDS Therapy. New York, Churchill Livingstone, 1999, pp 680–698.
39. Bowles NE, et al. The detection of viral genomes by polymerase chain reaction in the myocardium of pediatric patients with advanced HIV disease. J Am Coll Cardiol 34:857, 1999.
40. Lipshultz SE, et al. Predictive value of cardiac troponin T in pediatric patients at risk for myocardial injury. Circulation 96:2641, 1997.
41. Ottlinger M, et al. New developments in the biochemical assessment of myocardial injury in children: troponin T and I as highly sensitive and specific markers of myocardial injury. Prog Pediatr Cardiol 8:71, 1998.
42. Mair J. The utility of brain natriuretic peptides in patients with heart failure and coronary artery disease. In: Adams JE, et al (eds) Markers in Cardiology: Current and Future Clinical Applications. Armonk, NY, Futura, 2001, pp 235–262.
43. Chen HH, Burnett JC. The natriuretic peptides in heart failure: diagnostic and therapeutic potentials. Proc Assoc Am Physicians 111:406, 1999.
44. Tsutamoto T, Wada A, Maeda K, et al. Plasma brain natriuretic peptide level as a biochemical marker of morbidity and mortality in patients with asymptomatic or minimally symptomatic left ventricular dysfunction. Eur Heart J 20:1799, 1999.
45. Stein E. Laboratory surrogates for anti-atherosclerotic drug development. Am J Cardiol 87(suppl):21A, 2001.
46. Ridker PM. High-sensitivity C-reactive protein: a novel inflammatory marker for predicting the risk of coronary artery disease. In: Adams JE, et al (eds) Markers in Cardiology: Current and Future Clinical Applications. Armonk, NY, Futura, 2001, pp 173–184.
47. Ridker PM, Cushman M, Stampfer MJ, et al. Inflammation, aspirin, and the risk of cardiovascular disease in apparently healthy men. N Engl J Med 336:973, 1997.
48. Ridker PM, Hennekens CH, Buring JE, Rifai N. C-reactive protein and other markers of inflammation in the prediction of cardiovascular disease in women. N Engl J Med 342:836, 2000.
49. Rifai N, Tracy RP, Ridker PM. Clinical efficacy of an automated high-sensitivity C-reactive protein assay. Clin Chem 45:2136, 1999.
50. Haverkate F, Thompson SG, Pyke SD, et al. Production of C-reactive protein and risk of coronary events in stable and unstable angina. Lancet 349:462, 1997.
51. Dube MP, Sprecher D, Henry WK, et al. Adult AIDS Clinical Trial Group Cardiovascular Disease Focus Group: preliminary guidelines for the evaluation and management of dyslipidemia in adults infected with human immunodeficiency virus and receiving antiretroviral therapy: recommendations of the Adult AIDS Clinical Trial Group Cardiovascular Disease Focus Group. Clin Infect Dis 31:11216, 2000.
52. Orloff DG. Use of surrogate endpoints: a practical necessity in lipid-altering and antiatherosclerosis drug development. Am J Cardiol 87(suppl):35A, 2001.
53. Wilson PWF, D'Agostino RB, Levy D, et al. Prediction of coronary heart disease using risk factor categories. Circulation 97:1837, 1998.
54. Aoun S, Ramos E. Hypertension in the HIV-infected patient. Curr Hypertens Rep 2:478, 2000.
55. Anonymous. Drugs for non-HIV viral infections. Med Lett 41:113, 1999.
56. Rich MW. Heart failure disease management. 1 Critical review. J Card Fail 5:64, 1999.
57. Mller TD, Balady GJ, Fletcher GF. Exercise and its role in the prevention and rehabilitation of cardiovascular disease. Ann Behav Med 19:220, 1997.
58. Dracup K, Baker DW, Dunbar SB, et al. Management of heart failure. II. Counseling, education and lifestyle modification. JAMA 272:1442, 1994.
59. European Heart Failure Training Group. Experience from controlled trials of physical training in chronic heart failure: protocol and patient factors in effectiveness in the improvement in exercise tolerance. Eur Heart J 19:466, 1998.
60. Belardinelli R, Georgiou D, Cianci G, Purcaro A. Randomized, controlled trial of long-term moderate exercise training in chronic heart failure: effects on functional capacity, quality of life, and clinical outcomes. Circulation 99:1173, 1999.
61. Garg R, Yusuf S. Overview of randomized trials of angiotensin-converting enzyme inhibitors on mortality and morbidity in patients with heart failure. JAMA 273:1450, 1995.
62. Gheorghiade M, Benatar D, Konstam MA, et al. Pharmacotherapy for systolic dysfunction; a review of randomized clinical trials. Am J Cardiol 80(suppl 8B):14, 1997.
63. Yusuf S, Pepine CJ, Garces C, et al. Effect of enalapril on myocardial infarction and unstable angina in patients with low ejection fractions. Lancet 340:1173, 1992.
64. Packer M, Poole-Wilson PA, Armstrong PW, et al. Comparative effects of low and high doses of the angiotensin-converting enzyme inhibitor, lisinopril, on morbidity and mortality in chronic heart failure. Circulation 100:2312, 1999.
65. SOLVD Investigators. Effect of enalapril on survival in patients with reduced left ventricular ejection fractions and congestive heart failure. N Engl J Med 325:293, 1991.
66. Sharma D, Buyse M, Pitt B, Rucinska EJ. Meta-analysis of observed mortality data from all-controlled, double blind, multiple-dose studies of losartan in heart failure. Am J Cardiol 85:187, 2000.
67. Riegger GAJ, Bouzo H, Petr P, et al. Improvement in exercise tolerance and symptoms of congestive heart failure during treatment with candesartan cilexetil. Circulation 100:2224, 1999.
68. McKelvie R, Yusuf S, Pericak D, et al. Comparison of candesartan, enalapril, and their combination in congestive heart failure: randomized evaluation of strategies for left ventricular dysfunction (RESOLVD pilot study). Circulation 100:1056, 1999.
69. Hamroff G, Katz SD, Mancini D, et al. Addition of angiotensin II receptor blockade to maximal angiotensive-converting enzyme inhibition improves exercise capacity in patients with severe congestive heart failure. Circulation 99:990, 1999.
70. Kraus F, Rudolph C, Rudolph W. [Effectiveness of digitalis in patients with chronic heart failure and sinus rhythm. Review of randomized, double-blind and placebo controlled studies]. Wirksamkeit von Digitalis bei Patienten mit chronischer Herzinsuffizienz und Sinusrhythmus. Herz 18:95, 1993.
71. Digitalis Investigation Group. The effect of digoxin on mortality and morbidity in patients with heart failure. N Engl J Med 336:525, 1997.
72. Packer M, Carver JR, Rodeheffer RJ, et al. Effect of oral milrinone on mortality in severe chronic heart failure. N Engl J Med 325:1468, 1991.
73. CIBIS-II Investigators and Committees. The cardiac insufficiency bisoprolol study II (CIBIS-II): a randomised trial. Lancet 353:9, 1999.
74. MERIT-HF Study Group. Effect of metroprolol CR/XL in chronic heart failure: metoprolol CR/XL randomised intervention trial in congestive heart failure. Lancet 353:2001, 1999.
75. Lechat P, Packer M, Chalon S, et al. Clinical effects of β-adrenergic blockade in chronic heart failure: a meta-analysis of double-blind, placebo-controlled, randomized trials. Circulation 98:1184, 1998.
76. Anonymous. Which beta-blocker? Med Lett 43:9, 2001.
77. Packer M, O'Connor CM, Ghali JK, et al. Effect of amiodipine on morbidity and mortality in severe chronic heart failure. N Engl J Med 335:1107, 1996.

78. Pitt B, Zannad F, Remme WJ, et al. The effects of spironolactone on morbidity and mortality in patients with severe heart failure. N Engl J Med 341:709, 1999.
79. Piepoli M, Villani GQ, Ponikowski P, et al. Overview and meta-analysis of randomised trials of amiodarone in chronic heart failure. Int J Cardiol 66:1, 1998.
80. Amiodarone Trials Meta-Analysis Investigators. Effect of prophylactic amiodarone on mortality after acute myocardial infarction and in congestive heart failure: meta-analysis of individual data from 6500 patients in randomised trials. Lancet 350:1417, 1997.
81. Antiarrhythmic versus Implantable Defibrillators (AVID) Investigators. A comparison of antiarrhythmic-drug therapy with implantable defibrillators. 1. Patients resuscitated from near-fatal ventricular arrhythmias. N Engl J Med 337:1576, 1997.
82. Moss AJ, Hall WJ, Cannom DS, et al. Improved survival with an implanted defibrillator in patients with coronary disease at high risk for ventricular arrhythmia. N Engl J Med 335:1933, 1996.
83. Bigger JT, Coronary Artery Bypass Graft (CABG) Patch Trial Investigators. Prophylactic use of implanted cardiac defibrillators in patients at high risk for ventricular arrhythmias after coronary-artery bypass graft surgery. N Engl J Med 337:1569, 1997.
84. Teerlink JR, Jalaluddin M, Anderson S, et al. Ambulatory ventricular arrhythmias in patients with heart failure do not specifically predict an increased risk of sudden death. Circulation 101:40, 2000.
85. Connolly SJ. Prophylactic antiarrhythmic therapy for the prevention of sudden death in high-risk patients: drugs and devices. Eur Heart J 1 (suppl C):31, 1999.
86. Foster C, Murphy M, Ness A, et al. Primary prevention. Clin Evidence 4:51, 2000.
87. National Heart Committee. Guidelines for the management of mildly raised blood pressure in New Zealand. Wellington Ministry of Health, http://www.nzgg.org.nz/library/gl_complete/bloodpressure/table1.cfm, 1993.
88. Powell KE, Thompson PD, Caspersen CJ, Kendrick JS. Physical activity and the incidence of coronary heart disease. Annu Rev Public Health 8:253, 1987.
89. Berlin JA, Colditz GA. A meta-analysis of physical activity in the prevention of coronary heart disease. Am J Epidemiol 132:612, 1990.
90. Fraser GE, Strahan TM, Sabate J, et al. Effects of traditional coronary risk factors on rates of incident coronary events in a low-risk population: the Adventist health study. Circulation 86:406, 1992.
91. Folsom AR, Arnett DK, Hutchinson RG, et al. Physical activity and incidence of coronary heart disease in middle-aged women and men. Med Sci Sports Exerc 29:901, 1997.
92. Simonsick EM, Lafferty ME, Phillips CL, et al. Risk due to inactivity in physically capable older adults. Am J Public Health 83:1443, 1993.
93. Serman SE, D'Agostino RB, Cobb JL, Kannel WB. Does exercise reduce mortality rates in the elderly? Experience from the Framingham Heart Study. Am Heart J 128:965, 1994.
94. Rodriguez BL, Curb JD, Burchfiel CM, et al. Physical activity and 23-year incidence of coronary heart disease morbidity and mortality among middle-aged men: the Honolulu heart program. Circulation 89:2540, 1994.
95. Stender M, Hense HW, Doring A, Keil U. Physical activity at work and cardiovascular disease risk: results from the MONICA Augsburg study. Int J Epidemiol 22:644, 1993.
96. Gartside PS, Wang P, Glueck CJ. Prospective assessment of coronary heart disease risk factors: the NHANES I epidemiologic follow-up study (NHEFS) 16-year follow-up. J Am Coll Nutr 17:263, 1998.
97. Hakim AA, Curb JD, Petrovitch H, et al. Effects of walking on coronary heart disease in elderly men: the Honolulu heart program. Circulation 100:9, 1999.
98. Eaton CB. Relation of physical activity and cardiovascular fitness to coronary heart disease. II. Cardiovascular fitness and the safety and efficacy of physical activity prescription. J Am Board Fam Pract 5:157, 1992.
99. Blair SN, Kohl HW 3rd, Barlow CE, et al. Changes in physical fitness and all-cause mortality: a prospective study of healthy and unhealthy men. JAMA 273:1093, 1995.
100. Pate RR, Pratt M, Blair SN, et al. Physical activity and public health: a recommendation from the Centers for Disease Control and Prevention and the American College of Sports Medicine. JAMA 273:402, 1995.
101. Thompson PD. The cardiovascular complications of vigorous physical activity. Arch Intern Med 156:2297, 1996.
102. Oberman A. Exercise and the primary prevention of cardiovascular disease. Am J Cardiol 55:10, 1985.
103. Erikssen G, Liestol K, Bjornholt J, et al. Changes in physical fitness and changes in mortality. Lancet 352:759, 1998.
104. Shangold MM. Exercise in the menopausal woman. Obstet Gynecol 75(suppl):53S, 1990.
105. Bell MJ, Lineker SC, Wilkins AL, et al. A randomized controlled trial to evaluate the efficacy of community based physical therapy in the treatment of people with rheumatoid arthritis. J Rheumatol 25:231, 1998.
106. Agurs-Collins TD, Kumanyika SK, Ten Have TR, Adams-Campbell LL. A randomized controlled trial of weight reduction and exercise for diabetes management in older African-American subjects. Diabetes Care 20:1503, 1997.
107. Shepard RJ, Shek PN. Impact of physical activity and sport on the immune system. 11:133, 1996.
108. Cannon JG, Fielding RA, Fiatarone MA, et al. Increased interleukin-1b in human skeletal muscle after exercise. Am J Physiol 257:R451, 1989.
109. Boas SR, Joswiak ML, Nixon PA, et al. Effects of anaerobic exercise on the immune system in eight to seventeen year old trained and untrained boys. J Pediatr 129:846, 1996.
110. Nieman DC. Immune response to heavy exertion. J Appl Physiol 82:1385, 1997.
111. Osterback L, Qvarnberg Y. A prospective study of respiratory infections in 12 year old children actively engaged in sports. Acta Pediatr Scand 76:73, 1987.
112. Johnson JE, Anders GT, Blanton HM, et al. Exercise dysfunction in patients seropositive for the human immunodeficiency virus. Am Rev Respir Dis 141:618, 1990.
113. MacArthur RD, Levine SD, Birk TJ. Supervised exercise training improves cardiopulmonary fitness in HIV-infected persons. Med Sci Sports Exerc 25:684, 1993.
114. Mustafa T, Sy FS, Macera CA, et al. Association between exercise and HIV disease progression in a cohort of homosexual men. Ann Epidemiol 9:127, 1999.
115. Spence DW, Galantino ML, Mossberg KA, Zimmerman SO. Progressive resistance exercise: effect on muscle function and anthropometry of a select AIDS population. Arch Phys Med Rehabil 71:644, 1990.
116. Roubenoff R, et al. Feasibility of increasing lean body mass in HIV-infected adults using progressive resistance exercise [abstract]. Nutrition 13:271, 1997.
117. Rigsby LW, Dishman RK, Jackson AW, et al. Effects of exercise training on men seropositive for the human immunodeficiency virus-1. Med Sci Sports Exerc 24:6, 1992.
118. LaPierre A, Fletcher MA, Antoni MH, et al. Aerobic exercise training in an AIDS risk group. Int J Sports Med 12:S53, 1991.
119. Mosher PE, Nash MS, Perry AC, et al. Aerobic circuit training: effect on adolescents with well-controlled insulin-dependent diabetes mellitus. Arch Phys Med Rehabil 79:652, 1998.
120. Roubenoff R, Weiss L, McDermott A, et al. A pilot study of exercise training to reduce trunk fat in adults with HIV-associated fat redistribution. AIDS 13:1373, 1999.
121. US Department of Health and Human Services. The Health Benefits of Smoking Cessation: A Report of the Surgeon General. DHHS publication (CDC) 90-8416. Rockville, MD, US Department of health and Human Services, Public Health Service, Centers for Disease Control, 1990.
122. Doll R, Peto R, Wheatley K, et al. Mortality in relation to smoking: 40 years' observations on male British doctors. BMJ 309:901, 1994.
123. Rosenberg L. The risk of myocardial infarction after quitting smoking in men under 55 years of age. N Engl J Med 313:1511, 1985.
124. Rosenberg L. Decline in the risk of myocardial infarction among women who stop smoking. N Engl J Med 322:213, 1990.
125. Shinton R, Beevers G. Meta-analysis of relation between cigarette smoking and stroke. BMJ 298:789, 1989.
126. Ebrahim S, Davey Smith G. Lowering blood pressure: a systematic review of sustained non-pharmacological interventions. J Public Health Med 20:441, 1998.
127. Engstom G, Hedblad B, Janzon L. Hypertensive men who exercise regularly have lower rate of cardiovascular mortality. J Hypertens 17:737, 1999.

128. Appel LJ, Moore TJ, Obarzanek E, et al. A clinical trial of the effects of dietary patterns on blood pressure. N Engl J Med 336:1117, 1997.
129. Campbell NRC, Ashley MJ, Carruthers SG, et al. Lifestyle modifications to prevent and control hypertension. 3. Recommendations on alcohol consumption. Can Med Assoc J 160(suppl 9):13, 1999.
130. Graudal NA, Galloe AM, Garred P. Effects of sodium restriction on blood pressure, renin, aldosterone, catecholamines, cholesterols, and triglyceride. JAMA 279:1381, 1998.
131. Heart Outcomes Prevention Evaluation Study Investigators. Effects of an angiotensin-converting-enzyme inhibitor, ramipril, on cardiovascular events in high-risk patients. N Engl J Med 342:145, 2000.
132. Hansson L, Zanchetti A, Carruthers SG, et al. Effects of intensive blood pressure lowering and low-dose aspirin in patients with hypertension: principal results of the hypertension optimal treatment (HOT) trial. Lancet 351:1755, 1998.
133. Croog SH, Levine S, Testa MA, et al. The effects of antihypertensive therapy on quality of life. N Engl J Med 314:1657, 1986.
134. Katemdahl DA, Lawler WR. Variability in meta-analytic results concerning the value of cholesterol reduction in coronary heart disease: a meta-analysis. Am J Epidemiol 149:429, 1999.
135. Froom J, Froom P, Benjamin M, Benjamin BJ. Measurement and management of hyperlipidemia for the primary prevention of coronary heart disease. J Am Board Fam Pract 11:12, 1998.
136. LaRosa JC, He J, Vupputari S. Effect of statins on risk of coronary disease: a meta-analysis of randomized controlled trials. JAMA 282:2340, 1999.
137. Downs JR, Clearfield M, Weis S, et al. Primary prevention of acute coronary events with lovastatin in men and women with average cholesterol levels: results of the AFCAPS/TexCAPS. JAMA 279:1615, 1998.
138. Scandinavian Simvastatin Survival Study Group. Randomized trial of cholesterol lowering in 4444 patients with coronary heart disease: the Scandinavian Simvastatin Survival Study (4S). Lancet 344:1383, 1995.
139. Long-term Intervention with Pravastatin in Ischemic Disease (LIPID) Study Program. Prevention of cardiovascular events and death with pravastatin in patients with coronary heart disease and a broad range of initial cholesterol levels. N Engl J Med 339:1349, 1998.
140. Shepherd J, Cobbe SM, Ford I, et al. Prevention of coronary heart disease with pravastatin in men with hypercholesterolemia. N Engl J Med 333:1301, 1995.
141. Bucher HC, Griffith LE, Guyatt GH. Systematic review on the risk and benefit of different cholesterol-lowering interventions. Arterioscler Thromb Vasc Biol 19:187, 1999.
142. Anonymous. Colesevelam (Welchol) for hypercholesterolemia. Med Lett 42:102, 2000.
143. Kwah B, et al. Statins as a newly recognized type of immunomodulator. Nat Med 6:1399, 2000.
144. Palinski W. Immunomodulation: a new role for statins? Nat Med 6:1311, 2000.
145. Martinez E, Mocroft A, Garcia-Viejo MA, et al. Risk of lipodystrophy in HIV-1-infected patients treated with protease inhibitors: a prospective cohort study. Lancet 357:592, 2001.
146. Anonymous Drugs for HIV infection. Med Lett 42:1, 2000.
147. Piscitelli SC, Gallicano KD. Interactions among drugs for HIV and opportunistic infections. N Engl J Med 344:984, 2001.

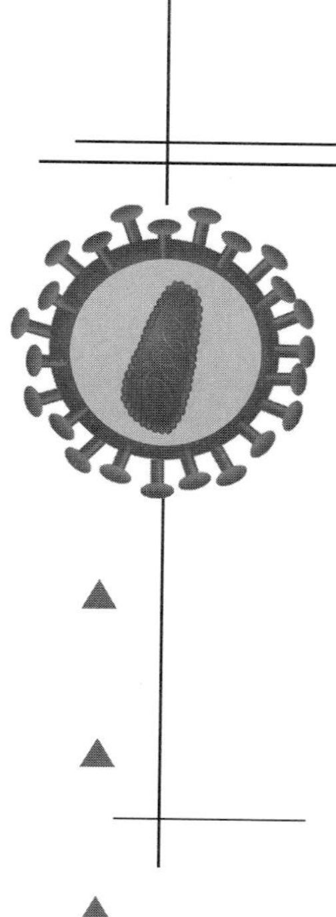

CHAPTER 60

Respiratory Disease

Laurence Huang, MD

Patients with human immunodeficiency virus (HIV) infection can develop respiratory dysfunction due to a wide variety of infectious, neoplastic, embolic, toxic, and cardiovascular disorders. Although the immediate focus is often directed at opportunistic infection, clinicians dealing with HIV-infected patients presenting with dyspnea, cough, chest pain, with or without fever, must approach the differential diagnosis methodically. They must recognize that patients with HIV infection may have pulmonary signs and symptoms that are totally unrelated to their HIV infection and may not be infectious or neoplastic; for example, they may have had asthma since childhood, congestive heart failure due to ischemic heart disease, or pulmonary emboli due to inactivity. Pulmonary function testing, a lung scan, empiric diuresis, or an echocardiogram may be the appropriate initial steps. If the clinical syndrome appears to be infectious, the causative organism may not be an opportunistic pathogen; patients with HIV infection are also susceptible to community-acquired pathogens (e.g., influenza or *Mycoplasma*) or hospital-acquired organisms (e.g., methicillin-resistant *Staphylococcus aureus* or extended-spectrum β-lactamase-producing enteric organisms). Thus a rational approach to respiratory dysfunction in patients with HIV infection should include the same considerations as any immunologically normal patient, as well as consideration for the processes that occur with special frequency or severity in patients with HIV infection (Table 60–1).

Clinicians should also recognize that HIV-infected persons may have preexisting or concurrent chronic pulmonary disease (e.g., asthma or chronic obstructive pulmonary disease). In addition, risk factors for HIV infection, such as injection drug use, may also contribute to pulmonary disease (e.g., endocarditis with septic pulmonary emboli, aspiration pneumonia secondary to altered mentation, noncardiogenic pulmonary edema, talc granulomatosis). Therefore in the proper clinical context, clinicians must also consider non-HIV-associated respiratory disorders.

This chapter presents an approach to lower respiratory tract and upper respiratory tract infections in this patient population.

▲ EPIDEMIOLOGIC PERSPECTIVE

The Pulmonary Complications of HIV Infection Study (PCHIS) was a prospective, observational cohort study that followed more than 1150 HIV-infected subjects for approximately 5 years at six sites across the United States prior to the era of HAART.[1,2] PCHIS documented that patients presenting to an outpatient clinic with respiratory illness more often had upper respiratory tract infections [including upper respiratory illnesses (URIs), sinusitis, and otitis media] and acute bronchitis than pneumonias due to bacteria or *Pneumocystis carinii*.[2] Over the course of the study, the annual incidence of upper respiratory tract infections and acute bronchitis in their cohort ranged from 35 to 52 episodes per 100 person-years and 13 to 14 episodes per 100 person-years, respectively. In fact, the overall incidence of acute bronchitis was higher than that for the next two most frequent diagnoses, bacterial pneumonia (range 3.9–7.3 episodes per 100 person-years) and *Pneumocystis carinii* pneumonia (PCP) (range 2.8–9.5 episodes per 100 person-years), combined. However, neither upper respiratory tract infections nor acute bronchitis typically necessitates hospitalization, whereas a considerable number of patients with bacterial pneumonia or PCP had to be admitted.

Table 60–1. CAUSES OF PULMONARY DYSFUNCTION SEEN WITH INCREASED FREQUENCY OR SEVERITY IN PATIENTS WITH HIV INFECTION

Opportunistic Infections
Bacteria
Streptococcus pneumoniae
Haemophilus influenzae
Staphylococcus aureus
Pseudomonas aeruginosa
Klebsiella pneumoniae
Rhodococcus equi
Mycobacterium tuberculosis
Atypical mycobacteria[a]
Fungi
Pneumocystis carinii
Cryptococcus neoformans
Histoplasma capsulatum
Coccidioides immitis
Penicillium marneffei
Viruses
CMV[a]
EBV
HSV
VZV
Protozoa
Toxoplasma gondii
Strongyloides stercoralis[b]
Neoplasms
Lymphoma
Kaposi sarcoma
Mantle cell lymphoma
Squamous cell carcinoma (?)
Other Disorders
Asthma
Pulmonary hypertension
Cardiomyopathy/congestive heart failure
Premature atherosclerosis/congestive heart failure?
Immune reconstitution syndrome
Alveolar hemorrhage
Sarcoid (?)

EBV, Epstein-Barr virus; HSV, herpes simplex virus; VZV, varicella-zoster virus.
[a]Cytomegalovirus (CMV) and *Mycobacterium avium* complex (MAC) are rarely the cause of pulmonary dysfunction in patients with HIV infection regardless of their CD4+ T-lymphocyte and neutrophil counts.
[b]Although disseminated *Strongyloides* is an AIDS-defining disease, it has rarely been documented in patients with HIV infection.

At San Francisco General Hospital, the most common pulmonary diseases observed among HIV-infected patients requiring hospitalization are bacterial pneumonia followed by PCP, both of which are significantly more common than the next most common diagnoses: tuberculosis, pulmonary Kaposi sarcoma, and cryptococcal pneumonia (unpublished data). In a year-long study of community-acquired pneumonia, Mundy and coworkers at Johns Hopkins Hospital and others have found that pneumonias due to bacteria (*Streptococcus pneumoniae*: 21% of all pneumonias in HIV-infected subjects) and *P. carinii* (27%) greatly exceeded those due to viruses, mycobacteria, and fungi (each < 5%).[3] Finally, PCHIS showed that the most common pulmonary diseases observed among HIV-infected patients requiring critical care were PCP followed by bacterial pneumonia.[4] These results from the multicenter PCHIS are similar to those reported from single institutions such as San Francisco General Hospital[5] and multicenter cohorts in Europe.[6]

The geographic location of the clinic or hospital may also influence the frequency of the diagnoses. In specific populations or geographic regions, mycobacterial and endemic fungal pneumonias are important considerations. Worldwide, tuberculosis is a leading cause of death. In endemic areas diseases caused by *Histoplasma capsulatum* or *Coccidioides immitis* are among the most frequent infections seen, whereas at San Francisco General Hospital they are rarely encountered. Table 60–2 lists diagnostic clues to the

Table 60–2. APPROACH TO RESPIRATORY DISEASE: DIAGNOSTIC CLUES

Clinical Setting
Ambulatory care/outpatient clinic: upper respiratory tract infections (including upper respiratory tract infection (URI), sinusitis, otitis media) > acute bronchitis > bacterial pneumonia +PCP[a]
Hospital: bacterial pneumonia > PCP > tuberculosis > pulmonary Kaposi sarcoma = cryptococcosis[b]
Intensive care unit: PCP > bacterial pneumonia[c]
Geographic Location
Mycobacterium tuberculosis
Endemic fungi (e.g., *Histoplasma capsulatum*, *Coccidioides immitis*)
CD4+ Lymphocyte Count
see Table 60–3
Patient Background
HIV transmission category
MSM: increased incidence of Kaposi sarcoma
IDU: increased incidence of bacterial pneumonia, tuberculosis, and IDU-related pulmonary complications
Habits: cigarette smoking—increased incidence of bacterial bronchitis, bacterial pneumonia, COPD, bronchogenic carcinoma
Travel and residence: assess risk for tuberculosis, endemic fungal diseases
Medical Background and Use of Prophylaxis
Prior disease increases incidence of recurrence: bacterial pneumonia, PCP, fungal pneumonias
Prophylaxis decreases incidence of disease: PCP, tuberculosis (if PPD+)
Symptoms and Signs
Respiratory symptoms: especially cough (productive or nonproductive) and symptom duration
Symptoms suggesting extrapulmonary or disseminated disease
Physical examination of chest: focal or nonfocal
Signs suggesting extrapulmonary or disseminated disease
Laboratory Tests
Arterial blood gas: nonspecific but useful for prognosis, management decisions (e.g., whether to hospitalize and whether corticosteroids are indicated for PCP)
White blood cell count: elevated or, if normal, elevated relative to baseline: bacterial pneumonia
Serum lactate dehydrogenase: elevated: nonspecific but classically seen in PCP
Chest Radiography
see Table 60–5

COPD, chronic obstructive pulmonary disease; IDU, injection drug users; MSM, men who have sex with men; PCP, *Pneumocystis carinii* pneumonia; PPD, purified protein derivative. URI, upper respiratory tract infection.
In HIV-infected persons, PPD is considered positive if ≥ 5 mm induration.
[a]Most frequent causes of respiratory illness among HIV-infected outpatients are from the multicenter Pulmonary Complications of HIV Infection Study.[2]
[b]Most frequent causes of pneumonia among HIV-infected persons hospitalized at San Francisco General Hospital 1996–1998 (Huang, unpublished data). PCP and *Streptococcus pneumoniae* were the two most common causes of community-acquired pneumonia among HIV-infected persons hospitalized at Johns Hopkins Hospital, 11/90 to 11/91.
[c]Most frequent causes of pneumonia among HIV-infected persons admitted to intensive care from the multicenter Pulmonary Complications of HIV Infection Study.[4]

causes of respiratory disease in patients with HIV infection.

▲ LOWER RESPIRATORY TRACT DISEASE: PNEUMONIA

One of the first issues with which clinicians must deal is whether to place a patient in isolation. Suspicion of tuberculosis, influenza, or respiratory syncytial virus (RSV) infection based on history, clinical presentation, radiography, or initial laboratory tests are examples of situations that would mandate respiratory (tuberculosis or influenza) or contact (RSV) isolation. Clinicians must be cognizant of the risk that transmissible respiratory pathogens pose to other patients, hospital staff, and visitors. It is far preferable to be liberal in the use of isolation precautions until the specific diagnosis is established than to risk the spread of transmissible pathogens.

HIV Transmission Category and Habits

A patient's HIV transmission category and habits influence the relative frequency of various HIV and non-HIV-associated pulmonary diseases (Table 60–2). Kaposi sarcoma is seen almost exclusively in men who report having sexual contact with other men (MSM).[7] Approximately 95% of the cases of HIV-associated Kaposi sarcoma occur in MSM; and although described in women, its occurrence is quite uncommon.[8] Bacterial pneumonia and tuberculosis are more common in HIV-infected patients who are injection drug users than in HIV-infected patients without a history of injection drug use. Hirschtick and colleagues in the PCHIS found that the rate of bacterial pneumonia was 11.1 episodes per 100 person-years among injection drug users, compared with 4.1 and 3.8 episodes per 100 person-years among MSM ($P < 0.001$) and female heterosexuals ($P = 0.003$), respectively.[9] Furthermore, injection or other illicit drug use can cause a variety of acute non-HIV-related pulmonary diseases (e.g., aspiration pneumonia secondary to central nervous system depression, endocarditis-related septic pulmonary emboli, drug-induced pulmonary edema) and a variety of chronic diseases (e.g., talc granulomatosis and pulmonary hypertension).[10]

As in the general population, HIV-infected patients who are cigarette smokers are at an increased risk of several respiratory illnesses. Bacterial bronchitis and pneumonia are more common in HIV-infected cigarette smokers than in HIV-infected nonsmokers or former smokers. This is especially true for persons with a CD4+ T-lymphocyte count of less than 200 cells/μl.[9] In addition, HIV-infected patients who report a long history of cigarette use may present with manifestations of chronic obstructive pulmonary disease (COPD) as the cause of their symptoms.[11] Most cases of lung cancer reported in HIV-infected patients have developed in persons with a history of cigarette smoking. One can speculate that the incidence of non-HIV-associated pulmonary conditions—many related to cigarette smoking—will increase among HIV-infected patients receiving highly active antiretroviral therapy (HAART) as they live longer and as the incidence of HIV-associated opportunistic infections (OIs) and neoplasms and the resulting mortality declines among them. As such, increased focus on strategies to reduce cigarette smoking is warranted.[12]

Travel and Residence

Tuberculosis is especially common in certain geographic areas and in certain populations.[13] HIV-infected patients who were born in or have traveled to a country with a high prevalence of tuberculosis and patients who are homeless, unstably housed, or previously incarcerated are at higher risk for exposure to *Mycobacterium tuberculosis*. Injection drug users, especially if anergic, are another population at increased risk for tuberculosis.[14] Patients who have a positive tuberculin skin test (defined as a ≥ 5 mm induration in HIV-infected persons), especially if recent converters, are also at increased risk for developing tuberculosis.[13, 15]

Travel to or residence in a geographic region that is endemic for fungi such as *Histoplasma capsulatum* or *Coccidioides immitis* is a strong determinant of the risk of exposure, infection, and ultimately disease. This may become increasingly important as the acquired immunodeficiency syndrome (AIDS) epidemic explodes in regions around the world that are host to fungi rarely if ever encountered in the United States (e.g., *Penicillium marneffei*).

Prior Illness and Use of Prophylaxis

Many HIV-associated OIs are recurrent. Recognition that bacterial pneumonias are common in HIV-infected patients and frequently recur led to the inclusion of recurrent pneumonia (i.e., more than two episodes within a 12-month period) as an AIDS-defining condition in the 1993 U.S. Centers for Disease Control and Prevention Expanded Surveillance Case Definition for AIDS.[16] Often patients with multiple, recurrent episodes of severe bacterial pneumonia develop airway damage or bronchiectasis, which in turn predisposes them to further bacterial infections.[11] I have seen numerous patients with severe bronchiectasis and recurrent bacterial infections that were the cause of repeated hospitalizations. Some such patients develop multidrug-resistant bacteria that are refractory to treatment.

Patients with prior PCP are at high risk for recurrence, and current recommendations advise secondary *P. carinii* prophylaxis unless antiretroviral therapy has produced a sustained CD4+ T-lymphocyte count of more than 200 cells/μl.[17,18] Similarly, patients with a history of cryptococcosis, coccidioidomycosis, or histoplasmosis are at high risk for relapse and should undergo maintenance therapy with fluconazole (cryptococcosis and coccidioidomycosis) or itraconazole (histoplasmosis).[18] Patients with a significant CD4+ T-lymphocyte count response to HAART might be able to discontinue secondary prophylaxis/maintenance therapy provided their cell count remains above the threshold associated with an increased risk of disease (e.g., 200 cells/μl for PCP). Data are currently being accumulated to determine whether maintenance therapy for fungal pneumonias can be safely discontinued if there is a satisfactory immunologic response to HAART.[18]

Chronic antimicrobial use clearly influences the likelihood of the targeted pathogen recurring, but it also affects the likelihood and the drug susceptibility of other organisms causing respiratory disease. For example, at San Francisco General Hospital, the dramatic rise in bacteria resistant to trimethoprim-sulfamethoxazole (TMP-SMZ) has coincided with use of TMP-SMZ for *P. carinii* prophylaxis.[19]

In HIV-infected patients, failure to adhere to recommended maintenance with the prescribed regimens frequently results in recurrent or relapsed disease. The corollary also can be used: Adherence to the prescribed regimen lessens the probability of disease, although even complete adherence to these regimens cannot completely prevent subsequent recurrence. HIV-infected patients, especially at the lowest CD4+ T-lymphocyte counts, may develop recurrent disease despite prophylaxis.

Current guidelines recommend pneumococcal vaccine and annual influenza immunization for all HIV-infected patients.[18] These preventive measures appear to be safe and effective in HIV-infected persons.[20–23] Their efficacy is best established in patients with CD4+ T-lymphocyte counts of more than 200 to 500 cells/μl and is likely to be diminished in patients with low CD4+ T-lymphocyte cell counts. One study of pneumococcal disease in Africa suggested increased morbidity and mortality among patients who received pneumococcal vaccine compared to those who did not.[22] These findings have not been satisfactorily explained or reproduced. Pneumococcal immunization should probably be repeated every 3 to 5 years and consideration given to repeat immunization for patients who were immunized prior to a rise in CD4+ T-lymphocyte counts induced by antiretroviral therapy.[23]

▲ **Table 60–3.** PRESENTATION OF BACTERIAL AND
▲ *PNEUMOCYSTIS CARINII* PNEUMONIA

Parameter	Bacteria	*Pneumocystis carinii*
CD4+ lymphocyte count	Any	≤ 200 cells/μl
Symptoms	Fever, chills or rigors	Fever
	Dyspnea	Dyspnea
	Pleuritic chest pain	
	Productive cough	Nonproductive cough
	Purulent sputum	
Symptom duration	Typically 3–5 days	Typically 2–4 weeks
Signs: lung examination	Focal findings	Often unremarkable
		Inspiratory crackles
Laboratory tests	WBC frequently elevated	WBC varies
	LDH varies	LDH frequently elevated
	ABG nonspecific[a]	ABG nonspecific
Chest radiography		
Distribution	Patchy, focal > multifocal	Diffuse > focal
Location	Unilateral, segmental/ lobar	Bilateral
Pattern	Consolidation	Reticular-granular
Associated findings		
Cysts	Rarely	15–20%
Pleural effusions	25–50%	Very rarely
Adenopathy	Rarely	Very rarely
Pneumothorax	Rarely	Occasionally
Normal radiograph	Never	Occasionally

ABG, arterial blood gases; LDH, lactate dehydrogenase; WBC, white blood cell count.

[a]Used to determine severity of disease and whether adjunctive corticosteroids are indicated.

Symptoms and Signs

As stated previously, the approach to respiratory disease in an HIV-infected patient begins with a thorough history and physical examination. Although nonspecific, constellations of particular symptoms and signs can often point to a specific diagnosis (Table 60–2).

The PCHIS demonstrated that respiratory symptoms are a frequent complaint in HIV-infected persons, and that symptoms increase in frequency as the CD4+ T-lymphocyte count decreases. In this study, subjects reported cough at 27% of more than 12,000 routine visits, dyspnea at 23%, and fever at 9% (Huang, unpublished data). These symptoms increased in frequency in the subset of subjects with a CD4+ T-lymphocyte count of less than 200 cells/μl.

All of the HIV-associated respiratory diseases may present with cough, dyspnea, and less frequently pleuritic chest pain. Particular aspects of these symptoms may be useful for suggesting a specific diagnosis. Most patients with bacterial bronchitis or pneumonia present with a cough productive of purulent sputum, whereas most patients with PCP note a dry, nonproductive cough.[11] In addition to the specific symptoms themselves, the duration of symptoms may also be useful. Bacterial pneumonias due to *Streptococcus pneumoniae* and *Haemophilus* spp. characteristically present with an acute onset and a symptom duration of 3 to 5 days. In contrast, PCP usually presents with a subacute, more insidious onset and a typical symptom duration of 2 to 4 weeks. Kovacs and coworkers found a median symptom duration of 28 days among 49 HIV-infected patients with PCP.[24] Thus, in an HIV-infected patient with a CD4+ T-lymphocyte count of less than 200 cells/μl (and hence at risk for both bacterial and *P. carinii* pneumonia), the presence of cough productive of purulent sputum of a few days' duration favors the diagnosis of bacterial infection (Table 60–3). In contrast, a nonproductive cough of a few weeks' duration strongly favors the diagnosis of PCP.

Clinicians should be aware of one caveat: Patients may have dual infections (bacterial infection and PCP). Afessa and colleagues reported that more than 10% of the 111 episodes of bacterial pneumonia reviewed were accompanied by PCP.[25] In my experience, a similar proportion (10%) of patients with PCP present with findings consistent with bacterial co-infection (Fig. 60–1). Although HIV-infected patients can present with multiple concurrent illnesses, extrapulmonary symptoms, when present, are often useful for suggesting a specific, unifying diagnosis, as many of the HIV-associated pulmonary diseases have important extrapulmonary manifestations. For example, the presence of

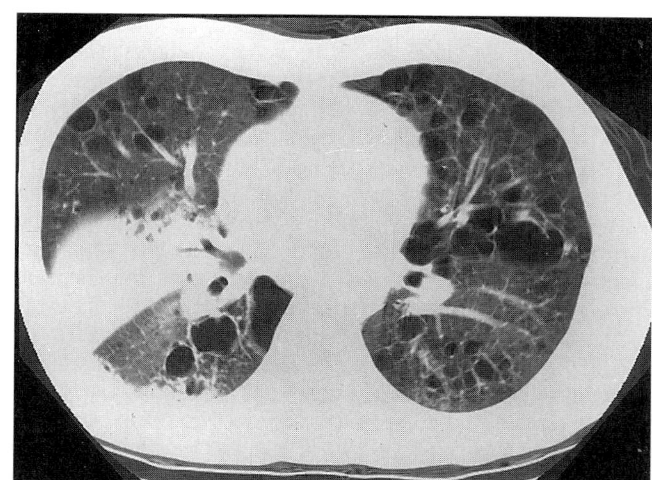

Figure 60–1. Chest computed tomographic (CT) scan of an HIV-infected patient, CD4+ T-lymphocyte count less than 200 cells/μl with multiple bilateral cysts secondary to *Pneumocystis carinii* and a focal alveolar consolidation secondary to *Streptococcus pneumoniae.*

headache in a patient with a CD4+ T-lymphocyte cell count of less than 200 cells/μl and respiratory complaints suggest the possibility of *Cryptococcus neoformans* meningitis and pneumonia. In fact, although the lungs are the portal of entry for *Cryptococcus*, many patients present with asymptomatic or minimally symptomatic pulmonary disease, and the diagnosis is only suggested by the presence of extrapulmonary symptoms. In a series of 106 patients with *C. neoformans* infection, 89 patients (84%) presented with meningitis; cough or dyspnea was present in fewer than one-third of these patients (n = 28, 31%).[26] In the National Institute of Allergy and Infectious Diseases Mycoses Study Group and the AIDS Clinical Trials Group study of treatment regimens for cryptococcal meningitis, 31% of the patients randomized to amphotericin B and 35% of those randomized to amphotericin B and flucytosine reported cough; 90% and 89% of the subjects, respectively, reported headache.

Knowledge of extrapulmonary disease can also be used occasionally to infer the pulmonary diagnosis without specific microbiologic or pathologic confirmation. For example, patients diagnosed with non-Hodgkin lymphoma from a biopsy of a nonpulmonary site who also have findings suggestive of thoracic involvement might potentially receive initial appropriate therapy for non-Hodgkin lymphoma and might have specific pulmonary diagnostic procedures reserved for situations where the pulmonary disease progresses despite this therapy.

Patients with pneumonia who are HIV-positive are usually febrile, tachycardic, and tachypneic. Evidence of systemic hypotension suggests a fulminant disease process (e.g., bacterial septicemia, the sepsis-like syndrome seen with disseminated histoplasmosis, or rarely PCP). Pulse oximetry provides a helpful estimate of the severity of the disease. The presence of exercise-induced oxygen desaturation is reported to be a sensitive (but not specific) indicator of PCP. Importantly, this simple test is often useful when making decisions regarding the need for hospitalization. Patients whose oxygen saturation declines on exertion are usually unable to care for themselves at home and are more likely to need respiratory support.

Patients with bacterial pneumonia often have focal lung examinations suggestive of consolidation, pleural effusion, or both, whereas patients with PCP may have bilateral inspiratory crackles (Table 60–3). Wheezing in a patient with a history of asthma suggests an exacerbation of that condition, whereas diminished breath sounds in a longtime cigarette smoker may indicate emphysema. Absent breath sounds suggest pneumothorax in a patient complaining of pleuritic chest pain, dyspnea, or both. Occasionally, abnormal findings on lung examination are the result of nonpulmonary disease. For example, rales in association with an S_3 cardiac gallop and elevated jugular venous pressure suggest a cardiac etiology for the respiratory complaints.

The remainder of the physical examination may also suggest an etiology for the respiratory symptoms. For example, in a patient whose CD4+ T-lymphocyte count is less than 200 cells/μl, an altered mental status may be secondary to *C. neoformans* meningitis, whereas a focal neurologic examination may be secondary to *T. gondii* encephalitis. Lymphadenopathy or hepatosplenomegaly suggests either disseminated mycobacterial or fungal disease or non-Hodgkin lymphoma. New cutaneous lesions may be manifestations of a disseminated fungal disease. The presence of mucocutaneous Kaposi sarcoma lesions may point toward pulmonary involvement with that disease. However, the absence of Kaposi sarcoma lesions on visual examination of the skin and mucous membranes does not preclude the possibility of significant visceral disease, including the lung. Huang and colleagues found that 15% of 168 patients with pulmonary Kaposi sarcoma diagnosed by bronchoscopy had no evidence of concurrent or preexisting mucocutaneous Kaposi sarcoma.[27]

Laboratory Tests

CD4+ T-Lymphocyte Counts

The CD4+ T-lymphocyte count is an excellent indicator of an HIV-infected patient's risk of developing a specific OI or neoplasm, and it remains an essential component of the approach to respiratory disease even during the era of HAART (Table 60–4). The CD4+ T-lymphocyte count is relevant to the occurrence of bacterial respiratory infections as well as more traditional OIs. Hirschtick and colleagues in the PCHIS found that the risk of bacterial pneumonia among subjects with a CD4+ T-lymphocyte count of less than 200 cells/μl was more than five and a half times greater than that for subjects whose count was more than 500 cells/μl[9]. In addition, as the CD4+ T-lymphocyte count decreases, the incidence of bacterial pneumonia accompanied by bacteremia or septicemia and of *Mycobacterium tuberculosis* infection accompanied by extrapulmonary or disseminated disease increase. It might also be noted that nonspecific interstitial pneumonitis (NSIP), whose clinical and chest radiographic features may be indistinguishable from PCP, differs from PCP in that NSIP may present at a CD4+ T-lymphocyte count of more than 200 cells/μl. In a

▲ **Table 60–4.** CD4+ LYMPHOCYTE COUNT RANGES FOR SELECTED
▲ RESPIRATORY DISEASES

Any CD4+ Lymphocyte Count
Upper respiratory tract infection
Acute bronchitis/sinusitis
Bacterial pneumonia (most often *Streptococcus pneumoniae*, *Haemophilus* spp.)
Mycobacterium tuberculosis pneumonia
Non-Hodgkin lymphoma
Bronchogenic carcinoma
Nonspecific interstitial pneumonitis
CD4+ Lymphocyte Count < 200 cells/μl
Pneumocystis carinii pneumonia
Cryptococcus neoformans pneumonia
Bacterial pneumonia accompanied by bacteremia or septicemia
Extrapulmonary or disseminated *M. tuberculosis*
CD4+ Lymphocyte Count < 100 cells/μl
Bacterial pneumonia due to *Pseudomonas aeruginosa*
Toxoplasma gondii pneumonia
Pulmonary Kaposi sarcoma
CD4+ Lymphocyte Count < 50 cells/μl
Histoplasma capsulatum: usually associated with disseminated disease
Coccidioides immitis: usually associated with disseminated disease
Aspergillus species (most often *A. fumigatus*) pneumonia
Cytomegalovirus pneumonia: usually associated with disseminated disease
Mycobacterium avium complex: usually associated with disseminated disease

series reported by Sattler and associates, the mean CD4+ T-lymphocyte count of 16 patients with nonspecific interstitial pneumonitis was 492 cells/μl[28].

At CD4+ T-lymphocyte counts of less than 200 cells/μl, PCP and *Cryptococcus neoformans* pneumonia become important diagnoses to consider, whereas neither is common in patients with counts that are significantly higher than 200 cells/μl. In a retrospective review of episodes of opportunistic pneumonia diagnosed at the Clinical Center of the National Institutes of Health, 46 of 49 patients (94%) diagnosed with PCP had a CD4+ T-lymphocyte count of less than 200 cells/μl.[29] The Multicenter AIDS Cohort Study demonstrated that subjects with a CD4+ T-lymphocyte count of less than 200 cells/μl had a nearly fivefold higher risk of developing PCP than subjects who had a count higher than 200 cells/μl at study entry.[30] Stansell et al. and the PCHIS confirmed these data and showed that 95% of the 145 cases of PCP occurred in subjects whose CD4+ T-lymphocyte count was less than 200 cells/μl (median count 29 cells/μl).[31] Darras-Joly et al. in a review of 76 patients with cryptococcal disease, found a mean CD4+ T-lymphocyte count of 46 cells/μl (range 2 to 220 cells/μl) in 65 patients with meningitis.[32] The median CD4+ T-lymphocyte counts among 381 patients with cryptococcal meningitis randomized to either amphotericin B alone or amphotericin B with flucytosine for initial treatment were 18 and 20 cells/μl, respectively.[33]

At CD4+ T-lymphocyte counts of less than 100 cells/μl, pulmonary diseases caused by *Pseudomonas aeruginosa*, *Toxoplasma gondii*, and Kaposi sarcoma are increasingly common. A study of 64 patients with pulmonary toxoplasmosis diagnosed by bronchoalveolar lavage (BAL) reported a mean CD4+ T-lymphocyte count of 40 cells/μl; 82% had a count of less than 50 cells/μl, and only 4% had a count of more than 200 cells/μl.[34] One series of 168 consecutive patients with pulmonary Kaposi sarcoma diagnosed by bronchoscopy reported a median CD4+ T-lymphocyte count of 19 cells/μl; 68% had a count below 50 cells/μl, and only 4% had a count above 200 cells/μl.[27] Finally, at CD4+ T-lymphocyte counts of less than 50 cells/μl, diseases may be caused by endemic fungi (*H. capsulatum, C. immitis*) and nonendemic fungi (*Aspergillus* spp.). Cytomegalovirus (CMV) and nontuberculous mycobacteria (*Mycobacterium kansasii*) also cause disease occasionally.

In many patients, especially those naive to antiretroviral drugs, the use of combinations of antiretroviral therapies has resulted in sustained increases in their CD4+ T-lymphocyte counts and concomitant declines in the incidence of OIs and mortality.[35,36] Often these CD4+ T-lymphocyte count increases are dramatic and cross from below to above characteristic thresholds associated with risk for a specific OI (e.g., 200 cells/μl for PCP). This raised questions as to which count (i.e., the current count above 200 cells/μl or the nadir count below 200 cells/μl) was the best indicator of a patient's risk for a specific OI. Numerous studies have indicated that the current CD4+ T-lymphocyte count is the best reflection of the risk for a specific OI.[37] For PCP, several studies have demonstrated that it is safe to discontinue primary or secondary *P. carinii* prophylaxis in HIV-infected subjects whose CD4+ T-lymphocyte count has risen from below to above 200 cells/μl.[17,38–44] However, I have seen one memorable case of PCP that occurred 5 years after the initial episode and that developed despite a count that had been higher than 200 cells/μl for more than 3 years while the patient was receiving HAART. This patient previously had been able to discontinue treatment successfully for disseminated *Mycobacterium avium* complex and disseminated fungal disease without relapse. Yet, despite a CD4+ T-lymphocyte count of 300 cells/μl just prior to the onset of PCP, PCP developed 4 months after secondary *P. carinii* prophylaxis was discontinued. Thus, although important, the CD4+ T-lymphocyte count should be a guide as to which pulmonary diseases are most common in that population. Exceptions to such guidelines occurred before the era of HAART, and exceptions continue to occur.

Arterial Blood Gases

Arterial blood gas (ABG) analysis is indicated for persons with clinical evidence of moderate to severe pulmonary disease (Table 60–2). Laboratory tests that may be useful for suggesting a specific diagnosis include the white blood cell (WBC) count and differential as part of the complete blood count and the serum lactate dehydrogenase (LDH) assay. Beyond their potential use as part of the diagnostic evaluation, these tests serve as prognostic markers and baseline values for subsequent measurements. Serial measurements are useful in any patient who fails to improve or who worsens despite apparent appropriate therapy. ABG analysis is useful for prognosis and for making clinical decisions regarding whether (and where) to admit the patient and whether adjunctive corticosteroids are indicated in patients with PCP.

White Blood Cell Count

Even for patients with HIV infection, the WBC count is frequently elevated in persons with bacterial infection. This elevation may be relative to the patient's baseline value; that is, an elevation from 2000 cells/μl to 6000 cells/μl suggests a bacterial process. Frequently, a left shift is also present in persons with bacterial infection. HIV-infected patients with neutropenia are at high risk for bacterial infections and fungal infections such as those caused by *Aspergillus* spp. Pancytopenia suggests the presence of an infectious or neoplastic process in the bone marrow.

Serum Lactate Dehydrogenase

Serum LDH is often (but not invariably) elevated in patients with PCP.[11] However, LDH may also be elevated in other pulmonary (including bacterial pneumonia and tuberculosis) and nonpulmonary conditions, making this test more useful for prognosis than diagnosis. Most of the studies reporting a high sensitivity of serum LDH for PCP consisted of hospitalized patients, some of whom had acute respiratory failure and were mechanically ventilated. The study that reported the lowest sensitivity examined outpatients presenting to an urgent care clinic.[45] This suggests that the severity of PCP and the patient population studied affect the diagnostic sensitivity of the test.

The degree to which serum LDH is elevated has been shown to correlate with prognosis and response to therapy.[11] Patients with PCP and an initial markedly elevated serum LDH level or a rising serum LDH level despite PCP treatment have a poor prognosis. Patients with PCP that is responding to treatment usually have a decline in their LDH toward the normal range.[46]

Imaging

Standard Chest Radiography

The characteristic chest radiographic findings for selected HIV-associated pulmonary diseases are presented in Table 60–5. For each disease, the findings from a large series ($n > 30$ cases) are presented as an overview. When no large series has been reported, summary data from smaller series are provided. Differences in the description of radiographic findings and the absence of a standardized approach to interpreting and presenting radiographic data limit the ability to combine studies on a specific pulmonary disease into a single summary table.

Bacterial pneumonia is the most common pulmonary disease among HIV-infected persons in the United States. The chest radiographic presentation is similar to that of the overall population: focal, segmental, or lobar consolidation. One study reported that of 55 patients with bacterial pneumonia 40% presented with focal, segmental, or lobar alveolar infiltrates, whereas 38% had diffuse reticulonodular infiltrates, 16% had focal reticulonodular infiltrates, and 5% had nodular or cavitary infiltrates on the chest radiograph.[47] Another study of 99 patients found that 54% of the patients with bacterial pneumonia had a lobar infiltrate, 17% had an interstitial infiltrate, 10% had a nodular infiltrate, and only 1% had a cavitary infiltrate on their radiograph. Pleural effusions were seen in 7% and intrathoracic adenopathy in 2%.[48] In this study, multivariate analysis demonstrated that the presence of a lobar infiltrate on chest radiograph was independently predictive of bacterial pneumonia. These studies, however, considered all bacterial pathogens together. Numerous reports as well as clinical experience demonstrate that the frequency of specific radiographic findings is dependent on the specific bacteria.

Studies suggest that radiographic presentations may differ among *Streptococcus pneumoniae*, *Haemophilus* spp., and *Pseudomonas aeruginosa*.[3,9,49] A review of all English-language articles and abstracts from 1981 to 1990 on *S. pneumoniae* disease in HIV-infected persons found that three-fourths of bacterial pneumonias due to *S. pneumoniae* presented with segmental, lobar, or multilobar consolidation on chest radiography.[50] Garcia-Leoni et al. reported that a classic lobar alveolar pattern was seen in 67% and a diffuse alveolar pattern in 10% of 21 patients with *S. pneumoniae* pneumonia.[51] Schlamm and Yancovitz found similar proportions in 34 patients with *H. influenzae* pneumonia; in this study, focal or diffuse lobar infiltrates were noted in 74%.[52] However, another series of 12 patients with *H. influenzae* pneumonia discovered that the presentation may be clinically and radiographically indistinguishable from that of PCP.[53] The patients in this series complained of nonproductive cough and dyspnea with a median symptom duration of 4 weeks. All presented with bilateral interstitial or mixed interstitial-alveolar infiltrates similar to PCP. Cordero et al. found that 35% of 26 patients with *H. influenzae* pneumonia presented with an interstitial pattern on chest radiograph.[54] A series of 16 patients with *P. aeruginosa* pneumonia showed that the pneumonia was community-acquired in 15 patients (94%).[55] Chest radiographs revealed cavitary infiltrates on admission in 50%, and an additional 19% presented with pulmonary infiltrates that subsequently cavitated. The frequency of cavitary infiltrates in *P. aeruginosa* pneumonia was also noted in a study of 25 patients: 24% had cavitary pneumonia.[56] Thus the presence of a cavitary pneumonia may be more suggestive of *Pseudomonas* than either *Streptococcus* or *Haemophilus*. However, the differential diagnosis of a pulmonary cavity is extensive and includes tuberculosis, endemic fungal diseases, and *Rhodococcus equi*.

Pneumonia due to bacteria such as *Legionella* spp., *Mycoplasma pneumoniae*, and *Chlamydia* spp. occurs in HIV-infected patients.[57–59] The frequency of these pathogens as causes of community-acquired pneumonia in HIV-infected patients appears to parallel that among HIV-uninfected patients. A study in Baltimore performed extensive diagnostic testing on 180 HIV-infected patients: *Legionella pneumophila* (3%), *Chlamydia pneumoniae* (4%), and *Mycoplasma pneumoniae* (<1%) were rarely detected.[3] The frequency of these pathogens matched that among the 205 HIV-uninfected patients (3%, 3%, and 1%, respectively) admitted during the same period.

Rhodococcus equi and *Nocardia* spp. (especially *N. asteroides*) have been described as causes of pneumonia in HIV-infected patients.[60,61] Neither is recognized often.

Pneumocystis carinii pneumonia remains a common AIDS-defining opportunistic infection in the United States.

▲ **Table 60–5.** CHARACTERISTIC CHEST RADIOGRAPHIC FINDINGS FOR SELECTED PULMONARY DISEASES[a]

Pulmonary Disease	Author (year)	No. of Patients	Distribution (%)	Pattern (%)	Associated Findings (%)
Bacteria[b]	Magnenat[47] (1991)	55		Alveolar (40%) Diffuse (38%) or focal (16%) reticulonodular Nodular/cavitary (5%)	
Bacteria[b]	Selwyn[48] (1998)	99	Focal (71%), Diffuse (29%)	Lobar (54%) Interstitial (17%) Nodular (10%)/ Cavitary (1%)	Pleural effusion (7%) Adenopathy (2%)
P. carinii[c]	DeLorenzo[62] (1987)	104	Bilateral (95%), Diffuse (48%)	Interstitial or mixed (87.5%) Alveolar (12.5%)	Cysts (7%) Honeycomb lesions (4%)
M. tuberculosis, CD4+ <200 cells/μl	Abouya[66] (1995)	45	Miliary (9%)	Cavitary (29%) Noncavitary (58%)	Adenopathy (20%) Pleural effusion (11%)
M. tuberculosis, CD4+ 200–399 cells/μl	Abouya[66] (1995)	36	Miliary (6%)	Cavitary (44%) Noncavitary (44%)	Adenopathy (14%) Pleural effusion (11%)
M. tuberculosis, CD4+ ≥400 cells/μl	Abouya[66] (1995)	30	Miliary (0%)	Cavitary (63%) Noncavitary (33%)	Adenopathy (0%) Pleural effusion (3%)
M. tuberculosis, CD4+ <200 cells/μl	Perlman[67] (1997)	98	Normal (9%)	Infiltrate (52%) Cavitary (7%) Interstitial (27%) Nodules(s) (18%)	Adenopathy (30%) Pleural effusion (7%)
M. tuberculosis, CD4+ ≥200 cells/μl	Perlman[67] (1997)	30	Normal (3%)	Infiltrate (67%) Cavitary (20%) Interstitial (17%) Nodules(s) (20%)	Adenopathy (7%) Pleural effusion (10%)
C. neoformans	Batungwanayo[78] (1994)	37	Diffuse (76%)	Interstitial or mixed (76%) Alveolar (19%) Nodular/nodules (5%)	Cavitation (11%) Adenopathy (11%) Pleural effusion (5%)
C. neoformans	Meyohas[91] (1995) (plus review)	17	Normal (6%)	Interstitial (76%) Alveolar (35%) Nodular (6%)	Cavitation (12%) Adenopathy (18%) Pleural effusion (24%)
Cytomegalovirus	Salomon[93] (1997)	18	Normal (33%)	Reticular-granular (33%) Alveolar (22%) Nodular (11%)	Cavitation (11%) Cyst (6%) Pleural effusion (33%) Adenopathy (11%)
Cytomegalovirus	Rodriguez-Barradas[92] (1996)	17	Bilateral (71%), Unilateral (29%)	Interstitial (82%) Alveolar (18%)	Pleural effusion (12%)
T. gondii	Rabaud[34] (1996)	43	Normal (23%), Bilateral (58%)	Interstitial (53%) Nodular (16%)	Pleural effusion (7%) Pneumothorax (2%)
Kaposi sarcoma	Gruden[122] (1995)	76	Normal (3%), Bilateral (96%), Diffuse or mid-lower lung zones (92%)	BWT± coalescence (95%) Nodules (78%)	Kerley B lines (71%) Pleural effusion (53%) Adenopathy (16%)
Non-Hodgkin lymphoma	Eisner[95] (1996)	38	Normal (3%)	Nodules (40%) or mass (24%), Lobar (40%), Reticular (24%)	Cavitation (3%) Pleural effusion (44%) Adenopathy (21%)

BWT, bronchial wall thickening; CD4+, CD4+ T-lymphocyte count.

[a]Chest radiograph presentations can vary significantly depending on a number of factors, including severity of disease and use of prophylaxis.

[b]The characteristic chest radiograph presentation is influenced by the specific bacteria (see text).

[c]Although the largest chest radiographic series, this study predates the widespread use of *P. carinii* prophylaxis. Multiple studies have documented "atypical" upper lung zone findings in patients receiving aerosolized pentamidine prophylaxis. At present it is unclear what, if any, effect oral prophylaxis regimens (trimethoprim-sulfamethoxazole, dapsone, and atovaquone) have on the chest radiographic presentation.

The classic PCP presentation is bilateral interstitial-reticular or granular opacities that are often diffuse. One large study of 104 patients with PCP revealed that 87.5% presented with an interstitial pattern (75.0%) or a mixed interstitial-alveolar pattern (12.5%); the remaining patients had an alveolar pattern.[62] In addition, 7% had thin-walled cysts (i.e., pneumatoceles), and 4% had honeycomb lesions. Infiltrates were bilateral in 95% and unilateral in 5%; they involved the entire lung in 48%. This study remains the largest radiology series of patients with PCP; it predates the widespread use of *P. carinii* prophylaxis. Since then, a number of reports have described the radiographic findings in patients receiving aerosolized pentamidine (AP) prophylaxis; these radiographs characteristically reveal an upper lung zone predominance that can mimic mycobacterial disease.[63] In my experience, however, this upper lung zone predominance can also be seen in patients who have never received AP prophylaxis, and the pattern seen (i.e., reticular or granular) is more important than the distribution for suggesting the diagnosis of PCP.[64] In the PCHIS study, 467 subjects presenting for evaluation of new or worsening respiratory complaints underwent chest radiography. In a multivariate analysis of the 174 subjects with an abnormal radiograph, the presence of interstitial infiltrates on the chest radiograph was an independent predictor of PCP.

Tuberculosis can present with a variety of chest radiographic findings, including upper lung-zone infiltrates often with cavitation, middle or lower lung zone consolidation mimicking bacterial pneumonia, miliary disease, nodule(s), pleural effusions, and intrathoracic adenopathy. Tuberculosis may also present with a normal chest radiograph. The frequency of these findings is influenced by the patient's CD4+ T-lymphocyte count. Jones and colleagues reported that mediastinal adenopathy was found in 13% of the 30 patients with a CD4+ T-lymphocyte count higher than 200 cells/μl compared with 36% of the 58 patients with a count less than 200 cells/μl ($P = 0.02$).[65] Abouya and coworkers reviewed the chest radiographic presentation of 111 patients with tuberculosis. The proportion of patients with cavitary infiltrates decreased as the CD4+ T-lymphocyte count decreased from more than 400 cells/μl to 200 to 399 cells/μl, and then to less than 200 cells/μl ($P < 0.05$), whereas the proportions with noncavitary infiltrates and intrathoracic adenopathy increased as the count decreased (both $P < 0.05$).[66] Perlman and colleagues in the Terry Beirn Community Programs for Clinical Research on AIDS (CPCRA) and the AIDS Clinical Trials Group (ACTG) pooled data from 128 patients with culture-positive tuberculosis.[67] When they combined their data with those from published studies, the authors found a significant association between the presence of infiltrates, cavitation (both more likely in patients with a CD4+ T-lymphocyte count of 200 cells/μl or more), and intrathoracic adenopathy (more likely in patients with a count of less than 200 cells/μl). Thus the radiographic key to the diagnosis of tuberculosis is knowledge of the patient's CD4+ T-lymphocyte count and an understanding of which patterns are more common at that count.

Pulmonary Kaposi sarcoma characteristically presents with bilateral opacities in a central or perihilar distribution and a middle/lower lung zone predominance. Linear densities, nodules, and pleural effusions are all common. In a study of 76 patients with HIV-related pulmonary Kaposi sarcoma, 95% of the chest radiographs had peribronchial cuffing and tram track opacities (45%) or had extensive perihilar coalescent opacities. Small nodules (50%) or nodular opacities (28%) were seen in 78%, Kerley B lines in 71%, and pleural effusions in 53% of the radiographs.[122] No patient presented with either Kerley B lines or pleural effusions without concurrent parenchymal findings. Sixteen percent of these patients had hilar or mediastinal lymph node enlargement.

Chest Computed Tomography

For most evaluations of symptomatic HIV-infected patients, a computed tomography (CT) scan is unnecessary because the clinical and chest radiographic presentation suggests a single diagnosis or a few diagnoses to consider.[68, 69] In my experience, high-resolution CT (HRCT) is extremely useful in cases of clinically suspected PCP in which the chest radiograph is normal or unchanged, a phenomenon that occurred in 39% of one reported series.[70] Most patients with respiratory symptoms suggestive of PCP whose radiograph is normal or unchanged do not have PCP. Subjecting these patients to diagnostic procedures such as bronchoscopy or to empiric PCP treatment with its associated toxicities is ill-advised. In these cases a sensitive test is needed to select which patients require diagnostic procedures or empiric therapy and, just as important, which patients can be observed without either of the above. The chest HRCT scan is one of several such tests. Patients with PCP and a normal chest radiograph have patchy areas of ground-glass opacities (GGOs) on HRCT.[68, 69] Although the presence of GGOs is nonspecific and may be seen with a number of pulmonary disorders, its absence strongly argues against the presence of PCP. In one study, none of the 40 HIV-infected patients with clinically suspected PCP, a normal or nonspecific chest radiograph, and an HRCT without GGOs had PCP diagnosed by BAL fluid examination or 60 days of clinical follow-up.[71] In fact, in my experience, no patient with a normal chest radiograph and an HRCT without GGOs has been diagnosed with PCP at San Francisco General Hospital.

Chest CT can also be useful for suggesting a diagnosis in cases in which the chest radiograph reveals multiple pulmonary nodules. A predominance of nodules smaller than 1 cm in diameter in a centrilobular distribution strongly suggests the presence of an opportunistic infection, whereas a predominance of nodules larger than 1 cm in diameter is suggestive of a neoplasm.[72, 73] In cases where the nodules are mostly smaller than 1 cm in diameter, the presence of intrathoracic adenopathy, especially if low attenuation (another potential use for CT) indicates that mycobacterial (or fungal) disease is probable. In cases in which the nodules are mostly larger than 1 cm, the finding of associated peribronchovascular thickening inevitably results in a diagnosis of pulmonary Kaposi sarcoma. Finally, chest CT scans are useful for guiding diagnostic procedures such as bronchoscopy, CT-guided transthoracic needle aspiration, and surgical procedures.

Gallium 67 Scans

Gallium scans are sensitive but nonspecific indicators of PCP. The sensitivity and specificity for PCP depend in part on the criteria used to define a positive scan. When a positive test is defined as any gallium uptake (1+) over the lung parenchyma, the sensitivity and specificity of gallium for PCP have been reported to be 99% and 50%, respectively.[74] However, using more stringent criteria and defining a positive test as one with uptake equal to (3+) or greater than (4+) that of the liver, the sensitivity of gallium for PCP decreases to 60% (although the specificity increases to 80%). In either case, given the inherent time delays for obtaining results from gallium scans and the availability of HRCT and pulmonary function tests, gallium scans are rarely used at San Francisco General Hospital for evaluating AIDS-related pulmonary disease.[75]

One situation where gallium scans can be extremely useful is for evaluation of a patient with suspected pulmonary Kaposi sarcoma in whom bronchoscopy fails to document endobronchial Kaposi sarcoma lesions. The reason for this is that Kaposi sarcoma, unlike opportunistic infections, non-Hodgkin lymphoma, and lymphocytic interstitial pneumonitis, is gallium-negative. Thus in an HIV-infected patient with mucocutaneous Kaposi sarcoma and a chest radiograph suggestive of pulmonary Kaposi sarcoma, a negative gallium scan is strongly suggestive of pulmonary Kaposi sarcoma. In a patient with known pulmonary Kaposi sarcoma who develops progressive respiratory complaints and a worsening chest radiograph, a negative gallium scan indicates that progressive Kaposi sarcoma is the probable etiology rather than a superimposed opportunistic infection.

Pulmonary Function Tests

In HIV-infected patients complaining of dry cough or dyspnea whose chest radiograph is normal, spirometry may diagnose airflow obstruction that may be responsive to bronchodilators.[76] In patients with PCP, pulmonary function testing often reveals decreased lung volumes and increased airflow. In addition, the diffusing capacity for carbon monoxide (DL_{co}) is a sensitive but nonspecific indicator of PCP, and a normal DL_{co} makes the diagnosis of PCP unlikely. Huang and colleagues in the PCHIS demonstrated that the combination of a chest radiograph followed by determination of the DL_{co} if the radiograph was normal or unchanged identified more than 97% of the 80 cases of PCP.[64] The sensitivity of a DL_{co} less than 75% of predicted after a normal or unchanged radiograph was 90% (specificity was 53%).

Although the DL_{co} can be useful for evaluating symptomatic patients, it has no role as a screening test to detect, for example, early PCP in asymptomatic individuals. In an evaluation of 64 patients who experienced more than a 20% decrease in their DL_{co} from a baseline value in the absence of new respiratory symptoms or new chest radiographic findings, none of the patients was found to have PCP or other opportunistic infection on sputum induction, bronchoscopy, or clinical follow-up.[77] Care should be taken, especially with HIV-infected patients given their varied clinical and radiographic presentations, to exclude a diagnosis of tuberculosis before pulmonary function testing.

Microbiologic Tests

Blood Culture

Because *Streptococcus pneumoniae* is the most frequent cause of bacterial pneumonia and pneumococcal pneumonia is often accompanied by bacteremia (especially when the CD4+ T-lymphocyte count is less than 200 cells/μl), blood cultures should always be obtained in cases of suspected bacterial pneumonia (Table 60–6). When positive, blood cultures are specific for the diagnosis and, in an era of increasing antibiotic resistance, the utility of drug susceptibility testing cannot be overemphasized.

Serology

The serum cryptococcal antigen (CRAG) is an extremely sensitive and specific test for the presence of cryptococcemia and cryptococcal meningitis. However, the serum CRAG assay may be negative in HIV-infected patients who

▲ **Table 60–6.** DIAGNOSTIC TESTS FOR SELECTED PULMONARY DISEASES

Pulmonary Disease	Serology or Blood Cultures	Sputum	BAL ± TBBX	Pleural Fluid	Important Other Sites[a]	Suggestive Tests
Bacteria	**Blood cultures (esp. *S. pneumoniae*)**	**Gram stain and culture**	Rarely quantitative cultures	Consider (esp. if concern for empyema)		
M. tuberculosis	**Blood cultures**	**AFB smear and culture × 3**	Occasionally BAL and TBBX	Consider (with biopsy)	Lymph nodes, bone marrow	
P. carinii	No	**Induced sputum examination**	**BAL ± TBBX** (depends on respective sensitivities at institution)	Rarely		HRCT-GGO; PFTs-↓ DL_{co}, gallium ↑ uptake; O_2 sat. ↓ with exercise
C. neoformans	**Serum CRAG[b] Blood cultures**	Occasionally	**BAL**	Rarely	Cerebrospinal fluid, skin	
Cytomegalovirus	?CMV-PCR	No	**TBBX**	No	Retina, GI tract	
T. gondii	*T. gondii* IgG, IgM	Occasionally	**BAL**	Rarely	Central nervous system	Head CT/MRI with multiple lesions
Kaposi sarcoma	?HHV-8	No	**Visualization of lesions ± TBBX**	No	Mucocutaneous	Gallium-negative
Non-Hodgkin lymphoma	No	No	**TBBX, Wang needle**	**Cytology, biopsy**	Extranodal disease	

Tests in **Boldface** are usual diagnostic tests of choice. Other tests should be considered if tests of choice are nondiagnostic.
AFB, acid-fast bacilli; BAL, bronchoalveolar lavage; CRAG, cryptococcal antigen; CT, Computed tomography; DL_{co}, diffusing capacity for carbon monoxide; GGO, ground-glass opacities; GI, gastrointestinal; HHV-8, human herpes virus-8 (Kaposi sarcoma herpes virus, KS-HV); HRCT, chest high-resolution computed tomography; MRI, Magnetic resonance imaging; PFTs, pulmonary function tests; TBBX, transbronchial biopsies;
[a]Many of the pulmonary diseases present with important extrapulmonary sites of involvement that may dominate the clinical presentation. In such cases, pulmonary disease (if classic presentation) may be presumed in selected patients if the diagnosis is established from another site.
[b]The serum CRAG may be negative in isolated cryptococcal pneumonia.

have isolated cryptococcal pneumonia. In a study of 37 HIV-infected patients with cryptococcal pneumonia, the serum CRAG was positive in only 8 of 26 patients (31%).[78] A serum CRAG assay should be performed on all patients with suspected cryptococcal disease; patients with a positive CRAG assay should have an evaluation to determine the extent of disease (i.e., lumbar puncture for possible meningitis), whereas those with a negative CRAG assay but respiratory complaints or chest radiograph findings should undergo further pulmonary evaluation (i.e., bronchoscopy with BAL) for possible isolated cryptococcal pneumonia.

The *Histoplasma capsulatum* polysaccharide antigen test is a sensitive and specific test for the presence of histoplasmosis. The antigen can be measured in blood and other fluids including BAL.[79] In a study of 64 patients with pulmonary toxoplasmosis, *Toxoplasma* immunoglobulin G (IgG) was positive in 55 of 60 cases (92%) for which prior serology results were available.[34] An additional three patients (5%) in this study seroconverted (IgA, IgM, and IgG all detected after previous negative results) at the time that toxoplasmosis was diagnosed, whereas the final two patients (3%) remained seronegative even after diagnosis. Thus a negative *Toxoplasma* IgG assay makes the diagnosis of toxoplasmosis unlikely but not unprecedented.

Sputum

The Infectious Diseases Society of America recommendation that a sputum Gram stain and culture be obtained for all patients with suspected community-acquired bacterial pneumonia is entirely appropriate for HIV-infected patients as well.[80–82] Similar to HIV-uninfected persons, the diagnostic sensitivity of sputum culture for bacteria is low. Hirschtick and colleagues demonstrated that sputum culture identified a specific bacterial pathogen in approximately 40% of cases of bacterial pneumonia,[9] and Mundy and associates were unable to identify any pathogen in 26% of cases of community-acquired pneumonia.[3]

Most patients with PCP have a dry, nonproductive cough. In patients able to expectorate an adequate specimen, the yield of expectorated (rather than induced) sputum for PCP is approximately 50%.[83] However, in most cases, sputum cannot be produced unless it is induced. This can be accomplished by inhaling hypertonic saline via a hand-held nebulizer. Sputum induction should be performed in a properly engineered room to minimize transmission of infectious microorganisms. Sputum induction is a sensitive diagnostic test for PCP, with a reported sensitivity ranging from 55% in early studies to 95% when specimens are carefully obtained, concentrated by centrifugation, and stained with fluorescent antibody.[84,85] There is no difference in the sensitivity of induced sputum examination for PCP between patients on aerosolized pentamidine and those on no prophylaxis; nor is there a difference in the sensitivity of induced sputum examination whether the PCP episode was a first or second episode. These results taken together imply that sputum induction can be used in a number of clinical settings and that its success is not limited to a few institutions, a specific staining technique, or a particular clinical situation. At San Francisco General Hospital and at the National Institutes of Health, the use of sputum induction has permitted 80% to 95% of the PCP cases to be definitively diagnosed without resorting to bronchoscopy.[84,85] In a review of 992 episodes of PCP over a 4-year period, sputum induction accounted for 800 of the 992 (80%) diagnoses.[84] In addition, induced sputum aided in the diagnosis of tuberculosis and fungal pneumonias, bacterial bronchitis, and bronchopneumonia. Thus sputum induction should be the initial diagnostic test for patients with pulmonary disease at institutions where it is available.

Sputum acid-fast bacilli (AFB) smear and culture are the foundations for the diagnosis of pulmonary tuberculosis. Sputum should be obtained on three consecutive days, ideally from the first morning specimen produced. Expectorated sputum is appropriate for patients with a productive cough, and sputum induction should be performed for those patients with a nonproductive or minimally productive cough. Several studies report that the sensitivity of sputum AFB smears and cultures in HIV-infected patients are similar to those seen in the overall population. The sensitivity of sputum AFB smears for *Mycobacterium tuberculosis* ranged from 50% to 60% in two large series; the sensitivity of sputum AFB smears in persons presenting with disseminated disease was 90%.[86,87] Thus, all patients with suspected tuberculosis, even if respiratory complaints are minimal and chest radiograph findings are absent, should have three sputum specimens submitted for AFB smears and culture.

One caveat regarding AFB smears and cultures: A positive sputum AFB smear can be due to a nontuberculous mycobacteria such as *M. kansasii*, *M. avium* complex, *M. chelonei*, or *M. gordonae*. The latter three organsims are rarely pathogenic.[88] The positive predictive value of a sputum AFB smear for *M. tuberculosis* depends in part on the relative frequencies of the other mycobacteria in that population.

Mycobacterium avium complex (MAC) and the identification of MAC from a single sputum or BAL specimen cannot be presumed to indicate that MAC is causing the pulmonary pathology. In fact, one review of 200 HIV-infected patients with disseminated MAC found evidence for pulmonary disease in only five individuals.[89] *Mycobacterium kansasii* has been reported to present in a clinical and radiographic pattern indistinguishable from that of tuberculosis.[90] *M. kansasii* should always be presumed to be a real pathogen when it is isolated. However, I have seen several cases where patients had *M. kansasii* cultured from sputum, yet the patients resolved their clinical complaints and chest radiograph findings without specific antimycobacterial therapy. *Mycobacterium gordonae* almost always represents a laboratory contaminant from a water source or from the laboratory. Nevertheless, any patient whose sputum smear reveals AFB must be approached as if it represents *M. tuberculosis*, and appropriate management (i.e., respiratory isolation if hospitalized, strong consideration for initiation of tuberculosis therapy) must be maintained until a definitive diagnosis is established. The use of molecular techniques such as direct amplification probes that are specific for *M. tuberculosis* can dramatically shorten the time until diagnosis. Finally, sputum AFB specimens should be sent for culture, regardless of the results of the AFB smear, and all *M. tuberculosis* isolates should be sent for drug susceptibility testing.

Sputum examination, culture, or both can be used occasionally to diagnose fungal pneumonias, including those due to *C. neoformans*, *H. capsulatum*, and *C. immitis*, but not invasive *Aspergillus* spp. disease. It can be used to diagnose *Toxoplasma gondii* and other parasitic pneumonias (e.g., *Strongyloides stercoralis*) as well.

Bronchoscopy

In general, bronchoscopy should be considered for any HIV-infected patient with pulmonary disease for which the severity warrants a prompt and accurate diagnosis, for patients with suspected pulmonary Kaposi sarcoma, for patients in whom the diagnosis is unclear despite less invasive diagnostic tests (e.g., sputum), and for those who are failing empiric therapy for a presumed pathogen.

Bronchoscopy with BAL is the gold standard diagnostic test for PCP and the initial test of choice at institutions where sputum induction is either unavailable or its sensitivity is low. Numerous studies have reported that the sensitivity of BAL for PCP is 95% to 98%. At San Francisco General Hospital we perform bronchoscopy with BAL for patients with suspected PCP whose induced sputum examination is negative. In a review of 992 cases of PCP diagnosed over a 4-year period, Huang and colleagues found that only two of the episodes (0.2%) were diagnosed by transbronchial biopsy (TBBX) alone; all of the remaining cases were diagnosed by sputum induction (n = 800) or BAL (n = 190).[84] This is not to imply that TBBX is an insensitive test for PCP; rather, it demonstrates that most cases of PCP can be diagnosed by other less invasive (e.g., sputum induction) or risky (e.g., BAL) procedures. To estimate the sensitivity of BAL for PCP, the authors of this study reviewed the medical records of 100 randomly selected patients who had both a negative induced sputum and a negative BAL fluid examination for *Pneumocystis carinii* and had no other diagnosis established. The authors found that two patients were diagnosed with PCP during the 60 days after their negative BAL; one was diagnosed 46 days after the negative BAL and the other 51 days after. These results suggest that BAL alone is sufficient to diagnose almost all cases of PCP and that it is both sensitive and specific. It is important to note, however, that there are institutional differences in the sensitivity of the BAL examination. At institutions where the yields of BAL and TBBX are complementary and procedure-related complications are rare, both procedures are warranted.

Bronchoscopy is an important test for diagnosing cryptococcal pneumonia, especially if the disease is limited to the lungs. Batungwanayo and coworkers reported that BAL fluid culture was positive in 27 of 33 HIV-infected patients (82%) with cryptococcal pneumonia.[78] These results are similar to those reported by Meyohas and colleagues in which 23 of 27 HIV-infected patients (85%) with pulmonary cryptococcosis had a positive BAL fluid culture.[91] In this study, two of the patients with a negative BAL fluid culture had a positive BAL CRAG assay, and the remaining two had pleural cryptococcosis that was diagnosed by pleural fluid culture and pleural fluid CRAG assay.

Bronchoscopy with visual inspection of the airways is the procedure of choice for the diagnosis of pulmonary Kaposi sarcoma.[27] In these patients, neither endobronchial biopsy nor TBBX adds to the yield when characteristic Kaposi sarcoma lesions are seen. However, the absence of visible Kaposi sarcoma lesions does not preclude their presence in more distal airways, nor does it preclude the possibility of parenchymal Kaposi sarcoma involvement. In these patients TBBX can occasionally establish the diagnosis, but a diagnosis of Kaposi sarcoma may be difficult for the pathologist to establish with TBBX because of the small size of the sample and the crush artifact the procedure produces. In some cases open lung biopsy is indicated.

The TBBX can improve the diagnostic yield for mycobacterial and fungal pneumonias. In addition, TBBX or open lung biopsy is required to establish the diagnosis of CMV pneumonia.[92,93] Tissue from TBBX should reveal evidence of CMV inclusions and virologic changes. The isolation of CMV from BAL fluid or lung tissue cannot distinguish between asymptomatic viral shedding and pneumonia.[94] Similarly, biopsy is an important tool for diagnosing pulmonary non-Hodgkin lymphoma.[95]

Occasionally, endobronchial lesions are encountered on bronchoscopic visualization.[96] The clinical presentation and endobronchial appearance of these lesions may suggest the correct diagnosis. In these cases, establishing an appropriate differential diagnosis at the time of visualization is important, as certain lesions require specific biopsy techniques, and several etiologies require special stains.

Other Procedures

Diagnostic thoracentesis should be considered for any HIV-infected patient with evidence of pleural effusion in whom other tests are nondiagnostic and for whom infection is a concern. In most cases pleural fluid culture, antigen testing, molecular probes, or cytology can establish the diagnosis. However, for patients with pleural effusion and suspected tuberculosis, the yield is improved with the addition of pleural biopsies.

Transthoracic needle aspiration with CT guidance is an important and useful diagnostic procedure for selected patients. HIV-infected patients with focal parenchymal lesions, most often peripheral nodules or masses that may be beyond the reach of a bronchoscope, are ideal candidates for CT-guided aspiration. In one study of 32 HIV-infected patients undergoing this procedure, a diagnosis was established in 27 patients.[97] Mediastinoscopy should be considered for patients with a mediastinal mass, adenopathy, or both.

Occasionally, despite all of these efforts, HIV-infected patients with pulmonary disease may elude a definitive diagnosis. In such patients, consideration should be given to open lung biopsy, although such procedures have a low yield for diagnosing treatable disease and thereby favorably affecting the prognosis.

Interpretation of Radiologic, Microbiologic, and Other Diagnostic Information

Clinicians must exercise considerable judgment to determine whether pneumonia is in fact present or organisms identified by the microbiology laboratory are the cause of the pulmonary dysfunction. As emphasized earlier, not all dyspnea, cough, hypoxia, or pulmonary infiltrates are due to pneumonia (i.e., pulmonary infection). Even if the constellation of symptoms, signs, and laboratory tests suggest that pneumonia is present, the microorganisms seen by direct microscopy or identified by culture or rapid tests may not be causative. Some organisms, such as *Pneumocystis*, *Cryptococcus*, *Histoplasma*, and *Legionella*, should almost always be considered pathogens and be treated as such. If CMV, MAC, *Aspergillus*, or *Streptococcus pneumoniae* is identified, it may represent a colonizer of the respiratory tract rather than the cause of disease. Whether such organisms should be treated or other processes sought is an issue that requires considerable judgment and cannot be determined by a simple formula or algorithm.

Pneumonia: Practical Case Scenarios

The following case scenarios illustrate how the CD4+ T-lymphocyte cell count and the chest radiograph interact to form a differential diagnosis that is further refined by information from the history, physical examination, and selected laboratory tests. Knowledge of the frequency of the various OIs and neoplasms in the demographic or regional setting assists the clinician in suggesting the most likely diagnosis. This, in turn, suggests a therapeutic approach.

Case Scenario 1: HIV-Infected Patient with CD4+ T-Lymphocyte Count Higher than 200 cells/μl

The differential diagnosis of pulmonary disease in an HIV-infected patient whose CD4+ T-lymphocyte count is higher than 200 cells/μl primarily includes those HIV-associated pulmonary diseases that can present in persons without underlying immunodeficiency: bacterial pneumonia, viral or atypical pneumonias, tuberculosis, non-Hodgkin lymphoma, fungal disease (Fig. 60–2). In most clinical settings in the United States, bacterial pneumonia is the most common HIV-associated pulmonary disease. Rarely, PCP or fungi can present when the CD4+ T-lymphocyte cell count is higher than 200 cells/μl. Because each of these illnesses has a characteristic chest radiograph presentation, the specific radiograph findings influence the diagnostic tests and management.

If the chest radiograph reveals a focal, segmental, or lobar infiltrate in an alveolar pattern, bacterial pneumonia is the most likely diagnosis (Fig. 60–3). The suspicion for bacterial pneumonia is increased if the patient reports an acute onset of symptoms, typically fevers, chills or rigors, pleuritic chest pain, and a cough productive of purulent sputum. Other suggestive factors include the presence of focal findings on lung examination, an elevated WBC count with a left shift, a history of cigarette or injection drug use, and a history of prior bacterial pneumonia. In this case the diagnostic approach typically includes sputum Gram stain, sputum and blood cultures for bacteria, and empiric therapy to cover the most common bacterial organ-

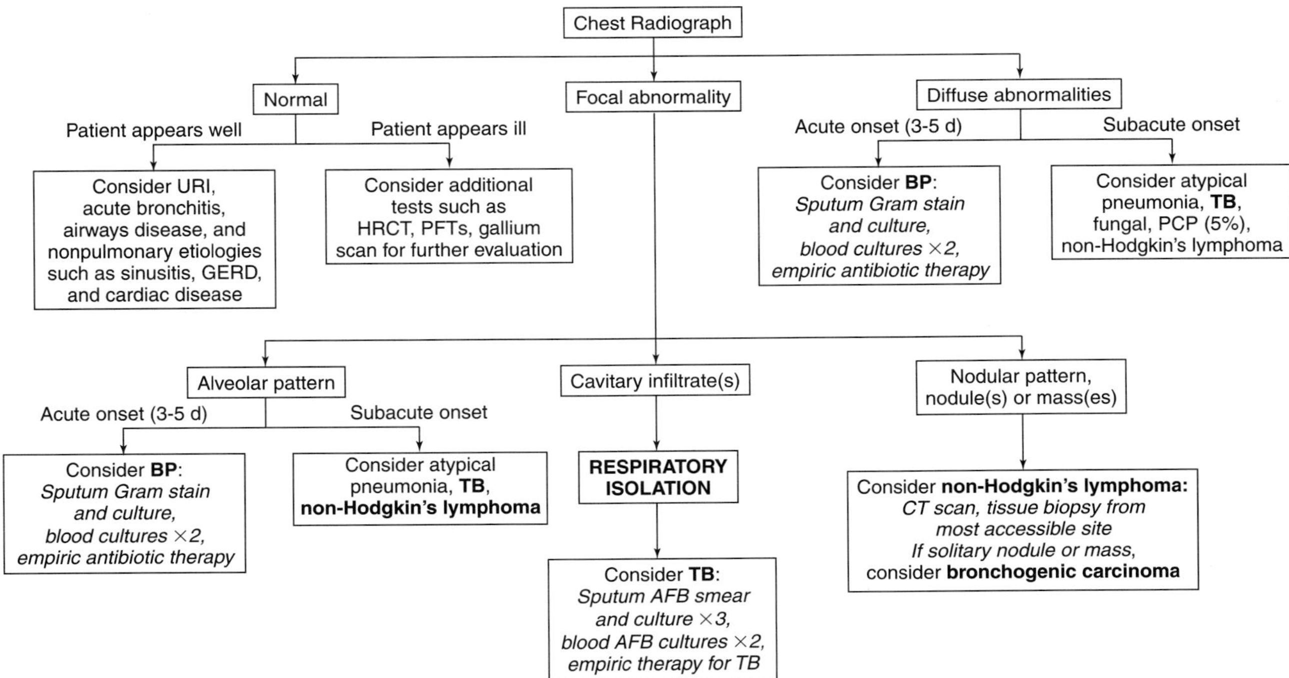

Figure 60–2. Diagnostic approach to an HIV-infected patient, CD4+ T-lymphocyte count of more than 200 cells/μl. AFB, acid-fast bacilli; BP, bacterial pneumonia; CT, chest computed tomography; GERD, gastroesophageal reflux disease; HRCT, chest high-resolution computed tomography; PCP, *Pneumocystis carinii* pneumonia; PFTs, pulmonary function tests; TB, tuberculosis; URI, upper respiratory tract infection.

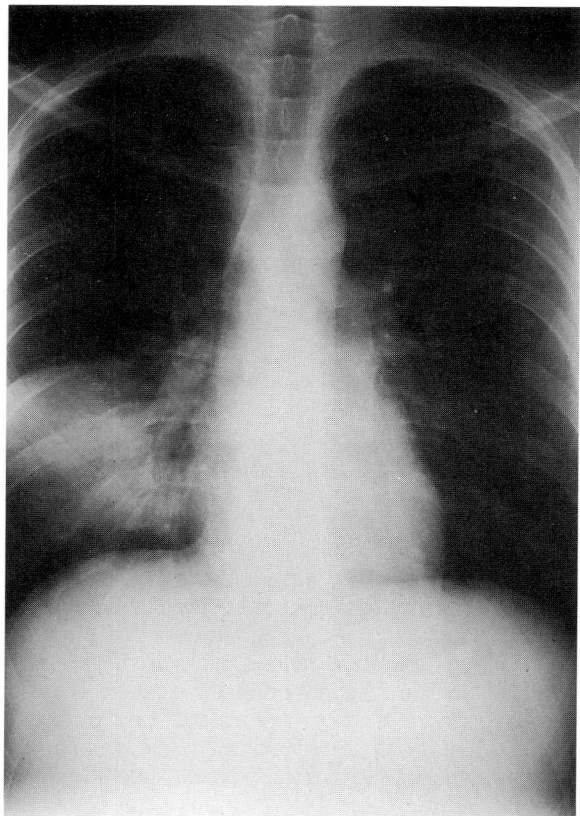

Figure 60–3. Chest radiograph of an HIV-infected person, CD4+ T-lymphocyte count of more than 200 cells/μl, revealing right middle lobe consolidation. Sputum and blood cultures were positive for *Streptococcus pneumoniae*.

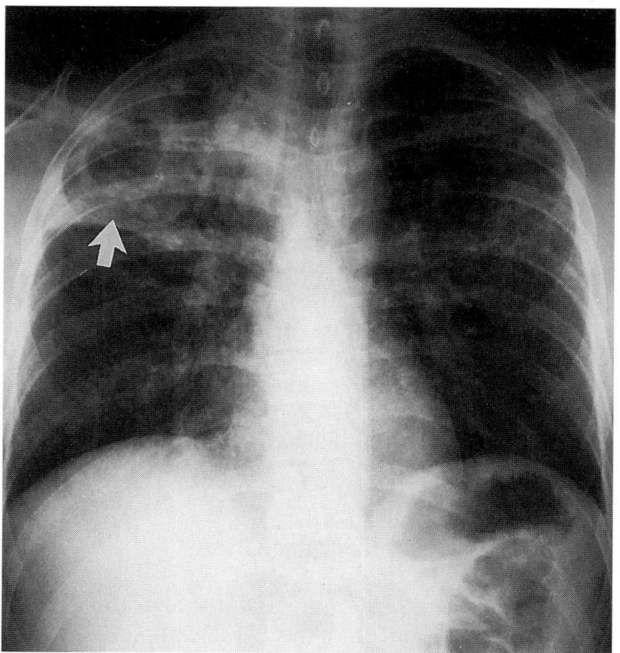

Figure 60–4. Chest radiograph of an HIV-infected person, CD4+ T-lymphocyte count of more than 200 cells/μl, revealing right upper lobe infiltrate, with areas of cavitation. Sputum acid-fast bacillus stain was positive, and multiple sputum cultures grew *Mycobacterium tuberculosis*.

isms, *S. pneumoniae* and *Haemophilus* spp. The presence of a pleural effusion should prompt consideration of thoracentesis.

If the chest radiograph reveals upper lung zone infiltrates with cavitation, tuberculosis is the primary consideration (Fig. 60–4). Suspicion for tuberculosis increases if the patient reports a subacute onset of fevers, cough, and constitutional complaints (night sweats, anorexia, weight loss), especially if the patient is at increased risk for exposure to *M. tuberculosis*. In this case, the diagnostic approach should include respiratory isolation (if the patient is hospitalized), examination of three sputum samples for AFB, sputum and blood cultures for mycobacteria, and empiric tuberculosis therapy with four drugs in addition to pyridoxine. For HIV-infected patients who are to receive concurrent therapy for HIV (with HAART) and tuberculosis, special attention must be paid to interactions between the protease inhibitors and nonnucleoside reverse transcriptase inhibitors and the rifamycins. These interactions frequently require dose adjustments from the standard antiviral and antituberculous doses. In such cases, expert consultation is often warranted. Clinicians should also be aware that "paradoxical reactions" to the initiation of therapy may occur; that is, the chest radiograph and pulmonary manifestations may worsen during the first few weeks despite effective antimycobacterial therapy. This phenomenon has been reported prior to the HIV era but has recently been noted when HAART is initiated (see Chapter 27). This syndrome appears to be caused by an improved immunologic response to AFB, not to antimicrobial failure.

Case Scenario 2: HIV-Infected Patient with CD4+ T-Lymphocyte Count Less than 200 cells/μl

As the CD4+ T-lymphocyte count declines, the number of possible pulmonary diagnoses to consider increases. Still, the combination of the CD4+ T-lymphocyte count and the chest radiograph often suggests a probable diagnosis (Fig. 60–5).

A number of possibilities and approaches exist if the chest radiograph is normal. In general, if the patient appears ill, additional tests are indicated to determine whether an occult pulmonary disease is present. As described, patients with PCP may have a normal chest radiograph; in these cases, chest HRCT may be useful. An HRCT with GGOs (Fig. 60–6) should prompt an evaluation for PCP (because this finding is not specific for PCP), whereas an HRCT without GGO makes the diagnosis unlikely.

If the chest radiograph reveals a focal infiltrate in an alveolar pattern (Figs. 60–2, 60–7), bacterial pneumonia is still the most likely diagnosis. However, if the patient presents with a subacute onset of symptoms and, especially if the patient has risk factors for exposure to *M. tuberculosis*, the possibility of tuberculosis must be strongly considered and sputum AFB specimens must be examined. In Figure 60–7, the key to the eventual diagnosis of tuberculosis was knowledge of the patient's CD4+ T-lymphocyte count (i.e.,

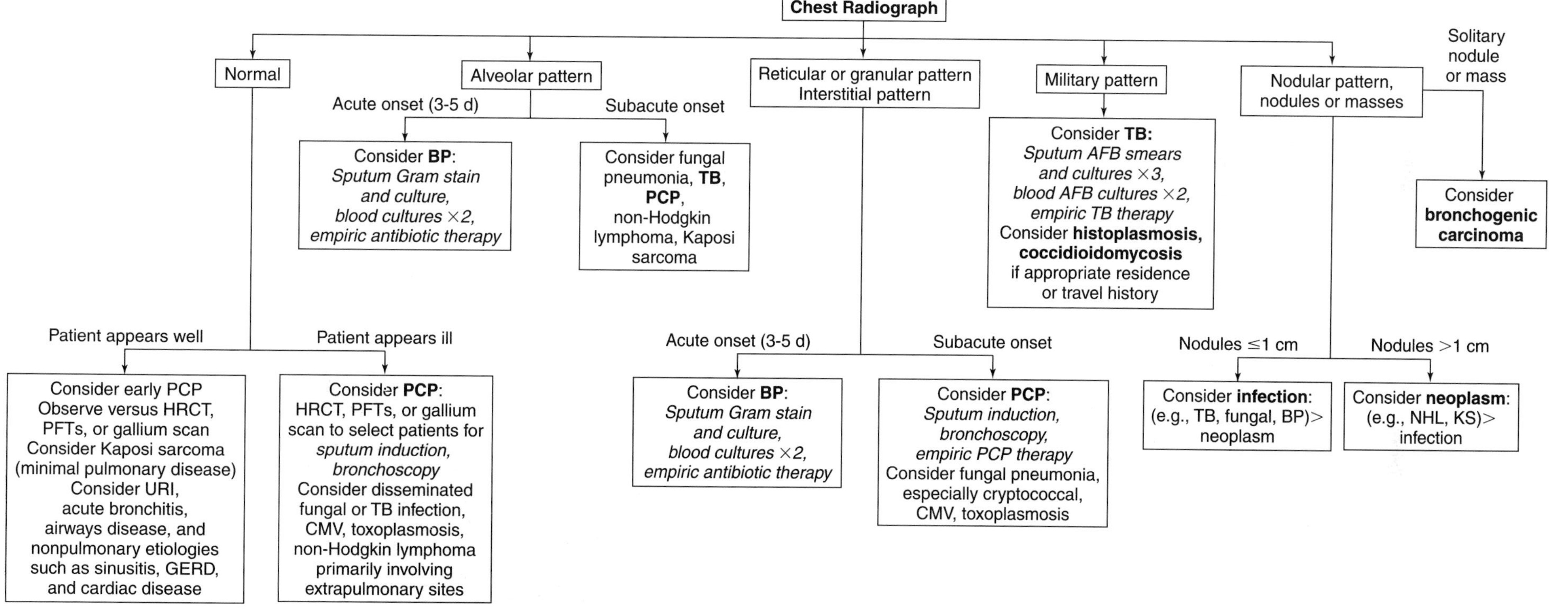

Figure 60–5. Diagnostic approach to an HIV-infected patient, CD4+ T-lymphocyte count of less than 200 cells/μl. *Some of the diagnoses occur when the CD4+ T-lymphocyte count is less than 100 cells/μl or even less than 50 cells/μl. AFB, acid-fast bacilli; BP, bacterial pneumonia; CMV, Cytomegalovirus; GERD, gastroesophageal reflux disease; HRCT, chest high-resolution computed tomography; KS, Kaposi sarcoma; NHL, non-Hodgkin lymphoma; PCP, *Pneumocystis carinii* pneumonia; PFTs, pulmonary function tests; TB, tuberculosis; URI, upper respiratory tract infection.

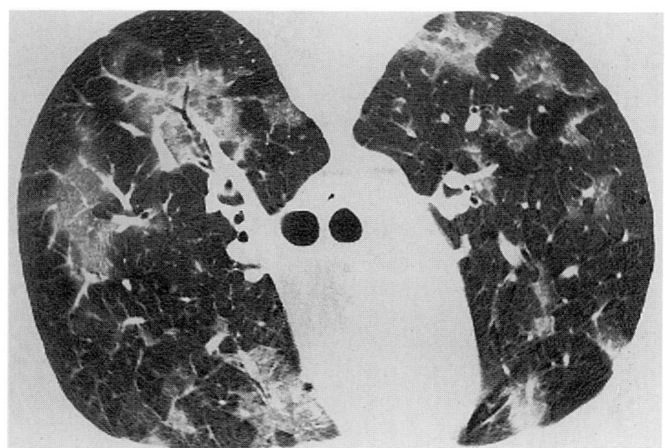

Figure 60–6. Chest high-resolution computed tomographic (HRCT) scan of an HIV-infected person, CD4+ T-lymphocyte count of less than 200 cells/μl, whose chest radiograph was normal. Because of a clinical suspicion for *Pneumocystis carinii* pneumonia (PCP), the patient underwent HRCT, which demonstrated the characteristic patchy ground-glass opacities of PCP. Induced sputum examination revealed *P. carinii.*

$<$200 cells/μl) and understanding that tuberculosis can present with middle or lower lung zone consolidation (or both) in these patients rather than the "classic" upper lung zone infiltrates with cavitation. Because of the higher incidence of mycobacteremia and disseminated or extrapulmonary disease, blood AFB cultures should be examined, and patients should have a careful physical examination for extrapulmonary sites of disease; for example, peripheral lymphadenopathy should prompt a lymph node aspirate or biopsy that may provide the diagnosis.

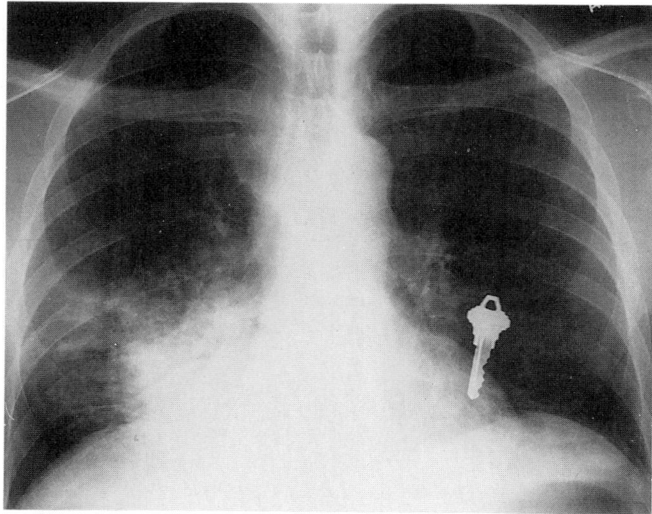

Figure 60–7. Chest radiograph of an HIV-infected person, CD4+ T-lymphocyte count of less than 200 cells/μl, revealing right lower lung consolidation with air bronchograms. Sputum culture grew *Mycobacterium tuberculosis* that was monorifampin-resistant. In this case the key to the diagnosis of tuberculosis was knowledge of the patient's CD4+ T-lymphocyte count and understanding that tuberculosis can present in this manner in such an individual.

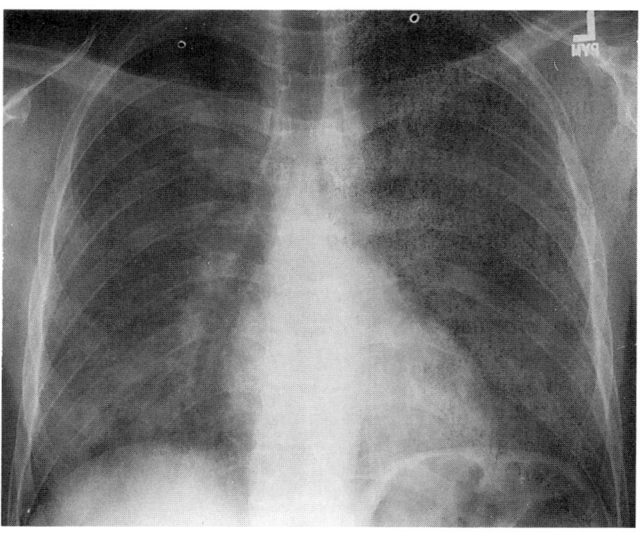

Figure 60–8. Chest radiograph of an HIV-infected person, CD4+ T-lymphocyte count of less than 200 cells/μl demonstrating the characteristic bilateral, reticular-granular opacities of *Pneumocystis carinii* pneumonia. Bronchoscopy with bronchoalveolar lavage fluid examination revealed *P. carinii.*

If the chest radiograph reveals bilateral interstitial-reticular or granular opacities (Fig. 60–8), PCP is the most likely diagnosis. Suspicion for PCP is increased if the patient reports a subacute onset of symptoms, typically fever, dyspnea, and a dry, nonproductive cough. Other suggestive factors include an elevated serum LDH. In this case, the diagnostic approach includes sputum induction/BAL and empiric PCP therapy. *C. neoformans* pneumonia also frequently presents below this CD4+ T-lymphocyte count range and with bilateral interstitial-reticular opacities. Cryptococcal infection is the leading diagnosis if the patient has evidence of concomitant neurologic dysfunction (e.g., headache, altered mental status). In this case, a serum CRAG assay is an excellent screening test and, if positive, should prompt analysis of cerebrospinal fluid. In addition, the diagnosis of cryptococcal disease can be made by fungal cultures of blood and respiratory specimens from sputum or bronchoscopy. Remember that the serum CRAG assay may be negative in isolated cryptococcal pneumonia.

A patient with a CD4+ T-lymphocyte count less than 50 cells/μl whose chest radiograph demonstrates a miliary pattern (Fig. 60–9) likely has either mycobacterial disease (e.g., miliary tuberculosis) or disseminated fungal disease. A history of risk factors for exposure to *M. tuberculosis* or residence in or travel to a geographic region that is endemic for certain fungal diseases may be useful when deciding which diagnosis is most likely and whether to begin empiric four-drug tuberculosis therapy or empiric amphotericin B.

Finally, a patient with a CD4+ T-lymphocyte count less than 100 cells/μl whose chest radiograph reveals bilateral, diffuse coalescent opacities in a central distribution (usually with associated smaller nodules, Kerley B lines, pleural effusions, and occasionally intrathoracic adenopathy) likely

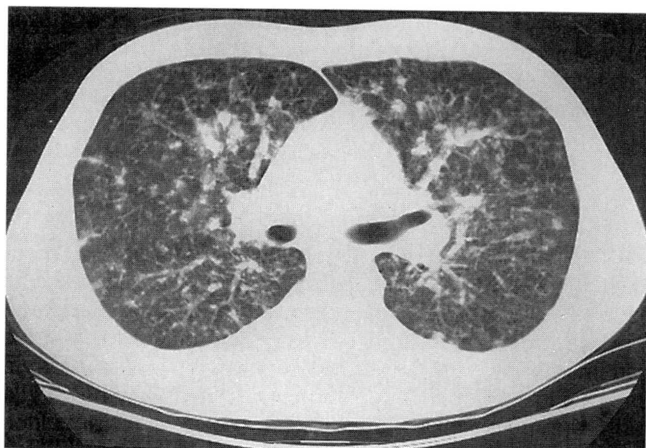

Figure 60–9. Chest computed tomographic (CT) scan of an HIV-infected person, CD4+ T-lymphocyte count of less than 50 cells/μl with a miliary pattern. This radiographic pattern is nonspecific and may be seen in disseminated mycobacterial, fungal, and occasionally *Pneumocystis carinii* infection. The diagnosis of *Coccidioides immitis* was suggested by a history of significant travel to the southwestern United States and was simultaneously confirmed by sputum, blood, and bronchoscopy cultures.

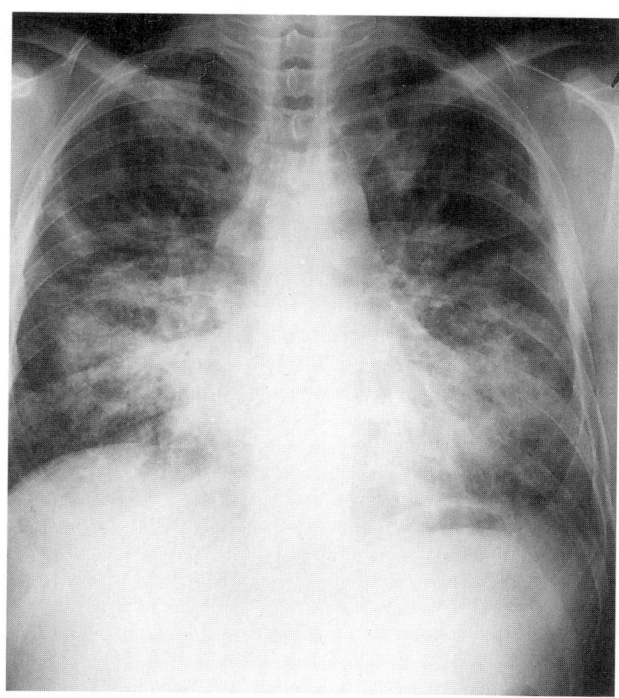

Figure 60–10. Chest radiograph of an HIV-infected person, CD4+ T-lymphocyte count of less than 100 cells/μl with the characteristic bilateral, middle and lower lung zone, predominantly central distribution of abnormalities of pulmonary Kaposi sarcoma. The patient had no evidence of mucocutaneous Kaposi sarcoma, and the diagnosis of pulmonary disease was made by bronchoscopy with visualization of the characteristic erythematous-violaceous Kaposi lesions throughout the visible airway (see Fig. 60–11).

has pulmonary Kaposi sarcoma (Fig. 60–10). This diagnosis is further supported by the presence of mucocutaneous Kaposi sarcoma lesions and can be confirmed by bronchoscopy and visualization of the characteristic Kaposi lesions (Fig. 60–11).

These case scenarios illustrate the most common HIV-related OIs and neoplasms. HIV-infected patients can develop a wide spectrum of pulmonary illnesses that include non-HIV-related conditions; HIV-related OIs due to bacterial, mycobacterial, fungal, viral, and parasitic pathogens; and HIV-related neoplasms. Usually, these diseases occur singly, but experience with HIV has reinforced the fact that occasionally diseases present simultaneously or develop rapidly one after another. Clinicians caring for HIV-infected patients must be vigilant for these situations and must have a low threshold for investigating any signs of clinical deterioration that may be due to a concurrent process that was missed initially.

Approach to Therapy

Without appropriate therapy, HIV-infected patients with certain types of pneumonia can progress rapidly to respiratory failure and death. Patients require a prompt evaluation and institution of treatment, especially those with low CD4+ T-lymphocyte counts, low neutrophil counts, or moderate, severe, or rapidly progressive disease. Unless disease is mild, or diagnostic facilities are unavailable, empiric therapy without any diagnostic evaluation is seldom justified. Specific therapy based on a well established diagnosis can avoid unnecessary drug toxicity and drug interactions, reduce unnecessary ecologic pressure that can produce drug-resistant pathogens, and avoid expensive delays in instituting appropriate therapy, delays that can adversely affect outcome.

Initial Therapy for Suspected Bacterial Pneumonia

The diagnostic evaluation of an HIV-infected patient with suspected bacterial pneumonia should include sputum Gram stain and culture. Although the Gram stain is simple to perform, it is insensitive. Most studies in non-HIV-infected persons have documented that the sensitivity of sputum Gram's stain for *S. pneumoniae* pneumonia is in the range of 50% to 60%, and that the specificity is higher than 80%.[82] Other factors that limit the sensitivity of sputum are the use of prior antimicrobials, the inability of the patient to produce an adequate specimen, and delays in transportation and processing. Blood cultures, which are specific, are nevertheless negative in most patients; therefore in many patients with bacterial pneumonia no definitive diagnosis is made, and empiric therapy is necessary.

The principles of the treatment of patients with community-acquired bacterial pneumonia are the same in HIV-infected as in HIV-uninfected persons. The choice of antimicrobial agent should be based on a number of factors, including the sputum Gram stain, the clinical and radiographic presentation, the severity of the pneumonia, and the patient's co-morbid conditions (e.g., COPD, alcohol use). Initial empiric therapy should include coverage against likely organisms (e.g., *S. pneumoniae*, *Haemophilus* spp.).

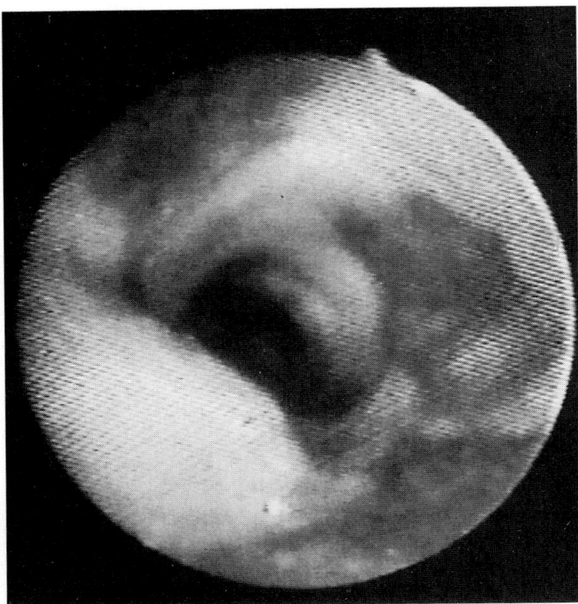

Figure 60–11. Characteristic Kaposi sarcoma lesions located in the trachea in an HIV-infected person, CD4+ T-lymphocyte count of less than 100 cells/μl. Concurrent bronchoalveolar lavage also revealed *Pneumocystis carinii* pneumonia.

Local or institutional drug-resistance patterns must be considered when selecting an antibiotic. For patients with CD4+ T-lymphocyte counts of less than 100 cells/μl, especially if associated with recent hospitalization, neutropenia, broad-spectrum antimicrobial use, or a chest radiograph with evidence of cavitation, consideration should be given to including coverage against *Pseudomonas aeruginosa*. The duration of therapy is similar in HIV-infected and non-HIV-infected persons, and the response rates appear to be comparable.

The Infectious Diseases Society of America (IDSA) guidelines for the management of community-acquired pneumonia in adults recommended antimicrobial choices for patients with bacterial pneumonia. Although these recommendations were designed to apply to nonimmunocompromised persons, they serve as a useful guide for HIV-infected patients.[82] In general, the guidelines recommend that outpatients with bacterial pneumonia receive a macrolide (e.g., azithromycin, clarithromycin, erythromycin), one of the newer fluoroquinolones (e.g., levofloxacin, moxifloxacin, gatifloxacin), or doxycycline. For patients admitted to the hospital, the guidelines recommend an extended-spectrum cephalosporin (e.g., ceftriaxone, cefotaxime) plus a macrolide or one of the newer fluoroquinolones alone. An extended-spectrum cephalosporin or β-lactam/β-lactamase inhibitor (e.g., ampicillin-sulbactam or piperacillin-tazobactam) plus either a macrolide or a fluoroquinolone is recommended for patients admitted to the intensive care unit for pneumonia.

Cordero and colleagues evaluated the prognosis and factors associated with mortality in 355 HIV-infected patients with community-acquired pneumonia.[98] They found that the mortality rate attributable to pneumonia was 9%. Patients meeting the American Thoracic Society criteria for severe pneumonia had a significantly higher mortality rate than those with nonsevere pneumonia (13% vs. 3.5%; $P = 0.02$). Multivariate analysis revealed that patients with (1) a CD4+ T-lymphocyte count less than 100 cells/μl, (2) septic shock, (3) cavities, (4) multilobar infiltrates, or (5) pleural effusions were at increased risk of death. Importantly, when these five predictors were assessed as a group, patients without any of the five risk factors were at a low risk for death (1.3%). This suggests that these criteria could be used to determine whether to admit an HIV-infected patient with community-acquired pneumonia or to treat the individual as an outpatient.

Approach to the Patient Who Is Failing PCP Therapy

Regardless of which approach (definitive diagnosis or empiric therapy) has been selected, a percentage of patients fail to improve despite apparent appropriate therapy. In these cases, there are several important factors to consider (Table 60–7).

The case of a patient with PCP who is worsening despite treatment with TMP-SMX is used to illustrate several of these considerations. First, how was the original diagnosis of PCP established? Strong consideration should be given to pursuing a definitive diagnosis, as several HIV-associated OIs can present in a fashion indistinguishable from that of PCP. Bronchoscopy is the procedure of choice, as it provides the maximal diagnostic yield. Occasionally, pa-

Table 60–7. DIAGNOSTIC APPROACH TO CLINICAL FAILURE OF PCP THERAPY

Review diagnosis
How was the initial diagnosis of PCP established?
Empiric? Strongly consider diagnostic procedure.
Induced sputum? Bronchoscopy?
Was there a concurrent process initially?
Review microbiology results and cultures.
Obtain or repeat sputum and blood cultures, serologies (e.g., serum CRAG).
Has another process supervened (consider infectious and noninfectious etiologies)?
Repeat diagnostic tests (e.g., chest radiograph).
Obtain or repeat sputum and blood cultures, serologies (e.g., serum CRAG).
Strongly consider diagnostic procedure.
Review treatment
Is the patient receiving the best PCP treatment?
Is the dose of the medication correct?
Is the patient receiving adjuvant corticosteroids?
Does the patient have nausea/vomiting or diarrhea? Switch to intravenous therapy.
Allow adequate time for initial therapy to work (usually 5–8 days).
Consider further evaluation
Consider bronchoscopy.
If initial diagnosis of PCP was empiric, bronchoscopy may confirm diagnosis or provide alternate diagnosis.
If initial diagnosis of PCP was obtained from induced sputum examination, bronchoscopy may provide higher yield for other infections or may provide a diagnosis of pulmonary Kaposi sarcoma.
If initial diagnosis of PCP was obtained from BAL examination, repeat bronchoscopy may provide evidence for new infection.

tients require elective intubation and transfer to an intensive care unit for this procedure to be performed.

Next, consideration should be given to the possibility of a concurrent pulmonary process, either infectious or noninfectious (e.g., noncardiogenic pulmonary edema, pulmonary embolism). A review of the microbiology results may reveal a coexistent infection. A chest radiograph should be repeated to evaluate for a supervening process. At this stage, sputum and blood cultures against bacteria, fungi, and mycobacteria should be obtained or repeated. A serum CRAG assay should be undertaken, as cryptococcal pneumonia frequently presents with a clinical and radiographic picture indistinguishable from that of PCP.

For patients with a CD4+ T-lymphocyte count below 50 cells/μl, ophthalmology consultation should be sought for a dilated retinal examination for CMV. Patients with evidence of CMV retinitis require induction therapy, which also treats presumed CMV pneumonitis. Alternatively, a definitive diagnosis of CMV pneumonitis may be pursued with transbronchial biopsy. The diagnosis depends on identifying multiple inclusion bodies. If the patient is known to have mucocutaneous Kaposi sarcoma, bronchoscopy may also provide a diagnosis of pulmonary Kaposi sarcoma by identifying endobronchial lesions.

Occasionally, a patient's "failure" to respond to PCP treatment is the result of noninfectious etiologies such as noncardiogenic edema, where a trial of diuresis may result in symptomatic and radiographic improvement. Concurrent with these considerations, a review of the patient's PCP therapy should consider whether the patient is receiving the "best" treatment option, whether adjuvant corticosteroids are warranted, and if the patient has nausea/vomiting or diarrhea whether a switch to an intravenous route is prudent.

Patients with PCP may have slow resolution of their disease, and it may be several days to a week or more until their clinical status improves. A general rule of thumb: The number of days a patient was symptomatic before treatment was begun is approximately the number of days it takes for resolution or near-resolution of the symptoms. Nevertheless, one expects a patient with PCP to manifest initial signs of improvement by day 7 to 10 of treatment. If a patient fails to improve after this time or there is progressive deterioration, an evaluation for an alternate process is recommended and a switch in PCP therapy may be indicated.

Finally, the specter of drug-resistant *Pneumocystis carinii* is often raised. Unfortunately, the lack of a standardized culture system for human *P. carinii* has limited our ability to confirm drug resistance in *P. carinii*. Several studies have reported that specific point mutations in the *P. carinii* dihydropteroate synthase gene—the enzymatic target of sulfamethoxazole and dapsone—are associated with an increased risk of TMP-SMX PCP treatment failure and increased mortality.[99–102] These results have been interpreted to imply that the *P. carinii* in these patients has developed "resistance" to TMP-SMX.

Immune Reconstitution Syndromes

The use of combinations of potent antiretroviral therapies has resulted in dramatic declines in AIDS deaths and OI rates. Among patients who have experienced dramatic, sustained rises in their CD4+ T-lymphocyte counts, primary and secondary OI prophylaxis and chronic maintenance therapy have been successfully discontinued. However, the initiation of combinations of potent antiretroviral therapies and the subsequent improvement in immune function has also resulted in several syndromes that have important clinical implications.[103] Interestingly, in some of the examples provided the use of antiretroviral therapy serves to exacerbate the disease transiently, whereas in others its use is seemingly solely responsible for the reported improvements. Finally, in some cases the use of antiretroviral therapy has been associated with the development of pulmonary disease that is host-mediated.

The transient worsening of clinical symptoms and signs and chest radiograph findings of tuberculosis after the initiation of appropriate antituberculous therapy have been well recognized. These "paradoxical" reactions are thought to represent an enhanced antituberculous immune response and usually resolve with continued therapy alone. HIV-infected patients who develop tuberculosis and receive concurrent antiretroviral and antituberculous therapies appear to have an increased incidence of paradoxical worsening. Narita and colleagues found that 36% of HIV-infected tuberculosis (TB) patients receiving these dual therapies developed a paradoxical reaction compared to 7% of HIV-infected TB patients who received TB therapy alone and 2% of TB patients without concomitant HIV infection.[104] Three-fourths of the patients who developed paradoxical reactions while on dual antiretroviral and antituberculous therapies developed hectic fevers, and three of the patients with severe paradoxical reactions required systemic corticosteroids for symptomatic relief. Fishman and colleagues noted transient worsening on serial chest radiographs in 45% of HIV-infected TB patients receiving dual HIV and TB therapies.[105] The radiographic worsening consisted of new or worsening parenchymal disease in 32%, new or worsening intrathoracic lymphadenopathy in 23%, and new or worsening pleural effusion in 19%. However, the diagnosis of paradoxical reaction must be one of exclusion. HIV-infected TB patients with suspected paradoxical reactions must also be thoroughly evaluated for progressive tuberculosis due to drug resistance or patient nonadherence and for the presence of a concurrent, superimposed opportunistic infection. A similar syndrome has been described for patients with PCP who, during acute PCP therapy, institute HAART.[106]

The use of potent antiretroviral therapy, often in the absence of specific chemotherapy, has resulted in clinical regression and occasionally complete resolution of Kaposi sarcoma (including pulmonary Kaposi sarcoma) lesions.[107–109] I have seen a handful of cases of clinically symptomatic pulmonary Kaposi sarcoma diagnosed by bronchoscopic visualization that responded to antiretroviral therapy alone. In these cases, subsequent chest radiographs and, in one patient, subsequent bronchoscopy demonstrated complete resolution of disease. One question of major clinical importance that remains largely unanswered is whether the addition of potent antiretroviral therapy to standard opportunistic infection treatment is beneficial—or potentially harmful if paradoxical reactions develop—in patients with OIs. Given the still significant mortality associated with respiratory failure due to opportunistic infections, this question is particularly important to HIV-associated pneumonias.

Improved immune function may also play a role in the development of host-mediated pulmonary disease. There are several reports of sarcoidosis or a sarcoidosis-like disease developing after the initiation of combinations of potent antiretroviral therapies.[110–113] In addition, I have seen a memorable case of subacute hypersensitivity pneumonitis to avian antigen that developed only when the patient's immune function improved on antiretroviral therapy.[114] Diseases in which the host immune response plays an essential role in pathogenesis can be expected to become more prevalent as more HIV-infected patients receive potent antiretroviral therapies.

▲ LOWER RESPIRATORY TRACT DISEASE: NEOPLASMS AND NONINFECTIOUS INFLAMMATORY DISORDERS

The initial evaluation of respiratory disease usually focuses on the diagnosis of HIV-associated OIs. This stems from the frequency of infectious complications, the need for their prompt treatment, and in the case of tuberculosis the concern for transmission to other persons, both HIV-infected and non-HIV-infected. However, HIV-infected patients are also susceptible to a number of noninfectious respiratory complications, whose aspects are summarized briefly.

Two HIV-associated malignancies, Kaposi sarcoma and non-Hodgkin lymphoma, may include pulmonary involvement. With both neoplasms, intrathoracic disease is usually a manifestation of disease already recognized elsewhere, but occasionally Kaposi sarcoma and non-Hodgkin lymphoma present with isolated pulmonary disease.

Kaposi Sarcoma

The most common HIV-associated malignancy is Kaposi sarcoma. One of the phenomena of the AIDS epidemic during the early 1980s was the veritable explosion in this previously rare disease. Although the incidence of Kaposi sarcoma has decreased dramatically since then, significant advances have been made in our understanding of its pathogenesis, including its association with human herpesvirus HHV-8.[115]

Almost all of the HIV-infected patients with Kaposi sarcoma are men who report having sex with other men. Pulmonary Kaposi sarcoma is detected clinically in approximately one-third of patients with known Kaposi sarcoma, with the proportion detected at autopsy approaching 50% to 75%.[7,116] Clinically symptomatic pulmonary Kaposi sarcoma presents at the lower range of CD4+ T-lymphocyte counts, but tracheobronchial lesions may be seen in patients with higher CD4+ T-lymphocyte counts who are undergoing bronchoscopy for other reasons. Most but not all patients with clinically diagnosed pulmonary Kaposi sarcoma have concomitant mucocutaneous disease.[27] Importantly, a significant proportion of patients with pulmonary Kaposi sarcoma also have concurrent opportunistic infection. Huang and colleagues found that 45 of the 168 patients (27%) with pulmonary Kaposi sarcoma had an accompanying OI, most frequently PCP.[27] These observations underscore the need to evaluate each patient with suspected or known pulmonary Kaposi's sarcoma for an OI. Patients with pulmonary Kaposi's sarcoma who develop opportunistic infection can also experience rapid progression of their Kaposi sarcoma.

Pulmonary Kaposi sarcoma characteristically presents with a nonproductive cough, dyspnea, and occasionally fever.[7,116] Chest pain and hemoptysis are noted less frequently. Rarely, Kaposi sarcoma lesions may involve the larynx or trachea to such an extent as to cause hoarseness or stridor. Symptoms are usually present for weeks or even months but may also progress rapidly in a manner indistinguishable from that of an OI.

As described previously, pulmonary Kaposi sarcoma characteristically presents with bilateral middle-lower lung zone opacities in a central or perihilar distribution (Fig. 60–10). Typical chest radiographic findings include linear densities (bronchial wall thickening), nodules or nodular opacities of varying size, Kerley B lines, pleural effusions, and intrathoracic adenopathy.[117] The latter finding may be underappreciated on the chest radiograph given the perihilar distribution of parenchymal disease. Chest CT scans often demonstrate the characteristic peribronchovascular distribution with associated nodules.[68,69]

The diagnosis of pulmonary Kaposi sarcoma is usually established by bronchoscopy. Finding characteristic endobronchial, reddish-purplish, flat or slightly raised lesions is sufficient to diagnose pulmonary disease in the proper clinical context (Fig. 60–11). Most patients with chest radiographic findings suggestive of pulmonary Kaposi sarcoma have endobronchial Kaposi sarcoma lesions seen below the level of the carina. However, the presence of these lesions does not preclude a concurrent infection, nor does their absence in the observable airway preclude more distal airway disease or parenchymal, pleural, or nodal involvement. In cases where there is a strong clinical suspicion for pulmonary Kaposi sarcoma but no endobronchial lesions are seen, transbronchial biopsies should be considered to establish the diagnosis. However, accurately and reliably identifying Kaposi sarcoma in a small piece of crushed transbronchoscopically obtained tissue is difficult; cytology is not helpful.

Patients with pleural effusions may be considered candidates for thoracentesis, primarily to exclude the presence of infection but also to provide symptomatic relief if the effusions are large. Although most Kaposi sarcoma effusions are exudative, effusions may be transudate or exudate, serous, serosanguineous, or even frankly bloody.[116] I have also seen several chylous effusions due to lymphatic obstruction from Kaposi sarcoma.

Non-Hodgkin Lymphoma

Intrathoracic involvement is more common in Kaposi sarcoma than in non-Hodgkin lymphoma. The incidence of HIV-associated Kaposi sarcoma is decreasing, whereas that of HIV-associated non-Hodgkin lymphoma appears to be increasing.[118] Most patients with non-Hodgkin lymphoma present with widely disseminated disease and extranodal involvement. Frequent extranodal sites include the liver, spleen, bone marrow, meninges, and gastrointestinal tract. Intrathoracic involvement is seen in a smaller proportion. The reported incidence of intrathoracic disease varies from 0% to 31% of non-Hodgkin lymphoma patients at the time of clinical diagnosis and is usually higher at the time of autopsy.[116] Occasionally, the lung is the only site involved. Non-Hodgkin lymphoma can present at a wide range of CD4+ T-lymphocyte counts. The median CD4+ T-lymphocyte count is approximately 100 cells/μl, and 75% of patients have a count less than 50 cells/μl.

When the lungs are involved, the most common symptoms are cough and dyspnea, with pleuritic chest pain and hemoptysis occurring less frequently. Eisner et al. found that these symptoms were present in 71%, 63%, 26%, and 11%, respectively, of the 38 patients reported.[95] B symptoms, such as fever, sweats, and weight loss, are also common features. Physical examination of the chest may reveal a variety of findings, including crackles, rhonchi, wheezes, decreased breath sounds, and egobronchophony.

The most common chest radiographic parenchymal findings are multiple nodular opacities or masses, lobar infiltrates, and diffuse interstitial infiltrates.[95,116,119] Occasionally, a solitary nodule or mass is seen. More rarely, endobronchial lesions have been reported.[96] Pleural effusions are the most common radiographic abnormality, occurring in 40% to 70% of cases, and they may occur in the absence of parenchymal disease.[95,116] The effusions may be unilateral or bilateral and may vary in size. Hilar and mediastinal adenopathy can be found in up to 60% of patients. Chest CT scans can be useful for deciding on the optimal diagnostic procedure.

The diagnosis of non-Hodgkin lymphoma requires demonstration of malignant lymphocytes on cytology or biopsy specimens. Most often needle aspiration or biopsy of an extrathoracic site establishes the diagnosis. Persons presenting with isolated intrathoracic involvement should undergo bronchoscopy with biopsies or CT-guided fine-needle aspiration. Other options include mediastinoscopy, thoracoscopy, and open lung biopsy. For patients with pleural effusions, pleural fluid cytology, biopsy, or both are often diagnostic.[116]

Bronchogenic Carcinoma

There is significant debate whether other malignancies that involve the lung (i.e., bronchogenic carcinoma) are also associated with HIV disease.[116] In contrast to Kaposi sarcoma and non-Hodgkin lymphoma, there is no increase in bronchogenic carcinoma seen in persons with other immunosuppressive disorders. Nevertheless, a number of reports have suggested that bronchogenic carcinoma is increased in frequency, occurs at a younger age, and has a more aggressive course in HIV-infected patients. One study that crossmatched the HIV/AIDS and cancer registries in Texas found a 6.5-fold increased incidence of bronchogenic carcinoma in HIV/AIDS patients compared to the U.S. population.[120] Johnson and colleagues in the PCHIS found a bronchogenic carcinoma rate of approximately 180 cases per 100,000 person-years in their HIV-infected cohort.[121] Other studies, however, found no significant increase. Nevertheless, one can expect the number of bronchogenic carcinomas in HIV-infected persons to increase as these individuals survive longer as a result of antiretroviral therapies and OI prophylaxis and as they reach an age where cancer rates are increased.

Most HIV-infected patients who develop bronchogenic carcinoma are cigarette smokers.[116] Although all pathologic types are seen, adenocarcinoma has been the most frequent type reported, similar to that seen in non-HIV-infected patients younger than 40 years of age who develop bronchogenic carcinoma. Bronchogenic carcinoma can develop at a wide range of CD4+ T-lymphocyte counts. In the PCHIS study, the range of CD4+ T-lymphocyte counts among the patients who developed lung cancer was 127 to 1026 cells/μl.[121] The characteristic presentation of bronchogenic carcinoma is familiar and includes respiratory symptoms such as cough occasionally with hemoptysis, dyspnea, and chest pain. Constitutional symptoms such as fatigue, anorexia, and weight loss may also be present. The chest radiographic presentation appears to include parenchymal nodules or masses, pleural effusion, and central parenchymal or hilar masses and mediastinal adenopathy.[122,123] Chest CT scans provide additional important details that are crucial for optimum diagnosis and management.

The diagnosis and treatment of bronchogenic carcinoma in an HIV-infected patient is similar to that in a non-HIV-infected individual. HIV infection should be considered an important concurrent underlying medical problem, much the same as one would consider underlying cardiopulmonary disease. Surgical resection should be considered for any patient whose staging and medical condition supports such an approach.[124,125]

Interstitial Pneumonitis

Although OI and, to a lesser extent, neoplasia dominate the clinical spectrum of HIV-associated pulmonary disease, occasionally patients present with signs and symptoms attributable to one of the interstitial pneumonitides: lymphocytic interstitial pneumonitis (LIP) or nonspecific interstitial pneumonitis (NIP).[126]

Lymphocytic Interstitial Pneumonitis

The most striking feature of HIV-associated LIP is the effect of age on its incidence. Early in the AIDS epidemic, one-third to one-half of AIDS-defining diagnoses in children were due to LIP. More recently, LIP accounted for 17% of these AIDS-defining diagnoses. In contrast, LIP is rare in adults. I have encountered but a handful of biopsy-proven LIP adult cases at San Francisco General Hospital, and there are only scattered case reports throughout the literature.[127]

The symptoms of LIP include slowly progressive dyspnea, nonproductive cough, and fever. Lung examination may be normal or may reveal inspiratory crackles. These clinical features are indistinguishable from an OI (e.g.,

PCP). In children, additional physical examination findings include clubbing, salivary gland enlargement, lymphadenopathy, and hepatosplenomegaly.

The chest radiograph presentation of LIP is nonspecific and characteristically shows bilateral reticulonodular "interstitial" infiltrates with a lower lung zone predominance.[128] Hilar or mediastinal adenopathy is occasionally seen and can potentially be used to distinguish LIP from PCP. Pulmonary function tests often reveal a restrictive ventilatory defect (decreased total lung capacity) and a decreased diffusing capacity. Chest CT scans may reveal small (2 to 4 mm) nodules often in a peribronchovascular distribution or diffuse areas of ground-glass opacification. Gallium scintigraphy may note diffuse pulmonary uptake, indistinguishable from that of PCP, although all patterns have been described. The diagnosis of LIP requires histologic confirmation by biopsy. Reports on treatment are limited, but corticosteroids have been used with success.[127]

Nonspecific Interstitial Pneumonitis

Nonspecific interstitial pneumonitis has been reported with various frequencies in HIV-infected patients. Because it is a histologic diagnosis, its incidence depends on the frequency that biopsy is performed during the diagnostic evaluation.[127]

The symptoms of NIP include dyspnea, nonproductive cough, and fever. Lung examination may be normal or may reveal inspiratory crackles. These clinical features are indistinguishable from those of PCP. However, NIP may present at CD4+ T-lymphocyte counts of more than 200 cells/μl, whereas PCP rarely does.[28,126,129] In one large series of 67 HIV-infected patients with NIP, the mean CD4+ T-lymphocyte count for patients with NIP was 492 cells/μl compared to 57 cells/μl for matched controls with PCP.[28]

The chest radiographic presentation of NIP is nonspecific and usually indistinguishable from that of PCP. As with PCP, NIP can present with a normal radiograph. One study of patients with NIP found that 16 of 36 patients (44%) with NIP had a normal radiograph.[130] The most common radiographic abnormality seen was a diffuse interstitial pattern. Other abnormalities include pleural effusions, alveolar infiltrates, and nodules. Pulmonary function tests often reveal a mildly decreased diffusing capacity.[126] The diagnosis of NIP requires histologic confirmation and exclusion of other etiologies.

▲ OTHER DISORDERS

Pulmonary Hypertension

Numerous reports of primary pulmonary hypertension (PPH) in HIV-infected patients are scattered throughout the literature.[131] The largest single series compared 20 HIV-infected patients with pulmonary hypertension to 93 non-HIV-infected patients with pulmonary hypertension.[132] At pulmonary hypertension diagnosis, the HIV-infected patients were significantly younger, and the proportion with New York Heart Association functional class III or IV was significantly lower (50% vs. 75%; $P < 0.01$). Pulmonary hypertension was thought to be the cause of death in 8 of the 10 HIV-infected patients who died within 1 year after the diagnosis of pulmonary hypertension. Pathologic findings resembled those of plexogenic pulmonary arteriopathy.

The characteristic clinical presentation is one of progressive dyspnea, with a nonproductive cough, chest pain, and syncope or near-syncope seen in a small number.[131] Physical examination usually reveals evidence of right heart failure, with bipedal edema being the most consistent finding. Chest radiographic findings include cardiomegaly and prominence of the pulmonary arteries. Our clinic has seen a number of cases of HIV-infected patients with pulmonary hypertension. In these patients, multiple potential factors (including injection drug use, cigarette use, history of underlying cardiac or pulmonary disease, and prior pulmonary opportunistic infections) have complicated the clinical picture and the classification of these patients as having primary pulmonary hypertension.

The chest radiograph or electrocardiogram with evidence of right ventricular hypertrophy often first suggests the diagnosis of pulmonary hypertension. Most commonly, the diagnosis is confirmed by echocardiogram. Patients diagnosed with pulmonary hypertension should undergo a thorough evaluation for secondary (potentially treatable) causes, including underlying cardiac disease (i.e., left ventricular failure, mitral or aortic valvular disease) and pulmonary disease (i.e., COPD, recurrent pulmonary emboli).

Treatment for HIV-infected patients with pulmonary hypertension should focus on oxygen supplementation (if the patient is hypoxemic); discontinuation of cigarette use, intravenous drug use, and other potential contributing factors; and aggressive treatment of underlying cardiopulmonary disease. More recently, HIV-infected patients with pulmonary hypertension have responded to continuous intravenous epoprostenol infusions,[133] and there is at least one report of the possible beneficial effects of potent antiretroviral therapy.[134] Nevertheless, the median time from diagnosis of pulmonary hypertension to death in the combined literature is approximately 6 months.

Bronchiolitis Obliterans Organizing Pneumonia

Bronchiolitis obliterans organizing pneumonia (BOOP) has been reported in a handful of HIV-infected patients.[135–139] The clinical and radiographic presentation, diagnosis, and clinical course with corticosteroid therapy were similar to cases of BOOP in non-HIV-infected persons.

Respiratory Bronchiolitis-Associated Interstitial Lung Disease

At San Francisco General Hospital, we have seen a handful of cases of respiratory bronchiolitis-associated interstitial lung disease in our HIV-infected cigarette smokers. Typically, these patients have been heavy smokers and presented with progressive cough followed by dyspnea. Physical examination may reveal inspiratory crackles. The chest radiograph shows bilateral, usually middle and lower lung zone reticular or granular opacities that resemble PCP. Similarly, chest HRCT has demonstrated multifocal areas of ground-glass opacification. The diagnosis has been confirmed by biopsy in most and inferred in a few HIV-infected patients. As this disorder is related to cigarette smoking, patients with respiratory bronchiolitis-associated interstitial lung disease must cease smoking.

Sarcoidosis

Sarcoidosis is one of the last disorders that one might expect to find among the pulmonary complications of HIV infection. In many respects, the coexistence of sarcoid and HIV is seemingly incompatible: Sarcoidosis is characterized by granuloma formation, which HIV infection inhibits. Moreover, sarcoid-induced alveolitis consists predominantly of CD4+ lymphocytes, whereas HIV-associated lymphocytic alveolitis consists chiefly of CD8+ lymphocytes. Nevertheless, several cases of sarcoidosis in HIV-infected patients have been reported.[140–143] In these cases, the clinical and radiographic presentation, diagnosis, and clinical course with corticosteroid therapy were similar to cases of sarcoidosis in non-HIV-infected persons.

▲ UPPER RESPIRATORY TRACT DISEASE

Sinusitis

Sinusitis is more common in HIV-infected persons than in immunocompetent ones.[144] Furthermore, it appears to increase in frequency as the CD4+ T-lymphocyte count declines. These episodes often alternate with episodes of bronchitis.[145] This “ping-pong” effect results in a chronic, relapsing condition that is challenging to clinicians and frustrating to patients.

The clinical presentation of sinusitis in HIV-infected persons is similar to that in immunocompetent persons. Patients often report frontal headaches with sinus or nasal congestion, fever, and postnasal drip or purulent nasal discharge. Physical examination may reveal sinus tenderness and occasionally even facial swelling. The diagnosis of sinusitis is usually established on clinical grounds, especially in a patient with prior radiographic evidence of disease and a characteristic presentation. Sinus radiographs can diagnose maxillary involvement, but sinus CT scanning is a more sensitive diagnostic test for nonmaxillary disease. The treatment for sinusitis in HIV-infected persons is similar to that in immunocompetent persons and often includes a combination of decongestants, nasal vasoconstrictors or nasal corticosteroids (or both), and for selected patients antibiotics. *Streptococcus pneumoniae* and *Haemophilus* spp. are the most common bacterial pathogens identified, so antibiotic therapy if indicated, should target these pathogens. However, patients with apparent refractory sinusitis may have more ominous etiologies: *Aspergillus*, *Mucor*, or *Fusarium* infections and lymphoma have been reported.[146–148] Erosion of bone adjacent to the sinuses in particular should prompt an aggressive diagnostic evaluation. In these patients, ENT consultation for invasive diagnostic and therapeutic procedures may be warranted.

Bronchitis

Similar to sinusitis, bronchitis is more common in HIV-infected persons than in immunocompetent ones.[2] Bronchitis also appears to increase in frequency as the CD4+ T-lymphocyte count declines, and recurrent infections occasionally lead to more permanent airway damage and bronchiectasis.

The clinical presentation of bronchitis in HIV-infected persons is similar to that in immunocompetent persons. Patients often report a cough that is usually productive of purulent sputum and fever. Physical examination may reveal coarse rhonchi. The chest radiograph is without infiltrate, but the presence of bronchial wall thickening or peribronchial cuffing should alert the clinician to the presence of underlying airways disease. Chest HRCT can be useful for demonstrating bronchiectasis. The treatment for bronchitis in HIV-infected persons is similar to that in immunocompetent persons, and issues regarding whether the episode is bacterial or viral in etiology pertain. HIV-infected patients with recurrent bronchitis or bronchiectasis who are cigarette smokers should be strongly encouraged to quit smoking, and preventive measures such as pneumococcal vaccine and an annual influenzae vaccine should be offered.

REFERENCES

1. Pulmonary Complications of HIV Infection Study Group. Design of a prospective study of the pulmonary complications of human immunodeficiency virus infection. J Clin Epidemiol 46:497, 1993.
2. Wallace JM, Hansen NI, Lavange L, et al. Respiratory disease trends in the pulmonary complications of HIV infection study cohort: Pulmonary Complications of HIV Infection Study Group. Am J Respir Crit Care Med 155:72, 1997.
3. Mundy LM, Auwaerter PG, Oldach D, et al. Community-acquired pneumonia: impact of immune status. Am J Respir Crit Care Med 152:1309, 1995.
4. Rosen MJ, Clayton K, Schneider RF, et al. Intensive care of patients with HIV infection: utilization, critical illnesses, and outcomes; Pulmonary Complications of HIV Infection Study Group. Am J Respir Crit Care Med 155:67, 1997.
5. Nickas G, Wachter RM. Outcomes of intensive care for patients with human immunodeficiency virus infection. Arch Intern Med 160:541, 2000.
6. Gill JK, Greene L, Miller R, et al. ICU admission in patients infected with the human immunodeficiency virus: a multicentre survey. Anaesthesia 54:727, 1999.
7. Aboulafia DM. The epidemiologic, pathologic, and clinical features of AIDS-associated pulmonary Kaposi's sarcoma. Chest 117:1128, 2000.
8. Haramati LB, Wong J. Intrathoracic Kaposi's sarcoma in women with AIDS. Chest 117:410, 2000.
9. Hirschtick RE, Glassroth J, Jordan MC, et al. Bacterial pneumonia in persons infected with the human immunodeficiency virus. Pulmonary Complications of HIV Infection Study Group. N Engl J Med 333:845, 1995.
10. O'Donnell AE, Selig J, Aravamuthan M, et al. Pulmonary complications associated with illicit drug use: an update. Chest 108:460, 1995.
11. Huang L, Stansell JD. AIDS and the lung. Med Clin North Am 80:775, 1996.
12. Niaura R, Shadel WG, Morrow K, et al. Human immunodeficiency virus infection, AIDS, and smoking cessation: the time is now. Clin Infect Dis 31:808, 2000.

13. Markowitz N, Hansen NI, Hopewell PC, et al. Incidence of tuberculosis in the United States among HIV-infected persons: the Pulmonary Complications of HIV Infection Study Group. Ann Intern Med 126:123, 1997.
14. Selwyn PA, Sckell BM, Alcabes P, et al. High risk of active tuberculosis in HIV-infected drug users with cutaneous anergy. JAMA 268:504, 1992.
15. Markowitz N, Hansen NI, Wilcosky TC, et al. Tuberculin and anergy testing in HIV-seropositive and HIV-seronegative persons: Pulmonary Complications of HIV Infection Study Group. Ann Intern Med 119:185, 1993.
16. Centers for Disease Control and Prevention. From the Centers for Disease Control and Prevention: 1993 revised classification system for HIV infection and expanded surveillance case definition for AIDS among adolescents and adults. JAMA 269:729, 1993.
17. Furrer H, Egger M, Opravil M, et al. Discontinuation of primary prophylaxis against *Pneumocystis carinii* pneumonia in HIV-1-infected adults treated with combination antiretroviral therapy. Swiss HIV Cohort Study. N Engl J Med 340:1301, 1999.
18. USPHS/IDSA. 1999 USPHS/IDSA guidelines for the prevention of opportunistic infections in persons infected with human immunodeficiency virus. U.S. Public Health Service (USPHS) and Infectious Diseases Society of America (IDSA), www.hivatis.org 48:1–59, 61–56, 1999.
19. Martin JN, Rose DA, Hadley WK, et al. Emergence of trimethoprim-sulfamethoxazole resistance in the AIDS era. J Infect Dis 180:1809, 1999.
20. Fuller JD, Craven DE, Steger KA, et al. Influenza vaccination of human immunodeficiency virus (HIV)-infected adults: impact on plasma levels of HIV type 1 RNA and determinants of antibody response. Clin Infect Dis 28:541, 1999.
21. Tasker SA, Treanor JJ, Paxton WB, et al. Efficacy of influenza vaccination in HIV-infected persons: a randomized, double-blind, placebo-controlled trial. Ann Intern Med 131:430, 1999.
22. French N, Nakiyingi J, Carpenter LM, et al. 23-Valent pneumococcal polysaccharide vaccine in HIV-1-infected Ugandan adults: double-blind, randomised and placebo controlled trial. Lancet 355:2106, 2000.
23. Dworkin MS, Ward JW, Hanson DL. Pneumococcal disease among human immunodeficiency virus-infected persons: incidence, risk factors, and impact of vaccination. Clin Infect Dis 32:794, 2001.
24. Kovacs JA, Hiemenz JW, Macher AM, et al. *Pneumocystis carinii* pneumonia: a comparison between patients with the acquired immunodeficiency syndrome and patients with other immunodeficiencies. Ann Intern Med 100:663, 1984.
25. Afessa B, Green B. Bacterial pneumonia in hospitalized patients with HIV infection: the Pulmonary Complications, ICU Support, and Prognostic Factors of Hospitalized Patients with HIV (PIP) study. Chest 117:1017, 2000.
26. Chuck SL, Sande MA: Infections with *Cryptococcus neoformans* in the acquired immunodeficiency syndrome. N Engl J Med 321:794, 1989.
27. Huang L, Schnapp LM, Gruden JF, et al. Presentation of AIDS-related pulmonary Kaposi's sarcoma diagnosed by bronchoscopy. Am J Respir Crit Care Med 153:1385, 1996.
28. Sattler F, Nichols L, Hirano L, et al. Nonspecific interstitial pneumonitis mimicking *Pneumocystis carinii* pneumonia. Am J Respir Crit Care Med 156:912, 1997.
29. Masur H, Ognibene FP, Yarchoan R, et al. CD4 counts as predictors of opportunistic pneumonias in human immunodeficiency virus (HIV) infection. Ann Intern Med 111:223, 1989.
30. Phair J, Munoz A, Detels R, et al. The risk of *Pneumocystis carinii* pneumonia among men infected with human immunodeficiency virus type 1: Multicenter AIDS Cohort Study Group. N Engl J Med 322:161, 1990.
31. Stansell JD, Osmond DH, Charlebois E, et al. Predictors of *Pneumocystis carinii* pneumonia in HIV-infected persons: Pulmonary Complications of HIV Infection Study Group. Am J Respir Crit Care Med 155:60, 1997.
32. Darras-Joly C, Chevret S, Wolff M, et al. *Cryptococcus neoformans* infection in France: epidemiologic features of and early prognostic parameters for 76 patients who were infected with human immunodeficiency virus. Clin Infect Dis 23:369, 1996.
33. Van der Horst CM, Saag MS, Cloud GA, et al. Treatment of cryptococcal meningitis associated with the acquired immunodeficiency syndrome: National Institute of Allergy and Infectious Diseases Mycoses Study Group and AIDS Clinical Trials Group. N Engl J Med 337:15, 1997.
34. Rabaud C, May T, Lucet JC, et al. Pulmonary toxoplasmosis in patients infected with human immunodeficiency virus: a French national survey. Clin Infect Dis 23:1249, 1996.
35. Palella FJ Jr, Delaney KM, Moorman AC, et al. Declining morbidity and mortality among patients with advanced human immunodeficiency virus infection: HIV Outpatient Study Investigators. N Engl J Med 338:853, 1998.
36. Sullivan JH, Moore RD, Keruly JC, et al. Effect of antiretroviral therapy on the incidence of bacterial pneumonia in patients with advanced HIV infection. Am J Respir Crit Care Med 162:64, 2000.
37. Kovacs JA, Masur H. Prophylaxis against opportunistic infections in patients with human immunodeficiency virus infection. N Engl J Med 342:1416, 2000.
38. Schneider MM, Borleffs JC, Stolk RP, et al. Discontinuation of prophylaxis for *Pneumocystis carinii* pneumonia in HIV-1-infected patients treated with highly active antiretroviral therapy. Lancet 353:201, 1999.
39. Weverling GJ, Mocroft A, Ledergerber B, et al. Discontinuation of *Pneumocystis carinii* pneumonia prophylaxis after start of highly active antiretroviral therapy in HIV-1 infection: EuroSIDA study group. Lancet 353:1293, 1999.
40. Kirk O, Lundgren JD, Pedersen C, et al. Can chemoprophylaxis against opportunistic infections be discontinued after an increase in CD4 cells induced by highly active antiretroviral therapy? AIDS 13:1647, 1999.
41. Mussini C, Pezzotti P, Govoni A, et al. Discontinuation of primary prophylaxis for *Pneumocystis carinii* pneumonia and toxoplasmic encephalitis in human immunodeficiency virus type I-infected patients: the changes in opportunistic prophylaxis study. J Infect Dis 181:1635, 2000.
42. Furrer H, Opravil M, Rossi M. Discontinuation of primary prophylaxis in HIV-infected patients at high risk of *Pneumocystis carinii* pneumonia: prospective multicentre study. AIDS 15:501, 2001.
43. Lopez Bernaldo de Quiros J, Miro J, Pena J. A randomized trial of the discontinuation of primary and secondary prophylaxis against *Pneumocystis carinii* pneumonia after highly active antiretroviral therapy in patients with HIV infection. N Engl J Med 344:159, 2001.
44. Ledergerber B, Mocroft A, Reiss P. Discontinuation of secondary prophylaxis against *Pneumocystis carinii* pneumonia in patients with HIV infection who have a response to antiretroviral therapy. N Engl J Med 344:168, 2001.
45. Katz MH, Baron RB, Grady D. Risk stratification of ambulatory patients suspected of *Pneumocystis* pneumonia. Arch Intern Med 151:105, 1991.
46. Garay SM, Greene J. Prognostic indicators in the initial presentation of *Pneumocystis carinii* pneumonia. Chest 95:769, 1989.
47. Magnenat JL, Nicod LP, Auckenthaler R, et al. Mode of presentation and diagnosis of bacterial pneumonia in human immunodeficiency virus-infected patients. Am Rev Respir Dis 144:917, 1991.
48. Selwyn PA, Pumerantz AS, Durante A, et al. Clinical predictors of *Pneumocystis carinii* pneumonia, bacterial pneumonia and tuberculosis in HIV-infected patients. AIDS 12:885, 1998.
49. Burack JH, Hahn JA, Saint-Maurice D, et al. Microbiology of community-acquired bacterial pneumonia in persons with and at risk for human immunodeficiency virus type 1 infection: implications for rational empiric antibiotic therapy. Arch Intern Med 154:2589, 1994.
50. Janoff EN, Breiman RF, Daley CL, et al. Pneumococcal disease during HIV infection: epidemiologic, clinical, and immunologic perspectives. Ann Intern Med 117:314, 1992.
51. Garcia-Leoni ME, Moreno S, Rodeno P, et al. Pneumococcal pneumonia in adult hospitalized patients infected with the human immunodeficiency virus. Arch Intern Med 152:1808, 1992.
52. Schlamm HT, Yancovitz SR. *Haemophilus influenzae* pneumonia in young adults with AIDS, ARC, or risk of AIDS. Am J Med 86:11, 1989.
53. Moreno S, Martinez R, Barros C, et al. Latent *Haemophilus influenzae* pneumonia in patients infected with HIV. AIDS 5:967, 1991.
54. Cordero E, Pachón J, Rivero A, et al. *Haemophilus influenzae* pneumonia in human immunodeficiency virus-infected patients: the Grupo Andaluz para el Estudio de las Enfermedades Infecciosas. Clin Infect Dis 30:461, 2000.

55. Schuster MG, Norris AH. Community-acquired *Pseudomonas aeruginosa* pneumonia in patients with HIV infection. AIDS 8:1437, 1994.
56. Dropulic LK, Leslie JM, Eldred LJ, et al. Clinical manifestations and risk factors of *Pseudomonas aeruginosa* infection in patients with AIDS. J Infect Dis 171:930, 1995.
57. Blatt SP, Dolan MJ, Hendrix CW, et al. Legionnaires' disease in human immunodeficiency virus-infected patients: eight cases and review. Clin Infect Dis 18:227, 1994.
58. Comandini UV, Maggi P, Santopadre P, et al. *Chlamydia pneumoniae* respiratory infections among patients infected with the human immunodeficiency virus. Eur J Clin Microbiol Infect Dis 16:720, 1997.
59. Tarp B, Jensen JS, Ostergaard L, et al. Search for agents causing atypical pneumonia in HIV-positive patients by inhibitor-controlled PCR assays. Eur Respir J 13:175, 1999.
60. Donisi A, Suardi MG, Casari S, et al. *Rhodococcus equi* infection in HIV-infected patients. AIDS 10:359, 1996.
61. Uttamchandani RB, Daikos GL, Reyes RR, et al. Nocardiosis in 30 patients with advanced human immunodeficiency virus infection: clinical features and outcome. Clin Infect Dis 18:348, 1994.
62. DeLorenzo LJ, Huang CT, Maguire GP, et al. Roentgenographic patterns of *Pneumocystis carinii* pneumonia in 104 patients with AIDS. Chest 91:323, 1987.
63. Kennedy CA, Goetz MB. Atypical roentgenographic manifestations of *Pneumocystis carinii* pneumonia. Arch Intern Med 152:1390, 1992.
64. Huang L, Stansell JD, Osmond D, et al. Performance of an algorithm to detect *P. carinii* pneumonia in HIV-infected patients. Chest 115:1025, 1999.
65. Jones BE, Young SM, Antoniskis D, et al. Relationship of the manifestations of tuberculosis to CD4 cell counts in patients with human immunodeficiency virus infection. Am Rev Respir Dis 148:1292, 1993.
66. Abouya L, Coulibaly IM, Coulibaly D, et al. Radiologic manifestations of pulmonary tuberculosis in HIV-1 and HIV-2-infected patients in Abidjan, Cote d'Ivoire. Tuber Lung Dis 76:436, 1995.
67. Perlman DC, el-Sadr WM, Nelson ET, et al. Variation of chest radiographic patterns in pulmonary tuberculosis by degree of human immunodeficiency virus-related immunosuppression: the Terry Beirn Community Programs for Clinical Research on AIDS (CPCRA); The AIDS Clinical Trials Group (ACTG). Clin Infect Dis 25:242, 1997.
68. Naidich DP, McGuinness G. Pulmonary manifestations of AIDS: CT and radiographic correlations. Radiol Clin North Am 29:999, 1991.
69. Hartman TE, Primack SL, Muller NL, et al. Diagnosis of thoracic complications in AIDS: accuracy of CT. AJR Am J Roentgenol 162:547, 1994.
70. Opravil M, Marincek B, Fuchs WA, et al. Shortcomings of chest radiography in detecting *Pneumocystis carinii* pneumonia. J Acquir Immune Defic Syndr 7:39, 1994.
71. Gruden JF, Huang L, Turner J, et al. High-resolution CT in the evaluation of clinically suspected *Pneumocystis carinii* pneumonia in AIDS patients with normal, equivocal, or nonspecific radiographic findings. AJR Am J Roentgenol 169:967, 1997.
72. Edinburgh KJ, Jasmer RM, Huang L, et al. Multiple pulmonary nodules in AIDS: usefulness of CT in distinguishing among potential causes. Radiology 214:427, 2000.
73. Jasmer RM, Edinburgh KJ, Thompson A, et al. Clinical and radiographic predictors of the etiology of pulmonary nodules in HIV-infected patients. Chest 117:1023, 2000.
74. Woolfenden JM, Carrasquillo JA, Larson SM, et al. Acquired immunodeficiency syndrome: Ga-67 citrate imaging. Radiology 162:383, 1987.
75. Kirshenbaum KJ, Burke R, Fanapour F, et al. Pulmonary high-resolution computed tomography versus gallium scintigraphy: diagnostic utility in the diagnosis of patients with AIDS who have chest symptoms and normal or equivocal chest radiographs. J Thorac Imaging 13:52, 1998.
76. Morris AM, Huang L, Bacchetti P, et al. Permanent declines in pulmonary function following pneumonia in human immunodeficiency virus-infected persons: the Pulmonary Complications of HIV Infection Study Group. Am J Respir Crit Care Med 162:612, 2000.
77. Kvale PA, Rosen MJ, Hopewell PC, et al. A decline in the pulmonary diffusing capacity does not indicate opportunistic lung disease in asymptomatic persons infected with the human immunodeficiency virus: Pulmonary Complications of HIV Infection Study Group. Am Rev Respir Dis 148:390, 1993.
78. Batungwanayo J, Taelman H, Bogaerts J, et al. Pulmonary cryptococcosis associated with HIV-1 infection in Rwanda: a retrospective study of 37 cases. AIDS 8:1271, 1994.
79. Wheat LJ, Connolly-Stringfield P, Williams B, et al. Diagnosis of histoplasmosis in patients with the acquired immunodeficiency syndrome by detection of *Histoplasma capsulatum* polysaccharide antigen in bronchoalveolar lavage fluid. Am Rev Respir Dis 145:1421, 1992.
80. Kvale PA, Hansen NI, Markowitz N, et al. Routine analysis of induced sputum is not an effective strategy for screening persons infected with human immunodeficiency virus for *Mycobacterium tuberculosis* or *Pneumocystis carinii:* Pulmonary Complications of HIV Infection Study Group. Clin Infect Dis 19:410, 1994.
81. Niederman MS, Bass JB Jr, Campbell GD, et al. Guidelines for the initial management of adults with community-acquired pneumonia: diagnosis, assessment of severity, and initial antimicrobial therapy: American Thoracic Society; Medical Section of the American Lung Association. Am Rev Respir Dis 148:1418, 1993.
82. Bartlett JG, Dowell SF, Mandell LA, et al. Practice guidelines for the management of community-acquired pneumonia in adults. Infectious Diseases Society of America. Clin Infect Dis 31:347, 2000.
83. Metersky ML, Aslenzadeh J, Stelmach P. A comparison of induced and expectorated sputum for the diagnosis of *Pneumocystis carinii* pneumonia. Chest 113:1555, 1998.
84. Huang L, Hecht FM, Stansell JD, et al. Suspected *Pneumocystis carinii* pneumonia with a negative induced sputum examination: is early bronchoscopy useful? Am J Respir Crit Care Med 151:1866, 1995.
85. Kovacs JA, Ng VL, Masur H, et al. Diagnosis of *Pneumocystis carinii* pneumonia: improved detection in sputum with use of monoclonal antibodies. N Engl J Med 318:589, 1988.
86. Greenberg SD, Frager D, Suster B, et al. Active pulmonary tuberculosis in patients with AIDS: spectrum of radiographic findings (including a normal appearance). Radiology 193:115, 1994.
87. Smith RL, Yew K, Berkowitz KA, et al. Factors affecting the yield of acid-fast sputum smears in patients with HIV and tuberculosis. Chest 106:684, 1994.
88. American Thoracic Society. Diagnosis and treatment of disease caused by nontuberculous mycobacteria. Am J Respir Crit Care Med 156:S1, 1997.
89. Kalayjian RC, Toossi Z, Tomashefski JF Jr, et al. Pulmonary disease due to infection by *Mycobacterium avium* complex in patients with AIDS. Clin Infect Dis 20:1186, 1995.
90. Witzig RS, Fazal BA, Mera RM, et al. Clinical manifestations and implications of coinfection with *Mycobacterium kansasii* and human immunodeficiency virus type 1. Clin Infect Dis 21:77, 1995.
91. Meyohas MC, Roux P, Bollens D, et al. Pulmonary cryptococcosis: localized and disseminated infections in 27 patients with AIDS. Clin Infect Dis 21:628, 1995.
92. Rodriguez-Barradas MC, Stool E, Musher DM, et al. Diagnosing and treating cytomegalovirus pneumonia in patients with AIDS. Clin Infect Dis 23:76, 1996.
93. Salomon N, Gomez T, Perlman DC, et al. Clinical features and outcomes of HIV-related cytomegalovirus pneumonia. AIDS 11:319, 1997.
94. Whitley RJ, Jacobson MA, Friedberg DN, et al. Guidelines for the treatment of cytomegalovirus diseases in patients with AIDS in the era of potent antiretroviral therapy: recommendations of an international panel: International AIDS Society—USA. Arch Intern Med 158:957, 1998.
95. Eisner MD, Kaplan LD, Herndier B, et al. The pulmonary manifestations of AIDS-related non-Hodgkin's lymphoma. Chest 110:729, 1996.
96. Judson MA, Sahn SA. Endobronchial lesions in HIV-infected individuals. Chest 105:1314, 1994.
97. Gruden JF, Klein JS, Webb WR. Percutaneous transthoracic needle biopsy in AIDS: analysis in 32 patients. Radiology 189:567, 1993.
98. Cordero E, Pachón J, Rivero A, et al. Community-acquired bacterial pneumonia in human immunodeficiency virus-infected patients: validation of severity criteria; the Grupo Andaluz para el Estudio de las Enfermedades Infecciosas. Am J Respir Crit Care Med 162:2063, 2000.
99. Ma L, Borio L, Masur H, et al. *Pneumocystis carinii* dihydropteroate synthase but not dihydrofolate reductase gene mutations correlate with prior trimethoprim-sulfamethoxazole or dapsone use. J Infect Dis 180:1969, 1999.
100. Helweg-Larsen J, Benfield TL, Eugen-Olsen J, et al. Effects of mutations in *Pneumocystis carinii* dihydropteroate synthase gene on out-

come of AIDS-associated *P. carinii* pneumonia. Lancet 354:1347, 1999.
101. Kazanjian P, Armstrong W, Hossler PA, et al. *Pneumocystis carinii* mutations are associated with duration of sulfa or sulfone prophylaxis exposure in AIDS patients. J Infect Dis 182:551, 2000.
102. Navin T, Beard CB, Huang L. Mutations in the *Pneumocystis carinii* dihydropteroate synthase gene do not affect outcome of *P. carinii* pneumonia in HIV-infected patients. Lancet 358:545, 2001.
103. Behrens GM, Meyer D, Stoll M, et al. Immune reconstitution syndromes in human immuno-deficiency virus infection following effective antiretroviral therapy. Immunobiology 202:186, 2000.
104. Narita M, Ashkin D, Hollender ES, et al. Paradoxical worsening of tuberculosis following antiretroviral therapy in patients with AIDS. Am J Respir Crit Care Med 158:157, 1998.
105. Fishman JE, Saraf-Lavi E, Narita M, et al. Pulmonary tuberculosis in AIDS patients: transient chest radiographic worsening after initiation of antiretroviral therapy. AJR Am J Roentgenol 174:43, 2000.
106. Wislez M, Bergot E, Antoine M, et al. Acute respiratory failure following HAART introduction in patient's treated for *Pneumocystis carinii* pneumonia. Am J Respir Crit Care Med 164:847, 2001.
107. Aboulafia DM. Regression of acquired immunodeficiency syndrome-related pulmonary Kaposi's sarcoma after highly active antiretroviral therapy. Mayo Clin Proc 73:439, 1998.
108. Lebbé C, Blum L, Pellet C, et al. Clinical and biological impact of antiretroviral therapy with protease inhibitors on HIV-related Kaposi's sarcoma. AIDS 12:F45, 1998.
109. Dupont C, Vasseur E, Beauchet A, et al. Long-term efficacy on Kaposi's sarcoma of highly active antiretroviral therapy in a cohort of HIV-positive patients; CISIH 92: Centre d'information et de soins de l'immunodéficience humaine. AIDS 14:987, 2000.
110. Naccache JM, Antoine M, Wislez M, et al. Sarcoid-like pulmonary disorder in human immunodeficiency virus-infected patients receiving antiretroviral therapy. Am J Respir Crit Care Med 159:2009, 1999.
111. Mirmirani P, Maurer TA, Herndier B, et al. Sarcoidosis in a patient with AIDS: a manifestation of immune restoration syndrome. J Am Acad Dermatol 41:285, 1999.
112. Gomez V, Smith PR, Burack J, et al. Sarcoidosis after antiretroviral therapy in a patient with acquired immunodeficiency syndrome. Clin Infect Dis 31:1278, 2000.
113. Blanche P, Gombert B, Rollot F, et al. Sarcoidosis in a patient with acquired immunodeficiency syndrome treated with interleukin-2. Clin Infect Dis 31:1493, 2000.
114. Morris AM, Nishimura S, Huang L. Subacute hypersensitivity pneumonitis in an HIV infected patient receiving antiretroviral therapy. Thorax 55:625, 2000.
115. Herndier B, Ganem D. The biology of Kaposi's sarcoma. Cancer Treat Res 104:89, 2001.
116. White DA. Pulmonary complications of HIV-associated malignancies. Clin Chest Med 17:755, 1996.
117. Gruden JF, Huang L, Webb WR, et al. AIDS-related Kaposi sarcoma of the lung: radiographic findings and staging system with bronchoscopic correlation. Radiology 195:545, 1995.
118. Dal Maso L, Serraino D, Franceschi S. Epidemiology of HIV-associated malignancies. Cancer Treat Res 104: 1, 2001.
119. Bazot M, Cadranel J, Benayoun S, et al. Primary pulmonary AIDS-related lymphoma: radiographic and CT findings. Chest 116:1282, 1999.
120. Parker MS, Leveno DM, Campbell TJ, et al. AIDS-related bronchogenic carcinoma: fact or fiction? Chest 113:154, 1998.
121. Johnson CC, Wilcosky T, Kvale P, et al. Cancer incidence among an HIV-infected cohort: Pulmonary Complications of HIV Infection Study Group. Am J Epidemiol 146:470, 1997.
122. Gruden JF, Webb WR, Yao DC, et al. Bronchogenic carcinoma in 13 patients infected with the human immunodeficiency virus (HIV): clinical and radiographic findings. J Thorac Imaging 10:99, 1995.
123. Bazot M, Cadranel J, Khalil A, et al. Computed tomographic diagnosis of bronchogenic carcinoma in HIV-infected patients. Lung Cancer 28:203, 2000.
124. Thurer RJ, Jacobs JP, Holland FW II, et al. Surgical treatment of lung cancer in patients with human immunodeficiency virus. Ann Thorac Surg 60:599, 1995.
125. Massera F, Rocco G, Rossi G, et al. Pulmonary resection for lung cancer in HIV-positive patients with low (< 200 lymphocytes/mm^3) CD4$^+$ count. Lung Cancer 29:147, 2000.
126. Ognibene FP, Masur H, Rogers P, et al. Nonspecific interstitial pneumonitis without evidence of *Pneumocystis carinii* in asymptomatic patients infected with human immunodeficiency virus (HIV). Ann Intern Med 109:874, 1988.
127. Schneider RF. Lymphocytic interstitial pneumonitis and nonspecific interstitial pneumonitis. Clin Chest Med 17:763, 1996.
128. Oldham SA, Castillo M, Jacobson FL, et al. HIV-associated lymphocytic interstitial pneumonia: radiologic manifestations and pathologic correlation. Radiology 170:83, 1989.
129. Griffiths MH, Miller RF, Semple SJ. Interstitial pneumonitis in patients infected with the human immunodeficiency virus. Thorax 50:1141, 1995.
130. Simmons JT, Suffredini AF, Lack EE, et al. Nonspecific interstitial pneumonitis in patients with AIDS: radiologic features. AJR Am J Roentgenol 149:265, 1987.
131. Mehta NJ, Khan IA, Mehta RN, et al. HIV-related pulmonary hypertension: analytic review of 131 cases. Chest 118:1133, 2000.
132. Petitpretz P, Brenot F, Azarian R, et al. Pulmonary hypertension in patients with human immunodeficiency virus infection: comparison with primary pulmonary hypertension. Circulation 89:2722, 1994.
133. Aguilar RV, Farber HW. Epoprostenol (prostacyclin) therapy in HIV-associated pulmonary hypertension. Am J Respir Crit Care Med 162:1846, 2000.
134. Opravil M, Pechère M, Speich R, et al. HIV-associated primary pulmonary hypertension: a case control study; Swiss HIV Cohort Study. Am J Respir Crit Care Med 155:990, 1997.
135. Allen JN, Wewers MD. HIV-associated bronchiolitis obliterans organizing pneumonia. Chest 96:197, 1989.
136. Leo YS, Pitchon HE, Messler G, et al. Bronchiolitis obliterans organizing pneumonia in a patient with AIDS. Clin Infect Dis 18:921, 1994.
137. Sanito NJ, Morley TF, Condoluci DV. Bronchiolitis obliterans organizing pneumonia in an AIDS patient. Eur Respir J 8:1021, 1995.
138. Zahraa J, Herold B, Abrahams C, et al. Bronchiolitis obliterans organizing pneumonia in a child with acquired immunodeficiency syndrome. Pediatr Infect Dis J 15:448, 1996.
139. Díaz F, Collazos J, Martinez E, et al. Bronchiolitis obliterans in a patient with HIV infection. Respir Med 91:171, 1997.
140. Coots LE, Lazarus AA. Sarcoidosis diagnosed in a patient with known HIV infection. Chest 96:201, 1989.
141. Lowery WS, Whitlock WL, Dietrich RA, et al. Sarcoidosis complicated by HIV infection: three case reports and a review of the literature. Am Rev Respir Dis 142:887, 1990.
142. Amin DN, Sperber K, Brown LK, et al. Positive Kveim test in patients with coexisting sarcoidosis and human immunodeficiency virus infection. Chest 101:1454, 1992.
143. Newman TG, Minkowitz S, Hanna A, et al. Coexistent sarcoidosis and HIV infection: a comparison of bronchoalveolar and peripheral blood lymphocytes. Chest 102:1899, 1992.
144. Porter JP, Patel AA, Dewey CM, et al. Prevalence of sinonasal symptoms in patients with HIV infection. Am J Rhinol 13:203, 1999.
145. Zurlo JJ, Feuerstein IM, Lebovics R, et al. Sinusitis in HIV-1 infection. Am J Med 93:157, 1992.
146. Upadhyay S, Marks SC, Arden RL, et al. Bacteriology of sinusitis in human immunodeficiency virus-positive patients: implications for management. Laryngoscope 105:1058, 1995.
147. Marks SC, Upadhyay S, Crane L. Cytomegalovirus sinusitis. a new manifestation of AIDS. Arch Otolaryngol Head Neck Surg 122:789, 1996.
148. Hunt SM, Miyamoto RC, Cornelius RS, et al. Invasive fungal sinusitis in the acquired immunodeficiency syndrome. Otolaryngol Clin North Am 33:335, 2000.

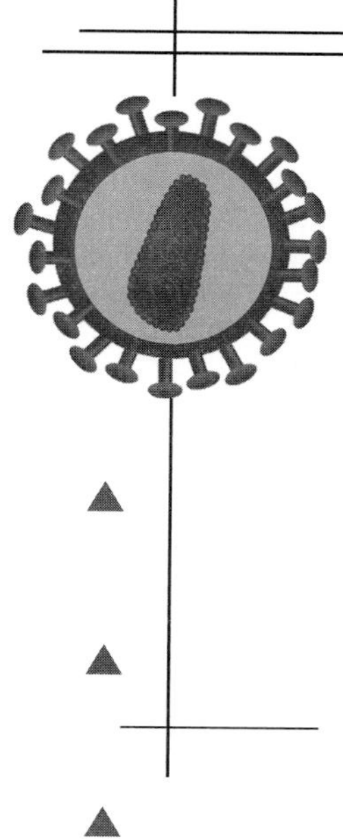

CHAPTER 61

Renal Disease

Jonathan A. Winston, MD
Paul E. Klotman, MD

Diseases of the kidney generally present as one of two clinical syndromes: acute renal failure or chronic renal failure. Both have become relatively common complications of human immunodeficiency virus type 1 (HIV-1) infection. Acute renal failure commonly occurs after ischemic injury and is often a component of a severe systemic inflammatory response syndrome. The spectrum of nephrotoxic renal injury has evolved with the introduction of new antimicrobial, antiretroviral, and antineoplastic agents. Drug-induced crystalluria and rhabdomyolysis are now relatively frequent drug-induced renal complications of HIV-1 infection. Several important forms of chronic kidney disease are associated with HIV-1 infection. This chapter reviews these disorders in detail and provides a clinical framework for diagnosis and treatment.

▲ ACUTE RENAL FAILURE

Acute renal failure (ARF) is defined as an abrupt, detectable fall in the glomerular filtration rate (GFR) in an individual with otherwise normal kidney function. Depending on the clinical setting, it may present as an otherwise asymptomatic increase in serum creatinine, or it may be associated with the clinical stigmata of an underlying systemic disease. The diagnostic approach is based on the context of the clinical setting, microscopic examination of the urine, and imaging studies that evaluate kidney structure and exclude urinary tract obstruction. Renal sonography is most effective and should be obtained in virtually all cases of ARF.

Ischemic ARF is common in seropositive hospitalized patients. In this setting, ARF may be due to hypoperfusion-induced ischemic injury in tubule cells and the renal microvasculature. The common clinical setting is sepsis, hypotension, or regional vasoconstriction. ARF may be oliguric or nonoliguric in nature. Nonoliguric ARF is more likely associated with nephrotoxic injury, but daily urinary volume exceeding 1 L/day does not exclude ischemic injury. Examination of the urine is a key to the diagnosis. Typically, with ischemic injury the urinary sediment contains numerous necrotic, pigmented (muddy-brown) tubule epithelial cells and casts. Hematuria or proteinuria suggests a parenchymal disease that is unrelated to ischemia, and other causes of kidney disease should be considered. HIV-associated mephropathy (HIVAN), acute glomerulonephritis, and hemolytic-uremic syndrome (HUS) frequently present as ARF.[1] Crystalluria suggests obstruction, either within the renal tubule or in the lower genitourinary (GU) tract. Eosinophiluria indicates drug-induced allergic interstitial nephritis. The diagnosis of ischemic injury can often be made with reasonable confidence using these clinical criteria. A kidney biopsy is rarely necessary.

In oliguric patients the chemical characteristics of the urine are important for distinguishing ischemic injury from prerenal azotemia.[2] The physiologic response to hypoperfusion is enhancement of renal salt and water reabsorption. Ischemic injury is therefore characterized by impaired urinary concentration ability (specific gravity about 1.010) and submaximal Na reabsorption [urinary Na concentration > 20 mEq/l; fractional Na excretion (FE_{Na}) > 1%]. Oliguria accompanied by preserved salt and H_2O handling (specific gravity > 1.018, urinary Na concentration < 10 mEq/L, and FE_{Na} < 1%) defines prerenal azotemia. An accurate diagnosis is important because correction of abnormal hemodynamics can prevent ischemic injury and promptly improve kidney function.

Two relatively new renal syndromes are assuming greater importance: drug-induced rhabdomyolysis and crystalluria. Rhabdomyolysis causes myoglobinuria-induced ARF. It can occur as a direct result of HIV-1 infection, in association with zidovudine (ZDV) administration, and complicating trauma, convulsions, and cocaine use. Several reports are now appearing that describe rhabdomyolysis when statins are prescribed for patients with protease inhibitor (PI)-induced dyslipidemia.[3] The magnitude of the problem, its pathogenesis, and prevention are areas of active investigation. Statins and PIs share a common metabolic pathway (CYP3A4), and the combination may result in high tissue drug levels. Rhabdomyolysis, however, has occurred with newer agents, (e.g., cerivastatin) that are metabolized via alternate pathways.[4] Myoglobinuria-induced renal failure is relatively unusual when creatine phospokinase (CPK) levels are appreciably lower than 10,000 U/L. Treatment is aimed at reducing urinary myoglobin solubility through a combination of intravenous hydration and urinary alkalinization.

Drug-induced crystalluria is observed in 20% to 40% of patients receiving indinavir.[5–7] The syndrome is recognized by leukocyturia, hematuria, and characteristic crystals seen by light microscopy. They appear as needle-shaped crystals, grouped in the form of fans or rectangles. Indinavir crystalluria is generally asymptomatic but can cause dysuria and colic. Obstructive uropathy may also occur. Chronic renal insufficiency due to interstitial fibrosis is a rare occurrence.[8] A hydration protocol of 1 to 2 L prior to drug ingestion has been advocated to prevent high intratubule concentrations of drug. Drug discontinuation is not necessary for asymptomatic disease or even colic. In patients with progressive renal impairment, it is prudent to discontinue the drug as the creatinine level approaches 2 mg/dl. Sulfadiazine also produces crystalluria.[9] The crystals are recognized as characteristic "shocks of wheat" under light microscopy. Treatment is with hydration and urinary alkalinization. Commonly used agents with direct nephrotoxic potential include aminoglycosides, amphotericin, acyclovir, ganciclovir, pentamidine, foscarnet, and trimethoprim-sulfamethoxazole. Rifampin and penicillins are relatively common causes of drug-induced interstitial nephritis.[10]

▲ CHRONIC RENAL INSUFFICIENCY

When describing the condition of chronic disease of the kidney, terms such as "chronic renal failure," "chronic renal insufficiency," and "chronic kidney disease" are often used interchangeably. Unfortunately, they tend to be imprecise and confusing. A variety of distinct diseases can damage the kidney, and each has characteristic clinicopathologic features. The focus should be on the etiology of disease, the magnitude of the reduction in the GFR, the likelihood of progression to end-stage renal disease (ESRD), the rate of progression to ESRD, and associated co-morbidities such as nephrotic syndrome, hypertension, cardiovascular disease, hyperkalemia, or metabolic bone disease. No single term accurately describes all these clinical features. Some advocate the term "chronic renal insufficiency (CRI)" as best to describe nonacute reductions in GFR. The degree of renal insufficiency can then be classified as mild (GFR 40 to 60 ml/min), moderate (20 to 40 ml/min), or advanced (< 20 ml/min).[11]

Hematuria

A detailed description of the clinical consequences of CRI is beyond the scope of this text but can be found in many excellent texts and reviews.[12] The severity of kidney disease may range from asymptomatic urinary abnormalities to severe reductions in GFR. Microscopic hematuria and mild proteinuria are examples of asymptomatic urinary abnormalities. By themselves they have little clinical impact, but their presence may indicate an early form of a serious disease. In the general population, microscopic hematuria (> 3 RBCs/hpf) is a useful sign for a variety of GU disturbances, the most important of which are occult neoplasms.

As is true for the general population, the underlying causes of hematuria in patients with HIV-1 infection are determined in part by the age of the population under study; their selection from an inpatient service, a general medical clinic, or a GU subspecialty clinic; and the presence of other GU symptoms. The prevalence of asymptomatic hematuria approaches 25% in a young, unselected cohort of HIV-1-infected individuals.[13] In this setting, a workup for medically important illness has proved unrewarding because most cases are mild and transient. Antiretroviral (ARV)-induced crystalluria has become a relatively frequent cause of microscopic hematuria, although leukocyturia is a more specific marker of the disorder. An opportunistic infection of the GU tract must be considered in the differential diagnosis, but this is unlikely in an otherwise asymptomatic patient. As in the general population, a selective diagnostic approach to hematuria is recommended for HIV-1 infected patients.[14] The extent of evaluation should be based on the individual's age, stage of HIV-1 infection, general medical status, and the presence of other symptoms. The risk of occult malignancy increases in patients approaching 50 years of age. In these older patients, a complete evaluation for microscopic hematuria is warranted, including renal imaging by intravenous pyelography (IVP) or computed tomography (CT) scans and cystoscopy. When hematuria is accompanied by proteinuria, underlying kidney disease is more likely.

Proteinuria

Daily urinary protein excretion ranging between 1000 and 3000 mg/day, when unaccompanied by other stigmata of chronic renal insufficiency, is referred to as asymptomatic proteinuria. When proteinuria exceeds 3 g/24 hr it is often accompanied by other components of the nephrotic syndrome: edema, hypoalbuminemia, and hypercholesterolemia. Nephrosis is complicated by anasarca, pleural effusions, immunoglobin G (IgG) deficiency, accelerated atherosclerosis and venous thrombosis, each of which requires specific therapy. Nephrologists take various approaches to establishing a renal diagnosis in patients with asymptomatic proteinura, but there is general agreement that a kidney biopsy is indicated for patients with the nephrotic syndrome. It is not clear whether the same clinical standards are being applied to HIV-1-infected individuals, and kidney biopsies are probably underutilized.

Renal Disease in HIV-Infected Patients

The spectrum of chronic renal diseases associated with HIV-1 infection is depicted in Table 61–1. HIVAN is most common. The disease is defined morphologically by collapse of the glomerular capillary tuft, glomerulosclerosis, and microcystic tubulointerstitial disease[15,16] (Fig. 61–1). The most striking epidemiologic characteristic is that approximately 90% of patients with HIVAN are of African descent. This racial predilection is observed not only in North America but has been confirmed in reports from Europe and Asia.[17–19] The US Renal Data System manages a comprehensive database for the ESRD program. According to this resource, 89% of patients who develop ESRD from HIVAN are of African descent.[20,21] This racial predisposition for kidney disease is second only to the racial clustering for sickle cell-associated renal disease. A better understanding of the genetic basis for HIVAN will likely provide important links to our understanding of the genetic basis of other kidney diseases in African Americans.

The racial predilection for HIVAN accounts for the differences in reported prevalence from various centers, which is highly dependent on the population under study. When reports of renal disease in HIV-1 infected subjects come from mainly Caucasian populations, such as those in studies from San Francisco, Italy, Asia, and northern Europe, HIVAN is not a frequent cause of chronic kidney disease.[22–25] When Blacks comprise a large proportion of the population under study, as in reports from New York, Washington, DC, Miami, and the African or Afro-Caribbean communities of Paris and London, HIVAN is by far the most common cause of renal disease in HIV-infected individuals.[17–19] HIVAN is now the third leading cause of ESRD in Blacks age 20 to 64 years old. It is a more common cause of renal failure than lupus nephritis, polycystic disease, or primary glomerulonephritis in this group.[20]

▲ Table 61–1. RENAL BIOPSIES IN HIV-1 INFECTION

Glomerular Disease
Focal segmental sclerosis—HIVAN (70%)
Membranoproliferative GN (10%)
Minimal change disease (6%)
Membranous nephropathy (5%)
Systemic lupus erythematosus (4%)
Amyloidosis (4%)
Tubulointerstitial Disease
Drug-induced
Idiopathic
Acute tubular necrosis
Lymphoma
Miscellaneous Disease
Hemolytic-uremic syndrome
IgA deficiency
Focal necrotizing GN
Postinfectious condition
Immunotactoid disorder

GN, glomerulonephritis; HIVAN, HIV-associated nephropathy; IgA, immunoglobulin A.

Adapted from D'Agati V, Appel GB. Renal pathology of human immunodeficiency virus infection. Semin Nephrol 18:406, 1998.

Clinical characteristics of HIVAN include the presence of heavy proteinuria (often in the nephrotic range) and varying degrees of renal insufficiency. Sonographic evaluation may reveal enlarged kidneys. The predictive value of these clinical characteristics has not been rigorously tested, and numerous reports confirm that the clinical impression is not always borne out by the biopsy findings.[26–28] The clinical course in most patients is marked by progression to ESRD within weeks to months. Maintenance of stable kidney function for a period much longer than 1 year after confirmation of the diagnosis is unusual. These data speak to the rapidly progressive nature of HIVAN and suggest that most cases are recognized late in the natural history of the disease.

Our understanding of disease pathogenesis has grown considerably over the past several years owing in large part to experiments performed in a murine model of the disease. Mice of the TG26 line contain copies of the HIV-1 proviral DNA pNL4-3d1443 under transcriptional control of the native promoter, the long terminal repeat (LTR). The transgene was generated by deletion of a 3 kb SphI/BalI fragment within pNL4-3 spanning the *gag* and *pol* genes, rendering the construct noninfectious and nonreplicating. Heterozygote mice develop a kidney disease that is both morphologically and functionally indistinguishable from HIVAN in humans.[29,30] Several important stages in disease pathogenesis have been studied.

Renal transgene expression precedes the development of nephropathy. Disease activity increases when transgene expression is induced ex vivo in kidney cultures. In this preparation there are no circulating factors to modify the disease, which supports a primary role for transgene expression in disease pathogenesis. Dysregulated cytokine expression and matrix accumulation does occur in vivo,[29,31] but these factors contribute to disease pathogenesis as modifying factors. Further support of a direct role for HIV-1 in pathogenesis is provided by cross-transplantation experiments. Kidney disease develops when kidneys from transgenic mice are transplanted into normal littermates, whereas normal kidneys transplanted into a transgenic host do not develop the disease.[32] Cellular markers of HIVAN have been identified. Renal tubule and glomerular epithelial cells express histochemical markers that characterize an immature, not a mature, cell type.[33,34] The HIV-1 transgene is expressed in these cells, which subsequently undergo proliferation and apoptosis.[32,35] These data identify the renal epithelial cells as primary targets of disease in the murine model.

For these events to be recapitulated in humans, epithelial cells must either become infected, or HIV-1 genes would have to be delivered to them by migrating infected mononuclear cells.[36] Support for direct infection comes from several experimental sources. Proviral DNA has been detected in microdissected glomeruli.[37] Tubule cells can be infected in vitro using co-culture techniques, and they express low levels of CD4 and chemokine receptors.[38] In situ

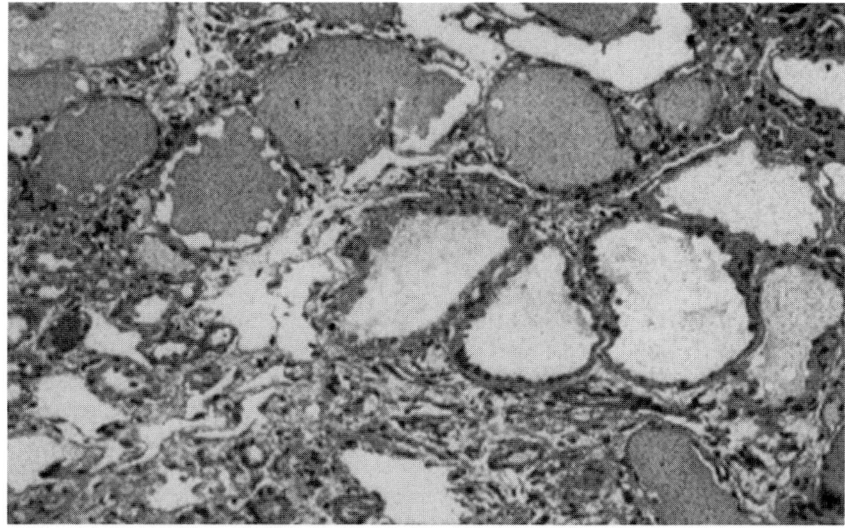

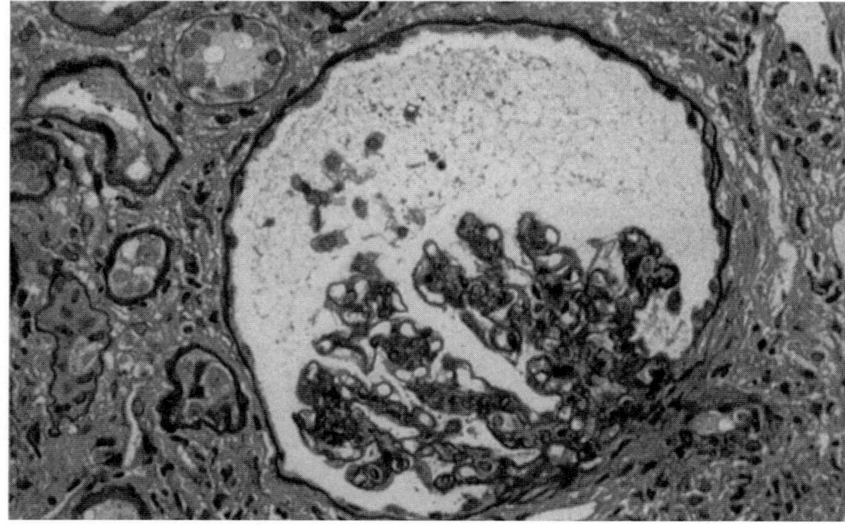

Figure 61–1. Light microscopic findings in HIV-associated nephropathy. *Top*, Characteristic microcystic tubule disease. Tubule lumens are dilated and filled with proteinaceous casts. Tubules are surrounded by interstitial edema, fibrosis, and inflammatory cells. *Bottom*, Characteristic retraction of the glomerular tuft. Several proliferating visceral epithelial cells can be seen in the urinary space.

hybridization studies have detected viral mRNA in podocytes, tubule epithelial cells, and infiltrating mononuclear cells[39] (Fig. 61–2). These data provide evidence in humans that HIVAN is a consequence of viral infection in tubule and glomerular epithelial cells. Infection is followed by a sequence of events that produce glomerular collapse and cystic tubule disease, although the exact host mechanisms remain unknown.

The studies in humans that detected viral mRNA in renal cells included a cohort of patients with kidney disease whose antiretroviral therapy and HIV-1 plasma viral load varied according to individual clinical circumstances. Renal viral mRNA was detectable in several patients who were receiving highly active retroviral therapy (HAART) and whose plasma viral RNA concentration was below the level of detection. This suggests that virus replicates in the kidney even when HAART has effectively decreased the pool of virus responsible for plasma RNA levels. One report described a patient with biopsy-proven HIVAN who presented during an acute retroviral syndrome and was therefore antiretroviral therapy-naive.[40] Studies were performed before and after initiation of HAART. Before HAART, the plasma viral load was 750,000 copies per milliliter, and kidney function was marked by nephrotic-range proteinuria and a reduced GFR. HAART reduced the plasma viral load to nondetectable levels and normalized the GFR and urinary protein excretion rate. Kidney biopsies before and during therapy demonstrated morphologic correlates of improved kidney function. DNA extracted from both biopsy specimens was assayed for the circular, unintegrated form of HIV-1 viral DNA. Circularized DNA was present before, but not during, therapy. This demonstrated that antiretroviral therapy aborted new rounds of renal cell infection. Viral mRNA, however, was detectable both before and during therapy. These observations suggest that in HIVAN the kidney is a persistent reservoir of HIV-1 RNA transcription during HAART.

Several critical questions remain. Why do Blacks get the disease and not Caucasians, and why do not all seropositive Blacks develop HIVAN? Although viral entry is the initial pathogenic step, it is not clear whether it is sufficient, by itself, to induce the disease. Factors that facilitate viral entry into kidney cells (e.g., genetic polymorphism of chemokine receptors) require further study, especially as

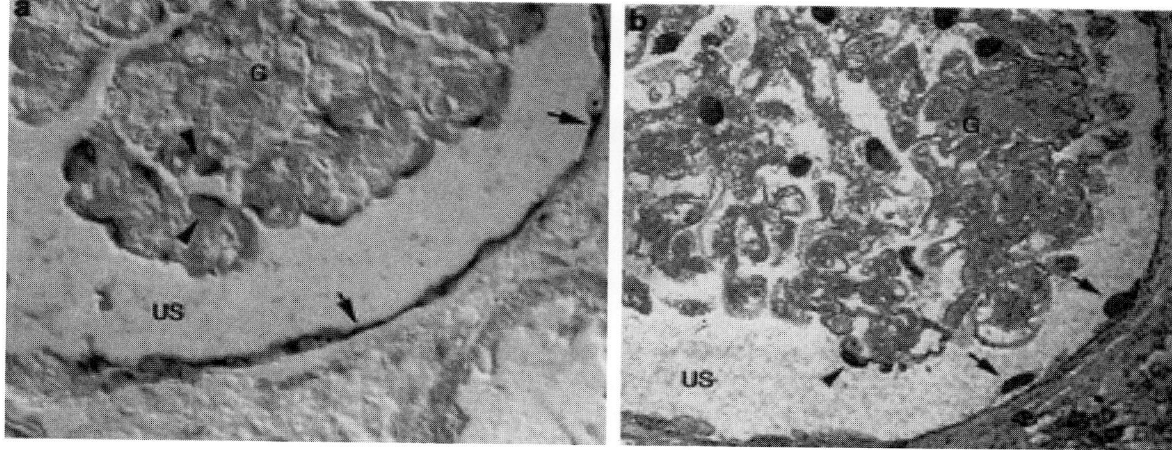

Figure 61–2. Detection of infected glomerular epithelial cells by mRNA in situ hybridization and DNA in situ polymerase chain reaction (PCR). *A*, Viral mRNA expression in podocytes (arrowheads) and the cytoplasm of parietal epithelial cells (arrows). *B*, In situ PCR demonstrates the presence of viral DNA in the same cells. (From Bruggeman LA, Ross MD, Tanji N, et al. Renal epithelium is a previously unrecognized site of HIV-1 infection. J Am Soc Nephrol 11:2079–2087, 2000, with permission.)

they may pertain to racial susceptibilities. Studies in the murine model hold promise to uncover important links between cell injury and glomerulosclerosis. This should be relevant to the pathogenesis and treatment of many forms of chronic kidney disease because sclerosis is a final common pathway. Studies in humans should be started that focus on the role of the kidney as a viral reservoir and whether interruption in therapy leads to the rapid formation of infectious virions.

Three classes of drugs have been advocated for the treatment of HIVAN: steroids, angiotensin-converting enzyme (ACE) inhibitors, and antiretroviral agents. Evidence for their respective efficacy is limited by deficiencies in study design and the limited array of effective antiretroviral therapy that had been available at the time of study. It is important to note that early in the epidemic, when AIDS was defined by the presence of opportunistic infections, survival in patients who developed kidney disease was limited to a range of weeks to months.[18,41] Subsequent to these early reports, but preceding the HAART era, mortality rates in patients with HIVAN approached 50% at 1 year and 70% at 3 years.[19] This was virtually identical to the overall acquired immunodeficiency syndrome (AIDS) mortality rates, independent of the presence of kidney disease.[26] A negative study in the pre-HAART era is difficult to interpret because of the high AIDS mortality rate. During the HAART era, a trend to improved survival for patients with kidney disease has been observed. It is difficult, however, to distinguish, an independent effect of therapy for kidney disease from the background of improved ARV therapy in general.

Steroids have been tested because they can reduce urinary protein excretion and improve the GFR in several forms of chronic kidney disease. Unfortunately, most studies using steroids for HIVAN were performed before the introduction of HAART. Several case reports described a benefit from steroids,[42–45] and an observational trial studied the effects of prednisone in 19 patients.[46] Most patients responded with a brief improvement in GFR or urinary protein excretion (or both), but by the end of the first year only two had survived without ESRD. Another group has reported their experience with steroids prior to the widespread use of HAART.[47] Steroids were dosed at 60 mg of prednisone for 1 month and gradually tapered over 2 to 4 months. Patients were not randomized but selected for treatment according to the individual physician's standards or preferences. Interpretation of the significance of these results becomes somewhat problematic. Kidney function did stabilize or improve more in the steroid-treated patients then in the untreated group. Although patients received prednisone, treatment was not associated with an increased risk of opportunistic infections during the follow-up period.

Agents that block the renin-angiotensin system, either converting enzyme inhibitors or the newer angiotensin receptor-blocking agents, have demonstrated efficacy in preventing progressive kidney failure. They have been tested in type 1 and 2 diabetes and in a cohort with advanced chronic renal insufficiency, irrespective of etiology.[48–51] Their mechanism(s) of action, although still unclear, is ascribed to reducing hydrostatic pressure in the glomerular capillary, altering glomerular basement membrane porosity (which lowers transcapillary protein flux), or reducing the renal generation of cytokines, such as transforming growth factor-β (TGFβ). Two studies have shown a benefit to the use of converting enzyme inhibitors in HIVAN.[52,53] Similar to the experience with steroids, however, these studies were performed prior to the HAART era and lacked randomized controls. Studies in the HIV transgenic mice seem to confirm the clinical impression that converting enzyme inhibitors may work, but this also requires further study. Transgenic mice given captopril in their drinking water survived longer than those given vehicle, although blood urea nitrogen levels and urinary protein excretion rates were unchanged.[54] The mechanism(s) of action of captopril in this setting remain unresolved.

The ability of antiretroviral therapy to improve kidney function in patients with HIVAN has become compelling. This is not surprising in light of the direct role of the virus in disease pathogenesis. Several studies have inferred that antiretroviral therapy reduces the rate of progression to ESRD.[52,55,56] Direct evidence for an effect is lacking because controlled trials that include an untreated arm are not justifiable; but there is evidence to support an effect of HAART on the natural history of the disease. First, the number of cases of ESRD due to HIVAN has stabilized despite an increase in the pool of patients living with AIDS since the introduction of HAART.[57] This indicates that the incidence of HIVAN has fallen or that the rate of progression to kidney failure has decreased. Retrospective reports indicate that the clinical course may have become less aggressive during the HAART era.[58] Finally, two reports have demonstrated unequivocal improvement in kidney structure and function when patients with HIVAN are treated with HAART early in the course of their kidney disease.[40,59] In these cases, treatment was initiated almost immediately after the onset of nephropathy, before glomerulosclerosis or interstitial fibrosis had developed. Usually, HIVAN is diagnosed later in the clinical course, so patients eligible for early treatment are difficult to identify. Once there is significant renal fibrosis, the overall effects of HAART may be less dramatic.

Other renal lesions are fairly common with HIV-1 infection, especially in Caucasians with chronic kidney disease. Their natural history, pathogenesis, and therapy are less well defined. Membranoproliferative glomerulonephritis is a pathologic term characterized by thickening of the glomerular basement membrane, proliferation of mesangial cells, and influx of mononuclear inflammatory cells. This disease is often the result of immune complexes. Evidence for this can be seen by electron microscopy with electron-dense immune deposits in the glomerular basement membrane. Immune complex disease associated with hepatitis C virus (HCV) co-infection is the most important cause of membranoproliferative glomerulonephritis in HIV-1 infection. This can be clinically indistinguishable from HIVAN, especially in injection drug users, who may present with heavy proteinuria and progress rapidly to ESRD.[60]

Treatment for HCV-induced glomerulonephritis has not been systematically studied. Prior to the identification of HCV, many of these cases were classified as mixed-essential cryoglobulinemia and were treated with steroids and plasmapheresis. Today, antiviral therapy with interferon-α and ribavirin are options, but their role in immune complex nephritis remains to be tested. Renal disease in association with HCV co-infection is assuming greater importance. The prevalence of proteinuria has been estimated to be as high 30% in patients with HIV-1 infection.[61] A positive test for hepatitis C antibody was associated with a greater risk of proteinuria. It seems likely that a spectrum of kidney diseases occur in HCV co-infected individuals, including HIVAN and membranoproliferative glomerulonephritis. The prevalence of these lesions, and others, in co-infected individuals must be better defined.

Several cases of glomerulonephritis have been described in which HIV proteins induce immune complex disease.[62,63] Appropriate therapy for this form of immune complex disease is uncertain. A hemolytic-uremic syndrome has been directly linked to HIV-1 infection,[64,65] and plasmapheresis is the treatment of choice. Membranous nephropathy, diabetes, amyloid, and systemic lupus erythematosus (SLE) have all been found on biopsies of seropositive patients, probably as a co-morbid condition rather than linked to HIV-1 infection. Steroids and alkylating agents are often used to treat lupus nephritis, and reports suggest that this therapy can be reasonably well tolerated in selected seropositive patients.[66,67]

Renal Biopsy

The clinician faces many diagnostic and therapeutic challenges when caring for individuals with chronic renal insufficiency and HIV-1 infection. The presence of hematuria and especially red blood cell casts in the urinary sediment indicates glomerulonephritis. Serologic tests for circulating immune complexes should be performed. Heavy proteinuria in patients who are Black or Hispanic suggests HIVAN, but a clinical diagnosis is not always accurate. In the general population, certain diseases, such as diabetic nephropathy, can be diagnosed on clinical grounds based on the positive predictive value of disease duration, proteinuria, and microvascular disease. A similar algorithm has not been validated for HIV-1-infected patients. A kidney biopsy is the most accurate way to establish the diagnosis. Indications for a biopsy in patients with HIV-1 infection should not be significantly different from that in other patients. The results provide a precise diagnosis, help establish a reasonable prognosis, and guide therapy. This can be especially useful in patients with renal disease for whom the criteria for initiating antiretroviral therapy are otherwise borderline. A diagnosis of HIVAN in this setting would favor such therapy because a response in kidney function is a realistic and important therapeutic goal.

If possible, the diagnosis of HIVAN should be established early in its course, before proteinuria reaches the nephrotic range. This is a time when it may be more amenable to treatment.[50,68] High risk patients should be screened for proteinuria and followed closely. Until new markers are identified, high risk patients are now defined as those who are either Black or Hispanic. Screening should be simple, and a urinalysis is a useful start. Urinary protein excretion should be quantified in patients whose dipstick proteinuria is 100 mg/dl or more. A 24-hour collection is precise but cumbersome. Measurement of urinary creatinine and protein concentrations in a randomly collected aliquot of urine is a convenient substitute. Normally, the urinary creatinine excretion rate is approximately 1 g/day and the protein excretion 100 to 200 mg/day. The ratio of their respective concentrations is approximately 0.1. A ratio of 1.0 indicates a urinary protein excretion rate of 1 g/day, and a ratio of 3.0 indicates nephrotic-range proteinuria.

The lowest level of proteinuria at which a biopsy is indicated is unknown, but our practice is to perform a biopsy when the daily protein excretion approaches 1000 mg. Generally, complications from a kidney biopsy are rare.[69] Transient microscopic hematuria, with or without CT evidence of a hematoma, occurs in virtually all patients and is therefore not considered an important complication. Transient gross hematuria occurs in 3% to 10% of cases and transfusions in 0.1% to 0.3%. Surgery or angiography with embolization of the bleeding vessel is necessary in 0.1% to 0.4% of cases. The latter procedure avoids nephrectomy, the incidence of which is roughly estimated at 0.06%.

In patients who have HIVAN, antiretroviral therapy should be initiated or intensified when clinically feasible. A randomized controlled trial to test the efficacy of converting enzyme inhibitors or steroids in this setting would provide invaluable information to clinicians. In the absence of such a trial, it is reasonable to use ACE inhibitors in patients whose response to antiretroviral drugs is not complete. Short-term steroids may be useful as salvage for those failing combination therapy.

Patients who progress to end-stage renal failure remain a special clinical challenge. Treatment must be initiated to control lipid abnormalities, Ca/PO_4 metabolism, and anemia. Hypertension must also be treated, although several reports indicate that hypertension is conspicuously absent in patients with HIVAN.[27] As the GFR falls, the therapeutic focus must shift to preparation for renal replacement therapy. Proper planning for hemodialysis, peritoneal dialysis, or kidney transplantation should be made well in advance of uremic symptoms. Kidney transplantation is a viable option in selected patients. Its safety and efficacy is currently under study through a cooperative research program sponsored by the National Institute of Allergy and Infectious Diseases (NIAID) and private industry.[70] Criteria for transplantation include undetectable viral RNA for at least 3 months, a CD4+ T-lymphocyte count of more than 200 cells per microliter, and no history of an opportunistic infection or neoplasm.

In patients who are likely to start hemodialysis, an arteriovenous fistula should be created months before an anticipated start date. Although this can be especially difficult in patients who are intravenous drug users because they often lack appropriate veins for fistula construction and medical follow-up is often inconsistent, venous mapping and close collaboration with vascular surgeons can increase the success rate of fistula creation. Fistulas are far superior to polytetrafluoroethylene (PTFE; Gore-Tex) grafts or percutaneous dialysis catheters because of reduced thrombosis and infection rates.[71] The long-term prognosis of patients with HIV on dialysis is determined by the stage of AIDS,[27,72] and these patients too must be aggressively treated with HAART. Survival on dialysis is improving and should continue to do so with the new antiviral drug therapies.[73,74] Current collaborative studies are underway to understand how antiretroviral drugs are prescribed in patients requiring dialysis and to develop standards of care for these patients.[75] Antiretroviral drug pharmacokinetics and dose adjustments during hemodialysis are the subject of a recent review.[76]

▲ CONCLUSIONS

Many forms of kidney disease are encountered in HIV-1-infected individuals. The clinical course of certain diseases, such as HIVAN, may be changing somewhat with the introduction of new antiretroviral therapies, but these therapies are also associated with new forms of drug-induced kidney disease. As the population ages, the prevalence of chronic renal insufficiency will likely increase. Not only is the risk pool for HIVAN increasing as patients with AIDS live longer, but HIV-1-infected patients may incur diseases more common in the aging population, such as chronic renal insufficiency due to type 2 diabetes, hypertension, and atherosclerotic vascular disease. The diagnostic approach is based on a careful history, physical examination, examination of the urine sediment, and renal imaging. Kidney biopsies should be performed to establish the precise diagnosis. Physicians should be proactive and screen for kidney disease in high risk patients. Multicenter clinical trials are necessary to define the spectrum of kidney diseases during the HAART era and the optimal therapy. This is especially true for HIVAN, which continues to be a major cause of morbidity and mortality.

REFERENCES

1. Peraldi MN, Maslo C, Akposso K, et al. Acute renal failure in the course of HIV infection: a single-institution retrospective study of ninety-two patients and sixty renal biopsies. Nephrol Dial Transplant 14:1578, 1999.
2. Brady HR, Brenner BM, Clarkson MR, Lieberthal W. Acute renal failure. In: Brenner BM (ed) The Kidney. Philadelphia, WB Saunders, 2000, pp 1201–1262.
3. Dube MP, Sprecher D, Henry WK, et al. Preliminary guidelines for the evaluation and management of dyslipidemia in adults infected with human immunodeficiency virus and receiving antiretroviral therapy: recommendations of the Adult AIDS Clinical Trial Group Cardiovascular Disease Focus Group. Clin Infect Dis 31:1216, 2000.
4. Mastroianni CM, d'Ettorre G, Forcina G, et al. Rhabdomyolysis after cerivastatin-gemfibrozil therapy in an HIV- infected patient with protease inhibitor-related hyperlipidemia. AIDS 15:820, 2001.
5. Kopp JB, Miller KD, Mican JA, et al. Crystalluria and urinary tract abnormalities associated with indinavir. Ann Intern Med 127:119, 1997.
6. Tashima KT, Horowitz JD, Rosen S. Indinavir nephropathy. N Engl J Med 336:138, 1997.
7. Wu DS, Stoller ML Indinavir urolithiasis. Curr Opin Urol 10:557, 2000.
8. Hanabusa H, Tagami H, Hataya H. Renal atrophy associated with long-term treatment with indinavir. N Engl J Med 340:392, 1999.
9. Becker K, Jablonowski H, Haussinger D. Sulfadiazine-associated nephrotoxicity in patients with the acquired immunodeficiency syndrome. Medicine (Baltimore) 75:185, 1996.
10. Rao TK. Acute renal failure syndromes in human immunodeficiency virus infection. Semin Nephrol 18:378, 1998.
11. Hsu CY, Chertow GM. Chronic renal confusion: insufficiency, failure, dysfunction, or disease. Am J Kidney Dis 36:415, 2000.
12. Anderson S, Tank JE, Brenner BM. Renal and systemic manifestations of glomerular disease. In: Brenner BM (ed) The Kidney. Philadelphia, WB Saunders, 2000, pp 1871–1900.
13. Cespedes RD, Peretsman SJ, Blatt SP. The significance of hematuria in patients infected with the human immunodeficiency virus. J Urol 154:1455, 1995.
14. Coburn M, Urological manifestations of HIV infection. AIDS Res Hum Retroviruses 14 (suppl 1):S23, 1998.
15. D'Agati V, Suh JI, Carbone L, et al. Pathology of HIV-associated nephropathy: a detailed morphologic and comparative study. Kidney Int 35:1358, 1989.
16. Cohen AH, Nast CC. HIV-associated nephropathy. a unique combined glomerular, tubular, and interstitial lesion. Mod Pathol 1:87, 1988.
17. Cantor ES, Kimmel PL, Bosch JP. Effect of race on expression of acquired immunodeficiency syndrome-associated nephropathy. Arch Intern Med 151:125, 1991.
18. Rao TK. Human immunodeficiency virus (HIV) associated nephropathy. Annu Rev Med 42:391, 1991.
19. Laradi A, Mallet A, Beaufils H, et al. HIV-associated nephropathy: outcome and prognosis factors. Groupe d' Etudes Nephrologiques d'Ile de France. J Am Soc Nephrol 9:2327, 1998.

20. US Renal Data System. USRDS 1999 Annual Data Report. Bethesda, The National Institutes of Health, National Institute of Diabetes and Digestive and Kidney Diseases, 1999.
21. Winston JA, Burns GC, Klotman PE. The human immunodeficiency virus (HIV) epidemic and HIV-associated nephropathy. Semin Nephrol 18:373, 1998.
22. Casanova S, Mazzucco G, Barbiano di Belgiojoso G, et al. Pattern of glomerular involvement in human immunodeficiency virus-infected patients: an Italian study. Am J Kidney Dis 26:446, 1995.
23. Praditpornsilpa K, Napathorn S, Yenrudi S, et al. Renal pathology and HIV infection in Thailand. Am J Kidney Dis 33:282, 1999.
24. Nochy D, Glotz D, Dosquet P, et al. Renal disease associated with HIV infection: a multicentric study of 60 patients from Paris hospitals. Nephrol Dial Transplant 8:11, 1993.
25. Humphreys MH. Human immunodeficiency virus-associated glomerulosclerosis. Kidney Int 48:311, 1995.
26. Winston JA, Klotman ME, Klotman PE. HIV-associated nephropathy is a late, not early, manifestation of HIV-1 infection. Kidney Int 55:1036, 1999.
27. D'Agati V, Appel GB. HIV infection and the kidney. J Am Soc Nephrol 8:138, 1997.
28. Feldman M, Jean-Jeromone K, Mohammed B, et al. Can HIV associated nephropathy be predicted on clinical grounds? J Am Soc Nephrol 9:146(A), 1988.
29. Kopp JB, Klotman JE, Adler SH, et al. Progressive glomerulosclerosis and enhanced renal accumulation of basement membrane components in mice transgenic for human immunodeficiency virus type 1 genes. Proc Natl Acad Sci USA 89:1577, 1992.
30. Klotman PE, Notkins AL. Transgenic models of human immunodeficiency virus type-1. Curr Top Microbiol Immunol 206:197, 1996.
31. Ray PE, Bruggeman LA, Weeks BS, et al. bFGF and its low affinity receptors in the pathogenesis of HIV-associated nephropathy in transgenic mice. Kidney Int 46:759, 1994.
32. Bruggeman LA, Dikman S, Meng C, et al. Nephropathy in human immunodeficiency virus-1 transgenic mice is due to renal transgene expression. J Clin Invest 100:84, 1997.
33. Barisoni L, Kriz W, Mundel P, D'Agati V. The dysregulated podocyte phenotype: a novel concept in the pathogenesis of collapsing idiopathic focal segmental glomerulosclerosis and HIV-associated nephropathy. J Am Soc Nephrol 10:51, 1999.
34. Barisoni L, Bruggeman LA, Mundel P, et al. HIV-1 induces renal epithelial dedifferentiation in a transgenic model of HIV-associated nephropathy. Kidney Int 58:173, 2000.
35. Schwartz EJ, Klotman PE, Pathogenesis of human immunodeficiency virus (HIV)-associated nephropathy. Semin Nephrol 18:436, 1998.
36. Klotman PE. HIV-associated nephropathy. Kidney Int 56:1161, 1999.
37. Kimmel PL, Ferreira-Centeno A, Farkas-Szallasi T, et al. Viral DNA in microdissected renal biopsy tissue from HIV infected patients with nephrotic syndrome. Kidney Int 43:1347, 1993.
38. Conaldi PG, Biancone L, Bottelli A, et al. HIV-1 kills renal tubular epithelial cells in vitro by triggering an apoptotic pathway involving caspase activation and Fas upregulation. J Clin Invest 102:2041, 1998.
39. Bruggeman LA, Ross MD, Tanji N, et al. Renal epithelium is a previously unrecognized site of HIV-1 infection. J Am Soc Nephrol 11:2079, 2000.
40. Winston JA, Bruggeman LA, Ross MD, et al. Nephropathy and establishment of a renal reservoir of HIV type 1 during primary infection. N Engl J Med 344:1979, 2001.
41. Rao TK. Clinical features of human immunodeficiency virus associated nephropathy. Kidney Int Suppl 35:S13, 1991.
42. Appel RG, Neill J. A steroid-responsive nephrotic syndrome in a patient with human immunodeficiency virus (HIV) infection. Ann Intern Med 113:892, 1990.
43. Briggs WA, Tanawattanacharoen S, Choi MJ, et al. Clinicopathologic correlates of prednisone treatment of human immunodeficiency virus-associated nephropathy. Am J Kidney Dis 28:618, 1996.
44. Watterson MK, Detwiler RK, Bolin P Jr. Clinical response to prolonged corticosteroids in a patient with human immunodeficiency virus-associated nephropathy. Am J Kidney Dis 29:624, 1997.
45. Smith MC, Pawar R, Carey JT, et al. Effect of corticosteroid therapy on human immunodeficiency virus- associated nephropathy. Am J Med 97:145, 1994.
46. Smith MC, Austen JL, Carey JT, et al. Prednisone improves renal function and proteinuria in human immunodeficiency virus-associated nephropathy. Am J Med 101:41, 1996.
47. Eustace JA, Nuermberger E, Choi M, et al. Cohort study of the treatment of severe HIV-associated nephropathy with corticosteroids. Kidney Int 58:1253, 2000.
48. Randomised placebo-controlled trial of effect of ramipril on decline in glomerular filtration rate and risk of terminal renal failure in proteinuric, nondiabetic nephropathy: the GISEN Group (Gruppo Italiano di Studi Epidemiologici in Nefrologia). Lancet 349:1857, 1997.
49. Brenner BM, Cooper ME, de Zeeuw D, et al. Effects of losartan on renal and cardiovascular outcomes in patients with type 2 diabetes and nephropathy. N Engl J Med 345:861, 2001.
50. Lewis EJ, Hunsicker LG, Bain RP, Rohde RD. The effect of angiotensin-converting-enzyme inhibition on diabetic nephropathy: the Collaborative Study Group. N Engl J Med 329:1456, 1993.
51. Lewis EJ, Hunsicker LG, Clarke WR, et al. Renoprotective effect of the angiotensin-receptor antagonist irbesartan in patients with nephropathy due to type 2 diabetes. N Engl J Med 345:851, 2001.
52. Kimmel PL, Mishkin GJ, Umana WO. Captopril and renal survival in patients with human immunodeficiency virus nephropathy. Am J Kidney Dis 28:202, 1996.
53. Burns GC, Paul SK, Toth IR, Sivak SL. Effect of angiotensin-converting enzyme inhibition in HIV-associated nephropathy. J Am Soc Nephrol 8:1140, 1997.
54. Bird JE, Durham SK, Giancarli MR, et al. Captopril prevents nephropathy in HIV-transgenic mice. J Am Soc Nephrol 9:1441, 1998.
55. Ifudu O, Rao TK, Tan CC, et al. Zidovudine is beneficial in human immunodeficiency virus associated nephropathy. Am J Nephrol 15:217, 1995.
56. Michel C, Dosquet P, Ronco P, et al. Nephropathy associated with infection by human immunodeficiency virus: a report on 11 cases including 6 treated with zidovudine. Nephron 62:434, 1992.
57. Schwartz EJ, Szczech L, Winston JA, Klotman PE. Effect of HAART on HIV-associated nephropathy. J Am Soc Nephrol 11:165A, 2000.
58. Szcech LA, Edwards LJ, Sanders LL, et al. Protease inhibitors are associated with a slowed progression of HIV-associated nephropathy. J Am Soc Nephrol 10:116(A), 1999.
59. Wali RK, Drachenberg CI, Papadimitriou JC, et al. HIV-1-associated nephropathy and response to highly active antiretroviral therapy [letter]. Lancet 352:783, 1998.
60. Cheng JT, Anderson HL Jr, Markowitz GS, et al. Hepatitis C virus-associated glomerular disease in patients with human immunodeficiency virus coinfection. J Am Soc Nephrol 10:1566, 1999.
61. Szczech LA, Gagne SJ, van der Horst C, et al. Predictors of proteinuria and renal failure among women with HIV infection. Kidney Int 61:195, 2002.
62. Kimmel PL, Phillips TM, Ferreira-Centeno A, et al. Brief report: idiotypic IgA nephropathy in patients with human immunodeficiency virus infection. N Engl J Med 327:702, 1992.
63. Kimmel PL, Phillips TM, Ferreira-Centeno A, et al. HIV-associated immune-mediated renal disease. Kidney Int 44:1327, 1993.
64. Eitner F, Cui Y, Hudkins KL, et al. Thrombotic microangiopathy in the HIV-2-infected macaque. Am J Pathol 155:649, 1999.
65. Sutor GC, Schmidt RE, Albrecht H. Thrombotic microangiopathies and HIV infection: report of two typical cases, features of HUS and TTP, and review of the literature. Infection 27:12, 1999.
66. Kudva YC, Peterson LS, Holley KE, et al. SLE nephropathy in a patient with HIV infection: case report and review of the literature. J Rheumatol 23:1811, 1996.
67. Chang BG, Markowitz GS, Seshan SV, et al. Renal manifestations of concurrent systemic lupus erythematosus and HIV infection. Am J Kidney Dis 33:441, 1999.
68. Burns GC, Visintainer P, Mohammed NB. Effect of angiotensin converting-enzyme inhibition on progression of renal disease and mortality in HIV-associated nephropathy. J Am Soc Nephrol 10:155(A), 1999.
69. Rose BD. Indications for and complications of renal biopsy. In: Rose BD (ed) Up to Date. Wellesly MA, Up to Date, 2000.
70. http://spitfire.emmes.com/study/hiv-k/.
71. Feldman HI, Kobrin S, Wasserstein A. Hemodialysis vascular access morbidity [editorial]. J Am Soc Nephrol 7:523, 1996.
72. Carbone L, D'Agati V, Cheng JT, Appel GB. Course and prognosis of human immunodeficiency virus-associated nephropathy. Am J Med 87:389, 1989.

73. Ahuja TS, Borucki M, Grady J. Highly active antiretroviral therapy improves survival of HIV-infected hemodialysis patients. Am J Kidney Dis 36:574, 2000.
74. Ifudu O, Mayers JD, Matthew JJ, et al. Uremia therapy in patients with end-stage renal disease and human immunodeficiency virus infection: has the outcome changed in the 1990s? Am J Kidney Dis 29:549, 1997.
75. Szczech L, Winston J, Rodriguez R, et al. Clinical characteristics and antiretroviral prescribing patterns among HIV-infected ESRD patients. J Am Soc Nephrol 12:348A, 2001.
76. Izzedine H, Launay-Vacher V, Baumelou A, Deray G. An appraisal of antiretroviral drugs in hemodialysis. Kidney Int 60:821, 2001.

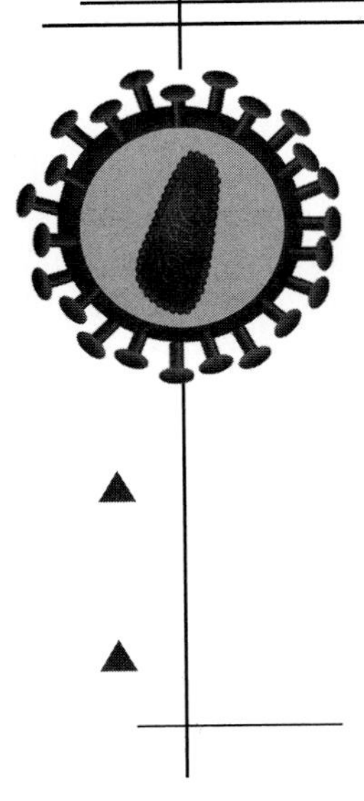

CHAPTER 62

Diabetes, Insulin Resistance, Lipid Disorders, and Fat Redistribution Syndromes

Colleen Hadigan, MD, MPH
Steven Grinspoon, MD

In 1997 the first reports of abnormal fat redistribution and abnormal glucose regulation began to appear among human immunodeficiency virus (HIV)-infected patients receiving highly active combination antiretroviral therapy (HAART). Initial studies included descriptions of posterior cervical fat accumulations, or "buffalo humps,"[1,2] abdominal adiposity,[3,4] and associated metabolic disturbances including hyperlipidemia and insulin resistance.[5] Significant subcutaneous fat atrophy has also been identified among many patients, often in combination with other aspects of fat redistribution (Table 62–1).[6,7]

The term "HIV lipodystrophy" has been used by many to describe this apparent syndrome of fat redistribution and metabolic disturbances (Table 62–2). The presentation of HIV-infected patients with changes in body fat distribution is reminiscent of congenital and acquired forms of lipodystrophy characterized by loss or absence of subcutaneous fat, relative hypertrophy of central adipose tissue, insulin resistance, and dyslipidemia. However, it is not clear whether there is a single syndrome of lipodystrophy with various phenotypic expressions or several independent alterations in fat and metabolism that may appear alone or in combination.

The etiology of fat redistribution, hyperlipidemia, and insulin resistance among patients with HIV infection is not known. The emergence of these findings coincided with the widespread introduction of protease inhibitor (PI) therapy, so initial investigations focused primarily on PI exposure. Subsequent epidemiologic studies have identified nondrug risk factors for the development of lipodystrophy such as age, the CD4+ T-lymphocyte nadir, and changes in body mass index;[8] moreover, nucleoside reverse transcriptase inhibitors (NRTIs) have been implicated in the development of subcutaneous fat atrophy.[6,9,10] Furthermore, PI-naive patients may present with symptoms of marked fat redistribution and evidence of metabolic abnormalities. The disturbances in fat redistribution and metabolism among HIV-infected patients cannot currently be explained by a single agent or class of agents, but there is mounting evidence that antiretroviral therapies play an active role in the development of lipodystrophy (Table 62–3).[11–13]

In this chapter we review the cardinal manifestations of HIV lipodystrophy: insulin resistance, dyslipidemia, fat redistribution. In each case we discuss the presentation and recognition of changes as well as potential strategies to reverse or minimize these metabolic abnormalities. Furthermore, we review the implications for cardiovascular disease risk and the long-term health implications of this metabolic syndrome.

INSULIN RESISTANCE AND DIABETES

Insulin resistance and the development of type 2 diabetes mellitus is increasingly recognized among HIV-infected patients, particularly those who experience changes in fat distribution.[7,14–16] Walli et al.[15] found that 54% of patients treated with a PI had impaired glucose tolerance (2-hour postchallenge glucose > 120 mg/dl). In a similar study using more stringent criteria for impaired glucose tolerance [World Health Organization (WHO) guidelines of 2-hour postchallenge glucose of 140 to 200 mg/dl], Behrens et al.[17] identified impaired glucose tolerance in 46% of PI-treated patients and 24% of PI-naive patients. Hadigan and colleagues[7] compared HIV-infected patients with fat redistribution, regardless of PI exposure, to healthy age-, gender-,

▲ **Table 62–1.** BODY COMPOSITION CHANGES IN HIV
▲ LIPODYSTROPHY

Subcutaneous fat atrophy
Facial fat atrophy
Gluteal fat wasting
Peripheral fat atrophy
Venomegaly of the extremities
Subcutaneous abdominal fat atrophy
Visceral abdominal fat hypertrophy
Dorsocervical fat hypertrophy
Submandibular fat hypertrophy
Breast hypertrophy

and body mass index (BMI)-matched controls from the Framingham Offspring Cohort and found marked hyperinsulinemia among the HIV-infected patients.

The HIV-infected patients with fat redistribution were significantly more likely than control subjects to have (1) impaired glucose tolerance (i.e., 2-hour postchallenge glucose level of 140 to 200 mg/dl) (HIV-infected 35.2% vs. control 5.2%, $P = 0.001$); (2) fasting hyperinsulinemia (fasting insulin level > 18 μU/ml; 26.5% vs. 6.1%, $P = 0.001$); and (3) previously unrecognized diabetes (2-hour post oral challenge glucose level > 200 mg/dl) (7.0% vs. 0.5%, $P = 0.01$) (Fig. 62–1). HIV-infected patients with fat redistribution also had notably increased waist/hip ratios (mean ± SEM: HIV-infected 0.97 ± 0.01 vs. control 0.90 ± 0.01; $P = 0.0001$); the large differences in the indices of insulin resistance remained statistically significant even after controlling for the differences in the waist/hip ratio between the two groups. Furthermore, insulin levels were uniformly elevated in patients regardless of PI exposure status. Combined, these data indicate that patients with HIV infection, particularly those exposed to PI treatment or with body fat redistribution, are at high risk of developing clinically significant glucose and insulin abnormalities.

The mechanism of insulin resistance among HIV-infected patients with fat redistribution is not known. Certainly, fat redistribution with visceral adiposity and reduced subcutaneous fat may contribute to insulin resistance, as is seen in cases of congenital and acquired lipodystrophy.[18] Visceral adiposity is associated with increased circulating levels of nonesterified fatty acids, which in turn may lead to the development of insulin resistance. This is one potential mechanism by which central fat accumulation contributes

▲ **Table 62–2.** METABOLIC ABNORMALITIES IN HIV
▲ LIPODYSTROPHY

Dyslipidemia
↑ Triglycerides
↓ HDL cholesterol
Modest ↑ LDL and total cholesterol
Insulin resistance
Impaired glucose tolerance
Diabetes
Cardiovascular disease markers
↑ Tissue plasminogen activator (tPA)
↑ Plasminogen activator inhibitor-1 (PAI-1)
? Decreased bone density

HDL, LDL, high and low density lipoprotein; PAI-1, plasminogen activator inhibitor-1; tPA, tissue plasminogen activator.

▲ **Table 62–3.** POTENTIAL MECHANISMS OF THE METABOLIC
▲ ABNORMALITIES IN HIV LIPODYSTROPHY

Direct effect of antiretroviral therapy
Protease inhibitors
Nucleotide reverse transcriptase inhibitors
Fat redistribution syndrome
Direct effects of HIV infection
↑ Triglycerides and ↓ HDL cholesterol
Immune reactivation syndrome following antiretroviral therapy
Hormonal factors
Hypogonadism
↓ Growth hormone

to insulin resistance and diabetes. Insulin resistance may also occur through loss of subcutaneous peripheral fat, which may limit peripheral glucose and triglyceride uptake. Indeed, both an increased waist/hip ratio and reduced thigh circumference (a marker of peripheral fat atrophy) were strong independent predictors of hyperinsulinemia in the cohort described by Hadigan et al.[7] Therefore fat redistribution, central adiposity, and abnormal lipolysis may play a direct role in glucose and insulin regulation in patients with HIV infection.

There is mounting evidence to support a direct effect of antiretroviral therapy, particularly PIs, on glucose and insulin metabolism. Mulligan et al.[13] demonstrated significant increases in fasting glucose (+9 mg/dl; $P = 0.014$) and fasting insulin levels (+12.2 U/ml; $P = 0.023$) after initiating a PI-containing regimen for as little as 3.5 months. These changes were apparent in the absence of any significant changes in fat distribution. Furthermore, Noor and colleagues[11] have completed a preliminary study to investigate the effect of PIs on insulin resistance, independent of HIV infection. Administration of indinavir to a group of HIV-negative healthy volunteers induced modest insulin resistance after 6 weeks,[11] again without notable changes in body fat distribution. Finally, Murata and colleagues[19] demonstrated a specific effect of PI therapy on GLUT-4, a membrane protein responsible for glucose transport into the cell. This mechanism may account, in part, for the metabolic effects of PI therapy. Thus the pathogenesis of the metabolic complications and insulin resistance among HIV-infected patients is likely multifactorial, resulting in part from changes in fat redistribution and in part from direct effects of antiretroviral therapies.

Cardiovascular Disease Risk Associated with Insulin Resistance

Insulin resistance and impaired glucose tolerance have been shown to predict elevated cardiovascular disease (CVD) risk in nondiabetic individuals without HIV infection.[20,21] Despres et al.[22] and Manson et al.[23] have shown that obesity and hyperinsulinemia increase the risk of CVD in men and women. Furthermore, an increased waist/hip ratio is associated with increased risk of CVD.[24] Therefore truncal obesity and insulin resistance may result in increased morbidity and mortality from cardiovascular-related disease among patients with HIV infection and these metabolic abnormalities.

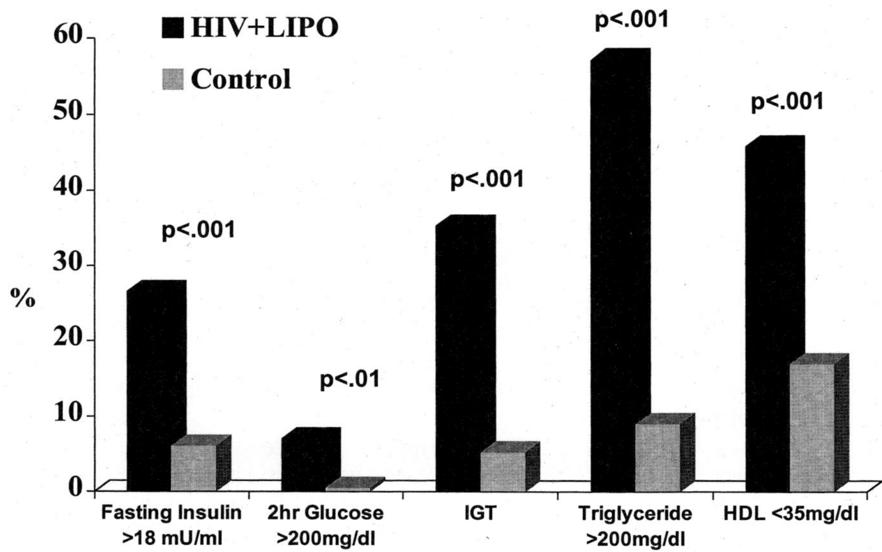

Figure 62–1. HIV lipodystrophy patients (n = 71) with metabolic abnormalities compared with the Framingham Cohort control subjects (n = 213) matched for age, gender, and body mass index.[7] IGT, impaired glucose tolerance defined as a 2-hour oral glucose tolerance test blood glucose level higher than 140 mg/dl. The P values represent results from chi-square analyses.

Concern over potentially increased CVD risk in association with metabolic disturbances in HIV-infected patients is supported by reports of premature cardiovascular events and elevated CVD markers. Maggi and colleagues[25] evaluated carotid arteries for premature lesions in PI-treated and PI-naive HIV-infected patients and compared them to HIV-negative control subjects. Premature carotid lesions were identified in 52.7% of PI-treated patients, 14.9% of PI naive patients, and only 6.4% of healthy controls. In this study, PI exposure, smoking, and the CD4+ T-lymphocyte count predicted the occurrence of carotid lesions.

In a large case-control study Klein and colleagues[26] identified increased rates of hospitalization for coronary heart disease among HIV-infected patients in the Kaiser Permanente health care system (n = 4541) compared to age- and gender-matched controls not known to have HIV infection (n = 41,000). The risk of a coronary heart disease event was 2.6 times greater among HIV-infected patients than among controls. Rates of coronary events were similar regardless of PI exposure. In a study by Mary-Krause and colleagues[27] rates of myocardial infarction increased significantly with increased duration of PI exposure among HIV-infected men. These data demonstrate that a higher than expected risk of CVD is present among HIV-infected patients and suggests that there may be an association with exposure to antiretroviral therapy.

Hyperinsulinemia and insulin resistance may be independent risk factors for CVD through impaired fibrinolysis and a prothrombotic state in HIV-infected patients with lipodystrophy. Meigs and colleagues[28] showed that both plasminogen activator inhibitor-1 (PAI-1) and tissue plasminogen activator (tPA) are highly correlated with insulin levels among non-HIV-infected adults, controlling for potential confounding variables such as age, BMI, lipid levels, and the waist/hip ratio in the Framingham Offspring Cohort. These data suggest a direct, independent effect of hyperinsulinemia to impair fibrinolysis in glucose-intolerant and diabetic subjects. An in vivo investigation in non-HIV-infected humans demonstrated increased expression of PAI-1 and tPA following local infusion of insulin,[29] further supporting a direct link between CVD risk and insulin resistance.

Increased tPA antigen predicts increased risk of coronary artery disease mortality among HIV-negative patients with a history of angina pectoris and CVD[30] as well as cerebral vascular events among individuals without a prior history of CVD.[31] Data indicate that patients with HIV infection and fat redistribution have markedly elevated PAI-1 and tPA antigen levels in association with significant hyperinsulinemia.[32] Among HIV-infected patients with fat redistribution, tPA and PAI-1 antigen levels were twice that of healthy age-, gender-, and BMI-matched control subjects (Fig. 62–2). These data combined with evidence of increased CVD-related morbidity among HIV-infected patients

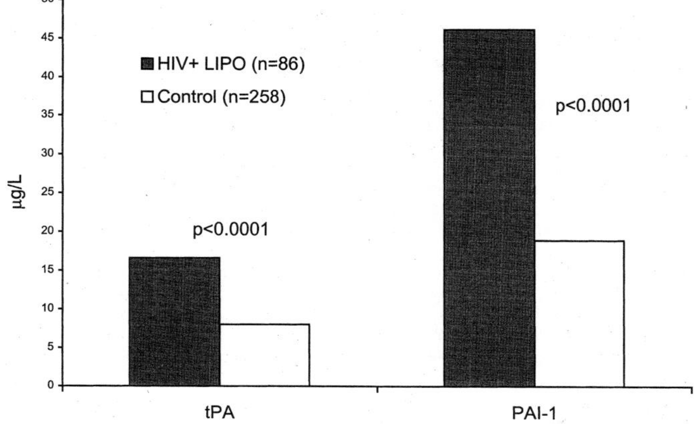

Figure 62–2. Tissue plasminogen activator (tPA) and plasminogen activator inhibitor-1 (PAI-1) antigen levels in patients with HIV lipodystrophy and healthy control subjects from the Framingham Offspring Cohort study. (Adapted from Hadigan C, Meigs JB, Rabe J, et al. Increased PAI-1 and tPA antigen levels are reduced with metformin therapy in HIV-infected patients with fat redistribution and insulin resistance. J Clin Endocrinol Metab 86:939–943, 2001.)

underscore the need for specific therapies to reduce insulin resistance and modulate CVD risk.

Management of Insulin Resistance

Routine performance of a fasting glucose assay is recommended for all HIV-infected patients with fat redistribution, particularly those who are obese, have a family history of diabetes, or are receiving PI therapy. It is important to note that most patients have a normal fasting blood glucose level, even though as many as 35% have impaired glucose tolerance and a small percentage have diabetes detectable with an oral glucose tolerance test.[7] Performance of a standard 75 g glucose tolerance test may be useful in patients to determine impaired glucose tolerance and the risk of developing diabetes mellitus. Measuring fasting insulin may also be useful but is not generally recommended outside the research setting.

The traditional approach to the management of a patient with insulin resistance in the absence of HIV infection or lipodystrophy is dietary modification, increased exercise, and sensible weight reduction or weight management, as indicated. Although there are currently no reported studies investigating the effects of diet and exercise to treat or prevent insulin resistance or diabetes associated with HIV and lipodystrophy, dietary and lifestyle counseling should be considered for all patients who present with such disturbances.

In HIV-negative hyperinsulinemic populations, the use of insulin-sensitizing agents has resulted in the successful reduction of fasting hyperinsulinemia and weight loss. Metformin (Glucophage) is particularly appropriate for use in patients with significant truncal adiposity and increased free fatty acid concentrations, in whom insulin resistance is in part attributable to increased hepatic glucose production. For example, the use of metformin improves glycemic control and weight in patients with type 2 diabetes mellitus.[33–35] In addition, metformin modestly lowers lipid levels. In patients with hyperlipidemia, metformin has been demonstrated to decrease triglyceride and low density lipoprotein (LDL) levels without adversely affecting other parameters. The modest 10% to 20% reduction in plasma triglyceride levels achieved with this agent may to be related to an associated decrease in hepatic very low density lipoprotein (VLDL) production. Development of lactic acidosis is a rare but potentially serious side effect of metformin, particularly in patients with renal dysfunction or heart failure.

The effects of metformin in HIV-infected patients with lipodystrophy were initially reported by Saint-Marc and Touraine.[36] In an open-label study, use of metformin, 850 mg three times a day for 8 weeks, was associated with significant reductions in fasting insulin levels, an insulin response to oral glucose challenge, weight and visceral abdominal fat among HIV-infected patients with insulin resistance, and central adiposity. Hadigan et al.[37] subsequently reported the results of a 12-week double-blind randomized placebo-controlled trial of metformin 500 mg twice daily (Fig. 62–3). The insulin area under the curve (AUC) following a 2-hour standard 75 g oral glucose challenge was significantly reduced in the metformin group compared with that in placebo-treated patients. Metformin treatment was also associated with reductions in weight, waist circumference, and diastolic blood pressure. It was well tolerated

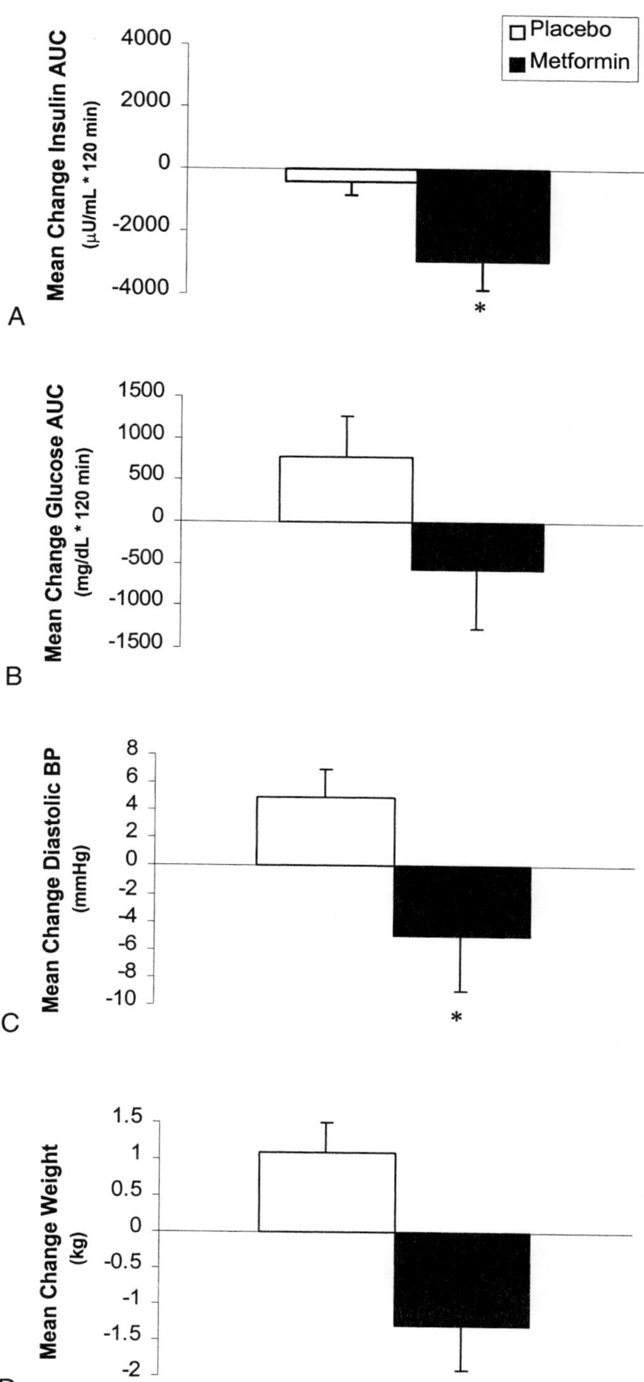

Figure 62–3. Change in (*a*) insulin area under the curve (AUC), (*b*) glucose AUC, (*c*) diastolic blood pressure, and (*d*) weight in HIV-infected patients treated with metformin ($n = 14$) compared to placebo ($n = 11$). $^*P \leq 0.01$. (From Hadigan C, Corcoran C, Basgoz N, et al. Metformin in the treatment of HIV Lipodystrophy. JAMA 284:472–477, 2000, with permission.)

and, in this relatively small study, did not result in increased lactic acid levels. Additional studies are needed to determine the long-term safety and efficacy of metformin before it can be generally endorsed for the treatment of insulin-resistant patients with HIV lipodystrophy.

Increased markers of CVD risk, such as tPA and PAI-1 antigen, have been identified in HIV-infected patients with fat redistribution.[32] These markers were elevated in association with increased insulin levels and may provide a mechanistic link between hyperinsulinemia and increased risk of CVD. Hadigan and colleagues[32] demonstrated that 12 weeks of metformin treatment reduced tPA antigen levels by 11% and PAI antigen levels by 16% (Fig. 62–4). In this way, metformin treatment may improve the overall cardiovascular risk profile in HIV-infected patients with fat redistribution and insulin resistance.

As stated previously, insulin resistance may also occur in patients with HIV infection through loss of subcutaneous fat, which may limit peripheral glucose and triglyceride uptake. Hadigan et al.[7] found that reduced thigh circumference, a marker of peripheral fat atrophy, was an independent predictor of hyperinsulinemia in HIV-positive patients with fat redistribution. Metformin, although a potent insulin-sensitizing agent, is not believed to restore peripheral adipogenesis but, rather, to act primarily via a reduction of hepatic insulin resistance. In contrast, a novel class of therapeutic agents, the thiazolidinediones, has been shown to promote adipogenesis, primarily through an action on peroxisome proliferator-activated receptor γ (PPARγ).[38,39] Although the thiazolidinediones have effects on both hepatic and peripheral insulin resistance, the dominant effect is to improve peripheral glucose uptake. For example, troglitazone was shown to increase peripheral glucose uptake significantly, with only modest effects on hepatic insulin sensitivity in a study of patients with type 2 diabetes mellitus.[40] In a nonrandomized pilot study of troglitazone, Walli et al.[41] reported improved insulin sensitivity among

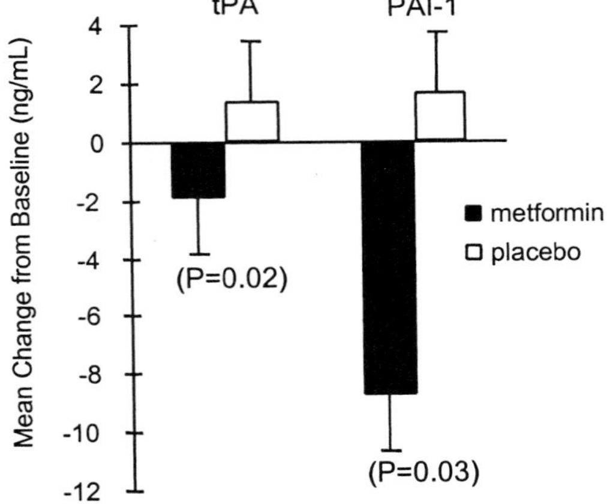

Figure 62–4. Mean change from baseline in tissue plasminogen activator (tPA) and plasminogen activator inhibitor-1 (PAI-1) antigen levels after 12 weeks of metformin (n = 14) compared to placebo (n = 11). (From Rabe J, et al. Increased PAI-1 and tPA antigen levels are reduced with metformin therapy in HIV-infected patients with fat redistribution and insulin resistance. J Clin Endocrinol Metab 86:939–943, 2001.)

patients with HIV infection and diabetes. However, troglitazone was recently withdrawn from the U.S. market by the Food and Drug Administration (FDA) for rare but significant hepatic toxicity.

Thiazolidinediones hold promise for the treatment of HIV-infected patients with fat redistribution and insulin resistance. In a series of clinical trials, rosiglitazone was efficacious in reducing hemoglobin A1c and fasting glucose in patients with diabetes, and it was not associated with liver toxicity or other serious adverse effects.[42,43] Thiazolidinediones may also reduce plasma triglyceride levels by 10% to 20% and increase high density lipoprotein (HDL) cholesterol by 5% to 10% in diabetic patients. Patients with diabetes have demonstrated weight increases and increased subcutaneous fat in response to thiazolidinediones, in contrast with metformin, which is associated with weight loss.[44] Therefore thiazolidinediones may also be efficacious for improving insulin sensitivity and promoting corrective fat redistribution in HIV-associated lipodystrophy. Clinical trials are underway to determine the safety and efficacy of thiazolidinediones in HIV-associated lipodystrophy.

Given the evidence supporting a direct link between PIs and insulin resistance in HIV-infected patients, one approach to the management of the metabolic abnormalities seen in these patients may be the initiation of PI-sparing regimens. Several studies have been conducted to evaluate the safety and efficacy of replacing a PI with a nonnucleoside reverse transcriptase inhibitor (NNRTI). Martinez and colleagues[45] prospectively evaluated 23 patients who decided to discontinue PI therapy because of changes in body fat distribution despite sustained virologic suppression (< 200 HIV-1 RNA copies per milliliter). Nevirapine was initiated to replace the PI, and after approximately 8 months patients experienced significant reductions in their waist/hip ratio (from 0.91 to 0.85; P = 0.048), glucose levels (15% reduction; P = 0.008), and fasting insulin resistance index (45% reduction; P = 0.0001). CD4+ T-lymphocyte counts remained unchanged, and all but one patient maintained virologic suppression after switching.

A similar study by Martinez et al.[46] evaluating a switch from PI to efavirenz demonstrated only a 28% reduction in the fasting insulin resistance index (P = 0.03), no improvement in glucose levels, and only a trend toward a decreased waist/hip ratio. In addition, 8 of 20 patients experienced neuropsychological side effects associated with efavirenz, and in 3 cases symptoms were severe and required discontinuation. Although studies of this nature demonstrate at least partial reversibility of some of the metabolic changes associated with lipodystrophy and PI therapy, the benefits of switching drug regimens may be of limited clinical significance, particularly in light of potential negative effects on suppression of HIV viral replication. Additional randomized switch trials with longer duration of follow-up are necessary to determine the role of PI switching in the management of metabolic complications in HIV treatment.

Supervised treatment interruptions (STIs) are currently being evaluated as a potential strategy to maximize virologic response in certain subsets of patients receiving HAART. In addition to improved virologic suppression, it is hoped that reduced incidence and severity of metabolic complications from HAART may be achieved through the careful use of STIs. Hatano and colleagues[47] evaluated metabolic parameters in 26 HIV-infected men who interrupted HAART for 5 to 10 weeks. Although patients experienced significant decreases in total cholesterol, LDL, and triglyceride levels, there were no significant changes in glucose or insulin levels or in anthropometric measurements. STI use remains investigational. The ability to maintain safe HIV virologic control in the setting of drug interruptions must be established and the effects of STIs on the development and treatment of lipodystrophy evaluated further before STI can be endorsed as a strategy for managing insulin resistance, dyslipidemia, and fat redistribution.

▲ LIPIDS

Lipid Abnormalities

Modest hypertriglyceridemia and low HDL are known to occur in HIV-infected patients. Grunfeld et al.[48] demonstrated increased triglyceride levels as a result of increased hepatic VLDL production and decreased triglyceride clearance in HIV-infected patients. In one study triglyceride levels correlated with interferon-α, suggesting that cytokines mediate some element of disordered lipid metabolism in HIV-infected patients.[49] However, other studies have not shown a direct effect of cytokines, and the role of cytokines in the dyslipidemia of HIV disease remains uncertain.

More recently, significant lipid abnormalities have been observed among HIV-infected patients receiving HAART.[13,50,51] Hypertriglyceridemia is the most common abnormality in such patients, but modest hypercholesterolemia is also seen. Hadigan et al.[7] demonstrated increased triglyceride, cholesterol, and LDL levels as well as an increased cholesterol/HDL ratio (an index of cardiac risk) in HIV-infected patients with fat redistribution compared to age- and BMI-matched subjects from the Framingham Offspring Cohort. Altogether, 57% of the HIV-infected subjects versus 42% of the control subjects demonstrated cholesterol levels higher than 200 mg/dl (P = 0.03). Similarly, 57% versus 9% (HIV-infected lipodystrophic versus control subjects) demonstrated a triglyceride level higher than 200 mg/dl (P = 0.001); and 22% versus 14% demonstrated LDL levels higher than 160 mg/dl (P = 0.16). In contrast, 46% versus 17% (HIV-infected versus control subjects) demonstrated an HDL level lower than 35 mg/dl (P = 0.001). Nonlipodystrophic, HIV-infected patients were compared to age- and BMI-matched control subjects, and low HDL levels were seen significantly more often in the HIV-infected patients than the controls; abnormalities in cholesterol and triglyceride were not seen.

Taken together, the data of Hadigan et al.[7] support prior work suggesting that low HDL is intrinsic to HIV disease, whereas fat redistribution and medications may contribute significantly to hypertriglyceridemia during the current era of HAART. For example, Miller et al.[3] demonstrated that triglyceride levels correlated with the degree of visceral fat in patients with HIV lipodystrophy, and direct effects of PIs on lipid metabolism have been demonstrated. Mulligan and colleagues[13] showed that changes in lipid levels occur

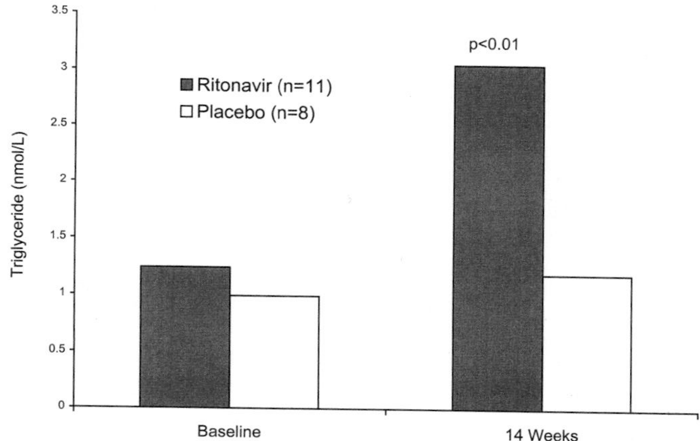

Figure 62–5. Mean triglyceride levels before and after 14 weeks of ritonavir (n = 11) compared to placebo (n = 8) among healthy HIV-negative volunteers. (Adapted from Purnell JQ, Zambon A, Knopp RH, et al. Effect of ritonavir on lipids and post-heparin lipase activities in normal subjects. AIDS 14:51–57, 2000, with permission.)

within 3 months of initiating PI therapy. A significant increase in triglyceride levels was seen in patients started on a PI compared to that in patients starting lamivudine. Furthermore, data suggest that individual PIs can affect lipid metabolism to greater and lesser extents. Papadapoulous and colleagues[52] and Chang and colleagues[53] demonstrated that ritonavir and ritonavir/saquinavir increase triglyceride levels to a greater degree then indinavir and nelfinavir.

To determine the direct effects of PIs on lipid metabolism independent of HIV disease, Purnell et al.[12] investigated the effects of a short course (2 weeks) of PI therapy in HIV-negative patients. In this randomized, placebo-controlled study, triglyceride levels increased approximately threefold in ritonavir-treated patients (Fig. 62–5). Total cholesterol also increased as a result of increased VLDL and intermediate density lipoprotein (IDL) but not LDL cholesterol. Postheparin hepatic lipase activity was decreased in the ritonavir-treated patients.

Management of Lipid Abnormalities

Some clinical data suggest that HIV-infected patients treated with PIs and those with evidence of fat redistribution should be monitored periodically for the development of dyslipidemia by measuring the fasting levels of cholesterol and triglyceride. Patients at risk for dyslipidemia include those with a family history of genetic dyslipidemia and patients receiving estrogen or consuming significant alcohol, in whom triglyceride levels are likely to be significantly increased. A number of lipid-lowering therapies are available for HIV-infected patients, but care should be exercised in the treatment of dyslipidemia because of potential interactions between certain anitretroviral agents and certain lipid-lowering agents, particularly the 3-hydroxy-3-methylglutaryl coenzyme A (HMG CoA) reductase inhibitors (see below). Furthermore, the specific therapy used for treating dyslipidemia in HIV-infected patients should be directed at the primary abnormality, (i.e., increased triglyceride and low HDL, increased cholesterol, or a mixed dyslipidemia).

Table 62–4. NATIONAL CHOLESTEROL EDUCATION PROGRAM (NCEP) III: CLASSIFICATION OF LDL, TOTAL, AND HDL CHOLESTEROL

Levels (mg/dl)	Comment
LDL cholesterol—Primary target of therapy	
< 100	Optimal
100–129	Near optimal/above optimal
130–159	Borderline high
160–189	High
≥ 190	Extremely high
Total cholesterol	
< 200	Desirable
200–239	Borderline high
≥ 240	High
HDL cholesterol	
< 40	Low
≥ 60	High

Adapted from the NIH-NHLBI ATP-III Guidelines, May 2001.

An AIDS Clinical Trial Group (ACTG) panel has recommended use of the National Cholesterol Education Program (NCEP) guidelines for the treatment of dyslipidemia in HIV-infected patients.[54] These guidelines evaluate the LDL cholesterol level and make therapeutic recommendations based on the absolute LDL level and the number of associated coronary artery disease (CAD) risk factors (Table 62–4; Fig. 62–6). For example, dietary therapy is recommended for patients with LDL levels higher than 160 mg/dl and fewer than two cardiac risk factors, whereas medication therapy would be initiated at an LDL level higher than 190 mg/dl in such patients.[55] A caveat in this regard is the fact that most laboratories calculate LDL indirectly from the cholesterol and triglyceride levels, but the standard equation to make this calculation is not valid when triglyceride levels are increased to higher than 400 mg/dl. Therefore direct measurement of LDL is recommended for patients with significantly increased levels of triglyceride. Epidemiologic data are inconsistent with respect to the potential risk of increased triglyceride levels on CAD. Increased triglyceride levels are often associated with low HDL, which may indirectly increase CAD risk in such patients. Severely increased triglyceride levels (> 1000 mg/dl) should always be treated to prevent the risk of pancreatitis.

Lipid-lowering therapy can be categorized into agents that primarily lower triglyceride levels (i.e., fibric acid and niacin) and those best used to lower the cholesterol level, such as the HMG CoA reductase inhibitors. Atorvostatin, an HMG CoA reductase inhibitor, simultaneously reduces cholesterol and triglyceride—to a greater degree than other HMG CoA reductase inhibitors. Fenofibrate is a lipid-lowering agent that may also be of use in lowering triglyceride in HIV-infected patients.[56] Henry[50] demonstrated effects of gemfibrozil and atorvostatin in comparison to diet and exercise in an initial study of hypertriglyceridemic HIV-infected patients. Diet and exercise lowered cholesterol and triglyceride levels by 11% and 21%, respectively, whereas gemfibrozil (600 mg PO bid) in combination with atorvostatin (10 mg PO qd) lowered cholesterol and triglyceride levels by 30% and 60%, respectively. The study by Henry[50] was nonrandomized, and baseline lipid levels were significantly lower, as expected, in patients undergoing diet and exercise.

In a randomized study, Miller et al.[57] demonstrated that gemfibrozil plus a low saturated fat diet lowered triglyceride levels 120 mg/dl compared to diet alone ($P = 0.06$). Diet and gemfibrozil administration are appropriate initial strategies for the management of severe hypertriglyceridemia in HIV-infected patients. In more refractory cases, atorvostatin may be considered an additional agent. However, the combination of HMG CoA reductase inhibitor and fibric acid inhibitor may lead to rhabdomyolysis and liver toxicity. Therefore creatine phosphokinase (CPK) levels and liver function tests should be monitored frequently if a fibric acid inhibitor and an HMG CoA reductase inhibitor are used in combination. Niacin is an excellent drug to lower triglyceride, increase HDL, and lower total cholesterol levels. However, use of niacin is often associated with bothersome flushing, increased liver transaminase levels, and aggravation of glucose intolerance.

Potential interactions between PIs and HMG CoA reductase inhibitors are important to recognize in HIV-infected patients. Fichtenbaum et al.[58] demonstrated a significant 32-fold increase in the simvastatin AUC concentrations in the presence of ritonavir and saquinavir. In contrast, the AUC for atorvostatin increased 4.5-fold in ritonavir/saquinavir-treated patients, whereas little effect was seen on pravastatin AUC concentrations. The authors recommended against the use of simvastatin in patients being treated with ritonavir/saquinavir and urged caution and low doses of atorvostatin if used with this combination of antiretroviral agents.

Given the available evidence that PI treatment may have a direct effect on lipid metabolism, interruption or replacement of the PI component of antiretroviral therapy has been investigated as a potential strategy to reverse hyperlipidemia. Martinez and colleagues[45] prospectively evaluated 23 patients who discontinued PI therapy owing to symptoms of lipodystrophy despite sustained virologic suppression (< 200 HIV-1 RNA copies per milliliter). Nevirapine was initiated to replace the PI; and after approximately 8 months patients experienced a 22% reduction in total cholesterol and a 57% reduction in triglycerides. These changes were seen in association with improved indices of insulin resistance and a decreased waist/hip ratio. However, subsequent reports (including a randomized trial comparing a switch to nevirapine versus continuation of PI[59]) failed to demonstrate a significant improvement in hyperlipidemia with the discontinuation of PI treatment. Similarly, switching to efavirenz after stopping a PI has not been as effective for reversing hypertriglyceridemia and hypercholesterolemia.[46,60] As previously described, Hatano et al.[47] showed significant reductions in cholesterol, LDL cholesterol, and triglycerides following interruption of HAART for a median of 7 weeks. Switching from PIs may well indeed improve triglyceride and cholesterol levels in HIV-infected patients, but such a course of action may be difficult in the well controlled patient with improved immunologic function. The treatment remains experimental.

Hyperlipidemia, especially hypertriglyceridemia and low HDL levels, are seen frequently in HIV-infected patients.

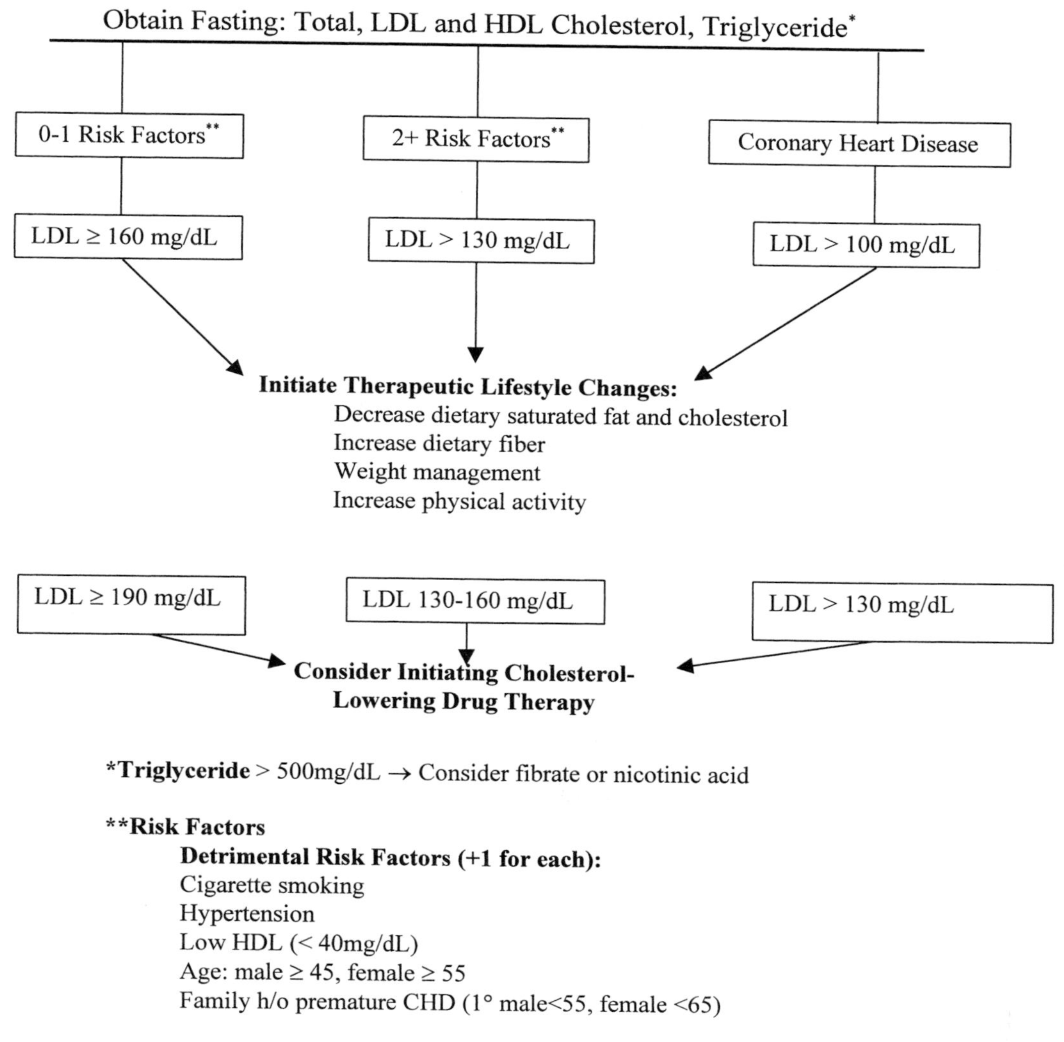

Figure 62–6. Assessment of hyperlipidemia in HIV-infected patients. (Adapted from the NIH-NHLBI ATP III Guidelines, May 2001.)

Dyslipidemia may be further exacerbated by direct effects of PIs and indirect effects mediated through fat redistribution in HAART-treated patients. Patients with severe dyslipidemia should be treated first with diet and then medications if necessary. Until further data become available, it is reasonable to use the NCEP treatment guidelines. However, special care should be taken to avoid interactions with PIs when using HMG CoA reductase inhibitors.

▲ FAT REDISTRIBUTION

Abnormalities

Abnormal hypertrophy of the dorsocervical fat pad, the "buffalo hump," was one of the first reported abnormalities of fat distribution among HIV-infected patients treated with combination antiretroviral therapy.[1,2,61] These reports were soon joined by descriptions of increased abdominal adiposity, breast hypertrophy, and subcutaneous fat atrophy.[4,62,63] Changes in fat redistribution may present as primary fat atrophy or primary central fat accumulation, but in most HIV-infected patients who experience changes in body fat these changes present in combination. In one series of 71 patients presenting for evaluation of fat redistribution, 15% had primarily lipoatrophy, 18% had primarily central fat hypertrophy without significant fat atrophy, and 66% had a combination of fat atrophy and hypertrophy.[7]

Alterations in fat redistribution can be highly distressing to patients who may experience marked changes in their appearance. These changes may threaten the anonymity of HIV-positive individuals and may contribute to noncompliance or discontinuation of antiretroviral therapy despite adequate HIV viral suppression.[64]

Much of the initial investigation in search of the cause of fat redistribution among HIV-infected patients was aimed at PI therapy, and studies compared patients who were PI-exposed to PI-naive patients. Exposure to NRTI therapy has also been implicated in the development of fat redistribution, particularly fat atrophy.[6,9,65] Mallal and colleagues[9] evaluated 277 patients participating in the Western Australian HIV Cohort Study and found that the development of fat atrophy was associated with increased age and longer duration of NRTI treatment, in addition to PI treatment. Stavudine exposure, in this study and others,[65] significantly increased the risk of developing fat atrophy. The exact mechanisms responsible for fat atrophy and visceral adiposity are not known, but drug effects on adipocyte cell differentiation[66,67] and adipocyte apoptosis have been proposed. Domingo et al.[68] performed subcutaneous fat cell biopsies on HIV-infected patients treated with a PI who were experiencing subcutaneous fat atrophy and truncal adiposity. Ten of eleven samples were positive for the presence of apoptosis of adipocytes, suggesting increased adipocyte cell death in the subcutaneous fat compartment.

Fat redistribution may contribute to metabolic disturbances noted in HIV-infected patients. Among HIV-negative individuals, an increased waist/hip ratio and central obesity are associated with increased risk of CAD.[24] Furthermore, visceral adiposity is highly correlated with insulin resistance. Seidell et al.[69] demonstrated a significant positive correlation between fasting insulin and visceral adiposity using computed tomography (CT) scans in healthy men with a wide range of body weight. Saint-Marc and colleagues[10] used cross-sectional abdominal CT imaging to evaluate HIV-infected patients participating in an observational cohort study assessing risk factors for changes in fat redistribution (LIPOCO study) (n = 154). Visceral abdominal fat was positively associated with fasting and 2 hour post glucose challenge insulin levels, regardless of the PI or NRTI status. These data indicate that changes in body fat distribution may contribute directly to the metabolic disturbances identified in patients with HIV infection independent of the pharmacologic effects of antiretroviral therapy. In addition, altered patterns of body fat distribution, particularly central adiposity, may further exacerbate the increased CVD risk profile among HIV-infected patients.

Management of Fat Redistribution

Fat distribution and redistribution may be assessed using various techniques to evaluate body composition. Visceral and subcutaneous fat may be precisely measured by using cross-sectional CT scans or magnetic resonance imaging (MRI) techniques, but these techniques need only be used in research settings at this time, as there are no data to suggest their utility in clinical practice. Dual energy x-ray absorptiometry (DEXA) is another radiographic technique that provides information on body fat distribution, lean body mass, and bone density. However, DEXA cannot distinguish between subcutaneous fat and fat in other body compartments. In contrast, serial measurements of the waist/hip ratio and waist circumference, which are readily obtainable in the clinical setting, may be useful for tracking the progression of fat redistribution and for identifying patients who may be at risk for developing metabolic complications.

As with insulin resistance and lipid abnormalities, treatment strategies to minimize or reverse fat redistribution are actively under investigation. In a pilot study of resistance training and aerobic exercise for HIV-infected patients with increased abdominal fat (n = 10), Roubenoff and colleagues[70] showed significant decreases in truncal fat after 16 weeks of exercise. Exercise may have additional benefits in reducing insulin resistance and improving lipid profiles and should be considered for all patients, particularly those with increased central adiposity.

The use of insulin-sensitizing agents in this population has also been shown to reduce abdominal fat.[36,37] Saint-Marc and Touraine[36] showed a 37% reduction in visceral abdominal adipose tissue (VAT) after 8 weeks of metformin therapy (Fig. 62–7). There was no significant effect of metformin on subcutaneous adipose tissue (SAT). Hadigan and colleagues[37] demonstrated significant reductions in waist circumference and BMI with metformin treatment; there was a trend toward a significant reduction in VAT (6% reduction for metformin-treated patients compared to an 8% increase in VAT for placebo-treated patients). Although the reduction was not significant, abdominal SAT also declined with metformin therapy. Therefore, although metformin has been shown to improve the metabolic profile and central adiposity of patients with fat redistribution and insulin resistance, it may not be beneficial for patients with primarily subcutaneous fat atrophy.

Metformin, although a potent insulin-sensitizing agent, is not believed to restore peripheral adipogenesis but, rather, to act primarily via a reduction of hepatic insulin resistance. In contrast, the thiazolidinediones have been shown to promote adipogenesis, primarily through an action on PPARγ.[71] Arioglu et al.[72] found that troglitazone, a thiazolidinedione, significantly improved the subcutaneous fat status in HIV-negative patients with congenital lipodystrophy, which is characterized by severe subcutaneous fat

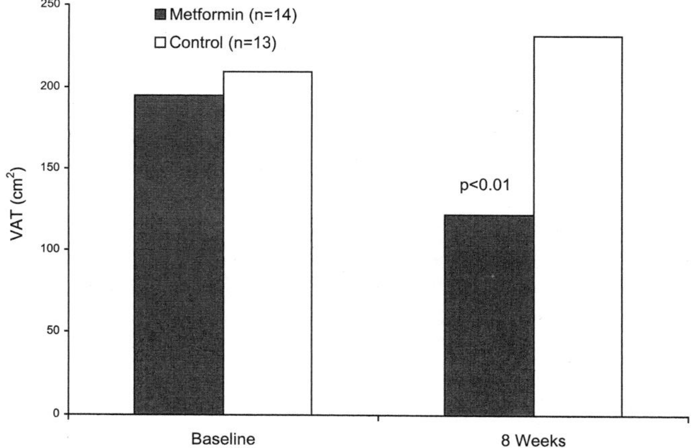

Figure 62–7. Mean cross-sectional visceral abdominal adipose tissue (VAT) measured by CT scan before and after 8 weeks of metformin treatment (850 mg three times daily) compared to control (no treatment). (Adapted from Saint-Marc T, Touraine JL. Effects of metformin on insulin resistance and central adiposity in patients receiving effective protease inhibitor therapy. AIDS 13:1000–1002, 1999, with permission.)

atrophy. Based on the clinical experience to date with rosiglitazone and its known effects to stimulate insulin sensitivity through PPARγ and promote adipogenesis, it is hypothesized that rosiglitazone may reverse insulin resistance and promote adipogenesis in patients with HIV, insulin resistance, and peripheral fat atrophy. Therapeutic trials of rosiglitazone to reverse subcutaneous fat loss and improve insulin resistance are planned by the ACTG.

Patient disfigurement secondary to fat redistribution has led some to seek treatment from plastic surgeons. To date only small case series have been reported, with little or no follow-up data on the use of plastic surgery techniques to correct fat redistribution. Wolfort and colleagues[73] described the result of two patients who underwent liposuction of the dorsocervical and submental fat pads and one patient who had liposuction of the abdomen and flanks. Patients reported satisfaction with the outcome, but no long-term follow-up information was presented. Carefully designed studies that control for antiretroviral exposure and evaluate the safety and efficacy of plastic surgery for lipodystrophy, including liposuction and fat transplantation, are imperative.

Growth hormone (GH) deficiency has been identified in association with central adiposity in both HIV-negative individuals[74] and HIV-infected patients with fat redistribution.[75] Rietschel and colleagues[75] found reduced mean GH concentrations and reduced basal and pulse amplitude GH concentrations among HIV-infected men with lipodystrophy compared to HIV-infected controls without lipodystrophy and to healthy men. Recombinant human GH (rhGH) has been used successfully in HIV-negative GH-deficient adults to reduce abdominal adiposity.[76] Therefore Wanke and colleagues[77] conducted a 12-week open-label trial of rhGH (6 mg/day SC) in 10 patients with HIV infection and fat redistribution. The waist/hip ratio, a measure of central adiposity, was significantly reduced with rhGH therapy. However, the use of rhGH may induce or exacerbate insulin resistance and glucose intolerance, and one patient in this trial developed hyperglycemia. Therefore the utility of rhGH for the treatment of lipodystrophy may be limited in this population with increased risk of insulin resistance and diabetes. Although rhGH treatment with lower doses may be useful, particularly in patients with primarily central adiposity, additional information from controlled trials is necessary to determine the long-term efficacy and safety of rhGH use to treat HIV-infected patients with fat redistribution.

Trials of antiretroviral switching and structured therapy interruptions have also been used to attempt reversal of fat redistribution. Martinez and colleagues[45] found significant reductions in the waist/hip ratio after 8 months in patients who switched from a PI-containing regimen to nevirapine. In addition, after 6 months of nevirapine, 91% of patients reported subjective improvement of body fat changes. Similarly, Barreiro et al.[59] found 50% of patients who switched from a PI to nevirapine reported improvements in body shape abnormalities after 6 months, whereas no patient who remained on a PI reported such improvement. Short-term interruption of HAART, however, has not been found to improve anthropometric measurements in patients with HIV infection and fat redistribution.[47]

▲ CONCLUSIONS

Lipodystrophy associated with HIV infection is estimated to affect most patients treated with potent combination antiretroviral therapy. Significant metabolic disturbances have been identified in association with fat redistribution in these patients including insulin resistance and hyperlipidemia. Preliminary investigations have demonstrated potential utility in the use of insulin-sensitizing agents and lipid-lowering therapies to ameliorate these metabolic disturbances. Furthermore, the use of PI-sparing treatment regimens and structured treatment interruption are under investigation as potential strategies to limit or prevent lipodystrophy. Patients with HIV infection who demonstrate fat redistribution and who develop hyperinsulinemia and dyslipidemia are at increased risk of CVD. However the long-term effects and the cardiovascular disease risks of these disturbances have not yet been fully appreciated.

REFERENCES

1. Lo JC, Mulligan K, Tai VW, et al. "Buffalo hump" in men with HIV-I infection. Lancet 351:871, 1998.
2. Roth VR, Kravcik S, Angel JB. Development of cervical fat pads following therapy with human immunodeficiency virus type-1 protease inhibitors. Clin Infect Dis 27:65, 1998.
3. Miller KD, Jones E, Yanovski JA, et al. Visceral abdominal-fat accumulation associated with use of indinavir. Lancet 351:871, 1998.
4. Dong KL, Bausserman LL, Flynn MM, et al. Changes in body habitus and serum lipid abnormalities in HIV-positive women on highly active antiretroviral therapy. J Acquir Immun Defic Syndr 21:107, 1999.
5. Carr A, Samaras K, Burton S, et al. A syndrome of peripheral lipodystrophy, hyperlipidemia and insulin resistance in patients receiving protease inhibitor therapy. AIDS 12:F51, 1998.
6. Carr A, Miller J, Law M, Cooper DA. A syndrome of lipoatrophy, lactic acidaemia and liver dysfunction associated with HIV nucleoside analogue therapy: contribution to protease inhibitor-related lipodystrophy syndrome. AIDS 14:F25, 2000.
7. Hadigan C, Meigs JB, Corcoran C, et al. Metabolic abnormalities and cardiovascular disease risk factors in adults with human immunodeficiency virus infection and lipodystrophy. Clin Infect Dis 32:130, 2001.
8. Lichtenstein K, Ward D, Delaney K, et al. Clinical factors related to the severity of fat redistribution in the HIV outpatient study (HOPS). In: XIII International AIDS Conference, Durban, South Africa, vol 2, 2000.
9. Mallal SA, John M, Moore CB, et al. Contribution of nucleoside analogue reverse transcriptase inhibitors to subcutaneous fat wasting in patients with HIV infection. AIDS 14:1309, 2000.
10. Saint-Marc T, Partisani M, Poizot-Martin I, et al. Fat distribution evaluated by computed tomography and metabolic abnormalities in patients undergoing antiretroviral therapy: preliminary results of the LIPOCO study. AIDS 14:37, 2000.
11. Noor M, Lo J, Mulligan K, et al. Metabolic effects of indinavir in healthy HIV-seronegative men. AIDS 15:F11, 2001.
12. Purnell JQ, Zambon A, Knopp RH, et al. Effect of ritonavir on lipids and post-heparin lipase activities in normal subjects. AIDS 14:51, 2000.
13. Mulligan K, Grunfeld C, Tai VW, et al. Hyperlipidemia and insulin resistance are induced by protease inhibitors independent of changes in body composition in patients with HIV infection. J Acquir Immune Defic Syndr 23:35, 2000.
14. Carr A, Samaras K, Thorisdottir A, et al. Diagnosis, prediction, and natural course of HIV-1 protease-inhibitor associated lipodystrophy, hyperlipidemia, and diabetes mellitus: a cohort study. Lancet 353:2093, 1999.
15. Walli RK, Herfort O, Michl GM, et al. Treatment with protease inhibitors associated with peripheral insulin resistance and impaired oral glucose tolerance in HIV-1 infected patients. AIDS 12:F167, 1998.

16. Hadigan C, Miller K, Corcoran C, et al. Fasting hyperinsulinemia and changes in regional body composition in hiv-infected women. J Clin Endocrinol Metab 84:1932, 1999.
17. Behrens G, Dejam A, Schmidt H, et al. Impaired glucose tolerance, beta cell function and lipid metabolism in HIV patients under treatment with protease inhibitors. AIDS 13:F63, 1999.
18. Ursich MJM, Fukui RT, Galvao MSA, et al. Insulin resistance in limb and trunk partial lipodystrophy (type 2 Kobberling-Dunnigan syndrome). Metabolism 46:159, 1997.
19. Murata H, Hruz PW, Mueckler M. The mechanism of insulin resistance caused by HIV protease inhibitor therapy. J Biol Chem 275:20251, 2000.
20. Feskens EJ, Kromhout D. Glucose tolerance and the risk of cardiovascular disease: the Zutphen Study. J Clin Epidemiol 45:1327, 1992.
21. Howard G, Bergman R, Wagenknecht LE, et al. Ability of alternative indices of insulin sensitivity to predict cardiovascular risk: comparison with the "minimal model". Insulin Resistance Atherosclerosis Study (IRAS) Investigators. Ann Epidemiol 8:358, 1998.
22. Despres JP, Lamarche B, Mauriege P, et al. Hyperinsulinemia as an independent risk factor for ischemic heart disease. N Engl J Med 334:952, 1996.
23. Manson JE, Colditz GA, Stampfer MJ, et al. A prospective study of obesity and risk of coronary heart disease in women. N Engl J Med 322:882, 1990.
24. Larsson L, Svardsudd K, Welin L, et al. Abdominal adipose tissue distribution, obesity, and risk of cardiovascular disease and death: 13 year follow up of participants in the study of men born in 1913. BMJ 288:1401, 1984.
25. Maggi P, Serio G, Epifani G, et al. Premature lesions of the carotid vessels in HIV-1-infected patients treated with protease inhibitors. AIDS 14:F123, 2000.
26. Klein D, Hurley L, Sorel M, Sidney S. Do protease inhibitors increase the risk for coronary heart disease among HIV positive patients—follow-up. Presented at the 8th Conference on Retroviruses and Opportunistic Infections, Chicago, 2001.
27. Mary-Krause M, Cotte L, Partisani M, et al. Impact of treatment with protease inhibitor (PI) on myocardial infarction (MI) occurrence in HIV-infected men. Presented at the 8th Conference on Retroviruses and Opportunistic Infections, Chicago, 2001.
28. Meigs JB, Mittleman MA, Nathan DM, et al. Hyperinsulinemia, hyperglycemia and impaired hemostasis: the Framingham Offspring Study. JAMA 283:220, 2000.
29. Carmassi F, Morale M, Ferrini L, et al. Local insulin infusion stimulates expression of plasminogen activator inhibitor-1 and tissue-type plasminogen activator in normal subjects. Am J Med 107:344, 1999.
30. Jansson JH, Olofsson BO, Nilsson TK. Predictive value of tissue plasminogen activator mass concentration on long-term mortality in patients with coronary artery disease: a 7-year follow-up. Circulation 88:2030, 1993.
31. Johansson L, Jansson JH, Boman K, et al. Tissue plasminogen activator, plasminogen activator inhibitor-1, and tissue plasminogen activator/plasminogen activator inhibitor-1 complex as risk factors for the development of a first stroke. Stroke 31:26, 2000.
32. Hadigan C, Meigs JB, Rabe J, et al. Increased PAI-1 and tPA antigen levels are reduced with metformin therapy in HIV-infected patients with fat redistribution and insulin resistance. J Clin Endocrinol Metab 86:939, 2001.
33. Wright A, Cull C, Holman R, et al. United Kingdom prospective diabetes study 24: a 6-year, randomized, controlled trial comparing sulfonylurea, insulin, and metformin therapy in patients with newly diagnosed type 2 diabetes that could not be controlled with diet therapy. Ann Intern Med 128:165, 1998.
34. Stumvoll M, Nurjhan N, Perriello G, et al. Metabolic effects of metformin in non-insulin-dependent diabetes mellitus. N Engl J Med 333:550, 1995.
35. Lee A, Morley JE. Metformin decreases food consumption and induces weight loss in subjects with obesity with type II non-insulin-dependent diabetes. Obes Res 6:47, 1998.
36. Saint-Marc T, Touraine JL. Effects of metformin on insulin resistance and central adiposity in patients receiving effective protease inhibitor therapy. AIDS 13:1000, 1999.
37. Hadigan C, Corcoran C, Basgoz N, et al. Metformin in the treatment of HIV lipodystrophy. JAMA 284:472, 2000.
38. Hallakou S, Doare L, Foufelle F, et al. Pioglitazone induces in vivo adipocyte differentiation in the obese Zucker fa/fa rat. Diabetes 46:1393, 1997.
39. Spiegelman BR. PPAR-gamma: adipogenic regulator and thiazolidinedione receptor. Diabetes 47:507, 1998.
40. Maggs DG, Buchanan TA, Burant CF, et al. Metabolic effects of troglitazone monotherapy in type 2 diabetes mellitus: a randomized, double-blind placebo-controlled trial. Ann Intern Med 128:176, 1998.
41. Walli R, Michl GM, Muhlbayer D, et al. Effects of troglitazone on insulin sensitivity in HIV-infected patients with protease inhibitor-associated diabetes mellitus. Res Exp Med (Berl) 199:253, 2000.
42. Rappaport E, Weill S, Patwardhan R. Once or twice daily rosiglitazone is effective first line treatment for type 2 diabetes. Presented at the 81st Annual Meeting of the Endocrine Society, San Diego, 1999.
43. Salzman A, Patel J. Rosiglitazone therapy is not associated with hepatotoxicity. Diabetes 48:S408, 1999.
44. Akazawa S, Sun F, Ito M, et al. Efficacy of troglitazone on body fat distribution in type 2 diabetes. Diabetes Care 23:1067, 2000.
45. Martinez E, Conget I, Lozano L, et al. Reversion of metabolic abnormalities after switching from HIV-1 protease inhibitors to nevirapine. AIDS 13:805, 1999.
46. Martinez E, Garcia-Viejo MA, Blanco JL, et al. Impact of switching from human immunodeficiency virus type 1 protease inhibitors to efavirenz in successfully treated adults with lipodystrophy. Clin Infect Dis 31:1266, 2000.
47. Hatano H, Miller KD, Yoder CP, et al. Metabolic and anthropometric consequences of interruption of highly active antiretroviral therapy. AIDS 14:1935, 2000.
48. Grunfeld C, Pang M, Doerrler W, et al. Lipids, lipoproteins, triglyceride clearance, and cytokines in human immunodeficiency virus infection and the acquired immunodeficiency syndrome. J Clin Endocrinol Metab 74:1045, 1992.
49. Grunfeld C, Pang M, Doerrler W. Circulating interferon alpha levels and hypertriglyceridemia in the acquired immunodeficiency syndrome. Am J Med 90:154, 1991.
50. Henry K. Lipid abnormalities associated with use of protease inhibitors: prevalence, clinical sequelae and treatment. Presented at the 12th World AIDS Conference, Geneva, 1998.
51. Carr AKS, Chisholm DJ, Cooper DA. Pathogenesis of HIV-1-protease-inhibitor-associated peripheral lipodystrophy, hyperlipidemia and insulin resistance. Lancet 352:1881, 1998.
52. Papadopoulos AI, Evangelopoulou EP, Niccolaidi NA, et al. Serum lipid changes in HIV-infected patients under combination therapy containing a protease inhibitor. Presented at the 12th World AIDS Conference, Geneva, 1998.
53. Chang E, Deleo M, Liu YT, et al. The effects of antiretroviral protease inhibitors (PIs) on serum lipids and glucose in HIV-infected patients. Presented at the 12th World AIDS Conference, Geneva, 1998.
54. Dube MP, Sprecher D, Henry WK, et al. Preliminary guidelines for the evaluation and management of dyslipidemia in adults infected with human immunodeficiency virus and receiving antiretroviral therapy: recommendations of the adult AIDS clinical trial group cardiovascular disease focus group. Clin Infect Dis 31:1216, 2000.
55. Program NCE. Second report of the expert panel on detection, evaluation, and treatment of high blood cholesterol in adults (Adult Treatment Panel II). Circulation 89:1329, 1994.
56. Thomas JC, Lopes-Virella MF, Del Bene VE, et al. Use of fenofibrate in the management of protease inhibitor-associated lipid abnormalities. Pharmacotherapy 20:727, 2000.
57. Miller J, Carr A, Brown D, Cooper DA. A randomized, double-blind study of gemfibrizol for the treatment of protease inhibitor-associated hypertriglyceridemia. Presented at the 8th Conference on Retroviruses and Opportunistic Infections, Chicago, 2001.
58. Fitchenbaum C, Gerber J, Rosenkrantz S, et al. Pharmacokinetic interactions between protease inhibitors and statins in HIV seronegative volunteers: ACTG Study A5047. AIDS 16:569, 2002.
59. Barreiro P, Soriano V, Blanco F, et al. Risks and benefits of replacing protease inhibitors by nevirapine in HIV-infected subjects under long-term successful triple combination therapy. AIDS 14:807, 2000.
60. Lafon E, Landman R, Quertainmont M, et al. LIPSTOP study: evolution of clinical lipodystrophy (LD) blood lipids, visceral (VAT) and subcutaneous (SAT) adipose tissue after switching from protease inhibitor (PI) to efavirenz (EFV) in HIV-1 infected patients.

In: XIII International AIDS Conference, Durban, South Africa, vol 2, 2000.

61. Miller KM, Daly PA, Sentochnik D, et al. Pseudo-Cushing's syndrome in HIV-infected men. Clin Infect Dis 27:68, 1998.
62. Gervasoni C, Ridolfo AL, Trifiro G, et al. Redistribution of body fat in HIV-infected women undergoing combined antiretroviral treatment. AIDS 13:465, 1999.
63. Carr A, Cooper DA. Lipodystrophy associated with an HIV-protease inhibitor. N Engl J Med 339:1296, 1998.
64. Kasper T, Arboleda C, Halpern M. The impact of patient perceptions of body shape changes and metabolic abnormalities on antiretroviral therapy, In: XIII International AIDS Conference, Durban, South Africa, vol 2, 2000.
65. Saint-Marc T, Partisani M, Poizot-MArtin I, et al. A syndrome of peripheral fat wasting (lipodystrophy) in patients receiving long-term nucleoside analogue therapy. AIDS 13:1659, 1999.
66. Zhang B, Macnaul K, Szalkowski D, et al. Inhibition of adipocyte differentiation by HIV protease inhbitors. J Clin Endocrinol Metab 84:4274, 1999.
67. Dowell P, Flexner C, Kwiterovich PO, Lane MD. Suppression of preadipocyte differentiation and promotion of adipocyte death by HIV protease inhibitors. J Biol Chem 275:41325, 2000.
68. Domingo P, Matias-Guiu X, Pugol RM, et al. Subutaneous adipocyte apoptosis in HIV-1 protease inhibitor associated lipodystrophy. AIDS 13:2261, 1999.
69. Seidell JC, Bjorntorp P, Sjostrom L, et al. Visceral fat accumulation in men is positively associated with insulin, glucose, and c-peptide levels, but negatively with testosterone levels. Metabolism 9:897, 1990.
70. Roubenoff R, Weiss L, McDermott A, et al. A pilot study of exercise training to reduce trunk fat in adults with HIV-associated fat redistribution. AIDS 13:1373, 1999.
71. Inzucchi SE, Maggs DG, Spollett GR, et al. Efficacy and metabolic effects of metformin and troglitazone in type II diabetes mellitus. N Engl J Med 338:867, 1998.
72. Arioglu E, Duncan-Morin J, Sebring N, et al. Efficacy and safety of troglitazone in the treatment of lipodystrophy. Ann Intern Med 133:263, 2000.
73. Wolfort FG, Cetrulo CL, Nevarre DR. Suction-assisted lipectomy for lipodystrophy syndromes attributed to HIV-protease inhibitor use. Plast Reconstr Surg 104:1814, 1999.
74. Vahl N, Jorgensen JO, Jurik AG, Christiansen JS. Abdominal adiposity and physical fitness are major determinants of the age associated decline in stimulated GH secretion in healthy adults. J Clin Endocrinol Metab 81:2209, 1996.
75. Rietschel P, Hadigan C, Corcoran C, et al. Assessment of growth hormone dynamics in human immunodeficiency virus-related lipodystrophy. J Clin Endocrinol Metab 86:504, 2001.
76. Cuneo RC, Judd S, Wallace JD, et al. The Australian multicenter trial of growth hormone (GH) treatment in GH-deficient adults. J Clin Endocrinol Metab 83:107, 1998.
77. Wanke C, Gerrior JJK, Coakley E, Albrech M. Recombinant human growth hormone improves the fat redistribution syndrome (lipodystrophy) in patients with HIV. AIDS 13:2099, 1999.

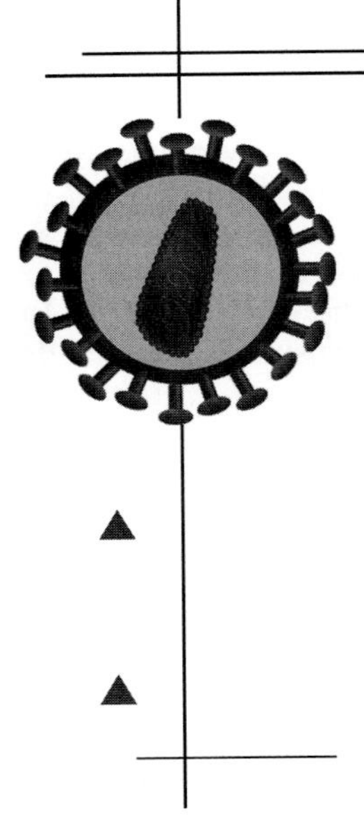

CHAPTER 63

Adrenal, Gonadal, and Thyroid Disorders

Joan C. Lo, MD
Morris Schambelan, MD

A variety of endocrine disorders have been reported in association with human immunodeficiency virus (HIV) infection and the acquired immunodeficiency syndrome (AIDS). Although direct viral infection may be responsible for organ dysfunction, most endocrine and metabolic perturbations are a consequence of systemic illness, opportunistic infections, neoplastic processes, body wasting, and HIV-related therapies. These abnormalities range from subclinical perturbations in hormone balance to overt glandular failure, and almost every endocrine organ system is affected. Moreover, although the clinical presentation may bear some similarity to that in immunocompetent individuals, many aspects appear to be unique to HIV-infected patients. The goals of this chapter are to review the adrenal, gonadal, and thyroid abnormalities associated with HIV infection and AIDS and to provide a general approach to the diagnosis and management of these disorders.

▲ ADRENAL GLAND

Adrenal Pathology

Pathologic involvement of the adrenal gland occurs commonly in AIDS, with abnormalities noted in as many as 68% of patients during postmortem examination.[1,2] Patients are typically asymptomatic, however, because clinical adrenal insufficiency is generally not evident until at least 80% to 90% of the adrenal gland has been destroyed.[3,4] Cytomegalovirus adrenalitis is the most frequent finding and has been reported in 40% to 50% of patients in whom an adrenal pathology report is available.[1,2,5] *Mycobacterium tuberculosis*, *Mycobacterium avium* complex, *Cryptococcus neoformans*, and *Toxoplasma gondii* also infect the adrenal gland, although most of these cases have not been associated with substantial adrenal destruction.[1,5] Other pathologic findings include hemorrhage, fibrosis, infarction, and focal necrosis.[5,6] Infiltration with Kaposi sarcoma or lymphoma occurs in a small number of patients and is generally not associated with clinical adrenal insufficiency.[5,7] One rather surprising finding has been the unusual occurrence of advanced adrenal carcinoma in three seropositive patients, but the relation of primary adrenal malignancy to HIV infection in these rare instances is not known.[8]

Alterations in Adrenal Function

In normal individuals, corticotropin-releasing hormone (CRH) is secreted by the hypothalamus and stimulates production of adrenocorticotropic hormone (ACTH) by the anterior pituitary gland. ACTH, in turn, stimulates production of cortisol by the adrenal cortex, and both hormones manifest a diurnal circadian rhythm. Homeostatic regulation of the hypothalamic-pituitary-adrenal (HPA) axis is maintained by cortisol feedback at the level of the hypothalamus and pituitary. In response to acute illness, infection, or stress, increased hypothalamic activation leads to an increase in circulating cortisol levels. The adrenal gland also produces aldosterone, which is primarily under regulation of the renin-angiotensin system.

Individuals infected with HIV commonly demonstrate an elevation in basal cortisol levels, frequently in association with lower levels of ACTH and the adrenal steroid dehydroepiandrosterone (DHEA).[9] Moreover, the adrenal reserve of the 17-deoxysteroids (corticosterone, deoxycorticosterone, 18-OH-deoxycorticosterone) appears to be impaired.[10] This shift in steroid metabolism may represent an adaptive response to systemic illness.[11] Alternatively, the increase in cortisol biosynthesis in the absence of an increase in ACTH suggests that nonpituitary factors (e.g., cytokines) may directly affect adrenocortical function.[9] Reports of increased ACTH and cortisol levels in some HIV-infected patients have led others to speculate that hypothalamic activation may occur,[12] although individuals with advanced HIV illness often demonstrate blunted pituitary-adrenal responsiveness to CRH infusion.[13] Increased ACTH levels may be also compensatory, particularly in patients with subclinical defects in adrenocortical function.[14] In addition, glucocorticoid resistance should be considered in patients with AIDS who present with hypercortisolism, ACTH elevation, and paradoxical addisonian features.[15]

Pituitary-adrenal function has also been studied in the setting of HIV-associated fat redistribution, particularly in patients who present with dorsocervical fat pad enlargement and visceral adiposity. Although these features are somewhat reminiscent of Cushing syndrome, overt hypercortisolism has not been found upon biochemical examination.[16–18] In addition, individuals with protease inhibitor (PI)-associated fat redistribution exhibit normal diurnal cortisol excretion as well as normal cortisol secretory dynamics after administration of ovine CRH.[18] Nevertheless, subtle changes in cortisol metabolism based on urinary steroid excretion profiles have been noted in these patients, although the significance of these findings is unclear.[18] Others have hypothesized that the lipodystrophic changes may be related to the increased cortisol/DHEA ratio observed in affected patients.[19] A rare exception to the above observations has been the development of exogenous Cushing syndrome reported in two patients treated with ritonavir and inhaled nasal fluticasone (a topical nasal glucocorticoid); the authors of that report postulated that ritonavir administration impaired the metabolism of fluticasone via effects on P_{450} metabolism, resulting in the high plasma levels of fluticasone observed and relative adrenal suppression.[20]

A number of drugs used to treat HIV-related disorders are known to affect adrenocortical function. For example, ketoconazole inhibits multiple steps in the pathway of cortisol biosynthesis and can cause clinical adrenal insufficiency, particularly in patients with limited adrenal reserve.[21] Rifampin increases the metabolic clearance of cortisol and may also lead to diminished cortisol levels in patients with limited adrenal reserve or those receiving glucocorticoid replacement therapy.[22] Megestrol acetate, a progestational agent with intrinsic glucocorticoid-like activity, has been shown to suppress the HPA axis and result in glucocorticoid deficiency when treatment is discontinued, particularly in patients who have had long-term therapy.[23,24] In one study of megestrol acetate treatment (800 mg/day) for HIV-associated wasting, the cortisol concentration decreased to nearly undetectable levels in virtually all patients in whom plasma megestrol acetate levels were higher than 150 ng/ml.[25] There have also been isolated reports of Cushing syndrome and diabetes mellitus in patients receiving megestrol acetate therapy.[24,26–28]

Diagnostic Approach and Therapy

Despite the abnormalities in adrenocortical function described above, most patients are asymptomatic and clinically significant adrenal impairment is relatively uncommon with HIV infection. However, glucocorticoid insufficiency in patients with AIDS is clearly more prevalent than in the general population, so it is important to perform tests of adrenal function in patients who present with features suggestive of adrenal insufficiency (Fig. 63–1). The signs and symptoms of adrenal insufficiency include weakness, orthostasis, nausea, abdominal pain, weight loss, hyponatremia and hypoglycemia, as well as hyperkalemia and metabolic acidosis in patients with primary adrenal failure. Hyperkalemia and renal sodium wasting have also been noted in patients receiving trimethoprim, an effect that is mediated through trimethoprim inhibition of the sodium channel in the distal nephron.[29]

The ACTH stimulation test provides the most direct means of assessing adrenal function. In patients with frank adrenal insufficiency, intravenous (or intramuscular) administration of cosyntropin (250 μg) results in little or no increase in plasma cortisol, whereas normal individuals generally achieve peak cortisol levels above 20 μg/dl (540 nmol/L). Basal glucocorticoid production is generally low in these patients, although the presence of low baseline cortisol levels alone should not be used for a definitive diagnosis. The ACTH stimulation test may not detect patients with impaired pituitary reserve, however, and in selected cases insulin-induced hypoglycemia or the metyrapone test is warranted to assess pituitary ACTH responsiveness specifically.[30]

Once the diagnosis of adrenal insufficiency has been established, it is important to distinguish between primary and secondary adrenal failure. Individuals with primary adrenal failure (Addison's disease) invariably present with high ACTH levels, and biochemical findings (hyperkalemia, metabolic acidosis) are generally consistent with concomitant mineralocorticoid deficiency. Aldosterone levels are low despite increased plasma renin levels. Adrenal computed tomography (CT) imaging may yield information about the etiology of adrenal disease in some patients,[31] although in many cases the findings are nondiagnostic. Conversely, ACTH levels are low to low normal (< 20 pg/ml by immunoradiometric assay) in patients with secondary hypoadrenalism due to pituitary ACTH deficiency. Such patients have normal levels of plasma renin and aldosterone.

Patients with documented adrenal insufficiency, based on failure to respond to stimulation with ACTH, should be treated with glucocorticoid replacement therapy. Hydrocortisone (20 to 30 mg/day) is generally administered in two divided doses, with higher doses in the morning to simulate normal circadian rhythmicity. In addition, fludrocortisone (0.05 to 0.10 mg/day) is usually added for mineralocorticoid replacement therapy in patients with primary adrenal insufficiency, although a small percentage of addisonian patients can be managed with cortisol and adequate dietary sodium intake alone. Larger doses of glucocorticoid are required for periods of stress, generally a two- to threefold increase for moderate stress coverage and maximal stress doses (hydrocortisone 100

SUSPECTED ADRENAL INSUFFICENCY
Weakness, fatigue
Orthostasis
Nausea, abdominal pain
Weight loss
Hyponatremia
Hypoglycemia
Hyperkalemia
Metabolic acidosis } In patients with ***primary*** adrenal insufficiency

↓

PERFORM ACTH STIMULATION TEST

- Administer 250 μg cosyntropin IV/IM, preferably in the morning
- Measure plasma cortisol level at T = 0 and 60 minutes
- Obtain baseline plasma ACTH level (at T = 0) if primary adrenal insufficiency is suspected. Baseline measurement of plasma renin activity and aldosterone is also recommended.

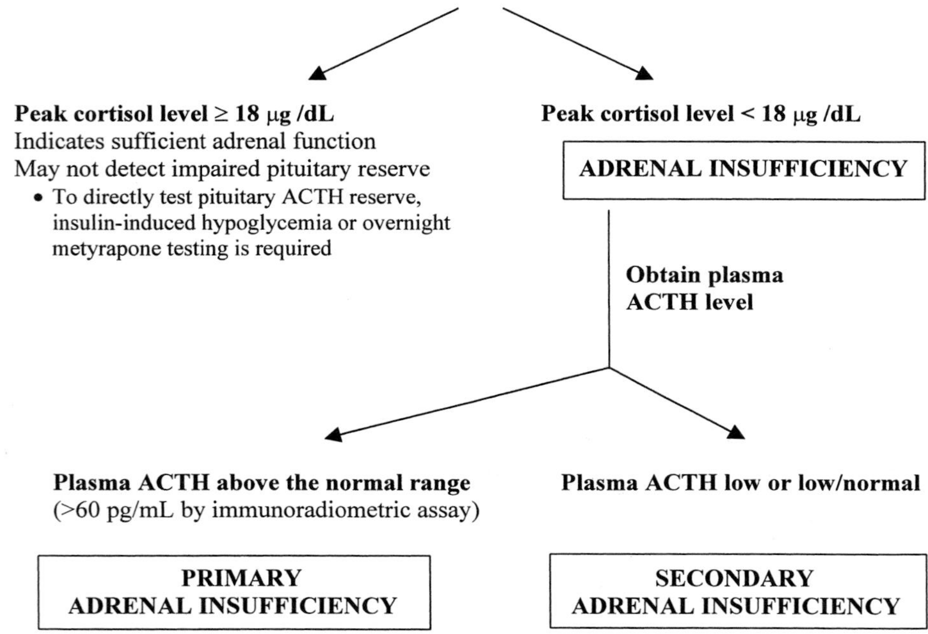

Figure 63–1. Diagnostic approach to patients with suspected adrenal insufficiency.

mg every 8 hours) for severe illness or trauma. The role of glucocorticoid therapy in patients with elevated basal cortisol levels who show somewhat diminished responsiveness to ACTH is less clear, however, and each case should be evaluated individually. A number of these patients respond to prolonged (72 hours) ACTH infusion,[10] suggesting that patients with a "borderline" response to acute ACTH stimulation may not require routine glucocorticoid maintenance therapy. However, some clinicians would give glucocorticoids to such patients at times of stress, provided the treatment is limited in duration, thereby avoiding the adverse consequences of prolonged steroid therapy. Routine glucocorticoid supplementation in patients with modest perturbations in the HPA axis is probably not warranted.

Special consideration should also be given to patients terminating pharmacologic glucocorticoid or megestrol acetate therapy because long-term treatment with these agents can lead to secondary adrenal insufficiency.[23,24] Although adrenal function generally recovers, the process can take months; and patients with subnormal ACTH stimulation test results may have to be maintained on low glucocorticoid replacement doses until a normal cortisol response is achieved.[32]

Dehydroepiandrosterone and HIV Infection

Dehydroepiandrosterone (DHEA) is a weak androgen produced by the adrenal gland. Although present in highest concentration during early adulthood, levels decline with advancing age and chronic illness, in contrast to cortisol levels, which remain relatively stable.[33,34] It has been postulated that the decline in DHEA levels may be responsible, in part, for the various immunologic, cognitive, and body composition changes associated with the aging process, leading to the widespread use of DHEA for its purported "fountain of youth" properties.[33] Furthermore, a number of preliminary studies support the role of DHEA as an immunomodulatory agent and have led to renewed interest in DHEA therapy in the HIV community.[35] The ratio of cortisol/DHEA levels has received increasing attention, largely based on the observation that an increased ratio is associated with an unfavorable shift in cytokine production that is synergistic with HIV infection.[36,37] Indeed, several cross-sectional studies in HIV-infected men suggest that low DHEA levels and elevated cortisol/DHEA ratios are associated with advanced HIV infection; and low DHEA levels, in particular, appear to be an independent predictor for progression to AIDS.[38–40] There is also some in vitro evidence that DHEA has inhibitory effects on HIV-1 replication and activation.[41–43] However, DHEA should not be used to treat HIV-infected patients until its efficacy has been proven in randomized clinical trials.

▲ TESTES AND OVARIES

Testicular Pathology

Examination of the testes at autopsy in men with AIDS indicate that a number of histopathologic changes occur, including hypospermatogenesis, basement membrane thickening, interstitial fibrosis, and tubular atrophy.[44–47] Multiple factors contribute to these findings, such as prolonged HIV illness, direct HIV cytopathic effects, chronic infection, fever, malnutrition, wasting, and the use of gonadotoxic and antiandrogenic drugs. Fewer than one-third of patients demonstrate specific testicular infection.[44,45] Direct testicular involvement by opportunistic infection is seen most commonly with cytomegalovirus, *Toxoplasma gondii*, and *Mycobacterium avium* complex.[44,45,47] Neoplastic processes affecting the testes occur infrequently, although Kaposi sarcoma and lymphoma of the testes have been observed in patients with evidence of disseminated disease.[7,47] Changes in semen quality have been reported in men with advanced HIV infection, including decreased sperm count and motility, reduced semen volume, increased abnormal sperm forms, and pyosemia.[48–50]

Alterations in Testicular Function

In normal individuals, gonadotropin-releasing hormone (GnRH) synthesized in the hypothalamus stimulates release of luteinizing hormone (LH) and follicle-stimulating hormone (FSH) from the anterior pituitary gland. LH, in turn, stimulates production of testosterone by testicular Leydig cells, and FSH promotes spermatogenesis in Sertoli cells. Both FSH and LH secretion are regulated by androgen concentrations; LH levels more directly reflect testosterone feedback, and FSH levels are predominantly regulated by inhibin produced by the Sertoli cells. Early in the course of HIV infection, total and free testosterone levels may be normal or slightly elevated[51,52]; an exaggerated LH response to infusion of GnRH has been observed in a subset of patients.[52] Thereafter, testosterone levels tend to fall with advanced HIV illness, generally as a consequence of both gonadal and extragonadal factors that lead to testicular dysfunction.[39,51,53] At that point, measurement of bioavailable or free testosterone levels may be the most sensitive indicator of hypogonadism, as sex hormone-binding globulin levels can be elevated in the setting of HIV infection[39,54,55] (Fig. 63–2).

With primary gonadal failure, FSH or LH levels (or both) are increased in the presence of decreased androgen production. Contributing factors include direct viral or opportunistic infection, prolonged fever, malignant infiltration, and administration of gonadotoxic agents, although the underlying cause is often not identified.[53,56] Ketoconazole inhibits steroidogenesis in the adrenal gland and testes, and prolonged treatment can lead to primary hypogonadism and gynecomastia, particularly at high doses.[21] The majority of HIV-infected patients with low circulating testosterone levels have secondary or central hypogonadism, which is established biochemically by detecting low or inappropriately normal serum FSH and LH concentrations in the presence of low testosterone levels. In most cases the etiology is not known but is likely multifactorial, as systemic illness, malnutrition, and wasting are common causes of central gonadotropin suppression.[7,53] A significant number of patients with the AIDS wasting syndrome have some degree of testosterone deficiency, and it has been suggested that the decline in circulating androgen levels may contribute to the critical loss of lean body mass.[55,57] In addition, systemic administration of glucocorticoids, megestrol acetate, and opiate drugs may also contribute to central hypogonadism,[58–60] as can previous treatment with anabolic androgenic steroids in cases in which recovery of the pituitary-gonadal axis is delayed. Direct pituitary destruction by opportunistic pathogens or malignant processes occurs rarely.[61,62]

Diagnostic Approach and Therapy

Once the diagnosis of hypogonadism has been established, pituitary gonadotropins (FSH, LH) should be measured to distinguish between primary and secondary (central) hypogonadism. A careful history should also be obtained to exclude reversible etiologies prior to initiating testosterone replacement. For patients with secondary hypogonadism who manifest other pituitary deficiencies, visual field defects, or additional findings suggestive of a central mass lesion, magnetic resonance imaging (MRI) of the pituitary and hypothalamus is warranted. However, it should be noted that the incidence of direct pituitary involvement by infectious, inflammatory, or malignant processes is extremely low.

Androgen replacement therapy is indicated in patients with symptomatic hypogonadism. Although bioavailable

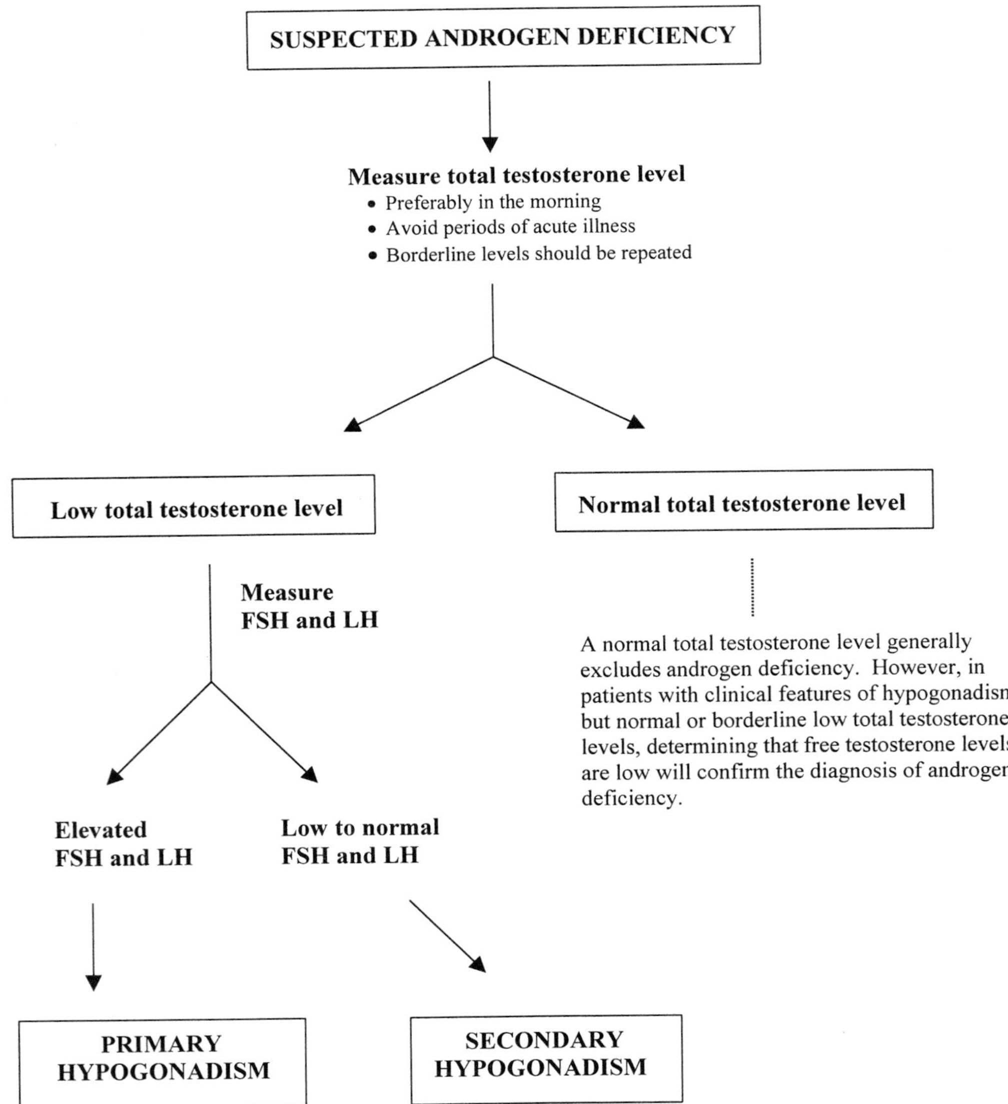

Figure 63–2. Diagnostic approach to male patients with suspected androgen deficiency.

testosterone levels are often subnormal and not extremely low, most individuals respond to replacement therapy with symptomatic improvement. Currently, there are three main routes of testosterone delivery. The testosterone esters enanthate and cypionate are the most widely used and provide a safe, effective, inexpensive approach to androgen replacement therapy. Starting doses range from 200 to 300 mg administered by intramuscular injection every 2 to 3 weeks (average dose 100 mg/week), although dosages may have to be adjusted for a clinical response. Because interval injections lead to large fluctuations in serum testosterone levels, some patients prefer treatment with smaller, more frequent doses (e.g., 100 mg/week). Generally, there is no role for routine determination of testosterone levels once replacement therapy has been initiated, except in cases where the appropriate dosing interval is difficult to determine. The newer transdermal testosterone delivery systems provide a more stable, continuous mode of testosterone administration and may be preferred in patients who experience disturbing fluctuations in energy level and sexual function. These transdermal systems require daily application and are more costly. Moreover, the skin patch can cause a local rash, although most patients are able to continue treatment with application of topical corticosteroids underneath the patch. A new testosterone gel formulation (Androgel) has become available and appears to be well tolerated,[63,64] although patients should realize that vigorous skin contact with a partner may lead to significant drug transfer, as a large proportion of the dose remains on the skin after application.[63] It should also be noted that the transdermal testosterone formulations may not deliver an adequate testosterone concentration at the recommended doses in every individual, so measurements to assess whether therapeutic levels are achieved might be considered. Testosterone replacement is contraindicated in men with known breast or prostate malignancies; and prostate-specific antigen (PSA) levels should be measured in older patients before and at least 3 months after testosterone treatment.[65]

Sexual dysfunction is prevalent among men with HIV infection, particularly in the setting of advanced HIV disease.[66] However, not all HIV-infected men are hypogonadal, because diminished libido and erectile dysfunction may be related to a variety of other factors, such as neurologic disease, systemic illness, medication effects, fatigue, and psychosexual issues.[66–69] Furthermore, there have been preliminary case reports of sexual dysfunction in the setting of PI treatment.[70,71] In many cases, sildenafil citrate (Viagra) has been used successfully to improve erectile function. Nevertheless, clinicians should be aware that sildenafil is metabolized by cytochrome P_{450} 3A4, the hepatic microsomal enzyme involved in the metabolism of various PIs (e.g., saquinavir, ritonavir, indinavir, nelfinavir). Co-administration of PIs with sildenafil have been shown to result in substantial elevation in the sildenafil concentration, particularly with indinavir and ritonavir, increasing the risk of sildenafil-related adverse events.[72,73] Thus only the lowest starting dose of sildenafil should be used and then with specific caution in patients receiving these PI concomitantly.[73]

Ovarian Pathology and Alterations in Ovarian Function

Because the ovaries have not been systematically examined during autopsy studies in women with AIDS, little is known regarding ovarian pathology in the setting of HIV infection. Thus far there has been one reported case of cytomegalovirus (CMV) oophoritis in a woman with disseminated CMV infection.[74]

Changes in menstrual function among women with HIV infection have been more carefully evaluated since the early 1990s. It has been suggested that rates of menstrual disturbances are increased in HIV-infected women without AIDS-defining illnesses,[75] although other studies indicate that infection with HIV and related immunosuppression do not have clinically significant effects on either menstruation or vaginal bleeding.[76,77] Data from two large cohorts also demonstrated that HIV serostatus per se has little overall effect on menstrual cycle length, variability, and rates of amenorrhea; however, among HIV-infected women, low CD4+ T-lymphocyte counts and high HIV viral loads were associated with polymenorrhea and increased cycle length.[78] The prevalence of amenorrhea is increased in women with AIDS wasting compared to women with AIDS who are weight-stable or manifest only mild weight loss,[79] findings that are not unexpected for women with a severe catabolic illness complicating their HIV infection. In addition, the use of narcotics, marijuana, and chronic alcohol consumption may similarly affect menstrual status and ovulation.[60] Among HIV-positive women who do report regular menstrual cycles, normal circulating levels of the ovarian hormones estradiol and progesterone have been observed during the follicular and luteal phases.[80]

During the era of highly active antiretroviral therapy (HAART), various body shape changes, including breast enlargement, abdominal obesity, and wasting of fat in the extremities and gluteal region, have been observed primarily but not exclusively in individuals receiving PI therapy.[81–83] These alterations in fat distribution have generally occurred in the absence of overt endocrine perturbations, except in one woman who also manifested hirsutism, polycystic ovaries, and an increased LH/FSH ratio, consistent with polycystic ovary syndrome.[84] A pilot study in nine women with HIV-associated fat redistribution found that circulating androgen levels were increased compared to those in HIV-infected women without fat redistribution and in seronegative controls.[85] These findings were accompanied by an increased LH/FSH ratio, higher fasting insulin levels, and dyslipidemia. However, most women with HIV-associated fat redistribution do not have typical features of androgen excess, and it remains to be established whether hyperandrogenism and other metabolic aspects of the polycystic ovary syndrome are prevalent among HIV-infected women with fat redistribution.

Treatment with ritonavir was associated with the development of hypermenorrhea and secondary anemia in at least four women.[86] In two of these women, the anemia was severe enough to require blood transfusion. There was no evidence of intermenstrual bleeding, and the pelvic examination was unremarkable. Although platelet counts were normal, one patient experienced hemoptysis, and the possibility of impaired hemostasis was raised. In a separate series of four patients, initiation of combination antiretroviral therapy that included either ritonavir, saquinavir, or indinavir (for HAART or post-HIV-exposure prophylaxis) was associated with the development of hyperprolactinemia and galactorrhea.[87] In three of these cases, use of concomitant medications known to increase serum prolactin levels was implicated, although symptom resolution was evident only after the PIs were discontinued. Whether these clinical findings are mediated directly by PIs or indirectly through the potentiation of other drug effects remains to be determined.

Diagnostic Approach and Therapy

The approach to treatment of ovarian failure in women with HIV infection should be the same as that for immunocompetent individuals. For peri- and postmenopausal women with symptoms of estrogen deficiency, hormone replacement therapy with estrogen (and a progestin in patients with an intact uterus) should be considered.[88] Estrogen replacement may also protect against the bone mineral loss associated with menopause. However, treatment with estrogen is contraindicated in patients with hormone-responsive tumors, such as breast and uterine malignancies. The degree of cardiovascular protection afforded by hormone replacement is somewhat controversial, based on data showing that there is no benefit of combined estrogen and progestin treatment in seronegative postmenopausal women with established coronary heart disease.[89]

Androgen replacement therapy and treatment with androgenic anabolic steroids have also been considered as a possible therapeutic strategy in HIV-infected women. Observations suggest that circulating total and free testosterone levels are lower in HIV-infected women (with and without HIV-associated weight loss) than in healthy seronegative controls.[90] Furthermore, preliminary studies indicate that low-dose twice-weekly transdermal administration of testosterone in these patients is generally well tolerated.[91,92] Among those with the AIDS wasting syndrome, physiologic testosterone therapy was associated with weight gain and improvement in quality-of-life parameters.[92] In a multicenter study among HIV-infected women with weight loss, administration of nandrolone decanoate also increased weight and lean body mass and appeared to have a tolerable safety profile.[93] For the postmenopausal woman, Estratest provides combined estrogen-androgen replacement; but the methyltestosterone component may contribute to hepatic dysfunction, and concomitant progestin treatment would still be necessary for women with an intact uterus to prevent endometrial hyperplasia.

▲ THYROID

Thyroid Pathology

Opportunistic infections of the thyroid occur infrequently in patients with AIDS. Reported pathogens include *Pneumocystis carinii*, CMV, *Cryptococcus neoformans*, *Aspergillus*, *Mycobacterium avium-intracellulare*, and *Mycobacterium tuberculosis*.[94–96] *P. carinii* thyroiditis has traditionally been the most common pathogen, occurring primarily among patients receiving aerosolized pentamidine for *P. carinii* pneumonia (PCP) prophylaxis.[94,97] Affected patients typically present with an enlarging neck mass (diffuse goiter or nodule) that is often tender on physical examination. Depending on the extent of follicular tissue destruction, *P. carinii* thyroiditis may be accompanied by hypothyroidism or transient hyperthyroidism.[97–99] Neoplastic infiltration of the thyroid seldom occurs in patients with AIDS. However, there have been a few isolated cases of Kaposi sarcoma involvement of the thyroid gland in patients with preexisting cutaneous manifestations, with clinical presentations ranging from asymptomatic thyroid nodules to diffuse glandular infiltration.[94,100,101] Presumably, thyroid lymphoma may also occur (as either primary or metastatic disease) based on observations in seronegative individuals, but to our knowledge only one case has been reported in the setting of HIV infection.[102]

Alterations in Thyroid Function

In the normal individual, thyrotropin-releasing hormone (TRH) from the hypothalamus stimulates the synthesis and release of thyroid-stimulating hormone (TSH) from the anterior pituitary gland. TSH, in turn, stimulates the secretion of thyroxine (T_4) and triiodothyronine (T_3) from the thyroid, which exert negative feedback at the level of both the pituitary and hypothalamus to maintain homeostasis. Although circulating T_4 concentrations are high relative to T_3, peripheral conversion to T_3 is required for activity. During the so-called sick euthyroid state, decreased conversion of T_4 to T_3 with enhanced deiodination of T_4 to reverse T_3 is seen, resulting in lower T_3 and increased reverse T_3 levels.[103,104] T_3 reduction is thought to be adaptive during illness, as the body attempts to conserve both protein stores and energy expenditure during a time of stress.[103] With severe nonthyroidal illness, both T_4 and T_3 levels may be low.[103,104] TSH levels may also fall, although they tend to increase above the normal range during the recovery phase of acute illness.

Abnormal thyroid homeostasis occurs frequently in patients with AIDS, usually in the absence of direct thyroid pathology. In general, findings similar to those in the sick euthyroid state are observed,[105] although T_3 levels are often higher and reverse T_3 levels lower than expected for chronic illness.[106] Because similar changes in free (unbound) T_3 levels are also seen, these findings cannot be attributed to the increased thyroid hormone-binding globulin levels observed with HIV infection.[107,108] This has led to the concern that inappropriate maintenance of T_3 levels may contribute to weight loss and body wasting.[106] However, most patients with AIDS do develop lower T_3 levels during secondary infection, anorexia, and weight loss.[106,107] Mild TSH elevations within the normal range have also been reported, with lower free T_4 levels and enhanced TSH responsiveness to TRH; these hypothyroid-like findings may be adaptive to the hypermetabolic changes associated with HIV infection.[109]

Effect of Drugs on Thyroid Function

Thyroid function may also be affected by medications used to treat HIV and associated opportunistic infections (Table 63–1). Both rifampin and ketoconazole increase the metabolic clearance of thyroid hormone through induction of

▲ Table 63–1. THERAPEUTIC AGENTS USED TO TREAT HIV-RELATED DISEASE AND THEIR EFFECTS ON ADRENAL, GONADAL, AND THYROID FUNCTION

Therapeutic Agent	Adrenal, Gonadal, and Thyroid Effects
Ketoconazole	Inhibits adrenal and gonadal steroid synthesis Adrenal insufficiency Hypogonadism Increases levothyroxine metabolism
Rifampin	Increases cortisol metabolism Increases levothyroxine metabolism
Megestrol acetate	Cushing syndrome Adrenal insufficiency (following withdrawal) Hypogonadism
Opiates	Hypogonadism
Marijuana	Hypogonadism
Androgenic steroids	Suppresses endogenous testicular function
Interferon-α	Autoimmune hyperthyroidism (Graves' disease) Autoimmune hypothyroidism (Hashimoto's thyroiditis) Subacute or destructive thyroiditis
Protease inhibitors (PI)	Immune restoration may unmask latent Graves' disease or other autoimmune thyroid disorders Ritonavir may increase levothyroxine metabolism Case reports / ? association with PI Sexual dysfunction Hypermenorrhea Hyperprolactinemia and galactorrhea

hepatic microsomal enzymes and can precipitate hypothyroidism in patients with diminished thyroid reserve.[94] Thus higher doses of thyroxine may be required in patients receiving replacement therapy.[110] Increased maintenance levothyroxine has also been reported in a hypothyroid patient treated with ritonavir, a known inducer of hepatic glucuronosyl transferase activity, presumably due to increased metabolism of levothyroxine through the glucuronidation pathway.[111]

Among patients with hepatitis C infection, treatment with interferon-α (INFα), a cytokine with antiviral and immunomodulatory properties, has been associated with the development of thyroid dysfunction. Initial presentations have ranged from thyrotoxicosis (Grave's disease) to frank hypothyroidism (Hashimoto's thyroiditis) due to autoimmune thyroid disease,[112–114] as well as subacute or destructive thyroiditis.[115–118] Individuals with evidence of preexisting thyroid autoantibodies appear to be at higher risk for INFα-induced autoimmune thyroid disease.[119–121] Other risk factors include the presence of specific human leukocyte antigen (HLA) subtypes, female gender, and the development of thyroid autoantibodies during the course of INFα treatment.[112,113,121,122] Thus it has been suggested that thyroid function and thyroid autoantibodies (e.g., thyroid peroxidase antibody) be monitored before, during, and up to 6 months after INFα treatment.[112,119] In the majority of cases thyroid function normalizes after discontinuation of INFα, although sustained thyroid disease has been observed and longer-term follow-up may be necessary.[112,114,119] For instance, the coexistence of anti-thyroglobulin and thyroid peroxidase autoantibodies at the end of treatment has been shown to be predictive for subsequent thyroid dysfunction, even years after INFα has been discontinued.[123]

During the era of HAART, several patients have presented with activation of Graves' disease in the setting of immune restoration, typically 1 to 2 years after initiation of potent antiretroviral therapy.[124,125] Based on the timing of thyroid autoantibody appearance and the rise in CD4+ T-lymphocyte count from nadir levels (compatible with thymic production of naive CD4+ T-lymphocytes), it has been hypothesized that thyroid-specific autoimmunity results from abnormal reconstitution of a markedly altered T-lymphocyte repertoire[125]; thus disease manifestation is usually delayed after initiation of HAART. This phenomenon might also lead to the development of Hashimoto's thyroiditis subsequent to HAART initiation. There has been one preliminary report suggesting that the prevalence of subclinical hypothyroidism is increased among patients receiving HAART owing to possible effects on thyroid hormone metabolism.[126]

Diagnostic Approach and Therapy

Overall, patients with AIDS demonstrate subtle alterations in thyroid function which, in many ways, parallel the changes seen with the euthyroid sick syndrome. The significance of these findings is unclear, however, and thyroid function studies should be interpreted in their clinical context. In general, measurement of serum TSH provides the most sensitive indicator of overt thyroid dysfunction, and free T_4 levels provide a more quantitative measure of hormone deficiency or excess. Symptoms and signs of hypothyroidism include cold intolerance, weight gain, fatigue, constipation, muscle cramps, dry skin, and myxedema. Often a goiter is present on physical examination, and thyroid indices are notable for increased TSH levels and subnormal free T_4 levels. Replacement therapy should be approached gradually to avoid exacerbation of AIDS-related cachexia in select patients,[94] and lower doses of levothyroxine (25 to 50 μg/day) are advised initially with dose titration every 4 to 6 weeks to achieve normal TSH levels.

Patients with hyperthyroidism typically present with symptoms of heat intolerance, irritability, fatigue, weight loss, sweats, palpitations, and an increased frequency of bowel movements. The diagnosis is confirmed by documentation of a suppressed TSH level in the setting of elevated thyroid hormone levels. A radioactive iodine uptake scan is generally required to distinguish among the common causes of hyperthyroidism, such as Graves' disease, toxic nodule(s), and subacute thyroiditis. The clinical management for each of these processes in patients with AIDS is similar to that for immunocompetent individuals. β-Adrenergic antagonists are prescribed initially to decrease symptoms related to tachycardia and, in the case of propanolol, decrease peripheral conversion of T_4 to T_3. Recommended therapeutic options for Graves' disease include antithyroid drugs (methimazole, propylthiouracil), thyroid ablation with radioactive iodine therapy, and rarely thyroid surgery. Patients with toxic nodules should receive radioactive iodine therapy, as the antithyroid drugs are used only as a temporizing measure. Patients with subacute thyroiditis typically present with hyperthyroid symptoms, a tender enlarged thyroid gland, elevated erythrocyte sedimentation rate, and reduced radioactive iodine uptake. These individuals should be treated with supportive care alone, as spontaneous resolution is generally the rule. However, a tender thyroid gland in a patient with advanced HIV disease should also prompt further investigation for an opportunistic infection of the thyroid.

As with immunocompetent individuals, solitary thyroid masses or nodules require evaluation by fine-needle aspiration biopsy to exclude the possibility of malignant disease. In addition, opportunistic infections and malignancies involving the thyroid gland should be considered in the differential diagnosis of any patient with AIDS who has an abnormal thyroid examination. For patients with *Pneumocystis carinii* thyroiditis, the diagnosis is established by Gomori methenamine silver staining of the fine-needle aspirate, which should be specifically requested in suspected cases.[97,99,127] Kaposi sarcoma of the thyroid is also diagnosed by fine-needle aspiration biopsy and should be considered in patients with preexisting cutaneous lesions or disseminated disease.

▲ CONCLUSIONS

A wide spectrum of adrenal, gonadal, and thyroid disorders are associated with HIV infection and AIDS. Although these disorders may reflect cytopathic changes induced by

HIV itself, they are more often a consequence of opportunistic infections, medications to prevent or treat these infections, malignancy, or therapies directed at slowing HIV-related disease progression. Every component of the endocrine system is susceptible, ranging from subtle biochemical aberrations to clinically manifest disease. A clearer understanding of these disorders is crucial to the appropriate diagnostic and therapeutic management of these patients. Clinicians caring for HIV patients should maintain a high suspicion for endocrine dysfunction; however, this vigilance should be balanced by the recognition that many subtle abnormalities do not require aggressive therapy.

Acknowledgments. This work was supported in part by grants from the National Institute of Diabetes and Digestive and Kidney Diseases (DK45833) and the National Center for Research Resources (RR00083) of the National Institutes of Health. Dr. Lo is a recipient of a Clinical Associate Physician Award from the National Center for Research Resources.

REFERENCES

1. Bricaire F, Marche C, Zoubi D, et al. Adrenocortical lesions and AIDS. Lancet 1:881, 1988.
2. Welch K, Finkbeiner W, Alpers CE, et al. Autopsy findings in the acquired immune deficiency syndrome. JAMA 252:1152, 1984.
3. Barker NW. The pathologic anatomy in twenty-eight cases of Addison's disease. Arch Pathol 8:432, 1929.
4. Sellmeyer DE, Grunfeld C. Endocrine and metabolic disturbances in human immunodeficiency virus infection and the acquired immune deficiency syndrome. Endocr Rev 17:518, 1996.
5. Glasgow BJ, Steinsapir KD, Anders K, et al. Adrenal pathology in the acquired immune deficiency syndrome. Am J Clin Pathol 84:594, 1985.
6. Reichert CM, O'Leary TJ, Levens DL, et al. Autopsy pathology in the acquired immune deficiency syndrome. Am J Pathol 112:357, 1983.
7. Dobs AS, Dempsey MA, Ladenson PW, et al. Endocrine disorders in men infected with human immunodeficiency virus. Am J Med 84:611, 1988.
8. Ferrozzi F, Bova D, Campodonico F, et al. Adrenal carcinomas in AIDS: report of three cases. Clin Imaging 21:375, 1997.
9. Villette JM, Bourin P, Doinel C, et al. Circadian variations in plasma levels of hypophyseal, adrenocortical and testicular hormones in men infected with human immunodeficiency virus. J Clin Endocrinol Metab 70:572, 1990.
10. Membreno L, Irony I, Dere W, et al. Adrenocortical function in acquired immunodeficiency syndrome. J Clin Endocrinol Metab 65:482, 1987.
11. Parker LN, Levin ER, Lifrak ET. Evidence for adrenocortical adaptation to severe illness. J Clin Endocrinol Metab 60:947, 1985.
12. Verges B, Chavanet P, Desgres J, et al. Adrenal function in HIV infected patients. Acta Endocrinol (Copenh) 121:633, 1989.
13. Lortholary O, Christeff N, Casassus P, et al. Hypothalamo-pituitary-adrenal function in human immunodeficiency virus-infected men. J Clin Endocrinol Metab 81:791, 1996.
14. Findling JW, Buggy BP, Gilson IH, et al. Longitudinal evaluation of adrenocortical function in patients infected with the human immunodeficiency virus. J Clin Endocrinol Metab 79:1091, 1994.
15. Norbiato G, Bevilacqua M, Vago T, et al. Cortisol resistance in acquired immunodeficiency syndrome. J Clin Endocrinol Metab 74:608, 1992.
16. Lo JC, Mulligan K, Tai VW, et al. "Buffalo hump" in men with HIV-1 infection. Lancet 351:867, 1998.
17. Miller KK, Daly PA, Sentochnik D, et al. Pseudo-Cushing's syndrome in human immunodeficiency virus-infected patients. Clin Infect Dis 27:68, 1998.
18. Yanovski JA, Miller KD, Kino T, et al. Endocrine and metabolic evaluation of human immunodeficiency virus-infected patients with evidence of protease inhibitor-associated lipodystrophy. J Clin Endocrinol Metab 84:1925, 1999.
19. Christeff N, Melchior JC, de Truchis P, et al. Lipodystrophy defined by a clinical score in HIV-infected men on highly active antiretroviral therapy: correlation between dyslipidaemia and steroid hormone alterations. AIDS 13:2251, 1999.
20. Chen F, Kearney T, Robinson S, et al. Cushing's syndrome and severe adrenal suppression in patients treated with ritonavir and inhaled nasal fluticasone. Sex Transm Infect 75:274, 1999.
21. Sonino N. The use of ketoconazole as an inhibitor of steroid production. N Engl J Med 317:812, 1987.
22. Kyriazopoulou V, Parparousi O, Vagenakis AG. Rifampicin-induced adrenal crisis in addisonian patients receiving corticosteroid replacement therapy. J Clin Endocrinol Metab 59:1204, 1984.
23. Leinung MC, Liporace R, Miller CH. Induction of adrenal suppression by megestrol acetate in patients with AIDS. Ann Intern Med 122:843, 1995.
24. Mann M, Koller E, Murgo A, et al. Glucocorticoidlike activity of megestrol: a summary of Food and Drug Administration experience and a review of the literature. Arch Intern Med 157:1651, 1997.
25. Schambelan M, Zackin R, Mulligan K, et al. Effect of testosterone on the response to megesterol acetate in patients with HIV-associated wasting: a randomized, double-blind placebo-controlled trial; ACTG 313 Study Team. In: Program and Abstracts of the 8th Conference on Retroviruses and Opportunistic Infections, Chicago, 2001, abstract 640.
26. Henry K, Rathgaber S, Sullivan C, et al. Diabetes mellitus induced by megestrol acetate in a patient with AIDS and cachexia. Ann Intern Med 116:53, 1992.
27. Steer KA, Kurtz AB, Honour JW. Megestrol-induced Cushing's syndrome. Clin Endocrinol (Oxf) 42:91, 1995.
28. Padmanabhan S, Rosenberg AS. Cushing's syndrome induced by megestrol acetate in a patient with AIDS. Clin Infect Dis 27:217, 1998.
29. Velazquez H, Perazella MA, Wright FS, et al. Renal mechanism of trimethoprim-induced hyperkalemia. Ann Intern Med 119:296, 1993.
30. Grinspoon SK, Biller BM. Clinical review 62: laboratory assessment of adrenal insufficiency. J Clin Endocrinol Metab 79:923, 1994.
31. Freda PU, Wardlaw SL, Brudney K, et al. Primary adrenal insufficiency in patients with the acquired immunodeficiency syndrome: a report of five cases. J Clin Endocrinol Metab 79:1540, 1994.
32. Stockheim JA, Daaboul JJ, Yogev R, et al. Adrenal suppression in children with the human immunodeficiency virus treated with megestrol acetate. J Pediatr 134:368, 1999.
33. Baulieu EE. Dehydroepiandrosterone (DHEA): a fountain of youth? J Clin Endocrinol Metab 81:3147, 1996.
34. Orentreich N, Brind JL, Vogelman JH, et al. Long-term longitudinal measurements of plasma dehydroepiandrosterone sulfate in normal men. J Clin Endocrinol Metab 75:1002, 1992.
35. Centurelli MA, Abate MA. The role of dehydroepiandrosterone in AIDS. Ann Pharmacother 31:639, 1997.
36. Clerici M, Bevilacqua M, Vago T, et al. An immunoendocrinological hypothesis of HIV infection. Lancet 343:1552, 1994.
37. Clerici M, Galli M, Bosis S, et al. Immunoendocrinologic abnormalities in human immunodeficiency virus infection. Ann NY Acad Sci 917:956, 2000.
38. Jacobson MA, Fusaro RE, Galmarini M, et al. Decreased serum dehydroepiandrosterone is associated with an increased progression of human immunodeficiency virus infection in men with CD4 cell counts of 200–499. J Infect Dis 164:864, 1991.
39. Laudat A, Blum L, Guechot J, et al. Changes in systemic gonadal and adrenal steroids in asymptomatic human immunodeficiency virus-infected men: relationship with the CD4 cell counts. Eur J Endocrinol 133:418, 1995.
40. Mulder JW, Frissen PH, Krijnen P, et al. Dehydroepiandrosterone as predictor for progression to AIDS in asymptomatic human immunodeficiency virus-infected men. J Infect Dis 165:413, 1992.
41. Henderson E, Yang JY, Schwartz A. Dehydroepiandrosterone (DHEA) and synthetic DHEA analogs are modest inhibitors of HIV-1 IIIB replication. AIDS Res Hum Retroviruses 8:625, 1992.
42. Yang JY, Schwartz A, Henderson EE. Inhibition of HIV-1 latency reactivation by dehydroepiandrosterone (DHEA) and an analog of DHEA. AIDS Res Hum Retroviruses 9:747, 1993.

43. Yang JY, Schwartz A, Henderson EE. Inhibition of 3′azido-3′deoxythymidine-resistant HIV-1 infection by dehydroepiandrosterone in vitro. Biochem Biophys Res Commun 201:1424, 1994.
44. Chabon AB, Stenger RJ, Grabstald H. Histopathology of testis in acquired immune deficiency syndrome. Urology 29:658, 1987.
45. De Paepe ME, Waxman M. Testicular atrophy in AIDS: a study of 57 autopsy cases. Hum Pathol 20:210, 1989.
46. Shevchuk MM, Nuovo GJ, Khalife G. HIV in testis: quantitative histology and HIV localization in germ cells. J Reprod Immunol 41:69, 1998.
47. Shevchuk MM, Pigato JB, Khalife G, et al. Changing testicular histology in AIDS: its implication for sexual transmission of HIV. Urology 53:203, 1999.
48. Krieger JN, Coombs RW, Collier AC, et al. Fertility parameters in men infected with human immunodeficiency virus. J Infect Dis 164:464, 1991.
49. Politch JA, Mayer KH, Abbott AF, et al. The effects of disease progression and zidovudine therapy on semen quality in human immunodeficiency virus type 1 seropositive men. Fertil Steril 61:922, 1994.
50. Crittenden JA, Handelsman DJ, Stewart GJ. Semen analysis in human immunodeficiency virus infection. Fertil Steril 57:1294, 1992.
51. Christeff N, Gharakhanian S, Thobie N, et al. Evidence for changes in adrenal and testicular steroids during HIV infection. J Acquir Immune Defic Syndr 5:841, 1992.
52. Merenich JA, McDermott MT, Asp AA, et al. Evidence of endocrine involvement early in the course of human immunodeficiency virus infection. J Clin Endocrinol Metab 70:566, 1990.
53. Poretsky L, Can S, Zumoff B. Testicular dysfunction in human immunodeficiency virus-infected men. Metabolism 44:946, 1995.
54. Martin ME, Benassayag C, Amiel C, et al. Alterations in the concentrations and binding properties of sex steroid binding protein and corticosteroid-binding globulin in HIV+ patients. J Endocrinol Invest 15:597, 1992.
55. Grinspoon S, Corcoran C, Lee K, et al. Loss of lean body and muscle mass correlates with androgen levels in hypogonadal men with acquired immunodeficiency syndrome and wasting. J Clin Endocrinol Metab 81:4051, 1996.
56. Croxson TS, Chapman WE, Miller LK, et al. Changes in the hypothalamic-pituitary-gonadal axis in human immunodeficiency virus-infected homosexual men. J Clin Endocrinol Metab 68:317, 1989.
57. Dobs AS, Few WL III, Blackman MR, et al. Serum hormones in men with human immunodeficiency virus-associated wasting. J Clin Endocrinol Metab 81:4108, 1996.
58. Engelson ES, Pi-Sunyer FX, Kotler DP. Effects of megestrol acetate therapy on body composition and circulating testosterone concentrations in patients with AIDS [letter]. AIDS 9:1107, 1995.
59. Wagner GJ, Rabkin JG. Testosterone, illness progression, and megestrol use in HIV-positive men [letter]. J Acquir Immune Defic Syndr Hum Retrovirol 17:179, 1998.
60. Smith CG, Asch RH. Drug abuse and reproduction. Fertil Steril 48:355, 1987.
61. Milligan SA, Katz MS, Craven PC, et al. Toxoplasmosis presenting as panhypopituitarism in a patient with the acquired immune deficiency syndrome. Am J Med 77:760, 1984.
62. Sullivan WM, Kelley GG, O'Connor PG, et al. Hypopituitarism associated with a hypothalamic CMV infection in a patient with AIDS [letter]. Am J Med 92:221, 1992.
63. Androgel. Med Lett 42:49, 2000.
64. Wang C, Berman N, Longstreth JA, et al. Pharmacokinetics of transdermal testosterone gel in hypogonadal men: application of gel at one site versus four sites: a General Clinical Research Center study. J Clin Endocrinol Metab 85:964, 2000.
65. Cofrancesco J Jr., Whalen JJ III, Dobs AS. Testosterone replacement treatment options for HIV-infected men. J Acquir Immune Defic Syndr Hum Retrovirol 16:254, 1997.
66. Tindall B, Forde S, Goldstein D, et al. Sexual dysfunction in advanced HIV disease. AIDS Care 6:105, 1994.
67. Meyer-Bahlburg HF, Exner TM, Lorenz G, et al. Sexual risk behavior, sexual functioning, and HIV-disease progression in gay men. J Sex Res 28:3, 1991.
68. Jones M, Klimes I, Catalan J. Psychosexual problems in people with HIV infection: controlled study of gay men and men with haemophilia. AIDS Care 6:587, 1994.
69. Newshan G, Taylor B, Gold R. Sexual functioning in ambulatory men with HIV/AIDS. Int J STD AIDS 9:672, 1998.
70. Martinez E, Collazos J, Mayo J, et al. Sexual dysfunction with protease inhibitors [letter]. Lancet 353:810, 1999.
71. Colebunders R, Smets E, Verdonck K, et al. Sexual dysfunction with protease inhibitors [letter]. Lancet 353:1802, 1999.
72. Merry C, Barry MG, Ryan M, et al. Interaction of sildenafil and indinavir when co-administered to HIV-positive patients. AIDS 13:F101, 1999.
73. Viagra (Sildenafil citrate). Prescribing information. New York, Pfizer, 2002.
74. Familiari U, Larocca LM, Tamburrini E, et al. Premenopausal cytomegalovirus oophoritis in a patient with AIDS [letter]. AIDS 5:458, 1991.
75. Chirgwin KD, Feldman J, Muneyyirci-Delale O, et al. Menstrual function in human immunodeficiency virus-infected women without acquired immunodeficiency syndrome. J Acquir Immune Defic Syndr Hum Retrovirol 12:489, 1996.
76. Ellerbrock TV, Wright TC, Bush TJ, et al. Characteristics of menstruation in women infected with human immunodeficiency virus. Obstet Gynecol 87:1030, 1996.
77. Shah PN, Smith JR, Wells C, et al. Menstrual symptoms in women infected by the human immunodeficiency virus. Obstet Gynecol 83:397, 1994.
78. Harlow SD, Schuman P, Cohen M, et al. Effect of HIV infection on menstrual cycle length. J Acquir Immune Defic Syndr 24:68, 2000.
79. Grinspoon S, Corcoran C, Miller K, et al. Body composition and endocrine function in women with acquired immunodeficiency syndrome wasting. J Clin Endocrinol Metab 82:1332, 1997. Erratum. J Clin Endocrinol Metab 82:3360, 1997.
80. Cu-Uvin S, Wright DJ, Anderson D, et al. Hormonal levels among HIV-1-seropositive women compared with high-risk HIV-seronegative women during the menstrual cycle: Women's Health Study (WHS) 001 and WHS 001a Study Team. J Womens Health Gend Based Med 9:857, 2000.
81. Herry I, Bernard L, de Truchis P, et al. Hypertrophy of the breasts in a patient treated with indinavir. Clin Infect Dis 25:937, 1997.
82. Gervasoni C, Ridolfo AL, Trifiro G, et al. Redistribution of body fat in HIV-infected women undergoing combined antiretroviral therapy. AIDS 13:465, 1999.
83. Dong KL, Bausserman LL, Flynn MM, et al. Changes in body habitus and serum lipid abnormalities in HIV-positive women on highly active antiretroviral therapy (HAART). J Acquir Immune Defic Syndr 21:107, 1999.
84. Wilson JD, Dunham RJ, Balen AH. HIV protease inhibitors, the lipodystrophy syndrome and polycystic ovary syndrome—is there a link? Sex Transm Infect 75:268, 1999.
85. Hadigan C, Corcoran C, Piecuch S, et al. Hyperandrogenemia in human immunodeficiency virus-infected women with the lipodystrophy syndrome. J Clin Endocrinol Metab 85:3544, 2000.
86. Nielsen H. Hypermenorrhea associated with ritonavir [letter]. Lancet 353:811, 1999.
87. Hutchinson J, Murphy M, Harries R, et al. Galactorrhoea and hyperprolactinaemia associated with protease- inhibitors [letter]. Lancet 356:1003, 2000.
88. Clark RA, Cohn SE, Jarek C, et al. Perimenopausal symptomatology among HIV-infected women at least 40 years of age [letter]. J Acquir Immune Defic Syndr 23:99, 2000.
89. Hulley S, Grady D, Bush T, et al. Randomized trial of estrogen plus progestin for secondary prevention of coronary heart disease in postmenopausal women: Heart and Estrogen/Progestin Replacement Study (HERS) Research Group. JAMA 280:605, 1998.
90. Sinha-Hikim I, Arver S, Beall G, et al. The use of a sensitive equilibrium dialysis method for the measurement of free testosterone levels in healthy, cycling women and in human immunodeficiency virus-infected women. J Clin Endocrinol Metab 83:1312, 1998. Erratum. J Clin Endocrinol Metab 83: 2959, 1998.
91. Javanbakht M, Singh AB, Mazer NA, et al. Pharmacokinetics of a novel testosterone matrix transdermal system in healthy, premenopausal women and women infected with the human immunodeficiency virus. J Clin Endocrinol Metab 85:2395, 2000.
92. Miller K, Corcoran C, Armstrong C, et al. Transdermal testosterone administration in women with acquired immunodeficiency syndrome wasting: a pilot study. J Clin Endocrinol Metab 83:2717, 1998.

93. Mulligan K, Zackin R, Clark RA, et al. Nandrolone decanoate increases weight and lean body mass in HIV-infected women with weight loss: a double-blind, placebo-controlled, multicenter trial: ACTG 329 Study Team. In: Program and Abstracts of the 8th Conference on Retroviruses and Opportunistic Infections, Chicago, 2001, abstract 641.
94. Heufelder AE, Hofbauer LC. Human immunodeficiency virus infection and the thyroid gland. Eur J Endocrinol 134:669, 1996.
95. Frank TS, LiVolsi VA, Connor AM. Cytomegalovirus infection of the thyroid in immunocompromised adults. Yale J Biol Med 60:1, 1987.
96. Kaw YT, Brunnemer C. Initial diagnosis of disseminated cryptococcosis and acquired immunodeficiency syndrome by fine needle aspiration of the thyroid: a case report. Acta Cytol 38:427, 1994.
97. Guttler R, Singer PA, Axline SG, et al. *Pneumocystis carinii* thyroiditis: report of three cases and review of the literature. Arch Intern Med 153:393, 1993.
98. Drucker DJ, Bailey D, Rotstein L. Thyroiditis as the presenting manifestation of disseminated extrapulmonary *Pneumocystis carinii* infection. J Clin Endocrinol Metab 71:1663, 1990.
99. Battan R, Mariuz P, Raviglione MC, et al. *Pneumocystis carinii* infection of the thyroid in a hypothyroid patient with AIDS: diagnosis by fine needle aspiration biopsy. J Clin Endocrinol Metab 72:724, 1991.
100. Krauth PH, Katz JF. Kaposi's sarcoma involving the thyroid in a patient with AIDS. Clin Nucl Med 12:848, 1987.
101. Mollison LC, Mijch A, McBride G, et al. Hypothyroidism due to destruction of the thyroid by Kaposi's sarcoma. Rev Infect Dis 13:826, 1991.
102. Samuels MH, Launder T. Hyperthyroidism due to lymphoma involving the thyroid gland in a patient with acquired immunodeficiency syndrome: case report and review of the literature. Thyroid 8:673, 1998.
103. Wartofsky L, Burman KD. Alterations in thyroid function in patients with systemic illness: the "euthyroid sick syndrome." Endocr Rev 3:164, 1982.
104. Cavalieri RR. The effects of nonthyroid disease and drugs on thyroid function tests. Med Clin North Am 75:27, 1991.
105. Raffi F, Brisseau JM, Planchon B, et al. Endocrine function in 98 HIV-infected patients: a prospective study. AIDS 5:729, 1991.
106. LoPresti JS, Fried JC, Spencer CA, et al. Unique alterations of thyroid hormone indices in the acquired immunodeficiency syndrome (AIDS). Ann Intern Med 110:970, 1989.
107. Grunfeld C, Pang M, Doerrler W, et al. Indices of thyroid function and weight loss in human immunodeficiency virus infection and the acquired immunodeficiency syndrome. Metabolism 42:1270, 1993.
108. Lambert M, Zech F, De Nayer P, et al. Elevation of serum thyroxine-binding globulin (but not of cortisol-binding globulin and sex hormone-binding globulin) associated with the progression of human immunodeficiency virus infection. Am J Med 89:748, 1990.
109. Hommes MJ, Romijn JA, Endert E, et al. Hypothyroid-like regulation of the pituitary-thyroid axis in stable human immunodeficiency virus infection. Metabolism 42:556, 1993.
110. Isley WL. Effect of rifampin therapy on thyroid function tests in a hypothyroid patient on replacement L-thyroxine. Ann Intern Med 107:517, 1987.
111. Tseng A, Fletcher D. Interaction between ritonavir and levothyroxine. AIDS 12:2235, 1998.
112. Koh LK, Greenspan FS, Yeo PP. Interferon-alpha induced thyroid dysfunction: three clinical presentations and a review of the literature. Thyroid 7:891, 1997.
113. Kakizaki S, Takagi H, Murakami M, et al. HLA antigens in patients with interferon-alpha-induced autoimmune thyroid disorders in chronic hepatitis C. J Hepatol 30:794, 1999.
114. Custro N, Montalto G, Scafidi V, et al. Prospective study on thyroid autoimmunity and dysfunction related to chronic hepatitis C and interferon therapy. J Endocrinol Invest 20:374, 1997.
115. Falaschi P, Martocchia A, D'Urso R, et al. Subacute thyroiditis during interferon-alpha therapy for chronic hepatitis C. J Endocrinol Invest 20:24, 1997.
116. Parana R, Cruz M, Lyra L, et al. Subacute thyroiditis during treatment with combination therapy (interferon plus ribavirin) for hepatitis C virus. J Viral Hepat 7:393, 2000.
117. Amenomori M, Mori T, Fukuda Y, et al. Incidence and characteristics of thyroid dysfunction following interferon therapy in patients with chronic hepatitis C. Intern Med 37:246, 1998.
118. Roti E, Minelli R, Giuberti T, et al. Multiple changes in thyroid function in patients with chronic active HCV hepatitis treated with recombinant interferon-alpha. Am J Med 101:482, 1996.
119. Fernandez-Soto L, Gonzalez A, Escobar-Jimenez F, et al. Increased risk of autoimmune thyroid disease in hepatitis C vs hepatitis B before, during, and after discontinuing interferon therapy. Arch Intern Med 158:1445, 1998.
120. Bell TM, Bansal AS, Shorthouse C, et al. Low-titre auto-antibodies predict autoimmune disease during interferon-alpha treatment of chronic hepatitis C. J Gastroenterol Hepatol 14:419, 1999.
121. Betterle C, Fabris P, Zanchetta R, et al. Autoimmunity against pancreatic islets and other tissues before and after interferon-alpha therapy in patients with hepatitis C virus chronic infection. Diabetes Care 23:1177, 2000.
122. Hsieh MC, Yu ML, Chuang WL, et al. Virologic factors related to interferon-alpha-induced thyroid dysfunction in patients with chronic hepatitis C. Eur J Endocrinol 142:431, 2000.
123. Carella C, Mazziotti G, Morisco F, et al. Long-term outcome of interferon-alpha-induced thyroid autoimmunity and prognostic influence of thyroid autoantibody pattern at the end of treatment. J Clin Endocrinol Metab 86:1925, 2001.
124. Gilquin J, Viard JP, Jubault V, et al. Delayed occurrence of Graves' disease after immune restoration with HAART. Lancet 352:1907, 1998.
125. Jubault V, Penfornis A, Schillo F, et al. Sequential occurrence of thyroid autoantibodies and Graves' disease after immune restoration in severely immunocompromised human immunodeficiency virus-1-infected patients. J Clin Endocrinol Metab 85:4254, 2000.
126. Grappin M, Piroth L, Verges B, et al. Increased prevalence of subclinical hypothyroidism in HIV patients treated with highly active antiretroviral therapy. AIDS 14:1070, 2000.
127. Walts AE, Pitchon HE. *Pneumocystis carinii* in FNA of the thyroid. Diagn Cytopathol 7:615, 1991.

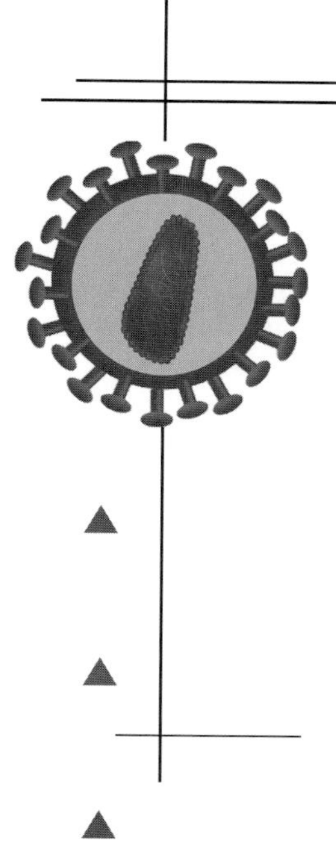

CHAPTER 64

Diseases of the Esophagus, Stomach, and Bowel

Klaus E. Mönkemüller, MD
C. Mel Wilcox, MD

Diseases of the gastrointestinal tract are among the most frequent complications of the acquired immunodeficiency syndrome (AIDS). Since the early 1990s more experience with gastrointestinal disorders in these patients has resulted in a better appreciation of the spectrum of potential etiologies, approach to evaluation and therapy, and indications for prophylaxis. Although our therapeutic armamentarium has been expanding to treat these problems, truly effective therapy for some opportunistic infections remains elusive. Fortunately, since the introduction of protease inhibitors and highly active antiretroviral therapy (HAART) during the mid-1990s there has been a constant decline of gastrointestinal opportunistic disorders in AIDS patients. The long-term prognosis for most gastrointestinal disorders is dictated primarily by the degree of underlying immunodeficiency.

▲ INFECTIONS OF THE ESOPHAGUS

Esophageal infections are common in patients with AIDS. At least one-third of these patients experience esophageal symptoms at some point during their illness. When evaluating a patient with esophageal complaints, a clear distinction must be established between dysphagia (sensation of food or pills "sticking" in the chest) and odynophagia (substernal pain after swallowing). Other esophageal signs and symptoms that can occur secondary to esophageal infections include esophagospasm (spontaneous substernal chest pain), singultus ("hiccups"), and hematemesis. In patients with esophageal infections the physical examination is relatively unrevealing, except for the presence of thrush, which suggests the presence of esophageal candidiasis. Oropharyngeal candidiasis is readily diagnosed by the characteristic multiple white-yellow plaques, which can be focal or completely coat the buccal mucosa. Occasionally, candidiasis manifests as mucosal erythema in the absence of recognizable plaques or angular cheilitis. It is important to differentiate oral hairy leukoplakia (nonremovable white plaques on the lateral aspect of the tongue) from thrush given the different etiologies and therapy.[1] The absence of thrush, however, does not exclude *Candida* esophagitis.[2] Another important fact is that the esophagus may be involved by multiple processes at the same time.[3,4] The main diagnostic tools employed to diagnose esophageal infections in HIV-infected patients are empiric therapy, barium esophagography, and endoscopy. The former is usually nonspecific and less sensitive. Upper endoscopy permits direct visualization of lesions and retrieval of tissue for analysis (Fig. 64–1).

Etiology

The most common infectious cause of esophagitis in patients with HIV infection is *Candida*. Although *Candida albicans* is by far the most common cause of candidiasis, several other non-*albicans* species, including *C. krusei*, *C. tropicalis*, *C. parapsilosis*, *C. glabrata*, and *C. dublinensis*, have been associated with oral and esophageal candidiasis in HIV-infected individuals,[5] particularly after prolonged antifungal drug therapy.[6,7] Heretofore, determining the specific *Candida* species was thought to be unnecessary. However, certain species are more often azole-resistant than others. The identification of *C. krusei*, for example, suggests that azole therapy is unlikely to be successful. In general, in vitro azole resistance in patients with AIDS corre-

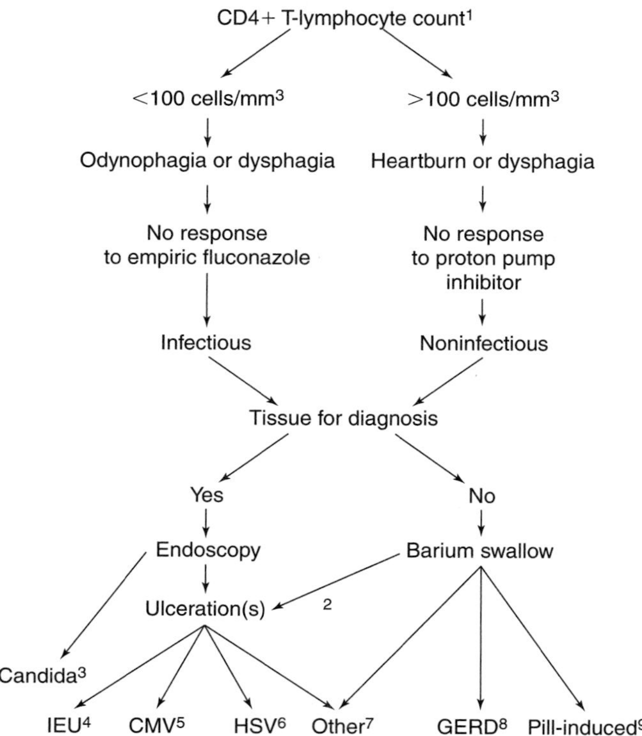

Figure 64–1. Suggested approach to esophageal symptoms in patients with AIDS. 1, CD4+ T-lymphocyte count is the major determining factor for the presence or absence of opportunistic infections. 2, Presence of ulcer on barium esophagogram requires endoscopy with biopsy. 3, *Candida albicans, C. krusei, C. tropicalis, C. parapsilosis, C. glabrata, C. guillermondi, C. dublinensis, C. inconspicua*. 4, Idiopatic esophageal ulcer. 5, Cytomegalovirus. 6, Herpes simplex virus (HSV) type 2. 7, Fungi: *Histoplasma capsulatum, Penicillium chrysogenum, Exophiala jeanselmani*. Viruses: Epstein-Barr virus, papovavirus, HSV-6. Bacteria: *Mycobacterium avium* complex, *M. tuberculosis, Rochalimae henselae, Nocardia asteroides, Actinomyces israelii*. Protozoa: *Pneumocystis carinii, Leishmania donovani*. 8, Gastroesophageal reflux disease. 9, Zalcitabine, zidovudine.

lates with azole treatment failure for oropharyngeal candidiasis.[8,9] The major risk factor associated with the development of resistance was the prophylactic daily or intermittent use of fluconazole within the last 6 months.[9] However, refractory mucosal candidiasis is now less common during the era of HAART.

Cytomegalovirus (CMV) is one of the most common opportunistic infections in patients with AIDS and typically occurs when the CD4+ T-lymphocyte count is less than 100 cells per cubic millimeter. In such patients the incidence of disease may approach 21% at 2 years.[10] Although the retina is the most common target for CMV, CMV esophagitis and colitis remain significant causes of morbidity. Involvement of the stomach and small bowel is less common.[11]

Herpes simplex virus (HSV) causes enteral disease occasionally. Because HSV infects primarily squamous mucosa, oropharyngeal, esophageal, and perianal involvement are the most common sites of disease. Oropharyngeal disease may be isolated or can occur in association with esophageal disease. In a large prospective study of 100 HIV-infected patients with ulcerative esophagitis, HSV esophagitis was identified in only 5%, compared to 50% for CMV.[12] Like CMV, the incidence of HSV disease increases as immunodeficiency worsens, with the greatest frequency occurring when the CD4+ T-lymphocyte count is less than 100 cells per cubic millimeter.[13]

An important cause of esophageal pain not clearly linked to a specific infection is HIV-associated idiopathic esophageal ulceration (IEU). These lesions can present at the time of seroconversion, although they typically occur when immunodeficiency is severe. The median CD4+ T-lymphocyte count in these patients is less than 50 cells per cubic millimeter. Several studies have identified HIV-infected inflammatory cells in the ulcer base of these lesions, suggesting an etiologic role for HIV.[14] However, HIV has not been identified in esophageal squamous mucosa but, rather, in inflammatory cells and has been found in HIV-infected patients with esophageal diseases other than IEU.[15] IEUs are almost as common as CMV esophagitis in patients with AIDS, comprising approximately 40% of esophageal ulcers in these patients.[12]

A variety of other infectious agents have been reported to involve the esophagus but are rare; the include protozoa (*Cryptosporidium, Pneumocystis carinii, Leishmania donovani, Trichomonas vaginalis*), bacteria (*Nocardia, Actinomyces*), mycobacteria (*Mycobacterium avium* complex, *M. tuberculosis*), fungi (*Histoplasma capsulatum, Penicillium chrysogenum, Exophiala jeanselmani*), and viruses (Epstein-Barr, human papillomavirus)[16] (Table 64–1). Esophagitis due to these entities is indistinguishable from that due to HSV or CMV.

Clinical Presentation

Esophageal candidiasis may be asymptomatic or may present as complete inability to swallow, with consequent dehydration, weight loss, and malnutrition. Dysphagia is the most frequent initial manifestation of esophageal candidiasis.[2] Less commonly, odynophagia, heartburn, or retrosternal pain is reported. The presence of fever, nausea, vomit-

▲ **Table 64–1.** ETIOLOGY OF ESOPHAGITIS IN AIDS PATIENTS

Fungi:	*Candida* species [*Penicillium chrysogenum, Pneumocystis carinii, Exophiala jeanselmani, Cryptococcus neoformans*, mucormycosis, *Aspergillus fumigatus*]
Viruses:	Cytomegalovirus (CMV), herpes simplex virus type II [Epstein-Barr virus, papovavirus, human herpesvirus (HHV-6)]
Idiopathic:	idiopathic esophageal ulcer
Pill-induced:	zalcitabine, zidovudine
Peptic:	gastroesophageal disease
Bacteria:	*Mycobacterium avium* complex [*Mycobacterium tuberculosis, Bartonella henselae, Nocardia asteroides, Actinomyces israelii*]
Protozoa:	[*Cryptosporidium parvum, Leishmania donovani, Trichomonas vaginalis*]
Tumors:	non-Hodgkin lymphoma, Kaposi sarcoma [squamous cell carcinoma, adenocarcinoma, lymphomatoid granulomatosis]

Rare entities are shown in brackets.

ing, and epigastric pain suggests another etiology. The only physical finding is oropharyngeal candidiasis (thrush).

Patients with CMV esophagitis usually present with odynophagia.[17] In contrast to *Candida* esophagitis, dysphagia is distinctly uncommon. Heartburn is uncommon; nausea, vomiting, and low grade fever may be reported. Concurrent oropharyngeal ulcerations are rare, whereas thrush is often present.

Esophagitis due to HSV presents similarly to CMV esophagitis. The most common manifestations of esophageal HSV are odynophagia and dysphagia (82%), chest pain (68%), and fever (44%).[18] Gastrointestinal bleeding is rare and is usually observed in patients with thrombocytopenia. Endoscopically, the presence of small vesicles is commonly seen in immunocompetent hosts, a finding unusual in human immunodeficiency virus (HIV)-infected patients. Ulcers of the oral mucosa, lips, and nares are often but not invariably present.

Patients with IEU present similarly to patients with ulcerative esophagitis from other causes. Severe odynophagia is almost uniformly present.

Diagnosis

Esophageal candidiasis is suspected clinically in the patient with moderately severe immunodeficiency (CD4+ T-lymphocyte count less than 100 cells per cubic millimeter) and esophageal symptoms, with or without thrush.[2] Thrush is absent in one-third of patients with esophageal candidiasis.[2] Barium esophagography is relatively insensitive and nonspecific for detecting mild esophagitis and should not be performed for diagnostic purposes. The most common radiographic finding of *Candida* esophagitis is diffuse mucosal irregularity resulting in a "shaggy" appearance mimicking diffuse ulceration. Endoscopy is the most sensitive diagnostic method. Multiple yellow-white plaques with the appearance of "cottage cheese" are pathognomonic for esophageal candidiasis. A definitive diagnosis rests on the identification of typical yeast forms in endoscopic mucosal biopsies, esophageal brushings, or balloon cytology. The detection of *Candida* by these methods does not exclude other disorders, as *Candida* may coexist with additional esophageal processes in up to 25% of symptomatic patients.[3,4] Cultures of the esophagus may provide specimens for drug susceptibility testing, but because *Candida* species can be cultured from patients without esophagitis such cultures are not as useful clinically.

On the barium esophagogram CMV may appear as one or multiple well circumscribed ulcers that may be shallow or deep. IEU is indistinguishable from CMV on barium swallow.[19] CMV results in large shallow or deep ulcerations that may be circumferential. The diagnosis of CMV disease is best established by identifying a viral cytopathic effect (intranuclear inclusions) in gastrointestinal mucosal biopsy specimens using routine hematoxylin and eosin (H & E) staining. The cytopathic effect of CMV is seen in endothelial cells and mesenchymal cells; thus it is imperative to obtain biopsy specimens from the ulcer base. Immunohistochemical stains of mucosal biopsies may be required to confirm the infection; viral culture of biopsy specimens is less sensitive and specific.[20] Blood cultures or serologic tests for CMV are not useful for diagnosing CMV gastrointestinal infection in HIV-infected patients.

A barium esophagram is seldom diagnostic of HSV esophagitis. On endoscopy, lesions involve the distal esophagus in 50% and the middle third in 12%, and they are diffuse in one-third of the cases.[18] The lesions appear as superficial ulcers in most patients, where they tend to be small and discrete; they can have a characteristic volcano shape. The presence of small vesicles, as seen in normal hosts, is uncommon in HIV-infected patients. Mucosal biopsy is the most specific diagnostic method. The H & E stain reveals characteristic inclusion bodies; cytology, culture, and in situ hybridization of biopsy material provide alternative information that can be helpful for establishing a diagnosis. Because HSV infects squamous epithelium, it is essential to biopsy the ulcer edge to identify the viral cytopathic effect.

Idiopathic esophageal ulceration appears endoscopically as one or multiple ulcers of variable depth with normal intervening mucosa. CMV esophagitis and IEU are indistinguishable clinically, radiographically, and endoscopically.[19] The diagnosis of IEU is one of exclusion; multiple biopsies (at least six) of the ulcer margins and ulcer base are necessary to exclude an infectious process.

Therapy

Given that esophageal candidiasis is the most common cause of esophageal infection in HIV-infected patients, it is common practice to administer an empirical trial of antifungal therapy in patients with esophageal complaints and thrush. A prospective study comparing empirical fluconazole to endoscopy for presumptive esophageal candidiasis in patients with AIDS showed that empirical fluconazole was a safe, cost-effective alternative to immediate endoscopy.[21] Fluconazole is administered with an oral or intravenous loading dose of 200 mg followed by 100 mg/day for 10 to 14 days. Failure to respond clinically in 3 to 7 days highlights the need for endoscopy to establish the correct etiology.

Although topical nystatin is effective for oropharyngeal candidiasis, clotrimazole troches have now largely replaced nystatin as the principal nonsystemic agent, given the ease of administration, palatability, negligible side effects, drug interactions, and effectiveness. Clinical cure is seen in 65% to 94% of patients following 14 days of clotrimazole therapy.[22,23] The use of systemic therapy with oral fluconazole for oropharyngeal candidiasis in HIV-infected patients achieves greater cure rates and lower relapse rates than clotrimazole troches[22,23] or nystatin.[24] Thus neither nystatin or clotrimazole is used by many clinicians. Single-dose therapy with fluconazole 150 mg is as efficacious as a 7-day treatment course for oral candidiasis.[25] Unlike oropharyngeal disease, nonsystemic therapy (e.g., nystatin) is largely ineffective for esophageal candidiasis.

Three systemic antifungal agents have been investigated and used extensively to treat esophageal candidiasis: ketoconazole, oral fluconazole, and itraconazole. At most centers fluconazole has become the drug of choice for esophageal candidiasis associated with AIDS. Randomized trials have shown fluconazole to have efficacy superior to that of ketoconazole for both oropharyngeal[26,27] and esophageal[28] candidiasis. The response rate of esophageal candidiasis to fluconazole tends to be rapid, with most patients experiencing significant clinical improvement within 5 days.[21,29] In a prospective randomized trial, Laine and colleagues[28] compared ketoconazole 200 mg/day to fluconazole 100 mg/day in 143 patients with AIDS and esophageal candidiasis. Endoscopic cure and symptom resolution were found in 91% and 85%, respectively, for fluconazole-treated patients compared with 52% and 65%, respectively, for ketoconazole-treated patients. Itraconazole capsules (200 mg/day) were found to be equivalent to ketoconazole 200 mg bid for oropharyngeal and esophageal candidiasis.[30] In the largest study reported to date, Barbaro et al.[31] randomized 2213 HIV-infected patients with a first episode of *Candida* esophagitis to either fluconazole or itraconazole. Clinical cure was achieved in 81% of fluconazole-treated patients compared to 75% of itraconazole-treated patients ($P < 0.001$), although there was no difference in clinical and endoscopic cure at the end of the follow-up period (1 year). Approximately 25% of patients in both groups required an increase in dosage at 2 weeks.

Monotherapy with flucytosine at 100 mg/kg/day PO appears to be inferior to fluconazole for the treatment of esophageal candidiasis.[32] Flucytosine is not recommended for therapy.

Oral suspensions of both fluconazole and itraconazole have been developed, and their efficacy appears similar to that of pills.[24,33] Results of comparative trials between fluconazole tablets and itraconazole suspension suggest equivalency in clinical response, mycologic eradication, and tolerability.[34]

Intravenous amphotericin B is highly effective against most *Candida* species. Because of its toxicity, this drug is used almost exclusively for candidiasis resistant to azole therapy. Lozenges containing amphotericin B and oral suspensions of amphotericin B have some efficacy and are available in Europe but not in the United States.[35] Low-dose amphotericin B (0.3 to 0.5 mg/kg/day for 7 to 14 days) is usually adequate therapy for oropharyngeal and esophageal candidiasis. Liposomal forms of amphotericin B are also effective and can be used if cost is not a factor and amphotericin B cannot be tolerated. Improved antiretroviral therapy, possibly by increasing the CD4+ T-lymphocyte count and thereby immune function, also leads to clearance of refractory thrush in some patients.

The incidence of azole-resistant mucosal candidiasis is increasing. Fichtenbaum et al.[9] conducted a study of the risk factors, natural history, and outcome of fluconazole-resistant mucosal candidiasis. The incidence of fluconazole-resistant mucosal candidiasis was 4.2 per 100 person-years. The researchers also found that the prognosis of these patients was worse than that of patients with nonresistant *Candida*.[9] The major risk factor associated with the development of resistance was the prophylactic daily or intermittent use of fluconazole within the last 6 months.[9] In patients with fluconazole-resistant mucocutaneous candidiasis, treatment options include itraconazole (oral suspension or intravenous[36] preparations), amphotericin, or caspofungin (see Chapter 37).

Despite the frequency of oropharyngeal and esophageal candidiasis in HIV-infected patients, primary prophylaxis is not recommended. Although fluconazole prophylaxis decreases the occurrence of disease,[37,38] it is not recommended because these disorders are not life-threatening, acute therapy of individual episodes is highly effective, and there is concern that widespread use of primary prophylaxis will exacerbate the problem of drug resistance and drug–drug interactions.[39] Therefore we do not recommend primary prophylaxis for oropharyngeal or esophageal candidiasis. Whereas primary prophylaxis for *Candida* is rarely provided, secondary prophylaxis can be given if patients have multiple and frequent recurrences of oropharyngeal or esophageal candidiasis. Oral fluconazole 50 to 100 mg/day or 150 mg once weekly is effective prophylaxis against recurrent oropharyngeal and esophageal candidiasis in patients with azole-sensitive disease.[40,41]

Treatment for gastrointestinal CMV disease is limited to intravenous therapy with ganciclovir, foscarnet, and more recently cidofovir. There are no specific studies using oral valganciclovir for enteric CMV disease. A number of open-label trials using intravenous ganciclovir in HIV-infected patients with gastrointestinal CMV disease have demonstrated clinical improvement in approximately 75% of patients.[42–44] Open-label trials of foscarnet have yielded comparable results.[45] The only placebo-controlled trial of ganciclovir, which evaluated colitis, found no clinically significant differences between the treatment groups probably because the treatment period was only 2 weeks.[46] The only randomized controlled study comparing ganciclovir to foscarnet for therapy of CMV esophagitis found no difference between the agents regarding clinical activity, but there was more toxicity with foscarnet.[47] Marked endoscopic improvement was observed in 73% of the foscarnet-treated patients and 70% of the ganciclovir-treated patients. The symptomatic response was also similar for the two treatments; 82% of patients who received foscarnet and 80% of those treated with ganciclovir had a complete or at least a good clinical response.[47] A randomized trial comparing ganciclovir to foscarnet in 48 AIDS patients with gastrointestinal CMV disease found similar clinical efficacy (73%) regardless of the location of the disease (esophagus versus colon), with endoscopic improvement documented in more than 80%.[48] The time to progression of disease was similar (13 to 16 weeks) despite the use of maintenance therapy. Side effects occurred in half the patients in both groups. Mönkemüller and Wilcox described one case of CMV esophagitis that resolved after initiation of HAART without specific anti-CMV therapy.[49] That report suggested that immune reconstitution secondary to HAART can be associated with clearance of an opportunistic gastrointestinal infection.

The decision to use either ganciclovir or foscarnet for gastrointestinal CMV disease in AIDS should be based on the experience of the physician and the differing toxicities of each agent. The efficacy, tolerability, and cost of ganciclovir have established it as first-line therapy for gastrointestinal CMV disease in the presence of AIDS. Our current policy for the therapy of gastrointestinal CMV disease is to administer intravenous ganciclovir, assuming there are no major contraindications to this agent such as neutropenia or thrombocytopenia. The usual induction dose is 10 to 15 mg/kg administered twice a day for 3 to 4 weeks. In our experience, esophageal disease tends to respond more rapidly than does colonic disease. The response to therapy is judged by alleviation of symptoms and improved endoscopic findings. Ophthalmologic examination is mandatory at the time of diagnosis in all patients to exclude retinal disease. If retinal disease is absent and a complete symptomatic and endoscopic response is documented following induction therapy, we stop therapy and observe for recurrent symptoms. For patients with persistently low CD4+ T-lymphocyte counts, the relapse rate for esophageal and colonic disease is similar (30% to 50%).[44,45,48] Endoscopic reexamination with biopsy of any mucosal abnormalities is important for patients with persistent symptoms following therapy. For those with frequent relapses of gastrointestinal disease, long-term once-daily maintenance intravenous administration is appropriate. Although there are no reported data regarding the efficacy of oral valganciclovir for either maintenance therapy or treatment of acute gastrointestinal disease, valganciclovir is likely to be effective in this setting and is a reasonable choice for treatment. Failure to respond to ganciclovir may be the result of low serum levels[50] or drug resistance.[51] As many as 32% of patients with gastrointestinal CMV disease do not have a favorable response to intravenous ganciclovir owing to toxicity or ineffectiveness.[51]

For patients with major contraindications or failure to respond to ganciclovir, foscarnet is usually effective.[45,46,52] The recommended dosing schedule is 90 mg/kg IV bid daily for 14 to 21 days. Salzberger et al.[53] demonstrated in an open label, randomized trial that a frequency reduction of fosarnet from 7 to 5 days a week for 3 weeks was associated with equal response and fewer side effects than using the medication daily for 21 days. Combination therapy of foscarnet (90 mg/kg bid daily) and ganciclovir (5 mg/kg bid daily)[54,55] may be as effective for ganciclovir failures.[56,57] A small study evaluated the safety of induction and maintenance therapy alternating ganciclovir (5 mg/kg every other day) and foscarnet (120 mg/kg every other day). There appears to be little benefit with their approach. The efficacy and incidence of side effects seemed to be equivalent to daily monotherapy or dual therapy.[54]

Randomized placebo-controlled studies of oral ganciclovir for primary prophylaxis have demonstrated a reduction in the incidence of retinal involvement.[58] No definitive data exist on the effectiveness of primary prophylaxis for decreasing gastrointestinal CMV disease in HIV-infected patients.[48]

For the patient with mild to moderate HSV esophagitis who is able to tolerate pills, oral administration of acyclovir 15 to 30 mg/kg/day is effective.[12,18] The drug is usually given in a dose of 400 mg PO five times a day for 2 weeks. Because absorption of oral acyclovir is inconsistent and may be as low as less than 30%,[59] valacyclovir 500 to 1000 mg bid PO has become the treatment of choice, especially for patients with more severe disease. Oral famciclovir is also highly effective against HSV. Intravenous administration of acyclovir should be applied when severe odynophagia limits oral intake or when the patient has not responded to high-dose oral therapy. Several studies have confirmed the safety and efficacy of intravenous foscarnet (40 mg/kg every 12 hours) for treating HSV disease and supported the utility of this agent as maintenance therapy for delaying recurrences.[60,61] Primary prophylaxis is not currently recommended; secondary prophylaxis with valacyclovir (500 to 1000 mg/day) is usually provided to patients with frequent relapses of oropharyngeal or esophageal disease.

Prospective studies of idiopathic esophageal ulcers have documented healing rates of more than 90% with oral corticosteroids.[62] The regimen most commonly employed is prednisone 40 mg/day tapering 10 mg/week for a 1-month treatment course.[62] Shorter courses of therapy may be effective for small ulcers. Although beneficial, intralesional injection of corticosteroids should be considered as second-line therapy.[14] The side effects of corticosteroids are well recognized; patients with AIDS may be more likely to develop CMV disease while on therapy.[63] Because oropharyngeal and esophageal candidiasis may complicate steroid use and confuse the therapeutic response, we routinely use short courses of azole therapy while the patients is receiving prednisone. The response to corticosteroids is rapid, with most patients experiencing significant pain relief within days.[62] Although not as well studied, thalidomide appears to be highly effective for IEU.[64,65] In doses of 200 to 300 mg/day, thalidomide has been documented to result in a clinical response and endoscopic cure in more than 90% of treated patients.[14,65] Thalidomide is well tolerated, with the main side effect being somnolence; administration of the drug at bedtime tends to overcome this problem. Peripheral neuropathy and skin rash are infrequent side effects. The major fear with thalidomide is inadvertent use during the first trimester of pregnancy, which consistently results in severe birth defects. Therefore most physicians do not prescribe this agent for women of childbearing age unless the patient is surgically sterile. The relapse rate of IEU is approximately 40% to 50% regardless of the initial therapy.[12,62]

▲ INFECTIONS OF THE STOMACH

Symptomatic and clinically significant opportunistic gastric infections are uncommon in patients with HIV infection. Although a number of opportunistic pathogens have been documented to infect the stomach in these patients, including cryptosporidia, *Toxoplasma gondii, Leishmania, Pneumocystis carinii, Treponema pallidium, Cryptococcus neoformans*, the most common opportunistic pathogen is CMV. All these infections may be asymptomatic or result in nausea and vomiting. Most present in the setting of disseminated disease and are associated with systemic symptoms (malaise, weakness, fever). Clues to the diagnosis may be found outside the gastrointestinal tract. Epigastric pain or gastrointestinal bleeding occur more frequently in the setting of ulcerative lesions such as peptic ulcer disease and CMV. The main diagnostic test for patients with these symptoms is upper endoscopy with biopsies.

Although earlier studies suggested that the prevalence of peptic ulcer disease and *Helicobacter pylori* infection were common in patients with HIV infection,[66] most studies performed since then have found that the prevalence of peptic ulcer disease and *H. pylori* is lower in HIV-infected patients.[67–70] Possible explanations for this phenomenon include hypochlorhydria, antibiotic use, and inadequate mucosal inflammatory response.[66–71] Varsky et al. studied 497 HIV-positive patients with upper digestive tract symptoms.[71] The investigators found that 5% of these patients had gastroduodenal ulcers (GDUs). *Helicobacter pylori* was detected in only 31% of patients with GDUs, whereas CMV was detected in 50% of these patients.[66] In HIV-infected patients with chronic active gastritis without a GDU, other organisms such as *Cryptosporidium* and CMV were more prevalent than *H. pylori.* Based on their findings it is recommended that endoscopic biopsies be performed to search of opportunistic pathogens in AIDS patients with upper digestive symptoms. Most studies from Europe, Australia, and the United States have found a low incidence of *H. pylori* in HV-infected patients.[66–69] In Italy, Cacciarelli et al. found that the prevalence of *H. pylori* in HIV-positive patients with a CD4+ T-lymphocyte count of less than 200 cells per cubic millimeter was significantly less than that of HIV-negative patients.[67] The authors also found that the number of peptic ulcers was significantly less in HIV-infected patients.[67] In New York, Marano et al. found *H. pylori* in only 15.9% of symptomatic HIV patients undergoing upper endoscopy, despite the presence of chronic active gastritis in 94.5% of them.[68] In Australia, Edwards et al. found that the prevalence of *H. pylori* was 3% in patients with AIDS, compared to 22% in non-HIV-infected patients.[69] Now that we are in the era of HAART, we must remember that improvement in the immune status of HIV-infected patients and "normalization" of their CD4+ T-lymphocyte counts may result in an incidence of peptic ulcer disease and *H. pylori* similar to that in nonimmunocompromised hosts. Mönkemüller et al. reported that the incidence of opportunistic gastrointestinal infections has declined, most likely secondary to the use of HAART.[70] During the same period they noted a rise in the number of nonopportunistic gastrointestinal disorders in these patients, including peptic ulcer disease.[70]

▲ ABDOMINAL PAIN

Abdominal pain is a common complaint among HIV-infected patients, with a reported incidence of 12%.[72] In the early stages of immunodeficiency, the causes of abdominal pain are similar to those of the nonimmunocompromised host. However as the immunodeficiency worsens, opportunistic pathogens (CMV, protozoa, mycobacteria, fungi, neoplasms) become a frequent cause of abdominal pain.

The diagnosis of abdominal pain can be a challenge given the broad spectrum of potential causes, including both opportunistic and nonopportunistic disorders.[72,73] In most cases a carefully performed history and physical examination in conjunction with the CD4+ T-lymphocyte count can help narrow the differential diagnosis. A thorough systematic evaluation is necessary to avoid overlooking potentially life-threatening conditions, such as hollow viscus perforation, appendicitis, intestinal obstruction, and toxic megacolon. It is also important to remember that multiple conditions associated with ongoing, chronic abdominal pain such as CMV enteritis and non-Hodgkin lymphoma (NHL) can suddenly result in an acute abdomen due to intestinal perforation and obstruction.[74,75] Treatment of abdominal pain is directed by the underlying etiology. A multidisciplinary comprehensive approach to pain management assists these individuals to achieve levels of comfort, function, and quality of life with this chronic and terminal illness.

Etiology

A cause of abdominal pain can be found in most HIV-infected patients, and treatment should be tailored accordingly. The most common causes of chronic abdominal pain in patients with advanced HIV disease (i.e., CD4+ T-lymphocyte count < 100 cells per microliter) are disseminated *Mycobacterium avium* complex (MAC), intestinal CMV disease, and neoplasms such as NHL and Kaposi sarcoma (KS) (Table 64–2).

Clinical Presentation

One of the largest studies evaluating the cause of abdominal pain in AIDS patients found that the predominant localization of abdominal pain had considerable value for establishing the final diagnosis.[74] In this study, upper abdominal pain most commonly resulted from gastric and duodenal involvement by nonopportunistic disorders such as pancreatitis and peptic ulcer disease and opportunistic processes such as CMV, KS, and NHL.[74] Right upper quadrant pain most commonly resulted from cholangiopathy or hepatitis. It is important not to limit the differential diagnosis to intraabdominal etiologies but to consider pulmonary, esophageal, and cardiac diseases as causes of upper abdominal pain (Table 64–2).

Accompanying symptoms such as nausea and vomiting or diarrhea are also helpful for determining the possible intraabdominal organ involved. Vomiting is common with partial or complete bowel obstruction, kidney stones, and gallbladder diseases, whereas it is rarely reported with colitis. Isolated vomiting suggests the presence of central nervous system involvement. Patients with a retroperitoneal process, such as pancreatitis or lymphadenopathy, may find relief by leaning forward; ingestion of food aggravates the pain in patients with gastric ulcerations; an inability to find a comfortable body position is common in the presence of nephrolithiasis; and patients with peritonitis prefer to lie quietly.[72–75] The presence of diarrhea suggests an intestinal source (colitis or enteritis). When abdominal pain is present in patients with enteritis, it is usually crampy and periumbilical in location. Symptoms such as nausea, vomiting, bloating, distension, and borborygmi are also commonly associated with small bowel diarrhea. In contrast, the pain in those with colitis tends to be localized to the lower abdominal quadrants, more commonly the left.[72–75]

Careful documentation of current medications is mandatory. Pancreatitis may occur as the result of the administration of pentamidine and trimethoprim-sulfamethoxazole (TMP-SMX) or the antiretroviral agents didanosine (ddI) and dideoxycytidine (ddC). The presence of diarrhea and abdominal pain in a patient with recent use of antibiotics

▲ **Table 64–2.** ETIOLOGY OF ABDOMINAL PAIN IN PATIENTS WITH HIV INFECTION

Epigastric
Acute and chronic pancreatitis (CMV, drug-induced, TMP-SMX)
Peptic ulcer disease (gastric ulcer, duodenal ulcer)
Gastritis (*Helicobacter pylori*, CMV, *Cryptococcus neoformans*, mucormycosis, cryptosporidia, *Leishmania donovani*)
Duodenitis (CMV, *L. donovani*, *Cryptococcus neoformans*, *Cryptosporidium parvum*)
Nonulcer dyspepsia)

Periumbilical
Enteritis (*viral:* CMV, rotavirus, astrovirus, picorna virus, coronavirus; *bacteria: Salmonella*, MAC, *M. tuberculosis; protozoa: Isospora belli*, cryptosporidia, microsporidia, *Cyclospora cayetanesis*, *Giardia lamblia; fungi: Cryptococcus neoformans* (duodenum)
Lymphoma

Right Upper Quadrant
Cholecystitis (gallstones and acalculous). Acalculous most frequently secondary to infections: CMV, *Isospora belli*, *Candida*, *cryptosporidia*, microsporidia, *Salmonella* spp., *Campylobacter fetus*
AIDS-cholangiopathy (CMV, MAC, *Salmonella* spp., *Enterobacter* spp., cryptosporidia, microsporidia, *Cyclospora cayetanensis*)
Shingles (varicella zoster)
Hepatitis (A,B,C,D, CMV, EBV)
Perihepatitis (*Chlamydia trachomatis, Neisseria gonorrhoeae), Bartonella*

Left Upper Quadrant
Splenic abscess
Pancreatic abscess (TB)
Pancreatitis (ddI, ddC, pentamidine, TMP-SMX, *Cryptosporidium*, *Campylobacter*, CMV, HIV)
Shingles

Right Lower Quadrant
Lymphoma
Appendicitis
Inflammatory bowel disease
Pelvic inflammatory disease
Ectopic pregnancy

Left Lower Quadrant
Colitis (infectious: *viral:* CMV, rotavirus, astrovirus, picobirna virus, coronavirus, adenovirus, HSV; *bacterial: Shigella, Campylobacter, Salmonella, Clostridium difficile, Mycobacterium avium, Mycobacterium tuberculosis, Bartonella henselae, Aeromonas hydrophila, protozoa: Entamoeba histolytica, Isospora belli, Cryptosporidium, Toxoplasma gondii, Schistosoma mansonii, Dientamoeba fragilis, Blastocystis hominis, microsporidia; fungi: Histoplasma capsulatum, Candida albicans, Cryptococcus neoformans, Pneumocystis carinii*
neoplastic: Kaposi's sarcoma (Herpesvirus 8), non-Hodgkin's lymphoma, idiopathic, drug-induced (acyclovir)
IBD (idiopathic, also can occur in association with KS)
Diverticulitis
IBS
Pelvic inflammatory disease
Ectopic pregnancy

Flanks
Kidney stones (drug-related: indinavir)
Pyelonephritis
Retroperitoneal lymphadenopathy (non-Hodgkin lymphoma, angioimmunoblastic lymphadenopathy, tuberculosis, MAC)

Suprapubic
Cervical cancer
Pelvic inflammatory disease
Ectopic pregnancy
Not localized to specific area:
- Toxic megacolon (CMV, *C. difficile, Cryptosporidium*, KS)
- Colonic perforation (CMV, histoplasmosis, idiopathic, diverticulum, neoplasm)
- Peritonitis
- Ileal perforation
- Neoplasm (lymphoma, Kaposi sarcoma)
- Adrenal failure

Diffuse
Peritonitis (TB, CMV, *Toxoplasma gondii, Cryptococcus neoformans, Histoplasma capsulatum*)
Bowel perforation
Intraabdominal lymphadenopathy (lymphoma, KS, MAC, TB, angioimmunoblastic lymphadenopathy, bartonellosis)
Adrenal failure-adrenalitis
Mesenteric fibrosis
Omental fibrosis (*H. capsulatum*)
IBS

HIV-infected patients are at similar risk of suffering from diseases and abdominal pain due to the same etiologies as nonimmunocompromised patients. This list highlights some conditions seen frequently in HIV-infected patients.
Microsporidia: *Enterocytozoon bieneusi, Encephalocytozoon (Septata) intestinalis, Encephalocytozoon cuniculi.*
EBV, Epstein-Barr virus; IBD, inflammatory bowel disease; IBS, irritable bowel syndrome; KS, Kaposi sarcoma; MAC, *Mycobacterium avium* complex.

suggests the possibility of *Clostridium difficile* colitis. Flank pain in a patient receiving indinavir may be the result of microlithiasis. Persistent nausea and abdominal pain has been associated with nucleoside-related hepatic steatosis or lactic acidosis.

On physical examination careful attention should be given to any extraabdominal findings, as conditions such as lower lobe pneumonia or pericarditis can result in upper abdominal pain. Fever, an important sign of infection in an immunocompetent person with abdominal pain, is an equally sensitive sign in AIDS patients. However, low-grade fever is a much less specific sign in AIDS patients because it may result from the HIV infection itself. Funduscopic examination is mandatory to exclude the presence of CMV retinitis; 20% with chronic diarrhea and abdominal pain from CMV have generalized CMV disease.[72–74] The skin should be closely examined for KS lesions, as 40% to 50% of patients with skin or lymph node involvement by KS also have gastrointestinal involvement. Jaundice suggests drug-induced liver disease, cholestatic hepatitis, or biliary tract obstruction secondary to infections or neoplasms (NHL, KS). The presence of lymphadenopathy in the neck and inguinal regions suggests a systemic process such as MAC, tuberculosis (TB), or NHL.[72,73] Decreased bowel sounds or high-pitched rushes is most often due to intestinal obstruction, whereas hyperactive bowel sounds are associated with diarrheal disorders. Tenderness on abdominal examination can be nonspecific, but localization to a specific quadrant can be helpful for pointing to the potentially affected organ (Table 64–2). Organomegaly can result from disseminated MAC, histoplasmosis, TB, bacillary angiomatosis, or tumors. Ascites may reflect underlying cirrhosis or represent a complication from TB, CMV enterocolitis, or toxoplasmosis. The anorectum should be examined carefully, as these patients can develop anal fissures and rectal ulcers.

Diagnostic Tests

Initial laboratory evaluation should include a white blood cell count and differential; assays for hemoglobin, liver and pancreatic enzymes, and albumin; coagulation studies; and urinalysis. Because of HIV-associated leukopenia, HIV-infected patients do not always exhibit leukocytosis as part of the systemic inflammatory response to intraabdominal processes such as cholecystitis, colitis, and pancreatitis.[76] Liver function tests are commonly abnormal and can be nonspecific, particularly when only minimally abnormal, or due to chronic viral hepatitis, drug-induced liver injury, or AIDS cholangiopathy.[72–75]

Plain abdominal radiographs are not generally helpful for evaluating abdominal pain but are useful for detecting free subdiaphragmatic air in the presence of viscus perforation, air-fluid levels in the presence of bowel obstruction, or "thumbprinting" due to severe colitis.[74] Ultrasonography (US) is the test of choice for evaluating right upper quadrant pain. We employ US for the patient without jaundice in whom AIDS cholangiopathy or gallbladder disease is suspected, reserving computed tomography (CT) for those with marked hepatomegaly, jaundice, suspected mass lesions, or peritoneal diseases. In addition, CT scans of the abdomen and pelvis should be performed in the ill-appearing patient with unexplained abdominal pain, where it may demonstrate appendicitis, pancreatitis, intraabdominal abscess, lymphadenopathy, or colitis.[77] Hydroxyiminodiacetic acid (HIDA) scanning is often diagnostic for acalculous cholecystitis, demonstrating an absence of uptake into the gallbladder despite imaging of the common bile duct.

Endoscopy

Endoscopy is a valuable tool for evaluating chronic abdominal pain in AIDS, especially in the presence of specific symptoms such as epigastric pain, diarrhea, nausea, and vomiting. Endoscopic retrograde cholangiopancreatography is the most sensitive means of diagnosing AIDS cholangiopathy.

Diagnostic Laparoscopy

Laparoscopy is useful for the evaluating of abdominal pain, hepatomegaly, fever of unknown origin, and ascites.[78–80] A diagnosis was established in 70% of patients and included MAC, TB, KS, histoplasmosis, cryptosporidiosis, chronic active hepatitis, and cirrhosis.

Therapy

Therapy should be directed by the cause of the abdominal pain. In most cases the treatment is medical; but when indicated, an aggressive surgical approach is warranted because the surgical morbidity and mortality rates are acceptable in these patients.[78–80] It is still unfortunate that on many occasions surgery has been delayed because of fear to operate, leading to worsening of the illness and the overall prognosis.

Once a life-threatening condition has been excluded and a diagnosis is established, consideration should be given to adding antispasmodics and specific medications for appropriate pain control. Lebovits et al. noted that various pain syndromes associated with HIV infection (e.g., neuropathies, chest and abdominal pain) were not managed appropriately.[81] They found that the most commonly used analgesic was acetaminophen alone or in combination with codeine used on an as-needed basis.[81] In HIV-infected patients with abdominal pain, we suggest that during and following the initiation of definitive treatment mild to moderate pain may be treated with a nonsteroidal antinflammatory drug (NSAID) or acetaminophen on a fixed-dosage schedule. Narcotic agents should be given in more severe cases or when there is no response to scheduled NSAID or acetaminophen. Tricyclic antidepressants should also be started at low dosages. Narcotics should be avoided when there is a partial or evolving bowel obstruction.

▲ DIARRHEA (ENTERITIS AND COLITIS)

Diarrhea is a frequent complaint among patients with HIV infection. Since the introduction of protease inhibitors (PIs) and HAART in 1996, there has been a constant decline in gastrointestinal opportunistic disorders associated with AIDS.[75] It is postulated that improvement in the immune status associated with the use of these medications as reflected by an increase in CD4+ T lymphocytes prevents the development of opportunistic disorders. The history indicates the possible sites of involvement (i.e., enteritis or colitis). Small bowel diarrhea ("enteritis") is manifested as large-volume (>2 L/day), watery stools frequently associated with dehydration, electrolyte disturbances, and malabsorption. Abdominal pain, when present, is usually crampy and periumbilical. Low-grade fever and nausea are also common. In contrast, colitis is characterized by frequent, small-volume stools that contain mucus, pus, and blood and frequently accompanied by "proctitis symptoms" (tenesmus or a feeling of incomplete evacuation and dyskesia or pain on defecation). Abdominal pain tends to be localized to the lower quadrants, more commonly on the left. The physical examination is rarely diagnostic for the specific etiology of the diarrhea but is extremely important for assessing the patient's general condition and hydration status. In addition, if the patient has chronic malabsorptive diarrhea, physical findings associated with specific nutrient deficiencies may become evident (e.g., ecchymosis with vitamin K deficiency). The list of diagnostic tests available for evaluating acute and chronic infectious diarrhea in HIV-infected patients is exhaustive, but it is rarely necessary to use more than a few of these tests. The approach to the HIV-infected patient with diarrhea is "stepwise," beginning with simple tests and gradually progressing to more invasive tests[82] (Table 64–3). A search for an etiology should always be attempted, as most causes of diarrhea are infectious and can be treated with specific antimicrobial agents.

When analyzing the stools, the first test should be a methylene blue stain to determine if fecal leukocytes are present. Their presence suggests an inflammatory (colonic) rather than a noninflammatory (small bowel) diarrhea. Stool cultures for *Salmonella*, *Shigella*, and *Campylobacter* should be done routinely, as well as a *Clostridium difficile* toxin screen. Routine stool stains should include a modified acid stain to look for cryptosporidia.[83]

Routine tests may be useful for evaluating the impact of the diarrhea on the host, such as malnutrition (hypoalbuminemia), hydration status, and electrolyte disturbances. The absolute CD4+ T-lymphocyte cell count is essential, as many organisms are causative only in the presence of severe immunodeficiency. Roentgenography plays an unimportant role in the evaluation of HIV-associated diarrhea. Endoscopy (esophagogastroduodenoscopy, flexible sigmoidoscopy, colonoscopy) are important and may be an integral part of the workup of patients suspected of having CMV or microsporidia and for patients with negative noninvasive studies.[83]

▲ **Table 64–3.** DIAGNOSTIC EVALUATION FOR DIARRHEA IN HIV-INFECTED PATIENTS

Acute Diarrhea (< 14 Days)
Step 1
- Stool methylene blue for leukocytes
- Stool culture for *Salmonella* spp.,[a], *Shigella* spp.,[a] and *Campylobacter jejunii*[a]; assay for *Clostridium difficile* toxin
- Stool microscopic examination for ova and parasites (*Giardia lamblia* and *Entamoeba histolytica*[b])
- Stool antibody testing (*Giardia lamblia*[c])

Step 2
- Flexible sigmoidoscopy
  - Inspection and endoscopic characterization of colon
  - Stool retrieval for cultures, ova and parasites, and *C. difficile* toxin (as above)

Chronic Diarrhea (> 14 Days)
Step 1
- Stool methylene blue for leukocytes
- Stool investigation for *Clostridium difficile* toxin
- Stool microscopic examination for ova and parasites (microsporidia,[d] cryptosporidia,[e] *Isospora belli*,[e] and *Cyclospora cayetanensis*)
- Blood cultures [*Mycobacterium avium* complex (MAC)]

Step 2
- Endoscopy with biopsies
  - Gastroduodenoscopy and duodenal biopsies (MAC, microsporidia)
- Flexible sigmoidoscopy or colonoscopy [cytomegalovirus (CMV), MAC, microsporidia, *Isospora belli, C. difficile*, inflammatory bowel disease]
- Biopsy specimens submitted for
  - Tissue stains[f]
  - Special tissue stains[g]
  - Culture of tissue[h]
  - Electron microscopy[i]

[a]Blood cultures (bacteremia by these bacteria is more common in HIV-infected patients).
[b]Hemophagocytosis needs to present to substantiate pathogenic *Entamoeba*.
[c]Electroimmunoassay (EIA) for *G. lamblia*.
[d]Gram stain, concentrated stool (zinc sulfate, Shether sucrose flotation).
[e]Modified Kinyoun acid-fast (*Cryptosporidium* and *Isospora belli*).
[f]Hematoxylin and eosin [CMV, herpes simplex virus (HSV), fungi], Giemsa or methenamine silver (*Candida, Histoplasma capsulatum*), Gram or methylene blue/azure II/basic fuchsin (microsporidia), Fite (Mycobacteria).
[g]In-situ hybridization, immunoperoxide stains (CMV, HSV, adenovirus).
[h]Bacteria and fungi.
[i]Microsporidia, adenovirus.

▲ INFECTIONS OF THE SMALL INTESTINE (ENTERITIS)

Etiology

In most series before the era of HAART, *Cryptosporidium parvum* was the most common protozoal infection causing diarrhea, identified in up to 11% of symptomatic patients.[84] The prevalence of infection has been markedly reduced with the advent of potent antiretroviral therapy. Outbreaks of cryptosporidiosis are well described in both immunocompetent and immunodeficient hosts, and they result from contamination of public water sources.[85] Microsporidia (*Enterocytozoon bieneusi* and *Encephalitozoon intestinalis*, formerly *Septata intestinalis*) involve a variety of organ systems causing either localized or disseminated

Table 64–4. ENTERIC PATHOGENS IN AIDS PATIENTS

Viruses
Cytomegalovirus
Astrovirus
Picornavirus
Coronavirus
Rotavirus
Herpesvirus
Adenovirus
Small round virus
HIV
Bacteria
Salmonella
Shigella
Campylobacter
Clostridium difficile
Mycobacterium avium complex
Treponema pallidum
Bartonella
Spirochaeta
Neisseria gonorrhoeae
Vibrio cholerae
Pseudomonas
Staphylococcus aureus
Parasites
Giardia lamblia
Entamoeba histolytica
Microsporidia
Enterocytozoon bieneusi
Septata intestinalis
Cyclospora
Cryptosporidium
Isospora belli
Blastocystis hominis
Fungi
Histoplasma
Candida albicans

disease[86] (Table 64–4). These parasites are common intestinal and biliary pathogens in patients with AIDS.[87] Kotler and Orenstein[87] found microsporidia in 39% of AIDS patients undergoing gastrointestinal evaluation for diarrhea. *E. bieneusi* is the cause of most cases of gastrointestinal disease.[86] Co-infection with these two microsporidia or with other pathogens has been reported.[88] This high prevalence of intestinal microsporidiosis is probably not related to an increasing incidence of disease but, rather, to greater recognition and improved diagnostic testing. *Isospora belli* is a rare gastrointestinal pathogen in HIV-infected patients in the United States, whereas it is endemic in many developing countries such as Haiti[86] and is an important cause of chronic diarrhea. As with other protozoa, it is primarily a small bowel pathogen. *Cyclospora*, another coccidial protozoon, has recently been recognized throughout the world as a gastrointestinal pathogen in immunocompetent patients and in patients with AIDS.[89] The prevalence of *Cyclospora* in developed and developing countries is unknown. A number of similarities exist in the microbiology, epidemiology, and clinical expression of *Cyclospora* and cryptosporidia. *Cyclospora* spp. have a morphologic appearance similar to that of cryptosporidia, although they are larger (8 to 10 μm vs. 4 to 6 μm). Giardiasis has no increased prevalence in HIV-infected patients, and the clinical presentation and diagnostic methods are similar to those for HIV-seronegative patients. *Mycobacterium avium* complex (MAC) has emerged as an increasingly important pathogen in AIDS.[90,91] Small intestinal disease is the most common site of luminal gastrointestinal involvement by MAC. It has been rarely reported to involve the esophagus, biliary tree, or colon.[92]

Rotavirus has been linked to both acute and chronic diarrhea.[93] Several unusual viruses have been identified in HIV-infected patients with chronic diarrhea including astrovirus, picornavirus, and coronavirus.[94] Although the true incidence of these viruses as gastrointestinal pathogens is unknown, it is probably low; and therapy is not currently available.

Clinical Presentation

In contrast to immunocompetent patients with cryptosporidiosis where spontaneous cure is uniform, in HIV-infected patients the natural history is much more variable.[85] This variability is due to the effect of immunodeficiency as patients with CD4+ T-lymphocyte counts higher than 180 cells per cubic millimeter usually have a self-limited illness.[95] In contrast, in patients with a CD4+ T-lymphocyte count of less than 50 cells per cubic millimeter the disease is often devastating, resulting in severe (voluminous) watery, nonbloody diarrhea with malabsorption, electrolyte disturbances, dehydration, and weight loss with a median survival of less than 12 weeks.[96] Abdominal cramps and weight loss are common. The parasite is distributed throughout the gastrointestinal tract, although most commonly it infects the small bowel. The diagnosis of cryptosporidiosis rests on the demonstration of oocysts in stool specimens (modified acid fast stain).

The most common clinical presentation of microsporidiosis is chronic, watery, nonbloody diarrhea of variable severity but infrequently voluminous. Substantial weight loss is uncommon. Abdominal pain and fever are not associated with intestinal involvement. In immunocompetent hosts the organism causes a self-limited illness characterized by crampy abdominal pain, flatulence, and diarrhea lasting 2 to 3 weeks.

Isosporiasis is typically a chronic illness characterized by profuse, nonbloody, watery diarrhea that may be indistinguishable from the diarrhea caused by microsporidia or cryptosporidia. Nausea and diffuse abdominal pain typically accompany the illness; fever and vomiting are uncommon. A malabsorption syndrome (steatorrhea and lactose intolerance) with weight loss of at least 10% often antedates the diagnosis.

The most frequent symptoms of giardiasis are flatulence, crampy abdominal pain, borborygmi, dyspepsia, and diarrhea. Fever and bloody stools are not associated with this infection.

Small bowel involvement by MAC is often diffuse. Massive infiltration of the small bowel mimicking Whipple's disease has been described and may account for the severe malabsorption seen in some patients.[97] The liver and spleen are the most common sites for dissemination.[98] The most common manifestations of intestinal MAC infection are abdominal pain, fever, night sweats, wasting, and anemia.[99]

Chronic watery diarrhea may result from small intestinal malabsorption.

Diagnosis

Cryptosporidiosis is diagnosed by stool analysis using a modified acid-fast stain. Although electron microscopy of small bowel biopsies is considered the gold standard for the diagnosis of microsporidiosis, studies have shown tissue stains (H & E, touch preparation with Giemsa, Brown-Brenn, Brown-Hopps, methylene blue azure II-basic fuchsin) of small bowel biopsies to have sensitivities of 77% to 83% with specificities approaching 100%.[100] When performing upper endoscopy, an attempt should be made to biopsy the most distal part of the small bowel, as microsporidia are mostly concentrated in the jejunum. The most commonly employed stool stain is a modified trichrome (chromotrope 2R) stain. The diagnosis of isosporiosis is best established using a modified Kinyoun acid-fast stool stain[96]; small bowel biopsy may also be diagnostic. *Cyclospora* are difficult to appreciate on routine microscopy of small bowel biopsies, although electron microscopy is often diagnostic. For the diagnosis of *Giardia*, it is well recognized that multiple stool tests (usually three) obtained on different days may be required, as intestinal shedding is sporadic[101]; moreover, only 40% of stools are positive in low excreters. Light microscopic detection of *Giardia* cysts (in semiformed stools) and trophozoites (in diarrheic stools) continues to be the mainstay of diagnosis. Fresh stool specimens should be examined or fixed with polyvinyl alcohol formalin and then stained with trichrome or iron hematoxylin. Cyst detection in stool can be increased by use of immunofluorescent antibody to cyst protein. Small bowel duodenal aspirate and biopsy may be diagnostic when stool testing is negative.

Positive blood cultures or bone marrow biopsy establish the diagnosis of disseminated MAC but do not establish the presence of active gastrointestinal disease. The presence of a positive stool culture suggests, but does not prove, gastrointestinal involvement; stool culture positivity is, however, a marker for subsequent disseminated disease.[102] Many laboratories, however, do not perform a MAC culture on stool.

Although many of these organisms (MAC, microsporidia, cryptosporidia) do not produce colitis per se, they may involve the colon. Thus the diagnosis can be established based on colonic mucosal biopsies obtained during flexible sigmoidoscopy or colonoscopy. We present a simplified but focused algorithm for the evaluation of diarrhea in AIDS in Figure 64–2.

Treatment

Numerous therapies have been used to treat intestinal cryptosporidiosis (see Chapter 29), most without success.[103] Several case reports have suggested that immune reconstitution, either through potent antiretroviral therapy[104,105] or improvements in nutritional status,[106] may result in a clinical remission. A novel therapy includes the use of bovine colostrum.[107]; case reports have demonstrated clinical improvement in 50% of patients following its use. The results of an open-label trial found a reduction in stool frequency and stool weight in patients receiving bovine immunoglobulin, although fewer than half of the patients had a reduction of 50% in stool weight or clearance of this pathogen from the stool.[108] Letrazuril, a drug with activity against coccidia, was found to have some efficacy in two small open-label studies.[109]

The agent most commonly advanced as treatment of cryptosporidiosis is paromomycin.[110–114] In a study of 35 patients, a complete symptomatic response was seen in 20% of patients, with a partial response observed in an additional 43%[110]; responders had more preserved immune function as assessed by the CD4+ T-lymphocyte count. In a prospective open-label trial of 24 patients, 22 (92%) had a clinical response, with a complete remission observed in 18.[112] Among the 22 responders, clearance of the organisms was noted on follow-up stool studies, small bowel biopsy, or both. Other studies, however, have found persistent oocyst excretion despite clinical improvement.[113] These results are in striking contrast to a randomized, double-blind placebo-controlled trial of 35 patients.[114] This study employed a 21-day placebo phase, but subsequently all patients then received an additional 21 days of active drug. A complete response was seen in 18% of the treated patients compared to 15% of the placebo patients. The findings from this study[114] are similar to our experience in that patients with the most severe disease (and most severe immunodeficiency) are the least likely to respond. For patients with a CD4+ T-lymphocyte count of less than 100 cells per microliter in whom therapy is clinically effective, long-term administration is required to prevent relapse, although relapse may still occur despite the continued therapy.[111,112] During the present era of HAART, it has been demonstrated that combination antiretroviral therapy that includes a PI can restore immunity to *E. bieneusi* and *C. parvum* in HIV-1 infected individuals, resulting in complete clinical, microbiologic, and histologic responses.[115] Therefore the therapy for patients with AIDS and chronic diarrhea may change dramatically, focusing more on approaches to restore these patients' immune status (i.e., with HAART) rather than treating the opportunistic disorder itself.[115]

Treatments for microsporidia are variably effective (see Chapter 30). Initial studies of metronidazole showed some efficacy,[116] although our experience has not been positive. Albendazole has shown promise in open-label trials,[117] with response rates of about 50% with a dose of 400 mg PO bid. Despite clinical improvement, the organisms persisted in the stool and small bowel biopsy specimens.[117] In contrast, studies of patients with *E. intestinalis* show response rates to albendazole of 66% to 100%, with some patients having clearance of the organism and no relapse.[118] With the recognition that two microsporidial species involve the bowel, it has become clear that albendazole is highly effective for *E. intestinalis* but largely ineffective for *E. bieneusi*. However, a recent study has shown that oral fumagillis is effective for *E. bieneusi*.[118a] This response difference emphasizes the importance of a species-specific diagnosis of intestinal microsporidiosis.

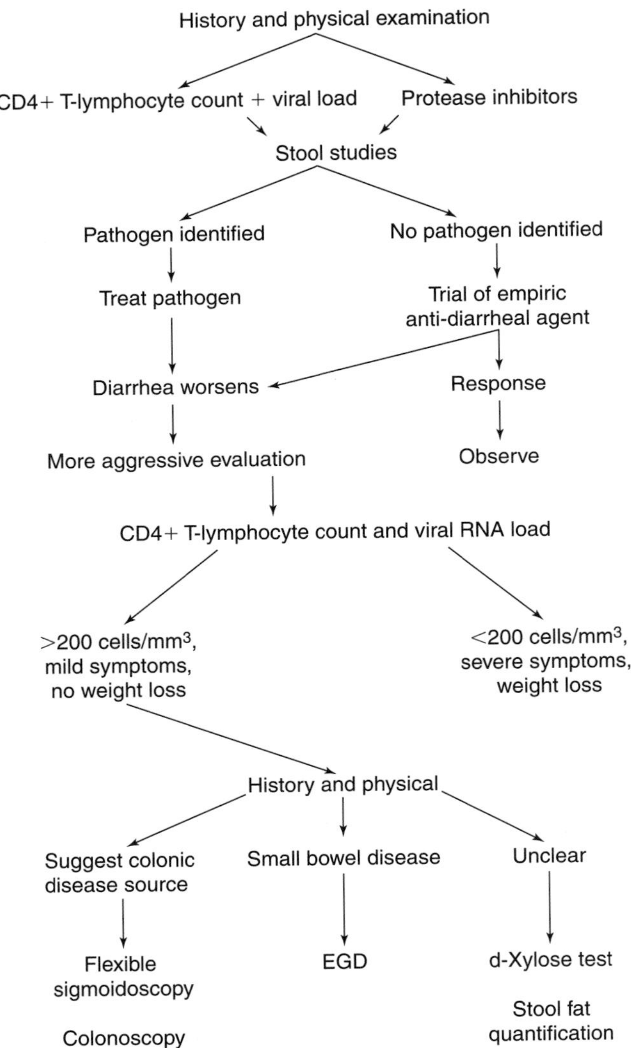

Figure 64–2. Diagnostic algorithm for evaluating diarrhea in the HIV-infected patient.

Atovaquone showed some efficacy for alleviating symptoms in a small open-label trial.[119]

In contrast to cryptosporidia and microsporidia, effective therapy is available for *Isospora belli* and *Cyclospora* (see Chapter 29). Cotrimoxazole or TMP-SMX results in cure in most patients. Because the relapse rate of isosporiasis is 50% once therapy is discontinued, lifelong suppressive therapy is required.[120] The widespread use of TMP-SMX for *Pneumocystis carinii* prophylaxis may be one explanation for the low incidence of these infections in developed countries. Therapy with metronidazole (500 mg bid × 5 to 7 days) is highly effective for treating giardiasis.

▲ INFECTIONS OF THE COLON (COLITIS)

The spectrum of pathogens causing colitis is similar to that in the normal host, except for CMV (Table 64–5). In earlier studies of diarrhea in HIV-infected patients, bacteria were frequently identified.[121] Unusual presentations of common bacterial diseases became apparent early in the AIDS epidemic where *Salmonella* sp.[122] or *Campylobacter* sp. bacteremia.[123] were reported as initial manifestations of AIDS. The infection was characterized by frequent relapses despite appropriate antimicrobial therapy. Currently, the prevalence of these infections as causes of diarrhea are not well known, although it is probably lower than in the past given the widespread use of TMP-SMX for *Pneumocystis Carinii pneumonia* (PCP) prophylaxis. *Clostridium difficile* colitis is an important cause of diarrhea in these patients because of their frequent exposure to antimicrobials and frequent hospitalizations—factors that have been linked to *C. difficile* disease.[124] CMV is the most common opportunistic cause of colonic disease. It usually presents as chronic diarrhea and is frequently associated with systemic disease (CMV retinitis). Adenovirus has been reported to cause diarrhea and colitis.[125] HIV-infected patients do not appear to have an increased susceptibility to *Entamoeba histolytica*.[126] Amebic colitis is distinctly uncommon.

Histoplasmosis infrequently involves the gastrointestinal tract in patients with AIDS (see Chapter 37). Gastrointestinal tract involvement occurs in about 5% of patients with

▲ **Table 64–5.** ETIOLOGY OF COLITIS IN HIV-INFECTED PATIENTS

Bacteria
Shigella, Campylobacter, Salmonella
Clostridium difficile
Mycobacerium avium complex
Mycobacterium tuberculosis
Bartonella henselae
Aeromonas hydrophila
Viruses
Cytomegalovirus
Herpes simplex virus
Adenovirus
Protozoa
Entamoeba histolytica
Isospora belli
Blastocystis hominis
Cryptosporidium
Microsporidia
Toxoplasma gondii
Fungi
Histoplasma capsulatum
Candida albicans
Cryptococcus neoformans
Pneumocystis carinii
Other
Inflammatory bowel disease
Kaposi sarcoma (herpesvirus 8)
Lymphoma

disseminated disease and occasionally is the first site of disease.[127] The colon is the most common site of involvement (80%).[127]

Clinical Presentation and Diagnosis

Salmonella gastroenteritis presents with watery diarrhea, abdominal pain, nausea, and vomiting. Some patients present with classic "colitis" symptoms: dysentery (mucopurulent, bloody diarrhea) and fever. *Salmonella* bacteremia should be sought in the patient with diarrhea and fever; and when identified, prolonged antimicrobial therapy should be given. Shigellosis and campylobacteriosis present in a fashion similar to that of *Salmonella* gastroenteritis. Stool cultures are usually diagnostic; blood cultures are useful and occasionally are positive when stool cultures are negative. Colitis may be identified by flexible sigmoidoscopy; mucosal biopsies should be performed in severely immunocompromised patients, as CMV colitis may appear endoscopically similar.[75]

Colonic CMV infection typically presents with chronic watery diarrhea, abdominal pain, wasting, anorexia, and fever. When the distal colorectum is involved, symptoms of proctitis may be reported. Gastrointestinal bleeding without diarrhea may be the initial manifestation of CMV colitis. Not infrequently perforation from small bowel ulcers or, less commonly, colonic ulcers occurs.[75] Physical findings are nonspecific. CMV colitis almost always occurs when the CD4+ T-lymphocyte count is less than 100 cells per microliter. Serologic studies for CMV antibody are not specific. Stool tests are negative, except for the presence of white blood cells. Abdominal radiographs are noncontributory unless the patient presents with toxic megacolon, where colonic dilation and "thumbprinting" of the mucosa may be observed. Barium enemas should not be used to evaluate colitis in HIV-infected patients. The main diagnostic tool is endoscopy with mucosal biopsies. In general, special histologic stains are not necessary for the diagnosis of CMV or other gastrointestinal opportunistic disorders so long as an experienced gastrointestinal pathologist examines the biopsy specimens.[128] Sigmoidoscopy is generally sufficient; however, CMV disease may be isolated to the right colon, thereby requiring full colonoscopy for diagnosis. Endoscopically, the most common appearance includes edema, submucosal hemorrhages, and multiple ulcerations. The viral cytopathic effect of CMV should be identified by histopathologic evaluation of multiple biopsy specimens to confirm the diagnosis.[75]

The clinical presentation and response to therapy of *C. difficile* colitis are no different in HIV-infected or HIV-uninfected patients.[124] In the appropriate clinical setting, detection of *C. difficile* toxin is diagnostic. Fecal leukocytes are usually present (60%) and are an important clue to the diagnosis. Flexible sigmoidoscopy is warranted in the patient in whom the disease is suspected but stool toxin is negative.

Amebiasis presents classically as "dysentery" with mucopurulent, bloody diarrhea, tenesmus, crampy abdominal pain, and fever. Amebiasis can also present as fulminant colitis with toxic megacolon, ameboma, and liver abscess. These more virulent presentations do not seem to be increased in the HIV-infected patient. Ameba are frequently found on routine stool studies from both asymptomatic and symptomatic homosexual men.[129] In these patients colonization with nonpathogenic ameba (nonpathogenic zymodemes) including *Entamoeba dispar*, *Entamoeba hartmanni*, and *Escherichia coli* are likely, as they are indistinguishable by light microscopy from pathogenic ameba.[129] One might anticipate that colonization, even with nonpathogenic strains, would cause significant disease in immunocompromised patients. Instead, a benign clinical course has been found. A number of symptomatic patients in whom amebae were identified had other potential pathogens, suggesting that a search for other pathogens is always appropriate in a symptomatic HIV-infected patient with diarrhea and amebic cysts in the stool. In addition, despite clearance of these protozoa from the stool, treatment has not been shown to cure the diarrhea reliably, suggesting that in most patients they do not represent pathogens (i.e., *E. dispar*).

Amebiasis is generally diagnosed by microscopic examination of a rectal swab or a wet mount of fresh stool. As with *Giardia*, multiple stool samples (three to six) may be required because of the intermittent shedding of the cysts and trophozoites. Serologic tests (indirect hemagglutination), agar cell diffusion, counterimmunoelectrophoresis, and enzyme immunoassay techniques are sensitive and specific in patients with invasive *Entamoeba histolytica*.

The most frequent symptoms of gastrointestinal histoplasmosis are fever, diarrhea, weight loss, and abdominal pain. The endoscopic appearance is that of a single segmental or constricting mass, but multiple ulcerations mimicking Crohn's disease have been described.[117] The diagnosis is made by identifying the fungus histologically and by culturing biopsy specimens.

Therapy

The antibiotic of choice for a presumed bacterial enterocolitis is a quinolone such as ciprofloxacin (500 mg PO bid). Potential drug–drug interactions must be carefully assessed. As with normal hosts infected with these organisms, the duration of therapy should be 7 to 10 days. Clinical experience with HIV-infected patients suggests that infections with *Shigella* sp. and *Campylobacter* sp. are occasionally recurrent after successful treatment and are more resistant to therapy. For the treatment of *C. difficile* diarrhea, two drugs are widely available and effective. Metronidazole (250 to 500 mg PO or IV tid for 7 to 10 days) represents first-line therapy. Vancomycin should be reserved for patients with a contraindication to or failure of metronidazole or when the disease is life-threatening; this agent is effective only when administered orally. Clinical cure can be obtained in essentially all patients. The relapse rate appears to be similar in HIV-infected and HIV-uninfected patients.[71]

The treatment of CMV gastrointestinal disease was discussed under Infections of the Esophagus.[43–48]

Metronidazole (750 mg tid × 14 days) is highly effective for invasive *Entamoeba histolytica*, and relapse after curative therapy is rare. Because metronidazole is not an effective agent for cysts (which remain in the gut lumen), use of a luminally acting agent to eradicate intestinal colonization is recommended for those with invasive amebiasis or for the asymptomatic "cyst excretor" who has a positive serology. Three major luminally active agents are available: iodoquinol (650 mg PO tid for 20 days), diloxanide furoate (500 mg PO tid for 10 days), and paromomycin (25 to 30 mg/kg/day in three divided doses for 7 days). All have efficacy rates of 85% to 95% for the eradication of cyst passage. There is no convincing evidence of an increased incidence of either *Dientamoeba fragilis* or *Blastocystis hominis* in AIDS patients.

Therapy for MAC has improved substantially over the last decade. Previously used multidrug regimens were poorly tolerated, were associated with significant side effects, and had low efficacy.[130] It has now been clearly established that a macrolide (clarithromycin)-containing multidrug regimen is superior to a non-macrolide-containing regimen for initial therapy of MAC disease.[131] Therapy and prophylaxis for gastrointestinal MAC is the same as for disseminated infection.

Amphotericin B is the drug of choice for colonic histoplasmosis, and the recommended dosing is the same as for disseminated histoplasmosis. A liposomal preparation is required in some patients. Secondary prophylaxis should be provided with itraconazole, fluconazole, or weekly amphotericin B.

Symptomatic Therapies for Diarrhea

For patients in whom antimicrobial therapy is ineffective or no specific cause for diarrhea is found despite multiple stool analysis and endoscopy with biopsies, symptomatic therapy is necessary. When the diarrhea is mild, bulking agents (bismuth or Kaopectate) may provide relief. With more severe diarrhea, medications to reduce intestinal transit are required. We routinely use diphenoxylate (Lomotil) in doses up to 10 tablets/day. Larger doses may cause anticholinergic side effects, as diphenoxylate is combined with atropine in Lomotil.

Despite the potential for abuse, narcotic agents are also highly effective agents. In patients with severe diarrhea, tincture of opium (paregoric) is highly effective. It is usually provided with a dropper that provides a morphine concentration of 0.4 mg/ml. The normal dose is 5 to 10 ml/day in divided doses, and the dose can be titrated up to 20 ml/day. Some patients experience somnolence or abdominal cramps, which tend to dissipate over time.

Octreotide, a somatostatin analogue, is an antisecretory agent with a variety of inhibitory functions throughout the gastrointestinal tract. Initial studies in patients with AIDS found that this drug provides effective control of diarrhea in about 50% of patients.[132–134] However, a large randomized placebo-controlled trial did not demonstrate efficacy of this agent in patients with and without identifiable pathogens.[135] The drug is given subcutaneously in doses of 50 to 500 μg tid. Side effects include decreased biliary motility (gallstones), diabetes, and steatorrhea, the latter of which can potentially exacerbate diarrhea. Although the drug has not been clearly proven effective, use in patients with severe diarrhea requiring hospitalization (e.g., *Cryptosporidia*) may be attempted. We define a clinical response as a reduction in stool frequency/volume of at least 50%.

REFERENCES

1. Weinert M, Grimes RM, Lynch DP. Oral manifestations of HIV infection. Ann Intern Med 125:485, 1996.
2. Wilcox CM, Straub RF, Clark WS. Prospective evaluation of oropharyngeal findings in human immunodeficiency virus-infected patients with esophageal ulcer. Am J Gastroenterol 90:1938, 1995.
3. Bonacini M, Young T, Laine L. The causes of esophageal symptoms in human immunodeficiency virus infection: a prospective study of 110 patients. Arch Intern Med 151:1567, 1991.
4. Wilcox CM. Evaluation of a technique to evaluate the underlying mucosa in patients with AIDS and severe *Candida* esophagitis. Gastrointest Endosc 42:360, 1995.
5. Coleman DC, Bennett DE, Sullivan DJ, et al. Oral *Candida* in HIV infection and AIDS: new perspectives/new approaches. Crit Rev Microbiol 19:61, 1993.
6. Sullivan DJ, Henman MC, Moran GP, et al. Molecular genetic approaches to identification, epidemiology and taxonomy of non-*albicans Candida* species. J Med Microbiol 44:399, 1996.
7. Coleman DC, Sullivan DJ, Bennett DE, et al. Candidiasis: the emergence of a novel species, *Candida dublinensis*. AIDS 11:557, 1997.
8. Troillet N, Durussel C, Bille J, et al. Correlation between in vitro susceptibility of *Candida albicans* and fluconazole-resistant oropharyngeal candidiasis in HIV-infected patients. Eur J Clin Microbiol Infect Dis 12:911, 1993.
9. Fichtenbaum CJ, Koletar S, Yiannotsos C, et al. Refractory mucosal candidiasis in advanced human immunodeficiency virus infection. Clin Infect Dis 30:749, 2000.
10. Gallant JE, Moore RD, Richman DD, et al. Incidence and natural history of cytomegalovirus disease in patients with advanced human immunodeficiency virus disease treated with zidovudine. J Infect Dis 166:1223, 1992.
11. Wilcox CM, Schwartz DA. Symtomatic cinical duodenitis: an important clinical problem in AIDS. J Clin Gastroenterol 14:293, 1992.

12. Wilcox CM, Schwartz DA, Clark WS. Causes, response to therapy, and long-term outcome of esophageal ulcer in patients with human immunodeficiency virus infection. Ann Intern Med 122:143, 1995.
13. Bagdades EK, Pillay D, Squire SB, et al. Relationship between herpes simplex virus ulceration and CD4+ cell counts in patients with HIV infection. AIDS 6:1317, 1992.
14. Kotler DP, Reka S, Orenstein JM, Fox CH. Chronic idiopathic esophageal ulceration in the acquired immunodeficiency syndrome. J Clin Gastroenterol 15:284, 1992.
15. Wilcox CM, Zaki SR, Coffield LM, et al. Evaluation of idiopathic esophageal ulcer for human immunodeficiency virus. Mod Pathol 8:568, 1995.
16. Mönkemüller KE, Wilcox CM. Diagnosis and treatment of esophageal ulcers in AIDS. Semin Gastroeneterol 10:1, 1999.
17. Raufman J-P. Odynophagia/dysphagia in AIDS. Gastroenterol Clin North Am 17:599, 1988.
18. Genereau T, Lortholary O, Bouchaud O, et al. Herpes simplex esophagitis in patients with AIDS: report of 34 cases. Clin Infect Dis 22:926, 1996.
19. Wilcox CM, Straub RA, Schwartz DA. Prospective endoscopic characterization of cytomegalovirus esophagitis in patients with AIDS. Gastrointest Endosc 40:481, 1994.
20. Goodgame RW, Genta RM, Estrada R, et al. Frequency of positive tests for cytomegalovirus in AIDS patients: endoscopic lesions compared with normal mucosa. Am J Gastroenterol 88:338, 1993.
21. Wilcox CM, Alexander LN, Clark WS, Thompson SE. Fluconazole compared with endoscopy for human immunodeficiency virus-infected patients with esophageal symptoms. Gastroenterology 110:1803, 1996.
22. Koletar SL, Russell JA, Fass RJ, Plouffe JF. Comparison of oral fluconazole and clotrimazole troches as treatment of oral candidiasis in patients infected with human immunodeficiency virus. Antimicrob Agents Chemother 34:2267, 1990.
23. Pons V, Greenspan D, Derbruin M, et al. Therapy for oropharyngeal candidiasis in HIV-infected patients: a randomized, prospective multicenter study of oral fluconazole versus clotrimazole troches. J Acquir Immune Defic Syndr 6:1311, 1993.
24. Pons V, Greenspan D, Lozada-Nur F, et al. Oropharyngeal candidiasis in patients with AIDS: randomized comparison of fluconazole versus nystatin oral suspensions. Clin Infect Dis 24:1204, 1997.
25. DeWit S, Goosens H, Clumeck N. Single-dose versus 7 days of fluconazole treatment for oral candidiasis in human immunodeficiency virus-infected patients: a prospective, randomized pilot study. J Infect Dis 168:1332, 1993.
26. DeWit SD, Weerts D, Goosens H, Clumeck N. Comparison of fluconazole and ketoconazole in oropharyngeal candidiasis in AIDS. Lancet 1:746, 1989.
27. Hernandez-Sampelayo T, Multicenter Study Group. Fluconazole versus ketaconazole in the treatment of oropharyngeal candidiasis in HIV-infected children. Eur J Clin Microbiol Infect Dis. 13:340, 1994.
28. Laine L, Dretler RH, Conteas CN, et al. Fluconazole compared with ketoconazole for the treatment of candida esophagitis in AIDS: a randomized trial. Ann Intern Med 117:655, 1992.
29. Wilcox CM. Time course of clinical response to fluconazole for *Candida* oesphagitis in AIDS. Aliment Pharmacol Ther 8:347, 1994.
30. Smith DE, Midgley J, Allan M, et al. Itraconazole versus ketaconazole in the treatment of oral and oesophageal candidosis in patients infected with HIV. AIDS 5:1367, 1991.
31. Barbaro G, Barbarini G, Caladeron W, et al. Fluconazole versus itraconazole for *Candida* esophagitis in acquired immunodeficiency syndrome. Gastroenterology 111:1169, 1996.
32. Barbaro G, Barbarini G, Di Lorenzo G. Fluconazole vs. flucytosine in the treatment of esophageal candidiasis in AIDS patients: a double-blind, placebo-controlled study. Endoscopy 27:377, 1995.
33. Laine L, Rabeneck LR. Prospective study of fluconazole suspension for the treatment of oesophageal candidiasis in patients with AIDS. Aliment Pharmacol Ther 9:553, 1995.
34. Wilcox CM, Darouiche RO, Laine L, et al. A randomized, double-blind comparison of itraconazole oral solution and fluconazole tablets in the treatment of esophageal candidiasis. J Infect Dis 176:227, 1997.
35. Dewsnup DH, Stevens DA. Efficacy of oral amphotericin B in AIDS patients with thrush clinically resistant to fluconazole. J Med Veter Mycol 32:389, 1994.
36. Vazquez JA. Options for the management of mucosal candidiasis in patients with AIDS and HIV infection. Pharmacotherapy 19:76, 1999.
37. Just-Nübling G, Gentshaw G, Meissner K, et al. Fluconazole prophylaxis of recurrent oral candidiasis in HIV-positive patients. Eur J Clin Microbiol Infect Dis 10:917, 1991.
38. Stevens DA, Greene SI, Lang OS. Thrush can be prevented in patients with acquired immunodeficiency syndrome and the acquired immunodeficiency syndrome-related complex: randomized, double-blind, placebo-controlled study of 100-mg oral fluconazole daily. Arch Intern Med 151:2458, 1991.
39. Gallant JE, Moore RD, Chaisson RE. Prophylaxis for opportunistic infections in patients with HIV infection. Ann Intern Med 120:932, 1994.
40. Marriott DJE. Fluconazole once a week as secondary prophylaxis against oropharyngeal candidiasis in HIV-infected patients: a double-blind placebo-controlled study. Med J Aust 158:312, 1993.
41. Leen CLS, Dunbar EM, Ellis ME, Mandal BK. Once-weekly fluconazole to prevent recurrence of oropharyngeal candidiasis in patients with AIDS and AIDS-related complex: a double-blind placebo-controlled study. J Infect 21:55, 1990.
42. Jacobson MA, O'Donnell JJ, Porteous D, et al. Retinal and gastrointestinal disease due to cytomegalovirus in patients with the acquired immune deficiency syndrome: prevalence, natural history, and response to ganciclovir therapy. Q J Med 67:473, 1988.
43. Dieterich DT, Chachoua A, Lafleur F, Worrell C. Ganciclovir treatment of gastrointestinal infections caused by cytomegalovirus in patients with AIDS. Rev Infect Dis 10:532, 1988.
44. Wilcox CM, Straub RF, Schwartz DA. Cytomegalovirus esophagitis in AIDS: a prospective study of clinical response to ganciclovir therapy, relapse rate, and long-term outcome. Am J Med 98:169, 1995.
45. Blanshard C. Treatment of HIV-related cytomegalovirus disease of the gastrointestinal tract with foscarnet. J Acquir Immune Defic Syndr 5(suppl 1):S25, 1992.
46. Dieterich DT, Kotler DP, Busch DF, et al. Ganciclovir treatment of cytomegalovirus colitis in AIDS: a randomized, double-blind, placebo-controlled multicenter study. J Infect Dis 167:278, 1993.
47. Parente F, Bianchi Porro G. Treatment of cytomegalovirus esophagitis in patients with acquired immunodeficiency syndrome: a randomized controlled study of foscarnet versus ganciclovir; the Italian Cytomegalovirus Study Group. Am J Gastroenterol 93:317, 1998.
48. Blanshard C, Benhamou Y, Dohin E, et al. Treatment of AIDS-associated gastrointestinal cytomegalovirus infection with foscarnet and ganciclovir: a randomized comparison. J Infect Dis 172:622, 1995.
49. Mönkemüller KE, Wilcox CM. Esophageal ulcer caused by cytomegalovirus: resolution during combination antiretroviral therapy for acquired immunodeficiency syndrome. South Med J 93:818, 2000.
50. Piketty C, Bardin C, Gilquin J, et al. Low plasma concentrations achieved with conventional schedules of administration of ganciclovir in patients with AIDS. J Infect Dis 174:188, 1996.
51. Crumpacker CS. Ganciclovir. N Engl J Med 335:721, 1996.
52. Dieterich DT, Poles MA, Dicker M, et al. Foscarnet treatment of cytomegalovirus gastrointestinal infections in acquired immunodeficiency syndrome patients who have failed ganciclovir induction. Am J Gastroenterol 88:542, 1993.
53. Salzberger B, Stoehr A, Jablonowski H, et al. Foscarnet 5 versus 7 days a week treatment for severe gastrointestinal CMV-diseases in HIV-infected patients. Infection 24:121, 1996.
54. Salzberger B, Stoehr A, Heise W, et al. Foscarnet and ganciclovir combination therapy for CMV disease in HIV-infected patients. Infection 22:197, 1994.
55. Peters M, Schurmann D, Bergmann F, et al. Safety of alternating ganciclovir and foscarnet maintenance therapy in human immunodeficiency virus (HIV)-related cytomegalovirus infections: an open-labeled pilot study. Scand J Infect Dis 26:49, 1994.
56. Dieterich DT, Poles MA, Lew EA, et al. Concurrent use of ganciclovir and foscarnet to treat cytomegalovirus infection in AIDS patients. J Infect Dis 167:1184, 1993.
57. Combination foscarnet and ganciclovir therapy vs. monotherapy for the treatment of relapsed cytomegalovirus retinitis in patients with AIDS: studies of the Ocular Complications of AIDS Research Group in collaboration with the AIDS Clinical Trials Group. Arch Ophthalmol 114: 23, 1996.

58. Spector SA, Mc Kinley, Lalezari JP, et al. Oral ganciclovir for the prevention of cytomegalovirus disease in persons with AIDS. N Engl J Med 334:1491, 1996.
59. Laskin OL. Clinical pharmacokinetics of acyclovir. Clin Pharmacokinet 8:187, 1983.
60. Safrin S. Treatment of acyclovir-resistant herpes simplex virus in patients with AIDS. J Acquir Immun Defic Syndr 5(suppl):S29, 1992.
61. Hardy W. Foscarnet treatment of acyclovir-resistant herpes simplex virus in patients with acquired immunodeficiency syndrome: preliminary results a controlled, randomized, regimen-comparative trial. Am J Med 92:S30, 1992.
62. Wilcox CM, Schwartz DA. Comparison of two corticosteroid regimens for the treatment of idiopathic esophageal ulcerations associated with HIV infection. Am J Gastroenterol 89:2163, 1994.
63. Nelson MR, Erskine D, Hawkins DA, Gazzard BG. Treatment with corticosteroids: a risk factor for the development of clinical cytomegalovirus disease in AIDS. AIDS 7:375, 1993.
64. Paterson DL, Georghiou PR, Allworth AM, Kemp RJ. Thalidomide as treatment of refractory aphthous ulceration related to human immunodeficiency virus infection. Clin Infect Dis 20:250, 1995.
65. Alexander LN, Wilcox CM. A prospective trial of thalidomide for the treatment of HIV-associated idiopathic esophageal ulcers. AIDS Res Hum Retroviruses 13:301, 1997.
66. Battan R, Raviglione MC, Palagiano A, et al. *Helicobacter pylori* infection in patients with acquired immunodeficiency syndrome. Am J Gastroenterol 85:1576, 1990.
67. Cacciarelli AG, Marano BJ Jr, Gualtieri NM, et al. Lower *Helicobacter pylori* infection and peptic ulcer disease prevalence in patients with AIDS and suppressed CD4 counts. Am J Gastroenterol 91:1783, 1996.
68. Marano BJ Jr, Smith F, Bonanno CA. *Helicobacter pylori* prevalence in acquired immunodeficiency syndrome. Am J Gastroenterol 88:687, 1993.
69. Edwards PD, Carrick J, Turner J, et al. *Helicobacter pylori*-associated gastritis is rare in AIDS: antibiotic effect or a consequence of immunodeficiency? Am J Gastroenterol 86:1761, 1991.
70. Mönkemüller KE, Call SA, Lazenby AJ, Wilcox CM. Declining prevalence of opportunistic gastrointestinal disease in the era of combination antiretroviral therapy. Am J Gastroenterol 95:457, 2000.
71. Varsky CG, Correa MC, Sarmiento N, et al. Prevalence and etiology of gastroduodenal ulcer in HIV-positive patients: a comparative study of 497 symptomatic subjects evaluated by endoscopy. Am J Gastroenterol 93:935, 1998.
72. Barone JE, Gingold BS, Arvanitis ML, et al. Abdominal pain in patients with AIDS. Ann Surg 204:619, 1986.
73. Sievert W, LaBrooy JT. HIV-related gastrointestinal disease. Med J Aust 158:175, 1993.
74. Thuluvath PJ, Connolly GM, Forbes A, et al. Abdominal pain in HIV infection. Q J Med 78:275, 1993.
75. Mönkemüller KE, Wilcox CM. Diagnosis and treatment of colonic disease in AIDS. Gastrointest Endosc Clin North Am 8:889, 1998.
76. Binderow SR, Cavallo RJ, Freed J. Laboratory parameters as predictors of operative outcome after major abdominal surgery in AIDS and HIV-infected patients. Am Surg 59:754, 1993.
77. Jeffrey RB, Nyberg DA, Bottles K, et al. Abdominal CT in acquired immunodeficiency syndrome. AJR Am J Roentgenol 146:7, 1986.
78. Lucas GW. Laparoscopy in the evaluation and treatment of patients with AIDS and acute abdominal complaints. Surg Endosc 11:1026, 1997.
79. Endres JC, Salky BA. Laparoscopy in AIDS. Gastrointest Endosc Clin North Am 8:975, 1998.
80. Tanner AG, Hartley JE, Darzi A, et al. Laparoscopic surgery in patients with immunodeficiency virus. Br J Surg 81:1647, 1994.
81. Lebovits AH, Lefkowitz M, McCarty D, et al. The prevalence and management of pain in patients with AIDS: a review of 134 cases. Clin J Pain 5:245, 1989.
82. Smith PD, Quinn TC, Strober W, et al. Gastrointestinal infections in AIDS. Ann Intern Med 116:63, 1992.
83. Blanshard C, Francis N, Gazzard BG. Investigation of chronic diarrhea in acquired immunodeficiency syndrome: a prospective study of 155 patients. Gut 39:824, 1996.
84. Connolly GM, Dryden MS, Shanson DC, Gazzard BG. Cryptosporidial diarrhea in AIDS and its treatment. Gut 29:593, 1988.
85. Goldstein ST, Juranek DD, Ravenholt O, et al. Cryptosporidiosis: an outbreak associated with drinking water despite state-of-the-art water treatment. Ann Intern Med 124:459, 1996.
86. Goodgame RW. Understanding intestinal spore-forming protozoa: cryptosporidia, microsporidia, *Isospora*, and *Cyclospora*. Ann Intern Med 124:429, 1996.
87. Kotler DP, Orenstein JM. Prevalence of intestinal microsporidiosis in HIV-infected pateints referred for gastroenterological evaluation. Am J Gastroenterol 89:1998, 1994.
88. Asmuth DM, DeGirolami PC, Federman M, et al. Clinical features of microsporidiosis in patients with AIDS. Clin Infect Dis 18:819, 1994.
89. Pape JW, Verdier R-I, Boncy M, et al. *Cyclospora* infection in adults infected with HIV: clinical manifestations, treatment, and prophylaxis. Ann Intern Med 121:654, 1994.
90. Hoover DR, Saah AJ, Bacellar H, et al. Clinical manifestations of AIDS in the era of *Pneumocystis* prophylaxis. N Engl J Med 329:1922, 1993.
91. Nightingale SD, Byrd LT, Southern PM, et al. Incidence of *Mycobacterium avium-intracellulare* complex bacteremia in human immunodeficiency virus-positive patients. J Infect Dis 165:1082, 1992.
92. Gray JR, Rabeneck L. Atypical mycobacterial infection of the gastrointestinal tract in AIDS patients. Am J Gastroenterol 84:1521, 1989.
93. Cunningham AL, Grohman GS, Harkness J, et al. Gastrointestinal viral infections in homosexual men who were symptomatic and seropositive for human immunodeficiency virus. J Infect Dis 158:386, 1988.
94. Grohmann GS, Glass RI, Pereira HG, et al. Enteric viruses and diarrhea in HIV-infected patients. N Engl Med 329:14, 1993.
95. Flanigan T, Whalen C, Turner J, et al. *Cryptosporidium* infection and CD4 counts. Ann Intern Med 116:840, 1992.
96. McGowan I, Hawkins AS, Weller IVD. The natural history of cryptosporidia diarrhea in HIV-infected patients. AIDS 7:349, 1993.
97. Benson C. Disseminated *Mycobacterium avium-intracellulare* complex in patients with AIDS. AIDS Res Hum Retroviruses 10:913, 1994.
98. Farhi DC, Mason UG, Horsburgh CR. Pathologic findings in disseminated *Mycobacterium avium-intracellulare* infection. Am J Clin Pathol 85:67, 1986.
99. Gordin FM, Cohn DL, Sullam PM, et al. Early manifestations of disseminated *Mycobacterium avium* complex disease; a prospective evaluation. J Infect Dis 176:126, 1997.
100. Kotler DP, Giang TT, Garro ML, Orenstein JM. Light microscopic diagnosis of microsporidiosis in patients with AIDS. Am J Gastroenterol 89:540, 1994.
101. Farthing MJG. Giardiasis. Gastroenterol Clin North Am 25:493, 1996.
102. Chin DP, Hopewell PC, Yajko DM, et al. *Mycobacterium avium* complex in the respiratory or gastrointestinal tract and the risk of *M. avium* complex bacteremia in patients with human immunodeficiency virus infection. J Infect Dis 169:289, 1994.
103. Armitage K, Flanigan T, Carey J, et al. Treatment of cryptosporidiosis with paromomycin. Arch Intern Med 152:2497, 1992.
104. Greenberg RE, Mir R, Bank S, Siegal FP. Resolution of intestinal cryptosporidiosis after treatment of AIDS with AZT. Gastroenterology 97:1327, 1989.
105. Foudraine NA, Weverling GJ, van Gool T, et al. Improvement in chronic diarrhoea in patients with advanced HIV-1 infection during potent antiretroviral therapy. AIDS 12:35, 1998.
106. Simon D, Weiss L, Tanowitz HB, Wittner M. Resolution of *Cryptosporidium* infection in an AIDS patient after improvement of nutritional and immune status with octreotide. Am J Gastroenterol 86:615, 1991.
107. Shield J, Melville C, Novelli V, et al. Bovine colostrum immunoglobulin concentrate for cryptosporidiosis in AIDS. Arch Dis Child 69:451, 1993.
108. Greenberg PD, Cello JP. Treatment of severe diarrhea caused by *Cryptosporidium parvum* with oral bovine immunoglobulin concentrate in patients with AIDS. J Acquir Immune Defic Syndr Hum Retrovirol 13:348, 1996.
109. Loeb M, Walach C, Phillips J, et al. Treatment with letrazuril of refractory cryptosporidial diarrhea complicating AIDS. J Acquir Immune Defic Syndr Hum Retrovirol 10:48, 1995.
110. White AC, Chappell CL, Hayat CS, et al. Paromomycin for cryptosporidiosis in AIDS: a prospective, double-blind trial. J Infect Dis 170:419, 1994.
111. Scaglia M, Atzori C, Marchetti G, et al. Effectiveness of aminosidine (paromomycin) sulfate in chronic *Cryptosporidium* diarrhea in AIDS patients: an open, uncontrolled, prospective clinical trial. J Infect Dis 170:1349, 1994.

112. Bissuel F, Cotte L, Rabodonirina M, et al. Paromomycin: an effective treatment for cryptosporidial diarrhea in patients with AIDS. Clin Infect Dis 18:447, 1994.
113. Clezy K, Gold J, Jones P. Paromomycin for the treatment of cryptosporidial diarrhoea in AIDS patients. AIDS 5:1146, 1991.
114. Hewitt RG, Yiannoutsos CT, Higgs ES, et al. Paromomycin: no more effective than placebo for treatment of cryptosporidiosis in patients with advanced human immunodeficiency virus infection. Clin Infect Dis 31:1084, 2000.
115. Carr A, Marriott D, Field A, et al. Treatment of HIV-1 associated microsporidiosis and cryptosporidiosis with combination antiretroviral therapy. Lancet 351:256, 1998.
116. Eeftinck Schattenkerk JKM, van Gool T, van Ketel RJ, et al. Clinical significance of small-intestinal microsporidiosis in HIV-1-infected individuals. Lancet 337:895, 1991.
117. Dore GJ, Marriott DJ, Hing MC, et al. Disseminated microsporidiosis due to *Septata intestinalis* in nine patients infected with the human immunodeficiency virus: response to therapy with albendazole. Clin Infect Dis 21:70, 1995.
118. Molina JM, Oksenhendler E, Beauvais B, et al. Disseminated microsporidiosis due to *Septata intestinalis* in patients with AIDS: clinical features and response to albendazole therapy. J Infect Dis 171:245, 1995.
118a. Molina JM, Tourneur M, Sarfati C, et al. Fumagillin treatment of intestinal microsporidiosis. N Engl J Med 346:1963, 2002.
119. Anwar-Bruni DM, Hogan SE, Schwartz DA, et al. Atovaquone is effective treatment for the symptoms of gastrointestinal microsporidiosis in HIV-1 infected patients. AIDS 10:619, 1996.
120. DeHovitz JA, Pape JW, Boncy M, Johnson WD Jr. Clinical manifestations and treatment of *Isospora belli* infection in patients with acquired immunodeficiency syndrome. N Engl J Med 315:87, 1986.
121. Rene E, Marche C, Regnier B, et al. Intestinal infections in patients with acquired immunodeficiency syndrome: a prospective study in 132 patients. Dig Dis Sci 34:773, 1989.
122. Smith PD, Macher AM, Bookman MA, et al. *Salmonella typhimurium* enteritis and bacteremia in the acquired immunodeficiency syndrome. Ann Intern Med 102:207, 1985.
123. Molina JM, Casin I, Hausfater P, et al. *Campylobacter* infections in HIV-infected patients: clinical and bacteriological features. AIDS 9:881, 1995.
124. Hutin Y, Molina JM, Casin I, et al. Risk factors for *Clostridium difficile*-associated diarrhoea in HIV-infected patients. AIDS 7:1441, 1993.
125. Janoff EN, Orenstein JM, Manischewitz JF, Smith PD. Adenovirus colitis in the acquired immunodeficiency syndrome. Gastroenterology 100:976, 1991.
126. Jessurun J, Barron-Rodriquez LP, Fernandez-Tinoco G, Hernandez-Avila M. The prevalence of invasive amebiasis is not increased in patients with AIDS. AIDS 6:307, 1992.
127. Halline AG, Maldonado-Lutomirsky, Ryoo JW, et al. Colonic histoplasmosis in AIDS: unusual endoscopic findings in two cases. Gastrointest Endosc 45:199, 1997.
128. Mönkemüller KE, Bussian AH, Lazenby AJ, Wilcox CM. Special histologic stains are rarely beneficial for the evaluation of HIV-related gastrointestinal infections. Am J Clin Pathol 114:387, 2000.
129. Burchard GD, Hufert FT, Mirelman D. Characterisation of 20 *Entamoeba histolytica* strains isolated from patients with HIV infection. Infection 19:44, 1991.
130. Kemper CA, Meng T-C, Nussbaum J, et al. Treatment of *Mycobacterium avium* complex bacteremia in AIDS with a four-drug oral regimen: rifampin, ethambutol, clofazimine, and ciprofloxacin. Ann Intern Med 116:466, 1992.
131. Shafran SD, Singer J, Zarowny DP, et al. A comparision of two regimens for the treatment of *Mycobacterium avium* complex bacteremia in AIDS: rifabutin, ethambutol, and clarithromycin versus rifampin, ethambutol, clofazimine, and ciprofloxacin. N Engl J Med 335:377, 1996.
132. Cello JP, Grendell JH, Basuk P, et al. Effect of octreotide on refractory AIDS-associated diarrhea: a prospective multicenter clinical trial. Ann Intern Med 115:705, 1991.
133. Compean DG, Jimenez JR, De La Garza FG, et al. Octreotide therapy of large-volume refractory AIDS-associated diarrhea: a randomized controlled trial. AIDS 8:1563, 1994.
134. Montaner JSG, Harris AG, Octreotide International Multicentre AIDS-Diarrhea Study Group. Octreotide therapy in AIDS-related, refractory diarrhea: results of a multicentre Canadian-European study [letter]. AIDS 9:209, 1995.
135. Simon DM, Cello JP, Valenzuela J, et al. Multicenter trial of octreotide in patients with refractory acquired immunodeficiency syndrome-associated diarrhea. Gastroenterology 108:1753, 1995.

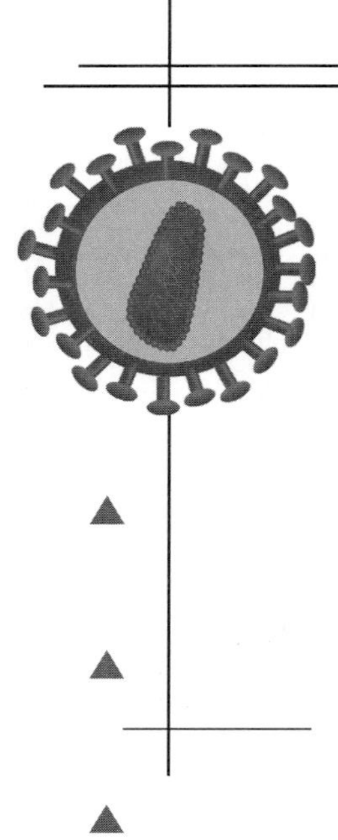

CHAPTER 65

Hepatic and Hepatobiliary Diseases

Raymond T. Chung, MD
Kenneth E. Sherman, MD, PhD

Diseases of the liver have become a major source of morbidity and mortality in patients with human immunodeficiency virus (HIV) infection. Use of highly active antiretroviral therapy (HAART) has effectively changed the spectrum of disease processes encountered by clinicians. Although immune reconstitution and prevention of severe acquired immunodeficiency has decreased the prevalence of most opportunistic infections, the high prevalence of chronic hepatotropic viruses in this population has become increasingly troublesome.[1] Furthermore, the very medications that improve life expectancy in HIV-infected patients may alter hepatic metabolism and produce features of direct and indirect hepatotoxicity.[2] Finally, some of the more common metabolic disorders of the liver assume increased importance because of their contribution to chronic liver disease. The evaluation and management of hepatic and hepatobiliary diseases has become a critical consideration for health care providers caring for patients with HIV infection.

▲ CLINICAL EVALUATION

History

Obtaining a detailed history related to liver disease is perhaps the most critical element of an evaluation of the patient with clinical or biochemical evidence of liver injury. Disease processes that must be considered include viral infections, medications, recreational drugs, toxic occupational exposures, vascular/thrombotic disorders, and inherited metabolic conditions. A detailed history of potential exposure to hepatotropic viruses is important for establishing a timeline for infection. This history should include the year of first exposure to intravenous drugs, nasal cocaine use, tattoos, body piercing, blood transfusion, and sexual exposures. Studies of injection drug users suggest that most of those with chronic hepatitis C (HCV) infection become infected during the first year of abuse. Risk of HCV was common in patients who received blood and blood products prior to 1991. Nearly all hemophilic men who required pooled factors are HCV-infected. High-risk sexual behavior is a clear risk for hepatitis B infection and probably for HCV as well.[3]

Medication history must be detailed and include all drugs started or stopped within a 3-month period. It is critical to include medications used transiently. For example, the use of common antibiotics such as amoxicillin-clavulinic acid (Augmentin) can cause severe cholestasis 2 to 12 weeks after a short drug course and is often missed by health care providers as a potential cause of liver injury.[4] Drug interactions must also be considered because some medications compete for active binding sites in hepatic mixed-function oxidase or cytochrome pathways, leading to toxic injury. Alcohol use alters the metabolism of many drugs by direct competition or enzyme induction in these pathways. Alcohol use should be estimated in terms of grams of ethanol ingested per day.

Family history is essential for establishing the possibility that the patient has an underlying inborn error of metabolism. A history of early cirrhosis (<45 years old) even in a relative described as an alcoholic should raise suspicion of a coexistent metabolic cause of injury. For instance, hereditary hemochromatosis and α_1-antitrypsin deficiency are quite common in certain ethnic groups.[5]

A review of the medical history for a patient with HIV infection must also include a detailed assessment of immunologic status. Patients with very low CD4+ T-lymphocyte counts (<50 cells/μl) are more susceptible to hepatic injury from infiltrative processes (Kaposi's sarcoma, non-Hodgkin's lymphoma, granulomatous disease) and less susceptible to injury from hepatitis B than those with a CD4+ T-lymphocyte count higher that 500 cells/μl. Patients who have undergone immune reconstitution may represent a special risk in terms of injury from hepatitis B[6] and hepatitis C. Because immune reconstitution is generally associated with use of highly active antiretroviral agents, which may independently cause liver toxicity, the health care provider must carefully document the timing of immunologic recovery as related to onset of liver injury.

Physical Examination

The physical examination may provide valuable information related to chronicity and occasionally to etiology. The HEENT (head, ears, eyes, nose, throat) examination should focus on the presence or absence of scleral icterus. Mild jaundice may be observed by experienced clinicians when the serum bilirubin level is 2 to 3 mg/dl. The sclera are examined first, but the underside of the tongue may also yield evidence of mild yellowing. This feature may be particularly useful in dark-skinned patients with muddy sclerae. The eyelids may show xanthomatous changes, which can occur with chronic cholestasis.

The abdomen must be carefully evaluated in patients suspected of having liver disease. Hepatomegaly with palpation tenderness suggests an acute process, though several series have reported a high prevalence of hepatic enlargement in patients with HIV. Preferential hypertrophy of the left lobe is often seen with chronic liver disease. The triad of hepatomegaly, pain on liver palpation, and ascites suggest the possibility of a vascular thrombosis of the hepatic vein (Budd-Chiari syndrome). The presence of ascites mandates a workup for the etiology, but nonhepatic causes (including severe malnutrition and nephrotic syndrome) must be considered in addition to end-stage liver disease. The presence of a caput on the anterior surface of the abdomen suggests portal hypertension, as does splenomegaly.

The skin examination should include evaluation for spider angiomas on the chest and back and palmar erythema. The latter is not specific for liver disease, however, and infact is seen in the absence of liver disease, particularly in women. The presence of excoriations raises the possibility of a severe cholestatic process associated with severe pruritus. Drug reactions may cause erythematous eruptions and urticaria.

Neurologic evaluation should include observation for a "flap" of the extended hand, which is seen in patients with late-stage liver disease and reflects the presence of hepatic encephalopathy. A number connection test to evaluate concentration is a valuable tool for clinical management of patients with encephalopathy.[7]

▲ BIOCHEMICAL TESTS

Liver Injury and Synthetic Function

Biochemical screening tests for liver disease generally include a panel of tests that help identify and categorize the type of liver injury. Common tests of liver injury and function can be divided into three groups: (1) tests of hepatocellular injury; (2) tests of cholestatic injury; and (3) tests of liver function capacity.[8,9]

The serum transaminase assay provides an indication of the likelihood and severity of active liver injury. The most sensitive, specific test for hepatocellular injury is the serum alanine aminotransferase (ALT, SGPT) assay. ALT is found predominantly in the cytoplasm of hepatocytes. Cell death leads to release of ALT into the serum, where its enzymatic activity is measured in a standardized reaction system. Most laboratories utilize local ranges of normal derived from "healthy" controls combined with the determination of an arbitrary cutoff for the upper limit of normal determined by the distribution of the "normal" sample population. It is important to understand that the likelihood of liver disease is proportional to the increase in ALT but not absolutely so. Thus not all patients with mildly increased ALT levels have discernible liver injury, and not all patients with ALT levels in the locally defined normal range lack liver injury. Women tend to have lower ALT levels than men, and standardization is often not gender-adjusted. Therefore the frequency of liver injury in women tends to be underestimated.

The other commonly reported serum transaminase is aspartate aminotransferase (AST, SGOT). This enzyme is present in hepatocytes but is found in high concentrations in muscle, erythrocytes, and other tissues as well. Therefore elevated AST levels are sometimes attributable to nonhepatic etiologies.

During the course of infection, up to 70% of patients with HIV infection have been reported to have abnormally high serum transaminase levels. This high prevalence has prompted a higher threshold for evaluating mild to moderately increased ALT/AST levels in HIV-infected patients. It is important to understand, though, that even mild chronic injury may result in fibrosis and eventual hepatic decompensation. An algorithm for evaluating patients with laboratory evidence of hepatocellular injury is shown in Figure 65–1.

Cholestatic injury is indicated by an elevated alkaline phosphatase level, an inducible enzyme produced by hepatocytes. Failure to excrete bile acids (as is seen with cholestasis) leads to induction of alkaline phosphatase, which is excreted into the serum. Alkaline phosphatase activity can be measured by a specific, well defined action on a substrate. Bile acid concentration may be increased by a variety of mechanisms including drug-induced canalicular transport dysfunction (e.g., chlorpromazine), small bile duct injury (e.g., primary biliary cirrhosis), large bile duct narrowing (e.g., acquired immunodeficiency syndrome [AIDS] cholangiopathy, cholangiocarcinoma), or following acute hepatocellular injury (posthepatitic cholestasis). Because alkaline phosphatase levels can also be due to abnormalities in bone, intestine, and salivary glands, confirmation of a liver source generally requires a concomitant elevation of γ-glutamyl transpeptidase (GGT) or 5′-nucleotidase. These liver enzymes are also induced by bile acids, and the GGT is induced by a variety of drugs and alcohol as well. It is important to note that increased GGT merely suggests cholestasis; it is *not* a marker of hepatocellular injury, as is

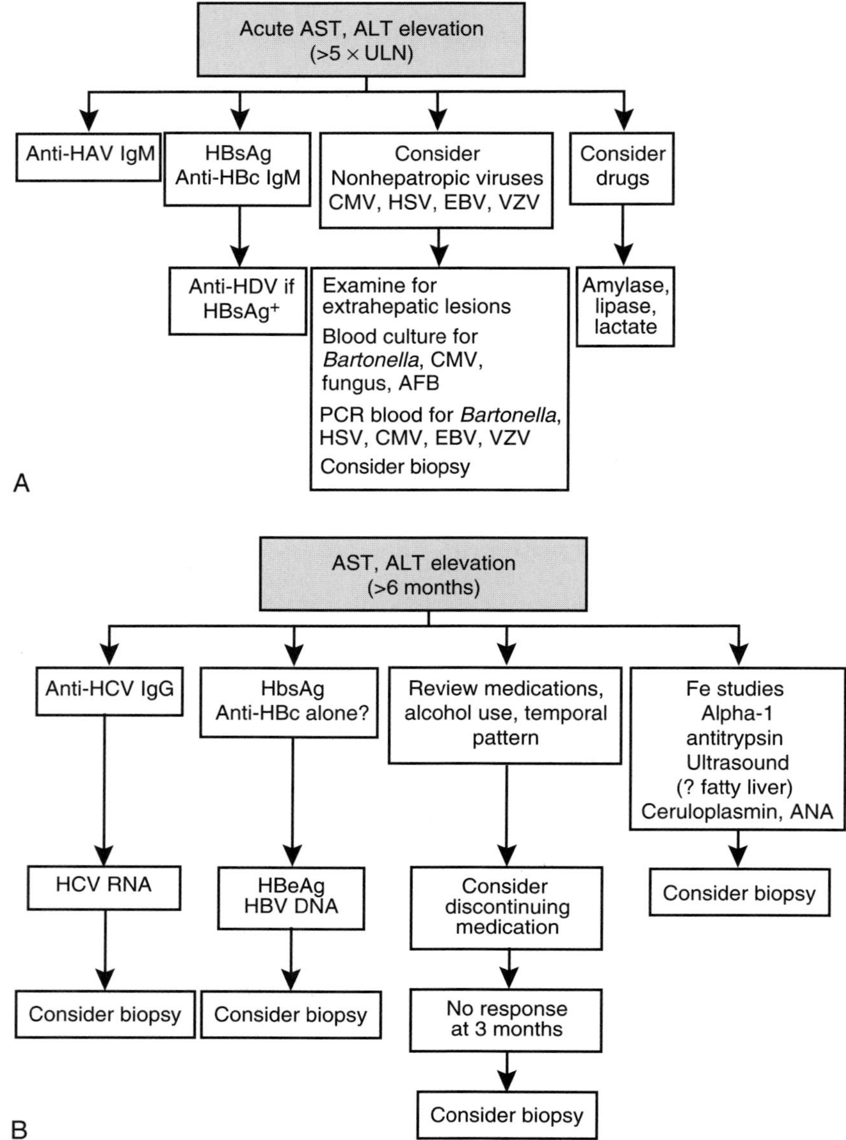

Figure 65–1. Algorithm for evaluating HIV-infected patients with increased serum transaminases consistent with a hepatocellular injury pattern. ALT, alanine aminotransferase; anti-HAV, hepatitis A antibody; anti-HDV, hepatitis D antibody; ART, antiretroviral therapy; AST, aspartate aminotransferase; HbeAg, hepatitis B "e" antigen; HbsAg, hepatitis B surface antigen; HBV DNA, hepatitis B DNA assay.

often mistakenly thought. The complete evaluation of patients with a cholestatic injury is described in Figure 65–2.

Frequently, the term "liver function tests" is used to describe basic biochemical tests of the liver; but this is a misrepresentation, as none of the above named tests measures liver function. Typical chemical profiles often include albumin, which *is* a measure of liver synthetic function. However, the serum albumin level may be abnormally low in patients with nephrotic-range proteinuria or in those with malnutrition. The prothrombin time (PT) is a more reliable measure of the liver's ability to manufacture clotting factors (II, VII, IX, X). Therefore, a prolonged PT is a measure of liver synthetic function, although it may also be abnormal because of severe cholestasis and malabsorption of fat-soluble vitamin K. Administration of parenteral vitamin K (10 mg SC or IV) corrects the PT within 3 days and therefore differentiates cholestasis from abnormal liver function due to a shortage of substrate. Specific measurements of liver function include studies of drug metabolism and clearance. Caffeine, bromsulphalein (BSP), and iodocyanine green clearance have all been utilized. Commercial test kits are available for evaluation of MEG-X, which is a metabolic by-product of liver metabolism of lidocaine. Unfortunately, these studies have not been helpful for discrim-

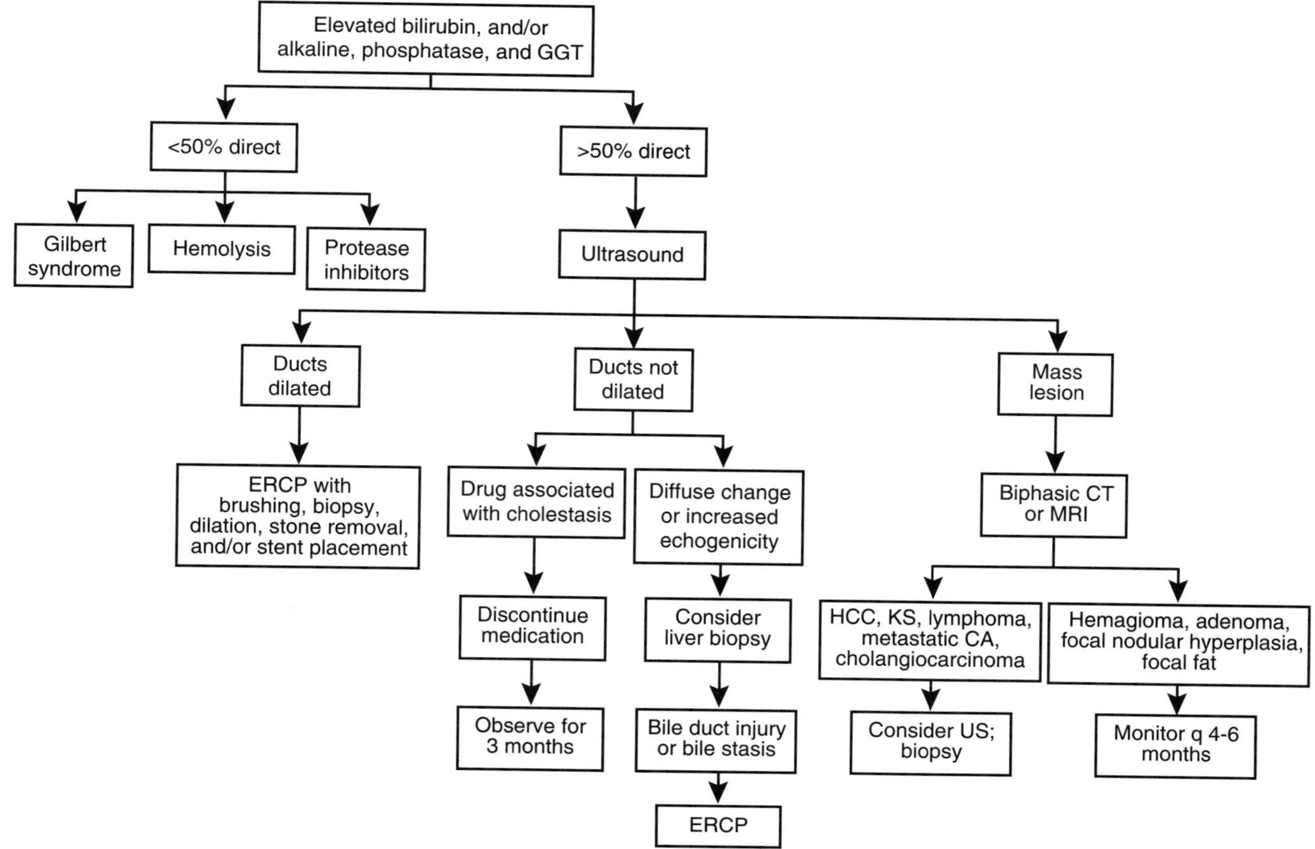

Figure 65–2. Algorithm for evaluating of HIV-infected patients with laboratory evidence of a cholestatic injury pattern. ERCP, endoscopic retrograde cholangiopancreatography; FNH, focal nodular hyperplasia; GOT, γ-glutamyltranspeptidase; HCC, hepatocellular carcinoma; KS, Kaposi's sarcoma; 5′NT, 5′-nucleotidase.

inating clinically relevant disease stages and are generally used only in the research setting.

Laboratory Evaluation for Disease Etiology

Although the tests described in the previous section define and classify liver injury, they do not necessarily identify specific etiologies. Some diagnoses are those of exclusion, combined with pertinent historical positives (e.g., drug injury), and others require specific biochemical or serologic tests to suggest or confirm the etiology. The range of diagnoses that must be considered is listed in Table 65–1.

The hepatotropic viruses represent the most important group of infectious agents. Their diagnoses are discussed in turn with specific reference to considerations in patients with HIV infection.

Acute hepatitis A virus (HAV) infection is identified by the appearance of immunoglobulin M (IgM) class antibodies against HAV. The assay turns positive shortly after the infection is established and is considered diagnostic of acute hepatitis A. Many clinical laboratories utilize a test that detects a combination of IgM and IgG antibodies, requiring further testing of IgM class antibody alone to distinguish between acute infection and past exposure. Therefore the clinician should request fractionation in cases of suspected acute hepatitis A. Prevention of hepatitis A is based on administration of a commercially available hepatitis A vaccine. A sometimes difficult decision for the clinician is whether to test for naturally acquired antibodies prior to vaccine administration. Prevaccination cutoff thresholds for anti-HAV testing based on its age-specific disease prevalence in the general population have been used, but this analysis is not available for patients with HIV infection.[10] As a general rule, patients with a high pretest probability of prior hepatitis A exposure (low socioeconomic strata, homosexual men with multiple partners) should be tested for antibody prior to vaccine use.

Hepatitis B virus (HBV) infection is generally diagnosed by the presence of circulating hepatitis B surface antigen (HBsAg). The infection is classified as acute or chronic by distinguishing whether IgM or IgG class antibodies are present directed against the virus core (anti-HBc), respectively. Tests for IgG, IgM, and both (total) are available. As with HAV diagnosis, the clinician should select the correct test for the clinical setting rather than relying on laboratory defaults. Patients with chronic hepatitis B should be evaluated for the degree of viral replication, which generally correlates with the degree of associated liver injury. Traditionally, the replicative state has been determined by

Table 65–1. DISEASES AFFECTING THE LIVER AND BILIARY TREE IN HIV INFECTION

Viral Hepatitis
Hepatotropic
Hepatitis A virus
Hepatitis B virus/hepatitis D virus
Hepatitis C virus
Nonhepatotropic
Cytomegalovirus
Herpes simplex virus
Epstein-Barr virus
Varicella-zoster virus
Human herpesvirus-6
Adenovirus
HIV
Fungal Liver Disease
Candida albicans
Histoplasma capsulatum
Parasitic Liver Disease
Leishmania donovani
Pneumocystis carinii
Microsporidia
Bacterial Liver Disease
Bacillary angiomatosis
Granulomatous Liver Disease
Mycobacterium tuberculosis
Mycobacterium avium complex
Toxic/Metabolic Liver Disease
Fatty liver, nonalcoholic steatohepatitis
Nucleoside reverse transcriptase inhibitors (NRTIs)
Protease inhibitors (PIs)
Nonnucleoside reverse transcriptase inhibitors (NNRTIs)
Alcohol
Other medications
Neoplastic Liver Disease
Kaposi's sarcoma
Non-Hodgkin's lymphoma
Hepatocellular carcinoma
AIDS Cholangiopathy
Sclerosing cholangitis
Papillary stenosis
Long extrahepatic bile duct strictures
Gallbladder Disease
Acalculous cholecystitis

testing the level of HBV DNA in serum using a branched-chain-based assay (Quantiplex) or a hybridization-based assay. Whereas qualitative polymerase chain reaction (PCR) assays are not acceptable alternatives because their inordinate level of sensitivity fails to define the replicative state, quantitative PCR assays (Monitor) may provide useful information. Hepatitis B "e" antigen (HBeAg) is generally associated with replicative levels of HBV DNA and may serve as a surrogate marker of replication. The presence of hepatitis B "e" antibody (HBeAb), conversely, is often a marker of a low or nonreplicative state. In patients with HIV infection, unique clinical scenarios uncommon in immunocompetent patients may occur. Data from at least one study suggest that a subset of patients with IgG anti-hepatitis B core (HBc) and without detectable HBsAg may harbor active HBV replication with associated liver injury.[11] These cases can be diagnosed only by using a sensitive PCR-based HBV DNA assay. With chronic HBV infection treated with lamivudine, a high rate of mutant virus breakthrough can be identified by the presence of HBV DNA by branched-chain or hybridization assays.[6] Testing for a specific mutation in a area called the YMDD motif is available in some research laboratories.

Hepatitis C virus infection can be detected by use of an enzyme-linked immunosorbent assay (ELISA or EIA). This test is highly sensitive, though false positives in patients with a low pretest probability of disease are common. False-negative reactions are sometimes observed in patients with HIV. The prevalence of this finding has been reported to range from 1.5% to nearly 10.0% in some series. Seroreversion associated with worsening immune function has also been described.[12] If HCV infection is strongly suspected and the HCV ELISA is negative, an HCV RNA test is indicated. Although HCV RNA detection represents the gold standard in terms of sensitivity and specificity, its accuracy and reliability have been low in some blind test panels of laboratories that routinely test for HCV RNA. Therefore the diagnosis and treatment intervention decisions should not be based on a single HCV RNA assay alone. Recombinant immunoblot assays (RIBA) may also serve to confirm infection in patients with a low pretest probability of infection.

Hepatitis D virus (HDV) infection is uncommon in the United States but much more prevalent in Mediterranean rim countries. Because it requires the presence of hepatitis B for its own replication, the diagnosis of HDV should be considered only in the presence of HBsAg. The presence of HDV antibody suggests active infection.

Hepatitis E virus (HEV) may be detected using commercial antibody assay kits. Uncommon in the United States and Western Europe, its prevalence has been shown to be increased in HIV-infected women in Brazil, though this may have been more related to socioeconomic status than to HIV.[13]

Other common liver diseases of adults that warrant investigation include α-antitrypsin deficiency (AAT) and hereditary hemochromatosis. The gene frequencies for defects in the AAT coding domain, which result in abnormal protein expression, exceed 5% in some populations. Initial testing makes use of a specific monoclonal antibody that binds serum AAT and can be used to determine the AAT level. Low levels are consistent with an AAT deficiency, which results from a conformational change in the protein. Confirmation of the diagnosis requires phenotyping on an isoelectric focusing gel. Wild-type AAT is classified as MM, based on its migration to the midpoint of the gel. Homozygote and heterozygote alleles migrate differently. The "Z" phenotype (pi type) is considered an important factor in chronic liver disease.

Hereditary hemochromatosis results from a gene defect in duodenal transport of iron by the protein HFE, which leads to excess iron absorption and end-organ injury in the liver and other organs. This excess iron results in increases in the iron storage protein ferritin, which suggests the presence of this disease. However, because ferritin is an acute-phase reactant, a more reliable index is iron saturation [Fe/total iron-binding capacity (TIBC)]. Saturations of more than 50% suggest the possible presence of hereditary hemochromatosis. Patients with hereditary hemochromatosis have substitution mutations in two loci in HFE, which can be tested by specific PCR amplification. Homozygosity for the *C282Y* mutation, seen in up to 90% of patients with hereditary hemochromatosis, or compound heterozygosity for *C282Y* and *H63D*, are associated with the disease. Tests for both of these mutations are available from specialized clinical laboratories. Ultimately, the level of iron storage and injury are determined by histologic evaluation of liver tissue. Quantitative evaluation of liver tissue permits calculation of an age-controlled index of hepatic iron content.

▲ LIVER IMAGING

A number of modalities for liver imaging are available to clinicians. The strengths and weaknesses of liver imaging methods in the context of HIV-positive patients mirror the characteristics in subjects without HIV infection. However, some liver disease processes are more prevalent in HIV patients, and the diagnosis may be enhanced by the correct choice of imaging study.

Liver/Spleen Scan and SPECT

Use of radionuclides such as technetium 99m-labeled sulfur colloid relies on the functional capacity of liver phagocytes to take up the label, retain and concentrate it during the scanning process, and be quantitatively measured by a photon camera. The methodology assumes that there is uniform uptake of the radionuclide in the liver parenchyma. Thus any disease process that alters the distribution or function of phagocytes alters the uptake pattern. Cysts, abscesses, and tumors fail to take up the sulfur colloid and appear as a "cold" spot on the subsequent image. Patients with portal hypertension demonstrate an altered pattern of uptake, with increased radionuclide in the spleen or bone marrow relative to the liver ("colloid shift"). Although ^{99m}Tc-labeled colloid studies are easily obtained in most centers, they have been largely supplanted by other imaging modalities in terms of accuracy, lesion discrimination, and resolution.

Traditional planar imaging efficacy may be improved by the use of single-photon emission computed tomography (SPECT), which permits three-dimensional evaluation of the radionuclide uptake. However, current computed tomography (CT) and magnetic resource imaging (MRI) scanning permit resolution at levels much higher than with SPECT. The role of SPECT in evaluating of fibrosis in HIV-infected patients with hepatitis C is under clinical investigation.

Biliary Scintigraphy

Using technetium 99m radiotracers attached to compounds that are taken up by hepatocytes and excreted into the biliary tract, biliary scintigraphy permits evaluation of bile excretion and creates images that define the biliary anatomy. A number of compounds have been studied, including *N;N*-(2,6-dimethylphenyl)carbamoylmethyl iminodiacetic acid (HIDA) and other diacetic acid derivatives. Patients with severe liver disease lack the functional capacity for radiotracer uptake and fail to "light up" the liver during the early phases of scanning. Following uptake, scanning during the excretion phase might reveal blockage in the biliary tree evidenced by a discrete cutoff of photon emission in the areas distal to the obstruction. These studies may have some value for identifying biliary obstruction, but endoscopic retrograde cholangiopancreatography (ERCP) and MR cholangiography have largely supplanted reliance on these imaging studies. Trials of hepatobiliary scintigraphy suggested a high correlation between biliary scintigraphy and ERCP in patients with AIDS-related cholangiopathy, but large clinical trials have not been reported.[14,15]

Ultrasonography and Doppler Ultrasonography

Sound pulses in the 2- to 5-MHz range are used to discern differences in soft tissues and fluids based on the "echo" return to a receiver probe. Transcutaneous ultrasonography has become an important noninvasive modality for assessing certain types of liver disease. Mass lesions can be discerned from normal liver tissue by the differences in the echogenicity of the lesion relative to its surroundings. A diffusely hyperechoic liver suggests the presence of an infiltrating process or a change in the water content of the hepatocytes. This finding may be observed in patients with diffuse fibrosis, fatty liver, or lymphoma. The bile ducts can be clearly visualized along with the gallbladder, and gallstones demonstrate a characteristic appearance with high echogenicity and shadowing. Ultrasonography is available in most clinical settings and is rapid and noninvasive—hence its popularity as a first-line choice for liver imaging, although the clinician must be aware of its limitations. It is highly operator-dependent and is often performed by technicians, with only selected images reviewed by radiologists, and the interpretation is highly subjective. Moreover, patients with truncal obesity may be too large to permit adequate penetration of the sound pulses to the liver below, and gas in the bowel may obscure the image. The resolution of ultrasound seans for discrete lesions is such that the reliability of detection is decreased for lesions less than 1 cm in diameter. The bile ducts represent an interface between the liver parenchyma and a fluid-filled tube. Ultrasonography excels in defining the size and path of bile ducts as small as 3 to 5 mm and is the screening test of choice for patients with cholestatic patterns of liver disease. It is also excellent for identifying the presence or absence of ascites.

It is important to note that ultrasonography is not useful for defining the presence of fibrosis or cirrhosis, and it rarely helps define the etiology of noncholestatic processes disease. Beale et al. found that 75% of 48 HIV-infected individuals had abnormal liver ultrasound scans. A diffusely hyperechoic liver was observed in 46% of patients, which was attributed mainly to steatosis. However, on biopsy nearly half of the patients had more than one histologic abnormality.[16] Albisetti et al. reported that significant hepatic steatosis on liver biopsy was suspected in only 70% of the pediatric HIV-infected cases reviewed.[17] The portability and low cost of ultrasonography have resulted in its extensive use for evaluating HIV-infected patients in developing countries with a high prevalence of AIDS.[18]

Doppler ultrasonography allows for the detection of frequency shifts, which permits sophisticated software packages to define the presence and direction of blood flow. This modality permits evaluation of waveforms, which can suggest portal hypertension and portal and hepatic vein thrombosis as a cause of liver injury.

Computed Tomography

Along with ultrasonography, CT imaging of the liver is the most important modality for evaluating masses, abscesses, cystic lesions, and infiltrative processes. Biphasic CT scans of the liver should generally be performed because identification and differentiation of mass lesions requires rapid imaging through the arterial and venous phases of contrast administration. Meta-analysis has shown that baseline CT without contrast was significantly inferior to biphasic or triphasic studies for identifying small mass lesions.[19] Therefore, noncontrast CT scans are not recommended for hepatic imaging.

Knollmann et al. described the results of abdominal imaging of 339 HIV-infected patients. This retrospective study reported that 82% of patients had abnormal imaging, including 11 patients with hepatic masses and 7 with ascites. Both findings were associated with decreased survival relative to the studied cohort.[20] Among 259 patients with HIV, hepatomegaly was reported in nearly 39%, and focal hepatic lesions were seen in 19%.[21]

Magnetic Resonance Imaging

Most major medical centers now utilize MRI as an imaging modality. The underlying physical principle relies on changes in the spin of water and lipid nuclei in a strong magnetic field that releases energy in the form of radio waves upon return to the baseline state. Therefore differences between tissues of similar density may be observed, even when CT or other modalities that rely on variable penetration of radiation fails to distinguish lesions or tissue planes. MRI is frequently used to help establish the presence and distribution of tumors and to evaluate vascular abnormalities. There is conflicting literature on the sensitivity of MRI versus biphasic CT for detecting small hepatocellular carcinomas.

Magnetic resonance cholangiography (MRC) is a variation of standard MRI that permits imaging of the biliary system. Studies comparing MRC to ERCP, which is the gold standard for biliary duct imaging, demonstrate a high correlation.[22] A prospective case-control study with blinding found that the mean sensitivity for detecting primary sclerosing cholangitis (PSC) for two observers was 86.5%, and the specificity was 94.5%. Results were similar for intrahepatic and extrahepatic PSC.[23] There is no literature evaluating the efficacy of MRC in HIV-infected patients with AIDS-related cholangiopathy, though it seems likely that similar efficacy might be observed.

Endoscopic Retrograde Cholangiopancreatography

Endoscopic retrograde cholangiopancreatography is regarded as the gold standard for evaluating the biliary duct system. Although somewhat invasive the procedure is generally tolerable and, in the hands of experienced endoscopists, highly efficacious for diagnosing strictures, papillary stenosis and AIDS cholangiopathy, small stones, and masses in the biliary tree (Fig. 65–3). Somewhat better diagnostically than MRC, it also offers the opportunity for immediate intervention, including stone removal, ductal dilation, sphincterotomy, and stent placement. Complications include pancreatitis in up to 5% of cases, though it is generally mild and self-limited. Some cases of severe pancreatitis continue to be observed, however.

Among patients with HIV infection, the literature supports use of ERCP for both diagnosis and intervention in patients with right upper quadrant pain and ultrasonographic evidence of ductal enlargement. Among 83 patients undergoing ERCP for abdominal pain or cholestatic liver enzyme abnormalities, 56 had AIDS-related cholangiopathy. Among patients who underwent ampullary biopsy, 62.5% had evidence of opportunistic infection.[24] A review of this subject by Walden suggested that patients with a prominent component of pain may benefit from ERCP with sphincterotomy, but those with asymptomatic cholestatic enzyme elevations are much less likely to benefit from in-

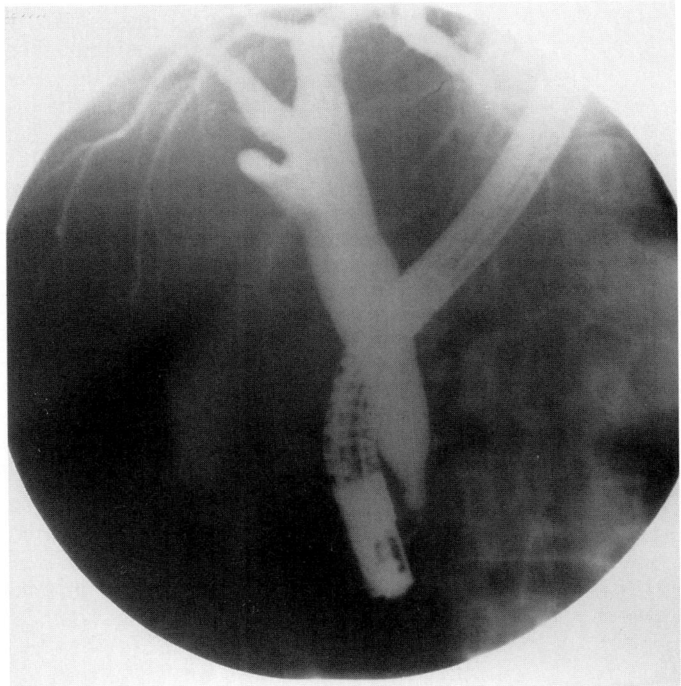

Figure 65–3. HIV-related papillary stenosis. Endoscopic cholangiogram from a 47-year-old woman with HIV presenting with episodic severe right upper quadrant abdominal pain. It reveals a diffusely dilated biliary tree and a smooth, stenotic distal common bile duct. There was no evidence of common bile duct stones. Endoscopic sphincterotomy produced immediate symptom relief. Multiple biopsies of the common duct and electron microscopy failed to reveal evidence of pathogens.

tervention.[25] Pancreatic ductal changes are common in patients diagnosed with AIDS cholangiopathy, and features suggestive of chronic pancreatitis may be observed in approximately half of these patients.[26]

▲ LIVER BIOPSY

Histologic evaluation of liver tissue remains the definitive study for determination of liver disease activity and degree of fibrosis. It also helps confirm the presence of processes suspected during the biochemical and serologic workup phase. Occasionally, liver biopsy identifies previously unsuspected findings in terms of etiology or co-morbidity. Most liver biopsies are performed by a percutaneous route, generally in the right upper quadrant in the midaxillary line, using an intercostal approach to enter the right lobe of the liver. The exact site varies and may be determined by percussion and palpation with or without ultrasound guidance. Liver biopsies may also be obtained at the time of laparoscopy under direct liver visualization or via a transjugular route. One editorial suggested that radiologic guidance be restricted to patients with a suspected tumor or hepatic mass, obesity, or the rare case when physical examination fails to define the precise location of the liver. For cases of decompensated disease with coagulopathy, ascites, or significant thrombocytopenia a transjugular approach is considered safer. All other cases may be performed by the percutaneous route, and physicians may or may not use ultrasound localization prior to biopsy.[27] Ultrasound guidance was not found to change morbidity or mortality in pediatric patients,[28] although Riley suggested that use of ultrasound prior to biopsy changed the management in 15.1% of cases[29]; moreover, an economic analysis supported the use of ultrasound prior to liver biopsy.[30]

The risk of complications from liver biopsy is highly variable based on the experience of the clinician, number of passes required, type of biopsy needle used, platelet count, prothrombin time, and type of lesion to be biopsied.[31] Serious complications are rare, although, death has been reported to occur at a rate of 9 per 100,000 cases and hemorrhage, pneumothorax, and biliary peritonitis at rates of 1 per 1000 to 3 per 1000 cases.[32,33]

There is little in the literature on the safety of liver biopsy in patients with HIV. A retrospective review of 248 liver biopsies in HIV antibody-positive patients reported a hemorrhage rate of 2.0%, which is higher than might be expected. The exceptionally high mortality rate (1.6%) was attributed to a high prevalence of thrombocytopenia and coagulation abnormalities in the cohort.[34] The higher risk of bleeding and death may also be attributable to a high prevalence of disease etiologies that may increase the risk of postbiopsy bleeding, including malignancies such as Kaposi's sarcoma and lymphoma and vascular abnormalities including peliosis due to bacillary angiomatosis. High risk cases (e.g., patients with thrombocytopenia, coagulopathy, liver lesions) with increased hemorrhage potential mandate screening and selection for safer biopsy approaches, such as transjugular liver biopsy.[35]

Deserving of special mention are patients with hemophilia who are frequently co-infected with HCV and HIV. There is often great reluctance to subject patients with heritable bleeding diatheses to liver biopsy, and the risk and cost of biopsy in hemophiliacs must be weighed against the value of the information obtained at liver biopsy. Current literature suggests that liver biopsy by the percutaneous or transjugular route can be performed safely in hemophiliacs following factor VIII replacement.[36,37]

The role of liver biopsy in patients with HIV infection has been controversial. Cappell et al. described the outcomes of liver biopsy in 36 patients with HIV. The leading indication was unexplained fever (83%) and abnormal liver enzymes (89%). Previously unidentified etiologies were found most frequently in patients with increased alkaline phosphatase, suggesting the presence of a cholestatic process. Most of these patients had granulomas associated with *Mycobacterium* infection. The patients in whom biopsy was helpful were those with leukocytosis, suggesting the presence of full-blown AIDS, and patients who were not known to have HIV infection prior to the biopsy.[38] Poles et al. reported on the findings of liver biopsies from 501 HIV-seropositive patients who underwent biopsy for indications similar to those described by Cappell et al. The most common diagnosis was mycobacterial infection (26.6% of the patients studied); 12% had chronic hepatitis. The study failed to determine if liver biopsy changed the treatment or the clinical diagnosis.[39] Similarly, a European study reported that among 24 patients with unexplained fever liver biopsy provided a microbiologic diagnosis in 54%.[40] Among children with HIV infection, liver biopsy was found to be useful for determining a diagnosis when there was a strong suspicion of mycobacterial infection or the child was jaundiced (or both).[41]

▲ ETIOLOGIES OF LIVER DISEASE IN PATIENTS WITH HIV

Viral Liver Disease

Hepatotropic Viruses

In view of the markedly high rates of co-infection with hepatitis B and C viruses in HIV-infected persons, it has become increasingly clear that the enhanced survival during the era of HAART will make chronic liver disease with these pathogens important sources of morbidity and mortality. These infections are considered in more detail in Chapter 46.

Hepatitis A Virus

Seroepidemiologic surveys for HAV infection reveal an increased overall prevalence in the HIV-infected population; among risk groups, men who have sex with men and injection drug users are at increased risk for infection. Although most cases of acute hepatitis with this fecal-oral pathogen are self-limited episodes and no more severe in the HIV-infected host than in the general population, individuals at particular risk are those who harbor chronic liver disease. Indeed, the risk of fatal acute hepatitis A is significantly increased in subjects with chronic HCV infection[42]; this has led to the recommendation that individuals with chronic HCV infection be actively immunized with a safe, effective HAV vaccine [Infections Disease Society of America (IDSA) guidelines]. HIV-infected individuals at continued risk for HAV infection should also be vaccinated.

Hepatitis B virus

Co-infection with hepatitis B virus occurs frequently in view of its shared routes of transmission with HIV. Up to 95% of persons with AIDS have serologic markers of prior HBV infection (anti-HBs+ or anti-HBc+) and 10% to 15% are chronic carriers (HBsAg+).[43,44] Although there is little evidence for a direct virologic interaction between HIV and HBV, the critical role of the immune system in mediating cell injury in chronic hepatitis B suggests that HIV alters its natural history. In support of this concept, the incidence of acute icteric hepatitis B is lower in the presence of HIV, and the risk of developing chronic HBV infection is increased substantially in patients with preexisting HIV.[45] Moreover, HIV appears to enhance and extend the period of HBV replication (HBeAg+, HBV DNA+) but without a concomitant increase in hepatic necroinflammatory activity. With advancing immunosuppression, markers of HBV replication appear to be reactivated. Evidence that HIV worsens the course of HBV-related liver disease is limited. One retrospective study showed higher histologic activity in HIV+/HBV+ individuals compared with HIV−/HBV+ individuals.[46] The same study saw an increased hepatic mortality rate (four of five deaths) among 25 HIV+/HBV+ persons compared with 6 of 121 deaths in HIV−/HBV+ persons over 31 months. However, most patients in this cohort were co-infected with HDV. There is little evidence that HBV worsens the course of HIV disease. One large-scale retrospective analysis demonstrated no influence on the mortality of co-infected patients compared with HBsAg− patients with HIV.[47]

Irrespective of whether HBV disease is hastened by HIV, alteration of the HIV treatment picture by introducing HAART increases the likelihood that HBV liver disease will become more problematic with control of HIV. Indeed, immune-mediated flares of HBV with successful pharmacologic reconstitution of the immune system have been described.[48] Furthermore, lamivudine withdrawal or *YMDD*-mutant breakthrough may precipitate acute liver injury in immunologically reconstituted patients with hepatitis B infection.[6]

The optimal management of chronic HBV disease is evolving (see Chapter 46), but it should be underscored that identification of HBV serologic status in individuals with HIV is essential to plan an optimal therapeutic program. Liver biopsy in individuals identified to harbor replicative HBV prior to initiation of HAART may be warranted in light of flares that could decompensate advanced HBV disease.

Hepatitis C Virus

It is estimated that the prevalence of HCV co-infection is about 16% across a broad cross section of a large U.S. HIV cohort (Sherman et al., unpublished data). Among injection drug users, co-infection rates of up to 92% have been cited.[49] When these rates are coupled with the known natural history of HCV (see Chapter 46), hepatic morbidity with this pathogen is a significant problem as the life expectancy of the HIV cohort is being extended. Because of the important role of the immune system in containing HCV, it is not surprising that HCV viremia levels are about 10-fold higher with HIV co-infection than with HCV infection alone.[50] These findings mirror those found in other immunocompromised populations, such as those undergoing liver transplantation.[51] However, no clear correlation of HCV RNA with CD4+ T-lymphocyte counts or definite relation between HCV and HIV levels has been established.

INFLUENCE OF HIV ON HCV-RELATED LIVER DISEASE

The most illuminating natural history studies have been performed in hemophiliacs, whose disease duration has been definable. Eyster et al.[52] found that 9% of co-infected hemophiliacs developed liver failure within 10 to 20 years after HCV infection compared with none of the HIV−/HCV+ group. In this cohort, the risk of liver failure was more than half the risk of developing AIDS. Subsequently, at least three other studies confirmed accelerated liver failure in those with HCV/HIV co-infection.[53–55] A possible explanation for this finding may lie in the observation that HIV co-infection accelerates HCV fibrosis progression compared with single infection with HCV.[56] Indeed, retrospective analyses indicate that since the inception of HAART mortality attributable to HCV-related end-stage liver disease has risen nearly fivefold.[57] The reciprocal relation is far less certain: Does HCV influence HIV disease progression? Three studies (one of them longitudinal) showed no influence of HCV on HIV progression, but the duration of HIV disease was not controlled.[58–60] One longitudinal study that did control for duration[61] followed 111 hemophiliacs co-infected during 1979 to 1985 and found that genotype 1 HCV strains predisposed to more rapid progression to AIDS and death than non-1 HCV. Another study found that clinical progression of HIV was also accelerated in HCV-co-infected versus HCV-negative subjects.[62] An evaluation of the Swiss HIV cohort during the post-HAART era also identified HCV as an important factor in increased progression to AIDS-defining complications.[63] These studies, which require confirmation, raise the intriguing possibility that HCV accelerates the effects of HIVs on the immune system. The mechanism for this finding is unclear but does not appear to be a rise in HIV viremia perse.

In summary, HIV co-infection increases HCV RNA levels and hastens progression to liver failure and death. HCV infection, particularly with genotype 1, *may* be associated with accelerated progression of HIV. The availability of HAART should permit examination of immune reconstitution-mediated hepatic flares. In this regard, several reports have found an early rise in ALT and HCV RNA levels followed by a return to baseline with continued treatment.[42,64] These data support the concept of a self-limited flare that is not readily attributable to drug hepatotoxicity. Nonetheless, vigilance should be practiced in this group until the data are more defined, and those individuals beginning HAART should be watched carefully for signs of hepatic decompensation. Because this phenomenon was described in subjects with advanced chronic HCV or cirrhosis, it may be important to risk-stratify co-infected persons with a liver biopsy prior to initiation of HAART.

ANTIVIRAL THERAPY FOR HCV IN HIV-CO-INFECTED PATIENTS

The cumulative data thus far suggest that interferon-α (IFNα) alone *rarely* produces sustained virologic responses in HIV/HCV-infected patients.[49] Rather, data demonstrating the superiority of a combination of IFNα and ribavirin (RBV) to IFNα alone offers optimism, especially for rapidly progressive HCV.[65,66] Small-scale results show increased viral clearance with IFN and RBV in co-infected persons. No randomized, controlled trials of a large number of co-infected subjects using IFN and RBV have been completed, nor has optimal timing of treatment of HCV infection with IFN and RBV been established. PEGylated interferon (IFN complexed with inert polyethylene glycol) has been developed to enhance IFN bioavailability by delaying clearance. When combined with RBV, PEGylated IFN achieves virologic sustained response rates of 54% in those with chronic HCV infections.[67]

Despite their potential promise, both IFN and RBV carry problematic adverse effects in the HIV-co-infected population especially with regard to bone marrow suppression and neuropsychiatric effects. In vitro, RBV antagonizes the phosphorylation of thymidine analogues, but thus far there has been no demonstration of an adverse effect of RBV on HIV disease control in individuals concomitantly receiving zidovudine or stavudine. The results of clinical trials using RBV in co-infected subjects will shed further light on this phenomenon in vivo. Whether ribavirin, a nucleoside analogue, produces mitochondrial toxicity, also awaits confirmation in ongoing trials.[68] Ultimately, the development of virus-specific agents that interrupt key viral functions will be critical to permit avoidance of these regimens. Cytokine-based immunomodulatory treatment with interleukins (IL-2 and IL-10) may also offer advantages in enhancing the host immune response and diminishing fibrosis, respectively.[69,70] These agents may have a role as adjuvants to IFN and RBV.

Other Viral Etiologies

Cytomegalovirus

Cytomegalovirus (CMV) infection, common in patients with HIV, can produce a wide range of clinical outcomes, including asymptomatic seropositivity to a fulminant, disseminated illness. It is a frequent finding in the livers of patients with AIDS, usually in the setting of multiorgan CMV disease. CMV can produce both an acute hepatitis-like illness and biliary tract disease. Clinical illness correlates with more advanced states of immunocompromise. There is usually mild elevation of the serum aminotransferases and occasionally predominant elevation of the serum alkaline phosphatase level. Histologic findings include a mild portal and periportal mononuclear infiltrate, sparse necrosis, and the presence of characteristic "owl's eye" intranuclear inclusions within hepatocytes, vascular endothelial cells, and biliary epithelium consistent with the broad cell tropism of this DNA virus. Less frequently, granulomatous reactions are seen. Serologic assays for diagnosis of active CMV disease are available but are of limited utility. Amplification assays and antigenemia assays usually reveal positive tests for viremia once CMV hepatitis has developed.[71] Treatment with intravenous ganciclovir is indicated for CMV hepatitis.

Herpes Simplex Virus and Other Herpes Viruses

Herpes simplex virus (HSV) can cause significant acute hepatitis in HIV-infected hosts as part of a disseminated infection, with an occasional fulminant or subfulminant presentation. Aminotransferase elevations may be severe and accompanied by disseminated intravascular coagulation. Histologic examination reveal's Cowdry type A intranuclear inclusions, but immunohistochemical staining may be required to distinguish HSV from CMV. Diffuse hepatocellular necrosis with sparse inflammatory reaction may be seen with severe hepatitis. Careful examination of the skin is therefore essential, as there is usually evidence of herpetic cutaneous lesions. Amplification assays for HSV DNA reveal high-titer viremia. Once the diagnosis is confirmed, prompt institution of intravenous acyclovir can be life-saving, particularly in patients with subfulminant or fulminant infection, among whom the case fatality rate is high.[72]

Other, less frequent herpetic agents implicated in liver disease in the HIV-infected person are varicella-zoster virus (VZV), Epstein-Barr virus, and human herpesvirus-6.[73] VZV hepatitis also presents in immunocompromised hosts as part of a disseminated syndrome with rash, fever, and pneumonitis. Treatment with intravenous acyclovir can shorten disease duration.[74]

Adenovirus

Disseminated adenovirus infection has been reported to cause acute hepatitis in HIV-infected persons. Clinically, the picture can be severe, with high fever, respiratory symptoms, enteritis, rash, and hepatomegaly. The mortality rate is high in immunocompromised patients.[75] Histologically, hepatocyte necrosis with massive hemorrhagic foci has been reported. "Smoky" intranuclear inclusions adjacent to areas of necrosis can also be seen. The diagnosis, which can be supported serologically, is made by recovering virus from body fluids or tissues. Treatment is supportive.

Human Immunodeficiency Virus

The p24 gag protein has been identified by immunohistochemistry in Kupffer cells and endothelial cells of the liver but not in hepatocytes.[76] Furthermore, HIV replication has been demonstrated in Kupffer cell cultures. It has been speculated that this is due to the presence of CD4 receptors present in both cell types, and the Kupffer cells (the macrophage-like cell type in the liver) may represent a reservoir for HIV. The clinical significance of these observations remains unclear but raises the possibility that HIV infection of the liver may serve as a portal of entry for other pathogens.

Fungal Liver Disease

Candidiasis

Candida species may cause invasive systemic infection with hepatic involvement in HIV-infected persons with advanced immunocompromise, especially in those who develop defects in neutrophil function.[77] The liver can become infected by *Candida albicans* in the setting of disseminated, multi-organ disease.[78] Disease is often overwhelming with high mortality rates.[78] With disseminated candidiasis involving the liver, clinical features include fever, abdominal pain and distension, nausea, vomiting, diarrhea, and tender hepatomegaly. The serum alkaline phosphatase level is almost invariably elevated, with variable elevations in serum aminotransferase and bilirubin levels. CT of the abdomen is the most sensitive test for detecting hepatic or splenic abscesses, which are often multicentric.[79] In cases diagnosed antemortem, liver biopsy or laparoscopy reveals macroscopic nodules, necrosis with microabscess formation, and characteristic yeast or hyphal forms of *Candida*.[79,80] The results of cultures of biopsy material are negative in most cases. Treatment with intravenous amphotericin B is warranted for disseminated candidiasis, but response rates to therapy are limited.

Histoplasmosis

Infection with *Histoplasma capsulatum* is acquired through the respiratory tract and in most cases is confined to the lungs. However, severely immunocompromised persons, such as those with AIDS, are predisposed to disseminated histoplasmosis. The liver can be invaded in both acute and chronic progressive disseminated histoplasmosis. Fever, oropharyngeal ulcers, hepatomegaly, and splenomegaly may be present in patients with chronic disease. Serum alanine aminotransferase and alkaline phosphatase levels are often elevated. Hepatosplenomegaly is present in approximately 30% of adults with acute disease, which is often the AIDS-defining illness.

Yeast forms can be identified in sections of liver biopsies with standard hematoxylin and eosin staining. The silver methenamine method is superior for detecting yeast forms in areas of caseating necrosis or granuloma formation (Fig. 65–4), but the organism is difficult to culture and almost never grows from biopsy specimens. Bone marrow biopsies produce a higher diagnostic yield than liver biopsy for stainable yeast.[81] Serologic testing for complement-fixing antibodies is therefore helpful for confirming the diagnosis. In immunocompromised persons who may not be capable of mounting an antibody response, detection of *H. capsulatum* antigens in urine and serum can be useful.[80] Treatment with intravenous amphotericin is warranted for disseminated disease.

Parasitic Liver Disease

Leishmaniasis

Visceral leishmaniasis is caused by *Leishmania donovani* and is endemic in the Mediterranean, central Asia, the former Soviet Union, the Middle East, China, India, Pakistan, Bangladesh, Africa, Central America, and South America.[82] Amastigotes are ingested by the sandfly (*Lutzomyia* in the New World, *Phlebotomus* in the Old World) and become fla-

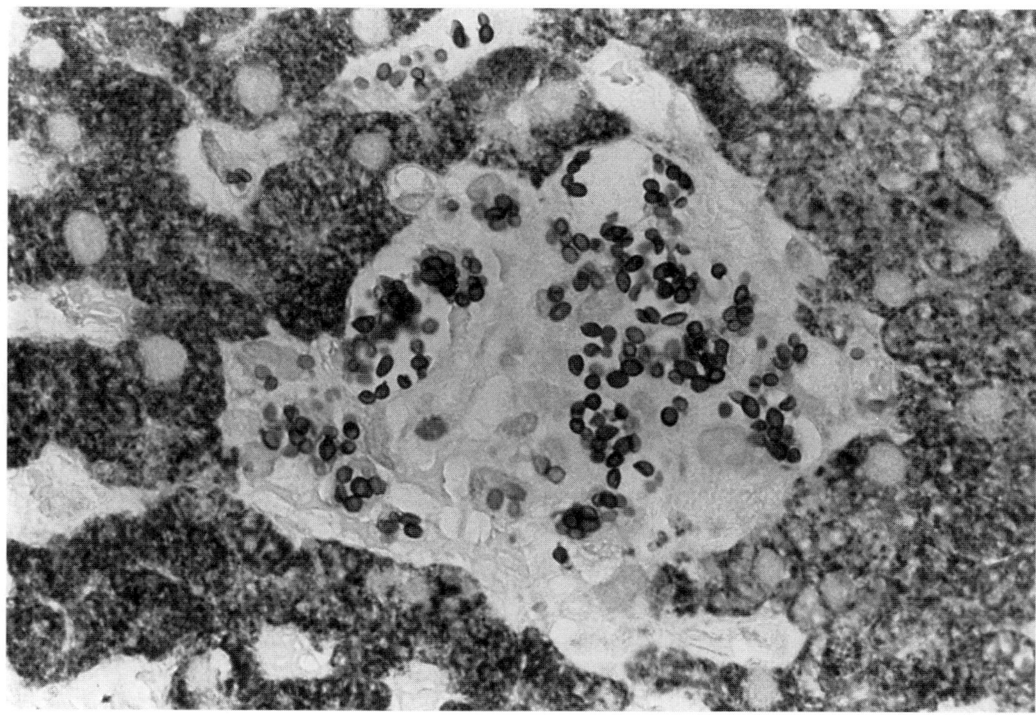

Figure 65–4. Liver biopsy from an HIV-infected patient with recurrent fevers and cholestatic injury pattern of the liver. Grocott silver stain shows a granuloma containing *Histoplasma* yeast forms.

gellated promastigotes. Following injection into the human host, the promastigotes are phagocytosed by macrophages in the reticuloendothelial system, where they multiply.

Visceral leishmaniasis can usually be found in mononuclear phagocytes of the liver, spleen, bone marrow, and lymph nodes. Proliferation of Kupffer cells is often seen, and amastigotes can be detected in these cells.[83] Occasionally, parasite-bearing cells aggregate in noncaseating granulomas.[84] Hepatocyte necrosis is mild compared with that seen in patients with cutaneous leishmaniasis. Healing is accompanied by fibrous deposition, and occasionally the liver takes on a cirrhotic appearance. However, complications of chronic liver disease are rare.

Visceral infection caused by *L. donovani* begins with a papular or ulcerative skin lesion at the site of the sandfly bite. Following an incubation period of 2 to 6 months (sometimes years), intermittent fevers, weight loss, diarrhea (of bacillary, amebic, or leishmanial origin), and progressive painful hepatosplenomegaly develop, often accompanied by pancytopenia and a polyclonal hypergammaglobulinemia. Secondary bacterial infections resulting from suppression of reticuloendothelial cell function are important causes of mortality and include pneumonia, pneumococcal infection, and tuberculosis.

Physical findings include hepatomegaly; often massive splenomegaly, jaundice, or ascites in severe disease; generalized lymphadenopathy; and muscle wasting. Cutaneous gray hyperpigmentation, which prompted the name kala-azar ("black fever"), is characteristically seen in India. Oral and nasopharyngeal nodules due to granuloma formation may also be seen.

The diagnosis is based on the history, physical examination, and microscopic demonstration of amastigotes in affected tissue samples. The highest yield (90%) comes from aspiration of the spleen. The yield of a liver biopsy is almost as high and less risky. The yield of bone marrow aspiration is 80% and that of lymph node aspirates 60%.[85] Serologic testing (ELISA, immunofluorescence, direct agglutination) can be used to support a presumptive diagnosis of visceral leishmaniasis. The leishmanin skin test (Montenegro test) is not helpful in the presence of acute visceral disease.

Pentavalent antimonial compounds are the drugs of choice for all forms of leishmaniasis. Parenteral sodium stibogluconate (Pentostam) is available through the Centers for Disease Control and Prevention for treatment of infections in the United States. γ-Interferon and allopurinol have been used in combination with antimonials in cases refractory to antimonials alone. Alternative parenteral agents include liposomal amphotericin B and aminosidine.[85] Treatment with antimonials should be administered for at least 4 weeks. However, patients with AIDS and leishmaniasis often fail to respond to or relapse following treatment with conventional regimens.[86] Miltefosine, a phosphocholine analogue administered orally, has shown promise against visceral leishmaniasis, with a reported cure rate of 97% in Phase 2 trials.[87]

Pneumocystis carinii

Hepatic involvement has been described frequently in patients with AIDS who present with disseminated extrapulmonary *Pneumocystis carinii* infection. In one study, *P. carinii* was found in 38% of cases.[88] It usually presents in persons who have received prophylactic aerosolized pentamidine or oral dapsone, which theoretically promotes emergence of extrapulmonary infection. Spread is also noted in lymph nodes, bone marrow, spleen, and liver, which is involved in 30% to 40% of extrapulmonary cases. Imaging studies may reveal low-attenuation lesions with rim-like calcifications. Biopsy discloses areas of granular necrosis without inflammation or nodules with a foamy eosinophilic exudate. Methenamine silver stains reveal cystic forms in necrotic areas. Treatment with intravenous pentamidine or trimethoprim-sulfamethoxazole, or TMP-SMX (Bactrim), is successful in up to 45% of cases.

Microsporidia

In addition to biliary involvement, hepatic infection with protozoa of the order Microsporidia has been described. Histologically, focal granulomas can be seen in portal tracts, and parasites are seen in histiocytes by Giemsa staining.

Bacterial Liver Disease

Bacillary angiomatosis is an infectious disorder that primarily affects persons with AIDS or other immunodeficiency states. The causative agents have been identified as the gram-negative bacilli *Bartonella henselae* and in some cases *Bartonella quintana*.[89] Infection is frequently associated with exposure to cats.

Bacillary angiomatosis is characterized most commonly by multiple blood-red papular skin lesions, but disseminated infection with or without skin involvement has also been described.[90] The causative bacilli can infect liver, lymph nodes, pleura, bronchi, bones, brain, bone marrow, and spleen. Additional manifestations include persistent fever, bacteremia, and sepsis. Hepatic infection should be suspected when serum aminotransferase levels are elevated in the absence of other explanations.

Hepatic infection in persons with bacillary angiomatosis may present as peliosis hepatis, or blood-filled cysts. Histologically, peliosis in patients with AIDS is characterized by an inflammatory myxoid stroma containing clumps of bacilli surrounding the blood-filled peliotic cysts. Diagnosis of *Bartonella* infection by polymerase chain reaction (PCR)-based methods is being used increasingly.[91]

Bacillary angiomatosis responds uniformly to therapy with erythromycin. For visceral infection, at least 6 weeks of treatment with erythromycin 2 g daily or doxycycline should be administered.

Granulomatous Liver Disease

Mycobacterium tuberculosis

Granulomas are commonly found in liver biopsy specimens (Fig. 65–5), and a wide variety of infectious, drug, and nonspecific etiologies have been implicated. Granulomas are

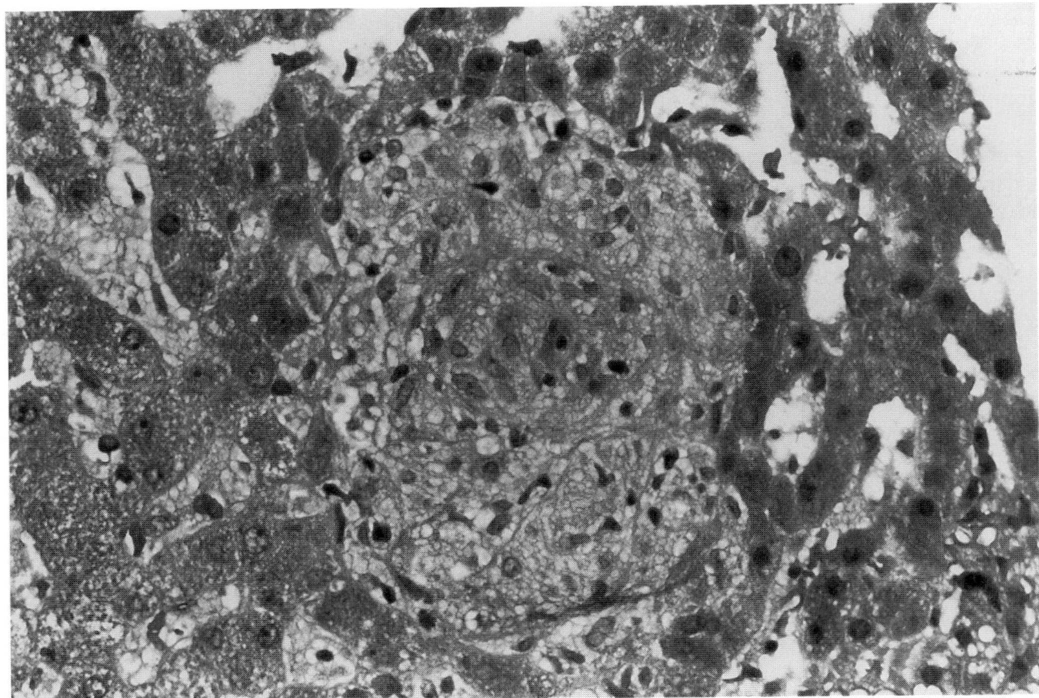

Figure 65–5. Liver biopsy from an HIV-infected patient with recurrent fever shows a nonspecific granuloma on H&E staining. Silver stains for fungal elements and stains for acid-fast bacilli were negative for organisms.

identified in the liver in about 25% of persons with pulmonary tuberculosis and 80% of those with extrapulmonary tuberculosis. Tuberculous granulomas can be distinguished from sarcoid granulomas by central caseation, acid-fast bacilli, and the presence of fewer granulomas with a tendency to coalesce.[92] Multiple granulomas in the liver may also be seen following vaccination with bacille Calmette Guérin, especially in persons with an impaired immune response. Patients with multiple granulomas due to tuberculosis rarely have clinically significant liver disease. Occasionally, tender hepatomegaly is found. Jaundice with elevated serum alkaline phosphatase levels may occur with miliary infections. The treatment of tuberculous granulomatous disease of the liver is the same as for active pulmonary tuberculosis, namely, four-drug therapy.[92]

Mycobacterium avium Complex

The most common pathogen producing granulomatous liver disease in HIV-infected individuals is *Mycobacterium avium* complex (MAC), which typically causes fatigue, malaise, low grade fever, night sweats, elevated serum alkaline phosphatase levels, and less frequently hepatomegaly. MAC is found in the liver of up to 80% of autopsy studies in patients who die of AIDS. Liver biopsy reveals poorly formed, noncaseating granulomas with foamy macrophages and a paucity of lymphocytes. Special stains (Ziehl-Nielsen and periodic acid-Schiff) combined with tissue cultures can be used to establish the diagnosis, but histologic examination is more sensitive.

Treatment of MAC infection has markedly improved. Significant benefit has been reported with combinations of three or four drugs given for more than 3 months.[93] The most common regimens contain a macrolide (e.g., clarithromycin or azithromycin) and two or three of the following: ethambutol, rifabutin, ciprofloxacin. Treatment can produce decreased mycobacterial load and symptomatic improvement as well as improved survival.[94,95]

Toxic and Metabolic Liver Disease

With the successful conversion of HIV to a chronic disease, liver disease has become an important source of morbidity and mortality in the HIV-infected population. In view of their shared routes of transmission, high co-infection rates with chronic viral hepatitis have been an important source of progressive liver disease and liver failure. Another major impediment to the successful initiation HAART has been treatment-limiting hepatotoxicity. This may be a consequence of the antiretroviral therapies themselves or the effect of these drugs on livers already injured by viral hepatitis or metabolic liver disease, particularly fatty liver. Additionally, many mediciations used for the management and prevention of AIDS-related processes may cause liver toxicity. A list of commonly encountered drugs and the patterns of injury observed are shown in Table 65–2.

Fatty Liver (Hepatic Steatosis, Nonalcoholic Steatohepatitis)

Macrovesicular fatty infiltration of the liver is the most common specific histologic finding in patients with HIV infection who undergo liver biopsy. It most commonly is

▲ **Table 65–2.** HEPATOTOXICITY OF DRUGS COMMONLY USED IN PATIENTS WITH HIV

Type of Drug	Pattern of Injury: Hepatocellular	Microvesicular Steatosis	Cholestatic	Granulomas	Mixed
Analgesics	Acetaminophen Ibuprofen Indomethacin Salicylates		Propoxyphene		Naproxen Piroxicam Sulindac
Anticonvulsants	Phenytoin	Valproate	Phenytoin	Phenytoin	Carbamazepine Phenobarbital
Antimicrobials	Acyclovir Amphotericin B Ethionamide Isoniazid Ketoconazole Metronidazole Penicillins Pentamidine Pyrazinamide Quinacrine Rifampin Sulfonamides Dapsone Tetracycline TMP-SMX 5-Flucytosine	Tetracycline (IV)	Albendazole Azithromycin Erythromycin Ketoconazole Rifampin Thiabendazole TMP-SMX	TMP-SMX	TMP-SMX
Antiretrovirals					
NRTIs		ddC d4T ddI AZT			
NNRTIs	Nevirapine Efavirenz				
PIs	Indinavir (increases in direct bilirubin) Saquinavir Nelfinavir Ritonavir (inhibits P_{450})				
Miscellaneous	Disulfiram Vitamin A Prochlorperazine		Anabolic steroids Chlorpromazine Contraceptive steroids Prochlorperazine		Chlordiazepoxide Diazepam

AZT, zidovudine; ddI, dideoxycytidine; ddI, didanosine; d4T, stavudine; TMP-SMX, trimethoprim-sulfamethoxazole.

found in association with multiple metabolic derangements, including weight loss or gain, obesity, diabetes, hyperlipidemias, hyperalimentation, and alcohol use. Macrovesicular steatosis is randomly distributed throughout the liver lobule, generally unaccompanied by inflammation. Steatosis can lead to hepatomegaly and elevations of serum alkaline phosphatase and aminotransferases. Imaging studies may demonstrate increased density. Treatment is generally directed at the underlying predisposition, if identifiable. In addition, consideration should be given to holding antiretroviral medications, which have also been associated with steatosis (see below), particularly the nucleoside analogues [zidovudine (AZT), stavudine (d4T), dideoxycytidine (ddC), didanosine (ddI)] and to a lesser extent protease inhibitors. In general, withholding antiretroviral therapy is recommended once grade 3 elevations of the liver function tests (LFTs) occur. However, with any chronic elevation of LFTs (more than 6 months), a liver biopsy should be strongly considered, even when imaging studies suggest the presence of fatty liver. A significant subset of those persons with fatty liver also have fibrosis and are at increased risk for the subsequent progression to cirrhosis. These patients cannot be identified by imaging studies. It is unclear whether steatosis resolves with successful control of HIV infection.

Nucleoside Analogue Reverse Transcriptase Inhibitors (AZT, d4T, ddI, ddC, 3TC)

The mode of action of nucleoside reverse transcriptase inhibitors (NRTIs) is competitive inhibition of the viral reverse transcriptase leading to premature viral chain termination. However, NRTIs have been associated with host mitochondrial toxicity. Mitochondria execute the key function of oxidative phosphorylation (OXPHOS) and generate ATP as energy for key cellular functions through the action of the electron transport chain. The mitochondrion is also the locus of fatty acid oxidation via medium-chain (MCAD) and long-chain (LCAD) acyl coenzyme A (coA) dehydrogenases. Mitochondrial proteins are encoded in large part by mitochondrial DNA (mtDNA), which is replicated separately by the mitochondrion-specific DNA polymerase γ. This is in contrast to nuclear DNA, which is replicated by DNA polymerases α, β, δ, and ε.

Because mtDNA has a high mutation rate, which is further accelerated by processes that enhance generation of reactive oxygen species, including chronic inflammation and aging, mitochondrial dysfunction related to drugs may occur at several levels. Toxicity would be expected to manifest as lactic acidosis (a result of enhanced pyruvate conversion to lactate) and microvesicular steatosis (a consequence of impaired fatty acid oxidation). Whereas phosphorylated nucleoside analogues have less affinity for cellular nuclear DNA polymerases, ddC, d4T, ddI, and to lesser extent AZT are potent inhibitors of DNA polymerase γ, leading ultimately to impaired oxidative phosphorylation. Clinical manifestations thus reflect blockade of OXPHOS and fatty acid oxidation, with lactic acidosis, microvesicular steatosis prevailing in the liver, anemia, myopathy, neuropathy, and pancreatitis elsewhere. The paradigm NRTI toxicity was due to 1-(2-deoxy-2-fluoro-b-D-arabinofuranosyl)-5-iodouracil (FIAU), an agent used to treat hepatitis B infection that produced irreversible lactic acidosis, liver failure, and death. An analogous effect has been reported with AZT (6/10,000 cases), with occasional severe toxicity (massive steatosis, enlarged irregular mitochondria).[96,97] Obese women were identified to be at particular risk for AZT hepatotoxicity,[98] raising the possibility that preexisting metabolic stress with fatty liver raises the risk by generating increased reactive oxygen species, lowering the threshold for mitochondrial dysfunction. AZT appears to exert further toxicity by also directly inhibiting cytochrome c oxidase and citrate synthase, two key enzymes in OXPHOS.[99] Dual nucleoside analogue therapy is associated with an approximately 5% incidence of grade 3 or 4 hepatotoxicity (ALT more than five times the upper limits of normal) in several studies.[2,100–102]

Protease Inhibitors (Indinavir, Ritonavir, Saquinavir, Nelfinavir)

Each protease inhibitor (PI) is associated with its own spectrum of hepatotoxic potential, despite similar mechanisms of action. A distinct histologic pattern may be associated with PI therapy, including hepatocyte ballooning, Kupffer cell activation, and pericellular zone 3 fibrosis. This was seen in 26% of liver biopsies performed in a cohort of 110 patients.[103] In addition, PIs may be associated with the syndrome of peripheral lipodystrophy, central adiposity, hyperlipidemia, and insulin resistance, which may itself be associated with hepatic steatosis.[48] The precise basis for this finding is not known but may relate to inhibition of cytoplasmic retinoic acid-binding protein (CRABP-1) and LDL receptor-related protein (LRP), which bear 60% homology with HIV protease. Under such conditions protease inhibitors may impair triglyceride clearance by the endothelial LRP–lipoprotein lipase complex, leading to lipidemia, insulin resistance, and fatty liver.

A prospective study of the AIDS-related virus (ARV) in 298 patients and found overall grade 3 or 4 toxicity in 10.4%, with no significant difference in patients treated with dual nucleoside analogues saquinavir, indinavir, or nelfinavir. However, ritonavir toxicity, seen in 30%, was the single most important variable predicting grade 3 or higher toxicity.[2]

Among PIs, indinavir is associated with asymptomatic indirect hyperbilirubinemia. There have been occasional reports of severe hepatitis. Histologic characterization has suggested a hypersensitivity reaction.[104] The frequency of grade 3 or higher hepatotoxicity with indinavir-containing regimens is 6%. Saquinavir and nelfinavir have a comparable incidence of hepatotoxicity (6%), but they are likely to cause liver injury as direct hepatotoxins. Ritonavir is a potent inhibitor of the P_{450} system. Its use has been associated with a significantly increased risk of grade 3 toxicity when used alone or in combination (27% to 32%); the mechanism is unclear.[2] It is noteworthy that coexistent viral hepatitis was associated with only a slight quantitative increase in higher grades of hepatotoxicity, suggesting that ritonavir toxicity is a more important factor.[2]

Nonnucleoside Reverse Transcriptase Inhibitors (Efavirenz, Nevirapine, Delavirdine)

The nonnucleoside reverse transcriptase inhibitors (NNRTIs)—efavirenz, neviropine, delavirdine—which inhibit HIV reverse transcriptase without blocking nucleotide chain incorporation, are theoretically at less risk of inhibiting mitochondrial DNA polymerase than nucleoside analogues. Studies suggest that the overall grade 3 to 4 toxicity rate is 2.4% to 3.6% for the NNRTIs, with the only grade 4 toxicities being associated with nevirapine.[105] Because of reports of severe hepatotoxicity, the U.S. Food and Drug Administration (FDA) has issued an alert for nevirapine. Caution is warranted, especially within the first 12 weeks of initiating therapy with this agent.

Alcohol and Liver Disease Progression

Alcohol accelerates disease progression in HIV/HCV-infected patients and appears to contribute as much to the rate liver disease progression as does low CD4 count.[56] Consumption of more than 50 g of alcohol daily appears to produce the same compression of the time to development of cirrhosis as a CD4 count of less than 200/μl.[56] Alcohol consumption should therefore be minimized in persons with HIV, especially those with preexisting chronic liver disease.

Role of Viral Hepatitis in Drug Hepatotoxicity

It is reasonable to speculate that chronic viral hepatitis lowers the threshold for antiretroviral hepatotoxicity through a number of mechanisms, including (1) increasing the formation of reactive oxygen species; (2) directly inducing steatosis, as has been demonstrated in a transgenic mouse model overexpressing HCV core protein[106]; or (3) inducing direct mitochondrial alterations, as has been suggested in an ultrastructural study of HCV-infected hepatocytes.[107]

Notwithstanding these considerations, the data are mixed regarding relative risk posed by preexisting HCV for hepatotoxicity. In one study the relative risk for hepatotoxicity was 2.8 in HCV$^+$ patients receiving three-drug HAART.[108] In the Johns Hopkins survey, the risk of hepatotoxicity was not increased by HCV in ritonavir users; however, the relative risk was increased by 3.7 in those receiving antiretroviral regimens not containing ritonavir.[2] Overall, 88% of the patients with HBV or HCV infection did not develop hepatotoxicity.[2] Several studies suggest that HAART can be continued safely in HCV-infected subjects despite a transient rise in aminotransferases and HCV RNA during the first 3 months of HAART,[64,109] suggesting that reactivation of HCV with immune reconstitution, not drug toxicity per se, explains these findings. Further studies are needed to help distinguish the HCV immune reconstitution phenomenon due to drug hepatotoxicity, so those patients with ALT flares who can be safely continued on treatment may be identified.

The risk of hepatotoxicity does appear to be higher in HIV^+ individuals receiving antituberculous therapy who are co-infected with HCV (relative risk with HCV alone 5, HIV alone 4, HCV/HIV 14.4).[110]

Several important questions remain in the face of an increasing problem with hepatic morbidity.

1. When can HAART be successfully continued in the presence of elevated LFTs?
2. Can pretreatment or simultaneous treatment for HCV permit successful reinitiation in co-infected persons who could not continue HAART because of toxicity?
3. Can an HCV reconstitution flare be noninvasively characterized?
4. Are there noninvasive baseline predictors for hepatotoxicity?

Neoplastic Liver Disease

Kaposi's Sarcoma

Kaposi's sarcoma, although more frequently encountered in the luminal gastrointestinal tract, can also present as a mass lesion of the liver. When the liver is involved, it is usually as part of a disseminated disease. Abdominal pain and hepatomegaly with disproportionate elevations of the serum alkaline phosphatase can be seen.

Non-Hodgkin's Lymphoma

With advancing immunodeficiency, HIV-infected persons are at risk for developing non-Hodgkin's lymphomas (NHLs), predominantly of the B cell type. These lymphomas present much more frequently extranodally in the HIV population. About 10% of NHLs in the HIV cohort involve the liver. Characteristic findings on ultrasound scans or CT scans (the preferred diagnostic modality) include the presence of a mass lesion(s). The diagnosis is confirmed by guided biopsy. The predominant laboratory abnormality is an elevated serum alkaline phosphatase level. Jaundice may be seen as a manifestation of more advanced lymphoma or associated with biliary occlusion by portal adenopathy. When present, jaundice is usually associated with high short-term mortality, as lymphomas are usually of high biologic grade and respond poorly to treatment.

Hepatocellular Carcinoma

With an increasing prevalence of chronic liver disease and cirrhosis in the HIV cohort, hepatocellular carcinoma (HCC), a frequent complication of HCV- and HBV-related cirrhosis, is being seen with higher frequency as well. HCC should be suspected when a known cirrhotic individual experiences hepatic decompensation. Imaging studies disclose the presence of a mass lesion that exhibits arterial phase enhancement on CT or MRI. Surveillance strategies include a semiannual serum α-fetoprotein assay and ultrasonography. It is unclear whether these strategies lead to decreased mortality among HIV-infected persons, as the only proven long-term cure for cirrhotic HCC is liver transplantation.

AIDS Cholangiopathy

Three overlapping clinical syndromes comprise AIDS cholangiopathy, which occurs late in HIV disease. Imaging studies suggest the diagnosis in most cases. Each syndrome can be diagnosed by ERCP. Signs and symptoms include fever, right upper quadrant abdominal pain, jaundice, and hepatomegaly. The predominant laboratory finding is an elevated serum alkaline phosphatase level. Aminotransferase elevations, when seen, are mild. The most commonly identified pathogens include *Cryptosporidium*, CMV, Microsporida, and MAC. Causality is not proven, however, as therapeutic approaches directed at these pathogens do not produce meaningful responses in the outcome of cholangiopathy.

1. Sclerosing cholangitis. The clinical and cholangiographic picture of this syndrome is analogous to that seen with idiopathic primary sclerosing cholangitis. It is characterized by focal strictures alternating with dilatations of the intrahepatic and extrahepatic biliary tree along with terminal pruning of the secondary or higher-order biliary radicles. The syndrome usually appears after AIDS is diagnosed. No medical therapy has been shown to be beneficial. In some cases dominant focal strictures respond to biliary stenting.
2. Papillary stenosis. This discrete entity can occur alone or in conjunction with sclerosing cholangitis. ERCP reveals narrowing of the distal common bile duct that may extend into the intraduodenal segment (Fig. 65–3). A dilated proximal CBD is common. This entity can be responsive to sphincterotomy, resulting in significantly diminished abdominal pain. Repeat sphincterotomy may be required.
3. Long extrahepatic bile duct strictures (with or without sclerosing cholangitis). This entity is likely a subset of sclerosing cholangitis and may respond to biliary stenting. Although stenting of large ducts may provide some decompression and pain relief, alkaline phosphatase levels may continue to rise as a result of progressive disease involving small intrahepatic bile ducts.

Acalculous Cholecystitis

Acalculous cholecystitis may be associated with a number of pathogens, including CMV, *Cryptosporidium*, *Isospora*, *Candida* sp., *Salmonella* sp., *Klebsiella*, *Campylobacter* sp., and *Serratia* spp. The presentation ranges from mild right upper quadrant pain to fulminant, gangrenous cholecystitis. Ultrasonography may reveal a thickened gallbladder wall, pericholecystic fluid, or ductal abnormalities. Technetium-HIDA scanning may be diagnostic by revealing an absence of gallbladder uptake. Both acute and chronic changes of cholecystitis can be seen pathologically. Under stable conditions, laparoscopic cholecystectomy can be performed with acceptable morbidity. More unstable patients may require open cholecystectomy.

▲ SUMMARY OF MANAGEMENT PRINCIPLES

Management of acute and chronic liver disease in patients with HIV infection is complex, partly because of the myriad linked etiologies that shade the decision process and partly the lack of sound scientific guidance due to the dearth of studies addressing this issue. The treatment algorithms provided herein describe a framework for the approach to patients. These are divided into acute (1a) and chronic (1b) hepatocellular injury patterns and cholestatic injury patterns (Fig. 65–2).

When a patient is first noted to have abnormal liver tests, it is often unclear whether the process is chronic or acute. However, serial enzyme profiles are available for some patients, and an acute process may be observed. As a general rule, acute elevations less than five times the upper limit of normal should be monitored to determine the trend. If the ALT/AST exceeds five times normal, it is reasonable to initiate a workup as shown in the acute AST/ALT elevation algorithm. A persistent transaminase abnormality lasting longer than 6 months should lead to initiation of a formal workup as shown in Figure 65–1. Key tests include evaluation for hepatitis B and C, medications and drugs associated with liver toxicity, and metabolic/autoimmune disorders. Liver biopsy is an important endpoint for all evaluations of chronic hepatitis.

Cholestatic processes that result in increased bilirubin, alkaline phosphatase, and GGT must be evaluated by a different process, as shown in Figure 65–2. As above, there are no absolute thresholds that determine whether to enter the diagnostic algorithm. However, bilirubin or alkaline phosphatase levels plus GGT that are more than two times normal deserve further evaluation. Isolated GGT abnormalities are most commonly due to induction by medications and do not generally require an extensive workup. Hyperbilirubinemia due to protease inhibitors (particularly indinavir) may be troubling to the patient and clinician but does not generally require additional evaluation if the process is identified early. Visible jaundice may lead to a change of protease inhibitor. For patients with jaundice, direct hyperbilirubinemia, and normal ducts, drug toxicity should be suspected. It is important to remember that cholestasis is slow to resolve, and months may pass before normalization after discontinuing the offending agent.

▲ ROLE OF LIVER TRANSPLANTATION

The treatment of last resort for end-stage nonmalignant liver disease is liver transplantation. Although AIDS is an absolute contraindication to transplantation, during the era of increased longevity associated with HAART this policy may undergo reconsideration for HIV-positive patients. One case of liver transplantation for a patient with HIV has been reported, specifically for HCV-related liver disease in a hemophiliac, with successful control of HIV on HAART 7 months after transplant.[111] More concerning is a recent report suggesting that four HCV/HIV-infected patients who underwent liver transplantation all died within 23 months of receiving the graft. This survival rate is significantly lower than the 70% three-year survival rate seen in most U.S. centers for HCV-infected patients.[112] The role of liver transplantation in the management of patients who develop end-stage liver disease requires further clarification in view of the disparity between the rapidly growing candidate list and the limited availability of donor organs. Active protocols for HCV/HIV-co-infected individuals with end-stage liver disease whose HIV is effectively suppressed are ongoing in a limited number of U.S. centers.

▲ CONCLUSIONS

Prolongation of survival in HIV-infected patients has led to increased prominence of liver disease from a variety of viral, metabolic, and toxic etiologies. Health care workers caring for such patients must become conversant with common causes of liver injury, diagnostic modalities, and treatment interventions. Use of diagnostic algorithms included herein can aid the clinician who has not previously managed patients with liver injury. Further research in this area is critical to long-term care and management of patients with HIV.

REFERENCES

1. Sulkowski MS, Mast EE, Seeff LB, Thomas DL. Hepatitis C virus infection as an opportunistic disease in persons infected with human immunodeficiency virus. Clin Infect Dis 30 (suppl 1):S77, 2000.
2. Sulkowski MS, Thomas DL, Chaisson RE, Moore RD. Hepatotoxicity associated with antiretroviral therapy in adults infected with human immunodeficiency virus and the role of hepatitis C or B virus infection. JAMA 283:74, 2000.
3. Alter MJ. Hepatitis C virus infection in the United States. J Hepatol 31:88, 1999.
4. Reddy KR, Brillant P, Schiff ER. Amoxicillin-clavulanate potassium-associated cholestasis. Gastroenterology 96:1135, 1989.
5. Olynyk JK, Cullen DJ, Aquilia S, et al. A population-based study of the clinical expression of the hemochromatosis gene. N Engl J Med 341:718, 1999.
6. Bessesen M, Ives D, Condreay L, et al. Chronic active hepatitis B exacerbations in human immunodeficiency virus-infected patients following development of resistance to or withdrawal of lamivudine. Clin Infect Dis 28:1032, 1999.
7. Conn HO. Trailmaking and number-connection tests in the assessment of mental state in portal systemic encephalopathy. Am J Dig Dis 22:541, 1977.
8. Sherman KE. Alanine aminotransferase in clinical practice: a review. Arch Intern Med 151:260, 1991.
9. Aranda-Michel J, Sherman KE. Tests of the liver: use and misuse. Gastroenterologist 6:34, 1998.
10. O'Connor JB, Imperiale TF, Singer ME. Cost-effectiveness analysis of hepatitis A vaccination strategies for adults. Hepatology 30:1077, 1999.
11. Hofer M, Joller-Jemelka HI, Grob PJ, et al. Frequent chronic hepatitis B virus infection in HIV-infected patients positive for antibody to

hepatitis B core antigen only: Swiss HIV Cohort Study. Eur J Clin Microbiol Infect Dis 17:6, 1998.
12. Ragni MV, Ndimbie OK, Rice EO, et al. The presence of hepatitis C virus (HCV) antibody in human immunodeficiency virus-positive hemophilic men undergoing HCV "seroreversion." Blood 82:1010, 1993.
13. Goncales NS, Pinho JR, Moreira RC, et al. Hepatitis E virus immunoglobulin G antibodies in different populations in Campinas, Brazil. Clin Diagn Lab Immunol 7:813, 2000.
14. Bair HJ, Behr T, Rubbert A, et al. ^{99m}Tc-trimethyl-BrIDA scintigraphy in HIV-related cholangiopathy. Nuklearmedizin 34:252, 1995.
15. Buscombe JR, Miller RF, Ell PJ. Hepatobiliary scintigraphy in the diagnosis of AIDS-related sclerosing cholangitis. Nucl Med Commun 13:154, 1992.
16. Beale TJ, Wetton CW, Crofton ME. A sonographic-pathological correlation of liver biopsies in patients with the acquired immune deficiency syndrome (AIDS). Clin Radiol 50:761, 1995.
17. Albisetti M, Braegger CP, Stallmach T, et al. Hepatic steatosis: a frequent nonspecific finding in HIV-infected children. Eur J Pediatr 158:971, 1999.
18. Tshibwabwa ET, Mwaba P, Bogle-Taylor J, Zumla A. Four-year study of abdominal ultrasound in 900 Central African adults with AIDS referred for diagnostic imaging. Abdom Imaging 25:290, 2000.
19. Catalano O, Cusati B, Sandomenico F, et al. [Multiple-phase spiral computerized tomography of small hepatocellular carcinoma: technique optimization and diagnostic yield.] Radiol Med (Torino) 98:53, 1999.
20. Knollmann FD, Maurer J, Grunewald T, et al. Abdominal CT features and survival in acquired immunodeficiency. Acta Radiol 38:970, 1997.
21. Radin R. HIV infection: analysis in 259 consecutive patients with abnormal abdominal CT findings. Radiology 197:712, 1995.
22. Macdonald GA, Peduto AJ. Magnetic resonance imaging and diseases of the liver and biliary tract. Part 2. Magnetic resonance cholangiography and angiography and conclusions. J Gastroenterol Hepatol 15:992, 2000.
23. Fulcher AS, Turner MA, Yelon JA, et al. Magnetic resonance cholangiopancreatography (MRCP) in the assessment of pancreatic duct trauma and its sequelae: preliminary findings. J Trauma 48:1001, 2000.
24. Teare JP, Daly CA, Rodgers C, et al. Pancreatic abnormalities and AIDS related sclerosing cholangitis. Genitourin Med 73:271, 1997.
25. Walden DT. Biliary problems in people with HIV disease. Curr Treat Options Gastroenterol 2:147, 1999.
26. Barthet M, Chauveau E, Bonnet E, et al. Pancreatic ductal changes in HIV-infected patients. Gastrointest Endosc 45:59, 1997.
27. Stotland BR, Lichtenstein GR. Liver biopsy complications and routine ultrasound. Am J Gastroenterol 91:1295, 1996.
28. Scheimann AO, Barrios JM, Al-Tawil YS, et al. Percutaneous liver biopsy in children: impact of ultrasonography and spring-loaded biopsy needles. J Pediatr Gastroenterol Nutr 31:536, 2000.
29. Riley TR. How often does ultrasound marking change the liver biopsy site? Am J Gastroenterol 94:3320, 1999.
30. Younossi ZM, Teran JC, Ganiats TG, Carey WD. Ultrasound-guided liver biopsy for parenchymal liver disease: an economic analysis. Dig Dis Sci 43:46, 1998.
31. Perrault J, McGill DB, Ott BJ, Taylor WF. Liver biopsy: complications in 1000 inpatients and outpatients. Gastroenterology 74:103, 1978.
32. Piccinino F, Sagnelli E, Pasquale G, Giusti G. Complications following percutaneous liver biopsy: a multicentre retrospective study on 68,276 biopsies. J Hepatol 2:165, 1986.
33. McGill DB, Rakela J, Zinsmeister AR, Ott BJ. A 21-year experience with major hemorrhage after percutaneous liver biopsy. Gastroenterology 99:1396, 1990.
34. Churchill DR, Mann D, Coker RJ, et al. Fatal haemorrhage following liver biopsy in patients with HIV infection. Genitourin Med 72:62, 1996.
35. McAfee JH, Keeffe EB, Lee RG, Rosch J. Transjugular liver biopsy. Hepatology 15:726, 1992.
36. Ahmed MM, Mutimer DJ, Elias E, et al. A combined management protocol for patients with coagulation disorders infected with hepatitis C virus. Br J Haematol 95:383, 1996.
37. Fried MW. Management of hepatitis C in the hemophilia patient. Am J Med 107:85S, 1999.
38. Cappell MS, Schwartz MS, Biempica L. Clinical utility of liver biopsy in patients with serum antibodies to the human immunodeficiency virus. Am J Med 88:123, 1990.
39. Poles MA, Dieterich DT. Hepatitis C virus/human immunodeficiency virus coinfection: clinical management issues. Clin Infect Dis 31:154, 2000.
40. Cavicchi M, Pialoux G, Carnot F, et al. Value of liver biopsy for the rapid diagnosis of infection in human immunodeficiency virus-infected patients who have unexplained fever and elevated serum levels of alkaline phosphatase or gamma-glutamyl transferase. Clin Infect Dis 20:606, 1995.
41. Lacaille F, Fournet JC, Blanche S. Clinical utility of liver biopsy in children with acquired immunodeficiency syndrome. Pediatr Infect Dis J 18:143, 1999.
42. Vento S, Garofano T, Renzini C, et al. Fulminant hepatitis associated with hepatitis A virus superinfection in patients with chronic hepatitis C. N Engl J Med 338:286, 1998.
43. Gordon SC, Reddy KR, Gould EE, et al. The spectrum of liver disease in the acquired immunodeficiency syndrome. J Hepatol 2:475, 1986.
44. Lebovics E, Dworkin BM, Heier SK, Rosenthal WS. The hepatobiliary manifestations of human immunodeficiency virus infection. Am J Gastroenterol 83:1, 1988.
45. Bodsworth NJ, Cooper DA, Donovan B. The influence of human immunodeficiency virus type 1 infection on the development of the hepatitis B virus carrier state. J Infect Dis 163:1138, 1991.
46. Housset C, Pol S, Carnot F, et al. Interactions between human immunodeficiency virus-1, hepatitis delta virus and hepatitis B virus infections in 260 chronic carriers of hepatitis B virus. Hepatology 15:578, 1992.
47. Scharschmidt BF, Held MJ, Hollander HH, et al. Hepatitis B in patients with HIV infection: relationship to AIDS and patient survival. Ann Intern Med 117:837, 1992.
48. Carr A, Samaras K, Chisholm DJ, Cooper DA. Pathogenesis of HIV-1-protease inhibitor-associated peripheral lipodystrophy, hyperlipidaemia, and insulin resistance. Lancet 351:1881, 1998.
49. Kim AY, Chung RT, Polsky B. Human immunodeficiency virus and hepatitis B and C coinfection: pathogenic interactions, natural history, and therapy. AIDS Clin Rev 263, 2000–01.
50. Eyster ME, Fried MW, Di Bisceglie AM, Goedert JJ. Increasing hepatitis C virus RNA levels in hemophiliacs: relationship to human immunodeficiency virus infection and liver disease. Multicenter Hemophilia Cohort Study. Blood 84:1020, 1994.
51. Chazouilleres O, Kim M, Combs C, et al. Quantitation of hepatitis C virus RNA in liver transplant recipients. Gastroenterology 106:994, 1994.
52. Eyster ME, Diamondstone LS, Lien JM, et al. Natural history of hepatitis C virus infection in multitransfused hemophiliacs: effect of coinfection with human immunodeficiency virus: the Multicenter Hemophilia Cohort Study. J Acquir Immune Defic Syndr 6:602, 1993.
53. Telfer P, Sabin C, Devereux H, et al. The progression of HCV-associated liver disease in a cohort of haemophilic patients. Br J Haematol 87:555, 1994.
54. Makris M, Preston FE, Rosendaal FR, et al. The natural history of chronic hepatitis C in haemophiliacs. Br J Haematol 94:746, 1996.
55. Lesens O, Deschenes M, Steben M, et al. Hepatitis C virus is related to progressive liver disease in human immunodeficiency virus-positive hemophiliacs and should be treated as an opportunistic infection. J Infect Dis 179:1254, 1999.
56. Benhamou Y, Bochet M, Di Martino V, et al. Liver fibrosis progression in human immunodeficiency virus and hepatitis C virus coinfected patients: the Multivirc Group. Hepatology 30:1054, 1999.
57. Bica I, McGovern B, Dhar R, et al. Increasing mortality due to end-stage liver disease in patients with human immunodeficiency virus infection. Clin Infect Dis 32:492, 2001.
58. Llibre JM, Garcia E, Aloy A, Valls J. Hepatitis C virus infection and progression of infection due to human immunodeficiency virus. Clin Infect Dis 16:182, 1993.
59. Quan CM, Krajden M, Grigoriew GA, Salit IE. Hepatitis C virus infection in patients infected with the human immunodeficiency virus. Clin Infect Dis 17:117, 1993.
60. Dorrucci M, Pezzotti P, Phillips AN, et al. Coinfection of hepatitis C virus with human immunodeficiency virus and progression to AIDS. Italian Seroconversion Study. J Infect Dis 172:1503, 1995.
61. Sabin CA, Telfer P, Phillips AN, et al. The association between hepatitis C virus genotype and human immunodeficiency virus disease progression in a cohort of hemophilic men. J Infect Dis 175:164, 1997.

62. Piroth L, Duong M, Quantin C, et al. Does hepatitis C virus co-infection accelerate clinical and immunological evolution of HIV-infected patients? AIDS 12:381, 1998.
63. Greub G, Ledergerber B, Battegay M, et al. Clinical progression, survival, and immune recovery during antiretroviral therapy in patients with HIV-1 and hepatitis C virus coinfection: the Swiss HIV Cohort Study. Lancet 356:1800, 2000.
64. Rutschmann OT, Negro F, Hirschel B, et al. Impact of treatment with human immunodeficiency virus (HIV) protease inhibitors on hepatitis C viremia in patients coinfected with HIV. J Infect Dis 177:783, 1998.
65. McHutchison JG, Gordon SC, Schiff ER, et al. Interferon alfa-2b alone or in combination with ribavirin as initial treatment for chronic hepatitis C. Hepatitis Interventional Therapy Group. N Engl J Med 339:1485, 1998.
66. Davis GL, Esteban-Mur R, Rustgi V, et al. Interferon alfa-2b alone or in combination with ribavirin for the treatment of relapse of chronic hepatitis C: International Hepatitis Interventional Therapy Group. N Engl J Med 339:1493, 1998.
67. Manns MP MJ, Gordon S, Rusti V, et al. PEGinterferon alfa-2B plus ribavirin compared to interferon alfa-2B plus ribavirin for the treatment of chronic hepatitis C: 24 week treatement analysis of a multicenter, multinational phase III randomized controlled trial. Hepatology 32:87A, 2000.
68. Lafeuillade A, Hittinger G, Chadapaud S. Increased mitochondrial toxicity with ribavirin in HIV/HCV coinfection. Lancet 357:280, 2001.
69. Uberti-Foppa C, De Bona A, Morsica G, et al. Recombinant interleukin-2 for treatment of HIV reduces hepatitis C viral load in coinfected patients. AIDS 13:140, 1999.
70. Nelson DR, Lauwers GY, Lau JY, Davis GL. Interleukin 10 treatment reduces fibrosis in patients with chronic hepatitis C: a pilot trial of interferon nonresponders. Gastroenterology 118:655, 2000.
71. Griffiths PD, Emery VC. Cytomegaloviruses. In: Richman DD, Whitley RJ, Hayden FG (eds) Clinical virology. New York, Churchill Livingstone, 1997, pp 445–470.
72. Kaufman B, Gandhi SA, Louie E, et al. Herpes simplex virus hepatitis: case report and review. Clin Infect Dis 24:334, 1997.
73. Knox KK, Carrigan DR. HHV-6 and CMV pneumonitis in immunocompromised patients. Lancet 343:1647, 1994.
74. Schiff G. Hepatitis caused by other viruses. In: Schiff ER, Sorrell MF, Maddrey WC (eds) Diseases of the Liver. Philadelphia, Lippincott-Raven, 1999, pp 869–877.
75. Hierholzer JC. Adenoviruses in the immunocompromised host. Clin Microbiol Rev 5:262, 1992.
76. Housset C, Boucher O, Girard P. Immunohistochemical evidence for HIV-1 infection of liver Kupffer cells. Hum Pathol 21:404, 1990.
77. Schaffner F. The liver in HIV infection. Prog Liver Dis 9:505, 1990.
78. Myerowitz RL, Pazin GJ, Allen CM. Disseminated candidiasis: changes in incidence, underlying diseases, and pathology. Am J Clin Pathol 68:29, 1977.
79. Semelka RC, Shoenut JP, Greenberg HM, Bow EJ. Detection of acute and treated lesions of hepatosplenic candidiasis: comparison of dynamic contrast-enhanced CT and MR imaging. J Magn Reson Imaging 2:341, 1992.
80. Phillips EH, Carroll BJ, Chandra M, et al. Laparoscopic-guided biopsy for diagnosis of hepatic candidiasis. J Laparoendosc Surg 2:33, 1992.
81. Cappell MS. Hepatobiliary manifestations of the acquired immune deficiency syndrome. Am J Gastroenterol 86:1, 1991.
82. Smith DH. Visceral leishmaniasis: human aspects. In: Giles HM (ed) Recent Advances in Tropical Medicine. Edinburgh, Churchill Livingstone, 1984, pp 79–87.
83. Gupta S. The liver in kala-azar. Ann Trop Med 50:252, 1956.
84. Moreno A, Marazuela M, Yebra M, et al. Hepatic fibrin-ring granulomas in visceral leishmaniasis. Gastroenterology 95:1123, 1988.
85. Murray HW, Pepin J, Nutman TB, et al. Tropical medicine. BMJ 320:490, 2000.
86. Dunn MA. Parasitic diseases. In: Schiff ER (ed) Diseases of the Liver, vol 8. Philadelphia, Lippincott, 1999, pp 1533–1548.
87. Jha TK, Sundar S, Thakur CP, et al. Miltefosine, an oral agent, for the treatment of Indian visceral leishmaniasis. N Engl J Med 341:1795, 1999.
88. Cohen O, Stoeckle M. Pneumocystis carinii infection in the acquired immunodeficiency syndrome. Arch Intern Med 151:1205, 1991.
89. Tompkins DC, Steigbigel RT. Rochalimaea's role in cat scratch disease and bacillary angiomatosis. Ann Intern Med 118:388, 1993.
90. Cotell SL, Noskin GA. Bacillary angiomatosis: clinical and histologic features, diagnosis, and treatment. Arch Intern Med 154:524, 1994.
91. Gasquet S, Maurin M, Brouqui P, et al. Bacillary angiomatosis in immunocompromised patients. AIDS 12:1793, 1998.
92. Alvarez SZ. Hepatobiliary tuberculosis. J Gastroenterol Hepatol 13:833, 1998.
93. Hoy J, Mijch A, Sandland M, et al. Quadruple-drug therapy for Mycobacterium avium-intracellulare bacteremia in AIDS patients. J Infect Dis 161:801, 1990.
94. Horsburgh CR, Metchock B, Gordon SM, et al. Predictors of survival in patients with AIDS and disseminated Mycobacterium avium complex disease. J Infect Dis 170:573, 1994.
95. Chin DP, Reingold AL, Stone EN, et al. The impact of Mycobacterium avium complex bacteremia and its treatment on survival of AIDS patients—a prospective study. J Infect Dis 170:578, 1994.
96. Chariot P, Drogou I, de Lacroix-Szmania I, et al. Zidovudine-induced mitochondrial disorder with massive liver steatosis, myopathy, lactic acidosis, and mitochondrial DNA depletion. J Hepatol 30:156, 1999.
97. Sundar K, Suarez M, Banogon PE, Shapiro JM. Zidovudine-induced fatal lactic acidosis and hepatic failure in patients with acquired immunodeficiency syndrome: report of two patients and review of the literature. Crit Care Med 25:1425, 1997.
98. Freiman JP, Helfert KE, Hamrell MR, Stein DS. Hepatomegaly with severe steatosis in HIV-seropositive patients. AIDS 7:379, 1993.
99. Pan-Zhou XR, Cui L, Zhou XJ, et al. Differential effects of antiretroviral nucleoside analogs on mitochondrial function in HepG2 cells. Antimicrob Agents Chemother 44:496, 2000.
100. Hammer SM, Katzenstein DA, Hughes MD, et al. A trial comparing nucleoside monotherapy with combination therapy in HIV-infected adults with CD4 cell counts from 200 to 500 per cubic millimeter: AIDS Clinical Trials Group Study 175 study team. N Engl J Med 335:1081, 1996.
101. Blackmore T, Gordon D. The Delta trial. Lancet 348:1238, 1996.
102. Randomised trial of addition of lamivudine or lamivudine plus loviride to zidovudine-containing regimens for patients with HIV-1 infection: the CAESAR trial. Lancet 349:1413, 1997.
103. Kemmer NM, Molina CP, Fuchs JE, et al. A distinctive histologic pattern of liver injury in HIV positive patients on HAART: a possible hepatotoxic effect of protease inhibitors. Hepatology 32:312A, 2000.
104. Brau N, Leaf HL, Wieczorek RL, Margolis DM. Severe hepatitis in three AIDS patients treated with indinavir. Lancet 349:924, 1997.
105. Palmon R, Tirelli R, Braun JF, et al. Hepatotoxicity associated with non-nucleoside reverse transcriptase inhibitors for the treatment of HIV and the effect of HBV or HCV infection. Hepatology 32:312A, 2000.
106. Moriya K, Fujie H, Shintani Y, et al. The core protein of hepatitis C virus induces hepatocellular carcinoma in transgenic mice. Nat Med 4:1065, 1998.
107. Barbaro G, Di Lorenzo G, Asti A, et al. Hepatocellular mitochondrial alterations in patients with chronic hepatitis C: ultrastructural and biochemical findings. Am J Gastroenterol 94:2198, 1999.
108. Rodriguez-Rosado R, Garcia-Samaniego J, Soriano V. Hepatotoxicity after introduction of highly active antiretroviral therapy. AIDS 12:1256, 1998.
109. Zylberberg H, Chaix ML, Rabian C, et al. Tritherapy for human immunodeficiency virus infection does not modify replication of hepatitis C virus in coinfected subjects. Clin Infect Dis 26:1104, 1998.
110. Ungo JR, Jones D, Ashkin D, et al. Antituberculosis drug-induced hepatotoxicity: the role of hepatitis C virus and the human immunodeficiency virus. Am J Respir Crit Care Med 157:1871, 1998.
111. Ragni MV, Bontempo FA. Increase in hepatitis C virus load in hemophiliacs during treatment with highly active antiretroviral therapy. J Infect Dis 180:2027, 1999.
112. Boyd AE, Taylor C, Norris S. Liver transplantation and HIV—a case series of 7 patients. In: 8th Conference on Retroviruses and Opportunistic Infections, 2001, p 578.

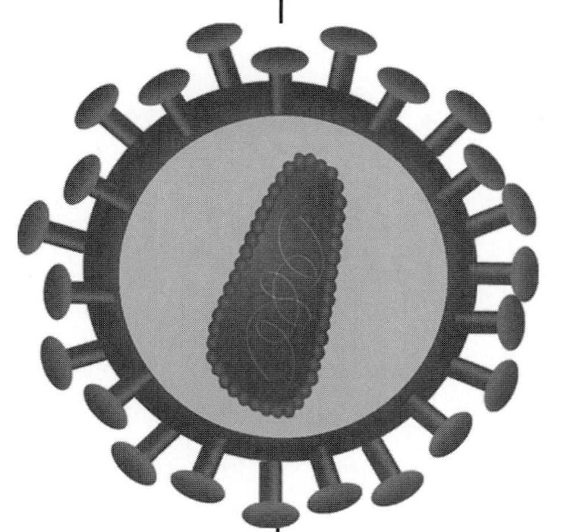

SECTION VIII

Drug Administration and Interactions

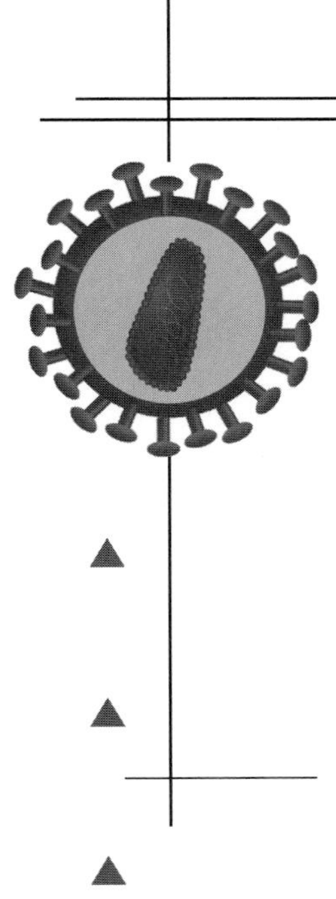

CHAPTER 66

Drug Administration and Interactions

Charles Flexner, MD
Stephen C. Piscitelli, PharmD

Pharmacology issues in the treatment of human immunodeficiency virus (HIV) infection have evolved from minor consideration points during the mid-1980s to recognition of their critical role in adherence, efficacy, and tolerability today. The era of highly active antiretrovirals therapy (HAART) has been characterized by drug regimens that are exceedingly potent, complicated, and burdensome and that are associated with a number of long-term toxicities. Many patients currently take at least three antiretroviral drugs for prophylaxis and treatment of opportunistic infections and often a variety of medications for supportive care of pain, depression, and other concomitant illnesses. Many patients are also receiving investigational agents or alternative medications (or both) from health food stores or acquired immunodeficiency syndrome (AIDS) buyers clubs. Although great strides have been made to improve formulations and pill burden, the late-stage patient may still require in excess of 10 or more medications and administration of 30 to 40 pills each day.

Selecting appropriate medications and constructing an effective antiretroviral regimen can be difficult in this era of polypharmacy. In addition to contending with drug resistance, the clinician is faced with food effects, proper spacing of medications, drug–drug interactions, overlapping toxicities, and patient adherence with the regimen. These factors, combined with pharmacokinetic, formulation, and storage issues, further complicate the care of the HIV-infected patient.

▲ FOOD EFFECTS

Food alters the absorption or bioavailability of several drugs commonly used in HIV-infected patients. Drug–food interactions can influence the scheduling of medications during the day and can profoundly affect the quality of life of patients. Dosing of antiretrovirals can be confusing for patients, who often have to schedule their meals around drug administration. For example, didanosine tablets and sachets are formulated with a buffer that requires administration on an empty stomach because low gastric pH leads to degradation of the drug.[1] Although not buffered, didanosine enteric coated capsules also must be given on an empty stomach because administration with food decreases the maximum concentration C_{max} and the area under the concentration–time curve (AUC) by 46% and 19%, respectively.[2] Bioavailability of the other nucleosides is not significantly affected by food, although peak absorption may be delayed. For example, a high-fat[3] or high-protein[4] meal slows the rate of absorption of zidovudine and may reduce the mean maximum concentration; but it does not significantly alter the overall extent of absorption.

Several protease inhibitor regimens are particularly problematic in terms of food effects. When used alone, indinavir must be given on an empty stomach or with a light meal containing less than 2 g of fat.[5] When combined with ritonavir, indinavir can be administered without regard to food.[6] Conversely, the bioavailability of both formulations of saquinavir (Invirase, Fortovase) is improved with high-calorie, high-fat foods, and these drugs must be given within 2 hours of a full meal. Lopinavir-ritonavir (Kaletra) and nelfinavir also require administration with food for optimal absorption. Although ritonavir capsule absorption is only somewhat increased in the presence of food, administration with a meal is recommended to decrease its gastrointestinal side effects.[7] A variety of HIV-related medications have specific food restrictions stemming from the

▲ **Table 66–1.** FOOD–DRUG INTERACTIONS WITH HIV-RELATED MEDICATIONS

Drug	Food Effect	Recommendation
Atovaquone	High-fat meal may increase bioavailability up to three-fold	Administer with food
Didanosine	Administration with food results in 55% increase in AUC	Administer on empty stomach at least 30 minutes before a meal
Ganciclovir (capsules)	High-fat meal results in 22% increase in AUC	Administer with food
Indinavir	High-fat caloric meal results in 77% increase in AUC	Administer on empty stomach or with low-fat, light meal
Itraconazole (capsules)	Significant increase in bioavailability when taken with a full meal	Administer with food
Itraconazole (solution)	Maximal absorption when taken under fasting conditions	Recommended without food if possible
Lopinavir	Increase in AUC when given with food	Administer with food
Nelfinavir	AUC two- to threefold higher when given with food	Administer with meal or light snack
Ritonavir	Food results in 15% increase in AUC	Recommended to be taken with meals
Saquinavir	Marked increase in AUC following high-fat meal	Administer within 2 hours after a full meal
Saquinavir	Grapefruit juice increases AUC by 50–200%	Use caution or avoid co-administration

AUC, area under the concentration–time curve.

possibility of increased or decreased absorption from the gastrointestinal tract; these restrictions are summarized in Table 66–1. A review of food restrictions should be an important part of patient counseling for a new or modified drug regimen.

▲ SPACING OF MEDICATIONS

The specific administration times for some antiretroviral durgs and how they are taken in relation to other medications may affect their absorption and activity. For example, the antacids in didanosine tablets and sachets may decrease the absorption of indinavir if the two are administered concomitantly.[8] Thus a minimum 30-minute separation is required. Because both agents are generally taken on an empty stomach, the patient may have to wait several hours before a full meal can be eaten. Didanosine is currently U.S. Food and Drug Administration (FDA)-approved for once-daily dosing, and this schedule may alleviate the problem. The new enteric coated formulation of didanosine does not alter indinavir's absorption, and they can be given concomitantly.

Concentrations of some protease inhibitors in dual combination may differ depending on whether they are given concomitantly or in a staggered fashion. A study in healthy volunteers evaluated single doses of a dual combination of protease inhibitors (saquinavir, ritonavir, nelfinavir) given simultaneously or when separated by 4 hours. The AUC of saquinavir was markedly lower when given 4 hours before ritonavir or nelfinavir compared to simultaneous dosing. Nelfinavir and ritonavir exposure did not appear to be affected by time separation.[9]

A number of dual protease inhibitor combinations are being evaluated for once-daily dosing.[10,11] Such regimens would be particularly useful for selected populations such as prison inmates, methadone clinics, and patients requiring directly observed therapy. Although these regimens would be more convenient, they might also require perfect adherence, as concentrations at the end of the 24-hour dosing interval may be near the 50% inhibitry concentration (IC_{50}) value. Therefore, a missed dose would result in suboptimal concentrations for a prolonged period, leading to increased risk of recurrent viral replication and drug resistance. Most protease inhibitors have large interpatient pharmacokinetic variability, so even with good adherence there may be a small proportion of patients with concentrations below the desired target at the end of a dosing interval.[5]

▲ DRUG INTERACTIONS

One of the greatest challenges for the HIV clinician is the recognition and management of drug interactions.[12] The HIV-infected patient often receives numerous medications and has a great potential for adverse drug interactions. Certain protease inhibitors combinations may also be used to take advantage of beneficial pharmacokinetic interactions.

A number of medications used in HIV-infected patients can produce adverse drug interactions[12] (Table 66–2). A review of product information for the 16 available antiretroviral agents reveals more than 200 potential drug interactions.[2,13–26] Although many of these interactions are minor in nature, some are potentially serious, leading to severe toxicity or treatment failure. Fortunately, most interactions can be easily recognized, prevented, and corrected. Minor alterations in scheduling or selection of an appropriate alternative are usually all that is required to avoid a potential interaction. Other drug interactions may be beneficial by increasing plasma concentrations of co-administered protease inhibitors.

Drug interactions can generally be classified as pharmacokinetic (i.e., affecting drug concentrations) or pharmacodynamic (i.e., affecting drug activity). Pharmacokinetic interactions involve changes in absorption, distribution, metabolism, or excretion, whereas pharmacodynamic interactions may involve additive, synergistic, or antagonistic effects.

Pharmacokinetic Interactions

Altered Drug Absorption

Impaired of drug absorption can lead to a marked reduction in the bioavailability of certain agents. One of the most common interactions affecting drug absorption is

▲ **Table 66–2.** CLINICALLY SIGNIFICANT DRUG INTERACTIONS IN HIV-INFECTED PATIENTS

Affected Drug	Interacting Drug(s)	Effect	Comment
APV IDV RTV NFV SQV	Rifampin	Protease inhibitor AUC decreased by 70–92%	Avoid concomitant use
APV IDV SQV LPV/RTV	Nevirapine Efavirenz	Protease inhibitor AUC decreased by 28–62%	Use with ritonavir or increase dose
Methadone	Efavirenz Nevirapine	Methadone concentrations decreased	Monitor for symptoms and adjust dose
Rifabutin	APV IDV NFV	Rifabutin AUC increased two- to threefold	Decrease dose to 150 mg/day; increase IDV dose to 1000 mg tid
Atorvastatin	RTV/SQV LPV/RTV	Atorvastatin AUC increased four- to fivefold	Use low dose and increase with caution
Simvastatin	RTV/SQV	Simvastatin AUC increased 32-fold	Avoid concomitant use
Pravastatin	RTV/SQV	Minimal change in pravastatin AUC	No dose adjustment necessary
Sildenafil	IDV SQV RTV	Sildenafil AUC increased 2- to 11-fold	Use 25 mg dose; with ritonavir do not repeat for 48 hours

APV, amprenavir; AUC, area under the concentration–time curve; IDV, indinavir; LPV, lopinavir; NFV, nelfinavir; RTV, ritonavir, SQV, saquinavir.

chelation, the binding of drugs to substances in the gastrointestinal tract. The concomitant administration of a fluoroquinolone antibiotic with a di- or trivalent cation such as calcium, magnesium, aluminum, or iron results in a more than 90% decrease in the AUC of the fluoroquinolone, possibly leading to therapeutic failure.[27–29] Didanosine formulations with a calcium and magnesium buffer (tablets) or citrate-phosphate buffer (sachet) can alter fluoroquinolone disposition. Concomitant administration of didanosine with ciprofloxacin has been shown to decrease the ciprofloxacin AUC from 15.5 to 0.26 μg/hr/ml.[30] A similar interaction would be expected with other products such as antacids, sucralfate, or iron preparations. Administration of these agents should be separated from the fluoroquinolone by at least 2 hours, and the fluoroquinolone should be administered first, followed by the cation, to ensure adequate absorption. The newer enteric coated formulation of didanosine does not alter ciprofloxacin pharmacokinetics and can be given concomitantly.[2]

A change in gastric pH may affect the absorption of azole antifungals such as ketoconazole and itraconazole. An acidic environment is required for absorption of ketoconazole; thus its administration should be avoided with concomitant histamine-2 antagonists, proton pump inhibitors, and antacids.[31,32] Administration of ketoconazole with sodium bicarbonate and cimetidine resulted in therapeutic failure in a patient with cryptococcal infection.[33] Fluconazole is an appropriate alternative in patients requiring agents that increase gastric pH or in those with achlorhydria because its absorption is not dependent on gastric pH.[34] For itraconazole capsules, a low pH is best for absorption, but the presence of food is more important for optimal absorption. Alternatively, it can be given with an acidic beverage such as Coca-Cola to improve absorption.[35] The oral solution of itraconazole is best absorbed on an empty stomach.[36]

Altered Drug Metabolism

Intestinal Metabolism and P-Glycoprotein

The cytochrome P_{450} (CYP) enzyme system consists of at least 12 families of enzymes common to all mammals and represents the major enzyme system involved in drug metabolism.[37] In humans, the CYP1, CYP2, and CYP3 families are primarily responsible for drug metabolism, with the CYP3A subfamily involved in the metabolism of the largest number of drugs, including most available protease inhibitors. CYP_{450}-mediated metabolism largely takes place in the liver, although CYP enzymes are also present in other sites including enterocytes in the intestinal wall.[38] Thus inhibitors of CYP3A4 may alter drug absorption or hepatic metabolism. The 20-fold increase in plasma concentrations of saquinavir produced by ritonavir is likely caused by inhibition of CYP3A4 at both sites.[39] Grapefruit juice contains various substances that inhibit CYP3A4-mediated metabolism only in the gut wall, mainly by selective down-regulation of CYP3A4 protein in the small intestine.[40] The AUC for saquinavir is increased by 1.5- to 2.5-fold during concomitant administration of grapefruit juice.[17] However, grapefruit juice should not be relied on to increase the plasma concentrations of protease inhibitors because the amounts of P_{450} inhibitors vary widely among brands and are affected by factors such as how much and how often the juice is consumed.[41]

P-Glycoprotein (P-gp) is the product of the *mdr1* gene first described as a mediator of resistance to cancer chemotherapy. Enterocytes in the intestinal mucosa are a major site for expression of P-gp, one of several membrane-bound proteins that increase efflux of drugs from cells.[42] P-gp appears to contribute to the low bioavailability of some drugs, including certain protease inhibitors. P-gp in the brush border cells of the intestine can pump drug back into the gastrointestinal lumen, decreasing absorption.

In the liver, P-gp pumps drug into bile; it is also present in the blood-brain barrier, where it can limit the uptake of drugs into the central nervous system (CNS). Several protease inhibitors are substrates for and inhibitors of P-gp. In theory, inhibiting P-gp could be used to increase protease inhibitor concentrations in target sites such as the CNS.[43] However, P-gp expression has a profound negative impact on HIV replication. In two separate sets of experiments, cells expressing P-gp produced at least 40- to 70-fold less HIV than control cells. This was thought to be due primarily to inhibition of HIV entry or membrane fusion.[44,45] The clinical implications of these findings highlight a dilemma regarding how (or whether) P-gp should be altered in HIV-infected patients: The presence of P-gp may lead to decreased intracellular drug concentrations, but the fact that P-gp expression may make the cell less susceptible to HIV infection might counteract these low drug concentrations.

Cytochrome P_{450} enyzmes and P-glycoprotein in the intestine and liver can present a barrier to absorption of orally administered drugs and have considerable impact on drug interactions. The overlap of tissue distribution and substrate specificity of CYP3A4 and P-glycoprotein complicates the definition of the specific mechanisms of some drug interactions. Many drugs that are modulators of P-glycoprotein are also inhibitors of CYP3A4.[46] The effect of these two pathways on antiretroviral drug concentrations remains a fertile area for additional research.

Enzyme Induction

Inducers increase the rate of hepatic metabolism, usually through increased transcription of mRNA; and they decrease serum concentrations of other drugs metabolized by the same hepatic isoenzyme. Rifampin and rifabutin are classic examples of enzyme inducers, causing decreases in plasma concentrations of concomitantly metabolized drugs. Both drugs can decrease concentrations of protease inhibitors. The Centers for Disease Control and Prevention (CDC) has issued guidelines for concomitant use of rifampin or rifabutin with HIV protease inhibitors in patients with tuberculosis.[47] Rifampin should be avoided with all single protease inhibitors but may be used with caution in patients receiving saquinavir plus ritonavir.[47] Patients receiving indinavir or nelfinavir should receive a reduced dose of rifabutin and a slightly increased PI dose.[47,48]

Nevirapine is a mild to moderate hepatic enzyme inducer and decreases the AUC of saquinavir and indinavir by 27% and 28%, respectively; but it has a minimal effect on ritonavir and nelfinavir.[49,50] It is currently recommended that the indinavir dose be increased to 1000 mg q8h with nevirapine, although clinical studies have not verified the effect of this combination on surrogate markers or clinical endpoints. Efavirenz is a mixed inducer/inhibitor, decreasing concentrations of amprenavir, saquinavir, and indinavir and necessitating an increased dose or the addition of ritonavir.[51]

Ritonavir and nelfinavir, also moderate enzyme inducers, can increase hepatic glucuronidation and CYP activity. The AUC of the oral contraceptive ethinyl estradiol is decreased by approximately 40% with these agents, necessitating an alternative form of birth control.[20,52] Ritonavir is also an inducer of CYP1A2, which is involved in the metabolism of theophylline.[53] Concomitant administration of ritonavir with theophylline has been reported to result in a 43% decrease in the theophylline AUC. Patients receiving this combination should be warned to watch for symptoms of reduced theophylline activity, and theophylline levels should be monitored.

Enzyme Inhibition

There are a number of CYP inhibitors that decrease the rate of hepatic metabolism and increase plasma concentrations of other drugs metabolized by the same isoenzyme. HIV protease inhibitors can be both CYP inhibitors and substrates, increasing the concentrations of some metabolized drugs and having their own concentrations increased by other CYP inhibitors. Most of the currently available protease inhibitors are primarily metabolized by CYP3A4.[5] These agents differ in the number and magnitude of potential drug interactions. Ritonavir is associated with the greatest number of drug interactions, and saquinavir is the weakest enzyme inhibitor and has less propensity to alter the concentrations of other drugs. The combination of lopinavir and ritonavir (Kaletra) has a drug interaction profile similar to that of ritonavir.[25] Amprenavir, nelfinavir, and indinavir inhibit CYP3A4 metabolism to a lesser extent than ritonavir. For example, all three drugs increase the rifabutin AUC approximately twofold, necessitating a 50% reduction in the rifabutin dose.[12] Ritonavir increases the rifabutin AUC fourfold, which may lead to clinically significant adverse effects.[54,55] Alternatives for patients taking protease inibitors and requiring *Mycobacterium avium* complex (MAC) prophylaxis include azithromycin and clarithromycin. The clarithromycin AUC is increased 77% with ritonavir and 53% with indinavir, although a dosage adjustment is unnecessary in patients with normal renal function.[56] Azithromycin is primarily excreted by the biliary route and does not interact with inhibitors of CYP.[57]

Deleterious Drug Interactions

The most serious potential interactions with CYP inhibitors involve concomitant administration with certain metabolized drugs, such as terfenadine and cisapride (both removed from the U.S. market), antiarrhythmics, and ergot alkaloids. In the case of cisapride and terfenadine, these combinations led to cardiotoxicity, with the potential for life-threatening arrhythmias.[58] Administration of protease inhibitors with some benzodiazepine sedative-hypnotics can result in exaggerated side effects such as oversedation.

Beneficial Drug Interactions

Drug interactions were initially viewed as a complication to be avoided in HIV-infected patients. The concept of using two protease inhibitors concomitantly to increase plasma concentrations or improve convenience was first recognized with the combination of saquinavir and ritonavir. Simultaneous administration of two protease inhibitors takes advantage of beneficial pharmacokinetic interactions and may circumvent many of the drugs' undesirable pharmacologic properties.[6] In addition, dual protease inhibitors decrease interpatient variability, making drug concentrations more predictable. Dual protease inhibitor regimens have now been widely prescribed and are included in reported treatment guidelines despite not being FDA-approved. A number of potentially beneficial metabolic drug interactions exist for combinations of two HIV protease inhibitors. One drug is used to inhibit the metabolism of the second agent, producing increased bioavailability, decreased clearance, or both. Two-way interactions also exist in which the pharmacokinetic profile of each drug benefits.

Ritonavir-Saquinavir

Saquinavir has a number of disadvantages, including poor bioavailability, three times a day dosing, and a pill burden of 18 capsules per day. However, when combined with even small doses of ritonavir, there is a marked increase in saquinavir bioavailability and a decrease in clearance, allowing twice-daily dosing and a decreased dose from 1800 mg tid to 400 mg bid. In a single-dose, crossover study in healthy volunteers, ritonavir increased the saquinavir AUC by 50- to 132-fold and increased the saquinavir C_{max} by 23- to 35-fold.[39] Because ritonavir is a P_{450} inducer and undergoes autoinduction during the first 10 to 14 days of therapy,[59] steady-state concentrations of saquinavir should be lower when these two drugs are combined. Multiple-dose pharmacokinetic interaction studies found that the steady-state saquinavir AUC was increased only 20- to 30-fold.[60]

The effect of the ritonavir dose on saquinavir plasma levels was evaluated in 120 patients receiving various saquinavir-ritonavir combinations.[61] Data from two dose-ranging trials of saquinavir-ritonavir given either twice daily or once daily were included in the analysis. A wide range of saquinavir doses (400 to 1800 mg) and ritonavir doses (100 to 400 mg) were evaluated. The investigators used multivariate linear and nonlinear regression to correlate steady-state saquinavir pharmacokinetic parameters (C_{min}, C_{max}, half-life) with saquinavir and ritonavir doses. This model showed a strong effect of ritonavir on saquinavir C_{max} and C_{min}, but these parameters were correlated only with saquinavir dosage, and the increase in saquinavir concentrations was similar for ritonavir dosages over the range of 100 to 400 mg twice daily. In this analysis there was not a dose-dependent effect of ritonavir on saquinavir concentrations.

The poor oral bioavailability of saquinavir (1% to 12%, depending on formulation and conditions) likely reflects extensive first-pass metabolism rather than poor absorption. The increase in saquinavir concentrations with ritonavir is the result of improved bioavailability, perhaps to as much as 100%, with little effect on postabsorptive systemic clearance. In addition to effects on intestinal CYP3A4, ritonavir is also an inhibitor of P-glycoprotein, and its dual effects on both CYP3A4 and P-gp may account for the large magnitude of ritonavir's effect on saquinavir oral bioavailability.[62]

Although the doses of 400 mg ritonavir/400 mg saquinavir twice daily has been commonly used for a number of years, dosing regimens that employ a lower dose of ritonavir to improve tolerability and reduce effects on plasma lipids are under evaluation. One single-dose study in healthy volunteers found that combining 200 mg of ritonavir with 600 mg saquinavir increased the saquinavir AUC by an average 74-fold, an effect similar to that seen with 400 mg ritonavir.[39] Clinically, a 1000 mg saquinavir/100 mg ritonavir bid dose is being evaluated as is 1600 mg saquinavir/100 mg ritonavir administered once daily.[11]

Ritonavir-Indinavir

When used as a sole protease inhibitor, indinavir has a number of limitations, including an every-8-hour dosing regimen, food restrictions, hydration requirements, and large interindividual pharmacokinetic variability.[5] The combination of indinavir, even with small doses of ritonavir, alleviates many of these disadvantages.

In a steady-state pharmacokinetic interaction study in healthy volunteers involving 14 days of ritonavir treatment, the combination of 200 or 400 mg ritonavir with 400 or 600 mg indinavir increased the indinavir AUC three- to sixfold compared to that seen with 800 mg indinavir alone.[63] This mechanism primarily involves inhibition of hepatic CYP3A4, with reduced first-pass metabolism making a minor contribution. Ritonavir increased the indinavir C_{max} up to 2-fold and the indinavir concentration 11- to 33-fold 8 hours after dosing.[63] Decreased ritonavir dose and increased indinavir dose were examined in a separate study.[64] In healthy volunteers administered ritonavir for 14 days, the 24-hour indinavir AUC with a 100 mg bid ritonavir/800 mg bid indinavir regimen was fourfold higher than with 800 mg q8h indinavir alone. In the same study, the 24-hour AUC of indinavir with a 400/400 mg bid ritonavir-indinavir regimen was 40% lower than with the 100/800 mg regimen and 55% lower than with a 200/800 mg regimen.[64] However, the mean 12-hour trough concentrations of the 400/400 mg regimen and the 100/800 mg regimen were nearly the same.

In two studies, co-administration of ritonavir and indinavir abolished the effect of food on indinavir bioavailability. A high-fat meal reduced the bioavailability of oral indinavir by up to 85%.[63] Doses of 100, 200, or 400 mg of ritonavir bid reversed the effect of a high- or low-fat meal on indinavir pharmacokinetics compared to 800 mg indinavir given in the fasted state.[64] Ritonavir could enhance indinavir oral bioavailability in the presence of food through inhibition of intestinal cytochrome P_{450} or drug transporters such as P-glycoprotein. This finding suggests that the deleterious effects of food on indinavir may be mediated by interaction with intestinal epithelial drug transporters or P_{450} complexes, processes potentially blocked by ritonavir.[6]

There is some concern that the high peak concentrations achieved with indinavir-ritonavir may lead to an increased risk of nephrolithiasis. In patients taking indinavir 800 mg q8h, a higher AUC and C_{max} were associated with increased risk of indinavir-induced nephrotoxicity in one study.[65] Increasing indinavir C_{max} and C_{min} were associated with an increase in nephrolithiasis in patients taking indinavir/ritonavir twice-daily combinations of 400/100, 400/400, 600/100, or 800/100 mg; these regimens were associated with short-term nephrotoxicity risks of 0%, 2%, 6%, or 10%, respectively.[66] Indinavir-ritonavir regimens of 400/400 mg bid were not associated with an increased incidence of nephrolithiasis compared to indinavir 800 mg q8h without ritonavir, although tolerability may be an issue with the higher ritonavir dose.[67]

Lopinavir-Ritonavir

Lopinavir-ritonavir (Kaletra) represents the first use of ritonavir in a co-formulated product to increase concentrations of a second protease inhibitor. Each dose of Kaletra contains 400 mg of lopinavir plus 100 mg of ritonavir (133/33 mg capsules × 3 capsules) given twice daily. Lopinavir is a highly active protease inhibitor, but its bioavailability is low and its clearance rapid when given alone. However, in combination with low doses of ritonavir, the AUC is increased by more than 100-fold[68] owing to inhibition of lopinavir's CYP3A4 metabolism in the liver and gastrointestinal tract. Ritonavir's effect on the lopinavir AUC was severalfold greater than ritonavir's effect on the saquinavir AUC.[6]

This beneficial pharmacokinetic interaction was confirmed in human volunteers; when dosed at 12-hour intervals (q12h) with ritonavir, mean trough concentrations of lopinavir were approximately 30-fold higher than the in vitro IC_{50} for HIV.[69] In 101 HIV-infected patients taking lopinavir 200 or 400 mg bid with ritonavir 100 or 200 mg bid plus two nucleoside analogues for 48 weeks, the HIV viral load was suppressed to less than 400 copies/ml in 93% to 100% of patients and to less than 50 copies/ml in 83% to 86%.[70]

The addition of efavirenz to lopinavir-ritonavir results in a decrease of 40% in the lopinavir AUC.[71] Although concentrations are still relatively high despite this reduction, the manufacturer suggests the dose be increased to 533/133 (four capsules) mg bid when combined with efavirenz or nevirapine to offset the enzyme induction effects of the nonnucleoside reverse transcriptase inhibitors (NNRTIs), especially if the patient is treatment-experienced and resistance is suspected.[25]

Amprenavir-Ritonavir

Amprenavir is a twice-daily protease inhibitor but has the disadvantage of an oral formulation requiring 16 capsules per day. The combination of amprenavir with varying ritonavir doses has been evaluated in a number of pharmacokinetic studies in patients and healthy volunteers. Administration of amprenavir with low-dose ritonavir increases the amprenavir AUC two- to threefold and increases the trough concentration by approximately fivefold.[72] In one study patients received amprenavir 1200 mg bid with ritonavir 200 or 500 mg bid. The patients receiving the higher ritonavir dose did not achieve higher amprenavir concentrations.[72] Thus increasing the ritonavir above 200 mg likely is associated only with more adverse effects and does not provide higher plasma concentrations.

A number of amprenavir-ritonavir regimens have been proposed based on pharmacokinetic studies in volunteers and simulation of plasma concentrations.[73] There are no clinical data, but many clinicians employ an amprenavir/ritonavir 600/100 mg bid regimen, although the amprenavir dose may need to be increased in treatment-experienced patients with suspected resistance. However, in patients also receiving nevirapine or efavirenz, ritonavir 100 mg bid does not appear to prevent a decrease in amprenavir concentrations from the enzyme-inducing properties of these NNRTIs. In a small study, patients receiving amprenavir 450 mg with ritonavir 200 mg bid were switched to a 600/100 mg regimen, and the amprenavir trough values decreased by 80%.[74] A separate study demonstrated no decrease in amprenavir C_{min} when efavirenz was added to an amprenavir-ritonavir regimen containing ritonavir 200 mg bid.[72] Thus it appears that a threshold dose of at least 200 mg of ritonavir is required to prevent NNRTI-induced drug interactions. Efavirenz also decreased the indinavir AUC by 30% when added to indinavir-ritonavir 800/100 mg bid.[75] The ritonavir dose should therefore be increased to 200 mg bid in dual protease inhibitor combinations with efavirenz or nevirapine.[25]

Once-daily dosing regimens of 1200 mg amprenavir/ 200 mg ritonavir have been evaluated in HIV-infected patients. At the end of a 24-hour dosing interval, amprenavir concentrations were approximately threefold higher with this regimen than with amprenavir 1200 mg bid alone.[76]

Ritonavir-Nelfinavir

Originally marketed as a three times a day regimen, nelfinavir was studied in combination with ritonavir to reduce its dosing frequency and the potential for once a day dosing. Although ritonavir does increase nelfinavir concentrations modestly, this combination is generally not widely used because of poor tolerability. Dose-limiting diarrhea or gastrointestinal adverse effects make it less attractive than other dual protease inhibitor combinations.[77]

A single-dose drug interaction study in healthy volunteers showed that ritonavir increased the nelfinavir AUC by 152%, whereas nelfinavir increased ritonavir's AUC by only 9%.[20] A steady-state pharmacokinetic interaction study in HIV-infected volunteers evaluated the combination of ritonavir 400 mg bid with nelfinavir 500 or 750 mg bid. After 5 weeks of dosing, ritonavir use was associated with a 162% increase in the 500 mg nelfinavir 24-hour AUC (dose-normalized) and a 62% increase in the 750 mg AUC compared to that of historical controls taking only nelfinavir 750 mg tid.[77] At the same time, the change in ritonavir's dose-normalized 24-hour AUC was +13% with nelfinavir 500 mg and −13% with the 750 mg regimen.

This pharmacokinetic interaction is more complicated than others because both drugs are CYP_{450} inducers as well as inhibitors.[6] The fact that nelfinavir's AUC did not increase significantly when the dose was increased from 500 to 750 mg bid may reflect increased induction with the higher nelfinavir dose. In addition, there was a trend for nelfinavir to reduce ritonavir's trough concentrations at the higher 750 mg nelfinavir dose.[77] This may have decreased the magnitude of ritonavir's beneficial impact on nelfinavir pharmacokinetics.

Nelfinavir is the only HIV protease inhibitor known to produce an active metabolite, the hydroxybutylamide M8 (AG1402), which is the major metabolite of nelfinavir in humans and has equipotent anti-HIV activity in vitro.[78] Ritonavir had a more significant beneficial impact on the pharmacokinetics of M8 than on nelfinavir itself. After 5 weeks of dosing, ritonavir use was associated with a 430% increase in the 500 mg M8 24-hour AUC and a 370% increase in the 750 mg M8 AUC compared to historical controls taking nelfinavir 750 mg tid alone.[6]

One study evaluated the effect of low-dose ritonavir (100 or 200 mg bid) on nelfinavir pharmacokinetics in healthy volunteers.[79] Overall, the AUC of nelfinavir was increased approximately 30% in both ritonavir dosing groups. The morning steady-state predose concentrations of nelfinavir were increased substantially in a dose-dependent fashion with 45% and 90% increases in the 100- and 200-mg arms, respectively. The half-life of nelfinavir was not altered by ritonavir, and the active nelfinavir M8 metabolite was increased by approximately 75% for C_{max} and 90% for AUC. The magnitude of the M8 increase was similar for both ritonavir doses.[79]

Nelfinavir-Saquinavir

In single-dose pharmacokinetic interaction studies, nelfinavir increased the saquinavir AUC by up to fivefold, with no effect of saquinavir on nelfinavir concentrations.[5] However, nelfinavir is an inducer of $CYP_{450}3A$, and at steady-state the magnitude of this interaction was substantially reduced. Combining nelfinavir 750 mg tid with the soft-gel formulation of saquinavir 800 mg tid produced a saquinavir AUC equivalent to 1200 mg tid at steady-state.[80] This combination was well tolerated and was highly active against HIV in patients who were also taking two nucleoside analogues.[81] However, this combination lacks many of the pharmacologic and clinical benefits of other dual protease inhibitor combinations. With a trend to convert all protease inhibitor regimens to twice a day, the three times a day dosing regimens of nelfinavir and saquinavir appear to be less relevant to clinical practice.

Nelfinavir-Indinavir

Combining nelfinavir with indinavir produced a 50% increase in the indinavir AUC and an 80% increase in the nelfinavir AUC in single-dose studies in healthy volunteers.[5] However, when these two drugs were administered to patients in a twice-daily steady-state regimen, there was little pharmacokinetic enhancement and a disappointing anti-HIV effect, with only 10 of 21 patients suppressing their plasma HIV RNA to less than 400 copies/ml (the lower limit of quantification) after 32 weeks.[82] Presumably, hepatic enzyme induction by nelfinavir resulted in reduced concentrations of both drugs and no real pharmacokinetic benefits.

Indinavir-Saquinavir

The indinavir-saquinavir combination was reported to be antagonistic when used to inhibit HIV replication in vitro.[83] Although the clinical relevance of this finding is unknown, this combination has not been pursued further in vivo, even though indinavir increased saquinavir concentrations fivefold in single-dose studies.

Other Antiretroviral Combinations

Other strategies for increasing concentrations of protease inhibitors through enzyme inhibition could include concomitant ketoconazole or delavirdine, both of which are CYP3A4 inhibitors. Delavirdine significantly increased the AUC of saquinavir by 520%, indinavir by 72%, and nelfinavir by 92%.[84,85]

Interactions with Herbal Therapies

Herbal remedies and nutritional supplements are widely used in HIV-infected patients, although little attention has been paid to the pharmacokinetic effects of these compounds, as they are thought to be benign. An increasing number of studies have shown that certain alternative therapies may cause clinically important drug interactions with agents used to treat HIV infection. In healthy volunteers, St. John's wort decreased the AUC of indinavir by more than 50%.[86] The mechanism of this interaction is complex and appears to be mediated by induction of both CYP3A4 and P-glycoprotein.[87,88] This herb should be avoided in patients taking protease inhibitors and NNRTIs. There are currently no data on whether ritonavir can reverse this interaction.

Garlic supplements are sometimes used by HIV-infected patients because of their touted effects on lowering cholesterol. Raw garlic and garlic supplements inhibit the activity of CYP3A4 in vitro and in animals, and case reports have documented ritonavir-related gastrointestinal toxicity in two people after they ingested uncooked garlic preparations with ritonavir.[89] A study in healthy volunteers showed that garlic capsules taken twice daily for 3 weeks led to a mean decrease in saquinavir concentrations of approximately 50% probably as a consequence of reduced bioavailibility.[90] Even after a 10-day washout period, AUC values returned to only 60% to 70% of baseline, suggesting a prolonged effect. Other herbs with reported in vitro effects on CYP_{450}-mediated metabolism include silymarin (milk thistle), ginseng, and skullcap, although clinical data are lacking.[91] Clinicians must include alternative medicines in their drug histories and consider them when adverse effects or treatment failures appear with no other cause.

Drug–Cytokine Interactions

Proinflammatory cytokines including interleukin-6 (IL-6), IL-1, and tumor necrosis factor-α (TNFα) are released during periods of stress, trauma, or infection. A number of in vitro and clinical studies have shown that IL-6 and TNFα inhibit cytochrome P_{450}-mediated metabolism. This mechanism is not competitive but is a metabolic interaction at the level of transcription of cytochrome P_{450} messenger RNA.[92]

Several immunodulating agents are being evaluated for the treatment of HIV infection. One of the best studied is IL-2. Its exogenous administration has been shown to increase CD4 cells but results in a profound release of proinflammatory cytokines that are a likely cause of its problematic side effect profile. In HIV-infected patients receiving a 5-day continuous infusion of IL-2, indinavir clearance significantly decreased and the AUC increased 75% compared with baseline values before IL-2 administration.[93] The short-term administration (< 5 days) of IL-2 makes this interaction less clinically significant, although drug–cytokine interactions should be considered as additional investigational cytokines are used more widely.

Altered Excretion

Drug interactions may also be caused by alterations in renal elimination. This can be a consequence of inhibited tubular secretion or impaired renal function. Probenecid and trimethoprim are inhibitors of renal tubular secretion, which may increase concentrations of some renally cleared drugs. The lamivudine AUC is increased by 44% with concomitant trimethoprim-sulfamethoxazole.[94] The acyclovir AUC is increased 40% with concomitant probenecid.[95] Inhibition of renal secretion may be a useful strategy to increase plasma concentrations of antimicrobials such as acyclovir, increase the likelihood of a successful response, or offset poor oral absorption.

Intracellular Interactions

The nucleoside reverse transcriptase inhibitors (NRTIs) are prodrugs that must undergo phosphorylation intracellularly to their active forms. These drugs are not generally affected by CYP_{450} interactions, but there may be competition for intracellular activation pathways that result in clinically relevant drug interactions. Ribavirin decreases the phosphorylation of zidovudine and stavudine in vitro, resulting in decreased intracellular concentrations of the active compound.[96,97] AIDS patients with hepatitis C may be treated with Rebetron, a ribavirin-interferon combination formulation that could result in decreased efficacy of zidovudine, although there have been no reported clinical studies assessing the importance of this interaction. Similarly, zidovudine may impair the intracellular phosphorylation of stavudine,[97] and this combination is associated with unfavorable clinical outcomes compared with other regimens containing two NRTIs.[98] Lamivudine inhibits zalcitabine phosphorylation, and this combination should be avoided.[99]

Recognizing and Circumventing Drug Interactions

Strategies for recognizing and avoiding drug interactions are shown in Table 66–3. A careful review of the patient's medication profile is essential to monitor for drug interactions. Patients should be asked to disclose all their medications because they may often seek treatment from more than one health care provider. Their medication history should include both prescription and nonprescription drugs, as well as any herbal, investigational, or alternative therapies. Clinicians should be familiar with those agents most commonly associated with drug interactions. Anyone receiving "red flag" drugs (e.g., rifampin, ritonavir, ketoconazole) requires extra attention. Patients should be given a list of drugs that should not be administered concomitantly.

Table 66–3. STRATEGIES FOR RECOGNIZING AND AVOIDING DRUG INTERACTIONS

Review of patient medication profiles
Full medication profile, including over-the-counter and "alternative" medications
Recognition of agents most commonly associated with interactions (e.g., protease inhibitors, ketoconazole, rifampin)
Recognition of agents with overlapping toxicities
Proper staggering and scheduling of medications
Knowledge of dietary restrictions with certain medications
Selection of agents with fewer drug interactions if clinically appropriate

Finally, drug interactions can be avoided by simplifying drug regimens whenever possible. Selection of a therapeutically equivalent agent with fewer drug interactions may be wise. Azithromycin could be substituted for erythromycin or clarithromycin if appropriate for the clinical situation. Similarly, it may be advantageous to replace ritonavir with another protease inhibitor for patients requiring medication with the potential for serious interactions. The care provider and the patient must work together to develop a tolerable regimen that meets therapeutic goals.

OVERLAPPING TOXICITIES

Many of the drugs used in the HIV-infected patient have similar toxicity profiles. Some common examples are shown in Table 66–4. Although it would be ideal to prescribe drugs with no overlapping adverse effects, the limited choices for antiretroviral therapy and opportunistic infection treatment often preclude it. In the nucleoside analogue class, stavudine, didanosine, and zalcitabine are all associated with the development of peripheral neuropathy. However, a clinical study examining the combination of stavudine and didanosine showed that only two patients developed peripheral neuropathy after 1 year of therapy.[100]

Table 66–4. COMMON EXAMPLES OF OVERLAPPING TOXICITIES OF HIV-RELATED MEDICATIONS

Bone Marrow Suppression
Co-trimoxazole
Cytotoxic chemotherapy (e.g., doxorubicin, cyclophosphamide, vinblastine)
Dapsone
Flucytosine
Ganciclovir
Interferon-α
Pentamidine
Sulfadiazine/pyrimethamine
Trimetrexate
Peripheral Neuropathy
Didanosine
Ethambutol
Isoniazid
Stavudine
Zalcitabine
Renal Dysfunction
Aminoglycosides
Amphotericin B
Cidofovir
Foscarnet

Regardless, patients receiving these drugs should be counseled on the signs and symptoms of peripheral neuropathy. Other examples include a flu-like syndrome with some recombinant cytokines (interferon, IL-2) or pancreatitis with didanosine and pentamidine. When the use of these combinations is unavoidable, the use of reduced dosages or supportive medications (i.e., antidiarrheals, antiemetics) should be considered to lessen certain adverse effects.

A common dilemma is trying to identify which drug is actually causing an adverse effect. For example, ritonavir, zidovudine, and didanosine are associated with nausea and other gastrointestinal side effects. One strategy involves stopping all medications until the side effects resolve and then adding drugs back sequentially as tolerated. Note that this strategy may be unwise for patients taking combination antiretroviral therapy. Alternatively, single drugs could be removed or substituted in the regimen to see if the gastrointestinal symptoms resolve. This situation may be more difficult in the case of neutropenia, in which the adverse effect could be caused by medications (Table 66–4) or by disease processes such as *Mycobacterium avium* infection. For particularly toxic combinations such as zidovudine and ganciclovir, supportive care with granulocyte colony-stimulating factor may be useful adjunctive therapy to allow continuation of the regimen.

▲ MEDICATION ADHERENCE

Health care providers generally assume that patients take most or all of their prescribed medication. Numerous studies indicate that adherence to prescribed medication regimens varies greatly, and that few patients take all of their prescribed doses of drug(s). Imperfect adherence has probably been a medical fact of life since the dawn of civilization.

Using the most accurate means available to assess adherence, studies with single drugs suggest that fewer than 10% of patients take all prescribed doses of medication. Most patients are moderately compliant, taking 70% to 90% of prescribed doses. About one-third of patients take less than 60% of prescribed doses.[101,102] These adherence estimates hold true in HIV-infected patients taking combination antiretroviral therapy[103] or treatment for opportunistic infections.[104] Adherence assessment of combination regimens is far more complicated because adherence behavior may be different for different agents prescribed at the same time.[105]

Even intelligent and highly motivated individuals with medical backgrounds have difficulty with adherence. A study in 36 medical students randomized to receive a twice-daily or thrice-daily placebo for 14 days found that the mean number of doses taken was only 71% of those prescribed,[106] a result similar to that seen in AIDS or epilepsy patients. Furthermore, fewer than 30% of dosing intervals were correct, regardless of the assigned regimen. The two most common reasons cited for improper compliance in this study were "hectic schedule" and "irregular routine."

Health care providers cannot predict with great precision which patients will be adherent and which will not. Patient self-reports and pill counts also provide unreliable and inaccurate information.[102,107,108] Socioeconomic factors, racial and ethnic background, and disease state, which seem as if they ought to be related to degree of adherence, generally are not.[109] Therefore care providers must anticipate noncompliance and, whenever possible, avert any problems it may cause.

Studies suggest that poor adherence may be a major factor in the development of resistance to HIV protease inhibitors.[110] Overall adherence rates of less than 80% were associated with a significant increase in the risk of treatment failure.[111,112] The risk of treatment failure increased with decreasing adherence rate in patients taking protease inhibitors plus two nucleoside analogues.[112] In one study, 78% of patients taking 95% or more of prescribed protease inhibitor doses had undetectable viral loads, whereas only 20% of those taking less than 80% of prescribed doses had undetectable viral loads.[112] Viral suppression dropped off substantially with each decile fall in adherence rate.[112] It should be noted that most subjects evaluated in these studies were taking only a single protease inhibitor without ritonavir enhancement, and therefore most were using a three times a day regimen. Whether similar stringent adherence requirements would occur with simplified dual protease inhibitor regimens remains to be demonstrated.

A number of interventions can promote better adherence.[103] Regimens involving fewer daily doses and fewer agents are easier to take. Once a day regimens promote adherence best; twice a day regimens are only marginally better than three times a day regimens in some studies,[102,105,106] although these studies were conducted in patients taking only a single medication. An additional consideration is that the consequences of noncompliance are more severe for agents dosed infrequently. For example, if a drug is dosed three times a day, the daily therapeutic coverage is reduced by 33% if a single dose is missed; however, if a drug is dosed once a day, then daily therapeutic coverage is reduced 100% if a single dose is missed.

Effective pharmacotherapy for AIDS in the future may benefit by incorporating means of improving adherence into medical practice. Previous studies in patients with epilepsy and hypertension show that adherence can often be improved by modifying the drug regimen, physician practice, and patient behavior (Table 66–5). Steps include increasing recognition of the problem, counseling and educating the patient about the importance of good adherence

▲ Table 66–5. STRATEGIES FOR IMPROVING MEDICATION ADHERENCE

Recognize and anticipate the problem.
Educate the patient about the importance of good adherence to the regimen.
Counsel the patient about the dangers of poor adherence.
Monitor the patient's adherence behavior.
Provide environmental cues for dosing.
Learn the patient's normal routine and incorporate dosing cues into that routine.
Provide positive feedback for clinical success.
Emphasize patient self-reliance.
Provide realistic therapeutic goals and expectations for the patient.
Use twice-a-day or once-a-day regimens whenever possible.
Minimize the number of agents prescribed.

and the dangers of poor adherence, providing environmental cues to habituate the taking of medicines, incorporating medication-taking into established routines, monitoring outcomes and providing feedback to reinforce success, minimizing polypharmacy, and using twice a day or once a day regimens whenever possible.

▲ THERAPEUTIC DRUG MONITORING

Therapeutic drug monitoring (TDM) refers to adjusting drug doses based on measured plasma concentrations to attain values within a "therapeutic window." Clinicians have used these principles for years to adjust doses of such drugs as theophylline, aminoglycosides, digoxin, and anticonvulsants. There is growing evidence that TDM is useful in some circumstances to ensure that HIV-infected patients have adequate blood concentrations for efficacy without producing toxicity. Some antiretroviral drugs share many of the characteristics of those that require monitoring plasma levels, including variable intersubject pharmacokinetics, serious consequences if there is a lack of effect or drug toxicity, documented relationships between concentration and effect or toxicity, and the availability of rapid, accurate assays. However, a number of inherent problems must be resolved before TDM becomes standard practice.

The beneficial role of TDM in HIV clinical practice remains to be demonstrated. Since the mid-1990s a number of studies have described relationships between antiretroviral drug concentrations and antiviral effect.[113–119] Results from two prospective, randomized trials of TDM in HIV-infected patients have been reported. ATHENA is an ongoing study of 600 patients randomized to TDM or no TDM. In treatment-naive patients, indinavir and nelfinavir doses were adjusted based on the "concentration ratio," a measure of the patient's drug level compared to the mean expected drug level in the population at any time during the dosage interval. The TDM group had a significantly improved clinical outcome at 1 year as defined by a viral load of less than 500 copies/ml and noncompleters being considered as treatment failures.[120,121] Improved outcome with TDM for indinavir was primarily driven by reduced toxicity leading to fewer discontinuations, and TDM of nelfinavir was primarily due to improved efficacy. Results in treatment-experienced patients are not yet available. Conversely, PharmAdapt, which used trough plasma protease inhibitor concentrations to modify salvage therapy, did not show a significant improvement in virologic outcomes at 12 weeks.[122] Modification of protease inhibitor therapy occurred for only 22% of patients receiving protease inhibitor TDM, and dosage modifications did not occur until 8 weeks into therapy. In addition, wild-type IC_{50} values were used as target concentrations in PharmAdapt, and this target may be too low.

Studies have evaluated the phenotype or "virtual" phenotype used along with the plasma concentration as a potential tool to optimize drug therapy. The ratio of the C_{min} (trough level) to the protein-adjusted IC_{50} is often called the inhibitory quotient (IQ). Preliminary trials demonstrate a correlation between the IQ and virologic outcome as measured by the viral load after 24 to 48 weeks; but larger, longer-term studies are needed to validate this approach.[123–125] These studies suggest that integration of the drug level and virus susceptibility to the drug may provide more complete information than either measurement alone. Ongoing trials are evaluating the IQ ratio as a useful monitoring tool in HIV-infected patients.

A number of practical and logistical challenges may limit the widespread use of TDM for antiretroviral therapy. A primary limitation of TDM is that it does not provide information on long-term adherence. Patients might not take the drugs correctly for weeks but then do so for the 2 to 3 days immediately before their clinic appointment if they know a TDM sample is to be examined. The drug concentration in such a patient appears to be adequate, although the patient may be failing therapy because of nonadherence. Intrapatient variability also appears to be large for some antiretroviral agents, suggesting that clinical decisions should be made only after two or more trough levels are measured, not after a single determination. The definition of a true "therapeutic range" must also be determined for each drug, knowing that the target value may be different for naive and treatment-experienced patients. Finally, accurate sample collection, timely processing, storage and shipping of plasma, and rapid turnaround times for assay results must be exsured. Ongoing clinical trials are determining if TDM can provide useful information for monitoring selected HIV-infected patients.

▲ PHARMACOKINETIC FACTORS

A number of pharmacokinetic factors (e.g., oral and systemic bioavailability, distribution, clearance) can be significant determinants in a patient's response to therapy. The importance of these factors as they apply to the administration of drugs for AIDS is emphasized in the next sections. The clinical pharmacokinetics of the available antiretroviral drugs are summarized in Chapter 67.

Distribution and Protein Binding

Drug distribution and tissue penetration are functions of several factors, including the drug's size its, lipophilicity, its affinity for plasma binding proteins, and if it is subject to active transport into or out of cells. For example, high-affinity binding to plasma proteins could affect a drug's ability to penetrate cells, which could affect a its antimicrobial activity.

Albumin, which accounts for about 50% of plasma protein, has a high binding capacity but generally low affinity for drugs. α_1-Acid glycoprotein (AAG) is a low-capacity, high-affinity drug-binding protein that may play a more important role in distribution. AAG is an inducible but minor component of plasma ($\leq$3% of total plasma protein). The addition of physiologic concentrations of AAG reduces the anti-HIV potency of a number of drugs in vitro by 10-fold or more,[126–129] which could contribute to reduced activity of such drugs under clinical circumstances.

For example, the HIV protease inhibitor SC-52151 bound to AAG with particularly high affinity[127] and failed to produce anti-HIV effects in Phase II clinical studies[130] despite achieving total drug concentrations well in excess of its 90% inhibitory concentration.[131] The use of AAG 2 mg/ml (a slightly supraphysiologic concentration) prevented penetration of radiolabeled SC-52151 into cells,[132] which probably contributed to its lack of activity in clinical studies because free drug concentrations were never high enough to exert an anti-HIV effect.[131] High-affinity AAG binding can be overcome if total drug concentrations are high enough to saturate protein-binding sites, as occurs with other highly AAG-bound drugs such as ritonavir.[133] This is of theoretical concern in HIV-infected patients because intercurrent infections and other illnesses may elevate AAG plasma concentrations and decrease free drug, although AAG concentrations remain in the normal range in asymptomatic patients with HIV infection.[131,134]

All of the available peptidomimetic HIV protease inhibitors are protein-bound in plasma to varying degrees, although the protein binding of indinavir is only about 60%, which has little or no effect on its disposition. Amprenavir, nelfinavir, ritonavir, and saquinavir are more than 90% bound to protein in plasma.[5] Plasma protein binding is quite low for most of the nucleoside analogues[135] and plays no significant role in their disposition. Displacement of one drug by another from its plasma protein binding sites may lead to transient changes in free drug concentrations, potentially affecting activity or toxicity.

Central Nervous System (CNS) Penetration

Penetration of drugs into the CNS is essential for activity in CNS disease. The relationship between plasma concentrations and CNS concentrations of drugs is complex, and activity against CNS infections often does not require that cerebrospinal fluid (CSF) concentrations be as high as simultaneous plasma concentrations. Studies with protease inhibitors have shown that even agents with marginal CSF penetration, such as saquinavir and indinavir, produce reductions in CSF viral load comparable to those produced in plasma.[136,137] The estimated fractional penetration of nelfinavir into CSF is less than 0.2%,[138] yet this drug is associated with remarkably good suppression of the CSF viral load.[139] Only 1 of 17 subjects receiving amprenavir had a higher CSF viral load than a plasma viral load in one study, and the magnitude of the difference in that single subject was small.[140] These findings suggest that the relatively low concentrations of free drug in the CSF are adequate to suppress HIV replication, or that CSF viral RNA may not adequately reflect virus replication in brain tissue.

Most nucleoside analogues penetrate the CNS to a limited extent, with CSF concentrations ranging from 10% to more than 30% of simultaneous plasma levels.[135] Higher fractional penetration has been reported for zidovudine, but in most studies assessment is based on limited CSF sampling, with only a single CSF–plasma pair used to ascertain the drug concentration ratio. The relationship between CNS penetration and activity in HIV-associated encephalopathy has not been well characterized, although higher doses of zidovudine are associated with improved response in patients with CNS disease.[141]

Genital Tract Penetration

Genital secretions are a potential vector for sexual transmission of HIV, and drugs that penetrate into these fluids more extensively might better inhibit replication and transmission of the virus. Antiretroviral drug concentrations in seminal plasma are generally much higher than in the CSF, and some antiretroviral agents appear to be concentrated more in semen than in blood.[142] Indinavir concentrations in semen equal the plasma concentration; ritonavir and saquinavir fractional penetration into seminal plasma is only 2% to 5%, perhaps reflecting the impact of plasma protein binding.[143]

Despite the differences in penetration into semen, indinavir, ritonavir, and saquinavir use has been associated with equivalent suppression of the viral load in the semen of treated patients.[143] Low concentrations of saquinavir or ritonavir are all that may be adequate to suppress HIV in the genital tract. Alternatively, HIV measured in semen could originate in and reflect virus concentrations in the blood. Penetration of antiretroviral agents into vaginal fluid is more difficult to quantify, and little information is available in the literature.

Drugs in the Pregnant Patient

Of increasing concern is administration of antiretroviral medication to pregnant patients (see Chapter 28). There are three situations in which this occurs: (1) an HIV-infected woman becomes pregnant while receiving standard pharmacotherapy; (2) a pregnant patient is newly diagnosed HIV-positive and is placed on antiretroviral drugs to prevent maternal–fetal transmission; and (3) a pregnant health care worker suffers an occupational exposure to HIV and receives antiretroviral drugs to prevent infection. Each of these cases presents a different set of risks and benefits for the woman and her unborn child. In the first two cases, transfer of antiretroviral drugs across the placenta is desirable to prevent fetal infection, especially during late stages of pregnancy. In the third case, fetal drug penetration may be undesirable because of potential fetal drug toxicity or teratogenicity.

Unlike the CNS, the placenta does not, in general, act as a functional barrier to drug penetration. Most drugs, especially those with reasonable oral bioavailability, cross the placenta to some degree. This is particularly true for lipophilic drugs; such compounds are large or highly ionized in plasma. Therefore they have limited penetration into extravascular compartments and reduced fetal penetration.

Animal and human studies of placental drug penetration found that fetal concentrations of nucleoside analogues such as zidovudine were half as high as that of concentrations in maternal plasma.[135] Although the placenta carries out some drug-metabolizing reactions, particularly glucuronidation, this is an inconsequential means of clearance for most drugs.

Penetration of drugs into breast milk is an important issue for women who are nursing. Like the placenta, mammary glands are no real barrier to drug penetration. Most orally available agents penetrate breast milk. Some lipophilic agents are actually concentrated in breast milk and may reach concentrations higher than those in maternal plasma. For example, zidovudine concentrations in breast milk are about 50% higher, on average, than those in maternal plasma.[144]

It is important to note that pregnancy may alter the apparent volume of distribution of some drugs by as much as 30% to 50%.[145] This is the consequence of increased body weight, total body water, and plasma volume, as well as changes in the concentration of certain plasma proteins. Drug concentrations in a pregnant woman may therefore be different if the drug dose is not altered. Fortunately, this does not require dose adjustment for most antiretroviral agents.

Drugs in Other Special Populations

Genetics can play an important role in drug disposition and effect. Human genetic polymorphisms are well known for several drug-metabolizing enzymes, including *N*-acetyltransferases and the CYP isoform 2C19. However, most gender and racial effects in pharmacokinetics are of a minor magnitude. Formal pharmacokinetic evaluation showed no significant difference in the disposition of zidovudine, for example, as a function of gender or race.[145] Medication adherence patterns and ingestion of concurrent medications that alter pharmacokinetics or pharmacodynamics appear to be much more important determinants of individual variability regarding drug disposition and drug responsiveness.

Pediatric pharmacokinetics are frequently different from those in adults, because renal and hepatic function change with age. This is especially true in neonates less than 1 month of age, in whom some drug-metabolizing enzymes (e.g., those involved in conjugation reactions) have not yet reached adult levels. For most drugs used in children older than 12 months of age, drug elimination as a function of body weight is equivalent to that in adults. For example, zidovudine clearance in infants more than 1 month old is not significantly different from that in adults.[146]

Liver disease can affect the clearance of all approved HIV protease inhibitors and NNRTIs, as elimination depends on hepatic cytochrome P_{450} activity. For some drugs, doses must be reduced in patients with moderate to severe hepatic impairment, as measured by the Child-Pugh classification. Dose adjustment should be based on published dosing guidelines. In general, mild liver impairment does not warrant dose adjustment. Moderate cirrhosis increased the AUC of amprenavir more than twofold compared to that in healthy volunteers; severe cirrhosis increased the amprenavir AUC more than threefold.[24] The AUC and half-life of indinavir were modestly altered in patients with mild to moderate hepatic insufficiency and cirrhosis.[19]

Nelfinavir pharmacokinetics were highly variable in five patients with liver disease compared to that in patients without liver disease. The calculated elimination half-life of nelfinavir was up to 20 hours, compared to 3.5 to 5.0 hours in patients without liver disease.[147] Formation of the nelfinavir M8 metabolite was reduced in these patients by approximately 10-fold compared to that in patients without liver disease.[147] Doses were adjusted in these patients to achieve concentrations that were within the range of those seen in patients without liver disease.

Amprenavir oral solution contains propylene glycol. This formulation should be used with caution in patients with hepatic impairment, as patients with liver disease may be at increased risk of propylene glycol toxicity.[24]

Critically ill patients represent another special population with potential changes in pharmacokinetics. Altered distribution or clearance of many drugs, including aminoglycosides, phenytoin, and pentobarbital, are well recognized in intensive care unit (ICU) patients.[148–150] It is important to note that absorption of oral medications is unpredictable in ICU patients, and some clinicians advocate discontinuing oral antiretroviral drugs. The later strategy is advocated because of the potential for suboptimal plasma concentrations, the fluctuations in renal and hepatic function, changes in volume distribution, and the complexity and changes in HIV-unrelated drugs, which can produce undesired and unpredictable drug interactions. Drug interactions may be an especially complex problem because of the large number of medications these critically ill patients receive. Many drugs used for prophylaxis of opportunistic infections are available in intravenous formulations (e.g., azithromycin, trimethoprim-sulfamethoxazole, fluconazole). If a critically ill patient does require prophylactic therapy, these medications could be continued intravenously in the ICU.

Antiretrovirals available as liquids (didanosine, zidovudine, stavudine, lamivudine, lopinavir, ritonavir, amprenavir, nelfinavir) can be given through feeding tubes to stable patients. For some medications, the contents of a capsule or crushed tablet are mixed with a small amount of fluid or enteral nutrition formulas and are administered through the tube. The absorption of antiretroviral drugs by this method of administration is unknown.

▲ FORMULATION ISSUES

Despite improved formulations of several antiretrovirals agents, many of the current drugs remain less than optimal in terms of patient convenience. A major problem is the actual number of capsules or tablets that must be swal-

▲ **Table 66–6.** NUMBER OF PILLS IN COMBINATION REGIMENS USING STANDARD DOSES

Daily Regimen	No. of Pills
Trizivir	2
COMB, NVP	4
COMB, EFV	5
COMB, IDV	8
d4T, 3TC, IDV	10
ZDV, ddI, NFV, TMP-SMX	15
ZDV, ddI, SAQ-SCG	24
d4T, 3TC, RTV, DLV	28
COMB, IDV, DLV, TMP-SMX, CLAR, FLU, GCV	36

CLAR, clarithromycin; COMB, Combivir; ddI, didanosine; d4T, stavudine; DLV, delavirdine; EFV, efavirenz; FLU, fluconazole; GCV, ganciclovir; IDV, indinavir; NFV, nelfinavir; NVP, nevirapine; RTV, ritonavir; SAQ-SGC, saquinavir soft gel capsules (Fortovase); TMP-SMX, trimethoprim-sulfamethoxazole (co-trimoxazole); 3TC, lamivudine; ZDV, zidovudine.

lowed throughout the course of the day. Approved protease inhibitors require from 6 capsules per day for indinavir or Kaletra® to 18 capsules per day for saquinavir (Fortovase formulation). Table 66–6 lists the number of pills for some common anti-HIV regimens. In patients taking two or more protease inhibitors, numerous pills per day may be required. Some recent improvements in formulation include the combination of zidovudine (300 mg) with lamivudine (150 mg) (Combivir) and the combination of zidovudine, lamivudine, and abacavir (Trizivir). This product represents the first triple-combination HAART regimen that requires only two tablets per day. This dramatically decreases the number of pills compared to the number when taking these drugs separately.

Didanosine is now available in a 200 mg tablet, and two of these tablets can be taken once daily. Didanosine can also be administered in an enteric coated capsule given once daily. A significant problem with the previous formulation of nelfinavir was that it was difficult to swallow. The new film-coated tablet has generally alleviated this problem.[20]

Two combination products also exist for the treatment of tuberculosis. Rifamate is a product containing 300 mg of rifampin and 150 mg of isoniazid; and Rifater contains 120 mg rifampin, 50 mg isoniazid, and 300 mg pyrazinamide. The use of these combination products provides a simple, convenient alternative if clinically warranted.

Many products are available in liquid formulations for use in pediatric patients or in adults with dysphagia. Antiretroviral agents with liquid or reconstitutable formulations include didanosine, stavudine, zidovudine, lamivudine, ritonavir, lopinavir, amprenavir, and nelfinavir. The taste of the ritonavir and amprenavir solutions are often described as unpleasant and so may cause administration problems. Ritonavir can be mixed with chocolate milk, Advera, or Ensure to mask the taste.[151] In addition, many of the medica-

▲ **Table 66–7.** STORAGE AND STABILITY OF ANTIRETROVIRAL DRUGS

Drug	Trade Name	Dosage Form	Storage and Stability
Abacavir	Ziagen	Tablets	Store at room temperature.
		Solution	Store at room temperature. May refrigerate, do not freeze.
Amprenavir	Agenerase	Capsules	Store at room temperature.
		Solution	Store at room temperature.
Delavirdine	Rescriptor	Tablets	Store in tightly closed containers at room temperature. Protect from high humidity. If dispersion in 3 oz water is prepared, consume within 1 to 2 hours.
Didanosine	Videx	Tablets	Store at room temperature in tightly closed bottles. If dispersed in water or apple juice, it is stable for 1 hour at room temperature.
		EC caps	Store at room temperature.
		Sachet	Store packets at room temperature. If dissolved in water, it is stable for 4 hours at room temperature.
		Suspension	Store bottles at room temperature. After mixing with antacid, store in refrigerator in tightly closed container for up to 30 days.
Efavirenz	Sustiva	Capsules	Store at room temperature.
Indinavir	Crixivan	Capsules	Sensitive to moisture; must be stored and dispensed in original container with desiccant.
Lamivudine	Epivir	Tablets	Store at room temperature in tightly closed bottles.
		Solution	Store at room temperature in tightly closed bottles.
Lopinavir/r	Kaletra	Capsules	If refrigerated, it is stable until expiration date. At room temperature, use within 2 months.
		Solution	If refrigerated, it is stable until expiration date. At room temperature, use within 2 months.
Nelfinavir	Viracept	Tablets	Store at room temperature.
		Oral powder	Store at room temperature. Once mixed with liquid, use within 6 hours.
Nevirapine	Viramune	Tablets	Store at room temperature in tightly closed bottles.
Ritonavir	Norvir	Capsules	Store in refrigerator; protect from light. Discard if left at room temperature for > 12 hours.
		Solution	Storage in refrigerator recommended but not required if used within 30 days and stored at room temperature. Keep in tightly closed, original container away from excessive heat.
Saquinavir	Fortovase	Capsules	Stored in refrigerator in pharmacy until dispensed. For patients, refrigerated capsules are stable until expiration date on label. If stored at room temperature, they are stable for up to 3 months.
Saquinavir	Invirase	Capsules	Store at room temperature in tightly closed bottles.
Stavudine	Zerit	Capsules	Store at room temperature in tightly closed bottles.
		Suspension	After reconstitution with water, store in refrigerator in tightly closed, original container for up to 30 days.
Zalcitabine	Hivid	Tablets	Store at room temperature in tightly closed bottles.
Zidovudine	Retrovir	Capsules	Store at room temperature and protect from moisture.
		Tablets	Store at room temperature.
		Solution	Store at room temperature.
Zidovudine/lamivudine	Combivir	Tablets	Store at room temperature.

r, ritonavir.

tions for opportunistic infections (e.g., azithromycin, clarithromycin, trimethoprim-sulfamethoxazole) are available as liquids.

▲ STORAGE OF ANTIRETROVIRAL DRUGS

Table 66–7 lists the storage requirements and stability of the FDA-approved antiretroviral drugs. Clinicians should remind patients to follow general precautions regarding storage of all medications.[152] Drugs must kept out of the reach of children and outdated medications discarded. In the absence of specific storage recommendations, medications should be kept in a cool, dry area away from excessive heat, light, and moisture. They should not be stored in places that may be damp, such as the bathroom or near the kitchen sink.

▲ CONCLUSIONS

Polypharmacy of HIV infection has led to clinical success and a host of complicated drug delivery issues. Pill burden, adherence, overlapping side effects, and proper medication scheduling are just some of the problems that must be addressed. Although these complex treatment regimens require a certain amount of patient self-motivation, there are various strategies the HIV clinician can employ to simplify regimens and optimize patient care. Medication profiles must be reviewed by the health care provider for duplication, drug interactions, and appropriateness of therapy. Patient counseling is critical for thorough explanations about how complicated regimens should be administered. Most importantly, each regimen should be individualized based on the patient's previous medication experience, history of side effects, willingness to understand and comply with the regimen, social factors, and overall quality of life. Although this is a daunting task for the patient and clinician, antiretroviral drugs can achieve long-term viral suppression and prolong life when administered correctly.

REFERENCES

1. Knupp CA, Milbrath R, Barbhaiya RH. Effect of time of food administration on the bioavailability of didanosine from a chewable tablet formulation. J Clin Pharmacol 33:568, 1993.
2. Videx EC (didanosine) product monograph. Princeton, NJ, Bristol Myers-Squibb, 2001.
3. Unadkat JD, Collier AC, Crosby SS, et al. Pharmacokinetics of oral zidovudine (azidothymidine) in patients with AIDS when administered with and without a high-fat meal. AIDS 4:299, 1990.
4. Sahai J, Gallicano K, Garber G, et al. The effect of a protein meal on zidovudine pharmacokinetics in HIV-infected patients. Br J Clin Pharmacol 33:657, 1992.
5. Flexner C. HIV protease inhibitors. N Engl J Med 338:1281, 1998.
6. Flexner C. Dual protease inhibitor therapy in HIV-infected patients: pharmacologic rationale and clinical benefits. Annu Rev Pharmacol Toxicol 40:649, 2000.
7. Lea AP, Faulds D. Ritonavir. Drugs 52:541, 1996.
8. Piscitelli SC, Flexner C, Minor JR, et al. Drug interactions in patients infected with human immunodeficiency virus. Clin Infect Dis 23:685, 1996.
9. Blaschke T, Flexner C, Sheiner L, et al. Effect of simultaneous or staggered dosing of saquinavir, ritonavir, and nelfinavir on pharmacokinetic interactions. In: Program and Abstracts of the 7th Conference on Retroviruses and Opportunistic Infections, 2000, San Francisco, abstract 76.
10. Saah A, Winchell M, Seniuk M, et al. Multiple-dose pharmacokinetics (PK) and tolerability of indinavir (IDV) and ritonavir (RTV) combinations in a once-daily regimen in healthy volunteers (Merck 089). In: Program and Abstracts from the 39th ICAAC; 1999, San Francisco, abstract 329.
11. Kilby JM, Sfakianos G, Gizzi N, et al. Safety and pharmacokinetics of once-daily regimens of soft-gel capsule saquinavir plus minidose ritonavir in human immunodeficiency virus-negative adults. Antimicrob Agents Chemother 44:2672, 2000.
12. Piscitelli SC, Gallicano KD. Interactions among drugs for HIV and opportunistic infections. N Engl J Med 344.984, 2001.
13. Retrovir (zidovudine) product monograph. Research Triangle Park, NC, Glaxo Smith Kline, 2000.
14. Hivid (zalcitabine) product monograph. Nutley, NJ, Roche Laboratories, 1994.
15. Zerit (stavudine) product monograph. Princeton, NJ, Bristol Myers-Squibb, 1994.
16. Epivir (lamivudine) product monograph. Research Triangle Park, NC, Glaxo Smith Kline, 2000.
17. Invirase (saquinavir) product monograph. Nutley, NJ, Roche Laboratories, 1997.
18. Norvir (ritonavir) product monograph. Abbott Park, IL, Abbott Laboratories, 1996.
19. Crixivan (indinavir) product monograph. West Point, PA, Merck & Co., 1996.
20. Viracept (nelfinavir) product monograph. La Jolla, CA, Agouron Pharmaceuticals, 1997.
21. Viramune (nevirapine) product monograph. Columbus, OH, Roxanne Laboratories, 1996.
22. Rescriptor (delavirdine) product monograph. Kalamazoo, MI, Pharmacia & Upjohn, 1997.
23. Sustiva (efavirenz) product monograph. Wilmington, DE, DuPont Pharmaceuticals, 2000.
24. Agenerase (amprenavir) product monograph. Research Triangle Park, NC, Glaxo Smith Kline, 2000.
25. Kaletra (lopinavir-ritonavir) product monograph. Abbott Park, IL, Abbott Laboratories, 2001.
26. Abacavir (Ziagen) product monograph. Research Triangle Park, NC, Glaxo Smith Kline, 2000.
27. Polk RE. Drug–drug interactions with ciprofloxacin and other fluoroquinolones. Am J Med 87(suppl 5A):8776S, 1989.
28. Noyes M, Polk RE. Norfloxacin and absorption of magnesium-aluminum. Ann Intern Med 109:168, 1988.
29. Lehto P, Kivisto KT. Effect of sucralfate on absorption of norfloxacin and ofloxacin. Antimicrob Agents Chemother 38:248, 1994.
30. Sahai J, Gallicano K, Oliveras RT, et al. Cations in the didanosine tablet reduce ciprofloxacin bioavailability. Clin Pharmacol Ther 53:292, 1993.
31. Piscitelli SC, Goss TF, Wilton JH, et al. Effects of ranitidine and sucralfate on ketoconazole bioavailability. Antimicrob Agents Chemother 35:1765, 1991.
32. Lake-Bakaar G, Tom W, Lake-Bakaar D, et al. Gastropathy and ketoconazole malabsorption in the acquired immunodeficiency syndrome. Ann Intern Med 109:471, 1988.
33. Van Der Meer JWM, Keuning JJ, Scheijgrond HW, et al. The influence of gastric acidity on the bio-availability of ketoconazole. J Antimicrob Chemother 6:552, 1980.
34. Blum RA, D'Andrea DT, Florentino BM, et al. Increased gastric pH and the bioavailability of fluconazole and ketoconazole. Ann Intern Med 114:755, 1991.
35. Lange D, Pavao JH, Wu J, et al. Effect of a cola beverage on the bioavailability of itraconazole in the presence of H_2 blockers. J Clin Pharmacol 37:535, 1997.
36. Van de Velde VJ, Van Peer AP, Heykants JJ, et al. Effect of food on the pharmacokinetics of a new hydroxypropyl-beta-cyclodextrin formulation of itraconazole. Pharmacotherapy 16:424, 1996.
37. Benet LZ, Kroetz DL, Sheiner LB. Pharmacokinetics: dynamics of drug absorption, distribution, and elimination. In: Hardman JG, Limbird LE (eds) The Pharmacological Basis of Therapeutics, 9th ed. New York, McGraw-Hill, 1996.
38. Kolars JC, Lown KS, Schmiedlin-Ren P, et al. CYP3A gene expression in human gut epithelium. Pharmacogenetics 4:247, 1994.

39. Hsu A, Granneman GR, Cao G, et al. Pharmacokinetic interactions between two human immunodeficiency virus protease inhibitors, ritonavir and saquinavir. Clin Pharmacol Ther 63:453, 1998.
40. Fuhr U. Drug interactions with grapefruit juice. Drug Saf 18:251, 1998.
41. Bailey DG, Arnold MJ, Spence JD. Grapefruit juice–drug interactions. Br J Clin Pharmacol 46:101, 1998.
42. Fojo AT, Ueda K, Slamon DJ, et al. Expression of multidrug-resistance gene in human tumors and tissues. Proc Natl Acad Sci USA 84:265, 1987.
43. Khaliq Y, Gallicano K, Venance S, et al. Effect of ketoconazole on ritonavir and saquinavir concentrations in plasma and cerebrospinal fluid from patients infected with human immunodeficiency virus. Clin Pharmacol Ther 68:637, 2000.
44. Lee CG, Ramachandra M, Jeang KT. Effect of ABC transporters on HIV-1 infection: inhibition of virus production by the MDR1 transporter. FASEB J 14:516, 2000.
45. Flexner C, Speck RR. Role of multidrug transporters in HIV pathogenesis. In: Eighth Conference on Retroviruses and Opportunistic Infections, Chicago, 2001, abstract S4.
46. Kim RB, Wandel C, Leake B, et al. Interrelationship between substrates and inhibitors of human CYP3A and P-glycoprotein. Pharm Res 16:408, 1999.
47. Centers for Disease Control and Prevention. Clinical update: impact of HIV protease inhibitors on the treatment of HIV-infected tuberculosis patients with rifampin. MMWR 45:921, 1996.
48. Hamzeh F, Benson C, Gerber J, et al. Steady-state pharmacokinetic interaction of modified-dose indinavir and rifabutin. In: Eighth Conference on Retroviruses and Opportunistic Infections, Chicago, 2001, abstract 742.
49. Murphy R, Gagnier P, Lamson M, et al. Effect of nevirapine on pharmacokinetics of indinavir and ritonavir in HIV-1 patients. In: Program and Abstracts of the 4th Conference on Retroviruses and Opportunistic Infections, Washington, DC. Alexandria, VA, Westover Management Group, 1997, p 374, abstract 374.
50. Sahai J, Cameron W, Salgo M, et al. Drug interaction between saquinavir and nevirapine. In: Program and Abstracts of the 4th Conference on Retroviruses and Opportunistic Infections, Washington, DC. Alexandria, VA, Westover Management Group, 1997, abstract 614.
51. Barry M, Mulcahy F, Merry C. Pharmacokinetics and potential interactions amongst antiretroviral agents used to treat patients with HIV infection. Clin Pharmacokinet 36:289, 1999.
52. Ouellet D, Hsu A, Qian J, et al. Effect of ritonavir on the pharmacokinetics of ethinyl estradiol in healthy female volunteers. In: Program and Abstracts of the XIth International Conference on AIDS, Vancouver, 1996, abstract Mo.B.1198.
53. Hsu A, Granneman GR, Witt G, et al. Assessment of multiple doses of ritonavir on the pharmacokinetics of theophylline. In: Program and Abstracts of the XIth International Conference on AIDS, Vancouver, 1996, abstract Mo.B.1200.
54. Cato A, Cavanaugh JH, Shi H, et al. Assessment of multiple doses of ritonavir on the pharmacokinetics of rifabutin. In: Program and Abstracts of the XIth International Conference on AIDS, Vancouver, 1996, abstract Mo.B.175.
55. Sun E, Heath-Chiozzi M, Cameron DW, et al. Concurrent ritonavir and rifabutin increases the risk of rifabutin-associated adverse effects. In: Program and Abstracts of the XIth International Conference on AIDS, Vancouver, 1996, abstract Mo.B.171.
56. Ouellet D, Hsu A, Granneman GR, et al. Assessment of the pharmacokinetic interaction between ritonavir and clarithromycin [abstract]. Clin Pharmacol Ther 59:143, 1996.
57. Honig PK, Wortham DC, Zamani K, et al. Comparison of the effects of the macrolide antibiotics erythromycin, clarithromycin, and azithromycin on terfenadine steady-state pharmacokinetics and electrocardiographic parameters. Drug Invest 7:148, 1994.
58. Paris DG, Parente TF, Bruschetta HR, et al. Torsades de pointes induced by erythromycin and terfenadine. Am J Emerg Med 12:636, 1994.
59. Hsu A, Granneman GR, Witt G, et al. Multiple-dose pharmacokinetics of ritonavir in human immunodeficiency virus-infected subjects. Antimicrob Agents Chemother 41:898, 1997.
60. Hsu A, Granneman GR, Bertz RJ. Ritonavir: clinical pharmacokinetics and interactions with other anti-HIV agents. Clin Pharmacokinet 35:275, 1998.
61. Kilby M, Hill AM, Buss N. The effect of ritonavir on increases in saquinavir plasma concentration is independent of ritonavir dosage: combined analysis of 120 subjects. In: Program and Abstracts of the 40th Interscience Conference on Antimicrobial Agents and Chemotherapy, Toronto, 2000, abstract 1650.
62. Drewe J, Gutmann H, Fricker G, et al. HIV protease inhibitor ritonavir: a more potent inhibitor of P-glycoprotein than the cyclosporine analog SDZ PSC 833. Biochem Pharmacol 57:1147, 1999.
63. Hsu A, Granneman GR, Cao G, et al. Pharmacokinetic interaction between ritonavir and indinavir in healthy volunteers. Antimicrob Agents Chemother 42:2784, 1998.
64. Saah AJ, Winchell G, Seniuk M, Deutsch P. Multiple-dose pharmacokinetics and tolerability of indinavir ritonavir combinations in healthy volunteers [abstract]. In: Program and Abstracts of the 6th Conference on Retroviruses and Opportunistic Infections, Chicago, 1999, p 136.
65. Burger D, Felderhof M, Phanupak P, et al. Both short-term virological efficacy and drug-associated nephrotoxicity are related to indinavir (IDV) pharmacokinetics in HIV-1 infected Thai patients. In: Program and Abstracts of the 8th Conference on Retroviruses and Opportunistic Infections, Chicago, 2001, abstract 730.
66. Lamotte C, Peytavin G, Perre P, et al. Increasing adverse events (AE) with indinavir (IDV) dosages and plasma concentrations in four different ritonavir (RTV)-IDV containing regimens in HIV-infected patients. In: Program and Abstracts of the 8th Conference on Retroviruses and Opportunistic Infections, Chicago, 2001, abstract 738.
67. Workman C, Whittaker W, Dyer W, Sullivan J. Combining ritonavir and indinavir decreases indinavir-associated nephrolithiasis [abstract]. In: Program and Abstracts of the 6th Conference on Retroviruses and Opportunistic Infections, Chicago, 1999, p 195.
68. Hurst M, Faulds D. Lopinavir. Drugs 60:1371, 2000.
69. Bertz R, Lam W, Brun S, et al. Multiple-dose pharmacokinetics of ABT-378/ ritonavir in HIV^+ subjects. In: 39th Interscience Conference on Antimicrobial Agents and Chemotherapy, San Francisco, 1999, abstract 327.
70. Gulick R, King M, Brun S, et al. ABT-378/ritonavir in antiretroviral naive HIV^+ patients: 72 weeks. In: 7th Conference on Retroviruses and Opportunistic Infections, San Francisco, 2000, abstract 515.
71. Bertz R, Lam W, Hsu A, et al. Assessment of the pharmacokinetic interaction between ABT-378/ritonavir and efavirenz in healthy volunteers and in HIV^+ subjects. In: Program and Abstracts of the 40th Interscience Conference on Antimicrobial Agents and Chemotherapy, Toronto, 2000, abstract 424.
72. Piscitelli S, Bechtel C, Sadler B, Falloon J. The addition of a second protease inhibitor eliminated amprenavir-efavirenz interactions and increase amprenavir concentrations [abstract]. In: 7th Conference on Retroviruses and Opportunistic Infections, San Francisco, 2000, p 90.
73. Sadler BM, Piliero P, Preston SL, et al. Pharmacokinetic drug interaction between amprenavir and ritonavir in HIV seronegative subjects after multiple, oral dosing. In: Program and Abstracts of the 7th Conference on Retroviruses and Opportunistic Infections, San Francisco, 2000, abstract 77.
74. Degen O, Kurowski M, Van Lunzen J, et al. Amprenavir (APV) and ritonavir (RTV): intraindividual comparison of different doses and influence of concomitant NNRTI on steady-state pharmacokinetics in HIV-infected patients. In: Program and Abstracts of the 8th Conference on Retroviruses and Opportunistic Infections, Chicago, 2001, abstract 739.
75. Aarnoutse RE, Burger DM, Hugen PWH, et al. A pharmacokinetic study to investigate the influence of efavirenz on a bid indinavir/ritonavir regimen in healthy volunteers. In: 40th Interscience Conference on Antimicrobial Agents and Chemotherapy, Toronto, 2000, abstract 423.
76. Wood R, Trepo C, Livrozet JM, et al. Amprenavir (APV) 600 mg/ritonavir (RTV) 100 mg bid or APV 1200 mg/RTV 200 mg qd given in combination with abacavir (ABC) and lamivudine (3TC) maintains efficacy in ART-naive HIV-1-infected adults over 12 weeks (APV20001). In: Program and Abstracts of the 8th Conference on Retroviruses and Opportunistic Infections, Chicago, 2001, abstract 332.
77. Flexner C, Hsu A, Kerr B, et al. Steady-state pharmacokinetic interactions between ritonavir (RTV), nelfinavir (NFV), and the nelfinavir active metabolite M8 (AG1402). Presented at the 12th World AIDS Conference, Geneva, 1998.

78. Zhang KE, Wu E, Patick AK, et al. Circulating metabolites of the human immunodeficiency virus protease inhibitor nelfinavir in humans: structural identification, levels in plasma, and antiviral activities. Antimicrob Agents Chemother 45:1086, 2001.
79. Kurowski M, Kaeser B, Mroziekiewicz A, et al. The influence of low doses of ritonavir on the pharmacokinetics of nelfinavir 1250 mg twice daily. In: Program and Abstracts of the 40th Interscience Conference on Antimicrobial Agents and Chemotherapy, Toronto, 2000, abstract 1639.
80. Kravcik S, Sahai J, Kerr B, et al. Nelfinavir mesylate increases saquinavir soft gel capsule exposure in HIV^+ patients. In: Program and Abstracts of the 4th Conference on Retroviruses and Opportunistic Infections, Washington, DC. Alexandria, VA, Westover Management Group, 1997, abstract 371.
81. Piroth L, Grappin M, Buisson M, et al. Randomized salvage therapy with saquinavir-ritonavir versus saquinavir-nelfinavir for highly experienced HIV-infected patients. In: Program and Abstracts of the 40th Interscience Conference on Antimicrobial Agents and Chemotherapy, Toronto, 2000, abstract 543.
82. Havlir DV, Riddler S, Squires K, et al. Coadministration of indinavir (IDV) and nelfinavir (NFV) in a twice daily regimen: preliminary safety, pharmacokinetic and anti-viral activity results. In: Program and Abstracts of 5th Conference on Retroviruses and Opportunistic Infections, Chicago, 1998, abstract 393.
83. Merrill DP, Manion DJ, Chou TC, Hirsch MS. Antagonism between human immunodeficiency virus type 1 protease inhibitors indinavir and saquinavir in vitro. J Infect Dis 176:265, 1997.
84. Cox SR, Ferry JJ, Batts DH, et al. Delavirdine and marketed protease inhibitors: pharmacokinetic interaction studies in healthy volunteers. In: Program and Abstracts of the 4th Conference on Retroviruses and Opportunistic Infections, Washington, DC. Alexandria, VA, Westover Management Group, 1997, abstract 372.
85. Cox SR, Schneck BD, Herman BD, et al. Delavirdine and nelfinavir: a pharmacokinetic drug interaction study in healthy adult volunteers. In: Program and Abstracts of the 5th Conference on Retroviruses and Opportunistic Infections, Chicago. Alexandria, VA, Westover Management Group, 1998, abstract 345.
86. Piscitelli SC, Burstein AH, Chaitt D, et al. St. John's wort and indinavir concentrations. Lancet 355:547, 2000.
87. Roby CA, Anderson GD, Kantor E, et al. St John's wort: effect on CYP3A4 activity. Clin Pharmacol Ther 67:451, 2000.
88. Johne A, Brockmoller J, Bauer S, et al. Pharmacokinetic interaction of digoxin with an herbal extract from St John's wort (Hypericum perforatum). Clin Pharmacol Ther 66:338, 1999.
89. Laroche M, Choudhri S, Gallicano K, Foster B. Severe gastrointestinal toxicity with concomitant ingestion of ritonavir and garlic [abstract]. Can J Infect Dis. 9(suppl A):471P, 1998.
90. Piscitelli SC, Burstein AH, Welden N, et al. Garlic supplements decrease plasma saquinavir concentrations. In: Program and Abstracts of the 8th Conference on Retroviruses and Opportunistic Infections, Chicago, 2001, abstract 743.
91. Piscitelli SC. Use of complementary medicines by patients with HIV infection: full sail into uncharted waters. www.medscape.com, May 2000.
92. Reiss WG, Piscitelli SC. Drug–cytokine interactions: mechanisms and clinical implications. Biodrugs 9:389, 1998.
93. Piscitelli SC, Vogel S, Figg WD, et al. Alteration in indinavir clearance during interleukin-2 infusions in HIV-infected patients. Pharmacotherapy 18:1212, 1998.
94. Moore KHP, Yuen GJ, Raasch RH, et al. Pharmacokinetics of lamivudine administered alone and with trimethoprim sulfamethoxazole. Clin Pharmacol Ther 59:550, 1996.
95. Laskin OL, De Miranda P, King DH, et al. Effects of probenecid on the pharmacokinetics and elimination of acyclovir in humans. Antimicrob Agents Chemother 21:804, 1982.
96. Sim SM, Hoggard PG, Sales SD, et al. Effect of ribavirin on zidovudine efficacy and toxicity in vitro: concentration-dependent interaction. AIDS Res Hum Retroviruses 14:1661, 1998.
97. Back D, Haworth S, Hoggard P, et al. Drug interactions with d4T phosphorylation in vitro [abstract]. In: Program and Abstracts of the XI International Conference on AIDS, Vancouver, 1996, p 88.
98. Havlir DV, Friedland G, Pollard R, et al. Combination zidovudine and stavudine therapy versus other nucleosides: report of two randomized trials (ACTG 290 and 298) [abstract]. In: 5th Conference on Retroviruses and Opportunistic Infections, Chicago, 1998, p 79.
99. Veal GJ, Hoggard PG, Barry MG, et al. Interaction between lamivudine and other nucleoside analogs for intracellular phosphorylation. AIDS 10:546, 1996.
100. Pollard RB, Peterson D, Hardy D, et al. Safety and antiretroviral effects of combined didanosine and stavudine therapy in HIV-infected individuals with CD4 counts of 200 to 500 cells/mm^3. J Acquir Immune Defic Syndr 22:39, 1999.
101. Evans L, Spelman M. The problem of noncompliance with drug therapy. Drugs 25:63, 1983.
102. Cramer JA, Mattson RH, Prevey ML, et al. How often is medication taken as prescribed? A novel assessment technique. JAMA 261:3723, 1989.
103. Chesney MA. Factors affecting adherence to antiretroviral therapy. Clin Infect Dis 30(suppl 2):S171, 2000.
104. Flexner C, Noe D, Benson C, et al. Adherence patterns in patients with symptomatic Mycobacterium avium complex (MAC) infection taking a twice-daily clarithromycin regimen [abstract 32324]. Int Conf AIDS 12:585, 1998.
105. Kasstrisios H, Flowers NT, Suarez JR, et al. Assessment of differential compliance in ACTG protocol 175 [abstract]. Clin Pharmacol Ther 55:191, 1994.
106. Kasstrisios H, Flowers NT, Blaschke TF. Introducing medical students to medication noncompliance. Clin Pharmacol Ther 59:577, 1996.
107. Rudd P, Byyny RL, Zachary V, et al. The natural history of medication compliance in a drug trial: limitations of pill counts. Clin Pharmacol Ther 46:169, 1989.
108. Waterhouse DM, Calzone KA, Mele C, et al. Adherence to oral tamoxifen: a comparison of patient self-report, pill counts, and microelectronic monitoring. J Clin Oncol 11:1189, 1993.
109. Cramer JA, Spilker B. Patient Compliance in Medical Practice and Clinical Trials. New York, Raven Press, 1991.
110. Vanhove GF, Schapiro JM, Winters MA, et al. Patient compliance and drug failure in protease inhibitor monotherapy [letter]. JAMA 276:1955, 1996.
111. Bangsberg DR, Hecht FM, Charlebois ED, et al. Adherence to protease inhibitors, HIV-1 viral load, and development of drug resistance in an indigent population. AIDS 14:357, 2000.
112. Paterson DL, Swindells S, Mohr J, et al. Adherence to protease inhibitor therapy and outcomes in patients with HIV infection. Ann Intern Med 133:21, 2000.
113. Schapiro JM, Winters MA, Stewart F, et al. The effect of high-dose saquinavir on viral load and $CD4^+$ T-cell counts in HIV-infected patients. Ann Intern Med 124:1039, 1996.
114. Molla A, Korneyeva M, Gao Q, et al. Ordered accumulation of mutations in HIV protease confers resistance to ritonavir. Nat Med 2:760, 1996.
115. Stein DS, Fish DG, Bilello JA, et al. A 24-week open-label phase I/II evaluation of the HIV protease inhibitor MK-639 (indinavir). AIDS 10:485, 1996.
116. Burger DM, Hoetelmans RM, Hugen PW, et al. Low plasma concentrations of indinavir are related to virological treatment failure in HIV-1 infected patients on indinavir-containing triple therapy. Antivir Ther 3:215, 1998.
117. Lorenzi P, Yerly S, Abderrakim K, et al. Toxicity, efficacy, plasma drug concentrations and protease mutations in patients with advanced HIV infection treated with ritonavir and saquinavir. AIDS 11:F95, 1997.
118. Acosta EP, Henry K, Weller D, et al. Indinavir pharmacokinetics and relationships between exposure and antiviral effect. Pharmacotherapy 19:708, 1999.
119. Fletcher CV, Fenton T, Powell C, et al. Pharmacologic characteristics of efavirenz and nelfinavir associated with virologic response in HIV-infected children. In: Program and Abstracts of the 8th Conference on Retroviruses and Opportunistic Infections, Chicago, 2001, abstract 259.
120. Burger DM, Hugen PWH, Droste J, et al. Therapeutic drug monitoring of indinavir in treatment naive patients improves therapeutic outcome after 1 year: results from ATHENA. In: 2nd International Workshop on Clinical Pharmacology of HIV Therapy, Noordwijk, The Netherlands, 2001, abstract 6.2a.
121. Burger DM, Hugen PWH, Droste J, et al. Therapeutic drug monitoring of nelfinavir 1250 bid in treatment naive patients improves therapeutic outcome after 1 year: results from ATHENA. In: 2nd Interna-

tional Workshop on Clinical Pharmacology of HIV Therapy, Noordwijk, The Netherlands, 2001, abstract 6.2b.
122. Clevenbergh P, Durant J, Garraffo R, et al. Usefulness of protease inhibitor therapeutic drug monitoring? PharmAdapt: a prospective multicentric randomized controlled trial: 12 week results. In: 8th Conference on Retroviruses and Opportunistic Infections, Chicago, 2001, abstract 260B.
123. Kempf D, Hsu A, Jiang P, et al. Response to ritonavir intensification in indinavir recipients is highly correlated with inhibitory quotient. In: Program and Abstracts of the 8th Conference on Retroviruses and Opportunistic Infections, Chicago, 2001, abstract 523.
124. Kempf D, Hsu A, Isaacson J, et al. Evaluation of the inhibitory quotient as a pharmacodynamic predictor of the virologic response to protease inhibitor therapy. In: 2nd International Workshop on Clinical Pharmacology of HIV Therapy, Noordwijk, The Netherlands, 2001, abstract 7.3.
125. Fletcher CV, Anderson PL, Kakuda TN, et al. A novel approach to integrate pharmacologic and virologic characteristics: an in vivo potency index for antiretroviral agents. In: Program and Abstracts of the 8th Conference on Retroviruses and Opportunistic Infections, 2001, Chicago, abstract 732.
126. Kageyama S, Anderson BD, Hoesterey BL, et al. Protein binding of human immunodeficiency virus protease inhibitor KNI-272 and alteration of its in vitro antiretroviral activity in the presence of high concentrations of protein. Antimicrob Agents Chemother 38:1107, 1994.
127. Bryant M, Getman D, Smidt M, et al. SC-52151, a novel inhibitor of the human immunodeficiency virus protease. Antimicrob Agents Chemother 39:2229, 1995.
128. Bilello JA, Bilello PA, Prichard M, et al. Reduction of the in vitro activity of A77003, an inhibitor of human immunodeficiency virus protease, by human serum α_1 acid glycoprotein. J Infect Dis 171:546, 1995.
129. Lazdins JK, Mestan J, Goutte G, et al. In vitro effect of α_1-acid glycoprotein on the anti-human immunodeficiency virus activity of the protease inhibitor CGP 61755: a comparative study with other relevant HIV protease inhibitors. J Infect Dis 175:1063, 1997.
130. Fischl MA, Richman DD, Flexner C, et al. Phase I study of the toxicity, pharmacokinetics, and activity of the HIV protease inhibitor SC-52151. J Acquir Immune Defic Syndr Hum Retrovirol 15:28, 1997.
131. Flexner C, Richman DD, Bryant M, et al. Effect of protein binding on the pharmacodynamics of an HIV protease inhibitor [abstract]. Antiviral Res 26:A282, 1995.
132. Sommadossi J, Schinazi RD, McMillan A, et al. A human serum glycoprotein profoundly affects antiviral activity of the protease inhibitor SC-52151 by decreasing its cellular uptake. In: Program and Abstracts of the 2nd National Conference on Human Retroviruses and Related Infections. Washington, DC, American Society for Microbiology, 1995, abstract LB4.
133. Molla A, Vasavanonda S, Kumar G, et al. Human serum attenuates the activity of protease inhibitors toward wild-type and mutant human immunodeficiency virus. Virology 250:255, 1998.
134. Hendrix CW, Flexner C, Szebeni J, et al. Dipyridamole's effect on zidovudine pharmacokinetics and short-term tolerance in asymptomatic HIV-infected subjects. Antimicrob Agents Chemother 38:1036, 1994.
135. Flexner C, Hendrix C. Pharmacology of antiretroviral agents. In: DeVita VT, Hellman S, Rosenberg SA (eds) AIDS Etiology, Diagnosis, Treatment, and Prevention, 4th ed. Philadelphia, Lippincott-Raven, 1997, p 479.
136. Moyle GJ, Sadler M, Buss N. Plasma and cerebrospinal fluid saquinavir concentrations in patients receiving combination antiretroviral therapy. Clin Infect Dis 28:403, 1999.
137. Collier AC, Marra C, Coombs RW, et al. Cerebrospinal fluid indinavir and HIV RNA levels in patients on chronic indinavir therapy. In: Program and Abstracts of the 35th Annual Meeting of the Infectious Diseases Society of America, San Francisco. Alexandria, VA, Infectious Diseases Society of America, 1997, abstract 22.
138. Aweeka F, Jayewardene A, Staprans S, et al. Failure to detect nelfinavir in the cerebrospinal fluid of HIV-1-infected patients with and without AIDS dementia complex. J Acquir Immune Defic Syndr 20:39, 1999.
139. Haas D, Clough L, Johnson B, et al. Quantification of nelfinavir and its active metabolite (M8) in CSF and plasma, and correlation with CSF HIV-1 RNA response. In: Program and Abstracts of the 7th Conference on Retroviruses and Opportunistic Infections, San Francisco, 2000, abstract 313.
140. Murphy R, Currier J, Gerber J, Antiviral activity and pharmacokinetics of amprenavir with and without zidovudine/3TC in the cerebral spinal fluid of HIV-infected adults. In: Program and Abstracts of the 7th Conference on Retroviruses and Opportunistic Infections, San Francisco, 2000, abstract 314.
141. Sidtis JJ, Gatsonis C, Price RW, et al. Zidovudine treatment of the AIDS dementia complex: results of a placebo-controlled trial: AIDS Clinical Trials Group. Ann Neurol 33:343, 1993.
142. Kashuba AD, Dyer JR, Kramer LM, et al. Antiretroviral-drug concentrations in semen: implications for sexual transmission of human immunodeficiency virus type 1. Antimicrob Agents Chemother 43:1817, 1999.
143. Taylor S, Back D, Drake S, et al. Antiretroviral drug concentrations in semen of HIV-infected men: differential penetration of indinavir (IDV), ritonavir (RTV), and saquinavir (SQV). In: Program and Abstracts of the 7th Conference on Retroviruses and Opportunistic Infections, San Francisco, 2000, abstract 318.
144. Ruff A, Hamzeh F, Lietman P, et al. Excretion of zidovudine (ZDV) in human breast milk. In: Program and Abstracts of the 34th Interscience Conference on Antimicrobial Agents and Chemotherapy, Orlando. Washington, DC, American Society for Microbiology, 1994, abstract I-11.
145. Fletcher CV, Acosta E, Strykowski JM. Gender differences in pharmacokinetics and pharmacodynamics. J Adolesc Health 15:619, 1994.
146. Mueller BU, Pizzo PA, Farley M, et al. Pharmacokinetic evaluation of the combination of zidovudine and didanosine in children with human immunodeficiency virus infection. J Pediatr 125:142, 1994.
147. Khaliq Y, Gallicano K, Sequin I, et al. Single and multiple dose pharmacokinetics of nelfinavir and CYP2C19 activity in human immunodeficiency virus-infected patients with chronic liver disease. Br J Clin Pharmacol 50:108, 2000.
148. Dasta JF, Armstrong DK. Variability in aminoglycoside pharmacokinetics in critically ill surgical patients. Crit Care Med 15:327, 1988.
149. Mlynarek ME, Peterson EL, Zarowitz BJ. Predicting unbound phenytoin concentrations in the critically ill neurosurgical patient. Ann Pharmacother 30:219, 1996.
150. Bayliff CD, Schwartz ML, Hardy GB. Pharmacokinetics of high dose pentobarbital in severe head trauma. Clin Pharmacol Ther 38:457, 1985.
151. Bertz R, Shi H, Cavanaugh J, et al. Effect of three vehicles, Advera, Ensure, and chocolate milk, on the bioavailability of an oral liquid formulation of Norvir. In: Abstracts of the 36th Interscience Conference on Antimicrobial Agents and Chemotherapy, New Orleans. Washington, DC, American Society for Microbiology, 1996, abstract A25.
152. USPDI Advice for the Patient: Drug Information in Lay Language. Rockville MD, United States Pharmacopoeia Convention, 1996.

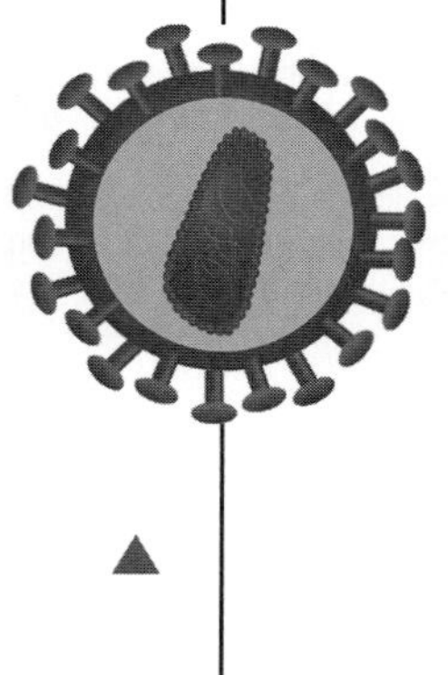

CHAPTER 67

AIDS-Related Medications

Stephen C. Piscitelli, PharmD
Alice K. Pau, PharmD

INDEX OF MEDICATIONS

ANTIRETROVIRALS

MYCOBACTERIUM AVIUM COMPLEX AND TUBERCULOSIS AGENTS

PNEUMOCYSTIS CARINII PNEUMONIA (PCP) AND TOXOPLASMOSIS AGENTS

ANTIFUNGALS

ANTI-CYTOMEGALOVIRUS, ANTI-HERPES SIMPLEX VIRUS, AND ANTI-VARICELLA-ZOSTER VIRUS AGENTS

BIOLOGICALS

MISCELLANEOUS

▲ DEFINITIONS OF FDA PREGNANCY RISK FACTOR CATEGORIES:

Category A: Controlled studies in women fail to show risk to fetus during first trimester (with no evidence of risk during later trimesters), and the possibility of fetal harm appears remote.

Category B: Either animal reproduction studies have not demonstrated a fetal risk (with no controlled studies in pregnant women) or animal reproduction studies have shown an adverse effect (other than a decrease in fertility) that was not confirmed in controlled studies of women during the first trimester (with no evidence of risk during later trimesters).

Category C: Either studies in animals have revealed adverse effects on the fetus (teratogenic, embryocidal, or other), with no controlled studies in pregnant women, or studies in women and animals are not available. Drugs should be given only if the potential benefit justifies the potential risk to the fetus.

Category D: There is positive evidence of human fetal risk, but the benefits from use in pregnant women may be acceptable despite the risk (e.g., if the drug is needed in a life-threatening situation or for a serious disease for which safer drugs cannot be used or are ineffective).

Category X: Studies in animals or humans have demonstrated fetal abnormalities, there is evidence of fetal risk based on human experience, or both; and the risk of the use of the drug in pregnant women clearly outweighs any possible benefit. The drug is contraindicated in women who are or may become pregnant.

▲ ABBREVIATIONS

AUC	Area under the concentration-time curve
C_{max}	Maximum concentration
CMV	Cytomegalovirus
CrCl	Creatinine clearance
CNS	Central nervous system
CSF	Cerebrospinal fluid
D5W	5% Dextrose in water
EC	enteric coated
GI	Gastrointestinal
HSV	Herpes simplex virus
IM	Intramuscular
IV	Intravenous
LFTs	Liver function tests
MAC	*Mycobacterium avium* complex
OTC	Over the counter
PCP	*Pneumocystis carinii* pneumonia
SC	Subcutaneous
$t_{1/2}$	Half-life
T_{max}	Time to maximum concentration
*T*oxo	Toxoplasmosis
USPHS	U.S. Public Health Service
VZV	Varicella-zoster virus

Prices are approximate and based on average wholesale price.

Antiretrovirals

Abacavir

Trade name: Ziagen (GlaxoSmithKline)

Available formulations:

300 mg tablets	$6.10
Trizivir (ZDV 300 mg/3TC 150 mg/abacavir 300 mg)	$13.30
20 mg/ml oral solution, 240 ml	$96.29

Class: Nucleoside analogue antiretroviral

Mechanism of action: Converted intracellularly to triphosphate, which is an inhibitor of HIV reverse transcriptase

Oral dose (adults): 300 mg bid

Storage and stability: Store at room temperature; oral solution may be refrigerated, do not freeze

PHARMACOKINETICS

T_{max}: 1 hour

Bioavailability: 83%

Half-life: 0.9 to 1.5 hours

CSF penetration: Approximately 18% of plasma concentration

Plasma protein binding: Approximately 50%

Metabolism/elimination: Primarily metabolized by alcohol dehydrogenase and glucuronyl transferase

Food effects: Can be taken without regard to meals

Breast milk: Animal studies indicate that abacavir is excreted in breast milk. USPHS recommends that HIV+ mothers not breastfeed to avoid transmission to infant

Dosage adjustment for organ failure: No studies performed in the presence of renal or hepatic impairment

Side effects: Systemic hypersensitivity reaction occurs in 3% to 5% of patients, associated with constitutional symptoms, fever, rash, gastrointestinal disturbances, or pulmonary symptoms. Abacavir should be discontinued and not rechallenged. Rechallenge reactions can be severe, even fatal. This reaction has also been reported in patients who discontinue abacavir for reasons other than a hypersensitivity reaction. Other side effects included asthenia, abdominal pain, diarrhea, nausea, vomiting, headache, hepatomegaly with steatosis, lactic acidosis

Pregnancy: Category C

Amprenavir

Trade name: Agenerase (GlaxoSmithKline)

Available formulations:

50 mg capsules	$0.44
150 mg capsules	$1.32
15 mg/ml oral solution, 240 ml	$31.72

Each capsule contains 109 IU of vitamin E; additional vitamin E supplements should be avoided

Oral solution contains propylene glycol, not recommended in children less than 4 years old, pregnant women, patients with renal or liver failure, and patients on metronidazole or disulfiram

Class: Protease inhibitor antiretroviral agent

Mechanism of action: Inhibition of HIV protease, which is responsible for cleaving viral polyproteins into functional protein necessary for production of replication-competent virions

Oral dose:

Adults: capsules 1200 mg bid or capsules 600 mg bid (when used with ritonavir 100 mg bid) or capsules 1200 mg qd (when used with ritonavir 200 mg qd)

Children: capsules: < 50 kg—20 mg/kg bid or 15 mg/kg tid

solution: < 50 kg—22.5 mg/kg bid or 17 mg/kg tid

Capsules and oral solution doses not interchangeable on a milligram per milligram basis

Storage and stability: Store at room temperature

PHARMACOKINETICS

T_{max}: 1 to 2 hours

Bioavailability: Not established

Half-life: 7 to 10 hours

CSF penetration: Not established

Plasma protein binding: 91% to 95%

Metabolism/elimination: Extensive hepatic metabolism by CYP3A4 metabolites excreted in feces; inhibitor of CYP3A4-mediated metabolism

Food effects: Can be taken without regard to meals but not with a high-fat meal

Breast milk: Animal studies indicate that amprenavir is excreted in breast milk. USPHS recommends that HIV+ mothers not breastfeed to avoid transmission to infant.

Dosage adjustment for organ failure: Dosage adjustment in hepatic impairment:

Child-Pugh Score	Dose
5–8	450 mg bid
9–12	300 mg bid

Side effects: Headache, nausea, vomiting, diarrhea, rash. Protease inhibitors have been associated with metabolic effects including hyperglycemia, increased triglycerides and cholesterol, and fat redistribution

Pregnancy: Category C

Delavirdine

Trade name: Rescriptor (Agouron)

Available formulations:

100 mg tablets	$0.79
200 mg tablets	$1.57

Class: Nonnucleoside antiretroviral

Mechanism of action: Inhibitor of HIV reverse transcriptase. Noncompetitive with nucleoside analogues acting at different sites

Oral dose (adults): 400 mg tid

Storage and stability: Keep in tightly closed container away from high humidity

PHARMACOKINETICS

T_{max}**:** 1 hour

Bioavailability: 85%, increased when in slurry of water

Half-life: increases with increased dose: 5.8 hours with 400 mg tid dose

CSF penetration: 0.4% of plasma concentration

Plasma protein binding: 98%

Metabolism/elimination: Extensively metabolized in liver by CYP3A4 and possibly CYP2D6. Inhibitor of CYP3A4-mediated metabolism

Food effects: Can be administered with or without food

Breast milk: Unknown. USPHS recommends that HIV+ mothers not breastfeed to avoid transmission to infant

Dosage adjustment for organ failure: Not investigated; minimal amount excreted in urine, suggesting that renal impairment would not require dose adjustments

Side effects: Rash in 18% and severe in 3.6%, usually appears within 1 to 3 weeks of therapy initiation; nausea; increased LFTs

Pregnancy: Category C

Didanosine (ddI)

Trade name: Videx (Bristol-Myers Squibb)

Available formulations:

25 mg buffered tablets	$0.47
50 mg buffered tablets	$0.95
100 mg buffered tablets	$1.89
150 mg buffered tablets	$2.84
200 mg buffered tablets	$3.79
2 g/100 ml pediatric powder	$34.70
4 g/200 ml pediatric powder	$78.61
100 mg sachet	$1.89
167 mg sachet	$3.16
250 mg sachet	$4.74
125 mg EC capsules	$3.60
200 mg EC capsules	$4.96
250 mg EC capsules	$6.19
400 mg EC capsules	$9.91

Class: Nucleoside analogue antiretroviral

Mechanism of action: Converted intracellularly to ddA triphosphate, which inhibits HIV reverse transcriptase

Buffered tablets (adults):
$>$ 60 kg: 200 mg bid (preferred) or 400 mg qd
$<$ 60 kg: 125 mg bid
Two tablets must be administered at each dose to ensure adequate buffering. Tablets should be chewed, crushed, or dispersed in water or clear apple juice

Sachet (adults):
$>$ 60 kg: 250 mg bid
$<$ 60 kg: 167 mg bid
Mix with 4 ounces of water; stir until dissolved

EC capsules:
$>$ 60 kg: 400 mg qd
$<$ 60 kg: 250 mg qd

Oral dose suspension (children): 200 mg/m^2/d, given bid
Suspension is dissolved in water and then mixed with equal amount of antacid

Storage and stability:
Tablets: Store at room temperature in tightly closed bottles. If dispersed in water or apple juice, stable for 1 hour at room temperature
Sachet: Store at room temperature. If dissolved in water, stable for 4 hours at room temperature
EC capsules: Store at room temperature
Suspension: Store bottles at room temperature. After mixing with antacid, store in refrigerator in tightly closed container for up to 30 days

PHARMACOKINETICS

T_{max}**:** 0.6 to 1.0 hour

Bioavailability: Buffered tablet and EC capsule 40%; sachet 30%

Half-life: 1.6 hours

CSF penetration: 21% of serum concentration (children 46%)

Plasma protein binding: Less than 5%

Metabolism/elimination: Primarily eliminated by renal excretion

Food effects: Requires administration on empty stomach at least 30 minutes before a meal

Breast milk: Unknown. The USPHS recommends that HIV+ women not breastfeed to avoid transmission to infants

Dosage adjustment for organ failure: Dosage reduction is recommended in patients with renal impairment.

Approximately 35% of ddI in the body is removed by dialysis. In patients with hepatic impairment, patients should be monitored closely for ddI toxicities

Side effects: Nausea, diarrhea, abdominal pain, peripheral neuropathy (12% to 34%, dose-related), pancreatitis, headache, rash, hepatomegaly with steatosis, lactic acidosis

Pregnancy: Category B. Fatal lactic acidosis has been reported in pregnant women treated with a combination of didanosine and stavudine

Efavirenz

Trade name: Sustiva (Bristol-Meyers Squibb)

Available formulations:

50 mg capsules $1.10
100 mg capsules $2.19
200 mg capsules $4.38
600 mg tablets $14.39

Class: Nonnucleoside antiretroviral

Mechanism of action: Inhibitor of HIV reverse transcriptase. Noncompetitive with nucleoside analogues acting at different sites

Oral dose:

Adults: 600 mg once daily, recommended to be given at bedtime

Children:

Weight (kg)	Dose (mg)
10 to <15	200
15 to <20	250
20 to <25	300
25 to <32.5	350
32.5 to <40	400
≥40	600

Storage and stability: Store at room temperature

PHARMACOKINETICS

T_{max}**:** 3 to 5 hours

Bioavailability: Not established

Half-life: 40 to 55 hours with multiple dosing

CSF penetration: 0.65% to 1.20% of plasma concentration

Plasma protein binding: More than 98%

Metabolism/elimination: Primarily hepatic metabolism by cytochrome P4503A4, a mild/moderate inducer of hepatic enzymes

Food effects: Administer on an empty stomach, food increases efavirenz absorption and may result in increased toxicities

Breast milk: Animal studies indicate that efavirenz is excreted in breast milk. USPHS recommends that HIV+ women not breastfeed to avoid transmission to infants

Dosage adjustment for organ failure: Not established

Side effects: Dizziness, paresthesias, headache, lightheadedness, confusion, vivid dreams (CNS-related symptoms may be minimized by administering drug at bedtime), nausea, rash, elevated LFTs, elevated serum lipids

Pregnancy: Category C. Efavirenz has been shown to cause major congenital anomalies in nonhuman primates

Indinavir

Trade name: Crixivan (Merck)

Available formulations:

200 mg capsules $1.29
333 mg capsules $2.14
400 mg capsules $2.58

Class: Protease inhibitor antiretroviral

Mechanism of action: Inhibition of HIV protease, which is responsible for cleaving viral polyproteins into functional protein necessary for production of replication-competent virions

Oral dose (adults): 800 mg every 8 hours

Storage and stability: Store in original, tightly closed container with desiccant

PHARMACOKINETICS

T_{max}**:** 0.8 hour

Bioavailability: 30%

Half-life: 1.5 to 2.0 hours

CSF penetration: 2.2% to 76.0% in limited number of patients

Plasma protein binding: Approximately 60%

Metabolism/elimination: Hepatic metabolism by CYP 4503A4; less than 20% excreted unchanged in urine; inhibitor of CY3A4-mediated metabolism

Food effects: High-caloric, high-fat meal reduces bioavailability. Administer on empty stomach or with a low-fat, light meal. Can administer with food when taken with ritonavir. Patients advised to drink at least 1.5 liters of fluid daily to avoid crystalluria and nephrolithiasis.

Breast milk: Available data suggest distribution into milk. USPHS recommends that HIV+ mothers not breastfeed to avoid transmission to infant

Dosage adjustment for organ failure: Minimal renal excretion suggests no alteration required for renal dysfunction. With severe hepatic disease, reduce dose to 600 mg every 8 hours

Side effects: Nausea, abdominal pain, bloating, nephrolithiasis, hyperbilirubinemia (8%), headache, dizziness, rash. Protease inhibitors have been associated with metabolic effects, including hyperglycemia, increased triglycerides and cholesterol, and fat redistribution.

Pregnancy: Category C

Lamivudine (3TC)

Trade name: Epivir (GlaxoSmithKline); Combivir (GlaxoSmithKline); Trizivir (GlaxoSmithKline)

Available formulations:

150 mg tablets	$4.54
10 mg/ml oral solution, 240 ml	$72.70
Combivir [zidovudine (ZVD)/lamivudine (3TC)]	$9.85
Trizivir (ZDV/3TC/abacavir)	$13.30

Class: Nucleoside analogue antiretroviral

Mechanism of action: Converted intracellularly to triphosphate metabolite, which is an inhibitor of HIV reverse transcriptase; also active against hepatitis B virus

Oral dose:

Adults, adolescents: 150 mg bid

Children: 3 to 12 years 4 mg/kg bid, maximum 150 mg bid

Storage and stability: Store at room temperature in tightly closed containers

PHARMACOKINETICS

T_{max}: Within 1 hour

Bioavailability: 86%

Half-life: 3 to 6 hours

CSF penetration: Unknown

Plasma protein binding: Less than 36%

Metabolism/elimination: Primarily eliminated unchanged in the urine

Food effects: Food delays absorption but not overall extent; give without regard to meals

Breast milk: Available data suggest that lamivudine is readily excreted in milk. USPHS recommends that HIV+ women not breastfeed to avoid transmission to infants

Dosage adjustment for renal failure: also see p. 949

CrCl (ml/m)	Dose
>50	150 mg bid
30–49	150 mg qd
15–29	150 mg first dose; 100 mg qd
5–14	150 mg first dose; 50 mg qd
<5	50 mg first dose; 25 mg qd

Side effects: Nausea, headache, malaise, nasal congestion, pancreatitis in children (14%), hepatomegaly with steatosis, lactic acidosis

Pregnancy: Category C

Lopinavir/Ritonavir

Trade name: Kaletra (Abbott)

Available formulations:

133 mg lopinavir/33 mg ritonavir	$3.76/cap
400 mg/100 mg/5 ml, 180 ml	$338.55/bottle

Class: Protease inhibitor antiretroviral

Mechanism of action: Inhibition of HIV protease, which is responsible for cleaving viral polyproteins into functional protein necessary for production of replication-competent virions

Oral dose:

Adults: 400/100 mg bid with food (533/133 mg bid with food if used with efavirenz or nevirapine)

Children

7 to < 15 kg	12/3 mg/kg bid
15 to 40 kg	10/2.5 mg/kg bid

Storage and stability: Capsules and solution stable in refrigerator until date on label. At room temperature, use within 2 months

PHARMACOKINETICS

T_{max}: 4 hours

Bioavailability: Not determined

Half-life: 5 to 6 hours

CSF penetration: Negligible

Plasma protein binding: Approximately 98% to 99%

Metabolism/elimination: Hepatic metabolism by CYP 4503A4; less than 3% excreted unchanged in urine; inhibitor of CY3A4-mediated metabolism primarily due to ritonavir component

Food effects: Food significantly increases plasma concentrations. Administer with food

Breast milk: Animal data suggest distribution into milk. USPHS recommends that HIV+ mothers not breastfeed to avoid transmission to infant

Dosage adjustment for organ failure: Minimal renal excretion suggests no alteration required for renal dysfunction. With hepatic disease, concentrations may be increased, and close monitoring is required

Side effects: Nausea, diarrhea, abdominal pain, asthenia, headache, elevated LFTs. Protease inhibitors have been associated with metabolic effects including hyperglycemia, increased triglycerides and cholesterol, and fat redistribution

Pregnancy: Category C

Nelfinavir

Trade name: Viracept (Agouron)

Available formulations:

250 mg tablets	$2.26
50 mg/g oral powder, 144 g	$59.45

Class: Protease inhibitor antiretroviral

Mechanism of action: Inhibition of HIV protease, which is responsible for cleaving viral polyproteins into functional protein necessary for production of replication-competent virions

Oral dose:

Adults: 750 mg tid or 1250 mg bid with food

Children: 20 to 30 mg/kg/dose tid with food

Storage and stability: Oral powder mixed with water, milk formulation, soy formulation. Store at room temperature; after mixing oral solution, stable for up to 6 hours

PHARMACOKINETICS

T_{max}: 2 to 4 hours

Bioavailability: 20% to 80%

Half-life: 3.5 to 5.0 hours

CSF penetration: Negligible

Plasma protein binding: More than 98%

Metabolism/elimination: Extensive hepatic metabolism by CYP3A4 and CYP2C19, with metabolites excreted in feces. Inhibitor of CYP3A4-mediated metabolism

Food effects: Bioavailability increased with food. Administer with meals or snack

Breast milk: Animal data suggest that nelfinavir is distributed into breast milk. USPHS recommends that HIV+ mothers do not breastfeed to avoid transmission to infant

Dosage adjustment for organ failure: Minimal renal excretion suggests no alteration required in renal dysfunction. Not studied in hepatic disease; close monitoring warranted

Side effects: Diarrhea, nausea, elevated LFTs, abdominal pain. Protease inhibitors have been associated with metabolic effects including hyperglycemia, increased triglycerides and cholesterol, and fat redistribution

Pregnancy: Category B

Nevirapine

Trade name: Viramune (Boeringer-Ingelheim/Roxanne)

Available formulations:

200 mg tablets	$4.64
10 mg/ml suspension, 240 ml	$60.34

Class: Nonnucleoside antiretroviral

Mechanism of action: Inhibitor of HIV reverse transcriptase. Noncompetitive with nucleoside analogues acting at different sites

Oral dose (adults): 200 mg qd for 14 days, then 200 mg bid. Do not increase dosage if rash appears during escalation phase. If therapy is stopped for more than 7 days, reinitiate dose escalation

Storage and stability: Store at room temperature in tightly closed bottles

PHARMACOKINETICS

T_{max}: Within 4 hours

Bioavailability: More than 90%

Half-life: 25 to 30 hours

CSF penetration: 45% of concentration in plasma

Plasma protein binding: 60%

Metabolism/elimination: Metabolized by CYP450 oxidative metabolism and glucuronidation; metabolites excreted in urine; inducer of CYP3A4-mediated metabolism

Food effects: Not affected by food; administer without regard to meals

Breast milk: Detectable in breast milk. USPHS recommends that HIV+ mothers not breastfeed to avoid transmission to infant

Dosage adjustment for organ failure: Not studied

Side effects: Rash (17%) usually appears within the first 6 weeks of therapy, potentially severe (7.6%). Hepatotoxicity—can be severe, close monitoring of LFTs is recommended, particularly during first 12 weeks of therapy. Nausea, fever, headache

Pregnancy: Category C

Ritonavir

Trade name: Norvir (Abbott)

Available formulations:

100 mg capsules	$1.85
80 mg/ml oral solution, 240ml	$311.65

Class: Protease inhibitor antiretroviral

Mechanism of action: Inhibition of HIV protease, which is responsible for cleaving viral polyproteins into functional protein necessary for production of replication-competent virions

Oral dose:

Adults: 600 mg bid; dose escalation required. Initiate with 300 mg bid and increase as tolerated over 2 weeks to 600 mg bid. Doses of 100 to 400 mg bid used as pharmacokinetic enhancer. Solution may be mixed with Advera, Ensure, or chocolate milk to increase palatability

Children: 400 mg/m^2; dose escalation required. Initiate with 250 mg/m^2 and increase in 50 mg/m^2 increments every 2 to 3 days

Storage and stability: Store capsules in refrigerator until dispensed. Ritonavir capsules can be left at room temperature for up to 30 days. Solution does not need refrigeration if used within 30 days; avoid exposure to extreme heat

PHARMACOKINETICS

T_{max}: 2 to 4 hours

Bioavailability: 60% to 80%

Half-life: 3 to 5 hours

CSF penetration: Negligible

Plasma protein binding: 98% to 99%

Metabolism/elimination: Extensive hepatic metabolism by hepatic CYP3A4, also CYP2D6 and CYP1A2 to a lesser extent; potent inhibitor of CYP3A4-mediated metabolism

Food effects: Recommended to be administered with food: 15% increase in AUC with food

Breast milk: Unknown. USPHS recommends that HIV+ mothers not breastfeed to avoid transmission to infant

Dosage adjustment for organ failure: Minimal renal excretion suggests no alteration required in renal dysfunction. Not studied in hepatic disease; close monitoring warranted.

Side effects: Predominantly GI side effects (nausea and vomiting, diarrhea, abdominal pain) especially during first month of treatment, circumoral paresthesias, taste perversion, elevated LFTs, hypertriglyceridemia. Protease inhibitors have been associated with metabolic effects including hyperglycemia, increased triglycerides and cholesterol, and fat redistribution

Pregnancy: Category B

Saquinavir

Trade name: Invirase (Roche); Fortovase (Roche)

Available formulations:

200 mg capsules (Invirase)	$2.24
200 mg soft gel capsules (Fortovase)	$1.15

Class: Protease inhibitor antiretroviral

Mechanism of action: Inhibition of HIV protease, which is responsible for cleaving viral polyproteins into functional protein necessary for production of replication-competent virions

Oral dose (adults):

Invirase: 600 mg tid

Fortovase: 1800 mg tid

Storage and stability:

Invirase: Store at room temperature.

Fortovase: refrigerated capsules stable to expiration date on label; at room temperature, use within 3 months

PHARMACOKINETICS

T_{max}: Approximately 3 hours

Bioavailability:

Invirase: approximately 4% with full meal.

Fortovase: food increases bioavailability threefold

Half-life: 1 to 2 hours

CSF penetration: Negligible

Plasma protein binding: 98%

Metabolism/elimination: Metabolized primarily by CYP3A4 in liver; extensive first-pass metabolism

Food effects: Must be administered within 2 hours of a full meal

Breast milk: Unknown. USPHS recommends that HIV+ mothers not breastfeed to avoid transmission to infant

Dosage adjustment for organ failure: Minimal renal excretion suggests no alteration required for renal dysfunction. Not studied for hepatic disease

Side effects: Nausea and vomiting, abdominal pain, diarrhea, elevated LFTs, headache. Protease inhibitors have been associated with metabolic effects including hyperglycemia, increased triglycerides and cholesterol, and fat redistribution

Pregnancy: Category B

Stavudine (d4T)

Trade name: Zerit (Bristol Myers Squibb)

Available formulations:

15 mg capsules	$4.24
20 mg capsules	$4.40
30 mg capsules	$4.60
40 mg capsules	$4.77
1 mg/ml oral solution, 200 ml	$55.77

Class: Nucleoside analogue antiretroviral

Mechanism of action: Converted intracellularly to d4T triphosphate, which inhibits HIV reverse transcriptase

Oral dose:

Adults: > 60 kg: 40 mg bid; < 60 kg: 30 mg bid

Children: < 30 kg: 1 mg/kg/dose every 12 hours

Storage and stability:

Capsules: store at room temperature in tightly closed bottles

Suspension: After reconstitution with water, store in refrigerator in tightly closed original container for up to 30 days

PHARMACOKINETICS

T_{max}: Within 1 hour

Bioavailability: 86%

Half-life: 1.0 to 1.4 hours

CSF penetration: 30% of serum levels

Plasma protein binding: Negligible

Metabolism/elimination: Primarily excreted renally (50%)

Food effects: AUC unchanged with food; give without regard to meals

Breast milk: Animal studies suggest stavudine is excreted in breast milk. USPHS recommends that HIV+ women not breastfeed to avoid transmission to infants

Dosage adjustment for organ failure: Adjust for renal dysfunction. Also see p. 949.

CrCl (ml/min)	> 60 kg	< 60 kg
> 50	40 mg bid	30 mg bid
26–50	20 mg bid	15 mg bid
10–25	20 mg qd	15 mg qd

Side effects: Peripheral neuropathy (15% to 21%), elevated LFTs, rapidly ascending neuromuscular weakness, gastrointestinal side effects, hepatomegaly with steatosis, lactic acidosis

Pregnancy: Category C. Fatal lactic acidosis has been reported in pregnant women treated with a combination of stavudine and didanosine

Tenofovir Disoproxil Fumarate (or Tenofovir DF or Tenofovir)

Trade name: Viread (Gilead)

Available formulations:

300 mg tablet	$13.60

Class: Nucleotide Analog Antiviral

Mechanism of action: Converted to tenofovir diphosphate which inhibits HIV reverse transcriptase by competing with deoxyadenosine 5′-triphosphate, leading to DNA chain termination; also has in vitro activities against hepatitis B virus

Dosages (adult): 300 mg qd

Storage and stability: Store at room temperature

PHARMACOKINETICS

T_{max}: 1 hour under fasting condition, and 2 hours when taken with food

Bioavailability: 27% under fasting condition, food increases by 40%

Half-life: 10–14 hours after administration with food

Metabolism/elimination: Primarily renal excretion by glomerular filtration and active tubular secretion

Food effects: Food increases oral absorption

Breast milk: not known

Dosage adjustment in organ failure: Not recommended in patients with CrCl <60 ml/min

Side effects: nausea, vomiting, headache, asthenia

Pregnancy: Category C

Zalcitabine (ddC)

Trade name: Hivid (Roche)

Available formulations:

0.375 tablets	$1.94
0.75 tablets	$2.43

Class: Nucleoside analogue antiretroviral

Mechanism of action: Converted intracellularly to ddC triphosphate, which inhibits HIV reverse transcriptase

Oral dose (adults): 0.75 mg tid

Storage and stability: Store in tightly closed bottles at room temperature

PHARMACOKINETICS

T_{max}: Within 1 hour

Bioavailability: 85%

Half-life: 1 to 3 hours

CSF penetration: CSF/plasma ratio approximately 20%

Plasma protein binding: 24%

Metabolism/elimination: 70% excreted renally

Food effects: May delay rate of absorption but not overall extent; give without regard to meals

Breast milk: Unknown. USPHS recommends that HIV+ women not breastfeed to avoid transmission to infants

Dosage adjustment for renal failure: also see p. 949

CrCl (ml/min)	Dose
10–40	0.75 mg q12h
< 10	0.75 mg qd

Side effects: Peripheral neuropathy (22% to 35%), pancreatitis, stomatitis, gastrointestinal complaints, hepatomegaly with steatosis, lactic acidosis

Pregnancy: Category C

Zidovudine (Azidothymidine, AZT)

Trade name: Retrovir (GlaxoSmithKline); Combivir (GlaxoSmithKline); Trizivir (GlaxoSmithKline)

Available formulations:

100 mg capsules	$1.77
300 mg tablets	$5.30
10 mg/ml syrup, 240 ml	$42.47
20 ml intravenous vials, 10 mg/ml	$19.14
Combivir (ZDV/3TC)	$9.85
Trizivir (ZDV/3TC/abacavir)	$13.30

Class: Pyrimidine nucleoside analogue antiretroviral

Mechanism of action: Converted intracellularly to zidovudine triphosphate, which is an inhibitor of HIV reverse transcriptase

Oral dose:

Adults: 600 mg/day in two or three divided doses

Children: 180 mg/m^2 every 6 hours (maximum 200 mg every 6 hours)

Neonates, for prevention of perinatal transmission: Starting within 12 hours after birth: 2 mg/kg po q6h × 6 weeks or 1.5 mg/kg IV over 30 minutes q6h

IV dose: 1 mg/kg infused over 1 hour every 4 hours

Storage and stability: Store at room temperature: protect from moisture

PHARMACOKINETICS

T_{max}: 0.5 to 1.5 hours

Bioavailability: 65%

Half-life: 1.1 hours (3.0 hours intracellularly)

CSF penetration: 60% of serum level

Plasma protein binding: 34% to 38%

Metabolism/elimination: Undergoes glucuronidation in liver; metabolite excreted in urine

Food effects: With zidovudine capsules, plasma concentrations decreased by more than 50%, although bioavailability determined by AUC unknown

Breast milk: Excreted in breast milk in similar concentration as serum. USPHS recommends that HIV+ women not breastfeed to avoid transmission to infants

Dosage adjustment for organ failure: Hemodialysis- or peritoneal dialysis: 100 mg every 6 to 8 hours recommended

Side effects: Subjective complaints (headache, nausea, malaise, anorexia), macrocytic anemia, granulocytopenia, myopathy, myositis, changes in nail and skin pigmentation, hepatomegaly with steatosis, lactic acidosis

Pregnancy: Category C. Indicated for reducing the risk of vertical transmission to fetus. Begin therapy between 14 and 34 weeks' gestation. Give intravenous therapy during labor and delivery (2 mg/kg over 1 hour, then 1 mg/kg continuous infusion until umbilical cord is clamped)

Investigational Antiretroviral Drugs

Name	Class	Dose	Pharmacokinetics	Safety
Atazanavir	Protease inhibitor	400 mg qd	Metabolized by CYP3A4, inhibitor of drug metabolism	Increased bilirubin, nausea, vomiting, diarrhea
T-20 Pentafuside (Roche)	Fusion inhibitor	12.5–22.0 mg/day SC	Limited data	Subcutaneous nodules

Dosing of Antiretrovirals in the Presence of Renal or Hepatic Insufficiency

NUCLEOSIDE REVERSE TRANSCRIPTASE INHIBITORS

Zidovudine

Renal Impairment, Hemodialysis or Peritoneal Dialysis
PO dose: 100 mg q6–8h
IV dose: 1 mg/kg q6–8h
Hepatic Impairment, Cirrhosis: Pharmacokinetic data suggest a 50% decrease in dose or doubling the interval. Product information states insufficient data

Didanosine Renal Impairment:

Crcl (ml/min)	> 60 kg	< 60 kg
Buffered tablets		
> 60	200 mg bid or 400 mg qd	125 mg bid or 250 mg qd
30–59	100 mg bid or 200 mg qd	75 mg bid or 125 mg qd
10–29	150 mg qd	100 mg qd
< 10	100 mg qd	75 mg qd
Sachets		
> 60	250 mg bid or 500 mg qd	167 mg bid or 334 mg qd
30–59	100 mg bid or 200 mg qd	75 mg bid or 150 mg qd
10–29	167 mg qd	100 mg qd
< 10	100 mg qd	100 mg qd
EC capsules		
> 60	400 mg qd	250 mg qd
30–59	200 mg qd	125 mg qd
10–29	125 mg qd	125 mg qd
< 10	125 mg qd	Not suitable

Hemodialysis: One-fourth the total daily dose once daily for anuric patients receiving dialysis
Hepatic Impairment: Insufficient data but consider dosage adjustment

Zalcitabine

Renal Impairment: see p. 948
Hepatic Impairment: Use with caution. If LFTs are more than five times normal, drug interruption is recommended

Stavudine

Renal Impairment: see p. 947
Hepatic Impairment: In the presence of clinically significant elevations in LFTs, interruption of therapy is recommended. After laboratory values normalize, reinstitute therapy at 20 mg q12h

Lamivudine

Renal Impairment: see p. 945
Hepatic Impairment: Lamivudine is primarily eliminated unchanged in the urine, so no change in dosing is necessary

Abacavir

Renal Impairment: Insufficient data; but because the drug is extensively metabolized in the liver, no change in dosing is probably necessary
Hepatic Impairment: No data available

NONNUCLEOSIDE REVERSE TRANSCRIPTASE INHIBITORS

Nevirapine

Standard dose: 200 mg qd × 14 days then 200 mg bid
Renal Impairment: Insufficient data; but because drug is extensively metabolized in the liver, no change in dosing is probably necessary
Hepatic Impairment: Interrupt therapy in patients experiencing moderate or severe liver function tests abnormalities. Nevirapine should not be reinstituted if other cause of liver abnormalities cannot be identified

Delavirdine

Standard dose: 400 mg tid
Renal Impairment: Insufficient data; but because drug is extensively metabolized in the liver, no change in dosing is probably necessary
Hepatic Impairment: No recommendations from manufacturer; however, because delavirdine is primarily metabolized in the liver, caution should be exercised and close monitoring is warranted

Efavirenz

Renal Impairment: Insufficient data; but because drug is extensively metabolized in the liver, no change in dosing is probably necessary
Hepatic Impairment: No recommendations from manufacturer; however, because efavirenz is primarily metabolized in the liver, caution should be exercised and close monitoring is warranted

PROTEASE INHIBITORS

Renal Impairment: Insufficient data; but because protease inhibitors are extensively metabolized in the liver, no change in dosing is probably necessary
Hepatic Insufficiency (Mild to Moderate):

Drug	Recommendation	
Saquinavir	None	
Ritonavir	None	
Indinavir	600 mg q8h	
Nelfinavir	None	
Amprenavir	Child-Pugh score	Dose
	5–8	450 mg bid
	9–12	300 mg bid
Lopinavir/ritonavir	None	

Food Effects on Antiretroviral Drugs

Antiretroviral	Effect of Food	Recommendation: Full or Empty Stomach
Zidovudine	Decrease in peak blood levels; overall exposure unaffected	Either
Didanosine	Marked decrease in blood levels	Empty stomach: 30 minutes before or 2 hours after a meal
Zalcitabine	None	Either
Stavudine	None	Either
Lamivudine	None	Either
Abacavir	None	Either
Tenofovir DF	Increase in blood levels	Administer with food
Saquinavir	Marked increase in blood levels	Administer within 2 hours after a meal
Ritonavir	Small increase in blood levels	Either, but recommended to be given with food
Nelfinavir	Increase in blood levels	Administer with food
Indinavir	Decrease in blood levels	Administer on empty stomach or with low-fat, low-protein food. Absorption not affected by food if administered with ritonavir
Amprenavir	None	Either; avoid a high-fat meal
Lopinavir/ritonavir	Increase in blood levels	Administer with food
Delavirdine	None	Either
Nevirapine	None	Either
Efavirenz	Increase in blood levels may increase CNS toxicities	Empty stomach

Mycobacterium avium Complex and Tuberculosis Agents

Amikacin

Trade name: Amikin (Bristol-Myers Squibb), Generic (Elkins)

Available formulations: Various preparations and strengths in single and multiple doses

Generic 250 mg/2 ml $65.00

Class: Aminoglycoside antibiotic

Mechanism of action: Binds to 30S ribosomal subunit, inhibiting protein synthesis

IV dose: 7.5 to 15.0 mg/kg/d. Administer over 60 minutes.

Storage and stability: Store vials at room temperature. After dilution, most admixtures are stable for 24 hours at room temperature

PHARMACOKINETICS

Half-life: Approximately 2 hours

CSF penetration: 10% to 20% of serum levels but may be higher with inflamed meninges

Plasma protein binding: 0% to 11%

Metabolism/elimination: Eliminated primarily by glomerular filtration

Breast milk: Unknown but recommended to be avoided

Dosage adjustment for organ failure: Dosage adjustment required for renal dysfunction. Creatinine clearance should be estimated and dosing interval adjusted to maintain peak and trough concentrations

Side effects: Nephrotoxicity, ototoxicity, arthralgia, fever, rash, eosinophilia

Pregnancy: Category D. Aminoglycosides can freely cross placenta. Its use has been associated with bilateral, irreversible deafness in neonates exposed to the drug in utero. One must weigh the benefit to the mother against the potential risks to the fetus.

Azithromycin

Trade name: Zithromax (Pfizer)

Available formulations:

250 mg tablets	$6.76
600 mg tablets	$16.21
1 g powder	$20.98
100 mg/5 ml suspension, 15 ml	$28.60
200 mg/5 ml suspension, 15 ml	$28.60
500 mg/vial for IV	$24.44

Class: Macrolide antibiotic

Mechanism of action: Binds to 50S ribosomal subunit, inhibiting protein synthesis

Oral dose (adults):

Treating MAC: 500 mg PO qd

Treating gonococcal urethritis: 1 g PO, single dose

MAC prophylaxis: 1200 mg once weekly

IV dose: 500 mg given over at least 1 hour for at least 1 to 2 days, then switch to PO *when appropriate*

Storage and stability:

Tablets: Store below 30°C

Suspension: Store at room temperature; administer within 10 days after reconstitution.

IV: reconstituted solution stable for 24 hours at room temperature. Admixtures in 250 or 500 ml of diluent are stable for 24 hours at room temperature or 7 days under refrigeration

PHARMACOKINETICS

T_{max}: Within 2 hours

Bioavailability: 34%

Half-life: 68 hours

CSF penetration: Negligible; extensive tissue and intracellular uptake

Plasma protein binding: 7% to 50%; concentration-dependent

Metabolism/elimination: Biliary excretion primarily as unchanged drug

Food effects: Decreased absorption of tablets by 43%; suspension not affected by food

Breast milk: Unknown

Dosage adjustment for organ failure: None

Side effects: Gastrointestinal side effects (loose stools, nausea, abdominal pain), rash, minor CNS disturbances, ototoxicity

Pregnancy: Category B

Clarithromycin

Trade name: Biaxin (Abbott); Biaxin-XL (Abbott)

Available formulations:

250 mg tablets	$3.57
500 mg tablets	$3.57
Oral suspensions	
125 mg/5 ml, 50 ml	$17.44
125 mg/5 ml, 100 ml	$32.25
250 mg/5 ml, 50 ml	$33.20
250 mg/5 ml, 100 ml	$61.48

Class: Macrolide antibiotic

Mechanism of action: Inhibits protein synthesis by binding to the 50S ribosomal subunit

Oral dose

Adults: 250 to 500 mg twice daily

Children: 7.5 mg/kg twice daily

MAC dose: 500 mg twice daily

Storage and stability: Store tablets and granules for suspension at room temperature in a well closed container and protected from light. Reconstituted suspension stored at room temperature and used within 14 days

PHARMACOKINETICS

T_{max}: 0.5 to 1.5 hours

Bioavailability: 50%

Half-life: 250 mg dose, 3 to 4 hours; 500 mg dose, 5 to 7 hours

CSF penetration: Unknown; extensive distribution into tissues, phagocytic cells

Metabolism/elimination: 20% to 30% excreted unchanged in urine; extensive hepatic metabolism. Active metabolite 14-OH-clarithromycin accounts for 20%

Food effects: Absorption unaffected by food

Breast milk: Unknown; caution should be exercised in nursing mothers

Dosage adjustment for organ failure: Dose should be reduced by half or the interval doubled in the presence of severe renal impairment (creatinine clearance < 30 ml/min) with or without hepatic disease

Side effects: Gastrointestinal adverse effects [nausea, vomiting, abdominal pain, diarrhea (11%)], infrequent reports of metallic taste, elevated LFTs, ototoxicity

Pregnancy: Category C

Clofazimine

Trade name: Lamprene (Geigy)

Available formulations: 50 mg capsules $0.17

Class: Antimycobacterial

Mechanism of action: Binds to mycobacterial DNA and inhibits growth through undefined mechanism

Oral dose (adults): 50 to 200 mg qd (*Not recommended for use in HIV-infected patients*)

Storage and stability: Store in tight containers at room temperature; protect from moisture

PHARMACOKINETICS

T_{max}: 4 to 12 hours

Bioavailability: 45% to 70%

Half-life: Estimated to be at least 70 days; retained in body for long periods

CSF penetration: Minimal or no penetration into CSF

Plasma protein binding: Unknown

Metabolism/elimination: Accumulation in body and excreted primarily unchanged in bile and feces; some partial metabolism to three metabolites

Food effects: Foods containing high fat and protein increase the AUC by 60%

Breast milk: Distributed into breast milk; should avoid breastfeeding because of potential for skin discoloration in infant

Dosage adjustment for organ failure: None

Side effects: Pinkish-brown skin discoloration (approximately 100% and dose-related), conjunctival discoloration, nausea, vomiting, abdominal pain

Pregnancy: Category C

Ethambutol

Trade name: Myambutol (Lederle)

Available formulations:

100 mg tablets	$0.59
400 mg tablets	$1.98

Class: Antimycobacterial

Mechanism of action: Appears to inhibit cell replication and metabolism by an unknown mechanism

Oral dose (adults): 15 to 25 mg/kg qd

Storage and stability: Store at room temperature. Protect from excessive moisture, heat

PHARMACOKINETICS

T_{max}: 2 to 4 hours

Bioavailability: 75% to 80%

Half-life: 3.3 hours

CSF penetration: Unknown

Plasma protein binding: 22%

Metabolism/elimination: Primarily eliminated unchanged in the urine (50%); partial oxidative metabolism in the liver and 20% excreted in feces unchanged

Food effects: Absorption is not affected by food

Breast milk: Distributed into milk in concentrations similar to those in plasma

Dosage adjustment for organ failure: Requires dosage adjustment in the presence of renal dysfunction

Side effects: Optic neuritis with decrease in visual acuity and fields, dermatitis, pruritus, headache, malaise

Pregnancy: Category B

Isoniazid

Trade name: Nydrazid Injection (Apothecon); Generic (various)

Available formulations:

100 mg tablets	$0.08
300 mg tablets	$0.09
50 mg/ml syrup, 480 ml	$22.65
100 mg/10 ml for IM	$16.93

Class: Antimycobacterial

Mechanism of action: Inhibition of mycolic acid synthesis; interference with metabolism of bacterial proteins, carbohydrates, and lipids

Oral dose (adults): 300 mg qd or 900 mg three times weekly

IM dose: 5 mg/kg up to 300 mg daily IM

Note: Concomitant pyridoxine recommended to avoid vitamin B_6 deficiency

Storage and stability: Protect from light, air, and excessive heat. Keep in well closed containers at room temperature

PHARMACOKINETICS

T_{max}: 1 to 2 hours

Bioavailability: 90%

Half-life: 1 to 4 hours

CSF penetration: 90% to 100% of plasma concentrations

Plasma protein binding: Minimal binding to plasma proteins

Metabolism/elimination: Metabolized primarily in liver by acetylation. Acetylator status is determined genetically: persons may be rapid or slow metabolizers, which affects AUC

Food effects: Food may slightly reduce isoniazid concentrations

Breast milk: Distributed into breast milk

Dosage adjustment for organ failure: Administer 50% of normal dose in slow acetylators with CrCl < 10 ml/min

Side effects: Peripheral neuritis, hepatic dysfunction, hepatitis, gastrointestinal complaints, vitamin B_6 deficiency, rash, fever

Pregnancy: Category C

Pyrazinamide

Trade name: Generic (Lederle)

Available formulations: 500 mg tablet $0.92

Class: Antimycobacterial

Mechanism of action: Unknown; bacteriostatic against *Mycobacterium tuberculosis*

Oral dose (adults): 15 to 30 mg/kg qd; twice weekly dosing at 50 to 70 mg/kg

Storage and stability: Store in well closed containers at room temperature

PHARMACOKINETICS

T_{max}: Within 2 hours

Half-life: 9 to 10 hours

CSF penetration: CSF and plasma concentration approximately equal

Plasma protein binding: 10%

Metabolism/elimination: Primarily renal excretion; 70% of dose excreted in urine within 24 hours

Food effects: Can be given with or without food

Breast milk: Small amounts excreted in breast milk

Dosage adjustment for organ failure: Dosage reduction recommended in patients with renal dysfunction

Side effects: Hyperuricemia, fever, hepatic dysfunction, gastrointestinal side effects, arthralgias, myalgias. May interfere with diabetic urine testing kits

Pregnancy: Category C

Rifabutin

Trade name: Mycobutin (Pharmacia & Upjohn)

Available formulations: 150 mg capsules $4.96

Class: Rifamycin antimycobacterial

Mechanism of action: Inhibits DNA-dependent RNA polymerase in certain bacteria; mechanism in MAC unknown

Oral dose (adults): 300 mg qd

Storage and stability: Store at room temperature

PHARMACOKINETICS

T_{max}: 2 to 4 hours

Bioavailability: Approximately 20%

Half-life: 45 hours

CSF penetration: Unknown

Plasma protein binding: 85%

Metabolism/elimination: Hepatic metabolism to multiple metabolites; 25-*O*-desacetyl metabolite has activity similar to parent drug. Metabolite excreted in feces and urine; substrate and inducer of CYP3A4-mediated metabolism

Food effects: Food may decrease the rate but not the extent of absorption

Breast milk: Unknown

Dosage adjustment for organ failure: Pharmacokinetics modified only slightly by renal and hepatic dysfunction

Side effects: Rash, gastrointestinal intolerance, neutropenia, thrombocytopenia, uveitis, discoloration of body fluids

Pregnancy: Category B

Rifampin

Trade name: Rifadin (Hoechst Marion Roussel), Rimactane (Ciba Geneva)

Available formulations:

150 mg capsules	$1.49
300 mg capsules	$2.11
600 mg IV vial	$79.38

Class: Rifamycin antimycobacterial

Mechanism of action: Inhibition of DNA-dependent RNA synthesis in susceptible bacteria

Oral dose:

Adults: 10 mg/kg (up to 600 mg) qd or two to three times weekly

Children: 10 to 20 mg/kg (up to 600 mg) qd

IV dose: 10 mg/kg (up to 600 mg) qd

Storage and stability:

Capsules: store in light-resistant container at room temperature

IV: Reconstitute with sterile water. Solution stable at room temperature for 24 hours. Further dilution with D5W; use within 4 hours

PHARMACOKINETICS

T_{max}: 2 to 4 hours

Bioavailability: Approximately 100%

Half-life: 3 hours; may decrease with prolonged therapy

CSF penetration: Wide distribution to body tissues; CSF levels 10% to 20% of serum concentrations with inflamed meninges

Plasma protein binding: 84% to 91%

Metabolism/elimination: Metabolized in liver by cytochrome P_{450}; excreted primarily in bile. Undergoes enterohepatic recirculation; potent inducer of CYP3A4-mediated metabolism

Food effects: Food may slightly reduce or delay absorption

Breast milk: Distributed into breast milk; nursing should be discontinued

Dosage adjustment for organ failure: Hepatic disease: use with caution under direct supervision; LFTs should be frequently monitored

Side effects: Nausea, abdominal cramps, heartburn, CNS disturbances, elevation of LFTs, discoloration of body fluids

Pregnancy: Category C

Streptomycin

Trade name: Generic (Pfizer)

Available formulations:
IV preparation 400 mg/ml, 2.5 ml ampule

Class: Aminoglycoside antibiotic

Mechanism of action: Binds to 30S ribosomal subunit, inhibiting protein synthesis

IM dose: Daily 15 mg/kg IM to maximum of 1 g, then 25 to 30 mg/kg IM two or three times weekly to maximum of 1.5 g

Storage and stability: Store ampules in the refrigerator

PHARMACOKINETICS

T_{max}: 1 hour

Half-life: 2.5 hours

CSF penetration: Negligible

Plasma protein binding: less than 10%

Metabolism/elimination: Eliminated primarily by glomerular filtration, with 80% to 95% of dose eliminated unchanged in urine

Breast milk: Small amounts excreted in breast milk

Dosage adjustment for organ failure: Requires adjustment in the presence of renal dysfunction. Significant removal by dialysis (25% to 50%)

Side effects: Nephrotoxicity, ototoxicity, edema, rash, paresthesias, fever, neuromuscular blockade

Pregnancy: Category D. Aminoglycosides can freely cross placenta. Its use has been associated with bilateral, irreversible deafness in neonates exposed to the drug in utero. Must weigh the benefit to the mother against the potential risks to the fetus

Pneumocystis carinii Pneumonia (PCP) and Toxoplasmosis Agents

Atovaquone

Trade name: Mepron (Glaxo Wellcome)

Available formulations: Suspension (750 mg/5 ml), 210 ml $637.09

Class: Antiprotozoal, anti-*Pneumocystis* agent

Mechanism of action: Inhibition of nuclear viral synthesis by inhibiting mitochondrial electron transport

Oral dose (adults):

For PCP treatment: 750 mg bid with food for 21 days

Prophylaxis: 1500 mg qd with food

For toxoplasmosis treatment: 1500 mg bid with food

Storage and stability: Store at room temperature; do not freeze

PHARMACOKINETICS

Bioavailability: 47%

Half-life: 67 to 78 hours

CSF penetration: Less than 1% of plasma concentration

Plasma protein binding: More than 99%

Metabolism/elimination: Little or no excretion in urine; enterohepatic recycling with elimination in feces

Food effects: Absorption enhanced twofold with food; administer with meals

Breast milk: Animal data suggest distribution into breast milk

Dosage adjustment for organ failure: Little or no excretion in urine

Side effects: Rash, nausea, diarrhea, headache, vomiting, fever, insomnia

Pregnancy: Category C

Clindamycin

Trade name: Cleocin (Pharmacia & Upjohn), Generic (various)

Available formulations:

150 mg capsules	$ 1.94
300 mg capsules	$ 3.88
600 mg/50 ml IV	$ 9.94
900 mg/50 ml IV	$ 12.75

Class: Antibacterial with activities against PCP and toxoplasmosis

Mechanism of action: Inhibits bacterial protein synthesis by attaching to the 50S subunit of bacterial ribosome

Dose:

PCP: 1200 to 1800 mg/day IV or PO in three or four divided doses together with primaquine × 14 to 21 days

Toxoplasmosis: 2400 to 4800 mg/day IV or PO in three or four divided doses together with pyrimethamine + leucovorin

Storage and stability:

Oral tablets: store at room temperature

Parenteral preparations: 150 mg/ml in 2, 4, and 6 ml vials

PHARMACOKINETICS

T_{max}: 45 minutes

Bioavailability: 90%

Half-life: 1.5 to 5.0 hours

CSF penetration: Poor, even in the presence of inflamed meninges

Plasma protein binding: 60% to 95%

Metabolism/elimination: Extensively metabolized to clindamycin sulfoxide and *N*-dimethyl clindamycin

Breast milk: Detectable in human breast milk after oral and intravenous doses

Dosage adjustment for organ failure: Adjustment recommended in patients with active liver disease. No adjustment necessary in patients with renal impairment or in those on hemodialysis or peritoneal dialysis

Side effects: Diarrhea, pseudomembranous colitis, rash, and ventricular arrhythmia reported after IV bolus of undiluted clindamycin solution

Pregnancy: Category B

Dapsone

Trade name: Generic (Jacobus)

Available formulations:
25 mg tablets $0.19
100 mg tablets $0.20

Class: Anti-Pneumocystis agent

Mechanism of action: Thought to interfere with folic acid synthesis by a mechanism similar to sulfonamides

Oral dose (adults): 50 to 100 mg qd

Storage and stability: Store in well closed containers at room temperature and protected from light

PHARMACOKINETICS

T_{max}**:** 2 to 8 hours

Bioavailability: Near-complete absorption from GI tract

Half-life: 10 to 50 hours

CSF penetration: Unknown

Plasma protein binding: 70% to 90%

Metabolism/elimination: Undergoes acetylation and hydroxylation in the liver (acetylation genetically determined); hydroxyalanine metabolite may be associated with hypersensitivity reactions

Food effects: Can be given without regard to meals

Breast milk: Excreted in high concentrations; avoid breastfeeding

Dosage adjustment for organ failure: None

Side effects: Fever, rash, anemia, pancytopenia, hepatitis, phototoxicity, gastrointestinal, peripheral neuropathy, G6PD deficiency-associated hemolysis, methemoglobinemia

Pregnancy: Category C

Pentamidine

Trade name: Pentam 300, NebuPent (Fujisawa); Generic (Abbott)

Available formulations:
Oral inhalation NebuPent 300 mg $98.75
Pentamidine isethionate 300 mg injection $98.75

Class: Antiprotozoal

Mechanism of action: Inhibition of protein and nucleic acid synthesis

Inhaled dose (adults): PCP prophylaxis 300 mg once a month (using Respirgard II nebulizer)

IM/IV dose: 3 to 4 mg/kg qd for 21 days; infuse IV over 1 to 2 hours

Storage and stability: Oral inhalation reconstituted with 6 ml sterile water; stable for 48 hours. IV preparation is reconstituted with sterile water and diluted with D5W 50 mg/250 ml; stable for 48 hours at room temperature. Protect from light

PHARMACOKINETICS

Half-life: 6.4 to 9.4 hours

CSF penetration: Minimal

Plasma protein binding: 69%

Metabolism/elimination: Extensive, prolonged uptake into tissues. Prolonged renal elimination over weeks appears to be the major route of elimination

Breast milk: Unknown

Dosage adjustment for organ failure: Half-life may be prolonged in patients with renal dysfunction

Side effects:

IV: hypotension and cardiac arrhythmia associated with rapid infusion

IM: sterile abscess or pain at injection site

IV or IM: nephrotoxicity, leukopenia, hypoglycemia, hyperglycemia, nausea, elevated LFTs, hypocalcemia, pancreatitis

Aerosol: fatigue, metallic taste, shortness of breath, dizziness, rash, cough, nausea, congestion, bronchospasm

Pregnancy: Category C

Primaquine Phosphate

Trade name: Generic (various)

Available formulations: 26 mg (15 mg base) tablet $0.81

Class: Antimalarial

Oral dose: PCP treatment: 15 to 30 mg base daily plus clindamycin 1200 to 3600 mg IV or PO per day × 14 to 21 days

Storage and stability: Store at room temperature

PHARMACOKINETICS

T_{max}**:** 1 to 2 hours

Bioavailability: 96%

Half-life: 4 to 7 hours

Metabolism/elimination: Extensively metabolized; 1% excreted renally

Breast milk: Unknown

Dosage adjustment for organ failure: No adjustment in renal failure. No recommendation for adjustment in hepatic failure, use with caution and monitor for toxicities.

Side effects: Acute hemolytic anemia in patients with G6PD deficiency, granulocytopenia, methemoglobinemia, abdominal pain, cramps

Pregnancy: Category C

Pyrimethamine

Trade name: Daraprim (GlaxoSmithKline)

Available formulations: 25 mg tablets $0.45

Class: Antitoxoplasmosis agent

Mechanism of action: Folic acid antagonist inhibition of dihydrofolate reductase

Oral dose (adults): Toxoplasmosis

Adults: 200 mg once, then 50 to 75 mg/day with sulfadiazine, then 25 to 50 mg/day

Children: 1 mg/kg/day divided into two doses, then 0.5 mg/kg/day

Note: Use with leucovorin 5 to 20 mg/day to reduce bone marrow suppression

Storage and stability: Store at room temperature in a dry place and protect from light

PHARMACOKINETICS

T_{max}: 2 to 6 hours

Bioavailability: Well absorbed

Half-life: 96 hours

CSF penetration: Unknown

Plasma protein binding: 87%

Metabolism/elimination: Metabolized hepatically to several metabolites, which are excreted in the urine

Food effects: Take with food or meals to minimize adverse GI effects

Breast milk: Approximately 5% of drug passed to infant in breast milk; discontinue nursing while on drug

Dosage adjustment for organ failure: Use with caution in the presence of hepatic disease

Side effects: Nausea and vomiting, anorexia, megaloblastic anemia, leukopenia, pancytopenia, skin rash

Pregnancy: Category C

Sulfadiazine

Trade name: Generic (various)

Available formulations: 500 mg tablets $1.02

Class: Antitoxoplasmosis agent

Mechanism of action: Interferes with the synthesis of tetrahydrofolic acid by altering PABA

Oral dose (adults):

Toxoplasmosis treatment: 1 to 1.5 g qid

Toxoplasmosis suppression: 0.5 to 0.75 g qid

Note: Use with pyrimethamine and leucovorin

Storage and stability: Store in well closed, light-resistant containers at room temperature

PHARMACOKINETICS

T_{max}: Within 4 hours

Bioavailability: More than 70%

Half-life: 7 to 17 hours

CSF penetration: 40% to 60% of serum levels

Plasma protein binding: 32% to 56% bound to plasma proteins

Metabolism/elimination: Partially metabolized in liver by acetylation; metabolites and 43% to 60% unaltered parent drug in urine

Food effects: Food may delay but does not decrease absorption

Breast milk: Distributed into breast milk

Dosage adjustment for organ failure: Use with caution in the presence of renal failure to avoid crystalluria; alkalinizing the urine may reduce the incidence

Side effects: Hypersensitivity reactions: fever, rash, marrow suppression, crystalluria

Pregnancy: Category C

Trimethoprim/Sulfamethoxazole (TMP/SMX)

Trade name: Bactrim (Roche); Septra (GlaxoSmithKline); Generics (various)

Available formulations:

Bactrim (SMX/TMP)	
400/80 mg tablet	$0.76
800/160 mg DS tablet	$1.25
Septra (SMX/TMP)	
400/80 mg tablet	$0.73
800/160 mg DS tablet	$1.21
Generic (SMX/TMP)	
400/80 mg tablet	$0.21
800/160 mg tablet	$0.38
Suspension (200 mg/40 mg/5 ml)	
100 ml	$9.05
150 ml	$12.94
200 ml	$17.26
480 ml	$42.82
IV (80 mg/ml and 16 mg/ml), 30 ml	$35.35

Class: Combination antibacterial, anti-*Pneumocystis* agent

Mechanism of action: Inhibition of sequential enzymes in pathway of folic acid synthesis

Oral dose (adults): PCP/Toxo prophylaxis: one DS tablet three times a week or qd

IV dose: PCP: 10 to 20 mg/kg/day (based on trimethoprim) divided into three or four doses given q6–8h; infuse over 60 to 90 minutes; once stabilized, can switch to equivalent oral dose to complete a 21-day course

Storage and stability:

Tablets/suspension: store in well closed, light-resistant containers at room temperature

IV: store vials at room temperature; admixtures with D5W stable for 2 to 6 hours depending on concentration

PHARMACOKINETICS

T_{max}: 1 to 4 hours; steady-state concentrations of TMP/SMX are approximately 1:20

Bioavailability: More than 90% for both agents

Half-life: TMP 8 to 11 hours; SMX 10 to 13 hours

CSF penetration: TMP 50% of plasma levels; SMX 40% of plasma levels

Plasma protein binding: TMP 44%; SMX 70%

Metabolism/elimination: 80% and 20% of TMP and SMX, respectively, are recovered unchanged in the urine. SMX metabolized by *N*-acetylation and conjugation

Food effects: Can be given without regard to meals

Breast milk: Both agents are distributed into breast milk

Dosage adjustment for organ failure: Recommended to reduce dose by 50% in patients with CrCl 15 to 30 m/min

Side effects: Nausea, vomiting, anorexia, rash, fever, hypersensitivity reactions, bone marrow suppression, headache, crystalluria. IV: thrombophlebitis

Pregnancy: Category C

Trimetrexate

Trade name: NeuTrexin (MedImmune)

Available formulations: 25 mg/5 ml IV vials $73.50

Class: Anti-pneumocystis agent

Mechanism of action: Inhibitor of dihydrofolate reductase

IV dose: 45 mg/m^2 qd over 60 to 90 minutes for 21 days, with PO or IV leucovorin 20 mg/m^2 q6h for 24 days or at least 72 hours after discontinuation of trimetrexate

Storage and stability: After reconstitution and dilution, stable for 24 hours. Store vials at room temperature and protect from light

PHARMACOKINETICS

Half-life: 11 to 16 hours

CSF penetration: CSF levels approximately 2% of plasma levels

Plasma protein binding: 80% to 98%

Metabolism/elimination: 10% to 30% excreted unchanged in urine; oxidative metabolism followed by conjugation to glucuronide or sulfate

Breast milk: Unknown; recommended to discontinue nursing while on drug

Dosage adjustment for organ failure: Modify dose based on hematologic parameters

Side effects: Neutropenia, anemia, thrombocytopenia, fever, rash, elevated LFTs, stomatitis

Pregnancy: Category D. Fetal harm may include skeletal, visceral, ocular, and cardiovascular abnormalities. One must weigh benefit of trimetrexate against potential harm to the fetus

Antifungals

Amphotericin B

Trade name: Fungizone (amphotericin B deoxycholate: Bristol-Myers Squibb); Abelcet (amphotericin B lipid complex: Liposome); Amphotec (amphotericin B colloidal dispersion: Sequus); AmBisome (liposomal amphotericin B: Fujisawa)

Available formulations:

Fungizone	50 mg/20 ml vial	$17.84
Abelcet	100 mg/20 ml vial	$200.00
Amphotec	50 mg/20 ml vial	$93.33
	100 mg/20 ml vial	$160.00
AmBisome	50 mg/vial	$188.40

Class: Polyene antifungal

Mechanism of action: Binds to sterols in fungal cell membrane leading to change in permeability

IV dose:

Fungizone: 0.25 to 1.5 mg/kg qd or qod by slow infusion over 2 to 6 hours. Test dose of 1 mg over 20 to 30 minutes may be given

Abelcet: 5 mg/kg/d at rate of 2.5 mg/kg/hr

Amphotec: 3 to 6 mg/kg/d over 2 hours

AmBisome: 3 to 5 mg/kg/d over 1 to 2 hours

PHARMACOKINETICS

Half-life: Terminal elimination half-life of 15 days

CSF penetration: Less than 2.5% of those in plasma

Plasma protein binding: More than 90%

Metabolism/elimination: Slow excretion by the kidneys over weeks to months; metabolism poorly understood. Extensive uptake by various tissues/organs including liver, spleen

Breast milk: Unknown

Dosage adjustment for organ failure: Dosage adjustment in the presence of renal failure suggested by decreasing dose or extending frequency

Side effects: Nephrotoxcity, infusion-related side effects (chills, rigors, fever, hypotension), electrolyte abnormailities, nausea, vomiting, muscle and joint pain, elevated LFTs, anemia

Pregnancy: Category B

Caspofungin Acetate

Trade name: Cancidas (Merck)

Available formulations:

70 mg vials	$463.75
50 mg vials	$360.00

Class: echinocandin antifungal

Mechanism of action: Inhibition of the synthese of β (1,3)D-glucan, which is an integral component of fungal cell wall synthesis

Spectrum of Antifungal Activities: *Aspergillus* spp., *Candida* spp.

Dosage for Invasive Aspergillosis:

Loading dose: 70 mg IV

Maintenance dose: 50 mg IV every 24 hour

Storage and stability: Store at room temperature—oral solution may be refrigerated, do not freeze

PHARMACOKINETICS

Half-lives: β-phase: 9 to 11 hours; γ-phase: 40 to 50 hours

Plasma protein binding: Approximately 97% bound to albumin

Metabolism/elimination: metabolized by hydrolysis and *N*-acetylation

Dosage adjustment in organ failure:

In moderate hepatic insufficiency (Child-Pugh score 7–9): maintenance dose at 35 mg every 24 hours

In severe hepatic insufficiency (Child-Pugh score >9): no experience

No dosage adjustment is necessary in patients with renal insufficiency; hemodialysis does not appreciably remove caspofungin acetate

Side effects: Histamine-related reactions such as skin rash, facial swelling, or pruritus. One case of anaphylaxis was reported in clinical trials. Other adverse effects: thrombophlebitis, nausea, vomiting, headache, flushing.

Pregnancy: Category C

Clotrimazole

Trade name: Mycelex (Bayer)

Available formulations: 10 mg troche $1.25

Class: Azole antifungal agent

Mechanism of action: Alters cell membrane permeability by binding with phospholipids

Oral dose (adults): One troche five times a day; dissolve slowly in the mouth

Storage and stability: Store at room temperature; avoid freezing

PHARMACOKINETICS

T_{max}: Clotrimazole present in saliva for 3 hours after dissolving troche

Bioavailability: Minimal absorption systemically

Breast milk: Minimal absorption suggests clotrimazole not present in significant amounts in breast milk

Dosage adjustment for organ failure: None

Side effects: Nausea, vomiting, unpleasant mouth sensations, pruritus, elevated LFTs

Pregnancy: Category C

Fluconazole

Trade name: Diflucan (Pfizer)

Available formulations:

50 mg tablets	$4.75
100 mg tablets	$7.47
150 mg tablets	$11.89
200 mg tablets	$12.22
50 mg/5 ml oral suspension, 35 ml	$30.54
200 mg/5 ml oral suspension, 35 ml	$110.95
(2 mg/ml) IV preparation, 100 ml	$88.27

Class: Triazole antifungal agent

Mechanism of action: Inhibits ergosterol production, necessary for synthesis of cell membrane

Oral dose

Adults: 50 to 400 mg qd

Children: 3 to 12 mg/kg/d

IV dose: Same as oral dose. Administered by IV infusion at a rate not exceeding 200 mg/hr

Storage and stability:

Tablets: tight container below 30°C

IV: reconstituted suspension is stable for 14 days at room temperature. IV products stored at room temperature. Protect from freezing

PHARMACOKINETICS

T_{max}: 1 to 2 hours

Bioavailability: More than 90%

Half-life: 32 to 40 hours for HIV-infected patients

CSF penetration: 50% to 94% of plasma concentrations

Plasma protein binding: 11% to 12%

Metabolism/elimination: Primarily renally excreted; 80% of dose excreted unchanged; inhibitor of CYP3A4-mediated metabolism

Food effects: Pharmacokinetics unaffected by food

Breast milk: Excreted in breast milk at concentrations similar to plasma; should be avoided in nursing mothers

Dosage adjustment for organ failure:

ClCr (ml/m)	Dose
< 50	50% of dose
Dialysis	Full dose after dialysis

Side effects: Nausea, headache, rash, vomiting, abdominal pain, diarrhea, elevated LFTs

Pregnancy: Category C. Craniofacial, cardiac, and limb defects reported in four infants born to mothers exposed to fluconazole during the first trimester of pregnancy

Flucytosine

Trade name: Ancobon (Roche)

Available formulations:

250 mg capsules	$3.51
500 mg capsules	$6.98

Class: Fluorinated pyrimidine antifungal

Mechanism of action: Deaminated to fluorouracil by cytosine deaminase; fluorouracil is an antimetabolite that interferes with RNA and protein synthesis

Oral dose (adults): 100 to 200 mg/kg/d divided into four doses

Storage and stability: Store in tight, light-resistant container at room temperature

PHARMACOKINETICS

T_{max}: 2 to 6 hours

Bioavailability: 75% to 90%

Half-life: 2.5 to 6.0 hours

CSF penetration: 60% to 100% of serum concentration

Plasma protein binding: 2% to 4%

Metabolism/elimination: 75% to 90% of dose excreted unchanged in urine

Food effects: Food affects the rate but not the extent of absorption

Breast milk: Unknown

Dosage adjustment for organ failure:

Renal impairment: requires dosage adjustment, maintain peak serum levels (2 hours after oral dose) at less than 100 μg/ml

Hemodialysis: 20 to 50 mg/kg immediately after dialysis, q48–72h

Side effects: Nausea, vomiting, diarrhea, bone marrow suppression, elevated LFTs, elevated serum creatinine

Pregnancy: Category C

Itraconazole

Trade name: Sporanox (Janssen)

Available formulations:

100 mg capsules	$7.07

10 mg/ml oral solution, 150 ml	$111.13
10 mg/ml IV preparation, 250 mg ampule	$176.23

Note: Capsules and solution are not interchangeable

Class: Triazole antifungal agent

Mechanism of action: Inhibits ergosterol production, necessary for synthesis of cell membrane

Oral dose (adults): 100 to 400 mg qd

Intravenous dose (adults): 200 to 400 mg qd

Storage and stability: Store at room temperature; protect from light and moisture; do not freeze solution

PHARMACOKINETICS

T_{max}: 3 to 5 hours (capsules)

Bioavailability: 55% (capsules)

Half-life: 21 hours

CSF penetration: Negligible

Plasma protein binding: 99.8%

Metabolism/elimination: Extensive hepatic metabolism to multiple metabolites including major metabolite (hydroxyitraconazole). Less than 1% of dose excreted renally. Inhibits CYP3A4-mediated metabolism

Food effects: Capsules require administration with food or cola beverage; suspension administered on empty stomach

Breast milk: Excreted into breast milk; should be avoided in nursing mothers

Dosage adjustment for organ failure: No change required in presence of renal dysfunction; use with caution in presence of hepatic disease

Side effects: Nausea, vomiting, diarrhea, dyspepsia, flatulence, rash, headache, dizziness, elevated in LFTs

Pregnancy: Category C

Ketoconazole

Trade name: Nizoral (Janssen)

Available formulations: 200 mg tablets $3.51

Class: Imidazole antifungal

Mechanism of action: Impairs synthesis of ergosterol, leading to increased permeability of fungal cell membrane

Oral dose:

Adults: 200 to 400 mg qd

Children: 3.3 to 6.6 mg/kg/d qd

Storage and stability: Protect from moisture; store in well closed containers

PHARMACOKINETICS

T_{max}: 1 to 2 hours

Bioavailability: Requires acidic pH for optimal absorption

Half-life: 8 hours

CSF penetration: Minimal

Plasma protein binding: 99%

Metabolism/elimination: Metabolized extensively in liver; 85% to 90% excreted in bile and feces. Inhibits CYP3A4-mediated metabolism

Food effects: Can be taken with food to minimize GI upset

Breast milk: Likely excretion into breast milk; should be avoided

Dosage adjustment for organ failure: Careful monitoring of LFTs required in patients with history of liver disease; not altered in renal failure; not dialyzable

Side effects: Nausea, vomiting, abdominal pain, decrease in testosterone, hepatotoxicity, elevated LFTs, adrenal insufficiency with high doses

Pregnancy: Category C

Nystatin

Trade names: Mycostatin (Apothecon); Nilstat (Lederle); Nystex (Savage); Generics (various)

Available formulations:

100,000 U/ml oral suspension

60 ml	$20.96
480 ml	$129.54
500,000 U tablets	$0.53
200,000 U troche	$1.01

Class: Polyene antifungal

Mechanism of action: Binds to sterols in cell membrane, resulting in changes in membrane permeability

Oral dose:

Adults: 400,000 to 600,000 U qid

Infants: 100,000 U qid

Storage and stability: Store at room temperature

PHARMACOKINETICS

Bioavailability: Negligible absorption

Metabolism/elimination: Eliminated unchanged in stool

Food effects: Topical agent, not affected by food

Breast milk: Not systemically absorbed

Dosage adjustment for organ failure: None

Side effects: Nausea and vomiting, diarrhea, oral irritation or sensitization, taste perversion

Pregnancy: Category C

Anti-Cytomegalovirus, Anti-Herpes Simplex Virus, and Anti-Varicella-Zoster Virus Agents

Acyclovir

Trade name: Zovirax (GlaxoSmithKline); Generic (various)

Available formulations:

200 mg capsules	$1.31
400 mg tablets	$2.54
800 mg tablets	$4.93
200 mg/5 ml oral suspension, 473 ml	$112.57
500 mg IV preparation	$60.10
1 g IV preparation	$120.21
5% ointment	
3 g	$20.69
15 g	$47.80

Class: Purine nucleoside analogue antiviral

Mechanism of action: Converted intracellularly to triphosphate metabolite, which interferes with DNA polymerase and inhibits viral DNA synthesis; active against HSV and VZV

Oral dose:

Adults:

HSV infections: 200 mg 5 times per day or 400 mg tid or 800 mg bid

Herpes zoster infections: 800 mg 5 times per day

Children: chickenpox 20 mg/kg per dose qid × 5 days

IV dose (zoster): Administer over 1 hour, 10 mg/kg q8h

IV dose (HSV): Administer over 1 hour, 5 mg/kg q8h

Storage and stability: Store in tight, light-resistant containers at room temperature. Reconstitute with sterile water. Dilute with IV solution to concentrations of 7 mg/ml or lower. Use reconstituted solution within 12 hours; after dilution, use within 24 hours

PHARMACOKINETICS

T_{max}: 1.5 to 2.5 hours

Bioavailability: 15% to 30%

Half-life: 2.1 to 3.5 hours

CSF penetration: 50% of serum concentration

Plasma protein binding: 9% to 33%

Metabolism/elimination: Excreted primarily in urine; 30% to 90% of dose recovered in urine

Food effects: Absorption is unaffected by food; give without regard to meals

Breast milk: Distribution into breast milk in concentrations similar to maternal plasma concentration

Dosage adjustment for organ failure: Adjust in the presence of renal dysfunction

Regimen	CrCl (ml/min/1.73 m²)	Adjusted Dose
200 mg PO q4h	< 10	200 mg q12h
400 mg PO q12h	< 10	200 mg q12h
800 mg PO q4h	10–25	800 mg q8h
	0–10	800 mg q12h
5–10 mg/kg	25–50	5–10 mg/kg q12h
IV q8h	10–25	5–10 mg/kg q24h
	0–10	2.5–5.0 mg/kg q24h

Side effects:

IV: phlebitis irritation at site, nausea and vomiting, itching, CNS changes, crystalluria, and renal failure associated with rapid IV infusion.

Oral: nausea and vomiting, diarrhea, headache, dizziness, rash, asthenia

Pregnancy: Category C

Cidofovir

Trade name: Vistide (Gilead)

Available formulations: IV: 75 mg/ml, 5 ml amp $762.00

Class: Antiviral

Mechanism of action: Converted to cidofovir diphosphate, which inhibits CMV DNA polymerase

IV dose (adults):

Induction: 5 mg/kg IV over 1 hour per week for 2 consecutive weeks

Maintenance: 5 mg/kg IV over 1 hour every other week

Note: Must be administered with probenecid: 2 g 3 hours prior to dose, then 1 g 2 and 8 hours after completion of the infusion (4 g total)

Hydration: Normal saline 1 L immediately before each infusion; if tolerated, another liter of normal saline is recommended during or immediately after cidofovir infusion

Storage and stability: Store vials at room temperature. Admixture in 100 ml normal saline stable in refrigerator for 24 hours

PHARMACOKINETICS

Half-life: 2.6 hours (intracellular half-life of metabolite 24 to 65 hours)

CSF penetration: Undetectable concentrations in CSF in limited number of patients

Plasma protein binding: Less than 6%

Metabolism/elimination: Eliminated primarily by renal excretion

Food effects: Food may decrease nausea and vomiting associated with probenecid

Breast milk: Unknown

Dosage adjustment for organ failure:
Reduce from 5 mg/kg to 3 mg/kg for an increase in creatinine of 0.3 to 0.4 mg/dl above baseline. Discontinue for an increase in creatinine of 0.5 mg/dl or more above baseline or development of 3+ proteinuria. Not recommended for patients with baseline serum creatinine higher than 1.5 mg/dl, CrCl 55 ml/min or less, or 2+ proteinuria or more

Side effects: Nephrotoxicity, proteinuria, neutropenia, nausea and vomiting, diarrhea, hypotony, abdominal pain, rash, fever, anemia, headache

Pregnancy: Category C

Famciclovir

Trade name: Famvir (SmithKline Beecham)

Available formulations:

125 mg tablets $ 3.38
250 mg tablets $ 3.68
500 mg tablets $ 7.38

Class: Antiviral

Mechanism of action: Prodrug of penciclovir, hydrolyzed in vivo to penciclovir and phosphorylated to penciclovir triphosphate, which inhibits viral DNA synthesis

Oral dose (adult):

Herpes zoster: 500 mg q8h × 7 days

Recurrent genital herpes: 250 to 500 mg bid × 7 days

HSV suppression: 250 mg bid

Storage and stability: Store at room temperature

PHARMACOKINETICS

T_{max}: 0.7 to 0.9 hour; rapid conversion to penciclovir

Bioavailability: 75%

Half-life: 2 to 3 hours (penciclovir)

CSF penetration: Unknown

Plasma protein binding: Less than 20%

Metabolism/elimination: Rapid conversion to penciclovir and 6-deoxypenciclovir; 73% of penciclovir excreted through the kidneys

Food effects: Food does not affect absorption; give without regard to meals

Breast milk: It is not known if famciclovir or penciclovir is distributed into milk in humans

Dosage adjustment for organ failure: Adjust for renal dysfunction

Dialysis: administer recommended dose after dialysis session

CrCl (ml/min)	Zoster Dose	Genital Herpes Dose
40–59	500 mg q12h	250–500 mg q12h
20–39	500 mg q24h	250–500 mg q24h
< 20	250 mg q24h	125–250 mg q24h

Side effects: Nausea, headache, vomiting, diarrhea, pruritus

Pregnancy: Category B

Fomivirsen

Trade name: Vitravene (Abbott)

Available formulations: 6.6 mg/ml, 2.5 ml vial $1000

Class: Antisense oligonucleotide against CMV

Mechanism of action: Phosphorothioate oligonucleotide, inhibits CMV through antisense mechanism

Intravitreal dose:

Induction: 300 μg/0.05 ml to affected eye each week × 2 weeks

Maintenance: 0.05 ml every 4 weeks

Storage and stability: Store at 35° to 77°F. Protect from heat and light

Pharmacokinetics: Human intraocular pharmacokinetic studies currently underway

Breast milk: Not known if fomvirisen is distributed to milk in humans

Dosage adjustment for organ failure: None

Side effects: Ocular inflammation, uveitis, iritis, vitreitis, increase intraocular pressure (usually transient), abnormal or blurry vision

Pregnancy: Category C

Foscarnet

Trade name: Foscavir (Astra)

Available formulations:

IV: 24 mg/ml, 250 ml $73.28
IV: 24 mg/ml, 500 ml $145.93

Class: Pyrophosphate analogue antiviral

Mechanism of action: Inhibition of viral DNA polymerase (does not require activation by kinases)

IV dose:

CMV induction: 90 mg/kg q12h (1.5 to 2.0 hours infusion) × 2 to 3 weeks *or* 60 mg/kg q8h (1 hour or longer infusion) × 2 to 3 weeks

CMV maintenance: 90 to 120 mg/kg/d over 2 hours

Storage and stability: Store 24 mg/ml solution at room temperature; do not freeze. In normal saline diluted to 12 mg/ml, stable for 30 days at 5°C

PHARMACOKINETICS

Half-life: 3 to 4 hours

CSF penetration: Approximately 70% of plasma concentrations

Plasma protein binding: 14% to 17%

Metabolism/elimination: 80% to 90% excreted unchanged in the urine; eliminated by both tubular secretion and glomerular filtration

Breast milk: Animal data suggest foscarnet is secreted in breast milk at concentrations higher than those in plasma

Dosage adjustment for organ failure:

CrCl (ml/min/kg)	Induction	Maintenance
> 1.4	60 mg q8h to 90 mg q12h	90 mg q24h to 120 mg q24h
> 1.0–1.4	45 mg q8h to 70 mg q12h	70 mg q24h to 90 mg q24h
> 0.08–1.00	50 mg q12h to 50 mg q12h	50 mg q24h to 65 mg q24h
> 0.6–0.8	40 mg q12h to 80 mg q24h	80 mg q48h to 105 mg q48h
> 0.5–0.6	60 mg q24h to 60 mg q24h	60 mg q48h to 80 mg q48h
> 0.4–0.5	50 mg q24h to 50 mg q24h	50 mg q48h to 65 mg q48h
< 0.4	Not recorded Not recorded	Not recorded Not recorded

Side effects: Nephrotoxicity, mineral and electrolyte disorders (hypocalcemia, hypophosphatemia, hypomagnesemia, hypokalemia), seizures, granulocytopenia, anemia, nausea, vomiting, headache, penile ulceration, thrombophlebitis (if peripheral IV used). Nephrotoxicity may be reduced with hydration (750 to 1000 ml), penile ulceration

Pregnancy: Category C

Ganciclovir

Trade name: Cytovene (Roche); Vitrasert (Chiron Vision)

Available formulations:

250 mg capsules	$4.00
500 mg capsules	$8.00
500 mg/10 ml IV vial	$35.67
4.5 mg ocular insert	$5000.00

Class: Guanine derivative nucleoside antiviral

Mechanism of action: Phosphorylated to triphosphate metabolite, which inhibits viral DNA synthesis

Oral dose (adults): 1 g tid with food (as maintenance therapy)

IV dose:

Induction: 5 mg/kg q12h × 14 to 21 days

Maintenance: 5 mg/kg qd or 6 mg/kg qd × 5 days a week

Note: Give IV infusions over 1 hour

Storage and stability: Store capsules and IV vials at room temperature. Reconstitute IV vial with sterile water; stable at room temperature for 12 hours. After dilution with normal saline or D5W, refrigerate solution and use within 24 hours

PHARMACOKINETICS

T_{max}: Capsules: 3 hours with food

Bioavailability: Capsules approximately 5% to 9%

Half-life: 2.5 to 4.8 hours; longer with oral dosing

CSF penetration: 24% to 70% of serum concentrations

Plasma protein binding: 1% to 2%

Metabolism/elimination: Eliminated primarily by renal excretion with more than 90% of dose recovered in the urine unmetabolized

Food effects: AUC increased by 22% with food; T_{max} and C_{max} increased

Breast milk: Unknown

Dosage adjustment for organ failure: Induction

CrCl (ml/min)	(mg/kg)	Capsules
50–69	2.50 q12h	1500 mg qd or 500 mg tid
25–49	2.50 q24h	1000 mg qd or 500 mg bid
10–24	1.25 q24h	500 mg qd
<10	1.25 3×/ week	500 mg 3× per week after dialysis

Side effects: Neutropenia, thrombocytopenia, anemia, CNS disturbances (headache, confusion, seizures), phlebitis. *Ocular insert*: retinal detachment, transient loss in visual acuity, vitreous hemorrhage, uveitis, cataracts, macular abnormalities

Pregnancy: Category C

Valacyclovir

Trade name: Valtrex (GlaxoSmithKline)

Available formulations:

500 mg tablets	$3.38
1 g tablets	$4.36

Class: Antiviral

Mechanism of action: Prodrug of acyclovir; rapidly absorbed and converted to acyclovir by first-pass metabolism. Produces concentrations three- to fivefold higher than similar acyclovir doses. Acyclovir inhibits viral DNA synthesis (see Acyclovir).

Oral dose (adults):

Herpes zoster: 1 g tid × 7 days
Recurrent genital herpes: 500 mg bid × 5 days

Storage and stability: Store at room temperature

PHARMACOKINETICS

T_{max}**:** Rapid conversion to acyclovir by first-pass metabolism; valacyclovir undetectable at 3 hours

Bioavailability: 54%

Half-life: 2.1 to 3.5 hours (acyclovir)

CSF penetration: 50% of serum concentration (acyclovir)

Plasma protein binding: 13.5% to 17.9%

Metabolism/elimination: Rapid conversion to acyclovir; valcyclovir levels not detectable by 3 hours. Acyclovir primarily excreted in urine; 30% to 90% of dose recovered in urine

Food effects: Food does not affect absorption; give without regard to meals

Breast milk: Acyclovir is distributed to breast milk in concentrations similar to those in maternal plasma

Dosage adjustment for organ failure: Adjust for renal dysfunction:

CrCl (ml/min)	Zoster	Genital Herpes
30–49	1 g q12h	500 mg q12h
10–29	1 g q24h	500 mg q24h
<10	500 mg q24h	500 mg q24h
Dialysis: administer recommended dose after dialysis session		

Side effects: Nausea, headache, vomiting, diarrhea, constipation, dizziness. Thrombotic thrombocytopenic purpura with hemolytic-uremic syndrome has been reported with doses of 8 g/day in immunocompromised patients, including advanced HIV patients

Pregnancy: Category B

Valganciclovir HCl

Trade name: Valcyte (Roche)

Available formulation:

450 mg tablet

Class: Antiviral Agent

Mechanism of action: L-valyl ester (prodrug) of ganciclovir. After oral administration, valganciclovir is rapidly converted to ganciclovir. Ganciclovir is converted to ganciclovir triphosphate intracellularly which produces its virustatic effect by inhibition of viral DNA synthesis.

Oral dose (adult dose in patients with normal renal function):

Induction therapy for CMV retinitis: 900 mg BID × 21 days with food

Maintenance therapy for CMV retinitis: 900 mg QD with food

Storage and stability: Room temperature

PHARMACOKINETICS

T_{max}**:** 1 to 3 hours (as ganciclovir)

Bioavailability: 60% (as ganciclovir)

Half-life: 4 hours

Plasma protein binding: 1–2% (for ganciclovir)

Metabolism/elimination: Valganciclovir is rapidly hydrolyzed to ganciclovir. Major route of elimination is through renal excretion

Food effects: High fat meal increases oral bioavailability of ganciclovir by 30%

Breast milk: No information available; because of the potential serious adverse events in infants, mothers should be instructed not to breastfeed if they are receiving valganciclovir tablet.

Dosage adjustment in organ failure:

CrCl (mL/min)	Induction Dose*	Maintenance Dose*
≥ 60	900 mg BID	900 mg QD
40–59	450 mg BID	450 mg QD
25–39	450 mg QD	450 mg QOD
10–24	450 mg QOD	450 mg TIW
≤ 10	Ganciclovir should be used instead of valganciclovir	

*Each dose should be given with food

Hemodialysis patients: Ganciclovir concentration is reduced by 50% after hemodialysis. Valganciclovir is not recommended as the daily dose is lower than 450 mg.

Side effects: Anemia, neutropenia, diarrhea, nausea, vomiting, abdominal pain, fever, headache, insomnia, sedation, seizure, confusion, retinal detachment

Pregnancy: Category C, teratogenic in animals. Valganciclovir is not recommended during pregnancy.

Biologicals

Erythropoietin

Trade name: Epogen (Amgen); Procrit (Ortho Biotech)

Available formulations:

2000 U/ml vial	$25
3000 U/ml vial	$37
4000 U/ml vial	$50
10000 U/ml vial	$125
40000 U/ml vial	$534.15

Class: Synthetic biological hematopoietic growth factor

Mechanism of action: Stimulation of erythropoiesis

SC/IV dose (adults): 50 to 100 units/kg/dose three times weekly with titration to response or 40000 units once weekly

Storage and stability: Store under refrigeration; do not freeze or shake

PHARMACOKINETICS

T_{max}: SC: 5 to 24 hours

Bioavailability: SC: 22% to 31% compared to IV, although serum levels persist after SC administration for 3 to 4 days

Half-life: *IV*: 4 to 13 hours in patients with renal failure; *SC*: approximately 28 hours

CSF penetration: Unknown

Metabolism/elimination: Metabolism and degradation not well defined; only small amounts recovered in urine

Breast milk: Not established

Dosage adjustment for organ failure: None; dosing guidelines established in renal failure patients. Continuous ambulatory peritoneal dialysis (CAPD): only 1% to 3% of dose removed in 24 hours

Side effects: Hypertension, iron deficiency, venous fistula clotting, polycythemia, nausea, arthralgias, seizures, increased risk of thrombosis

Pregnancy: C

Filgrastim

Trade name: Neupogen (Amgen)

Available formulations: 300 μg/ml vial, 1 ml $180.40
480 μg/ml vial $315.10

Class: Recombinant hematopoietic growth factor

Mechanism of action: Promotion of proliferation and maturation of neutrophil precursors

IV/SC dose (adults): Initiate at 5 μg/kg/d and titrate to response. For IV administration, give as a short infusion (15 to 30 minutes)

Storage and stability: Store under refrigeration, use within 24 hours of preparation. Do not freeze or shake. Discard if left at room temperature for more than 6 hours.

PHARMACOKINETICS

T_{max}: SC dosing 2 to 6 hours

Bioavailability: SC: approximately 70%

Half-life: 1.5 to 7.0 hours

Metabolism/elimination: Not well established, although neutrophil endocytosis and degradation is thought to be involved

Breast milk: Not established

Dosage adjustment for organ failure: None

Side effects: Bone pain, nausea, elevated LFTs, increased uric acid

Pregnancy: Category C

Growth Hormone

Trade name: Serostim (Serono)

Available formulations: 6 mg vial $252

Class: Recombinant human growth hormone

Mechanism of action: Anabolic and anticatabolic agent that binds to receptors on various cells and interacts with other human hormones

SC dose (adults):

> 55 kg	6 mg qd
45–55 kg	5 mg qd
35–45 kg	4 mg qd
> 35 kg	0.1 mg/kg qd

Storage and stability: Store at room temperature. After reconstituting with sterile water, store under refrigeration and use within 24 hours

PHARMACOKINETICS

Bioavailability: 70% to 90%

Half-life: Approximately 4 hours

CSF penetration: Unknown

Metabolism/elimination: Glomerular filtration and enzymatic cleavage by renal cells; liver may also play a role in metabolism

Breast milk: Not determined

Dosage adjustment for organ failure: Not established

Side effects: Musculoskeletal discomfort, tissue swelling, arthralgias, myalgias, nausea, elevated LFTs, pancreatitis

Pregnancy: Category B

Interferon-α

Trade name: Roferon A (Roche), Intron A (Schering-Plough)

Available formulations: Various: 3 million to 50 million units/vial Approximately $35/3 million units

Class: Recombinant antitumor, antiviral, and immunomodulatory cytokine

Mechanism of action: Various intracellular mechanisms including induction of specific enzymes, suppression of cell proliferation, augmentation of cytotoxicity and phagocytosis, and inhibition of viral replication

Dose (adults): Kaposi sarcoma: 30 MIU/m^2 tiw IM or SC. Reduce dosage based on adverse effects

For Hepatitis B infection: 10 MIU tiw IM or SC or 5 MIU/day IM or SC × 24 to 48 weeks

For Hepatitis C infection: 3 MIU tiw IM or SC × 16 weeks

Storage and stability: Store both powder and reconstituted solution under refrigeration

PHARMACOKINETICS

T_{max}: 3 to 12 hours

Bioavailability: 80%

Half-life: 3.7 to 8.5 hours

Metabolism/elimination: Primarily metabolized by enzymes in the kidney

Breast milk: Animal studies suggest excretion into human milk

Dosage adjustment for organ failure: Use caution in patients with liver disease

Side effects: Flu-like symptoms, nausea, diarrhea, bone marrow suppression, elevated LFTs, depression, abnormal thyroid function

Pregnancy: Category C

Pegylated interferon alfa-2b

Trade name: PEG-Intron (Schering)

Available formulations:

100 μg/mL	$250.30
160 μg/mL	$262.62
240 μg/mL	$276.37
300 μg/mL	$290.19

Class: Immunomodulatory cytokine, antiviral

Mechanism of action: not yet established

Dosages (adult):

37–45 kg	40 μg subcutaneously once a week
46–56 kg	50 μg subcutaneously once a week
57–72 kg	64 μg subcutaneously once a week
73–88 kg	80 μg subcutaneously once a week
89–106 kg	96 μg subcutaneously once a week
107–136 kg	120 μg subcutaneously once a week
137–150 kg	150 μg subcutaneously once a week

Storage and stability: PEG-Intron powder should be stored at room temperature. After reconstitution, the solution should be used immediately or may be kept in the refrigerator at 2–8°C for up to 24 hours.

PHARMACOKINETICS

T_{max}: 15–44 hours

Half-life: 40 hours after multiple dosing

Metabolism/elimination: 30% renally eliminated

Breast milk excretion: not known

Dosage adjustment in organ failure: Use with caution in patients with creatinine clearance < 50 ml/min.

Side effects: Flu-like syndrome, injection site reactions, nausea, anorexia, neuropsychiatric toxicities (depression, insomnia, suicidal ideation, aggressive behavior), neutropenia, thrombocytopenia, pancreatitis, exacerbation of autoimmune disorders, hypothyroidism

Pregnancy: Category C

Interleukin-2 (Aldesleukin)

Trade name: Proleukin (Chiron)

Available formulations: 22 million unit vial $645

Class: Recombinant cytokine

Mechanism of action: Various effects on the immune system including T-lymphocyte proliferation, increased natural killer (NK) cell function, and increased interferon-γ production

SC dose (adults): Investigational for HIV infection: up to 15 IU/day SC given twice daily for 5 days every 8 weeks

Storage and stability: After reconstitution with sterile water, stable for 24 hours in refrigerator

PHARMACOKINETICS

T_{max}: SC: 2 to 4 hours

Bioavailability: SC: approximately 65%

Half-life: 1 to 3 hours

Metabolism/elimination: Primarily metabolized by enzymes in the renal tubules

Breast milk: Unknown

Dosage adjustment for organ failure: Not established

Side effects: Flu-like syndrome, rash, fever, renal and hepatic dysfunction, nausea and vomiting, myalgias, congestion, phlebitis (IV), hypothyroidism, CNS abnormalities (insomnia, headache, depression), vascular leak syndrome

Pregnancy: Category C. Animal reproduction studies have not been performed. Use during pregnancy only when benefit clearly outweighs risk

Miscellaneous

Albendazole

Trade name: Albenza (GlaxoSmithKline)
Available formulations: 200 mg tablets $1.10
Class: Anthelmintic
Mechanism of action: Inhibition of tubulin polymerization resulting in loss of cytoplasmic microtubules
Oral dose (adult):
$>$ 60 kg: 400 mg bid
$<$ 60 kg: 15 mg/kg/d divided bid
Storage and stability: Store at room temperature

PHARMACOKINETICS

T_{max}: 2 to 5 hours
Bioavailability: Unknown
Half-life: 8 to 12 hours (sulfoxide)
CSF penetration: 20% to 50% of plasma
Plasma protein binding: 70%
Metabolism/elimination: Hepatic metabolism to the sulfoxide metabolite, then undergoes further metabolism to the sulfone and other metabolites; primarily excreted in bile
Food effects: Administration with a high-fat meal results in fivefold or higher concentrations
Breast milk: Excreted into milk in animal studies
Dosage adjustment for organ failure: Closely monitor patients with hepatic disease
Side effects: Elevated LFTs, abdominal pain, nausea, vomiting, headache, leukopenia (monitor white blood cells)
Pregnancy: Category C

Dronabinol

Trade name: Marinol (Roxane)
Available formulations:

2.5 mg capsules	$3.19
5 mg capsules	$6.32
10 mg capsules	$13.13

Class: Cannabinoid antiemetic
Mechanism of action: CNS active agent with multiple effects including central sympathomimetic activity
Oral dose (adult):
Antiemetic: 5 mg/m^2 1 to 3 hours before chemotherapy, then q2-4h for 4 to 6 doses/day
Appetite stimulation: 2.5 to 5.0 mg bid before meals
Storage and stability: Store in well sealed containers in cool place

PHARMACOKINETICS

T_{max}: 2 to 4 hours
Bioavailability: Poor and erratic GI absorption; 90% to 95% absorbed but only 10% to 20% reaches systemic circulation due to first-pass metabolism
Half-life: 25 to 36 hours
CSF penetration: Large volume of distribution, high lipid solubility, and CNS effects suggest extensive uptake into brain
Plasma protein binding: 97% to 99%
Metabolism/elimination: Extensive first-pass liver metabolism yielding multiple metabolites; major active metabolite (11-OH-Δ-9-THC) found in equal concentrations in plasma as parent drug. Primarily excreted in bile
Food effects: Can be given without regard to meals
Breast milk: Excreted in breast milk; nursing not recommended
Dosage adjustment for organ failure: No adjustment for renal failure
Side effects: Sedation, tachycardia, mood changes, hallucinations, depersonalization
Pregnancy: Category C

Megestrol

Trade name: Megace (Bristol-Myers Squibb)
Available formulations:

20 mg tablets	$0.76
40 mg tablets	$1.35
40 mg/ml oral suspension, (237 ml)	$144.10

Class: Synthetic progestin
Mechanism of action (cachexia): Thought to act as appetite stimulant and to alter metabolism by interfering with mediators of cachexia
Oral dose (adult): 800 mg once daily

Storage and stability: Store in well closed containers at room temperature; protect from heat

PHARMACOKINETICS

T_{max}**:** 3 to 5 hours

Bioavailability: Well absorbed from GI tract but bioavailability unknown

Half-life: 30 hours

CSF penetration: Unknown

Metabolism/elimination: Undergoes hepatic metabolism to free steroids and glucuronidated conjugates. Primarily excreted by kidneys (65%)

Food effects: Unknown

Breast milk: Nursing mothers should discontinue megestrol therapy due to potential harm to infants

Dosage adjustment for organ failure: No data available

Side effects: Gastrointestinal effects (10%), decreased libido, impotence (5%), rash (6%), CNS-related effects (insomnia, headache, confusion), breakthrough bleeding, adrenal insufficiency

Pregnancy: Category X. Contraindicated during pregnancy

Paromomycin

Trade name: Humatin (Monarch)

Available formulations: 250 mg capsules $2.68

Class: Aminoglycoside antibiotic

Mechanism of action: Not significantly absorbed; acts directly on intestinal lumen; binds to 30S ribosomal subunit inhibiting bacterial protein synthesis

Oral dose (adult):

Intestinal amebiasis: 25 to 35 mg/kg/d in three divided doses × 5 to 10 days

Cryptosporidium: some success reported with 500 mg qid × 4 weeks

Storage and stability: Store in airtight containers

PHARMACOKINETICS

Bioavailability: Minimal or negligible absorption from GI tract; approximately 100% of dose excreted unchanged in feces

Breast milk: Excretion into breast milk not expected owing to poor oral absorption

Dosage adjustment for organ failure: None

Side effects: Abdominal cramps, nausea, diarrhea, superinfection

Pregnancy: Negligible absorption suggests low risk to fetus

Ribavirin (oral)

Trade name: Rebetol (with Intron A—Rebetron Combination Therapy)

Available formulations:

200 mg capsules $10.29

Class: Nucleoside analog antiviral

Mechanism of action: not yet established

Dosages (adult):

≥ 75 kg	600 mg qAM, 600 mg qPM
< 75 kg	400 mg qAM, 600 mg qPM

Storage and stability: When separated from Intron A, can be stored at room temperature. Together with Intron A—refrigerate at 2 to 8°C

PHARMACOKINETICS

T_{max}**:** 3 hours (after multiple dosing)

Bioavailability: 64%

Half-life: 298 hours after multiple dosing

Metabolism/elimination: metabolized via (1) a reversible phosphorylation pathway; and (2) a degradative pathway; then ribavirin and its metabolites are excreted renally

Food effects: High fat meal increases AUC by 70%, clinical significance not known; recommended to take with or without food

Breast milk: not known

Dosage adjustment in organ failure: Use with caution in patients with creatinine clearance < 50 ml/min. Ribavirin is not recommended in patients with severe renal impairment

Side effects: hemolytic anemia, depression, insomnia, psychosis, hallucination, pulmonary symptoms such as dyspnea, and pancreatitis have all been associated with the cost of Rebetron Combination Therapy

Pregnancy: Category X–should not be used in pregnant women

Thalidomide

Trade name: Thalomid (Celgene)

Available formulations: 50 mg capsules $7.84

Class: Immunomodulator

Mechanism of action: Multiple effects on the immune system including inhibition of neutrophil chemotaxis, monocyte phagocytosis, and secretion of tumor necrosis factor decreased immunoglobulin M levels, decreased T-helper lymphocytes, and increased T-suppressor lymphocytes

Oral dose (adult): HIV aphthous ulcers: 200 mg/day

Storage and stability: Store in tight containers away from excessive heat, light, and moisture

PHARMACOKINETICS

T_{max}**:** 2 to 4 hours

Bioavailability: Animal data 67% to 93%

Half-life: 6 to 9 hours

CSF penetration: Unknown, but wide distribution into various tissues

Metabolism/elimination: Extensive hepatic metabolism with multiple metabolites. Less than 1% of dose excreted unchanged in the urine

Breast milk: Unknown

Dosage adjustment for organ failure: No recommendations

Side effects: CNS [drowsiness, dizziness, mood alterations, peripheral neuropathy (may be severe and irreversible)], nausea, constipation, pruritus, fever, rash

Pregnancy: Category X. Known teratogen. Use caution in women of childbearing potential and discontinue therapy in pregnant patients

APPENDIX

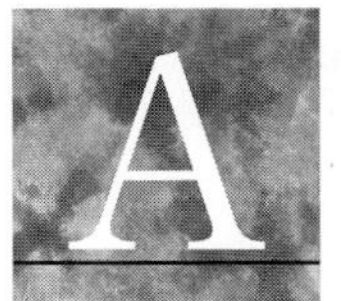

HIV/AIDS-Related Internet Resources

Richard A. Colvin, MD, PhD

The internet and proliferation of personal computers have allowed information to be shared among scientists, clinicians, and patients at a speed and to an extent not imagined even 20 years ago. Together, the internet and the world wide web have become invaluable, ubiquitous tools for clinicians, scientists, and patients to communicate about research, patient care, and problems with questions about their diseases or current therapies.[1–3]

In this section, a framework is presented as a guide to acquired immunodeficiency syndrome (AIDS)-related resources on the internet. Categorizing the important web sites is difficult, and anyone interested in AIDS can likely find interesting information in *all* of the categories listed below. The best way to get a sense of the resources available on the world wide web is to spend time on a computer looking at the various web pages and then linking to other sites, many of which are not listed here. All of the sites described below have been found to be useful, up to date, and accurate.

Index and Comprehensive Sites (Table 1)

Index and comprehensive web sites are listed in Table A–1. Some of these sites are human immunodeficiency virus (HIV)- and AIDS-specific, and others are general medical sites that give significant attention to HIV and AIDS. They are good launch points when searching for answers to specific questions.

Johns Hopkins (http://hopkins-aids.edu): The John Hopkins AIDS Service is an extremely useful site that provides HIV-related updates, the full text of Bartlett's *Medical Management of HIV Infection*, and access to HIV experts who answer questions from clinicians and patients. It also has links to other HIV-related sites.

HIV Insite (http://hivinsite.ucsf.edu): HIV Insite is a product of the University of California at San Francisco. Insite provides news, a textbook, and links to other HIV sites. It additionally offers support for those infected with HIV.

AEGIS (http://www.aegis.com): AEGIS provides news about HIV and AIDS. It has links to online HIV resources including the Centers for Disease Control and Prevention (CDC) Daily Update and AIDS Treatment News, easily accessible information about all HIV drugs, and sections for the newly infected.

JAMA AIDS Section (http://www.ama-assn.org/special/hiv): The JAMA site provides news, conference news, continuing medical education (CME) credits, and reviews.

International Association of Physicians in AIDS Care (http://www.iapac.org): The IAPAC site offers news about HIV and AIDS from around the world as well as conference listings and news.

HealthCite (http://www.healthcite.com): HealthCite is designed as a portal to health-related information on the internet. It has extensive links to many HIV-related sites and is a useful place to start searching for HIV-related information on the web.

Intelihealth (http://www.intelihealth.com): This Harvard Medical School- and University of Pennsylvania-sponsored site has information and news on many diseases and conditions. It has basic information and news about HIV and AIDS as well as access to search engines across the internet and MEDLINE.

Medscape (http://www.medscape.com): Medscape is a free commercial site that requires registration. It offers news about many medical specialties. In addition to news about conferences, it provides a guide to antiretroviral agents and *The AIDS Reader*.

Patient Sites

Perhaps the most interesting development the internet has brought to the world of medicine is the change in the patient–doctor relationship. It has come about owing to the plethora of clinical information available to patients on the world wide web (Table A–2). Patients now have easy access to the primary literature as well as reviews and anecdotes from others living with the same condition.

AEGIS (http://www.aegis.com): In addition to the news that Aegis brings daily to the world wide web, it offers reviews of drugs and basic information for those newly in-

▲ **Table A–1.** GENERAL MEDICAL WEB SITES AND HEALTH CARE INDEXES

Site	Address on www	Producer	Corporate Sponsors?
Johns Hopkins	http://hopkins-aids.edu	Johns Hopkins University	Yes
HIV Insite	http://hivinsite.ucsf.edu	University of California at San Francisco	Yes
AEGIS	http://www.aegis.com	AEGIS; nonprofit site	Yes
JAMA AIDS Section	http://www.ama-assn.org/special/hiv	American Medical Association	Yes
International Association of Physicians in AIDS Care	http://www.iapac.org	International Association of Physicians in AIDS Care	Yes
HealthCite	http://www.healthcite.com	HealthCite.com; commercial site	No
Intelihealth	http://www.intelihealth.com	Harvard Medical School, University of Pennsylvania School of Medicine and Dentistry	Yes
Medscape	http://www.medscape.com	Medscape.com; commercial site	Yes

fected. It has links to sites and phone numbers that offer assistance to those in need.

The Body (http://www.thebody.com): The Body is an HIV- and AIDS-specific site that offers news and information from experts. It offers useful news and commentaries from experts attending all significant meetings. The Body offers links to other important HIV sites as well, including POZ magazine, AIDS Treatment News, and U.S. government sites.

National AIDS Treatment Advocacy Project (NATAP) (http://www.natap.org): NATAP is an HIV community-run organization devoted to disseminating and explaining new information about therapeutics and treatment strategies for HIV and hepatititis C virus (HCV) infections. It is an excellent educational site for patients and providers alike, with timely news from conferences.

Gay Men's Health Crisis (http://www.gmhc.org): The GMHC was one of the first grass roots organizations created in response to the AIDS crisis during the early 1980s. Their web site continues to be devoted to education and support.

Project Inform (http://www.projinf.org): Project Inform was an early HIV education/activist organization and continues to provide excellent material for patients and their physicians. The site also contains a useful list of links.

Physician and Patient Care Sites

As is the case for patients, there is a plethora of information for physicians on the web devoted to the clinical practice of HIV and AIDS care (Table A–3).

Basic Information

Johns Hopkins AIDS Service: One of the immediately useful sections of the Johns Hopkins site is the text of the *Medical Management of HIV Infection* by John Bartlett and Joel Gallant (http://www.hopkins-aids.edu/publications/publications.html). Other sections on the site offer access to clinicians with extensive experience treating HIV-positive patients.

International AIDS Society—USA (www.iasusa.org/): This site provides treatment guidelines and publishes *Topics in HIV Medicines*. Articles and guidelines are written by some of the most prominent physicians and scientists working on HIV/AIDS and related issues.

AIDS Treatment News (http://www.immunonet.org/immune/atn.nsf/homepage): AIDS Treatment News, useful for both clinicians and patients, provides news from conferences and early data from clinical trials. It is published by long-time AIDS activist John James and does not accept corporate sponsorship. AIDS Treatment News is also available through links on AEGIS and The Body.

HIV/AIDS Clinical Guidelines (http://www.hivatis.org): HIVATIS has treatment guidelines, clinical trials information, and links to other web sites. It is also extremely useful for patients, as it has a glossary of clinical terms.

Clinical Trials

The internet has been used as an effective communication device for informing investigators of the progress of trials and for recruiting participants in the trials (Table A–4).

▲ **Table A–2.** WEB SITES DEVOTED TO PATIENTS

Web Site	Web Address	Producer	Corporate Sponsors?
AEGIS	http://www.aegis.com	AEGIS; nonprofit site	Yes
The Body	http://www.thebody.com	The Body; commercial site	Yes
National AIDS Treatment Advocacy Program	http://www.natap.org	National AIDS Treatment Advocacy Project; nonprofit organization	Yes
Gay Men's Health Crisis	http://www.gmhc.org	Gay Men's Health Crisis; nonprofit organization	Yes
Project Inform	http://www.projinf.org	Project Inform; nonprofit organization	Yes

▲ **Table A–3.** PATIENT CARE/CLINICIAN SITES

Web Site	Web Address	Producer	Corporate Sponsors?
International AIDS Society—USA	http://www.iasusa.org/	International AIDS Society—USA	No
Johns Hopkins AIDS Service	http://www.hopkins-aids.edu/publications/publications.html	Johns Hopkins University	Yes
AIDS Treatment News	http://www.immunonet.org/immune/atn.nsf/homepage	AIDS Treatment News; nonprofit publisher	No
HIV/AIDS Treatment Information Service (ATIS)	http://www.hivatis.org	U.S. federal government	No
HIV Forum	http://www.hivforum.org	George Washington University	Yes

The Forum for Collaborative HIV Research of George Washington University (http://hivforum.org) has treatment guidelines and patient outcomes research available for clinicians and patients.

AIDS Clinical Trial Information Service (ACTIS) (http://www.actis.org): ACTIS is a service of the U.S. Department of Health and Human Services. It posts interim and final results of AIDS-related clinical trials in the AIDS Trials Results Database. It also allows users to access the National Library of Medicine (NLM) databases and provides links to AIDS Clinical Trial Group (ACTG) and Community Programs for Clinical Research on AIDS (CPCRA) sites.

Adult AIDS Clinical Trial Group (http://aactg.s-3.com/): This is the website of the ACTG. It has pages for the public listing clinical trials and private pages for scientists who are members of the ACTG.

National Institutes of Health Clinical Trials (http://clinicaltrials.gov): This U.S. National Institutes of Health (NIH) site lists all NIH-sponsored trials and briefly describes them. It notes whether the trial is recruiting subjects, in progress, or completed, with links to results.

AMFAR (http://www.amfar.org): The AMFAR site lists trials by location, classes of drugs being tested, specific drugs being tested, and trial dates. Each trial has a summary with links to abstracts and descriptions of the drugs being used in the trial.

Canadian HIV Trials Network (http://www.hivnet.ubc.ca/ctn.html): This Canadian site lists trials that are enrolling or completed in Canada.

Initio (http://www.ctu.mrc.ac.uk/initio): Initio is the website of a large multicenter, multicountry, European-based trial with many treatment protocols for previously untreated HIV-positive patients.

▲ **Table A–4.** CLINICAL TRIAL SITES

Web Site	Web Address
AIDS Clinical Trial Information Service	http://www.actis.org
NIH Clinical Trials Site	http://clinicaltrials.gov
AMFAR	http://www.amfar.org
Canadian HIV Trials Network	http://www.hivnet.ubc.ca/ctn.html
Initio	http://www.ctu.mrc.ac.uk/initio

Research Sites and Databases

Biologists have been using resources on the world wide web for years for ongoing research projects. These sites are useful to AIDS researchers who have expanded and created specific tools to foster the understanding of HIV biology and therapy (Table A–5). The NLM provides access to MEDLINE, AIDSLINE, AIDSDRUGS, and AIDSTRIALS through PubMed (http://ncbi.nlm.nih.gov). These databases allow access to the available scientific and clinical literature about HIV and AIDS. In addition to the general databases from the NLM, HIV-specific databases are available that are particularly useful to AIDS researchers.

HIV Sequence Databank (http://hiv-web.lanl.gov): The HIV Sequence database, maintained in Los Alamos National Laboratory, is a collection of all known HIV sequence data. The site has a list of all known HIV drug resistance mutations as well and links to the HIV Immunology Database, also maintained at Los Alamos. There are a number of sequence analysis tools and tutorials on the site that allow searches and alignment of sequences. The immunology database contains T and B cell epitope maps as well as listings of HIV-specific cytotoxic T-lymphocyte (CTL) clones.

HIV RT and Protease Sequence databank (http://hivdb.stanford.edu/hiv/): This website is a resource for researchers studying treatment and evolutionary change in the HIV reverse transcriptase and protease genes. It contains almost every known sequence of these genes. The site also has a useful program for technicians performing genotypic HIV resistance studies.

HIV Protease Database (http://www.ncifcrf.gov/HIVdb): The protease database was created by the National Cancer Institute and contains many solved and de-

▲ **Table A–5.** RESEARCH AND DATABASE SITES

Web Site	Web Address
MEDLINE	http://ncbi.nlm.nih.gov
HIV sequence databank	http://hiv-web.lanl.gov
HIV ATIS	http://www.hivatis.org
HIV RT and protease database	http://hivdb.stanford.edu/hiv/
HIV protease database	http://www.ncifcrf.gov/HIVdb
AIDS reagent program	http://www.aidsreagent.org
Anti-HIV compound list	http://www.niaid.nih.gov/daids/dtpdb

▲ **Table A–6.** GOVERNMENT SITES

Web Site	Web Address
NIAID	http://www.niaid.nih.gov/research/daids/htm
CDC National Prevention Information Network	http://www.cdcnpin.org
World Health Organization/UNAIDS	http://www.unaids.org
U.S. Food and Drug Administration	http://www.fda.gov.oashi/aids/hiv.html
HIV/AIDS Treatment Information Service	http://www.hivatis.org
AIDS Clinical Trial Information Site	http://www.actis.org

rived three-dimensional structures of HIV-1, HIV-2, and semian immunodeficiency virus (SIV) proteases for use when designing new drugs and for gaining insight into structure–function relations.

AIDS Reagent Program (http://www.aidsreagent.org): The AIDS Reagent Program of the NIH and National Institute of Allergy and Infectious Diseases (NIAID) predates the world wide web and provides registered users with immunologic, biochemical, and biologic material for use in AIDS and AIDS-related research. The ability to access the AIDS Reagent Program by the world wide web has made it much more efficient to use.

Anti-HIV Compound List (http://www.niaid.nih.gov/daids/dtpdb): This NIH/NIAID database contains a list of all known anti-HIV compounds with references and links to other sites. Its introductory material shows the HIV life cycle and the mechanism of activity for various classes of drugs.

Government Sites

Many of the sites listed in Table A–6 are HIV- and AIDS-related. They emphasize dissemination of information to patients, clinicians, and scientists and are maintained by the NIH. The sites listed below focus on information for HIV and AIDS funding and prevention.

NIAID (http://www.niaid.nih.gov/research/daids.htm): The NIAID site provides information about funding sources and links to many of the sites described above.

CDC National Prevention Information Network (http://www.cdcnpin.org)

World Health Organization/UNAIDS (http://www.unaids.org): The UNAIDS site provides up-to-date news on the worldwide epidemic and what is being done to slow the spread of HIV around the world.

U.S. Food and Drug Administration (http://www.fda.gov/oashi/aids/hiv.html): The U.S. Food and Drug Administration (FDA) AIDS site has lists of HIV therapies, clinical trials, HIV history, and links to many other HIV- and AIDS-related sites.

Journals

Many journals are now available online (Table A–7). Some of them are free of charge, and others are free when accessed through a network with a site license. Many medical

▲ **Table A–7.** JOURNAL SITES

Web Site	Web Address
AIDS	http://www.aidsonline.com/
AIDS Patient Care and STDs	http://www.liebertpub.com/apc/default.htm
AIDS Research and Human Retroviruses	http://www.liebertpub.com/AID/default1.asp
Annals of Internal Medicine	http://www.acponline.org/journals/annals/annaltoc.htm
Antimicrobial Agents and Chemotherapy	http://intl-aac.asm.org/
Antiviral Chemistry & Chemotherapy	http://www.intmedpress.com/IMPWeb/Journals/AVCC/avcchome.htm
Antiviral Therapy	http://www.intmedpress.com/IMPWeb/Journals/AVT/avthome.htm
British Medical Journal	http://www.bmj.com/
Cell	http://www.cell.com/
Clinical Infectious Diseases	http://www.journals.uchicago.edu/CID/home.htm
Emerging Infectious Diseases	http://www.cdc.gov/ncidod/eid/index.htm
HIV Clinical Trials	http://www.thomasland.com/_nonsearch/hctissues.htm
International Journal of STDs and AIDS	http://www.catchword.co.uk/titles/rsm/09564624/contp1-1.htm
Journal of Acquired Immune Deficiency Syndromes	http://www.jaids.com
Journal of the American Medical Association	http://jama.ama-assn.org
Journal of the Association of Nurses in AIDS Care	http://www.sagepub.com/Shopping/Journal.asp
Journal of Immunology	http://www.jimmunol.org/
Journal of Infectious Diseases	http://www.journals.uchicago.edu/JID/
Journal of Virology	http://jvi.asm.org
Lancet	http://www.thelancet.com/
Morbidity and Mortality Weekly Report	http://www.cdc.gov/mmwr
Nature	http://www.nature.com/
Nature Medicine	http://medicine.nature.com/
New England Journal of Medicine	http://www.nejm.org/content/index.asp
Pediatrics	http://www.pediatrics.org/
Proceedings of the National Academy of Sciences of the United States of America	http://www.pnas.org/
Science	http://science-mag.aaas.org/

▲ **Table A–8.** MEETING WEB SITES

Web Site	Web Address
IAPAC list of clinical meetings	http://www.iapac.org/clinmgt/conferences/conflist.html
13th Meeting on AIDS 2000	http://www.aids2000.com
Conference on Retroviruses and Opportunistic Infections	http://www.retroconference.org
ICAAC	http://www.asm.org/mtgsrc/mtgs.htm
Meeting reviews at The Body (reviews every major HIV meeting)	http://www.thebody.com/confs/confcov.html
AIDS Vaccine 2001 (a biennial international conference to present basic, clinical, and public health data relevant to AIDS vaccines)	http://www.AIDSvaccine2001.org

center libraries have thus accumulated electronic libraries containing numerous medical and scientific journals. Most of the journals allow the user to download copies of articles to their computer in the PDF format. The PDF format can be read by the Acrobat Reader, which allows the user to display and print the article in its original published form. The web addresses of journals related to HIV and AIDS are listed in Table A–7. Some require a subscription or site license for access to the full text of articles, but all allow viewing the table of contents and usually allow the user to search back issues for topics of interest. In addition to that list, the NLM, through PubMed, provides access to the full text of many other scientific journals.

Clinical and Scientific Meetings

Many sites offer reviews and highlights of meetings (Table A–8).

Online Support and E-mail Lists

HIV Insite (http://hivinsite.ucsf.edu)

The Body (http://thebody.com/help.htm): The help page at The Body provides links to many other web sites and phone numbers for people who wish to talk directly.

E-mail lists (http://www.support-lists.com/listManage.cgi): This web site hosts many e-mail lists that offer support for HIV-positive people, people with hemophilia, and physicians and lawyers who take care of HIV-positive people.

Conclusions

The emergence and convergence of the AIDS epidemic and the world wide web have changed health care, the doctor–patient relationship, and the way scientific inquiry is conducted. Because of the extent of the architecture on the world wide web, this section can only provide an outline of the information available. Readers who wish to explore more sites may want to begin with a general site, such as AEGIS, and follow links that are of particular interest.

REFERENCES

1. Leiner BM, Cerf VG, Clark DD, et al. A brief history of the internet. 2000. http://www.isoc.org/internet-history/brief.html.
2. Mayr D. See; think; the history of the net. 2000. http://members.magnet.at/daymr/history.htm.
3. Shafer RW, Deresinski SC. Human immune deficiency virus on the web: a guided tour. Clin Infect Dis. 31:568, 2000.

APPENDIX

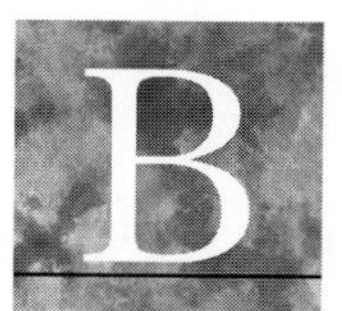

Antiretroviral Adult Dosage Guidelines

Alice K. Pau, PharmD

Table B–1. ADULT ANTIRETROVIRAL DOSAGE GUIDELINES

Antiretroviral Drugs	Adult Dosages	Renal Function Adjustment	Food and Other Considerations
Nucleoside/Nucleotide Reverse Transcriptase Inhibitors			
Abacavir (ABC, Ziagen) Yellow, capsule-shaped tablets, 300 mg Oral solution, 20 mg/ml	300 mg bid (2 tabs/day) *Hypersensitivity Registry: 1-800-270-0425*	Not necessary	Can be taken with or without food. Oral solution: room temperature or refrigerate, *do not* freeze.
Didanosine (ddI) Videx Buffered tablets, White, round tablets, 25, 50, 100, 150 mg, 200 mg (for once-daily dosing only) Sachets, 167, 250 mg Pediatric suspension, 2, 4 g powder, final solution 10 mg/ml Videx-EC White, opaque capsules, 125, 200, 250, 400 mg	**≥60 kg** *Buffered tablets,* 2–100 mg bid *or* 2–200 mg qd, *or* *Enteric coated capsules,* 1–400 mg EC cap qd, *or* *Sachet,* 250 mg bid **<60 kg** 1–100 mg + 1–25 mg bid *or* 1–100 mg tablet + 1–150 mg tablet qd *or* 1–200 mg tablet + 1–50 mg tablet, *or* 1–250 mg EC capsule qd *or* Sachet, 167 mg bid	**≥60 kg** CrCl / Tablets / EC capsules / Sachet 30–59 / 100 mg bid or 200 mg qd / 200 mg qd / 100 mg bid 10–29 / 150 mg qd / 125 mg qd / 167 mg qd <10 / 100 mg qd / 125 mg qd / 100 mg qd **<60 kg** CrCl / Tablets / EC capsules / Sachet 30–59 / 150 mg qd or 75 mg bid / 125 mg qd / 100 mg bid 10–29 / 100 mg qd / 125 mg qd / 100 mg qd <10 / 75 mg qd / Use tablet / 100 mg qd **CAPD or hemodialysis patient** Use same dose as CrCl < 10 ml/min	*All preparations:* take on an empty stomach: ≥0.5 hr before or ≥2 hr after meals. Space apart from PIs (see EC capsule), tenofovir and delavirdine. *Buffered tablets:* Always take two tablets with each dose. Chew thoroughly before swallowing or dissolve in water or apple juice (stable for 1 hour). *Sachets:* Dissolve in a glass of water. Stable for 4 hr after dissolution. *Pediatric suspension:* Mix with antacid as directed. Store in refrigerator; stable for up to 30 days. *EC capsules:* Can be taken together with indinavir. Space apart from other PIs.
Lamivudine (3TC, Epivir) Gray, diamond shape tablets, 300 mg White, diamond shape tablets, 150 mg Oral solution, 10 mg/ml	150 mg bid or 300 mg bid	CrCl / Dose 30–49 / 150 mg qd 15–29 / 150 mg × 1, then 100 qd 5–14 / 150 mg × 1, then 50 qd <5 / 50 × 1, then 25 qd No data on hemodialysis	No specific food considerations.
Stavudine (d4T, Zerit) Dark orange capsules, 40 mg Light & dark orange capsules, 30 mg Light brown capsules, 20 mg Light yellow & dark red capsules, 15 mg Oral solution, 1 mg/ml	**≥60 kg:** 40 mg bid **<60 kg:** 30 mg bid	CrCl / ≥60 kg (Dose) / <60 kg (Dose) 26–50 / 20 mg q12h / 15 mg q12h ≤25 / 20 mg q24h / 15 mg q24h No data on hemodialysis	No specific food considerations. Oral suspension: store in refrigerator after reconstitution; stable for up to 30 days.
Tenofovir DF (Viread) Light blue almond-shaped tablets, 300 mg	300 mg once daily	*Not recommended* for CrCl <60	Take with food; take at least 2 hr before or 1 hr after ddI
Zalcitabine (ddC, Hivid) White, oblong tablets, 0.75 mg Beige, oblong tablets, 0.375 mg	0.75 mg tid	CrCl / Dose 10–40 / 0.75 mg bid <10 / 0.75 mg qd No data on hemodialysis	No specific food considerations.
Zidovudine (ZDV, AZT, Retrovir) Blue & white capsules, 100 mg White round tablets, 300 mg Oral syrup, 50 mg/5 ml IV, 10 mg/ml	300 mg tid 200 mg bid, *or* 100 mg 5 × per day	100 mg tid in patients with severe renal impairment Hemodialysis: 100 mg tid	Not to be taken with meals if possible—but not absolutely necessary (≥30 min before or 2 hr after meals).
Combivir (ZDV 300 mg/ 3TC 150 mg) White, oblong tablet	One tablet bid	*Not recommended* in patients where dosage adjustment is required (i.e., those with renal insufficiency) low body weight (<50 kg), or experiencing dose-limiting side effects	No specific food consideration.

Trizivir (ABC 300 mg/ZDV 300 mg/3TC 150 mg) Pale blue, oblong tablet	One tablet bid	*Not recommended* in patients with renal insufficiency where dosage adjustment is required	No specific food considerations.
Nonnucleoside Reverse Transcriptase Inhibitors			
Delavirdine (Rescriptor) White, oblong tablets, 100, 200 mg	400 mg tid	Not necessary Hemodialysis: no effect	With or without food. Avoid taking with antacids, ddI, or H_2-blockers. Acidic beverages ↑ absorption. Can mix tablets in 3 oz of water to make a dispersion (drink promptly).
Efavirenz (Sustiva, Stocrin) Yellow, capsule-shaped tablet, 600 mg Gold capsules, 200 mg White capsules, 100 mg Gold & white capsules, 50 mg	600 mg qd (usually qhs or a couple of hours before bedtime)	Not necessary	Take on an empty stomach; food increases concentrations and toxicities
Nevirapine (Viramune) White oval tablets, 200 mg Oral suspension, 50 mg/5 ml	200 mg qd × 14 days, then 200 mg bid Repeat dose escalation recommended if therapy interrupted	Not necessary Hemodialysis: data not available	No specific food considerations.
Protease Inhibitors			
Amprenavir (Agenerase) White capsules, 50, 150 mg Oral solution, 15 mg/ml *Note*: capsules & solution are not interchangeable on a mg/mg basis	1200 mg q12h *or* 600 mg q12h + ritonavir 100 mg q12h, *or* 1200 mg qd + ritonavir 200 mg qd	Not necessary Dosage adjustment recommended in patients with liver failure	No food restriction. Each 150 mg capsule contains 109 IU of vitamin E, vitamin E supplementation should be discontinued. Oral solution contains a large amount of propylene glycol—contraindicated in children under age 4 years, pregnant women, patients with renal or hepatic failure, patients treated with disulfiram or metronidazole.
Indinavir (Crixivan) Off-white capsules, 200, 333, 400 mg	800 mg q8h	Not necessary No data on dialysis	Empty stomach or with light, low-fat meals. Drink 1–2 liters of fluid per day.
Lopinavir (Kaletra) Lopinavir/ritonavir (133/33 mg per capsule) Orange soft gel capsules Oral solution, lopinavir/ritonavir (400/100 mg per 5 ml)	Lopinavir/ritonavir (400/100 mg) (3 capsules bid) Lopinavir/ritonavir (533/133 mg) (4 capsules bid) if used with efavirenz or nevirapine in treatment-experienced patients where reduced lopinavir susceptibility is suspected	Not necessary	Take with food. Take 2 hr before or 1 hr after ddI. Oral solution contains 42.4% alcohol.
Nelfinavir (Viracept) Light blue capsule-shaped tablets, 250 mg Oral powder, 50 mg/g (scoop)	750 mg tid or 1250 mg bid	Not necessary Hemodialysis: not likely to affect clearance	Take with food or light snack
Ritonavir (Norvir) Off-white soft gel capsules, 100 mg Oral solution, 600 mg/7.5 ml	600 mg bid (titration from 300 to 400 mg bid to full dose in <2 weeks) 100–400 mg bid if used as PK enhancer for another PI	Not necessary Hemodialysis: not likely to affect clearance	With meals if possible. At least 2.5 hr apart from ddI. Oral solution can be taken with Ensure, chocolate milk, or Advera.
Saquinavir Soft Gel Cap (Fortovase) Beige, opaque, soft gelatin capsules, 200 mg **Saquinavir Hard Gel Cap (Invirase)** Yellow & green capsules, 200 mg	*Fortovase*: 1200 mg tid *Invirase*: as single PI: 600 mg tid—not recommended *Not recommended to be used as single PI in presence of efavirenz*	Not necessary Hemodialysis: not likely to affect clearance	Take with a meal or up to 2 hours after a meal.

EC, enteric coated; PI, protease inhibitor; CrCl, creatinine clearance (mL/min); PK, pharmacokinetic.

Table B–2. ANTIRETROVIRAL COMBINATION DOSAGE ADJUSTMENT

Drug	Amprenavir (APV or A)	Indinavir (IDV or I)	Lopinavir/r (LPV/r)	Nelfinavir (NFV or N)	Ritonavir (RTV or R)	Saquinavir (SQV or S)	Delavirdine (DLV or D)	Efavirenz (EFV or E)	Nevirapine (NVP or N)
Amprenavir	—	No modification	APV 750 bid[a] LPV/r 4 caps bid	No data	R-100/A-600 bid[a] *or* R-200/A-1200 qd	No data	No data	APV 1200 tid[a] No modification for APV if used w/ RTV 200 mg bid or full-dose NFV	APV 1200 tid[a] No modification for APV if used w/ RTV 200 mg bid or full-dose NFV
Indinavir	No modification	—	IDV 600–800 bid[a]	No data	R-100/I-800 bid[a] R-200/I-800 bid[a] R-400/I-400 bid[a]	No data	I-1200/D-600 bid[a]	IDV 1000 mg q8h if IDV used as sole PI	IDV 1000 mg q8h if IDV used as sole PI
Lopinavir/r	APV 750 bid[a] LPV/r 4 caps bid	IDV 600–800 bid[a]	—	NFV 750 bid	Additional RTV not generally recommended	SQV 800 bid	No data	LPV/r 4 caps bid	LPV/r 4 caps bid
Nelfinavir	No data	No data	NFV 750 bid[a]	—	N-750/R-400 bid[a]	SQV 800 tid *or* SQV 1200 bid	No data	No modification	NFV 750–1000 tid *or* NFV1250–1500 bid
Ritonavir	R-100/A-600 bid[a] *or* R-200/A-1200 qd	R-100/I-800 bid[a] R-200/I-600 bid[a] R-200/I-800 bid[a] R-400/I-400 bid[a]	Additional RTV not generally recommended	N-500–750/ R-400 bid[a]	—	R-400/S-400 bid *or* R-200/S-800 bid[a] *or* R-100/S-1600 qd[a] *or* R-200/S-1200 qd[a]	No modification	No modification	No modification
Saquinavir	No data	No data	SQV 800 bid[a]	SQV 800 tid or SQV 1200 bid	R-400/S-400 bid R-200/S-800 bid[a] R-100/S-1600 qd[a] R-200/S-1200 qd[a]	—	SQV 800 tid	Not recommended if SQV is sole PI	No data
Delavirdine	No data	I-1200/D-600 bid[a]	No data	No data	No modification	SQV 800 tid	—	No data	No data
Efavirenz	APV 1200 tid No modification for APV if used w/ RTV 200 mg bid or full-dose NFV	IDV 1000 mg q8h if used as sole PI	LPV/r 4 capsules bid	No modification	No modification	Not recommended if SQV is sole PI	No data	—	No modification
Nevirapine	APV 1200 tid No modification for APV if used w/ RTV 200 mg bid or full-dose NFV	IDV 1000 mg q8h if used as sole PI	LPV/r 4 capsules bid	NFV 750–1000 tid *or* NFV 1250–1500	No modification	No data	No data	No modification	—

LPVr, lopinavir/ritonavir; PI, protease inhibition; w/, with. Dosages represent dosing adjustments due to pharmacokinetic interactions. The doses differ from current FDA-approved doses.
[a]Regimens with favorable pharmacokinetic data, clinical efficacy data are yet to be determined.

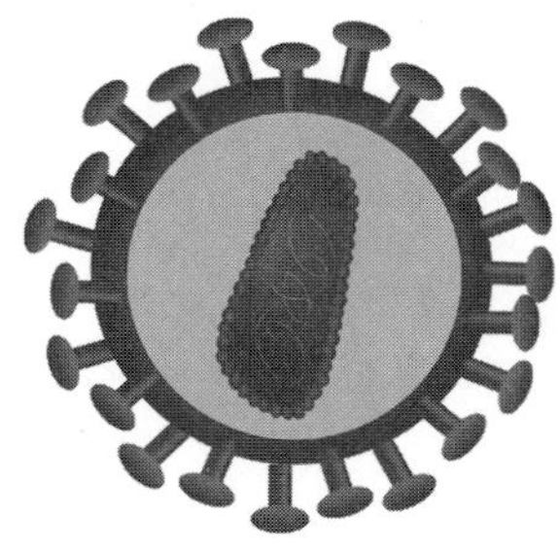

Index

Page numbers followed by the letter f refer to figures and those followed by t refer to tables.